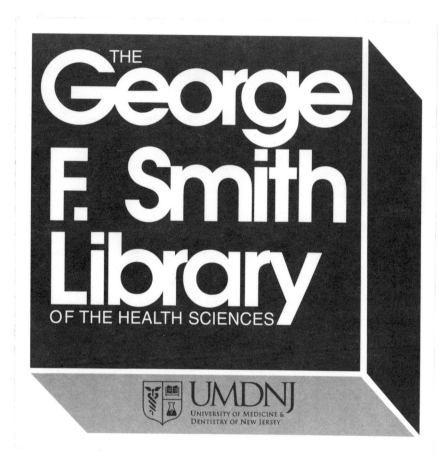

Histology for Pathologists

THIRD EDITION

Histology for Pathologists

THIRD EDITION

EDITOR

STACEY E. MILLS, MD

W.S. Royster Professor of Pathology
Director of Surgical Pathology and Cytopathology
University of Virginia Health System
Charlottesville, Virginia

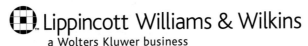
. Lippincott Williams & Wilkins
a Wolters Kluwer business
Philadelphia · Baltimore · New York · London
Buenos Aires · Hong Kong · Sydney · Tokyo

Acquisitions Editor: Jonathan W. Pine, Jr.
Managing Editor: Anne E. Jacobs
Project Manager: Alicia Jackson
Senior Manufacturing Manager: Benjamin Rivera
Marketing Manager: Angela Panetta
Creative Director: Doug Smock
Cover Designer: Joseph DePinho
Production Service: Black Dot Group
Printer: RR Donnelley–Willard

© 2007 by LIPPINCOTT WILLIAMS & WILKINS, a WOLTERS KLUWER business
530 Walnut Street
Philadelphia, PA 19106 USA
LWW.com

1st Edition, © 1992 Raven Press
2nd Edition, © 1997 Lippincott-Raven Publishers

Library of Congress Cataloging-in-Publication Data

Histology for pathologists. —3rd ed./editor, Stacey E. Mills.
    p. ; cm.
  Includes bibliographical references and index.
  ISBN 978-0-7817-6241-0
  ISBN 0-7817-6241-3 (alk. paper)
  1. Histology. 2. Histology, Pathological. I. Mills, Stacey E.
  [DNLM: 1. Histology. 2. Pathology. QS 504 H6765 2007]

  QM551.H667 2007
  611'.018—dc22

                                                                        2006018492

Care has been taken to confirm the accuracy of the information presented and to describe
generally accepted practices. However, the authors, editors, and publisher are not responsible
for errors or omissions or for any consequences from application of the information in this
book and make no warranty, expressed or implied, with respect to the currency, completeness,
or accuracy of the contents of the publication. Application of the information in a particular
situation remains the professional responsibility of the practitioner.

The authors, editors, and publisher have exerted every effort to ensure that drug selection
and dosage set forth in this text are in accordance with current recommendations and practice
at the time of publication. However, in view of ongoing research, changes in government
regulations, and the constant flow of information relating to drug therapy and drug reactions,
the reader is urged to check the package insert for each drug for any change in indications and
dosage and for added warnings and precautions. This is particularly important when the
recommended agent is a new or infrequently employed drug.

Some drugs and medical devices presented in the publication have Food and Drug
Administration (FDA) clearance for limited use in restricted research settings. It is the
responsibility of the health care provider to ascertain the FDA status of each drug or device
planned for use in their clinical practice.

To purchase additional copies of this book, call our customer service department at (800)
638-3030 or fax orders to (301) 223-2320. International customers should call (301) 223-2300.

Visit Lippincott Williams & Wilkins on the Internet: at LWW.com. Lippincott Williams &
Wilkins customer service representatives are available from 8:30 AM to 6 PM, EST.

10 9 8 7 6 5 4 3 2 1

Contents

Contributors

GRAZIELLA ABU-JAWDEH, MD
Associate Pathologist
Department of Pathology
North Shore Medical Center
Salem, Massachusetts

KRISTEN A. ATKINS, MD
Assistant Professor
Department of Pathology
University of Virginia Health System
Charlottesville, Virginia

KAROLY BALOGH, MD
Associate Professor
Department of Pathology
Harvard Medical School
Staff Pathologist
Department of Pathology
Beth Israel Deaconess Medical Center
Boston, Massachusetts

LUCIA L. BALOS, MD
Assistant Professor of Pathology
Department of Pathology
and Anatomical Sciences
University of New York at Buffalo
School of Medicine
and Biomedical Sciences
Director of Anatomic Pathology
Department of Pathology
Kaleida Health
Buffalo, New York

JOSÉ E. BARRETO, MD
Associate Professor
Department of Pathology
Instituto de Patologia e Investigacion
Professor, Department of Pathology
Facultad de Medicina
Universidad Catolica
Villarrica, Paraguay

NICOLE A. BELSLEY, MD
Fellow in Cytopathology
Department of Pathology
Massachusetts General Hospital
Boston, Massachusetts

KURT BENIRSCHKE, MD
Professor Emeritus, Pathology
and Reproductive Medicine
Department of Pathology
University of California, San Diego
La Jolla, California
Pathologist, Department of Pathology
San Diego Medical Center
San Diego, California

REX C. BENTLEY, MD, PhD
Associate Professor
Department of Pathology
Duke University Medical Center
Durham, North Carolina

GERALD J. BERRY, MD
Professor, Department of Pathology
Stanford University Medical Center
Director of Cardiac Pathology
Associate Director of Surgical Pathology
Stanford University Hospital
Stanford, California

MARGARET E. BILLINGHAM, MB, BS, FRCPath
Professor Emerita of Pathology
Department of Pathology
Stanford University Medical School
Stanford, California

JAQUES BOSQ, MD
Assistant Professor of Pathology
Department of Histopathology "A"
Institut Gustave-Roussy
Villejuif Cedex, France

JOHN S. J. BROOKS, MD, MRCPath
Professor and Vice Chair
Department of Pathology and
Laboratory Medicine
University of Pennsylvania Medical
School
Chair of Pathology
Pennsylvania Hospital of the University
of Pennsylvania Health System
Philadelphia, Pennsylvania

PETER G. BULLOUGH, MD
Professor, Department of Pathology and
Laboratory Medicine
Weill Medical College
Cornell University
Director of Laboratory Medicine
Hospital for Special Surgery
New York, New York

PETER C. BURGER, MD
Professor of Pathology, Neurosurgery,
and Oncology
Department of Pathology
The Johns Hopkins University School
of Medicine
Baltimore, Maryland

MARIA LUISA CARCANGIU, MD
Director of Anatomic Pathology
Department of Pathology
Istituto Nazionale Tumori
Milan, Italy

J. AIDAN CARNEY, MD, PhD, FRCPI, FRCP
Professor Emeritus of Pathology
Emeritus Consultant in Pathology
Department of Laboratory Medicine
and Pathology
Mayo Clinic
Rochester, Minnesota

DARRYL CARTER, MD
Professor Emeritus of Pathology
Department of Pathology
Yale University School of Medicine
New Haven, Connecticut

ODILE CASIRAGHI, MD
Department of Histopathology "A"
Institut Gustave-Roussy
Villejuif Cedex, France

WILLIAM L. CLAPP, MD
Associate Professor
Department of Pathology, Immunology,
and Laboratory Medicine
University of Florida College of
Medicine
Chief, Anatomic Pathology
Department of Pathology and
Laboratory Medicine Service
North Florida/South Georgia Veterans
Health System
Gainesville, Florida

PHILIP B. CLEMENT, MD
Professor of Pathology and Laboratory
Medicine
University of British Columbia
Consultant Pathologist
Department of Pathology and
Laboratory Medicine
Division of Anatomic Pathology
Vancouver General Hospital
Vancouver, British Columbia
Canada

THOMAS V. COLBY, MD
Consultant in Pathology
Department of Pathology
Mayo Clinic Arizona
Scottsdale, Arizona

CHRISTOPHER J. COLD, MD
Anatomic Pathologist
Marshfield Laboratory
Department of Anatomic Pathology
Saint Joseph's Hospital
Marshfield, Wisconsin

LAURA C. COLLINS, MD, MBBS
Assistant Professor of Pathology
Harvard Medical School
Staff Pathologist
Department of Pathology
Beth Israel Deaconess Medical Center
Boston, Massachusetts

JULIAN CONEJO-MIR, MD, PhD
Professor and Chairman of
Dermatology
Virgen del Rocio University Hospital
University of Seville
Sevilla, Spain

BYRON P. CROKER, MD, PhD
Professor, Department of Pathology,
Immunology, and Laboratory Medicine
University of Florida
Chief, Pathology and Laboratory
Medicine Service
North Florida/South Georgia Veterans
Health System
Gainesville, Florida

ANTONIO L. CUBILLA, MD
Professor Emeritus
Department of Pathology
Facultad de Ciencias Medicas
Director of Pathology
Instituto de Patologia e Investigacion
Asunción, Paraguay

THOMAS J. CUMMINGS, MD
Associate Professor
Department of Pathology
Duke University Medical Center
Durham, North Carolina

JULIA DAHL, MD
Chief Medical Officer
Mosaic Gastrointestinal Research and
Education Consortium
Laboratory Director
Mosaic Gastrointestinal Pathology
Services, PLLC
Germantown, Tennessee

YOGESHWAR DAYAL, BS, MB, MD
Clinical Professor
Department of Pathology
Tufts University School of Medicine
Senior Pathologist
Department of Pathology
New England Medical Center
Hospitals
Boston, Massachusetts

RONALD A. DeLELLIS, MD
Professor and Associate Chair
Department of Pathology and
Medicine
Brown Medical School
Pathologist-in-Chief
Department of Pathology
Rhode Island Hospital
Providence, Rhode Island

FRANCO G. DeNARDI, MD, FRCP(C)
Department of Anatomical Pathology
Henderson General Hospital
Department of Pathobiology and
Molecular Medicine
McMaster University
Hamilton, Ontario
Canada

CLAUS FENGER, MD, PhD
Professor, Chief Pathologist
Department of Clinical Pathology
Odense University Hospital
Odense, Denmark

HENRY F. FRIERSON, JR., MD
Professor, Department of Pathology
University of Virginia Health System
Charlottesville, Virginia

GREGORY N. FULLER, MD, PhD
Professor, Department of Pathology
Chief, Section of Neuropathology
The University of Texas
M.D. Anderson Cancer Center
Houston, Texas

GIULIO GABBIANI, MD, PhD
Professor, Department of Pathology
and Immunology
University of Geneva–CMU
Geneva, Switzerland

**PATRICK J. GALLAGHER, MD, PhD,
FRCPath**
Reader in Pathology
School of Medicine
University of Southampton
Consultant Cardiovascular Pathologist
Department of Cellular Pathology
Southampton University Hospitals
Southampton, United Kingdom

TERRY L. GRAMLICH, MD
Director of Hepatopathology
AmeriPath Institute of Gastrointestinal
Pathology and Digestive Disease
Oakwood Village, Ohio

JOEL K. GREENSON, MD
Professor of Pathology
Department of Pathology
University of Michigan Medical School
University of Michigan Health System
Ann Arbor, Michigan

NANCY S. HARDT, MD
Clinical Professor
Department of Pathology
University of Florida
Shands at the University of Florida
Gainesville, Florida

REID R. HEFFNER, JR., MD
Professor, Department of Pathology and
Anatomical Sciences
University at Buffalo School of
Medicine
Buffalo, New York

MICHAEL R. HENDRICKSON, MD
Professor of Pathology
Co-Director of Surgical Pathology
Department of Pathology
Stanford University Medical Center
Stanford, California

BORIS HINZ, PhD
Laboratory of Cell Biophysics
Swiss Federal Institute of Technology
Lausanne, Switzerland

SEUNG-MO HONG, MD, PhD
Research Associate
Department of Pathology
University of Virginia
Charlottesville, Virginia

EVA HORVATH, PhD
Department of Laboratory Medicine
St. Michael's Hospital
University of Toronto
Toronto, Ontario
Canada

RALPH H. HRUBAN, MD
Professor of Pathology and Oncology
Director, The Sol Goldman Pancreatic
Cancer Research Center
Pathologist, Department of Pathology
The Johns Hopkins Hospital
Baltimore, Maryland

RICHARD L. KEMPSON, MD
Professor of Pathology, Emeritus Active
Department of Pathology
Stanford University
Stanford, California

DAVID S. KLIMSTRA, MD
Professor, Department of Pathology and
Laboratory Medicine
Weill Medical College
Cornell University
Attending Pathologist and Chief of
Surgical Pathology
Department of Pathology
Memorial Sloan-Kettering Cancer
Center
New York, New York

GORDON K. KLINTWORTH, MD, PhD
Professor or Pathology
Joseph A. C. Wadsworth Research
Professor of Ophthalmology
Duke University Medical Center
Durham, North Carolina

KALMAN KOVACS, MD, PhD
Department of Laboratory Medicine
St. Michael's Hospital
University of Toronto
Toronto, Ontario
Canada

KEVIN O. LESLIE, MD
Professor of Pathology
Mayo Clinic College of Medicine
Consultant, Department of Laboratory
Medicine and Pathology
Mayo Clinic Arizona
Scottsdale, Arizona

STEVEN H. LEWIS, MD, FCAP, FACOG
Adjunct Associate Professor of
Pathology and Obstetrics and
Gynecology
University of South Florida
Tampa, Florida

MIN LI, MD, PhD
Associate Pathologist
Department of Pathology
St. Luke's Hospital
Bethlehem, Pennsylvania

RICARDO V. LLOYD, MD, PhD
Professor of Pathology
Department of Laboratory Medicine
and Pathology
Consultant, Department of Laboratory
Medicine and Pathology
Mayo Clinic
Rochester, Minnesota

M. BEATRIZ S. LOPES, MD
Professor of Pathology and
Neurological Surgery
University of Virginia School of
Medicine
Director of Neuropathology & Autopsy
Department of Pathology
University of Virginia Health Services
Charlottesville, Virginia

**FERNANDO MARTÍNEZ-MADRIGAL,
MD**
Department of Pathology
Hospital General "Dr. Miguel Silva"
Hospital General de Zona No.1
IMSS and the Medical Faculty of the
Universidad Michoacana de
San Nicolas de Hidalgo
Morelia, Michoacán
Mexico

JOHN E. McNEAL, MD
Clinical Professor of Urology and
Pathology
Department of Urology
Stanford University School of Medicine
Stanford, California

CHRIS J. L. M. MEIJER, MD, PhD
Professor, Department of Pathology
VU University Medical Center
Amsterdam, The Netherlands

**LESLIE MICHAELS, MD, FRCPath,
FRCP(C), DPath**
Professor Emeritus
Department of Histopathology
Royal Free & University College
London Medical School
London, United Kingdom

STACEY E. MILLS, MD
W.S. Royster Professor of Pathology
Department of Pathology
University of Virginia
Director of Surgical Pathology &
Cytopathology
University of Virginia Health System
Charlottesville, Virginia

ATTILIO ORAZI, MD, FRCPath (ENGL)
Professor of Pathology and Laboratory
Medicine
Indiana University School of Medicine
Director of Pathology Laboratory
Medicine
Clarian Pathology Laboratory
Indianapolis, Indiana

CARFLOS ORTIZ-HIDALGO, MD
Professor of Histology
Universidad Panamericana
Chairman, Department of Surgical
Pathology
The American British Cowdray (ABC)
Medical Center
Mexico City, Mexico

CHRISTOPHER N. OTIS, MD
Associate Professor
Department of Pathology
Tufts University School of Medicine
Boston, Massachusetts
Director of Surgical Pathology
Baystate Medical Center
Springfield, Massachusetts

**DAVID A. OWEN, MB, BCH, FRCPath,
FRCPC**
Professor, Department of Pathology and
Laboratory Medicine
University of British Columbia
Consultant Pathologist
Vancouver General Hospital
Vancouver, British Columbia
Canada

LIRON PANTANOWITZ, MD
Assistant Professor
Department of Pathology
Tufts University School of Medicine
Boston, Massachusetts
Director of Informatics
Department of Pathology
Baystate Medical Center
Springfield, Massachusetts

PETER J. PERNICONE, MD
Director of Surgical Pathology
Laboratory
Department of Pathology
Florida Hospital Medical Center
Orlando, Florida

PATRICIA M. PEROSIO, MD
Staff Pathologist
Department of Pathology
Montgomery Hospital Medical Center
Norristown, Pennsylvania

ROBERT E. PETRAS, MD
Staff Pathologist
Clinical Associate Professor
Department of Pathology
Northeastern Ohio Universities
College of Medicine
Rootstown, Ohio
National Director for Gastrointestinal
Pathology Services
AmeriPath, Inc.
Oakwood Village, Ohio

MARTHA BISHOP PITMAN, MD
Associate Professor of Pathology
Harvard Medical School
Director, Fine Needle Aspiration Biopsy
Service
Department of Pathology
Massachusetts General Hospital
Boston, Massachusetts

LUIS REQUENA, MD, PhD
Professor and Chairman of
Dermatology and Dermatopathology
Fundación Jimenez Diaz
Ciudad Universitaria
Universidad Autonoma de Madrid
Madrid, Spain

VICTOR E. REUTER, MD
Vice Chairman
Department of Pathology
Memorial Sloan-Kettering
Cancer Center
Professor of Pathology
Weill Medical College
Cornell University
New York, New York

**ROBERT H. RIDDELL, MD, FRCPath,
FRCPC**
Professor, Department of Laboratory
Medicine & Pathobiology
University of Toronto
Pathologist
Department of Pathology & Laboratory
Medicine
Mount Sinai Hospital
Toronto, Ontario
Canada

STANLEY J. ROBBOY, MD
Professor of Pathology
Professor of Obstetrics and
Gynecology
Chief, Diagnostic Services
Departments of Pathology and
Obstetrics and Gynecology
Duke University Medical Center
Durham, North Carolina

JUAN ROSAI, MD
Professor of Pathology
Istituto Nazionale Tumori
Director, Consultation Center
Centro Consulenze Anatomia
Patologica Oncologica
Centro Diagnostico Italiano (CDI)
Milan, Italy

ANDREW E. ROSENBERG, MD
Associate Professor
Department of Pathology
Harvard Medical School
Associate Pathologist
Chief, Bone and Soft Tissue Pathology
Massachusetts General Hospital
Boston, Massachusetts

SANFORD I. ROTH, MD
Senior Lecturer
Department of Pathology
Harvard Medical School
Consultant, Department of Pathology
Massachusetts General Hospital
Boston, Massachusetts

BERND W. SCHEITHAUER, MD
Professor, Department of Pathology
Mayo Medical School
Consultant, Department of Laboratory
Medicine and Pathology
Mayo Clinic
Rochester, Minnesota

STUART J. SCHNITT, MD
Professor, Department of Pathology
Harvard Medical School
Director, Division of Anatomic
Pathology
Department of Pathology
Beth Israel Deaconess Medical Center
Boston, Massachusetts

WALTER SCHÜRCH, MD
Professor, Department of Pathology
Hôtel-Dieu Hospital
University of Montreal (CHUM)
Montreal, Quebec
Canada

THOMAS A. SEEMAYER, MD
Emeritus Professor
Department of Pathology and
Microbiology
University of Nebraska Medical Center
Omaha, Nebraska

EDWARD B. STELOW, MD
Assistant Professor
Department of Pathology
University of Virginia Health System
Charlottesville, Virginia

ARIEF A. SURIAWINATA, MD
Assistant Professor
Department of Pathology
Dartmouth Medical School
Pathologist, Department of Pathology
Dartmouth Hitchcock Medical Center
Lebanon, New Hampshire

SAUL SUSTER, MD
Professor and Vice Chair
Department of Pathology
The Ohio State University
Director of Anatomic Pathology
Department of Pathology
The Ohio State University Hospitals
Columbus, Ohio

SWAN N. THUNG, MD
Professor, Departments of Pathology
and Gene and Cell Medicine
Mount Sinai School of Medicine
Director of Hepatopathology Division
Department of Pathology
Mount Sinai Medical Center
New York, New York

ARTHUR S. TISCHLER, MD
Professor, Department of Pathology
Tufts University School of Medicine
Senior Pathologist
Department of Pathology
Tufts New England Medical Center
Boston, Massachusetts

THOMAS D. TRAINER, MD
Professor Emeritus
Department of Pathology
University of Vermont
College of Medicine
Fletcher Allen Health Care
Burlington, Vermont

LAWRENCE TRUE, MD
Professor, Department of Pathology
University of Washington
School of Medicine
Staff Pathologist
Department of Pathology
University of Washington Medical
Center
Seattle, Washington

CARLOS D. URMACHER, MD
Vice President and Chief Medical
Officer
Department of Pathology
CBLPath Inc.
Rye Brook, New York

PAUL van der VALK, MD, PhD
Professor, Department of Pathology
Head, Department of Neuropathology
VU University Medical Center
Amsterdam, The Netherlands

ALLARD C. van der WAL, MD, PhD
Consultant Pathologist
Department of Pathology
Academisch Medisch Centrun
Amsterdam, The Netherlands

J. HAN J. M. van KRIEKEN, MD
Department of Pathology
University Nijmegen Medical Center
Nijmegen, The Netherlands

ELSA F. VELAZQUEZ, MD
Assistant Professor
Department of Pathology
Harvard Medical School
Attending Pathologist
Department of Pathology
Brigham and Women's Hospital
Boston, Massachusetts

**ROY O. WELLER, BSC, MD, PhD,
FRCPATH**
Emeritus Professor of Neuropathology
Department of Clinical Neurosciences
University of Southampton School of
Medicine
Emeritus Consultant in
Neuropathology
Department of Cellular Pathology
(Neuropathology)
Southampton University Hospital
Southampton, United Kingdom

BRUCE M. WENIG, MD
Chairman, Department of Pathology
and Laboratory Medicine
Beth Israel Medical Center
and St. Luke's and Roosevelt Hospitals
New York, New York
Professor of Pathology
Albert Einstein College of Medicine
Bronx, New York

**SUNITHA N. WICKRAMASINGHE,
SCD, PhD, FRCP, FRCPath**
Professor Emeritus of Hematology
Department of Hematology
University of London
Imperial College
London, England
Visiting Professor of Hematology
University of Oxford
Oxford, England
Consultant Hematologist
Department of Hematology
St. Mary's Hospital
London, England

**EDWARD J. WILKINSON, MD, FCAP,
FACOG**
Professor and Vice Chairman
Department of Pathology
University of Florida
Vice Chairman of Pathology
Shands at the University, of Florida
Gainesville, Florida

SAMUEL A. YOUSEM, MD
Professor, Department of Pathology
University of Pittsburgh School of
Medicine
Vice Chair, Anatomic Pathology
Services
Department of Pathology
University of Pittsburgh Medical
Center–Presbyterian Campus
Pittsburgh, Pennsylvania

Preface

The third edition of *Histology for Pathologists* builds on the tradition of its two predecessors as a text to bridge the gap between the histology of normality and pathology. Dr. Stephen S. Sternberg, who first recognized the need for this text, shepherded the first two editions through production, and made this work a "must have" for practicing pathologists, has retired as editor. It is a great honor to replace him on the third edition and continue his legacy.

It is axiomatic that in order to understand the abnormal, one must first have a clear understanding of the normal. Although normal histology appears static, at least when viewed over the life span of humans, our understanding of normality evolves at a considerably more rapid rate. Accordingly, the third edition is greatly revised and completely reorganized. Where appropriate, immunohistochemical features of normal tissues are presented, using the latest available markers. Several new chapter authors have been added and many new color illustrations are provided.

Considerable effort has been expended to improve the illustrations held over from prior editions. At the time of the second edition, apoptosis was a relatively new discovery and merited a separate chapter. This now well-accepted concept is discussed in detail in individual chapters of the third edition. Although the text emphasizes normality, as in prior editions, prepathologic conditions are briefly considered in many chapters. More importantly, emphasis is placed on normal processes that may be confused with pathologic conditions. It is this pathologic perspective that sets *Histology for Pathologists* apart from standard histology texts written by anatomists.

As in the prior two editions, our goal for the third edition remains to provide a text that both the neophyte pathology trainee and experienced anatomic pathologist will find of considerable value in their professional careers.

Stacey E. Mills, MD

Preface to the First Edition

Histology textbooks exist in abundance. Some are classics of their kind and have gone through innumerable editions over many years. They have served pathologists well, for the most part, especially in terms of strict tissue and cell histology. There is, however, a borderline between histology and pathology in which information for the pathologist is often lacking.

With this textbook we made an attempt to fill the gap. The significance and function of many histological structures in terms of pathological interpretation is often absent or obscure. In particular, variations of the norm related to such variables as age, sex, and race are often not clarified in conventional textbooks. For example, the chapter on paraganglia notes that the connective tissue between the lobules in the carotid body increases with age. Another example related to age is in the pediatric kidney chapter, where it is noted that the glomeruli of fetuses are disproportionately large and are rarely seen in a state of histological "immaturity." While the chapter on the myofibroblast details the location, staining, ultrastructure, and cytoskeletal protein composition of this unusual cell, we also learn of its importance in the desmoplastic reaction in cancerous tissue and, most importantly, that it is not found in carcinomas which are still in situ.

Some gross observations occasionally will be found as lagniappe, such as the notation that in patients with congenital absence of a kidney, the ipsilateral adrenal will be round rather than angulated. Another example would be that there is a crease in the earlobe associated with coronary artery disease.

Variations in staining reactions are considered, such as the failure of factor VIII to stain renal glomerular vessels. One finds that intestinal endocrine cells can be detected with hematoxylin and eosin (sic) stains by the infranuclear location of the granules. Uncommonly known fixation artifacts are uncovered; for example, the prickle-cell layer (with so-called intercellular bridges) is actually a retraction artifact of the plasma membranes with the desmosomes remaining relatively fixed.

In most chapters, "prepathological" considerations are emphasized, while in others the developed pathological alterations related to the norm represent the major thrust of the chapter.

Some comments will be perceived as gratuitous, such as the remark in the penis chapter to the effect that "the prepuce could be a mistake of nature." Furthermore, we learn that the "collagen fibers are wavy in the flaccid state and become straight during erection."

The pathology neophyte as well as the many esteemed and experienced pathologists will find helpful information in this book.

Stephen S. Sternberg, MD

Acknowledgments

My contributions to this text would not have been possible without the unending support of many family members, friends, and colleagues. I would like to dedicate this work to my wife, Linda, and our daughters, Elizabeth and Anne, for always being there when I needed them and for teaching me more than they will ever know about all things beyond pathology; to my early mentors in pathology, Ben Sturgill, Shannon Allen, and Bob Fechner who got me started on the right path; and to all my colleagues and our trainees at the University of Virginia from whom I continue to learn and hope to do so for a long time.

Stacey E. Mills, MD

CUTANEOUS TISSUE

Normal Skin

Min Li   Carlos D. Urmacher

INTRODUCTION

The skin accounts for about 15% of the total body weight and is the largest organ of the body. It is composed of three layers: (a) epidermis, (b) dermis and (c) the subcutaneous adipose tissue. Each component has its unique and complex structure and function (1–3), with variation according to age, gender, race, and anatomic location. Functions of the skin are extremely diverse. It serves as a mechanical barrier against external physical, chemical, and biological noxious substances and as an immunologic organ. It participates in body temperature and electrolyte regulation. It is an important organ of sensuality and psychological well-being. In addition, it is a vehicle that expresses not only primary diseases of the skin, but also diseases of the internal organs. An understanding of the skin's normal histology is essential to the understanding of pathologic conditions.

EMBRYOLOGY

Epidermis

Embryologically, the ectoderm gives rise to epidermis and its appendages. The mesoderm provides the mesenchymal elements of the dermis and subcutaneous fat (4,5).

At first, the embryo is covered by a single layer of ectodermal cells. By the sixth to eighth week of development, it differentiates into two layers, the basal layer and an overlying second layer called periderm. The surface of the periderm is covered by microvilli and is in contact with the amniotic fluid. The mitotic activity of the basal layer predominates over that of the periderm, and soon the basal layer becomes the germinative layer. Additional rows of cells develop from this proliferating layer, forming a multilayer of cells between ectoderm and periderm (5). By the twenty-third week, keratinization has taken place in the upper stratum, and the cells of the periderm have already been shed (5–7). Interestingly, it has been demonstrated that many of the cell junction proteins are expressed in the early two-layered embryonic epidermis and as early as the eighth week of estimated gestational age (8). By the end of the first trimester, the dermal epidermal junction with its component is ultrastructually similar to that of mature skin (9). Thus, the characteristic neonatal epidermis is well developed by the fourth month.

The majority of cells in the epidermis are keratinocytes (90 to 95%). The rest of the epidermal cells are nonkeratinocytes (5 to 10%), and they include melanocytes, Langerhans cells, and Merkel cells. The nonkeratinocytes are seen in the epidermis of 8- to 10-week-old embryos. The precursor cells of melanocytes migrate from the neural crest to the dermis and then to the epidermis, where they differentiate into melanocytes during the first three months of development. During this migration, melanocytes can reside in other organs and tissue. Ultrastructually, recognizable melanosomes in melanocytes may be seen in the fetal epidermis at 8 to 10 weeks of gestational age (10).

Langerhans cells are derived from the CD34+ hematopoietic precursor cell of the bone marrow. The characteristic cytoplasmic marker, the Birbeck granule, is seen ultrastructurally in 10-week-old embryos (11). The expression of a more characteristic immunohistochemical marker, CD1a is completed by 12 to 13 weeks of estimated gestational age (12,13).

Merkel cells can also be seen in the epidermis of 8- to 10-week-old embryos. The origin of Merkel cells is debatable. Some have suggested a neural crest derivation (14), whereas others suggest epidermal origin through a process of differentiation from neighboring keratinocytes (15–18). Merkel cells in the epidermis are initially numerous and later diminish with increasing gestational age, which suggests their role in growth and development (19).

Dermis

The dermis is derived from the primitive mesenchyme underlying the surface ectoderm. The papillary and reticular dermis is recognized by 15 weeks of intrauterine life (20,21).

As described by Breathnach (20), three types of cells are recognized in 6- to 14-week old embryos. Type I cells are stellate-dendritic cells with long slender processes. These are the most numerous primitive mesenchymal cells and probably give rise to the endothelial cells and the pericytes. Type II cells have less extensive cell processes; the nucleus is round, and the cytoplasm contains large vacuoles. They are classified as phagocytic macrophages of yolk-sac origin. Type III cells are round with little or no membrane extension, but they contain numerous vesicles, some with an in-

ternal content suggestive of granule-secretory type of cells. These cells could be melanoblasts on their way to the epidermis, or they could be precursors of mast cells; Schwann cells associated with neuroaxons, but lacking basal lamina, are also identified during this period.

The type II mesenchymal cells are rarely seen after week 14 of development. However, another cell type with ultrastructure of histiocyte or macrophage is frequently seen during this time. Well-formed mast cells are also seen in the dermis.

In 14 to 21 weeks of development, fibroblasts are numerous and active. Fibroblasts are recognized as elongated spindle cells with abundant rough endoplasmic reticulum. They are the fundamental cell of the dermis and synthesize all types of fibers and ground substance (1). Type III collagen fibers are abundantly present in the matrix of fetus, whereas type I collagen fibers are more prominent in adult skin (21). Elastic fibers appear in the dermis after the collagen fiber during the twenty-second week of gestational age; and, by week 32, a well-developed network of elastic fiber is formed in the dermis (5).

Initially, the dermis is organized into somites, but soon this segmental organization ends and the dermis of the head and neck and extremities organizes into dermatomes along the segmental nerves that are being formed (22). From the twenty-fourth week to term, fat cells develop in the subcutaneous tissue from the primitive mesenchymal cells.

Epithelial Skin Appendages

Most epithelial cells of skin appendages derive from follicular epithelial stem cells localized in the basal layer of epidermis at the prominent bulge region of the developing human fetal hair follicles. Furthermore, such multipotent stem cells may represent the ultimate epidermal stem cell (23). In 10-week-old embryos, a group of mesenchymal cells of the developing dermis aggregate beneath a budding group of tightly packed basal cells (24). These epidermal cells grow both downward to the dermis and upward through the epidermis to form the opening of the hair canal. As the growing epithelial cells reach the subcutaneous fat, the lower portion becomes bulbous and partially encloses the mesenchymal cells, descending with them to form the dermal papillae of the hair follicle. The descending epidermal cells around the dermal papillae constitute the matrix cells from which the hair layers and inner root sheath will develop. The outer root sheath derives from downward growth of the epidermis. The first hairs appear by the end of the third gestational month as lanugo hair around the eyebrow and the upper lip. The lanugo hair is shed around the time of birth. The developing hair follicle gives rise to the sebaceous and apocrine glands.

The sebaceous glands originate as epithelial buds from the outer root sheath of the hair follicles and are developed at approximately the thirteenth to fifteenth gestational week (25). Differentiated sebaceous gland with a hair protruding through the skin surface are present at the eighteenth week of gestational age (26). They respond to maternal hormones and are well developed at the time of birth.

The apocrine glands also develop as epithelial buds from the outer sheath of the hair follicles in 5- to 6-month-old fetuses (22,24) and continue into late embryonic life as long as new hair follicles develop.

The eccrine glands develop from the fetal epidermis independent of the hair follicles (22). Initially, they are seen as regularly spaced undulations of the basal layer. At 14 to 15 weeks, the tips of the primordial eccrine glands have reached the deep dermis, forming the eccrine coils (27). At the same time, the eccrine epithelium grows upward into the epidermis. The primordial eccrine epithelium acquires a lumen by the seventh to eighth fetal month, and thus the first eccrine unit is formed. Both ducts and secretory portions are lined by two layers of cells. The two layers in the secretory segment undergo further differentiation; the luminal cells into tall columnar secretory cells, and the basal layer into secretory cells or myoepithelial cells (5). The first glands are formed on the palms and soles by the fourth month, then in the axillae in the fifth month, and finally on the rest of the hairy skin (28).

PHYSIOLOGY

Epidermis

The skin not only serves as a physical barrier between internal organs and the environment, but also functions as an active immune organ (29). Langerhans cells, the antigen-presenting cells of the epidermis, function as immunologic cells by recognizing antigens on the skin and presenting them to naive T lymphocytes. They become mature after contact with the antigen (30). Melanocytes produce melanin from the substrate tyrosine, using tyrosinase, and store it in melanosomes. Mature melanosomes are then transported to adjacent keratinocytes, where they provide protection against the harmful effects of solar radiation.

The keratinocytes are responsible for the process of keratinization. The formation of keratin filaments, in association with desmosomes, hemidesmosomes, and the basement membrane provides the structural integrity of the epidermis (31). Keratinocytes produce immunologic molecules, such as interleukins, interferons, and growth factors (32). It is recognized that the epidermal keratinocytes have immune properties.

Different types of keratin intermediate filaments are expressed in fetal and adult skin, and this process is, in part, regulated by apoptosis.

Apoptosis

Apoptosis, or programmed cell death, is the mechanism by which cells are deleted in normal tissue (33) and is the process responsible in establishing the final normal architecture of adult skin (34).

Terminal differentiation of the epidermis into a stratified squamous layer can be considered a specialized form of apoptosis (34). Apoptosis also participates in the cycling of the hair follicle (35–37) and is the principal mechanism by which catagen hair is formed (38–40). The bcl-2 proto-oncogen is a protein that blocks apoptosis and is expressed in basal cell keratinocytes and in the dermal papillae, protecting the latter from apoptosis (38).

Apoptosis affects individual cells—not groups of cells, as in necrosis (33). The basic morphologic changes include fragmentation of the nucleus, chromatin compaction, and budding of the cells to produce membrane-bound apoptotic bodies, which are ingested by neighboring cells. No inflammation is seen with the process of apoptosis (33).

By light microscopy, apoptotic cells are seen as isolated cells with bright eosinophilic cytoplasms and dark, pyknotic and fragmented nuclei (Figure 1.1).

In routine hematoxylin-eosin (H&E)–stained sections, apoptotic bodies are seen in a large variety of inflammatory and neoplastic diseases, such as graft-versus-host disease, lichen planus, erythema multiforme, squamous carcinoma, and malignant melanoma.

Recent study suggests that the mitogen-activated protein kinase signal transduction pathways are important in regulating the balance between keratinocyte cell proliferation, survival, apoptosis, and cell differentiation. Furthermore, it is suggested that extracellular regulated kinases induce keratinocyte proliferation and survival, whereas p38

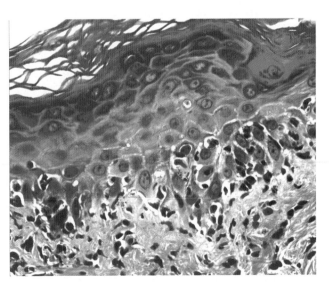

Figure 1.1 Apoptotic cell in a case of erythema multiforme. Note the eosinophilic cytoplasm and condensed nucleus.

mitogen-activated protein kinase promote differentiation and apoptosis (41).

Dermis

The dermis is a supportive, connective tissue composed of cells, fibrous molecules, and ground substance (1). The mesenchymal component of dense fibrous connective tissue provides the mechanical support, rigidity, and thickness to the skin. Collagenous and elastic fibers are closely associated with each other in the dermis. Collagen presumably provides the skin with tensile strength, whereas elastin posseses the retractile properties of the skin (42). The dermis also has immunologic functions because it contains dendritic cells, lymphocytes, other migrant leukocytes, mast cells, and tissue macrophages. Mast cells react to inflammatory process and also participate in wound healing.

Except for the epidermis, the skin is rich in a vascular network. In addition to providing nutrients to the skin, blood vessels are involved in thermal regulation, wound healing, immune response, and control of blood pressure. The lymphatic system is important in regulating the pressure of interstitial fluid (1).

The skin is supplied with autonomic nerves and sensory nerves. Small and large nerve plexuses participate in the innervations, which are responsible for the detection of touch, pressure, vibration, pain, temperature, and itching, as well as sweat secretion and piloerection.

Eccrine and Apocrine Glands

The most important function of the eccrine glands is in the processes of thermoregulation and electrolytic balance (43). The eccrine glands are the true sweat glands, and their function begins in the neonatal period. Eccrine glands produce colorless and odorless hypotonic sweat composed of predominantly water and the same electrolytes that are present in the plasma. There are two types of secretory cells, clear and dark cells. The clear cells of the eccrine coil, responding predominantly to cholinergic stimuli, and to a lesser degree to sympathetic stimulation (44–46), produce an isotonic sweat. When it reaches the duct, sodium and chloride ions are reabsorbed, delivering a hypotonic solution to the surface. The function of the dark cells is still not known with certainty. It has been suggested that they permit reabsorption of sodium, potassium, and chloride (24) and may secrete sialomucin (47) to the sweat.

In addition, the eccrine duct has the important function of delivering parenteral or orally administered drugs to the surface of the skin (48). Ductal epithelium also participates in the process of wound healing (22).

The major function of the myoepithelial cells is mechanical support against a high hydrostatic pressure. The contraction of myoepithelial cells aids in delivery of sweat to the skin surface (49).

The exact role of apocrine glands and the mechanisms regulating apocrine secretory process in humans are still under investigation. Apocrine glands might also play a role in thermal regulation (50,51). In nonhuman mammals, apocrine glands are found over the entire skin surface; they are believed to serve as identifying or sexual organs (24). Apocrine secretion has a milky color and is sterile and odorless; however, when it reaches the surface of the skin, the action of regional microorganisms on the apocrine secretion makes it odorous (24). The most abundant odor component, known to be E-3-methyl-2-hexanoic acid (E-3M2H), is liberated from nonodorous apocrine secretion by microorganisms (52).

Alteration in the rate and amount of sweat secretion manifests as anhidrosis, hypohidrosis, and hyperhidrosis (53,54). Cystic fibrosis (44,49) is the disorder with alterations in the electrolyte composition of eccrine sweat. Few morphologic changes are seen in association with these diseases.

LIGHT MICROSCOPY

Epidermis

The epidermis is a stratified keratinizing squamous epithelium that dynamically renews itself but maintains its normal thickness by the process of desquamation. The cells in the epidermis include: (a) keratinocytes, (b) melanocytes, (c) Langerhans cells, and (d) Merkel cells. In addition, the epidermis contains the openings for the eccrine ducts (acrosyringium) and hair follicles. Recent immunohistochemical studies have demonstrated that the epidermis contains free nerve axons in association with Langerhans cells (55).

Keratinocytes

The keratinocytes of the epidermis are stratified into four orderly layers from bottom to top: (a) the basal layer (stratum basalis, germinativum); (b) the squamous layer (prickle cell layer, or stratum spinosum); (c) the granular layer (stratum granulosum); (d) the cornified, or horny, layer (stratum corneum) (Figure 1.2). In histologic sections, the dermoepidermal junction has an irregular contour because of the upward extension of the papillary dermis to form the dermal papillae. The portion on the epidermis separating the dermal papillae are the rete ridges (Figure 1.3).

The Basal Layer

Basal cells are the mitotically active cells that give rise to the other keratinocytes. In histologic sections, basal cells are seen as a single layer of cells above the basement membrane that show some variation in size, shape, and melanin

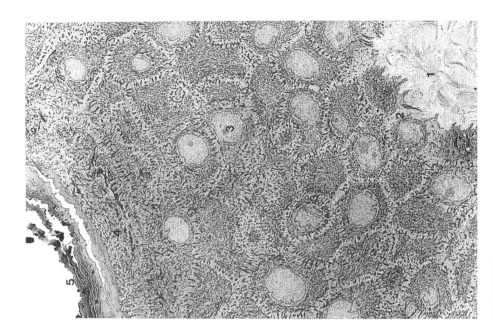

Figure 1.2 Electron micrograph of normal epidermis and portion of papillary dermis (×2,100). (*1*, papillary dermis; *2*, basal cells; *3*, squamous layer; *4*, granular layer; *5*, cornified layer)

content. Basal cells are columnar or cuboidal, with a basophilic cytoplasm. The nucleus is round or oval, with coarse chromatin and indistinct nucleolus. Basal cells contain melanin in their cytoplasm as a result of pigment transfer from neighboring melanocytes. Basal cells are connected to each other and to keratinocytes by specialized regions (known as desmosomes) located in the plasma cell membranes. They are aligned perpendicular to the subepidermal basement membrane and attached to it by modified desmosomes, hemidesmosomes (1).

Dermatitis involving the basal layer produces vacuolar alteration of the basal cells, which may progress to the

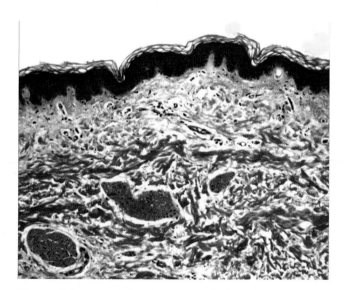

Figure 1.3 Normal skin showing stratified epidermis with rete ridges, papillary dermis and reticular dermis (H&E).

formation of subepidermal vesicles as seen in diseases such as graft-versus-host disease, lupus erythematosus, and erythema multiforme.

The Squamous Layer

The squamous layers are composed of approximately five to ten layers of cells with keratinocytes larger than the basal cells. The suprabasal keratinocytes are polyhedral, have a somewhat basophilic cytoplasm, and with a round nucleus. Again, melanin is seen scattered in many of these keratinocytes, where it provides protection from the damaging effect of ultraviolet light. The more superficial cells are larger, flattened, eosinophilic, and oriented parallel to the surface. The keratinocytes contain one or two conspicuous nucleoli and tonofilaments within the cytoplasm.

The squamous layer is also called the spinous or prickle cell layer because of the characteristic appearance by light microscopy of short projections extending from cell to cell. These projections are the result of retraction of the plasma membrane during tissue processing whereas the desmosomes remain relatively fixed and correlate with intercellular bridges.

Desmosomes are composed of a variety of polypeptides; desmogleins and desmocollins as transmembrane constituents and the desmoplakin, plakoglobin and plakophilin as cytoplasmic components (5). In addition, other intercellular junctions (such as gap junctions and adherens junctions) are distinct from desmosomes in composition and distribution and provide alternative cell-to-cell adhesion mechanisms (56). An intercellular space of constant dimension (57) is present between each cell; acid and neutral mucopolysaccharides are present in the intercellular spaces as indicated by special stains (5). The pemphigus antigens are localized in the cell membranes (58) or in the desmosomes of these cells (59). Antibodies to desmosomal proteins are used as additional markers for the study of neoplasm (60).

It is important to recognize that occasionally cells with clear or pale cytoplasms are seen in the squamous layer. These cells must be distinguished from the neoplastic cells of Paget's disease. Benign clear cells have a pyknotic nucleus surrounded by a clear halo and a narrow rim of clear cytoplasm (Figure 1.4). They lack the pleiomorphism, nuclear morphology, and intensity of the chromatin staining seen in Paget's cells (Figure 1.5). These benign clear cells are often seen in the epidermis of the nipple, the accessory nipple (61,62), and the pubic regions or in the milk line distribution (63). In the nipple, these clear cells, also called Toker cells, have been considered to be nonneoplastic mammary elements (61), although some authors hypothesized that these cells might be the precursors of mammary or extramammary Paget's diseases (62,64). Those outside of the nipple are considered to be the result of either abnormal keratinization or aberrant derivatives of eccrine or apocrine sweat gland epithelial cells (65–67). They may present as hypopigmented macules or papules in a rare disorder called clear cell papulosis (63,67). The immunohistochemical and mucin staining pattern of benign clear cells may resemble that of Paget's cells. Therefore, they must be distinguished on a morphologic basis from the neoplastic cells.

Common inflammatory changes seen in the squamous layer are: (a) spongiosis—intercellular edema (*e.g.*, allergic contact dermatitis); (b) acanthosis—thickening of the epi-

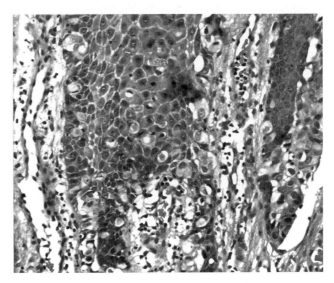

Figure 1.5 Paget's cells in extramammary Paget's disease.

dermis (*e.g.*, psoriasis); (c) atrophy—thinning of the epidermis (*e.g.*, discoid lupus erythematosus); (d) acantholysis—detachment of keratinocytes because of changes involving intercellular junctions (*e.g.*, pemphigus); and (e) dyskeratosis—abnormal keratinization (*e.g.*, squamous carcinoma).

The Granular Layer

The granular layer is composed of one to three layers of flattened cells lying parallel to the skin surface. The cytoplasm contains intensely basophilic-stained granules known as the keratohyalin granules. In contrast, trichohyalin granules (produced by the inner root sheath of hair follicles) are stained red on routine H&E-stained sections. The keratohyalin granules are histidine-rich and are the precursors to the protein flaggrin, which promotes aggregation of keratin filaments in the cornified layer. The granular layer is rich in lysosomal enzyme, which is crucial for the autolytic changes in the granular layer (68). The increase (*e.g.*, lichen planus) and decrease (*e.g.*, psoriasis) in the thickness of the granular layer can be used as a clue in the diagnosis of different pathologic entities.

Keratinocytes located between the squamous layer and the granular layer contain small membrane-coating granules known as lamellar granules (also called Odland bodies or keratosomes. They are composed of the acid hydrolase and of neutral sugars conjugated with proteins and lipids. These granules are present both intra- and extracellularly, are approximately 300 nm in diameter, and are not visible by light microscopy. Their functions are to provide epidermal lipids, increase the barrier property of the cornified layer against water loss, and aid in the desquamation process. This interface between the squamous and granular layer is also the site of synthesis and storage of cholesterol (57,69).

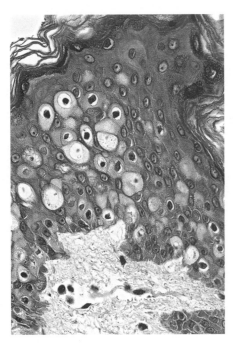

Figure 1.4 Clear cells of the nipple epidermis.

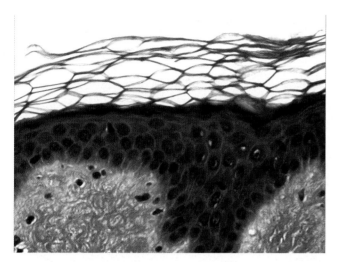

Figure 1.6 Basket-weave pattern of the cornified layer (also in Figure 1.3).

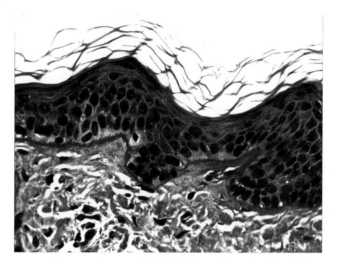

Figure 1.7 PAS-positive basement membrane.

The Cornified Layer

The cornified layer is composed of multiple layers of polyhedral eosinophilic keratinocytes that lack a nucleus and cytoplasmic organelles. These cells are the most differentiated cells of the keratinization system. They are composed entirely of high-molecular weight keratin filaments. In formalin-fixed section, the cornified layers are arranged in a basket-weave pattern (Figure 1.6). These cells eventually shed from the surface of the skin. The process of keratinization takes 20 to 45 days.

In histologic sections taken from the skin of the palms and soles, a homogenous eosinophilic zone, known as the stratum lucidum is present in the lowest portion of the cornified layer (above the granular layer). This additional layer is rich in protein-bound lipids contained in the lamellar granules (5), energetic enzymes and SH groups secreted by the granular cells in molecular structure (70).

Common abnormalities of the cornified layer are: (a) hyperkeratosis—increased thickness in the cornified layer (*e.g.*, ichythyosis); (b) parakeratosis—presence of nuclei in the cornified layer (as usually seen in actinic keratosis); and (c) presence of fungal organisms (superficial dermatophytosis).

Basement Membrane Zone

The basement membrane zone separates the epidermal basal layer from the dermis. It is seen by light microscopy as a continuous, undulating and thin periodic acid-Schiff (PAS)-stained layer (Figure 1.7). By electron microscopy, the basal cells are attached to the basal lamina by hemidesmosomes (57). Ultrastructurally, the basement membrane zone is composed of four distinct structures, from top to bottom (Figure 1.8) (57,71):

1. The plasma membrane of the basal cells containing the hemidesmosomes. Bullous pemphigoid antigen 1 is localized in the intracellular component of hemidesmosomes.

2. The lamina lucida, an electron-lucent area with anchoring filaments containing various laminin isoforms (1,72). Bullous pemphigoid antigen 2 (type XVII collagen) is associated with the transmembrane component of hemidesmosome-anchoring filament complexes in

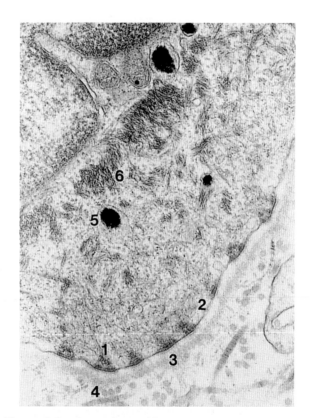

Figure 1.8 Ultrastructure of basement membrane (×37,800). (*1*, hemidesmosome; *2*, lamina lucida; *3*, lamina densa; *4*, lamina reticularis; *5*, melanin; *6*, tonofilaments)

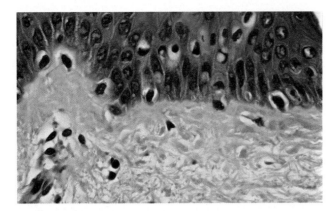

Figure 1.9 Melanocytes in the basal layer, composed of ovoid nuclei within a clear space.

the lamina lucida. It is also the site of the blister in dermatitis herpetiformis (73).

3. The lamina densa, an electron-dense area composed of mainly type IV collagen.
4. The sublamina densa zone, or pars fibroreticularis, contains mainly the anchoring fibrils (74) (type VII collagen) that attach the basal lamina to the connective tissue of the dermis. Antibodies against epidermolysis bullosa aquisita react with the carboxy terminus of type VII collagen (75,76).

Inflammatory conditions of the basement membrane can be seen by light microscopy as thickening (*e.g.*, discoid lupus erythematosus) or by the formation of subepidermal vesicles (*e.g.*, bullous pemphigoid).

Melanocytes

Melanocytes are dendritic cells that derive from the neural crest. During migration from the neural crest, melanocytes may localize in other epithelia. In the epidermis, the melanocytes are localized in the basal layer, and their dendritic processes extend in all directions. The dendritic nature of normal melanocytes is usually not seen in routine H&E-stained sections. In H&E preparations, melanocytes are composed of elongated or ovoid nuclei surrounded by a clear space (Figure 1.9). They are usually smaller than the neighboring basal keratinocytes. Melanocytes do not contain tonofilaments and do not attach to basal cells with desmosomes (5,77). However, anchoring filaments extend from the plasma membrane of these melanocytes to the basal lamina. Laminin-5, a component of anchoring filaments, may be a ligand for melanocyte attachment to the basement membrane in vivo (78). In addition, melanocytes that are close to the basal lamina have structures resembling hemidesmosomes of basal keratinocytes (79).

Melanocytes produce and secrete melanin. Melanin can be red (pheomelanin) or yellow-black (eumelanin) (80,81). The most important function of melanin is to pro-

tect against the injurious effects of non-ionizing ultraviolet irradiation.

Melanin is formed through a complex metabolic process in which tyrosinase is the main catabolic enzyme, using tyrosine as substrate. The synthesis of melanin takes place in melanosomes, lysosome-related organelles. In the early stages of development, melanosomes are membrane-limited vesicles, located in the Golgi-associated endoplasmic reticulum. The maturation of melanosomes undergoes four stages. Stage I melanosomes are round without melanin. These are seen in balloon cell melanoma. Stage II through stage IV melanosomes are ellipsoidal with numerous longitudinal filaments (5). Melanin deposits start at stage II. In stage III, melanin deposits are prominent. Stage IV melanosomes are fully-packed, with melanin obscuring the internal structures.

The developing melanosomes, with their content of melanin, are transferred to the neighboring basal keratinocytes and hair follicular cells. The mechanism of melanin transfer is a complex process (82,83), with the end result being phagocytosis of the tip of melanocytic dendrites by the keratinocytes (Figure 1.10) in a process called pigment donation (84). The "epidermal melanin unit" refers to one melanocyte with associated 36 keratinocytes to which the melanocytes deliver melanosomes (1).

The number of melanocytes in normal skin is constant in all races, the ratio being one melanocyte for every 4 to 10 basal keratinocytes (77,80). Thus, the color of the skin is determined by the number and size of melanosomes present both in keratinocytes and melanocytes—and not by the number of melanocytes. The number of melanocytes decreases with age. As a result, the availability of melanin to keratinocytes diminishes, so the skin becomes lighter in color and the incidence of skin cancer increases.

Melanin is both argentaffin and argyrophilic. It can be recognized by Fontana-Masson silver stains. In addition,

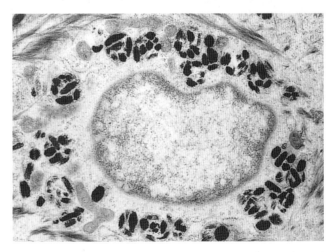

Figure 1.10 Electron micrograph showing membrane-bound phagocytized melanin in keratinocyte (×19,200).

melanocytes and their dendritic processes are identified by the dopa reaction in histologic slides prepared from frozen sections and in paraffin-embedded sections with immuno-histochemical stains with S-100 protein. The latter is highly sensitive but not specific for cells of melanocytic lineage. The S-100 protein can be detected in various types of cells, such as Langerhans cells, schwann cells, eccrine, and apocrine gland cells. Melanocytes can also be identified with monoclonal antibodies to Melan A/MART-1 (Melanoma Antigens Recognized by T cells-1), a melanocytic differentiation marker. The MART-1 antigen is expressed in normal melanocytes, common nevi, Spitz nevi, and malignant melanoma (5). Under normal conditions, the melanoma-associated antigen HMB-45 does not react with adult melanocytes (85). It is expressed in embryonic melanocytes, hair bulb melanocytes and activated melanocytes (86). It is usually seen reacting with most melanoma cells, Spitz nevi, the junctional component of common nevi, and dysplastic nevi.

A decrease or absent number of melanocytes is seen in vitiligo. In albinism, there is a defect in the synthesis of melanin, but the number of melanocytes is normal in a skin biopsy. Melanocytic hyperplasia is seen in lentigo, benign and malignant melanocytic neoplasm, and as a reaction pattern in a variety of neoplastic and nonneoplastic conditions (*e.g.,* dermatofibroma). In a freckle, there is an increase in pigment donation to adjacent keratinocytes rather than melanocytic hyperplasia (84).

Langerhans Cells (LCs)

Langerhans cells (LCs), discovered by Paul Langerhans in 1868, are mobile, dendritic, antigen-presenting cells present in all stratified epithelium and predominantly in the mid to upper part of the squamous layer. In H&E-stained sections, LCs can be suggested as they appear to lie within lacunae having darkly stained nuclei with indented, reniform shape at high magnification (Figure 1.11). As with melanocytes, their dendritic nature cannot be seen in routine sections. Langerhans cells can be recognized by histoenzymatic stains for adenosine triphosphatase (ATPase); they can also be detected in formalin-fixed, paraffin-embedded tissue using immunoreactivity for S-100 protein and, more specifically, the antibody to the CD1a antigen (Figure 1.12). With histoenzymatic and immunohistochemical stains, the extensive dendritic nature of LCs becomes evident.

By electron microscopy, LCs show no desmosomes, tonofilaments, or melanosomes. They contain small vesicles, multivesicular bodies, lysosomes, and the characteristic Birbeck granule (Figure 1.13) (87), a rod-shape organelle varying in size from 100 nm to1 μm (88). It has a centrally striated density and an occasional bulb at one end with a unique tennis racquet appearance. Their function is still undetermined. Langerin is a protein implicated

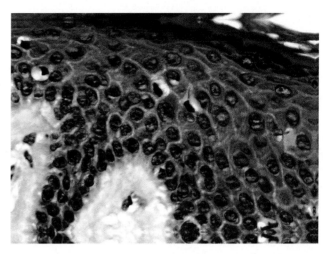

Figure 1.11 H&E section of possible Langerhans cells composed of elongated nuclei surrounded by a clear space in the mid-epidermis.

in Birbeck granule biogenesis and represents a key molecule to trace LCs and study their function (89,90).

Langerhans cells are also present in epithelia, lymphoid organs, and dermis and are increased in the skin in a variety of inflammatory conditions, such as contact dermatitis, where they can be seen as minute nodular aggregates in the epidermis. Langerhans' cell granulomatosis is a reactive lesion most commonly seen in bones but also appearing at other sites.

Merkel Cells (MCs)

Merkel cells (MCs), first described by F.S. Merkel in 1875, are scattered and irregularly distributed in the basal cell layer in the epidermis. They may group together in clusters coupled with enlarged terminal sensory nerve fibers to form slowly adapting mechanoreceptors; within the epidermis, they mediate tactile sensation (91–93). They are

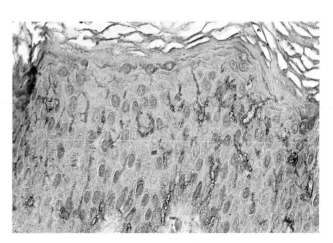

Figure 1.12 CD1a-specific reaction of Langerhans cells. Note the dendritic processes.

located in higher concentration in the glabrous skin of the digits, lips, and oral cavity (9), in the outer root sheath of hair follicles (94), and in the tactile hair disks (95).

Merkel cells are not recognized in routine histologic preparations. Electron microscopy and immunostaining are required for their identification. By electron microscopy, MCs are attached to adjacent keratinocytes by desmosomes. They have scant cytoplasms, invaginated nuclei, a parallel array of cytokeratin filaments in the paranuclear zone, and the characteristic membrane-bound dense core granules that are often, but not always, related to unmyelinated neurites.

By immunostaining techniques, normal and neoplastic MCs may express neuron-specific enolase, chromogranin, synaptophysin, neural cell adhesion molecule, and various neuropeptides and other substances (96–98). However, the expression of these substances in MCs is heterogenous and variable. The constant pattern seen in MCs is the presence of paranuclear aggregates of cytokeratins (16,98,99), which include low-molecular weight keratins 8, 18, 19, and 20. The most specific cytokeratin is CK20 because, in addition to MCs, they are expressed in simple epithelial cells and not in adjacent keratinocytes (100,101) (Figure 1.14).

Pilar Unit

The pilar unit is composed of the hair follicle, sebaceous gland, arrector pili muscle, and (when present) eccrine gland and apocrine gland.

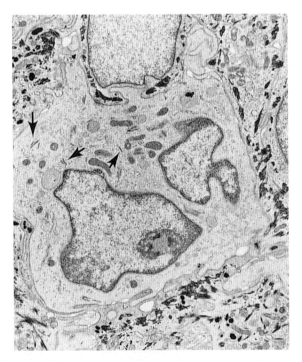

Figure 1.13 Electron micrograph of a Langerhans cell containing Birbeck granules (*arrows*) and multisegmented nucleus (×8,000).

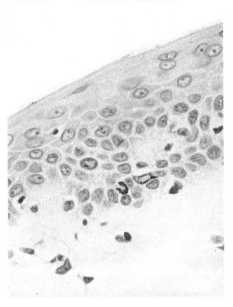

Figure 1.14 Cytokeratin-20 staining a Merkel cell in the basal layer of the epidermis.

Hair Follicle

The hair follicle is divided into three segments from top to bottom: (a) the infundibulum, which extends from the opening of the hair follicle in the epidermis to the opening of the sebaceous duct; (b) the isthmus, which extends from the opening of the sebaceous duct to the insertion of the arrector pili muscle; and (c) the inferior segment, which extends to the base of the follicle. The inferior segment is bulbous and encloses a vascularized component of the dermis referred to as follicular (dermal) papilla of the hair follicle (Figure 1.15).

The microanatomy and function of the hair follicle is very complex. The cells of the hair matrix differentiate along six cell linings. Beginning from the innermost layer, they are: (a) the hair medulla; (b) hair cortex; (c) hair cuticle; and (d) three concentric layers of the inner root sheath, which are the cuticle of the inner root sheath, Hexley's layer, and Henle's layer.

The inner root sheath of the hair follicle is surrounded by the outer root sheath (Figure 1.16), which is composed of clear cells. These glycogen-rich cells are seen in some of the neoplasm with hair follicular differentiation (*e.g.*, trichilemmoma). A PAS-positive basement membrane separates the outer root sheath from the surrounding connective tissue. Thus, the hair shaft is formed from the bulb region that occupies the hair follicular canal.

Dendritic melanocytes are present only in the upper half of the bulb, whereas inactive (amelanotic) melanocytes are present in the outer root sheath. These melanocytes can become active after injury, migrating into the upper portion of the outer root sheath and to the regenerating epidermis (5).

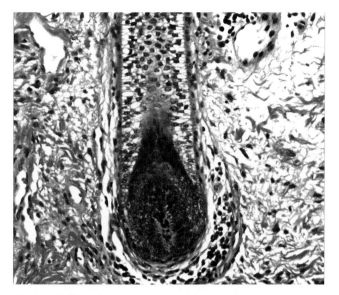

Figure 1.15 Inferior segment of the hair follicle, showing the hair papilla.

At the level of the isthmus, the cells of the inner root sheath disintegrate and disappear, whereas the cells of the outer root sheath begin an abrupt sequence of keratinization. This process is called trichilemmal keratinization (102). Trichohyalin granules are red in routine H&E-stained sections, as opposed to the blue granules of the keratohyalin of epidermal keratinization and of the epithelium of the follicular infundibulum of the hair follicle. The staining features of these granules permit neoplasms and cysts to be distinguished from either pilar or epidermal origin.

Under normal circumstances, microorganisms like *Staphylococcus epidermis*, yeasts of *Pityrosporum* (Figure 1.17), and the *Demodex folliculorum* (Figure 1.18) mites are encountered in the follicular infundibulum.

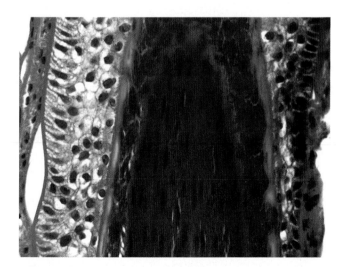

Figure 1.16 Hair follicle showing the hair shaft (*center*) surrounded by the inner root sheath, which contains trichohyalin granules. The outer root sheath is composed of clear cells.

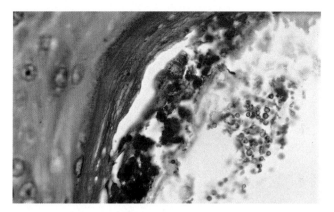

Figure 1.17 Yeasts of *Pityrosporum* in the follicular infundibulum.

The mantle hair of Pinkus (103) is a hair follicle in which proliferation of basaloid epithelioid cells emanating from the infundibulum is seen. Sebaceous proliferation is present in those cords (Figure 1.19). The significance of this hair follicle is not known.

The hair growth is in lifelong cyclic transformation. Hormones and their receptors play prominent roles in hair cycle regulation (104). Three phases are recognized: (a) anagen—active growth phase; (b) catagen—involuting phase (apoptosis-driven regression); and (c) telogen—relative resting phase. The histologic features previously described correspond to the anagen hair.

During the catagen phase, mitosis and melanin synthesis cease at the level of the hair bulb. The hair bulb is then replaced by a cornified sac formed by retraction of the outer root sheath around the hair bulb, and a club hair is formed. A thick glassy basement membrane surrounds the hair follicle. Apoptosis of single cells in the outer root sheath is a characteristic finding during the catagen phase (40).

During the telogen phase, the club hair and its cornified sac retract even further to the insertion of the arrector pili muscle, leaving behind the dermal papilla, which is

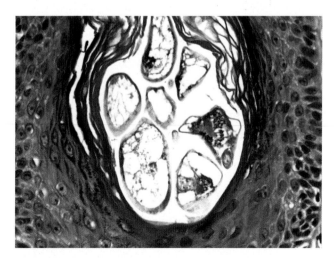

Figure 1.18 *Demodex folliculorum* mites in the follicular infundibulum.

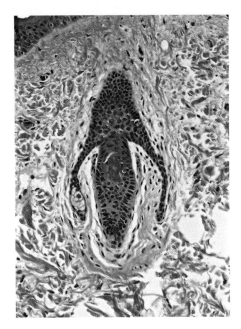

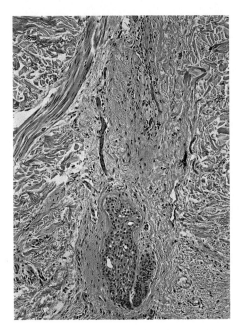

Figure 1.19   Mantle hair of Pinkus with lateral extensions containing sebaceous cells.

Figure 1.20   Catagen–telogen hair follicle located entirely within the dermis.

connected to the retracted hair follicle by a fibrous tract (Figure 1.20) (24). When the cycle is complete, a new anagen phase begins with the formation of new hair matrix.

The duration of the normal hair cycle varies. The anagen phase is measured in years for the scalp, but it is measured in shorter periods of time for the anagen cycle in other regions of the body. The length of the hair is also related to the amount of the anagen hair. More than 80% of hair present in normal scalp is anagen hair. The catagen phase takes two to three weeks, and the telogen phase may last a few months.

The color of normal hair depends on the amount and distribution of the melanin in the hair shaft (24). Normal human epidermal melanocytes may synthesize both eumelanin and pheomelanin (105). The melanins in black hair are eumelanin (characterized by the presence of ellipsoidal eumelanosomes), while those in red hair are mainly pheomelanin (ascribed to spherical pheomelanosomes) (105,106). Fewer melanosomes are produced in the bulbar melanocytes of blond hair. A relative absence of melanin and fewer melanosomes are seen in gray hair. Multiple internal or external regulatory factors are involved in hair pigmentation. There might be some correlation between tryptophan content and tyrosinase expression with hair color (107,108).

Another structure related to the pilar unit is the hair or pilar disk (the Haarscheibe). The Haarscheibe is a specialized spot in close vicinity to hairs. This structure is usually not recognized on routine histologic section. It may present as an acanthotic elevation of the epidermis, limited by two elongated rete ridges laterally (1). The epidermis in this area has more Merkel cells in the basal layer, and the dermal component is well vasculized, containing myelinized nerve fibers in contact with Merkel cells (22,95). It is considered as a highly sensitive, slowly adapting mechanoreceptor (1,109).

Sebaceous Glands

The sebaceous glands are holocrine glands associated with hair follicles. Their secretions are made of disintegrated cells. The palms and soles are the only regions devoid of sebaceous glands. Sebaceous glands are prominent in facial skin. They are also seen in the buccal mucosa, vermilion of the lip (Fordyce's spot), prepuce, labia minora, and, at times, in the parotid gland.

The sebaceous glands are lobulated structures composed of multiple acini in some locations like the head and neck; in other sites, such as chest, they are composed of a single acinus. The periphery of the lobules contains the germinative cells, which are cuboidal and flat with large nucleoli and basophilic cytoplasms without lipid droplets. As differentiation occurs, several inner layers show lipid droplet accumulation in the cytoplasm until they fill the cell.

The more differentiated cells (sebocytes) have a characteristic multivacuolated cytoplasm (Figure 1.21). The nucleus is centrally located and scalloped due to the lipid imprints. The more differentiated cells disintegrate and discharge the cellular debris (sebum) into the excretory duct, which opens into the hair follicle in the lower portion of the infundibulum. The excretory duct is short, shared by several lobules, and lined by keratinized squamous epithelium.

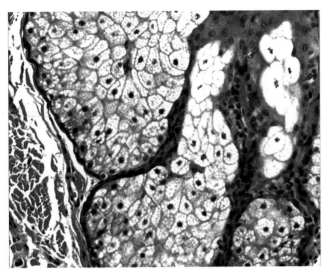

Figure 1.21 Sebaceous glands with peripheral germinative cells and, toward the center, the differentiated vacuolated cells.

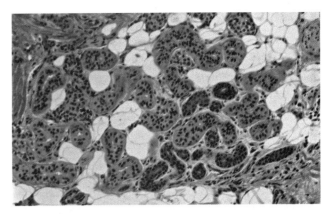

Figure 1.22 Eccrine lobule containing fat, glands, and ducts.

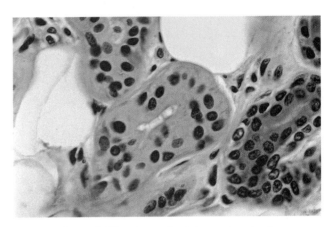

Figure 1.23 Clear cells of the eccrine glands.

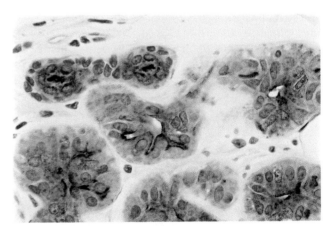

Figure 1.24 Intercellular canaliculi (anti-CEA).

Within sebaceous glands, the germinative cells express appreciable quantities of keratins. Mature sebocytes demonstrate cytoplasmic reactivity for high-molecular weight keratins and epithelial membrane antigen (1).

Eccrine Glands

The eccrine glands are the true sweat glands responsible for thermoregulation. They are found in higher concentration in palms, soles, forehead, and axillae and have dual secretory and excretory functions.

The secretory portion of an eccrine gland is a convoluted tube located in the dermis, in the interface with the subcutaneous tissue, and, rarely, within the subcutaneous tissue. In cross-sections, it appears that several glandular structures with a central lumen form the secretory coils. These are seen as lobular structures often surrounded by fat even when located within the dermis (Figure 1.22).

Three types of cells are identified in the eccrine coil: clear cells, dark cells, and myoepithelial cells. The clear cells are easily seen H&E-stained sections (Figure 1.23). They rest directly on the basement membrane and on the myoepithelial cells. Clear cells are composed of pale or finely granular cytoplasms with a round nucleus usually seen in the center of the cell. Deep invaginations of the luminal membranes of adjacent clear cells form intercellular canaliculi lined with microvilli (Figure 1.24) (110). The intercellular canaliculi often persistent in neoplasms derived from eccrine glands. The clear cells contain abundant mitochondria and variable amount of PAS-positive, diastase-labile glycogen.

The dark cells border the lumen of the glands. Electron microscopy shows that they contain abundant secretory granules that have glycogen-staining characteristics. They contain sialomucin (PAS-positive, diastase-resistant (PASD) mucopolysaccharides) and high concentration of

proteins (5,111). The dark cells are difficult to identify in routine H&E-stained sections. However, the acid-fast, PASD, and S-100 protein stains will highlight the granularity of the cells (Figure 1.25) (22).

The myoepithelial cells are contractile spindle cells that surround the secretory coil (Figure 1.26). In turn, they are surrounded by a PAS-positive basement membrane. Elastic

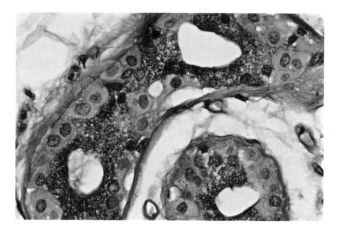

Figure 1.25 Dark cells with granular cytoplasm (acid-fast stain).

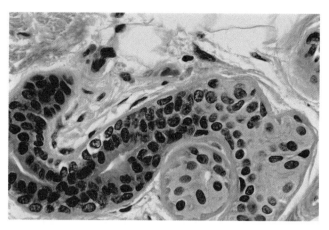

Figure 1.27 Eccrine duct. Note the abrupt transition from the secretory portion.

fibers, fat, and small nerves are present in the adjacent stroma.

The excretory component of the eccrine gland is composed of three segments: (a) a convoluted duct in close association with the secretory unit (Figure 1.27); (b) a straight dermal component; and (c) a spiral intraepidermal portion, the acrosyringium, which opens onto the skin surface (Figure 1.28). The transition between the secretory and excretory component is abrupt. Both convoluted and straight dermal ducts are histologically identical. They are narrow tubes with a slitlike lumina lined by double layers of cuboidal cells. The luminal cells have a more granular eosinophilic cytoplasm and a larger round nucleus than the peripheral row of cells. The peripheral cells are rich in mitochondria.

The luminal cells produce a layer of tonofilaments near the luminal membrane that are often referred to as "the cuticular border," which is a PASD eosinophilic cuticle (5). This cuticular border often persists in the eccrine neoplasm (*e.g.,* eccrine poroma). There are no myoepithelial cells and peripheral hyalin basement membrane zone in the eccrine ducts (5).

The intraepidermal segment of eccrine duct, known as acrosyringium has a unique symmetrical and helicoidal course in the epidermis with its length correlated to the thickness of the epidermis (43). It consists of a single layer of luminal cells and two or three rows of concentrically oriented outer cells. The presence of keratohyalin granules in acrosyringium in the lower levels of the squamous layer indicates that they keratinize independently. The intraepidermal lumen is lined by acellular eosinophilic cuticle before keratinization (5,24). Melanin granules are absent.

Apocrine Glands

The apocrine gland (Figure 1.29) has a coiled secretory portion and an excretory (ductal) component. The secretory portion is much longer than its eccrine counterpart; and it may reach 200 μm in diameter, compared to 20 μm for the eccrine glands (77). The secretory glands are located in the

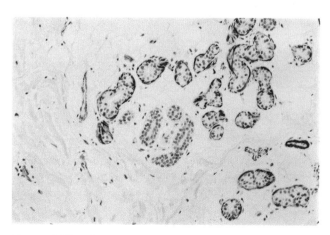

Figure 1.26 Glands, but not the ducts, are surrounded by myoepithelial cells (anti-HHF35).

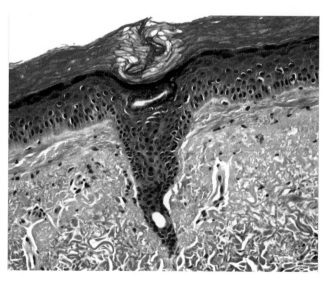

Figure 1.28 Acrosyringium.

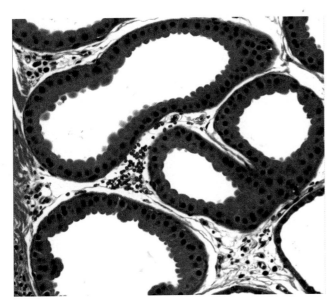

Figure 1.29 Secretory apocrine glands.

are located in the subcutaneous fat or in the deep dermis. They are lined by one layer of cuboidal, columnar, or flat cells (luminal cells), and an outer layer of myoepithelial cells, which is surrounded by a PAS-positive basement membrane. The luminal cells are composed of eosinophilic cytoplasm, which may contain lipid, iron, lipofuscin, PASD granules (24), and a large nucleus located near the base of the cell. Detached fragments of apical cytoplasm are found in the lumen of the glands. The secretion from apocrine glands releases secretory materials accompanied with loss of part of cytoplasm (112), although other forms of secretion have been observed, including melocrine (granular contents within numerous vesicles are released without loss of cytoplasm) and holocrine type (the entire cell is secreted into the glandular lumen) (50,112).

Similar to the eccrine duct, the excretory (ductal) component of the apocrine gland has a double layer of cuboidal cells. Microvilli are identified on the surface of the luminal cells and keratin filaments are in their cytoplasms, the latter giving the eosinophilic hyalin appearance to the inner lining of the duct. No myoepithelial cells and peripheral basement membrane are identified in the excretory duct. Apocrine glands are always connected to a pilosebaceous follicle. The intrafollicular or intraepidermal portion of apocrine duct is straight other than the spiral as seen in acrosyringium (5).

Apocrine glands are mostly located in the axillary, anogenital areas, mammary region, eyelids (Moll's glands), and external ear canal (ceruminous glands), and their presence is characteristic in Nevus sebaceous Jadassohn.

A third type of sweat gland, so-called "apoeccrine glands" of the human axillae (113), are composed of a dilated secretory portion that, by electron microscopy, is in-distinguishable from the apocrine glands; however, they retain the intercellular canaliculi, as well as the dark cells of the eccrine glands. The duct does not open in the hair follicle but in the epidermis. These glands, which develop from eccrine glands during puberty, account for as much as 45% of all axillary sweat glands in a young person. Recently, it was reported that the obstruction of intraepidermal apoeccrine sweat ducts by apoeccrine secretory cells might be the possible causes of Fox-Fordyce disease (114).

The most useful marker of sweat gland differentiation is carcinoembryonic antigen (CEA), found mainly in the luminal borders of secretory cells of eccrine glands and excretory eccrine ducts and, to a less extent, on apocrine glands. Gross cystic disease fluid protein-15 (GCDFP-15) and epithelial membrane antigen (EMA) are also detected in both eccrine and apocrine sweat glands (1,115). Myoepithelial cells lining the secretory sweat glands express smooth muscle actin and keratin K17 (1).

Dermis

The dermis is a dynamic, supportive connective tissue harboring cells, fibrous tissue, and ground substances with adnexal structures and vascular and nerve plexuses running through it (1). The dermis (Figure 1.30) consists of two zones: the papillary dermis and reticular dermis. The adventitial dermis (116) combines the papillary and the periadnexal dermis.

The papillary and periadnexal dermis can be recognized by a loose meshwork of thin, poorly organized collagen composed of predominantly type III collagen (117–119) mixed with some type I collagen and a delicate branching network of fine elastic fibers. The papillary dermis also contains abundant ground substance, fibroblasts and the capillaries of the superficial arterial and venous plexuses.

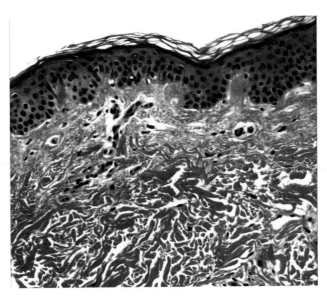

Figure 1.30 Dermis with papillary and thick reticular dermis.

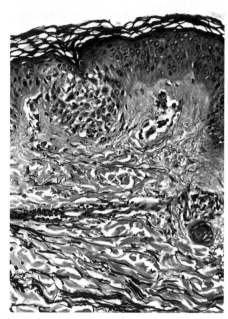

Figure 1.31 Distribution of elastic fibers. Elastin fibers are thin and branching in the papillary dermis and thick and fragmented in the reticular dermis.

The reticular dermis is thicker than the papillary dermis and is composed of multiple layers of well-organized thick bundles of collagens, predominantly type I collagen, mostly arranged parallel to the surface (117–119). These layers are built from overlapping of individual fibers of uniform size. The plates are oriented randomly in different directions (120). There are also thick elastic fibers with fragmented appearance detected by special elastic tissue stains (Figure 1.31). Some ground substance and the vessels of the deep plexuses are also present in the reticular dermis.

The resident cells in the dermis mainly include dermal dendritic cells, fibroblasts, and mast cells (1). Dermal dendritic cells are a group of cells with immunophenotypic and functional heterogeneity located in the dermis and possessing a dendritic morphology (121). There are multiple subsets of dendritic cells. At least three types of dermal dendritic cells are recognized as distinct cell types with unique immunophenotype in vivo (122,123).

1. Factor XIIIa+ dermal dendrocytes are in the perivascular distribution in the papillary dermis and around sweat glands (1,122). Dermal dendrocytes, also known as dendrophages (126), express some markers of mononuclear macrophages (124) and have phagocytic function (125).
2. CD34+ dendritic cells are present in the mid- and deep dermis around adnexae (1,122).
3. The dermis harbors a true dendritic cell population, also in a perivascular distribution. These are Langerhans' cell–like dendritic cells involved in dermal antigen presentation, expressing HLA-DR and CD1a except for lack of Birbeck granules (123,127,128).

Fibroblasts are the dynamic and fundamental cells of the dermis, synthesizing all types of fibers and ground substances (1,119). They appear as spindle-shaped or stellate cells, which are not reliably differentiated from other dermal spindle-shaped cells and dendritic cells in H&E-stained sections. Ultrastructurally, they contain prominent, well-developed rough endoplasmic reticulum.

Mast cells are derived from bone marrow CD34+ progenitor cells and are sparsely distributed in the perivascular and periadnexal dermis. They are recognized by a darkly stained ovoid nucleus and granular cytoplasm, which is highlighted by Giemsa and toluidine blue stains. Mast cells are positive with tryptase and c-kit (CD117) immunohistochemical stains (129–131). Mastocytosis is characterized by abnormal growth and accumulation of mast cells in various organs with heterogenous manifestation. Urticaria pigmentosa is the most common cutaneous manifestation of mastocytosis (132,133).

Macrophages are also seen in the normal dermis; they become visible when pigments or other ingested material is present in the cytoplasm of the cells.

Besides fibrous tissue and cellular components, the dermis also contains amorphous ground substance filling the spaces between fibers and dermal cells. It mainly consists of glycosaminoglycans or acid mucopolysaccharides (the nonsulfated acid mucopolysaccharides [predominantly hyaluronic acid] and, to a lesser degree, sulfated acid mucopolysaccharide [largely chondroitin sulfate]]) (1,5). The ground substance is present in small amounts and is seen as empty spaces between collagen bundles in routine H&E-stained sections; it also is hardly identified with Alcian blue and toluidine blue special stains. In pathologic conditions such as lupus erythematosus, granuloma annulare, and dermal mucinosis, the excessive quantity of ground substance produced can be seen without the aid of special stains as strings of bluish material.

Subcutaneous Tissue

Subcutaneous tissue, also called subcutis or hypodermis, is crucial in thermal regulation, insulation, provision of energy, and protection from mechanical injuries. It is composed of mature adipose tissue arranged into lobules. The mature adipocytes within the lobules are round cells rich in cytoplasmic lipids, which compress the nucleus to the side of the cell membrane. The adipocytes express S-100 protein and vimentin in immunohistochemical stains (123). These lobules of mature adipocytes are separated by the thin bands of dermal connective tissue that constitute the interlobular septa (Figure 1.32). Thus, inflammatory changes involving the subcutaneous tissue can be divided into septal panniculitis (*e.g.*, erythema nodosum) and lobular panniculitis (*e.g.*, panniculitis associated with pancreatitis) (24).

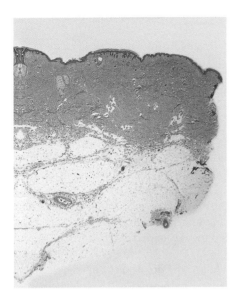

Figure 1.32 Septa and lobules of subcutaneous fat.

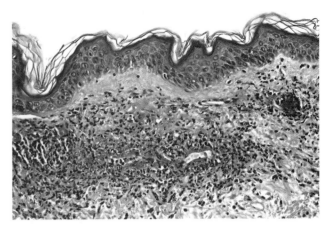

Figure 1.33 Vasculitis. Case of leukocytoclastic vasculitis showing damage to the capillary wall.

Blood Vessels, Lymphatics, Nerves, and Muscle

The large arteries that supply the skin are located in the subcutaneous tissue, usually within the interlobular septa, and are accompanied by large veins. Smaller arteries, venules, and capillaries constitute the main vasculature seen in the dermis and within the lobules of the subcutaneous fat.

A network of these smaller vessels is located in the papillary dermis (superficial plexus) and in the deep reticular dermis (deep plexus). Superficial vascular plexuses separate the papillary dermis from the reticular dermis, whereas the deep vascular plexuses define the boundary between the reticular dermis and subcutaneous tissue. The division of superficial and deep plexuses is important in the classification and recognition of many inflammatory diseases of the skin in which characteristic infiltrates are located around the superficial, deep, or superficial and deep plexuses. Blood endothelial cells express von Willebrand factor (factor VIII-related antigen), vimentin, CD34, and CD31 antigens (1,123).

Vasculitis is the inflammatory process that involves the blood vessels. It is important to remember that strict criteria are applied for the diagnosis of cutaneous vasculitis, and they include: (a) the presence of inflammatory cell infiltrate within the vessel wall, and (b) the presence of vascular injury, in a spectrum from edema and extravasations of red blood cells, leukocytoclasis, thrombi within the lumina of these blood vessels to fibrinoid necrosis and/or destruction of the blood vessel wall (Figure 1.33). The presence of fibrinoid necrosis of the vessel wall is essential for diagnosis of true vasculitis. Perivascular inflammation alone is not a sign of vasculitis.

Mainly in the acral skin, special arteriovenous anastomosing structures known as glomera are present in the reticular dermis. Each glomus is composed of an arterial segment (the Sucquet-Hoyer canals) connected directly with venous segments. Each Sucquet-Hoyer canal is surrounded by four to six layers of glomus cells, which are considered as vascular smooth muscle cells serving as a spincter. Glomus is involved in thermal regulation (1,5).

The lymphatics of the skin (134) accompany the venules and are also located in the deep and superficial plexuses. Unless valves are seen within these vessels, their recognition in routine sections is impossible. Under normal conditions, they are surrounded by a cuff of elastic fibers. In contrast to blood endothelial cells, lymphatic endothelium do not react with antibodies to von Willebrand factor (factor VIII-related antigen) and CD34 (123).

Large nerve bundles are seen in the subcutaneous fat and in the deep reticular dermis; however, small nerve fibers are present throughout the skin, reaching the papillary dermis. As mentioned earlier, recent immunohistochemical studies have demonstrated that the epidermis contains free nerve axons in association with Langerhans cells (55).

In sections of the palm and sole, some sensory nerves form nerve ending organs. Meissner corpuscles are seen in the papillary dermis, which is composed of several parallel layers of Schwann cells containing an axon; they function as rapid mechanical receptors for the sense of touch. In weight-bearing areas, the Vater-Pacini corpuscles consist of concentrically arranged Schwann cells with an axon and are located in the deep dermis and subcutaneous fat. They serve as receptors for sense of deep pressure and vibration (Figure 1.34).

Smooth muscle is represented in the skin by the arrector pili muscles, which arise in the connective tissue of the dermis and insert into hair follicles below the sebaceous glands. Melanocytes of congenital nevus are often seen within the arrector pili muscle. Smooth muscle is also seen in the skin of external genitalia (tunica dartos) and in the areolae.

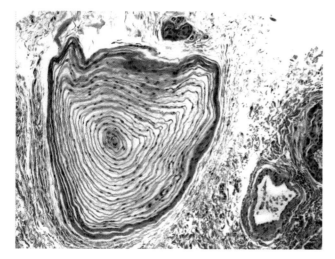

Figure 1.34 Vater-Pacini corpuscle.

Strands of striated muscle are found in the skin of the neck, face, and particularly the eyelids as muscle of expression.

HISTOLOGIC DIFFERENCES OF SKIN WITH AGE

Newborns and Children

The epidermis of newborns and children is usually of the same thickness as in adults, with the exception of the acral skin. There is a greater density of melanocytes and Langerhans cells.

The dermis is more cellular than in the adult with a higher concentration of ground substance. The number of eccrine glands is higher at birth, while apocrine glands are not well developed until after puberty (135). The sebaceous glands are developed in children, but sebaceous secretion begins at puberty under the influence of androgen stimulation (136).

The adipocytes of the subcutaneous tissue in newborns and children are thin-walled and larger than the adult adipocytes. In addition to white fat as seen in adults, infants possess brown fat, which initially comprises up to 5% of body weight then diminishes with age to virtually disappear by adulthood. Brown adipocytes are rich in mitochondria and contain multiple lipid droplets of varying size in the cytoplasm with centrally located nuclei. Brown fat contains an abundance of blood-filled capillaries and is of particular importance in neonates because it has the ability to produce heat (thermogenesis) by degrading fat molecules into fatty acids (137,138).

Elderly

In the elderly, the histologic differences are mainly due to atrophy and to reduction of most cutaneous elements (139–141). The cells of the epidermis are arranged haphazardly because of aberrant proliferation of the basal cell layer, which may predispose to the development of neoplasms (142). There is a marked decrease in the number of melanocytes and in the number of melanosomes, leading to reduced pigmentation (140,143) and, consequently, more exposure to the damaging effects of ultraviolet light. The Langerhans cells also decrease in number and function with advanced age (140,143), which increases the damaging effects of contactants and partially contributes to age-associated deterioration of immune function (144).

In the elderly, the dermis is thinned, relatively acellular, and avascular. The dermal collagen, elastin, and ground substance are altered and reduced (139,142). Elastic fibers show structural and biochemical alterations that change the elasticity of the skin. Collagen bundles are thicker but stiffer. The net effect is that age-associated alterations make the dermis less stretchable, less resilient, and prone to wrinkling (145). Fibroblasts, dendritic cells, and mast cells are also reduced in number.

Because of the reduction in the cutaneous vascular supply, there is a decrease in inflammatory response, absorption, and cutaneous clearance (146).

Both eccrine and apocrine glands are also reduced, with diminished secretions in the elderly. Sebaceous glands increase in size and manifest clinically as sebaceous hyperplasia, but paradoxically their secretory output is lessened by decreased activity (139,147).

With age, the number and rate of growth of hair follicles decreases, vellus hair will develop into terminal hairs in un-

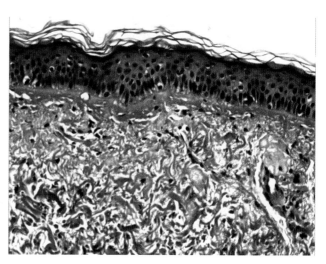

Figure 1.35 Solar elastosis in the dermis.

usual sites, such as the ear, nose, and nostrils, resulting in possible cosmetic problems. There is also a decreased functioning of Meissner's and Vater-Pacini corpuscles (148). Finally, there is diminished subcutaneous tissue especially in the face, shins, hands, and feet, but it increases in other areas, particularly the abdomen in men and the thighs in women (139).

The pathologic hallmark of extrinsic aging is solar elastosis (Figure 1.35), whereas wrinkling is due to the intrinsic factors mentioned previously (149).

HISTOLOGIC VARIATIONS ACCORDING TO ANATOMIC SITES

Regional variations of the normal histomorphology are important to recognize so as to avoid misinterpretation of variation as abnormality.

The normal scalp and other densely hair-containing regions show hair follicles extending through the dermis into the subcutaneous fat (Figure 1.36). This is usually not seen in areas with less concentration of hair. Abundant vellus hair is seen in sections taken from the skin of the ear. The skin of the face shows characteristically many pilosebaceous units (Figure 1.37), and large sebaceous glands are seen on the nose.

The squamous layer of the eyelid epidermis is thin and composed of two to three layers of cells and basoloid epithelial buds. Modified apocrine glands (Moll's glands) and vellus hairs are seen in the dermis.

Sections taken from the skin of the trunk, especially the back, show a normally thickened reticular dermis when compared to other sites (Figure 1.38). Unawareness of this normal variation may lead to the erroneous diagnosis of processes producing thick collagen, such as scleroderma.

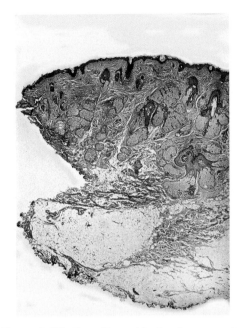

Figure 1.37   Skin of face with pilosebaceous units.

The skin around the umbilicus also shows thick and fibrotic dermis (Figure 1.39).

The palms and soles contain stratum lucidum and show a thick, compact cornified layer with loss of the characteristic basket-weave pattern (Figure 1.40). In addition, there are numerous eccrine units, nerve end organs, and glomus structures seen in the dermis. There are no pilosebaceous units. Sections of the skin of the lower leg may show thicker blood vessels in the papillary dermis as a result of gravity and stasis (Figure 1.41). Smooth muscle fibers are seen in the dermis of the skin of external genitalia and areola of the nipple. Cutaneous-mucosal junctions may lack granular and cornified layers, and cells of the squamous layers are larger, with higher glycogen content.

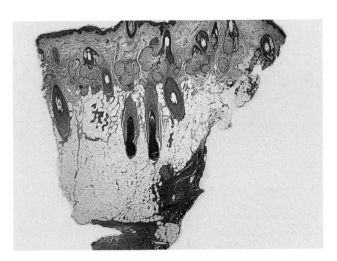

Figure 1.36   Section of scalp showing hair follicles extending into the subcutaneous tissue.

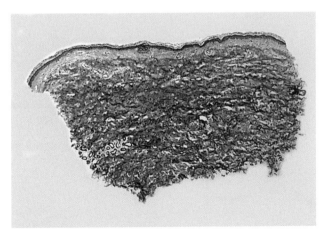

Figure 1.38   Section of skin of the back showing the normal reticular dermis.

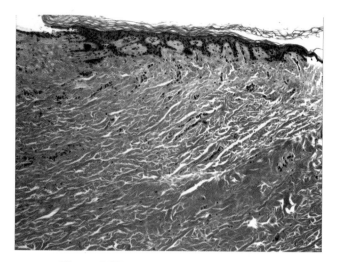

Figure 1.39   Umbillicus with dermal fibrosis.

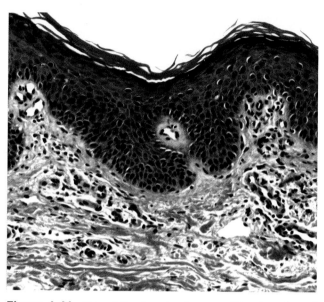

Figure 1.41   Skin of the leg showing a proliferation of small thickened blood vessels secondary to stasis.

PATHOLOGIC CHANGES FOUND IN BIOPSIES AND INTERPRETED AS "NORMAL" SKIN

Biopsies taken from clinically abnormal skin lesions may be interpreted histologically as normal because of the presence of subtle changes. The following are some examples.

- Dermatophytosis is seen in the cornified layer (Figure 1.42) of an otherwise normal skin.
- A thick or absent granular layer may indicate an abnormal process of keratinization like psoriasis or an ichthyosiform dermatosis.Vitiligo (Figure 1.43, 1.44) may give the histologic impression of normal skin unless one searches for melanocytes.

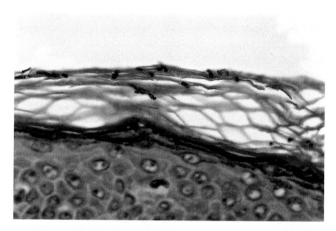

Figure 1.42   Superficial dermatophytosis (PAS stains).

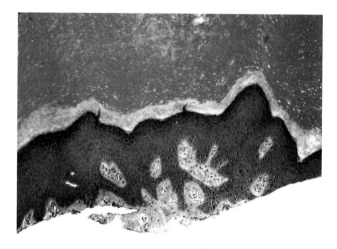

Figure 1.40   Histologic section of the palm with compact cornified layers and stratum lucidum.

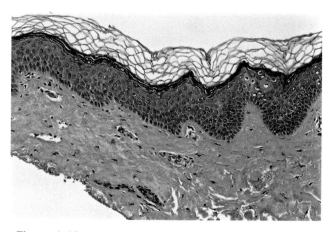

Figure 1.43   Vitiligo. Note the absence of basal melanocytes.

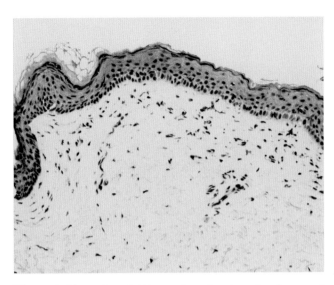

Figure 1.44 Vitiligo. S-100 protein stains show the absence of basal melanocytes.

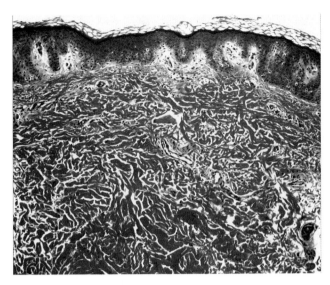

Figure 1.46 Urticaria shows only dermal edema.

■ Macular and lichen amyloidosis (Figure 1.45) may be overlooked because the pink globules of amyloid seen in the papillary dermis can be mistaken for normal dermis.

■ Urticaria (Figure 1.46) produces only edema, which in routine sections is seen as separation of the collagen bundles in the dermis. Similar changes are seen in the case of dermal mucinosis, in which deposition of mucinous material may be inconspicuous in routine sections. Special stains for mucin will be helpful.

■ In telangiectasia macularis eruptive perstans, a subtype of cutaneous mastocytosis, the changes may be quite subtle and are composed of dilated blood vessels in the upper dermis with a scant infiltrate of mast cells. The infiltrate must be confirmed with appropriate stains for mast cells.

■ Trichotillomania is a hair pulling habit resulting in areas of alopecia. Although histologic changes can be numer-

ous (24), at times hair follicles devoid of hair are the only changes seen, which give an impression of normal skin in the biopsy material.

■ Some degenerative disease of skin, such as anetoderma, can represent only as partial loss of elastic fibers in the dermis, which will be demonstrated by special stains of elastic tissue.

■ The so-called "connective tissue nevus" representing a hamartoma with an overproduction of collagen bundles and increased, normal or decreased elastic tissue in the dermis is another condition that can be erroneously interpreted as normal skin.

Other conditions that might be missed as "normal skin" include café-au-lait spots, cutis laxa (elastolysis), myxoedema, scleromyxedema, and more. Therefore, the clinical information combined with careful histological examination, sometimes special stains, or immunohistochemical studies of the biopsy material is crucial to avoid misinterpretation of skin disorders as normal tissue.

SPECIMEN HANDLING

Once the biopsy is done, the specimen should be placed in formalin fixative immediately for the purpose of routine histological examination. Specimens needed for direct immunofluorescent study ideally should be placed in Michel's medium or, alternatively, put in saline-moistened gauze if it is going to be processed within 24 hours. Specimens required for flow cytometry, molecular studies, and electron microscopy are sent fresh in saline-soaked gauze; they should be processed as soon as possible. If the specimens are excisional biopsies or larger surgical material,

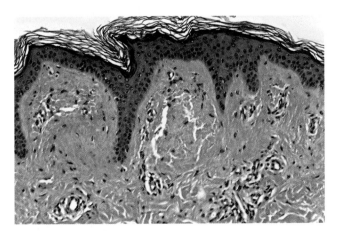

Figure 1.45 Lichen amyloidosis composed of pink globules in the papillary dermis.

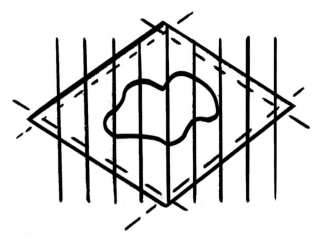

Figure 1.47 The entire neoplasm in the center of the lesion is examined by "bread-loafing" the specimen; the deep margin is also evaluated. The lateral margins are included in each section submitted for histologic evaluation, or they can be submitted separately by cutting them along the depicted interrupted lines.

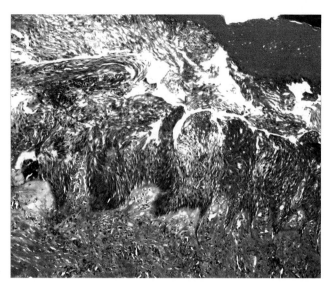

Figure 1.48 Cautery effect with vertical elongation of keratinocytes; such a sample is difficult to evaluate.

proper sharing of the specimen is done, always with consideration that histology has priority if no prior diagnosis exists for that particular patient.

Punch and shave biopsies are described grossly and either embedded intact or sectioned, depending on the size of the biopsy. Then the specimen is embedded on "edge" (vertical). Five levels are usually obtained for histologic examination.

Excisional biopsies and surgical specimens obtained for neoplasm are described grossly, and the entire deep and lateral margins of the specimen are inked prior to sectioning. The margins are evaluated by cutting along all margins or, most commonly, by entirely "bread loafing" the specimen (Figure 1.47). The entire neoplasm is also evaluated using the bread-loafing technique.

ARTIFACTS

Poor histologic preparation as a result of artifacts will hamper the evaluation of slides by the pathologists. These artifacts can be the result of a variety of factors.

1. Fixation problems such as poor or no fixation of the specimen prior to cutting, old solutions being used, insufficient fixation time, or inadequate volume of fixative (ideally, the specimen must be properly fixed in a solution 15 to 20 times the volume of the specimen) (150).
2. Improper monitoring of the multiple steps involved in the preparation of a slide, such as cutting, temperature of the water bath, freshness of the staining solutions employed, and other factors.
3. Artifacts produced at the time of excision, such as cautery (Figure 1.48) and excessive squeezing of the specimen.

4. Specimens stored at low temperatures, giving freezing artifacts (Figure 1.49).
5. Artifacts characteristically seen in certain pathologic processes, such as tissue holes in basal cell carcinoma (Figure 1.50) and the lack of epidermis in sections from toxic epidermolytic necrolysis.

STAINING METHODS

The majority of the skin lesions can be diagnosed with well-prepared H&E-stained sections. However, they will not provide an adequate answer in all cases. A comprehensive review of "special stains" is beyond the scope of this chapter because every case is different and may require a specific approach. The following are the most common stains used in our laboratory in the study of cutaneous tissue.

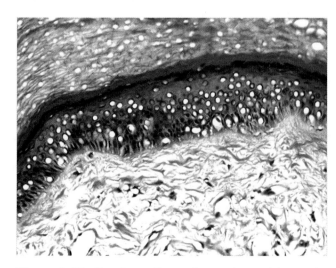

Figure 1.49 Freezing artifacts of a specimen with vacuolar changes in the epidermis.

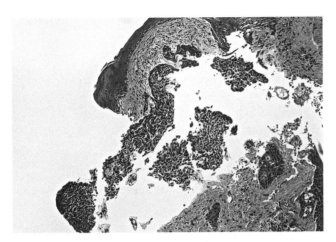

Figure 1.50 Tissue defects in a basal cell carcinoma, which appear in the spaces after multiple sections were performed.

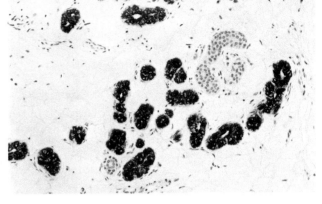

Figure 1.51 CAM 5.2 immunostaining. The secretory glands but not the ducts are stained.

Histochemical Stains

1. PAS: to study the thickness of the basement membrane, for glycogen (diastase liable) and fungal organisms (diastase resistant)
2. Gomori's methanamine silver: for fungal organisms and cutaneous *Pneumocystis carinii*
3. Ziehl-Nielsen and Fite stains: for acid-fast organisms
4. Gram's stains: for bacteria
5. Steiner and Warthin-Starry stains: in cases of bacillary angiomatosis and for spirochetes
6. Giemsa: for mast cells and protozoan organisms, such as *Leishmania*
7. Mucicarmine: for mucin
8. Alcian blue: for acid mucopolysaccharides (pH 2.5) and sulfated mucopolysaccharides (pH 0.5)
9. Congo red: for amyloid
10. Elastic van Gieson (EVG): for elastic fibers
11. Fontana-Masson: for melanin
12. Von Kossa: for calcium

Immunofluorescence

Immunofluorescence plays an important place in the diagnosis and evaluation of skin disorders such as lupus erythematosus and autoimmune blistering diseases. Either direct immunofluorescence using tissue or indirect immunofluorescence using serum of patients is available for diagnosis of skin diseases. Direct immunofluorescent studies are performed on cryostat sections of skin specimen using fluorescein isothiocyanate–conjugated antisera to examine for the presence of immunoglobulins A, G, and M, as well as fibrinogen and complement.

Immunohistochemical Stains

Immunohistochemical stains are used widely now in combinations of H&E-stained sections for diagnosis of difficult cases, such as poorly differentiated malignant tumors, spindle cell neoplasms, and lymphoproliferative malignancies. Most of the times, these stains are used in panels and not as single preparations. The most commonly used in our laboratory are:

1. Epithelial markers: Cytokeratin CAM 5.2 (Figure 1.51) (low-molecular weight cytokeratin), a combination of cytokeratins AE1/AE3 (low- and intermediate-molecular weight keratin, carcinoembryonic antigen (CEA), and epithelial membrane antigen (EMA): They are used in the differential diagnosis of epithelial tumors, adnexal tumors, and Paget's disease.
2. Melanocytic markers: S-100 protein, Melan A/MART-1, and HMB-45.
3. Mesenchymal markers:
   - Vimentin: dendritic cells, macrophages;
   - Factor XIIIa: fibroblast-like mesenchymal cells, dermal dendrocytes;
   - Factor VIII-associated antigen, CD31 and CD34: endothelial cells; CD34 in combination with Factor XIIIa are useful markers in the diagnosis of dermatofibrosarcoma protuberans (151);
   - HHF35 (muscle specific actin), smooth muscle actin and desmin: muscle differentiation;
   - S-100 protein: nerve, fat, and cartilage.
4. Lymphoid markers: all available CD markers for the characterization of lymphoid proliferations and other hematologic conditions are used.
5. Histiocytic markers: CD68 (KP-1) and lysozymes
6. Langerhans cells and Langerhans cell granulomatosis: CD1a and S-100 protein.
7. Neuroendocrine cells: neurospecific enolase (NSE), chromogranin and synaptophysin. These markers are also expressed in Merkel cell carcinoma; however, cytoplasmic stains for cytokeratin CK20 is most characteristic.
8. Cell proliferation marker: Ki-67 is an excellent marker for determining the so-called growth fraction of a given

cell population (152). Higher staining intensity in malignant lesions might be correlated with significant proliferative capabilities in tumor; Ki-67 labeling may have some value in the differentiation between benign and malignant lesions (153,154).

REFERENCES

1. Kanitakis J. Anatomy, histology and immunohistochemistry of normal human skin. *Eur J Dermatol* 2002;12:390–399.
2. Montagna W, Parakkal PF. *The Structure and Function of the Skin.* 3rd ed. New York: Academic Press; 1974.
3. Montagna W, Freedberg IM, eds. Cutaneous biology 1950–1975. *J Invest Dermatol* 1976;67:1–230.
4. Mckee P. *Pathology of the Skin.* 2nd ed. London: Mosby–Wolfe; 1996.
5. Murphy GF. Histology of the skin. In: Elder DE, Elenitsas R, Johnson, BL Jr, Murphy GF, eds. *Lever's Histopathology of the Skin.* 9th ed. Philadelphia: Lippincott Williams & Wilkins; 2005.
6. Breathnach AS. Embryology of human skin. A review of ultrastructural studies. *J Invest Dermatol* 1971;57:133–143.
7. Holbrook KA, Odland GF. The fine structure of developing human epidermis: light, scanning and transmission electron microscopy of the periderm. *J Invest Dermatol* 1975;65:16–38.
8. Hentula M, Peltonen J, Peltonen S. Expression profiles of cell-cell and cell-matrix junction proteins in developing human epidermis. *Arch Dermatol Res* 2001;293:259–267.
9. Smith LT, Sakai LY, Burgeson RE, Holbrook KA. Ontogeny of structural component at the dermal-epidermal junction in human embryonic and fetal skin: the appearance of anchoring fibrils and type VII collagen. *J Invest Dermatol* 1988;90:480–485.
10. Sagebiel RW, Rorsman H. Ultrastructural identification of melanocytes in early human embryos [abstract]. *J Invest Dermatol* 1970;54:96.
11. Foster CA, Holbrook KA, Farr AG. Ontogeny of Langerhans cells in human embryonic and fetal skin: expression of HLA-DR and OKT-6 determinants. *J Invest Dermatol* 1986;86:240–243.
12. Foster CA, Holbrook KA. Ontogeny of Langerhans cells in human embryonic and fetal skin: cell densities and phenotypic expression relative to epidermal growth. *Am J Anat* 1989;184:157–164.
13. Foster CA, Holbrook KA, Farr AG. Ontogeny of Langerhans cells in human embryonic and fetal skin: expression of HLA-DR and OKT-6 determinants. *J Invest Dermatol* 1986;86:240–243.
14. Winkelmann RK, Breathnach AS. The Merkel cell. *J Invest Dermatol* 1973;60:2–15.
15. Gould VE, Moll R, Moll I, Lee I, Franke WW. Neuroendocrine (Merkel) cells of the skin: hyperplasias, dysplasias and neoplasias. *Lab Invest* 1985;52:334–353.
16. Moll R, Moll I, Franke WW. Identification of Merkel cells in human skin by specific cytokeratin antibodies: changes of cell density and distribution in fetal and adult plantar epidermis. *Differentiation* 1984;28:136–154.
17. Ochiai T, Suzuki H. Fine structural and morphometric studies of the Merkel cell during fetal and postnatal development. *J Invest Dermatol* 1981;77:437–443.
18. Moll I, Lane AT, Franke WW, Moll R. Intraepidermal formation of Merkel cells in xenografts of human fetal skin. *J Invest Dermatol* 1990;94:359–364.
19. Boot PM, Rowden G, Walsh N. The distribution of Merkel cells in human fetal and adult skin. *Am J Dermatopathol* 1992;14:391–396.
20. Breathnach AS. Development and differentiation of dermal cells in man. *J Invest Dermatol* 1978;71:2–8.
21. Smith LT, Holbrook KA, Madri JA. Collagen types I, III, and V in human embryonic and fetal skin. *Am J Anat* 1986;175:507–521.
22. Mehregan AH, Hashimoto K, Mehregan DA, Mehregan DR. Normal structure of the skin. In: Mehregan AH, Hashimoto K, Mehregan DA, Mehregan DR, eds. *Pinkus' Guide to Dermatohistopathology.* 6th ed. Norwalk, CT; Appleton & Lange; 1995.
23. Lavker RM, Sun TT, Oshima H, et al. Hair follicle stem cells. *J Investig Dermatol Symp Proc* 2003;8:28–38.
24. Ackerman AB. Skin, structure and function. In: Ackerman AB, ed. *Histologic Diagnosis of Inflammatory Skin Diseases.* Philadelphia: Lea & Febiger; 1978.
25. Downig DT, Stewart ME, Strauss JJ. Biology of sebaceous glands. In: Fitzpatrick TB, Eisen AZ, Wolff K, Freedberg IM, Austen KF, eds. *Dermatology in General Medicine.* Vol 1. 3rd ed. New York: McGraw-Hill; 1987:185–190.
26. Muller M, Jasmin JR, Monteil RA, Loubiere R. Embryology of the hair follicle. *Early Hum Dev* 1991;26:159–166.
27. Hashimoto K, Gross BG, Lever WF. The ultrastructure of the skin of human embryos. I. The intraepidermal eccrine sweat duct. *J Invest Dermatol* 1965;45:139–151.
28. Montagna W. Embryology and anatomy of the cutaneous adnexa. *J Cutan Pathol* 1984;11:350–351.
29. Salmon JK, Armstrong CA, Ansel JC. The skin as an immune organ. *West J Med* 1994;160:146–152.
30. Girolomoni G, Caux C, Lebecque S, Dezutter-Dambuyant C, Ricciardi-Castagnoli P. Langerhans cells: still a fundamental paradigm for studying the immunobiology of dendritic cells. *Trends Immunol* 2002;23:6–8.
31. Smack DP, Korge BP, James WD. Keratin and keratinization. *J Am Acad Dermatol* 1994;30:85–102.
32. Bos JD, Kapsenberg ML. The skin immune system: progress in cutaneous biology. *Immunol Today* 1993;14:75–78.
33. Kerr JFR, Winterford CM, Harmon BV. Apoptosis. Its significance in cancer and cancer therapy. *Cancer* 1994;73:2013–2026.
34. Polakowska RR, Piacentini M, Bartlett R, Goldsmith LA, Haake AR. Apoptosis in human skin development: morphogenesis, periderm, and stem cells. *Dev Dyn* 1994;199:176–188.
35. Weedon D, Strutton G. Apoptosis as the mechanism of the involution of hair follicles in catagen transformation. *Acta Derm Venereol (Stockh)* 1981;61:335–339.
36. McCall CA, Cohen JJ. Programmed cell death in terminally differentiating keratinocytes: role of endogenous endonuclease. *J Invest Dermatol* 1991;97:111–114.
37. Tamada Y, Takama H, Kitamura T, et al. Identification of programmed cell death in normal human skin tissues by using specific labeling of fragmented DNA. *Br J Dermatol* 1994;131:521–524.
38. Stenn KS, Lawrence L, Veis D, Korsmeyer S, Seiberg M. Expression of the bcl-2 protooncogene in the cycling adult mouse hair follicle. *J Invest Dermatol* 1994;103:107–111.
39. Seiberg M, Marthinuss J, Stenn KS. Changes in expression of apoptosis-associated genes in skin mark early catagen. *J Invest Dermatol* 1995;104:78–82.
40. Weedon D, Strutton G. The recognition of early stages of catagen. *Am J Dermatopathol* 1984;6:553–555.
41. Eckert RL, Efimova T, Dashti SR, et al. Keratinocyte survival, differentiation, and death: many roads lead to mitogen-activated protein kinase. *J Investig Dermatol Symp Proc* 2002;7:36–40.
42. Masellis M. Deep burns of the knee: joint capsule reconstruction with dermis graft. *Annals of Burns and Fire Disasters* 1997;10:3–11.
43. Scrivener Y, Cribier B. Morphology of sweat glands. *Morphologie* 2002;86:5–17.
44. Sato K, Kang WH, Saga K, Sato KT. Biology of sweat glands and their disorders. I. Normal sweat gland function. *J Am Acad Dermatol* 1989;20:537–563.
45. Sato K, Sato F. Individual variations in structure and function of human eccrine sweat gland. *Am J Physiol* 1983;245:R203–R208.
46. Uno H. Sympathetic innervation of sweat glands and piloerector muscles of macaques and human beings. *J Invest Dermatol* 1977;69:112–120.
47. Headington JT. Primary mucinous carcinoma of skin: histochemistry and electron microscopy. *Cancer* 1977;39:1055–1063.
48. Shah VP, Epstein WL, Riegelman S. Role of sweat in accumulation of orally administered griseofulvin in skin. *J Clin Invest* 1974;53:1673–1678.
49. Sato K, Kang WH, Saga K, Sato KT. Biology of sweat glands and their disorders. II. Disorders of sweat gland function. *J Am Acad Dermatol* 1989;20:713–726.

50. Gesase AP, Satoh Y. Apocrine secretory mechanism: recent findings and unresolved problems. *Histol Histopathol* 2003;18:597–608.

51. Porter AM. Why do we have apocrine and sebaceous glands? *J R Soc Med* 2001;94:236–237.

52. Zeng C, Spielman AI, Vowels BR, Leyden JJ, Biemann K, Preti G. A human axillary odorant is carried by apolipoprotein D. *Proc Natl Acad Sci USA* 1996;93:6626–6630.

53. Wenzel FG, Horn TD. Nonneoplastic disorders of the eccrine glands. *J Am Acad Dermatol* 1998;38:1–17.

54. Cheshire WP, Freeman R. Disorders of sweating. *Semin Neurol* 2003;23:399–406.

55. Hosoi J, Murphy GF, Egan CL, et al. Regulation of Langerhans cell function by nerves containing calcitonin gene-related peptide. *Nature* 1993;363:159–163.

56. Ishiko A, Matsunaga Y, Masunaga T, Aiso S, Nishikawa T, Shimizu H. Immunomolecular mapping of adherens junction and desmosomal components in normal human epidermis. *Exp Dermatol* 2003;12:747–754.

57. Holbrook KA, Wolff K. The structure and development of skin. In: Fitzpatrick TB, Eisen AZ, Wolff K, Freedberg IM, Austen KF, eds. *Dermatology in General Medicine*. 3rd ed. New York: McGraw-Hill; 1987.

58. Wolff K, Schreiner E. Ultrastructural localization of pemphigus autoantibodies within the epidermis. *Nature* 1971;229:59–61.

59. Stanley JR, Klaus-Kovtun V, Sampaio SAP. Antigenic specificity of fogo selvagem autoantibodies is similar to North American pemphigus foliaceus and distinct from pemphigus vulgaris autoantibodies. *J Invest Dermatol* 1986;87:197–201.

60. Moll R, Cowin P, Kapprell HP, Franke WW. Desmosomal proteins: new markers for identification and classification of tumors. *Lab Invest* 1986;54:4–25.

61. Toker C. Clear cells of the nipple epidermis. *Cancer* 1970;25:601–610.

62. Willman JH, Golitz LE, Fitzpatrick JE. Clear cells of Toker in accessory nipples. *J Cutan Pathol* 2003;30:256–260.

63. Kumarasinghe SP, Chin GY, Kumarasinghe MP. Clear cell papulosis of the skin: a case report from Singapore. *Arch Pathol Lab Med* 2004;128:e149–152.

64. Marucci G, Betts CM, Golouh R, Peterse JL, Foschini MP, Eusebi V. Toker cells are probably precursors of Paget cell carcinoma: a morphological and ultrastructural description. *Virchows Arch* 2002 Aug;441(2):117–123. Epub 2002 Feb 01.

65. Kuo TT, Chan HL, Hsueh S. Clear cell papulosis of the skin. A new entity with histogenetic implications for cutaneous Paget's disease. *Am J Surg Pathol* 1987;11:827–834.

66. Tschen JA, McGavran MH, Kettler AH. Pagetoid dyskeratosis: a selective keratinocytic response. *J Am Acad Dermatol* 1988;19:891–894.

67. Kim YC, Mehregan DA, Bang D. Clear cell papulosis: an immunohistochemical study to determine histogenesis. *J Cutan Pathol* 2002;29:11–14.

68. Lazarus GS, Hatcher VB, Levine N. Lysosomes and the skin. *J Invest Dermatol* 1975;65:259–271.

69. Elias PM. Epidermal lipids, barrier function, and desquamation. *J Invest Dermatol* 1983;80(suppl):44s–49s.

70. Zirra AM. The functional significance of the skin's stratum lucidum. *Morphol Embryol* (Bucur) 1976;22:9–12.

71. Katz SI. The epidermal basement membrane zone—structure, ontogeny, and role in disease. *J Am Acad Dermatol* 1984;11:1025–1037.

72. Foidart JM, Bere EW Jr, Yaar M, et al. Distribution and immuno-electron microscopic localization of laminin, a noncollagenous basement membrane glycoprotein. *Lab Invest* 1980;42:336–342.

73. Smith JB, Taylor TB, Zone JJ. The site of blister formation in dermatitis herpetiformis is within the lamina lucida. *J Am Acad Dermatol* 1992;27:209–213.

74. Leblond CP, Inoue S. Structure, composition, and assembly of basement membrane. *Am J Anat* 1989;185:367–390.

75. Woodley DT, Burgeson RE, Lunstrum G, Bruckner-Tuderman L, Reese MJ, Briggaman RA. Epidermolysis bullosa acquisita antigen is the globular carboxyl terminus of type VII procollagen. *J Clin Invest* 1988;81:683–687.

76. Shimizu H, McDonald JN, Gunner DB, et al. Epidermolysis bullosa acquisita antigen and the carboxy terminus of type VII collagen have a common immunolocalization to anchoring fibrils and lamina densa of basement membrane. *Br J Dermatol* 1990;122: 577–585.

77. Elder DE, Johnson BL Jr, Elenitsas R, eds. Histology of the skin. In: Elder DE, Johnson BL Jr, Elenitsas R, eds. *Lever's Histopathology of the Skin*. 9th ed. Baltimore: Lippincott Williams & Wilkins: 2004:35.

78. Scott GA, Cassidy L, Tran H, Rao SK, Marinkovich MP. Melanocytes adhere to and synthesize laminin-5 in vitro. *Exp Dermatol* 1999;8:212–221.

79. Tarnowski WM. Ultrastructure of the epidermal melanocyte dense plate. *J Invest Dermatol* 1970;55:265–268.

80. Nordlund JJ, Sober AJ, Hansen TW. Periodic synopsis on pigmentation. *J Am Acad Dermatol* 1985;12:359–363.

81. Quevedo WC Jr, Fitzpatrick TB, Szabo G, et al. Biology of the melanin pigmentary system. In: Fitzpatrick TB, Eisen AZ, Wolff K, Freedberg IM, Austen KF, eds. *Dermatology in General Medicine*. Vol I. 3rd ed. New York: McGraw-Hill; 1987.

82. Seiberg M. Keratinocyte-melanocyte interactions during melanosome transfer. *Pigment Cell Res* 2001;14:236–242.

83. Barral DC, Seabra MC. The melanosome as a model to study organelle motility in mammals. *Pigment Cell Res* 2004;17:111–118.

84. Murphy GF. Structure, function and reaction patterns. In: Murphy GF, ed. *Dermatopathology*. Philadelphia: WB Saunders; 1995.

85. Gown AM, Vogel AM, Hoak D, Gough F, McNutt MA. Monoclonal antibodies specific for melanocytic tumors distinguish subpopulations of melanocytes. *Am J Pathol* 1986;123:195–203.

86. Kanitakis J. Immunohistochemistry of normal skin. In: Kanitakis J, Vassileva S, Woodley D, eds. *Diagnostic Immunohistochemistry of the Skin. An Illustrated Text*. London: Chapman & Hall Med; 1998:38–51.

87. Birbeck NS, Breathnach AS, Everall JD. An electron microscope study of basal melanocytes and high-level clear cells (Langerhans cells) in vitiligo. *J Invest Dermatol* 1961;37:51–64.

88. Niebauer G, Krawczyk W, Wilgram GF. The Langerhans cell organelle in Letterer Siwe's disease. *Arch Klin Exp Dermatol* 1970;239:125–137.

89. Valladeau J, Dezutter-Dambuyant C, Saeland S. Langerin/CD207 sheds light on formation of birbeck granules and their possible function in Langerhans cells. *Immunol Res* 2003;28:93–107.

90. Mc Dermott R, Ziylan U, Spehner D, et al. Birbeck granules are subdomains of endosomal recycling compartment in human epidermal Langerhans cells, which form where Langerin accumulates. *Mol Biol Cell* 2002;13:317–335.

91. Halata Z, Grim M, Baumann KI. The Merkel cell: morphology, developmental origin, function. *Cas Lek Cesk* 2003;142:4–9.

92. Halata Z, Grim M, Bauman KI. Friedrich Sigmund Merkel and his "Merkel cell," morphology, development, and physiology: review and new results. *Anat Rec A Discov Mol Cell Evol Biol* 2003;271:225–239.

93. Tachibana T, Nawa T. Recent progress in studies on Merkel cell biology. *Anat Sci Int* 2002;77:26–33.

94. Santa Cruz DJ, Bauer EA. Merkel cells in the outer follicular sheath. *Ultrastruct Pathol* 1982;3:59–63.

95. Camisa C, Weissmann A. Friedrich Sigmund Merkel Part II. The cell. *Am J Dermatopathol* 1982;4:527–535.

96. Gu J, Polak JM, Van Noorden S, Pearse AG, Marangos PJ, Azzopardi JG. Immunostaining of neuron-specific enolase as a diagnostic tool for Merkel cell tumors. *Cancer* 1983;52:1039–1043.

97. Leff EL, Brooks JSJ, Trojanowski JQ. Expression of neurofilament and neuron-specific enolase in small cell tumors of skin using immunohistochemistry. *Cancer* 1985;56:625–631.

98. Rosen ST, Gould VE, Salwen HR, et al. Establishment and characterization of a neuroendocrine skin carcinoma cell line. *Lab Invest* 1987;56:302–312.

99. van Muijen GNP, Ruiter DJ, Warnaar SO. Intermediate filaments in Merkel cell tumors. *Hum Pathol* 1985;16:590–595.

100. Wang NP, Zee S, Zarbo RJ, Bacchi CE, Gown AM. Coordinate expression of cytokeratins 7 and 20 defines unique subsets of carcinomas. *Appl Immunohistochem* 1995;3:99–107.

101. Moll I, Kuhn C, Moll R. Cytokeratin 20 is a general marker of cutaneous Merkel cells while certain neuronal proteins are absent. *J Invest Dermatol* 1995;104:910–915.

102. Headington JT. Transverse microscopic anatomy of the human scalp. A basis for a morphometric approach to disorders of the hair follicle. *Arch Dermatol* 1984;120:449–456.

103. de Viragh PA. The 'mantle hair of Pinkus'. A review on the occasion of its centennial. *Dermatology* 1995;191:82–87.

104. Alonso LC, Rosenfield RL. Molecular genetic and endocrine mechanisms of hair growth. *Horm Res* 2003;60:1–13.

105. Nakagawa H, Imokawa G. Characterization of melanogenesis in normal human epidermal melanocytes by chemical and ultrastructural analysis. *Pigment Cell Res* 1996;9:175–178.

106. Jimbow K, Ishida O, Ito S, Hori Y, Witkop CJ Jr, King RA. Combined chemical and electron microscopic studies of pheomelanosomes in human red hair. *J Invest Dermatol* 1983;81:506–511.

107. Biasiolo M, Bertazzo A, Costa CV, Allegri G. Correlation between tryptophan and hair pigmentation in human hair. *Adv Exp Med Biol* 1999;467:653–657.

108. Burchill SA, Ito S, Thody AJ. Effects of melanocyte-stimulating hormone on tyrosinase expression and melanin synthesis in hair follicular melanocytes of the mouse. *J Endocrinol* 1993;137:189–195.

109. Smith KR Jr. The Haarscheibe. *J Invest Dermatol* 1977;69:68–74.

110. Baron DA, Briggman JV, Spicer SS. Tubulocisternal endoplasmic reticulum in human eccrine sweat glands. *Lab Invest* 1984;51:233–243.

111. Sbarbati A, Osculati A, Morroni M, Carboni V, Cinti S. Electron spectroscopic imaging of secretory granules in human eccrine sweat glands. *Eur J Histochem* 1994;38:327–330.

112. Schaumburg-Lever G, Lever WF. Secretion from human apocrine glands: an electron microscopic study. *J Invest Dermatol* 1975;64:38–41.

113. Sato K, Leidal R, Sato F. Morphology and development of an apoeccrine sweat gland in human axillae. *Am J Physiol* 1987;252: R166–R180.

114. Kamada A, Saga K, Jimbow K. Apoeccrine sweat duct obstruction as a cause for Fox-Fordyce disease. *J Am Acad Dermatol* 2003;48: 453–455.

115. Saga K. Histochemical and immunohistochemical markers for human eccrine and apocrine sweat glands: an aid for histopathologic differentiation of sweat gland tumors. *J Investig Dermatol Symp Proc* 2001;6:49–53.

116. Reed RJ, Ackerman AB. Pathology of the adventitial dermis. Anatomic observations and biologic speculations. *Hum Pathol* 1973;4:207–217.

117. Meigel WN, Gay S, Weber L. Dermal architecture and collagen type distribution. *Arch Dermatol Res* 1977;259:1–10.

118. Junqueira LC, Montes GS, Martins JE, Joazeiro PP. Dermal collagen distribution. A histochemical and ultrastructural study. *Histochemistry* 1983;79:397–403.

119. Sorrell JM, Caplan AI. Fibroblast heterogeneity: more than skin deep. *J Cell Sci* 2004;117(pt 5):667–675.

120. McNeal JE. Scleroderma and the structural basis of skin compliance. *Arch Dermatol* 1973;107:699–705.

121. Nestle FO, Nickoloff BJ. A fresh morphological and functional look at dermal dendritic cells. *J Cutan Pathol* 1995;22:385–393.

122. Narvaez D, Kanitakis J, Faure M, Claudy A. Immunohistochemical study of CD34-positive dendritic cells of human dermis. *Am J Dermatopathol* 1996;18:283–288.

123. Kanitakis J. Immunohistochemistry of normal human skin. *Eur J Dermatol* 1998;8:539–547.

124. Headington JT. The dermal dendrocyte. *Adv Dermatol* 1986;1: 159–171.

125. Headington JT, Cerio R. Dendritic cells and the dermis: 1990. *Am J Dermatopathol* 1990;12:217–220.

126. Nickoloff BJ, Griffiths CE. Not all spindled-shaped cells embedded in a collagenous stroma are fibroblasts: recognition of the "collagen-associated dendrophage." *J Cutan Pathol* 1990;17: 252–254.

127. Sepulveda-Merrill C, Mayall S, Hamblin AS, Breathnach SM. Antigen-presenting capacity in normal human dermis is mainly subserved by CD1a+ cells. *Br J Dermatol* 1994;131:15–22.

128. Meunier L, Gonzalez-Ramos A, Cooper KD. Heterogeneous populations of class II MHC+ cells in human dermal cell suspensions. Identification of a small subset responsible for potent dermal antigen-presenting cell activity with features analogous to Langerhans cells. *J Immunol* 1993;151:4067–4080.

129. Walls AF, Jones DB, Williams JH, Church MK, Holgate ST. Immunohistochemical identification of mast cells in formaldehyde-fixed tissue using monoclonal antibodies specific for tryptase. *J Pathol* 1990;162:119–126.

130. Arber DA, Tamayo R, Weiss LM. Paraffin section detection of the c-kit gene product (CD117) in human tissues: value in the diagnosis of mast cell disorders. *Hum Pathol* 1998;29:498–504.

131. Longley BJ, Reguera MJ, Ma Y. Classes of c-KIT activating mutations: proposed mechanisms of action and implications for disease classification and therapy. *Leuk Res* 2001;25:571–576.

132. Metcalfe DD, Akin C. Mastocytosis: molecular mechanisms and clinical disease heterogeneity. *Leuk Res* 2001;25:577–582.

133. Valent P, Horny HP, Escribano L, et al. Diagnostic criteria and classification of mastocytosis: a consensus proposal. *Leuk Res* 2001;25:603–625.

134. Ryan TJ, Mortimer PS, Jones RL. Lymphatics of the skin. Neglected but important. *Int J Dermatol* 1986;25:411–419.

135. Johnson BL, Honig PJ, Jaworsky C. In: Johnson BL, Honig PJ, Jaworsky C, eds. *Pediatric Dermatopathology*. Newton, MA: Butterworth-Heinemann; 1994.

136. Pochi PE, Strauss JS, Downing DT. Age-related changes in sebaceous gland activity. *J Invest Dermatol* 1979;73:108–111.

137. Klaus S. Functional differentiation of white and brown adipocytes. *Bioessays* 1997;19:215–223.

138. Klaus S. Adipose tissue as a regulator of energy balance. *Curr Drug Targets* 2004;5:241–250.

139. Fenske NA, Lober CW. Structural and functional changes of normal aging skin. *J Am Acad Dermatol* 1986;15(pt 1):571–585.

140. Kurban RS, Bhawan J. Histologic changes in skin associated with aging. J Dermatol Surg Oncol 1990;16:908–914.

141. Smith L. Histopathologic characteristics and ultrastructure of aging skin. *Cutis* 1989;43:414–424.

142. Patterson JAK. Structural and physiologic changes in the skin with age. In: Patterson JAK, ed. *Aging and Clinical Practice: Skin Disorders, Diagnosis and Treatment*. New York: Igaku-Shoin; 1989.

143. Montagna W, Carlisle K. Structural changes in ageing skin. *Br J Dermatol* 1990;122(suppl 35):61–70.

144. Sauder DN. Effect of age on epidermal immune function. *Dermatol Clin* 1986;4:447–454.

145. Lavker RM, Zheng PS, Dong G. Morphology of aged skin. *Clin Geriatr Med* 1989;5:53–67.

146. Balin AK, Pratt LA. Physiological consequences of human skin aging. *Cutis* 1989;43:431–436.

147. Bolognia JL. Aging skin. *Am J Med* 1995;98:99S–103S.

148. Cerimele D, Celleno L, Serri F. Physiological changes in ageing skin. *Br J Dermatol* 1990;122(suppl 35):13–20.

149. Rongioletti F, Rebora A. Fibroelastolytic patterns of intrinsic skin aging: pseudoxanthoma-elasticum-like papillary dermal elastolysis and white fibrous papulosis of the neck. *Dermatology* 1995;191:19–24.

150. Mondragon G, Nygaard F. Routine and special procedures for processing biopsy specimens of lesions suspected to be malignant melanomas. *Am J Dermatopathol* 1981;3:265–272.

151. Altman DA, Nickoloff BJ, Fivenson DP. Differential expression of factor XIIIa and CD34 in cutaneous mesenchymal tumors. *J Cutan Pathol* 1993;20:154–158.

152. Scholzen T, Gerdes J. The Ki-67 protein: from the known and the unknown. *J Cell Physiol* 2000;182:311–322.

153. Li LX, Crotty KA, McCarthy SW, Palmer AA, Kril JJ. A zonal comparison of MIB1-Ki67 immunoreactivity in benign and malignant melanocytic lesions. *Am J Dermatopathol* 2000;22: 489–495.

154. Abdelsayed RA, Guijarro-Rojas M, Ibrahim NA, Sangueza OP. Immunohistochemical evaluation of basal cell carcinoma and trichepithelioma using Bcl-2, Ki67, PCNA and P53. *J Cutan Pathol* 2000;27:169–175.

Nail

Julian Conejo-Mir   *Luis Requena*

2

INTRODUCTION

Fingernails are an important epithelial mini-organ system of the hand, with a complex anatomical structure well described in the last decades. They are important in certain animals for the apprehension and capture of prey. In primates and humans, the nails have two different functions: as a protective plate and to enhance sensation of the fingertip. The protection function of the fingernail is commonly known, but the sensation function is equally important. The fingertip has many nerve endings in it allowing us to receive volumes of information about objects we touch. The nail acts as a counterforce to the fingertip providing even more sensory input when an object is touched.

Although most pathological specimens from the nail show well-known changes such as psoriasis, lichen planus, and the characteristic malignant tumors, a broad spectrum of other changes may be found. For the pathologist, knowledge of the normal histology and its more common variations is important in establishing a correct diagnosis.

Unfortunately, much of the literature on the nail can be troublesome and confusing because a great profusion of names and concepts exists and has changed over the years; also, many newer concepts of the embryology, physiology, genetics, immunohistochemistry, and nail growth mechanism find their way slowly into textbooks. This chapter emphasizes those observations and theories related to clinical pathology.

HISTORY

Historical interest can be traced to the works of Galen in the second century BC when he noticed the nail's resemblance to hair structure. However, the real study of the nail begins at the end of the nineteenth century, mostly by Germans like Zander (1), Kolliker (2), and Unna (3). The first studies dealt with embryology and anatomy and their comparison to birds and primates (1,4,5). After the initial spark of interest, the nail literature was enriched by many authors, both on the embryology and the anatomy of the human nail (6,7). Because of the technical shortcomings of their time, the authors interpreted the nail plate as formed entirely by the matrix cells and concluded that other adjacent structures did not contribute in the formation of the plate.

During the 1950s, Lewis (8) challenged this view and published his idea of the "nail unit," consisting of a dorsal, intermediate, and ventral nail, with differentiation based on the use of a silver-proteinate stain. In 1963, Zaias (9) extended the concept of the nail unit, including the proximal nail fold, the matrix, the nail bed, and the hyponychium, all of which contribute to the formation of the nail.

During the last 25 years, most studies on the nail have fundamentally tried to explain its biochemistry and physiology, with emphasis on analyzing nail growth; also considered were ultrastructure and, most recently, the immunohistochemistry of the nail. At the same time, new conditions, particularly tumors, unknown until a few years ago, have been described from the point of ungual structures, especially keratoacanthomas, merkelomas (Merkel cell tumors), and subungual Bowen's disease. In the last five years, however, publications have been very scarce following the great proliferation of papers in previous years.

Difficult biopsy access, as well as the complicated orientation and specimen handling (with the resulting difficulties of interpretation), are the main reasons why there are few histologic and histopathologic studies on the nail.

EMBRYOLOGY

Whereas the embryonic development of the fetal skin has been divided into eight stages, using scanning electron microscopy (10), the embryonic development of the nail shows only five stages (11,12): (a) plate phase; (b) fibrillar phase; (c) granular phase; (d) squamous phase; and (e) definitive nail phase, or end phase (Table 2.1).

The earliest recognizable fingers are seen in 42- to 45-day-old embryos (16 mm crown-rump), while the toes lag somewhat and are seen at 52 to 54 days of age (18.5 mm) (13). Studies using optical microscopy showed that the ungual morphogenesis begins at the embryonal age of 10 weeks, with a smooth, shiny quadrangular surface delineated by continuous shallow grooves. This surface of the phalanx is the primary nail base of Zander (1) or primary nail field of Zaias (9), delimited proximally by a transversal groove (the proximal nail groove).

Studies we performed using scanning electron microscopy showed that the formation of the nail begins very early, at the embryonal age of seven weeks, with an accumulation of strongly active cells, abundant mitosis, and cellular damage, followed by necrosis, with the presence of T lymphocytes in the primary nail base (Figure 2.1). This phenomenon, named apoptosis, occurs in all the

TABLE 2.1

COMPARISON OF THE DIFFERENT STAGES OF NAIL DEVELOPMENT WITH THE EPIDERMIS OF THE EMBRYO USING SCANNING ELECTRON MICROSCOPY

Nail Unit[a]	Embryonic/Fetal Skin[b]	Development
Plaque phase	Indifferent epithelium phase	7–10 weeks
	Flattened surface phase	
	Elevated surface phase	
Fibrillar phase	Incipient bleb formation phase	2.5–3 months
Granular phase	Single bleb formation phase	3–4 months
Squamous phase	Complex bleb formation phase	4–5 months
Definitive nail phase	Cornification phase	Up to 5 months

[a]Suchard R. Des modifications des cellules de la matrice et du lit de l'ongle dans quelques cas pathologiques. *Arch Physiol (Paris)* 1882;2:445.
[b]Holbrook KA, Odland GF. The fine structure of the developing human epidermis: light, scanning, and transmission electron microscopy of the periderm. *J Invest Dermatol* 1975;65:16–38.

epidermal accumulated cells following a transversal band in the dorsal area of the distal third of the fingers. Apoptosis of these epidermal cells is the most important step in the nail's development because it permits an immediate epidermal invagination identical to the one in the hair follicle except for one difference: in the hair follicle, the process starts at the age of 2.5 to 3 months. We observed apoptosis in nail development in this first phase only. Yet, the two processes are so identical that sometimes the layers of the nail have been compared with those of the hair follicle. The result is the formation of a transversal groove, which subsequently becomes the proximal nail fold.

An interesting feature of the first stages is the excessive size of the primitive nail plate (2.5 to 3 months), nearly occupying the total distal third part of the finger. This plate stays attached to its surroundings through some periungual-fixing filaments (Figure 2.2). At the age of 11 weeks, all the proximal and lateral nail folds are already formed. The transversal distal fold, corresponding to the hyponychium, is completely keratinized at the age of 3.5 months (Figure 2.3). Afterward, the epidermal cells of the nail field suffer a process of keratin formation that is different from the rest of the embryo. The result is a keratinized structure, covering the whole nail bed from the age of 14 weeks on and sometimes confused by some authors with a false nail (Figure 2.4) (8,9). The production of the true nail plate starts from the matrix cells, located in the proximal nail groove and the most proximal portion of the nail bed. Its presence in the

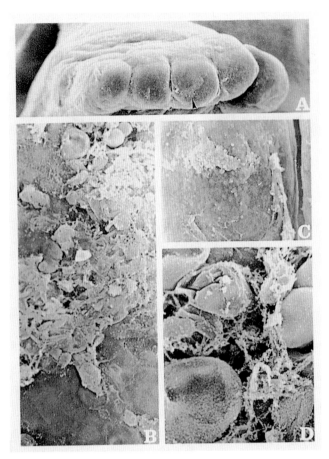

Figure 2.1 Development of the human nail exhibited through scanning electron microscopy (13). **A.** Plaque phase: foot of 7-week-old human embryo. The fingers are already defined but have no interphalangeal folds (×50). Distally on the third toe, you can see poorly structured material accumulated (*arrow* in **A**) that corresponds to apoptotic cells. **B and C.** These apoptotic cells limit the future proximal nail fold (**B**, ×500; **C**, ×100). **D.** Close-up view of the apoptotic cells: amorphous extracellular material appears with numerous vesicles of keratohyalin, which are in different phases of their evolution (×1500).

descending at an angle into the subjacent primitive mesenchymal tissue. The superficial part of this wedge of epithelial cells will become the proximal nail fold, and the deeper part will eventuate in the dorsal and intermediate nail matrices. At the junction between the superficial and deeper parts, there is a crease of cornified cells that will be the cuticle of the fully developed nail. At this stage of development, the primitive mesenchymal tissue underlying the future nail is a highly cellular tissue with abundant ground substance. At this time, the future distal phalanx is represented by primitive cartilaginous tissue with the earliest evidences of focal calcification. Distally, the primitive epithelium forms another cluster of cells with a distal ridge that will become the hyponychium.

From the fifth month on, the definitive nail plate starts to grow in a distal sense until it reaches the hyponychium at the time of birth. The growth mechanism of the definitive nail is discussed later in the section entitled Nail Growth.

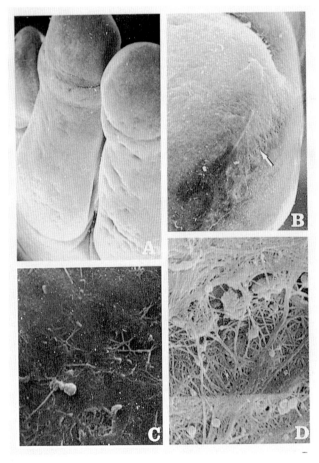

Figure 2.2 Fibrillar phase. Fingers of the hand of a 3-month-old embryo. **A.** The ungual region is perfectly delimited by the proximal nail fold (×40). **B.** The ungual region is delimited by multiple fibrillar formations (×150). **C.** Different morphology is seen in the nail bed surface (×2400). **D.** Detail of the fibrillar attachment of the nail region to the neighboring tissue (×2400).

proximal fold is visible from the fifth month of intrauterine life onward, the histochemical confirmation of its formation being the presence of sulfhydryl radicals (14).

The nail unit at this stage shows grooves form by invaginations of primitive ectoderm in regions that will become nail folds. These grooves delimit rectangular areas at distal aspects of dorsa of fingers and toes where nail plates will be situated subsequently. These areas are covered by primitive epithelium that, approximately at the fourteenth week of intrauterine-life (Figure 2.5), appears composed of a basal layer of primitive germinative cells, three or four layers of primitive keratinocytes with clear or pale cytoplasm, and a thin and eosinophilic acellular layer at the surface. This primitive epithelium covering the dorsum of a distal phalanx develops two clusters of epithelial cells at their proximal and distal ends. The proximal bud of primitive epithelial basaloid cells proliferates backward and downward,

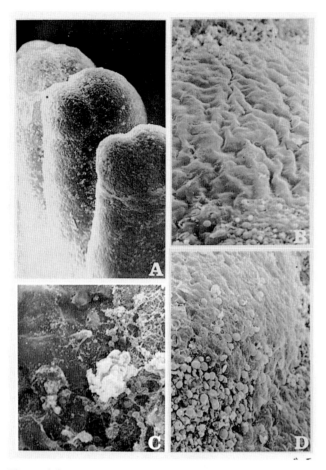

Figure 2.3 Granular phase. Fingers of the hand of 4.5-month-old embryo. **A.** All fingers show a granular aspect (×40). **B.** The nail bed has an undulating surface covered by keratin scales (×400). **C. and D.** The hyponychium zone is occupied by numerous keratohyalin vesicles (**C**, ×400; **D**, ×150).

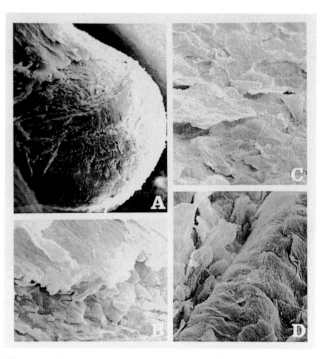

Figure 2.4 Squamous phase **A.** Index finger of 5.5-month-old fetus (×200). **C.** The keratinization process is complete in the nail bed surface, simulating a false nail (×500). **B.** The cuticle (×500) and **D.** The hyponychium are also completely developed (×500).

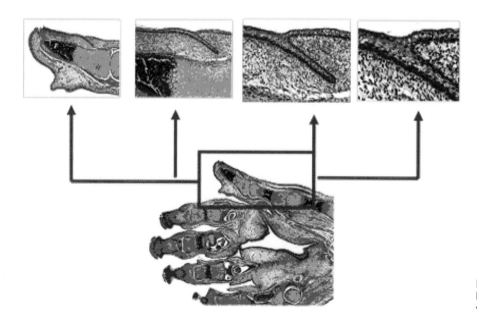

Figure 2.5 Sagittal section of a fetus hand of 16 weeks, with special close up views of the nail matrix area.

GENETICS AND NAIL KERATINS

Epithelial cells possess three cytoskeletal systems: actin microfilaments, microtubules, and keratin intermediate filaments. The protective structural role of keratins was clearly revealed in the early 1990s, when mutations in human keratin genes were discovered in a variety of human genetic diseases characterized by fragility and/or overgrowth (hyperkeratosis) of specific epithelial tissues (15). It is not precisely known how mutations in these keratins lead to hyperkeratosis of the nail, but fragility of the underlying nail bed keratinocytes presumably leads to release of cytokines and other inflammatory factors that act upon the proliferative cells of the nail matrix and produce overgrowth of the nail (16).

Keratins are a large family of intermediate filament proteins encoded by more than 50 distinct genes in humans (17). About half of these are the epithelial keratins that are found in soft epithelial tissues of the human body. The rest are the trichocyte or high-sulphur hard keratins of which hair and nail is composed. Both epithelial keratins and hard keratins can be further subdivided into type I and type II proteins on the basis of their size, charge, and amino acid sequence characteristics (18). Recent work has shown that the human hair keratin family consists of nine type I and six type II members, whose genes are organized as distinct clusters within the type I and type II epithelial keratin gene domains on chromosomes 17q21.2 and 12q13.3, respectively (16). The functional type I (*K9–K23; Ha1–Ha8*) and type II keratin genes (*K1–K8; Hb1–Hb6*) are each clustered on distinct chromosomes in the human and mouse genomes. The pairwise and differentiation-related regulation of most type I and type II keratin genes provides a unique handle to track differentiation within epithelial tissue (19). A family-wide, crucial function of keratin filaments is to endow epithelial cells with the ability to withstand mechanical and other forms of stress.

Accordingly, mutations in keratin genes are responsible for a number of genetically based fragility disorders involving specific cell types in skin and other epithelia (20,21). Among type I keratin genes, *K17* stands out in multiple ways. In mouse embryonic skin, it is first expressed in ectodermal cells committing to a nonepidermal cell fate (i.e., all appendages and periderm) in response to mesenchymal induction (22). Concomitant with skin maturation, *mK17* expression becomes restricted to specific cell layers and compartments within all major types of epithelial appendages. Both *hK17* and *mK17* can be coregulated with distinct type II keratin genes (e.g., *K5, K6a, K6b, K6hf*) in mature epithelial settings (23). In addition to its constitutive expression in epithelial appendages, *K17* expression is induced in mature interfollicular epidermis subjected to various types of acute challenges (e.g., injury, ultraviolet light exposure, inflammation) or during diseases (e.g., psoriasis, basal cell carcinoma). Mutations affecting a particular segment of *hK17*'s coding sequence can cause distinct disorders of the skin, related to ectodermal dysplasias (15).

Several genodermatoses, such as Darier's disease, X-linked dyskeratosis congenita (DC), and pachyonychia congenita (PC), are associated with characteristic nail changes (24). A causative gene for Darier's disease, which resides at 12q23-q24.1, encodes the sarco/endoplasmic reticulum Ca^{2+}-ATPase type 2 isoform. Mutations in *XAP101* gene, which maps to Xq28, are responsible for DC. Thus, mutations in *DKC1* gene encoding dyskerin have been also found (25). Pachyonychia congenita is a group of autosomal dominant ectodermal dysplasias, whose most obvious phenotype is hypertrophic nail dystrophy leading to a phenotype of grossly thickened nail. There are two main types of PC: the Jadassohn–Lewandowsky form (type 1) and the Jackson–Lawler form (type 2). The epithelia affected in pachyonychia congenita type 1 express the keratin pair K6a and K16, and the condition is caused by dominant-negative mutations in these genes (26). The pachyonychia congenita type 2 variant is caused by mutations in keratins K6b and K17 (27). All the tissues affected in pachyonychia congenita type 2 express K6b and K17(28–30).

GROSS ANATOMY

It was first noted early in the twentieth century that the nail unit was comparable in several respects to a hair follicle sectioned longitudinally and laid on its side. The epithelial components of the hair follicle and nail apparatus are differentiated epidermal structures that may be involved jointly in several ways as congenital and hereditary anomalies and acquired conditions such as alopecia areata, lichen planus, iatrogenic causes, and fungal infection (31).

Various types of differently keratinizing epidermis make up the nail. What commonly is termed "the nail plate" is the horny end product of the most important epidermal component, the matrix. Usually, this nail plate is slightly convex or flat, rectangular, and of varying size between approximately 1×1 and 2×3 cm, depending on the finger (Figures 2.6–2.8). In the hand, this is usually 25 to 50% of the dorsal surface of the fingertips, whereas in the big toe it occupies about 75%. The nail is translucent and becomes rosy from the underlying vascular network. However, change of colors (erythronychia, melanonychia) can be observed in the nail plate and may indicate inflammatory diseases (lichen planus, lupus erythematosus); benign or malignant neoplasms, main subungual melanoma; and scarring of the dermis or epidermis (32). The white appearance of nails in leukonychia seems to be a result of an abnormal keratinization of cells originating from the proximal nail matrix, which leads to the presence of abundant intracellular vacuoles and to a lesser compactness of keratins. Genes mapping within this chromosomal region include the genes coding for type II (basic) cytokeratins and

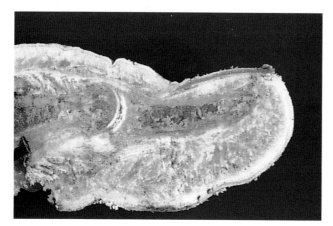

Figure 2.6 Sagittal section of an adult thumb, in which it is possible to observe the relations of the nail unit with the adjacent tissues.

hard keratins, and the gene defect resides on chromosome 12q13 (33).

In the proximal portion of the nail, there is an arch called the lunula. The thickness of the nail plate is 0.5 mm in women and 0.6 mm in men (34). The nail plate is delimited by three folds: two lateral and one proximal (Figure 2.9). If the nail plate is avulsed, the grooves become visible where the nail plate rested. These potential spaces are only real spaces in abnormal conditions of the nail, as in paronychia. In the lateral nail grooves, the epidermal lining does not contribute to the formation of the nail plate except in the most proximal portions, where it becomes continuous with the epidermis of the proximal groove or matrix.

The proximal nail fold is the most important one, since, as we shall note later, its contribution to the formation of the nail plate is fundamental (35). This fold shows two portions: a dorsal portion, lodging the matrix, and a ventral

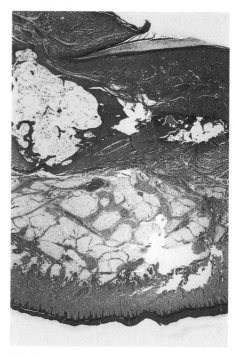

Figure 2.8 Histological sagittal section of a finger (H&E, ×10).

portion. Twenty-five percent of the total surface of the nail plate is located under the ventral portion of the proximal nail fold. The terminal tendon of the digital extensor is closely related with this area, and the thin nature and proximity with the nail matrix must be kept in mind during surgery (36).

A white crescent-shaped lunula can project from under the proximal nail fold. It is usual on the thumbs and common on other fingers and on large toenails. The lunula

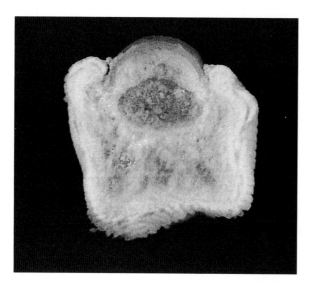

Figure 2.7 Cross section of an adult finger. The nail plate lies on nail bed, and the lateral border is overlapped by lateral nail fold.

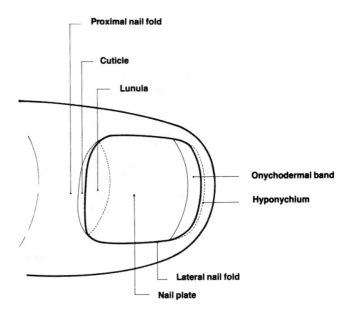

Figure 2.9 Schematic nail diagram, including nomenclature.

is the most distal portion of the matrix and determines the shape of the free edge of the nail plate. The color of the lunula is partly due to the effect of light scattered by the nucleated cells of the keratogenous zone of the matrix and partly to the thicker layer of epithelial cells making up the matrix (35,37).

At the point of separation of the nail plate and the nail bed, the subungual epidermis may be modified as the sole-horn (38). In humans, this structure may only be vestigial, its original significance only being evident from comparative anatomical studies. However, in certain diseases, it could be the seat of distal subungual hyperkeratosis or parakeratosis; for example, in pachyonychia congenita and pityriasis rubra pilaris (39). The distal limit of the ungual layer is the hyponychium, which determines the formation of the distal fold, a keratinized structure that continues until the fingertips. A subungual extension of the hyponichium and obliteration of the distal groove is named the pterygium inversum unguis (40). This term was coined because of the similarity between the behavior of the hyponychium and the eponychium in classic cases of pterygium unguis.

On close examination, two further distal zones can often be identified: the distal yellow-white margin and, immediately proximal to this, the onychodermal band (41). This band is a barely perceptible narrow transverse band, 0.5 to 1.5 mm wide, that is more prominent in acrocyanosis. The exact anatomical basis for the onychodermal band is not known, but it appears to have a different blood supply from the main body of the nail bed (42). It is possible to explore it through a strong compression of the distal zone of the finger, leaving behind a white band. The band's color can occasionally be modified by diseases (39,43).

Several studies have been published about the exploration of the nail apparatus. Although ultrasound

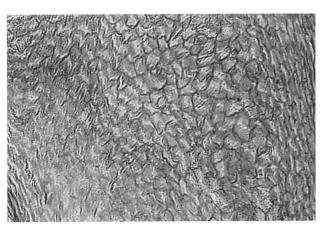

Figure 2.10 Horizontal section of the dorsal nail plate. Corneocytes show a polydedral disposition with rounded corners; the cells do not contain nuclei or elements (VVG stain, ×200).

transmission can be useful for studying the nail plate thickness (44), magnetic resonance imaging (MRI) permits the detection of subungual lesions smaller than 1 mm in diameter (45).

MICROSCOPIC ANATOMY

The Nail Plate

Microscopically, the nail plate consists of closely packed, adherent, interdigitating corneocytes lacking nuclei or organelles (Figures 2.10–2.11). Many intercellular links, including tight, intermediate, and desmosomal junctions, are present (46). The nail plate is made-up of three layers: a thin dorsal layer, a thick intermediate layer, and the ventral

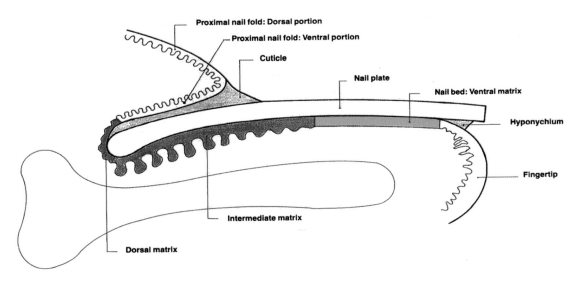

Figure 2.11 Schematic diagram of a sagittal section through the nail unit.

layer from the nail bed. The cells of the surface of the nail plate overlap, slanting from proximal-dorsal to distal-volar. For this reason, the dorsal surface of the nail plate is smooth, whereas the palmar surface is irregular, showing longitudinal striations. This can also be observed with optical microscopy, scanning electron microscopy (47), and x-ray microdiffraction (48). With this latter technique, Garson et al. (48) demonstrated three different layers in the nail plate that are characterized by different orientations of the keratin molecules from the outer to the inner side of human nail. These layers were associated with the histological dorsal, intermediate, and ventral plates. The hairlike type α-keratin filaments (81 Å in diameter) are only present in the intermediate layer (accounting for approximately two-thirds of the nail width) and are perfectly oriented perpendicularly to the growth axis in the nail plane. Keratin filaments of stratum corneum (epidermis) type, found in the dorsal and ventral cells, are oriented in two privileged directions; parallel and perpendicular to the growth axis. This "sandwich" structure in the corneocytes and the strong intercellular junctions gives the nail high mechanical rigidity and hardness, both in the curvature direction and in the growth direction. Lipid bilayers (49 Å thick) parallel to the nail surface fill certain ampullar dilations of the dorsal plate and intercellular spaces in the ventral plate. Using x-ray microdiffraction, Garson et al. also showed that onychomycosis disrupts the keratin structure, probably during the synthesis phase. No keratohyalin granules were seen, but acidophilic masses, called pertinax bodies of Lewis and Montgomery, are occasionally seen in older age groups.

Hamilton et al. (49) believed that the progressive increase in the thickness of the nail plate with age is attributable to the increasing size of the cells in the plate, consecutive to the frictional loss of nail; however, Johnson and Shuster (50) studied 20 normal great toenails to find the determinant of final nail thickness and length at its point of detachment at the onychodermal band. They confirmed that the increase of nail thickness with age is independent of the frictional traumatisms on the plate. Cutting tests showed that fracture of the nail plate occurred because the energy to cut nails transversely, at approximately 3 kJ/m^2, was about half that needed (approx. 6 kJ/m^2) to cut them longitudinally (51).

Corneocytes of the human nail plate have been studied by Germann et al. (52). Corneocytes of the dorsal nail plates of normal nails are irregular and polyhedral, nonnucleated, and with distinctly irregular networks. These horny cells from nail plates increase in size with age: babies have small cells, adults have significantly larger cells, and aged subjects have significantly larger cells than the younger adults. These authors also commented that the faster-than-normal growing nail plates yield smaller cells; for example, corneocytes from psoriatic patients are smaller than normal, whereas corneocytes from slow-growing nails, such as from persons having lichen planus or dyskeratosis congenita, are larger than normal.

Frequent gap junctions were observed near the area where lamellar granules were discharging their contents, and it was suggested that a certain substance might be able to pass through the nail plate using such intercellular channels. Perhaps such channels explain the greater permeability of the nail plate to polar molecules compared with the permeability of the skin (53). The water content of human nail plates has been determined using a portable near-infrared spectrometer with an InGaAs photodiode array detector and PLS regression by Egawa et al. (54).

Transonychial water loss (TOWL) in vivo has been studied by Nuutinen et al. (55). These authors have demonstrated that TOWL values decrease with age and patients with eczema, psoriasis, and onychomycosis have significantly lowered TOWL values compared with healthy subjects.

The biochemical composition of the nail plate has been widely studied. Calcium, found as the phosphate in hydroxyapatite crystals, is an important component of the nail plate; it is intracelluarly bound to phospholipids, particularly in the dorsal and ventral nail plate (56). Calcium concentration is approximately 0.1% of the weight, 10 times greater than in hair (57). However, some authors believe that the proportion of calcium in the nail contributes little to the hardness of the nail plate in human beings (39,58). Also, it is possible that calcium is not an intrinsic part of the nail but is incorporated from extrinsic sources, such as soaps; the nail is relatively porous, and calcium could enter as ionic calcium or bound to fatty acids. Other metals such as copper, manganese, zinc, and iron are also found in small quantities in the nail plate, although their function is still unknown (58,59). Lipids are also an important component of the nail plate. Helmdach et al. (59) have demonstrated that nail plate lipid composition varies with age and sex: the lipid composition of the fertile years shows distinct profiles compared to that of childhood and old age, suggesting an influence of sex hormones on nail lipogenesis.

The existence of sulfhydryl and disulfide groups has been demonstrated in the nail plate. During early embryonic life, there is a very high concentration of the sulfhydryl groups (9), which decreases as the delivery date approaches and stabilizes at about the age of 3 years (14). These sulfurous radicals are formed at the expense of amino acids, such as cystine. Quantification of cysteine and cystine can be performed by hydrolysis (60). Total sulfur concentration is similar in the dorsal and intermediate plates. Compared with hair, the nail plate also contains glutamic acid, serine, and less tyrosine (57–60).

In certain diseases, the quantity of various organic and metallic components of the nail plate can be increased. A brief listing is presented for reference: total nonprotein nitrogen, urea nitrogen, ammonia nitrogen, and uric acid in gout (61); creatinine in chronic renal failure (62); sodium in cystic fibrosis (63,64); calcium in older subjects

(48,57); copper in Wilson's disease (65); arsenic as biomarker to arsenic exposure in the endemic areas (66) ; and morphine, 6-acetylmorphine, and cocaine in drug abusers (67).

An analysis of the keratin of the nail plate revealed the following (68): (a) α-fibrillar, low-sulfur protein; (b) globular, high-sulfur matrix protein; and (c) high-glycine–tyrosine-rich matrix protein. All these fractions are also present in hair. The hardness of nail is due to the high-sulfur matrix protein, contrasting with the relatively soft keratin of the epidermis.

Proximal Nail Fold

The proximal nail fold is an invaginating, wedge-shaped fold of the skin on the dorsum of the distal digit, and the nail plate arises from under this fold (Figure 2.12). The proximal nail fold consists of two layers of epidermis: the ventral portion overlying the newly formed nail plate and the dorsal portion that forms the dorsum of the finger epidermis. The keratinization process in both portions does not differ from that of the epidermis elsewhere, possessing a granular layer that is absent in all parts of the nail matrix.

The dorsal portion of the proximal nail fold consists of a continuation of the epidermis and dermis of the dorsal digit with sweat glands but no follicles or sebaceous glands. At the distal tip, a thick corneal layer called the cuticle

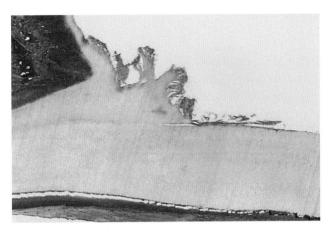

Figure 2.13 Detail of the cuticle. At the distal tip, the proximal nail fold shows a thick corneal layer (cuticle) on the dorsal surface of the nail plate.

shows on the dorsal surface of the nail plate (Figure 2.13). Its function is the protection of the nail base, particularly the germinative matrix. Loss of the cuticle often allows acute and chronic inflammatory and infective processes to involve the nail matrix, leading to secondary nail plate dystrophies.

The ventral portion is thick-skinned, has no appendages, and is closely attached on the dorsal surface of the nail plate. The epithelium of the ventral surface of the proximal nail fold has been called the eponychium (9,37,39). Diseases that affect the ventral portion of the proximal nail fold can affect the newly formed nail plate. For this reason, some authors think that the proximal nail fold contributes to form the superficial layer of the nail plate. In particular, the apparition of pits and grooves (Beau's line) on the nail is due to parakeratotic and growth detention phenomena, respectively, in the ventral portion of the proximal nail fold.

Matrix

The ventral surface of the proximal nail fold forms the roof of the proximal nail groove; the nail matrix forms its floor, and the nail plate lies between the two. The matrix is divided into three parts (8,9,39): dorsal, intermediate, and ventral. Of these, the dorsal and, above all, the intermediate portions play an important role in nail plate formation. In particular, the true matrix is the intermediate portion. For this reason, when we discuss the histology of the matrix, we are fundamentally referring to the intermediate portion. The ventral portion corresponds to the nail bed; the controversy about its participation in the formation of the definitive nail plate is discussed in the section entitled Nail Growth.

The main body of the matrix is composed of epithelial cells, with melanocytes, Merkel cells, and Langerhans cells scattered among the epithelial cells.

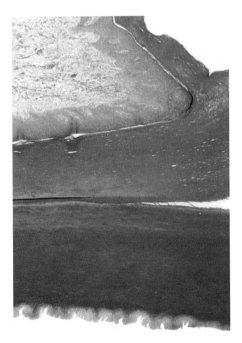

Figure 2.12 Proximal nail fold with its two portions: *dorsal portion*, with identical histologic pattern to the skin of the dorsum of the distal digit; *ventral portion*, overlying the nail plate. Note the great thickness of the stratum corneum of this epithelium (MF stain, ×63).

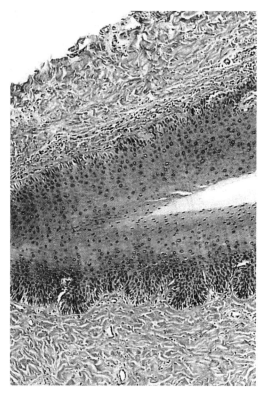

Figure 2.14 Histologic appearance of the matrix angle, formed by the ventral portion of the nail fold and the dorsal and intermediate matrix.

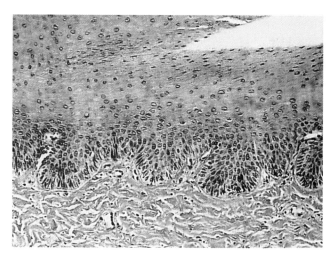

Figure 2.15 Detail of matrix epithelium. This zone shows an acanthotic epithelium, with germinative basal cells keratinocytes and scarce melanocytes.

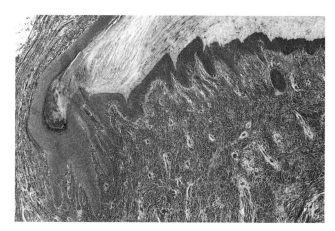

Figure 2.16 Detail of the matrix zone, in which one can observe the abrupt keratinization.

Epithelial Cells

The matrix is an easily identified thick squamous epithelium, situated immediately below the ventral portion of the proximal nail fold (Figure 2.14). Its main feature is its thickness, with between 8 and 15 mamelons (protuberances) (Figure 2.15). Its undulation can be seen for only a few millimeters, flattening itself in the area corresponding to the nail bed. As in the epidermis of the skin, the matrix possesses a very active germinative basal layer of immature basaloid cells, producing keratinocytes which differentiate, harden, die, and contribute to the nail plate (Figure 2.16). The nail plate is formed by a process that involves flattening of the basal cells of the matrix, fragmentation of nuclei, and condensation of the cell cytoplasm to form horny flat cells. An important histologic feature is the lack of granular layer. Acanthosis and papillomatosis are only seen in the nail unit in the matrix and, distally, in the hyponychium (Table 2.2).

TABLE 2.2
HISTOLOGIC CHARACTERISTIC FEATURES OF EACH ZONE OF THE NAIL UNIT

Nail Area	Epithelium	Granular Layer	Horny End Product
Proximal nail fold	Similar to normal skin or slightly acanthotic	Present	Cuticle
Matrix	Acanthotic	Absent	Nail plate
Nail bed	Flat	Absent	Lower layer of the nail plate
Hyponychium	Acanthotic	Present	Horny layer in the under surface of the distal nail, similar to cuticle

Melanocytes

The nail matrix possesses melanocytes, just as the hair matrix does. The matrix of Caucasian patients contains sparse, poorly developed melanocytes (Figures 2.17, 2.18, 2.19) (69). It is difficult to observe melanocytes in the proximal matrix zone using light microscopy, but their number is progressively increased distally. Nevertheless, the number of melanocytes is always less than in normal skin (69–73).

There are distinct differences in the distribution of melanocytes in adult skin and nail matrix. Immunostaining of nail matrix melanocytes revealed that they are not singly interspersed between the keratinocytes of the basal layer, but they are frequently arranged in small clusters among the suprabasal layers of the nail matrix (73,74). A similar pattern of distribution of melanocytes has been described in fetal skin and in fetal skin equivalents, in which the melanocytes are grouped and localized both basally and suprabasally. The suprabasal location of nail matrix melanocytes may be a consequence of differences in the distribution of adhesion molecules in the nail epithelium (73,74).

Higashi and Saito (75) demonstrated that the number of melanocytes and the intensity of the dopa reaction in them were much greater in the distal than the proximal matrix. The melanocyte count in normal epidermis was reported to be 400 per 2.784 mm^2 (74,75), while the range was 208 to 576 in the distal areas of the intermediate nail matrix (75).

Ultraviolet rays and trauma are factors that could influence a more extensive distribution in the distal zone (73,74). In some races such as Japanese, the matrix contains several

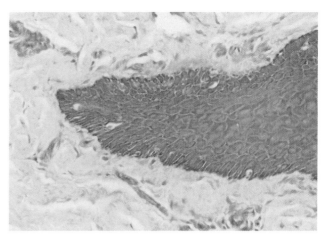

Figure 2.18 Melanocytes of the nail matrix, are negative with cytokeratin antibody stain. Observe its scarce number in the nail matrix (cytokeratin antibody, ×10).

hundred well-developed melanocytes per millimeter (75). Also, it seems that melanocytes of the nail matrix in Oriental races have larger dendritic processes than Caucasians.

Pigment, therefore, arrives in the nail plate as in the keratinized cells of the stratum corneum and hair cortex (76). Nail pigmentation is most evident in African Americans, in whom it is commonly seen as longitudinal linear streaks, although this anomalous distribution of pigmentation can also be seen in pathological states such as subungual pigmented nevi and melanomas in the matrix zone (77). Abundant melanosomas of these subjects have a protective effect against ultraviolet radiation, since variations in racial pigmentation are due to the number and size of melanosomes produced (78).

The location of melanocytes in the matrix is directly related to the location of pigmented bands, most of which originate in the distal matrix and do not cross the lunula (73). Longitudinal melanonychia in AIDS patients is a common finding. Although this pigmentary nail change

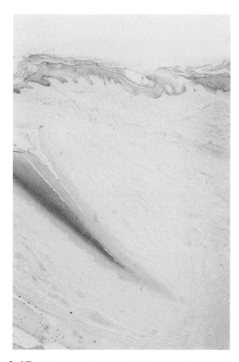

Figure 2.17 Observe the notable hyperpigmentation of the basal layer in the pulp of the finger in contrast with the absence of pigmentation in the nail matrix (Fontana's stain, ×4).

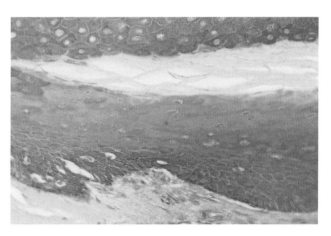

Figure 2.19 Melanocytes of the lunula, not staining with cytokeratin antibody in contrast with positive epithelial cells. Note its location in basal and suprabasal epithelial layers (cytokeratin antibody, ×20).

can be related to the zidovudine oral treatment, in other cases it seems to be independent and associated with elevated levels of α-melanocyte-stimulating hormone (α-MSH) (79). Cancer chemotherapeutic agents often induce nail changes, and nail pigmentation is probably the most frequently observed nail abnormality. The mechanism of drug-induced hyperpigmentation is not fully understood, but this is most probably due to increased melanogenesis in matrix melanocytes. Beau's lines, transverse leuconychia, and onychomedesis are the result of nail matrix toxicity and can be seen after intensive or combined chemotherapy. Nail bed toxicity, as manifested in apparent leuconychia or onycholysis, may be seen in association with nail bed hemorrhage, which may be exacerbated by concurrent thrombocytopenia. Acute paronychia has also been described after treatment with methotrexate (80).

Langerhans and Merkel Cells

Langerhans and Merkel cells have also been identified in the matrix (70), although their signification is unknown. Studies of the Langerhans cells in the nail matrix are almost absent. Nevertheless, interesting studies about the Merkel cells have been recently published. Moll and Moll (81) studied the Merkel cells (MCs) in ontogenesis of human nails, using immunohistochemical stains with cytokeratins 18 and 20 in human fetuses of 9 to 22 weeks of life. These authors have concluded the number of MCs are detected very early (nine weeks) in the matrix primordium. However, MCs were found to decrease in number with aging of the fetuses: MCs were only seen in the proximal nail fold at 12 to 15 weeks and were essentially absent from the epithelium of the ventral matrix and nail bed in the adult.

Lunula

The intermediate matrix continues forward with a visible, white half-moon-shaped area called the lunula. The lunula is shown to be linked to a well-defined area in the underlying dermis with a specific histology and microvascularization. Although always present, it cannot be seen in some fingers but is most visible in the thumbs. The typical white color is related to some histologic features of this area. Lewin (34) confirmed that the opacity of the proximal nail plate, the relative avascularity of the subepidermal layer, and the loose texture of the dermal collagen are responsible for its color. Samman (82,83) thought that it was a combination of incomplete keratinization in the nail plate and loose connective tissue in the underlying tissue. Zaias (84) believed that the nail plate would be thinner in the lunula because it coincides with the keratogenous zone, the zone of cytoplasmic condensation in the matrix just before cells form the nail plate. The length of the subnail matrix area distal to the free edge of the proximal nail fold is highly correlated with the length of the lunula (85).

Other special histologic features of this zone of the matrix, including a different chemical composition of the nail plate and a different distribution of the dermal fibers, have been related to the typical white color of the lunula (86,87), although not one of these factors has been confirmed. We do not even know the exact function of the lunula.

Nail Bed

The nail bed begins where the intermediate matrix ends, and some authors prefer to designate the ventral matrix as the site (39,86). A histologic appreciation of the end of the intermediate matrix and the beginning of the nail bed is very easy. The nail bed epidermal layer is usually a flat epithelium no more than three- or four-cells thick and without melanocytes (Figures 2.20–2.22). The transition zone from living keratinocytes to dead ventral nail plate cells is abrupt, occurring in the space of one horizontal cell layer in a manner very similar to what occurs in the Henle layer of the internal root sheath of the hair follicle (87).

During its early development, the nail bed exhibits a keratinization process differing from the adult's, with a prominent granular layer at 17 to 20 weeks of development. However, after birth, the nail bed, like the matrix, keratinizes without a granular layer. It is less active than the matrix, with a longer turnover time than the matrix and skin (88). A thin parakeratotic keratin is produced, apparently dragged forward by the nail plate growing over it rather than becoming incorporated into the nail.

In the nail bed, the dermis fits into the longitudinal and parallel nail bed ridges in tongue-and-groove fashion. The fine capillaries of the nail bed run in these parallel dermal ridges, and disruption of these accounts for the splinter hemorrhages commonly seen in normal and disease states (42). There is no fat tissue in the nail bed, although scattered dermal fat cells may be visible microscopically.

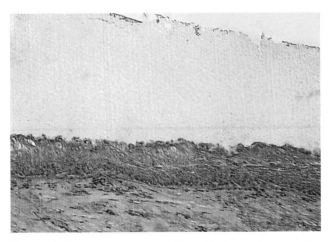

Figure 2.20 Nail bed. Note the flat epithelium with an interdigitated upper zone.

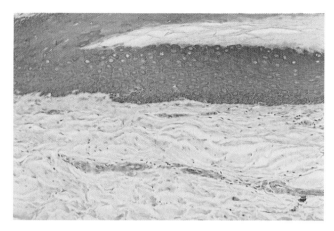

Figure 2.21 Melanocytes are absent in the nail bed (cytokeratin antibody stain, ×10).

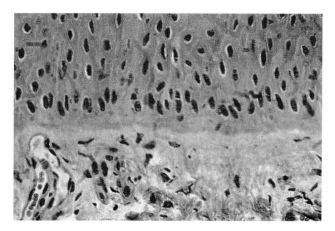

Figure 2.22 Detail of the nail bed zone. The epithelium shows a few active germinative cells at the basal layer. In the upper dermis, it is possible to observe larger vessels than in the normal skin.

The nail bed epidermis moves distally toward the hyponychium. The cells that appear to be the germinative population lie near the lunula, so close together that they may be confused as belonging to one population. The distal movement from this position may also help explain why during development the nail bed epidermis seems to lose keratohyalin granule layers from a proximal-to-distal direction concomitantly with the formation of the primitive nail plate (89).

In some pathologic states, the nail bed shows a granular layer in which the activity in the nail bed is greatly increased, such as occurs in onychogryphosis, pachyonychia congenita, and psoriasis (90); in these cases, the horny cells produced push the nail plate upward and give it a claw-like appearance.

Histochemical studies of the nail bed prove the presence of bound phospholipids in the nail bed epidermis (Table 2.3). Bound cysteine can be detected in the transition zones: acid phosphatase and nonspecific esterase are absent in the dorsal and intermediate zones (39,56).

Immunohistochemical studies have demonstrated that nail bed expressed all the target antigens found in the normal nonappendageal basement membrane. In particular, there was normal expression of the epidermal-associated antigens, the 230- and 180-kDa bullous pemphigoid antigens, and the α6β4 integrin. There was also normal expression of the lamina lucida antigens LH39, GB3, and laminin. Sinclair et al. (91) pointed out that the dermal-associated components, namely the 285-kDa linear immunoglobulin A (IgA) antigen, the extracellular matrix glycoproteins chondroitin sulphate, type VII collagen and its closely associated proteins, and the poorly characterized antigen for LH24 and LH39 were all normally expressed. All the former molecules were also found in the proximal nail fold, nail matrix, and hyponychium.

The presence of antimicrobial peptides in nails (mainly cathelicidin LL-37, demonstrated by immunostaining and which has activity against relevant nail pathogens) may account for the ability of the nail unit to resist infection

TABLE 2.3

HISTOCHEMISTRY OF THE NAIL[a]

| | Matrix | | Nail Bed | | Nail Plate | | | Nail Folds—Hyponychium | | | |
	Dorsal	Intermediate	Basal Layer	Malpighian Layer	Ventral	Intermediate	Dorsal	Basal Layer	Malpighian Layer	Keratinized Layer	Dermis
Glycogen	−	−	−	±	−	−	−	−	±	−	
Mucopolysaccharide	+	+	±	+	++	−	+	±	+	±	+
Ribonucleic acid	+	+	+	+	−	−	−	+	+	−	
Sulfhydryl groups					++	++	+		+	+	
Acid phosphatase	+		±	±	+	++	−	+	+	+	
Alkaline phosphatase	−		−		−	−	−		+		+
Amylophosphorylase	+	+	+		−	−					
Cholinesterase											+

[a]Baran R. Dawber RPR, eds. *Diseases of the Nail and Their Management.* Oxford: Blackwell Scientific; 1984:1–21. Jarrett A, Spearman RI. The histochemistry of the human nail. *Arch Dermatol* 1966;94:652–657.

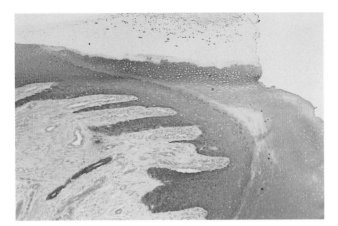

Figure 2.23 Panoramic view of the hyponychium (cytokeratin stain, ×10).

in the absence of direct access to the cellular immune system (92).

Hyponychium

The most distal portion of the nail bed is the hyponychium, representing the union between the nail bed and the fingertips (Figure 2.23); its histologic characteristics are rather peculiar. This transition zone presents a notable change of appearance after a few millimeters because the epithelium undergoes keratinization similar to that of the epidermis (Figure 2.24). The result is marked acanthosis and hyperplasia with the crests oriented almost horizontally; this is associated with normal appendages (Figure 2.25). An area of abundant keratohyalin granules is present, and the horny layer produced tends to accumulate under the free edge of the nail plate, producing a keratin horn similar to the cuticle. The hyponychium is the first site of keratinization in the nail unit (8,9,11–13) and of all epidermis in the embryo (93). The function of this anatomical formation is to render the nail bed impermeable to protect it from external agents (94). If this

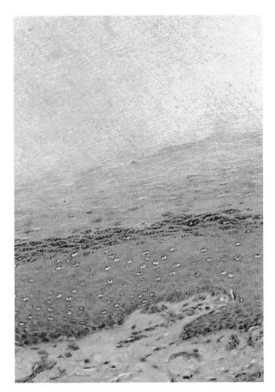

Figure 2.25 Detail of the hyponychium zone. Note the great keratin layer under the nail plate and the visible granular layer. The epithelium shows an acanthotic aspect, with transversal papillae.

structure fails, dermatophyte invasions will be frequent, producing onychomycosis (95).

Terry (41) describes an intermediate zone between the nail bed and the hyponychium, which he called the onychodermal band. Terry speculated that this area, normally from 0.5 to 1.5 mm wide, had a blood supply different from the remainder of the nail bed, a fact later confirmed by other authors (42). For this reason, the color is paler than the pink nail bed and has a slightly amber tinge with a translucent quality. The onychodermal band occasionally changes its color, especially in cirrhosis and other chronic diseases (39,43).

Lateral Nail Folds

The lateral nail folds have a structure similar to the adjacent skin but are normally devoid of dermatoglyphic markings and folliculo sebaceous units. Acanthosis and hyperplasia of the epithelium are present, similar to that of the hyponychium. Keratinization within the nail folds proceeds by keratohyalin formation in the granular layer (Figure 2.26). The epidermal lining of these grooves does not contribute to the formation of the nail plate except in the most proximal portions of the grooves, where it becomes continuous with the epidermis of the proximal nail fold or matrix.

When the lateral border of the nail plate pathologically breaks this fold, abundant granulation tissue forms, constituting the onychocryptosis, a frequent pathologic alteration of the great toenail.

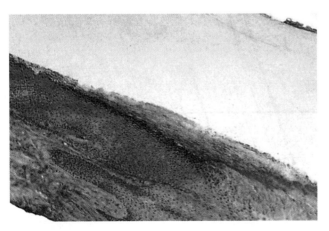

Figure 2.24 Hyponychium zone. The most important feature of this zone is the great accumulation of keratin under the distal nail plate.

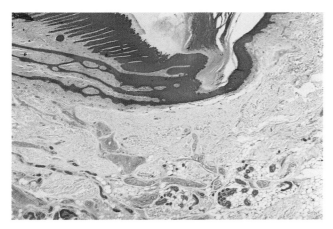

Figure 2.26 Lateral nail fold. Observe its acanthotic epithelial layer and the presence of eccrine glands in the middle dermis (cytokeratin antibody, ×4).

IMMUNOHISTOCHEMISTRY OF THE NAIL UNIT

Nail Plate

The cornified envelope of the epidermis is formed by several precursor proteins, including involucrin, keratolinin, loricrin, pancornulin, sciellin, 195-kDa protein, keratin, and filiagrin. Baden and Kvedar (96) used monoclonal antibodies to demonstrate that pancornulin is present in the nail fold and proximal matrix, and sciellin is detectable in the nail fold, matrix, and bed. Similarly, in studies of human nails (which contain hard keratins), the use of immunofluorescence, immunoblotting, and PCR (polymerase chain reaction) have shown that trichohyalin, a 200-kDa protein of the inner root sheath and medulla, was present in the ventral matrix but not in the nail bed; a few scattered cells stained for trichohyalin were observed within the nail plate (97).

Heid et al. (98) studied the keratin expression patterns observed in the human fetal nail matrix and revealed that the nail develops from both skin- and hair-type differentiating cells. Kitahara and Ogawa (99) demonstrated that AE13 antibody reacted with the dorsal nail matrix. Because AE13 antibody recognized hard keratins that are characteristic of differentiation in hair, these results show that adult nail develops in such a way that hair-type differentiation is confined to the ventral nail matrix, supporting the Heid et al. study's results (100,101).

Keratinocytes

Expression of keratins in the different compartments within the nail unit have been demonstrated in some recent articles (102–112). The characteristics of the different keratins found at different sites could be relevant to our understanding of the biology of the normal nail and changes seen in several diseases.

Analysis of human nail plate by gel electrophoresis demonstrates a range of keratins of two characteristic types, as we commented formerly (see Genetics and Nail Keratins). Soft, or epithelial, keratins represent the major structural intermediate filament isolated from human skin but constitute only 10 to 20% of the keratin found in nail (99). Hard keratins, characteristic of hair and nail differentiation, exist in the same acid-base heterodimer configuration as soft epithelial keratins but have additional resistance. Molecular classification of hard keratin proteins on gel electrophoresis describes eight major (Ha1–4 and Hb1–4) and two minor (Hax and Hbx) proteins, all of which are probably present in human nail (103). This family has been extended by genomic analysis into at least seven type I Ha keratins and six type II Hb keratins. Further keratins and their isoforms are likely to be discovered. In addition to the hard keratins, epithelial keratins isolated from the nail plate include K1, K10, K5, K14, K6, K16, K17 and K19 from fetal nail (102,103) (Figure 2.27).

Ha1 is one of the major hard keratins found in nail, where hard keratin represents 80 to 90% of nail keratin. Keratins K5, K14, K1, and K10 were also detected in the nail. Since Berker et al. (102) have found a low expression of the differentiation-specific keratins K1 and K10 in the keratogenous zone of the ventral matrix, this feature was not demonstrated by other authors (104).

Keratins K6, K16, and K17 are normally found in hyperproliferative epidermis, such as in psoriasis or in wound healing (105). Studies of proliferative compartments in the nail unit suggest that the nail bed is not a major contributor to the nail plate. It may be that the ventral aspect of the proximal nail fold and not the nail bed is the source of nail plate K6 and K16, and the matrix and not the nail bed provides K17. Keratin K14 is synthesized in the basal layer, and K14 protein was detected throughout the epithelium, as has been noted in other tissues. However, the marker of basal keratin conformation, LH6, was also seen throughout the nail bed. This is unusual and may reflect the absence of the expression of the suprabasal keratins K1 and K10, which are thought to obscure the epitopes detected by LH6 in normal stratified epithelium. This persistence of LH6 antigen is also seen in the outer root sheath of the hair follicle; because this is also the site of expression of K16, K6, and K17 (106), the data support the analogy drawn between the nail bed and outer root sheath (107). However, expression of K1 and K10 is found to a degree in the upper outer root sheath superficial to the level of the sebaceous gland.

The absence of K1 and K10 from the nail bed correlates with a reduction in terminal differentiation. Lack of cornification is also seen in mucosal epithelium in combination with the presence of K16 and K17. However, mucosal differentiation is defined by the presence of K4 and K13, which was absent in the nail bed (108). The exact significance of these keratins remains to be established.

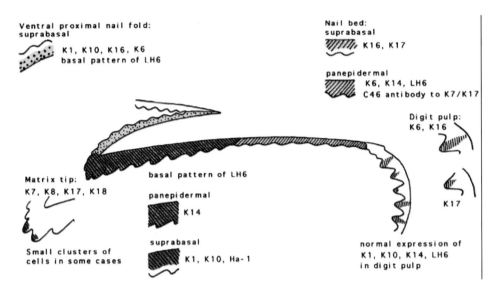

Figure 2.27 Keratin expression in the normal nail unit: markers of regional differentiation. Taken from De Berker D, Wojnarowska F, Sviland L, Westgate GE, Dawber RPR, Leigh IM. Keratin expression in the normal nail unit: markers of regional differentiation. *Br J Dermatol* 2000;142: 89–96.

Additional molecular studies have demonstrated the homology between hair and nail keratins (109). Retinoic acid–inducible gene-1 was originally identified as an orphan G-protein coupled receptor (oGPCR) induced by retinoic acid. Three highly homologous oGPCR (GPCR5B, GPCR5C, and GPCR5D) have since been classified into the RAIG1 family. Inoue et al. (109) studied the unique tissue distribution of GPCR5D and its mechanism of expression by in situ hybridization in hair shafts, nail, and filiform papillae of the tongue. They found that GPCR5D is expressed in differentiating cells that produce hard keratin, including cortical cells of the hair shaft, the keratogenous zone of the nail, and in a central region of the filiform papillae of the tongue. GPCR5D transcript is expressed in hair follicles during mid- and late anagen, and catagen but not at telogen and early anagen phases. The differentiation-inducer, all-*trans* retinoic acid, induces GPCR5D expression in cultured hair bulb cells. Because the tissue distribution of GPCR5D indicates a relationship with hard keratins that constitute the major structural proteins of hard epithelial tissues, they investigated the effect of GPCR5D on acid hard keratins.

Analyses of cultured cells showed that transient overexpression resulted in suppression of *Ha3* and stimulation of *Ha4* hair keratin gene expression. The expression was maintained in the hair follicles of *whn*-deficient (nude) mice, suggesting that this gene is regulated by a signal pathway different from that of hair keratin synthesis. These data provide a framework for understanding the molecular mechanisms of GPCR5D function in hard keratinization.

For the expression of hard keratin by matrical keratinocytes is primordial the influence of matrical fibroblasts. Okazaki et al. (110) demonstrated that, even in non–nail-matrical keratinocytes, expression of hard keratin could be induced by nail-matrical fibroblasts. These investigators constructed three different skin equivalents: (a) ventral keratinocytes (from the ventral side of the digit) were cocultured with ventral fibroblasts (group A); (b) ventral keratinocytes were cocultured with nail-matrical fibroblasts (group B); and

(c) nail-matrical keratinocytes were cocultured with ventral fibroblasts (group C). Immunohistochemical examinations with antihard keratin antibody (HKN-7) revealed hard keratin expression in groups B and C. The HKN-7-positive cells were distributed continuously in the entire epithelial strata or in the suprabasal layer in group B, whereas HKN-7-positive cells were distributed spottily in group C. This study indicated extrinsic hard keratin induction in non–nail-matrical keratinocytes by nail-matrical fibroblasts and suggests that non–nail-matrical epidermal grafts may be effective in the treatment of de-epithelialized nail injuries. In addition, it is possible that lost nails could be reconstructed with grafts of tissue-engineered nail equivalent.

Human carcinoembryonic antigen (CEA) and CEA-related molecules play an important role in adhesion of the nail plate to the nail bed. Egawa et al. (111) demonstrated that a CEA family antigen with NCA (CD66c)-like immunoreactivity was strongly expressed in the nail. A strong expression of the NCA-like antigen was only seen in the keratinocytes distributed in the upper epithelial cell layers of the major central portions of the nail bed, to which the nail plate is firmly bonded; expression was stronger at the more distal portion of the nail bed and was absent in the nail matrix, the hyponychium, and the lateral folds. The results are interesting because the nail plate is firmly bonded to the nail bed, less so proximal to the matrix margin, and it has been shown that the bed epithelium travels at the same speed as the nail plate, indicating that the bed epithelium has a proximal site of origin and a distal end.

Plasminogen activator inhibitor type 2 (PAI-2) was detected in the differentiating cells of the matrix and nail bed (112). These authors, using transfected cell lines that express high levels of PAI-2, have suggested that this inhibitor may confer protection against programmed cell death. This consistent, selective distribution of PAI-2 in the postmitotic, maturing cells prior to terminal keratinization and death suggests that (a) PAI-2 may be considered as a differentiation marker for many epithelial cell types, and

(b) PAI-2 is appropriately positioned to protect epithelial cells from premature demise (112).

Merkel Cells

Lacour et al. (113), in a double indirect immunofluorescence and immunoelectron microscopic study with the monoclonal antibody Troma-1, have only found MCs in the proximal nail fold of the adults, with a concentration greater than 50 MCs/mm².

Immunohistochemically, keratins K8 and K18 have been used as markers of MCs (81). Merkel cells have neuroendocrine characteristics and are of uncertain function, although their prominence in the nail unit in the early stages of fetal development has been noted, and a role in ontogenesis has been proposed. The number and location of cells demonstrating K8 and K18, which included the rete ridges of the digit pulp, suggested that these cells were MCs rather than they contributing directly to nail plate formation.

Melanocytes

Tosti et al. (114) have recently studied the melanocyte characterization of the normal nail matrix using immunohistochemistry techniques. These authors found nail matrix melanocytes reacted with the antibodies anti-PEP-1, anti-PEP-8, and anti-TMP-1, which recognize the tyrosinase-related protein-1, the tyrosinase-related protein-2 (DOPA-chrome tautomerase), and the tyrosinase-related protein encoded by *pMT4* (Table 2.4). This confirms that, even if normally quiescent, nail matrix melanocytes possess the key enzymes responsible for the formation of melanin pigment (115).

Expression of integrins in the nail matrix have been studied by Cameli et al. (116). These authors found that $\alpha2\beta1$ and $\alpha3\beta1$ expression differ in nail matrix epithelium. In the nail matrix, these integrins are not only expressed on the basal layer, but also on the fourth to fifth suprabasal layers, with suprabasal expression gradually decreasing from the distal to proximal matrix (Table 2.5). As in the normal human epidermis, $\alpha1$, $\alpha4$, and $\alpha5$ integrins subunits are not expressed in the nail matrix; in the same way, ICAM-1, the ligand of LFA1, was negative in the matrix cells. The expression of $\beta1$ subunits in the suprabasal layers of the nail matrix indicates a very strong cohesion between nail matrix cells, thus probably revealing them to be an essential prerequisite for the development of a compact nail plate. Cultures of nail matrix cells may represent a useful model to study the biologic properties of nail structure (117).

ULTRASTRUCTURAL ANATOMY

Very few studies of the normal ultrastructural morphology of the nail exist (10–13,46,47,69–72,76,89) because of varied difficulties (70): (a) achieving proper fixation and

TABLE 2.4

IMMUNOSTAINING OF HUMAN NAIL MELANOCYTES[a]

Antibody	Reactive to	Species	Nail Matrix Melanocytes
Anti-PEP-1	Tyrosinase-related protein-1	Rabbit	++
Anti-PEP-8	Tyrosinase-related protein-2 (DOPA-chrome tautomerasa)	Rabbit	+
HMB-45	Glycoconjugate present in immature melanosomes	Mouse	++
TMH-1	Tyrosinase-related protein encoded by *pMT4*	Mouse	+

[a]Tosti A, Cameli N, Piraccini BM, Fanti PA, Ortonne JP. Characterization of nail matrix melanocytes with anti-PEP1, anti-PEP8, TMH-1 and HMB-45 antibodies. *J Am Acad Dermatol* 1994;31:193–196.

TABLE 2.5

INTEGRIN EXPRESSION IN HUMAN NAIL MATRIX[a]

	Alpha-1	Alpha-2	Alpha-3	Alpha-4	Alpha-5	Alpha-6	Alpha-v	Beta-1	Beta-4	ICAM-1
Basal membrane zone	–	–	–	–	–	+++	–	–	+++	–
Basal layer	–	++	++	–	–	++	++	++	++	–
Suprabasal layer (Ventral matrix)	–	++	++	–	–	–	+	++	–	–
Suprabasal layers (Dorsal matrix)	–	+	+	–	–	–	+	+	–	–
Keratogenous zone	–	–	–	–	–	–	–	–	–	–

[a]Cameli N, Picardo M, Tosti A, Perrin C, Pisani A, Ortonne JP. Expression of integrins in human nail matrix. *Br J Dermatol* 1994;130:583–588.

adequate penetration of epoxy resin into the nail plate; (b) obtaining ultrathin sections; and (c) securing the high-voltage electron beam necessary to penetrate through extraordinarily hard tissue (because of the availability of 100 to 200 kV machines).

The proximal end of the human toenail is composed of several layers of epithelial cells. Hashimoto and coworkers (69–72) make the distinction between a proximal dorsal, apical, and ventral matrix, although noting that there are few differences between them. They found that the cells composing the proximal matrix were: (a) relatively small, elongated basal cells attached to the basal lamina; (b) relatively large, round, or polygonal squamous cells filling the more central portion of the matrix; (c) melanocytes; (d) Langerhans cells; and (e) Merkel cells.

Moreover, there exists a system of attachment to the dermis, showing the surface of the basal cell with frequent fingerlike elongations that interdigitate with the papillary dermis (Figure 2.28). This results in the formation of numerous micropapillae, with bundles of very fine fibrils (11 to 12 μm). The subjacent dermis of the matrix zone shows poor vascularity and scarce collagen fibers, with abundant basic matrix.

The basal cells are very active, with frequent mitotic figures. They showed an elongated nucleus and cytoplasm with numerous, slender projections (villi) intricately interdigitated with neighboring cells. Tonofibrils were also seen as a perinuclear ring with an interposition of the nuclear clear zone in which the majority of mitochondria, transferred melanosomes, and occasional centrioles are located. The suprabasal matrix cells are also round, with fre-

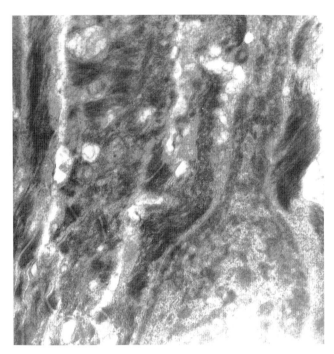

Figure 2.29 Detail of the basal layer of the matrix. Extensive condensation of cytokeratin. The nuclei show the habitual shape of normal skin at this epidermal level (×12,000).

quent mitotic figures. Generally, the long axes of these cells were oriented axiodistally, suggesting the direction of their migration. Large intercellular spaces were often seen between these suprabasal cells. The extensive interdigitation of the peripheral villi as seen in the basal cells disappeared, and multiple desmosomal junctions alone connected these cells (Figures 2.29 and 2.30).

Abundant desmosomes can be seen in the intermediate layers with high condensations of intermediate fibrils. The aspect of the intermediate layer of the nail matrix is similar to the upper layers of the normal epidermis (Figure 2.31). The cells have lost their organelles, and their cytoplasm is nearly filled with tonofibrils. For this reason, the keratinization process is very abrupt, passing from three to four cellular lines to completely keratinized corneocytes.

OTHER TISSUES OF THE NAIL UNIT

Dermis

The dermal component of the nail structures is a very specialized tissue, unique in that it is limited by the underlying phalanx and closely associated with its vasculature and nerve supply. There is no subcutaneous tissue, as previously noted.

Dermis, epithelium, and nail plate in the nail bed present special histologic features due to the great traction that is supported. The dermis is very thick with a dense collagen layer. These fibers are vertically situated in the proximal zone of the nail bed (Figure 2.32) and inclined at an angle of 45 degrees in the zone adjacent to the hyponychium

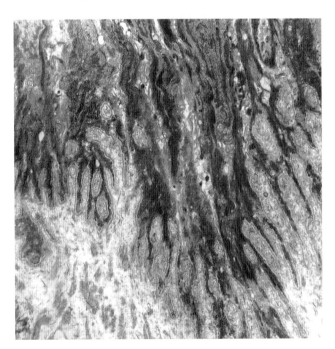

Figure 2.28 Ultrastructural appearance of the dermoepidermal junction of the intermediate matrix. The basal layer shows an accentuated digitiform distribution, with multiple intermediate filaments (×7000).

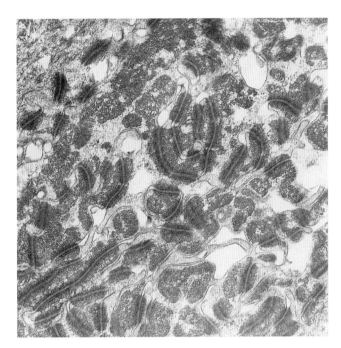

Figure 2.30 Detail of the desmosomal junctions of the suprabasal layer. They are bigger and more abundant than in a normal epidermis (×12,000).

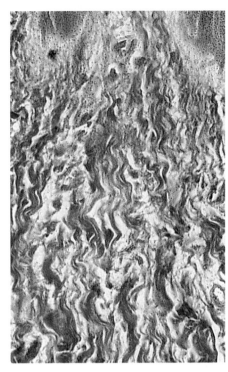

Figure 2.32 Collagen fibers of the proximal nail bed. Observe the peculiar vertical disposition (reticulin stain, ×400).

(Figure 2.33). Their mission is to attach the nail plate directly with the phalangeal periosteum. Conversely, the nail plate and nail bed are quite firmly attached to each other, more so than the nail plate to the matrix, and this seems to be accomplished by the striking, deep longitudinal ridges and furrows of the nail surface of the nail plate. The nail

bed has a unique, longitudinal, tongue-and-groove spatial arrangement of papillary dermal papillae and epidermal rete ridges. This feature is easily observed in transverse sections, in which this arrangement is appreciated as a serrated interdigitation of the ventral surface of the nail, papillae, and rete. These furrows can be seen very well macroscopically just after avulsion of the nail plate, but they are also beautifully shown microscopically by a scanning electron microscope (Figures 2.34 and 2.35) (89).

There are few studies about the nerve supply of the nail. The matrix and nail bed present sparse nerve endings and few Vater-Pacini (118) and Meissner corpuscles (119). Intraepithelial nerve fibers were described at the beginning

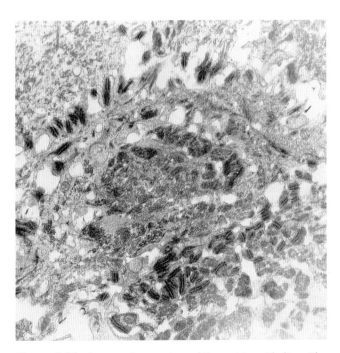

Figure 2.31 Intermediate stratum of the matrix epithelium. The intermediate filaments of cytokeratin show a special disposition in the nail matrix (×4400).

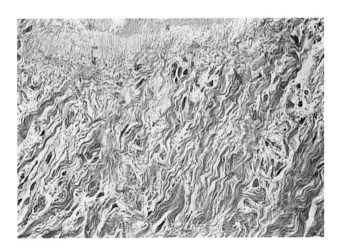

Figure 2.33 Collagen fibers of the distal nail bed. Observe the peculiar inclined disposition (VVG stain, ×200).

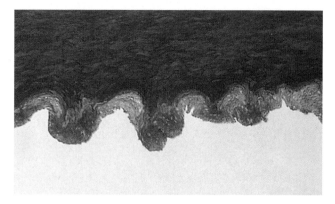

Figure 2.34 Transverse section of the nail plate. Note the serrated lower surface of the nail plate (MF stain,×200).

of this century (118), but other authors (120) were unable to confirm the description. Experimental studies have established that, for digit-tip regrowth, the major nerve supply is not needed but the nail organ is needed. Nail organs of regrowing fetal digit-tips have been shown to produce Msx, a transcription factor associated with limb bud outgrowth (121). In the same way, it is plausible that nail bed epithelium, acting like an inductive wound epithelium in newts, provides growth factors in mammals that can substitute for those generated by nerve in newt limbs (124).

The hyponychium is the area with greater abundance of nerve endings of the nail and with abundant Meissner and Merkel-Ranvier corpuscles, as in the lateral nail folds (120). This histologic feature gives the hyponychium an important role in the fine sensibility of the finger.

Bone

The nail apparatus includes the subjacent bone. Although the bone has been ignored during the last years, a recent study of postamputational repair following digit-tip amputation revealed an unexpected correlation between nail regrowth and bone regrowth. In this way, Zhao and Neufeld (123) have studied this relationship, observing that in the absence of nail, bone did not regrow at distal levels, and, conversely, when the nail was surgically retained, bone regrew from proximal levels.

Blood Supply

The nail has a rich vascularization that deserves separate mention. The arterial blood supply of the nail bed and matrix is derived from paired digital arteries. The most important studies have been published by Flint in 1955 (124), Ryan in 1973 (125), and Smith et al. in 1991 (126), concluding that the main supply passes into the pulp space of the distal phalanx before reaching the dorsum of the digit. An accessory supply arises further back on the digit and does not enter the pulp space. The digital arterial system manifests three characteristic anatomic features: arched anastomotic arteries in the deep dermis; more superficial terminal arteries branching to supply the rete (127), and the great tortuosity of the arterial architecture subjacent to the nail apparatus (Figure 2.36). The arteries possess inner longitudinal and outer circular coats of smooth muscle (Figure 2.37). Oxygen-sensitive microelectrodes (tip diameter of 5 μm) to measure the distribution of P_{O2} in dermal papillae of the fingernail folds of healthy human subjects have been developed by Wang et al. (128).

The vasculature in the nail bed is unique in that it must supply a vascular structure between two hard surfaces, the nail plate and the bone. Studies with scanning electron microscopy revealed special vascular patterns of nail microcirculation (129). In the eponychium and perionychium, the vascular villi followed the direction of nail growth. In the face of the eponychium in contact with the nail, a wide-

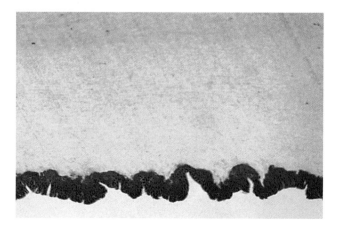

Figure 2.35 Avulsed nail plate. Observe the sinusoidal form of the nail bed epithelium attached to the lower surface of the nail plate.

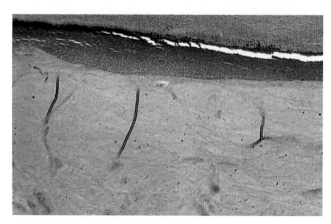

Figure 2.36 Vascular system of the nail bed. This zone has a rich vascular supply, with numerous vertical arteries (branches of the arched arteries of the deep dermis) (MF stain,×47).

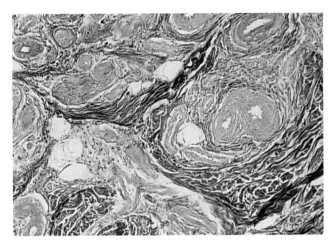

Figure 2.37 Detail of the rich vascular supply of the nail bed (reticulin stain, ×158).

mesh net of capillaries was evident. In the nail bed, the vessels were arranged in many longitudinal trabeculae parallel to the major axis of the digit. In the root of the nail, many columnar vessels characterized by multiple angiogenic buttons on their surface may be observed.

The venous drainage is achieved by two veins, one on each side of the nail plate, in the proximal nail folds (127). The capillary network is easily seen in the proximal nail fold with a magnifying lens and is seen in more detail with an ophthalmoscopic or capillary microscope. It is essentially the same as the network of the skin, but the capillary loops are more horizontal and visible throughout their length. Certain diseases (e.g., connective tissue disorders, macroglobulinemia, cryoglobulinemia, psoriasis, antiphospolipid syndrome) can modify its normal structure and a simple clinical examination or use of widefield nailfold microscopy can be very useful as an aid in diagnosis (130–133). A special vascular formation is present in the distal zone of the nail bed: the glomus bodies. This vascular structure has the mission of regulating the peripheral temperature by means of arteriovenous shunts (134).

NAIL GROWTH

The rate of growth of the nail plate has been studied extensively. Normal nail growth varies between 0.1 and 1.12 mm per day, or 1.9 to 4.4 mm per month (135,136). This growth, however, is not the same in all fingers or toes. For example, fingernails grow faster than toenails. Whereas a normal fingernail grows out completely in approximately six months, a normal toenail takes 12 to 18 months to do the same (83). Nails grow faster when regenerating after avulsion (39).

Several physiological circumstances can cause variations in the nail growth (Table 2.6). Nail growth is quicker in

males (39), during the day, during pregnancy (137), in persons who bite their nails (43), and in summer or warm climates (138). Conversely, nails grow more slowly in females, during the night, in toes, in winter, after age 20 (139), and during lactation (137).

Nail growth is also altered in several diseases (Table 2.6) (140–145). Nails grow quicker with psoriasis (140), pityriasis rubra pilaris (94), etretinate treatment (141), and hyperthyroidism (39); nails grow slower in cases of immobilization or paralysis (142), local ischemic conditions (135), cytostatic therapy (39,83), denutrition (143), hypothyroidism (139), and yellow nail syndrome (144). In the case of a sudden decrease in nail growth, for example, in acute infections (136), a transverse band will appear afterward, depressed in the proximal line called Beau's line. However, patients with unilateral toenail onychomycosis did not support the hypothesis that slow nail growth rate is a predisposing factor for this onychomycosis (145). The absence of K1 and K10 from healthy nail bed may also be related to the adherence of the overlying nail. In simple terms, the nail plate might be interpreted as the suprabasal layer of the nail bed, containing keratins not produced by the nail bed but affording barrier function or some other properties associated with K1, K10, and Ha1. The presence of these overlying keratins might be responsible for the lack of a granular layer and associated absence of K1 and K10. In diseases such as onychomycosis and psoriasis, where nail plate adherence is lost, a granular layer forms alongside expression of K1 and K10. (99–101,145)

The rate of growth of the nail plate is determined by the turnover rate of the matrix cells. Shortly after death, matrix cells do not incorporate tritiated thymidine in their nuclei; the cells appear to be incapable of DNA synthesis and cell division, and, therefore, the nail does not grow (88). Previous reports of nail growth after death are, in fact, erroneous. Apparent growth, caused by severe postmortem drying and shrinking of the soft tissues around the nail plate, is what was observed (146).

The question of where the nail plate is formed is still controversial (147). The first theories at the beginning of the century pointed toward a complete formation by the matrix (148). Years later, Lewis (8), however, concluded that the nail plate was the product of three different matrices on the basis of staining of the nail plate with a silver-protein stain and the morphology of keratinizing cells. Lewis's hypothesis was supported by differential staining of the nail plate (8), by differential interference contrast microscopy (69–72), and by ultrastructural observation of keratohyalin granules in embryonic nail (69). Lewis's hypothesis, however, has been extensively reviewed. Zaias and Alvarez (88) used radioautography to show that the nail plate was formed exclusively by the matrix in normal conditions; Samman (149) and Norton (147) confirmed it by following the incorporation of H-labeled glycine and thymidine in

---

TABLE 2.6

PHYSIOLOGICAL AND PATHOLOGICAL VARIATIONS THAT INFLUENCE NAIL GROWTH (SD, SYNDROME)

Physiological		Pathological	
Increased	**Decreased**	**Increased**	**Decreased**
Men	Women	Psoriasis	Fever
Daytime	Night	Pityriasis rubra pilaris	Poor nutrition
Summer	Winter	Hyperthyroidism	Hypothyroidism
Pregnancy	First day of life	A-V shunts	Decreased blood supply
Third digit	First and fifth digits	Idiopathic onycholysis in women	Kwashiorkor
Right hand*	Left hand*	Epidermolytic hyperkeratosis	Beau's lines
Youth	Old age	Hyperpituitarism	Denervation/Immobilization
Nail biting		Morgagni-Stewart-Morel sd.	Acute infection
Avulsion		Brittle nail sd.	Chronic disease
		Medications: calcium, vitamin D,	Smoking
		benoxaprofen, biotin, cysteine, oral	Onychomycosis
		contraceptives, L-dopa, fluconazole,	Yellow nail sd.
		itraconazole, terbinafine, etretinate	Lichen planus
			Relapsing polychondritis
			Medications: methotrexate,
			azathioprine, cyclosporine,
			lithium, retinoids,
			sulfonamides, heparin

*In a person's dominant right hand.

---

human toenails; and Caputo and Dadati (46) reported that, ultrastructurally, the nail plate was a homogeneous structure with no evidence of formation from three different matrices. To add one final bit to the confusion, Samman (149) suggests that, although under normal conditions the nail plate is made exclusively by the matrix, in certain pathologic conditions the nail bed adds a ventral nail to the undersurface of the nail plate. Finally, Kato (150) published a case with an ectopic nail at the palmar tip, with a vertical growth. In this case, the proximal nail fold promotes upward growth of the nail plate in absence of a proper nail bed.

Some recent authors believe that the nail bed epithelium produces a significant 20% portion of the nail plate and thus include the nail bed in the generative portion of the nail (151). Interestingly, indirect immunofluorescence studies in the fetal nail by means of pan-anti-type I and II hair keratin antibodies revealed a positive staining in a broad band of suprabasal cells of the nail bed epithelium. However, exclusion of hair keratins hHa1, hHb5, hHb1, hHb6 and hHa4 from the adult nail bed epithelium clearly identifies the matrix as the sole origin of the nail plate (152). It has previously been speculated that a few so-called "horn cells" may be added by the nail bed epithelium to the underside of the nail plate. Although our study confirmed the occurrence of clearly visible K5/17-positive nail bed cells in the lower nail plate, we believe that these cells represent sectioning artefacts. Our transverse nail sections, stained for either K5/17 or hHb5, show that the boundary between the nail bed epithelium and the nail plate is extremely undulated and that the resulting narrow-spaced folds and ridges exhibit a distinctly varying height. Therefore, it is evident that already slight deviations from a vertical angle of section through the nail bed region may reveal K5-positive cells in the nail plate, which in reality stem from the tip of an adjacent epithelial fold of the bed epithelium. Collectively these data emphasize that the nail bed epithelium does not actively contribute to the formation of the nail plate. (Figure 2.38).

An important controversy is why nails grow out instead of up. Kligman (153,154) postulated that the cul-de-sac of the proximal nail groove forced the cells of the matrix to grow out. To confirm his theory he transplanted nail matrix to the forearm, producing a vertical cylinder of hard keratin that had histologic characteristics of the nail. Hashimoto et al. (69) stated later that the long axis of matrix cells in embryonic nail was directed upward and distally.

Another important question is why the nail bed accompanies the nail plate in its growth. A well-known fact is that a hemorrhage that occurs between the plate and bed will grow forward with the plate. If the plate merely moved over the bed, the blood would not move; therefore, the upper part of the bed must move out with the plate. Some authors, such as Krantz (155), Kligman (153,154), and Zaias (84), tried to study this phenomenon in an experimental way. Of all theories, the one by Zaias is most acceptable at present: he believes that the proximal nail bed moves out, either by pressure by advancing plate or because of trauma, but that the distal nail bed and hyponychium do not move. Similarly

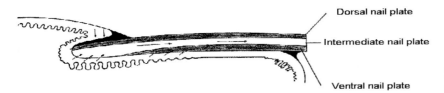

Dorsal nail plate

Intermediate nail plate

Ventral nail plate

Figure 2.38 Schematic diagram of nail growth.

controversial is the existence of a thin dorsal nail plate, which has been postulated on the basis of differential staining properties of the nail plate (156); a differential distribution of phospholipid, sulfhydryl, and disulphide groups (157); and ultrastructural observations (118). Moreover, the keratin pattern of the thin dorsal nail is different from that of the lower nail in that, in addition to hair keratins as a major constituent and the epithelial keratin pairs K5/K14 and K6/K16/K17 as minor components, it also contained low amounts of K1/10 (152).

HANDLING AND PROCESSING OF THE NAIL

The major problems of processing the nail unit are the difficulty of tissue selection and the need for proper orientation of the specimen. These problems are the reason for the small number of histologic studies.

The first important point is how to take a biopsy of the nail unit (153–165). The best way of studying a biopsy of the nail is to ascertain that it includes the complete thickness of the nail unit (which means nail plate, bed, and subjacent dermis); these can be sectioned transversely. If a punch biopsy is taken, it should be done by boring firmly through the nail plate and into the underlying tissue to obtain a specimen with the plate attached. If one wishes to eliminate the nail plate before taking the biopsy, special care has to be taken about nail avulsion because if it has been avulsed without care, the epithelium of the bed or matrix may become separated and the undersurface may remain attached to the plate and distort the true histopathologic picture. The ideal biopsy technique for the nail is a longitudinal biopsy (159), which includes the hyponychium, the nail bed, matrix with overlying plate, and the proximal nail fold and cuticle. The specimen may be taken from the center of the nail apparatus or from the lateral edge (161,162), or it may be modified to provide elliptical excision of a tumor of the nail bed (163,164).

The second point is the orientation of the specimen for cutting. In all cases, the surgeon should alert the pathologist on the submission form as to the way the specimen was obtained, whether a particular orientation is needed, and whether a piece of the nail plate is included.

The third point is how to treat the specimen in the laboratory. If the nail plate is present in the specimen, it will be too hard for ready cutting with a microtome unless some method of softening is used. A special fixative of

5% trichloroacetic acid and 10% formalin will leave the plate softer (161). Alternatively, the specimen can be placed in distilled water for a few hours before placing in formalin (162). Another helpful technique for softening the hard keratin of the nail plate was proposed by Luna (165):

1. Fix specimen in 10% formalin for 24 hours.
2. Place specimens in the following solution until completely dekeratinized. Change solution every 2 days for best results.
   - Mercuric chloride — 4.0 g
   - Chromic acid — 0.5 g
   - Nitric acid, concentrated — 10.0 mL
   - Ethyl alcohol, 95% — 50.0 mL
   - Distilled water — 200.0 mL
3. Wash in running water for three hours.
4. Dehydrate, clear, and impregnate with paraffin, or process as desired.

With this technique, the preservation of the cytologic characteristics of the epithelial cells of the nail matrix and nail bed is not as good as with the previous one, but it is very helpful for softening the hardest nail specimens.

REFERENCES

1. Zander R. Untersuchungen uber den verhornungsprogress: 1. Die histogenese des Nagels beim menschiichen fetus. *Arch Anat Entwicklungsmech* 1886;273.
2. Kolliker A. Die entwicklung des menschlichen Nagels. *Z Wiss Zool* 1988;1:1–12.
3. Unna PG. Entwicklungsgeschichte und anatomie. In: von Ziemssen, HW. *Handbuch der Speciellen Pathologie und Therapie.* Vol. 14. Leipzig: 1883.
4. Boas JEV. Ein Beitrag zur Morphologie der Nägel, Krallen, Hufe und Klauen der Säugetiere. *Morphol Jb* 1883;9:389–399.
5. Henle J. *Das Wachstum des Menschlichen Nagels und des Pferdehufs.* Göttingen: Dieterich; 1884.
6. Branca A. Notes sur la structure de l'ongle. *Ann Dermatol Syphiligr (Paris)* 1910; 1:353–371.
7. Clark WE, Buxton LH. Studies in nail growth. *Br J Dermatol* 1938;50:221.
8. Lewis BL. Microscopic studies of fetal and mature nail and surrounding soft tissue. *AMA Arch Dermatol Syphilol* 1954;70: 733–747.
9. Zaias N. Embryology of the human nail. *Arch Dermatol* 1963;87: 37–53.
10. Holbrook KA, Odland GF. The fine structure of the developing human epidermis: light, scanning, and transmission electron microscopy of the periderm. *J Invest Dermatol* 1975;65:16–38.
11. Conejo-Mir JS, Ambrosiani J, Dorado M. Analisis de la morfogénesis ungueal. *Estudio con Microscopio Electronico de Barrido en el Embrion Humano.* Barcelona: lsdin, 1985;1–8.
12. Conejo-Mir JS, Ambrosiani J, Dorado M, Camacho F, Genis BJM. *Human Nail Development: A Scanning Electron Microscopy Study.*

Abstract book of the Meeting of the American Society of Dermatopathology. Washington, DC; 1988.

13. Suchard R. Des modifications des cellules de la matrice et du lit de l'ongle dans quelques cas pathologiques. *Arch Physiol (Paris)* 1882;2:445.

14. Ogura R, Knox JM, Griffin AC, Kusuhara M: The concentration of sulfhydryl and disulfide in human epidermis, hair and nail. *J Invest Dermatol* 1962;38:69–75.

15. Irvine AD, McLean WH. Human keratin diseases: the increasing spectrum of disease and subtlety of phenotype-genotype correlation. *Br J Dermatol* 1999;140,815–828.

16. De Berker D, Wojnarowska F, Sviland L, Westgate GE, Dawber RP, Leigh IM: Keratin expression in the normal nail unit: markers of regional differentiation. *Br J Dermatol* 2000;142:89–96.

17. Hesse M, Magin TM, Weber K. Genes for intermediate filament proteins and the draft sequence of the human genome: novel keratin genes and a surprisingly high number of pseudogenes related to keratin genes 8 and 18. *J Cell Sci* 2001;114,2569–2575.

18. Smith TA, Strelkov SV, Burkhard P, Aebi U, Parry DAD: Sequence comparisons of intermediate filament chains: evidence of a unique functional/structural role for coiled-coil segment 1A and linker L1. *J Struct Biol* 2002;137:128–145.

19. Fuchs E. Keratins and the skin. *Annu Rev Cell Dev Biol* 1995; 11:123–153.

20. Coulombe PA, Omary MB. "Hard" and "soft" principles defining the structure, function and regulation of keratin intermediate filaments. *Curr Opin Cell Biol* 2002;14:110–122.

21. Wong P, Coulombe PA. Loss of keratin 6 (K6) proteins reveals a function for intermediate filaments during wound repair. *J Cell Biol* 2003;163:327–337.

22. McGowan KM, Coulombe PA. Onset of keratin 17 expression coincides with the definition of major epithelial lineages during skin development. *J Cell Biol* 1998;143:469–486.

23. Wang Z, Wong P, Langbein L, Schweizer J, Coulombe PA: The type II epithelial keratin 6 hf (K6hf) is expressed in the companion layer, matrix and medulla of anagen-stage hair follicles. *J Invest Dermatol* 2003;121:1276–1283.

24. Smith FJD. Keratin 17 defect in late-onset pachyonychia. *J Invest Dermatol* 2004;122:268–271.

25. Ding YG, Zhu TS, Jiang W, et al. Identification of a novel mutation and a de novo mutation in DKC1 in two Chinese pedigrees with dyskeratosis congenita. *J Invest Dermatol* 2004;123: 470–473.

26. Bowden PE, Haley JL, Kansky A, Rothnagel JA, Jones DO, Turner RJ: Mutation of a type II keratin gene (K6a) in pachyonychia congenita. *Nature Genet* 1995;10:363–365.

27. Smith FJE, Jonkman MF, van Goor H, et al. A mutation in human keratin K6b produces a phenocopy of the K17 disorder pachyonychia congenita type 2. *Human Mol Genet* 1998;7: 1143–1148.

28. Available at: http://www.interfil.org. Accessed January 25, 2006.

29. Available at: http://www.genome.cse.ucsc.edu/. Accessed January 25, 2006.

30. Available at: http://www.marshmed.org/genetics/. Accessed January 25, 2006.

31. Baran R, Dawber RP, Haneke E. Hair and nail relationship. *Skinmed* 2005;4:18–23.

32. De Berker DA, Perrin C, Baran R. Localized longitudinal erythronychia: diagnostic significance and physical explanation. *Arch Dermatol* 2004;140:1253–1257.

33. Norgett EE, Wolf F, Balme B, et al. Hereditary "white nails": a genetic and structural study. *Br J Dermatol* 2004;151:65–72.

34. Lewin K. The normal fingernail. *Br J Dermatol* 1965;77:421–430.

35. Pinkus F. The development of the integument. In: Keibel F, Mall F, eds. *Manual of Human Embryology*. Philadelphia: Lippincott; 1910:243–291.

36. Schweitzer TP, Rayan GM. The terminal tendon of the digital extensor mechanism: Part I, anatomic study. *J Hand Surg Am* 2004;29:898–902.

37. Le Gros Clark WB. The problems of the claw in primates. *Proc Zool Soc Lond* 1936;I:1–24.

38. Pinkus F. Der Nagel. In: *Jadassohns Handbuch, der Haut- und Geschlechtskrankheiten*. Berlin:Springer-Verlag; 1927.

39. Baran R, Dawber RPR, eds. *Diseases of the Nail and Their Management*. Oxford: Blackwell Scientific; 1984:1–21.

40. Caputo R, Cappio F, Rigoni C, et al. Pterygium inversum unguis. Report of 19 cases and review of the literature. *Arch Dermatol* 1993;129:1307–1309.

41. Terry RB. The onychodermal hand in health and disease. *Lancet* 1955;1:179–18l.

42. Martin BF, Platts MM. A histological study of the nail region in normal human subjects and in those showing splinter hemorrhages of the nail. *J Anat* 1959;93:323–330.

43. Raffle EJ. Terry's nails. *Lancet* 1984;1:1131.

44. Finlay AY, Moseley H, Duggan TC. Ultrasound transmission time: an in vivo guide to nail thickness. *Br J Dermatol* 1987;117:765–770.

45. Goettmann S, Drape JL, Idy-Peretti I, et al. Magnetic resonance imaging: a new tool in the diagnosis of tumors of the nail apparatus. *Br J Dermatol* 1994;130:701–710.

46. Caputo R, Dadati E. Preliminary observations about the ultrastructure of the human nail plate treated with thioglycolic acid. *Arch Klin Exp Dermatol* 1968; 231:344–354.

47. Forslind B, Thyresson N. On the structure of the normal nail. A scanning electron microscope study. *Arch Dermatol Forsch* 1975;251:199–204.

48. Garson JC, Baltenneck F, Leroy F, et al. Histological structure of human nail as studied by synchrotron X-ray microdiffraction. *Cell Mol Biol* 2000;46:1025–1034.

49. Hamilton JB, Terada H, Mestler GE. Studies of growth throughout the lifespan in Japanese. Growth and size of nails and their relationship to age, sex, hereditary and other factors. *J Gerontol* 1955;10:401–415.

50. Johnson M, Shuster S. Determinants of nail thickness and length. *Br J Dermatol* 1994;130:195–198.

51. Farren L, Shayler S, Ennos AR. The fracture properties and mechanical design of human fingernails. *J Exp Biol* 2004;207 (pt 5):735–741.

52. Germann H, Barran W, Plewig G. Morphology of corneocytes from human nail plates. *J Invest Dermatol* 1980;74:115–118.

53. Walters KA, Flynn GL, Marvel JR. Physicochemical characterization of the human nail: I. Pressure sealed apparatus for measuring nail plate permeabilities. *J Invest Dermatol* 1981; 76:76–79.

54. Egawa M, Fukuhara T, Takahashi M, Ozaki Y. Determining water content in human nails with a portable near-infrared spectrometer. *Appl Spectrosc* 2003;57:473–478.

55. Nuutinen J, Harvima I, Lahtinen MR, Lahtinen RT. Water loss through the lip, nail, eyelid skin, scalp skin and axillary skin measured with a closed-chamber evaporation principle. *Br J Dermatol* 2003;148:839–842.

56. Jarrett A, Spearman RI. The histochemistry of the human nail. *Arch Dermatol* 1966;94:652–657.

57. Pautard FGE. Mineralization of keratin and its comparison with the enamel matrix. *Nature* 1963;199:531–540.

58. Forslind B, Wroblewski R, Afzelius BA. Calcium and sulphur location in human nail. *J Invest Dermatol* 1976;67:273–290.

59. Helmdach M, Thielitz A, Ropke EM, Gollnick H. Age and sex variation in lipid composition of human fingernail plates. *Skin Pharmacol Appl Skin Physiol* 2000;13:111–119.

60. Sass JO, Skladal D, Zelger B, Romani N, Utermann B. Trichothiodystrophy: quantification of cysteine in human hair and nails by application of sodium azide-dependent oxidation to cysteic acid. *Arch Dermatol Res* 2004;296:188–191.

61. Bolliger A, Gross R. Non-keratin of human toenails. *Aust J Exp Biol Med Sci* 1953;127–130.

62. Levitt JI. Creatinine concentration of human fingernail and toenail clippings. Application in determining the duration of renal failure. *Ann Intern Med* 1966;64:312–327.

63. Goldblum RW, Derby S, Lerner AB. The metal content of skin, nails and hair. *J Invest Dermatol* 1953;20:13–18.

64. Kopito L, Mahmoodian A, Townley RRW, Khaw KT, Shwachman H. Studies in cystic fibrosis: analysis of nail clippings for sodium and potassium. *N Engl J Med* 1965;272:504–509.

65. Martin GM. Copper content of hair and nails of normal individuals and of patients with hepatolenticular degeneration. *Nature* 1964;202:903–904.

66. Mandal BK, Ogra Y, Anzai K, Suzuki KT. Speciation of arsenic in biological samples. *Toxicol Appl Pharmacol* 2004;198:307–318.

67. Cingolani M, Scavella S, Mencarelli R, Mirtella D, Froldi R, Rodriguez D. Simultaneous detection and quantitation of morphine, 6-acetylmorphine, and cocaine in toenails: comparison with hair analysis. *J Anal Toxicol* 2004;28:128–131.

68. Gillespie JM, Frenkel MJ. The diversity of keratins. *Comp Biochem Physiol* 1974;47B:339–346.

69. Hashimoto K, Gross BG, Nelson R, Lever WF. The ultrastructure of the skin of human embryos. III. The formation of the nail in 16–18-week-old embryos. *J Invest Dermatol* 1966;47:205–217.

70. Hashimoto K. Ultrastructure of the human toenail. l. Proximal nail matrix. *J Invest Dermatol* 1971;56:235–246.

71. Hashimoto K. Ultrastructure of the human toenail. II. Keratinization and formation of the marginal band. *J Ultrastruct Res* 1971;36:391–410.

72. Hashimoto K. Ultrastructure of the human toenail. III. Cell migration, keratinization and formation of the intercellular cement. *Arch Dermatol Forsch* 1971;240:1–22.

73. Higashi N. Melanocytes of nail matrix and nail pigmentation. *Arch Dermatol* 1968;97:570–574.

74. Scott GA, Haake AR. Keratinocytes regulate melanocyte number in human fetal and neonatal skin equivalents. *J Invest Dermatol* 1991;97:776–781.

75. Higashi N, Saito T. Horizontal distribution of dopa-positive melanocytes in the nail matrix. *J Invest Dermatol* 1969;53:163–165.

76. Jimbow K, Takahashi M, Sato S, Kukita A. Ultrastructural and cytochemical studies on melanogenesis in melanocytes of normal human hair matrix. *J Electron Microsc (Tokyo)* 1971;20:87–92.

77. Feibleman CE, Stoll H, Maize JC. Melanomas of the palm, sole and nail bed: a clinicopathologic study. *Cancer* 1980;46:2492–2504.

78. Baran R, Juhlin L. Photoonycholysis. *Photodermatol Photoinmunol Photomed* 2002;18:202–208.

79. Gallais V, Lacour JP, Perrin C, Ghanem G, Bodokh I, Ortonne JP. Acral hyperpigmented macules and longitudinal melanonychia in AIDS patients. *Br J Dermatol* 1992;126:387–391.

80. Uyttendaele H, Geyer A, Scher RK. Drugs and nails. *J Eur Acad Dermatol Venereol* 2004;18:124–125.

81. Moll I, Moll R. Merkel cells in ontogenesis of human nails. *Arch Dermatol Res* 1993;285:366–371.

82. Samman PD. The ventral nail. *Arch Dermatol* 1961;84:1030–1033.

83. Samman PD. *The Nails in Disease*. 3rd ed. London: Heinemann Medical Books; 1978.

84. Zaias N. The movement of the nail bed. *J Invest Dermatol* 1967;48:402–403.

85. Drape JL, Wolfram-Gabel W, Idy-Peretti I, et al. The lunula: a magnetic resonance imaging approach to the subnail matrix area. *J Invest Dermatol* 1996;106:1081–1085.

86. Dawber RPR, Baran R. The nails. In: Rook A, Wilkinson DS, Ebling FJG, Champion RH, Burton JL, eds. *Textbook of Dermatology*. Oxford: Blackwell Scientific; 1986:2039–2044.

87. Burrows MT. The significance of the lunula of the nail. *Johns Hopkins Hosp Res* 1919;18:357–361.

88. Zaias N, Alvarez J. The formation of the primate nail plate. An autoradiographic study in squirrel monkeys. *J Invest Dermatol* 1968;51:120–136.

89. Meyer JC, Grundmann HP. Scanning electron microscopic investigation of the healthy nail and its surrounding tissue. *J Cutan Pathol* 1984;11:74–79.

90. Omura EF. Histopathology of the nail. *Dermatol Clin* 1985;3:531–541.

91. Sinclair RD, Wojnarowska F, Leigh IM, Dawber RP. The basement membrane zone of the nail. *Br J Dermatol* 1994;131:499–505.

92. Dorschner RA, Lopez-Garcia B, Massie J, Kim C, Gallo RL. Innate immune defense of the nail unit by antimicrobial peptides. *J Am Acad Dermatol* 2004;50:343–348.

93. Holbrook KA. Human epidermal embryogenesis. *Int J Dermatol* 1979;18:329–356.

94. Runne U, Orfanos CE. The human nail: structure, growth and pathological changes. *Curr Probl Dermatol* 1981;9:102–149.

95. Zaias N. Onychomycosis. *Arch Dermatol* 1972;105:263–274.

96. Baden HP, Kvedar JC. Epithelial cornified envelope precursors are in the hair follicle and nail. *J Invest Dermatol* 1993;101(suppl1):72S–74S.

97. O'Keefe EJ, Hamilton EH, Lee SC, Steinert P. Trichohyalin: a structural protein of hair, tongue, nail and epidermis. *J Invest Dermatol* 1993;101(suppl 1):65S–71S.

98. Heid HW, Moll I, Franke WW. Pattern of expression of trichocytic and epithelial cytokeratins in mammalian tissues. II. Concomitant and mutually exclusive synthesis of trichocytic and epithelial cytokeratins in diverse human and bovine tissues (hair follicle, nail bed and matrix, lingual papilla, thymic reticulum). *Differentiation* 1988;37:215–230.

99. Kitahara T, Ogawa H. The extraction and characterization of human nail keratin. *J Dermatol Sci* 1991;2:402–406.

100. Kitahara T, Ogawa H. Cultured nail keratinocytes express hard keratins characteristic of nail and hair in vivo. *Arch Dermatol Res* 1992;284:253–256.

101. Kitahara T, Ogawa H. Coexpression of keratins characteristic of skin and hair differentiation in nail cells. *J Invest Dermatol* 1993;100:171–175.

102. De Berker D, Wojnarowska F, Sviland L, Westgate GE, Dawber RPR, Leigh IM. Keratin expression in the normal nail unit: markers of regional differentiation. *Br J Dermatol* 2000;142:89–96.

103. Heid HW, Moll I, Franke WW. Patterns of expression of trichocytic and epithelial cytokeratins in mammalian tissues. II. Concomitant and mutually exclusive synthesis of trichocytic and epithelial cytokeratins in diverse human and bovine tissues (hair follicle, nail bed and matrix, lingual papilla, thymic reticulum). *Differentiation* 1988;37:215–230.

104. Perrin C, Langbein L, Schweizer J. Expression of hair keratins in the adult nail unit: an immunohistochemical analysis of the onychogenesis in the proximal nail fold, matrix and nail bed. *Br J Dermatol* 2004;151:362–371.

105. Kitahara T, Ogawa H. Cellular features of differentiation in the nail. *Microsc Res Tech* 1997;38:436–442.

106. Lane EB, Wilson CA, Hughes BR, Leigh IM. Stem cells in hair follicles. Cytoskeletal studies. *Ann NY Acad Sci* 1991;642:197–213.

107. Stark HJ, Breitkreutz D, Limat A, et al. Keratins of the human hair follicle: "hyperproliferative" keratins consistently expressed in outer root sheath cells in vivo and in vitro. *Differentiation* 1987;35:236–248.

108. McLean WH Irwin, Epithelial Genetics Group. Genetic disorders of palm skin and nail. *J Anat* 2003;202:133–141.

109. Inoue S, Nambu T, Shimomura T. The RAIG family member, GPRC5D, is associated with hard-keratinized structures. *J Invest Dermatol* 2004;122:565–573.

110. Okazaki M, Yoshimura K, Fujiwara H, Suzuki Y, Harii K. Induction of hard keratin expression in non-nail-matrical keratinocytes by nail-matrical fibroblasts through epithelial-mesenchymal interactions. *Plast Reconstr Surg* 2003;111:286–290.

111. Egawa K, Kuroki M, Inoue Y, Ono T. Nail bed keratinocytes express an antigen of the carcinoembryonic antigen family. *Br J Dermatol* 2000;143:79–83.

112. Lavker RM, Risse B, Brown H, et al. Localization of plasminogen activator inhibitor type 2 (PAI-2) in hair and nail: implications for terminal differentiation. *J Invest Dermatol* 1998;110:917–922.

113. Lacour JP, Dubois D, Pisani A, Ortonne JP. Anatomical mapping of Merkel cells in normal human adult epidermis. *Br J Dermatol* 1991;125:535–542.

114. Tosti A, Cameli N, Piraccini BM, Fanti PA, Ortonne JP. Characterization of nail matrix melanocytes with anti-PEP1, anti-PEP8, TMH-1 and HMB-45 antibodies. *J Am Acad Dermatol* 1994;31(pt 1):193–196.

115. Guerrero-Fernandez J, Garcia-Ascaso MT, Guerrero Vazquez J. Pigmentation band on toenail [in Spanish]. *An Pediatr (Barc)*. 2004;61:455–456.

116. Cameli N, Picardo M, Tosti A, Perrin C, Pisani A, Ortonne JP. Expression of integrins in human nail matrix. *Br J Dermatol* 1994;130:583–588.

117. Picardo M, Tosti A, Marchese C, et al. Characterization of cultured nail matrix cells. *J Am Acad Dermatol* 1994;30:434–440.

118. Doigel AS. Die nerbenendigungen im nagelbett des Menschen. *Arch Mikros Anat* 1904;64:173–188.

119. Martino L. Sulia innervazione dell'apparato ungueale. *Boll Soc Ital Biol Sper* 1942;1;7:488–489.
120. Winkelmann RK. *Nerve Endings in Normal and Pathologic Skin.* Springfield, IL: Charles C Thomas; 1960:100.
121. Reginelli AD, Wang YQ, Sassoon D, Muneoka K. Digit tip regeneration correlates with regions of Msx1 (Hox7) expression in fetal and newborn mice. *Development* 1995;121:1065–1076.
122. Mohammad KS, Neufeld DA. Denervation retards but does not prevent toetip regeneration. *Wound Repair Regen* 2000;8:277–281.
123. Zhao W, Neufeld DA. Bone regrowth in young mice stimulated by nail organ. *J Exp Zool* 1995;271:155–159.
124. Flint MH. Some observations on the vascular supply of the nail bed and terminal segments of the finger. *Br J Plastic Surg* 1955;8:186–195.
125. Ryan TJ. The blood vessels of the skin. In: Jarret A, ed. *The Physiology and Pathophysiology of the Skin.* Vol 2. London: Academic Press; 1973:612:658–659.
126. Smith DO, Oura C, Kimura C, Toshimori K. Artery anatomy and tortuosity in the distal finger. *J Hand Surg Am* 1991;16:297–302.
127. Hale AR, Burch GE. The arteriovenous anastomoses and blood vessels of the human finger. *Medicine (Baltimore)* 1960;39:191–240.
128. Wang W, Winlove CP, Michel CC. Oxygen partial pressure in outer layers of skin of human finger nail folds. *J Physiol* 2003;549:855–863.
129. Sangiorgi S, Manelli A, Congiu T, et al. Microvascularization of the human digit as studied by corrosion casting. *J Anat* 2004;204:123–131.
130. Ross JB. Nail fold capillaroscopy: a useful aid in the diagnosis of collagen vascular diseases. *J Invest Dermatol* 1966;47:282–285.
131. Gilje O, Kierland R, Baldes EJ. Capillary microscopy in the diagnosis of dermatologic diseases. *J Invest Dermatol* 1974;22:199–206.
132. Ohtsuka T, Yamakage A, Miyachi Y. Statistical definition of nail-fold capillary pattern in patients with psoriasis. *Int J Dermatol* 1994;33:779–782.
133. Vaz JL, Dancour MA, Bottino DA, Bouskela E. Nailfold videocapillaroscopy in primary antiphospholipid syndrome (PAPS). *Rheumatology* 2004;43:1025–1027.
134. Mehregan AH. *Pinkus' Guide to Dermatohistopathology.* 4th ed. Norwalk, CT: Appleton-Century-Crofts; 1986:563–564.
135. Bean WB. Nail growth: 30 years of observation. *Arch Intern Med* 1974;134:497–502.
136. Sibinga MS. Observations on growth of fingernails in health and disease. *Pediatrics* 1959;24:225–233.
137. Halban J, Spitzer MZ. On the increased growth of nails in pregnancy. *Monatsschr Gerburtshilfe Gynaekol* 1929;82:25.
138. Geoghegan B, Roberts DF, Sampford MR. A possible climatic effect on nail growth. *J Appl Physiol* 1958;13:135–138.
139. Orentreich N, Markofsky J, Vogelman JH. The effect of aging on the rate of linear nail growth. *J Invest Dermatol* 1979;73:126–130.
140. Landherr G, Braun-Falco O, Hofmann C, Plewig G, Galosl A. Fingernagelwachstum bei Psoriatikem unter puvatherapie. *Hautarzt* 1982;33:210–213.
141. Baran R. Action thérapeutique et complications due rétinoïde sur l'appareil unguéal. *Ann Dermatol Vénéréol* 1982;109:367–371.
142. Fleckman P. Anatomy and physiology of the nail. *Dermatol Clin* 1985;3:373–381.
143. Geyer AS, Onumah N, Uyttendaele H, Scher RK. Modulation of linear nail growth to treat disease of the nail. *J Am Acad Dermatol* 2004;50:229–234.
144. Pavlidakey GP, Hashimoto K, Blum D. Yellow nail syndrome. *J Am Acad Dermatol* 1984;11:509–512.
145. Yu HJ, Kwon HM, Oh DH, Kim JS. Is slow nail growth a risk factor for onychomycosis? *Clin Exp Dermatol* 2004;29:415–418.
146. Zaias N. Nails. components, growth and composition of the nail. In: Demis DJ, Dobson RL, McGuire J, eds. *Clinical Dermatology.* Vol. 1. New York: Harper & Row; 1980:1–6.
147. Norton LA. Incorporation of thymidine-methyl-H3 and glycine-2-H3 in the nail matrix and bed of humans. *J Invest Dermatol* 1971;56:61–68.
148. Unna PG. Entwicklungsgeschichte und anatomie. In: von Ziemssen, HW *Handbuch der Speciellen Pathologie und Therapie.* Vol 14. Leipzig: 1883.
149. Samman PD. The human toe nail. Its genesis and blood supply. *Br J Dermatol* 1959;71:296–302.
150. Kato N. Vertically growing ectopic nail. *J Cutan Pathol* 1992;19:445–447.
151. Johnson M, Comaish JS, Shuster S. Nail is produced by the normal nail bed: a controversy resolved. *Br J Dermatol* 1991;125:27–29.
152. De Berker D, Mawhinney B, Sviland L. Quantification of regional matrix nail production. *Br J Dermatol* 1996;134:1083–1086.
153. Kligman AM. Nails. In: Pillsbury DM, Shelley WB, Kligman AM, eds. *Dermatology.* Philadelphia: WB Saunders; 1956:80–86.
154. Kligman AM. Why do nails grow out instead of up? *Arch Dermatol* 1961;84:313–315.
155. Krantz W. Beitrag zur anatomie des nagels. *Dermatol Z* 1937;239–242.
156. Achten G, Andre J, Laporte M. Nails in light and electron microscopy. *Semin Dermatol* 1991;10:54–64.
157. Lynch MH, O'Guin WM, Hardy C, Mak L, Sun TT. Acidic and basic hair/nail ("hard") keratins: their colocalization in upper cortical and cuticle cells of the human hair follicle and their relationship to "soft" keratins. *J Cell Biol* 1986;103(pt 2): 2593–2606.
158. Parent D, Achten G, Stoofs-Vamhoof F. Ultrastructure of the normal human nail. *Am J Dermatopathol* 1985;7:529–535.
159. Baran R, Sayag J. Nail biopsy: why, when, where, how? *J Dermatol Surg* 1976;2:322–324.
160. Bennet RG. Technique of biopsy of nails. *J Dermatol Surg* 1976;2:325–326.
161. Stone OJ, Barr RJ, Herten RJ. Biopsy of the nail area. *Cutis* 1978;21:257–260.
162. Scher RK. Biopsy of the matrix of a nail. *J Dermatol Surg Oncol* 1980;6:19–21.
163. Scher RK. Longitudinal resection of nails for purposes of biopsy and treatment. *J Dermatol Surg Oncol* 1980;6:805–807.
164. Rich P. Nail biopsy: indications and methods. *J Dermatol Surg Oncol* 1992;18:673–682.
165. Luna LG. Preparation of tissues. In: Luna LG. *Manual of Histologic Staining Methods of the Armed Forces Institute of Pathology.* 3rd ed. New York: McGraw-Hill Book Company; 1968: 1–12.

BREAST

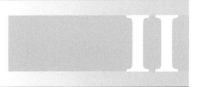

II

Breast

Laura C. Collins   *Stuart J. Schnitt*

INTRODUCTION

Remarkable advances in breast imaging over the past decade have provided a variety of noninvasive means to assist in the evaluation of patients with breast disorders (1–4). Nevertheless, at the present time, histologic examination of tissue specimens remains the cornerstone for the diagnosis of breast diseases, and an understanding of normal breast histology is essential for accurate evaluation of such specimens. It should be noted, however, that what constitutes "normal" histology in the breast varies according to gender, age, menopausal status, phase of the menstrual cycle, pregnancy, and lactation, among other factors. Therefore, determination of whether a given breast specimen is normal or shows pathologic alterations must take these variables into consideration.

EMBRYOLOGY

Development of the human mammary gland begins during the fifth week of gestation, at which time thickenings of the ectoderm appear on the ventral surface of the fetus. These mammary ridges, also known as milk lines, extend from the axilla to the groin. Except for a small area in the pectoral region, the bulk of these ridges normally regress as the fetus continues to develop. Failure of regression of other portions of the milk lines can result in the appearance in postnatal life of ectopic mammary tissue or accessory nipples anywhere along the milk lines; this phenomenon is most commonly encountered in the axilla, inframammary fold, and vulva (5–7).

The earliest stages of breast development are largely independent of sex steroid hormones (8). After the fifteenth week of gestation, the developing breast exhibits transient sensitivity to testosterone, which acts primarily on the mesenchyme. Under the influence of testosterone, the mesenchyme condenses around an epithelial stalk on the chest wall to form the breast bud, the site of mammary gland development. Solid epithelial columns then develop within the mesenchyme, and these ultimately give rise to the lobes or segments of the mammary gland. Portions of the fetal papillary dermis encase the developing epithelial cords and eventually give rise to the vascularized fibrous connective tissue that surrounds and invests the mammary ducts and lobules. The more collagen-rich reticular dermis extends into the breast to form the sus-pensory ligaments of Cooper, which attach the breast parenchyma to the skin. Portions of the mesenchyme differentiate into fat within the collagenous stroma between the twentieth and thirty-second weeks of gestation. During the last eight weeks of gestation, the epithelial cords canalize and branch, forming lobuloalve-olar structures as a result of mesenchymal paracrine ef-fects. A depression in the epidermis, the mammary pit, forms at the convergence of the lactiferous ducts. The nip-ple forms by evagination of the mammary pit near the time of birth.

During the last few weeks of gestation the fetal mam-mary gland is responsive to maternal and placental steroid hormones, and, as a result, the epithelial cells in the acinar units exhibit secretory activity. At the time of birth, withdrawal of the maternal and placental sex steroids stimulates prolactin secretion, which in turn stimulates colostrom secretion. At this time, both male and female neonates exhibit palpable enlargement of the breast bud. As the serum levels of maternal and placental sex steroid hormones and prolactin decline during the first month of life, secretory activity ends, and the gland regresses and becomes inactive. At this stage, and until pu-berty, the breast consists primarily of lactiferous ducts that exhibit some branching without evidence of progressive alveolar differentiation, although some rudimentary lob-ular structures may persist.

Another feature that may be seen in the fetal breast is extramedullary hematopoiesis, and this may persist in the periductal stroma until 4 months of age (9) (Figure 3.1).

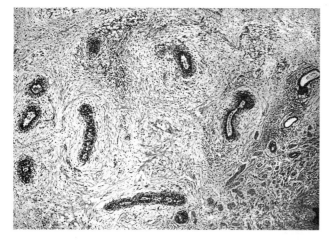

Figure 3.1 Breast tissue from an infant showing ducts embed-ded in a loose connective tissue stroma. The stromal mononuclear cells are hematopoietic elements, indicative of persistent ex-tramedullary hematopoiesis. (Courtesy of Theonia Boyd, M.D, Children's Hospital, Boston, MA)

ADOLESCENCE

Adolescent breast development in the female begins with the onset of puberty and the cyclic secretion of estrogen and progesterone. However, a variety of other steroid and peptide hormones are also required for proper mammary gland development (8) (Table 3.1). The ducts elongate, branch, and develop a thickened epithelium due primar-ily to the influence of estrogen (10) (Figure 3.2). The pro-cess of ductal growth and branching is largely indepen-

TABLE 3.1	
MAJOR STEROID AND PEPTIDE HORMONAL INFLUENCES ON THE BREAST (ADAPTED FROM MCCARTY AND NATH (8))	
Hormone	**Effects**
Estrogen	Required for ductal growth and branching during adolescence
	Required for lobuloalveolar growth during pregnancy
	Required for induction of progesterone receptor
	Not necessary for maintenance of secretion or lactation
Progesterone	Required for lobuloalveolar differentiation and growth
	Probable mitogen in normal estrogen-primed breast
	Not necessary for ductal growth and branching
Testosterone	Stimulates breast mesenchyme during fetal development
	Causes mesenchymal destruction of mammary epithelium during critical period of testosterone sensitivity
Glucocorticoids	Required for maximal ductal growth
	Enhances lobuloalveolar growth during pregnancy
Insulin	Enhanced ductal-alveolar growth
	Enhances protein synthesis in mammary epithelium
	Required for secretory activity (with glucocorticoids and prolactin)
Prolactin	Stimulates epithelial growth after parturition
	Required for initiation and maintenance of lactation
Human placental lactogen	Able to substitute for prolactin in epithelial growth and differentiation
	Stimulates alveolar growth and lactogenesis in second half of pregnancy
Growth hormone	Required for ductal growth and branching during adolescence
	May contribute to lobuloacinar growth during pregnancy
Thyroid hormone	Increases epithelial response to prolactin
	May enhance lobuloacinar growth

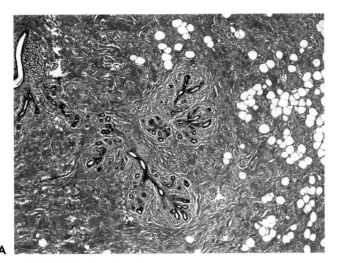
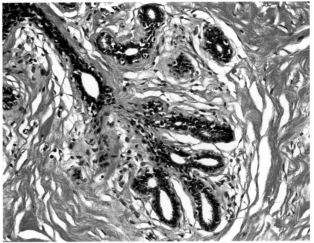

Figure 3.2 Adolescent breast tissue composed of branching ducts with rudimentary lobule development (type 1 lobules). The stroma consists a mixture of fibrous connective tissue and adipose tissue. **A.** Scanning magnification. **B.** High power.

dent of progesterone. There is an increase in the density of periductal connective tissue, also as a result of relative estrogen dominance. Deposition of stromal adipose tissue occurs, and it is this adipose tissue that is largely responsible for the enlargement and protrusion of the breast disk at this time. Cyclical exposure to progesterone following exposure to estrogen during ovulatory cycles promotes lobuloacinar growth, as well as connective tissue growth. Although the majority of breast development occurs during puberty, this process continues into the third decade, and terminal differentiation of the breast is only induced by pregnancy.

The adolescent male breast is composed of fibroadipose tissue and ducts lined by low cuboidal cells.

THE ADULT FEMALE BREAST

The size of the breast is greatly influenced by the individual's body habitus since the breast is a major repository for fat; it can range in size from 30 g to more than 1000 g. The breast lies on the anterior chest wall over the pectoralis major muscle and typically extends from the second to the sixth rib in the vertical axis and from the sternal edge to the midaxillary line in the horizontal axis. Breast tissue also projects into the axilla as the tail of Spence. The breast extends laterally over the serratus anterior muscle and inferiorly over the external oblique muscle and the superior rectus sheath. The breast lies within a space in the superficial fascia, which is continuous with the cervical fascia superiorly and the superficial abdominal fascia of Cooper inferiorly. The only boundary of the breast that is anatomically well-defined is the deep surface where it abuts the pec-

toralis fascia. However, despite this macroscopic demarcation, microscopic foci of glandular tissue may extend into and even through the pectoral fascia and may traverse the other anatomic boundaries described above. The clinical significance of this observation is that even total mastectomy does not result in removal of all glandular breast tissue. Bundles of dense fibrous connective tissue, the suspensory ligaments of Cooper, extend from the skin to the pectoral fascia and provide support to the breast.

The adult female breast consists of a series of ducts, ductules, and lobular acinar units embedded within a stroma that is composed of varying amounts of fibrous and adipose tissue. The stroma comprises the major portion of the nonlactating adult breast, and the relative proportions of fibrous tissue and adipose tissue vary with age and among individuals (Figure 3.3).

The ductal-lobular system of the breast is arranged in the form of segments, or lobes. While these segments can be readily appreciated by injecting the ductal system with dyes or radiologic contrast agents (Figure 3.4), they are anatomically poorly defined, and no obvious boundaries can be appreciated between these segments during surgery, upon gross inspection of mastectomy specimens, or on histologic examination. In addition, these segments show considerable individual variation with regard to their distribution, and the ramifications of individual segments may overlap. The segmental nature of some neoplastic processes in the breast, particularly ductal carcinoma in situ, is now widely appreciated, and surgical resection of the involved segment is an important therapeutic goal. Unfortunately, since it is not possible for the surgeon to define intra-operatively the boundaries of the involved segment, performing a "segmentectomy" to remove the entirety of a diseased segment is at this time more of a theoretical concept than a practically attainable goal.

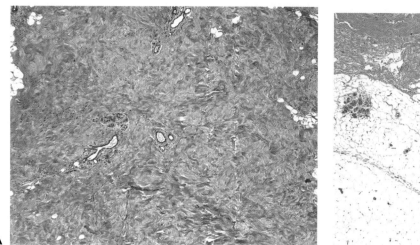
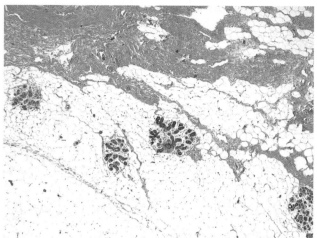

Figure 3.3 The stroma is the predominant component of the nonlactating breast and consists of varying amounts of collagen and adipose tissue. **A.** Low-power view of breast with dense, fibrotic stroma. **B.** Low-power view of breast with predominantly fatty stroma.

Each segment consists of a branching structure that has been likened to a flowering tree (11) (Figure 3.5). The lobules represent the flowers, draining into ductules and ducts (twigs and branches), which, in turn, drain into the collecting ducts (trunk) that open onto the surface of the nipple. Just below the nipple, the ducts are expanded to form lactiferous sinuses. The sinuses terminate in cone-shaped ampullae just below the surface of the nipple.

The actual number of segments in the breast and their relationship to each other has long been a matter of debate. Most textbooks indicate that there are 15 to 20 ductal orifices on the nipple surface and suggest that this corresponds to the number of ductal systems, segments, or lobes in the breast (5,6,12,13). In contrast, a number of mammary duct injection studies have suggested that there are only between five and ten discrete breast ductal systems or segments in each breast. The discrepancy between the number of ductal orifices on the nipple and the actual number of breast segments or ductal systems may be explained by the fact that some of the orifices on the nipple represent openings of

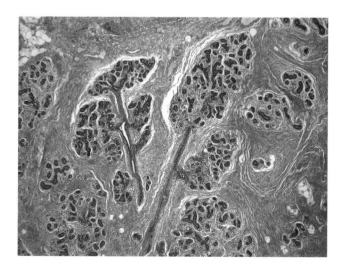

Figure 3.4 Ductogram (galactogram). Performed by injecting contrast material into an orifice of a lactiferous duct at the nipple, a ductogram demonstrates the complex ramifications of a single mammary ductal system (also known as a segment or lobe).

Figure 3.5 Microanatomy of normal adult female breast tissue showing extralobular ducts, terminal ducts, and lobules, the latter composed of groups of small glandular structures, the acini.

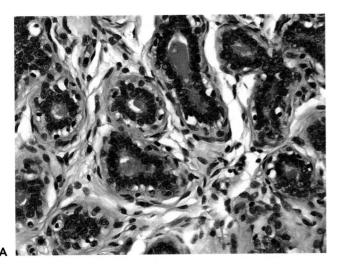
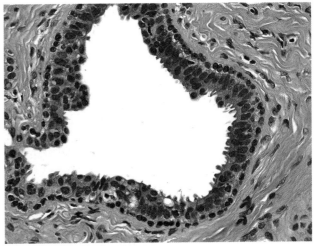

A
B

Figure 3.6 The mammary ductal-lobular system is lined by a dual cell population, an inner epithelial cell layer and an outer layer of myoepithelial cells. **A.** High-power view of a lobule. The myoepithelial cells surrounding the acinar epithelial cells are variably conspicuous. **B.** High-power view of an extralobular duct, showing distinct epithelial and myoepithelial cell layers.

sebaceous glands or other nonductal tubular structures that do not contribute to the ductal-lobular anatomy of the breast. Another possibility is that some lactiferous ducts bifurcate immediately prior to entering the nipple or end blindly (13). The issue of anastomoses between ductal systems is also unresolved. One recent study indicated that, while ductal systems may lie in close proximity to one another and even intertwine within a particular quadrant, they do not interconnect (13). However, anastamoses between ductal systems have been reported by others (14).

The epithelium throughout the ductal-lobular system is bilayered, consisting of an inner (luminal) epithelial cell layer and an outer (basal) myoepithelial cell layer. The importance of this double cell layer cannot be overemphasized because it is one of the main guides used to dis-

tinguish benign from malignant lesions (15). The luminal epithelial cells of the resting breast ducts and lobules are cuboidal to columnar in shape and typically have pale eosinophilic cytoplasm and relatively uniform oval nuclei. These epithelial cells express a variety of low-molecular weight cytokeratins, including cytokeratins 7, 8, 18, and 19 (16–20). The outer (or myoepithelial) cell layer, although always present, is variably distinctive (Figure 3.6). Myoepithelial cells range in appearance from barely discernible, flattened cells with compressed nuclei to prominent epithelioid cells with abundant clear cytoplasm. In some cases, the myoepithelial cells have a myoid appearance featuring a spindle cell shape and dense, eosinophilic cytoplasm, reminiscent of smooth muscle cells (Figure 3.7). Even when inconspicuous on

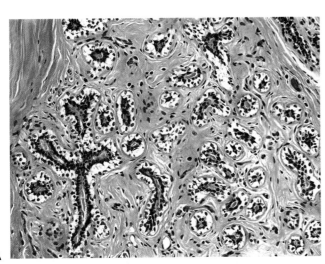
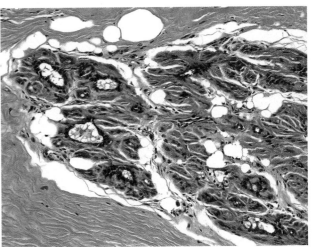

A
B

Figure 3.7 Myoepithelial cells can vary in their histologic appearance. **A.** Myoepithelial cells in this lobule show prominent cytoplasmic clearing. **B.** In this lobule, the myoepithelial cells show myoid features.

toxylin- and eosin-stained sections, myoepithelial cells can readily be demonstrated using immunohistochemical stains for a variety of markers, including S-100 protein, actins, calponin, smooth muscle myosin heavy chain, p63, and CD10, among others (21–23) (Figure 3.8). However, these markers vary in both sensitivity and specificity for myoepithelium. Myoepithelial cells also express high molecular weight cytokeratins 5/6, 14, and 17 (16–20,24). Recent work has documented the presence of a third cell type in normal breast tissue. These cells are dispersed individually and irregularly throughout the ductal-lobular system, express the basal cytokeratin CK5, and are thought to be progenitor cells capable of differentiating into both glandular epithelial cells and myoepithelial cells (19). However, the presence of such progenitor cells has not yet been universally accepted (25).

A basal lamina consisting of type IV collagen and laminin surrounds the mammary ducts, ductules, and acini (17,26). This basal lamina is present outside of the myoepithelial cell layer and serves to demarcate the breast ductal-lobular system from the surrounding stroma (Figure 3.9). Beyond the basal lamina, the extralobular ducts exhibit a zone of fibroblasts and capillaries. Elastic tissue is normally present in variable amounts around ducts and is generally more prominent in older than in younger women. Elastic fibers are not typically seen around the terminal ducts or acini.

The lobule, together with its terminal duct, has been called the terminal duct lobular unit (TDLU). This represents the structural and functional unit of the breast. During lactation, epithelial cells in both the terminal duct and lobule undergo secretory changes. Thus, the terminal ducts are responsible for both secretion and transport of the se-

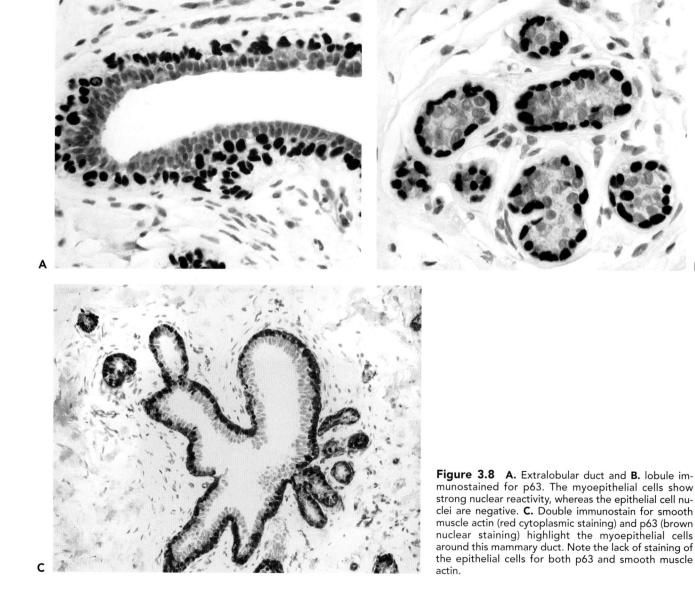

A

B

C

Figure 3.8 **A.** Extralobular duct and **B.** lobule immunostained for p63. The myoepithelial cells show strong nuclear reactivity, whereas the epithelial cell nuclei are negative. **C.** Double immunostain for smooth muscle actin (red cytoplasmic staining) and p63 (brown nuclear staining) highlight the myoepithelial cells around this mammary duct. Note the lack of staining of the epithelial cells for both p63 and smooth muscle actin.

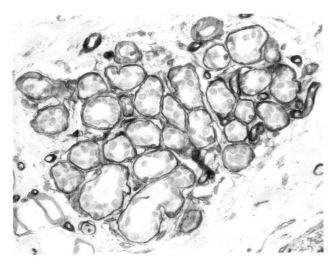

Figure 3.9 Immunostain for type IV collagen highlights the basal lamina around the acini of a lobule.

cretions to the extra-lobular portion of the ductal system (12). Subgross anatomic studies have shown that most lesions originally termed "ductal" (e.g., cysts, ductal epithelial hyperplasia, and ductal carcinoma in situ) actually arise from the TDLU, which "unfolds" with coalescence of the acini to produce larger structures resembling ducts. The majority of pathologic changes in the breast, including in situ and invasive carcinomas, are generally considered to arise from the TDLU (11,27). Indeed, the only common lesion thought to arise from the large- or medium-sized duct rather than from the TDLU is the solitary intraductal papilloma (Figure 3.10).

The normal lobule consists of a variable number of blind-ending terminal ductules, also called acini, each with its typical double cell layer. The lobular acini are invested by a loose, fibrovascular intralobular stroma with varying numbers of lymphocytes, plasma cells, macrophages, and

mast cells. This specialized intralobular stroma is sharply demarcated from the surrounding denser, more highly collagenized, paucicellular interlobular stroma and stromal adipose tissue (Figure 3.11). One feature of note that is sometimes encountered in the extralobular stroma is the presence of multinucleated giant cells (28). Their significance is unknown; and, while they may present a disturbing appearance, they should not be mistaken for the malignant cells of an invasive carcinoma (Figure 3.12).

The size of mammary lobules and number of acini per lobule are extremely variable. Russo et al. (29–31) have described four lobule types. Type 1 lobules are the most rudimentary and are most prevalent in prepubertal and nulliparous women, comprising 65 to 80% of the lobules in this group (Figure 3.2). These lobules are comprised primarily of ducts with sprouting alveolar buds. Type 1 lobules gradually evolve to more mature structures (type 2 and type 3 lobules) through the development of additional alveolar buds. The number of alveolar buds per lobule increases from approximately 11 in type 1 lobules to 47 and 80 in type 2 and 3 lobules, respectively. In the parous, premenopausal woman, type 3 lobules are most prevalent, comprising 70 to 90% of the lobular elements. Type 4 lobules are those seen during pregnancy and lactation. Of interest, Russo et al. (31) have reported that type 1 lobules predominate in the breasts of women with breast cancer, regardless of pregnancy history. They have also provided experimental evidence suggesting that type 1 and 2 lobules are more susceptible to malignant transformation than are type 3 lobules upon exposure to chemical carcinogens (32). It should be noted, however, that type 1, 2, and 3 lobules commonly co-exist in the same breast and that the utility of distinguishing among them in clinical practice remains to be defined.

The lobules exhibit morphologic changes during the menstrual cycle, and these are seen in both the epithelial

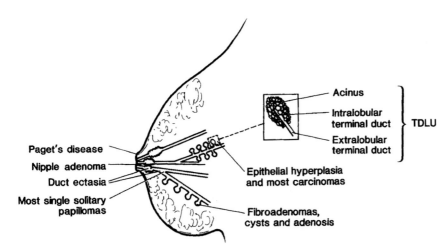

Figure 3.10 A schematic representation of the breast, indicating the sites of origin of pathologic lesions. (Reprinted from Schnitt SJ, Millis RR, Hanby AM, Oberman HA. The breast. Mills SE, Carter D, Greeson JK, Oberman HA, Reuter VE, Stoler MH eds. *Sternberg's Diagnostic Surgical Pathology.* 4th ed. Philadelphia: Lippincott Williams & Wilkins; 2004; 323–398.)

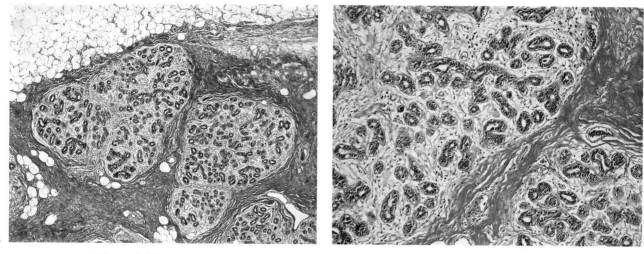

Figure 3.11 Intralobular and extralobular stroma. **A.** Low-power view of several lobules that are invested by loose, intralobular stroma. The interlobular stroma is composed primarily of dense collagen with admixed adipose tissue. **B.** Higher power view contrasts loose intralobular stroma with more collagenized interlobular stroma.

and stromal components (33–36). These changes are summarized in Table 3.2. While the changes that occur during the menstrual cycle are variable among lobules in the same breast, even among immediately adjacent lobules, a dominant morphologic pattern is typically present in each phase. However, these menstrual cycle–related changes are subtle when compared with the dramatic alterations seen during pregnancy and lactation and when compared with the menstrual cycle-related changes seen in the endometrium.

Occasionally, the TDLU epithelial cells show prominent clear cell change in the cytoplasm. This may be seen in both premenopausal and postmenopausal women and

appears to be unrelated to pregnancy or exogenous hormone use (37).

The nipple-areola complex is a circular area of skin that exhibits increased pigmentation and contains numerous sensory nerve endings. The nipple is placed centrally and is elevated above the surrounding areola. The tip of the nipple contains 15 to 20 orifices. However, as discussed earlier, the number of such openings may not correlate directly with the number of breast segments. In the nonlactating breast, these duct openings typically possess keratin plugs. The areola surface exhibits numerous small, rounded elevations, the tubercles of Montgomery.

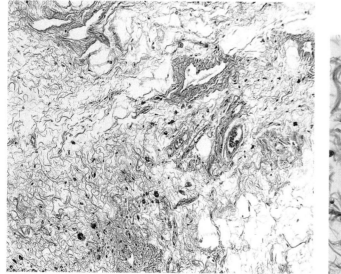
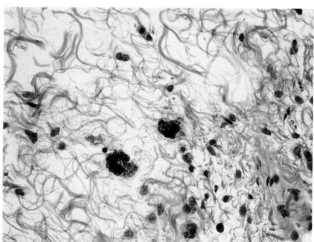

Figure 3.12 Multinucleated stromal giant cells. **A.** Low-power view showing multinucleated giant cells scattered in the stroma. **B.** High power illustrates cytologic detail. These cells have a mesenchymal phenotype. Despite their worrisome histologic appearance, they have no known clinical significance.

TABLE 3.2

HISTOLOGIC CHANGES IN LOBULES DURING THE MENSTRUAL CYCLE (ADAPTED FROM MCCARTY AND NATH (8))

Menstrual Cycle Phase	Epithelium	Acinar Lumina	Intralobular Stroma
Early follicular	*Cells*: single cell type (small, polygonal cells with pale eosinophilic cells); myoepithelial cells inconspicuous *Orientation*: poor *Secretion*: none *Mitoses/apoptosis*: rare	Largely closed and inapparent	Dense, cellular, with plump fibroblasts
Late follicular	*Cells*: three cell types, including luminal basophilic cells, intermediate pale cells (as seen in early follicular phase), and myoepithelial cells with clear cytoplasm *Orientation*: radial around lumen *Secretion*: none *Mitoses/apoptosis*: rare	Well defined	Less cellular and more collagenized than in early luteal phase
Early luteal	*Cells*: three cell types, including luminal basophilic cells with minimal apical snouting, intermediate pale cells, and myoepithelial cells with prominent cytoplasmic vacuolization and ballooning *Orientation*: radial around lumen *Secretion*: slight *Mitoses/apoptosis*: rare	Open, enlarged compared to follicular phase, with slight secretion	Loose
Late luteal	*Cells*: three cell types, including luminal basophilic cells with prominent apical snouting, intermediate pale cells and myoepithelial cells with prominent cytoplasmic vacuolization *Orientation*: radial around lumen *Secretion*: active apocrine secretion from luminal cells *Mitoses/apoptosis*: frequent (peak of mitotic activity)	Open, with secretion	Loose, edematous, congested blood vessels
Menstrual	*Cells*: two cell types, including luminal basophilic cells with scant cytoplasm and less apical snouting than in late luteal phase, and myoepithelial cells with extensive cytoplasmic vacuolization *Orientation*: radial around lumen *Secretion*: resorbing *Mitoses/apoptosis*: rare	Distended with secretion	Dense, cellular

Both the nipple and areola are covered by keratinizing, stratified squamous epithelium, and this extends for a short distance into the terminal portions of the lactiferous ducts. The epidermis of the nipple-areola complex may contain occasional clear cells that are cytologically benign and that must not be confused with Paget's cells (38,39) (Figure 3.13). Some of these cells represent clear keratinocytes, whereas others are thought to be derived from epidermally located mammary ductal epithelium (39).

The proximal ramifications of the mammary ductal system that are present in the dermis of the nipple typically have a pleated or serrated contour (Figure 3.14). These ducts are surrounded by a stroma rich in circular and longitudinal smooth muscle bundles, collagen, and elastic fibers (Figure 3.15). Occasionally, lobules may be seen in the nipple (40). Simple mammary ducts are also present throughout the dermis of the areola, even at its periphery, and these may extend to within less than 1 mm of the basal layer of the epidermis (41).

While the nipple-areola complex lacks pilosebaceous units and hairs except at the periphery of the areola, the dermis contains numerous sebaceous glands. Some of

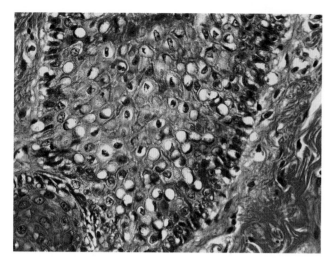

Figure 3.13 Clear cells in nipple epidermis. In some cells, the clearing is extreme, with formation of large intracytoplasmic vacuoles. These cells should not be mistaken for the cells of Paget's disease.

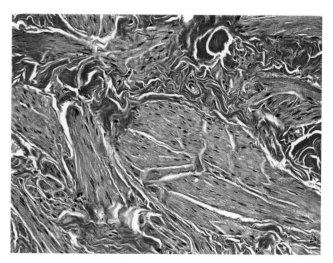

Figure 3.15 High-power view of nipple dermis/stroma, demonstrating prominent bundles of smooth muscle fibers.

these glands open directly onto the surface of the nipple and areola, whereas others drain into a lactiferous duct or share a common ostium with a lactiferous duct. The tubercles of Montgomery represent a unit consisting of a sebaceous apparatus and an associated lactiferous duct (42) (Figure 3.16). During pregnancy, these tubercles become increasingly prominent. Apocrine sweat glands may also be seen in the dermis of the nipple and areola.

Another finding that may occasionally be encountered within the breast parenchyma is the presence of intramammary lymph nodes (43,44). These lymph nodes may be identified as an incidental finding in breast tissue removed because of another abnormality, or they may be seen as densities on mammograms (45).

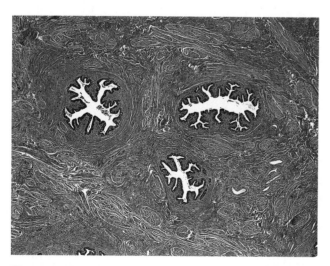

Figure 3.14 Cross section through the nipple. The irregular, pleated or serrated contour of the nipple ducts is evident.

PREGNANCY AND LACTATION

It is not until pregnancy that full development of the breast occurs in humans. During pregnancy, epithelial cell proliferation resumes. There is a dramatic increase in the number of lobules, as well as in the number of acinar units within each lobule secondary to epithelial cell proliferation and lobuloalveolar differentiation under the influence of estrogen, progesterone, prolactin, and growth hormone; growth is further enhanced by adrenal glucocorticoids and insulin. This lobular development and expansion occurs at the expense of both the intralobular and extralobular stroma. By the end of the first trimester, there is grossly evident breast enlargement, superficial venous dilatation, and increased pigmentation of the areola.

During the second and third trimesters, lobular growth continues, and the acinar units begin to appear monolayered. The myoepithelial cells in the acini are difficult to discern at this time due to the increase in size and volume of the epithelial cells, but they remain clearly evident in the extralobular ducts. The cytoplasm of the epithelial cells becomes vacuolated, and secretion accumulates in the greatly expanded lobules. After parturition, the lactating breast is characterized by distension of the lobular acini as a result of accumulated abundant secretory material and prominent epithelial cell cytoplasmic vacuolization. Many of the epithelial cells have a bulbous or hobnail appearance and protrude into the acinar lumina (Figure 3.17). Myoepithelial cells remain attenuated and inconspicuous. The florid changes seen in pregnancy and lactation can be alarming to the inexperienced observer; areas of infarction, which occasionally occur in the pregnant breast, may compound the problem (46).

When lactation ceases, the lobules involute and return to their normal resting appearance. Involution usually pro-

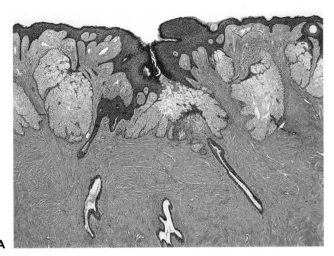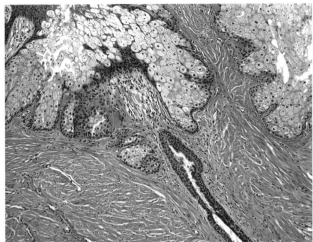

A   B

Figure 3.16 Montgomery's areolar tubercle. **A.** Low power view. **B.** Higher power view. These tubercles are units composed of a lactiferous duct and associated sebaceous gland.

ceeds unevenly and takes several months. Involuting lobules are irregular in contour and are frequently infiltrated by lymphocytes and plasma cells (47,48). Occasionally, an isolated lobule showing secretory changes may be seen in the breasts of women who are not pregnant. Although this is often called a residual lactating lobule, it may occur in the nulliparous woman as well.

MENOPAUSE

During the postmenopausal period, with the reduction of estrogen and progesterone levels, there is involution and atrophy of the mammary TDLUs, with reduction in the size and complexity of the acini, and there is loss of the specialized intralobular stroma (49,50). Ducts may become

variably ectatic. The postmenopausal breast is characterized by a marked reduction in glandular tissue and collagenous stroma, often with a concomitant increase in stromal adipose tissue. The end stage of menopausal involution is typified by remnants of the TDLUs, typically composed of ducts with atrophic acini, surrounded by hyalinized connective tissue or embedded within adipose tissue with little or no surrounding stroma (Figure 3.18).

BLOOD SUPPLY

The principal arterial supply to the breast is provided by the internal mammary and lateral thoracic arteries. Perforating branches of the internal mammary artery provide the blood supply to approximately 60% of the breast, mainly the

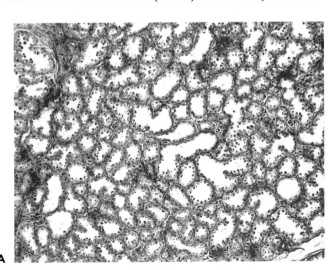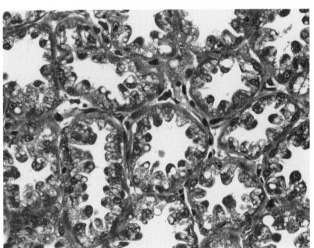

A   B

Figure 3.17 Lactating breast tissue. **A.** There are numerous acini in this lobule, and these are enlarged and dilated. There is minimal intervening stroma. **B.** Higher power view illustrates prominent epithelial cell enlargement, cytoplasmic vacuolization, and protrusion of cells into the acinar lumen. Some of the cells have a hobnail appearance. Myoepithelial cells are inconspicuous.

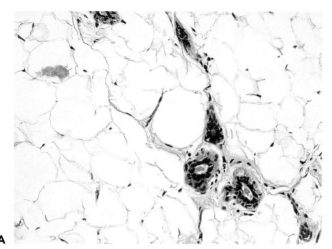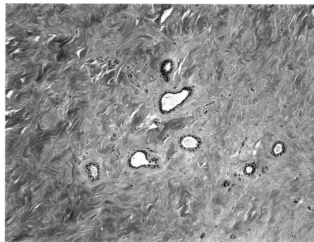

A   B

Figure 3.18 Postmenopausal breast tissue. **A.** This sample consists primarily of fatty stroma with a few atrophic ductules. **B.** In this specimen, a few residual, atrophic lobular acini are evident in a fibrotic stroma, which has replaced the normal, loose intralobular stroma.

medial and central portions. Approximately 30% of the breast, mainly the upper and outer portions, receives blood from the lateral thoracic artery. Branches of the thoracoacromial, intercostal, subscapular, and thoracodorsal arteries make minor contributions to the mammary blood supply (7).

Venous drainage of the breast, as in other locations, shows considerable individual variation but largely follows the arterial system. There is a superficial venous complex that runs transversely from lateral to medial in the subcutaneous tissue. These vessels then drain into the internal thoracic vein. Deep venous drainage of the breast is via three routes: the perforating branches of the internal thoracic vein, branches of the axillary vein, and tributaries of the intercostal veins, which drain posteriorly into the vertebral veins and the vertebral plexus (5,51).

LYMPHATIC DRAINAGE

Lymphatic drainage of the breast occurs through four routes: cutaneous, axillary, internal thoracic, and posterior intercostal lymphatics. The cutaneous lymphatic drainage system consists of both a superficial plexus of channels that lie within the dermis overlying the breast and a deeper network of lymphatic channels that runs with the mammary ducts in the subareolar area. Most of these cutaneous channels drain to the ipsilateral axilla. Cutaneous lymphatics from the inferior aspect of the breast may drain to the epigastric plexus and ultimately to the lymphatic channels of the liver and intra-abdominal lymph nodes.

There are three lymphatic drainage pathways in the mammary parenchyma. The most important drainage basin for lymphatic flow from the breast is the axilla, and the axillary lymph nodes receive the vast majority of the lymph drained.

The internal thoracic lymphatic route carries less than 10% of the lymphatic flow from the breast and ultimately terminates in the internal mammary lymph nodes (7). Drainage eventually empties into the great veins via the thoracic duct, the lower cervical nodes, or the jugular-subclavian confluence. The third and least important route of mammary lymphatic drainage are the posterior intercostal lymphatics, which drain into the posterior intercostal lymph nodes. An understanding of the lymphatic drainage of the breast is of particular importance in the current era of sentinel lymph node biopsy since this explains the occasional finding of sentinel lymph nodes outside of the axilla (5,7,8).

THE ADULT MALE BREAST

The adult male breast, like the female breast, is composed of glandular epithelial elements embedded in a stroma that is composed of varying amounts of collagen and adipose tissue. However, in contrast to the adult female breast, the epithelial elements of the male breast normally consist of branching ducts without lobule formation.

BIOLOGIC MARKERS, IMMUNOPHENOTYPE, AND MOLECULAR BIOLOGY

Estrogen Receptor and Progesterone Receptor

It is now known that there are at least two different estrogen receptors (ER), ERα and ERβ; ERα has been far more extensively studied. Using immunohistochemistry, ERα expression can be demonstrated in the nuclei of both ductal and lobular epithelial cells, with a higher proportion in

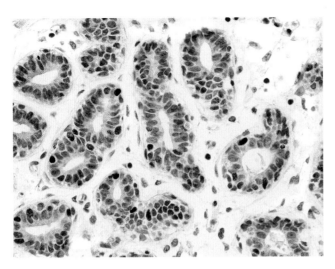

Figure 3.19 Immunostain for estrogen receptor-α (ERα) in a normal lobule. A minority of epithelial cells show nuclear staining.

lobules than in ducts. However, even in the lobules, only a small proportion of the cells show ERα immunoreactivity. Most often, ERα-positive cells in the lobules are distributed singly, admixed with and surrounded by ERα-negative cells (52) (Figure 3.19). Furthermore, there is considerable heterogeneity in staining for ERα among lobules in the same breast. Of interest, in breast tissue from premenopausal women, there is generally an inverse relationship between expression of ERα and markers of cell proliferation. In particular, most ERα-positive cells do not show expression of the proliferation related antigen Ki-67, and Ki-67-positive cells are typically ERα-negative. The proportion of ERα-positive cells gradually increases with age but remains relatively stable after the menopause. The incidence of lobules showing contiguous patches of ERα-positive cells also increases with age and with involutional changes (52). In addition, the proportion of ERα-positive proliferating cells increases with age (53). In premenopausal women, ERα expression varies with the phase of the menstrual cycle, being higher in the follicular than in the luteal phase (54). Myoepithelial cells do not show ERα immunoreactivity.

Recent studies have indicated that a second form of ER, ERβ, is also expressed in normal breast tissue. Expression of ERβ has been observed not only in epithelial cells of ducts and lobules, but also in myoepithelial cells, endothelial cells, and stromal cells (54,55). The expression of this form of ER does not seem to vary with the phase of the menstrual cycle. It has been speculated that the relative levels of ERβ and ERα may be important in determining the risk of breast cancer development, and that higher levels of ERβ relative to ERα are protective against neoplastic progression in the breast (55). However, additional studies are needed to more clearly elucidate the role of ERβ in normal breast physiology and in breast cancer pathogenesis.

Expression of progesterone receptor (PR) has not been as extensively studied in normal breast tissue as has ER.

Like ERα, PR is expressed in the nuclei of ductal and lobular epithelium. However, in contrast to ERα expression, PR expression does not seem to vary with the menstrual cycle phase (54).

Other Biomarkers and Immunophenotypic Features

Expression of a wide variety of biomarkers has been studied in benign breast tissue (56) and a comprehensive review of these is beyond the scope of this chapter. However, a few of these merit brief mention. Rarely, normal breast epithelium may show HER2 protein overexpression, *p53* protein accumulation, or *p53* mutations, but, the clinical significance of these findings is uncertain.

The anti-apoptotic protein bcl-2 is consistently expressed by normal breast epithelial cells (57). The S-100 protein is strongly expressed by normal myoepithelial cells and variably expressed by mammary epithelial cells (58). Epithelial cells also show variable expression for casein (59), α-lactalbumin (60), gross cystic disease fluid protein-15 (61), and c-kit (CD117) (62), among other proteins. As noted earlier, cytokeratins 7, 8, 18, and 19 (16–20) are typically expressed by epithelial cells, whereas myoepithelial cells express cytokeratins 5/6, 14, and 17 (16–20,24).

Molecular Markers

The ability to evaluate DNA, RNA, and protein using the modern tools of molecular biology, particularly when guided by such techniques as laser capture microdissection (63), will greatly enhance our understanding of breast tumorigenesis and may even serve to redefine what constitutes "normal." For example, a number of studies have shown that histologically normal TDLUs can exhibit an abnormal genotype, characterized by loss of heterozygosity (64) or allelic imbalance (65,66) at various chromosomal loci. At this time, however, the significance of these genetic alterations in histologically normal breast tissue remains to be determined. Studies of normal breast tissue using these techniques will also help define the presence and nature of progenitor cells or stem cells and their role in breast development and carcinogenesis (19,67), as well as patterns of gene and protein expression that distinguish normal from abnormal breast tissue and cells (68–71).

CONCLUSION

The histologic features of the normal breast are dynamic and vary with age and hormonal milieu, among other factors. An understanding of normal breast histology is essential to permit the reliable distinction between physiologic changes and pathologic alterations.

REFERENCES

1. Jochelson M. Breast cancer imaging: the future. *Semin Oncol* 2001;28:221–228.
2. Leung JW. New modalities in breast imaging: digital mammography, positron emission tomography, and sestamibi scintimammography. *Radiol Clin North Am* 2002;40:467–482.
3. Koomen M, Pisano ED, Kuzmiak C, Pavic D, McLelland R. Future directions in breast imaging. *J Clin Oncol* 2005;23:1674–1677.
4. Hylton N. Magnetic resonance imaging of the breast: opportunities to improve breast cancer management. *J Clin Oncol* 2005;23:1678–1684.
5. Rosen P. Anatomy and physiologic morphology. In: *Rosen's Breast Pathology*. 2nd ed. Philadelphia: Lippincott Williams & Wilkins; 2001:1–21.
6. Tavassoli FA. Normal development and anomalies. In: Tavassoli FA, ed. *Pathology of the Breast*. 2nd ed. Stamford, CT: Appleton & Lange; 1999:1–25.
7. Osborne MP. Breast anatomy and development. In: Harris JR, Lippman ME, Morrow M, Osborne CK, eds. *Diseases of the Breast*. 3rd ed. Philadelphia: Lippincott Williams & Wilkins; 2004:3–13.
8. McCarty KS, Nath M. Breast. In: Sternberg SS, ed. *Histology for Pathologists*. Philadelphia: Lippincott-Raven; 1997:71–82.
9. Anbazhagan R, Bartek J, Monaghan P, Gusterson BA. Growth and development of the human infant breast. *Am J Anat* 1991;192:407–417.
10. Monaghan P, Perusinghe NP, Cowen P, Gusterson BA. Peripubertal human breast development. *Anat Rec* 1990;226:501–508.
11. Jensen HM. Breast pathology, emphasizing precancerous and cancer-associated lesions. In: Bulbrook RD, Taylor DJ, eds. *Commentaries on Research in Breast Disease*. Vol 2. New York: Alan R. Liss; 1981:41–86.
12. Page DL, Anderson TJ. *Diagnostic Histopathology of the Breast*. Edinburgh: Churchill Livingstone; 1987.
13. Love SM, Barsky SH. Anatomy of the nipple and breast ducts revisited. *Cancer* 2004;101:1947–1957.
14. Ohtake T, Kimijima I, Fukushima T, et al. Computer-assisted complete three-dimensional reconstruction of the mammary ductal/lobular systems: implications of ductal anastomoses for breast-conserving surgery. *Cancer* 2001;91:2263–2272.
15. Schnitt SJ, Millis RR, Hanby AM, Oberman HA. The breast. In: Mills SE, Carter D, Greenson JK, Oberman HA, Reuter VE, Stoler MH, eds. *Sternberg's Diagnostic Surgical Pathology*. 4th ed. Philadelphia: Lippincott Williams & Wilkins; 2004:323–398.
16. Jarasch ED, Nagle RB, Kaufmann M, Maurer C, Bocker WJ. Differential diagnosis of benign epithelial proliferations and carcinomas of the breast using antibodies to cytokeratins. *Hum Pathol* 1988;19:276–289.
17. Bocker W, Bier B, Freytag G, et al. An immunohistochemical study of the breast using antibodies to basal and luminal keratins, alpha-smooth muscle actin, vimentin, collagen IV and laminin. Part I: Normal breast and benign proliferative lesions. *Virchows Arch A Pathol Anat Histopathol* 1992;421:315–322.
18. Heatley M, Maxwell P, Whiteside C, Toner P. Cytokeratin intermediate filament expression in benign and malignant breast disease. *J Clin Pathol* 1995;48:26–32.
19. Bocker W, Moll R, Poremba C, et al. Common adult stem cells in the human breast give rise to glandular and myoepithelial cell lineages: a new cell biological concept. *Lab Invest* 2002;82:737–746.
20. Abd El-Rehim DM, Pinder SE, Paish CE, et al. Expression of luminal and basal cytokeratins in human breast carcinoma. *J Pathol* 2004;203:661–671.
21. Yazji H, Gown AM, Sneige N. Detection of stromal invasion in breast cancer: the myoepithelial markers. *Adv Anat Pathol* 2000;7:100–109.
22. Barbareschi M, Pecciarini L, Cangi MG, et al. p63, a p53 homologue, is a selective nuclear marker of myoepithelial cells of the human breast. *Am J Surg Pathol* 2001;25:1054–1060.
23. Moritani S, Kushima R, Sugihara H, Bamba M, Kobayashi TK, Hattori T. Availability of CD10 immunohistochemistry as a marker of breast myoepithelial cells on paraffin sections. *Mod Pathol* 2002;15:397–405.
24. Nielsen TO, Hsu FD, Jensen K, et al. Immunohistochemical and clinical characterization of the basal-like subtype of invasive breast carcinoma. *Clin Cancer Res* 2004;10:5367–5374.
25. Clarke CL, Sandle J, Parry SC, Reis-Filho JS, O'Hare MJ, Lakhani SR. Cytokeratin 5/6 in normal human breast: lack of evidence for a stem cell phenotype. *J Pathol* 2004;204:147–152.
26. Barsky SH, Siegal GP, Jannotta F, Liotta LA. Loss of basement membrane components by invasive tumors but not by their benign counterparts. *Lab Invest* 1983;49:140–147.
27. Wellings SR, Jensen HM, Marcum RG. An atlas of subgross pathology of the human breast with special reference to possible precancerous lesions. *J Natl Cancer Inst* 1975;55:231–273.
28. Rosen PP. Multinucleated mammary stromal giant cells: a benign lesion that simulates invasive carcinoma. *Cancer* 1979;44:1305–1308.
29. Russo J, Russo IH. Development of the human mammary gland. In: Neville MC, Daniel CW, eds. *The Mammary Gland: Development, Regulation, and Function*. New York: Plenum Press; 1987:67–93.
30. Russo J, Rivera R, Russo IH. Influence of age and parity on the development of the human breast. *Breast Cancer Res Treat* 1992;23:211–218.
31. Russo J, Romero AL, Russo IH. Architectural pattern of the normal and cancerous breast under the influence of parity. *Cancer Epidemiol Biomarkers Prev* 1994;3:219–224.
32. Russo J, Mills MJ, Moussalli MJ, Russo IH. Influence of human breast development on the growth properties of primary cultures. *In Vitro Cell Dev Biol* 1989;25:643–649.
33. Vogel PM, Georgiade NG, Fetter BF, Vogel FS, McCarty KS Jr. The correlation of histologic changes in the human breast with the menstrual cycle. *Am J Pathol* 1981;104:23–34.
34. Longacre TA, Bartow SA. A correlative morphologic study of human breast and endometrium in the menstrual cycle. *Am J Surg Pathol* 1986;10:382–393.
35. Ramakrishnan R, Khan SA, Badve S. Morphological changes in breast tissue with menstrual cycle. *Mod Pathol* 2002;15:1348–1356.
36. Anderson TJ. Normal breast: myths, realities, and prospects. *Mod Pathol* 1998;11:115–119.
37. Tavassoli FA, Yeh IT. Lactational and clear cell changes of the breast in nonlactating, nonpregnant women. *Am J Clin Pathol* 1987; 87:23–29.
38. Toker C. Clear cells of the nipple epidermis. *Cancer* 1970;25:601–610.
39. Kohler S, Rouse RV, Smoller BR. The differential diagnosis of pagetoid cells in the epidermis. *Mod Pathol* 1998;11:79–92.
40. Rosen PP, Tench W. Lobules in the nipple. Frequency and significance for breast cancer treatment. *Pathol Annu* 1985;20(pt 2):317–322.
41. Schnitt SJ, Goldwyn RM, Slavin SA. Mammary ducts in the areola: implications for patients undergoing reconstructive surgery of the breast. *Plast Reconstr Surg* 1993;92:1290–1293.
42. Smith DM Jr, Peters TG, Donegan WL. Montgomery's areolar tubercle. A light microscopic study. *Arch Pathol Lab Med* 1982;106:60–63.
43. Egan RL, McSweeney MB. Intramammary lymph nodes. *Cancer* 1983;51:1838–1842.
44. Jadusingh IH. Intramammary lymph nodes. *J Clin Pathol* 1992;45:1023–1026.
45. Svane G, Franzen S. Radiologic appearance of nonpalpable intramammary lymph nodes. *Acta Radiol* 1993;34:577–580.
46. Oberman HA. Breast lesions confused with carcinoma. In: McDivitt R, Oberman HA, Ozello I, eds. *The Breast*. Baltimore: Williams & Wilkins; 1984:1–3.
47. Battersby S, Anderson TJ. Proliferative and secretory activity in the pregnant and lactating human breast. *Virchows Arch A Pathol Anat Histopathol* 1988;413:189–196.
48. Battersby S, Anderson TJ. Histological changes in breast tissue that characterize recent pregnancy. *Histopathology* 1989;15:415–419.
49. Hutson SW, Cowen PN, Bird CC. Morphometric studies of age related changes in normal human breast and their significance for evolution of mammary cancer. *J Clin Pathol* 1985;38:281–287.

50. Cowan DF, Herbert TA. Involution of the breast in women aged 50–104 years: a histopathologic study of 102 cases. *Surgical Pathology* 1989;2:323–333.

51. McCarty KS, Nath M. Breast. In: Sternberg SS, ed. *Histopathology for Pathologists*. 2nd ed. Philadelphia: Lipincott-Raven; 1997:71–82.

52. Shoker BS, Jarvis C, Sibson DR, Walker C, Sloane JP. Oestrogen receptor expression in the normal and pre-cancerous breast. *J Pathol* 1999;188:237–244.

53. Shoker BS, Jarvis C, Clarke RB, et al. Estrogen receptor-positive proliferating cells in the normal and precancerous breast. *Am J Pathol* 1999;155:1811–1815.

54. Shaw JA, Udokang K, Mosquera JM, Chauhan H, Jones JL, Walker RA. Oestrogen receptors alpha and beta differ in normal human breast and breast carcinomas. *J Pathol* 2002;198:450–457.

55. Shaaban AM, O'Neill PA, Davies MP, et al. Declining estrogen receptor-beta expression defines malignant progression of human breast neoplasia. *Am J Surg Pathol* 2003;27:1502–1512.

56. Krishnamurthy S, Sneige N. Molecular and biologic markers of premalignant lesions of human breast. *Adv Anat Pathol* 2002;9:185–197.

57. Siziopikou KP, Prioleau JE, Harris JR, Schnitt SJ. bcl-2 expression in the spectrum of preinvasive breast lesions. *Cancer* 1996;77:499–506.

58. Egan MJ, Newman J, Crocker J, Collard M. Immunohistochemical localization of S100 protein in benign and malignant conditions of the breast. *Arch Pathol Lab Med* 1987;111:28–31.

59. Earl HM, McIlhinney RA, Wilson P, Gusterson BA, Coombes RC. Immunohistochemical study of beta- and kappa-casein in the human breast and breast carcinomas, using monoclonal antibodies. *Cancer Res* 1989;49:6070–6076.

60. Bailey AJ, Sloane JP, Trickey BS, Ormerod MG. An immunocytochemical study of alpha-lactalbumin in human breast tissue. *J Pathol* 1982;137:13–23.

61. Mazoujian G, Pinkus GS, Davis S, Haagensen DE Jr. Immunohistochemistry of a gross cystic disease fluid protein (GCDFP-15) of the breast. A marker of apocrine epithelium and breast carcinomas with apocrine features. *Am J Pathol* 1983;110:105–112.

62. Chui X, Egami H, Yamashita J, et al. Immunohistochemical expression of the c-kit proto-oncogene product in human malignant and non-malignant breast tissues. *Br J Cancer* 1996;73:1233–1236.

63. Simone NL, Paweletz CP, Charboneau L, Petricoin EF III, Liotta LA. Laser capture microdissection: beyond functional genomics to proteomics. *Mol Diagn* 2000;5:301–307.

64. Deng G, Lu Y, Zlotnikov G, Thor AD, Smith HS. Loss of heterozygosity in normal tissue adjacent to breast carcinomas. *Science* 1996;274:2057–2059.

65. Larson PS, de las Morenas A, Cupples LA, Huang K, Rosenberg CL. Genetically abnormal clones in histologically normal breast tissue. *Am J Pathol* 1998;152:1591–1598.

66. Larson PS, de las Morenas A, Bennett SR, Cupples LA, Rosenberg CL. Loss of heterozygosity or allele imbalance in histologically normal breast epithelium is distinct from loss of heterozygosity or allele imbalance in co-existing carcinomas. *Am J Pathol* 2002;161:283–290.

67. Dontu G, Al-Hajj M, Abdallah WM, Clarke MF, Wicha MS. Stem cells in normal breast development and breast cancer. *Cell Prolif* 2003;36(suppl 1):59–72.

68. Sgroi DC, Teng S, Robinson G, LeVangie R, Hudson JR Jr, Elkahloun AG. In vivo gene expression profile analysis of human breast cancer progression. *Cancer Res* 1999;59:5656–5661.

69. Perou CM, Jeffrey SS, van de Rijn M, et al. Distinctive gene expression patterns in human mammary epithelial cells and breast cancers. *Proc Natl Acad Sci U S A* 1999;96:9212–9217.

70. Emmert-Buck MR, Strausberg RL, Krizman DB, et al. Molecular profiling of clinical tissue specimens: feasibility and applications. *Am J Pathol* 2000;156:1109–1115.

71. Espina V, Geho D, Mehta AI, Petricoin EF III, Liotta LA, Rosenblatt KP. Pathology of the future: molecular profiling for targeted therapy. *Cancer Invest* 2005;23:36–46.

MUSCULOSKELETAL SYSTEM

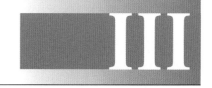

Bone

4

Andrew E. Rosenberg   Sanford I. Roth

INTRODUCTION

Bone tissue along with cartilage, fibrous tissue, fat, blood vessels, nerves, and hematopoietic elements form individual bones. In humans, there are 206 separate bones, which together with their articulations form the skeleton. Anatomically, the skeleton can be divided into the *axial* skeleton, which includes the skull, vertebral column, ribs, sternum, and hyoid, and the *peripheral* (or *appendicular*) skeleton, which consists of the upper and lower limbs and the pelvis (Figure 4.1). The *acral* skeleton refers to the bones of the hands and feet.

Bone, whether referring to an organ or a type of connective tissue, is composed of a unique biphasic blend of organic and inorganic elements. The quality, quantity, and architectural arrangement of these components determine its ultimate form and function and confer important biological properties. The contributions of bone to mineral homeostasis are vital to life, and its structural characteristics are essential to locomotion and organ protection. Additionally, bones form the framework of our bodies, thereby giving it size and shape and provide a nurturing storehouse for the hematopoietic elements.

BONE—THE ORGAN: GROSS AND MICROSCOPIC ANATOMY

Bones are rigid (but not brittle), lightweight, usually cylindrical structures, that have a relatively high tensile strength. Tan-white and smooth-surfaced, they are the hardest and strongest structures of the body, being as strong as cast iron but one-third of the weight as a result of their unique structure. Bones are reinforced, asymmetric, hollow structures designed to provide a maximum strength-to-weight ratio (Figure 4.2).

Individual bones are classified according to their size and shape. There are bones that are flat (bilaminar plates), those that are cuboid, and the most common group are bones that are tubular, both long and short (Figure 4.1). Tubular bones are further subdivided anatomically along their long axis into the epiphysis (extends from the base of the articular surface to the region of the growth plate), the metaphysis (extends from the region of the growth plate to where the diameter of the bone becomes significantly narrow), and the diaphysis or shaft (extends from the base of one metaphysis to the base of the opposing metaphysis) (Figure 4.3). In immature or growing bones, the metaphysis is

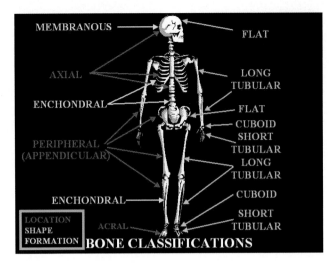

Figure 4.1 Diagram of the skeleton illustrating the different shapes and sizes of bones, as well as their method of formation.

separated from the epiphysis by a cartilaginous growth plate, or physis (1). Apophyses, such as the greater and lesser trochanters of the femur, are protuberances that form at large tendoligamentous insertion sites. The medical and forensic determination of skeletal age and growth utilizes the amount and localization of bone ossification, the formulation and size of the secondary ossification centers, and the degree and amount of remodeling (see below).

Despite their differences in size and shape, all bones are of similar composition and generally have a periosteum, cortex, and medullary canal that contains variable amounts of cortical (compact) and cancellous bone, fatty and hematopoietic marrow (Figure 4.2), blood vessels, and nerves. For any given bone, the quantity and arrangement of cortical or cancellous bone is directly related to the biome-

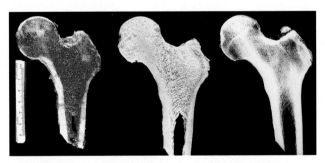

Figure 4.2 Gross (*left*) and macerated (*center*) longitudinally cut specimen and the accompanying x-ray (*right*) of a proximal femur, including the head, neck, and upper diaphysis sectioned in the frontal plane. The cortex defines the outer limits of the bone and is thickest along the medial surface (*left*) of the neck and diaphysis, where load bearing is greatest. The medullary cavity is filled with bony trabeculae and red hematopoietic and yellow fatty marrow. The trabeculae are aligned along the lines of stress; this is especially prominent in the medial portion. The horizontal line at the base of the head on the x-ray represents the accrual of bone that occurred during closure of the epiphyseal growth plate.

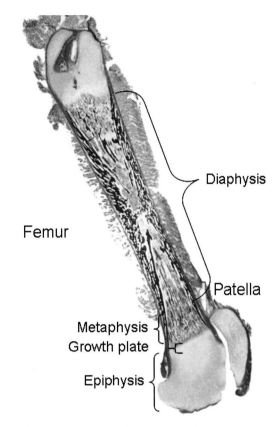

Figure 4.3 Whole mount of an immature femur and patella. The long bone is composed of the proximal and distal epiphyses, metaphyses and growth plates, and the intervening diaphysis.

chanical requirements (Wolff's law). For instance, bones exposed to the largest torsional forces are usually long bones, and they are composed roughly of 80% cortical bone and 20% cancellous bone. In contrast, bones that predominately transmit weight-bearing forces, such as the vertebral bodies, consist of 80% cancellous bone and 20% cortical bone.

Woven and Lamellar Bone

Histologically, bone tissue, regardless of whether it is cortical or cancellous, normal or part of a pathologic process, is categorized into woven and lamellar types based on the organization of its type I collagen fibers. In woven bone, the collagen fibers are arranged in an irregular feltwork (Figure 4.4), while in lamellar bone they are deposited in parallel arrays (Figure 4.5).

Woven bone is fabricated during periods of rapid bone growth; it composes the developing bony skeleton during embryogenesis and portions of bones in the growing infant and adolescent. It may also be the predominant type of bone that is formed in a variety of reactive (fracture-callus, infection-involucrum) and neoplastic (Codman's triangle, matrix of bone forming neoplasms) conditions. Woven bone is hypercellular, and the osteocytes and their lacunae

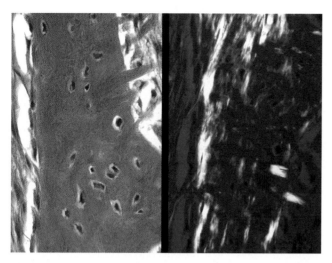

Figure 4.4 Woven bone seen on hematoxylin- and eosin-stained slide (*left*) and with polarized light (*right*). The collagen fibers are oriented in all planes. There are many osteocytes, and their long axes follow the direction of the neighboring collagen fibers.

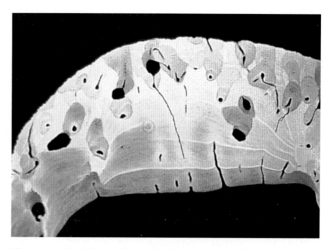

Figure 4.6 Microradiograph of the cortex of a 2-month old female. There are various degrees of mineralization, with the radiolucent being the most recently deposited and the radiodense portions representing the oldest.

are large and appear to be distributed in a haphazard fashion as the long axes of the cells parallel the feltlike direction of the neighboring collagen fibers (Figure 4.4). The mineral content of woven bone is higher than that of lamellar bone, and more than 50% of it is deposited outside of the collagen fibers. Overall, this structural organization enables woven bone to resist forces equally in all directions and facilitates rapid formation, mineralization, and resorption. These factors explain why woven bone is weaker, less rigid, and more flexibile than lamellar bone.

Normally, the entire mature skeleton is composed solely of lamellar bone. Lamellar bone, in contrast to woven bone, is synthesized more slowly, is less cellular, and the

osteocytes and their lacunae are smaller and distributed in a more organized fashion along the more regular collagen lamellae (Figure 4.5). Additionally, the process of mineralization of lamellar bone differs from that of woven bone in that it occurs more slowly and continues long after the organic matrix is initially deposited. Furthermore, the mineral deposits are localized almost exclusively within the collagen fibers and are first deposited within the spaces, or "hole regions," between the ends of adjacent collagen fibers (2,3). Subsequently, the mineral content increases as a result of enlargement and increase in the number of the apatite crystals. Microradiographs of undemineralized sections reveal varying densities, with the oldest bone being most heavily mineralized (Figure 4.6). Since the mineral and collagen fibers are well-organized and intimately bound to one another, lamellar bone has greater rigidity and tensile strength and less elasticity than woven bone.

Both lamellar and woven bone are made by osteoblasts in discrete quantities or units, which are fastened to one another by cement or reversal lines. Cement lines are thin and intensely basophilic on conventional histologic slides, and comparatively little is known about them. Recent studies, however, have shown that they are collagen poor, have less mineral, an increased calcium-to-phosphorus ratio compared to hydroxyapatite, and are richer in sulfur than is the surrounding bone matrix (4,5). Some investigators have suggested that cement lines represent a residuum of mineralized "ground substance" that is secreted during the initial reversal phase in the formation of new bone (6).

Cortical (Compact) Bone

Cortical bone, also known as dense compact bone, is hard and tan-white (Figures 4.2, 4.7). Its thickness depends on its location and mechanical requirements, being thickest in

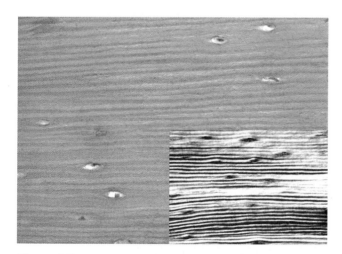

Figure 4.5 Lamellar bone as seen on hematoxylin- and eosin-stained slide and with polarization (inset). The collagen fibers are arranged in parallel arrays. There are comparatively fewer osteocytes, and they oriented in the same direction as the collagen fibers.

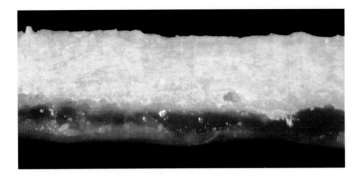

Figure 4.7 Longitudinal section through cortical bone. The cortex is tan-white and solid. The round hole within it represents the pathway of the nutrient artery.

areas exposed to large torsional and weight-bearing forces, such as the middiaphysis of the femur or tibia, and thinnest where the transmission of weight-bearing forces is paramount, as seen adjacent to articular surfaces and in vertebral bodies (Figure 4.2).

During the early stages of growth and development, cortical bone is constructed entirely of woven bone. Over time, it is gradually remodeled until it is composed of pure lamellar bone in the mature skeleton. Adult cortical bone is composed of three different architectural patterns of lamellar bone: circumferential, concentric, and interstitial (Figure 4.8). The circumferential lamellae form outer and inner envelopes to the cortex and consist of several subperiosteal and endosteal layers that are oriented parallel to the long axis of the bone. They are the first cortical lamellae to be deposited, and in young individuals comprise almost the entire cortex. As mechanical stresses on the bone increase, many of the circumferential lamellae (except for several lamellae just beneath the periostum and along the endosteum) are replaced by the concentric lamellae of the haversian systems (Figures 4.8–4.12).

Haversian systems, or osteons, are created by osteoclastic resorption of the circumferential lamellae that usually begins on the endosteal surface of the cortex, and less

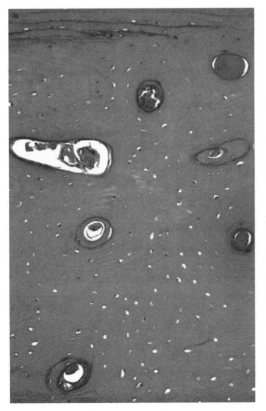

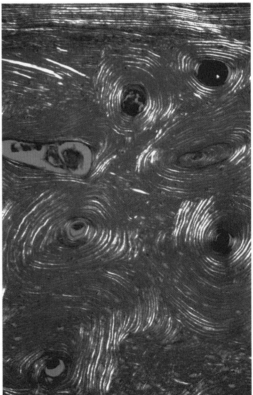

A   **B**

Figure 4.8 Cross sections of cortex with circumferential, concentric, and interstitial lamellae. The circumferential lamellae are beneath the periosteum, the concentric lamellae surround the haversian canals containing blood vessels, and the interstitial lamellae fills the intervening spaces (**A,** H&E; **B,** polarized light).

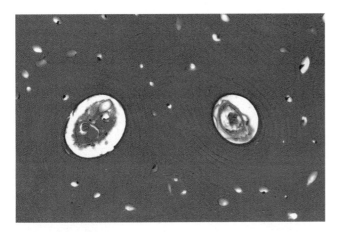

Figure 4.9 Two adjacent mature haversian systems containing the central canal, blood vessels, and surrounding concentric lamellae. Empty lacunae are seen in areas of the interstitial lamellae.

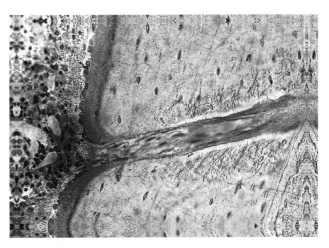

Figure 4.11 A forming Volkmann's canal coursing through the cortex of the bone. The canal is angled with respect to the bone lamellae and is filled with connective tissue. Osteoid and osteoblasts, indicating new bone formation, are present around the endosteal opening of the canal, but none are seen in the canal. The cortex shows circumferential lamellar bone with regularly placed osteocytes. (Undemineralized bone section.)

frequently on the periosteal surface. As the bone resorption proceeds, it penetrates into the cortex and forms a canal (Volkmann's canal) perpendicular or at an angle to the long axis of the bone (Figures 4.10, 4.11). The numerous osteoclasts located in the head of the canal form the "cutting cone," and the canal they generate is filled with vessels, nerves, and mesenchymal cells (including stem cells) enmeshed in a loose connective tissue stroma. Within a short distance, the osteoclastic activity becomes concentrated on one side of the canal; and, as a consequence, the direction of the cutting cone becomes aligned with the long axis of the bone. The burrowing osteoclasts elongate the canal, and in their wake newly formed osteoblasts deposit lamellae of bone in a targetlike, or concentric, fashion. The collagen fibers in any one lamella are oriented parallel to each other; however, their pitch is slightly different from those in adjacent lamellae, and this enhances the

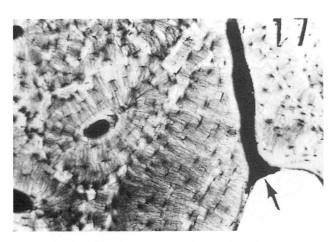

Figure 4.10 Ground, unstained section of mineralized, compact, cortical bone. The arrow points to a Volkmann's canal arising from the endosteum. Canaliculi connect cells in adjacent circumferential lamellae. (This slide was prepared by Glimcher MJ, Roth SI, Schiller AL, as part of a course in Pathophysiology of Bone for the Harvard Medical School, Boston, MA.)

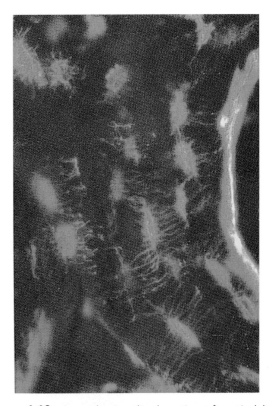

Figure 4.12 An undemineralized section of cortical bone, stained in vivo, with tetracycline. A layer of tetracycline appears at the mineralization front of the haversian system where new bone is being formed. The osteocyte lacunae and the canaliculi of their connecting dendritic processes are visible as bright green areas. (Unstained, fluorescent light.)

biomechanical strength of the cortex. In due course, the accrual of concentric lamellae reduces the diameter of the haversian canal so that in the end it is small and contains nutritional blood vessels and nerve twigs (Figure 4.8).

Individual haversian systems are relatively self-contained metabolic units because nutritional support of their cells, especially the bone cells, depends upon the process of diffusion from their central vessels. Consequently, osteocyte viability is not sustainable beyond a certain distance from the vessels, which imposes a biologic limit on the maximal number of lamellae contained within any haversian system. Also, the integrated network of osteocytes is generally limited to the osteon within which it develops, as osteocytic cytoplasmic processes generally contact only those that dwell in the same system, with cement lines defining the physical boundaries of every haversian system (Figures 4.10, 4.12).

Mature haversian canals are long and cylindrical, range from 25 to 125 μm in diameter (average 50 μm), and are widest nearest the medullary cavity. They form an intricate, branching, spiraling, and interconnecting network that courses thoughout the cortex. The number of haversian systems in a particular bone is variable and is determined by age, the amount of mechanical stress and weight that the bone is subjected to over time, and other biological and genetic factors (6,7).

Between the haversian systems are the interstitial lamellae, which are somewhat irregular, geometric-shaped units of lamellar bone (Figure 4.9). They fill the spaces between active haversian systems and help "glue," or anneal, them to one another, which is important in maintaining cortical integrity. The osteocytes confined to the interstitial lamellae may lose their access to nutritional sources and consequently undergo necrosis, leaving behind empty lacunae.

The endosteum is the loose areolar connective tissue that immediately abuts the osteoblasts along the inner surface of the cortex and along the medullary surfaces of the trabeculae.

Cancellous (Trabecular, or Spongy) Bone

Cancellous bone, also known as trabecular or spongy bone, is tan-white and fenestrated. It is composed of interconnecting plates and struts of trabecular bone and is located within the medullary cavity (Figure 4.2). In the adult, it is the fourth type of lamellar bone, and the lamellae are oriented parallel to the long axis of the bone (Figure 4.13). In developing bone, it is composed of significant amounts of woven bone; and, when initially formed, it contains a central core of calcified cartilage (primary spongiosa). Cancellous bone is deposited in relation to lines of mechanical stress (Wolff's law) to provide added support and distribute large weight-bearing forces along a variety of different pathways (Figure 4.2). Accordingly, cancellous bone is most abundant in the weight-bearing ends of bones, such as the epiphyses and vertebral bodies, and is present in only small amounts in the middiaphysis of tubular bones. Small

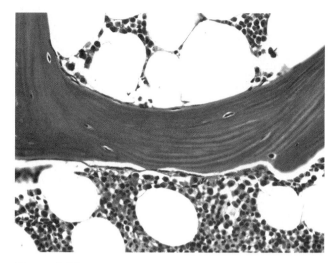

Figure 4.13 A mature trabeculum composed of lamellar bone. The lamellae are oriented in the same direction as the trabeculum.

trabeculae are avascular, while larger ones may contain haversian systems, including concentric lamellae. The surfaces of mature trabeculae are typically lined by endosteum composed of quiescent osteoblasts or surface-lining cells (Figure 4.14). In three dimensions, the trabeculae are usually interconnecting plates (Figure 4.15). The global surface area of cancellous bone is very large, which facilitates remodeling and the ability of the skeleton to rapidly respond to the metabolic demands of the body. The mature trabeculae are heavily mineralized with a thin (1–3 μm) layer of osteoid beneath the inactive flattened osteoblasts.

Periosteum

The periosteum consists of a thin layer of tan-white connective tissue that covers the outer surface of all cortices. In children it is relatively loosely attached, whereas in adults it is firmly anchored to the bone. The periosteum is composed of an outer fibrous layer and an inner cellular (cambium)

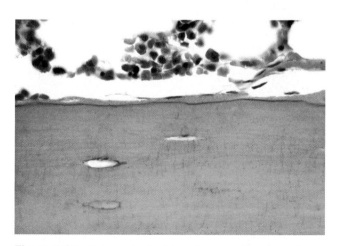

Figure 4.14 Quiescent osteoblasts lining a trabecular surface.

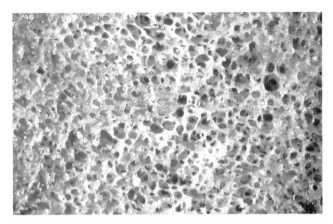

Figure 4.15 Gross photograph of a macerated portion of cancellous bone. The trabeculae are interconnecting plates.

layer (Figure 4.16). The fibrous layer contains fibroblasts and broad collagen fibers that are continuous with those of the joint capsule, tendons, and muscle fascia. At tendoligamentous insertion sites, the collagen fibers of the tendoligamentous structure pierce the periosteum and become anchored in the bone (Sharpey's fibers). Spindle-shaped

fibroblasts and osteoprogenitor cells occupy the cambium layer, which is generally the most cellular during growth and development. The number of osteoprogenitor cells present depends on the age of the individual and the amount of bone cell activity in any particular region; they are especially numerous during periods of active bone formation.

Vascular Supply and Innervation

Bones are vascular organs and require a vascular supply for viability. Bones receive their blood supply from three main sources: (a) large nutrient arteries (one to two per bone), (b) metaphyseal and epiphyseal vessels, and (c) periosteal vessels. Nutrient arteries enter long bones in the diaphysis, traverse the cortex through foramina, and divide into ascending and descending branches within the medullary cavity. Smaller branch arteries, arterioles, capillaries, venules, and veins (Figure 4.17) course throughout the medullary cavity, nourish the fatty and hematopoietic marrow, and extend into haversian canals, where they supply the inner two-thirds of the cortex. At the ends of growing bones, they terminate as small arteries that give rise to capillary loops at the bases of epiphyseal growth plates. The epiphyseal and metaphyseal vessels access bone through small apertures and provide blood flow to regions of the epiphysis and metaphysis in the mature skeleton and to the secondary centers of ossification during active enchondral ossification. The periosteal vessels are small and are believed to nourish the outer third of the cortex. The venous drainage system bone is composed of medullary sinusoids that empty into a central venous sinus, which merges with nutrient veins.

Bones are innervated largely by nonmylineated nerves that are derived from the autonomic nervous system, and their function is to control blood flow. Larger nerve branches are usually associated with arterial vessels (Figure

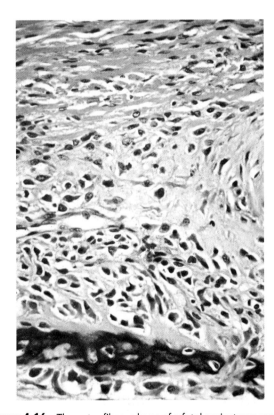

Figure 4.16 The outer fibrous layer of a fetal periosteum consists of thick bundles of horizontally oriented collagen fibers. The inner cellular cambium layer contains spindle-shaped, osteoprogenitor cells. The maturing osteoblasts steadily become more polyhedral and acquire increasing amounts of amphophilic cytoplasm. A portion of intramembraneous woven bone is seen forming the new cortex.

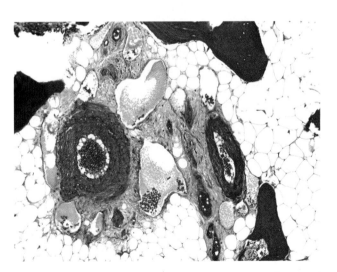

Figure 4.17 Small arteries, surrounded by dilated capillaries and nerves in an area of fatty marrow.

4.17), whereas small groups of fibers can be found adjacent to vessels in haversian systems. Nerves supplying the periosteum contain sensory elements and are the source of the sensation of bone pain.

BONE—THE TISSUE: ORGANIC AND INORGANIC COMPONENTS

The special biphasic amalgamation of organic and inorganic materials found in bone distinguishes it from all other tissues in the body. The organic component consists of proteins and bone cells, and the inorganic element is a specialized, calcium-poor form of apatite, resembling hydroxyapatite $[Ca_{10}(PO_4)_6(OH)_2]$ in which the hydroxyl residues are replaced by phosphate and carbonate ions. The integration of the mineral phase with the organic matrix (primarily collagen) provides bone with hardness, strength, and limited elasticity (2).

Organic Components

Proteins

The organic component accounts for approximately 35% of the wet weight of bone; and, of this, collagen is responsible for 90%. Collagen is the primary structural protein of bone, and the overwhelming majority (90%) is type I (8); type V collagen is present in much smaller amounts, and there are only trace quantities of collagens III, XI, and XIII (9). Type III

collagen may be increased in pathologic conditions (10). The numerous large type I collagen molecules are produced by osteoblasts; aside from their contribution to structural support, they also anchor many of the other constituents (11).

The noncollagenous proteins are grouped according to their function as adhesion proteins, calcium-binding proteins, mineralization proteins, enzymes, cytokines, growth factors, and receptors. These proteins mediate all aspects of bone cell activity and are extremely important to the biological success of bone as a tissue. Many of these substances are synthesized and secreted by osteoblasts, and others are derived and concentrated from the serum. The most abundant of the osteoblast-produced noncollagenous proteins is osteocalcin, which functions as a regulator of mineralization. Osteocalcin is made solely by osteoblasts, and its quantification in serum has made it an important clinical marker of bone formation (11).

Osteoprogenitor Cells

Osteoprogenitor cells are derived from tissue-bound mesenchymal stem cells that have developed into fibroblastic colony-forming units (F-CFU) (12–16). They are located in the periosteum, the haversian system, and the Volkmann's and medullary canal. Osteoprogenitor cells are primitive determined mesenchymal cells that have the capacity to produce only osteoblasts. The process of osteoblast differentiation and maturation is complex and involves a variety of different factors (Figure 4.18). By light microscopy, osteoprogenitor cells appear as generic spindle cells and do

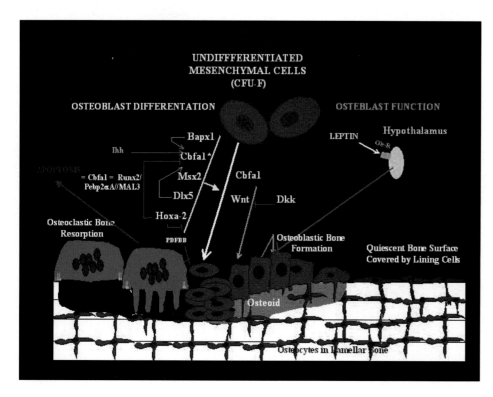

Figure 4.18 Diagram of osteoblast formation and metabolism. (*Bagpipe*, the vertebrate homologue of the *Drosophila* gene; *Bapx1*, a member of the NK2 class of homeobox genes; *Cbfa1*, core binding factor α1; *F-CFU*, colony-forming unit fibroblasts; *Dlx5*, homeodomain transcription factor; *Dkk*, Wnt antagonist Dickkopf2; *HOX2a*, homeobox gene; *Ihh*, Indian hedgehog gene; *MSx2*, homeodomain protein; *Ob-R*, leptin receptor; *PDFBB*, prostate-derived factor BB; *BMP*, a member of the bone morphogenic protein; *RUNX2/Pebp2aA//MAL3*, runt homology domain protein; *Wnt*, secreted glycoproteins that function as ligands for members of the Frizzled family of seven transmembrane-domain receptors.)

not have any distinguishing morphologic features; therefore, they cannot be identified with certainty in ordinary histologic sections (Figure 4.16). Because bone can be formed in skin, soft tissue, muscle, and viscera, in both experimental and pathologic conditions, osteoprogenitor cells or induceable stem cells are likely present in these sites as well.

Osteoblasts

Osteoblasts are vital to bone tissue and are the cells responsible for the production, transport, and arrangement of most of the components of the organic matrix (osteoid). Additionally, they initiate and regulate matrix mineralization and use autocrine and paracrine mechanisms to control the activity of neighboring osteoblasts, osteocytes, and osteoclasts (3,12,14,17). Immunohistochemical and biochemical studies reveal the presence of alkaline phosphatase, osteopontin, and osteocalcin within their cytoplasm, constitutively expressed RANKL (see section entitled Osteoclasts), and receptors for parathyroid hormone (PTH), prostoglandins, vitamin D$_3$, estrogens, and cytokines, including colony-stimulating factor 1 (CFS-1), on their cell membranes (8,18–21).

Osteoblasts cover all bone surfaces, where their lifespan may range from months to many years. Their metabolic state is closely related to their morpholgy; they are spindle-shaped when quiescent and large and polyhedral when rapidly producing bone. Metabolically active osteoblasts vary in size from 10 to 80 μm (average 20–30 μm) and have abundant amphophilic to basophilic cytoplasm that is in intimate contact with the bone (Figures 4.19, 4.20). Multiple cytoplasmic processes extend from the cells into and through the bone, contacting adjacent osteoblasts and osteocytes via nexus (gap) junctions. The nucleus is polarized away from the matrix surface and often has a conspicuous nucleolus and a prominent perinuclear halo that represents

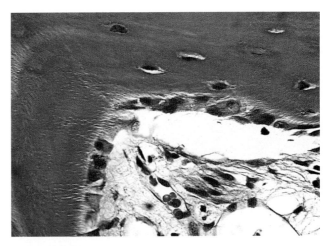

Figure 4.20 Metabolically active osteoblasts forming lamellar bone. The thin layer of osteoid cannot be identified in this demineralized sections. At the right of the micrograph, the osteoblasts are becoming inactive, flattening, and being incorporated into the bone as osteocytes. The osteocytes of the lamellar bone are spindle-shaped. The dendrites are identifiable extending from the osteoblast bodies into the bone where they are seen as clear streaks perpendicular to the bone surface represent the canaliculi containing the dendrites of the osteocytes and osteoblasts.

a well-developed Golgi apparatus. The cells flatten and elongate as their synthetic activity diminishes and remain lining the resting bone surfaces (Figures 4.14, 4.20).

Ultrastructurally, the cytoplasm of productive osteoblasts contains extensive, granular endoplasmic reticulum, a large prominent Golgi apparatus, and numerous mitochondria and lysosomes (8,9,14,22). In contrast, the cytoplasm of inactive osteoblasts resembles that of quiescent fibroblasts (14).

Osteocytes

Osteoblasts enveloped by matrix become osteocytes, and their half-life is estimated to be as long as 25 years (23). The cell body, nucleus, and surrounding scant cytoplasm reside within a lacunar space. The nuclei are comparatively small and are not always visible in every plane of section; therefore, in most slides of bone tissue, random lacunae appear empty. Osteocytes have numerous long and delicate cytoplasmic processes (dentrites), similar to the neuritic processes (axons) of neurons (Figures 4.12, 4.21). These cell processes traverse the matrix through small tunnels termed *canaliculi* and provide a very large surface area of contact between the osteocyte and the matrix and extracellular fluid that bathes each cell (22). Osteocyte cell processes connect to those of neighboring osteocytes and to surface osteoblasts via gap junctions. Gap junctions facilitate the transfer of small molecules and biologically generated electrical potentials from cell to cell. In this manner, osteocytes communicate with one another and form a complex and integrated network throughout bone tissue.

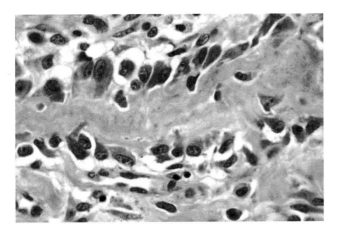

Figure 4.19 Metabolically active osteoblasts lining a trabeculum of woven bone. Some osteoblasts are in various stages of being surrounded by matrix and becoming osteocytes.

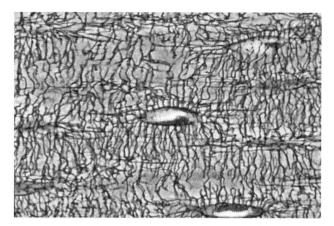

Figure 4.21 Osteocytes within lacunar space. Numerous cell processes course through the matrix and contact those of neighboring osteocytes.

The number, size, shape, and position of osteocytes varies according to the type of bone they inhabit. In woven bone, they are numerous, large, and plump (Figure 4.4). Their arrangement appears disorganized because their long axes parallel the direction of the neighboring collagen fibers, which in sections of woven bone appears random. In lamellar bone, osteocytes are comparatively fewer in number, smaller, more spindle-shaped, and appear in sections to be more regularly organized because the cells are oriented in the same direction as the surrounding lamellae (Figure 4.5).

The repertoire of biological activity possessed by osteocytes helps them maintain bone tissue and allows bone to be responsive to the mechanical and metabolic demands of the body. For instance, osteocytes are mechanosensory cells that translate mechanical forces into biological activity (23,24). The detection of physical forces stimulates osteocytes to produce and release intercellular messengers that target precursor cells, osteoblasts, and osteoclasts (23). These cells, in turn, respond by remodeling the bone regionally and allowing it to change its mass and structure according to demands of the external physical environment (Wolff's law) (25,26). The widespread distribution of osteocytes and their cell processes is fundamental to another important role of theirs, namely, mineral homeostasis (27). Osteocytes generate and respond to microfluxes in ion concentrations and mediate the exchange of calcium and other ions between the bone matrix and extracellular fluid. In certain conditions, they may even be able to rapidly release calcium and phosphorus from the mineralized matrix by a process termed *osteocytic osteolysis*, which manifests histologically as enlarged lacunar spaces (28). All in all, their aggregate activity likely influences the systemic metabolism of calcium and phosphous (27).

Osteoclasts

Osteoclasts are terminally differentiated, multinucleated cells responsible for bone resorption. They are mobile effector cells that have a lifespan of only several weeks. By the time they are recognizable by light microscopy, they are mature and biologically active and can be found residing within resorption pits (Howship's lacunae) produced by their digestion of mineralized bone matrix (Figure 4.22).

Osteoclasts are 40 to 100 μm in diameter and are polarized with one portion of the cell membrane intimately attached to the bone and the remainder exposed to the extracellular fluid in its microenvironment. The segment of cell membrane that actually adheres or seals to bone is laden with $\alpha_V\beta_3$ integrins. The integrins bind to specific extracellular bone matrix proteins (vitronectin, osteopontin, and bone sialoprotein) previously deposited by osteoblasts, and in this manner the osteoclast can anchor to the bone surface. A network of interconnecting actin filaments that produces a clear area in the cytoplasm links the sealing zone of the osteoclast cell membrane to the nuclei (14,29). On average, osteoclasts have 4 to 20 nuclei (8), though the number may range from 2 to as many as 100. In normal circumstances, however, the amount is usually not greater than 12. The nuclei and adjacent prominent Golgi apppartus tend to congregate away from the bone-resorbing surface, and are surrounded by abundant amphophilic cytoplasm.

The cytoplasm in the vicinity of the resorbing surface is rich in tartrate-resistant acid phosphatase, carbonic anhydrase, and membrane-bound lysosomes. The adjacent cell membrane, which also directly apposes the bone-resorbing surface, has numerous fingerlike extensions that effectively increase its surface area and form the so-called brush border.

The lysosomes fuse with the brush border and release their contents into the resorption pit, which begins the actual process of bone digestion. Metabolic activation of osteoclasts is initiated by anchorage, and this process gen-

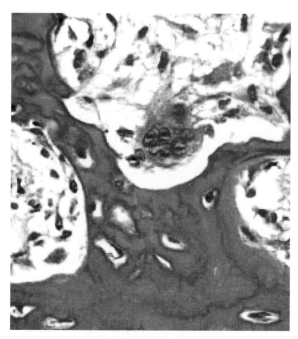

Figure 4.22 Osteoclast located within a resorption pit on a trabeculum (Howship's lacunae).

erates a stimulatory signal that is transmitted to the nuclei by the actin network. The nuclei, now activated, orchestrate the complex and transitory cytoplasmic and cell membrane modifications required for bone digestion. Importantly, mineralized bone or cartilage is more efficiently resorbed by osteoclasts than is nonmineralized bone or cartilage. Focal, or partial, demineralization of collagen fibers appears to be one of the first steps in matrix resorption and is followed by catabolism of noncollagenous proteins and, lastly, the degradation of collagen fibers themselves. Once osteoclast activity ceases and the cell moves to another targeted site, macrophages meander into the base of the resorption pit and phagocytize the organic remnants.

Osteoclasts are derived from mononuclear, hematopoietic progenitor cells of the granulocytic-macrophage colony-forming (GM-CFU) and macrophage colony-forming units (M-CFU) (16,29–42) (Figure 4.23). The mononuclear pre-osteoclasts undergo primary fusion to form multinucleated osteoclasts, which are capable of acquiring and shedding nuclei throughout their short lifespans (40). A variety of cy-

tokines and growth factors are critical to their development, maturation, and activity and include interleukin (IL)-1, IL-3, IL-6, IL-11, tumor necrosis factor (TNF), granulocyte-macrophage colony-stimulating factor (GM-CSF), and macrophage colony-stimulating factor (M-CSF) (43). These factors work by either stimulating osteoclast progenitor cells or participating in a paracrine system in which osteoblasts and marrow stromal cells play a central role.

This system is essential to bone metabolism, and its mediators include the molecules RANK (receptor activator for nuclear factor κβ), RANK ligand (RANKL), and osteoprotegerin (OPG) (43). RANK is a member of the TNF family of receptors expressed mainly on cells of macrophage/monocytic lineage, such as preosteoclasts. When this receptor binds its specific ligand (RANKL) through cell-to-cell contact, a series of signal cascades are activated and osteoclastogenesis is initiated. RANKL is produced by and expressed on the cell membranes of osteoblasts and marrow stromal cells. It's expression may be influenced by other osteotropic factors, and its major role in bone metabolism is stimulation of

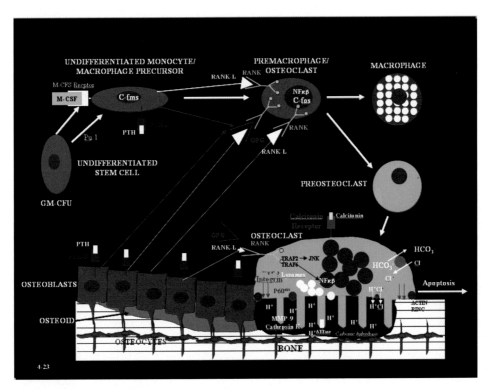

Figure 4.23 Diagram of the formation of osteoclasts and their relationship to osteoblasts and undifferentiated mesenchymal cells. ($\alpha_V\beta_3$, $\alpha_V\beta_3$ integrin; *C-fms*, gene for M-CSF receptor; *C-fos* (murine osteosarcoma viral oncogene homolog); *CFU-GM*, colony-forming unit for the granulocyte-macrophage series; *Cl⁻*, chloride ion; *CSF-1*, colony-stimulating factor-1; *H⁺*, hydrogen ion; *H⁺AT-Pase*, H⁺-adenosine triphosphatase; *HCO3⁻*, carbonate ion; *IL-1*, interleukin-1; *JNK*, c-Jun N-terminal kinase; *M-CSF*, monocyte-macrophage colony-stimulating factor; *MMP-9*, matrix metaloproteinase 9; *NFκβ*, nuclear factor kappa beta; *OPG*, osteoprotegerin; *ORA, XX; P6OCˢʳᶜ*, protein tyrosine kinase; *PTH*, parathyroid hormone; *PTH-R*, Parathyroid Hormone Receptor; *Pu.1*, a member of the ets family that is exclusively expressed by hematopoietic cells; *RANK*, receptor activator factor of nuclear factor kappa beta; *RANKL*, RANK ligand/osteoclast differentiation factor; *TNFR*, tumor necrosis factor receptor; *TRAF2*, tumor necrosis factor receptor–associated factor 2; *TRAF6*, tumor necrosis factor receptor–associated factor 6.

osteoclast formation, differentiation, activation, and survival. The actions of RANKL can be blocked by another member of the TNF family of receptors, osteoprotegerin, which is a soluble protein produced by a number of tissues, including bone, hematopoietic marrow cells, and immune cells. Osteoprotegerin inhibits osteoclastogenesis by acting as a decoy receptor that binds to RANKL, thus preventing the interaction of RANK with RANKL. The interplay between bone cells and these molecules permits osteoblasts and stromal cells to control osteoclast development. This ensures the tight coupling of bone formation and resorption vital to the success of the skeletal system and provides a mechanism for a wide variety of biologic mediators (hormones, cytokines, growth factors) to influence the homeostasis of bone tissue.

Inorganic Component

Mineral

The primary mature inorganic mineral of bone is a calcium deficient varient of hydroxyapatite [$Ca_{10}(PO_4)_6(OH)_2$], in which the hydroxyl groups have been largely replaced by phosphate and carbonate groups (44). There is minimal water in the mature crystals (44). It is the body's major reservoir for calcium and phosphate and contains more than 99% of the body's calcium and 85% of the body's phosphorus (1,9,44). Also harbored within the bone crystals are 95% of the body's sodium, 50% of the body's magnesium, and trace amounts of other essential minerals (1,9,44).

The process of mineralization varies according to the type of tissue. In cartilage and possibly woven bone, it begins with the production of numerous small vesicles (matrix vesicles) derived from chondroblasts and osteoblasts (1,2,45). The matrix vesicles are 2 to 4 μm in diameter and are the sites where mineral is first observed. Although there is some uncertainty regarding the initial structure and composition of the mineral, crystals of hydroxyapatite, as well as amorphous calcium phosphate and brushite have been identified (2,3,12,18,45–48). The primary crystals serve as a nidus for the deposition of larger aggregates, which are then deposited in and around the collagen fibers.

In lamellar bone, matrix vesicles are not present, and the process of mineralization is controlled by osteoblasts. The regulatory steps are complex and incompletely understood, though numerous proteins, growth factors, and cytokines are involved (2,3,12). Mineralization begins with the deposition of mineral in the spaces ("holes") between the ends of adjacent collagen molecules. It is still unclear whether the first deposits are hydroxyapatite, amorphous calcium phosphate, or a nonapatite crystalline calcium phosphate (octocalcium phosphate, [$Ca_8(HPO_4)_2PO_4)_4$·$5H_2O$]) (44). Regardless of their initial form, the aggregates grow and form crystalline bone apatite. Initially, the crystals are situated within the collagen fibrils, but eventually they also develop outside the fibrils and fibers (44). The shapes of the mature crystals are are not known with certainty. High resolution transmission electron microscopy shows that they have the features of thin plates, whereas, studies with small-angle x-ray scattering suggest that they are needlelike (44). Once the crystals are deposited in bone, they remain there for days to years, only to be dissolved at a future time during bone resorption, when the calcium and phosphorous are released into the extracellular fluid and become available for other biological activities.

Mineralization of osseous organic matrix takes approximately two weeks, therefore, the surfaces of bone are covered by a layer of unmineralized bone, called osteoid (Figures 4.11, 4.19, 4.20). The width of this layer is dependent on the relative rate of bone formation. In inactive regions, the bone is nearly fully mineralized and is covered by a thin osteoid seam (1–5 μm in thickness), whereas, in foci of rapid bone deposition, the osteoid layer may be more than several times thicker. The actual zone of mineralization can be detected by the systemic administration of the antibiotic tetracycline, which binds to the bone at the mineralization front and can be visualized with flourescent microscopy (Figure 4.12).

BONE FORMATION, GROWTH, AND REMODELING

From the time that skeleton formation begins in the embryo until the stage that adult stature is attained, the bones of the body undergo a marked increase in size, refinement of their shape, and enhancement of their contour. Bone is a rigid structure that cannot grow interstitially and only enlarges by the apposition of new bone on its surface. Appositional growth alone is adequate for portions of the skeleton that enlarge slowly during maturation, such as the skull, and the diameter of long bones; however, it is insufficient for bones that must increase in size at a more rapid rate, such as the length of long and short tubular bones of the extremities, the vertebrae, and the ribs. Cartilage, in contrast, exhibits both appositional and interstitial growth; that is, it increases its volume and enlarges in all dimensions by adding new cells and elaborating freshly synthesized extracellular matrix. Consequently, the growth in length of tubular bones in embryos and prepubertal children occurs as growing cartilage is replaced by bone, with the majority of the increase in bone length derived from the cartilage primordium represented in the anlage and growth plate (physis). In the case of callus, bone formation occurs both intramembranously in the fibrous callus and by enchondral cartilage replacement.

The genetic code for skeletal morphogenesis is encrypted in the homeobox genes. Homeobox genes contain the DNA library of a repository of transcriptional regulators essential for growth and differentiation. The expression of homeobox genes occurs in a specific order and temporal sequence; and, regarding the skeletal system, their activation results in the generation of localized cellular condensations of primitive mesenchyme at the sites of future bones. The mesenchymal condensations are the earliest precursors of individual bones and are critical to the formation of the skeleton. They begin to develop just prior to day 40 of gestation and, depending upon their anatomic location, are derived from cells that migrate from the cranial neural crest (craniofacial skeleton), paraxial mesoderm (axial skeleton), or the lateral plate mesoderm (appendicular skeleton) (49). Shortly after being formed, usually by the seventh week of gestation, the mesenchymal cells in the condensations begin to alter their genetic expression and assume the morphology of matrix-forming cells. Those cells that mature into chondrocytes form a cartilage model or anlage of the future bone, which is fundamental to the process of enchondral ossification, whereas those that develop directly into osteoblasts produce bone via the mechanism of intramembranous ossification. The mature bone tissue formed from either enchondral or intramembranous ossification are grossly and histologically indistinguishable.

Enchondral Ossification

Initially, the newly formed cartilage anlage is avascular and has the crude shape of the adult bone (Figure 4.24). The mesenchyme surrounding the anlage forms the perichondrium (Figure 4.25), which is the precursor to the periosteum that develops once ossification begins (see below). This process is initiated in each bone at a specific time, and this temporal sequence is the same in all humans.

Growth of the anlage occurs both interstitially and appositionally as a result of the proliferation of chondrocytes and the accumulation of secreted extracellular matrix (Figures 4.25–4.27). The matrix is composed of proteoglycans and type II collagen with smaller amounts of collagen types IX, X,

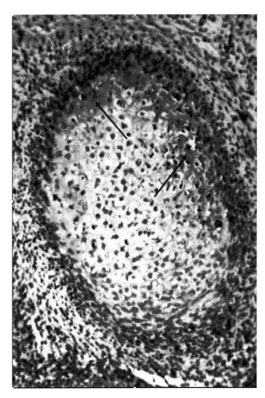

Figure 4.25 Cross section of the cartilage anlage of the embryonic femur. The chondrocytes are regular with little hypertrophy. The perichondrium is composed of undifferentiated spindle cells with little intervening stroma, surrounded by a loose mesenchymal tissue.

XI, and XIII (2). As this process continues, three events occur at very nearly the same time in every bone (50):

- The mesenchymal stems cells of the perichondrium, located around the midportion of the cartilaginous shaft, produce a layer of osteoblasts that deposit a collar of woven mineralized bone on the surface of the anlage. This heralds the transformation of the perichondrium into periosteum. The periosteum, osteoblasts, and the thin

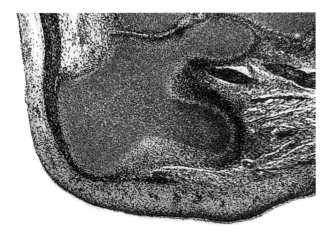

Figure 4.24 Cartilage anlage of the os calcis (calcaneus). The cartilage model is the approximate shape of the adult bone. The attachment site of the Achilles tendon and the tibial-calcaneal joint are present.

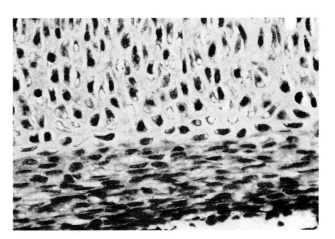

Figure 4.26 Cartilage anlage of femur in an embryo. The perichondrium is in intimate contact with the cartilage.

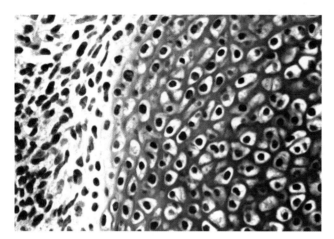

Figure 4.27 Cells of mesechymal condensation surrounding an area in which they have differentiated into hyalin cartilage anlage. The chondrocytes show early hypertrophy.

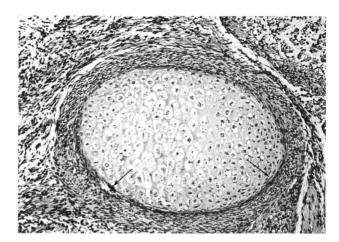

Figure 4.29 Cross section of the diaphysis of an embryonic femur. The thin, collarlike primary center of ossification is between the hypertrophying chondrocytes and the periosteal cells.

surface layer of bone form the primary center of ossification and delineate the middle region of the diaphysis (Figures 4.28–4.31).

■ The chondrocytes in the center of the anlage shaft become encased by the periosteal shell of bone and begin to hypertrophy and swell (Figures 4.27–4.31). The cell enlargement is accompanied by an increase in intracellular glycogen and in the perichondrocyte depostion of type X

collagen, and soon thereafter the chondrocytes undergo apoptotic necrosis (51–54). Concurrently, the surrounding matrix mineralizes, largely via matrix vesicles, although some crystallization may occur within collagen fibers.

■ A capillary network originating from periosteal vessels forms and, with the aid of osteoclastic (chondroclastic) resorption, penetrates the woven bone of the primary center of ossification (Figure 4.32) into the mineralized cartilage. The capillaries are the precursor to the future nutrient vessels and are accompanied by pericytes and other primitive mesenchymal cells, including osteoprogenitor and osteoclast progenitor cells.

As the cartilaginous core of the bone undergoes continued resorption, osteoblasts derived from perivascular stem cells deposit layers of osteoid on the residual longitudinally ori-

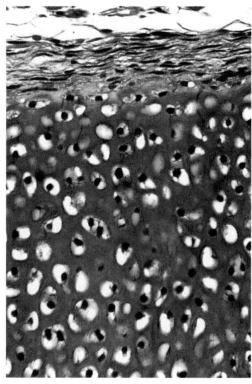

Figure 4.28 The early periosteum about the diaphysis of a cartilage anlage, showing the perichondrium surrounding the hypertrophied chondrocytes.

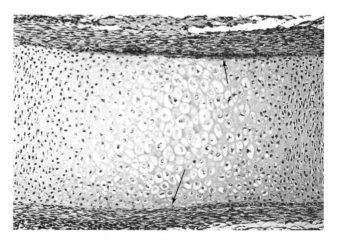

Figure 4.30 Longitudinal section of the primary center of ossification in an embryonic femur. The cellular layer of the periosteum is producing osteoblasts, which have formed a layer of pink osteoid. The outer spindle cells of the periosteum are oriented longitudinally along the femoral shaft. The underlying chondrocytes show hypertrophy.

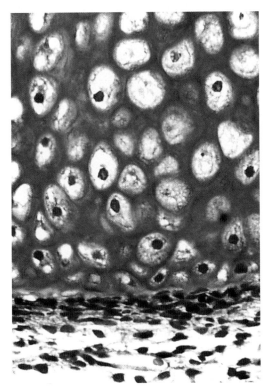

Figure 4.31 Primary center of ossification. A thin pink layer of osteoid, containing flattened osteocytes, separates the hypertrophied chondrocytes from the periosteal osteoblasts.

ented struts of mineralized cartilage. These trabeculae, composed of a central cartilaginous core covered by a rim of bone, are the first (or primary) trabeculae formed, and together they form the primary spongiosa. The spaces that develop as a consequence of the cartilage resorption then coalesce and form the medullary cavity, which is initially filled with loose connective tissue. Eventually, it becomes occupied by varying

amounts of adipose tissue and hematopoietic elements. This complex process begins within the center of the shaft and progresses toward both ends of the bone. When complete with primary trabeculae and an adjacent secondary center of ossification (see below), this is recognized as the fully developed growth plate (the physis) (Figures 4.33–4.36).

The fully developed growth plate is structured and has been divided into five merging regions that correspond to different stages of chondrocyte maturation (Figures 4.34, 4.36). As the chondrocytes pass through the different stages, they do not literally move within the matrix but mature in the position they occupy when first formed. Important regulators of this sequence of chondrocyte growth and maturation are the *Indian hedgehog* gene and parathyroid hormone–related protein (PTHrP) (54–56). The zones include: (a) a region of resting or reserve chondrocytes located nearest the ends of the bone; (b) a region of proliferating chondrocytes that become arranged in spiral columns; (c) a region of chondrocyte hypertrophy; (d) a region of chondrocyte apoptotic necrosis and matrix mineralization; and (e) a region of cartilage resorption by osteoclasts (chondroclasts) that tunnel into the mineralized matrix and leave behind residual longitudinal struts of cartilage that parallel the long axis of the bone. The orientation of the struts is determined by the preexisting columnar arrangement of the chondrocytes in the proliferative and hypertrophied zones (Figures 4.34, 4.36). These cartilaginous struts act as scaffolding for newly deposited woven bone. These struts of mineralized cartilage covered by newly formed woven bone are the primary trabeculae (Figures 4.36–4.38). The rate of growth differs for each physeal plate and is greatest in the growth plate of the distal femur,

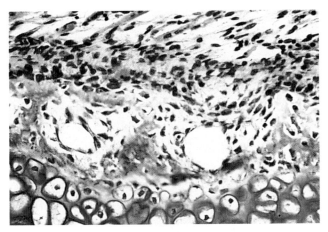

Figure 4.32 Primary center of ossification with capillary proliferation indicating the early formation of the nutrient artery. Between these capillaries, new trabecular membranous woven bone is being formed: in the cambium layer of the periosteum. The outer fibrous layer of the periosteum is more cellular than in the adult.

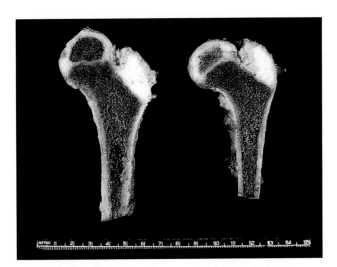

Figure 4.33 Gross photograph of the femoral heads of 3.5-year-old male. The secondary centers of ossification in the femoral heads are separated from the primary centers by the epiphyseal growth plates (the physes). The secondary center of ossification of the apophysis of the greater trochanter has not as yet formed. The metaphyses and diaphyses resemble their adult shapes.

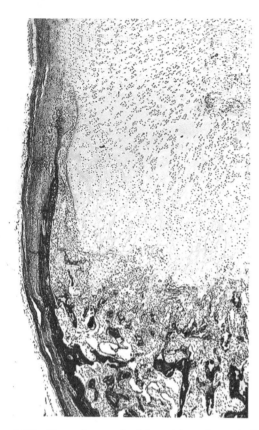

Figure 4.34 Photomicrograph of the epiphyseal growth plate of the costochondral junction from a 2-month-old male. The growth plate is surrounded by the ring of Ranvier. No secondary center is present. Primary trabeculae with central cartilaginous cores are seen in the metaphysis and upper diaphysis.

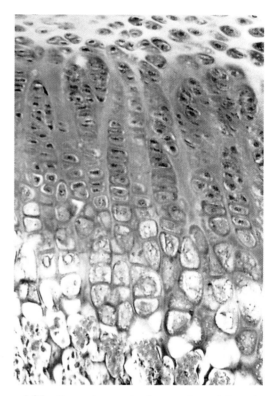

Figure 4.36 Photomicrograph of a maturing epiphyseal growth plate, showing the reserve zone (*top*), the proliferating zone, the hypertrophied zone, and zone of mineralization of the cartilage. The primary trabeculae are oriented vertically and are supporting the base of the growth plate.

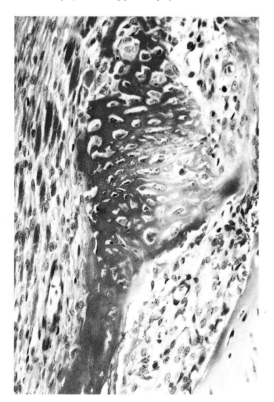

Figure 4.35 Ring of Ranvier, composed of bone that forms by the process of intramembranous ossification beneath the periosteum on the left and delineates the peripheral portion of the epiphyseal growth plate near the metaphysis.

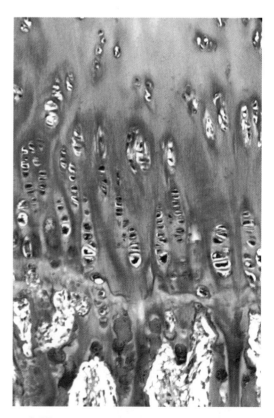

Figure 4.37 Junction between the mineralized cartilage columns and the primary trabeculae with the mineralized cartilage cores covered by a layer of woven bone.

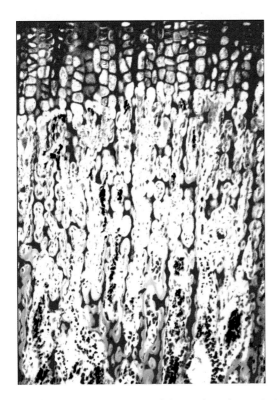

Figure 4.38 Longitudinal section of the epiphyseal growth plate, showing the zone of mineralization of the cartilage (orange) and the cartilage struts are being covered by a thin layer of osteoid (blue-green). Capillaries with numerous erythrocytes (green) are present between the primary bone trabeculae. (Goldner's stain.) (This slide was prepared by Glimcher MJ, Roth SI, Schiller AL, as part of a course in the Pathophysiology of Bone for the Harvard Medical School, Boston, MA.)

followed by that of the proximal tibia. In diseases in which mineralization of the cartilage is impaired (rickets), removal of the cartilage is handicapped, and the zone of hypertrophy becomes massively and irregularly thickened. While most tubular long bones have two epiphyseal growth plates, other bones (such as the ribs and some of the phalanges, carpals, tarsals, metacarpals, and metatarsals) have only a single physis. The growth plates, located at the diaphyseal-epiphyseal junctions of the bones, are delineated peripherally by a circumferential, thin collar of membrane bone that is a continuation of the primary center of ossification and is called the ring of Ranvier (Figures 4.34, 4.35) (57).

Concurrent with continued appositional and interstitial growth of epiphyseal and growth plate cartilage are dramatic changes in the cortex. As the bone increases in diameter, subperiosteal bone is deposited while the bone along the endosteum is resorbed so that the cortical thickness remains proportionally uniform and the medullary cavity enlarges. The bone that first forms the cortex is woven in nature; but, within the first several years of life, the fabricated bone is lamellar. Variation in the rate of formation and resorption changes the shape of the bone. This

is most pronounced in a region just distal to the base of the growth plate, known as the "cut back" zone. The cut back zone is rich in subperiosteal osteoclasts, which reduce the diameter of the bone to that of the diaphysis, and this results in "funnelization" of the bone. At the same time, the cortical thickness is maintained or increases by appositional new bone formation on the endosteal surface of the cortex. During growth and development, the diameter of the diaphysis continues to enlarge and in specific sites becomes asymmetric. This process is dynamic and not only determines the eventual diameter of the bone but controls the thickness and contour of the cortex. The increase in diaphyseal diameter is the result of periosteal osteoblastic bone formation. The thickness of the cortex is maintained by endosteal osteoclastic bone resorption. Conditions altering the balance of bone formation and resorption may cause abnormally thickened or significantly thinned (osteoporotic) cortices.

In most long bones, a similar process subsequently develops in the middle of the epiphysis, and this region is the secondary center of ossification (Figures 4.33, 4.39). A few long bones have a similar growth center in the apophyses. The maturation and replacement of the cartilage anlage in a secondary center is identical to that which occurs in the diaphysis except that the maturation proceeds from the center centrifugally, toward the periphery. This means that the growing area of the secondary center is, at first, a sphere. Eventually, the enlarging primary and secondary centers of ossification approach one another, entrapping a cylindrical segment of residual cartilage anlage and delineating the final form of the physis.

Continued growth of the primary and secondary centers of ossification results in the mergence of their reserve zones. At this time, a plate of bone demarcating the

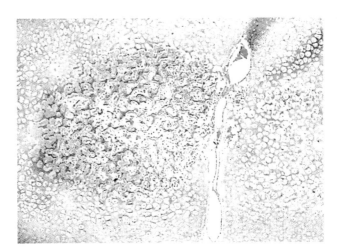

Figure 4.39 Photomicrograph of the secondary center of ossification of the femoral head. The nutrient vessels from the ligamentum teres are seen. Osteoid (green) is seen on the cartilage trabeculae (orange) in the spherical center. (Goldner's stain.)

secondary center from the forming growth plate is deposited. From then on, the centrifugal growth of the epiphysis is hemispheric. The cartilage located at the base of the true articular cartilage is responsible for progressive epiphyseal enlargement, and it has the architectural organization of a physis. Variation in the subarticular growth results in concordant shapes of the ends of the adjacent bones about the joint spaces. The epiphysis receives its nutrition primarily from blood vessels within the bone and its adjacent periosteum, whereas, the true articular cartilage is nourished by synovial fluid.

In the apophyseal cartilage, located on the surface of the bone, a secondary-like center of ossification appears and is responsible for the development of apophyseal bone of the iliac crests, the greater and lesser trochanters of the femur (Figure 4.34), and the tibial tuberosities, to name a few.

Once enchondral ossification is well underway at the growth plate, modeling of the newly formed bone begins. The primary spongiosa undergoes complete osteoclastic resorption, and secondary trabeculae composed solely of lamellar bone are deposited. The expanding medullary cavity becomes largely free of spicules of cancellous bone in much of the diaphysis and fills with adipose tissue and the hematopoietic marrow. Subperiosteal bone deposition and endosteal resorption of the cortex maintains a proper, tubular shape, and mechanical forces exerted by weight bearing and muscle attachments alter the rate of these processes in specific regions, which help sculpt the contour of the bone.

Several hormones, including parathyroid hormone, growth hormone, somatomedins, thyroid hormone, androgens, estrogens, and adrenal cortical hormones, are essential regulators of bone growth. At puberty, low doses of androgens and estrogens cause an increase in cell division in the proliferative zone of the growth plate and the secondary center of ossification. This is accompanied by an increase in the rate of cartilage maturation, mineralization, osteoclastic removal, and formation of primary trabeculae. In toto, these effects produce the so-called growth spurt seen at puberty. As estrogen and androgen levels increase and growth hormone and somatomedin levels fall off, chondrocyte proliferation decreases while maturation and bone formation proceed. This leads to a diminution or thinning of the growth plate, and eventually all of the cartilage of the growth plate undergoes complete enchondral ossification, leaving little or no evidence of its previous existence. At this time, the growth plate is considered closed, and all additional bone growth is appositional (Figure 4.40) (1,14). Cessation of growth of the secondary centers of ossification occurs in a similar fashion. However, a remnant of mineralized growth cartilage, which is the tide mark cartilage, persists at the base of the articular surface. It is demarcated from the true articular cartilage by a thin undulating layer of more densely mineralized matrix, known as the tidemark (Figure 4.41). The biologic potential of the tidemark cartilage persists as increases in hormones, such as growth hormone in the setting of acromegaly, can re-

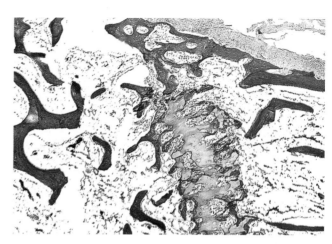

Figure 4.40 Closing epiphyseal growth plate in a 16-year-old boy. The periphery of the plate has been bridged by bone connecting the diaphysis and the secondary center of ossification. Cellular proliferation in the physis has ceased while the maturation process continues. The secondary center of ossification is at the top of the micrograph above the remnant of the physis.

activate the process of enchondral ossification and produce additional growth in the adult. In normal circumstances, however, the vestige of the growth cartilage remains dormant and functions as an anchor of the true articular cartilage to the subchondral bone plate.

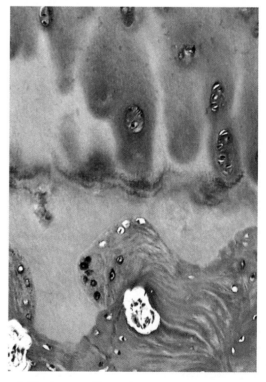

Figure 4.41 Section of base of articular cartilage in the region of the tidemark. The tidemark separates the articular nonmineralized cartilage (above) from the mineralized cartilage remnant of the physis and the lamellar bone of the subchondral plate (below).

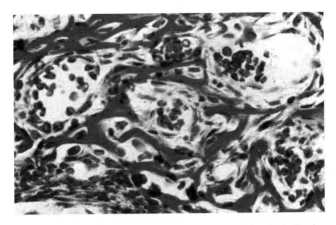

Figure 4.42 Intramembranous bone from a fetal skull. The osteoblasts are large along the randomly formed trabeculae. The osteocytes and their lacunae are large, round, and irregularly spaced in the trabeculae. (Trichrome stain.)

Intramembranous Ossification

Intramembranous ossification, or bone growth, refers to the process of bone formation in which the tissue occupying the site of the future bone or bone tissue is a fibrouslike membrane. The membrane is rich in osteoprogenitor cells and in normal situations forms the mesenchymal condensations in the developing embryo, the periosteum in the fetus, child, and adult, and the thin layer of fibrous tissue adjacent to all active bone-forming sites. The osteoprogenitor cells within the membrane produce offspring that differentiate into mature osteoblasts that directly deposit bone matrix (Figures 4.19, 4.42). Large portions of the flat bones of the skull, including the frontal, parietal, occipital, and temporal bones, form by this process (1,14). Also, since the cortices of all bones are largely created by osteoblasts derived from the cambium layer of the periosteum, all bones, in at least some part, are formed by intramembranous ossification. Growth of membranous bone occurs only by the apposition of new bone, and the medullary cavites of membranous bones are created and maintained by endosteal osteoclastic activity. Initially, the marrow spaces of these bones are composed of highly vascularized loose connective tissue, which is eventually replaced by adipose and hematopoietic tissues.

Modeling and Remodeling

The processes of bone formation and resorption are tightly coupled, and their balance determines skeletal mass at any point in time (58). As the skeleton grows and enlarges (undergoes modeling) during childhood and young adulthood, bone formation predominates, whereas after the third or fourth decades bone resorption prevails. The breakdown and renewal of bone fundamental to the formation and maintenance of the skeleton is called remodeling.

Remodeling is a dynamic process involving the removal and replenishment of both cortical and trabecular bone; it continues throughout life to maintain bone mass, skeletal integrity, and skeletal function. (39,59). This process is complex and at least partially controlled by the central nervous system through hormones (such as leptins) and by mechanically induced microdamage. It depends on the integrated actions of osteoblasts, osteocytes, and osteoclasts (60). Together these cells form the functional or basic multicellular unit of bone (BMU, or bone remodeling unit of Frost) and, in adults, are responsible for remodeling approximately 10% of the skeleton on an annual basis (Figures 4.43, 4.44) (61). This feat is accomplished by approximately 1 million BMUs that are active at any one time, and which likely first target sites that are experiencing fatigue and microdamage (33). The process may begin on any bony surface and incorporates three phases of cell activity: activation, bone resorption, and bone formation (62).

Many pathologic conditions of bone result from abnormalities in bone remodeling (1,9). These disorders may be generalized, in the form of a metabolic bone disease, or localized to small regions of the skeleton or individual bones. For instance, the diminished bone mass in postmenopausal osteoporosis, hyperparathyroidism, and hyperthyroidism results from increased osteoclastic bone resorption, which is not adequately compensated for by an appropriate amount of new bone formation. The lytic lesions in early Paget's disease or those caused by metastases and myeloma result from localized increased osteoclastic bone resorption, which is significantly greater in amount than any new bone that is deposited. The goal of therapy for this broad spectrum of diseases is to restore bone mass, balance bone formation and resorption, and protect and maintain strutural integrity.

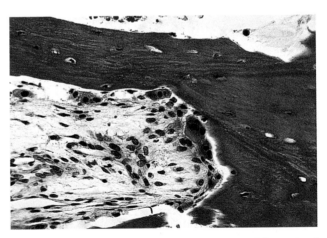

Figure 4.43 Basic multicellular unit (bone remodeling unit of Frost) of bone. Osteoclasts form the leading edge of the bone resorption ("the cutting cone"), and just behind them are mononuclear macrophages and osteoblasts. The newly created space is filled with a vascular loose connective tissue.

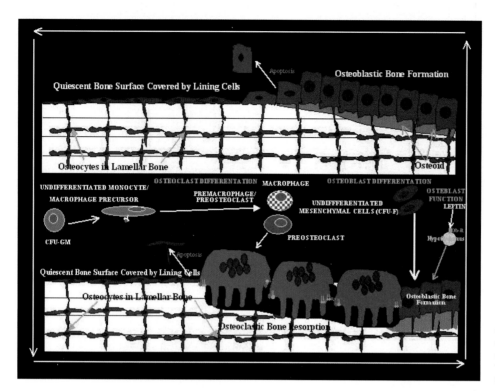

Figure 4.44 Drawing of the basic multicellular unit (bone remodeling unit of Frost) of bone. The resting osteoblasts are replaced by osteoclasts. New osteoblastic bone fills the resorbed lacunae of the haversian canal.

REFERENCES

1. Howell D, Dean D. The biology, chemistry, and biochemistry of the mammalian growth plate. In: Coe FL, Favus MJ, eds. *Disorders of Bone and Mineral Metabolism.* New York: Raven Press; 1992:313–353.
2. Glimcher MJ. Mechanism of calcification: role of collagen fibrils and collagen-phosphoprotein complexes in vitro and in vivo. *Anat Rec* 1989;224:139–153.
3. Glimcher MJ. The nature of the mineral component of bone and the mechanism of calcification. In: Coe FL, Favus MJ, eds. *Disorders of Bone and Mineral Metabolism.* New York: Raven Press; 1992:265–286.
4. Huffer WE. Morphology and biochemistry of bone remodeling: possible control by vitamin D, parathyroid hormone, and other substances. *Lab Invest* 1988;59:418–442.
5. Burr DB, Martin RB. Errors in bone remodeling: toward a unified theory of metabolic bone disease. *Am J Anat* 1989;186:186–216.
6. Schaffler MB, Burr DB, Frederickson RG. Morphology of the osteonal cement line in human bone. *Anat Rec* 1987;217:223–228.
7. Ortner DJ. Aging effects on osteon remodeling. *Calcif Tissue Res* 1975;18:27–36.
8. Baron R. General principles of bone biology. In: Favus MJ, ed. *Primer on the Metabolic Bone Diseases and Disorders of Mineral Metabolism.* 5th ed. Washington, DC: American Society for Bone and Mineral Research; 2003:1–8.
9. Robey P, Bianco P, Termine JD. The cellular biology and molecular biochemistry of bone formation. In: Coe FL, Favus MJ, eds. *Disorders of Bone and Mineral Metabolism.* New York: Raven Press; 1992:241–263.
10. Veis A, Sabsay B. The collagen of mineralized matrices. In: Peck W, ed. *Bone and Mineral Research.* Vol. 5. Amsterdam: Elsevier; 1988: 1–63.
11. Young MF. Bone matrix proteins: their function, regulation, and relationship to osteoporosis. *Osteoporos Int* 2003;14(suppl 3):S35–S42.
12. Lian, J, Stein GS, Canalis E, Robey PG, Boskey A. Bone formation: Osteoblast lineage cells, growth factors, matrix proteins, and the mineralization process. In: Favus MJ, ed. *Primer on the Metabolic Bone Diseases and Disorders of Mineral Metabolism.* 4th ed. Philadephia: Lippincott Williams & Wilkins; 1999:14–29.
13. Manolagas SC, Jilka, RL. Bone marrow, cytokines, and bone remodeling. Emerging insights into the pathophysiology of osteoporosis. *N Engl J Med* 1995;332:305–311.
14. Marks SC Jr, Popoff, SN. Bone cell biology: the regulation of development, structure, and function in the skeleton. *Am J Anat* 1988;183:1–44.
15. Friedenstein A. Stromal mechanisms of bone marrow: cloning in vitro and retransplantation in vivo. In: Thienfelder S, ed. *Immunology of Bone Marrow Transplantation.* Berlin: Springer-Verlag; 1980:19–29.
16. Jotereau FV, Le Douarin NM. The development relationship between osteocytes and osteoclasts: a study using the quail-chick nuclear marker in endochondral ossification. *Dev Biol* 1978;63:253– 265.
17. Leblond CP. Synthesis and secretion of collagen by cells of connective tissue, bone, and dentin. *Anat Rec* 1989;224:123–138.
18. Lian J, Stein GS, Aubin JE. Bone formation: maturation and functional activities of osteoblast lineage. In: Favus MJ, ed. *Primer on the Metabolic Bone Diseases and Disorders of Mineral Metabolism.* 5th ed. Washington, DC: American Society for Bone and Mineral Research. 2003:13–27.
19. Jilka RL. Are osteoblastic cells required for the control of osteoclast activity by parathyroid hormone? *Bone Miner* 1986;1:261–266.
20. Marks SC Jr. Osteoclast biology: lessons from mammalian mutations. *Am J Med Genet* 1989;34:43–54.
21. Rouleau MF, Mitchell J, Goltzman D. In vivo distribution of parathyroid hormone receptors in bone: evidence that a predominant osseous target cell is not the mature osteoblast. *Endocrinology* 1988;123:187–191.
22. Baron R. Anatomy and ultrastructure of bone. In: Favus MJ, ed. *Primer on the Metabolic Bone Diseases and Disorders of Mineral Metabolism.* 4th ed. Philadelphia: Lippincott Williams & Wilkins; 1999:3–10.
23. Knothe Tate ML, Adamson JR, Tami AE, Bauer TW. The osteocyte. *Int J Biochem Cell Biol* 2004;36:1–8.

24. Iqbal J, Zaidi M. Molecular regulation of mechanotransduction. *Biochem Biophys Res Commun* 2005;328:751–755.

25. Wolff J. Die Lehre von der functionellen Knochengestalt. *Arch f. path. Anat.* 1899;155: 256–315.

26. Wolff J. Gesetz der Transformation der Knochen. Berlin: Hirschwald; 1892.

27. Cullinane DM. The role of osteocytes in bone regulation: mineral homeostasis versus mechanoreception. *J Musculoskelet Neuronal Interact* 2002;2:242–244.

28. Belanger LF. Osteocytic osteolysis. *Calcif Tissue Res* 1969;4:1–12.

29. Raisz L. Mechanisms and regulation of bone resorption by osteoclastic cells. In: Coe FL, Favus MJ, eds. *Disorders of Bone and Mineral Metabolism.* New York: Raven Press;1992:287–311.

30. Friedenstein, A. Determined and inducible osteogenic precursor cells. In: Elliott K, Fitzsimons D, eds. *Hard Tissue Growth, Repair and Remineralization.* Ciba Foundation Symposium. 11th ed. Amsterdam: Elsevier-Excerpta Medica; 1973:169–185.

31. Fallon MD, Teitelbaum SL. The interpretation of fluorescent tetracycline markers in the diagnosis of metabolic bone diseases. *Hum Pathol* 1982;13:416–417.

32. Chambers T. The origin of the osteoclast. In: Peck W, ed. *Bone and Mineral Research.* Vol. 6. Amsterdam: Elsevier; 1989:1–25.

33. Mundy G, Roodman D. Osteoclast ontogeny and function. In: Peck W, ed. *Bone and Mineral Research.* Vol. 5. Amsterdam: Elsevier; 1987:209–279.

34. Walker DG. Congenital osteopetrosis in mice cured by parabiotic union with normal siblings. *Endocrinology* 1972;91:916–920.

35. Walker DG. Osteopetrosis cured by temporary parabiosis. *Science* 1973;180:875.

36. Walker DG. Bone resorption restored in osteopetrotic mice by transplants of normal bone marrow and spleen cells. *Science* 1975;190:784–785.

37. Walker DG. Spleen cells transmit osteopetrosis in mice. *Science* 1975;190:785–787.

38. Walker DG. Control of bone resorption by hematopoietic tissue. The induction and reversal of congenital osteopetrosis in mice through use of bone marrow and splenic transplants. *J Exp Med* 1975;142:651–663.

39. Dempster D. Bone remodeling. In: Coe FL, Favus MJ, eds. *Disorders of Bone and Mineral Metabolism.* New York: Raven Press; 1992:355–380.

40. Stout SD, Teitelbaum SL. Histomorphometric determination of formation rates of archaeological bone. *Calcif Tissue Res* 1976;21:163–169.

41. Reddy SV. Regulatory mechanisms operative in osteoclasts. *Crit Rev Eukaryot Gene Expr* 2004;14:255–270.

42. Quinn JM, Gillespie MT. Modulation of osteoclast formation. *Biochem Biophys Res Commun* 2005;328:739–745.

43. Blair HC, Robinson LJ, Zaidi M. Osteoclast signalling pathways. *Biochem Biophys Res Commun* 2005;328:728–738.

44. Glimcher MJ. The nature of the mineral phase of bone: biological and clinical implications. In: Avioloi L, Krane S, eds. *Metabolic Bone Disease and Clinically Related Disorders.* 3rd ed. San Diego: Academic Press; 1998:23–50.

45. Robey P, Boskey A. Extracellular matrix and biomineralization of bone. In: Favus MJ, ed. *Primer on the Metabolic Bone Diseases and Disorders of Mineral Metabolism.* 5th ed. Washington, DC: American Society for Bone and Mineral Research; 2003:38–45.

46. Canalis E. Osteogenic growth factors. In: Favus MJ, ed. *Primer on the Metabolic Bone Diseases and Disorders of Mineral Metabolism.* 5th ed. Washington, DC: American Society for Bone and Mineral Research; 2003:28–31.

47. Posner AS. The mineral of bone. *Clin Orthop Relat Res* 1985:200:87–89.

48. Posner A. Bone mineral and the mineralization process. In: Peck W, ed. *Bone and Mineral Research.* Vol. 6. Amsterdam: Elsevier; 1988:65–116.

49. Olsen BR. Bone morphogenesis and embryological development. In: Favus MJ, ed. *Primer on the Metabolic Bone Diseases of Mineral Metabolism.* 5th ed. Philadelphia: Lippincott Williams & Wilkins; 2003:9–13.

50. Mundy G, Chen D, Oyajobi BO. Bone remodeling. In: Favus MJ, ed. *Primer on the Metabolic Bone Diseases and Disorders of Mineral Metabolism.* 5th ed. Washington, DC: American Society for Bone and Mineral Research; 2003:46–58.

51. Linsenmayer TF, Eavey RD, Schmid TM. Type X collagen: a hypertrophic cartilage-specific molecule. *Pathol Immunopathol Res* 1988;7:14–19.

52. Poole AR, Matsui Y, Hinek A, Lee ER. Cartilage macromolecules and the calcification of cartilage matrix. *Anat Rec* 1989;224:167–179.

53. Poole AR, Pidoux I. Immunoelectron microscopic studies of type X collagen in endochondral ossification. *J Cell Biol* 1989;109:2547–2554.

54. Provot S, Schipani E. Molecular mechanisms of endochondral bone development. *Biochem Biophys Res Commun* 2005;328:658–665.

55. van der Eerden BC, Karperien M, Wit JM. Systemic and local regulation of the growth plate. *Endocr Rev* 2003;24:782–801.

56. Kronenberg HM. Developmental regulation of the growth plate. *Nature* 2003;423:332–336.

57. Shapiro F, Holtrop ME, Glimcher MJ. Organization and cellular biology of the perichondrial ossification groove of ranvier: a morphological study in rabbits. *J Bone Joint Surg Am* 1977;59:703–723.

58. Olsen BR, Reginato AM, Wang W. Bone development. *Annu Rev Cell Dev Biol* 2000;16:191–220.

59. Canalis E, McCarthy T, Centrella M. The regulation of bone formation by local growth factors. In: Peck W, ed. *Bone and Mineral Research.* Vol. 6. Amsterdam: Elsevier; 1989:27–56.

60. Takeda S. Central control of bone remodeling. *Biochem Biophys Res Commun* 2005;328:697–699.

61. Pogoda P, Priemel M, Rueger JM, Amling M. Bone remodeling: new aspects of a key process that controls skeletal maintenance and repair. *Osteoporos Int* 2005;16(suppl 2):S18–S24.

62. Eriksen EF. Normal and pathological remodeling of human trabecular bone: three dimensional reconstruction of the remodeling sequence in normals and in metabolic bone disease. *Endocr Rev* 1986;7:379–408.

Joints

5

Peter G. Bullough

INTRODUCTION

Bone, cartilage, ligaments, and tendons have primarily a mechanical function: providing movement, stability, and protection. Unlike the liver or kidneys, which are composed mainly of cellular elements with a metabolic function, the connective tissues are mostly formed of an extracellular material (or matrix) made up of substances to resist the tensile and compressive forces to which they are subjected.

THE NORMAL JOINT

The ends of contiguous bones together with their soft tissue components, including cartilage, ligaments, and synovium, constitute a functioning unit: the joint. There are three types of joints. The most common is the diarthrodial joint, which is a cavitated movable connecting unit between two bones. (Hyalin cartilage covers the articulating surfaces of the diarthrodial joints, with the exception of the sternoclavicular and temporomandibular joints, which are covered by fibrocartilage.) The second type is the amphiarthrodial joint, typified by the intervertebral disk and characterized by limited mobility. The third type is the

fibrous synarthrosis, such as the skull sutures, which are nonmovable joints and will not be discussed further.

Diarthrodial Joint

Histology makes more sense when we have an understanding of both the function and dysfunction (i.e., the pathology) of the joint. In the diarthrodial joint normal function is characterized by: the maintenance of stability during use; freedom of the opposed articular surfaces to move painlessly over each other within the required range of motion; and an equitable distribution of load across joint tissues. Conversely clinical joint dysfunction is characterized by instability, loss of motion, maldistribution of load, and pain.

The three interdependent aspects of normal joint function depend on the shape of the joint, the mechanical properties of the extracellular matrices of the various tissues, and the integrity of the neuromuscular control.

The Shape

Perhaps the most obvious feature of any joint is the shape of its articulating surfaces. In general, one surface is convex and the other concave. The convex side of the articulation

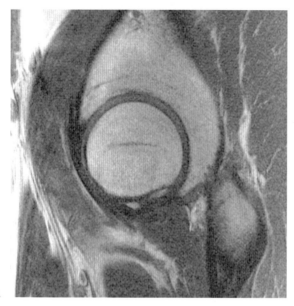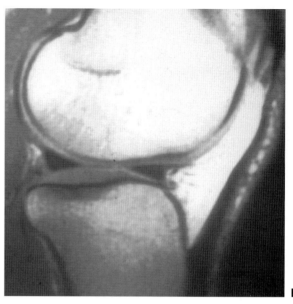

A   B

Figure 5.1 A. Sagittal section through the hip joint seen by MRI shows a close fit between the acetabulum and femoral head. **B.** Lateral MRI of a normal knee shows the gross incongruity of the articular surfaces. This is partially corrected by the interposed menisci, which act as load-bearing structures.

usually has a larger surface than the concave side. These complementary shapes permit the normal range of motion, as well as providing stability and equitable loading during use.

In some joints at first sight the articular surfaces appear to fit exactly (i.e., they appear congruent) (e.g., the hip and the ankle) (1). However, in other joints (e.g., the knee and finger joints), it is readily apparent that the surfaces are incongruent (Figure 5.1).

In a movable joint, congruence in all positions of the joint would necessitate that all joint surfaces were either perfectly spherical or cylindrical, which obviously they are not. Therefore no joint can be congruent in all positions (though in every joint there is usually a position in which it is *most* congruent) (2).

In some joints, of which the knee is a notable example, the gross incongruencies of the opposed surfaces are partially compensated for by the interposed, pliable intra-articular fibrocartilaginous menisci (3). The menisci constitute an important component contributing to joint morphology and function and cannot be removed or damaged without significant consequences.

In many joints, perhaps most, the initial contact between the opposed articular surfaces seems to be at the periphery of the joint. However, because the tissues that make up the articulating surfaces (particularly the cartilage but also the bone) undergo elastic deformation when loaded, the surfaces come into increasing contact as the load increases, thereby distributing the load more equitably (Figure 5.2).

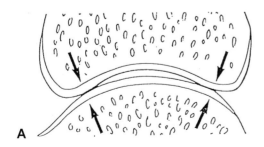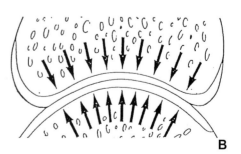

A   B

Figure 5.2 A. Light load. At rest and under light load, limited contact at the joint periphery assures access for synovial fluid to the joint space. **B.** Increased load. With increasing load, deformation of the bone and cartilage allow increased contact of the cartilage surfaces and an equitable distribution of the load. Cyclical loading permits circulation of the synovial fluid in the joint and between the articular surfaces to provide for the metabolic needs of the cartilage.

The incongruence, the deformation of the joint space under load, and the movement of the joint provide for the circulation and mixing of the synovial fluid, which, because the articular cartilage has no blood supply, are essential to the metabolism of the chondrocytes.

The Mechanical Properties of the Extracellular Matrices

In 1743, William Hunter (4) noted that:

> The articulating cartilages are most happily contrived to all purposes of motion in those parts. By their uniform surface, they move upon one another with ease; by their soft, smooth and slippery surface, mutual abrasion is prevented; by their flexibility, the contiguous surfaces are constantly adapted to each other and the friction diffused equally over the whole; by their elasticity, the violence of any shock, which may happen in running, jumping, etc. is broken and gradually spent; which must have been extremely pernicious, if the hard surfaces of bones had been immediately contiguous.

These mechanical properties of articular cartilage (as of all other connective tissues) are determined by the extracellular matrices.

In each of the different connective tissues (bone, cartilage, ligament, etc.), as well as in each particular anatomic structure, the matrices have a unique composition and structural organization that provide for mechanical function at that locus. Disturbances in the structure and/or composition of the extracellular matrix of articular cartilage may result in joint dysfunction, and we should add that, since the joint also includes the bone beneath the cartilage as well as the capsule and ligaments, alterations in the mechanical properties of bone or disruption of the ligaments could have equally disastrous effects on joint function. Clearly some knowledge of the matrix components is necessary to an understanding of connective tissue diseases.

The connective tissue matrices are mostly synthesized and to some extent broken down by their intrinsic cells (e.g., fibroblasts, osteoblasts, osteoclasts, chondrocytes). In maintaining the physicochemical and mechanical properties of tissues, the metabolism of these cells must be subject to highly sensitive feedback systems involving both local and systemic factors.

Collagen fibers, the principal extracellular component of connective tissues, are made up of bundles of fibrils, which in turn, are composed of stacked molecules formed from polypeptide chains arranged in a helical pattern. Fourteen different types of collagen molecule are now known, and these vary both in size and configuration (5).

Type I collagen is both the most common form of collagen and the major form of collagen found in skin, fascia, tendon, ligaments, and bone. Many other types of collagen are also aligned in a staggered array to form collagen fibrils. However there are also nonfiber-forming collagens that have varying functions, such as acting as binding sites for other matrix components (type IX collagen) or facilitating calcification (type X collagen) (6).

Articular hyalin cartilage has a unique type of collagen, type II, which is structurally characterized by three triple helical α-1 (II) chains. The type II fibrillar network gives articular cartilage its tensile strength and, together with the proteoglycans, is essential for maintaining the tissues volume and shape (7).

The fibrillar collagens provide tensile strength. However, connective tissues are also subjected to compression. In bone, the compressive load is resisted by hydroxyapatite. In cartilage, it is the filler between the collagen fibers that provides the compressive strength of the tissue, as well as its viscoelastic properties. This filler is composed of large negatively charged macromolecular proteoglycan aggregates.

Proteoglycans (PGs) are a group of heterogenous molecules, consisting of protein chains and attached carbohydrates, which have a sticky gel-like quality. The major PG in cartilage is aggrecan (8), containing a protein core of Mr 2.15×10^5 to which carbohydrate side chains (keratan and chondroitin sulfate) are attached. The core protein, which contains three globular domains, interacts with hyaluronic acid, and this interaction is stabilized by link protein. As many as 200 aggrecan molecules bind to one hyaluronic acid chain (Mr $1-2 \times 10^6$) to form an aggregate (Mr 5×10^7 to 5×10^8).

The highly charged PG molecules attract water and swell considerably. However, within the cartilage, the expansion of the PGs is restricted by the collagen network to approximately 20% of the maximum possible; this creates a swelling pressure within cartilage tissue. When cartilage is loaded, some water is extruded and PGs are further compressed. Removal of the load permits the imbibing of water into the tissue, together with essential nutrients, until the swelling pressure of the PGs is again balanced by the tensile resistance of the collagen network.

Aggrecan shows an age-related decrease in size and enrichment in keratan sulfate relative to chondroitin sulfate, and these changes may relate to the observed age-dependent change in the stiffness and water content of the cartilage (9).

In addition to aggrecan, the extracellular matrix of cartilage contains many noncollagenous proteins and proteoglycans, whose precise functions are only just beginning to be understood. These molecules may serve a structural or regulatory role—and in some cases may do both—because degradation products of some of the structural molecules are known to influence the chondrocyte. The recognition of genetic disorders in which synthesis of the matrix molecules is perturbed has aided greatly in our understanding of their functional role, but the reason for many site- and age-related restrictions in expression remains unclear. This is an area where there is still a wealth of information to be mined (10).

In a mature joint, cyclic hydrostatic fluid pressure through the entire cartilage thickness is comparable in magnitude to the applied joint pressure. Prolonged

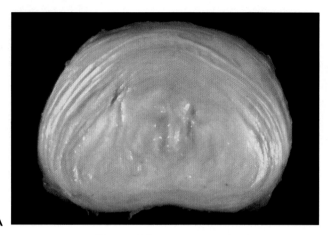

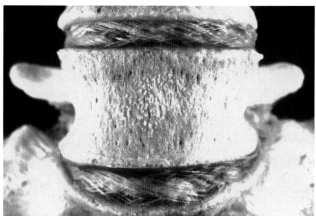

A   B

Figure 5.3 **A.** Photograph of an intervertebral disk seen in cross section. Note the layers of circumferential fibers that make up the annulus fibrosus and the well demarcated bulging central mass of the nucleus pulposus. Note also the decreasing width of the annulus from anterior (*top*) to posterior (*bottom*). **B.** In this desiccated specimen of the lower lumbar spine, the alternating oblique orientation of the collagen fibers in the annulus can be appreciated.

physical activity can cause the total cartilage thickness to decrease about 5%, although the consolidation strains vary tremendously in the superficial, transitional, and radial zones. The superficial zone can experience significant fluid exudation and consolidation (compressing strains) in the range of 60%, while the radial zone experiences relatively little fluid flow and consolidation. The topological variation in the microscopic appearance and quantitative biochemistry of articular cartilage is influenced by the local mechanical loading of chondrocytes in the different zones. Patterns of stress, strain, and fluid flow created in the joint result in spatial and temporal changes in the rates of synthesis and degradation of matrix proteins. When viewed over the course of a lifetime, even subtle differences in these cellular processes may be expected to affect the micro- and macromorphology of articular cartilage.

Capsular, Pericapsular Tissues, and Muscular Control

Any consideration of functional joint anatomy must include the capsule of the joint with its synovial lining; the ligamentous conjoining of the articulating surfaces; and the neuromuscular control of joint motion. Through the perception of touch, temperature, pain, and position, sensory feedbacks monitor our movements. Correct joint function is thus dependent on intact ligaments, muscles, and nerves. As recognized by Charcot a breakdown of neuromuscular coordination can lead to profound arthritis (11).

Amphiarthrodial Joint

The intervertebral disk can be divided into two components: the outermost fibrous ring (annulus fibrosus) and the innermost gelatinous core (nucleus pulposus).

The annulus, when viewed from above, is seen to contain fibrous tissue layers arranged in concentric circles. Each layer extends obliquely from vertebral body to vertebral body, with the fibers of one layer running in a direction opposite to that of the adjacent layer. This arrangement of alternating oblique layers provides for motion that is universal in direction (rotation, flexion and extension but restricted in degree (Figure 5.3).

The fibers of the annulus are attached by Sharpey's fibers to the bony endplates of the adjacent vertebral bodies. The fibrous lamellae are stronger and more numerous in the anterior and lateral aspects of the disk than in the posterior aspect, where they are sparser and thinner. The anterior annulus is therefore almost twice the thickness of the posterior annulus. This variation probably reflects the additional protection offered by the posterior elements of the vertebral bodies. As a result of the variation in thickness of the annulus, the nucleus pulposus typically occupies an

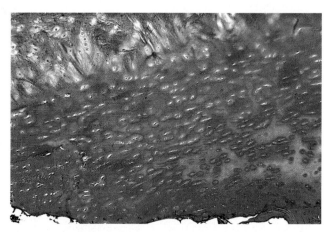

Figure 5.4 The nucleus pulposus of the disk (*top*) is separated from the bone (*bottom*) by a dense layer of hyaline cartilage, as demonstrated in this photomicrograph (H&E stain, ×4 objective).

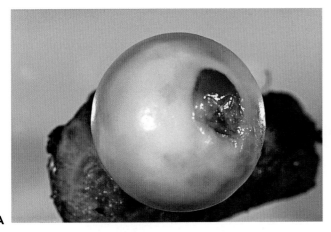
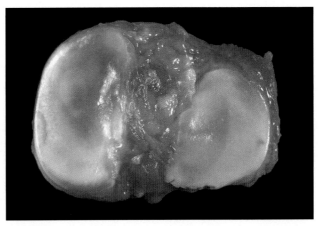

Figure 5.5 A. A femoral head, resected from a 16-year-old, demonstrates the blue-white translucency of young healthy cartilage. **B.** For comparison, the tibial plateau of a 50-year-old. The cartilage is smooth and healthy in appearance but is more yellowish in color and opaque in quality than that of the 16-year-old.

eccentric position within the disk space, being closer to the posterior margin.

The tissue of the nucleus is separated from that of the bone above and below by a clearly defined layer of hyalincartilage which extends to the inner margins of the insertion of the annulus (Figure 5.4).

On microscopic examination, the nucleus pulposus shows a varying number of stellate and fusiform cells suspended in a loose fibromyxoid matrix rich in proteoglycans.

Because no blood vessels are present in most of the adult disk tissue, nutrients must travel by diffusion from capillary beds at the disk margins. A restricted flow of nutrients to the nucleus and inner annulus may contribute to disk degeneration in the adult.

It should be noted that disk height, in general, is not the same in all segments of the spine, the cervical and thoracic disks being flatter than those of the lumbar region. There is also a variation in disk height from front to back, relative to the curvature of the spine. With age, the disk gets thinner as a result of age-related dehydration of the disk.

THE NORMAL JOINT TISSUES

Articular Cartilage

Morphology

The articular ends of the bones are covered by hyalin cartilage, which is a nerveless, bloodless, firm, and yet pliable tissue. Hyalin cartilage deforms under pressure but recovers its original shape on removal of pressure (12). In growing children, cartilage is the most obvious precursor of the bony skeleton, and it is the means by which the bones increase in length by the mechanism of endochondral ossification through the medium of the cartilaginous growth plate (physis).

In young people, hyalin cartilage is translucent and bluish-white; in older individuals, it is opaque and slightly yellowish (13) (Figure 5.5). This change in the appearance of the articular cartilage with advancing age is also seen in other connective tissues and is probably related to a number of factors, including dehydration of the tissues, increased numbers of cross linkages in the collagen, and the possible accumulation of pigment.

On microscopic examination, articular cartilage is characterized by its abundant glassy (hyalin) extracellular matrix with isolated, relatively sparse cells located in well-defined spaces (lacunae) (Figure 5.6). It is usually

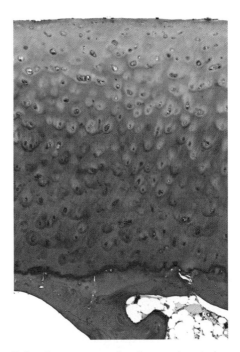

Figure 5.6 Photomicrograph of normal articular cartilage obtained from the femoral condyle of a middle-aged individual (H&E stain, ×4 objective).

described as having four layers (or zones): superficial, intermediate, deep, and calcified. In the superficial layer, the cells are flat. In the intermediate zone, the cells have a tendency to form radial groups that apparently follow the pattern of collagen disposition. In the deep zone, the cells are hypertrophied; and in the calcified zone (i.e., the zone adjacent to the bone), the cells are nonviable and the matrix is heavily calcified (Figures 5.7 and 5.8).

Within the mineralized bone matrix, the cells are connected with one another by means of cytoplasmic processes; however, no such syncytial arrangement is present within the cartilage. The chondrocytes are dependent upon the diffusion of solutes through the extracellular matrix for their metabolism. Since the matrix of the deep calcified zone of the articular cartilage effectively blocks the passage of solutes from the subchondral bone, the articular cartilage is thus dependent on the diffusion of nutrients and the exchange of metabolites from the synovial fluid through the articular surface (14).

In the late nineteenth century, Hultkranz (15) demonstrated that the precisely organized fibrous system within normal articular cartilage is readily demonstrable by the simple expedient of pricking the articular surface with a pin. When this is done, a split results; if the pricking is repeated all over the surface, a pattern of split lines is revealed that is constant for each joint from individual to individual (16) (Figure 5.9).

When the superficial layer of the cartilage is pared away and the exposed surface pricked, only small round holes appear instead of fissures. If the cut edge of the cartilage is pricked, a vertical split line is produced, and this occurs in all planes of section (Figure 5.10). If the fissures reflect the internal fiber arrangement of the cartilage, then at the articular surface the fibers run parallel to the surface and in the general direction of the split line, and in the deeper layers of the cartilage the fibers are predominantly vertical (17).

A combination of polarizing microscopy, transmission electron microscopy, and scanning electron microscopy have confirmed that the principal orientation of collagen fibers in articular cartilage is vertical through most of its thickness and horizontal at the surface (17) (Figure 5.11).

Electron microscopic studies have shown that, in the surface layer of normal articular cartilage, the collagen fibers are closely packed, of fine diameter, and mostly oriented parallel to the joint surface. The collagen content of cartilage progressively diminishes from the superficial to

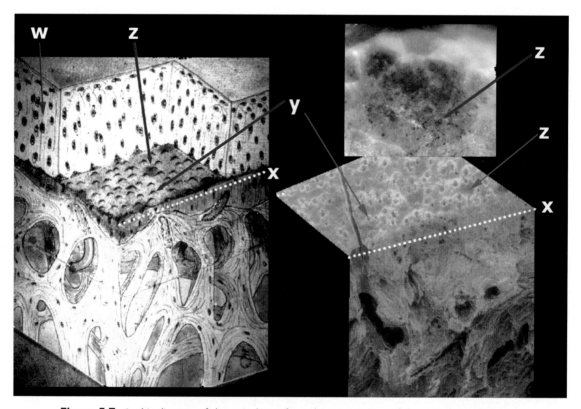

Figure 5.7 In this diagram of the articular surface, the organization of the articular surface seen on Figure 5.6 is shown diagrammatically. This distribution of the collagen arcades described by Benninghoff has been drawn in (**w**). Noncalcified articular cartilage has been removed to reveal the surface of the tidemark (**x**). The small "volcanic" structures (**y**) represent the location of the cells in the calcification front. The vessels that penetrate the calcification cartilage (**z**) are seen just beneath the calcification front. A dissection (*upper right*) shows the vessels when the cartilage has been pared away, and a scanning electron photomicrograph (*lower right*) shows the section from which the diagram was reconstructed.

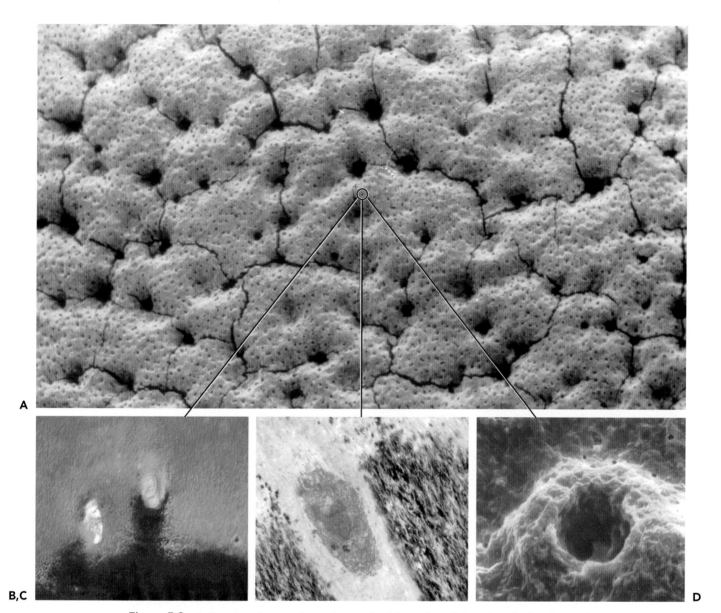

Figure 5.8 **A.** Scanning electron photomicrograph of the surface of the tidemark after the uncalcified articular cartilage had been digested away. The small dots represent chondrocytes embedded in the mineralization front (tidemark). The larger voids result from underlying vessels close to the tidemark. The cracks are preparation artifact. **B.** The appearance of chondrocytes embedded in this surface is shown in a cross sectional image of an H&E section, photomicrographed using polarized light. The same sample (as in **B**) is shown in **C.** as in a transmission electron and in **D.** as a higher power scanning image. It is hypothesized that this layer of embedded chondrocytes regulates the rate of active calcification at the tidemark.

the deep layer. In deep layers, collagen fibers are more widely separated, thicker in diameter, and are vertically aligned in such a fashion as to form a web of arch-shaped structures (18) (Figure 5.12). The collagen fibers are continuous with those in the calcified layer of cartilage but not with underlying subchondral bone. The morphology of the collagen-fibril network influences the local stresses and strains in the articular cartilage (19).

The menisci of the knee are composed mainly of collagen, although some PG is also present. Microscopic examination of carefully oriented sections has shown that the principal

orientation of the collagen fibers in the menisci is circumferential to withstand the circumferential tension within the meniscus during normal loading of the knee joint. The few small radially disposed fibers probably act as ties to resist any longitudinal splitting of the menisci that might result from undue compression (20) (Figure 5.13).

The precise organization of collagen in the cartilage, in the annulus of the intervertebral disc, and in the menisci is also present in all the connective tissues of the body (e.g., Langer's lines in the skin) and serves a mechanical function in all of these locations.

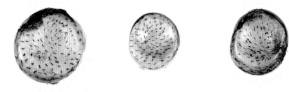

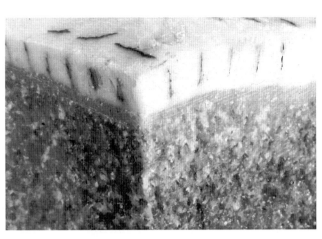

Figure 5.9 Photograph of the articular surfaces of three radial heads from three different individuals after the surfaces have been pricked with a pin whose tip had been dipped in India ink. Note the resulting pattern of split lines, which is unique for each joint in the body. Note that the pattern is similar from individual to individal.

Figure 5.10 Photograph of a portion of articular cartilage that has been sectioned vertically to show the cut edge and the underlying bone. The direction of pin pricks made on the surface can be seen; additional pin pricks have been made on the cut edge, all of which resulted in vertical splits.

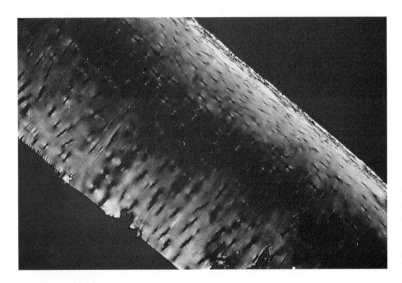

Figure 5.11 In this polarized-light photomicrograph, the surface collagen fibers can be visualized as blue, the deeper collagen fibers (which are perpendicular) as yellow. Collagen cannot be seen in the intermediate area because the fibers in this zone are decussating as in the model of Benninghoff's arcade shown in Figure 5.7 (×4 objective).

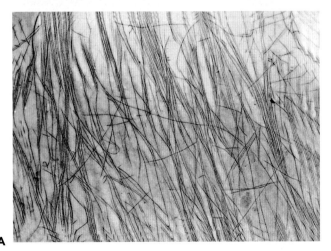

A

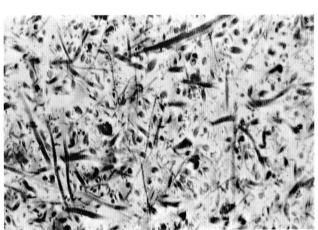

B

Figure 5.12 **A.** A transmission electron micrograph taken from tissue cut parallel to the surface collagen layer demonstrates thin closely packed and oriented fibers (×10,000). **B.** Transmission electron micrograph, taken from tissue obtained from the midzone of the cartilage and cut randomly, demonstrates variable fiber thickness and more widely separated fibers than are seen at the surface (×10,000).

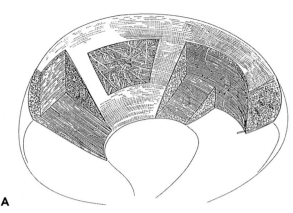

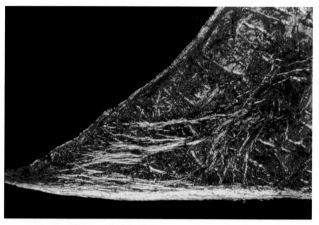

A   B

Figure 5.13 **A.** A drawing to illustrate the distribution of collagen fibers in the meniscus. The majority of the fibers are circumferentially distributed to resist the tension generated in the meniscus when the knee is under compressive load. The radially distributed fibers are most obvious on the tibial surface of the meniscus. (Modified from: Bullough PG, Munuera L, Murphy J, Weinstein AM. The strength of the menisci of the knee as it relates to their fine structure. *J Bone Joint Surg Br* 1970;52:564–567 with permission). **B.** Photomicrograph of a cross section of meniscus seen with polarized light. The tibial surface is the bottom edge where most of the fibers are radially arranged (×1 objective).

The distribution of PGs in the cartilage matrix is also related to the mechanical requirements. It varies quantitatively and possibly qualitatively from joint to joint, geographically within a single articular surface, and also as a function of age. (In general, PG distribution is more even in children than in adults.) The surface layers of the cartilage contain much less PG than do the deeper layers. In the deeper layers, there is a higher concentration of staining with safranin O and methylene blue around the cells (the pericellular matrix) than between the cells (the intercellular matrix) (21) (Figure 5.14).

Besides the PG aggregates, the articular cartilage contains other extracellular matrix proteins. Chondrocalcin (type X collagen) is a protein probably involved in the calcification process. Anchorin (type IX collagen) is a protein on the surface of chondrocytes involved in binding of these cells to extracellular matrix components, possibly transmitting altered stress in type II fibers to chondrocytes. Fibronectin, thrombomodulin, and cartilage oligomeric high Mr matrix protein are all found in cartilage, but their precise functions are not yet established.

In histologic sections stained with hematoxylin and eosin, the junction between the calcified cartilage and the noncalcified cartilage is marked by a basophilic line known as the tidemark (Figure 5.15). This basophilic line is not seen in the developing skeleton but is clearly visible in the

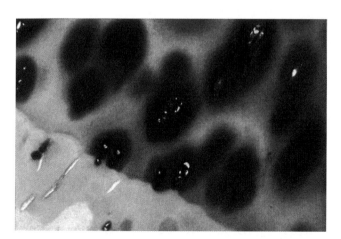

Figure 5.14 Portion of cartilage showing intense metachromasia around the chondrocytes in the deep part of the noncalcified cartilage. This represents staining of the proteoglycan. There is much less staining in the interterritorial matrix than around the cell. Even less staining is seen in the calcified cartilage (methylene blue stain, ×25 objective).

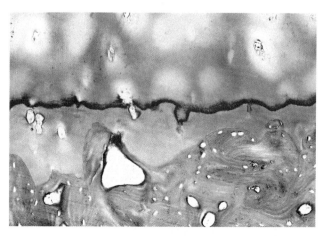

Figure 5.15 Photomicrograph of the deep and calcified layers of the articular cartilage. The deep layer is separated from the calcified layer by a basophilic line referred to as the "tidemark," which represents the mineralizing front (H&E stain, ×4 objective).

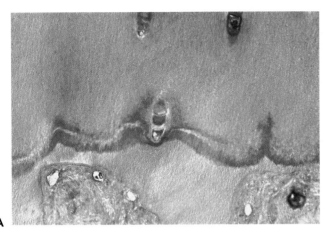
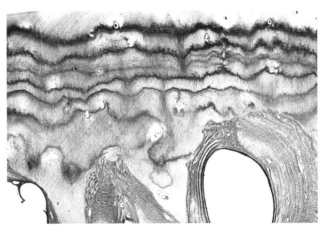

A   **B**

Figure 5.16   A. Photomicrograph demonstrating accelerated mineralization with a replicated tidemark. The mineralization front is almost certainly under cellular control; here, a chondrocyte is seen caught up in the tidemark (H&E stain, ×25 objective). **B.** In most areas of normal cartilage, only one tidemark is observed. However, in an early stage of osteoarthritis, seen here, multiple tidemarks indicating rapid advance of the mineralization front can often be seen (H&E stain, ×10 objective).

adult. In older individuals (over 60), replication of the tidemark is usually evident, and in osteoarthritic joints replication may be marked (Figure 5.16). Mechanical failure in the deep cartilage rarely, if ever, gives rise to separation at the bone cartilage interface. However, when failure occurs, it is often seen as a horizontal cleft at the tidemark, presumably because of the considerable change in the rigidity of the cartilage at this junction.

At its base, adult articular cartilage is bordered by the subchondral bone plate, and the calcified cartilage tissue is keyed into the irregular surface of the underlying bone, somewhat like a jigsaw puzzle. Because the cartilage adjacent to the bone is calcified and has a rigidity similar to that of bone, the keying is rigid (Figure 5.17).

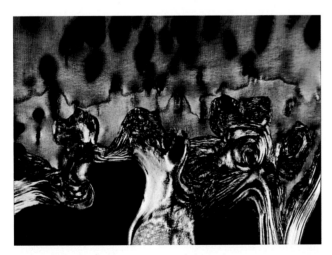

Figure 5.17   In this photomicrograph, taken with polarized light, the irregularity of the interface between the subchondral bone and the overlying calcified cartilage is obvious. The functional keying of the bone and cartilage depends on the two tissues having equal rigidity (×4 objective).

The insertions of ligaments and tendons are also calcified, and their insertions into the bone are effected by a similar keying. Because the insertions of ligament and tendons into the bone are generally studied in dry bone specimens, the bone markings we see are in fact the calcified portion of the ligament or tendon. Because the sites of such insertions are approximately the same from individual to individual, there is a tendency to think of them as static structures. However, since in the child growth is taking place continuously and in the adult bone turnover is continuously taking place (albeit slowly), it follows that the insertions of ligaments and tendons must participate in this dynamic process. (Our knowledge of anatomy is for the most part based upon the dissection of the dead; but, for morphology to be understood, time must be put into the equation. Life is characterized by continuous growth and change.)

The chondrocytes embedded in the cartilage matrix are responsible for synthesis and maintenance of the extracellular matrix of the tissue. The chondrocytes vary in size, shape, and number per unit volume of tissue, both from the superficial to the deep layers and in different anatomic locations (22) (Figure 5.18). Generally, cells at the cartilage surface are flatter, smaller, and orientated parallel with the cartilage surface. They also have a greater density than the cells deeper in the matrix (23). In the middle zones, chondrocytes are more spherical and arranged in columns. This vertical arrangement of cells probably reflects some interaction with the highly organized arrangement of collagen fibers in cartilage and suggests the possibility of movement of chondrocytes within the matrix substance as the collagen fibers are being laid down. (An analogy would be the precise organization of a spider's web that necessitates the movement of the spider.)

An interesting ultrastructural feature of chondrocytes is a nonmotile monocilium, which may have a mechan-

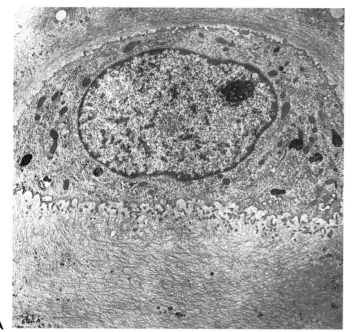

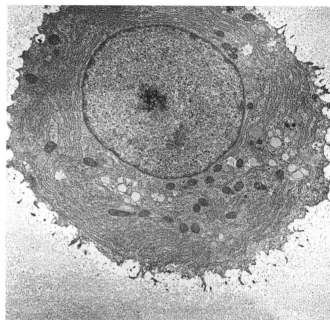

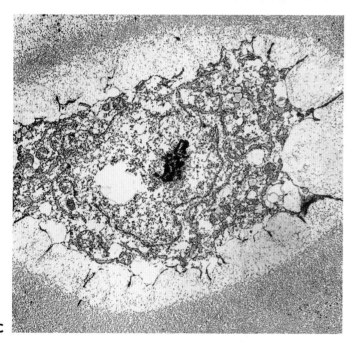

Figure 5.18 **A.** Electron micrographs to illustrate the typical appearance of chondrocytes at the **A.** surface, **B.** mid-zone, and **C.** deep-zone of articular cartilage. At the surface the cells typically show more cell processes on the inferior surface. The Golgi and endoplasmic reticulum are less well developed than in the mid-zone. In the deep zone, the cells are degenerate, with disaggregated chromatin in the nucleus and vacuolization and fragmentation of the cytoplasm (all approximately ×10,000).

otransductory function in regulation of matrix synthesis (24). This monocilium has been more frequently observed in young cartilage and reactive or reparative cartilage (25).

Chondrocytes are encased in a specialized layer of matrix distinctly different from the bulk of extracellular matrix. This layer is rich in proteoglycans, has some hyaluronic acid, and contains relatively little collagen. Around this paucicollagenous layer is a basketlike structure composed of cross-linked fibrillar collagen encapsulating the cell or sometimes groups of cells, and this provides a protective framework. Collagen type VI is found in this region.

In chondrocytes, mitochondria are sparse—probably as a result of their comparatively low rates of oxygen consumption. Cells in the deeper uncalcified zone have the most prominent endoplasmic reticulum and Golgi apparatus, indicating active protein synthesis as well as sulfation of proteoglycan carbohydrate side chains. The cell membrane shows numerous short, as well as some longer, branched cytoplasmic processes, but they make no connection with the processes of other chondrocytes. In the extracellular matrix adjacent to the chondrocytes that lie above the tidemark, as in the hypertrophic zone of the growth plate, small

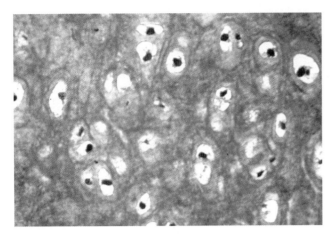

Figure 5.19 Photomicrograph of ear cartilage. Although the cells resemble those seen in hyalin cartilage, the matrix contains many elastic fibers that appear red in this section (phloxine and tartrazine stain, ×25 objective).

membrane-bound vesicles are visible. These may play a role in the calcification of cartilage matrix (26).

In addition to hyalin cartilage, of which articular cartilage is composed, two other forms of cartilage can be histologically recognized. Fibrocartilage is a tissue in which the matrix contains PG aggregates and a high proportion of type I collagen, the fibers of which are usually visible by transmitted light microscopy. Fibrocartilage may be found in the menisci of the knee, the annulus fibrosus, at the insertions of ligaments and tendons into the bone, and on the inner side of tendons as they angle around pulleys (e.g., at the malleoli). In all of these locations, the structures are subjected to compressive forces as well as tension. The second type of nonhyalin cartilage, elastic cartilage, contains a high proportion of elastin in the matrix and is found in the ligamentum flavum, external ear, and epiglottis (Figure 5.19). Compared to collagen, elastin has much greater elasticity; this is particularly important in the yellow ligaments, which make possible the flexion of the spinal canal.

Both the fibrocartilage and elastic cartilage incorporate the term "cartilage" because the cells are rounded and lie in lacunae, which give them a superficial microscopic resemblance to the cells of hyalin cartilage. However, the mechanical functions of these tissues are very different from those of hyalin cartilage. Hyalin cartilage is mainly subjected to and resists compressive forces, whereas both fibrocartilage and elastic cartilage function principally as resisters of tension, with some element of compression.

Cartilage Turnover and Articular Remodeling

Wolff's law states that both bone density and bone architecture correlate with the magnitude and direction of applied load. At the articular end of a bone, this implies that the subchondral bone trabeculae must also undergo a self-regulated modeling that maintains a joint shape capable of optimal

load distribution. In other words, the shape of bones, *including their articular ends*, reflects a dynamic state that incorporates a feedback dependent on mechanical stress.

Endochondral ossification is an important mechanism for both growth and bone modeling. This is exemplified in the epiphyseal growth plate where calcified cartilage is invaded by blood vessels from the metaphyseal bone and is then replaced by bone tissue synthesized by osteoblasts lying close to the blood vessels.

Studies of adult joints have shown that replacement of the calcified layer of articular cartilage by bone tissue involves a similar process. Blood vessels from the subarticular bone penetrate the calcified cartilage, and new bone is laid down alongside the channels created by this process; thus the calcified cartilage is slowly replaced by new subarticular bone (Figure 5.20).

Replacement of the calcified layer of cartilage by bone might be expected to result in thinning and eventual disappearance of the calcified cartilage. However, histologic study of articular cartilage from subjects of various ages shows that the calcified cartilage remains much the same thickness throughout life. This is because the calcification front (tidemark) continues to advance into the noncalcified cartilage at a slow rate, which is in equilibrium with the rate of absorption of the calcified cartilage from the subarticular bone (27). Since the thickness of the articular cartilage does not significantly change during life, it can be postulated that articular cartilage is not a static tissue, as it was long believed to be. The extracellular matrix and the chondrocytes are being replaced throughout life; and, through these mechanisms, the joint undergoes continuous modeling. It seems likely that programmed cell death (apoptosis) plays an important role in this process in a similar way to what Mitrovic (28) has demonstrated in joint formation during limb development (29).

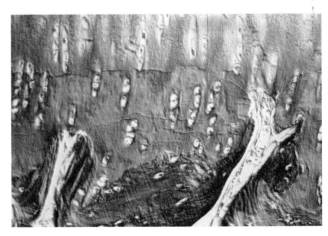

Figure 5.20 In this photomicrograph, two vessels can be seen that have extended into the calcified layer of cartilage. Around the circumference of each of these vessels, a thin layer of lamellar bone can be appreciated. By means of continuing endochondral ossification, the articular bone end is continuously modeled (H&E stain, ×10 objective).

Heterogeneity of articular cartilage, including morphological, biochemical, and biomechanical variations, can be observed within different regions of a normal weight-bearing joint. Considerable variation in cartilage thickness over an articular surface is present in most joints. A variation in stiffness in different areas of the femoral head has been related both to PG content and to the amount of water held by the tissue (30). The stiffness of the cartilage is the main factor that determines stress in the tissue and, together with the thickness of the cartilage, has the largest effect on the stress in the calcified cartilage and underlying cancellous bone (31).

An example of the normal geographic variation in articular cartilage can be readily observed in the human tibial plateau, as well as in other animals, where there are distinct morphological differences between the articular cartilage that is covered by the meniscus and that which is not (32).

These differences consist of a rough surface and soft matrix in the uncovered area as compared to the smooth, firm tissue that is covered by the meniscus. In adult human knee joints at autopsy, it has been found that articular cartilage that was not covered by meniscus (even as young as 17 years of age) always showed matrix softening and superficial fibrillation (33). The morphologic and biochemical findings in these two distinct articular areas as studied in the adult dog are summarized in Figure 5.21.

It has been postulated that these naturally occurring variations in matrix structure and mechanical properties are related to joint loading. In the normally functioning knee, load is transmitted through the meniscus and onto the tibial cartilage underlying the meniscus, whereas the exposed cartilage, that which is not covered by the meniscus, remains relatively unloaded. Similar areas of possible disuse atrophy have been described around the rim of the radial head, in

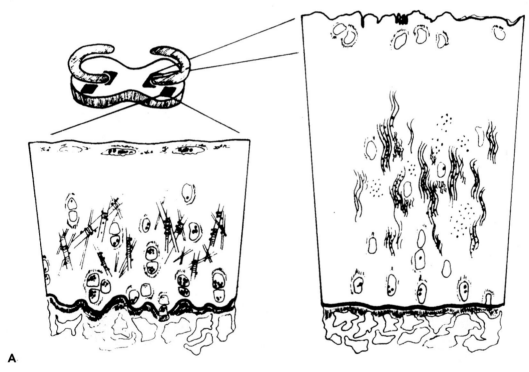

A

B

Figure 5.21 Morphological and chemical differences seen in the tibial articular cartilage under the meniscus, as compared with that not covered by the meniscus. **A.** In the covered area, the surface is smooth, and on the surface there is an amorphous electron-dense layer; the chondrocytes are flattened. With respect to lipid, there is an increased intracellular accumulation in all three layers. Increased accumulation of extracellular lipid is noted at the surface, and there are increased numbers of extracellular matrix vesicles in the deep zone. In electron microscopy sections, collagen appears as randomly oriented fibers of varying diameter but with thicker mean diameter than seen in B; there is regular binding of proteoglycan to the collagen fibrils; and the concentration of proteoglycans per wet weight is increased. The tidemark is irregular. **B.** In the uncovered area, the surface is irregular, there is a detached electron-dense layer, and the chondrocytes are rounded. The concentration of water per unit volume is increased. Collagen appears in wavy aggregated bundles with thinner mean diameters that vary but little from each other, and binding of proteoglycan to the collagen fibrils is ill defined. Proteoglycan can be extracted more easily from the cartilage matrix. The tidemark is smooth. In both the covered and the uncovered areas, the cell size is the same histologically, and there is the same amount of DNA per dry weight of cartilage tissue. (Modified from: Bullough PG, Yawitz PS, Tafra L, Boskey AL. Topographical variations in the morphology and biochemistry of adult canine tibial plateau articular cartilage. *J Orthop Res* 1985;3:1–16 with permission.)

the roof of the acetabulum, and on the perifoveal and inferomedial aspects of the femoral head (34).

The extracellular matrix of the cartilage and of the other connective tissues is synthesized by their intrinsic cells under the control of both local and systemic factors. Both in vivo and in vitro studies have demonstrated that changes in the immediate environment of the joint lead to alterations of the cartilage matrix (35). Thus, immobilization or unloading of a joint results in decreased synthesis of glycosaminoglycans. Conversely, exercise appears to increase synthesis (36). These experimentally induced variations are in agreement with naturally observed topographic variations in joints that have been ascribed to normally occurring patterns of joint loading.

In general, it seems that low levels of mechanical stress (i.e., below the physiologic range) are associated with enhanced catabolic activity, whereas stress within the physiologic range is associated with more anabolic activity. Under conditions of supraphysiologic stress the chondrocytes are unable to adapt. In other words, there is a window of physiologic stress above or below which the chondrocytes cannot maintain an adequate functional matrix.

Although a number of factors have been implicated in the transduction of mechanical stimuli to metabolic events, the exact mechanism still remains unclear.

Histomorphogenesis of Articular Cartilage

Recent studies suggest that the histomorphogenesis of articular cartilage is regulated during skeletal development by the intermittent forces and motions acting at the site of diarthrodial joints. A key feature in this development is the formation of the superficial, transitional, radial, and zones through the cartilage thickness. The histomorphological and mechanical characteristics of these zones have been correlated with the distribution of pressures, deformations, and pressure-induced fluid flow created in vivo (31). However, unlike muscle and bone, the thickness of articular cartilage does not appear to adapt to mechanical stimulation (38).

Synovial Membrane

The synovial membrane lines the inner surface of the joint capsule and all other intra-articular structures, with the exception of articular cartilage and the meniscus. In addition to lining the joints, synovial membrane lines (a) the subcutaneous and subtendinous sacs known as bursae, which permit freedom of movement over a limited range for the structures adjacent to the bursae, and (b) the sheaths that form around tendons wherever they pass under ligamentous bands or through osseofibrous tunnels.

Synovial membrane consists of two components. The first of these is the cellular lining (or intimal layer) bound-

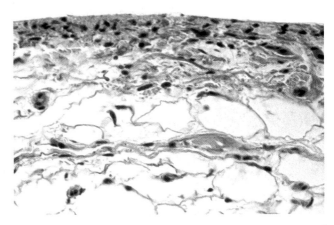

Figure 5.22 Photomicrograph of normal synovium. The ratio of fat-to-fibrous tissue varies depending on the joint and the location within the joint (H&E, ×10 objective).

ing the joint space. This surface is smooth, moist, and glistening, with a few small villi and fringelike folds. The second component is a subintimal, supportive, or backing layer (39).

Along the edge facing the synovial cavity, microscopic examination of synovial membrane reveals a single row or sometimes multiple rows of closely packed cells with large elliptical nuclei (Figure 5.22). Beneath the surface layer in the subintima, there is vascularized fibro-adipose tissue that contains some histiocytes, and mast cells.

Electron microscopic studies reveal two principal types of synovial lining cells, designated by Barland as Types A and B. (Many cells have features of both types and have been called intermediate.) The less common cell (Type A) has many of the features of a macrophage, and there is good evidence that it is structurally adapted for phagocytic functions. The more common Type B cells are richly endowed with rough endoplasmic reticulum, contain Golgi systems, and often show pinocytotic vesicles. Normal synovial intima contains 25% Type A and 75% Type B cells (40).

The synovial membrane has three principal functions: secretion of synovial fluid hyaluronate (Type B cells); phagocytosis of waste material derived from the various components of the joint (Type A cells); and regulation of the movement of solutes, electrolytes, and proteins from the capillaries into the synovial fluid, thus providing for the metabolic requirement of the joint chondrocytes and possibly also providing a regulatory mechanism for maintenance of the matrix through the role of various mediators.

Ligaments and Tendons

Ligaments, which are structures that join together two adjacent bones, are formed mainly of collagen. The arrangement of the collagen bundles within a particular ligament depend on the required movements within the joint; and, because these movements are complex, the arrangement of the collagen bundles is similarly complex.

The collagen fibers of the ligament are calcified where they enter the bone, and the calcified portion of the ligament interdigitates and locks onto the underlying bone in the same way as does the calcified cartilage (vide supra). Just adjacent to the calcified portion of the ligament, the extracellular matrix of the ligament will be found to contain some proteoglycan; and, in association with this finding, the cells will be found to be contained within lacunaelike chondrocytes (41). The reason for this is that generally tendons enter the bone at an acute angle; for this reason a shear force acts on the ligament at its insertion and the normal tension in the ligament is complicated by an added compressive force (Figure 5.23).

Tendons are specialized connective tissue structures that enable muscles to concentrate or extend their action. The Achilles tendon is a good example of a tendon that concentrates the power of several bulky muscles to one limited area of insertion; the long tendons of the hands and feet exemplify the function of extending the effect of distant muscles. Many muscles have no obvious tendinous insertions; for example the paravertebral and the gluteal muscles have short fan shaped fibrous insertions, which hardly justify their description as tendons.

The majority of cells within normal tendons are relatively inactive fibrocytes scattered in a sparse longitudinal pattern between the collagen bundles (Figure 5.24). There is a slight gradient in the cell population, the proximal (muscular) portion of the tendon being more cellular than its distal

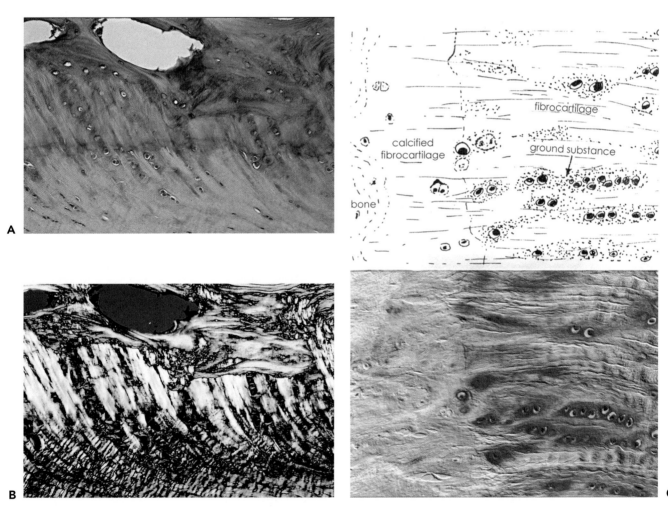

Figure 5.23   A. Photomicrograph of a ligamentous insertion using transmitted white light (H&E stain, ×10 objective). **B.** Polarized light. The portion of the ligament that interfaces with the bone is calcified, and the edge of the calcified portion of the ligament is marked by a basophilic line (tidemark) that represents the mineralization front. Note the similarity with the bone cartilage interface illustrated in Figure 5.17. **C.** A higher powered view to demonstrate the rounded cells lying in lacunae, which are seen at the insertion site of both ligaments and tendons (fibrocartilaginous metaplasia). The red staining in the matrix indicates the presence of proteoglycans (safranin O stain, ×25 objective).

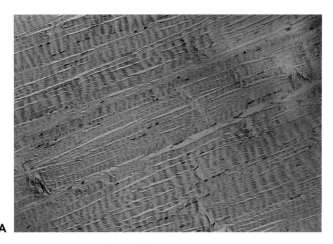
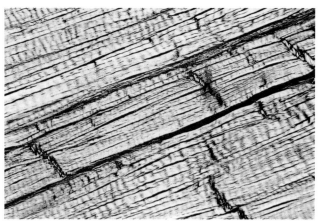

A   B

Figure 5.24   Photomicrograph of the same field of a tendon that has been photographed in transmitted light in **A** and in polarized light in **B**. Both images demonstrate the scant and elongated fibroblasts lying between the dense parallel collagen bundles characteristic of tendon (H&E stain, ×4 objective).

insertion. The surfaces of the flexor tendons of the hand which glide within a synovial sheath, are covered by a single layer of synovial cells (the endotenon) and a similar layer covers the parietal surface of the fibrous tendon sheath (the epitenon). In the palm of the hand the tendons are covered by a fine vascular adventitia (paratenon) nourished by vessels from the deep palmar arch (42).

The feeding arteries to the tendons of the hands and feet, both the vessels in the vinculae, and the vessels in the palmar or plantar paratenon are long, coiled vessels that can stretch as the tendons move. (The flexor tendons may glide some 6 cm between full flexion and full extension.)

Human tendons are poorly innervated. Apart from the nerve fibers associated with blood vessels and the free nerve endings in the region of the vinculae, there are very few nerve endings in the tendon proper.

Wherever a tendon turns a corner, or has to bend in association with neighboring joints, it is restrained under a pulley, or retinacular system, and is lubricated in this region by means of a synovial sheath. Because of the compression that occurs in these locations, just as at the insertion of the tendon or ligament, there is some cartilaginous metaplasia with the accumulation within the tissue of PGs that resist the compressive component of the load.

THE ARTHRITIC JOINT

Clinical arthritis is the consequence of a breakdown in the joint's normal function; that is to say, it involves loss of capacity for the articulating surfaces to move over one another easily, loss of joint stability, and almost always pain.

The loss of freedom of motion may be the result of a change in joint shape that results in severe incongruities or, on the other hand, a change in the tissue matrices that affects

their mechanical properties. Instability may result from alterations in ligamentous support and neuromuscular control. Pain may originate in the bone as a result of maldistribution of load; in the synovium as a result of reactive synovitis; or in the muscle as a consequence of reflex spasm.

Malfunction of a joint results from acute or chronic morbid conditions that produce either:

- Anatomic alterations in the shape of the articulating surfaces (e.g., a transarticular or subarticular fracture, increased modeling activity, Paget's disease, or acromegaly) (43).
- Loss of structural integrity of the cartilage tissue or of the support structures around the joint (e.g., by enzymatic destruction in inflammatory arthritis [septic or rheumatic arthritis] or, more commonly, traumatic injury).
- Alterations in the mechanical properties of the tissue matrices making up the joint (e.g., brittle collagen as occurs in ochronosis).

During the past century, several types of arthritis have been well delineated on the basis of their characteristic clinical presentations and their morbid anatomy. These include the infectious arthritides, both granulomatous (TB) and pyogenic (septic); the metabolic arthritides (e.g., gout, pseudogout, and ochronosis); and the arthritis that complicates many cases of aseptic subchondral bone necrosis (44). The various "rheumatic syndromes" have been classified according to their clinical and immunologic characteristics; histologically, these inflammatory arthritides show chronic synovitis and a destructive pattern involving the bone, cartilage, and periarticular structures. However, they are difficult to differentiate from each other solely by microscopic examination.

Even when these various etiologies have been considered, there remain a large number of cases of arthritis affecting especially certain small joints of the hands and feet and some larger joints, of which the hip and knee are most commonly involved. These cases, which run a chronic course, are essentially noninflammatory and usually occur in older individuals. The clinical presentation and morbid anatomy in these cases are similar enough for all of them to be classified under the general appellation of *osteoarthritis* or *degenerative joint disease*. In the majority of cases, the etiology is unclear; however, the important role of mechanical trauma is not in dispute. The onset of osteoarthritis in middle age can often be traced in sport-related injuries in adolescence and young adulthood. Repetitive impact loading, such as occurs in running on hard surfaces with poorly designed shoes, is recognized as contributing to knee arthritis. A study designed to understand the relationship between impactor energy and mass on injury modalities in the canine knee has shown that injuries were typically more frequent and more severe with the largest mass at each energy level. Histologic analysis of the patellae revealed cartilage injuries at low energy, with deep injuries in the underlying bone at higher energies (45).

Alteration in Shape

A change in joint shape is characteristic of most forms of arthritis. In the inflammatory arthritides tissue loss results from destruction. On the other hand, although bone and cartilage loss play an important part in the osteoarthritic process, it is the addition of new bone and cartilage in the form of osteophytes, particularly at the joint periphery and sometimes beneath the articular surface, that forms one of the characteristic features of the disease.

We now recognize that a change in joint shape—either sudden, as with a fracture, or gradual, as in acromegaly or other metabolic disturbances such as Paget's disease—may play an important role in the etiology of arthritis. In other words a change in the shape of the joint is an expected result of arthritis, but a change in shape may also be the cause of arthritis.

TISSUE RESPONSE TO INJURY

Regardless of the etiology, joint injury is characterized by certain basic cellular and tissue responses.

- There is usually macroscopic and microscopic evidence of both degeneration and of repair in the cells and in the extracellular matrix. (In the extracellular matrix, the changes may result from direct physical injury, from alteration in the cellular synthesis of the matrix, or from enzymatic breakdown of the matrix constituents. These changes are probably most apparent in the surface cartilage (46).
- In the vascularized tissues, injury is followed by an acute and then by a chronic inflammatory response. As a result, the necrotic injured tissue is removed and replaced by proliferative vascular tissue (granulation tissue). The inflammatory response results in "repair" of injured tissue by fibrous scar. Independently of scarring, a second mode of repair involves regeneration of tissue similar to that which was injured originally. In nonvascularized tissue, such as cartilage, an inflammatory response and subsequent scarring cannot occur, but this does not preclude tissue regeneration. Note that cartilage injury always eventually invokes an inflammatory response since some vascularized tissues (i.e., bone and/or synovium) are inevitably involved.

Cartilage

Macroscopic (naked eye) evidence of injury to cartilage is evident only in the extracellular matrix, mainly the collagenous component; one of the earliest findings is a disruption of the collagen fibers at the surface, which, instead of being smooth, becomes rough and/or eroded (47). The local stresses and strains in the collagen fibrils, which cause the damage, cannot be determined dependably without taking the local arcadelike collagen-fibril structure into account (21). Three patterns of macroscopic alteration involving the cartilage surface and, to a variable degree, the underlying cartilage tissue can be identified: fibrillation (generally age related), erosion (ulceration), and cracking (probably trauma related) (48).

The term *fibrillation* is used to describe replacement of the normally smooth, shiny surface by a surface similar to cut velvet. This type of transformation can be observed both on very thick cartilage, such as the patella, and on very thin cartilage, such as that found in the interphalangeal joints. The "pile" of the fibrillated area may be short or shaggy. The junction between the fibrillated area and the adjacent normal appearing cartilage is morphologically usually well defined and generally distinct (Figure 5.25). A recent study has concluded that both microscopic magnetic resonance imaging and polarized light microscopy can detect quantitative changes in collagen fiber architecture in early osteoarthritis and also resolve topographical variation in cartilage microstructure of canine tibial plateau (49).

In this regard, continuing collaborative studies of morphology, including imaging studies, biochemistry, and biomechanics, are urgently needed.

For the morphologist, there appear to be two patterns of fibrillation. Well-defined areas of fibrillation affecting particular locations in certain joints are present in everyone from an early age (35). It is suggested by this author that these areas may be related to underloading of the cartilage. In osteoarthritic joints, there are areas of fibrillation that appear in different areas of the joint than those previously mentioned and that appear to be secondary to mechanical abrasion of the cartilage surface. The microscopic

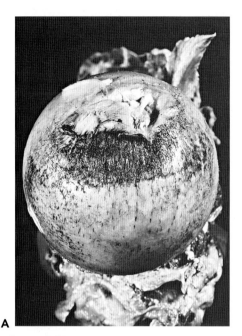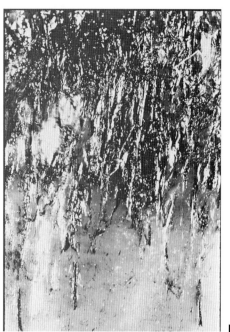

A   B

Figure 5.25   **A.** Photograph to demonstrate superficial fibrillation of the cartilage on the femoral head in the perifoveal region. The fibrillated cartilage has been highlighted by India ink. **B.** In a close up photograph, pin splits in the cartilage seem to follow the orientation of the collagen fibers in the fibrillated area.

characterization of these two distinct types of fibrillation is incomplete, but perhaps the latter is distinguished by deeper clefts and a greater tendency for the chondrocytes to form proliferating clones.

Cartilage ulceration, or solution of the surface, is characteristic of progressive degenerative changes in the joint. The base of the erosion appears initially to be either contoured or smooth. Tissue damage may eventually be so extensive as to completely denude the bone surface of its covering cartilage layer (eburnation).

The last form of structural lesion in this group, which is distinctly less common than either fibrillation or ulceration, is deep cracking of the cartilage. These cracks extend vertically deep into the cartilage and microscopically often have a deep horizontal component. Perhaps these result from severe impact loading (Figure 5.26).

In considering the pathogenesis of these three histologic types of cartilage matrix damage in the early stages of osteoarthritis, it is important to recognize that they may affect the opposed articular surfaces in different areas and to different degrees. This is in marked contrast to eburnation, in which both of the opposed surfaces are affected. It therefore appears that in many cases fibrillation and other cartilage alteration cannot be ascribed simply to abrasion.

An increase in the ratio of water to PG in the cartilage matrix leads to softening of the cartilage (chondromalacia), and this may be evidence of insufficient loading of the joint. Chondromalacia and fibrillation usually occur

together, but chondromalacia may be present before there is any obvious gross evidence of fibrillation.

Injury at a cellular level is recognizable only microscopically. Necrosis can be identified when only the ghost outlines of the chondrocytes remain. This ghosting, usually scattered but focal in distribution, is a common finding in arthritis. Less often, all of the chondrocytes are seen to be necrotic (Figure 5.27).

Just as the effect of injury to the articular cartilage is reflected by the histologic response of both matrix and cells,

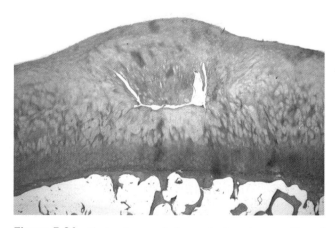

Figure 5.26   Photomicrograph demonstrating deep cracking of the cartilage matrix. The lesion shown is characteristic of a blister-like lesion, which is seen in many cases of chondromalacia patellae (H&E stain, ×4 objective).

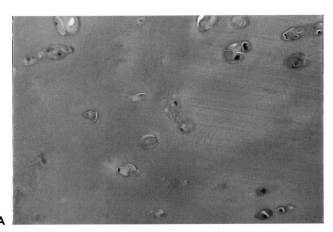
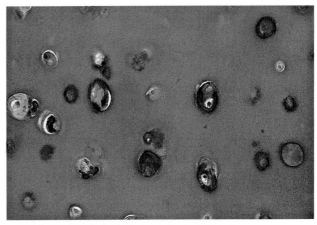

A

B

Figure 5.27 **A.** A photomicrograph to demonstrate focal chondrocyte necrosis. In cases of degenerative arthritis, focal areas of necrosis (such as seen here) are common. Rarely, the necrosis is extensive. In inflammatory arthritis, chondrocyte necrosis is also common and often associated with an irregular lysis of the matrix around the necrotic cells, the so-called Weichselbaum's lacunae (H&E stain, ×10 objective). **B.** Photomicrograph to demonstrate focal calcification around necrotic chondrocytes in the deep zone of the cartilage (H&E stain, ×25 objective).

so too is the subsequent reparative cartilage regeneration. Within the preexisting cartilage matrix, there is focal cell proliferation with clumps, or clones, of chondrocytes. When the tissue is stained with toluidine blue, there is often intense metachromasia of the matrix around these clumps of proliferating chondrocytes, evidence of increased PG synthesis. This process can be thought of as "intrinsic" repair (50) (Figure 5.28).

In a damaged joint, cartilage repair may also be initiated from either or both of two possible sites, either the joint margin or the subchondral bone. Extrinsic repair of cartilage, which develops from the joint margin, can be seen as a cellular layer of cartilage extending over, and sometimes dissecting into, the existing cartilage. This extrinsically repaired cartilage is usually much more cellular than the preexisting articular cartilage, and the chondrocytes are evenly distributed throughout the matrix (Figure 5.29).

On microscopic examination this type of repair cartilage can easily be overlooked. However, examination under polarized light will clearly demonstrate the discontinuity between the collagen network of the repair cartilage and that of the preexisting cartilage (Figure 5.30), as well as the denser thicker collagen fibers of the repair cartilage.

In arthritic joints in which loss of the articular cartilage has denuded the underlying bone, especially in cases of osteoarthritis, there are frequently small pits in the bone surface from which protrude small nodules of firm white

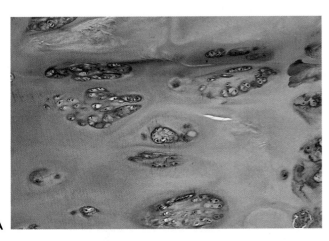
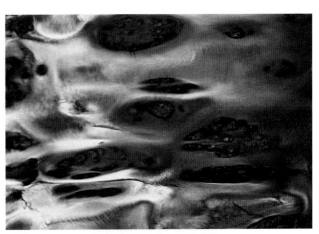

A

B

Figure 5.28 **A.** Photomicrograph to demonstrate clones of regenerating chondrocytes. Note the basophilia around the clones, which correspond to increased proteoglycan synthesis by the cells (H&E stain, ×10 objective). **B.** When examined by polarized light, the proliferating clones are visibly displacing the existing collagen matrix.

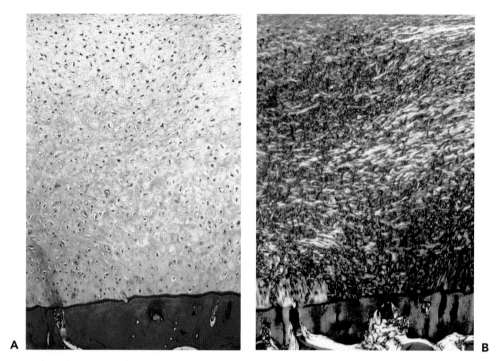

Figure 5.29 **A.** A section through the articular surface of an arthritic joint demonstrates extrinsic reparative fibrocartilage, which extends to the tidemark of the original articular hyaline cartilage (H&E stain, ×10 objective). **B.** The same field photographed with polarized light shows the discontinuity of the collagen between the calcified zone and the reparative cartilage.

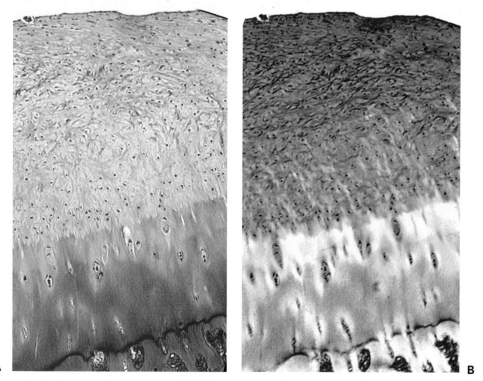

Figure 5.30 **A.** Photomicrograph showing reparative cartilage extending over preexisting damaged cartilage (H&E stain, ×4 objective). **B.** Same field photographed with polarized light.

tissue. On microscopic examination, these nodules have the appearance of fibrocartilage arising in the marrow spaces of the subchondral bone. They may extend over the previously denuded surface to form a more or less continuous layer of repair tissue. Most specimens obtained from cases of osteoarthritis reveal both intrinsic and extrinsic repair of cartilage (51).

Bone

Arthritis is a disease that affects not only the articular cartilage, but also the underlying bone and the structures around the joint.

As the articular cartilage is eroded from the surface, the underlying bone is subjected to increasingly localized overloading. In subarticular bone that has been denuded, there is proliferation of osteoblasts and formation of new bone, which occurs both on the surfaces of existing intact trabeculae and around microfractures (52) (Figure 5.31). In x-rays of arthritic joints, this new bone appears as increased density or sclerosis.

A further result of increased local stress is that the bone at the articulating surface is likely to undergo focal pressure necrosis (Figure 5.32). (This superficial necrosis is different both in its etiology and pathogenesis from that associated with "primary" subchondral infarction, which itself leads to secondary osteoarthritis. However, in clinical practice, differentiation between the two may be difficult, especially in the late stages of primary subchondral infarction.) (53)

Subarticular cysts are usually seen only where the overlying cartilage is absent. Such cysts are common in cases of osteoarthritis and are believed to result from transmission of intra-articular pressure through defects in the articulating bony surface into the marrow spaces of the subchondral

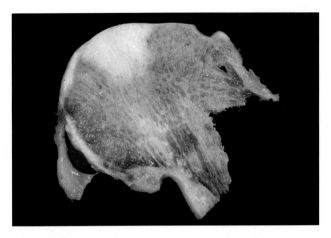

Figure 5.32 A section through an osteoarthritic femoral head shows a large wedge shaped area of necrosis of the superior portion of the head.

bone (54). The cysts increase in size until the pressure within them is equal to the intra-articular pressure.

Cysts may also occur because of focal tissue necrosis (55). (In cases of arthritis due to rheumatoid disease or gout, periarticular radiologic "cysts" may be associated with erosion of the marginal subchondral bone by the diseased synovium.)

Separated fragments of bone and cartilage from a damaged joint surface may become incorporated into the synovial membrane and digested, or they may remain free as loose bodies in the joint cavity. Under certain circumstances, proliferation of cartilage cells occurs on the surface of these loose bodies and consequently they grow larger (Figure 5.33). As they grow, their centers become necrotic and calcified. In histologic sections it is possible to visualize periodic extension of this central calcification in the form of concentric rings, which increase in number as the loose body grows larger. Sometimes the loose bodies reattach to the synovial membrane at a later stage, in which case they are invaded by blood vessels. Endochondral ossification then occurs, and the loose bodies again develop a viable bony core.

There is some degree of loose body formation in many cases of arthritis, but they are especially prominent in Charcot's joints and in other types of rapidly destructive osteoarthritis. Occasionally, in cases of osteoarthritis, the loose bodies are so numerous that they must be distinguished from those that occur in primary synovial chondromatosis (56).

Ligaments

Microscopic evidence both of lacerations and of repair by scar tissue is common in the ligamentous and capsular tissue around an arthritic joint. These changes are readily recognized by the use of polarized microscopy, where the

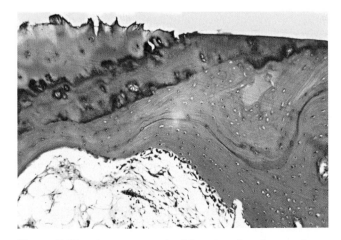

Figure 5.31 Photomicrograph of the edge of an eburnated area of bone in a case of osteoarthritis. There is a very prominent layer of osteoblasts covering the sclerotic bone that underlies the area denuded of cartilage (H&E stain, ×4 objective).

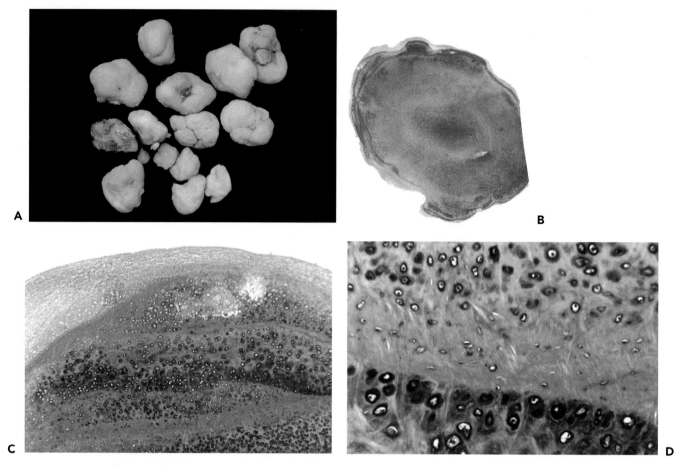

Figure 5.33 **A.** Gross photograph of multiple loose bodies in a case of osteoarthritis of the hip joint. **B.** Low-power photograph of a cross section of a loose body showing concentric growth rings (H&E stain, ×1 objective). **C.** Photomicrograph showing crowded proliferating chondrocytes and a growth ring (H&E stain, ×4 objective). **D.** Photomicrograph to show benign proliferating chondrocytes (H&E stain, ×25 objective).

alterations in the organization of the collagen are made very clear (Figure 5.34). Whether these lacerations preceded the arthritic process or whether they are a consequence of it cannot usually be determined by microscopic examination.

Synovial Membrane

Injury and breakdown of cartilage and bone result in increased amounts of breakdown product and particulate debris within the joint cavity. This is removed from the synovial fluid by phagocytic cells (the Type A cells) of the synovial membrane. In consequence, the membrane becomes both hypertrophic and hyperplastic, and the breakdown products of the cartilage and bone matrix frequently evoke an inflammatory response (Figure 5.35).

For this reason, some degree of chronic inflammation can be expected in the synovial membrane of arthritic joints, even when the injury has been purely a mechanical one. Inflammation is especially prominent where there has been rapid breakdown of the articular components as evi-

denced by the presence in the synovium of bone and cartilage detritus.

Histologic studies have shown that there may be a similarity between the degree of inflammatory response as seen in some cases of severe osteoarthritis and that of rheumatoid arthritis (57). However, in osteoarthritis the synovial inflammation is likely to be the result of cartilage breakdown, whereas in rheumatoid arthritis the synovial inflammation is the cause of cartilage breakdown.

Extension of the hyperplastic synovium onto the articular surface of the joint (i.e., a pannus) is a common finding even in osteoarthritis, particularly in the hip (Figure 5.36). However, the extent and the aggressiveness of this pannus with respect to underlying cartilage destruction is much less marked in osteoarthritis than in rheumatoid arthritis.

Since, under normal conditions, the synovial membrane is responsible for the nutrition of articular cartilage, it might be expected that the chronically inflamed and scarred synovial membrane of an arthritic joint would function less effectively than that of a normal joint. Disturbance in synovial nutrient function, as well as increased enzy-

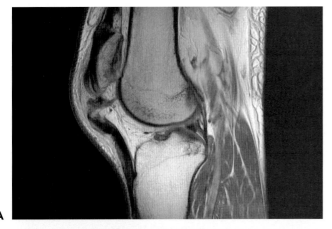

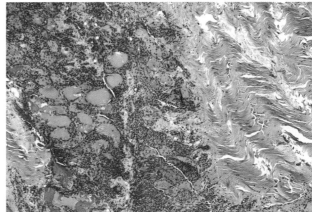

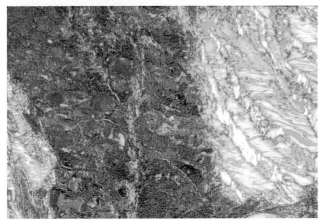

Figure 5.34 **A.** A magnetic resonance image of a knee shows rupture of the patellar ligament. **B.** Photomicrograph to demonstrate an area in a ligament where a laceration has occurred. The well-oriented collagen of the lacerated ligament is clearly demarcated from the resultant defect, which can be seen to have been filled with a vascularized cellular fibrous scar tissue (H&E stain, ×10 objective). **C.** Same field photographed with polarized light.

matic activity, may very well contribute to the chronicity of the arthritic process.

The hypertrophied and hyperplastic synovium associated with arthritis is also likely to be traumatized as it extends into the joint cavity. Evidence of bleeding into the joint, with subsequent hemosiderin staining of the synovial membrane, is a common histologic finding and may occasionally be marked. When this is the case, and despite their similar color, the orange-brown staining of the fine villous synovium seen at operation should not be confused with the swollen papillary synovium of pigmented villonodular synovitis.

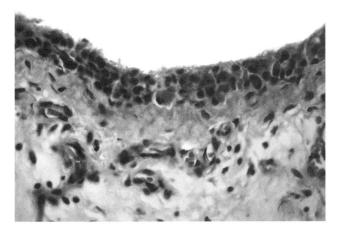

Figure 5.35 Photomicrograph of the synovium removed from the joint of a patient with a moderate degree of osteoarthritis reveals not only a hypertrophy of the synovial lining cells, but also hyperplasia that has resulted in a piling up of the synoviocytes. In the subsynovial tissue, there is increased vascularity and a mild chronic inflammatory infiltrate (H&E stain, ×25 objective).

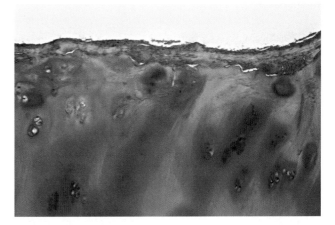

Figure 5.36 Photomicrograph of a portion of the articular surface of a femoral head in a case of osteoarthritis. A fibrous pannus extends over the articular surface (H&E stain, ×10 objective).

Synovial Fluid

Examination of synovial fluid is extremely helpful in the diagnosis of arthritis, both for determining the cause and the stage of the disease. Whatever the cause of arthritis, the synovial fluid is altered.

Normal synovial fluid, a dialysate of plasma to which hyaluronic acid produced by the Type B cells of the synovial lining is added, is viscous, pale yellow, and clear. Even in large joints the volume is small.

In cases of inflammatory arthritis, there is an increased volume of synovial fluid with a high count of inflammatory cells. The amount of hyaluronic acid is markedly diminished, leading to a typical decrease in viscosity. On the other hand, in degenerate forms of arthritis the amount of hyaluronic acid is increased, resulting in an extremely viscous fluid. There is also an increase in volume, although not to the same degree as that which is seen in the inflammatory arthritides.

REFERENCES

1. Hammond BT, Charnley J. The sphericity of the femoral head. *Med Biol Eng* 1967;5:445–453.
2. Bullough P, Goodfellow J, O'Conner J. The relationship between degenerative changes and load-bearing in the human hip. *J Bone Joint Surg Br* 1973;55:746–758.
3. Bullough PG, Walker PS. The distribution of load through the knee joint and its possible significance to the observed patterns of articular cartilage breakdown. *Bull Hosp Joint Dis* 1976;37:110–123.
4. Hunter W. On the structure and disease of articulating cartilages. *Phil Trans* 1743;42:514–521.
5. Eyre DR. Collagens and cartilage matrix homeostasis. *Clin Orthop Relat Res* 2004; 427(suppl):S118–S122.
6. Mayne R, Irwin MH. Collagen types in cartilage. In: Kuettner KE, Schleyerbach R, Hascall VC, eds. *Articular Cartilage Biochemistry.* New York: Raven Press; 1986:23.
7. Eyre DR, Wu JJ, Woods P. Cartilage-specific collagens: structural studies. In: Kuettner KE, Schleyerbach R, Peyron JG, Haskell VC, eds. *Articular Cartilage and Osteoarthritis.* New York: Raven Press; 1992:119–132.
8. Watanabe H, Yamada Y, Kimata K. Roles of aggrecan, a large chondroitin sulfate proteoglycan, in cartilage structure and function. *J Biochem (Tokyo)* 1998;124:687–693.
9. Kiani C, Chen L, Wu YJ, Yee AJ, Yang BB. Structure and function of aggrecan. *Cell Res* 2002;12:19–32.
10. Roughley PJ. Articular cartilage and changes in arthritis: noncollagenous proteins and proteoglycans in the extracellular matrix of cartilage. *Arthritis Res* 2001;3:342–347.
11. Smith MM, Gosh P. Experimental models of osteoarthritis. In: Moskowitz RW, Howell DS, Goldberg VM, Mankin HJ, eds. *Osteoarthritis:Diagnosis and Medical/Surgical Management.* 3rd ed. Philadelphia: WB Saunders; 2001:171–200.
12. Kempson GE. Mechanical properties of articular cartilage. In: Freeman MAR, ed. *Adult Articular Cartilage.* 2nd ed. London: Pitman Medical; 1973.
13. Van der Korst JK, Skoloff L., Miller EJ. Senescent pigmentation of cartilage and degenerative joint disease. *Arch Pathol* 1968;86:40–47.
14. Maroudas A, Bullough P, Swanson SA, Freeman MAR. The permeability of articular cartilage. *J Bone Joint Surg Br* 1968;50:166–177.
15. Hultkranz W. Ueber die Spaltrichtungen der Gelenkknorpel. Verhandlungen der Anatomischen Gesellschaft. 1898;12:248.
16. Bullough P, Goodfellow J. The significance of the fine structure of articular cartilage. *J Bone Joint Surg Br* 1968;50:852–857.
17. Benninghoff A. Form und Bau der Gelenkknorpel in ihren Beziehungen zur Funktion. II. Der Aufbau des Gelenkknorpels in seinen Beziehungen zur Funktion. *Z Zellforsch Mikrosk Anat* 1925;2:783–862.
18. Muir H, Bullough P, Maroudas A. The distribution of collagen in human articular cartilage with some of its physiological implications. *J Bone Joint Surg Br* 1970;52:554–563.
19. Wilson W, van Donkelaar CC, van Rietbergen B, Ito K, Huiskes R. Stresses in the local collagen network of articular cartilage: a poroviscoelastic fibril-reinforced finite element study. *J Biomech* 2004;37:357–366.
20. Bullough PG, Munuera L, Murphy J, Weinstein AM. The strength of the menisci of the knee as it relates to their fine structure. *J Bone Joint Surg Br* 1970;52:564–567.
21. Maroudas A, Evans H, Almeida L. Cartilage of the hip joint. Topographical variation of glycosaminoglycan content in normal and fibrillated tissue. *Ann Rheum Dis* 1973;32:1–9.
22. Stockwell RA, Meachim G. The chondrocytes. In: Freeman MAR, ed. *Adult Articular Cartilage.* London: Pitman Medical; 1973.
23. Stockwell RA. The interrelationship of cell density and cartilage thickness in mammalian articular cartilage. *J Anat* 1971;109:411–421.
24. Wilsman NJ. Cilia of adult canine articular chondrocytes. *J Ultrastruct Res* 1978;64:270–281.
25. Stockwell RA. The ultrastructure of cartilage canals and the surrounding cartilage in the sheep fetus. *J Anat* 1971;109(pt 3):397–410.
26. Anderson HC. Calcification processes. *Pathol Annu* 1980;15(pt 2):45–75.
27. Boskey AL, Bullough PG, Dmitrovsky E. The biochemistry of the mineralization front. *Metab Bone Dis Relat Res* 1980;2S:61–67.
28. Mitrovic D. Regression of normally constituted articular cavities in paralyzed chick embryos [in French]. *C R Acad Sci Hebd Seances Acad Sci D* 1972;274:288–291.
29. Mori C, Nakamura N, Kimura S, Irie H, Takigawa T, Shiota K. Programmed cell death in the interdigital tissue of the fetal mouse limb is apoptosis with DNA fragmentation. *Anat Rec* 1995;242:103–110.
30. Kempson GE. *Mechanical Properties of Human Articular Cartilage.* [doctoral thesis]. London:University of London; 1970.
31. Dar FH, Aspden RM. A finite element model of an idealized diarthrodial joint to investigate the effects of variation in the mechanical properties of the tissues. *Proc Inst Mech Eng H* 2003;217:341–348.
32. Bullough PG, Yawitz PS, Tafra L, Boskey AL. Topographical variations in the morphology and biochemistry of adult canine tibial plateau articular cartilage. *J Orthop Res* 1985;3:1–16.
33. Bennet GA, Waine H, Bauer W. *Changes in the Knee Joint at Various Ages: With Particular Reference to the Nature and Development of Degenerative Joint Disease.* New York: Commonwealth Fund; 1942.
34. Goodfellow JW, Bullough PG. The pattern of ageing of the articular cartilage of the elbow joint. *J Bone Joint Surg Br* 1967;49:175–181.
35. Palmoski MJ, Brandt KD. Effects of static and cyclic compressive loading on articular cartilage plugs in vitro. *Arthritis Rheum* 1984;27:675–681.
36. Palmoski M, Perricone E, Brandt KD. Development and reversal of a proteoglycan aggregation defect in normal canine knee cartilage after immobilization. *Arthritis Rheum* 1979;22:508–517.
37. Wong M, Carter DR. Articular cartilage functional histomorphology and mechanobiology: a research perspective. *Bone* 2003;33:1–13.
38. Eckstein F, Faber S, Muhlbauer R, et al. Functional adaptation of human joints to mechanical stimuli. *Osteoarthritis Cartilage* 2002;10:44–50.
39. Henderson B, Pettipher ER. The synovial lining cell: biology and pathobiology. *Semin Arthritis Rheum* 1985;15:1–32.
40. Barland P, Novikoff AB, Hamerman D. Electron microscopy of the human synovial membrane. *J Cell Biol* 1962;14:207–220.
41. Cooper RR, Misol S. Tendon and ligament insertion. A light and electron microscopic study. *J Bone Joint Surg Am* 1970;52:1–20.

42. Lundborg G, Myrhage R. The vascularization and structure of the human digital tendon sheath as related to flexor tendon function. An angiographic and histological study. *Scand J Plast Reconstr Surg* 1977;11:195–203.

43. Johanson NA. Endocrine arthropathies. *Clin Rheum Dis* 1985;11: 297–323.

44. Bullough PG, DiCarlo EF. Subchondral avascular necrosis: a common cause of arthritis. *Ann Rheum Dis* 1990;49:412–420.

45. Atkinson PJ, Ewers BJ, Haut RC. Blunt injuries to the patellofemoral joint resulting from transarticular loading are influenced by impactor energy and mass. *J Biomech Eng* 2001;123: 293–295.

46. Rieppo J, Toyras J, Nieminen MT, et al. Structure-function relationships in enzymatically modified articular cartilage. *Cells Tissues Organs* 2003;175:121–132.

47. Collins DH. *The Pathology of Articular and Spinal Diseases.* London: Edward Arnold, 1949.

48. Heine J. Über die Arthritis deformans. *Virchows Arch Path Anat* 1926;260:521–663.

49. Alhadlaq HA, Xia Y, Moody JB, Matyas JR. Detecting structural changes in early experimental osteoarthritis of tibial cartilage by microscopic magnetic resonance imaging and polarised light microscopy. *Ann Rheum Dis* 2004;63:709–717.

50. Nakata K, Bullough PG. The injury and repair of human articular cartilage: a morphological study of 192 cases of coxarthrosis. *Nippon Seikeigeka Gakkai Zasshi* 1986;60:763–775.

51. Macys JR, Bullough PG, Wilson PD Jr. Coxarthrosis: a study of the natural history based on a correlation of clinical, radiographic, and pathologic findings. *Semin Arthritis Rheum* 1980;10: 66–80.

52. Christensen SB. Osteoarthrosis. Changes of bone, cartilage and synovial membrane in relation to bone scintigraphy. *Acta Orthop Scand Suppl* 1985;214:1–43.

53. Franchi A, Bullough PG. Secondary avascular necrosis in coxarthrosis: a morphologic study. *J Rheumatol* 1992;19:1263– 1268.

54. Landells JW. The bone cysts of osteoarthritis. *J Bone Joint Surg Br* 1953;35-B:643–649.

55. Rhaney K, Lamb DW. The cysts of osteoarthritis of the hip: a radiological and pathological study. *J Bone Joint Surg Br* 1955;37-B:663–675.

56. Villacin AB, Brigham LN, Bullough PG. Primary and secondary synovial chondrometaplasia: histopathologic and clinicoradiologic differences. *Hum Pathol* 1979;10:439–451.

57. Ito S, Bullough PG. Synovial and osseous inflammation in degenerative joint disease and rheumatoid arthritis of the hip. Histometric study. Proceedings of the 25th Annual ORS 1979;199.

Myofibroblast

6

Walter Schürch   Thomas A. Seemayer   Boris Hinz
Giulio Gabbiani

DISCOVERY OF THE MYOFIBROBLAST

The myofibroblast was discovered in 1971 in electron micrographs from contracting (healing) experimental granulation tissue (1). Soon thereafter, its biochemical, pharmacologic, and immunohistochemical features were delineated (2–5). Since these early days, the list of pathologic conditions in which this cell has been identified has grown considerably (6–8). Looking back, it is somewhat surprising that such a pivotal element of diverse fundamental processes had not been defined earlier (9).

The road to discovery stems from interest in the process of wound healing as traced from the time of fossils to the ancient world (10). Indeed, the fate of civilizations rested on the ability of people to recover from wounds inflicted through battle or disease. Nearly a century ago, Carrel and Hartmann hypothesized that contractile forces were present in granulating wounds (11). For years it was believed, even taught, that collagen was the element essential for wound contraction. Dogma changed (slowly) with two reports in the mid-1950s. In one, experiments established that wound contraction was normal in guinea pigs rendered scorbutic

(12). In the other, fibroblasts, under appropriate conditions, could be induced to contract in vitro (13). These findings cast doubt on the contractility of collagen and suggested that cells were central to tissue contraction.

In 1969, Majno and colleagues performed seminal experiments that established that histamine caused postcapillary venular interendothelial gaps that brought about vascular leakage (14). In electron micrographs, such endothelial cells were shrunken, distorted, and with notched nuclei. On this basis, they reasoned that gap formation might be produced by active endothelial contraction (14). This suggestion, made before the establishment of the concept that nonmuscle cells contain contractile proteins, was not easily accepted; in turn, it stimulated work based on the possibility that endothelial and other mesenchymal cells could exert contractile activities.

A few years later, the ultrastructural observation was made that the cytoplasm of granulation tissue fibroblasts was loaded with bundles and aggregates of microfilaments (1), a feature typical of smooth muscle cells. On this basis, the possibility that these modified fibroblastic cells were responsible for granulation tissue contraction was relatively easy to suggest (1); however, acceptance took some time (15). Further experiments, employing pharmacologic agents known to effect cellular contraction/relaxation, established that granulating wounds indeed contained contractile cells, and the term *myofibroblast* was proposed (2). Subsequently, myofibroblasts were found to be capable of being decorated by human smooth muscle antibodies (4); these were then shown to be specifically directed against actin (5). Shortly thereafter, myofibroblasts were identified within nodules of Dupuytren's disease (16) and in human granulation tissue (17) and shown to transmit their contractile forces from cell to cell through intermediate (adherens) junctions and from cell to stroma by means of microtendons, the whole being synchronized by intercellular gap junctions (18). The microtendon, an apparatus connecting myofibroblasts to the surrounding extracellular matrix, was named *fibronexus* (19).

In the late 1970s, Tremblay (20) described the presence of myofibroblasts in the stroma of invasive mammary carcinomas. The neoplasms in which these myofibroblasts had been noted were firm and retracted, unassociated with an inflammatory infiltrate. Because myofibroblasts are normally not present in mammary stroma, it was suggested that they contributed to the retraction phenomena and desmoplasia, which characterized these neoplasms (20). It was then reasoned that such contractile cells might be contained in diverse carcinomas characterized by retraction and desmoplasia. Accordingly, a series of invasive and metastatic carcinomas was examined ultrastructurally. Myofibroblasts were present in the stroma of each tumor and were particularly numerous in those that were hard, sclerotic, and retracted (21). Within several years, the spatial distribution of such cells within invasive and metastatic carcinomas was described (22,23), and it was proposed that similarities between the process of wound healing and the stromal response to neoplastic invasion might exist (22).

In the following years detailed studies of intermediate filament proteins and actin isoforms of myofibroblasts in various settings and conditions were performed; this led to the finding that myofibroblasts from diverse pathologic settings were heterogeneous in their content of intermediate filaments and actin isoforms (24,25). The presence of α-smooth muscle actin, the actin isoform characteristic of vascular smooth muscle cells, was suggested as the marker of the myofibroblastic phenotype (25). In these works, it was shown that there is a correlation between the phenotypic modulation of myofibroblasts and the clinical behavior of lesions containing these cells. In particular, it was shown that myofibroblasts in granulation tissue of normally healing wounds express α-smooth muscle actin only temporarily (25), whereas myofibroblasts with a smooth muscle phenotype persist in hypertrophic scars, fibrocontractive diseases, quasi-neoplastic proliferative conditions, and within the stroma of certain neoplasms (24,26).

More recently, it was shown that transforming growth factor β1 (TGF-β1) is the most important stimulator of myofibroblastic differentiation (27,28), as well as of collagen production by this cell (29). For TGF-β1 to be active, the ED-A splice variant of cellular fibronectin must be present in the extracellular matrix (30). This provided the first hint of the mechanisms controlling the modulation of the myofibroblastic phenotype. It was also shown that myofibroblasts undergo apoptosis during the transition between granulation tissue and scar tissue (31). The possibility that myofibroblasts could arise from such specialized mesenchymal cells as hepatic perisinusoidal stellate cells (32), mesangial (33) and renal tubular cells (34), and mesothelial cells (35) was demonstrated. Quite unexpectedly, the hematogenous origin of myofibroblasts in several human and experimental pathologic settings was recently established (36,37).

In 2005, some 34 years after the initial discovery and four decades after the quest began, the myofibroblast is recognized as a central element in normal and abnormal wound healing, in diverse reactive proliferative conditions, and within the stroma of certain invasive and metastatic neoplasms.

The sections that follow more fully characterize the myofibroblast, describe the settings in which it is found, and relate recent studies that provide further insight into the biology of this unique cell.

CHARACTERIZATION OF THE MYOFIBROBLAST

Ultrastructural

As initially described in granulation tissue and nodules of Dupuytren's disease (1,16), myofibroblasts share morphologic features in common with fibroblasts and smooth muscle cells.

Fibroblasts of adult animals and humans display a slender fusiform and smooth, contoured nucleus, a well-developed Golgi area, numerous and often dilated cisternae of rough endoplasmic reticulum, scattered mitochondria, and small numbers of microfilaments, the latter sometimes arranged in discrete bundles beneath the plasma membrane. Cell contours are generally smooth or display a few short cytoplasmic extensions. Plasmalemmal attachment plaques, dense patches or dense bands (38,39), basal lamina, pinocytotic vesicles, intercellular junctions, and cell-to-stroma attachment sites are absent.

Smooth muscle cells are enveloped by a continuous basal lamina. Their plasma membrane is studded with plasmalemmal attachment plaques or so-called membrane-associated dense bodies, dense plaques, dense patches or dense bands (39), and numerous pinocytotic vesicles. Intercellular gap junctions and adherens junctions are present

(40). The cytoplasm is laden with bundles of microfilaments, usually disposed parallel to the long axis of the cell, among which numerous dense bodies are interspersed. The material of the dense bodies appears similar to the one forming the dense bands, which are attached to the cell membrane in certain vascular smooth muscle cells. Some dense bodies are in continuity with dense bands. Dense bodies and dense bands probably correspond to Z-lines of striated muscle fibers. In both structures, α-actinin has been demonstrated by immunohistochemical techniques (41,42). Force transmission from the contractile apparatus to the cell membrane in smooth muscle cells occurs via the insertion of bundles of actin filaments into the dense bands (38). Transmission of the contractile force occurs also across cell membranes of smooth muscle cells and from cell membranes to the stroma. Although it seems clear that the traction generated by the myofilaments is transmitted to the dense bands, the exact mechanism of the transmission of the traction across the cell membrane is not fully understood. The fibronectin receptor as a transmembrane receptor glycoprotein complex (43–46) has extracellular binding sites for fibronectin (47), suggesting specific interactions between cytoplasmic actin filaments and extracellular fibronectin fibers across the plasma membrane at cell-to-matrix attachment sites. A close association between bundles of cytoplasmic actin filaments (stress fibers) and bundles of extracellular fibronectin fibrils has been observed in transformed fibroblasts and in myofibroblasts of granulation tissue in vivo; this structure, designated fibronexus, is specialized for enhanced cell-to-matrix connections (48,49). Contractile forces from cell to cell are transmitted through adherens or intermediate junctions, which are symmetrical structures formed by two complementary dense bands that match each other in adjacent smooth muscle cells (38). Their nuclei are elongated with blunt ends and are deformed by shallow invaginations. In contrast to fibroblasts, the Golgi area and the rough endoplasmic reticulum are poorly developed.

Myofibroblasts (Figure 6.1 A–E) disclose irregular, often stellate, cellular outlines with numerous and long cytoplasmic extensions and are connected by intermediate or adherens junctions (Figure 6.1D) (50) and by gap junctions (Figure 6.1E), the latter considered as low-resistance pathways for intercellular communications (18). In addition, myofibroblasts are partly enveloped by a basal lamina and display plasmalemmal attachment plaques, dense patches or dense bands, and pinocytotic vesicles (Figure 6.1C). They are also connected by microtendons to the extracellular matrix by cell-to-stroma attachment sites through the fibronexus, a transmembrane complex of intracellular microfilament bundles in apparent continuity with extracellular fibronectin fibers (Figure 6.1B) (19,49). At the surface of myofibroblasts, three types of fibronexus are observed: (a) plaquelike; (b) tracklike; and (c) tandem associations (49). These cell-to-stroma attachment sites are well-developed and numerous in myofibroblasts compared with their attenuated appearance in smooth muscle cells. Myofibroblasts contain numerous bundles of cytoplasmic microfilaments (stress fibers), usually arranged parallel to the long axis of the cell and among which are interspersed numerous dense bodies (Figure 6.1A). As in vascular smooth muscle cells, these structures may be in continuity with dense bands or plasmalemmal attachment plaques. Rough endoplasmic reticulum and Golgi area are well developed. The nucleus displays deep indentations (Figure 6.1A), an ultrastructural feature that has been correlated with cellular contraction in several systems (51–54). Several nuclear bodies are usually present, and nucleoli are conspicuous. Myofibroblasts generally are surrounded by substantial amounts of extracellular matrix.

A precise definition of the myofibroblast is an issue of major importance for the surgical pathologist. In our opinion, a myofibroblast can only be defined by ultrastructure, since immunohistochemical studies reveal that myofibroblasts have a heterogeneous and complex pattern of protein expression. The three essential ultrastructural elements that define a myofibroblast are: (a) stress fibers (i.e., bundles of micro- (myo-) filaments with interspersed dense bodies running parallel to the long axis of the cell, commonly located beneath the cell membrane); (b) well-developed cell-to-stroma attachment sites (fibronexus); and (c) intercellular intermediate and gap junctions (55,56). This definition has now been accepted by several major textbooks (57–59) in regard to the issue of myofibroblasts in tumor pathology. We do not deny that the light and immunohistochemical microscopic differences between smooth muscle cells and myofibroblasts may be subtle, especially when considering degrees of differentiation of smooth muscle and myofibroblastic proliferations. Nonetheless, the myofibroblast is defined as a highly differentiated cell by ultrastructure alone.

Histologic

Although morphologically defined with the electron microscope, myofibroblasts disclose several typical histologic traits that permit their presumptive recognition in routine paraffin or (even better) in plastic sections in settings in which they previously were identified by ultrastructure. The cells are usually large, spindle-shaped, and often stellate (spiderlike) with several long cytoplasmic extensions, and they possess distinct acidophilic to amphophilic and fibrillar cytoplasm with cablelike condensations (stress fibers) running through the subplasmalemmal cytoplasm parallel to the long axis. The nuclei often are indented or reveal strangulations of nuclear segments, a feature thought to reflect cellular contraction, and contain finely granular, regularly dispersed chromatin and conspicuous nucleoli (Figure 6.2). Well-differentiated myofibroblasts with the previously mentioned traits are observed in poorly-collagenized and edematous areas of various settings in which they were

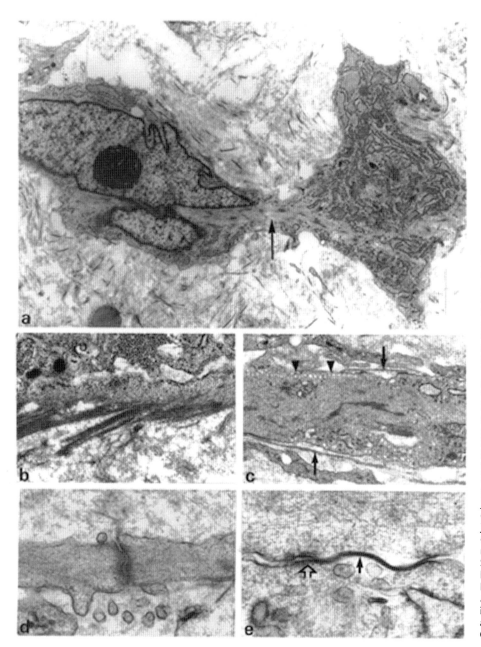

Figure 6.1 Ultrastructural characterization of the myofibroblast. **A.** Typical myofibroblast with irregular shape and cytoplasmic extensions, well-developed rough endoplasmic reticulum, and bundle of cytoplasmic microfilaments (*arrow*) with numerous dense bodies running through the cytoplasm (stress fibers) giving rise to "strangulation" of a nuclear segment. (Source: Schürch W, Seemayer T, Lagacé R, Gabbiani G. The intermediate filament cytoskeleton of myofibroblasts. *Virchows Arch A.* 1984; 403:323–336.) **B.** Microtendons in apparent continuity with bundles of cytoplasmic microfilaments (cell-to-stroma attachment sites; i.e., fibronexus). **C.** Cytoplasm of myofibroblast demonstrating basal lamina (*arrows*), pinocytotic vesicles (*arrowheads*), and plasmalemmal attachment plaques. **D.** Intermediate or adherens junction between two cytoplasmic extensions of myofibroblasts. **E.** Gap junction (*arrow*), followed by intermediate junction (*open arrow*) joining two myofibroblasts. (Source: Schürch W, Skalli O, Gabbiani G. Cellular biology of Dupuytren's disease. In McFarlane RM, McGrouther DA, Flint MH, eds. *Biology and Treatment*. Edinburgh: Churchill Livingstone: 1990: 31–47.) (Uranyl acetate and lead citrate; A, ×9900; B, ×25,000; C, ×18,200; D, ×39,000; E, ×78,000.)

originally described; for example, in granulation tissue, in zones of early invasive carcinomas, in invasive and metastatic carcinomas characterized by retraction and desmoplasia, and in several other proliferative conditions. In heavily collagenized zones, myofibroblasts are difficult to recognize with the light microscope since they correspond ultrastructurally to poorly-developed myofibroblasts or fibroblasts.

It is possible that in the near future myofibroblasts might be clearly recognized and defined by immunohistochemical examination of the complex stress fiber–associated cell-to-matrix junctions, using multiple labeling techniques and employing confocal laser microscopy on paraffin sections (for illustrations see Figure 6.3 and 6.4).

Immunohistochemical

For a better understanding and appreciation of the various cytoskeletal phenotypes of myofibroblasts, a detailed description of cytoskeletal proteins of muscular tissues, particularly smooth muscle cells, is presented.

Specific cytoskeletal proteins have been defined during the differentiation of muscular tissues (60–63). These proteins have served as reliable markers of cellular adaptation to physiologic and pathologic conditions (64).

Desmin is a muscle differentiation marker that appears early in embryogenesis (65,66). This intermediate filament, however, does not permit one to distinguish between different muscle types (67). Moreover, desmin is present in

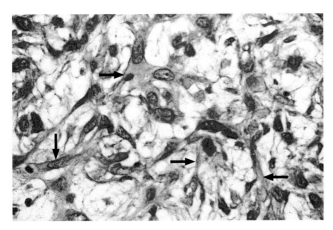

Figure 6.2 Histological aspect of myofibroblasts from the exudativo-productive layer of human granulation tissue, approximately 15 days old. Myofibroblasts disclose stellate, spiderlike shapes with long cytoplasmic extensions and distinct fibrillar cytoplasm with cablelike (*arrows*) subplasmalemmal condensations (stress fibers) (hematoxylin-phloxine-saffron).

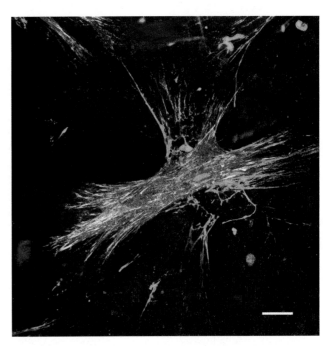

Figure 6.4 Fibronexus organization in myofibroblasts placed in three-dimensional collagen gels. Rat lung myofibroblasts were cultured in restrained collagen gels and immunostained for α-smooth muscle actin (red) in stress fibers, vinculin (green) in cell-matrix adhesions, and ED-A fibronectin (blue) in the extracellular matrix. The image has been reconstructed from the overlay of 10 optical sections of 0.2 μm acquired with a laser scanning confocal microscope; yellow color indicates colocalization of α-smooth muscle actin and vinculin; white shows colocalization of both proteins with ED-A fibronectin. Note that extracellular fibronectin fibrils are co-orientated with intracellular stress fibers; they also penetrate in the surrounding extracellular matrix in the continuation of stress fibers. This organization corresponds to the fibronexus originally described by means of electron microscopy. (Bar, 20 μm.)

stromal cells of several organs, which traditionally were considered fibroblastic in nature (68). When smooth muscle cells are cultured, desmin disappears (69). Smooth muscle myosin is a precise marker of smooth muscle differentiation. This contractile protein, however, disappears rapidly from smooth muscle cells in several conditions in vivo and also early in culture (69,70). These findings suggest that smooth muscle myosin is a more reliable marker of smooth muscle differentiation than smooth muscle origin. Vascular smooth muscle cells are heterogeneous with respect to intermediate filament proteins. Most contain vimentin as their sole detectable intermediate filament; a lesser proportion also expresses desmin (71–75). Parenchymal smooth muscle cells of the respiratory, gastrointestinal, and genitourinary tracts represent a homogeneous population in which desmin is almost the exclusive intermediate filament protein (76–78).

With regard to actin expression, at least six isoforms are defined in mammals (79–81): two nonmuscle actins (β and γ), two smooth muscle actins (α and γ) and two sarcomeric actins (α-cardiac and α-skeletal). The emergence of distinct muscle and cytoplasmic actin isoforms is phylogenetically ancestral, dating before chordates (82,83). The nonmuscle actins, the so-called cytoplasmic actins, are considered the archetypes (80) because of their presence in all nonmuscle cells, including eukaryotic unicellular organisms. According to amino acid patterns, α-skeletal actin represents the most

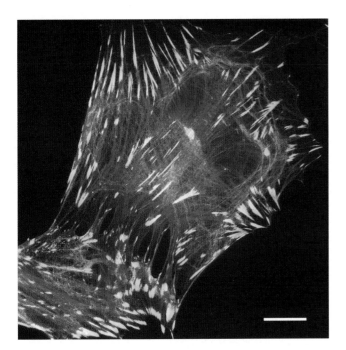

Figure 6.3 Stress fiber–associated cell-to-matrix and cell-to-cell junctions in cultured myofibroblasts. Rat lung myofibroblasts were cultured on planar glass substrates and immunostained for α-smooth muscle actin (red) as a component of contractile stress fibers, paxillin (green) as a component of cell-matrix focal adhesions, and β-catenin (blue) as a marker for cell-cell adherens junctions. Myofibroblasts form large, "supermature" focal adhesions with the extracellular matrix and adherens junctions with adjacent cells; both structures are located at the terminal portion of α-smooth muscle actin–positive stress fibers. (Bar, 20 μm.)

differentiated isoform (80). At the protein level, α-skeletal actin is most closely related to α-cardiac actin, whereas α-smooth-muscle actin is more closely related to the cytoplasmic actins. Some years ago it was suggested that both α-cardiac and α-smooth muscle actin represent embryonic or fetal actin isoforms, as they are expressed during skeletal myogenesis (60). Two-dimensional gel electrophoresis resolves only three isoforms: β and γ (nonmuscle and muscle actins) and the α-actins (smooth, striated skeletal, and striated cardiac). The biochemical identification of the six actin isoforms requires chemical analysis of the amino-terminal tryptic peptide in cellular extracts. The six actin isoforms may also be determined by RNA extraction and Northern blot hybridization using specific probes (84) and, more recently, with specific antibodies for the six actin isoforms (85). Vascular smooth muscle cells are characterized by a predominance of the α-smooth muscle actin isoform. In contrast, parenchymal smooth muscle cells contain large amounts of the γ-smooth muscle actin isoform (79–81,86). The pattern of α-, β- and γ-actin isoform expression varies in smooth muscle tissues of adult mammals (86). This pattern varies also during nonneoplastic pathologic conditions, such as atheromatosis (87,88), but changes only slightly in uterine leiomyomas, compared with normal myometrium (86). During the early months of life, 50% of cells in the aortic media lack α-smooth muscle actin, whereas α-smooth muscle actin–negative cells constitute less than 1% in the adult. These findings demonstrate that, at least in arteries, differentiation of smooth muscle cells is completed after birth (67). These observations collectively suggest that the pattern of α-actin isoform expression and, particularly, the expression of α-smooth muscle actin in vascular smooth muscle cells are related to the degree of smooth muscle differentiation.

Pericytes resemble vascular smooth muscle cells (89). In a meticulously executed treatise published in 1923, Zimmermann showed that pre- and postcapillary pericytes are connected to vascular smooth muscle cells (90). In 1991, an elegant study showed that pre- and postcapillary pericytes indeed expressed α-smooth muscle actin, whereas the midcapillary pericytes fail to express this actin isoform (91). Pericytes were also shown to resemble vascular smooth muscle cells by their intermediate filament expression. Both cell types express vimentin or vimentin and desmin (92). In addition, the intermediate filament composition of pericytes discloses species and tissue differences similar to those observed in vascular smooth muscle cells (71–74).

Myofibroblasts in normal tissue, granulation tissue, and pathologic tissues disclose five cytoskeletal phenotypes: phenotype V, represented by cells expressing only vimentin; phenotype VA, represented by cells expressing vimentin and α-smooth muscle actin; phenotype VAD, represented by cells expressing vimentin, α-smooth muscle actin, and desmin; phenotype VD, represented by cells expressing vimentin and desmin; and phenotype VA (D) M, representing myofibroblasts expressing vimentin, α-smooth muscle actin, and smooth muscle myosin heavy chains, with and without desmin. The five phenotypes are readily defined in frozen and paraffin sections using immunohistochemistry, employing single, double, or triple staining techniques. Myofibroblasts of the various immunophenotypes may also express the β-and γ-cytoplasmic actins, although it is more common that they express α-smooth muscle actin. This has led to the misconception that, for a cell to be classified as a myofibroblast, it must express α-smooth muscle actin. This is not true, as cells other than myofibroblasts express α- smooth muscle actin. There are situations in which cells have the ultrastructural characteristics of myofibroblasts (e.g., stress fibers) but do not express α-smooth muscle actin; for example, interstitial cells in alveolar septa and the early phase of granulation tissue (93,94). (For illustration see below.) Considering these data, it is apparent that the distinction between smooth muscle cells and myofibroblasts remains complex at the immunohistochemical level and that no single immunophenotype is distinctive for myofibroblasts.

Biochemical

Myofibroblasts possess not only contractile forces, but also synthetic properties. Four major groups of macromolecules comprise the extracellular matrix: (a) collagens; (b) glycoproteins (e.g., fibronectins, laminins, tenascin); (c) proteoglycans (e.g., aggrecan, synchrons, perlecan, decorin); and, (d) elastins with their associated proteins (95). Myofibroblasts possess synthetic properties for several extracellular matrix components: collagens type I, III, IV and V (29, 96–98), glycoproteins (99), and proteoglycans such as fibronectin, laminin, and tenascin (100). In addition, liver myofibroblasts in the murine schistosomiasis model secrete lysyl oxidase, an enzyme that initiates the first step in the cross-linking of collagen and elastin, a crucial function for the stabilization of the extracellular matrix (101,102).

Concerning collagen synthesis in granulating wounds, the collagen initially produced is type III. This form of collagen imparts a measure of plasticity to the wound in the early phase of healing. When granulation tissue is resorbed following wound closure, myofibroblasts disappear through the process of apoptosis (see below) and the more rigid type I collagen is biochemically identified (97,98). In similar fashion, the proliferative cellular phase of palmar fibromatosis and the young edematous mesenchyme of areas corresponding to early stromal invasion of breast carcinomas, both rich in myofibroblasts, contain increased amounts of type III collagen (26,103,104). Increased amounts of type V collagen are biochemically identified in desmoplastic human breast carcinomas, apparently also produced by myofibroblasts (98).

Pharmacologic

Strips of granulation tissue exposed in vitro to a variety of pharmacological agents contract and relax in a manner analogous to smooth muscle. Prostaglandin F_1, bradykinin, serotonin, endothelin-1, histamine, angiotensin, norepinephrine, epinephrine and vasopressin initiate contraction. The intensity of the response depends on the origin, age, and initial degree of contraction of the granulation tissue tested. Prostaglandins E_1 and E_2 and papaverine induce relaxation in tissues in a contracted state (2,3,17). Cytocholasin B abolishes the contraction of granulation tissue, probably as the result of microfilament disruption (105). Trocinate (β-diethylaminoethylphenylthioacetate), another inhibitor of smooth muscle contraction, has been reported to decrease contraction when applied topically on rabbit wounds (106).

Strips of cirrhotic liver, when exposed to smooth muscle stimulating agents, contract significantly when compared with strips of normal liver (107). Pronounced myofibroblastic interstitial fibrosis is also produced in lungs of bleomycin-injected rats. When strips of these fibrotic lungs are exposed to acetylcholine, epinephrine, and a K^+-depolarizing solution, the force developed is approximately twice that of normal lung tissue strips (108). The relative reactivity to various stimulating agents of myofibroblasts from diverse sources varies; thus, acetylcholine causes contraction of strips of fibrotic lungs but not of granulation tissue from a skin wound or a granuloma pouch, and serotonin induces retraction of the granuloma pouch but not strips from a skin wound (3). In addition to this heterogeneity in the pharmacological reactivity of granulation tissue strips from various sources, there are also differences between the response of strips of granulation tissue and strips of smooth muscle; the former reach their peak contraction slower but maintain it longer than the latter.

Whereas the various enumerated agents were shown to reveal their activity on granulation tissue in vitro, the exact mechanism leading to myofibroblast contraction in vivo remains to be elucidated. In this context, it is noteworthy that when hepatic stellate cells are subjected to in vivo ischemia reperfusion injury, they exhibit a de novo temporary increase of α-smooth muscle actin expression. A similar phenomenon takes place during the initial phases of liver transplantation in humans (109). Likely, this represents a response to ischemic injury.

Endothelin-1 was originally isolated from the conditioned medium of cultured porcine endothelial cells and was shown to be the most potent vasopressor substance yet characterized (110). Endothelin-1 may be an endogenous modulator of myofibroblast-mediated contraction because it causes reversible and concentration-dependent contraction of granuloma pouch granulation tissue, the 21-day granulation tissue being the most responsive. This response can be inhibited by calcium antagonists (111,112). The vasopressor effect of endothelin-1 possibly is controlled and mediated through the action of cytokines, among others, TGF-β (113,114), which, in turn, is able to induce α-smooth muscle actin expression in fibroblasts and myofibroblasts. More recently it has been shown that the intracellular administration of the N-terminal peptide of α-smooth muscle actin, the actin isoform responsible for myofibroblast contraction (see below), decreases force generation by myofibroblasts in vitro and inhibits wound contraction in vivo (115); this may represent a useful tool for the control of tissue retraction and remodeling during several pathological situations.

In Vitro Culture Studies

When myofibroblasts from various sources (granulating wounds, Dupuytren's disease, and invasive breast cancer) are cultured, they maintain to a certain extent their unique resemblance to fibroblasts and smooth muscle cells. Cultured fibroblasts may express different phenotypic features, and a spectrum of differentiation steps has been described (116). In particular, primary passaged fibroblastic cells in culture express α-smooth muscle actin (68,79,117). Cytoskeletal proteins such as desmin and smooth muscle myosin heavy chains are also variably expressed by cultured fibroblasts derived from different organs or pathologic tissues, but expression is generally low and absent in several populations (118). Myofibroblasts cultured from skin wound granulation tissue maintain some biologic features different from those of dermal fibroblasts (119). If the growth rate and the actin concentration of cultured fibroblasts from normal dermis and myofibroblasts of human granulation tissue are compared, myofibroblasts grow slower than fibroblasts (120) and contain a significantly higher concentration of actin (121). Wound-healing fibroblasts were shown to develop greater contractile properties than dermal fibroblasts (122). Similarly, fibroblastic cells cultured from Dupuytren's nodules maintain biologic features different from those of normal dermis or fascial fibroblasts yet are similar to those of neoplastic or embryonic fibroblasts (123). However, it is important to state that the percentage of cells exhibiting myofibroblast features in culture does not necessarily reflect their proportion in the tissue of origin. When fibroblast cultures from various species, including man, were established using cloning and subcloning techniques, a certain percentage of cells was positive for α-smooth muscle actin (118). This concept of fibroblast heterogeneity is now well-established in vitro (124) and in vivo [see review by Schmitt-Gräff et al. (8)]. Alpha-smooth muscle actin is expressed by fibroblasts cultured from the lens of the eye, mammary gland, perisinusoidal cells of the liver, and glomerular mesangial cells, sites where stromal cells normally expressing this protein do not occur (125–128) but which may give rise to reactive stromal cells expressing α-smooth muscle actin in pathologic conditions. It is likely that α-smooth muscle actin expression in cultured fibroblasts stems from the culture conditions imposed upon the fibroblasts. Fibroblastic modulation to a myofibroblast phenotype in vitro may thus reflect a cellular response to their altered biochemical and mechanical environment, somewhat analogous to that which occurs in wounds.

Myofibroblast Development: A Two-Stage Model

Fibroblasts cultured on planar culture dishes rapidly attach to the wall of the container and move across its surface; adherence and mobility are attributed to the de novo development of a system of microfilament bundles called stress fibers (129). These may measure up to 2 μm in diameter and connect to the extracellular matrix at sites of focal adhesions (130) and to adjacent cells at sites of adherens junctions (50) (Figure 6.3). Initially, stress fibers are mainly composed of cytoplasmic actins, as shown by immunofluorescence and immunoelectron microscopy with specific antibodies (131–133). Several studies have shown that stress fibers also contain actin-associated proteins such as myosin, tropomyosin, α-actinin, and filamin (7). The formation of stress fibers and cell-matrix adhesions is in sharp contrast to the cortical arrangement of actin in fibroblasts in most normal connective tissues and represents the first step in the development of the myofibroblast phenotype. The term *protomyofibroblast* was recently proposed for fibroblasts with contractile stress fibers that do not (yet) express α-smooth muscle actin (134).

Development of the protomyofibroblast is predominantly controlled by the mechanical properties of the extracellular matrix [for reviews see (134,135)] and requires the permanent feedback between intracellular and extracellular tension. Stress fiber formation in fibroblasts on rigid glass or plastic surfaces is increased after contractile activity stimulation and is lost upon application of inhibitors of contraction (136). In contrast, fibroblasts grown on compliant substrates fail to develop protomyofibroblastic features even in the presence of contraction agonists (137). When embedded in a three-dimensional gel of newly polymerized collagen, fibroblasts acquire a dendritic morphology similar to that in normal dermis (138); they extend and retract long processes, possibly to explore and organize the new environment (139). In free-floating collagen gels the forces developed by such processes lead to collagen gel condensation (139). However, since collagen fibers are free to move, overall matrix stress does not develop, and fibroblasts maintain their dendritic appearance (139). In contrast, collagen reorganization in restrained gels produces matrix stiffening and increases global stress, inducing alignment of fibroblasts along the lines of tension and the formation of stress fibers (134,139) (Figure 6.4). Similarly,

after stress-release of restrained collagen gels, protomyofibroblasts rapidly loose stress fibers and matrix contacts (140). Importantly, fibroblasts are capable of adjusting their contractile activity according to the external load; controlled stress-release of collagen gels in a culture increases fibroblast contractile activity, whereas gel stretching leads to fibroblast relaxation, a phenomenon that has been termed *tensional homeostasis* (141).

A similar mechanism of protomyofibroblast development appears to apply in vivo. In most normal connective tissues, fibroblasts are protected from external tensile stress by their surrounding matrix (134). This situation changes dramatically with an altered microenvironment, such as when a dermal wound is provisionally filled with a clot of fibrin and blood platelets, which, in conjunction with white blood cells, release a variety of cytokines (142,143). These changes stimulate fibroblasts to migrate into the wound bed, where they proliferate and initiate restoration of the dermis by secreting and organizing the dermal matrix. The increasing number of migrating fibroblasts enhances matrix rigidity by applying tractional forces to the newly formed granulation tissue, ultimately leading to the development of stress fibers.

A number of recent studies have demonstrated that mechanical stress is a prerequisite for the second step of myofibroblast development, signaled by the expression of α-smooth muscle actin in stress fibers (134,68). In vitro, the level of α-smooth muscle actin expression increases with increasing matrix rigidity, as demonstrated by growing differentiated myofibroblasts in collagen substrates or on polyacrylamide elastomers exhibiting different degrees of stiffness (144,145). In vivo, application of mechanical stress to granulation tissue fibroblasts by splinting the wound edges with a plastic frame accelerates expression of α-smooth muscle actin compared to normally healing wounds; stress release by removal of the frame rapidly leads to the disassembly of stress fibers and loss of α-smooth muscle actin expression (146).

In addition to mechanical stress, transformation of the protomyofibroblast into the differentiated myofibroblast requires the concerted action of cytokines and specific components of the extracellular matrix. It is increasingly accepted that TGF-β1 is the major growth factor inducing myofibroblast differentiation (27,147,148) from fibroblastic cells (147,149) and mesangial cells (33,150). More recently, thrombin (151) and endothelin-1 (152) have been shown to induce myofibroblast differentiation, the latter either directly or in coculture with epidermal cells (153). It has been demonstrated in experimental animals that the subcutaneous administration of granulocyte macrophage–colony stimulating factor (GM-CSF) promotes the development of granulation tissue rich in α-smooth muscle actin–positive myofibroblasts (154,155); this action, however, is indirect and could be mediated by TGF-β. TGF-β–mediated expression of α-smooth muscle actin depends upon the presence of the fibronectin splice variant ED-A fibronectin (30) in the extracellular matrix (Figure 6.4). This clearly demonstrates the complex interplay of diffusible and immobilized factors in promoting the development of differentiated myofibroblasts. Other cytokines and/or growth factors have been shown to facilitate or inhibit myofibroblast development and proliferation. Nerve growth factor (156) facilitates the process, however, it is not known whether this action is independent of TGF-β1; interferon-γ inhibits the process (118).

Mechanisms of Force Generation and Transmission

Several observations suggest that stress fibers are the force-generating elements in wound contraction, since they contract upon addition of adenosine triphosphate to glycerinated fibroblasts (13,157,158). As well, microinjection experiments revealed that stress fibers are functionally analogous to skeletal muscle fibers (158,159). Several models have been developed to study the contractile activity of fibroblastic cells in vitro. Using two-dimensional deformable silicone substrates, fibroblasts have been shown to produce long-lasting wrinkles of the substrate, suggesting the production of continuous isometric tension (160). This technique has been greatly improved over the past years by employing different elastic polymers and mathematical models to calculate cell-generated forces from substrate distortions [for a review see (161)]. In a more tissuelike approach to assess the dynamics of wound contraction, fibroblasts are cultured in collagen or fibrin matrices that are either free-floating and retracting over days or mechanically restrained for days and then stress released, leading to contraction within minutes [for review see (139)]. Importantly, stress fibers and matrix adhesion (i.e., the myofibroblastic phenotype) only develop in mechanically restrained gels. Hence, the choice of the appropriate collagen model facilitates study of the traction forces of migrating fibroblasts or stress fiber-mediated contraction.

Similar to what occurs in smooth muscle, stress fiber contraction may be regulated by elevated levels of intracellular Ca^{2+}, leading to activation of myosin light chain kinase and phosphorylation of the myosin light chain. However, experimental and clinical observations show that granulation tissue retraction, in contrast to rapid and reversible contraction of smooth muscle, is the result of a continuous isometric force exerted on the surrounding connective tissue. This retraction is then stabilized by deposition of newly synthesized matrix components and thus becomes irreversible (134). In the last few years, the work of several laboratories has suggested that the isometric tension produced by stress fibers is regulated by Rho/Rho-kinase, which in its active form leads to long lasting tensile activity by the inhibition of myosin phosphatase (162).

Phosphatase inhibitors stimulate myofibroblast contraction in vitro in the absence of any other contraction agonist (163). In contrast, increasing intracellular Ca^{2+} with ionophore has no contractile effect, indicating that activation of myosin light chain kinase alone is not sufficient to promote myofibroblast tension development (164). More recently it has been reported that thrombin activation of human lung myofibroblast tension development is mediated by protein kinase Cε and RhoA and depends on the activation of Ca^{2+}-mediated and Rho-kinase signaling pathways (151).

During the past several years, it has become evident that the expression of α-smooth muscle actin in stress fibers is instrumental in force generation by myofibroblasts. Compared with α-smooth muscle actin–negative fibroblasts, myofibroblasts develop higher contractile force as demonstrated using deformable silicone substrates (164,165) and contracting collagen gels (165,166). Stable transfection with α-smooth muscle actin confers upon fibroblasts a higher contractile activity compared with transfection with cytoplasmic or sarcomeric actin isoforms; this effect is exerted in the absence of any change in the expression of other contractile proteins, such as smooth muscle or non-muscle myosin (165). The mechanism by which α-smooth muscle actin promotes myofibroblast-enhanced contractile activity has not been defined; however, it is inhibited in vitro and in vivo and by the intracellular delivery of the α-smooth muscle actin–specific N-terminal sequence AcEEED (115).

The force generated by stress fibers is transmitted to the extracellular matrix at sites of cell-matrix adhesions (130). In vivo, myofibroblasts form a specialized adhesion complex, the fibronexus (49), which is characterized by a firm co-alignment of intracellular actin fibers with extracellular fibronectin fibrils (Figure 6.1B); these in turn are connected to collagen in the wound matrix (19). In vitro, differentiated myofibroblasts communicate with the extracellular matrix through specialized "supermature focal adhesions" (145,167), which have a diameter of 6 to 30 μm and strongly express the cytoplasmic proteins vinculin, paxillin, and tensin and the transmembrane integrins αvβ3 and α5β1 (145,167). This is in contrast to smaller focal adhesions (FAs) (2–6 μm) of α-smooth muscle actin-negative fibroblasts that do not exhibit significant levels of tensin and α5β1 integrin or to fibrillar adhesions that are generally negative for vinculin, paxillin and αvβ3 integrin (130,168). Focal adhesion supermaturation depends on the high contractile activity developed by α-SMA–containing stress fibers (145), analogous to the maturation of classical FAs from nascent focal complexes in response to up-regulated cell contractile activity (136). It has been proposed that supermature focal adhesions are particularly efficient in promoting tissue contraction (134,135) by providing high adhesion to the substrate (145) and by immobilizing the cells in the wound bed (169).

TISSUE DISTRIBUTION OF MYOFIBROBLASTS

Normal Tissues

Myofibroblasts were described in normal human and animal tissues on the basis of ultrastructural and/or immunohistochemical evidence of smooth muscle differentiation. The normal settings in which myofibroblasts were observed include the external theca of the rat ovarian follicle (170); developing human palatal mucosa (171); rat, rabbit, and human intestinal mucosa (172–174); rat and mouse adrenal capsule (175), human, lamb, and monkey pulmonary alveolar septa (176); rat testicular stroma (68); rat testicular capsule (177); human theca externa of the ovary (178); Wharton's jelly of human umbilical cord (179); bovine endometrial caruncle (180); and periodontal ligament of the mouse (181) and rat (182), where they facilitate tooth eruption. Stromal cells with myoid features were also identified in rat and human lymph nodes and in the

human spleen (183). Another group of stromal cells with myoid features include hepatic perisinusoidal cells (184), those in the human uterine submucosa (185) and human bone marrow (186), glomerular mesangial cells of mouse, rat, and human (187), and, possibly, pre-and postcapillary pericytes (89,91).

Immunohistochemical studies disclosed heterogeneous cytoskeletal phenotypes among all of these stromal cells (myofibroblasts) in terms of intermediate filament protein, smooth muscle actin, and smooth muscle myosin expression; these include V, VD, VA (D) M, VA, and VAD phenotypes (188,189). This cytoskeletal heterogeneity could reflect different functional needs since all of these stromal cells seem to participate in visceral contraction or extracellular matrix remodeling, a view supported by the observation that stromal cells with myoid features are generally present in organs requiring contraction or high degrees of remodeling (190). Another recently advanced interpretation proposes that most spindle cells in normal tissues cited as being myofibroblasts might be closer to pericytes,

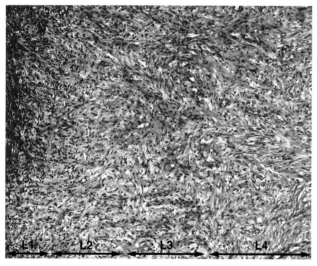

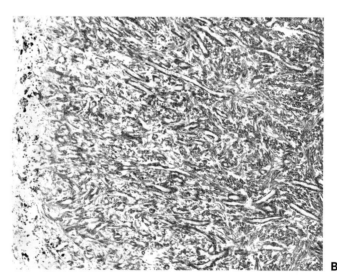

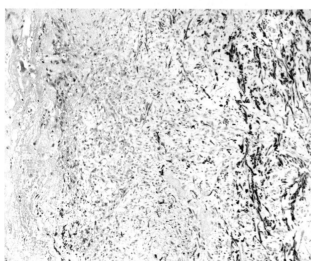

Figure 6.5 Human chronic granulation tissue from pleural empyema. **A.** The four layers *(L1–L4)* are clearly discernible: L1, alterative; L2, exudative; L3, exudativo-productive; L4, cicatrizing (hematoxylin-phloxine-saffron). **B.** Most myofibroblasts from the exudative and exudativo-productive layer (L2 and L3) reveal intense immunostaining for α-smooth muscle actin (phenotype VA) (avidin-biotin-complex-peroxidase). Note that myofibroblastic cells change their orientation within the different layers. Within the exudative layer, their long axis is perpendicular to the surface, whereas in the exudativo-productive layer their long axis is often oblique to the surface. Within the cicatrizing layer, myofibroblastic cells are oriented parallel to the surface, which indicates that the modulation of cellular orientation serves to transmit contractile forces to effect wound closure. **C.** In the cicatrizing layer (L4), numerous myofibroblasts express desmin (phenotype VAD). (B and C are step-sections.)

smooth muscle cells (191), or stromal cells with myoid features of variable degrees that correspond to functional demands. As shall be seen in the following sections, myofibroblasts and/or stromal cells with myoid features are not stable in terms of cytoskeletal phenotypes. In normal, abnormal, and pathologic conditions, the phenotype V may change into phenotype VA, VAD, VD, and, eventually, into VA (D) M, but terminal smooth muscle differentiation (smooth muscle metaplasia) is never attained. Thus, the myofibroblast remains an enigmatic cell, one that appears and disappears after completion of its functions or, exceptionally, one that may persist in certain pathologic conditions.

Granulation Tissue

Granulation tissue (Figures 6.5–6.7) consists of a bed of fibroblastic cells separated by a collagenous matrix containing capillary buds, fibrin, and inflammatory cells. According to the relative predominance of each constituent, four layers are classically distinguished: (a) alterative; (b) exudative; (c) exudativo-productive; and (d) cicatrizing (Figure 6.6A). Granulation tissue fibroblasts characteristically disclose ultrastructural features of myofibroblasts. They are most numerous and best developed within the exudativo-productive layer and become progressively replaced toward the deepest cicatrizing layer by fibroblasts. The orientation of the myofibroblasts varies in the different layers of granulation tissue. In the exudative layer, the long axis is perpendicular to the surface, whereas in the exudativo-productive and cicatrizing layers, the long axis is parallel to the surface (Figure 6.6A). These data suggest that the spatial orientation of myofibroblasts in granulating wounds varies, possibly to

maximize the transmission of contractile forces and thereby effect wound closure. When the collagenous matrix is analyzed, type III collagen predominates. When granulation tissue is resorbed following wound closure, myofibroblasts disappear (25,97,192) and the more rigid type I collagen is identified (96).

Analysis of cytoskeletal proteins by immunohistochemical methods reveals that myofibroblasts from normal healing wounds never express desmin or smooth muscle myosin heavy chains during the process of wound closure in the experimental animal (25). Smooth muscle differentiation in early granulation tissue is absent and myofibroblasts are often poorly-developed and correspond to V cells (Figure 6.5). Smooth muscle differentiation of myofibroblasts, however, becomes temporarily apparent because myofibroblasts express α-smooth muscle actin (VA cells) (Figure 6.7A and B) in increasing amounts from the eighth to the fifteenth day; this protein is located within bundles of microfilaments (stress fibers), as illustrated by immunoelectron microscopic techniques (Figure 6.7C and D). This actin isoform disappears progressively from myofibroblasts and is not detectable after the thirtieth day by immunohistochemical and immunoelectron microscopic methods. These results clearly indicate that granulation tissue myofibroblasts temporarily acquire a VA phenotype. This is valid when wound repair is accomplished by primary intention. When repair is accomplished by secondary intention in chronic granulation tissue (e.g., chronic gastric ulcer, cutaneous ulceration, or pleural empyema), myofibroblasts of the VAD phenotype may be detectable (Figure 6.6B and C).

The study of the ontogenesis of wound healing reveals that many species possess the unique ability to heal wounds without scarring (193–198). Estes et al. (199),

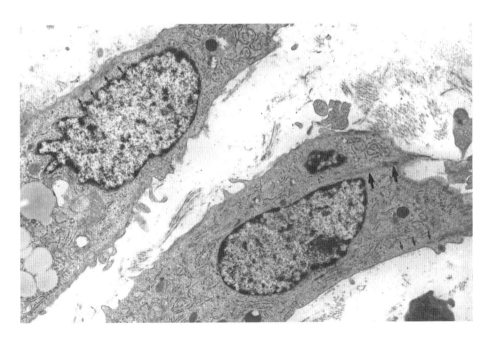

Figure 6.6 Human granulation tissue, approximately 5 days old, composed of phenotype V myofibroblasts. These cells disclose subplasmalemmal bundles of microfilaments with few dense bodies (*small arrows*) and also intracytoplasmic bundles of microfilaments with dense bodies (*large arrows*) corresponding to stress fibers in formation (uranyl acetate and lead citrate, ×12,500).

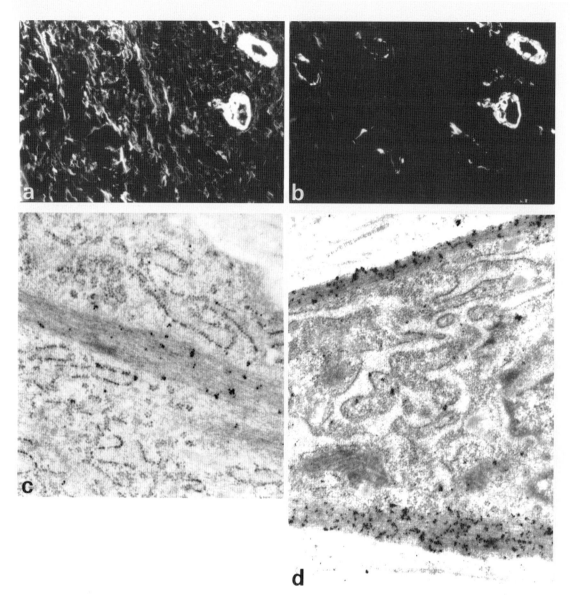

Figure 6.7 Experimental granulation tissue from the rat, 15 days old. **A.** Double immunofluorescent staining for α-smooth muscle actin (A). **B.** Double immunofluorescent staining for desmin. Myofibroblastic cells reveal intense staining for α-smooth muscle actin (A) but are negative for desmin (B). Vascular smooth muscle cells are positive both for α smooth muscle actin and desmin. **C.** Immunoelectron microscopic localization of α-smooth muscle actin within intracytoplasmic bundles of microfilaments, that is, stress fibers. **D.** Immunoelectron microscopic localization of α-smooth muscle actin in subplasmalemmal bundles of microfilaments. (C, ×31,000; D, ×28,400.)

examining fetal wounds in the fetal lamb, recently showed that there are differences between early and late gestational wound healing. In the lamb, term gestation is approximately 145 days. Early gestational wounds (75 days) healed without scarring by repair of the epidermis, reconstitution of epidermal appendages, and remodeling of the dermal collagenous network. In contrast, late gestational wounds (100 and 120 days) healed with scarring through formation of granulation tissue containing myofibroblasts that were mostly derived from local resident fibroblasts. The situation appears to be different in healing corneal wounds, in which corneal keratocytes transform into repair corneal fibroblasts or myofibroblasts (200–202).

Pathologic Tissues

Upon analysis of the many pathologic conditions in which myofibroblasts have been described, three fundamental processes emerge: (a) responses to injury and repair phenomena or situations related to inflammation and tissue remodeling; (b) quasineoplastic proliferative conditions; and (c) the stromal response to neoplasia (6,203). This concept, enunciated some 25 years ago, appears valid to this day (6).

Responses to Injury and Repair Phenomena

Responses to injury and repair phenomena comprise human and experimental cirrhosis (204–206), tenosynovitis (207), radiation-induced pseudosarcoma of skin (208), burn contracture (209), ischemic contractures of intrinsic muscles of the hand (210), renal interstitial fibrosis during obstructive nephropathy (211), pulmonary sarcoidosis (212), giant cell granuloma of jaws (213), schistosomal liver fibrosis (214), regenerating tendon (215), fibrous capsule around silicon mammary implants (216,217), nodular hyperplasia of the liver (218), ganglia of soft tissue (219), hypertrophic scars (220), cataract (221), bleomycin-induced pulmonary interstitial fibrosis in the rat (222), fibrous heart plaque in the carcinoid syndrome (223), atherosclerotic lesions in humans and experimental animals (224–227), localized and systemic scleroderma (228), and experimental hydronephrosis (229). When cytoskeletal proteins of these conditions are analyzed most reactive cells correspond to the VA, some to the VAD, and few to the VD and VA (D) M phenotype (188,192).

A recent report proposed that a reactive myofibroblastic proliferation with increased deposition/formation of extracellular matrix might be responsible for the progressive and irreversible obstruction of airways in chronic bronchial asthma (230). In asthma, it appears that epithelial-mesenchymal interactions may play an important role in its pathogenesis. Epithelial injury and subepithelial collagen deposition are characteristic of asthma. It was proposed that epithelial cell proliferation increases after airway injury in asthmatics, that epithelial cells stimulate lung myofibroblast collagen production, and that both processes are modulated by allergen-recruited inflammatory cells, proinflammatory cytokines, growth factors, and mediator-generating enzymes. Beneath the damaged bronchial epithelium, there is an increase in the number of subepithelial myofibroblasts that deposit interstitial collagens, causing thickening and increased density of the subepithelial basement membrane (231–233).

Focal segmental glomerular hyalinosis/sclerosis (FSGS) is another state which might belong to the group of responses to injury and repair phenomena (Figure 6.8A–I). The condition is associated with significant proteinuria and hypertension; many patients develop chronic renal failure, requiring dialysis and eventual renal transplantation. In FSGS, mesangial cells, which normally express only cytoplasmic actins and therefore correspond to myofibroblasts with a V phenotype, may gradually acquire a VA phenotype, expressing α-smooth muscle actin as revealed by immunohistochemical techniques (Figure 6.8D). Moreover, they develop stress fibers as observed by ultrastructural examination

(Figure 6.8I). These findings are similar to those in experimental immune complex nephritis in which mesangial expression of smooth muscle actin correlates with mesangial cell proliferation (33). In FSGS, mesangial cells expressing α-smooth muscle actin become progressively apparent in the early stage of the disease (podocytosis; Figure 6.8C and D) (234). Their numbers increase as the lesion progresses to the hyalinosis stage (Figure 6.8E and F). At the stage of sclerosis, the number of mesangial cells immunostained for α-smooth muscle actin is reduced, somewhat analogous to that which occurs over time in wound healing (Figure 6.8G and H).

In abnormally healing wounds (hypertrophic scars and keloids), one observes several important differences. Hypertrophic scars always exhibit nodular structures in which fibroblastic cells, small vessels, and fine randomly organized collagen fibers are present. Within these nodules, numerous myofibroblasts of the VA phenotype and, in lesser numbers, myofibroblasts of the VAD phenotype are identified (Figure 6.9A–H). Exceptionally, myofibroblasts of the VA (D) M phenotype are observed. Keloids contain large thick bands of closely packed cell fibers and rare nodular structures, the latter containing few or no VA cells (235,236). VAD cells are not observed within classical keloids (231), however VA and VAD cells are frequently observed in relatively small keloids of Caucasians (237).

Quasi-neoplastic Proliferative Conditions

This group embodies the poorly-understood but very important and frequent soft tissue proliferations included under the broad heading of fibromatoses, as well as many other soft tissue proliferations (often mimicking sarcomas) that share a predominant myofibroblastic composition and a variable proliferative potential yet do not disseminate or metastasize (6,203).

Myofibroblasts constitute the principal cellular components of superficial and deep musculoaponeurotic fibromatoses (238). Superficial (fascial) fibromatoses include palmar fibromatosis [Dupuytren's disease (16,103,239–241)], plantar fibromatosis [Ledderhose's disease (16)], penile fibromatosis [Peyronie's disease (240)], and knuckle pads (243). Deep musculoaponeurotic fibromatoses comprise extra-abdominal, abdominal and intra-abdominal variants, collectively named desmoid tumors (238). To this group belong the infantile fibromatoses (244). Other soft tissue proliferations predominantly composed of myofibroblasts are nodular fasciitis (245), proliferative fasciitis (246), proliferative myositis (247), giant fibroma of oral mucosa (248), dermatofibroma (249), elastofibroma (250), plasma cell granuloma of the lung (251), digital fibroma of infancy (252), and juvenile nasopharyngeal angiofibroma (253). Myofibroblasts are also present in cardiac myxomas (254) and in uterine plexiform tumors (255).

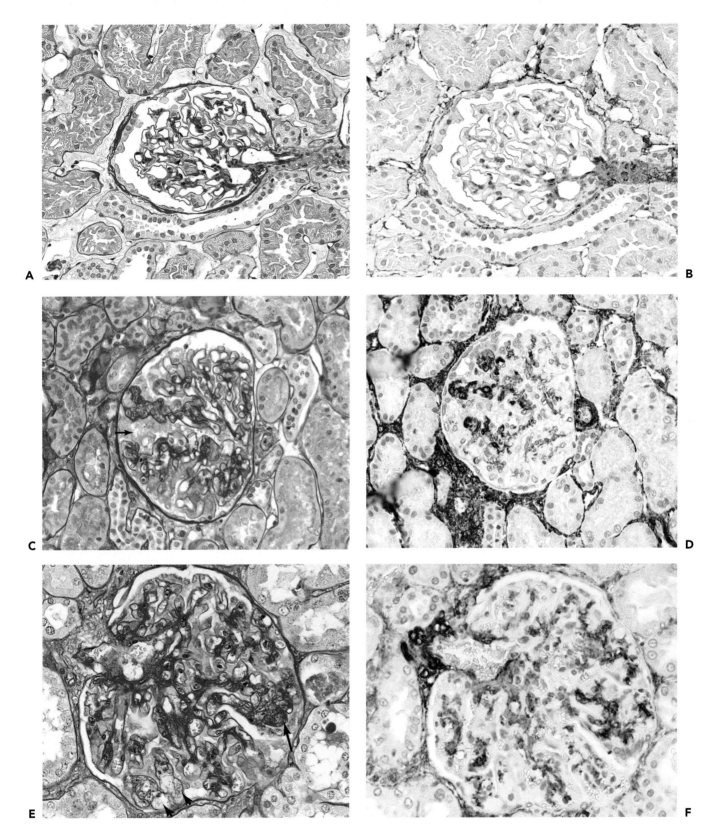

Figure 6.8 Evolution of focal segmental glomerular hyalinosis/sclerosis using step-sections stained with PAS and α-smooth muscle actin. **A. and B.** Normal glomerulus; B is without significant immunostaining of mesangial cells for α-smooth muscle actin. **C. and D.** Early stage of focal segmental hyalinosis characterized by vacuolar degeneration of podocytes with hyalin PAS-positive droplets and increased mesangial matrix in two glomerular segments; that is, podocytosis (*arrow*). Mesangial cells of the two glomerular segments disclose significant immunostaining for α-smooth muscle actin (D). **E. and F.** Typical segmental lesion with hyaline endomembranous PAS-positive deposit (*arrow*) and foam cells (*arrowheads*). Mesangial cells disclose significant immunostaining for α-smooth muscle actin.

136

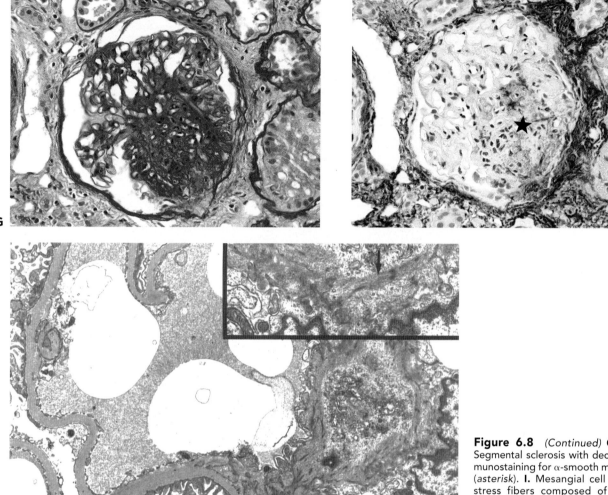

G

H

I

Figure 6.8 *(Continued)* **G. and H.** Segmental sclerosis with decreased immunostaining for α-smooth muscle actin (*asterisk*). **I.** Mesangial cell disclosing stress fibers composed of microfilaments with dense bodies (*arrow*), enhanced in inset (uranyl acetate and lead citrate, ×8000; inset ×15,150).

Dupuytren's Disease

Among quasineoplastic proliferations, Dupuytren's fibromatosis has been studied extensively by morphologic, immunohistochemical, and biochemical techniques (24,26,256,257). Cytoskeletal proteins have been widely used as markers of differentiation for neoplastic and quasineoplastic proliferations and as markers of adaptation to physiologic situations, particularly for muscular and related soft tissue proliferations (24,26,64).

According to Luck (258), the nodules of Dupuytren's disease are assigned to three different phases, depending on the histologic pattern: (a) proliferative phase; (b) involutional phase; and (c) residual phase (Figure 6.10A–D). Patients with Dupuytren's disease often present multiple nodules showing considerable variation in their histologic appearance. The classification is, therefore, based on the predominant histologic pattern (105,259).

Sections from proliferative phase nodules feature high cellular density, decreasing from the center to the periphery (Figure 6.10A). They are well-vascularized and display a poorly-collagenized appearance. Ultrastructurally, they are composed of myofibroblasts with numerous and long cytoplasmic extensions, joined by numerous gap and adherens junctions (Figure 6.11A and inset). Their plasma membrane displays focal deposition of basal lamina, plasmalemmal attachment plaques, and pinocytotic vesicles, as well as cell-to-stroma attachment sites in the form of fibronexus (49). The cytoplasm features a well-developed rough endoplasmic reticulum and Golgi apparatus and numerous stress fibers, the latter usually oriented parallel to the long axis of the cell (Figure 6.11A). The nucleus is typically indented and often contains one or several nuclear bodies. The extracellular matrix is composed of a few mature collagen fibers (64 nm periodicity) admixed

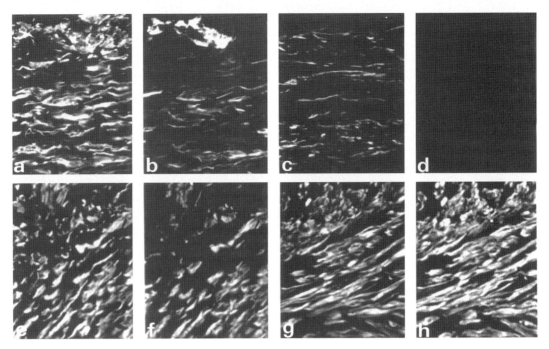

Figure 6.9 Double immunofluorescent staining of two hypertrophic scars (**A–D and E–H**) with antibodies to vimentin (A and E), α-smooth muscle actin (B and F), α-smooth muscle actin (C and G), and desmin (D and H). One hypertrophic scar (A–D) contains V and VA cells, and the other, from a site of smallpox vaccination (E–H), contains mainly VAD cells. Note that most small blood vessels are positive for vimentin and α-smooth muscle actin. (Source: Sappino AP, Schürch W, Gabbiani G. Differentiation repertoire of fibroblastic cells: expression of cytoskeletal proteins as marker of phenotypic modulations. *Lab Invest* 1990;63:144–161.)

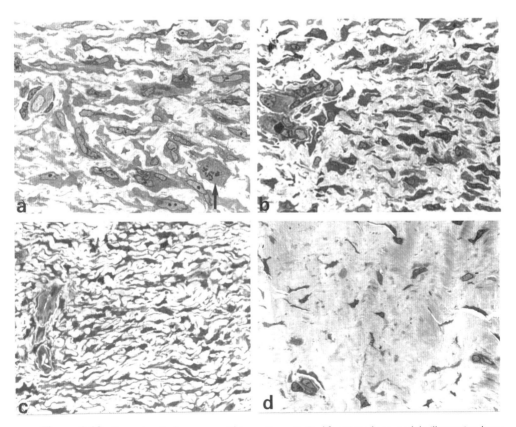

Figure 6.10 Dupuytren's disease: semithin sections. **A.** Proliferative phase nodule illustrating large elongated cells with numerous cytoplasmic extensions and indented nuclei, some in cell division (*arrow*). **B. and C.** Involutional phase nodule composed of aligned spindle cells that display fewer, shorter, and smaller cytoplasmic extensions than in A. **D.** Residual phase nodule showing slender spindle cells in a poorly-vascularized and densely collagenous matrix. (Toluidine blue-stain.) (Source: Schürch W, Skalli O, Gabbiani G. Cellular biology of Dupuytren's disease. In: McFarlane RM, McGrouther DA, Flint MH, eds. *Dupuytren's Disease: Biology and Treatment.* London: Churchill Livingstone; 1990:31–47.)

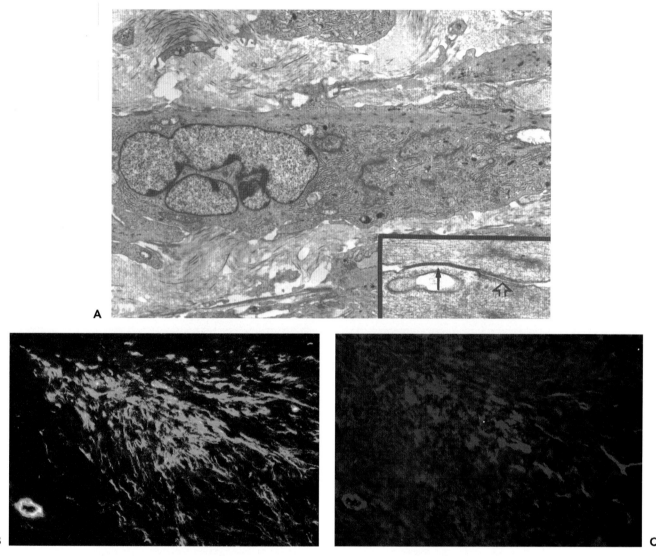

Figure 6.11 Dupuytren's disease: proliferative phase nodule. **A.** Transmission electron micrograph of proliferative phase nodule. Note large typical myofibroblast with cytoplasmic extensions, well-developed rough endoplasmic reticulum and Golgi areas, and prominent cytoplasmic bundle of microfilaments with numerous dense bodies oriented parallel to the long axis of the cell. The nucleus is indented. The extracellular matrix contains few mature collagen fibers. **Inset:** Gap junction between two myofibroblasts (*arrow*) followed by an intermediate junction (*open arrow*). (Uranyl acetate and lead citrate: ×7500; inset, ×72,000.) **B. and C.** Double immunofluorescent staining for α-smooth muscle actin (B) and desmin (C). The majority of the proliferating cells comprising the nodule correspond to VA cells, while lesser numbers of cells express VAD and V phenotypes.

with indistinct granular and basal lamina-like material (Figure 6.11A).

Involutional phase nodules also feature high cellularity, but the cells are smaller than those of the proliferative phase and tend to be aligned in the same direction (Figure 6.10B–C). Ultrastructurally, these nodules are composed of myofibroblasts that are also connected by gap and adherens junctions. These intercellular junctions, however, seem to be less numerous than in proliferative phase nodules. The most striking difference with proliferative phase nodules is the increased amount of collagen that envelopes myofibroblasts.

By immunoelectron microscopy, α-smooth muscle actin is localized within bundles of microfilaments of myofibroblasts of the proliferative and involutional phase nodules.

Residual phase nodules are hypocellular and the slender and aligned cells are surrounded by thick bands of collagen, giving them a tendonlike appearance (Figure 6.10D). By ultrastructure, these nodules are composed of mature fibroblasts (Figure 6.12A), some containing discrete subplasmalemmal bundles of microfilaments without dense bodies. Occasional poorly-developed adherens-type junctions (Figure 6.12A and inset) connect the fibroblasts, but

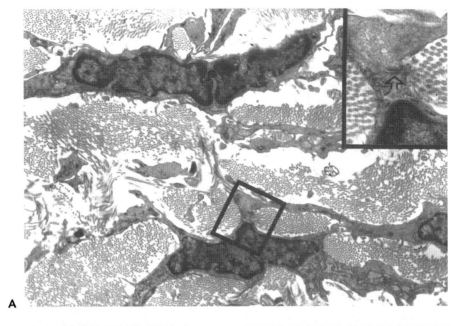

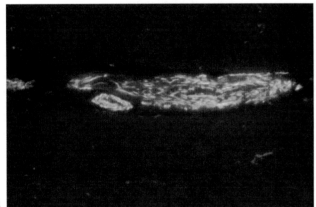

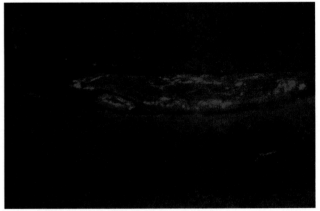

Figure 6.12 Dupuytren's disease: residual phase nodule. **A.** Transmission electron micrograph illustrating slender fibroblasts with smooth contoured nuclei embedded in a dense collagenous matrix and joined by poorly-differentiated junction (*open arrow,* **inset**) (uranyl acetate and lead citrate, ×12,150; inset, ×40,500). **B. and C.** Double immunofluorescent staining for α-smooth muscle actin (B) and desmin (C). Cells comprising the residual phase nodule correspond to V cells. A few isolated cells express only VAD or VA phenotypes.

gap junctions are no longer observed. The slender fibroblasts show smooth, contoured nuclei and are embedded in a dense collagenous matrix formed by thick bands of tightly packed collagen fibers. In conclusion, significant ultrastructural differences exist between proliferative, involutional, and residual phase nodules in Dupuytren's disease in relation to the cells, intercellular junctions, and composition of the extracellular matrix.

When the collagenous matrix of Dupuytren's disease is analyzed by immunohistochemical techniques, proliferative phase nodules reveal a predominance of type III collagen, whereas in the residual fibroblastic phase, type I collagen predominates (103). Differences between proliferative

and residual phase nodules are also defined in the vascularization. In proliferative phase nodules, capillaries are numerous and feature, ultrastructurally, large and prominent pericytes that display distinct smooth muscle differentiation; whereas in residual phase nodules, capillaries are few in number and are surrounded by small and inconspicuous pericytes that are devoid of a well-developed microfilamentous apparatus (26). Analogous to wound healing, the cicatrizing process within proliferative and involutional phase nodules is centripetal, being completed within residual phase nodules.

When immunohistochemical techniques are employed to study the cellular phases of Dupuytren's disease the following results are obtained. Cells of the proliferative phase nodules always express vimentin, which is associated in approximately 80% of the cells with α-smooth muscle actin (68) and in about 20 to 40% with desmin when double-labeling immunofluorescence techniques are performed (Figure 6.11B–C). Rarely, isolated cells positive for vimentin, α-smooth muscle actin, and smooth muscle myosin heavy chains with or without desmin are present [VA (D) M phenotype] (189). In involutional phase nodules, desmin-positive cells are less numerous or even absent, whereas α-smooth muscle actin-positive cells are still present, albeit in lesser numbers. In residual phase nodules few or no α-smooth muscle actin–positive cells persist, and the remaining slender cells express solely vimentin (Figure 6.12B–C). Accordingly, cells comprising the nodules of Dupuytren's disease express different cytoskeletal phenotypes: (a) phenotype V; (b) phenotype VAD; (c) phenotype VA; and (d) phenotype VD. In most proliferative phase nodules of Dupuytren's disease and also in the cellular areas of musculoaponeurotic fibromatoses, the number of VA cells considerably exceeds the number of VAD and VD cells (24). At the heavily collagenized interphase of involutional and residual nodules, the number of VAD and VD cells decreases progressively and is replaced by an almost pure population of V cells (24,26,257). Despite their heterogeneity in intermediate filament proteins and actin isoforms, myofibroblasts from Dupuytren's disease (69,256) express usually only nonmuscle myosins. Exceptionally, isolated cells expressing smooth muscle myosin heavy chains [VA (D) M phenotypes] are observed (189). In these tissues, the extracellular matrix around myofibroblasts is strongly stained with antibodies to fibronectin but not to laminin (256,260).

Other Quasi-Neoplastic Proliferative Conditions

A heterogeneous cytoskeletal composition is also observed in myofibroblasts of dermatofibromas, which reveal at least three cytoskeletal phenotypes: VA, VAD, and V cells, with a predominance of VA cells in cellular dermatofibromas and an almost exclusive composition of V cells in fibrous dermatofibromas (261). Whether myofibroblasts of the VA (D) M phenotype exist has not yet been determined. By ultrastructure, cellular dermatofibromas are composed of well-developed myofibroblasts, joined by gap and intermediate junctions, and admixed with variable numbers of fibroblasts and macrophages. Fibrous dermatofibromas, in contrast, are composed almost exclusively of fibroblasts and feature only small numbers of poorly developed myofibroblasts.

This heterogeneous cellular and cytoskeletal phenotypic composition of dermatofibromas permits one to distinguish them from dermatofibrosarcoma protuberans, which represents a pure fibroblastic neoplasm—both at the ultrastructural level and with regard to the cytoskeletal immunophenotype (261). Furthermore, the heterogeneous cytoskeletal composition of dermatofibroma identifies this lesion definitively as a quasineoplastic reactive and proliferative condition, whereas dermatofibrosarcoma protuberans represents a fibroblastic neoplasm (261).

Nodular and proliferative fasciitis are predominantly composed of myofibroblasts with similar cytoskeletal phenotypes of VA and rare VAD cells, the latter being more prominent in the proliferative variant (Figure 6.13A–C).

Infantile myofibromatosis reveals a predominance of VA cells with limited numbers of VAD cells. By ultrastructure, in contrast to other fibromatoses, smooth muscle differentiation appears to be more prominent than in conventional fibromatoses, although typical myofibroblasts are numerous, a feature that justifies the term *infantile myofibromatosis*. Furthermore, massive apoptosis has been documented in infantile myofibromatosis and is proposed as a putative mechanism of regression of this proliferative myofibroblastic lesion (262).

Stromal Response to Neoplasia

Legions of medical students have been taught that many invasive and metastatic carcinomas are characterized by hard consistency and retraction and are often fixed to adjacent tissues. Typical examples are invasive ductal mammary carcinomas, associated with skin and or nipple retraction (Figure 6.14A), annular stenosing colon carcinomas (Figure 6.14B), gastric linitis plastica, the so-called frozen pelvis in advanced gynecological carcinomas, the "woody hard" nodule of invasive prostatic carcinoma, and metastatic carcinoma in matted lymph nodes fixed to surrounding tissues and the overlying skin. The hard consistency and the retraction phenomena are due to the desmoplastic stromal reaction and contracting myofibroblasts.

Myofibroblasts are particularly numerous within the stroma of desmoplastic and retracted primary invasive and metastatic carcinomas (6,20–23,263), and the retraction associated with such carcinomas is attributed to the contractile forces generated by stromal myofibroblasts. Myofibroblasts are usually not observed in the stroma contiguous to in situ carcinomas (Figures 6.15A–B, 6.16A–B) (6,23), suggesting that invasion beyond the basal lamina is required to evoke a myofibroblastic stromal reaction. On occasion, stromal cells expressing α-smooth muscle actin are observed around in situ ductal breast carcinoma (personal observation, Figure 6.15C–D). By ultrastructure, the periductal stromal cells expressing α-smooth muscle actin may disclose the typical morphologic features of myofibroblasts with well-developed stress fibers and fibronexus. This early myofibroblastic stromal reaction around ducts of in situ carcinomas is not uniform in a given case but may change from one duct to another (Figure 6.17A–B). Myofibroblasts have also been described in squamous intraepithelial lesions of the uterine cervix, close to the basal lamina, in increasing numbers and intensity of staining

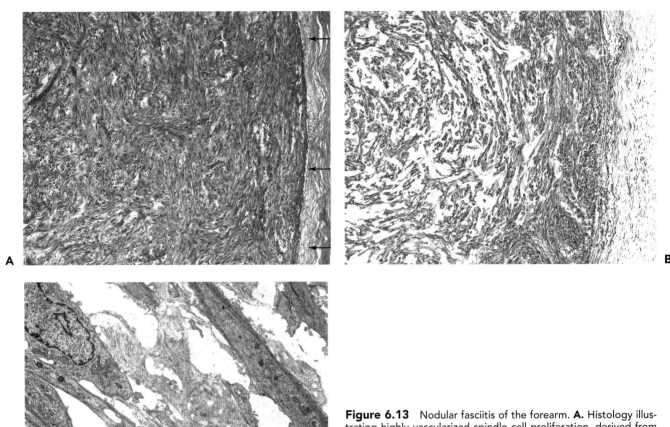

A

B

C

Figure 6.13   Nodular fasciitis of the forearm. **A.** Histology illustrating highly vascularized spindle cell proliferation, derived from the subcutaneous fascia (*arrows*) (hematoxylin-phloxine-saffron). **B.** The majority of the spindle cells and vascular smooth muscle cells express α-smooth muscle actin (VA cells). **C.** By ultrastructure, most of the stromal cells within the nodule correspond to typical myofibroblasts. (Uranyl acetate and lead citrate, ×6900.)

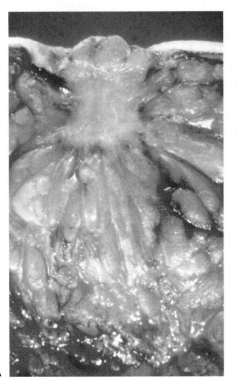

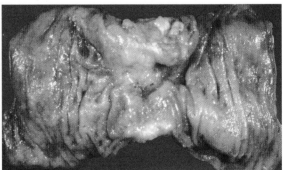

A

B

Figure 6.14   Gross appearance of infiltrating ductal carcinoma of the breast and of infiltrating colon carcinoma. **A.** Note irregular stellate shape of the carcinoma and retraction of the cut surface and the nipple. **B.** The colon carcinoma features annular stenosis. The carcinoma invaded the pericolic fibroadipose tissue.

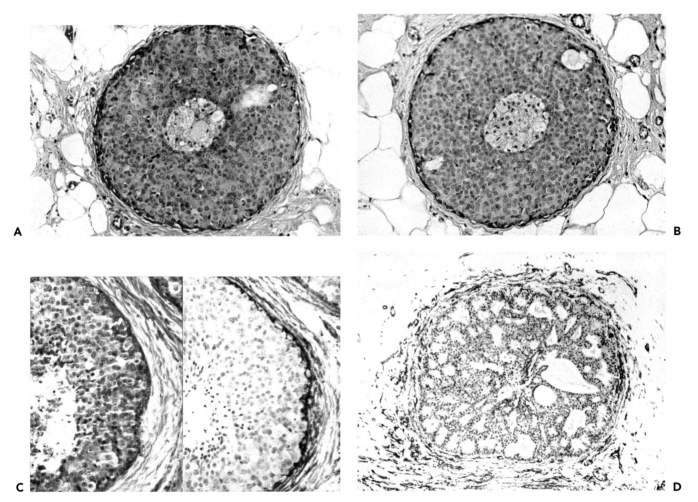

Figure 6.15 In situ breast carcinoma. **A. and B.** Step-sections of in situ cribriform carcinoma, disclosing continuous layer of myoepithelial cells as revealed by immunostaining for α-smooth muscle actin. Periductal stromal cells lack immunostaining for α-smooth muscle actin (B). **C.** Step-sections of comedocarcinoma: Numerous periductal stromal cells disclose significant staining for α-smooth muscle actin. **D.** In situ cribriform carcinoma with numerous periductal stromal cells stained for α-smooth muscle actin. (A and C–left part: hematoxylin-phloxine-saffron.)

from low-grade to high-grade variants, using immunohistochemical techniques (264).

Stromal cells with myofibroblastic features are notably absent or equivocally present within carcinomas lacking significant retraction and desmoplasia (Figure 6.18A–C) (23).

Myofibroblasts are not uniformly distributed within desmoplastic carcinomas. When their spatial relation to other components of breast carcinomas is analyzed, they are most numerous within the young mesenchymal stroma, areas corresponding to early stromal invasion, or, more consistently, in the peripheral invasive cellular front of mammary carcinomas (Figures 6.19A–F, 6.20A) (23). In the central sclerotic area of such neoplasms, myofibroblasts are poorly-developed or absent; this possibly is a reflection of apoptosis (Figures 6.19G–H, 6.20B) (23). Similarly, myofibroblasts are numerous in the cellular, edematous, and poorly collagenized stroma of other invasive and metastatic carcinomas (23).

Three types of myofibroblastic stromal reactions are observed within infiltrating ductal mammary carcinomas: (a) precocious (Figure 6.19A–B), myofibroblasts precede the carcinoma cells by some distance into adjacent tissue; (b) synchronous (Figure 6.19C–D), myofibroblasts appear spatially among the carcinoma cells; and (c) late (Figure 6.19E–F), myofibroblasts are identified central to the peripheral invasive cellular front of the carcinoma cells (23). These three types of myofibroblastic stromal reactions are observed in different areas of the invading front of most infiltrating ductal carcinomas of the breast, the synchronous stromal reaction being usually predominant (23). When the collagenous matrix is analyzed, increased amounts of type III collagen are present within the young mesenchyme, areas with numerous myofibroblasts. In contrast, type I collagen is most prominent within the central sclerotic zone of breast carcinomas (106), areas in which myofibroblasts are replaced by fibroblasts (Figure 6.19G–H) (22,23).

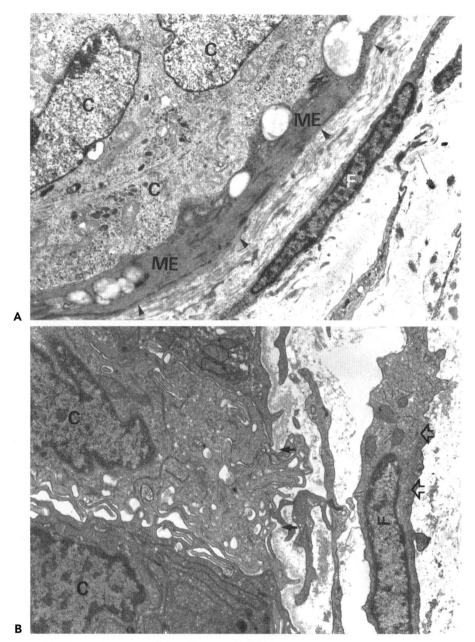

Figure 6.16 Ultrastructure of in situ ductal carcinoma of the breast. **A.** A continuous layer of my-oepithelial cells *(ME)* and a continuous basal lamina *(arrowheads)* separate the carcinoma cells *(C)* from the surrounding stroma. The stromal fibroblast *(F)* discloses smooth cellular and nuclear con-tours; the cytoplasm is scant and devoid of bundles of microfilaments. **B.** Ultramicroinvasive ductal carcinoma. A carcinoma cell *(C)* protrudes with a cytoplasmic extension into the periductal stroma through a gap within the basal lamina *(arrows)*. The periductal fibroblast reveals abundant cytoplasm and discloses aggregates of microfilaments with attenuated dense bodies *(open arrows)*. (Uranyl ac-etate and lead citrate, A, ×11,250; B, ×13,500). (Source: Schürch W, Lagacé R, Seemayer TA. Myofibroblastic stromal reactions in retracted scirrhous carcinomas of the breast. *Surg Gynec Oncol* 1982;154:351–358.)

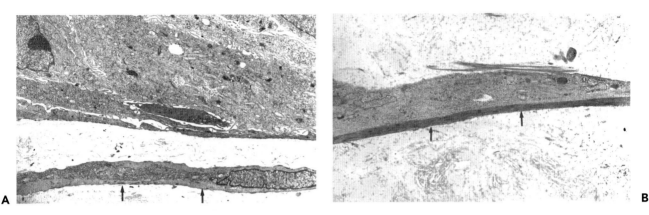

Figure 6.17   A. and B. Ultrastructure of in situ ductal carcinoma of the breast. In situ carcinoma with periductal myofibroblasts with well-developed stress fibers (*arrows*) (uranyl acetate and lead citrate; A, ×7875; B, ×12,500).

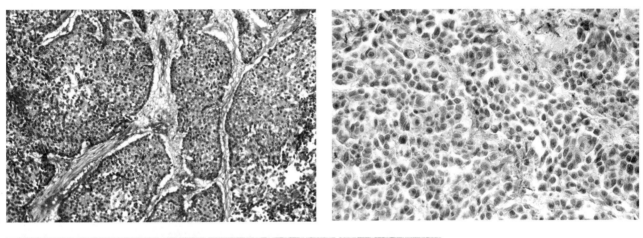

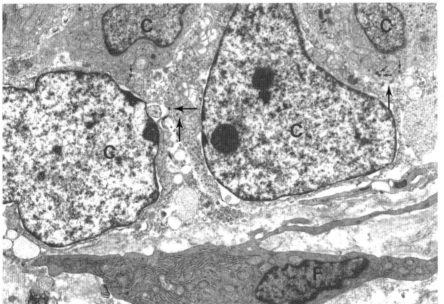

Figure 6.18 Oat-cell carcinoma of the lung. **A.** Histological aspect illustrating clusters of small neoplastic cells separated by small connective tissue septa (hematoxylin-phloxine-saffron). **B.** Stromal cells reveal no significant staining for α-smooth muscle actin (avidin-biotin-complex-peroxidase). **C.** Transmission electron micrograph illustrating neoplastic cells (*C*) with scattered electron-dense neurosecretory-type granules (*arrows*) in close proximity to a fibroblast (*F*) with a smooth, contoured nucleus devoid of microfilaments (uranyl acetate and lead citrate, ×10,300).

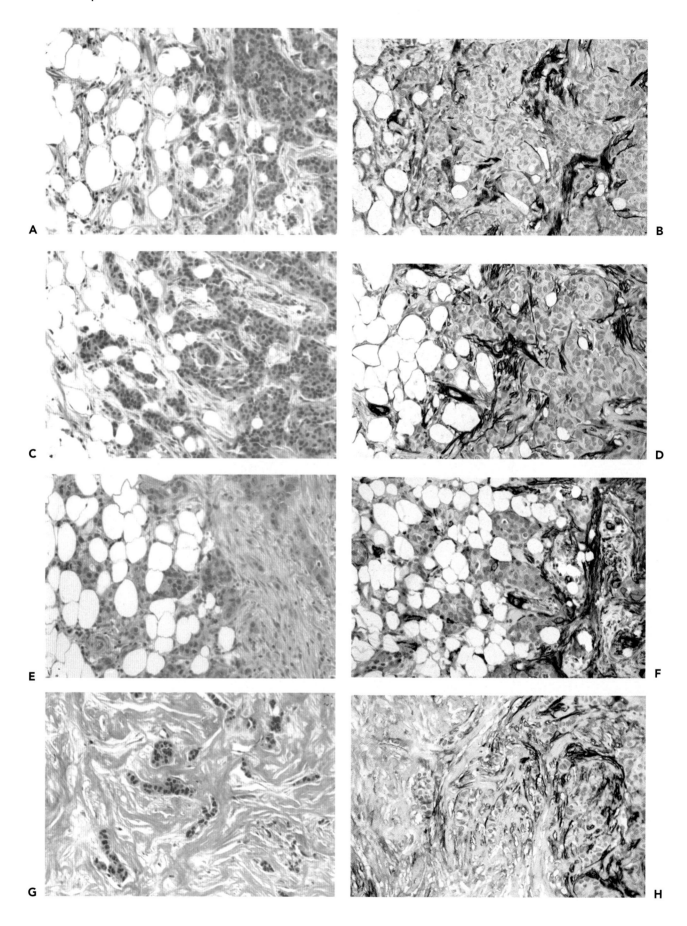

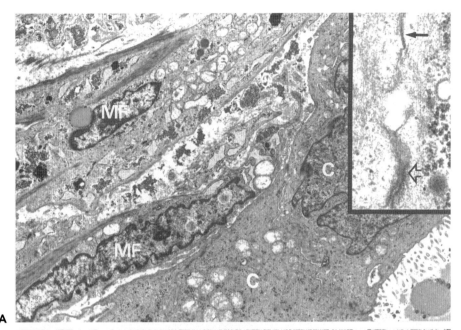

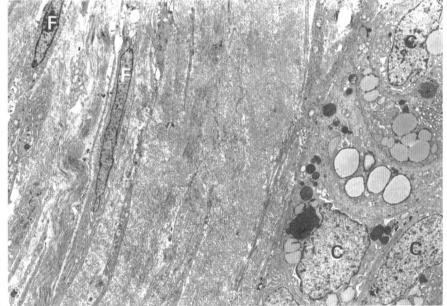

Figure 6.20 Ultrastructural aspect of ductal-infiltrating carcinoma of the breast. **A.** Peripheral invasive cellular front revealing numerous typical stromal myofibroblasts *(MF)* with notched nuclei and bundles of cytoplasmic microfilaments with dense bodies around neoplastic cells *(C)* adjacent to an acinus, which is in the lower right corner. **Inset:** Stromal myofibroblasts are joined by gap *(arrow)* and intermediate junctions *(open arrow)*. (Source: Schürch W, Seemayer TA, Lagacé R, Gabbiani G. The intermediate filament cytoskeleton of myofibroblasts. *Virchows Arch A* 1984;403:323–336.) **B.** Central sclerotic area illustrating stromal cells *(F)* with smooth contoured nuclei devoid of abundant cytoplasmic microfilaments and separated by thick bands of mature collagen around clusters of carcinoma cells*(C)*. (Source: Schürch W, Seemayer TA, Lagacé R. Stromal myofibroblasts in primary invasive and metastatic carcinomas. *Virchows Arch A* 1981;391:125–139.) (Uranyl acetate and lead citrate, A, ×8400; inset, ×60,000; B, ×5000.)

Figure 6.19 Ductal-infiltrating carcinoma of the breast with stromal desmoplasia, step-sections stained with hematoxylin-phloxine-saffron and with antibodies to α-smooth muscle actin. **A. and B.** Precocious stromal reaction; stromal cells precede carcinoma cells by some distance into the adjacent fatty tissue. The majority of these stromal cells express α-smooth muscle actin (B). **C. and D.** Synchronous stromal reaction; stromal cells are distributed amongst the carcinoma cells. Most of these stromal cells express α-smooth muscle actin (D). **E. and F.** Late stromal reaction; stromal cells appear central to the peripheral invasive front of carcinoma cells and express α-smooth muscle actin (F). **G. and H.** Central sclerotic area of ductal-infiltrating carcinoma. Clusters of carcinoma cells are surrounded by thick bands of collagen (G). At the border of the invasive cellular front of the carcinoma, a decrease of the immunostaining of the stromal cells toward the central area *(left to right side)* is observed. (A, C, E and G, hematoxylin-phloxine-saffron; B, D, F, and H, avidin-biotin-complex-peroxidase.)

Many pulmonary carcinomas, especially peripheral adenocarcinomas, are associated with some degree of scarring and are often associated with pleural retraction. If this process is pronounced, the term *scar carcinoma* is applied to these neoplasms. In 1962, Carroll (265) reported that the presence of elastic fibers and anthracotic pigment in scars suggested that they had been present prior to the development of the neoplasm. The more recent literature suggests that scarring represents a desmoplastic stromal reaction in response to neoplastic invasion rather than a preexistent condition. In favor of this latter interpretation is the presence of increased amounts of type III collagen within pul-

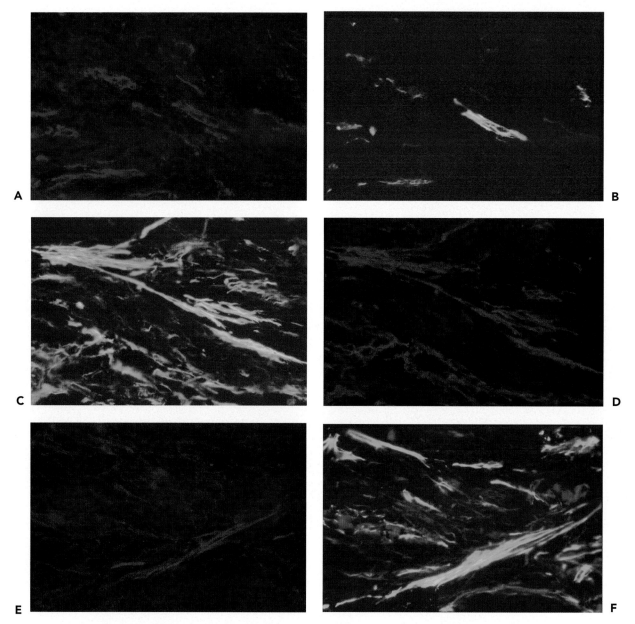

Figure 6.21 Step-sections of peripheral invasive cellular front of ductal breast carcinoma revealing V, VA, VAD, and VA (D) M myofibroblasts. **A. and B.** Double immunofluorescent staining for α-smooth muscle actin (A) and desmin (B). Stromal cells expressing α-smooth muscle actin (VA cells) are more numerous than those expressing α-smooth muscle actin and desmin (VAD cells). **C. and D.** Double immunofluorescent staining for α-smooth muscle actin (C) and smooth muscle myosin heavy chain (D). Stromal cells expressing α-smooth muscle actin (VA cells) are slightly more numerous than those expressing smooth muscle myosin heavy chain [VA (D) M cells]. **E. and F.** Double immunofluorescent staining for desmin (E) and myosin heavy chain (F). Stromal cells expressing smooth muscle myosin heavy chain (VM cells) are far more numerous than those that express desmin [VA (D) M cells]. In conclusion, the peripheral invasive front of ductal breast carcinomas contains predominantly VA cells, followed by VA (D) M cells.

monary carcinomas with marked scarring (266), as is seen in early invasive zones of mammary carcinoma (104). In addition, the majority of stromal cells in scar carcinomas of the lung reveal ultrastructural features of myofibroblasts (267), suggesting that pulmonary carcinomas with scarring are neoplasms with a desmoplastic stromal reaction, analogous to many invasive and metastatic carcinomas elsewhere.

Analysis of cytoskeletal proteins, including intermediate filaments, actin isoforms, and smooth muscle myosin heavy chains reveals phenotypic heterogeneity of stromal cells in invasive and metastatic carcinomas. Areas with numerous myofibroblasts, corresponding to early stromal invasion of breast carcinomas, contain a predominance of VA cells admixed with variable numbers of VAD, VA (D) M, and V cells (Figure 6.21A–F), suggesting that certain stromal cells undergo a form of cytodifferentiation not too dissimilar from smooth muscle metaplasia (VA (D) M cells). In contrast, sclerotic areas disclose numerous V cells with occasional VA cells. No VAD and VA (D) M cells are observed (results not shown).

Myofibroblasts have also been described in sarcomas where they generally constitute a small fraction of the cell population (268–270). They were identified in all cases of malignant fibrous histiocytomas and well-differentiated sclerosing liposarcomas (270). Though most numerous in areas of desmoplasia, in no instance did myofibroblasts constitute the dominant cellular constituent of either neoplasm (Figure 6.22) (270). Myofibroblasts have been identified with lesser frequency and in smaller numbers in fibrosarcoma, synovial sarcoma, malignant hemangiopericytoma, and neuroblastoma. No myofibroblasts were observed in a wide assortment of diverse sarcomas in which desmoplasia was not a feature.

Myofibroblasts have been identified in nodular sclerosing Hodgkin's disease at the nodule-stromal interphase, which is usually heavily collagenized (271). These areas contain numerous VA and V cells with very occasional VAD cells (Figure 6.23). Whether this contributes to the relatively favorable prognosis of this variant of Hodgkin's disease is an open question.

Neoplasms of Myofibroblasts: Benign and Malignant

Finally, several reports describe myofibroblastic neoplasms. In our opinion, neoplastic transformation of the myofibroblast, in the extreme is possible (272) but certainly remains an uncommon event. The plethora of articles related to this matter, particularly in the mid- and late-1990s, stems from the criteria employed to define this cell. The

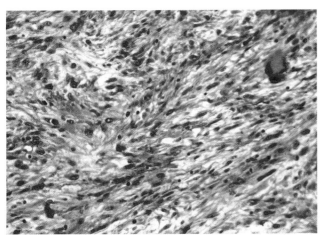

A

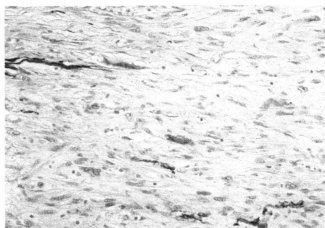

B

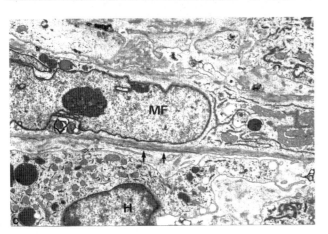

C

Figure 6.22 Malignant fibrous histiocytoma (storiform-pleomorphic type). **A.** Histological aspect illustrating spindle cell tumor with storiform pattern and isolated pleomorphic cells (hematoxylin-phloxine-saffron). **B.** Few spindle cells disclose immunostaining for α-smooth muscle actin (avidin-biotin-complex-peroxidase). **C.** Transmission electron micrograph illustrating a typical myofibroblast *(MF)* with cytoplasmic bundle of microfilaments; the cell is partly enveloped by a basal lamina *(arrows)* (uranyl acetate and lead citrate, ×25,000).

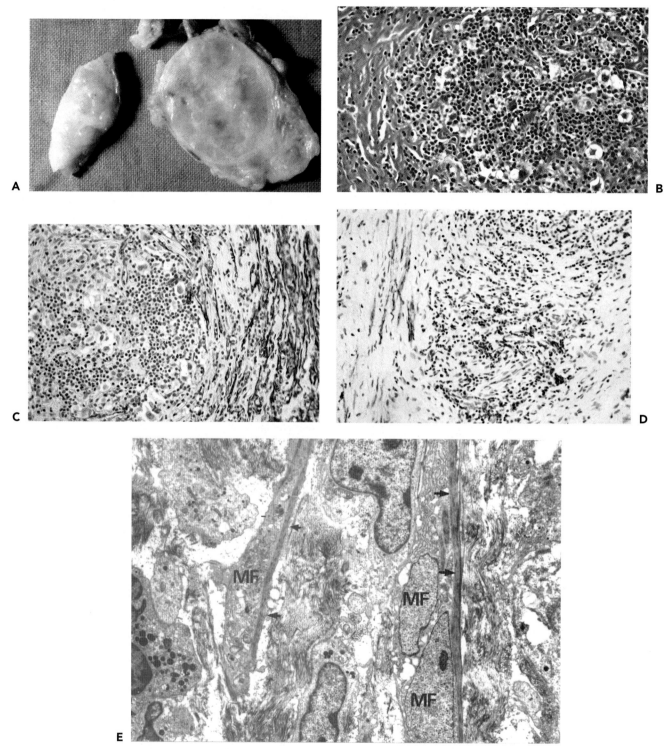

Figure 6.23   Nodular sclerosing Hodgkin's disease. **A.** Gross aspect of cut surface of lymph node demonstrating nodules surrounded by thick connective tissue septa (lymph node cirrhosis). (Courtesy of Dr. Roger Gareau, Department of Pathology, Hôtel-Dieu Hospital, University of Montreal, Montreal, Quebec, Canada.) **B.** Histologic aspect illustrating nodules of atypical lymphoid nodules with some lacunar cells. The nodules are enveloped by dense collagenous containing numerous spindle cells (hematoxylin-phloxine-saffron). **C.** Several spindle cells around the nodule express α-smooth muscle actin (VA cells). **D.** Few spindle cells express desmin (VAD cells). All internodular stromal cells express antivimentin (results not shown). **E.** Transmission electron micrograph from internodular stroma illustrating numerous typical myofibroblasts *(MF)* with bundles of cytoplasmic microfilaments and dense bodies *(arrows)*. (Uranyl acetate and lead citrate, ×5000.)

myofibroblast is presently defined solely at the ultrastructural level; its definition at the light microscopic and immunohistochemical levels is less precise and, on occasion, imprecise. A significant number of reports describe myofibroblastic neoplasms; some were considered as sarcomas (273–279), and many more were described as benign myofibroblastomas or tumors of similar character with an assortment of designations (280–291).

The benign myofibroblastic proliferations are generally well-circumscribed lesions, contrary to the poorly circumscribed and often infiltrating quality of reactive and quasineoplastic proliferative conditions; for example, fibromatoses, nodular and proliferative fasciitis, and proliferative myositis, lesions replete with myofibroblasts. Although thought to be composed of myofibroblasts, most of the benign myofibroblastomas were not evaluated ultrastructurally; in the few cases for which this technique was employed, typical myofibroblasts were not found. For similar reasons one might cast a jaundiced eye on the presence of myofibroblasts in mammary myofibroblastomas (289,290), the palisaded myofibroblastoma, the intranodal hemorrhagic spindle-cell tumors with amianthoid fibers of lymph nodes (288,291), soft tissue myofibroblastomas (284), angiomyofibroblastomas of the vulva (281,282), angiomyofibroblastoma-like tumors of the male genital tract (285), meningeal myofibroblastomas (287), and pulmonary myofibroblastic tumors (280). Immunohistochemically, the proliferating cells composing the so-called myofibroblastomas and related neoplasms disclose heterogeneous cytoskeletal phenotypes, such as positive reaction for α-smooth muscle actin and absence of reactivity for desmin in the palisaded myofibroblastoma (291) and intranodal hemorrhagic spindle-cell tumors of lymph nodes (288) and staining for desmin associated with a negative reaction for α-smooth muscle actin in angiomyofibroblastoma of the vulva (281). The so-called myofibroblastomas and all other related neoplasms most likely represent myogenic stromal tumors, a designation proposed by Bégin (292), possibly derived from myogenic stromal cells that have variable degrees of smooth muscle differentiation (rather than myofibroblastic neoplasms) because myofibroblasts, using strict ultrastructural criteria, either were not identified or were rare (Figure 6.24).

Sarcomas composed entirely or partially of cells that disclose some degree of morphologic or immunohistochemical features of myofibroblasts but lack the typical ultrastructural traits of myofibroblasts could well belong to the group of myogenic sarcomas (63). One has to remember that for a cell to be classified as a myofibroblast it need not express α-smooth muscle actin (134). In fact, whether or not a cell expresses α-smooth muscle actin has no bearing on whether or not it is a myofibroblast. In our opinion, while myofibroblastic sarcomas may exist, they are rare and their identification requires electron microscopy (57,58).

Finally, to conclude this controversial issue, it might be well to cite Juan Rosai (59):

> Cells with myofibroblastic (myoid) features can be found in a large number of benign and malignant soft tissue lesions, which means that we are in danger of creating a waste-basket category, just as large if not larger than that of malignant fibrous histiocytoma. Therefore, if there is to be a category of myofibroblastic tumors, it would be wise to reserve it for lesions that are composed almost entirely of cells having the hybrid features of myofibroblasts and which do not fit the criteria of already established entities.

Now, a few words concerning inflammatory myofibroblastic tumor (IMT). In the 2002 World Health Organization (WHO) classification of soft tissue tumors, IMT is presented as a clinical/pathologic entity, albeit one that is genetically heterogeneous. Its synonyms are numerous: plasma cell granuloma, plasma cell pseudotumor, inflammatory myofibrohistiocytic proliferation, omental mesenteric myxoid hamartoma, inflammatory pseudotumor, and inflammatory fibrosarcoma. The entity appears to have emerged in a manner reminiscent of malignant fibrous histiocytoma (293). That this tumor discloses predominant myofibroblastic differentiation is questionable. Classically, these tumors present in the lung, mesentery, and omentum of children or adolescents and may be accompanied by fever, weight loss, fatigue, anemia, thrombocytosis, polyclonal hyperglobulinemia, and an elevated erythrocyte sedimentation rate (294). Histologic sections reveal a polymorphous mixture of cells, including spindle cells, plasma cells, lymphocytes, eosinophils, and occasional ganglion-like cells. The spindle cells in 50% of the tumors express cytoplasmic ALK protein, and this correlates with rearrangments of the ALK receptor tyrosine kinase gene at 2p23, as detected by fluorescent in situ hybridization (FISH). This genetic aberration is most commonly seen in pediatric IMT tumors but is not specific for the condition. In addition to anaplastic lymphoma kinase (ALK) expression, p80 is consistently expressed in IMT (295). Most of the tumors are biologically benign; however, up to 25% of the nonpulmonary tumors may recur and, in rare instances, the tumor may metastasize.

Thus, in our opinion, most of the described myofibroblastic sarcomas described are not unequivocally composed of myofibroblasts. That said, we have to admit that a few conditions (particularly malignant neoplasms) composed of spindle cells disclosing ultrastructural features of myofibroblasts have been described, but they are rare (57,296). As for IMT, whether or not this is a specific entity in which the myofibroblast is the principal cell is an open question.

MULTIPLE ORIGINS OF THE MYOFIBROBLAST

Considering the many conditions in which myofibroblasts occur, their heterogeneous cytoskeletal composition, and

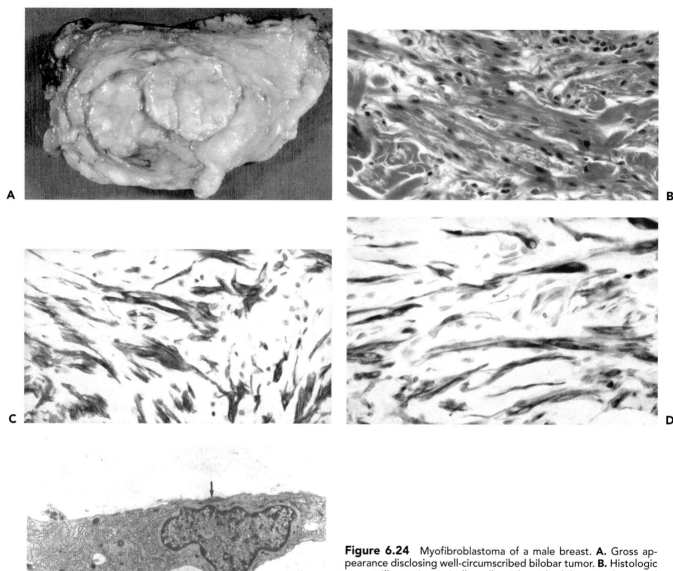

Figure 6.24 Myofibroblastoma of a male breast. **A.** Gross appearance disclosing well-circumscribed bilobar tumor. **B.** Histologic aspect illustrating spindle cells with acidophilic cytoplasm and bland nuclei (hematoxylin-phloxine-saffron). **C. and D.** Intense immunostaining for α-smooth muscle actin and desmin. **E.** Ultrastructural aspect disclosing discrete smooth muscle differentiation. Short bundle of microfilaments and segment of basal lamina (*arrow*). (Uranyl acetate and lead citrate, ×17,750.)

the various functions attributed to them, it seems difficult at first glance to assume a common origin for these cells. In 1867, Cohnheim (297) proposed the vascular theory, which states that leukocytes are transformed into fibroblasts during the process of wound healing. Several subsequent studies, however, provided evidence that granulation tissue fibroblasts arise rather from local connective tissue cells (298–301). As we shall see below, circulating leukocytes and resident tissue fibroblasts are now recognized as precursors to the myofibroblasts found in granulation tissue.

Amongst connective tissue cells that could transform into myofibroblasts, any mesenchymal cell is a potential candidate: foremost is the fibroblast, followed by the

pericyte and the smooth muscle cell (302). With the accumulated knowledge of cytoskeletal proteins and actin isoforms in these three cell types, both in vivo and in vitro, all of these cells could be considered as possible progenitors of myofibroblasts.

Granulation tissue myofibroblasts are principally derived from local fibroblasts (25,260,303). Within experimental and human granulation tissues, myofibroblasts temporarily express a marker of smooth muscle differentiation, α-smooth muscle actin, which disappears after wound closure (25). This suggests that differentiation of myofibroblasts toward smooth muscle cells is only partial, at least during normal wound healing, because myofibroblasts in this condition never express desmin or smooth muscle myosin heavy chain isoforms.

Recently, the cytoskeletal features of myofibroblasts during wound healing, Dupuytren's disease, and the stroma of mammary carcinomas were investigated. In these three conditions, myofibroblasts disclosed a progressive differentiation toward the smooth muscle phenotype (189). Whereas myofibroblasts during wound healing express only α-smooth muscle actin, myofibroblasts in Dupuytren's disease express smooth muscle myosin heavy chains, at least in some cases. An important proportion of myofibroblasts within the stroma of all cases of mammary carcinomas express, in addition to α-smooth muscle actin, desmin and smooth muscle myosin heavy chain isoforms. This suggests that fibroblastic cells are capable of proceeding well along the lines of smooth muscle cell differentiation. However myofibroblasts have not been shown to express smoothelin (304–306), a terminal smooth muscle cell differentiation marker, in any of the pathologic states examined (305). Hence, smoothelin expression may be used as a discrimination marker between the two cells.

Ultrastructural data provide evidence that during pathologic or culture conditions, fibroblasts and smooth muscle cells acquire morphologic features resembling myofibroblasts (87,307–311), suggesting that both cell types might be progenitors of myofibroblasts. Indeed, an extensive study on the modulation of mesenchymal cells within the mammary gland stroma when placed in culture in a microenvironment mimicking conditions observed in vivo indicates that although most myofibroblasts are derived from fibroblasts, a certain proportion are derived from vascular smooth muscle cells and a lesser proportion from pericytes (312). With the caveat that it is difficult to extrapolate in vitro data to in vivo situations, this work supports the concept of a heterogeneous origin of myofibroblastic cells.

A vascular origin of the myofibroblast was also proposed on the basis of morphologic observations. It was suggested that desmin-positive cells migrate from the wall of vessels to the tissue (257). A possible source of myofibroblasts expressing vimentin and desmin also are the stromal cells of various organs positive for desmin but negative for α-smooth muscle actin (67,183,184,313). The possibility that myofibroblasts arise from specialized mesenchymal cells of certain organs has found a convincing confirmation in recent years. An abundant clinical and experimental literature has shown that, during the onset of experimental and human hepatic fibrosis and cirrhosis, perisinusoidal stellate cells of the liver are the most likely source of myofibroblastic cells (32,314–316). The conditions facilitating the modulation of perisinusoidal stellate cells into myofibroblasts have been studied, and extracellular matrix components and cytokines have been suggested as possible initiators (317–320,149). Similarly, glomerular mesangial cells have been shown to acquire myofibroblastic features, including the expression of α-smooth muscle actin and col-

lagen, in several experimental and human pathologic situations (33,229,321,322). Lung septal fibroblasts, which normally possess contractile features without expressing α-smooth muscle actin (323), can be induced to express this protein and collagen type I mRNA upon pathologic stimuli, such as bleomycin treatment (324,29).

Recently, advances have been made demonstrating that myofibroblasts can originate from circulating precursors and also be the product of epithelial-mesenchymal transitions. Buccala et al. (36) have identified a leukocyte subpopulation, named fibrocyte, with fibroblast-like properties. Peripheral blood fibrocytes can rapidly enter the site of injury at the same time as circulating inflammatory cells. It has been suggested that circulating fibrocytes may represent an important source of myofibroblasts during healing of extensive burn wounds, where it may be difficult for fibroblasts to migrate from the wound edge (37). This study has also shown that fibrocyte development is systematically elevated in burn patients. Furthermore, TGF-β1, which is elevated in the serum of burn patients (325), stimulates the modulation of peripheral blood mononuclear cells into collagen-producing cells, underlying the well-known role of this cytokine in the differentiation of the myofibroblast (326,27). It has been also shown that bone marrow–derived myofibroblasts contribute to the stroma reaction, at least in experimental situations (325). Another location in which fibrocytes contribute to myofibroblast population is the bronchial submucosa during the development of asthma (327). Epithelial-mesenchymal transition plays an important role in myofibroblast accumulation taking place in kidney interstitial fibrosis, the source of myofibroblasts being tubular epithelial cells, (34) and in dialysis-induced peritoneal fibrosis, the source of myofibroblasts being mesothelial cells (35).

Thus, it appears that several cells, including fibroblasts, vascular smooth muscle cells, pericytes, perisinusoidal stellate cells in the liver, renal tubular epithelial cells, mesangial cells, bloodborne cells (fibrocytes), and mesothelial cells, can modulate (upon appropriate stimulation) into a myofibroblastic phenotype. It should be stressed, however, that the major source of myofibroblasts in whatever setting they appear is the resident fibroblast.

MECHANISMS OF MYOFIBROBLAST REGRESSION

Granulation tissue formation involves the replication and migration of fibroblasts from normal tissues to the area of inflammation and the modulation of at least a proportion of them to the myofibroblastic phenotype. Angiogenesis takes place in a coordinated way, and granulation tissue acquires its typical features. When the wound closes, a gradual evolution toward scar tissue takes place that involves the disappearance of vascular cells and myofibroblasts with a proportional increase of extracellular matrix components. This phenomenon, which ends with the establishment of a scar, is more or less rapid according to the species, the location of granulation tissue, and the type of inflammation (7). When granulation tissue cells are not eliminated, there is the development of pathologic scarring (i.e., hypertrophic scars and keloids), which are distinct clinical and pathologic conditions (232), both characterized by a relative high degree of cellularity.

Recently, using several morphologic and biochemical techniques, it has been shown that the reduction in cell number (myofibroblasts and vascular cells) observed during the transition between granulation tissue and scar formation is achieved to a great extent through apoptosis (Figure 6.25) (31); whether the lack of apoptosis plays a role in the establishment of hypertrophic scar and keloid remains to be explored. It appears that apoptosis of granulation tissue cells takes place essentially after wound closure and affects myofibroblasts and vascular cells over a

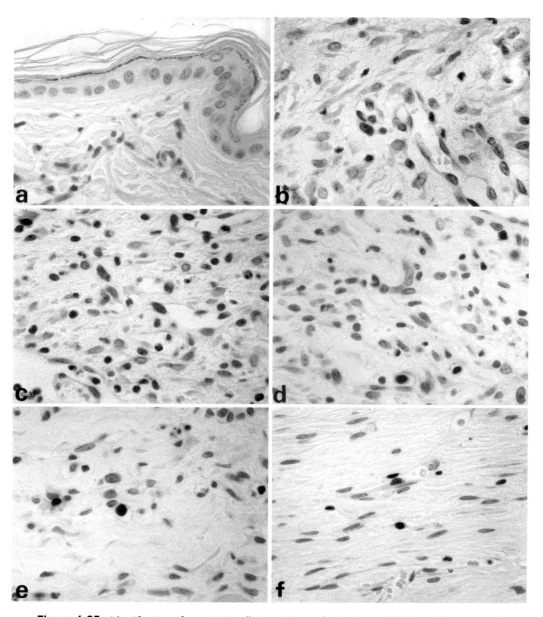

Figure 6.25 Identification of apoptotic cells in rat tissues by in situ end labeling of fragmented DNA. **A.** Normal rat skin, no apoptotic cells are detected. **B.** Twelve-day-old wound tissue. **C.** Sixteen-day-old wound tissue. **D.** Twenty-day-old wound tissue. **E.** Twenty-five-day-old wound tissue. **F.** Thirty-day-old wound tissue. At 12 days, when α-smooth muscle actin expression is maximal, there is no nuclear staining for apoptotic cells; after this, the number of labeled cells increases, with a maximum at 20 days (D). Thereafter (E and F), the number of labeled cells decreases. (A–F, ×1000.)

period of time, rather than occurring as a single and massive wave of cellular apoptosis. This observation is in line with the gradual resorption of granulation tissue after wound closure and with the observation that dead cells are digested by macrophages and surrounding cells. It appears that granulation tissue cell apoptosis can be accelerated significantly by the application of a viable cutaneous flap (328). This observation underlines the importance of cell communication between normal connective tissue and granulation tissue. These reports suggest that, at least during normal wound healing, the process of myofibroblast differentiation generally ends with cell death; thus, myofibroblasts can be considered terminally differentiated cells.

The question that remains to be answered is the stimulus that leads to apoptosis during wound healing. The loss of mechanical stress seems to be an important signal for differentiated myofibroblasts to de-differentiate and/or disappear. At the end of normal wound healing the extracellular matrix is reconstituted and assumes the mechanical load, thereby releasing embedded myofibroblasts from stress. Myofibroblast apoptosis has been induced by the stress-release of wound granulation tissue after removal of a flap coverage with splinting characteristics in vivo (329) and by the relaxation of attached collagen gels (330,331) in vitro. Fibroblasts in mechanically unrestrained floating versus anchored collagen matrices also show differences in cell proliferation and DNA synthesis. After contraction of floating collagen matrices there is a marked decline in DNA synthesis; the cell cycle becomes arrested and cell regression begins. In contrast, fibroblastic cells in anchored matrices continue to proliferate and to synthesize DNA.

Recently gene products regulating cell death have been identified (332–337). In fibroblasts, the c-myc protein (338) and interleukin-1–converting enzyme, the mammalian homologue of the *Caenorhabditis elegans* gene *ced-3* (339), have been shown to induce apoptosis. In turn, it has been shown that the bcl-2 protein is capable of blocking apoptosis (340); however, fibroblasts lack bcl-2 expression, as assessed by antibody staining. A possible mechanism for apoptosis induction could be via the direct action and/or withdrawal of cytokines or growth factors (341–343). Several factors have been shown to increase the rate of wound healing, including platelet-derived growth factor (PDGF) (344), TGF-β (344–346), and tumor necrosis factor (TNF) (347). These factors may be present in the normal healing wound, released by platelets and inflammatory cells (348,349). It is probable that, as the wound heals and resolves, there is a decrease in the level of these factors. A possible explanation for the death of at least a subpopulation of myofibroblasts and vascular cells could be that they are growth-factor dependent. Alternatively, factors selectively causing the death of myofibroblasts and vascular cells might be liberated after epithelialization has been completed. Additional work is necessary to identify these hypothetical factors, but it appears that apoptosis is the

mechanism through which vascular and myofibroblastic cells are gradually eliminated from normally healing granulation tissue.

CONCLUDING REMARKS

For this third edition, every section has been updated. In addition, several new topics have been added to reflect recent developments; additional photographs have been submitted; the reference list has been expanded.

Since the 1971 discovery of the myofibroblast in granulating wounds, one cannot help but be fascinated with the subject as the body of knowledge related to this pivotal cell expands, largely through the contributions of cellular and molecular biology.

It would appear that following induction of a large skin wound, resting fibroblasts are triggered through the effects of mechanical forces and possibly yet unknown cytokines released at the wound site to assume a proto-myofibroblastic phenotype characterized by the presence of stress fibers that contain cytoplasmic actin isoforms. These cells continue to modulate and eventually assume a myofibroblastic phenotype characterized by α-smooth muscle actin incorporation into stress fibers and the formation of specialized "supermature" focal adhesions. This process is regulated by TGF-β1 and ED-A cellular fibronectin and results in connective tissue remodeling with an increase of extracellular matrix synthesis, collagen type III in particular, and tissue retraction (i.e., wound contraction). Recent studies strongly indicate that the forces generated by myofibroblast stress fibers produce isometric tension; this is different from the reversible contraction taking place in smooth muscle cells and involves the Rho/Rho-kinase pathway, as well as regulated activity of myosin phosphatase.

As wound healing approaches completion, genes that encode for apoptotic proteins are expressed to initiate myofibroblastic cell death; the formerly cellular wound is then converted into a poorly cellular scar. Commensurate with this, there is a shift from collagen type III to collagen type I gene expression and synthesis, resulting in the deposition of type I collagen that provides strength to the developing scar. Furthermore, cytokines that stimulate extracellular matrix synthesis early on are repressed once wound closure is completed and a functional basement membrane has been synthesized; this suggests the existence of a feedback loop (350). It is likely that deviations from this finely orchestrated process contribute to the development of hypertrophic scars and keloids.

Regarding the diverse assortment of quasineoplastic myofibroblastic proliferative processes, the cellular/molecular mechanisms central to their pathogenesis remain essentially unexplored.

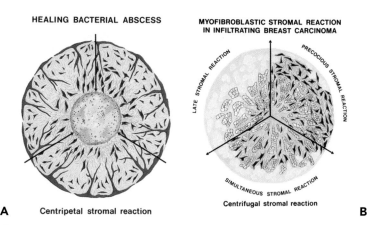

Figure 6.26 Schematic illustration of the stromal reaction. **A.** In a healing bacterial abscess, the cicatrizing layer is at the periphery, and the two layers containing myofibroblasts (exudativo-productive and exudative, respectively) are developing toward the center. **B.** In infiltrating ductal breast carcinoma, the cicatrizing area is in the center and myofibroblasts are disposed variably in the peripheral invasive cellular front of the carcinoma; precocious (preceding the invasive carcinoma cells), simultaneous (amongst the invasive carcinoma cells), and late (following the invasive carcinoma cells). In normal wound healing the stromal reaction is centripetal; whereas in invasive ductal breast carcinomas, the stromal reaction is centrifugal, indicating that cancers are wounds that do not heal.

Turning to the myofibroblastic response associated with diverse invasive and metastatic carcinomas, it was originally proposed that this represented an expression of host response to the cancer. The hypothesis appears valid today, although one could posit whether this is beneficial since many of these cancers, despite the attending desmoplasia, continue to exact lives. Yet, death, in these settings, stems largely from the ability of the neoplastic cell to enter vascular channels and disseminate. It remains possible that these myofibroblasts, while affecting contraction and elaborating collagens and other extracellular matrix components, also release enzymes that permit tissue and vascular invasion. Recently, the mechanisms regulating the cross talk between tumor cells and stroma myofibroblasts have started to be clarified (351). Thus, it appears that the concomitant production of growth factors and/or cytokines (such as TGF-β, hepatocyte growth factor, or stromal cell–derived factor-1) and synthesis of extracellular matrix components (such as tenascin) by stromal myofibroblasts stimulates the invasive activity of malignant epithelial cells (352,353,354). If one considers that during development connective tissue remodeling plays an important role in epithelial morphogenesis (353), it is possible to conceive that cross talk between stroma and epithelium regulates both physiologic and pathologic epithelial organization. Clearly, future studies of human cancer should focus not only on the neoplastic cell, but also on the regulation of extracellular matrix synthesis and the cell-to-extracellular matrix interactions of tumors (i.e., the stroma).

Twenty-four years ago (22), we proposed that similarities might exist between the process of wound healing and the stromal response to neoplastic invasion. This assumption may also be extended to quasineoplastic proliferative conditions (e.g., Dupuytren's disease). During normal wound healing and within nodules of Dupuytren's disease and possibly other quasineoplastic proliferations, the myofibroblastic/fibroblastic reaction appears to be centripetal (Figure 6.26A), whereas within neoplastic invasion this reaction is centrifugal (Figure 6.26B), indicating that cancers are wounds that do not heal (355). The underlying cellular/molecular mechanisms explaining these fundamental differences, including the presence, delay, or absence of apoptosis, remain to be explored.

Finally, we conclude, as in the 1997 edition, with a most intriguing report uncovered in a literature search of TGF-β. It would appear that fetal skin wounds in a murine model heal without scarring; such wounds, apart from that contained in platelets, are devoid of TGF-β (356). Once again, one is reminded of the lessons to be learned by study of the events of early life.

ACKNOWLEDGMENTS

This work was supported in part by the Cancer Research Society Inc., Montreal, Canada, the Swiss National Science Foundation (Grant No. #31-61.336.00 to GG and 3100A0-102150/1 to BH), and the Macdonald Stewart Foundation, Montreal, whose benefactors, Mrs. Liliane Stewart and the late David M. Stewart, have generously supported the Department of Pathology of the Hôtel-Dieu Hospital of Montreal over many years. We thank Mr. Som Chatterjee and Ms. Myrielle Vermette for skillful technical assistance and Mr. Jean-Jacques Dufour for the photographic work.

REFERENCES

1. Gabbiani G, Ryan GB, Majno G. Presence of modified fibroblasts in granulation tissue and their possible role in wound contraction. *Experientia* 1971;27:549–550.
2. Majno G, Gabbiani G, Hirschel BJ, Ryan GB, Statkov PR. Contraction of granulation tissue in vitro: similarity to smooth muscle. *Science* 1971;173:548–550.
3. Gabbiani G, Hirschel BJ, Ryan GB, Statkov PR, Majno G. Granulation tissue as a contractile organ. A study of structure and function. *J Exp Med* 1972;135:719–734.
4. Hirschel BJ, Gabbiani G, Ryan GB, Majno G. Fibroblasts of granulation tissue: immunofluorescent staining with antismooth muscle serum. *Proc Soc Exp Biol Med* 1971;138:466–469.
5. Gabbiani G, Ryan GB, Lamelin JP, et al. Human smooth muscle autoantibody. Its identification as antiactin antibody and a study of its binding to "nonmuscular" cells. *Am J Pathol* 1973;72: 473–488.
6. Seemayer TA, Lagacé R, Schürch W, Thelmo WL. The myofibroblast: biologic pathologic, and theoretical considerations. *Pathol Annu* 1980;15(pt 1):443–470.
7. Skalli O, Gabbiani G. The biology of the myofibroblast relationship to wound contraction and fibrocontractive diseases. In: Clark RAF, Henson PM, eds. *The Molecular and Cellular Biology of Wound Repair*. New York: Plenum Press; 1988:373–402.
8. Schmitt-Gräff A, Desmoulière A, Gabbiani G. Heterogeneity of myofibroblast phenotypic features: an example of fibroblastic cell plasticity. *Virchows Arch* 1994;425:3–24.
9. Majno G. The story of the myofibroblasts. *Am J Surg Pathol* 1979;3:535–542.
10. Majno G. *The Healing Hand: Man and Wound in the Ancient World.* Cambridge: Harvard University Press, 1975.
11. Carrel A, Hartmann A. Cicatrization of wounds. I. The relation between the size of the wound and the rate of its cicatrization. *J Exp Med* 1916;24:429–450.
12. Abercrombie M, Flint MH, James DW. Wound contraction in relation to collagen formation in scorbutic guinea pigs. *J Embryol Exp Morphol* 1956;4:167–175.
13. Hoffmann-Berling H. Adenosintriphosphat als betriebsstoff von zellbewegungen. *Biochim Biophys Acta* 1954;14:182–194.
14. Majno G, Shea SM, Leventhal M. Endothelial contraction induced by histamine-type mediators: an electron microscopic study. *J Cell Biol* 1969;42(3):647–672.
15. Gabbiani G. *Curr Contents: Citation Classics* 1988;31:16.
16. Gabbiani G, Majno G. Dupuytren's contracture: fibroblast contraction? An ultrastructural study. *Am J Pathol* 1972;66:131–146.
17. Ryan GB, Cliff WJ, Gabbiani G, et al. Myofibroblasts in human granulation tissue. *Hum Pathol* 1974;5:55–67.
18. Gabbiani G, Chaponnier C, Hüttner I. Cytoplasmic filaments and gap junctions in epithelial cells and myofibroblasts during wound healing. *J Cell Biol* 1978;76:561–568.
19. Singer II, Kawka DW, Kazazis DM, Clark RA. In vivo co-distribution of fibronectin and actin fibers in granulation tissue: immunofluorescence and electron microscope studies of the fibronexus at the myofibroblast surface. *J Cell Biol* 1984;98: 2091–2106.
20. Tremblay G. Stromal aspects of breast carcinoma. *Exp Mol Pathol* 1979;31:248–260.
21. Seemayer TA, Lagacé R, Schürch W, Tremblay G. Myofibroblasts in the stroma of invasive and metastatic carcinoma: a possible host response to neoplasia. *Am J Surg Pathol* 1979;3:525–533.
22. Schürch W, Seemayer TA, Lagacé R. Stromal myofibroblasts in primary invasive and metastatic carcinomas. A combined immunological, light and electron microscopic study. *Virchows Arch A Pathol Anat Histopathol* 1981;391:125–139.
23. Schürch W, Lagacé R, Seemayer TA. Myofibroblastic stromal reaction in retracted scirrhous carcinoma of the breast. *Surg Gynecol Obstet* 1982;154:351–358.
24. Skalli O, Schürch W, Seemayer TA, et al. Myofibroblasts from diverse pathologic settings are heterogeneous in their content of actin isoforms and intermediate filament proteins. *Lab Invest* 1989;60:275–285.
25. Darby I, Skalli O, Gabbiani G. *Alpha*-smooth muscle actin is transiently expressed by myofibroblasts during experimental wound healing. *Lab Invest* 1990;63:21–29.
26. Schürch W, Skalli O, Gabbiani G. Cellular biology of Dupuytren's disease. In: McFarlane RM, McGrouther DA, Flint MH, eds. *Dupuytren's Disease*. London: Churchill Livingstone; 1990.
27. Desmoulière A, Geinoz A, Gabbiani F, Gabbiani G. Transforming growth factor-beta 1 induces alpha-smooth muscle actin expression in granulation tissue myofibroblasts and in quiescent and growing cultured fibroblasts. *J Cell Biol* 1993;122: 103–111.
28. Rønnov-Jessen L, Petersen OW. Induction of alpha-smooth muscle actin by transforming growth factor-beta1 in quiescent human breast gland fibroblasts. *Lab Invest* 1993;68:696–707.
29. Zhang K, Rekhter MD, Gordon D, Phan SH. Myofibroblasts and their role in lung collagen gene expression during pulmonary fibrosis. A combined immunohistochemical and in situ hybridization study. *Am J Pathol* 1994;145:114–125.
30. Serini G, Bochaton-Piallat ML, Ropraz P, et al. The fibronectin domain ED-A is crucial for myofibroblastic phenotype induction by transforming growth factor-beta1. *J Cell Biol* 1998;142: 873–881.
31. Desmoulière A, Redard M, Darby I, Gabbiani G. Apoptosis mediates the decrease in cellularity during the transition between granulation tissue and scar. *Am J Pathol* 1995;146:56–66.
32. Friedman SL. The cellular basis of hepatic fibrosis. Mechanisms and treatment strategies. *N Engl J Med* 1993;328:1828–1835.
33. Johnson RJ, Iida H, Alpers CE, et al. Expression of smooth muscle cell phenotype by rat mesangial cells in immune complex nephritis. Alpha-smooth muscle actin is a marker of mesangial cell proliferation. *J Clin Invest* 1991;87:847–858.
34. Kalluri R, Neilson EG. Epithelial-mesenchymal transition and its implications for fibrosis. *J Clin Invest* 2003;112:1776–1784.
35. Yanez-Mo M, Lara-Pezzi E, Selgas R, et al. Peritoneal dialysis and epithelial-to-mesenchymal transition of mesothelial cells. *N Engl J Med* 2003;348:403–413.
36. Bucala R, Spiegel LA, Chesney J, Hogan M, Cerami A. Circulating fibrocytes define a new leukocyte subpopulation that mediates tissue repair. *Mol Med* 1994;1:71–81.
37. Yang L, Scott PG, Giuffre J, Shankowsky HA, Ghahary A, Tredget EE. Peripheral blood fibrocytes from burn patients: identification and quantification of fibrocytes in adherent cells cultured from peripheral blood mononuclear cells. *Lab Invest* 2002; 82:1183–1192.
38. Gabella G. Structural apparatus for force transmission in smooth muscles. *Physiol Rev* 1984;64:455–477.
39. Somlyo AV. Ultrastructure of vascular smooth muscle. In: Bohr DF, Somlyo AP, Sparks HV, eds. *The Handbook of Physiology: The Cardiovascular System, Vol II: Vascular Smooth Muscle*. Bethesda, Md: American Physiological Society, 1980;33–67.
40. Hüttner I, Kocher O, Gabbiani G. Endothelial and smooth muscle cells. In: Camilleri JP, Berry CL, Fiessinger JN, Bariety J, eds. *Diseases of the Arterial Wall*. New York: Springer-Verlag; 1989:3–41.
41. Schollmeyer JE, Goll DE, Robson RM, Stromer MH. Localization of alpha actinin and tropomyosin in different muscles [abstract]. *J Cell Biol* 1973;59:306.
42. Schollmeyer JE, Furcht LT, Goll DE, Robson RM, Stromer MH. Localization of contractile proteins in smooth muscle cells and in normal and transformed fibroblasts. In: Goldman R, Pollard T, Rosenbaum J, eds. *Cell Motility*. Vol A. Cold Spring Harbor, NY: Cold Spring Harbor Laboratory; 1976:361–388.
43. Brown PJ, Juliano RL. Expression and function of a putative cell surface receptor for fibronectin in hamster and human cell lines. *J Cell Biol* 1986;103:1595–1603.
44. Hasegawa T, Hasegawa E, Chen WT, Yamada KM. Characterization of a membrane-associated glycoprotein complex implicated in cell adhesion to fibronectin. *J Cell Biochem* 1985;28:307–318.
45. Knudsen KA, Horwitz AF, Buck CA. A monoclonal antibody identifies a glycoprotein complex involved in cell-substratum adhesion. *Exp Cell Res* 1985;157:218–226.
46. Rogalski AA, Singer SJ. An integral glycoprotein associated with the membrane attachment sites of actin microfilaments. *J Cell Biol* 1985;101:785–801.

47. Horwitz A, Duggan K, Buck C, Beckerle MC, Burridge K. Interaction of plasma membrane fibronectin receptor with talin: a transmembrane linkage. *Nature* 1986;320;531–533.

48. Hynes RO, Yamada KM. Fibronectins: multifunctional modular glycoproteins. *J Cell Biol* 1982;95(pt 1):369–377.

49. Singer II. The fibronexus: a transmembrane association of fibronectin-containing fibers and bundles of 5nm microfilaments in hamster and human fibroblasts. *Cell* 1979;16:675–685.

50. Hinz B, Gabbiani G. Cell-matrix and cell-cell contacts of myofibroblasts: role in connective tissue remodeling. *Thromb Haemost* 2003;90:993–1002.

51. Bloom S, Cancilla PA. Conformational changes in myocardial nuclei of rats. *Circ Res* 1969;24:189–196.

52. Franke WW, Schinko W. Nuclear shape in muscle cells. *J Cell Biol* 1969;42:326–331.

53. Lane BP. Alterations in the cytologic detail of intestinal smooth muscle cells in various stages of contraction. *J Cell Biol* 1965;27:199–213.

54. Majno G, Shea SM, Leventhal M. Endothelial contraction induced by histamine-type mediators. An electron microscopic study. *J Cell Biol* 1969;42:647–672.

55. Schürch W, Seemayer TA, Gabbiani G. The myofibroblast: a quarter century after its discovery. *Am J Surg Pathol* 1998;22:141–147.

56. Eyden B. The fibronexus in reactive and tumoral myofibroblasts: further characterization by electron microscopy. *Histol Histopathol* 2001;16:57–70.

57. Weiss SW, Goldblum JR, eds. *Enzinger and Weiss's Soft Tissue Tumors.* 4th ed. St. Louis: Mosby; 2001:416.

58. Erlandson RA. In: Weidner N, Cote RJ, Suster S, Weiss LM, eds. *Modern Surgical Pathology. Role of Electron Microscopy in Modern Diagnostic Surgical Pathology.* Philadelphia: WB Saunders; 2003:83.

59. Rosai J. *Rosai and Ackerman's Surgical Pathology.* Mosby; 2004:2254.

60. Caplan AI, Fiszman MY, Eppenberger HM. Molecular and cell isoforms during development. *Science* 1983;221:921–927.

61. Schürch W, Skalli O, Seemayer TA, Gabbiani G. Intermediate filament proteins and actin isoforms as markers for soft tissue tumor differentiation and origin. I. Smooth muscle tumors. *Am J Pathol* 1987;128:91–103.

62. Schürch W, Skalli O, Lagacé R, Seemayer TA, Gabbiani G. Intermediate filament proteins and actin isoforms as markers for soft-tissue tumor differentiation and origin. III. Hemangiopericytomas and glomus tumors. *Am J Pathol* 1990;136:771–786.

63. Schürch W, Bégin LR, Seemayer TA, et al. Pleomorphic soft tissue myogenic sarcomas of adulthood. A reappraisal in the mid-1990s. *Am J Surg Pathol* 1996;20:131–147.

64. Rungger-Brändle E, Gabbiani G. The role of cytoskeletal and cytocontractile elements in pathologic processes. *Am J Pathol* 1983;110:361–392.

65. Babaï F, Skalli O, Schürch W, Seemayer TA, Gabbiani G. Chemically induced rhabdomyosarcomas in rats. Ultrastructural, immunohistochemical, biochemical features and expression of alpha-actin isoforms. *Virchows Arch B Cell Pathol Incl Mol Pathol* 1988;55:263–277.

66. Babaï F, Musevi-Aghdam J, Schürch W, Royal A, Gabbiani G. Coexpression of alpha-sarcomeric actin, alpha-smooth muscle actin and desmin during myogenesis in rat and mouse embryos. I. Skeletal muscle. *Differentiation* 1990;44:132–142.

67. Skalli O, Bloom WS, Ropraz P, Azzarone B, Gabbiani G. Cytoskeletal remodeling of rat aortic smooth muscle cells in vitro: relationships to culture conditions and analogies to in vivo situations. *J Submicrosc Cytol* 1986;18:481–493.

68. Skalli O, Ropraz P, Trzeciak A, Benzonana G, Gillessen DG, Gabbiani G. A monoclonal antibody against alpha-smooth muscle actin: a new probe for smooth muscle differentiation. *J Cell Biol* 1986;103(pt 2):2787–2796.

69. Benzonana G, Skalli O, Gabbiani G. Correlation between the distribution of smooth muscle or non muscle myosins and α-smooth muscle actin in normal and pathological soft tissues. *Cell Motil Cytoskeleton* 1988;11:260–274.

70. Larson DM, Fujiwara K, Alexander RW, Gimbrone MA Jr. Myosin in cultured vascular smooth muscle cells: immunofluorescence and immunochemical studies of alterations in antigenic expression. *J Cell Biol* 1984;99:1582–1589.

71. Schmid E, Osborn M, Rungger-Brändle E, Gabbiani G, Weber K, Franke WW. Distribution of vimentin and desmin filaments in smooth muscle tissue of mammalian and avian aorta. *Exp Cell Res* 1982;137:329–340.

72. Gabbiani G, Schmid E, Winter S, et al. Vascular smooth muscle cells differ from other smooth muscle cells: predominance of vimentin filaments and a specific α-type actin. *Proc Natl Acad Sci U S A* 1981;78:298–302.

73. Frank ED, Warren L. Aortic smooth muscle cells contain vimentin instead of desmin. *Proc Natl Acad Sci U S A* 1981;78:3020–3024.

74. Osborn M, Caselitz J, Puschel K, Weber K. Intermediate filament expression in human vascular smooth muscle and in arteriosclerotic plaques. *Virchows Arch A Pathol Anat Histopathol* 1987;411:449–458.

75. Travo P, Weber K, Osborn M. Co-existence of vimentin and desmin type intermediate filaments in a subpopulation of adult rat vascular smooth muscle cells growing in primary culture. *Exp Cell Res* 1982;139:87–94.

76. Schmid E, Tapscott S, Bennett GS, et al. Differential location of different types of intermediate-sized filaments in various tissues of the chicken embryo. *Differentiation* 1979;15:27–40.

77. Lazarides E. Intermediate filaments as mechanical integrators of cellular space. *Nature* 1980;283:249–256.

78. Franke WW, Schmid E, Freudenstein C, et al. Intermediate-sized filaments of the prekeratin type in myoepithelial cells. *J Cell Biol* 1980;84:633–654.

79. Vandekerckhove J, Weber K. At least six different actins are expressed in a higher mammal: an analysis based on the amino acid sequence of the amino-terminal tryptic peptide. *J Mol Biol* 1978;126:783–802.

80. Vandekerckhove J, Weber K. The complete amino acid sequence of actins from bovine aorta, bovine heart, bovine fast skeletal muscle, and rabbit slow skeletal muscle. A protein-chemical analysis of muscle actin differentiation. *Differentiation* 1979;14:123–133.

81. Vandekerckhove J, Weber K. Actin typing on total cellular extracts: a highly sensitive protein-chemical procedure able to distinguish different actins. *Eur J Biochem* 1981;113:595–603.

82. Hennessey ES, Drummond DR, Sparrow JC. Molecular genetics of actin function. *Biochem J* 1993;291(pt 3):657–671.

83. Miwa T, Manabe Y, Kurokawa K, et al. Structure, chromosome location, and expression of the human smooth muscle (enteric type) gamma-actin gene: evolution of six human actin genes. *Mol Cell Biol* 1991;11:3296–3306.

84. Schürch W, Bochaton-Piallat ML, Geinoz A, et al. All histological types of primary human rhabdomyosarcoma express alpha-cardiac and not alpha-skeletal actin messenger RNA. *Am J Pathol* 1994;144:836–846.

85. Chaponnier C, Gabbiani G. Pathological situations characterized by altered actin isoform expression. *J Pathol* 2004;204:386–395.

86. Skalli O, Vandekerckhove J, Gabbiani G. Actin-isoform pattern as a marker of normal or pathological smooth-muscle and fibroblastic tissues. *Differentiation* 1987;33:232–238.

87. Kocher O, Skalli O, Bloom WS, Gabbiani G. Cytoskeleton of rat aortic smooth muscle cells. Normal conditions and experimental intimal thickening. *Lab Invest* 1984;50:645–652.

88. Gabbiani G, Kocher O, Bloom WS, Vandekerckhove J, Weber K. Actin expression in smooth muscle cells of rat aortic intimal thickening, human atheromatous plaque, and cultured rat aortic media. *J Clin Invest* 1984;73:148–152.

89. Skalli O, Pelte MF, Peclet MC, et al. Alpha-smooth muscle actin, a differentiation marker of smooth muscle cells is present in microfilamentous bundles of pericytes. *J Histochem Cytochem* 1989;37:315–321.

90. Zimmermann KW. Der feine Bau der Blutkapillaren. *Z Anat Entwicklungsgesch* 1923;68:29–109.

91. Nehls V, Drenckhahn D. Heterogeneity of microvascular pericytes for smooth muscle type alpha-actin. *J Cell Biol* 1991;113:147–154.

92. Fujimoto T, Singer SJ. Immunocytochemical studies of desmin and vimentin in pericapillary cells of chicken. *J Histochem Cytochem* 1987;35:1105–1115.

93. Hinz B, Mastrangelo D, Iselin CE, Chaponnier C, Gabbiani G. Mechanical tension controls granulation tissue contractile

activity and myofibroblast differentiation. *Am J Pathol* 2001;159: 1009–1020.

94. Kapanci Y, Ribaux C, Chaponnier C, Gabbiani G. Cytoskeletal features of alveolar myofibroblasts and pericytes in normal human and rat lung. *J Histochem Cytochem* 1992;40:1955–1963.

95. Loreal O, Clement B, Deugnier Y. Hepatic fibrogenesis. *Rev Prat* 1997;47(5):482–6. French.

96. Gabbiani G, LeLous M, Bailey AJ, Bazin S, Delaunay A. Collagen and myofibroblasts of granulation tissue. A chemical, ultrastuctural and immunologic study. *Virchows Arch B Cell Pathol* 1976;21:133–145.

97. Rudolph R, Guber S, Suzuki M, Woodward M. The life cycle of the myofibroblast. *Surg Gynecol Obstet* 1977;145:389–394.

98. Barsky SH, Rao CN, Grotendorst GR, Liotta LA. Increased content of type V collagen in desmoplasia of human breast carcinoma. *Am J Pathol* 1982;108:276–283.

99. Gressner AM, Bachem MG. Cellular sources of noncollagenous matrix proteins: role of fat-storing cells in fibrogenesis. *Semin Liver Dis* 1990;10:30–46.

100. Berndt A, Kosmehl H, Katenkamp D, Tauchmann V. The appearance of the myofibroblastic phenotype in Dupuytren's disease is associated with a fibronectin, laminin, collagen type IV and tenascin extracellular matrix. *Pathobiology* 1994;62:55–58.

101. Sommer P, Gleyzal C, Raccurt M, et al. Transient expression of lysyl oxidase by liver myofibroblasts in murine schistosomiasis. *Lab Invest* 1993;69:460–470.

102. Jourdan-Le Saux C, Gleyzal C, Garnier JM, Peraldi M, Sommer P, Grimaud JA. Lysyl oxidase cDNA of myofibroblast from mouse fibrotic liver. *Biochem Biophys Res Commun* 1994;199:587–592.

103. Meister P, Gokel JM, Remberger K. Palmar fibromatosis- "Dupuytren's contracture." A comparison of light electron and immunofluorescence microscopic findings. *Pathol Res Pract* 1979;164:402–412.

104. Lagacé R, Grimaud JA, Schürch W, Seemayer TA. Myofibroblastic stromal reaction in carcinoma of the breast: variations of collagenous matrix and structural glycoproteins. *Virchows Arch A Pathol Anat Histopathol* 1985;408:49–59.

105. Wessells NK, Spooner BS, Ash JF, et al. Microfilaments in cellular and developmental processes. *Science* 1971;171:135–143.

106. Madden JW, Morton D Jr, Peacock EE Jr. Contraction of experimental wounds. I. Inhibiting wound contraction by using a topical smooth muscle antagonist. *Surgery* 1974;76:8–15.

107. Irlé C, Kocher O, Gabbiani G. Contractility of myofibroblasts during experimental liver cirrhosis. *J Submicrosc Cytol Pathol* 1980;12:209–217.

108. Evans JN, Kelley J, Low RB, Adler KB. Increased contractility of isolated lung parenchyma in an animal model of pulmonary fibrosis induced by bleomycin. *Am Rev Respir Dis* 1982;125:89–94.

109. Rubbia-Brandt L, Mentha G, Desmoulière A, et al. Hepatic stellate cells reversibly express alpha-smooth muscle actin during acute hepatic ischemia. *Transplant Proc* 1997;29:2390–2395.

110. Yanagisawa M, Kurihara H, Kimura S, et al. A novel potent vasoconstrictor peptide produced by vascular endothelial cells. *Nature* 1988;332:411–415.

111. Appleton I, Tomlinson A, Chandler CL, Willoughby DA. Effect of endothelin-1 on croton oil-induced granulation tissue in the rat. A pharmacologic and immunohistochemical study. *Lab Invest* 1992;67:703–710.

112. Thiemermann C, Corder R. Is endothelin-1 the regulator of myofibroblast contraction during wound healing? *Lab Invest* 1992;67:677–679.

113. Kurihara H, Yoshizumi M, Sugiyama T, et al. Transforming growth factor-beta stimulates the expression of endothelin mRNA by vascular endothelial cells. *Biochem Biophys Res Commun* 1989;159:1435–1440.

114. Hahn AW, Resink TJ, Kern F, Bühler FR. Effects of endothelin-1 on vascular smooth muscle cell phenotypic differentiation. *J Cardiovasc Pharmacol* 1992;20(suppl 12):S33–S36.

115. Hinz B, Gabbiani G, Chaponnier C. The NH2-terminal peptide of alpha-smooth muscle actin inhibits force generation by the myofibroblast in vitro and in vivo. *J Cell Biol* 2002;157:657–663.

116. Bayreuther K, Rodemann HP, Hommel R, Dittmann K, Albiez M, Francz PI. Human skin fibroblasts in vitro differentiate along a terminal cell lineage. *Proc Natl Acad Sci U S A* 1988;85:5112–5116.

117. Leavitt J, Gunning P, Kedes L, Jariwalla R. Smooth muscle alpha-actin is a transformation-sensitive marker for mouse NIH 3T3 and rat-2 cells. *Nature* 1985;316:840–842.

118. Desmoulière A, Rubbia-Brandt L, Abdiu A, Walz T, Macieira-Coelho A, Gabbiani G. Alpha-smooth muscle actin is expressed in a subpopulation of cultured and cloned fibroblasts and is modulated by gamma-interferon. *Exp Cell Res* 1992;201:64–73.

119. Vande Berg JS, Rudolph R, Woodward M. Growth dynamics of cultured myofibroblasts from human breast cancer and non-malignant contracting tissues. *Plast Reconstr Surg* 1984;73: 605–618.

120. Vande Berg JS, Rudolph R, Woodward M. Comparative growth dynamics and morphology between cultured myofibroblasts from granulating wounds and dermal fibroblasts. *Am J Pathol* 1984;114:187–200.

121. Vande Berg JS, Rudolph R, Poolman WL, Disharoon DR. Comparative growth dynamics and actin concentration between cultured human myofibroblasts from granulating wounds and dermal fibroblasts from normal skin. *Lab Invest* 1989;61:532–538.

122. Germain L, Jean A, Auger FA, Garrel DR. Human wound healing fibroblasts have greater contractile properties than dermal fibroblasts. *J Surg Res* 1994;57:268–273.

123. Azzarone B, Failly-Crepin C, Daya-Grosjean L, Chaponnier C, Gabbiani G. Abnormal behavior of cultured fibroblasts from nodule and nonaffected aponeurosis of Dupuytren's disease. *J Cell Physiol* 1983;117:353–361.

124. Dugina V, Alexandrova A, Chaponnier C, Vasiliev J, Gabbiani G. Rat fibroblasts cultured from various organs exhibit differences in alpha-smooth muscle actin expression, cytoskeletal pattern, and adhesive structure organization. *Exp Cell Res* 1998;238:481–490.

125. Schmitt-Gräff A, Pau H, Spahr R, Piper, HM, Skalli O, Gabbiani G. Appearance of alpha-smooth muscle actin in human eye lens cells of anterior capsular cataract and in cultured bovine lens-forming cells. *Differentiation* 1990;43:115–122.

126. Rønnov-Jessen L, van Deurs B, Celis JE, Petersen OW. Smooth muscle differentiation in cultured human breast gland stromal cells. *Lab Invest* 1990;63:532–543.

127. Rockey DC, Friedman SL. Cytoskeleton of liver perisinusoidal cells (lipocytes) in normal and pathological conditions. *Cell Motil Cytoskeleton* 1992;22:227–234.

128. Elger M, Drenckhahn D, Nobiling R, Mundel P, Kriz W. Cultured rat mesangial cells contain smooth muscle alpha-actin not found in vivo. *Am J Pathol* 1993;142:497–509.

129. Buckley IK, Porter KR. Cytoplasmic fibrils in living cultured cells. A light and electron microscope study. *Protoplasma* 1967;64: 349–380.

130. Geiger B, Bershadsky A, Pankov R, Yamada KM. Transmembrane crosstalk between the extracellular matrix-cytoskeleton crosstalk. *Nat Rev Mol Cell Biol* 2001;2:793–805.

131. Goldman RD. The use of heavy meromyosin binding as an ultra-structural cytochemical method for localizing and determining the possible functions of actin-like microfilaments in nonmuscle cells. *J Histochem Cytochem* 1975;23:529–542.

132. Goldman RD, Lazarides E, Pollack R, Weber K. The distribution of actin in non-muscle cells. The use of actin antibody in the localization of actin within the microfilament bundles of mouse 3T3 cells. *Exp Cell Res* 1975;90:333–344.

133. Willingham MC, Yamada SS, Davies PJ, Rutherford AV, Gallo MG, Pastan I. Intracellular localization of actin in cultured fibroblasts by electron microscopic immunochemistry. *J Histochem Cytochem* 1981;29:17–37.

134. Tomasek JJ, Gabbiani G, Hinz B, Chaponnier C, Brown RA. Myofibroblasts and mechano-regulation of connective tissue remodelling. *Nat Rev Mol Cell Biol* 2002;3:349–363.

135. Hinz B, Gabbiani G. Mechanisms of force generation and transmission by myofibroblasts. *Curr Opin Biotechnol* 2003;14:538–546.

136. Chrzanowska-Wodnicka M, Burridge K. Rho-stimulated contractility drives the formation of stress fibers and focal adhesions. *J Cell Biol* 1996;133:1403–1415.

137. Pelham RJ Jr, Wang Y. Cell locomotion and focal adhesions are regulated by substrate flexibility. *Proc Natl Acad Sci U S A* 1997;94:13661–13665.

138. Silver FH, Siperko LM, Seehra GP. Mechanobiology of force transduction in dermal tissue. *Skin Res Technol* 2003;9:3–23.

139. Grinnell F. Fibroblast biology in three-dimensional collagen matrices. *Trends Cell Biol* 2003;13:264–269.

140. Mochitate K, Pawelek P, Grinnell F. Stress relaxation of contracted collagen gels: disruption of actin filament bundles, release of cell surface fibronectin, and down-regulation of DNA and protein synthesis. *Exp Cell Res* 1991;193:198–207.

141. Brown RA, Prajapati R, McGrouther DA, Yannas IV, Eastwood M. Tensional homeostasis in dermal fibroblasts: mechanical responses to mechanical loading in three-dimensional substrates. *J Cell Physiol* 1998;175:323–332.

142. Martin P. Wound healing: aiming for perfect skin regeneration. *Science* 1997;276:75–81.

143. Werner S, Grose R. Regulation of wound healing by growth factors and cytokines. *Physiol Rev* 2003;83:835–870.

144. Arora PD, Narani N, McCulloch CA. The compliance of collagen gels regulates transforming growth factor-beta induction of alpha-smooth muscle actin in fibroblasts. *Am J Pathol* 1999;154: 871–882.

145. Hinz B, Dugina V, Ballestrem C, Wehrle-Haller B, Chaponnier C. Alpha-smooth muscle actin is crucial for focal adhesion maturation in myofibroblasts. *Mol Biol Cell* 2003;14:2508–2519.

146. Hinz B, Mastrangelo D, Iselin CE, Chaponnier C, Gabbiani G. Mechanical tension controls granulation tissue contractile activity and myofibroblast differentiation. *Am J Pathol* 2001;159: 1009–1020.

147. Roberts AB, Sporn MB, Assoian RK, et al. Transforming growth factor type beta: rapid induction of fibrosis and angiogenesis in vivo and stimulation of collagen formation in vitro. *Proc Natl Acad Sci U S A* 1986;83:4167–4171.

148. Ignotz RA, Massagué J. Transforming growth factor-beta stimulates the expression of fibronectin and collagen and their incorporation into the extracellular matrix. *J Biol Chem* 1986;261:4337–4345.

149. Friedman SL, Yamasaki G, Wong L. Modulation of transforming growth factor beta receptors of rat lipocytes during the hepatic wound healing response. Enhanced binding and reduced gene expression accompany cellular activation in culture and in vivo. *J Biol Chem* 1994;269:10551–10558.

150. Border WA, Ruoslahti E. Transfoming growth factor-beta in disease: the dark side of tissue repair. *J Clin Invest* 1992;90:1–7.

151. Bogatkevich GS, Tourkina E, Abrams CS, Harley RA, Silver RM, Ludwicka-Bradley A. Contractile activity and smooth muscle alpha-actin organization in thrombin-induced human lung myofibroblasts. *Am J Physiol Lung Cell Mol Physiol* 2003;285: L334–L343.

152. Shi-Wen X, Chen Y, Denton CP, et al. Endothelin-1 promotes myofibroblast induction through the ETA receptor via a rac/phosphoinositide 3-kinase/Akt-dependent pathway and is essential for the enhanced contractile phenotype of fibrotic fibroblasts. *Mol Biol Cell* 2004;15:2707–2719.

153. Shephard P, Hinz B, Smola-Hess S, Meister JJ, Krieg T, Smola H. Dissecting the roles of endothelin, TGF-beta and GM-CSF on myofibroblast differentiation by keratinocytes. *Thromb Haemost* 2004;92:262–274.

154. Vyalov S, Desmoulière A, Gabbiani G. GM-CSF-induced granulation tissue formation: relationships between macrophage and myofibroblast accumulation. *Virchows Archiv B Cell Pathol Incl Mol Pathol* 1993;63:231–239.

155. Rubbia-Brandt L, Sappino AP, Gabbiani G. Locally applied GM-CSF induces the accumulation of alpha-smooth muscle actin containing myofibroblasts. *Virchows Archiv B Cell Pathol Incl Mol Pathol* 1991;60:73–82.

156. Micera A, Vigneti E, Pickholtz D, et al. Nerve growth factor displays stimulatory effects on human skin and lung fibroblasts, demonstrating a direct role for this factor in tissue repair. *Proc Natl Acad Sci U S A* 2001;98:6162–6167.

157. Isenberg G, Rathke PC, Hülsmann N, Franke WW, Wohlfarth-Bottermann KE. Cytoplasmic actomyosin fibrils in tissue culture cells: direct proof of contractility by visualization of ATP-induced contraction in fibrils isolated by laser micro-beam dissection. *Cell Tissue Res* 1976;166:427–443.

158. Kreis TE, Birchmeier W. Stress fiber sarcomeres of fibroblasts are contractile. *Cell* 1980;22(pt 2):555–561.

159. Burridge K. Are stress fibres contractile? *Nature* 1981;294: 691–692.

160. Harris AK, Stopak D, Wild P. Fibroblast traction as a mechanism for collagen morphogenesis. *Nature* 1981;290:249–251.

161. Beningo KA, Wang YL. Flexible substrata for the detection of cellular traction forces. *Trends Cell Biol* 2002;12:79–84.

162. Katoh K, Kano Y, Amano M, Onishi H, Kaibuchi K, Fujiwara K. Rho-kinase: mediated contraction of isolated stress fibers. *J Cell Biol* 2001;153:569–584.

163. Parizi M, Howard EW, Tomasek JJ. Regulation of LPA-promoted myofibroblast contraction: role of Rho, myosin light chain kinase, and myosin light chain phosphatase. *Exp Cell Res* 2000;254:210–220.

164. Wrobel LK, Fray TR, Molloy JE, Adams JJ, Armitage MP, Sparrow JC. Contractility of single human dermal myofibroblasts and fibroblasts. *Cell Motil Cytoskeleton* 2002;52:82–90.

165. Hinz B, Celetta G, Tomasek JJ, Gabbiani G, Chaponnier C. Alpha-smooth muscle actin expression upregulates fibroblast contractile activity. *Mol Biol Cell* 2001;12:2730–2741.

166. Arora PD, McCulloch CA. Dependence of collagen remodelling on alpha-smooth muscle actin expression by fibroblasts. *J Cell Physiol* 1994;159:161–175.

167. Dugina V, Fontao L, Chaponnier C, Vasiliev J, Gabbiani G. Focal adhesion features during myofibroblastic differentiation are controlled by intracellular and extracellular factors. *J Cell Sci* 2001;114(pt 18):3285–3296.

168. Cukierman E, Pankov R, Yamada KM. Cell interactions with three-dimensional matrices. *Curr Opin Cell Biol* 2002;14: 633–639.

169. Rønnov-Jessen L, Petersen OW. A function for filamentous alpha-smooth muscle actin: retardation of motility in fibroblasts. *J Cell Biol* 1996;134:67–80.

170. O'Shea JD. An ultrastructural study of smooth muscle-like cells in the theca externa of ovarian follicles of the rat. *Anat Rec* 1970;167:127–131.

171. Boya J, Carbonell AL, Martinez A. Myofibroblasts in human palatal mucosa. *Acta Anat (Basel)* 1988;131:161–165.

172. Güldner FH, Wolff JR, Keyserling DG. Fibroblasts as a part of the contractile system in duodenal villi of rat. *Z Zellforsch Mikrosk Anat* 1972;135:349–360.

173. Kaye GI, Lane N, Pascal RR. Colonic pericryptal fibroblast sheath: replication, migration, and cytodifferentiation of a mesenchymal cell system in adult tissue. II. Fine structural aspects of normal rabbit and human colon. *Gastroenterology* 1968;54: 852–865.

174. Sappino AP, Dietrich PY, Skalli O, Widgren S, Gabbiani G. Colonic pericryptal fibroblasts. Differentiation pattern in embryogenesis and phenotypic modulation in epithelial proliferative lesions. *Virchows Arch A Pathol Anat Histopathol* 1989;415:551–557.

175. Bressler RS. Myoid cells in the capsule of the adrenal gland and in monolayers derived from cultured adrenal capsules. *Anat Rec* 1973;177:525–531.

176. Kapanci Y, Assimacopoulos A, Irlé C, Zwahlen A, Gabbiani G. "Contractile interstitial cells" in pulmonary alveolar septa: a possible regulator of ventilation-perfusion ratio? Ultrastructural, immunofluorescence, and in vitro studies. *J Cell Biol* 1974;60: 375–392.

177. Gorgas K, Böck P. Myofibroblasts in the rat testicular capsule. *Cell Tissue Res* 1974;154:533–541.

178. Czernobilsky B, Shezen E, Lifschitz-Mercer B, et al. Alpha smooth muscle actin (alpha-SM actin) in normal human ovaries, in ovarian stromal hyperplasia and in ovarian neoplasms. *Virchows Arch B Cell Pathol Incl Mol Pathol* 1989;57:55–61.

179. Parry EW. Some electron microscope observations on the mesenchymal structures of full-term umbilical cord. *J Anat* 1970;107(pt 3):505–518.

180. Tabone E, Andujar MB, DeBarros SS, Dos Santos MN, Barros CL, Graca DL. Myofibroblast-like cells in non-pathological bovine endometrial caruncle. *Cell Biol Int Rep* 1983;7:395–400.

181. Beertsen W, Everts V, van den Hooff A. Fine structure of fibroblasts in the periodontal ligament of the rat incisor and their possible role in tooth eruption. *Arch Oral Biol* 1974;19: 1087–1098.

182. Beertsen W. Migration of fibroblasts in the periodontal ligament of the mouse incisor as revealed by autoradiography. *Arch Oral Biol* 1975;20:659–666.

183. Toccanier-Pelte MF, Skalli O, Kapanci Y, Gabbiani G. Characterization of stromal cells with myoid features in lymph nodes and spleen in normal and pathologic conditions. *Am J Pathol* 1987;129:109–118.

184. Yokoi Y, Namihisa T, Kuroda H, et al. Immunocytochemical detection of desmin in fat-storing cells (Ito cells). *Hepatology* 1984;4:709–714.

185. Glasser SR, Julian J. Intermediate filament protein as a marker of uterine stromal cell decidualization. *Biol Reprod* 1986;35:463–474.

186. Charbord P, Lerat H, Newton I, et al. The cytoskeleton of stromal cells from human bone marrow cultures resembles that of cultured smooth muscle cells. *Exp Hematol* 1990;18:276–282.

187. Becker CG. Demonstration of actomyosin in mesangial cells of the renal glomerulus. *Am J Pathol* 1972;66:97–110.

188. Desmoulière A, Gabbiani G. Modulation of fibroblastic cytoskeletal features during pathological situations: the role of extracellular matrix and cytokines. *Cell Motil Cytoskeleton* 1994;29:195–203.

189. Chiavegato A, Bochaton-Piallat ML, D'Amore E, Sartore S, Gabbiani G. Expression of myosin heavy chain isoforms in mammary epithelial cells and in myofibroblasts from different fibrotic settings during neoplasia. *Virchows Arch* 1995;426:77–86.

190. Sappino AP, Schürch W, Gabbiani G. Differentiation repertoire of fibroblastic cells: expression of cytoskeletal proteins as marker of phenotypic modulations. *Lab Invest* 1990;63:144–161.

191. Eyden BP, Ponting J, Davies H, Bartley C, Torgersen E. Defining the myofibroblast: normal tissues, with special reference to the stromal cells of Wharton's jelly in human umbilical cord. *J Submicrosc Cytol Pathol* 1994;26:347–355.

192. Desmoulière A, Gabbiani G. The role of the myofibroblast in wound healing and fibrocontractive diseases. In: Clark RAF, ed. *The Molecular and Cellular Biology of Wound Repair*. 2nd ed. New York: Plenum Press; 1996:391–423.

193. Burrington JD. Wound healing in the fetal lamb. *J Pediatr Surg* 1971;6:523–528.

194. Goss AN. Intra-uterine healing of fetal rat oral mucosal, skin and cartilage wounds. *J Oral Pathol* 1977;6:35–43.

195. Adzick NS, Harrison MR, Glick PL, et al. Comparison of fetal, newborn, and adult wound healing by histologic, enzyme-histochemical, and hydroxyproline determinations. *J Pediatr Surg* 1985;20:315–319.

196. Rowsell AR. The intra-uterine healing of foetal muscle wounds: experimental study in the rat. *Br J Plast Surg* 1984;37:635–642.

197. Krummel TM, Nelson JM, Diegelmann RF, et al. Fetal response to injury in the rabbit. *J Pediatr Surg* 1987;22:640–644.

198. Adzick NS, Longaker MT. Scarless fetal healing: therapeutic implications. *Ann Surg* 1992;215:3–7.

199. Estes JM, Vande Berg JS, Adzick NS, MacGillivray TE, Desmoulière A, Gabbiani G. Phenotypic and functional features of myofibroblasts in sheep fetal wounds. *Differentiation* 1994;56:173–181.

200. Chakravarti S, Wu F, Vij N, Roberts L, Joyce S. Microarray studies reveal macrophage-like function of stromal keratocytes in the cornea. *Invest Ophthalmol Vis Sci* 2004;45:3475–3484.

201. Pei Y, Sherry DM, McDermott AM. Thy-1 distinguishes human corneal fibroblasts and myofibroblasts from keratocytes. *Exp Eye Res* 2004;79:705–712.

202. Anderson S, DiCesare L, Tan I, Leung T, SundarRaj N. Rho-mediated assembly of stress fibers is differentially regulated in corneal fibroblasts and myofibroblasts. *Exp Cell Res* 2004;298:574–583.

203. Seemayer TA, Schürch W, Lagacé R. Myofibroblasts in human pathology. *Hum Pathol* 1981;12:491–492.

204. Bhathal PS. Presence of modified fibroblasts in cirrhotic livers in man. *Pathology* 1972;4:139–144.

205. Cassiman D, Libbrecht L, Desmet V, Denef C, Roskams T. Hepatic stellate cell/myofibroblast subpopulations in fibrotic human and rat livers. *J Hepatol* 2002;36:200–209.

206. Rudolph R, McClure WJ, Woodward M. Contractile fibroblasts in chronic alcoholic cirrhosis. *Gastroenterology* 1979;76:704–709.

207. Madden JW. On "the contractile fibroblast." *Plast Recontsr Surg* 1973;52:291–292.

208. Woyke S, Domagala W, Olszewski W, Korabiec M. Pseudosarcoma of the skin. An electron microscopic study and comparison with fine structure of the spindle-cell variant of squamous carcinoma. *Cancer* 1974;33:970–980.

209. Larson DL, Abston S, Willis B, et al. Contracture and scar formation in the burn patient. *Clin Plast Surg* 1974;1:653–656.

210. Madden JW, Carlson EC, Hines J. Presence of modified fibroblasts in ischemic contracture of the intrinsic musculature of the hand. *Surg Gynecol Obstet* 1975;140:509–516.

211. Nagle RB, Kneiser MR, Bulger RE, Benditt EP. Induction of smooth muscle characteristics in renal interstitial fibroblasts during obstructive nephropathy. *Lab Invest* 1973;29:422–427.

212. Judd PA, Finnegan P, Curran RC. Pulmonary sarcoidosis: a clinico–pathological study. *J Pathol* 1975;115:191–198.

213. El-Labban NG, Lee KW. Myofibroblasts in central giant cell granuloma of the jaws: an ultrastructural study. *Histopathology* 1983;7:907–918.

214. Grimaud JA, Borojevic R. Myofibroblasts in hepatic schistosomal fibrosis. *Experientia* 1977;33:890–892.

215. Postacchini F, Natali PG, Accinni L, Ippolito E, de Martino C. Contractile filaments in cells of regenerating tendon. *Experientia* 1977;33:957–959.

216. Rudolph R, Woodward M. Spatial orientation of microtubules in contractile fibroblasts in vivo. *Anat Rec* 1978;191:169–181.

217. Zimman OA, Robles JM, Lee JC. The fibrous capsule around mammary implants: an investigation. *Aesthetic Plast Surg* 1978;2:217–234.

218. Callea F, Mebis J, Desmet VJ. Myofibroblasts in focal nodular hyperplasia of the liver. *Virchows Arch A Pathol Anat Histol* 1982;396:155–166.

219. Ghadially FN, Mehta PN. Multifunctional mesenchymal cells resembling smooth muscle cells in ganglia of the wrist. *Ann Rheum Dis* 1971;30:31–44.

220. Baur PS, Larson DL, Stacey TR. The observation of myofibroblasts in hypertrophic scars. *Surg Gynecol Obstet* 1975;141:22–26.

221. Novotny GE, Pau H. Myofibroblast-like cells in human anterior capsular cataract. *Virchows Arch A Pathol Anat Histopathol* 1984;404:393–401.

222. Woodcock-Mitchell J, Adler KB, Low RB. Immunohistochemical identification of cell types in normal and in bleomycin-induced fibrotic rat lung. Cellular origin of interstitial cells. *Am Rev Respir Dis* 1984;130:910–916.

223. Lagacé R, Delage C, Boutet M. Light and electron microscopic study of cellular proliferation in carcinoid heart disease. *Recent Adv Stud Cardiac Struct Metab* 1975;10:605–616.

224. Thomas WA, Jones R, Scott RF, Morrison E, Goodale MF, Imai H. Production of early atherosclerotic lesions in rats characterized by proliferation of "modified smooth muscle cells." *Exp Mol Pathol* 1963;52(suppl 1):40–61.

225. Flora G, Dahl E, Nelson E. Electron microscopic observations on human intracranial arteries. Changes seen with aging and atherosclerosis. *Arch Neurol* 1967;17:162–173.

226. Wissler RW. The arterial medial cell, smooth muscle, or multifunctional mesenchyme? *Circulation* 1967;36:1–4.

227. Gabbiani G, Badonnel MC. Contractile apparatus in aortic endothelium of hypertensive rat. *Recent Adv Stud Cardiac Struct Metab* 1975;10:591–601.

228. Sappino AP, Masouyé I, Saurat JH, Gabbiani G. Smooth muscle differentiation in scleroderma fibroblastic cells. *Am J Pathol* 1990;137:585–591.

229. Diamond JR, van Goor H, Ding G, Engelmyer E. Myofibroblasts in experimental hydronephrosis. *Am J Pathol* 1995;146:121–129.

230. Gabbrielli S, Di Lollo S, Stanflin N, Romagnoli P. Myofibroblast and elastic and collagen fiber hyperplasia in the bronchial mucosa: a possible basis for the progressive irreversibility of airway obstruction in chronic asthma. *Pathologica* 1994;86:157–160.

231. Gizycki MJ, Adelroth E, Rogers AV, O'Byrne PM, Jeffery PK. Myofibroblast involvement in the allergen-induced late response in mild atopic asthma. *Am J Respir Cell Mol Biol* 1997;16:664–673.

232. Holgate ST, Davies DE, Lackie PM, Wilson SJ, Puddicombe SM, Lordan JL. Epithelial-mesenchymal interactions in the pathogenesis of asthma. *J Alllergy Clin Immunol* 2000;105(pt 1):193–204.

233. Hastie AT, Kraft WK, Nyce KB, et al. Asthmatic epithelial cell proliferation and stimulation of collagen production: human asthmatic epithelial cells stimulate collagen type III production by human lung myofibroblasts after segmental allergen challenge. *Am J Respir Crit Care Med* 2002;165:266–272.

234. Bariéty J. *La biopsie rénale.* In: Droz D, Lanz B, eds. La biopsie rénale dans la hyalinose segmentaire et focale des glomérules. Paris, France; Publisher: Editions INSERM. 1996:109–134.

235. Schürch W, Seemayer TA, Gabbiani G. Myofibroblasts. In: Sternberg SS, ed. *Histology for Pathologists.* New York: Raven Press; 1992:109–144.

236. Ehrlich HP, Desmoulière A, Diegelmann RF, et al. Morphological and immunochemical differences between keloid and hypertrophic scar. *Am J Pathol* 1994;145:105–113.

237. Santucci M, Borgognoni L, Reali UM, Gabbiani G. Keliods and hypertrophic scars of Caucasians show distinctive morphologic and immunophenotypic profiles. *Virchows Arch* 2001;438:457–463.

238. Enzinger FM, Weiss SW. Fibromatoses. In: Enzinger FM, Weiss SW, eds. *Soft Tissue Tumors.* 3rd ed. St Louis: CV Mosby; 1994:201–229.

239. Chiu HF, McFarlane RM. Pathogenesis of Dupuytren's contracture: a correlative clinical-pathological study. *J Hand Surg (Am)* 1978;3:1–10.

240. Navas-Palacios JJ. The fibromatoses. An ultrastructural study of 31 cases. *Pathol Res Pract* 1983;176:158–175.

241. Ushijima M, Tsuneyoshi M, Enjoji M. Dupuytren type fibromatoses. A clinicopathologic study of 62 cases. *Acta Pathol Jpn* 1984;34:991–1001.

242. Ariyan S, Enriquez R, Krizek TJ. Wound contraction and fibrocontractive disorders. *Arch Surg* 1978;113:1034–1046.

243. Allen PW. The fibromatoses: a clinicopathologic classification based on 140 cases. *Am J Surg Pathol* 1977;1:255–270.

244. Chung EB, Enzinger FM. Infantile myofibromatosis. *Cancer* 1981;48:1807–1818.

245. Wirman JA. Nodular fasciitis, a lesion of myofibroblasts: an ultrastructural study. *Cancer* 1976;38:2378–2389.

246. Chung EB, Enzinger FM. Proliferative fasciitis. *Cancer* 1975;36:1450–1458.

247. Povysil C, Matejovsky Z. Ultrastructural evidence of myofibroblasts in pseudomalignant myositis ossificans. *Virchows Arch A Pathol Anat Histol* 1979;381:189–203.

248. Weathers DR, Campbell WG. Ultrastructure of the giant-cell fibroma of the oral mucosa. *Oral Surg Oral Med Oral Pathol* 1974;38:550–561.

249. Stiller D, Katenkamp D. Cellular features in desmoid fibromatosis and well-differentiated fibrosarcomas: an electron microscopic study. *Virchows Arch A Pathol Anat Histol* 1975;369:155–164.

250. Ramos CV, Gillespie W, Narconis RJ. Elastofibroma. A pseudotumor of myofibroblasts. *Arch Pathol Lab Med* 1978;102:538–540.

251. Buell R, Wang NS, Seemayer TA, Ahmed MN. Endobronchial plasma cell granuloma (xanathomatous pseudotumor): a light and electron microscopic study. *Hum Pathol* 1976;7:411–426.

252. Bhawan J, Bacchetta C, Joris I, Majno G. A myofibroblastic tumor. Infantile digital fibroma (recurrent digital fibrous tumor of childhood). *Am J Pathol* 1979;94:19–36.

253. Taxy JB. Juvenile nasopharyngeal angiofibroma: an ultrastructural study. *Cancer* 1977;39:1044–1054.

254. Ferrans VJ, Roberts WC. Structural features of cardiac myxomas. Histology, histochemistry, and electron microscopy. *Hum Pathol* 1973;4:111–146.

255. Fisher ER, Paulson JD, Gregorio RM. The myofibroblastic nature of the uterine plexiform tumor. *Arch Pathol Lab Med* 1978;102:477–480.

256. Tomasek JJ, Schultz RJ, Episalla CW, Newman SA. The cytoskeleton and extracellular matrix of the Dupuytren's disease "myofibroblast": an immunofluorescence study of a nonmuscle cell type. *J Hand Surg (Am)* 1986;11:365–371.

257. Shum DT, McFarlane RM. Histogenesis of Dupuytren's disease: an immunohistochemical study of 30 cases. *J Hand Surg (Am)* 1988;13:61–67.

258. Luck JV. Dupuyten's contracture: a new concept of the pathogenesis correlated with surgical management. *J Bone Joint Surg Am* 1959;41-A:635–664.

259. Iwasaki H, Müller H, Stutte HJ, Brennscheidt U. Palmar fibromatosis (Dupuytren's contracture). Ultrastructural and enzyme histochemical studies of 43 cases. *Virchows Arch A Pathol Anat Histopathol* 1984;405:41–53.

260. Eddy RJ, Petro JA, Tomasek JJ. Evidence for the nonmuscle nature of the "myofibroblast" of granulation tissue and hypertrophic scar. An immunofluorescence study. *Am J Pathol* 1988;130:252–260.

261. Matte C, Cadotte M, Schürch W. Intermediate filament proteins and actin isoforms of dermatofibrosarcoma protuberans and dermatofibroma. *Lab Invest* 1990;62(1):64A(abst. 373).

262. Fukasawa Y, Ishikura H, Takada A, et al. Massive apoptosis in infantile myofibromatosis. A putative mechanism of tumor regression. *Am J Pathol* 1994;144:480–485.

263. Ohtani H, Sasano N. Myofibroblasts and myoepithelial cells in human breast carcinoma. An ultrastructural study. *Virchows Arch A Pathol Anat Histol* 1980;385:247–261.

264. Cintorino M, Bellizzi de Marco E, Leoncini P, et al. Expression of α-smooth-muscle actin in stromal cells of the uterine cervix during epithelial neoplastic changes. *Int J Cancer* 1991;47:843–846.

265. Carroll R. The influence of lung scars on primary lung cancer. *J Pathol Bacteriol* 1962;83:293–297.

266. Madri JA, Carter D. Scar cancers of the lung: origin and significance. *Hum Pathol* 1984;15:625–631.

267. Barsky SH, Huang SJ, Bhuta S. The extracellular matrix of pulmonary scar carcinomas is suggestive of a desmoplastic origin. *Am J Pathol* 1986;124:412–419.

268. Gabbiani G, Kaye GI, Lattes R, Majno G. Synovial sarcoma. Electron microscopic study of a typical case. *Cancer* 1971;28:1031–1039.

269. Gabbiani G, Fu YS, Kaye GI, Lattes R, Majno G. Epithelioid sarcoma. A light and electron microscopic study suggesting a synovial origin. *Cancer* 1972;30:486–499.

270. Lagacé R, Schürch W, Seemayer TA. Myofibroblasts in soft tissue sarcomas. *Virchows Arch A Pathol Anat Histol* 1980;389:1–11.

271. Seemayer TA, Lagacé R, Schürch W. On the pathogenesis of sclerosis and nodularity in nodular sclerosing Hodgkin's disease. *Virchows Arch A Pathol Anat Histol* 1980;385:283–291.

272. Taccagni G, Rovere E, Masullo M, Christensen L, Eyden B. Myofibrosarcoma of the breast: review of the literature on myofibroblastic tumors and criteria for defining myofibroblastic differentiation. *Am J Surg Pathol* 1997;21:489–496.

273. Churg AM, Kahn LB. Myofibroblasts and related cells in malignant fibrous and fibrohistiocytic tumors. *Hum Pathol* 1977;8:205–218.

274. D'Andiran G, Gabbiani G. A metastasizing sarcoma of the pleura composed of myofibroblasts. In: Fenoglio CM, Woolf CM, eds. *Progress in Surgical Pathology.* New York: Masson Publishing; 1980:31–40.

275. Eyden BP, Christensen L, Tagore V, Harris M. Myofibrosarcoma of subcutaneous soft tissue of the cheek. *J Submicrosc Cytol Pathol* 1992;24:307–313.

276. Eyden BP, Ponting J, Davies H, Bartley C, Torgersen E. Defining the myofibroblast: normal tissues, with special reference to the stromal cells of Wharton's jelly in human umbilical cord. *J Submicrosc Cytol Pathol* 1994;26:347–355.

277. Mentzel T, Dry S, Katenkamp D, Fletcher CD. Low-grade myofibroblastic sarcoma: analysis of 18 cases in the spectrum of myofibroblastic tumors. *Am J Surg Pathol* 1998;22:1228–1238.

278. Eyden BP, Banerjee SS, Harris M, Mene A. A study of spindle cell sarcomas showing myofibroblastic differentiation. *Ultrastruct Pathol* 1991;15:367–378.

279. Fisher C. Myofibroblastic malignancies. *Adv Anat Pathol* 2004;11:190–201.

280. Alobeid B, Beneck D, Sreekantaiah C, Abbi RK, Slim MS. Congenital pulmonary myofibroblastic tumor: a case report with

cytogenetic analysis and review of the literature. *Am J Surg Pathol* 1997;21:610–614.

281. Fletcher CD, Tsang WY, Fisher C, Lee KC, Chan JK. Angiomyofibroblastoma of the vulva. A benign neoplasm distinct from aggressive angiomyxoma. *Am J Surg Pathol* 1992;16: 373–382.

282. Fukunaga M, Nomura K, Matsumoto K, Doi K, Endo Y, Ushigome S. Vulval angiomyofibroblastoma. Clinicopathologic analysis of six cases. *Am J Clin Pathol* 1997;107:45–51.

283. Ghadially FN, McNaughton JD, Lalonde JM. Myofibroblastoma: a tumor of myofibroblasts. *J Submicrosc Cytol* 1983;15: 1055–1063.

284. Herrera GA, Johnson WW, Lockard VG, Walker BL. Soft tissue myofibroblastomas. *Mod Pathol* 1991;4:571–577.

285. Laskin WB, Fetsch JF, Mostofi FK. Angiomyofibroblastomalike tumor of the male genital tract: analysis of 11 cases with comparison to female angiomyofibroblastoma and spindle cell lipoma. *Am J Surg Pathol* 1998;22:6–16.

286. Ockner DM, Sayadi H, Swanson PE, Ritter JH, Wick MR. Genital angiomyofibroblastoma. Comparison with aggressive angiomyxoma and other myxoid neoplasms of skin and soft tissue. *Am J Clin Pathol* 1997;107:36–44.

287. Prayson RA, Estes ML, McMahon JT, Kalfas I, Sebek BA. Meningeal myofibroblastoma. *Am J Surg Pathol* 1993;17: 931–936.

288. Suster S, Rosai J. Intranodal hemorrhagic spindle-cell tumor with "amianthoid" fibers. Report of six cases of a distinctive mesenchymal neoplasm of the inguinal region that simulates Kaposi's sarcoma. *Am J Surg Pathol* 1989;13:347–357.

289. Thomas TM, Myint A, Mak CK, Chan JK. Mammary myofibroblastoma with leiomyomatous differentiation. *Am J Clin Pathol* 1997;107:52–55.

290. Wargotz ES, Weiss SW, Norris HJ. Myofibroblastoma of the breast. Sixteen cases of a distinctive benign mesenchymal tumor. *Am J Surg Pathol* 1987;11:493–502.

291. Weiss SW, Gnepp DR, Bratthauer GL. Palisaded myofibroblastoma. A benign mesenchymal tumor of lymph node. *Am J Surg Pathol* 1989;13:341–346.

292. Bégin LR. Myogenic stromal tumor of the male breast (so-called myofibroblastoma). *Ultrastruct Pathol* 1991;15:613–622.

293. Fletcher CD, Unni KK, Mertens F, eds. *Pathology and Genetics of Tumors of Soft Tissue and Bone. World Health Organization Classification of Tumors.* Lyon, France: IARC; 2002:91–93.

294. O'Brien JE, Stout AP. Malignant fibrous xanthomas. *Cancer* 1964;17:1445–1455.

295. Cessna MH, Zhou H, Sanger WG, et al. Expression of ALK1 and p80 in inflammatory myofibroblastic tumor and its mesenchymal mimics: a study of 135 cases. *Mod Pathol* 2002;15:931–938.

296. Eyden B. Electron microscopy in the study of myofibroblastic lesions. *Semin Diagn Pathol* 2003;20:13–24.

297. Cohnheim J. Ueber Entzündung und Eiterung. *Virchows Arch Path Anat* 1867;40:1–79.

298. Arey LB. Wound healing. *Physiol Rev* 1936;16:327–406.

299. Grillo HC. Derivation of fibroblasts in healing wound. *Arch Surg* 1964;88:218–224.

300. Allgöwer M. *The Cellular Basis of Wound Repair.* Springfield, IL: Charles C Thomas, 1956.

301. Ross R, Everett NB, Tyler R. Wound healing and collagen formation. VI. The origin of the wound fibroblast studied in parabiosis. *J Cell Biol* 1970;44:645–654.

302. Crocker DJ, Murad TM, Geer JC. Role of the pericyte in wound healing. An ultrastructural study. *Exp Mol Pathol* 1970;13: 51–65.

303. Oda D, Gown AM, Vande Berg JS, Stern R. The fibroblast-like nature of myofibroblasts. *Exp Mol Pathol* 1988;49:316–329.

304. van der Loop FT, Gabbiani G, Kohnen G, Ramaekers FC, van Eys GJ. Differentiation of smooth muscle cells in human blood vessels as defined by smoothelin, a novel marker for the contractile phenotype. *Arterioscler Thromb Vasc Biol* 1997;17: 665–671.

305. Christen T, Verin V, Bochaton-Piallat M, et al. Mechanisms of neointima formation and remodeling in the porcine coronary artery. *Circulation* 2001;103:882–888.

306. van der Loop FT, Schaart G, Timmer ED, Ramaekers FC, van Eys GJ. Smoothelin, a novel cytoskeletal protein specific for smooth muscle cells. *J Cell Biol* 1996;134:401–411.

307. Chamley JH, Campbell GR, McConnell JD, Gröschel-Stewart U. Comparison of vascular smooth muscle cells from adult human, monkey and rabbit in primary culture and subculture. *Cell Tissue Res* 1977;177:503–522.

308. Moss NS, Benditt EP. Spontaneous and experimentally induced arterial lesions. I. An ultrastructural survey of the normal chicken aorta. *Lab Invest* 1970;22:166–183.

309. Mosse PR, Campbell GR, Wang ZL, Campbell JH. Smooth muscle phenotypic expression in human carotid arteries. I. Comparison of cells from diffuse intimal thickenings adjacent to atheromatous plaques with those of the media. *Lab Invest* 1985;53:556–562.

310. Olivetti G, Anversa P, Melissari M, Loud AV. Morphometric study of early postnatal development of the thoracic aorta in the rat. *Circ Res* 1980;47:417–424.

311. Poole JC, Cromwell SB, Benditt EP. Behavior of smooth muscle cells and formation of extracellular structures in the reaction of arterial walls to injury. *Am J Pathol* 1971;62:391–414.

312. Rønnov-Jessen L, Petersen OW, Koteliansky VE, Bissell MJ. The origin of the myofibroblasts in breast cancer. Recapitulation of tumor environment in culture unravels diversity and implicates converted fibroblasts and recruited smooth muscle cells. *J Clin Invest* 1995;95:859–873.

313. Franke WW, Moll R. Cytoskeletal components of lymphoid organs. I. Synthesis of cytokeratins 8 and 18 and desmin in subpopulations of extrafollicular reticulum cells of human lymph nodes, tonsils and spleen. *Differentiation* 1987;36:145–163.

314. Ramadori G, Veit T, Schwogler S, et al. Expression of the gene of the α-smooth muscle-actin isoform in rat liver and in rat fat-storing (ITO) cells. *Virchows Arch B Cell Pathol Incl Mol Pathol* 1990;59:349–357.

315. Schmitt-Gräff A, Krüger S, Bochard F, Gabbiani G, Denk H. Modulation of alpha smooth muscle actin and desmin expression in perisinusoidal cells of normal and diseased human livers. *Am J Pathol* 1991;138:1233–1242.

316. Blazejewski S, Preaux AM, Mallat A, et al. Human myofibroblast-like cells obtained by outgrowth are representative of the fibrogenic cells in the liver. *Hepatology* 1995;22:788–797.

317. Milani S, Herbst H, Schuppan D, Riecken EO, Stein H. Cellular localization of laminin gene transcripts in normal and fibrotic human liver. *Am J Pathol* 1989;134:1175–1182.

318. Milani S, Herbst H, Schuppan D, Surrenti C, Riecken EO, Stein H. Cellular localization of type I, III, and IV procollagen gene transcripts in normal and fibrotic human liver. *Am J Pathol* 1990;137:59–70.

319. Takahara T, Nakayama Y, Itoh H, et al. Extracellular matrix formation in piecemeal necrosis: immunoelectron microscopic study. *Liver* 1992;12:368–380.

320. Nagy P, Schaff Z, Lapis K. Immunohistochemical detection of transforming growth factor-β1 in fibrotic liver diseases. *Hepatology* 1991;14:269–273.

321. Goumenos DS, Brown CB, Shortland J, El Nahas AM. Myofibroblasts, predictors of progression of mesangial IgA nephropathy? *Nephrol Dial Transplant* 1994;9:1418–1425.

322. Boukhalfa G, Desmoulière A, Rondeau E, Gabbiani G, Sraer JD. Relationship between α-smooth muscle actin expression and fibrotic changes in human kidney. *Exp Nephrol* 1996;4:241–247.

323. Kapanci Y, Ribaux C, Chaponnier C, Gabbiani G. Cytoskeletal features of alveolar myofibroblasts and pericytes in normal human and rat lung. *J Histochem Cytochem* 1992;40: 1955–1963.

324. Vyalov SL, Gabbiani G, Kapanci Y. Rat alveolar myofibroblasts acquire α-smooth muscle actin expression during bleomycin-induced pulmonary fibrosis. *Am J Pathol* 1993;143:1754–1765.

325. Tredget EE, Shankowsky HA, Pannu R, et al. Transforming growth factor-beta in thermally injured patients with hypertrophic scars: effects of interferon alpha-2b. *Plast Reconstr Surg* 1998;102:1317–1330.

326. Ishii G, Sangai T, Oda T, et al. Bone-marrow-derived myofibroblasts contribute to the cancer-induced stromal reaction. *Biochem Biophys Res Commun* 2003;309:232–240.

327. Schmidt M, Sun G, Stacey MA, Mori L, Mattoli S. Identification of circulating fibrocytes as precursors of bronchial myofibroblasts in asthma. *J Immunol* 2003;171:380–389.

328. Garbin S, Pittet B, Montandon D, Gabbiani G, Desmoulière A. Covering by a flap induces apoptosis of granulation tissue myofibroblasts and vascular cells. *Wound Repair Regen* 1996; 4:244–251.

329. Carlson MA, Longaker MT, Thompson JS. Granulation tissue regression induced by musculocutaneous advancement flap coverage. *Surgery* 2002;131:332–337.

330. Grinnell F, Zhu M, Carlson MA, Abrams JM. Release of mechanical tension triggers apoptosis of human fibroblasts in a model of regressing granulation tissue. *Exp Cell Res* 1999;248: 608–619.

331. Fluck J, Querfeld C, Cremer A, Niland S, Krieg T, Sollberg S. Normal human primary fibroblasts undergo apoptosis in three-dimensional contractile collagen gels. *J Invest Dermatol* 1998;110: 153–157.

332. Evans VG. Multiple pathways to apoptosis. *Cell Biol Int* 1993;17:461–476.

333. Lee S, Christakos S, Small MB. Apoptosis and signal transduction: clues to a molecular mechanism. *Curr Opin Cell Biol* 1993;5:286–291.

334. Schwartzman RA, Cidlowski JA. Apoptosis: the biochemistry and molecular biology of programmed cell death. *Endocrinol Rev* 1993;14:133–151.

335. White E. Death-defying acts: a meeting review on apoptosis. *Genes Dev* 1993;7:2277–2284.

336. Williams GT, Smith CA. Molecular regulation of apoptosis: genetic controls on cell death. *Cell* 1993;74:777–779.

337. Martin SJ, Green DR, Cotter TG. Dicing with death: dissecting the components of the apoptosis machinery. *Trends Biochem Sci* 1994;19:26–30.

338. Evan GI, Wyllie AH, Gilbert CS, et al. Induction of apoptosis in fibroblasts by c-myc protein. *Cell* 1992;69:119–128.

339. Miura M, Zhu H, Rotello R, Hartwieg EA, Yuan J. Induction of apoptosis in fibroblasts by IL-1β-converting enzyme, a mammalian homolog of the *C. elegans* cell death gene ced-3. *Cell* 1993;75:653–660.

340. Reed JC. Bcl-2 and the regulation of programmed cell death. *J Cell Biol* 1994;124:1–6.

341. Laster SM, Wood JG, Gooding LR. Tumor necrosis factor can induce both apoptic and necrotic forms of cell lysis. *J Immunol* 1988;141;2629–2634.

342. Robaye B, Mosselmans R, Fiers W, Dumont JE, Galand P. Tumor necrosis factor induces apoptosis (programmed cell death) in normal endothelial cells in vitro. *Am J Pathol* 1991;138: 447–453.

343. Moulton BC. Transforming growth factor-β stimulates endometrial stromal apoptosis in vitro. *Endocrinology* 1994;134: 1055–1060.

344. Pierce GF, Mustoe TA, Senior RM, et al. In vivo incisional wound healing augmented by platelet-derived growth factor and recombinant c-sis gene homodimeric proteins. *J Exp Med* 1988;167: 974–987.

345. Mustoe TA, Pierce GF, Thomason A, Gramates P, Sporn MB, Deuel TF. Accelerated healing of incisional wounds in rats induced by transforming growth factor-β. *Science* 1987;237: 1333–1336.

346. Beck LS, DeGuzman L, Lee WP, Xu Y, Siegel MW, Amento EP. One systemic administration of transforming growth factor-β1 reverses age- or glucocorticoid-impaired wound healing. *J Clin Invest* 1993;92:2841–2849.

347. Schultz GS, White M, Mitchell R, et al. Epithelial wound healing enhanced by transforming growth factor-α and vaccinia growth factor. *Science* 1987;235:350–352.

348. Mooney DP, O'Reilly M, Gamelli RL. Tumor necrosis factor and wound healing. *Ann Surg* 1990;211:124–129.

349. Martin P, Hopkinson-Woolley J, McCluskey J. Growth factors and cutaneous wound repair. *Prog Growth Factor Res* 1992;4:25–44.

350. Streuli CH, Schmidhauser C, Kobrin M, Bissell MJ, Derynck R. Extracellular matrix regulates expression of the TGF-β1 gene. *J Cell Biol* 1993;120:253–260.

351. Micke P, Ostman A. Tumour-stroma interaction: cancer-associated fibroblasts as novel targets in anti-cancer therapy? *Lung Cancer* 2004;45(suppl 2):S163–S175.

352. De Wever O, Nguyen QD, Van Hoorde L, et al. Tenascin-C and SF/HGF produced myofibroblasts in vitro provide convergent pro-invasive signals to human colon cancer cells through RhoA and Rac. *Faseb J* 2004;18:1016–1018.

353. Doljanski F. The sculpturing role of fibroblast-like cells in morphogenesis. *Perspect Biol Med* 2004;47:339–356.

354. Orimo A, Gupta PB, Sgroi DC, et al. Stromal fibroblasts in invasive human breast carcinomas promote tumor growth and angiogenesis through elevated SDF-1/CXCL12 secretion. *Cell* 2005;121:335–348.

355. Dvorak HF. Tumors: wounds that do not heal. Similarities between tumor stroma generation and wound healing. *N Engl J Med* 1986;315:1650–1659.

356. Whitby DJ, Ferguson MW. Immunohistochemical localization of growth factors in fetal wound healing. *Dev Biol* 1991;147: 207–215.

Adipose Tissue

7

John S.J. Brooks   Patricia M. Perosio

INTRODUCTION

In compiling this chapter, our intention was to provide practicing surgical pathologists with both a description of normal and abnormal adipose tissue and a reference source. We were inclusive in our approach and considered all bodily lesions containing mature fat appropriate for discussion regardless of site. The section on development should provide a deeper understanding for the diagnostician and a starting point for the researcher. Collected and detailed as a group are the fatty infiltrations of organs, the inflammations affecting fat, the hamartomas and mesenchymomas, and the lipomas and variants thereof. Up-to-date definitions are provided where necessary. Importantly, we have also summarized clinical and genetic syndromes in which fat cells may participate. Unusual but distinctive histologies are enumerated, such as may occur in starvation, pancreatic fat necrosis, and true lipodystrophy. All topics are well-referenced, hopefully providing the reader with a valuable resource. In short, we have attempted to describe as many lesions as possible, not just primary fatty entities, but also anything extraneous within adipose tissue or confused with it.

WHITE FAT

Prenatal Development

The morphology of developing adipose tissue has been studied in detail. By examining serial sections obtained from 805 human fetuses of various ages, Poissonnet et al. (1) have determined that prior to the second trimester of pregnancy, adipose tissue primordia cannot be identified by light microscopy. After 14 weeks' gestation, aggregates of mesenchymal cells are seen condensed around proliferating primitive blood vessels. They refer to these findings as stage II in the development of adipose tissue (Figure 7.1). Prior to this time, future adipose tissue is characterized by loose spindle cells and ground substance (stage I). Later on, capillaries continue to proliferate into a rich network, around which preadipocytes become stellate and organized into a mesenchymal lobule (stage III). These preadipocytes do not contain lipid. With further development, fine lipid vacuoles characteristic of stage IV accumulate within cytoplasm (Figure 7.2). Continued proliferation of the components of the lobule results in the formation of densely packed aggregates of vacuolated fat cells with a rich capillary vascular network. Finally, condensation of perilobular mesenchyme at the periphery of the lobule results in formation of fibrous interlobular septa in stage V. This process occurs over the 10-week period between the 14- and 24-week gestation period. From approximately 24 to 29

weeks, the number of fat lobules is relatively constant. Continued growth occurs mainly due to proliferation of capillaries and adipocytes, causing an increase in the size of the fat lobules (Figure 7.2).

The same sequence of development of adipose tissue occurs at all sites throughout the body (2). The earliest white fat lobules appear first in the face, neck, breast, and abdominal wall at 14 weeks' gestation. By 15 weeks, they are also evident over the back and shoulders. Development in the upper and lower extremities and anterior chest begins around the sixteenth week. By the end of the twenty-third week, a layer of subcutaneous fat completely covers the extremities.

There is a very close association of adipocyte development and angiogenesis. Fat appears first in well-vascularized regions, such as the shoulder joint, before differentiation can be identified in the less well-supplied adjacent subcutaneous tissue. There is also an important physiologic significance to this close anatomic relationship. Lipoprotein lipase, the hormone responsible for transfer of triglyceride from circulating lipoproteins to adipose tissue, is synthesized by adipocytes and transferred to the luminal surface of the capillary endothelium (3). Thus, this close spatial relationship provides efficient transfer of enzyme and lipid.

Because of this close developmental association of capillaries and adipocytes, some have proposed that the adipocyte precursor, or preadipocyte, actually is derived from endothelial cells (4). Others have felt the preadipocyte may be a perivascular reticulum cell, perivascular fibroblast-like cell, or undifferentiated mesenchymal cell. The presumptive adipocyte precursor has been characterized ultrastructurally in the newborn rat (5). The preadipocyte is

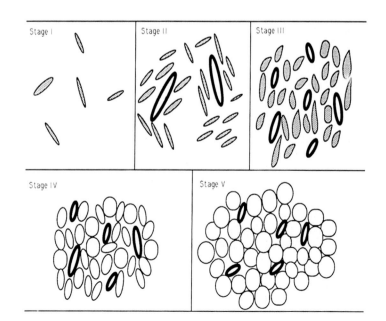

Figure 7.1 Developmental stages of adipose tissue. Stage I: Stellate cells (*stippled*) embedded in amorphous ground substance. Stage II: As angiogenesis begins, mesenchymal cells (*stippled*) condense around the blood vessels (*bold ovals*). Stage III: A rich capillary network develops from each vessel, forming a glomerulus-like network around which each lobule forms. The preadipocytes become more stellate. Stage IV: With accumulation of lipid, these adipocytes, with multiple small lipid droplets, become closely packed around the capillaries. Stage V: Further accumulation of lipid with many unilocular cells (*clear circles*) is evident. The perilobular mesenchyme condenses into interlobular septa at this stage.

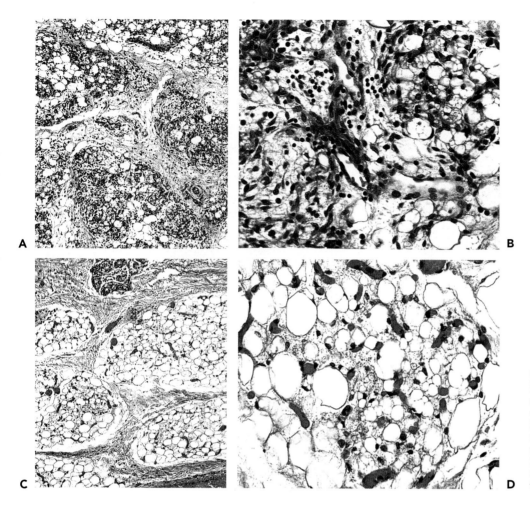

Figure 7.2 Fetal fat. **A.** Fat lobules from a 25-week fetus with a myxoid quality and prominent vasculature. **B.** At high power, both univacuolated and multivacuolated cells are noted together with small capillaries. **C. and D.** By 37 weeks, the lobules are more developed (C) and many of the cells are univacuolated (D).

a spindle cell with four to five cytoplasmic extensions along its long axis and abundant rough endoplasmic reticulum (ER). Lipid accumulates first as small droplets adjacent to the nucleus. As more lipid appears, it coalesces into a single large vacuole, and the cell takes on an oval then, finally, a round shape. The amount of rough ER decreases as the cell matures. Although cell shape and abundance of rough ER were taken as supportive evidence for the common origin of the preadipocyte and the fibroblast, which has a similar ultrastructural appearance, these similarities may have been a coincidence. The immature adipocyte needs to synthesize and excrete lipoprotein lipase—thus the abundant rough ER. Fibroblasts synthesizing and secreting procollagen would be expected to have a similar array of organelles.

As the preadipocyte accumulates lipid to become an adipocyte, both multilocular and unilocular adipocytes can be seen. Multilocular adipocytes predominate at first. With further lipid accumulation, more cells assume the unilocular appearance characteristic of mature adipocytes. Thus, attempts to differentiate brown from white adipocyte tissue at the light microscopic level, which rely on the presence of multivacuolated cells to characterize and identify brown

fat, are not reliable. Reliance on ultrastructural and biochemical differences helps to distinguish between these different forms of adipose tissue.

Molecular Biology

Through work on the adipocytic neoplasm known as myxoid liposarcoma (MLS), at least one gene involved in adipocytic differentiation has been identified. The translocation t(12;16)(q13;p11) of that tumor disrupts the normal function of the *CHOP* gene found at 12q13. First, the *CHOP* gene was shown to be rearranged in nearly all MLS (6), and, subsequently, the actual breakpoint was cloned (7,8). The *CHOP* gene, also known as *GADD153*, encodes a member of the CCAAT/enhancer binding protein (C/EBP) family and has a DNA binding domain. It appears to be involved in normal adipocyte differentiation because the protein it produces may be a dominant inhibitor of other C/EBP transcription factors known to be important in cell proliferation (9). Members of this C/EBP group are highly expressed in fat and are involved in the differentiation of fibroblasts into adipocytes and in the growth arrest of terminally differentiated adipocytes (6). *CHOP* itself is induced in the differentiation of 3T3-L1 cells to adipocytes. In the neoplasm, the translocation results in a fusion gene involving *CHOP* and *TLS* (translocated in liposarcoma), an RNA binding gene with much similarity structurally and functionally to the *EWS* gene of Ewing's sarcoma. Presumably, the lack of the normal inhibitory function of an intact *CHOP* gene allows the fatty tumor to proliferate unchecked. The use of both Southern blots and fluorescent in situ hybridization (FISH) techniques in detecting the rearranged gene will have usefulness in the diagnosis of fatty tumors. Likewise, when it becomes commercially available, antibody to the CHOP protein might be used immunohistochemically to detect such tumors.

Apoptosis, or programmed cell death, probably occurs in adipocytic tissues, but studies localizing the bcl-2 protein in human fetal tissues fail to mention its detection in fat (10).

Postnatal Development

At birth, the average-size infant has approximately 5 billion adipocytes (11). This represents only 16% of the total number of adipocytes in adults. Adipose tissue continues to grow in parallel with general growth throughout the first 10 years of life. Fat cells enlarge significantly during the first six months of life without much increase in cell number (12). Until puberty, the cell size remains fairly constant while the number of adipocytes progressively increases. At puberty, there is a substantial increase in adipocyte size and number (12). Although at the end of puberty, the total number of adipocytes is similar to the adult, new adipocytes may continue to form throughout life (13). Studies on adult rats have shown that overfeeding results in proliferation of adipocyte precursors and development of new fat cells (14). De novo adipocyte formation can be triggered by overdistension of existing fat cells and the mass of stored triglycerides (15). Loss of fat cells may also occur and has been shown in overweight women following several years of strict dietary restriction (16).

Gender Differences

The differences in body fat content noted between men and women begins in early childhood. Young girls are fatter than boys. Studies on fetuses, however, have not noted differences in the pattern of distribution or quantity of fat in prenatal life (1). The distribution of adipose tissue, however, even in prenatal life is not homogeneous throughout the body. Gender differences in the distribution of adipose tissue following puberty are well-known and thought to be related to steroid hormone secretion (12). In humans, estrogens and progesterone induce an increase in trochanteric fat. The localization of more fat in the lower body in women results in the so-called gynecoid habitus. These same deposits are reduced by androgens in men, resulting in an android distribution of fat. The percentage of body fat also differs in men and women. Males reach a peak in body fat content during early adolescence, whereas women continue to accumulate fat relative to body weight throughout the teen years.

Functions

White adipose tissue is the body's largest energy store, and it possesses the enzymes necessary for the uptake and release of triglycerides. Briefly, triglycerides circulate in the blood in the form of chylomicrons from the intestine and very low density lipoproteins from the liver (17). Lipoprotein lipase present on the luminal surface of endothelial cells hydrolyzes the triglyceride to release free fatty acids. This enzyme is synthesized by adipocytes and transferred to the endothelial cells. Most of the free fatty acids are taken up by the fat cells and reesterified to glycerol phosphate within the adipocyte to form triacylglycerol, which is then stored within the cell's lipid droplet. The fat is mobilized through the action of hormone-sensitive lipase, which hydrolyzes stored triglycerides. The released free fatty acids may be reesterified or released to the circulation and bound to albumin for transfer to other cells.

Until recently the main endocrine function of adipose tissue was thought to be the conversion of androstenedione to estrone, the major source of estrogen in men and postmenopausal women. The aromatase action, however, has been localized to the stromal cell fraction of adipose tissue and not the adipocyte (18). More recently a dynamic role of adipose tissue has emerged with expression of several hormones, growth factors, and cytokines identified in adipocytes, stromal cells, and macrophages that are localized to adipose tissue. These include leptin, a regulator of energy expenditure and appetite; interleukin-6, which may play a role in the metabolic syndrome; and several important regulators of glucose and lipid metabolism, the complement cascade, and the fibrinolytic system.

Leptin, the protein product of the *ob* gene, is synthesized exclusively by adipocytes and acts on the hypothalamus to increase energy expenditure and decrease appetite (19). This pathway is well-established in rats. In humans, fasting lowers serum leptin levels and increases appetite (20). Unfortunately elevated or rising levels of leptin do not show the reverse effect, and leptin has not been shown to have an anti-obesity action in humans. The majority of obese individuals have elevated serum leptin levels, proportional to the amount of adipose tissue, and it is postulated that humans are leptin resistant (21). Leptin receptors are present on most tissues, and leptin may play a role outside the adipose tissue to accelerate wound healing, increase vascular tone, and inhibit bone formation (22).

Cytokines are secreted by adipocytes, stromal cells, and resident macrophages. Interleukin-6 (IL-6) is made by adipocytes and macrophages, and adipose tissue accounts for approximately 30% of circulating IL-6 in humans (23).

Like leptin, serum IL-6 levels are highly correlated with percent body fat. The IL-6 released from intra-abdominal stores enters the portal circulation. Hepatic triglyceride secretion is stimulated by IL-6, and this may contribute to the hypertriglyceridemia seen with visceral obesity (22). Interleukin-6 also stimulates hepatic secretion of acute phase reactants, increases platelet number and activity, and increases expression of endothelial adhesion molecules. There are ongoing investigations of the role this cytokine (which is derived in large part from adipose tissue) plays in the metabolic syndrome and the risk of cardiovascular disease in obesity.

Adipocytes also secrete C3 and adipsin, the proteins of the alternate complement pathway (24). Plasminogen activator inhibitor-1 (PAI-1) is a potent inhibitor of the fibrinolytic system and favors the development of thromboemboli. Insulin induces expression of PAI-1 by adipocytes, and elevated levels are seen with obesity (25).

Regulation

White adipose tissue contains numerous receptors for hormones, cytokines, catecholamines, and lipoproteins. Catecholamines acting through α-2 receptors inhibit lipolysis, and a predominance of α-2 receptors in gluteal fat of women is thought to impact maintenance of these fat stores despite weight loss (17). Regional differences in lipoprotein lipase levels (LPL) also occur in women. Gluteal fat in premenopausal women tends to have high LPL levels, and these regions contain larger fat cells. Such regional differences disappear after menopause and are not present in obese men (26,27). This suggests that the sex steroids also play a role in adipose tissue distribution and activity. Both androgens and estrogen modulate *ob* gene expression and control adipose tissue development (28,29). Androgens are antiadipogenic and estrogens proadipogenic. These may play a role in the regional differences in fat distribution and the development of the android and gynecoid patterns of obesity.

Insulin stimulates lipogenesis and glucose uptake while inhibiting fat breakdown. Insulin and glucocorticoids stimulate DNA synthesis in cultured human adipocytes and conversion of preadipocytes to mature adipocytes. These effects are enhanced on cells obtained from obese, as compared to lean, people. Estradiol-17β has also been shown to stimulate division of cultured preadipocytes obtained from both men and women. Progesterone acts in vitro to stimulate both preadipocyte division and LPL activity (30). This dual role facilitates triglyceride accumulation in women. Fibroblast growth factor 1, secreted by adipose-derived microvascular endothelial cells, stimulates preadipocyte differentiation and acculumlation of triglycerides (31).

Tumor necrosis factor alpha (TNF-α) and IL-6 have the opposite effect and are implicated along with leptin in the weight loss and anorexia of chronic wasting illnesses and cancer (32,33). TNF-α is expressed in preadipocytes and acts to block differentiation to mature adipocytes through CCAAT/enhancer binding protein alpha (C/EBP-α) (34). It also suppresses lipoprotein lipase and stimulates the mobilization of fatty acids. The TNF-α induces the release of IL-6 and leptin from adipose tissue, and the action of these cytokines is closely interrelated.

In addition to adipocyte function, fat cell size and number are also regulated. Numerous studies using tritiated thymidine incorporation as a marker for cell division in adipose tissue have been done in rats to identify mitotically active cells within fat. Mature lipid-laden adipocytes are generally considered to be incapable of cell differentiation because of the absence of mitotic figures seen histologically in normal adipose tissue. Sampling fat from rats injected with tritiated thymidine at 1 day and 3 days of age, which are then sacrificed at various times up to 5 months of age, has shown that the number of labeled cells in subcutaneous fat initially rises due to cell proliferation. The concentration of radioactivity then falls, probably as a result of a dilutional effect resulting from continued cell division (35). This study, however, failed to distinguish adipocyte from stromal labeling. Similar studies had been performed on rats in which the subcutaneous tissue is separated into stromal and adipose components. In one study, the specific radioactivity of the adipocyte fraction did not increase until two to five days after injection (36). Thus, they concluded that DNA synthesis occurs in nonlipid-laden cells or preadipocytes. As these cells accumulate lipid, labeled cells are detected within the adipocyte fraction.

Gross Aspects

Fatty tissue is typically a homogeneous, bright cadmium-like yellow, with a glistening and greasy surface texture, and finely divided by faint septa. Any variation in color indicates a pathologic process: white to white/yellow in fat necrosis, paler yellows in many lipomas, reddish tinge to orange/yellow in angiolipoma, definite gray/white to whitish streaks in spindle cell lipoma, and white/yellow to white nodules in liposarcoma.

Histology

Microscopically, a mature white fat cell is spherical and measures up to 120 μm in diameter (37). The cytoplasm is compressed at the perimeter of the cell, and only a thin rim of cell membrane is evident on hematoxylin-eosin (H&E)–stained sections. Reticulin and periodic acid-Schiff (PAS) stains highlight the adipocyte basement membrane (Figure 7.3). The cytoplasm is displaced by a single lipid vacuole, and the cells are fairly uniform in size (Figure 7.4). The nucleus, although oval, is thin and small with finely distributed chromatin; when seen in profile, a central minute clear vacuole may be seen within the nucleus (Figure 7.4). Normal subcutaneous fat is finely divided into ill-defined lobules by thin bands of collagen (Figure 7.5).

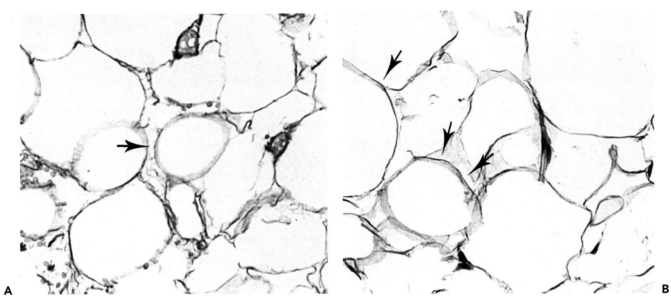

Figure 7.3 Normal adult adipocyte. **A.** On a reticulin stain, each adipocyte is outlined by reticulin (*arrow*), which is present outside the cytoplasm. **B.** The same is true on PAS stain, where the basement membrane is highlighted (*arrows*) and encompasses the pale residue of cytoplasm remaining after fixation and embedding.

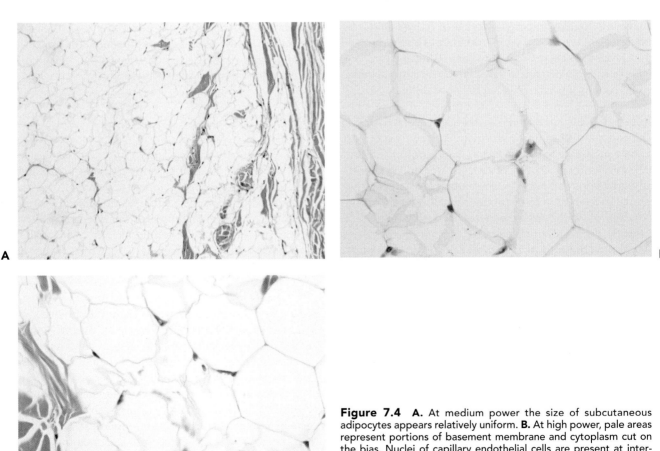

Figure 7.4 **A.** At medium power the size of subcutaneous adipocytes appears relatively uniform. **B.** At high power, pale areas represent portions of basement membrane and cytoplasm cut on the bias. Nuclei of capillary endothelial cells are present at intersections between multiple cells. **C.** In contrast to other nuclei, an ideal section of an adipocyte nucleus shows a pale character due to its thin nature and the common central vacuole, or "Locherne." The wrinkled cell outlines are an artifact occasionally seen, the result of improper fixation.

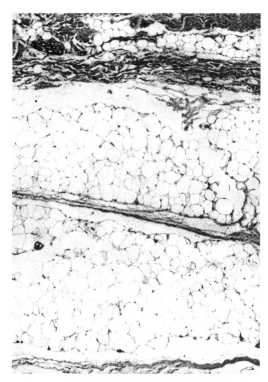

Figure 7.5 Adult subcutaneous fat lobule with associated microvasculature; note the thin and delicate fibrous tissue septa.

Ultrastructure

The ultrastructure of developing adipocytes has previously been discussed. In brief, a spindle shape with abundant endoplasmic reticulum and small spherical mitochondria characterizes preadipocytes (37). Lipid accumulates as small perinuclear inclusions that coalesce to form larger lipid droplets. The mitochondria become filamentous and the endoplasmic reticulum less prominent. In a mature adipocyte, the nucleus is flattened against the cytoplasmic membrane by a large lipid droplet. There is only a thin, tenuous rim of cytoplasm that surrounds it. Pinocytotic vesicles are seen in variable numbers but are very numerous following periods of starvation. Adjacent to the cell membrane are deposits of basement membrane. Capillaries are closely opposed to the adipocyte basement membrane. Only rarely have nerves been identified adjacent to white fat cells, although they may be seen in intercellular collagenous septa.

BROWN FAT

Prenatal Development

The development of brown adipose tissue has been studied in animal models. The brown adipocyte precursors are spindle cells closely related to a network of capillaries (38).

As the cells and vessels proliferate, they are organized into lobules by connective tissue septa. As the cells accumulate lipid, they initially are unilocular. However, with further lipid accumulation, multiple cytoplasmic lipid vacuoles appear. As in white fat, the close association of developing adipocytes and blood vessels has led some to speculate that adipocytes actually develop from endothelial cells. Although similar ultrastructural features are cited as supportive evidence of theory, more recent investigations have attributed these similarities to a common origin from undifferentiated mesenchyme. In fact, ultrastructural and biochemical studies that have examined developing brown adipose tissue have shown that unique features such as large mitochondria and a unique mitochondrial protein are found early in development and distinguish brown from white fat.

Fetal necropsy studies have identified lobules of developing brown fat in the human fetus (39). The largest of these are from the posterior cervical, axillary, suprailiac, and perirenal regions. Those in the neck and axillae are closely associated with the major blood vessels of these regions in such a way that they extend along the course of the cervical blood vessels into the root of the neck. The suprailiac collections lie deep to the abdominal muscles, yet superficial to the peritoneum, and invest the anterior abdominal wall to the diaphragm. Intermediate-sized brown fat pads are seen in the interscapular paralateral trapezius and deltoid regions. Small collections are evident in the intercostal area. In this study, no difference was noted in distribution between the sexes or among the races. The amount of brown fat increases in proportion to growth throughout life. Deposits are well-established by the fifth month of gestation.

Postnatal Development

The presence of brown fat beyond the neonatal period in humans has been debated. An autopsy study by Heaton (40), however, has identified lobules of brown fat throughout life to the eighth decade. Brown fat is most widely distributed in young children and, over the next several decades, gradually disappears from most sites. In children under age 10, identifiable deposits of brown fat were identified in the interscapular region, around the neck vessels and muscles, around the structures of the mediastinum, and adjacent to the lung hila. Intra-abdominal and retroperitoneal deposits were noted around the kidneys, pancreas, spleen, mesocolon, and omentum, as well as in the anterior abdominal wall. The extremities were not sampled. Although brown fat disappeared from most areas, it was found to persist around the kidneys, adrenals, and aorta and within the mediastinum and neck throughout adult life. As in fetal life, no difference in distribution based on gender was noted.

Function

The main function of brown adipose tissue is heat production. It has been estimated that the maximal aerobic capacity per gram of tissue is almost 10 times that of skeletal muscle (41). It has been estimated that even in humans the small quantities of brown fat present are capable of raising heat production by over 20% (42). The production of heat is closely related to the active sympathetic innervation of brown fat and stimulation by norepinephrine. Release of norepinephrine results in the production of cyclic adenosine monophosphate (AMP) and lipolysis to release free fatty acids (43). These undergo oxidation within the mitochondria to produce adenosine triphosphate (ATP). Brown fat mitochondria contain a unique uncoupling protein, also known as thermogenin, which uncouples the oxidation of fatty acids from generation of ATP (44,45). The resultant energy is dissipated as heat. In small rodents and hibernating animals, brown fat is activated by cold temperatures to produce heat, resulting in what is known as nonshivering thermogenesis. Teleologically, this would be useful in those at risk for hypothermia. Thus, neonates, unable to alter the external environment in order to maintain body temperature, would be expected to have relatively more active brown fat than adults. In addition, brown fat accumulation and activation may play a role in weight regulation. Experimentally overfed rats show a compensatory increase in brown fat activation in metabolic rate, minimizing weight gain (46). Many types of obesity in laboratory mice and rats are related to defective regulation of brown adipose tissue, including that seen in ob/ob mice (47). In contrast, exaggerated leanness may be associated with excessive brown adipose tissue responsiveness to external factors, such as sympathetic stimulation. Although brown adipose tissue is present in humans, its role in weight regulation, obesity, and thermal regulation in adults remains controversial (48). Increased amounts of periadrenal brown fat in malnourished people at autopsy suggest a compensatory increase in nonshivering thermogenesis to maintain body temperature in those with diminished subcutaneous fat and cachexia (49).

Regulation

Unlike white fat, brown fat is highly innervated and regulated by sympathetic stimulation. Nerves enter each lobe and branch within the interlobular septa, running along the vessels to terminate on the fat cells (50). Brown fat cells have numerous β1- and β2-adrenoreceptors that regulate lipolysis and thermogenesis (43). The α-adrenoreceptors, although present, probably do not act directly in heat production. Norepinephrine also may act to increase the number and character of brown fat cells. Using continuous infusions of norepinephrine, Mory et al. (51) have shown that such chronic sympathetic stimulation results in

increased cellularity, increased protein content, and increased mitochondrial density in brown fat. Because of this close association of sympathetic activity and brown fat activity, several investigators have used pheochromocytoma as a model to study brown fat activities in humans. These studies have provided evidence supportive of early autopsy studies. Functional brown adipose tissue was identified in adults with pheochromocytomas that had similar biochemical features to the better-characterized brown adipose tissue of rodents (52).

Hormones also play a role in brown fat regulation, but it is minor in comparison to the sympathetic system. Thyroid hormone, although active in regulating metabolic rate, has little importance in diet-induced or nonshivering thermogenesis (43). Insulin stimulates glucose intake into brown adipose tissue. Both cortisol and gonadal steroid hormones inhibit thermogenesis, thus promoting energy conservation.

Histology

The term *brown fat* was applied to this tissue because of its characteristic gross appearance. It is incorrect to refer to it as "fetal" fat because it is present throughout life. The abundant vascularity and numerous mitochondria within the cells impart a characteristic reddish-brown color to the tissue. Brown fat has a glandular lobulated appearance. This is in contrast to the more diffuse growth pattern of white fat. Histologically, brown fat is organized into lobules of cells that are made up of adipocytes, capillaries, nerves, and connective tissue. These are surrounded by a thin, fibrous capsule containing blood vessels, nerves, and scattered white adipose cells (53). The cells are polygonal in shape, with a mixture of multivacuolated and univacuolated cells (Figure 7.6). The occurrence of both cell types is emphasized, and

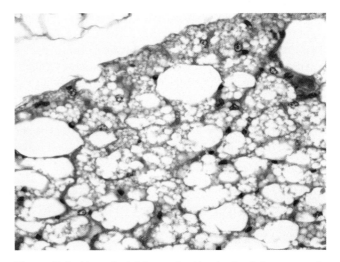

Figure 7.6 Normal adult brown fat. Nearly all cells have centrally placed nuclei and multivacuolated cytoplasm. Rare cells (*top left*) are nonvacuolated. An arborizing thin capillary network is noted.

their presence in developing white fat initially confused studies on its origin. The multivacuolated cell, characteristic of brown fat, has a highly granular cytoplasm with numerous lipid inclusions. Its granular appearance is due to the numerous mitochondria necessary for thermogenesis. The nucleus is spherical and often centrally located, although a large lipid inclusion may displace it toward the periphery of the cell or, rarely, to the extreme perimeter (as in white fat). Small nucleoli are common. The unilobular cells are indistinguishable histologically from the mature signet-ring cell–type white adipocytes but are different ultrastructurally. On average, the size of the brown fat cells is smaller than white adipocytes, approximately 25 to 40 μm. In animals that hibernate, marked seasonal variation in cell size has been noted. Both exposure to cold and starvation result in lipid depletion, causing reduction in cell size and wrinkling of the cell membrane.

Brown adipose cells are surrounded by a network of collagen fibers that contain numerous minute nerve axons and blood vessels. Nonmyelinated axons terminate on the fat cells, providing an avenue for direct sympathetic regulation. The vascularity is quite prominent with numerous capillaries coursing between the adipocytes. It is estimated in rats that the vascularity of brown fat is four to six times greater than that of white fat (53).

HISTOCHEMISTRY

Enzyme Histochemistry

In development, enzyme histochemistry within developing adipocytes is related to the stage of adipocyte differentiation. In fact, in some systems, such as the rat, it is clear that enzymatic differentiation of adipocytes precedes morphologic differentiation (54,55). In regions destined to become adipose tissue, undifferentiated morphology is initially present without a capillary bed and without any enzymatic capacity. Subsequently, immature cells or what can be termed "preadipocytes" exist in the form of spindle cells within an area containing a capillary bed. These cells lack any lipid or a basal lamina and have a large complement of enzymatic activity; but they lack the capability to release fat as a result of the absence of esterase (lipase). In mature lobules, adipocytes in the form of rounded cells now contain lipid, a basal lamina, and a well-developed capillary bed; the entire complement of enzymatic activity is present, including NADH-tetrazolium reductase, ADPH-tetrazolium reductase, and glucose 6-phosphate dehydrogenase (G6PDH). Malate dehydrogenase (NADP) activity is acquired only by late-stage adipocytes (54). Hausman and Thomas (54) demonstrated the presence of such enzymatic differentiation before the assumption of an obviously rounded cell shape consistent with an adipocyte.

Lipoprotein lipase is an enzyme found at high concentration in fatty tissues. It is involved in the transport of serum triglycerides into adipocytes in the form of fatty acids. However, it can be found in other tissues such as skeletal muscles (56,57) and cardiac muscle (58), where it may be localized to endothelial cells. Concentration in fat is directly related to the serum insulin concentration.

Lipid Histochemistry

Lipids in adipose tissue are generally identified using various stains, such as oil red O and Sudan IV (59–65). It should be noted that lipids are lost in formaldehyde after prolonged fixation, and, thus, cases to be tested using frozen cryostat sections of fixed material should be obtained as soon as possible. Of the two time-honored lipid stains mentioned, oil red O gives the more intense stain and is more rapid to perform. Sudan black B may stain nonlipid substances (such as coagulated proteins) nonspecifically. As a rule, neutral fats are detected using these fat stains. However, a differential staining pattern between neutral fats and fatty acid components and phospholipids can be obtained with the Nile blue sulfate stain (66); with this stain, neutral fat stains pink to red, and fatty acids and phospholipids stain bluish. The lipid composition of fatty tissues may also be investigated using new techniques such as the hot-stage polarizing-light microscopic method (67).

The normal composition of lipid in white adipose tissue consists of 99% triglyceride in the form of neutral fat and less than 1% in the form of phospholipid, cholesterol, and fatty acids (53). In less-differentiated adipocytes, such as those found in liposarcomas, there is a shift away from neutral fat to phospholipids and cholesterol (66). Unfortunately, lipid stains appear to have little use in the everyday examination of adipocyte lesions. The droplets seen on the stains may represent nonspecific staining, and a variety of other mesenchymal lesions may contain lipid (64). An exception is the distinction between lesions with artificial vacuoles, such as epithelioid smooth muscle lesions, which are negative with fat stains.

Intracellular Lipid in Nonadipocytes

Lipid may accumulate in a variety of other cell types and in nonadipocytic tumors.

Steatosis

According to *Stedman's Medical Dictionary* (68), steatosis has two main meanings: adiposis and fatty degeneration (e.g., steatosis cordis = fatty degeneration of heart). These terms (and the terms used in a variety of pathology texts) are unclear, and the distinction between intracellular lipid accumulation and adipocyte infiltration of organs is not made. When nonadipocytes store lipid intracellularly, the phrase *lipid accumulation* is accurate; in the liver, the term *steatosis* is used; and, in major pathology texts (69,70), the term appears to be applied solely to the hepatocyte. However, intracytoplasmic lipid can be found within other solid organs, such as the heart [in the myocardial fibers in hypoxia (69)] and the kidney [in the renal tubule in diabetes, poisonings, Reye's syndrome (71)]. Theoretically, there is no reason why these processes cannot be referred to as myocardial or renal tubular steatosis. Regardless, in referring to intracellular lipid accumulation, terms such as *lipid accumulation* or *steatosis* are preferable to unclear and archaic designations, such as *adiposis* or *fatty degeneration*. Discussion of adipocyte infiltration of organs is found later (see the section entitled Syndromes Associated With Fatty Lesions (including Lipomatosis).

Lipid accumulation may occur in the placenta after prolonged parenteral nutrition; there, it takes the form of foamy vacuoles within the syncytial and Hofbauer cells of the chorionic villi (72).

Aside from adipocytes, lipid in the form of cholesterol and cholesterol esters may be identified in cells with a steroid-producing function in organs, such as the adrenal, ovary, and testis (and tumors thereof). In addition, other types of lipid are found within a variety of tumors. In practice, it is generally thought that a lipid stain (e.g., oil red O) can aid in the differential diagnosis of certain tumors. For example, it is well-known that renal cell carcinomas typically contain lipid (73), and most pathologists have the impression that many other tumors do not. However, it is clear from studies four decades ago (74) that fat stains are positive in the majority of cancers (Table 7.1). Thus, there are problems with the use of the fat stain in the diagnosis of carcinoma, and caution should be exercised in interpretation. Furthermore, although some clear cell lesions in the differential diagnosis of renal cancer contain glycogen (benign sugar tumor of lung) (75), others such as xanthoma of bone (76) contain lipid—and thus a fat stain is of no assistance.

TABLE 7.1
OIL RED O–POSITIVE CARCINOMAS[a]

Squamous cell carcinoma	Ovarian carcinoma
Gastric carcinoma	Breast carcinoma
Lung carcinomas	Prostatic carcinoma
Renal cell carcinoma	Thyroid carcinoma
Lymphoma, large cell	Myeloma

[a] For the majority of cancer types, a high percentage of the tumors listed showed a positive reaction.
Source: Elizalde N, Korman S. Cytochemical studies of glycogen, neutral mucopolysaccharides, and fat in malignant tissues. *Cancer* 1968;21:1061–1068.

IMMUNOHISTOCHEMISTRY

Currently, there is no commercially available specific immunohistochemical marker for adipose tissue. However, an adipocyte lipid-binding protein, p422 or aP2, is a protein expressed exclusively in preadipocytes late in adipogenesis. Preliminary studies with an antibody to aP2 demonstrate that it stains only lipoblasts and brown fat cells and is capable of identifying liposarcomas selectively (77). This may be quite useful diagnostically in the future.

Adipocytes and tumors thereof stain positively for vimentin; and, in our experience, adipocytic tumors have been negative for cytokeratin, desmin, and muscle-specific actin. In 1983, Michetti et al. (78) were the first to describe S-100 immunoreactivity in adipocytes, specifically of rat origin. The S-100 protein was extracted and shown to be identical to that found in the rat brain. Ultrastructurally, S-100 reactivity was widely dispersed within adipocyte cytoplasm but was not found within mitochondria, lipid droplets, or most of the endoplasmic reticulum. In a similar ultrastructural study, Haimoto et al. (79) identified S-100 protein in the plasma membranes, in membranes of microvesicles, and within polysomes. The Golgi apparatus was negative for this marker, although some reactivity was found within the rough endoplasmic reticulum. During the process of lipolysis in fat cells, Haimoto et al. (79) noted a change in the distribution of S-100 antigen and suggested that S-100 protein molecules interact with free fatty acids, indicating that this protein may act as a carrier protein for free fatty acids.

The S-100 protein is a highly acidic calcium-binding protein of molecular weight 21,000. It consists of two polypeptide chains (α and β) and may occur as dimers in three ways: S-100a (α, β), S-100b (β, β), or S-100ao (α, α) (80). When fat cells have been analyzed, they have been shown to contain only S-100b (β form), like Schwann cells (80,81). In the routine practice of immunohistochemistry, adipose tissue reacts in a variable fashion (Figure 7.7), accounting for some negative reactions observed by Kahn et al. (82). Although lipomas and liposarcomas are reported to be frequently positive with S-100 (83–86), in our experience, this has not been true. Regardless of fixation with formalin or Bouin's solution, very few liposarcomas have exhibited S-100 immunoreactivity.

Adipocytic lesions do not stain with antibodies to neuron-specific enolase (87).

Obesity

Human obesity is thought to be approximately 60% genetic in origin, with multiple genetic and environmental factors involved (88). The role of brown adipose tissue (BAT) was briefly alluded to earlier, and new research continues to underscore its importance. For example, in transgenic mice engineered to lack BAT, obesity develops routinely (89). In

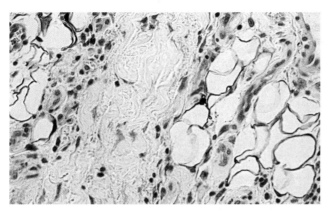

Figure 7.7 S-100 immunohistochemistry. Reactivity is seen both in the nuclei and in the cytoplasm surrounding the lipid droplets. Such S-100–positive results appear to vary considerably from case to case, probably reflecting fixation differences.

mice, the genetics of obesity are more clear than in humans. A team at the Rockefeller University led by Dr. Friedman first reported the identification of the *ob* mouse gene and showed that mutations of it are associated with the development of obesity (90). These same researchers have located the human counterpart (*OB* gene) (90) and mapped its location to chromosome 7 (91). The human protein produced by this gene has 84% homology with the mouse protein, appears to be a hormone secreted by adipose tissue, and likely functions as part of a pathway to regulate body fat. If, indeed, a defective hormone is responsible for some forms of obesity, then there is an immediate therapy available in the form of fully intact native hormone. In 1995, several research groups (92–94) have shown that injection of the ob protein into mice causes the animals to lose weight and maintain their weight loss. Even obesity due to a nongenetic defect like excess diet fat is corrected by the ob protein, now called leptin.

Finally, the receptor for this protein has been identified recently and shown to be nonfunctional in obese animals (95). Clearly, there have been major advances constituting a breakthrough in obesity research, and the fruits of this research should affect human therapy soon.

ADIPOCYTE LESIONS

Terminology

In contrast to other human tissue cell types, the terms *hypertrophy* and *hyperplasia* are not usually applied to the adipocyte. It is stressed here, however, that adipocyte hypertrophy (or increased fat cell size) is a recognized phenomenon and is found, for example, in obesity. Enlarged, or hypertrophic, fat cells (>120 μm or so) can also be identified in neoplasia (lipoma and liposarcoma) where cells

appear to have three or four times the normal diameter (e.g., >300 μm). Hyperplasia (or an increased number of adipocytes), in contrast to widespread belief, is a definite occurrence. Again, it is common in obese patients, but it may also be seen in organ-based infiltrations; these are a type of site-specific adipocyte hyperplastic processes. Mature adipocytes are incapable of regeneration, and new fat cells are added through in situ mesenchymal cell differentiation recruited from primitive perivascular cells. No disease or change involving adipocytes can appropriately be termed a degeneration (as mentioned earlier), other than liquefaction with necrosis. Atrophy of adipocytes may be seen in malnutrition, starvation, or as the effect of chemotherapy (see the section entitled Atrophy). The appearance of mature fat cells as small foci in unusual places is termed *metaplasia* and is discussed in a later section. Localized new growths of either pure adipocytes or mixtures of adipocytes in other tissue constitute neoplasia and are presumably clonal entities.

Degeneration

In the condition sclerema adiposum neonatorum, the subcutaneous fat is grossly and microscopically abnormal. Rubbery plaques are due to fat necrosis and degenerative individual fat cells with intracellular needle-shaped crystals (96). This fat crystallization is brown and can be highlighted by polarization. Such crystals apparently may also be identified in up to 30% of stillbirths as a general degeneration following intrauterine demise (96). In another disease, Neu Laxova syndrome, a defect in lipid metabolism causes a lard-like appearance to the adipose tissue and is lethal.

Atrophy

The changes in fat lobules during starvation or malnutrition are particularly noticeable in the subcutaneous region or the omentum. Individual fat cells are reduced in size and fat content, and those without much lipid take on a rounded or epithelioid appearance (97). In the extreme, lobules of these epithelioid cells can simulate tumor nodules histologically (Figure 7.8). The cytoplasm is variable in amount and is eosinophilic or granular with or without small lipid vacuoles of differing size, depending on the severity of the malnutrition. Some cells have a multivacuolated appearance. The intervening region between cells is constituted by homogeneous eosinophilic or amphophilic myxoid ground substance (Figure 7.8) that is probably an extract of serum, although stimulation of proteoglycan matrix by the process of starvation (98) is possible. As part of this involution process, lipofuscin is deposited within the shrinking cells (Figure 7.8). Importantly, each lobule retains its overall oval shape, although markedly reduced in size and considerably separated from other lobules (Figure 7.8). In extreme cachexia, only streaks of tissue remain.

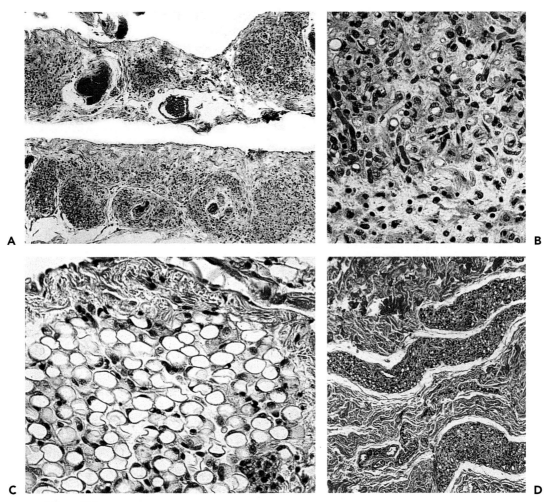

Figure 7.8 A. The extreme atrophy seen here in the omentum of a patient with anorexia nervosa may mimic tumor deposits. **B.** At high power, shrunken eosinophilic cells are seen with occasional vacuoles and lipofuscin pigment. **C.** In less severe starvation, these omental adipocytes are well-recognized, although much smaller than normal size; again, note the presence of pigment. **D.** In the skin, severe cachexia secondary to a cancer resulted in marked involution of the cutaneous fat lobules, which appear only as elongated streaks.

Nearly identical changes can also be seen in the white adipose tissue of fasted animals. As the cells gradually lose their lipid, the single lipid droplet breaks up into multiple vacuoles. Gradually, all lipid disappears. These cells become small and ovoid in shape, sometimes measuring only 15 μm in diameter (99). There is an apparent expansion of pericellular collagen in such a way that these cells appear as clusters of mesenchymal cells in fibrous stroma. Ultrastructurally, multiple pinocytotic vesicles are seen clustered along the entire cell membrane (53). Lipid is not seen within these vesicles, and their significance is unknown.

In the bone marrow, chemotherapy causes changes referred to as serous atrophy or gelatinous transformation (100,101). The majority of the fat cells have been destroyed, leaving scattered adipocytes of varying size remaining. No lobular appearance is present in the marrow, but the interstitial compartment is composed of the same eosinophilic myxoid substance described previously, again probably consisting of serum fluid and proteins. Droplets of lipid scattered about are also found and, upon regeneration, may appear as foci of lipogranulomas.

Although the microscopic features of the starvation effect on human brown fat have not been described, animals maintained on a dextrose-thiamine diet are known to show distinct morphologic changes in brown fat (37). The mitochondria are disrupted and large, irregular electron-dense inclusions are seen within the mitochondrial matrix. The cristae may assume a mosaic pattern with compartmentalization of the material. These cells revert to normal after 24 hours of a normal diet. Similar changes in white fat mitochondria have not been seen with starvation, suggesting that the active mitochondria of brown fat are particularly labile and sensitive to dietary changes.

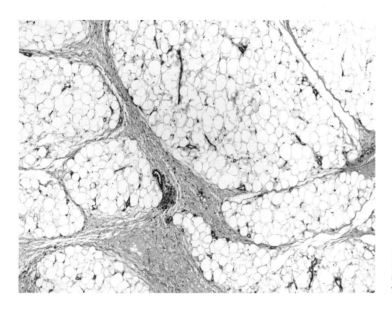

Figure 7.9 Accentuated fat lobules in ischemia of the lower extremity. Loose myxoid connective tissue widens the septa between lobules; edema and a mild inflammatory infiltrate are present.

Cellulite

The term cellulite is applied to the external skin when it exhibits linear depressed streaks (mattress phenomenon) or frank dimpling. Cellulite is typically found on the thigh and buttocks and is more common in females; it can be divided into incipient cellulite and full-blown cellulite. The former results from an uneven undersurface of the dermal-hypodermal interface, with fibrous tissue surrounding the protruding papillae adiposa; vertical fibrous strands of uneven thickness divide the hypodermal fat (102). In contrast, full-blown cellulite consists of a delicate meshwork of collagen fibers produced by increased hypodermal pressure of fat accumulation and increasing fat volume. Scattered CD34+ fibroblasts are seen in both forms of cellulite. Unlike women, men have a more smooth, strand-free dermal interface in the thigh and buttock areas (102).

Ischemia

Little is written about the effect of ischemia on the adipocyte. We have observed changes in the subcutaneous fat of legs removed for atherosclerotic vascular disease. They consist of accentuation of the lobular architecture by thickening of the fibrous septa; wider and more myxoid in quality, the septa are edematous and also contain scattered inflammatory cells (Figure 7.9). Actual necrosis was not observed.

Metaplasia

As surgical pathologists, we most frequently encounter adipocytic metaplasia, usually calcified, in cardiac valves (Figure 7.10). There is little in the literature or textbooks on this phenomenon. The emergence of mature adipose tissue seems to parallel the appearance of osteoblasts forming bone within the calcific deposits. Once adipose tissue is present, bone marrow precursors may become resident, presumably from circulating cells, and cause hematopoiesis. Metaplasia is not limited to this site and may be encountered in calcified large vessels or elsewhere, such as in laryngeal cartilage undergoing ossification. We have even seen it in small ossified bronchioles. A similar phenomenon of hematopoiesis without adipose tissue and bone has been reported within acoustic neuromas (103).

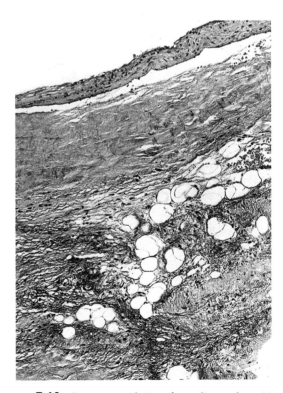

Figure 7.10 Fatty metaplasia of cardiac valve. Mature adipocytes are found in a myxoid background but are more commonly seen in association with calcification or ossification.

LIPODYSTROPHY

Although there are several different entities referred to in the past under this name, some (idiopathic intestinal lipodystrophy, or Whipple's disease) are infectious and others (mesenteric lipodystrophy; see section entitled Mesenteritis) are inflammatory disorders without fundamental changes in the fat cells themselves. The one example of a true lipodystrophy is called membranous lipodystrophy, a relatively new clinical entity characterized by abnormal fat cells, bone cysts with pathologic fractures, and leukodystrophy of the brain (104–106). The marrow fat is particularly affected (104), but the "membranocystic" lesions are also present to a lesser degree in the subcutaneous adipose tissue (106). The characteristic and pathognomonic finding is the highly shrivelled, undulating outline of individual fat cell membranes, giving them hyalin eosinophilic convolutions or "arabesque profiles." Multiple small cysts are found, apparently formed by fusion of ruptured adipocytes. Young adults are affected in Japan and Finland primarily, but five cases have been seen in the United States (105). Its etiology and pathogenesis are unknown; it is probably related to an enzyme deficiency (104). A secondary form of membranous lipodystrophy has been described in association with lupus erythematosus and morphea profunda (107). Interestingly, the membranous changes in fat characteristic of lipodystrophy can also be seen in normal fat affected by radiation therapy (108).

ADIPOCYTES IN ORGANS

Fatty Infiltration

As distinct from lipid accumulation or steatosis (see section entitled Steatosis), fatty infiltration is defined as the presence of mature adipose tissue in sites not normally containing fat. This is a disorder or condition relating to adipocyte cell growth and, therefore, the term *fatty degeneration* is a misnomer and incorrect. In some situations, such as within extremity muscle groups, the process of fatty infiltration is often related to atrophy of the involved site (109). This association between fatty infiltration and atrophy or involution is also noted in other organs [thymus (110), bone marrow (111), and kidney (112)], and apparently signifies the propensity for adipocytes to fill a vacuum, in a sense, left by atrophic processes (97). Whatever the stimulus may be, the adipocytes probably arise from pleuripotent mesenchymal cells adjacent to blood vessels (97). The reversal of this relationship is found in the parathyroid gland, where there is an inverse relationship between parenchymal cells and adipocytes, to the point where no adipocytes are present in complete parathyroid hyperplasia.

Nonatrophic organs can also accumulate fat cells (lipomatosis), and the classic examples are the heart and pancreas (69). In these locations, no parenchymal damage is discerned, and the process is a type of accidental lipogenesis (97). In the case of the pancreas, normal parenchymal histology and function are present even though the pancreas may be nearly invisible grossly (69,113). This type of pancreatic lipomatosis is correlated with age and obesity and also occurs in diabetics (113). The amount of pancreatic tissue is thought to be either completely normal (69) or partially depleted (113). However, true pancreatic atrophy with resultant lipomatosis also exists as a rare condition known as Schwachman syndrome (113) [see Table 7.2 in section entitled Syndromes Associated with Fatty Lesions (Including Lipomatosis)]. Fatty infiltration of the heart is most often an innocuous condition with no effect on the myocardial fiber or cardiac function (69). However, there are rare exceptions in which severe adipocity has resulted in cardiac rupture (97). Another clinically important lesion is termed *lipomatous hypertrophy of the interatrial septum* (114), a focal enlargement that may cause sudden death, arrhythmias, or congestive failure (115,116). Be mindful that the occasional appearance of fat in endocardial biopsies in no way indicates cardiac perforation (117).

Isolated fat cells can be found within lymph nodes in childhood, but enlarged nodes with prominent fatty infiltration mainly occur in adults, particularly in obesity (118). Common in the abdomen and retroperitoneum, such "lipolymph nodes" can be mistaken for lipomas (118) or be interpreted as positive in a lymphangiogram for lymphoma or Hodgkin's disease (personal observation), mimicking lymphoma relapse (119). Rarely, a lipoma or angiomyolipoma occurs in the liver (120), but those lesions should not be confused with the hepatic pseudolipoma (121). This pseudolipoma is often found as a bulge on the surface of the liver and probably represents capture of previously detached appendices epiploicae. In the mouth, fat is one of the components contributing to macroglossia in certain conditions (122).

The Ito cells of the liver are fat-containing cells along the sinuses and are a variation on normal histology (123); they may become prominent in the condition known as lipopeliosis (124) and may be involved in the benign neoplasm called spongiotic pericytoma (125).

FAT BIOPSY FOR AMYLOID

It is becoming increasingly popular to perform a subcutaneous fat biopsy for the diagnosis of amyloidosis. In such instances, the Congo red stain may reveal amyloid around blood vessels and, occasionally, between adipocytes (126–128). This procedure is at least as sensitive as the rectal biopsy (128), can identify up to 84% of cases (127), can be combined with other studies to determine amyloid type (126), and is a safe and innocuous way to make the diagnosis (127).

Biopsy analysis of adipose tissue may become important in the future, to assess a given individual's storage content of toxic chemicals. A variety of industrial and environmental hydrocarbons are stored predominantly in fat, and subcutaneous adipose tissue deposits may be analyzed and results correlated with the development of diseases such as neoplasia.

INFLAMMATIONS

Fat Necrosis

Three histologically distinct types of fat necrosis exist: the ordinary variety secondary to trauma and other inflammation, that associated with pancreatitis, and infarction of fat. Histologically, ordinary fat necrosis is typified by the presence of epithelioid histiocytes, foamy macrophages, and giant cells in adipose tissue, often surrounding and isolating individual adipocytes (Figure 7.11). Lymphocytes and plasma cells are also found in small numbers. Occasionally, unusual crystalloids may be seen (129). Fat cells become destroyed, and the released lipid may fuse to result in a single droplet larger than the average cell or in minute droplets. This process may resolve with mild fibrosis or, if extensive, may cause cyst formation with eventual dense fibrosis and even calcification at the periphery. Such cysts with central liquefaction may be located on the buttocks and be the final result of trauma, secondary to an injection. Just beneath the cyst wall, necrotic outlines of adipocytes are usually present, signifying the origin of the end-stage cyst in fat necrosis.

An unusual type of fat necrosis forming cystic spaces has been designated *membranous fat necrosis* by Poppiti et al.

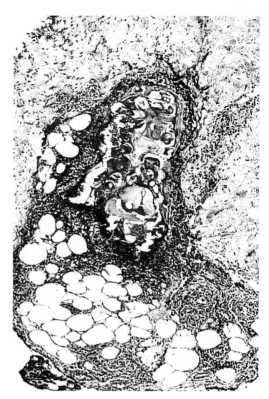

Figure 7.12 Fat necrosis, pancreatic type. In contrast to regular fat necrosis, numerous neutrophils are found, together with central liquefaction. The central material may give either an eosinophilic or basophilic appearance, and disrupted cell membranes can be appreciated.

(130). In this example, actual cysts are formed that contain pseudopapillary structures and central debris. Although the fat cell outlines are normal in appearance, the formation of these cysts resembles that seen in membranous lipodystrophy. Membranous fat necrosis can also occur secondary to radiation therapy (108).

Fat necrosis secondary to acute pancreatitis is histologically distinctive (Figure 7.12). Rather than consisting of a histiocytic infiltrate, the pancreatic fat necrosis is accompanied by an infiltrate of neutrophils predominantly, and liquefaction of fat is apparent (131,132). In the center of the lesion, the infarctlike outlines of fat cells can be seen, and fat cell membranes are ruptured, releasing their contents into a central eosinophilic or basophilic material. The entire region is bordered by an acute inflammatory infiltrate. The process is thought to be secondary to the action of pancreatic lipolytic enzymes in the serum acting on susceptible foci.

The infarction type of fat necrosis, in which eosinophilic outlines of fat cells without nuclei or inflammation are present histologically, may be seen in lipomas and in detached peritoneal tissue originating from appendices epiploicae. The lipomas containing infarction may be pedunculated with twisting, causing compromise of blood flow.

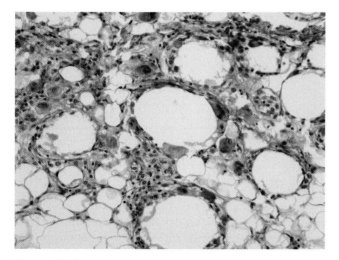

Figure 7.11 Fat necrosis, ordinary type. Multinucleated histiocytic giant cells surround a large lipid vacuole formed by fusion of destroyed adipocytes. Scattered lymphocytes and monocytes occupy expanded spaces between cells at top.

Calciphylaxis

Another disorder that often manifests itself as skin and sub-cutaneous fat necrosis is called calciphylaxis; here, the characteristic vascular necrosis with calcium precipitation will aid in the diagnosis (133). It is a painful and often lethal complication of dialysis and renal failure (134). Small vessels (including arterioles in the fat) show mural calcification and necrosis, along with thrombosis and necrosis of surrounding tissues. In some cases, an association with primary hyperparathyroidism has been reported (135).

Panniculitis

Numerous diseases and conditions may cause an inflammatory infiltrate of the subcutaneous adipose tissue, namely, a panniculitis; readers are referred to a variety of textbooks on skin pathology for an in-depth enumeration of these. Only a few relevant points are made here. First, the condition called Weber-Christian disease, or febrile nodular nonsuppurative panniculitis of the subcutaneous fat, was described early in this century and is consistently referred to in discussions of this topic. However, it became clear in the 1960s and 1970s that this disease was not a clinically distinct entity, but rather had many separate etiologies, including steroid withdrawal, diabetes mellitus, tuberculosis, pancreatic disease, and systemic lupus erythematosus (136). Thus, it is generally agreed today that Weber-Christian "disease" was a clinical description of a presentation for numerous diseases and is a term to be avoided (137).

Panniculitis, as a rule, can be divided into those that are septal and those that involve the lobules of adipose tissue (137). The character of the infiltrate is important, and note should be made of the presence of eosinophils (138), neutrophils and granulomas (139), histiocytes with lymphophagocytosis (140), or other specific changes (141). Autoimmune diseases such as scleroderma (142) and lupus (143) may be causative, indicating the importance of historical detail. Unusual causes, such as α 1-antitrypsin deficiency (137), have a characteristic histology, as does pancreatic fat necrosis (described in other texts). Even withdrawal from steroids may cause a panniculitis (144).

Mesenteritis

Inflammation of the mesenteric fat is a recognizable clinical entity that has more recently been termed *mesenteric panniculitis* to signify the active inflammatory stage and *retractile mesenteritis* to signify the fibrotic stage (145). Other terms complicate the literature, but it is generally held that they all refer to the same disease process and spectrum: liposclerotic mesenteritis, sclerosing mesenteritis, mesenteric lipodystrophy (ML), and Weber-Christian disease of the mesentery [see recent review by Kelly and Hwang (146)].

The process consists of a chronic inflammatory infiltrate of lymphocytes, plasma cells, foamy histiocytes, and giant cells, along with recognizable fat necrosis, edema, and a variable amount of fibrosis and calcification. Myofibroblasts proliferate and are directly involved in the pathogenesis of the retractile disease (146). While it most often thickens the mesentery (type 1 ML), it can appear as a single tumefaction at the mesenteric base (type 2 ML) or as multiple discrete nodules (type 3 ML) (147). Other space-occupying lesions, such as inflammatory pseudotumors, xanthogranulomatosis (see below), and fibromatosis, are in the differential diagnosis (119). Affected patients are usually middle-aged and predominantly male, and they complain of vague abdominal discomfort and weight loss, with over one-half presenting with fever. Nearly one-half of them are, oddly enough, asymptomatic (146). Rare cases have been fatal, but the prognosis is generally excellent. Mass lesions regress within 2 years in about two-thirds of the patients, and any pain disappears in three-quarters of them (145). Steroids are commonly given to treat the disease, but it is unclear whether the course of the disease or the progression to fibrosis is changed (145).

Retroperitoneal xanthogranulomatosis can be due to a primary inflammatory process of the kidney, or it can represent involvement of the retroperitoneum by the mesenteritis. Many foamy histiocytes and lymphocytes are seen. Rarely, it can be associated with Erdheim-Chester disease (multisystem fibroxanthomas with bone pain and sclerotic bone lesions) (148).

Lipogranuloma

Small collections of epithelioid histiocytes with lipid droplets are commonly encountered in lymph nodes, draining the gastrointestinal tract (mesenteric, porta hepatis, retroperitoneal), and in the liver, spleen, and bone marrow. They do not imply a pancreatitis (in which necrosis should be present) or other pathologic process and are completely incidental.

TUMORS AND TUMORLIKE LESIONS

Brown Fat Lesions

Hibernoma

The only pathologic lesion of brown fat known to date is the hibernoma, the neoplastic counterpart given its name by Gery (149). Although many of the cells in the hibernoma are multivacuolated, some cells lack vacuoles completely and are eosinophilic and granular in appearance. Both of these cell types have a centrally placed nucleus. Importantly, univacuolated cells with peripherally placed nuclei resembling white adipocytes can be identified, as they can in normal brown fat (149,150). The red-brown color of a hibernoma is the result of the increased vascularity in numerous mitochondria. The ultrastructure of hibernoma is similar to brown fat (151); and, indeed, when cellular organelles are compared, the ultrastructure suggested to a number of authors (149,150) is that brown fat and white fat are two distinct tissues, with different ultrastructural features.

Concerning location, many hibernomas arise in sites corresponding to the distribution of normal brown fat—interscapular area, neck, mediastinum, and axilla (149); other cases have been reported in the abdominal wall, thigh, and popliteal space (149), all sites considered devoid of brown fat (152). Generally medium-sized tumors (5 to 10 cm), hibernomas may obtain a huge dimension [23 cm (153)] and are often present for years prior to excision. The tumors typically occur in young adults with a median age of 26 years, much younger than patients with ordinary lipoma (149). Interestingly, endocrine activity has been noted within these tumors, with steroid hormones (including cortisol and testosterone) detected (154). Hibernomas do not recur, but whether malignant hibernomas exist has been a controversial topic. A case having atypical mitoses and bizarre nuclei was reported by Enterline et al. (155), and a similar case with ultrastructural features was documented by Teplitz et al. (156).

White Fat Lesions

Adipose Tissue within Nonfatty Lesions

Almost any malignant tumor may invade and incorporate mature fat cells. Occasionally, however, the presence of fat cells within mesenchymal proliferation can be confusing. For example, nodular fasciitis may incorporate individual fat cells that can appear smaller than normal, mimicking lipoblasts (136). Likewise, a very prominent component of adipose tissue accompanies intramuscular angiomatosis and lymphangiomatosis of the extremities (152). Benign teratomas of the ovary (157) and lung (158,159) occasionally contain mature adipose tissue as an incidental finding. So-called fibrous polyps of the esophagus (160) also contain adipose tissue. Other nonlipomatous tumors that may contain fat include the pleomorphic adenoma of the salivary gland and the benign spindle cell breast tumor described by Toker et al. (161). This lesion may be what has been described recently as a myofibroblastoma (162) with the incorporation of adipose tissue.

Perhaps by a process of cellular metaplasia, fat may also be found occasionally in the endometrium (163) or in epithelial tumors of various types (see below).

Ectopic Adipose Tissue

Ectopic fat either in cardiac valves or within organs was discussed earlier in the Metaplasia and Fatty Infiltration sections. Oddly enough, ectopic fat may occur in the dermis, where it causes a pedunculated appearance; this has been termed *nevus lipomatosis superficialis* or, more recently, *pedunculated lipofibroma* (164).

Hamartomas Containing Fat Cells

Many of us are aware that the benign pulmonary "chondroma," or "hamartoma," may contain fat (158). In fact, approximately 75% of these lesions do (165), and the presence of such a tissue foreign to the lung parenchyma supports the concept that these lesions are benign mesenchymomas (158,165). Occasionally, the lipomatous component may be so dominant as to suggest a lipoma (165,166).

Amazingly, adipose tissue can be a component of many other unusual lesions. It may be coupled with vascular, fibrous, and myofibroblastic components in multiple congenital mesenchymal hamartomas [multiple sites (167)]; with undifferentiated spindle cells and fibroblasts in the fibrous hamartoma of infancy [mainly in shoulder and axillary regions (168–170)]; with fibrous tissue and mature nerve in the sometimes congenital fibrolipomatous hamartoma of nerve with or without macrodactyly [palm, wrist, or fingers (171–173)]; or with smooth muscle and vessels in the angiomyolipoma (174,175). These hamartomatous lesions of tuberous sclerosis will be discussed further. In another oddity, adipose tissue is one component of human tails and pseudotails (176), along with skin and other tissues.

Massive Localized Lymphedema

In morbidly obese patients, huge subcutaneous masses as large as 50 cm may form, clinically mimicking liposarcoma (177–178). Pedunculated masses of adipose tissue show dilated lymphatics and edema and thus this condition is known as massive localized lymphedema (MLL). Grossly, the fat is marbled in appearance secondary to coarse bands of fibrous tissue intersecting fat lobules. Microscopically, the adipose tissue is dissected by fibrosis simulating sclerosing liposarcoma; however, the lesion is superficial, and there are no atypical stromal cells nor lipoblasts. In the edematous septa, scattered myofibroblasts are noted. Aside from the often postsurgical abdominal sites reported initially, MLL may also occur in the thigh, scrotum, and inguinal regions and be associated with hypothyroidism (178).

Mesenchymomas

Adipose tissue is a nearly constant component of benign mesenchymomas—growth that should be redefined as having more than two mesenchymal elements. LeBer and Stout (179) required the presence of at least two different mesenchymal elements to make a diagnosis of mesenchymoma. However, we believe the trend has evolved in favor of more than two elements, and those lesions with only two elements currently appear to be designated separately as chondrolipoma, fibrolipoma, and so on (152,180). This seems appropriate since the secondary element, usually in a lipoma, is frequently a very focal finding (as it may be in a liposarcoma). Thus, aside from lesions with focal "metaplasia," lesions with three or more elements can be designated true mesenchymomas. For instance, a description of a trigeminal neurilemmoma (181) was really a mesenchymoma with cartilage, bone, hemangioma, schwannoma, and adipose tissue. Also, a thoracic tumor with smooth muscle, angiomatoid spaces, fibrous tissue, and adipose tissue is another mesenchymoma, reported in association with hemihypertrophy (182). Angiomyolipoma is another example of a benign mesenchymoma and is frequently found in the kidney, where approximately 40% are associated with tuberous sclerosis (175). Although the fat seen here is practically always mature, rarely lipoblast-like cells may be seen in these (152,183). Angiomyolipomas have also been reported in other sites, such as lymph nodes (184).

Lipomas

The distinction between adipose tissue lobules and true lipoma occasionally arises in the practice of surgical pathology, necessitating a strict definition of lipoma. Although lipoma is well described in two major texts (152,180), definitions are concise without detail. Lipoma is herein defined as a superficial or deep-circumscribed and expansile benign neoplasm composed of mature adipose tissue, which is commonly (but need not be) encapsulated. Such a definition emphasizes its well-differentiated and clonal nature (see following) and serves to distinguish most lipomas from normal fat and prominent posttraumatic skin folds, or "fat fractures" (185). As Allen (180) emphasizes, the capsule may be quite thin and poorly defined. Nonetheless, it is a crucial requirement for superficial tumors; deep lesions, on the contrary, are often nonencapsulated. When a subcutaneous lipoma is excised in a piecemeal fashion, the lesion may be diagnosed by noting the presence of portions of capsular fibrous tissue in the form of a circular arc of collagen of varying width at the edge of tissue fragments. In the absence of a clear-cut capsule or fragments thereof, a diagnosis of a superficial lipoma cannot be made.

Clinically, the majority of lipomas seen in surgical pathology are subcutaneous tumors typically in the middle-aged to elderly patient. Males and females are probably equally affected, and there are no racial differences. Most tumors are located on the trunk or upper extremities; if other sites are encountered, consideration should be given to one of the lipoma subtypes (e.g., forearm for angiolipoma, neck for spindle and pleomorphic types). Lipomas probably outnumber all other soft tissue tumors combined (152). Interesting facts about lipomas include (a) a nearly static size after the initial growth period (152); (b) the relative rarity of lesions on the hands, feet, face, and lower leg despite the presence of fat (152); (c) hardness after the application of ice, a diagnostic sign (152); (d) the lack of size reduction in starvation (152,180); (e) a definite, but low, recurrence rate [1 to 4% (152,180)]; (f) an unknown etiology; (g) a possible relation to potassium intake (186); and (h) a possible association with an increased incidence of cancer [46% (187)].

Many lesions of the subcutaneous region come to surgical pathology labeled as lipomas; and, not uncommonly, a portion of these actually turn out to be something else that is frequently more interesting.

When one views normal fat histologically, the size of fat cells appears to vary somewhat due to the sectioning plane; however, the variation is relatively small [80 to 120 μm (personal observation); Figure 7.4]. In lipomas [including atypical lipoma (188)], there is a tendency for cell size to vary more widely, with larger cells (e.g., >300 μm) being apparent. Practically, this means that a medium-power view will often disclose a two- to fivefold size range (Figure 7.13). Normal fat has a netlike structure of fibrous tissue, wherein such dispersed fibrous bands or septa dissect the adipose tissue randomly. The fibrous tissue is thicker in quality in bodily regions exposed to pressure, such as the hands, feet, and buttocks (97). This netlike fibrous tissue arrangement is recapitulated within lipomas (Figure 7.14), particularly at the periphery where small lobules are often found. A high degree of vascularity is a feature associated with lipogenic malignancy, but we should be aware that this refers to a visible network of capillaries, often in strings and branching arrays. However, normal adipose tissue and lipomas are likewise highly vascular, except the capillary vascular bed is more difficult to visualize. A PAS stain of a lipoma, for example, can highlight the minute but diffuse capillaries, particularly at the junctions between cells, where they are made more difficult to see due to compression. A delicate reticulin

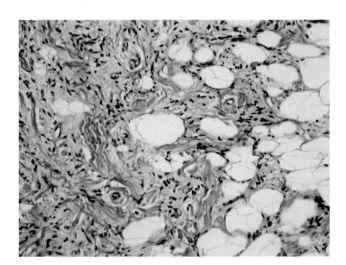

Figure 7.13 Variation in fat cell size in spindle cell lipoma. Some adipocytes are three to five times the size of a normal adipocyte; compare with Figure 7.4. Increased numbers of spindle cells together with collagen bands characterize this lipoma subtype, although the size variation seems to be present in all unusual types of lipoma.

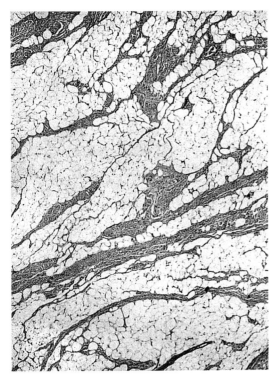

Figure 7.14 Lipoma with accentuated lobulation. In certain sites such as the buttock, foot, and hand (*depicted here*), thick fibrous septa are noted throughout; these correspond to the thicker septa within the normal adipose tissue in these regions.

network is also present in lipomas, contributed to by the basement membranes of both lipocytes and capillaries; each lipocyte is completely encircled by reticulin in a manner similar to normal fat cells (Figure 7.3). Normally, lipomas have a low degree of cellularity and no nuclear atypia; the presence of either is cause for concern. Sometimes increased cellularity is due to a diffuse low-grade form of fat necrosis (Figure 7.15). The ultrastructure of lipoma recapitulates that of its normal counterpart (189).

Myxoid Change

In rare lipomas, the mature fat cells are separated by varying amounts of a loose basophilic ground substance, probably proteoglycan (Figure 7.16). When prominent, the lesion may be designated a *myxolipoma* or *myxoid lipoma* (152,180). The myxoid quality often raises the possibility of a myxoid liposarcoma. However, these areas contain only widely scattered bland cells and are never hypercellular. Furthermore, the plexiform capillary network so typical of the malignant tumor is absent, as are lipoblasts. As Enzinger and Weiss (152) observed, rare cells may be vacuolated but contain bluish mucoid material.

Intramuscular Lipoma

Deep lipomas may be either intermuscular or intramuscular, with the latter unencapsulated tumors being the more common. Intramuscular lipomas (190), also known as infiltrating lipomas, involve the large muscles of the extremities (particularly the thigh, shoulder, and upper arm) or the paraspinal muscles. For extremity lesions, an inapparent mass may become visible upon voluntary contraction. Microscopically, the lipocytes are typically mature, and mitoses or atypical nuclei are not found. Muscle fibers are widely dispersed throughout the lesion (Figure 7.17). Any unusual features should raise the suspicion of a well-differentiated liposarcoma (191). Often, intramuscular lipomas extend beyond the muscle fascia to involve the intervening connective tissue space. Therefore, it is often difficult to completely excise such lesions, and the recurrence rate is higher than that for ordinary subcutaneous lipoma. This has been particularly true for paraspinal intramuscular lipomas.

Intramuscular angiolipomas are lesions considered to be intramuscular hemangiomas with a variable fat content (152).

Lipoma arborescens is a special type of lipoma occurring in a joint: it has a characteristic villiform gross appearance,

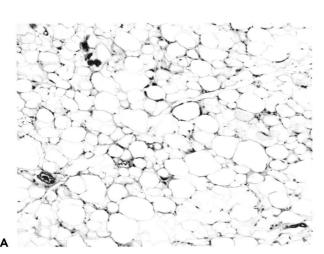

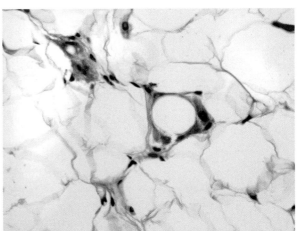

A   B

Figure 7.15 Lipoma. **A.** In some tumors, an increased cellularity at medium power may cause concern, but it is frequently due to a mild but diffuse fat necrosis. **B.** The lipocytes are falsely enlarged by the histiocytes without much other inflammation.

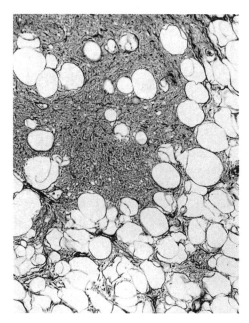

Figure 7.16 Lipoma with myxoid change. Features that differentiate this from myxoid liposarcoma are the lack of branching capillary vessels and significant cellularity in the myxoid component.

and the patients typically have a highly painful knee (180). The mere presence of adipose tissue on a synovial biopsy is not synonymous with this entity.

Other Elements in Lipomas

Aside from the ordinary lipoma, extraneous elements of various types can be associated with an adipose tissue benign proliferation, including combinations with epithelial or other mesenchymal components.

Mesenchymal Components

Perhaps the most common mesenchymal component associated with the lipoma is, as surgical pathologists are aware, benign cartilaginous metaplasia (Figure 7.18). So-called chondrolipomas may occur in almost any site of the body,

including the breast (192) and mediastinum (193). Although the term *benign mesenchymoma* has been applied to such lesions, the chondroid metaplasia is practically always an extremely minor component in the form of very small isolated islands of cartilage; therefore, the designation of mesenchymoma appears to be an exaggeration (as it is when cartilaginous metaplasia occurs in liposarcoma). Allen (194) also prefers to avoid the term *mesenchymoma*.

Lipochondromatosis is a recently reported entity that involves the tendons and synovium of the ankle region as a mass lesion (195). Rarely benign osteoid is also found in lipomas, either solely or coupled with cartilage (196). Some of these osteolipomas are in contact with periosteum and may be termed *periosteal lipoma* (196). Smooth muscle lesions, particularly of the uterus, may be combined with adipose tissue to produce lipoleiomyomas (197) and lipoleiomyomatosis (198). Prominent blood vessels are a frequent component of superficial small subcutaneous tumors called angiolipomas (152). These lesions are interesting, as they may be multiple, cause pain due to frequent microthrombi, and give rise to the differential diagnosis of Kaposi's sarcoma when the angiomatoid component completely overcomes the lipocytic component (Figure 7.19). These fat-poor variants are designated cellular angiolipomas (199). In such instances, the diagnosis is made by finding rare-to-scattered mature fat cells, usually at the periphery of the lesion.

Some lipomas contain an increased content of fibrous tissue. These usually superficial tumors have been called fibrolipomas. However, it is likely that the amount of fibrous

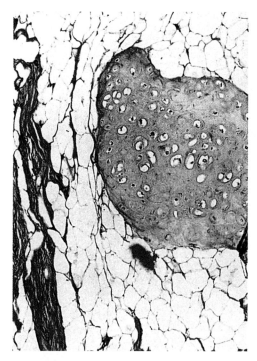

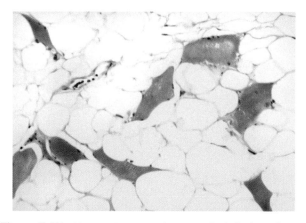

Figure 7.17 Lipoma, intramuscular type. The light fat cells proliferate between dark individual skeletal muscle fibers in this commonly unencapsulated tumor (trichrome stain).

Figure 7.18 Chondrolipoma. Small nodules of mature cartilage are present, often very focally; this combination alone should not be labeled a mesenchymoma.

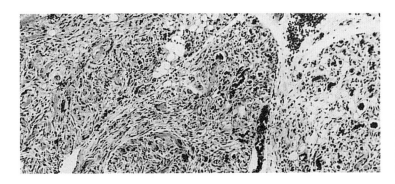

Figure 7.19 Angiolipoma. In this unusual example, the rarity of adipocytes (*top middle*) makes the tumor resemble a deep Kaposi's-like lesion; the location, circumscription, frequent microthrombi (*center*), and isolated islands of fat cells at the periphery aid in the diagnosis.

tissue in a lipoma is directly related to its anatomic site of origin (Figure 7.14). Dense thicker fibrous tissue is typically found in lipomas of the pressure-bearing regions of the body such as the hands, feet, and buttocks; the lobular architecture accentuated by such fibrous bands may be apparent grossly.

Epithelial Components

In some superficial lipomas, eccrine glands may be incorporated into the lesion. Eccrine glands may be found at the junction of dermal collagen; the subcutaneous fat and lipomas arising in this region can cause displacement of these glands, well within the substance of the lipoma. This phenomenon has been noted in locations such as the hand and buttock (personal observation).

Adipose tissue may accompany adenomas (i.e., lipoadenomas) of the thyroid (200) and parathyroid (201). Aside from lipoadenomas, other lesions of the thyroid gland may contain fat—including colloid nodules, lymphocytic thyroiditis, and papillary carcinomas (202,203). Another unusual phenomenon is the formation of the thymolipoma (204). As listed in Table 7.2 [see section entitled Syndromes Associated with Fatty Lesions (Including Lipomatosis)], an unusual lipomatous syndrome is described that consists of thyrolipoma, thymolipoma, and pharyngeal lipoma (205).

Lymphocytes in Lipomas

Occasionally, one may observe a dense perivascular lymphocytic infiltrate in scattered vessels within and outside ordinary lipomas. Although not generally described, the authors have observed this phenomenon several times and investigated the patients; they have not exhibited evidence of chronic lymphocytic leukemia or autoimmune disease. Perhaps this may represent a localized host reaction to the proliferation.

Special Lipoma Types

In the spindle cell (206–208) and pleomorphic (209,210) lipomas, the fat cells appear variable in size at low power. In spindle cell lipoma (Figure 7.13), the spindle cell content may vary from scanty to abundant, and the nuclei of the spindle cells are wavy, resembling nerve sheath le-

sions. Dense fibrous tissue is also found sometimes with a keloidal quality. Similar cells may be seen in pleomorphic lipoma, which has, in addition, characteristic floret tumor giant cells (Figure 7.20). Both of these lesions are encapsulated and have characteristic locations commonly limited to the head and neck of elderly males. They may be related entities (211). Interestingly, immunoreactivity for androgen receptor has recently been demonstrated in the fibroblast-like spindle cells of spindle cell lipoma (Brooks, personal data).

The chondroid lipoma is a well-circumscribed lesion with two elements: mature adipose tissue and focal or prominent areas containing strands and nests of eosinophilic vacuolated cells resembling chondroblasts or lipoblasts. A hyalinized myxoid matrix is also seen. This tumor is S-100 protein, vimentin, and CD68-positive, and may be cytokeratin-positive. It occurs mainly in women in the superficial soft tissues or skeletal muscle of extremities, head, and neck. While worrisome in appearance, the lesion does not recur or metastasize (212,213).

Finally, an unusual fatty tumor of the mediastinum with elastic tissue has been described as elastofibrolipoma (214).

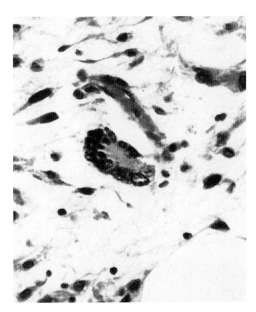

Figure 7.20 Floret cell. The wreath of nuclei at the periphery characterizes this cell, which is classically present in pleomorphic lipoma but may occur in some liposarcomas.

Lipoblastoma

Frequently a congenital lesion, the lipoblastoma (215–221) is a benign solitary proliferation of fat, retaining the lobular architecture of developing fetal white adipose tissue. Nearly 90% of these superficial lesions occur before the age of 3 (152). Interestingly, lesions tend to mature with the age of the patient. Tumors may be predominantly myxoid with spindle cells, predominantly lipocytic, or mixed; all types have a prominent capillary bed and are often encapsulated. When mature fat cells are present, they are typically in the central portion of the lobules, in turn surrounded by collagen. In contrast, the presence of maturing adipocytes in myxoid liposarcoma is frequently found at the periphery of the lobule (220). Thus, while these tumors bear a resemblance to myxoid liposarcoma, there are clear differences, and the lobular accentuation with collagen is quite typical (Figure 7.21), as is the age at presentation. Rare cells resembling brown fat or hibernoma cells have been identified in lipoblastoma (219). If these lesions are single, they should be termed *lipoblastoma* (216) and not *lipoblastomatosis* (218,221); that was the original designation given appropriately by Vellios et al. in 1958 for a diffuse form (215).

Lipoblastomatosis

Lipoblastomatosis is the proper designation for the less common diffuse form of lipoblastoma. About one-third of the patients have diffuse tumors, which (in contrast to the solitary form) are usually deeply situated, more poorly circumscribed, infiltrating muscle, and with a higher tendency to recur (216).

CYTOGENETICS OF LIPOMAS

Chromosomal karyotypes of lipomas have been studied (222–229) and reveal nonrandom changes involving chromosomes 3 and 12, indicative of clonality. The balanced translocation t(3;12) is a common finding (224,225), with breakpoints described at probably identical locations—q27;q13 (223) and q28;q14 (222). The breakpoint on chromosome 12 is very close to the one described in the t(12;16) translocation in myxoid liposarcomas (224). This balanced translocation involving chromosome 12 is seen in roughly 50% of lipomas (225) and may involve other chromosomes such as 21 and 7 (225). Another one-third of lipomas show a ring chromosome (225) originally described by Heim et al. (226) as a possible rearrangement of chromosome 3; this may be a marker for lipogenic tumors. Rarely, chromosome 6 has shown an abnormality (229). Interestingly, subgroups of lipomas may show different cytogenic changes (227).

Likewise, clonal chromosomal changes are noted in lipoblastoma with the abnormality at 8q11-q13 (230).

SYNDROMES ASSOCIATED WITH FATTY LESIONS (INCLUDING LIPOMATOSIS)

The word *lipomatosis* may appropriately refer to two separate conditions: the presence of multiple subcutaneous lipomas and the infiltration of organs or sites such as the pelvis (231,232) by adipose tissue. The bilateral multiple symmetrical lipomatosis (MSL) syndrome [Madelung's disease (233–237)] is said to be frequently accompanied by a high intake of alcohol (180). However, there is increasing evidence that there is no association of MSL with alcohol abuse (238), that there may be a constitutional mitochondrial dysfunction (239), that mitochondrial DNA may be abnormal (240), that patients have plasma lipid anomalies (241), and that the cells involved may be distorted brown fat cells supportive of a neoplastic nature to MSL (242).

Lipomatosis may involve a single portion of the body, such as the face (243), the spinal epidural area (244–247), the mesentery (248), the mediastinum and abdomen (249), the mediastinum alone (250), the brain (251, 252), and the

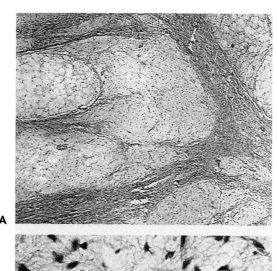
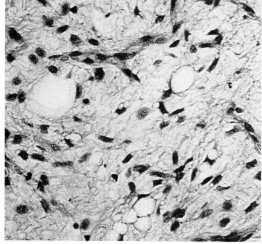

Figure 7.21 Lipoblastoma. **A.** At low power, a distinctly lobulated appearance can be observed. In some lobules, differentiation has started in the center. **B.** Within the myxoid lobules, small lipoblasts and spindle cells are found. The spindle cells are similar to those in developing fat (see Figure 7.2B).

kidney (253), as well as subcutaneous tissue (254). Syndromes relating to many of these are delineated in Table 7.2.

Lipomas, either as single or multiple tumors, may be part of a variety of syndromes (Table 7.2), some of which are autosomal dominant [Gardner's syndrome (255,256), MEA type 1 (257,258), Bannayan's syndrome (259), or tuberous sclerosis (260)]. Pathologists may find it interesting to note that lipomatous lesions may also occur in Cowden's disease (261), Beckwith's hemihypertrophy (180), and as fat within a pulmonary "hamartoma" in Carney's syndrome (262,263).

Furthermore, adipose tissue lesions may be found in association with other clinical syndromes as well (264,265,269). The listing in Table 7.2 is meant to be as complete as possible for informational purposes. The lipodystrophies (membranous and intestinal or mesenteric) were discussed earlier.

MIMICS OF FAT CELLS

Mature Fat Cells

Pathologists visualize adipocytes as clear cells or "white holes" on routine sections. Therefore, other cells or processes with this white hole appearance may be confused with them. Some lesions are fairly obvious—like the vacuolated lymphadenopathy of lymphangiogram effect.

TABLE 7.2	
SYNDROMES ASSOCIATED WITH FATTY PROCESSES	
Syndrome	**Description**
Diffuse mammary steatonecrosis	Fat necrosis with infarction and lipogranulomatous reaction; found in patients with large pendulous breasts (97)
Acute pancreatitis	Disseminated focal areas of fat necrosis in the subcutis; may also occur with pancreatic carcinoma (97)
Retractile mesenteritis	Fibrosis and retraction of mesentary with distortion of intestinal loops; the outcome of mesentary panniculitis/isolated mesenteric lipodystrophy (97,146)
Weber-Christian disease (avoid term)	Historic term for a clinical syndrome with chronic inflammation, fat necrosis, and scattered acute inflammatory cells in the subcutis— "nonsuppurative panniculitis" with recurrent lesions and febrile illness; this is now known to be due to a variety of separate diseases and is a term to be avoided (136,137)
Beradinelli's lipodystrophy	A minor part of a complex disorder including gigantism, hyperlipidemia, fatty cirrhosis of liver, muscular hypertrophy, and hyperpigmentation; familial (97)
Dercum's disease	Multiple lipomas with pain and tenderness (79,97,152,180)
Fröhlich's syndrome	Sexual infantilism with obesity and symmetrical or asymmetrical lipomas (a form of hypopituitarism)
Madelung's disease	Symmetrical lipomatosis; associated with alcohol intake (180,233–237)
Gardner's syndrome	Familial intestinal polyposis; subcutaneous lipomas may occur (255,256)
Multiple endocrine adenomotosis I (MEA 1)	Subcutaneous lipomas occur (257); a case of liposarcoma reported (258)
Schwachman syndrome	Lipomatous atrophy of the pancreas with prominent lipomatosis, maldigestion, neutropenia, and growth retardation (113)
Trite's syndrome	A combination of thymolipoma, thyrolipoma, and pharyngeal lipoma (205)
Carney's syndrome	Pulmonary hamartomas (which often contain fat), gastric smooth muscle tumors, and paraganglioma (262,263)
Tuberous sclerosis	Angiomyolipomas of kidney, other tumors, and hamartomas; occasionally diffuse lipomatosis (260)
Beckwith's hemihypertrophy	Congenital asymmetry, some with associated Wilms' tumor, occasional benign mesenchymoma with adipose tissue (182)
Familial multiple lipomas	Multiple subcutaneous lipomas (268)
Bannayan's syndrome	Autosomal dominant disorder with macrocephaly, lipomas, hemangiomas, and intracranial tumors (259)
Laurence-Moon-Biedl syndrome	Congenital optic nerve atrophy, polydactyly, mental defect, and occasional adrenal lipomas (267)
Carpal tunnel syndrome	Occasionally caused by tendon sheath lipoma (264)
Fishman's syndrome	Encephalocraniocutaneous lipomatosis (251,252)
Goldenhar-Gorlin syndrome	Oculoauriculo-vertebral dysplasia with CNS lipomas (266)
Cowden's disease	GI polyposis with orocutaneous hamartomas; angiolipomas have been observed (260)
Spinal epidural lipomatosis	Fatty infiltration of epidural space (244,247); occasionally secondary to steroids (247)
Membranous lipodystrophy	Abnormal subcutaneous and bony fat with bone cysts, pathologic fractures, and leukodystrophy of brain (104–106)

Dilated superficial lymphatics if closely clustered, as they may be in a nasal polyp, remind one of adipocytes at medium power. The submucosal cystic spaces of pneumatosis cystoides intestinalis (270) are composed of gas with a lining of inflammatory cells, histiocytes, and giant cells. Cysts very similar in histology are occasionally noted within ovarian teratomas; here, it is probably a reaction to internal rupture. Likewise, small gaseous cysts without any lining in the intestinal mucosa truly mimic lipocytes in an entity termed *pseudolipomatosis* (270). Similar clear but artifactual vacuoles in the skin have been called pseudolipomatosis cutis (271). Termed *villous edema* in placental texts, this artifact of chorionic villi gives them a pseudolipomatous appearance. Lipid-filled sinusoidal Ito cells in the liver simulate small adipocytes in vitamin A toxicity (272).

Lipoblasts

The response to the lipidlike substance silicone after the rupture of a breast implant can cause concern: when the response to the silicone is marked with sheets of histiocytes containing a single dominant vacuole, the cells resemble lipoblasts and the lesion may be mistaken for liposarcoma.

Tumors with vacuoles also cause the pathologist to consider a lipocytic origin. Metastases to the skin or subcutaneous region of signet-ring carcinoma or signet-ring melanoma (273) (Figure 7.22) may resemble lipoblasts, and other helpful features such as nesting or spindling are not always present. Lymphomas of both B- and T-cell origin exhibiting a vacuolated or signet-ring appearance have recently been described (274–278), may mimic liposarcoma (278), and should be in the differential diagnosis of cutaneous, nodal, or retroperitoneal tumors.

Mesenchymal tumors such as epithelioid smooth muscle lesions and fibrohistiocytic neoplasms (Figure 7.23) can

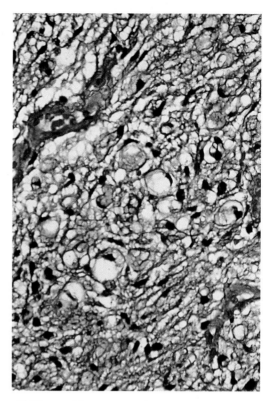

Figure 7.23 Lipoblast mimic. In fibrohistiocytic tumors like myxoid dermatofibrosarcoma and myxoid malignant fibrous histiocytoma, cells with a vacuolated appearance may be confused with lipoblasts; however, the vacuole contains a wispy bluish coloration due to the presence of proteoglycan matrix.

be vacuolated as well, due to an artifact and proteoglycan material, respectively. These two tumor groups, particularly in the form of gastrointestinal (GI) stromal malignancies (leiomyosarcomas) and myxoid malignant fibrous histiocytoma, probably account for the largest number of lesions mistaken for liposarcoma. In the GI tumors, the perinuclear vacuole coupled with a cellular epithelioid morphology can closely mimic the round cell or cellular myxoid liposarcoma. In myxoid fibrohistiocytic tumors of various types, vacuolated cells superficially simulate the lipoblast, but closer inspection reveals a delicate basophilic substance in the cytoplasm, apparently due to matrix production by the tumor cells (Figure 7.23). Unusual paragangliomas with vacuoles (279,280) may also be puzzling. Other lesions most often simulating lipocytes are those of endothelial origin because a true and often large vacuole is produced. Such cells may be identified in the histiocytoid hemangioma (281), in other epithelioid angiomas (282,283), in the spindle cell hemangioendothelioma (Figure 7.24) (284), in epithelioid hemangioendothelioma (285), and in some poorly differentiated angiosarcomas (Figure 7.25). In contrast to most large lipoblasts, the large vacuoles in endothelial tumors show a central septation. Chordomas, particularly with a sacral presentation, may be confused with a lipocytic tumor due to the prominent

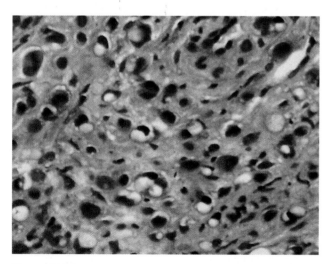

Figure 7.22 Adipocyte mimic. Subcutaneous metastases from either signet-ring carcinoma or melanoma (*seen here*) may rarely imitate a lipocytic tumor.

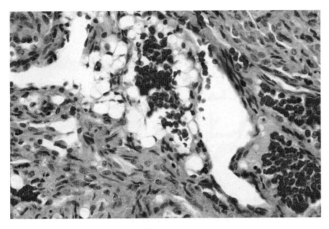

Figure 7.24 Adipocyte mimic. Large vacuolated cells can be found in the spindle cell hemangioma, but they are endothelial in nature and often line vascular spaces as seen here.

vacuolization of the physaliphorous cells. Mesotheliomas may also be vacuoled mimicking liposarcoma (286).

The best defense against a misdiagnosis of another tumor as a lipocytic one is strict adherence to the definition of a lipoblast: a cell, occasionally large but usually small, with a vacuole or vacuoles indenting the nucleus. The requirement for nuclear indentation assures an intracellular/cytoplasmic location for the vacuole and also excludes the semicircular nuclei around small vascular channels. Extracellular vacuoles are a common phenomenon, particularly in lesions with areas of mucoid matrix, and are often mistaken for a true intracellular finding; however, the nucleus is never affected since the substance is noncytoplasmic.

True liposarcomatous differentiation may be rarely identified in nonfatty malignancies such as medulloblastoma (287), cystosarcoma phyllodes (288), and even mesothelioma (289).

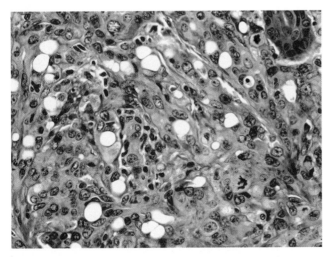

Figure 7.25 Adipocyte mimic. In some poorly differentiated angiosarcomas, vacuolated endothelial cells also resemble fat cells; however, note the presence of occasional septated vacuoles (*center*), a feature typical for proliferating endothelial cells and unlike adipocytes.

REFERENCES

1. Poissonnet CM, Burdi AR, Bookstein FL. Growth and development of human adipose tissue during early gestation. *Early Hum Dev* 1983;8:1–11.
2. Poissonnet CM, Burdi AR, Garn JM. The chronology of adipose tissue appearance and distribution in the human fetus. *Early Hum Dev* 1984;10:1–11.
3. Robinson DS. In: Florkin M, Stotz EH, eds. *Comparative Biochemistry.* Vol. 18 Amsterdam: Elsevier; 1970:51–116.
4. Hausman GJ, Champion DR, Martin RJ. Search for the adipocyte precursor cell and factors that promote its differentiation. *J Lipid Res* 1980;21:657–670.
5. Napolitano L. The differentiation of white adipose cells: an electron microscope study. *J Cell Biol* 1963;18:663–679.
6. Aman P, Ron D, Mandahl N, et al. Rearrangement of the transcription factor gene CHOP in myxoid liposarcomas with t(12;16)(q13;p11). *Genes Chromosomes Cancer* 1992;5:278–285.
7. Crozat A, Aman P, Mandahl F, Ron D. Fusion of CHOP to a novel RNA-binding protein in human myxoid liposarcoma. *Nature* 1993;363:640–644.
8. Rabitts TH, Forster A, Larson R, Nathan P. Fusion of the dominant negative transcription regulator CHOP with a novel gene FUS by translocation t(12;16) in malignant liposarcoma. *Nature Genet* 1993;4:175–180.
9. Ladanyi M. The emerging molecular genetics of sarcoma translocations. *Diagn Mol Pathol* 1995;4:162–173.
10. LeBrun DP, Warnke RA, Cleary ML. Expression of bcl-2 in fetal tissues suggests a role in morphogenesis. *Am J Pathol* 1993;142:743–753.
11. Martin RJ, Ramsay T, Hausman GJ. Adipocyte development. *Pediatr Ann* 1984;13:448–453.
12. Poissonnet CM, LaVelle M, Burdi AR. Growth and development of adipose tissue. *J Pediatr* 1988;113(pt 1):1–9.
13. Hirsch J, Batchelor B. Adipose tissue cellularity in human obesity. *Clin Endocrinol Metab* 1976 5:299–311.
14. Faust IM. Factors which affect adipocyte formation in the rat. In: Bjorntorp P, Cairella M, Howard AN, eds. *Recent Advances in Obesity Research III. Proceedings of the 3rd International Congress on Obesity.* London: John Libbey; 1981:52–57.
15. Bjorntorp P. Adipocyte precursor cells. In: Bjorntorp P, Cairella M, Howard AN, eds. *Recent Advances in Obesity Research III. Proceedings of the 3rd International Congress on Obesity.* London: John Libbey;1981:58–69.
16. Sjostrom L, William-Olsson T. Prospective studies on adipose tissue development in man. *Int J Obes* 1981;5:597–604.
17. Kolata G. Why do people get fat? *Science* 1985;227:1327–1328.
18. Hirsch J, Fried SK, Edens NK, Leibel RL. The fat cell. *Med Clin North Am* 1989;73:83–96.
19. Cinti S, Frederich RC, Zingaretti C, De Matteis R, Flier JS, Lowell BB. Immunohistochemical localization of leptin and uncoupling protein in white and brown adipose tissue. *Endocrinology* 1997;138:797–804.
20. Hukshorn CJ, Saris WH. Leptin and energy expenditure. *Curr Opin Clin Nutr Metab Care* 2004;7:629–633.
21. Jequier E. Leptin signaling, adiposity, and energy balance. *Ann N Y Acad Sci* 2002;967:379–388.
22. Fruhbeck G, Gomez-Ambrosi J, Muruzabal FJ, Burrell MA. The adipocyte: a model for integration of endocrine and metabolic signaling in energy metabolism regulation. *Am J Physiol Endocrinol Metab* 2001;280:E827–E847.
23. Wisse BE. The inflammatory syndrome: the role of adipose tissue cytokines in metabolic disorders linked to obesity. *J Am Soc Nephrol* 2004;15:2792–2800.
24. Choy LN, Rosen BS, Spiegelman BM. Adipsin and an endogenous pathway of complement from adipose cells. *J Biol Chem* 1992;267:12736–12741.
25. Birgel M, Gottschling-Zeller H, Rohrig K, Hauner H. Role of cytokines in the regulation of plasminogen activator inhibitor-1 expression and secretion in newly differentiated subcutaneous human adipocytes. *Arterioscler Thromb Vasc Biol* 2000;20:1682–1687.

26. Rebuffe-Scrive M, Enk L, Crona N, et al. Fat cell metabolism in different regions in women. Effect of menstrual cycle, pregnancy, and lactation. *J Clin Invest* 1985;75:1973–1976.

27. Fried SK, Kral JB. Sex differences in regional distribution of fat cell size and lipoprotein lipase activity in morbidly obese patients. *Int J Obes* 1987;11:129–140.

28. Bjorntorp P. The regulation of adipose tissue distribution in humans. *Int J Obes Relat Metab Disord* 1996;20:291–302.

29. Kopelman PG. Effects of obesity on fat topography: metabolic and endocrine determinants. In: Kopelman PG, Stock MJ eds. *Clinical Obesity.* Oxford, UK: Blackwell Science; 1998:158–175.

30. Bjorntorp P. Fat cell distribution and metabolism. *Ann NY Acad Sci* 1987;499:66–72.

31. Hutley L, Shurety W, Newell F, et al. Fibroblast growth factor 1: a key regulator of human adipogenesis. *Diabetes* 2004;53:3097–3106.

32. Hube F, Hauner H. The role of TNF-a in human adipose tissue: prevention of weight gain at the expense of insulin resistance? *Horm Metab Res* 1999;31:626–631.

33. Strassmann G, Fong M, Kenney JS, Jacob CO. Evidence for the involvement of interleukin 6 in experimental cancer cachexia. *J Clin Invest* 1992;89:1681–1684.

34. Stephens JM, Pekala PH. Transcriptional repression of GLUT4 and C/EBP genes in 3T3-L1 adipocytes by tumor necrosis factor-alpha. *J Biol Chem* 1991;266:21839–21845.

35. Hellman B, Hellerstrom C. Cell renewal in the white and brown fat of the rat. *Acta Pathol Microbiol Scand* 1961;51:347–353.

36. Hollenberg CH, Vost A. Regulation of DNA synthesis in fat cells and stromal elements from rat adipose tissue. *J Clin Invest* 1969;47:2485–2498.

37. Napolitano L. The fine structure of adipose tissues. In: Reynold AE, Cahill GF, eds. *Handbook of Physiology. Section 5: Adipose Tissue.* Washington, DC: American Physical Society; 1965:109–123.

38. Nnodim JO. Development of adipose tissue. *Anat Rec* 1987; 219:331–337.

39. Merklin RJ. Growth and distribution of human fetal brown fat. *Anat Rec* 1974;178: 637–646.

40. Heaton JM. The distribution of brown adipose tissue in the human. *J Anat* 1972;112(pt 1):35–39.

41. Girardier L. Brown fat: an energy dissipating tissue. In: Girardier L, Stock MJ, eds. *Mammalian Thermogenesis.* London: Chapman and Hall, 1983:50–98.

42. Rothwell NJ, Stock MJ. Brown adipose tissue. In: Baker PF, ed. *Recent Advances in Physiology.* Volume 10. Edinburgh: Churchill Livingstone; 1984:349–384.

43. Rothwell NJ, Stock MJ. Whither brown fat? *Biosci Rep* 1986;6: 3–18.

44. Bouillaud F, Combes-George M, Ricquier D. Mitochondria of adult human brown adipose tissue contain a 32 000-Mr uncoupling protein. *Biosci Rep* 1983;3:775–780.

45. Cunningham S, Leslie P, Hopwood D, et al. The characterization and energetic potential of brown adipose tissue in man. *Clin Sci (Lond)* 1985;69:343–348.

46. Rothwell NJ, Stock MJ. A role for brown adipose tissue in diet-induced thermogenesis. *Nature* 1979;281:31–35.

47. Himms-Hagen J. Brown adipose tissue thermogenesis: interdisciplinary studies. *FASEB J* 1990;4:2890–2898.

48. Blaza S. Brown adipose tissue in man: a review. *J R Soc Med* 1983;76:213–216.

49. Santos GC, Araujo MR, Silveira TC, Soares FA. Accumulation of brown adipose tissue and nutritional status: a prospective study of 366 consecutive autopsies. *Arch Pathol Lab Med* 1992;116: 1152–1154.

50. Cottle WH. The innervation of brown adipose tissue. In: Lindberg O, ed. *Brown Adipose Tissue.* New York: Elsevier; 1970:155–178.

51. Mory G, Bouillaud F, Combes-George M, Ricquier D. Noradrenaline controls the concentration of the uncoupling protein in brown adipose tissue. *FEBS Lett* 1984;166:393–396.

52. Ricquier D, Nechad M, Mory G. Ultrastructural and biochemical characterization of human brown adipose tissue in pheochromocytoma. *J Clin Endocrinol Metab* 1982;54:803–807.

53. Afzelius BA. Brown adipose tissue: its gross anatomy, histology, and cytology. In: Lindberg O, ed. *Brown Adipose Tissue.* New York: Elsevier; 1970:1–31.

54. Pearse AG. *Histochemistry: Theoretical and Applied.* Vol 2. 3rd ed. Baltimore: Williams & Wilkins; 1972.

55. Hausman GJ. Anatomical and enzyme histochemical differentiation of adipose tissue. *Int J Obes* 1985;9(suppl 1):1–6.

56. Lithell J, Boberg J, Hellsing K, Lundqvist G, Vessby B. Lipoprotein-lipase activity in human skeletal muscle and adipose tissue in the fasting and the fed states. *Atherosclerosis* 1978;30:89–94.

57. Lithell H, Hellsing K, Lundqvist G, Malmberg P. Lipoprotein-lipase activity of human skeletal-muscle and adipose tissue after intensive physical exercise. *Acta Physiol Scand* 1979;105:312–315.

58. Fielding CJ, Havel RJ. Lipoprotein lipase. *Arch Pathol Lab Med* 1977;101:225–229.

59. Zugibe FT. *Diagnostic Histochemistry.* St. Louis: CV Mosby; 1970.

60. Pearse AG. *Histochemistry: Theoretical and Applied.* Vol. 2. 3rd ed. Baltimore: Williams & Wilkins; 1972.

61. Pearse AG. *Histochemistry: Theoretical and Applied.* Vol. 2. 3rd ed. Baltimore: Williams & Wilkins; 1972.

62. Sheehan DC, Hrapchak BB. *Theory and Practice of Histotechnology.* St. Louis: CV Mosby; 1973.

63. Filipe MI, Lake BD, eds. *Histochemistry in Pathology.* Edinburgh: Churchill Livingstone; 1983.

64. Spicer SS, ed. *Histochemistry in Pathologic Diagnosis.* New York: Marcel Dekker; 1987.

65. Hausman GJ. Techniques for studying adipocytes. *Stain Technol* 1981;56:149–154.

66. Popper H, Knipping G. A histochemical and biochemical study of a liposarcoma with several aspects on the development of fat synthesis. *Pathol Res Pract* 1981;171:373–380.

67. Waugh DA, Small DM. Methods in laboratory investigation: identification and detection of in situ cellular and regional differences of lipid composition and class in lipid-rich tissue using hot stage polarizing light microscopy. *Lab Invest* 1984;51:702–714.

68. Stedman TL. *Stedman's Medical Dictionary.* 21st ed. Baltimore: Williams & Wilkins; 1966.

69. Robbins SL, Cotran RS, Kumar V. *The Pathologic Basis of Disease.* 3rd ed. Philadelphia: WB Saunders; 1984.

70. Rubin E, Farber JL. eds. *Pathology.* Philadelphia: Lippincott; 1988.

71. Heptinstall RH. *Pathology of the Kidney.* 2nd ed. Boston: Little, Brown & Co; 1974.

72. Jasnosz KM, Pickeral JJ, Graner S. Fat deposits in the placenta following maternal total parenteral nutrition with intravenous lipid emulsion. *Arch Pathol Lab Med* 1995;119:555–557.

73. Bennington JL. Proceedings: Cancer of the kidney: etiology, epidemiology, and pathology. *Cancer* 1973;32:1017–1029.

74. Elizalde N, Korman S. Cytochemical studies of glycogen, neutral mucopolysaccharides and fat in malignant tissues. *Cancer* 1968; 21:1061–1068.

75. Andrion A, Mazzucco G, Gugliotta P, Monga G. Benign clear cell (sugar) tumor of the lung: a light microscopic, histochemical, and ultrastructural study with a review of the literature. *Cancer* 1985;56:2657–2663.

76. Bertoni F, Unni KK, McLeod RA, Sim FH. Xanthoma of bone. *Am J Clin Pathol* 1988;90:377–384.

77. Bennett JH, Shousha S, Puddle B, Athanasou NA. Immunohistochemical identification of tumours of adipocytic differentiation using an antibody to aP2 protein. *J Clin Pathol* 1995;48:950–954.

78. Michetti F, Dell'Anna E, Tiberio G, Cocchia D. Immunochemical and immunocytochemical study of S-100 protein in rat adipocytes. *Brain Res* 1983;262:352–356.

79. Haimoto H, Kato K, Suzuki F, Nagura H. The ultrastructural changes of S-100 protein localization during lipolysis in adipocytes. An immunoelectron-microscopic study. *Am J Pathol* 1985;121:185–191.

80. Takahashi K, Isobe T, Ohtsuki Y, Akagi T, Sonobe H, Okuyama T. Immunochemical study of the distribution of alpha and beta subunits of S-100 protein in human neoplasms and normal tissues. *Virchows Arch Cell Pathol* 1984;45:385–396.

81. Nakazato Y, Ishida Y, Takahashi K, Suzuki K. Immunohistochemical distribution of S-100 protein and glial fibrillary acidic protein in normal and neoplastic salivary glands. *Virchows Arch A Pathol Anat Histopathol* 1985;405:299–310.

82. Kahn HJ, Marks A, Thom H, Baumal R. Role of antibody to S100 protein in diagnostic pathology. *Am J Clin Pathol* 1983;79: 341–347.

83. Nakajima T, Watanabe S, Sato Y, Kameya T, Hirota T, Shimosato Y. An immunoperoxidase study of S-100 protein distribution in normal and neoplastic tissues. *Am J Surg Pathol* 1982;6:715–727.

84. Cocchia D, Lauriola L, Stolfi V, Tallini G, Michetti F. S-100 antigen labels neoplastic cells in liposarcoma and cartilaginous tumours. *Virchows Arch A Pathol Anat Histopathol* 1983;402:139–145.

85. Weiss SW, Langloss JM, Enzinger FM. Value of S-100 protein in the diagnosis of soft tissue tumors with particular reference to benign and malignant Schwann cell tumors. *Lab Invest* 1983;49:299–308.

86. Hashimoto H, Daimaru Y, Enjoji M. S-100 protein distribution in liposarcoma. An immunoperoxidase study with special reference to the distinction of liposarcoma from myxoid malignant fibrous histiocytoma. *Virchows Arch A Pathol Anat Histopathol* 1984;405:1–10.

87. Haimoto H, Takahashi Y, Koshikawa T, Nagura H, Kato K. Immunohistochemical localization of gamma-enolase in normal human tissues other than nervous and neuroendocrine tissues. *Lab Invest* 1985;52:257–263.

88. Stunkard AJ, Wadden TA, eds. *Obesity: Theory and Therapy.* 2nd ed. New York: Raven Press; 1993.

89. Lowell BB, Susulic VS, Hamann A, et al. Development of obesity in transgenic mice after genetic ablation of brown adipose tissue. *Nature* 1993;366:740–742.

90. Zhang Y, Proenca R, Maffei M, Barone M, Leopold L, Friedman JM. Positional cloning of the mouse obese gene and its human homologue. *Nature* 1994;372:425–432.

91. Green ED, Maffei M, Braden VV, et al. The human obese (OB) gene: RNA expression pattern and mapping on the physical, cytogenetic, and genetic maps of chromosome 7. *Genome Res* 1995;5:5–12.

92. Pelleymounter MA, Cullen MJ, Baker MB, et al. Effects of the obese gene product on body weight regulation in ob/ob mice. *Science* 1995;269:540–543.

93. Halaas JL, Gajiwala KS, Maffei M, et al. Weight-reducing effects of the plasma protein encoded by the obese gene. *Science* 1995;269:543–546.

94. Campfield LA, Smith FJ, Guisez Y, Devos R, Burn P. Recombinant mouse OB protein: evidence for a peripheral signal linking adiposity and central neural networks. *Science* 1995;269:546–549.

95. Chua SC Jr, Chung WK, Wu-Peng XS, et al. Phenotypes of mouse diabetes and rat fatty due to mutations in the OB (leptin) receptor. *Science* 1996;271:994–996.

96. Raife T, Landas SK. Intracellular crystalline material in visceral adipose tissue: a common autopsy finding [abstract]. *Am J Clin Pathol* 1990;94:511.

97. Tedeschi CG. Pathologic anatomy of adipose tissue. In: Renold AE, Cahill GF, eds. *Handbook of Physiology. Section 5: Adipose Tissue.* Baltimore: Waverly Press; 1965.

98. Manthorpe R, Helin G, Kofod B, Lorenzen I. Effect of glucocorticoid on connective tissue of aorta and skin in rabbits. Biochemical studies on collagen, glycosaminoglycans, DNA and RNA. *Acta Endocrinol (Copenh)* 1974;77:310–324.

99. Napolitano LM. Observations on the fine structure of adipose cells. *Ann NY Acad Sci* 1965;131:34–42.

100. Seaman JP, Kjeldsberg CR, Linker A. Gelatinous transformation of the bone marrow. *Hum Pathol* 1978;9:685–692.

101. Wittels B. Bone marrow biopsy changes following chemotherapy for acute leukemia. *Am J Surg Pathol* 1980;4:135–142.

102. Pierard GE, Nizet JL, Pierard-Franchimont C. Cellulite: from standing fat herniation to hypodermal stretch marks. *Am J Dermatopath* 2000;22:34–37.

103. Gruskin P, Canberry JN. Pathology of acoustic neuromas. In: House WF, Leutje CM, eds. *Acoustic Tumors.* Baltimore: University Park Press; 1979:85–148.

104. Wood C. Membranous lipodystrophy of bone. *Arch Pathol Lab Med* 1978;102:22–27.

105. Bird TD, Koerker RM, Leaird BJ, Vlcek BW, Thorning DR. Lipomembranous polycystic osteodysplasia (brain, bone and fat disease): a genetic cause of presenile dementia. *Neurology* 1983;33:81–86.

106. Kitajima I, Suganuma T, Murata F, Nagamatsu K. Ultrastructural demonstration of Maclura pomifera agglutinin binding sites in the membranocystic lesions of membranous lipodystrophy (Nasu–Hakola disease). *Virchows Arch A Pathol Anat Histopathol* 1988;413:475–483.

107. Chun SI, Chung KY. Membranous lipodystrophy: secondary type. *J Am Acad Dermatol* 1994;31:601–605.

108. Coyne JD, Parkinson D, Baildam AD. Membranous fat necrosis of the breast. *Histopathology* 1996;28:61–64.

109. Adams RD. *Diseases of Muscle: A Study in Pathology.* 3rd ed. New York: Harper & Row; 1975.

110. Rosai J, Levine GD. Tumors of the thymus. In: of Atlas of Tumor Pathology. 2nd series, fascicle 13. Washington, DC: Armed Forces Institute of Pathology; 1976.

111. Rywlin AM. *Histopathology of the Bone Marrow.* Boston: Little, Brown & Co; 1976:19.

112. Ackerman LV, Rosai J. *Surgical Pathology.* 5th ed. St Louis: CV-Mosby; 1974:649.

113. Seifert G. Lipomatous atrophy and other forms. In: Kloppel G, Heitz PU, eds. *Pancreatic Pathology.* New York: Churchill Livingstone; 1984.

114. Heggtveit HA, Fenoglio JJ, McAllister HA. Lipomatous hypertrophy of the interatrial septum: An assessment of 41 cases. *Lab Invest* 1976;34:318.

115. McAllister HA, Fenoglio JJ. *Tumors of the Cardiovascular System.* Washington, DC: Armed Forces Institute of Pathology; 1978:44–46.

116. Rokey R, Mulvagh SL, Cheirif J, Mattox KL, Johnston DL. Lipomatous encasement and compression of the heart: antemortem diagnosis by cardiac nuclear magnetic resonance imaging and catheterization. *Am Heart J* 1989;117 952–953.

117. Waller BF, ed. *Pathology of the Heart and Great Vessels.* New York: Churchill Livingstone; 1988.

118. Symmers WSC. The lymphoreticular system. In: Symmers WSC, ed. *Systemic Pathology.* Vol. 2. Edinburgh: Churchill Livingstone, 1978:647–651.

119. Smith T. Fatty replacement of lymph nodes mimicking lymphoma relapse. *Cancer* 1986; 58:2686–2688.

120. Takayasu K, Shima Y, Muramatsu Y, et al. Imaging characteristics of large lipoma and angiomyolipoma of the liver. Case reports. *Cancer* 1987;59:916–921.

121. Pounder DJ. Hepatic pseudolipoma. *Pathology* 1983;15:83–84.

122. Shafer WG, Hine MK, Levy BM. Development disterbances of oral and paraoral structures. *A Textbook of Oral Pathology.* 4th ed. Philadelphia: WB Saunders; 1983:24–25.

123. Ramadori G. The stellate cell (Ito-cell, fat-storing cell, lipocyte, perisinusoidal cell) of the liver. New insights into pathophysiology of an intriguing cell. *Virchows Arch B Cell Pathol Incl Mol Pathol* 1991;61:147–158.

124. Cha I, Bass N, Ferrell LD. Lipopeliosis: an immunohistochemical and clinicopathologic study of five cases. *Am J Surg Pathol* 1994;18:789–795.

125. Stroebel P, Mayer F, Zerban H, Bannasch P. Spongiotic pericytoma: a benign neoplasm deriving from the perisinusoidal (Ito) cells in rat liver. *Am J Pathol* 1995;146:903–913.

126. Orfila C, Giraud P, Modesto A, Suc JM. Abdominal fat tissue aspirate in human amyloidosis: light, electron, and immunofluorescence microscopic studies. *Hum Pathol* 1986;17:366–369.

127. Duston MA, Skinner M, Shirahama T, Cohen AS. Diagnosis of amyloidosis by abdominal fat aspiration: analysis of four years' experience. *Am J Med* 1987;82:412–414.

128. Gertz MA, Li CY, Shirahama T, Kyle RA. Utility of subcutaneous fat aspiration for the diagnosis of systemic amyloidosis (immunoglobulin light chain). *Arch Intern Med* 1988;48:929–933.

129. Keen CE, Buk SJ, Brady K, Levison DA. Fat necrosis presenting as obscure abdominal mass: birefringent saponified fatty acid crystalloids as a clue to diagnosis. *J Clin Pathol* 1994;47:1028–1031.

130. Poppiti RJ Jr, Margulies M, Cabello B, Rywlin AM. Membranous fat necrosis. *Am J Surg Pathol* 1986;10:62–69.

131. Bennett RG, Petrozzi JW. Nodular subcutaneous fat necrosis: a manifestation of silent pancreatitis. *Arch Dermatol* 1975;111:896–898.

132. Hughes PS, Apisarnthanarax P, Mullins F. Subcutaneous fat necrosis associated with pancreatic disease. *Arch Dermatol* 1975;111:506–510.

133. Fischer AH, Morris DJ. Pathogenesis of calciphylaxis: study of three cases and literature review. *Hum Pathol* 1995;26:1055–1064.

134. Wilmer WA, Magro CM. Calciphylaxis: emerging concepts in prevention, diagnosis, and treatment. *Semin Dial* 2002;15:172–86.
135. Mirza I, Chaubay D, Gunderia H, Shih W, El-Fanek H. An unusual presentation of calciphylaxis due to primary hyperparathyroidism. *Arch Pathol Lab Med* 2001;125:1351–1353.
136. Macdonald A, Feiwel M. A review of the concept of Weber–Christian panniculitis with a report of five cases. *Br J Dermatol* 1968;80:355–361.
137. Sweatt HL, Hardman WJ, Solomon AR. Non-neoplastic diseases of the skin. In: Mills SE, ed. *Sternberg's Diagnostic Surgical Pathology*. 4th ed. New York: Lippincott Williams Wilkins; 2004:40–43.
138. Winkelmann RK, Frigas E. Eosinophilic panniculitis: a clinicopathologic study. *J Cutan Pathol* 1986;13:1–12.
139. Blaustein A, Moreno A, Noguera J, de Moragas JM. Septal granulomatous panniculitis in Sweet's syndrome: report of two cases. *Arch Dermatol* 1985;121:785–788.
140. Suster S, Cartagena N, Cabello-Inchausti B, Robinson MJ. Histiocytic lymphophagocytic panniculitis: an unusual extranodal presentation of sinus histiocytosis with massive lymphadenopathy (Rosai–Dorfman disease). *Arch Dermatol* 1988;124:1246–1249.
141. Alegre VA, Winkelmann RK, Aliaga A. Lipomembranous changes in chronic panniculitis. *J Am Acad Dermatol* 1988;19(pt 1):39–46.
142. Vincent F, Prokopetz R, Miller RA. Plasma cell panniculitis: a unique clinical and pathologic presentation of linear scleroderma. *J Am Acad Dermatol* 1989;21(pt 2):357–360.
143. Izumi AK, Takiguchi P. Lupus erythematosus panniculitis. *Arch Dermatol* 1983;119:61–64.
144. Silverman RA, Newman AJ, LeVine MJ, Kaplan B. Poststeroid panniculitis: a case report. *Pediatr Dermatol* 1988;5:92–93.
145. Sleisenger MH, Fordtran JS, eds. *Gastrointestinal Disease: Pathophysiology, Diagnosis, Management*. 3rd ed. Philadelphia: WB Saunders; 1983.
146. Kelly JK, Hwang WS. Idiopathic retractile (sclerosing) mesenteritis and its differential diagnosis. *Am J Surg Pathol* 1989;13:513–521.
147. Scully RE, Galdabini JJ, McNeely BU. Lipodystrophy of mesentery (Case 30-1976). *N Engl J Med* 1976;295:214–218.
148. Eble JN, Rosenberg AE, Young RH. Retroperitoneal xanthogranulomatosis in a patient with Erdheim–Chester disease. *Am J Surg Pathol* 1994;18:843–848.
149. Seemayer TA, Knaack J, Wang NS, Ahmed MN. On the ultrastructure of hibernoma. *Cancer* 1975;36:1785–1793.
150. Dardick I. Hibernoma: a possible model of brown fat histogenesis. *Hum Pathol* 1978;9:321–329.
151. Gaffney EF, Hargreaves HK, Semple E, Vellios F. Hibernoma: distinctive light and electron microscopic features and relationship to brown adipose tissue. *Hum Pathol* 1983;14:677–687.
152. Enzinger FM, Weiss SW. *Soft Tissue Tumors*. 2nd ed. St. Louis: CV Mosby; 1988.
153. Rigor VU, Goldstone SE, Jones J, Bernstein R, Gold MS, Weiner S. Hibernoma. A case report and discussion of a rare tumor. *Cancer* 1986;57:2207–2211.
154. Allegra SR, Gmuer C, O'Leary GP Jr. Endocrine activity in a large hibernoma. *Hum Pathol* 1983;14:1044–1052.
155. Enterline HT, Lowry LD, Richman AV. Does malignant hibernoma exist? *Am J Surg Pathol* 1979;3:265–271.
156. Teplitz C, Farrugia R, Glicksman AS. Malignant hibernoma does exist. *Lab Invest* 1980;42:59A.
157. Talerman A. Germ cell tumors of the ovary. In: Kurman R, ed. *Blaustein's Pathology of the Female Genital Tract*. 3rd ed. New York: Springer-Verlag; 1987:689.
158. Dail DH. Uncommon tumors. In: Dale DH, Hammar SP, eds. *Pulmonary Pathology*. New York: Springer-Verlag; 1988:847–972.
159. Ali MY, Wong PK. Intrapulmonary teratoma. *Thorax* 1964;19:228–235.
160. Lee RG. Esophagus. In: Sternberg SS, ed. *Diagnostic Surgical Pathology*. New York: Raven Press; 1989:928.
161. Toker C, Tang CK, Whitely JF, Berkheiser SW, Rachman R. Benign spindle cell breast tumor. *Cancer* 1981;48:1615–1622.
162. Wargotz ES, Weiss SW, Norris HJ. Myofibroblastoma of the breast: sixteen cases of a distinctive benign mesenchymal tumor. *Am J Surg Pathol* 1987;11:493–502.
163. Nogales FF, Pavcovich M, Medina MT, Palomino M. Fatty change in the endometrium. *Histopathology* 1992;20:362–363.
164. Nogita T, Wong TY, Hidano A, Mihm MC Jr, Kawashima M. Pedunculated lipofibroma: a clinicopathologic study of thirty-two cases supporting a simplified nomenclature. *J Am Acad Dermatol* 1994;31(pt 1):235–240.
165. Tomashefski JF Jr. Benign endobronchial mesenchymal tumors: their relationship to parenchymal pulmonary hamartomas. *Am J Surg Pathol* 1982;6:531–540.
166. Palvio D, Egeblad K, Paulsen SM. Atypical lipomatous hamartoma of the lung. *Virchows Arch A Pathol Anat Histopathol* 1985;405:253–261.
167. Benjamin SP, Mercer RD, Hawk WA. Myofibroblastic contraction in spontaneous regression of multiple congenital mesenchymal hamartomas. *Cancer* 1977;40:2343–2352.
168. Enzinger FM. Fibrous hamartoma of infancy. *Cancer* 1965;18:241–248.
169. Reye RD. A consideration of certain subdermal fibromatous tumours of infancy. *J Pathol Bacteriol* 1956;72:149–154.
170. Fletcher CD, Powell G, van Noorden S, McKee PH. Fibrous hamartoma of infancy: a histochemical and immunohistochemical study. *Histopathology* 1988;12:65–74.
171. Silverman TA, Enzinger FM. Fibrolipomatous hamartoma of nerve: a clinocopatholigic analysis of 26 cases. *Am J Surg Pathol* 1985;9:7–14.
172. Silverman TA, Enzinger FM. Fibrolipomatous hamartoma of nerve: a clinicopathologic analysis of 26 cases. *Am J Surg Pathol* 1985;9:7–14.
173. Aymard B, Bowman-Ferrand F, Vernhes L, Floquet A, Floquet J, Morel O, Merle M, Delagoutte JP. Hamartome lipofibromateux des nerfs périphériques. Etude anatomo-clinique de 5 cas dont 2 avec étude ultrastructurale. *Ann Pathol* 1987;7:320–324.
174. Price EB Jr, Mostofi FK. Symptomatic angiomyolipoma of the kidney. *Cancer* 1965;18:761–774.
175. McCullough DL, Scott R, Seybold HM. Renal angiomyolipoma (hamartoma): review of the literature and report on 7 cases. *J Urol* 1971;105:32–44.
176. Dao AH, Netsky NG. Human tails and pseudotails. *Hum Pathol* 1984;15:449–453.
177. Farshid G, Weiss SW. Massive localized lymphedema in the morbidly obese: a histologically distinct reactive lesion simulating liposarcoma. *Am J Surg Pathol* 1998;22:1277–1283.
178. Wu D, Gibbs J, Corral D, Intengan M, Brooks JJ. Massive localized lymphedema: additional locations and association with hypothyroidism. *Hum Pathol* 2000:31:1162–1168.
179. LeBer MS, Stout AP. Benign mesenchymomas in children. *Cancer* 1962;15:595–605.
180. Allen P. *Tumors and Proliferations of Adipose Tissue*. New York; Masson, 1981.
181. Kasantikul V, Brown WJ, Netsky MG. Mesenchymal differentiation in trigeminal neurilemmoma. *Cancer* 1982;50:1568–1571.
182. Majeski JA, Paxton ES, Wirman JA, Schrieber JT. A thoracic benign mesenchymoma in association with hemihypertrophy. *Am J Clin Pathol* 1981;76:827–832.
183. Rosai J. Case presentation at the European Society of Pathology meeting in Porto, Portugal; September 1989.
184. Brecher ME, Gill WB, Straus FH. Angiomyolipoma with regional lymph node involvement and long-term follow-up study. *Hum Pathol* 1986;17:962–963.
185. Meggitt BF, Wilson JN. The battered buttock syndrome—fat fractures: a report on a group of traumatic lipomata. *Br J Surg* 1972;59:165–169.
186. Wilson JE. Lipomas and potassium intake. *Ann Intern Med* 1989;110:750–751.
187. Solvonuk PF, Taylor GP, Hancock R, Wood WS, Frohlich J. Correlation of morphologic and biochemical observations in human lipomas. *Lab Invest* 1984;51:469–474.
188. Azumi N, Curtis J, Kempson R, Hendrickson M. Atypical and malignant neoplasms showing lipomatous differentiation: a study of 111 cases. *Am J Surg Pathol* 1987;11:161–183.
189. Fu YS, Parker FG, Kaye GI, Lattes R. Ultrastructure of benign and malignant adipose tissue tumors. *Pathol Annu* 1980;15(pt 1):67–69.

190. Kindblom L, Angervall L, Stener B, Wickbom I. Intermuscular and intramuscular lipomas and hibernomas. A clinical, roentgenologic, histologic and prognostic study of 46 cases. *Cancer* 1974;33:754–762.

191. Evans HL, Soule EH, Winkelmann RK. Atypical lipoma, atypical intramuscular lipoma, and well differentiated retroperitoneal liposarcoma: a reappraisal of 30 cases. *Cancer* 1979;43:574–584.

192. Marsh WL Jr, Lucas JG, Olsen J. Chondrolipoma of the breast. *Arch Pathol Lab Med* 1989;113:369–371.

193. Lim YC. Mediastinal chondrolipoma. *Am J Surg Pathol* 1980;4:407–409.

194. Allen P. Letter to the case. *Pathol Res Pract* 1989;184:444–445.

195. Hayden JW, Abellera RM. Tenosynovial lipochondromatosis of the flexor hallucis, common toe flexor, and posterior tibial tendons. *Clin Orthop Relat Res* 1989;245:220–222.

196. Katzer B. Histopathology of rare chondroosteoblastic metaplasia in benign lipomas. *Pathol Res Pract* 1989;184:437–445.

197. Honore LH. Uterine fibrolipoleiomyoma: report of a case with discussion of histogenesis. *Am J Obstet Gynecol* 1978;132:635–636.

198. Brescia RJ, Tazelaar HD, Hobbs J, Miller AW. Intravascular lipoleiomyomatosis: a report of two cases. *Hum Pathol* 1989;20:252–256.

199. Hunt SJ, Santa Cruz DJ, Barr RJ. Cellular angiolipoma. *Am J Surg Pathol* 1990;14:75–81.

200. DeRienzo D, Truong L. Thyroid neoplasms containing mature fat: a report of two cases and review of the literature. *Mod Pathol* 1989;2:506–510.

201. Perosio P, Brooks JJ, LiVolsi VA. Orbital brown tumor as the initial manifestation of a parathyroid lipoadenoma. *Surg Pathol* 1988;1:77–82.

202. Gnepp DR, Ogorzalek JM, Heffess CA. Fat-containing lesions of the thyroid gland. *Am J Surg Pathol* 1989;13:605–612.

203. Bruno J, Ciancia EM, Pingitore R. Thyroid papillary adenocarcinoma; lipomatous-type. *Virchows Arch A Pathol Anat Histopathol* 1989;414:371–373.

204. Otto HF, Loning T, Lachenmayer L, Janzen RW, Gurtler KF, Fischer K. Thymolipoma in association with myasthenia gravis. *Cancer* 1982;50:1623–1628.

205. Trites AE. Thyrolipoma, thymolipoma and pharyngeal lipoma: a syndrome. *Can Med Assoc J* 1966;95:1254–1259.

206. Enzinger FM, Harvey DA. Spindle cell lipoma. *Cancer* 1975;36:1852–1859.

207. Angervall L, Dahl I, Kindblom LG, Save-Soderbergh J. Spindle cell lipoma. *Acta Pathol Microbiol Scand A* 1976;84:477–487.

208. Fletcher CD, Martin-Bates E. Spindle cell lipoma: a clinicopathological study with some original observations. *Histopathology* 1987;11:803–817.

209. Shmookler BM, Enzinger FM. Pleomorphic lipoma: a benign tumor simulating liposarcoma: a clinicopathologic analysis of 48 cases. *Cancer* 1981;47:126–133.

210. Azzopardi J, Iocco J, Salm R. Pleomorphic lipoma: a tumour simulating liposarcoma. *Histopathology* 1983;7:511–523.

211. Beham A, Schmid C, Hödl S, Fletcher CD. Spindle cell and pleomorphic lipoma: an immunohistochemical study and histogenetic analysis. *J Pathol* 1989;158:219–222.

212. Meis JM, Enzinger FM. Chondroid lipoma. A unique tumor simulating liposarcoma and myxoid chondrosarcoma. *Am J Surg Pathol* 1993;17:1103–1112.

213. Kindblom LG, Meis-Kindblom JM. Chondroid lipoma: an ultrastructural and immunohistochemical analysis with further observations regarding its differentiation. *Hum Pathol* 1995;26:706–715.

214. De Nictolis M, Goteri G, Campanati G, Prat J. Elastofibrolipoma of the mediastinum: a previously undescribed benign tumor containing abnormal elastic fibers. *Am J Surg Pathol* 1995;19:364–367.

215. Vellios F, Baez J, Schumacker HB. Lipoblastomatosis: a tumor of fetal fat different from hibernoma; report of a case, with observations on the embryogenesis of human adipose tissue. *Am J Pathol* 1958;34:1149–1159.

216. Chung EB, Enzinger FM. Benign lipoblastomatosis: an analysis of 35 cases. *Cancer* 1973;32:482–492.

217. Bolen JW, Thorning D. Benign lipoblastoma and myxoid liposarcoma: a comparative light- and electron-microscopic study. *Am J Surg Pathol* 1980;4:163–174.

218. Alba Greco M, Garcia RL, Vuletin JC. Benign lipoblastomatosis: ultrastructure and histogenesis. *Cancer* 1980;45:511–515.

219. Chaudhuri B, Ronan SG, Ghosh L. Benign lipoblastoma: report of a case. *Cancer* 1980;46:611–614.

220. Hanada M, Tokuda R, Ohnishi Y, Takami M, Takahashi T, Kimura M. Benign lipoblastoma and liposarcoma in children. *Acta Pathol Jpn* 1986;36:605–612.

221. Dudgeon DL, Haller JA Jr. Pediatric lipoblastomatosis: two unusual cases. *Surgery* 1984;95:371–373.

222. Turc-Carel C, Dal Cin P, Rao U, Karakousis C, Sandberg AA. Cytogenetic studies of adipose tissue tumors: I. A benign lipoma with reciprocal translocation t(3;12)(q28;q14). *Cancer Genet Cytogenet* 1986;23:283–289.

223. Heim S, Mandahl N, Kristoffersson U, et al. Reciprocal translocation t(3;12)(q27;q13) in lipoma. *Cancer Genet Cytogenet* 1986;23:301–304.

224. Sandberg AA, Turc-Carel C. The cytogenetics of solid tumors. Relation to diagnosis, classification and pathology. *Cancer* 1987;59:387–395.

225. Heim S, Mitelman F. *Cancer Cytogenetics.* New York: Alan R. Liss; 1987:240–241.

226. Heim S, Mandahl N, Kristoffersson U, et al. Marker ring chromosome—a new cytogenetic abnormality characterizing lipogenic tumors? *Cancer Genet Cytogenet* 1987;24:319–326.

227. Heim S, Mandahl N, Rydholm A, Willen H, Mitelman F. Different karyotypic features characterize different clinicopathologic subgroups of benign lipogenic tumors. *Int J Cancer* 1988;42:863–867.

228. Turc-Carel C, Dal Cin P, Boghosian L, Leong SP, Sandberg AA. Breakpoints in benign lipoma may be at 12q13 or 12q14. *Cancer Genet Cytogenet* 1988;36:131–135.

229. Sait SN, Dal Cin P, Sandberg AA, et al. Involvement of 6p in benign lipomas. A new cytogenetic entity? *Cancer Genet Cytogenet* 1989;37:281–283.

230. Dal Cin P, Sciot R, De Wever I, Van Damme B, Van den Berghe H. New discriminative chromosomal marker in adipose tissue tumors. The chromosome 8q11–q13 region in lipoblastoma. *Cancer Genet Cytogenet* 1994;78:232–235.

231. Bechtold R, Shaff MI. Pelvic lipomatosis with ureteral encasement and recurrent thrombophlebitis. *South Med J* 1983;76:1030–1032.

232. Henriksson L, Liljeholm H, Lonnerholm T. Pelvic lipomatosis causing constriction of the lower urinary tract and the rectum. Case report. *Scand J Urol Nephrol* 1984;18:249–252.

233. Shugar MA, Gavron JP. Benign symmetrical lipomatosis (Madelung's disease). *Otolaryngol Head Neck Surg* 1985;93:109–112.

234. Keller SM, Waxman JS, Kim US. Benign symmetrical lipomatosis. *South Med J* 1986;79:1428–1429.

235. Cinti S, Enzi G, Cigolini M, Bosello O. Ultrastructural features of cultured mature adipocyte precursors from adipose tissue in multiple symmetric lipomatosis. *Ultrastruct Pathol* 1983;5:145–152.

236. Enzi G. Multiple symmetric lipomatosis: an updated clinical report. *Medicine (Baltimore)* 1984;63:56–64.

237. Pollock M, Nicholson GI, Nukada H, Cameron S, Frankish P. Neuropathy in multiple symmetric lipomatosis. Madelung's disease. *Brain* 1988;111(pt 5):1157–1171.

238. Boozan JA, Maves MD, Schuller DE. Surgical management of massive benign symmetric lipomatosis. *Laryngoscope* 1992;102:94–99.

239. Berkovic SF, Andermann F, Shoubridge EA, et al. Mitochondrial dysfunction in multiple symmetrical lipomatosis. *Ann Neurol* 1991;29:566–569.

240. Klopstock T, Naumann M, Schalke B, et al. Multiple symmetric lipomatosis: abnormalities in complex IV and multiple deletions in mitochondrial DNA. *Neurology* 1994;44:862–866.

241. Deiana L, Pes GM, Carru C, Campus GV, Tidore MG, Cherchi GM. Extremely high HDL levels in a patient with multiple symmetric lipomatosis. *Clin Chim Acta* 1993;223:143–147.

242. Zancanaro C, Sbarbati A, Morroni M, et al. Multiple symmetric lipomatosis. Ultrastructural investigation of the tissue and preadipocytes in primary culture. *Lab Invest* 1990;63:253–258.

243. DeRosa G, Cozzolino A, Guarino M, Giardino C. Congenital infiltrating lipomatosis of the face: report of cases and review of the literature. *J Oral Maxillofac Surg* 1987;45:879–883.

244. Quint DJ, Boulos RS, Sanders WP, Mehta BA, Patel SC, Tiel RL. Epidural lipomatosis. *Radiology* 1988;169:485–490.

245. Vazquez L, Ellis A, Saint-Genez D, Patino J, Nogues M. Epidural lipomatosis after renal transplantation—complete recovery without surgery. *Transplantation* 1988;46:773–774.

246. Doppman JL. Epidural lipomatosis. *Radiology* 1989;171:581–582.

247. Kaplan JG, Barasch E, Hirschfeld A, Ross L, Einberg K, Gordon M. Spinal epidural lipomatosis: a serious complication of iatrogenic Cushing's syndrome. *Neurology* 1989;39:1031–1034.

248. Siskind BN, Weiner FR, Frank M, Weiner SN, Bernstein RG, Luftschein S. Steroid-induced mesenteric lipomatosis. *Comput Radiol* 1984;8:175–177.

249. Enzi G, Digito M, Marin R, Carraro R, Baritussio A, Manzato E. Mediastino-abdominal lipomatosis: deep accumulation of fat mimicking a respiratory disease and ascites. Clinical aspects and metabolic studies in vitro. *Q J Med* 1984;53:453–463.

250. Shukla LW, Katz JA, Wagner ML. Mediastinal lipomatosis: a complication of high dose steroid therapy in children. *Pediatr Radiol* 1988;19:57–58.

251. Al-Mefty O, Fox JL, Sakati N, Bashir R, Probst F. The multiple manifestations of the encephalocraniocutaneous lipomatosis syndrome. *Childs Nerv Syst* 1987;3:132–134.

252. Brumback RA, Leech RW. Fishman's syndrome (encephalocraniocutaneous lipomatosis): a field defect of ectomesoderm. *J Child Neurol* 1987;2:168–169.

253. Arora PK. Re: Non-operative diagnosis of renal sinus lipomatosis simulating tumour of the renal pelvis [letter]. *Br J Urol* 1989;63:445.

254. Rubinstein A, Goor Y, Gazit E, Cabili S. Non-symmetric subcutaneous lipomatosis associated with familial combined hyperlipidaemia. *Br J Dermatol* 1989;120:689–694.

255. Scully RE, Galdabini JJ, McNeely BU. Case records of the Massachusetts General Hospital. Weekly clinicopathological exercise. Case 53-1976 (Gardner's syndrome). *N Engl J Med* 1976;295:1526–1532.

256. Scully RE, Galdabini JJ, McNeely BU. Case records of the Massachusetts General Hospital. Weekly clinicopathological exercises. Case 47-1978 (Gardner's syndrome). *N Engl J Med* 1978;299:1237–1244.

257. Snyder N III, Scurry MT, Diess WP. Five families with multiple endocrine adenomatosis. *Ann Intern Med* 1972;76:53–58.

258. Johnson GJ, Summerskill WH, Anderson VE, Keating FR Jr. Clinical and genetic investigation of a large kindred with multiple endocrine adenomatosis. *N Engl J Med* 1967;277:1379–1385.

259. Higginbottom MC, Schultz P. The Bannayan syndrome: an autosomal dominant disorder consisting of macrocephaly, lipomas, hemangiomas, and a risk for intracranial tumors. *Pediatrics* 1982;69:632–634.

260. Klein JA, Barr RJ. Diffuse lipomatosis and tuberous sclerosis. *Arch Dermatol* 1986;122:1298–1302.

261. Weinstock JV, Kawanishi H. Gastrointestinal polyposis with orocutaneous hamartomas (Cowden's disease). *Gastroenterology* 1978;74(pt 1):890–895.

262. Carney JA. The triad of gastric epithelioid leiomyosarcoma, functioning extra-adrenal paraganglioma, and pulmonary chondroma. *Cancer* 1979;43:374–382.

263. Carney JA. The triad of gastric epithelioid leiomyosarcoma, pulmonary chondroma, and functioning extra-adrenal paraganglioma: a five-year review. *Medicine (Baltimore)* 1983;62:159–169.

264. Kremchek TE, Kremchek EJ. Carpal tunnel syndrome caused by flexor tendon sheath lipoma. *Orthop Rev* 1988;17:1083–1085.

265. Juhlin L, Strand A, Johnsen B. A syndrome with painful lipomas, familial dysarthria, abnormal eye-movements and clumsiness. *Acta Med Scand* 1987;221:215–218.

266. Aleksic S, Budzilovich G, Greco MA, et al. Intracranial lipomas, hydrocephalus and other CNS anomalies in oculoauriculo-vertebral dysplasia (Goldenhar–Gorlin syndrome). *Childs Brain* 1984;11:285–297.

267. Oochi N, Rikitake O, Maeda T, Yamaguchi M. A case of Laurence–Moon–Biedl syndrome associated with bilateral adrenal lipomas and renal abnormalities. *Nippon Naika Gakkai Zasshi* 1984;73:89–93.

268. Humphrey AA, Kinsley PC. Familial multiple lipomas: report of a family. *Arch Derm Syph* 1938;37:30–34.

269. Temtamy SA, Rogers JG. Macrodactyly, hemihypertrophy, and connective tissue nevi: report of a new syndrome and review of the literature. *J Pediatr* 1976;89:924–927.

270. Petras RE. Nonneoplastic intestinal diseases. In: Mills SE, ed. *Sternberg's Diagnostic Surgical Pathology.* 4th ed. New York: Lippincott Wilkins; 2004:1519–1520.

271. Trotter MJ, Crawford RI. Pseudolipomatosis cutis: superficial dermal vacuoles resembling fatty infiltration of the skin. *Am J Dermatopathol* 1998;20:443–447.

272. Russell RM, Boyer JL, Bagheri SA, Hruban Z. Hepatic injury from chronic hypervitaminosis a resulting in portal hypertension and ascites. *N Engl J Med* 1974;291:435–440.

273. Sheibani K, Battifora H. Signet-ring cell melanoma. A rare morphologic variant of malignant melanoma. *Am J Surg Pathol* 1988;12:28–34.

274. Iossifides I, Mackay B, Butler JJ. Signet-ring cell lymphoma. *Ultrastruct Pathol* 1980;1:511–517.

275. Hanna W, Kahn HJ, From L. Signet ring lymphoma of the skin: ultrastructural and immunohistochemical features. *J Am Acad Dermatol* 1986;14(pt 2):344–350.

276. Cross PA, Eyden BP, Harris M. Signet ring cell lymphoma of T cell type. *J Clin Pathol* 1989;42:239–245.

277. Uccini S, Pescarmona E, Ruco LP, Baroni CD, Monarca B, Modesti A. Immunohistochemical characterization of a B-cell signet ring cell lymphoma. Report of a case. *Pathol Res Pract* 1988;183:497–504.

278. Mathur DR, Ramdeo IN, Sharma SP, Singh H. Signet ring cell lymphoma simulating liposarcoma—a case report with brief review of literature. *Indian J Cancer* 1988;25:52–55.

279. Jacobs DM, Waisman J. Cervical paraganglioma with intranuclear vacuoles in a fine needle aspirate. *Acta Cytol* 1987;31:29–32.

280. Spagnolo DV, Paradinas FJ. Laryngeal neuroendocrine tumour with features of a paraganglioma, intracytoplasmic lumina and acinar formation. *Histopathology* 1985;9:117–131.

281. Rosai J, Gold J, Landy R. The histiocytoid hemangiomas. A unifying concept embracing several previously described entities of skin, soft tissue, large vessels, bone, and heart. *Hum Pathol* 1979;10:707–730.

282. Barnes L, Koss W, Nieland M. Angiolymphoid hyperplasia with eosinophilia: a disease that may be confused with malignancy. *Head Neck Surg* 1980;2:425–434.

283. Kung IT, Gibson JB, Bannatyne PM. Kimura's disease: a clinicopathological study of 21 cases and its distinction from angiolymphoid hyperplasia with eosinophilia. *Pathology* 1984;16:39–44.

284. Weiss SW, Enzinger FM. Spindle cell hemangioendothelioma. A low-grade angiosarcoma resembling a cavernous hemangioma and Kaposi's sarcoma. *Am J Surg Pathol* 1986;10:521–530.

285. Weiss SW, Enzinger FM. Epithelioid hemangioendothelioma: a vascular tumor often mistaken for a carcinoma. *Cancer* 1982;50:970–981.

286. Shimazaki H, Aida S, Iizuka Y, Yoshizu H, Tamai S. Vacuolated cell mesothelioma of the pericardium resembling liposarcoma: a case report. *Hum Pathol* 2000;31:767–770.

287. Chimelli L, Hahn MD, Budka H. Lipomatous differentiation in a medulloblastoma. *Acta Neuropathol (Berl)* 1991;81:471–473.

288. Powell CM, Rosen PP. Adipose differentiation in cystosarcoma phyllodes. A study of 14 cases. *Am J Surg Pathol* 1994;18:720–727.

289. Krishna J, Haqqani MT. Liposarcomatous differentiation in diffuse pleural mesothelioma. *Thorax* 1993;48:409–410.

Skeletal Muscle

8

Reid R. Heffner, Jr.   Lucia L. Balos

INTRODUCTION

Skeletal muscle is the largest organ in the body by weight and volume. There are hundreds of individual muscles comprising the skeletal musculature. The functions of these muscles encompass not only the movement of skeletal components, but also swallowing, respiration, and maintaining posture. The variation in the gross anatomy of these muscles is considerable. More to the point for our purposes are the histologic characteristics of muscle in general and the site-specific variations such as fiber size and fiber-type proportions. Since the anatomic pathologist is increasingly called upon to interpret microscopic findings in muscle as they relate to disease, a familiarity with the histology of normal muscle is the basis of any accurate assessment of this kind. Today, an understanding of muscle histology in a modern context depends upon some knowledge of developmental biology and molecular biology.

EMBRYOLOGY

The development of skeletal muscle is orchestrated in the unborn baby by a host of genes, many of which are yet unknown. These genes have the function of regulating the transformation of mesenchyme into muscle tissue and of reorganizing previously formed tissue through processes like apoptosis. We will have more to say about the molecular biology of muscle development after a discussion of some basic embryology. Skeletal muscle develops embryologically from somatic mesodermal tissue. The paraxial mesoderm is first apparent on day 17 and is the origin of the somites that are completely formed by day 30. At this time, a series of 42 to 44 pairs of rounded somites can be found adjacent to the notochord in the midline. By the fourth week, the mesodermal somites separate into the dermatomes and segmental myotomes. The latter give rise to the muscles of the body wall. The dorsal division of myotomes, the epimeres, represent the origin of the back muscles, while the ventral division hypomeres differentiate into the lateral and ventral muscles of the body wall, including the intercostals, abdominal obliques, and strap muscles of the neck. The muscles of the extremities arise from the limb buds that form from the lateral plate mesoderm that is also the origin of the bone, tendon, ligaments, and blood vessels. In the human embryo the mesenchyme of the limb buds appears at about the fourth week of gestation and is subject to induction by the somites. At the end of the eighth week, the primordia of individual muscles can be appreciated. Muscle tissue is not derived directly from the lateral plate mesoderm (as was previously thought) but from somitic mesoderm, which invades the limb bud in week 5 (1). Differentiation of the limb musculature follows a cephalocaudad and proximal-to-distal progression. In each limb, the somitic mesenchyme subdivides into a dorsal and ventral mass with respect to the skeletal elements. The extensor, abductor, and supinator muscles are derived from the dorsal mass, whereas the flexor, adductor, and pronator muscles originate from the ventral mass (2).

The most immature muscle cells are myoblasts. These are small, round, mononucleate cells with prominent nucleoli and evidence of mitotic activity. Myoblast cytoplasm contains no microscopically detectable filaments, but ribosomes can be identified. Masses of proliferating myoblasts represent the source of myotubes, the next step in myogenesis (3). Myotubes appear to arise as a result of fusion of the more primitive myoblasts (4). Myoblast fusion has been shown to depend upon a plasma membrane glycoprotein with a molecular weight of 38 KDa (5). This surface marker presumably allows fusing myoblasts to recognize each other. The 38-KDa membrane protein is also found on immature myotubes and satellite cells. Ultrastructurally, myoblasts are seen to have contact with each other through filopodia. Adjacent myoblasts are often joined by gap junctions (6). Fusing myoblasts become longitudinally oriented, a process which requires fibronectin (7). At this stage of myogenesis, groups of primitive muscle cells, including myoblasts and myotubes, are enclosed by a common basement membrane. In each cluster, there is usually one larger primary myotube. Between groups of cells are aggregates of interstitial cells (8).

Myotubes differ from myoblasts by the presence of multiple nuclei and cytoplasmic filaments. Filaments first form at the peripheral portions of the sarcoplasm and consist of 10 nm fibroblast-like fibrils that disappear during maturation (9). Immunohistochemical techniques also demonstrate the presence of desmin and vimentin within myotubes. More mature secondary myotubes have a larger diameter, increased numbers of nuclei that are central in cross sections, and more prominent myofilaments (Figure 8.1). These cells also begin to show evidence of contractile activity. Secondary myotubes eventually give rise to muscle fibers. As they approach this stage of development, secondary myotubes cease fusing and develop acetylcholine receptor protein on the cell surface. At first receptor protein is diffusely distributed on the cell surface, but it later becomes focused into so-called hot spots where motor endplates will develop (10).

Muscle fibers differ from myotubes in that their nuclei are peripheral and their filaments are organized into sarcomeres. Muscle fibers also develop a sarcotubular system, and in time they become innervated. Immature muscle fibers often acquire multiple innervation sites, all but one of which eventually disappears.

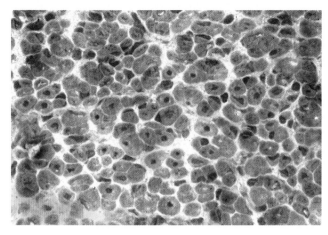

Figure 8.1 Myotube stage of muscle development. Myotubes typically have large central nuclei (trichrome).

The number of myotubes continues to decline after the twenty-first week of gestation so that at the time of birth myotubes are no longer conspicuous histologically. As myotubes become fewer in number, the muscle fibers undergo histochemical differentiation, which begins in the fifth month of development. Between fifteen and twenty weeks of gestation, a primitive progenitor of the checkerboard pattern emerges in which all myotubes and myofibers have high ATPase and oxidative enzyme activity (11). By twenty weeks gestation, approximately 10% of fibers are larger in diameter, with both high oxidative enzyme activity and reduced ATPase activity. These fibers, which are basophilic in H&E stains, are the so-called Wohlfart B fibers and are the earliest example of type 1 fibers to be detected in developing muscle (12). The remaining 90% of fibers (Wohlfart type A) correspond to type 2 fibers with enhanced ATPase activity. Although type 2A and 2B fibers are not yet visible, a few type 2C fibers that stain dark in both acid and alkaline ATPase reactions are apparent. These fibers typically immunostain with antibodies to both fast and slow myosin. The more mature checkerboard histochemical pattern, which is stimulated by the innervation of fibers, is almost completed between 26 and 30 weeks of gestation (13). At birth the histochemical mosaic begins to resemble that of mature adult muscle. Approximately 80% of fibers are clearly identified as type 1 or type 2. The remaining 20% are undifferentiated fibers that have both abundant oxidative enzyme activity and stain darkly in routine ATPase reactions. A few Wohlfart type B fibers remain at birth. Type 2C fibers are not encountered.

As mentioned earlier, the development of skeletal muscle is under the control of several categories of genes and their products (14). Among these categories are transcription factors and signaling molecules such as growth factors and their receptors. A comprehensive discussion of this subject would not be appropriate, but a few illustrative examples will be given in recognition of the fact that these molecular events in the embryo will soon be relevant in the understanding and diagnosis of muscle disease, especially the congenital myopathies and dystrophies.

One of the important influences in the early stages of segmentation when the segmental identity of the somites is established is the expression of *Hox* genes, a family of homeobox genes that act as transcription factors involved in craniocaudal segmentation of the body. Myogenesis originates with a population of mesenchymal cells that become devoted to a lineage of myogenic cells. The molecular basis of this transition rests with an array of myogenic regulatory factors, MyoD, myogenin, Myf-5, and MRF-4, which are basic helix-loop-helix proteins. Both Myf-5 and another transcription factor, Pax-3, activate MyoD (myogenic determining factor), which leads to the formation of mononuclear myoblasts. Meanwhile, myoblasts in the myotome of the somite continue to replicate and are kept in the cell cycle by growth factors such as fibroblast growth factor (FGF-8). Myogenin expression is controlled by Myf-5 and MyoD; along with myoblast recognition and adherence mechanisms that rely on adhesion molecules like M-cadherin, myogenin expression promotes myotube fusion. In turn, MRF-4 is responsible for differentiation into myofibers.

POSTNATAL AND DEVELOPMENTAL CHANGES

During the prenatal period and childhood, muscle fibers continue to increase in length until full growth is attained. Muscle fibers lengthen in response to growth of the skeleton by virtue of two fundamental changes in the sarcomeres. Existing sarcomeres lengthen, producing longitudinal fiber growth (15). This mechanism may account for up to a 25% increase in fiber length and indicates that there is a relative "excess" of sarcomeres that may elongate during periods of rapid growth of the skeleton. Muscle fibers also undergo real longitudinal growth with the addition of new sarcomeres, which involves the synthesis of contractile proteins (16). New sarcomeres are known to be added at the end of fibers, usually at the myotendinous junctions (17). There is also evidence to suggest that new sarcomeres are not only added at the end of fibers, but within internal segments as well. Whether the actual number of muscle fibers is augmented after birth is the subject of a current debate. Until recently the myofiber population was thought to be relatively stable after birth and throughout adult life (18). The studies of Adams and DeReuck (19) and others, however, seem to suggest a gradual rise in the number of fibers between birth and the end of the fifth decade. In some muscles, the total increase in fibers may reach 80 to 100% of the neonatal level. The mechanism accounting for an increase in the fiber population probably involves a population of dividing stem cells that subsequently undergo fusion to produce new mature fibers. A major aspect of growth of muscle fibers after birth relates to an increase in transverse dimension. In general, between birth and adulthood there is a five-fold increase in muscle fiber diameters (20). For example, in the leg muscles, the average diameter of mature fibers is 45 μm as compared to 7 μm at birth. The enlargement in fiber diameters does not proceed at an even rate from birth to early adulthood, when fibers obtain a maximum diameter. Instead, fiber diameters increase at a relatively slow rate until puberty, when a burst of growth occurs. As an example, in the gastrocnemius, fibers more than triple in size from age 12 (average 19 μm) to age 21 (average 62 μm) years.

A major revision in the histochemical profile of muscle occurs after birth. In the term infant, a checkerboard staining pattern is clearly evident in alkaline ATPase reactions. However, fiber typing is often not distinct in oxidative enzyme reactions (Figure 8.2). The emergence of type 1, 2A, and 2B fibers in oxidative preparations occurs during infancy. Undifferentiated fibers having both abundant oxidative enzyme and ATPase activity represent approximately 20% of fibers at birth. These gradually differentiate into type 1 and type 2 fibers during the first year of life. The fate of Wohlfart B fibers, comprising about 1% of myofibers at birth, is unknown. They are not seen in biopsies of children past the age of 12 months.

The connective tissue elements of muscle are much more prominent at birth, particularly the perimysial components. Immediately after birth the perimysium may account for up to 20% of the cross-sectional area of muscle tissue. During early childhood, the perimysium and other connective tissue components rapidly shrink to less than 5% of the cross-sectional area, in part because of the enlargement of the muscle fibers. In the immediate postnatal period, blood vessels (especially arteries) appear excessively thickened as a result of the presence of abundant smooth muscle elements.

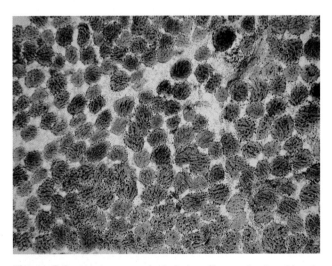

Figure 8.2 Newborn muscle. Indistinct fiber typing is evident in oxidative enzyme reactions (NADH-TR).

Expansion of the luminal diameter of blood vessels in the first year of life gives the vascular elements an adult appearance. The noncontractile, supporting connective tissue contains abundant collagen and scattered fibroblasts. Foci of hematopoiesis remain after birth, containing stem cells, erythroblasts, and myelocytes. These foci are more likely to be seen in the distal muscles of the extremities. They disappear within one month after birth.

APOPTOSIS

Our scientific knowledge of apoptosis in skeletal muscle is at a rudimentary stage, but the medical literature is beginning to address apoptosis as a regulatory process in the normal development of muscle and in its relationship to selected pathologic conditions (21).

During embryologic life, both neurons and skeletal muscle are affected by the process of apoptosis. A great deal more is known about programmed cell death in nerve cells, including motor neurons, than in muscle. A review of the earlier literature discussing natural neuronal death has been published by Hamburger (22). A recent article by Sohal (23) addresses the subject of embryonic development of motor neurons and muscles, culminating in the establishment of mature nerve-muscle relationships. During embryogenesis, a necessary remodeling of muscles occurs through apoptosis, which removes "unwanted" cells or structures to make room for further maturation. In the chick embryo, programmed cell death clearly occurs as the myofibers are developing. The large diameter primary myotubes are preferentially affected. The cytological features suggesting apoptosis include misshapen nuclei and irregular chromatin condensations along the nuclear envelope (24). It has been shown that, in rat embryos, macrophages play an important role in the removal of dead fibers (25). In human fetal muscle, the programmed cell death of both primary and mature myotubes occurs between 10 and 16 weeks of gestation (26).

A body of information regarding apoptotic events in postnatal and adult muscle is beginning to accumulate. Such diverse conditions as disuse, exercise, ischemia, aging, and certain myopathies are being examined. Skeletal muscle apoptosis differs from most other tissues in several ways. Muscle cells are multinucleated, and their mitochondrial composition varies with fiber type and other factors such as exercise. Muscle cells contain two separate mitochondrial populations, subsarcolemmal and intermyofibrillar. It is unclear at the moment whether the expression of pro- and antiapoptotic agents differ in the two populations. Because it is a multinucleated cell, the muscle fiber does not always undergo apoptosis in same fashion as other cell types. Damage limited to individual myonuclei seems to be more common than death of the entire cell. In denervation, myonuclear loss leads to fiber atrophy instead of cell death. Finally, the elevated expression of endogenous caspase in-

hibitors in muscle seems to confer relatively greater resistance to apoptosis.

ANATOMY

There are 434 voluntary muscles in the human body (27). They comprise 25% of the total body weight at birth and 40 to 50% of the total weight in adults. Not surprisingly, a greater muscle mass is encountered in males than in females. Individual muscles vary greatly in size. For example, the smallest muscle in the body, the stapedius, measures only 2 mm in length. On the other hand, the sartorius and other large muscles of the extremities measure up to 2 feet in length (61 cm). Skeletal muscles are composed of varying numbers of muscle fibers (e.g., 10,000 in lumbricals and 1,000,000 in gastrocnemius) (28). These are connected at both ends to tendons or the epimysium.

Because the fibers work in conjunction with each other, they are aligned in the same direction. Few skeletal muscles are modeled after the lumbricals, where all the fibers are arranged in a fusiform structure that tapers at either end at the site of tendinous insertion (29). The more familiar unit is a parallelogram composed of muscle fibers that insert at both ends on a flat tendon composed of dense collagen. In a parallel muscle, the fascicles are parallel to the longitudinal axis of the muscle, as in the thyrohyoid. In oblique muscles, a tendon typically runs within the muscle or on its surface, and the muscle fibers insert obliquely on the tendon. Oblique muscles are most often pennate or featherlike. Some are bipennate, much like a feather in which there is a central shaft from which a series of barbs radiate on either side. Such muscles have a central tendinous structure from which two sets of parallel muscle fibers radiate (e.g., peroneus longus). Other muscles are simple pennate, in which only one set of parallel muscle fibers attaches obliquely on a shaftlike tendon (e.g., extensor digitorum longus). Muscles are designated as complex pennate when the muscle consists of multiple parallelograms attaching to several tendons in the muscle mass. Not all skeletal muscles follow precisely the model of parallel or pennate design. They may be triangular like the pectoralis minor or spiral in structure like the forearm supinators. Although most muscles are attached to and are involved in moving bony skeletal structures, some voluntary muscles (such as those of the larynx and esophagus) do not have attachments to bone.

The blood supply to individual skeletal muscles has not been extensively studied and is therefore incompletely understood. It is known that the arterial supply to muscles varies somewhat with the individual. In general, the skeletal muscles are subserved by several rather than a single artery, which renders them rather resistant to ischemia from an embolus or from disease of a single vessel. Much of our understanding regarding the pattern of vascularization in human muscle is derived from studies performed by Blomfield (30). The vascular supply to skeletal muscle falls into one of five categories.

1. The blood supply is derived from a single nutrient artery that divides in a longitudinal fashion within the muscle itself. The gastrocnemius is an example of such a system.
2. The muscle is supplied by several separate arteries entering the muscle along its length. Anastomoses are formed within the muscle between the territories of each artery. This pattern is typical of the soleus.
3. The blood supply arises from a single main artery that enters the belly of the muscle and subsequently forms a radiating pattern of collaterals, as in the biceps brachii.
4. In muscles like the tibialis anterior, a pattern of anastomosing arcades is derived from a series of penetrating arteries. This vascular pattern is considered to be the most efficient form of vascularization.
5. A less efficient form of the anastomosing arcade pattern is the rectangular pattern of anastomoses formed by a series of penetrating arteries. This so-called quadrilateral pattern is seen in the extensor hallucis longus muscle.

Once a main artery enters the muscle substance, it branches into a number of primary intramuscular arteries that ramify in the epimysium and perimysium. The primary arteries, with a diameter which ranges from 80 to 360 μm, give rise to numerous secondary arterioles that run parallel to the direction of the muscle fibers. The secondary arterioles often connect to primary arteries, forming artery-to-artery anastomoses. The secondary arterioles, which range in diameter from 50 to 100 μm, typically have a thin adventitia composed of fibroblasts and collagen. The smooth muscle coat is much thinner than that of the primary arteries, usually having only two to three layers of cells. The internal elastica is prominent and continuous. The secondary arterioles branch to form terminal arterioles, which measure 15 to 50 μm in diameter. Their smooth muscle coat is usually only one layer of cells. The internal elastica becomes discontinuous and is lost in smaller vessels. The distal portions of the terminal arterioles have precapillary sphincters, which are formed from the smooth muscle cells of the media. These sphincters are found in blood vessels with an inner diameter of less than 15 μm. Footlike processes between the smooth muscle cells and the endothelium may be seen in the region of the sphincters.

As in other tissues, the arterioles end in an elaborate system of capillaries. In contrast to most other organs, in muscle a relatively small number of capillaries are open at rest (31). During muscle activity there is a considerable increase in the number of open capillaries. A marked difference in capillary density is observed in different muscles, as well as in trained versus untrained subjects. Studies of capillary density reveal that the average single muscle fiber is surrounded by 1.7 capillaries (32). Capillary density may also be expressed as the number of capillaries per fiber, which on average in cross sections is 0.7.

The density of capillaries also reflects oxygen consumption within muscle. Therefore increased numbers of capillaries are evident where larger numbers of type 1 fibers are present. This phenomenon is less evident in humans than in animals such as the cat, in which muscles are composed chiefly or totally of one fiber type. Thus in the cat soleus muscle, which is composed almost entirely of type 1 fibers, the density of capillaries is 1,600 per mm^2. In the gastrocnemius, a muscle with far fewer type 1 fibers, the capillary density is 600 per mm^2 (33). The capillaries within skeletal muscle travel primarily in a longitudinal direction, although they are frequently linked by short transverse branches.

Ultrastructurally, capillaries are composed of endothelial cells surrounded by a basement lamina. Occasional pericytes are encountered outside the basement membrane. Endothelial cells typically contain numerous pinocytotic vesicles. Where endothelial cells are joined, they lack tight junctions. Hence the capillary endothelium is freely permeable to tracers such as horseradish peroxidase. The capillary pericytes are essentially smooth muscle cells that contain large numbers of filaments. The pericytes are innervated by small-diameter unmyelinated nerve fibers. The basement membrane (which lies between the endothelium and pericytes) measures 20 to 30 nm, although some thickening and reduplication of the basal lamina occurs in older patients.

The nerve supply to individual skeletal muscles often enters the surface of the muscle at the belly and is accompanied by one or more major penetrating arteries. Within the main nerve trunk are myelinated and unmyelinated axons. Contributions to the nerve are made from myelinated efferent motor fibers that innervate the muscle fibers; somatic afferent sensory fibers from muscle spindles, Golgi tendon organs, and Pacinian corpuscles; and unmyelinated autonomic efferent fibers. At least 50% of the fibers are sensory in function. The motor fibers that innervate the myofibers demonstrate a bimodal size distribution. The large diameter α fibers innervate fast motor units, while the β fibers are distributed to slow motor units and some intrafusal fibers of the muscle spindle. The very small diameter γ fibers supply the remainder of the muscle spindle fibers. The large motor fibers are relatively uniform in diameter, measuring between 10 and 15 μm. The small motor fibers vary from 2 to 7 μm in diameter.

As the distal motor axon approaches the muscle fiber, it is transformed into the terminal axon, which represents the proximal portion of the neuromuscular junction, or motor endplate (MEP). The neuromuscular junction, measuring about 50 μm in diameter, is composed of the presynaptic (PRS) portion or terminal axon and the postsynaptic (POS) portion, which is formed by a unique region in the muscle fiber (Figure 8.3). The PRS and POS domains are separated by a specialized, 50-nm wide intercellular space, the synaptic cleft.

The myelinated motor nerve terminates at the PRS region as an unmyelinated axonal segment that is enveloped

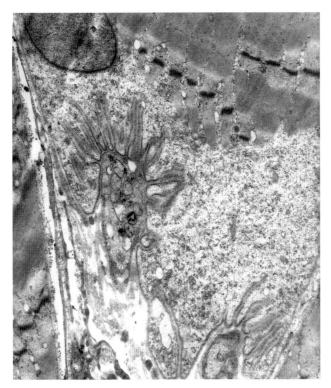

Figure 8.3 Electron micrograph of motor endplate (MEP). Ultrastructurally, the MEP consists of a terminal axon and a postsynaptic region formed by a specialized portion of the muscle fiber. The surface of the fiber is undulating, representing the postjunctional folds.

by the teloglia, the distal projections of Schwann cells. The terminal axon and teloglia are covered by a layer of endoneurium, the sheath of Henle, which becomes continuous with the endomysium of the muscle fiber in the area of MEP. Numerous synaptic vesicles, each 45 to 50 nm in diameter, are found in the terminal axon. The vesicles are most plentiful around thickened zones of increased electron density at the presynaptic membrane. Studies utilizing freeze-fracture electron microscopy have demonstrated that parallel pairs of double rows of intramembranous particles, measuring 10 nm in diameter, are located at these electron dense zones (34). The particles are considered to represent voltage-sensitive calcium channels known as active zones.

At the POS region of the muscle fiber, the cell surface is elevated to form the hillock of Doyère, or sole plate. Within the sole plate, the sarcoplasm is granular, and a cluster of sarcolemmal nuclei is often seen. Nuclei in this location are plump and vesicular. The terminal axon ramifies in the sole plate as a series of branches called telodendria, which indent the surface of the fiber, producing gutters or troughs. The surface of the fiber at the MEP is undulating and redundant, creating the complex of postjunctional folds that can be demonstrated by supravital staining as the subneural apparatus of Couteaux. The spaces between the folds denote the secondary synaptic clefts. As a result of the formation of these clefts, the surface area of the POS membrane is increased to approximately 10 times the surface area of the

PRS. The postsynaptic membrane of the folds is thicker and more densely stained at the crests than in the depths of the clefts. By electron microscopy, the juxtaneural membrane at the crests of the folds contains irregularly spaced densities measuring 11 to 14 nm in diameter. In freeze-fracture preparations, on the P face of the membrane, the crests are studded with rows of particles that are similar in size to these densities (about 10 nm) (35). These large intramembranous particles are considered to represent the acetylcholine receptor, a pentameric 275 KDa glycoprotein (36).

LIGHT MICROSCOPY

Familiarity with the normal structure of skeletal muscle provides a useful background for the pathologist in the evaluation of muscle biopsies. Other sources offering a more comprehensive discussion of the light microscopy, histochemistry, and electron microscopy of normal muscle than is possible here are found in the literature (37–48). The muscle fiber is a multinucleated, syncytial-like unit shaped like a long, narrow cylinder. The normal adult myocyte is not perfectly round but is polygonal, producing a multi-faceted profile in cross section. The nuclei are usually located subsarcolemmally, numbering four to six per cell when sectioned transversely. For each millimeter of fiber length, there are approximately 30 nuclei (49). In routine sections the sarcolemmal nuclei are slender and flat, with an orientation that is parallel to the long axis of the fiber. These nuclei measure 5 to 12 μm in length and 1 to 3 μm in width. Their chromatin is fine and dustlike. The nucleoli are small and not visible in many fibers. In paraffin sections stained with H&E, the sarcoplasm is light pink and textured in cross sections (Figure 8.4). In frozen sections that are often routine in biopsies submitted for diagnosis, muscle tissue is stained with Gomori's rapid trichrome (RTC). Here the fibers and connective tissue stain green while nuclei are blue-black. In some cases the mitochondria can be identified, especially in

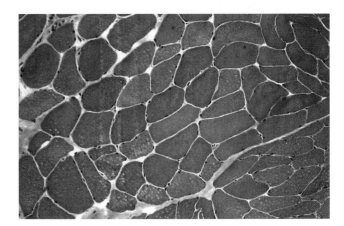

Figure 8.4 Cross section of muscle. The sarcoplasm is textured and the sarcolemmal nuclei are peripheral in location (H&E).

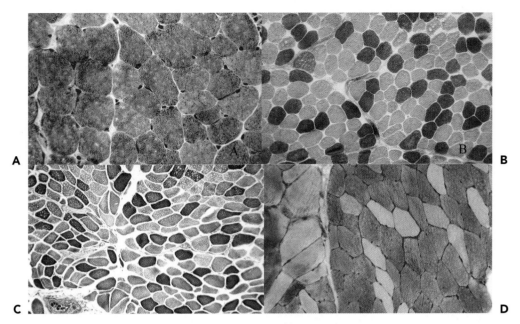

Figure 8.5 **A.** Reverse trichrome stain. Mitochondria appear as red granular areas, especially prominent in the subsarcolemmal regions of the fiber. **B.** Normal muscle. In the standard ATPase reaction, type 1 fibers are light and type 2 fibers are dark (ATPase, pH9.4, eosin counterstain). **C.** Normal muscle. In oxidative enzyme reactions, type 1 fibers are very dark, and type 2 fibers are intermediate or light in staining intensity (NADH-TR). **D.** With PAS stain, variable staining of fibers reflects glycogen content and crudely approximates fiber type distribution (PAS).

type 1 fibers, as tiny red granules within the sarcoplasm (Figure 8.5A). The cross-striations must be viewed in longitudinal sections and are difficult to see in any detail without special stains. They are best demonstrated in PAS and PTAH stains or in resin-embedded material where alternating dark and light bands are evident (Figure 8.6). The diameter of fibers is determined by several factors (see the section entitled Gender, Training, and Aging).

Proximal muscles, where power rather than finely coordinated movement is required, have a fiber population with a larger mean diameter (85–90 μm), while those of smaller, distal, and ocular muscles are composed of thinner fibers (20 μm). Fiber size in males exceeds that in females, probably in part because of androgenic hormonal influences and more strenuous physical demands. In both genders, exercise promotes fiber hypertrophy. Muscle fibers are smaller in children and in the elderly than in young active adults, although comprehensive normative data at these ages are not easy to find (50–52).

Red muscle, having a larger mitochondrial and lipid content and higher capillary density, depends on aerobic respiration and is designed for postural function or sustained activity. The color of red muscles is actually due to relatively greater myoglobin content than white muscles, which contain fewer mitochondria but abundant glycogen, rendering it better suited to anaerobic respiration and to sudden and intermittent contraction. In vertebrates, particularly in birds, red (e.g., soleus) can easily be distinguished

from white (e.g., pectoralis) muscles upon external inspection, since an entire muscle in such species may be composed of either red or white fibers. Human muscles, on the other hand, contain both fiber types, which typically assume a mixed mosaic arrangement reminiscent of checkerboard. Depending on anatomic location and function, the proportion of type 1 and type 2 fibers varies, but a typical muscle contains approximately twice as many type 2 fibers (60–65%) as type 1 fibers (35–40%).

The demonstration of the histochemical properties of the muscle fibers comprising a biopsy, which is known as

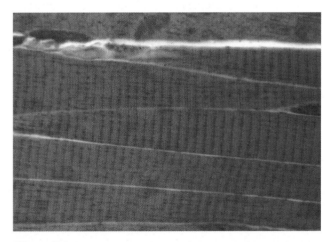

Figure 8.6 Resin section. Sarcomere pattern is shown in longitudinal section (toluidine blue).

TABLE 8.1		
FIBER TYPING		
Stain/Reaction	**Type 1 Fibers**	**Type 2 Fibers**
ATPase, pH 9.4	Light	Dark
NADH-TR	Dark	Light
PAS/phosphorylase	Light	Dark
Oil red O	Dark	Light

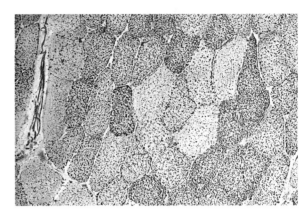

Figure 8.7   Lipid content of fibers is demonstrated with oil red O stain. Oxidative fibers have a more dense lipid concentration (oil red O).

fiber typing, is accomplished by applying histochemical techniques (Table 8.1). Fiber typing is not possible in routine H&E-stained slides and is only appreciated in using histoenzymatic reactions performed on frozen sections. In our laboratory, two complementary histochemical procedures are employed for the detection of fiber types. The most reliable method for this purpose is the myofibrillar ATPase reaction. By changing the pH during the procedure, a spectrum of staining reactions can be produced. In the standard or alkaline ATPase reaction, which is conducted at a pH of 9.4, two fiber types are seen. Type 2 fibers are dark in staining intensity, whereas type 1 fibers are pale (Figure 8.5B). Fibers of intermediate staining intensity are not observed in the alkaline incubation.

If the pH of the incubating solution is brought into the acidic range (pH 4.6) in what is sometimes known as the reverse ATPase reaction, two populations of type 2 fibers emerge. Type 2A fibers are virtually unstained and type 2B fibers are intermediately stained, while type 1 fibers are extremely dark. All the oxidative enzyme reactions, like the NADH-TR used in our laboratory, merely reflect the mitochondrial content of the muscle fibers. Intensely stained fibers are designated as oxidative (type 1) and lighter fibers as type 2 (Figure 8.5C). Most oxidative enzyme reactions further subdivide type 2 fibers into two categories. Type 2B fibers are poorly stained in contrast to type 2A fibers, which exhibit a staining intensity that is intermediate between type 1 and 2B. Although all muscle fibers contain glycogen and the companion enzyme phosphorylase, they are more abundant in type 2 (glycolytic) fibers. The PAS stain, a crude method of detecting glycogen, and the histochemical reaction for phosphorylase can be used as a means of fiber typing (Figure 8.5D). However, staining with these techniques is not totally reliable for fiber typing. We only use the phosphorylase reaction to investigate possible cases of enzyme deficiency (McArdle's disease). Type 1 fibers are rich in lipid, which can be visualized in fat stains such as the oil red O (Figure 8.7); but, like the PAS stain, fat stains are not as reliable for fiber typing as are enzyme reactions.

Striated muscles are partitioned into fascicles, each of which is invested by a connective tissue sheath known as the perimysium. Within this sheath, the intramuscular nerves, primary arteries, secondary and terminal arterioles,

and veins travel throughout the muscle. At the innervation zone in the belly of the muscle, intramuscular nerve bundles or twigs are especially numerous (Figure 8.8). Up to 10 myelinated nerve fibers may be present in an individual twig, which is surrounded by a thin mantle of perineurial connective tissue. The myelinated nerve fibers are perhaps best demonstrated in trichrome-stained sections, preferably the RTC, in which the bright red–colored myelin sheaths resemble doughnuts surrounding the unstained axons. Tangential sections of twigs may be mistaken for areas of focal fibrosis or abnormal vascular structures. The perimysium is a framework that lends stability to the fascicles, in part by its attachment to the epimysium. The epimysium forms septa that sequester groups of fascicles, as well as the fascia that encircles the entire muscle and merges with the dense collagenous connective tissue of the tendons.

Within each fascicle, the perimysium gives way to a normally unobtrusive network, the endomysium. Each muscle fiber may appear to be partly or completely invested by endomysium, a mesenchymal matrix composed of collagen,

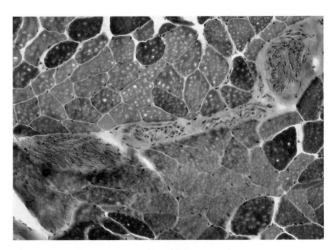

Figure 8.8   Intramuscular nerves. Nerve twigs contain axons surrounded by red-staining myelin sheaths (trichrome).

elastic, and reticulin fibers that support the preterminal arterioles and capillary blood supply to the fascicles. Where the muscle-tendon junction has interdigitations of the cell membrane, the interface is enlarged, transferring tension into shear stress. Two transmembrane proteins, the dystrophin-glycoprotein complex and α7β1 integrin, are especially abundant at the myotendinous junction (53). It is believed that the dystrophin-glycoprotein complex maintains the integrity of the sarcolemma while α7β1 integrin, a receptor for laminin-2, plays a role in the organization of the basement membrane at the myotendinous junction. At the interface between muscle and either fascia or tendon, the muscle fibers become variable, often small in size, and internal nuclei are more abundant. As they attach to the tendon or fascia, the fibers are separated by dense collagenous trabeculae (Figure 8.9). Since the normal histology of these regions may easily be misinterpreted as evidence of pathologic change, the muscle biopsy should be obtained from the belly of the muscle, avoiding the tendinous insertions. A deep rather than a superficial biopsy is preferred to avoid the fascia.

Several specialized structures are found within the connective tissue supporting framework. Muscle spindles, first described by Hassal and later by Kolliker were once considered to be a pathologic finding (54). Spindles are now known to be mechanoreceptors that sense the length and tension of skeletal muscle, governing integrated muscle activity. Although they are encountered in virtually all muscles, they are more frequently detected in smaller muscles devoted to finely coordinated activities, such as those of the hand. They are more numerous in distal than in girdle muscles. Quantitative studies have shown that 70 to 100 muscle spindles may be located in an individual muscle. Muscle spindles tend to lie in the deeper portions of the muscle, particularly in the muscle belly. They are often found where type 1 fibers are more plentiful.

As the name implies, muscle spindles are fusiform in shape with a swollen center and tapering ends. They measure 3 to 4 mm in length and 200 μm in diameter. A thin fibrous capsule represents the outer boundaries of the muscle spindle. The capsule is an extension of the perimysium, where spindles are usually located. In certain muscles such as those of the eye, face, and mouth, the capsule merges with the perimysium and is somewhat indistinct. The capsule is composed of 10 to 15 layers of flattened pavement cells that are specialized fibroblasts. The pavement cells are tightly adherent and separated only by thin layers of delicate collagen fibrils. The pavement cells are epithelial-like in that each is surrounded by a basement membrane. As one proceeds from the equatorial region of the spindle toward the poles, the number of layers of pavement cells progressively diminishes.

Within the capsule are 3 to 15 intrafusal fibers in the typical muscle spindle (Figure 8.10). Generally the number of intrafusal fibers is less in small muscles than in larger axial muscles. Two distinct populations of intrafusal fibers are found, both of which are smaller in diameter than the extrafusal fibers. The larger bag fibers, usually one to three per spindle, measure about 20 μm in diameter. The chain fibers number two to seven per spindle, with a diameter of 10 μm or less. The bag fibers are longer, sometimes extending beyond the polar ends of the capsule. They measure 4 to 8 mm in length. The chain fibers are shorter, measuring 2 to 4 mm. The bag fibers are recognized in the equatorial region of the spindle by the presence of large aggregations of nuclei. Away from the equatorial region, the nuclei remain internal or central in the bag fibers but are far less numerous. The smaller chain fibers are distinguished by a row of central nuclei, which extends along the length of the fiber. In histochemical stains, there are two types of bag fibers. Bag 1 fibers reveal considerable oxidative enzyme activity and are pale in ATPase reactions. On the other hand, bag 2 fibers, which also have high oxidative enzyme

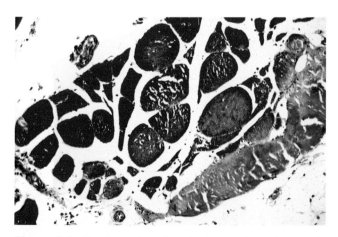

Figure 8.9 Tendinous insertion. At the interface, the muscle fibers normally vary in size and are partly surrounded by connective tissue (trichrome).

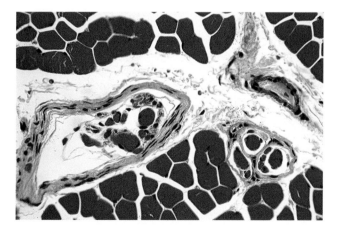

Figure 8.10 Muscle spindle. A fibrous capsule encloses a nerve twig and several intrafusal fibers, which are normally smaller than the extrafusal fibers (trichrome).

activity, reveal intermediate staining in ATPase reactions. Chain fibers, although they possess high oxidative enzyme activity, stain darkly in ATPase reactions and are considered by many to be type 2 fibers (55).

The innervation of muscle spindles, which is both motor and sensory, is complex and will only be summarized here (56). The intrafusal efferent fibers are derived from branches of β and γ efferent axons. The β axons appear to terminate primarily on nuclear bag fibers. The γ fibers supply both nuclear bag and chain intrafusal fibers. It is not uncommon for intrafusal fibers to have polyneural innervation. Two types of sensory innervation are seen in the muscle spindle. The larger diameter group Ia afferent fibers emanate from the equator. They originate as the annulospiral endings, a series of neural coils and spirals that attach to the nuclear bag and chain fibers. Smaller diameter group II afferent fibers come from the paraequatorial regions of the spindle and are associated mainly with the so-called flower spray endings of Ruffini. The majority of these endings project from the nuclear chain fibers. The secondary, or flower spray, endings consist of a branching network that enwraps the intrafusal fiber between its polar and equatorial regions.

The Golgi tendon organ is an encapsulated sensory nerve terminal that is located at the junction of muscle with tendon or aponeurosis. The location of these structures allows them to sense changes in muscle tension. They have an inhibitory function in the event of strong muscle contraction. These fusiform structures measure about 1.5 mm in length and 120 μm in diameter. They consist of one or more fascicles of collagen fibrils that are attached to tendon or aponeurosis and enveloped by a multilamellar capsule (Figure 8.11). Each structure is connected to 20 to 30 muscle fibers. The Golgi tendon organ is innervated by a myelinated Ib afferent axon, measuring 7 to 15 μm in diameter. The afferent nerve typically divides and arborizes around the individual collagen bundles.

Pacinian corpuscles are distributed widely in the subcutaneous tissues of the body, although they may also be encountered within the muscular fascial planes and adjacent to tendons or aponeuroses. They are seldom seen within muscle tissue itself. In the center of the pacinian corpuscle is a central rodlike nerve terminal innervated by fast-conducting group I or II afferent axons. The central axon is surrounded by a capsule composed of concentric layers of cells (Figure 8.12). The elongated cells forming the capsule are surrounded by basal lamina and separated by fine collagen fibrils. Pacinian corpuscles are receptor organs that are sensitive to vibration.

ULTRASTRUCTURE

The ultrastructural examination of skeletal muscle is conventionally performed on sections oriented longitudinally, wherein deviations from the orderly striated architecture

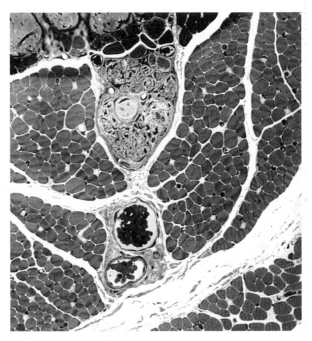

Figure 8.11 Golgi tendon organ. Fascicles of collagen surrounded by several nerve bundles (resin section, toluidine blue).

are more easily detected than in cross sections. The sarcoplasm of each muscle fiber is divided into multiple parallel subunits, the myofibrils, which are minute, cylindroid contractile structures measuring approximately 1 μm in diameter. Myofibrils are segmented into a series of identical sarcomeres that are equal in length, whether the muscle is contracted or at rest, and are aligned in register with the sarcomeres of surrounding myofibrils. The unique periodicity of the fine structure of the muscle fiber is a function of the regimentation of this contractile system. The rectangular

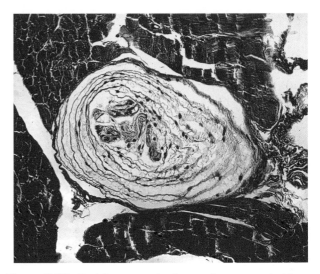

Figure 8.12 Pacinian corpuscle. A central nerve terminal is surrounded by a capsule composed of concentric layers of cells (H&E).

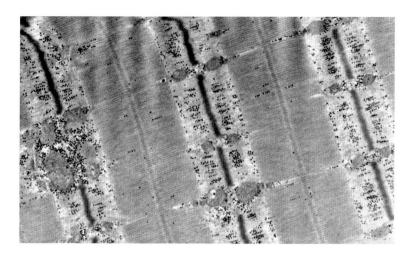

Figure 8.13 Ultrastructurally, the several myofibrils can be seen in register. Each is composed of a series of sarcomeres that contain A, I, and Z band regions (EM).

banding pattern within each sarcomere is produced by the arrangement of the filaments (Figure 8.13). The Z band, which forms the lateral boundaries of the sarcomere, is an electron-dense bar-shaped structure oriented perpendicular to the long axis of the myofibril. The distance between consecutive Z bands represents the sarcomere length, an average of 2.5 to 3.0 μm. The I bands are the most electron-lucent portions of the sarcomere and stand in dramatic contrast to the dark Z bands that bisect them. The I bands are shorter in length than the moderately dense A bands located at the center of the sarcomeres. Within each sarcomere are stacks of parallel filaments that, under the electron microscope, appear to be of two types. The thicker filaments measure 15 nm in diameter and are principally composed of myosin. The thinner filaments, containing chiefly actin, are 8 nm in diameter. The thin filaments are attached to the Z band and extend across the I band, where only thin filaments are found. They penetrate the A band in which alternating thick and thin filaments are visualized. Thick filaments on the other hand, are restricted to the A band region of the sarcomere and determine its length.

The sarcoplasmic organelles are more concentrated around the sarcolemmal nuclei and between the myofibrils. The mitochondria are somewhat variable in shape and size, although the majority are oval or elliptical in configuration and 1.0 μm in greatest dimension. They are most easily recognized adjacent to the Z bands where their long axes are parallel to those of the myofibrils. Both mitochondria and lipid vacuoles are more conspicuous in oxidative fibers.

Glycogen, composed of granules with a diameter of 15–30 nm, is more abundant in glycolytic fibers, particularly in the I band region of the sarcomere. The sarcoplasmic reticulum (SR) and the transverse (T) tubules together comprise the sarcotubular complex. The SR, which is analogous to the endoplasmic reticulum of other cells, is an elaborate system of tubules that, by branching in all directions, surrounds the myofibrils. In contrast to the SR, which has no communica-

tion with the extracellular space, the T tubules arise as invaginations from the cell membrane. They are observed at regular intervals along the length of the fiber, particularly at the junction of the A and I bands. The T tubules encircle the myofibrils and are disposed in a predominantly transverse direction. Branches of the sarcotubular complex join together as triads at the A-I band junctions. Here, pairs of terminal cisterns derived from the SR are positioned on either side of a central T tubule. In this location, the SR tubules appear as hollow, membrane-bound profiles, while the T tubules are somewhat more electron dense.

Satellite cells are a population of myoblastic stem cells that are a source of nuclei during muscle growth, particularly hypertrophy. Satellite cells also have the capacity to synthesize new muscle after myocyte injury. These primitive, indeterminate cells can, under appropriate circumstances, be transformed into blastic elements that serve as an important source of fiber regeneration. Satellite cells represent approximately 10% of the myonuclei seen in cross sections of muscle. There is a decline in the number of satellite cells as a result of the aging process so that they constitute only 2 to 3% of myofiber nuclei in older individuals. Satellite cells are small, mononuclear, fusiform cells that are situated beneath the basement membrane of neighboring muscle fibers (57). They cannot be reliably distinguished from the muscle fiber nuclei under the light microscope. Satellite cells are not randomly distributed along the length of the muscle fiber and are more numerous in certain locations such as the sole plates of the neuromuscular junction and the polar regions of the muscle spindles. Ultrastructurally, the nuclei of satellite cells differ somewhat from the nuclei of muscle fibers. They are more elongated, their nuclear chromatin is peripherally dense, and nucleoli are lacking. The satellite cell nuclei are usually asymmetrical within the cytoplasm, which contains only a few filaments without evidence of sarcomere formation. The sarcoplasm also contains free ribosomes, microtubules, and centrioles, which may be associated with cilia.

Where the cell membranes of the satellite cell and muscle fiber are opposed, numerous pinocytotic vesicles are seen.

SPECIAL TECHNIQUES

Perhaps more than any other tissue, skeletal muscle in humans has been studied using a wide variety of specialized techniques, in part because human muscle biopsies are frequently collected in such a way as to make both fresh, unfixed tissue and material for special studies available. In addition to routine histochemical methods that are focused primarily on the identification of fiber types, a number of other histochemical procedures have been employed for the study of both normal and abnormal skeletal muscle. An array of histochemical techniques have been developed to provide greater understanding of muscle metabolism (37,39,40,46). Among these are histochemical techniques to identify various enzymes involved in glycoge metabolism and glycolysis. Familiar examples are histochemical stains for phosphorylase and phosphofructokinase. Other histochemical procedures have been developed to study mitochondrial function. The most widely used is the histochemical stain for cytochrome oxidase. In the workup of human disease, histochemical analysis of muscle tissue can be supplemented by biochemical analysis, specifically when histochemical techniques are unavailable. It is also best, whenever possible, to confirm histochemical findings with biochemical studies. Biochemical analysis has been particularly useful in the study of mitochondrial disease, examining such parameters as the respiratory chain. Molecular techniques are being used with increasing frequency in elucidating normal muscle development as well as muscle disease. A number of abnormal conditions can now be diagnosed using molecular strategies. These include Duchenne dystrophy and other dystrophinopathies (58) and certain mitochondrial disorders in which there is a defect in the mitochondrial genome (59). As mentioned above, it seems likely that the genes that are being discovered in developmental biology one day will contribute to our understanding and diagnosis of muscle disease.

Several techniques have been adapted for the study of intramuscular blood vessels. For example, capillaries are particularly well seen in histochemical procedures for alkaline phosphatase. Capillaries are also nicely demonstrated in immunohistochemical stains for factor VIII.

Immunohistochemistry is an emerging field in pathology that has begun to find a niche in the study of muscle. As already described, muscle fiber typing can be done in frozen sections using histochemical stains such as ATPase. Antibodies to fast and slow myosins are now available for the identification of type 1 and type 2 muscle fibers in fixed tissue (Figure 8.14) (60). It is also possible to subdivide type 2 fibers into types 2A and 2B using myosin antibodies.

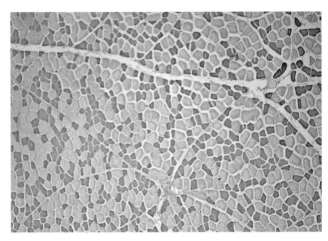

Figure 8.14 Checkerboard pattern is seen with dark type 2 fibers and pale type 1 fibers (immunostain for fast myosin).

Fibers undergoing regeneration can be detected by immunohistochemical methods. Regenerating fibers contain fetal myosins and react using antibodies to vimentin and desmin. Recently visualization of the membrane-associated proteins, dystrophin, and the family of sarcoglycans (α-δ), has become practical (Figure 8.15). Antibodies to dystrophin, as well as to some of the dystrophin-associated glycoproteins, permit the diagnosis of Duchenne dystrophy, selected other dystrophinopathies, and the some of the limb girdle muscular dystrophies (61). In fact, it is now possible to identify an array of myopathies using immunohistochemistry to study disease-related proteins (Table 8.2).

The nerve supply to muscle, including the intramuscular nerve twigs and MEPs, cannot be adequately studied in routine samples. The anatomic location of nerve endings and endplates is variable, depending on the muscle selected. They may be restricted to a narrow band across the muscle, or they may be more widely distributed throughout the

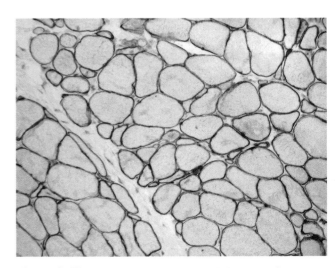

Figure 8.15 Sarcolemmal regions are darkly stained (immunostain for dystrophin).

TABLE 8.2
IMMUNOHISTOCHEMICAL IDENTIFICATION OF PROTEINS IN SKELETAL MUSCLE DISEASE

Protein	Muscle Disease
Dystrophin	Duchenne muscular dystropy; Becker type muscular dystrophy
Lamin A/C	LGMD 1B
Dysferlin	LGMD 2B
Sarcoglycans	LGMD 2C-2F
Fukutin	Congenital muscular dystrophy
Merosin	Congenital muscular dystrophy
Tropomyosin	Nemaline myopathy
Myotubulin	Centronuclear myopathy
Desmin	Desmin storage myopathy

LGMD, limb girdle muscular dystrophy

muscle tissue. Some investigators prefer to biopsy shorter muscles, maximizing the chance of finding the intramuscular nerves. The external intercostal muscle has been used for this reason. Many limb muscles have a single band of terminal motor innervation that corresponds to the so-called motor point. The motor point can be identified with the use of an electrical stimulator. After the administration of local anesthesia and incision of the skin, the muscle is stimulated using a metallic electrode before any tissue is removed. The nerve endings can be located at sites where a single fascicle rather than the whole muscle contracts after stimulation with a very weak current. Once the innervation zone is established electrically, the biopsy is removed. Using a variety of techniques, different portions of the muscle innervation can be subsequently evaluated.

Vital staining with methylene blue has been used to demonstrate the intramuscular nerve twigs as well as the endplates (62). This technique requires that the muscle be injected with a methylene blue solution before the muscle sample is actually taken. An undesirable complication of this technique is muscle pain, which many patients experience during the injection of the dye. In order to preserve the staining of the nerve endings, the biopsy must be oxygenated for one hour. This technique is obviously complicated and not recommended for most laboratories. A simpler but less elegant technique for the demonstration of nerve twigs is the staining of muscle with silver methods such as Bodian's stain. The postjunctional portion of the endplate can be stained histochemically for acetylcholinesterase activity (63). The reaction product is not restricted to the postjunctional membrane, and consequently this is a relatively crude method of studying endplates.

More precise methods of studying endplates involve the use of α-bungarotoxin and freeze-fracture electron microscopy. Alpha-bungarotoxin is derived from cobra venom and binds specifically with the actelycholine

receptor. Immunoperoxidase techniques using α-bungarotoxin allow direct ultrastructural visualization of the postjunctional region of the MEP (64). With the use of freeze-fracture preparations, both the active zones of the presynaptic membrane and the acetylcholine receptors of the postsynaptic membrane can be studied in greater detail (65). In certain rare disorders of the neuromuscular junction, freeze-fracture microscopy may be a useful ancillary diagnostic tool.

The nearly crystalline arrangement of filaments within muscle fibers renders them a suitable subject for x-ray diffraction studies. Diffractograms have provided considerable insight into the architecture and structure of the myofilaments (66). A major advantage of x-ray diffraction is its application to living muscle cells. Recently x-ray diffraction has been enhanced by the use of increasingly powerful x-ray sources and electronic signal detectors that have replaced photographic film. Reflection signals from a living muscle fiber can be adjusted to reveal equatorial reflections from the regular lateral spacing of the filaments or meridional reflections originating from the arrangement of subunits in the direction of the fiber axis, depending on the angle of the diffractogram and the camera light.

Finally, morphometric analysis of muscle tissue is indicated in the event that normal or abnormal findings, such as variations in fiber diameters, are minimal and subtle. In the past, morphometry has been performed manually, using an eyepiece micrometer, but this procedure is time-consuming and tedious. More recently, it has been possible to conduct sophisticated morphometric analysis electronically, using a computer-assisted image analyzer (67). Automated image analysis can be adapted for quantitative measurements on photographs of microscopic sections, but systems also exist for totally automated analysis of images taken directly from microscopic slides or other types of tissue preparations.

FUNCTION

Muscle has at least two major functions. In addition to the obvious role in locomotion, skeletal muscle is also an important participant in general protein metabolism. The reader will recall that muscles are a significant repository of protein for many systemic metabolic requirements. Protein metabolism depends upon a number of factors in a healthy person. These include the rate of protein synthesis and breakdown, which in turn are determined by diet, hormonal influences, growth, and muscular activity. In general, protein synthesis and degradation are governed by the dietary intake of amino acids.

However, the aspect of muscle function that is most familiar relates to contraction, subsequent movement, and locomotion. It is this aspect of skeletal muscle function on which we will concentrate. When a muscle undergoes contraction, it usually exerts force on a movable structure. Isotonic contraction refers to movement that changes the lengths of muscle fibers. If movement does not take place and fiber lengths do not shorten, the contraction is considered to be isometric. The sustained activity of the calf muscles, which do not change length while a person is standing erect, exemplifies isometric contraction. As a rule, a single muscle does not act alone functionally. The coordinated actions of several muscles are usually necessary in the performance of movement. The prime movers are those muscles directly responsible for the desired motion. Antagonists, muscles with opposite action, control the smoothness of the motion. Sometimes agonists and antagonists contract together to stabilize the joint.

An understanding of muscle contraction is predicated on the concept of the motor unit. In simple terms, the motor unit consists of the anterior horn cell that resides in the spinal cord, its motor axon, the intramuscular branches of the main axon (nerve twigs), and the muscle fibers innervated by the twigs. Each motor unit consists of an average of 50 to 100 muscle fibers. The interface between each muscle fiber and its terminal axon is the motor endplate or neuromuscular junction.

There are at least seven critical steps in the process of muscle contraction, each of which will be briefly described (68).

1. The first step is initiated by the excitation and discharge of the motor neuron or anterior horn cell within the spinal cord. The neuronal discharge is associated with a nerve impulse, or action potential, that is propagated along the axon to its terminal. Nerve conduction is an active process so that the impulse travels along the nerve at a constant amplitude and velocity. The impulse is due to a change in ion concentration across the cell membrane that ultimately depends upon alterations in membrane ion channels. Commensurate with depolarization, the voltage-gated sodium channels open, permitting a massive influx of sodium ions.

2. It is useful to remember that the neuromuscular junction consists of presynaptic (PRS) and postsynaptic (POS) regions that are separated by a narrow, intercellular synaptic cleft. The process of neuromuscular transmission is heralded by a depolarization of the PRS axon terminal of the motor nerve, which promotes an elevation of intracellular calcium. Calcium ions gain access to the axoplasm through calcium channels in the PRS membrane. In turn, the synaptic vesicles, which contain acetylcholine (ACh), fuse with the axon membrane. This fusion is calcium dependent and leads to a release of ACh into the extracellular space.

3. Acetylcholine molecules then cross the synaptic cleft and bind to the nicotinic acetylcholine receptors (AChR) on the POS membrane of the muscle fiber. The binding of ACh to the AChR increases the sodium and potassium conductance of the muscle membrane. As a result, there is an influx of sodium ions that is accompanied by a depolarizing potential, representing the endplate potential.

4. The motor endplate potential is transmitted along the entire muscle fiber surface to initiate the contractile response. Since the T tubules are an extension of the sarcolemma, depolarization spreads along the T tubules, which ramify within the sarcoplasm. Depolarization of the transverse tubular membrane activates the SR by means of the dihydropyridine receptors. These are voltage sensors that respond to the T tubule action potential. They are located next to the calcium channels in the T tubule membranes that trigger the release of calcium from the adjacent SR. Calcium is released from the SR through specific calcium channels known as ryanodine receptors (69).

5. Once calcium is released from the SR, it rapidly diffuses through the sarcoplasm. Calcium ions initiate contraction by binding to troponin C. In muscle at rest, troponin I is tightly bound to actin so that tropomyosin covers the sites where myosin can bind to actin. This troponin-tropomyosin complex inhibits the interaction between actin and myosin filaments. When calcium ion binds to troponin C, tropomyosin is displaced laterally, uncovering the binding sites for the myosin heads.

6. The molecular basis of muscle contraction involves the shortening of the contractile elements resulting from a sliding of the thin filaments across the thick filaments. The sliding of actin and myosin filaments occurs when the myosin heads bind to actin to form a crossbridge. X-ray crystallography has revealed that each myosin head has an actin-binding site and an ATP-binding site. The site that binds ATP is cleftlike; but, when ATP is bound and hydrolyzed by ATPase, the conformation of the myosin head changes, and the cleft appears to close. During this conformational change, the rotation of the angle of the crossbridge produces a movement called the power stroke, which advances the myosin filaments along the actin molecules. Every power stroke shortens the muscle approximately 1%. During contraction, numerous power strokes occur each second through crossbridge cycling and involve about 500 myosin heads on each thick filament.

7. Following contraction, the muscle relaxes as calcium ions are pumped back into the SR and calcium is released from troponin. This inhibits the interaction between actin and myosin.

Muscle is sometimes conceptualized as machinery that converts chemical energy into mechanical work. Muscle contraction requires large amounts of energy, which is derived from the intermediary metabolism of lipids and carbohydrates. The metabolism of these energy sources, which lead to the production of ATP, is beyond the scope of this chapter.

GENDER, TRAINING, AND AGING

Some of the earliest studies addressing differences between males and females with regard to muscle fiber size and composition were conducted by Brooke and his colleagues (70). In a seminal study of the biceps muscle in six patients, they established certain principles which remain generally true concerning gender differences in skeletal muscle. Individual muscle fibers are larger in males than in females for several reasons. Explanations include the fact that males are generally bigger than females, being taller and heavier, with a larger muscle mass for body size. Males are also more active and frequently engage in more strenuous physical exertion. Androgens are also thought to play a role in the size of muscle fibers in males, since it is known that testosterone supplements produce muscle fiber hypertrophy. In males, type 2 fibers are usually larger than type 1 fibers, in contrast to females where type 1 fibers tend to be of equal or greater diameter. An excellent summary of this subject was published by Bennington (67) who showed that some of the differences between males and females are dependent upon the muscles sampled. For example, studies of the biceps muscle essentially verify the findings of Brooke et al. However, examination of the vastus lateralis indicates no significant difference in diameter between type 1 and type 2 fibers in males. Another interesting conclusion from these studies addresses the question of fiber type predominance in the two sexes. With regard to the biceps muscle, males have a much higher percentage of type 2 fibers, whereas females have almost equal numbers of each. On the other hand, in the vastus lateralis, both males and females have similar proportions of type 1 and type 2 fibers.

The effect of exercise and training on skeletal muscle has been examined in a host of investigations over the past 25 years. The results of many of these studies are conflicting, but certain general principles have emerged. It is clear that exercise and training of any type causes an increase in muscle fiber diameters. Activities that are basically anaerobic in nature promote hypertrophy of type 2 fibers, a common finding in sprinters. In long distance runners, for whom aerobic metabolism is more important, type 1 fibers tend to be larger. Most authorities agree that power training such as weight lifting results in remarkable hypertrophy of type 2 fibers and less, if any, enlargement of type 1 fibers.

A more controversial topic is whether there is a change in fiber type composition after long periods of training. It is well known that sprinters tend to have larger numbers of type 2 fibers than sedentary controls and long distance runners tend to have more type 1 fibers than untrained counterparts. Many investigators tend to believe that these two groups of runners have genetically determined fiber type composition and little, if any, conversion of fiber types takes place during training. However, some studies have shown that while conversion from type 1 to type 2 fibers probably does not occur, certain activities such as endurance running may be responsible for the conversion of type 2B to type 2A fibers over prolonged periods of time (71). Animal studies have shed minimal light on these questions, in part because animal muscle responds differently to exercise and training than does human muscle. In fact, animal experiments have more often clouded the issues of exercise and fiber composition instead of resolving the controversy.

During the process of aging, there is a functional and structural decline in skeletal muscle beginning in the sixth decade and accelerating after the age of 70 years (72). By the age of 75 years, there is a 30 to 50% decline in muscle strength, the cause of which is complex. Because of the alterations in the composition of their connective tissues, associated with decreased elasticity and flexibility, and because many older patients have joint disease of varying severity, the elderly become less active with a corresponding reduction in muscle volume and contractile strength. Some experts view this condition as a form of disuse. Their conclusions are supported by the fact that aging individuals, like young patients who do not use their muscles (for example, as a result of immobilization in a cast), have selective atrophy of type 2 fibers (Figure 8.16). The effect of poor nutrition in the elderly has not been extensively studied, although it is well known that cachexia is also accompanied by atrophy of type 2 fibers.

A second problem in the elderly population is an insidious damage to the motor units, specifically to the anterior horn cells in the spinal cord. It has repeatedly been shown that with advancing age there is a progressive loss of anterior horn cells. Due to degenerative spine disease, there is also injury to nerve roots, with subsequent radiculopathy. The integrity of the muscle fiber is closely related to the maintenance of its nerve supply. Any sustained interruption of trophic influences from the motor neuron or nerve will culminate in atrophy of the denervated muscle fiber. In acutely denervated muscle, randomly distributed small fibers are seen. When sectioned transversely, atrophic fibers

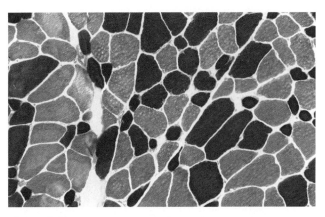

Figure 8.16 Type 2 fiber atrophy (ATPase, pH 9.4, eosin counterstain).

are characteristically angular or ensate. They appear flattened and bipolar with tapering ends. Most or all of the atrophic fibers are dark in alkaline ATPase reactions and are of glycolytic type. At this stage, selective atrophy of type 2 fibers is commonly the only pathologic abnormality, so that the proper diagnosis of denervation requires corroborative clinical information. With progressive denervation, the proportion of atrophic type 1 and type 2 fibers tends to equalize. As long as atrophic fibers remain scattered and are not yet grouped together, from a diagnostic perspective, the pattern of atrophy is nonspecific.

The esterase stain is very useful under these circumstances because denervated fibers are extremely dark in esterase preparations, whereas atrophic fibers in other conditions are not. Atrophic fibers are also excessively dark in oxidative enzyme reactions, but such staining applies to fiber atrophy of almost any cause. Small dark fibers are probably explained by the fact that mitochondria are relatively spared in the atrophic process and occupy a proportionately greater volume of sarcoplasm. The affinity of atrophic fibers for oxidative enzyme stains means that the ATPase reaction is preferable for accurate fiber typing of small fibers, no matter what the pathogenesis of fiber atrophy is.

Prima facie evidence of advanced denervation is a progression from random fiber atrophy to grouped atrophy in which multiple collections of small, angular or ensate fibers are present in the biopsy sample (Figure 8.17). As a consequence of chronic denervation and of reinnervation (73), the normal checkerboard staining profile observed in histoenzymatic reactions is effaced. In an effort to reestablish the nerve supply to denervated muscle fibers, intact intramuscular nerves undergo collateral sprouting, and new synapses are formed with atrophic fibers. As

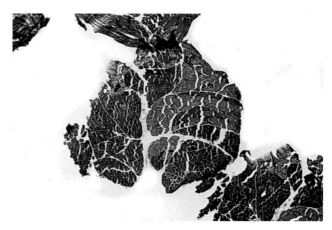

Figure 8.18 Chronic denervation with reinnervation. Type grouping has altered the normal checkerboard staining profile (NADH-TR).

motor units enlarge, reinnervated fibers occupying a large area are converted to one histochemical type. The phenomenon of type grouping (Figure 8.18) is explained by the fact that all muscle fibers within a single motor unit are of the same type—either type 1 or type 2—and the motor neuron, through the trophic influences of its axon and collaterals, governs the histochemical properties of its fibers. The plasticity of muscle fibers allows conversion from one histochemical type to the other when there is reinnervation by a motor neuron of the opposite type. Along with type grouping, target fibers are pathognomic of denervation (74).

Despite their unique specificity, regrettably bone fide target fibers are present in less than 25% of cases of neurogenic atrophy. Although targets and cores are similar morphologically, they differ in three ways. While both tend to occur singly within a fiber, the target is larger in diameter. The target is limited in length, only extending across a few sarcomeres, in contrast to the core, which may run the entire length of the fiber. Most important is the three-zone architecture of the target fiber (Figure 8.19). The central zone, indistinguishable at the ultrastructural level from the unstructured core, is surrounded by an intermediate zone that forms an intensely stained rim in oxidative enzyme reactions. By definition, the intermediate zone, difficult to identify in most other stains, is absent from a core. It is a zone of transition between the central zone of severe sarcoplasmic disruption and the third zone, which represents the normal portion of the muscle fiber. Targetoid fibers, which lack the intermediate zone of increased oxidative enzyme activity, are morphologically identical to core fibers. The term *core* is conventionally used in cases of congenital central core disease, and the term *targetoid* is applied to cores that are found in any other condition. In our experience, targetoid fibers are more commonly encountered in neurogenic atrophy than any other condition and are more frequently seen than target fibers.

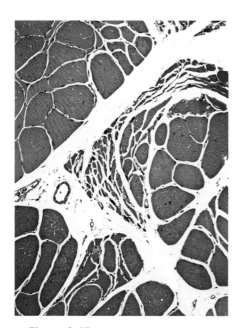

Figure 8.17 Grouped atrophy (H&E).

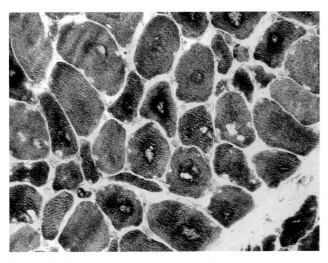

Figure 8.19 Neurogenic atrophy. Target fibers have an inner, un-stained zone surrounded by a rim of increased enzyme activity (NADH-TR).

ARTIFACTS

The most common artifacts are related to unsuspected or inadvertent injury to the muscle specimen, irreverent handling at the time of removal, or to improper tissue sectioning and staining. When they are linear in configuration, needle tracts, such as those produced during electromyography (EMG) studies, may easily be recognized. More often, needle tracts are cut tangentially so that the pathologist may be misled by a histologic picture of myopathy exemplified by fiber necrosis, regeneration, inflammation, and interstitial fibrosis (Figure 8.20). This kind of artifact is generally traceable to poor communication between the physician requesting the biopsy and the individual performing the procedure, who is unaware of the previous intramuscular injections.

Large numbers of neutrophils are occasionally observed within the intramuscular blood vessels. Typically, these cells are marginated and may have begun to penetrate the vascular walls and enter the perimysium or endomysium. In the absence of other pathologic changes within the

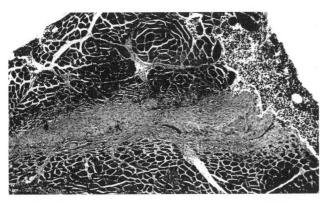

Figure 8.20 Needle tract. Area of injury contains necrotic fibers and a small focus of lymphocytic inflammation (H&E).

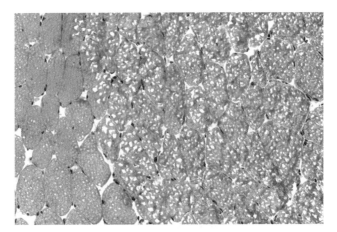

Figure 8.21 Vacuolar artifact. Improper freezing has caused numerous clear holes to form within the fibers (NADH-TR).

specimen, the presence of neutrophils usually means that the muscle has been crushed during the biopsy procedure or it has been infiltrated with anesthetic agent.

Even with the best technical expertise available, muscle tissue is sufficiently fragile that most laboratories find vacuolization of muscle fibers produced during freezing is unavoidable in 10 to 20% of specimens. Vacuolization can be minimized by using proper techniques that permit rapid freezing and by proper specimen storage to prevent thawing. Mild vacuolar artifacts may be tolerable, but large vacuoles that disrupt the sarcoplasm are especially troublesome (Figure 8.21). Larger vacuoles may interfere with accurate biopsy interpretation by distorting the pathologic changes in the sample or by simulating the picture of vacuolar myopathy, such as glycogen or lipid storage disease.

Muscle that is unprotected by isometric clamping is vulnerable to contraction artifact. During uncontrolled contraction, a series of segmental contractions occur along the length of the muscle fiber as the contractile elements are pulled beyond the confines of their respective sarcomeres. This phenomenon is best observed in longitudinal sections where dark hypercontracted regions are punctuated by pale, ghostlike zones of myofibrillar disruption (Figure 8.22). In transverse orientation, these disrupted segments are seen as irregular fissures in the sarcoplasm. Contraction artifact is particularly undesirable when electron microscopic studies are needed, even if the artifact is subtle and cannot be appreciated at the light microscopic level. The detection of ultrastructural abnormalities, which is dependent on the normal alignment of the myofibrils and myofilaments, is compromised by the distortion of sarcomeric structures. Tissue within the teeth of the clamp is sometimes submitted for processing. This tissue, if not entirely crushed and easily recognized as such, may be compressed, producing an artifact that looks like fiber atrophy. A clue to artifact is the difference in fiber diameters in the rest of the biopsy specimen and the clamped fibers, all of which are uniformly small and angular.

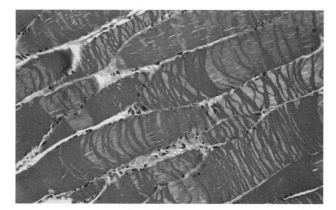

Figure 8.22 Contraction artifact. Dark contraction bands and lucent zones of fiber disruption are seen in longitudinally oriented fibers (H&E).

Dark staining of the sarcoplasm in random fibers is often due to variations in section thickness. Fibers adjacent to the connective tissue of the perimysium are especially susceptible to this artifact. Inconsistencies of section thickness may be recognized when linear, bandlike regions of intense staining are visible within muscle fibers. Excessively pale histochemical reactions can result from the degradation of enzyme systems in the sarcoplasm. Artifacts are distinguished from legitimate abnormal staining if all histochemical reactions in the biopsy are pale. In our experience, this artifact is most often attributable to delayed freezing of the specimen because of a delay in transport. Laboratories that accept consultation specimens from institutions other than their own should be aware of this problem in order to reduce the time required for transportation.

Another transportation-related artifact is seen in specimens shipped in ice when the ice melts, leaving the exposed fresh tissue floating in water. This situation results in a disfiguring and distracting artifact in frozen sections stained with RTC. The normal green staining of the tissue is distorted by irregular red-stained areas that interfere with interpretation of a biopsy (Figure 8.23).

DIFFERENTIAL DIAGNOSIS

Several findings in skeletal muscle biopsies are normal or are minor variations that may be mistaken for pathologic change. These include internal nuclei, ring fibers, hyalin fibers, excessive endomysial connective tissue, perivascular inflammation, variations in fiber diameters, and ragged red fibers.

One of the most common pathological abnormalities in muscle biopsies is nuclear internalization (Figure 8.24). Quantitative analyses have demonstrated that the nuclei are peripherally located in 97 to 99% of normal muscle fibers, which means that up to 3% of fibers with internal nuclei is a normal finding. In many different conditions, an increase in internal nuclei is found, typically affecting 5 to 10% of fibers and particularly those that are mildly atrophic. Nuclear internalization has no specific diagnostic significance and appears to be a reaction to virtually any type of injury. The diagnosis of myotonic dystrophy should be strongly considered if the majority of fibers contain internal nuclei.

One must exercise caution in interpreting the significance of ring fibers in specimens disrupted by contraction artifact because, in this situation, ring fibers are not a genuine pathologic change. In properly processed, uncontracted muscle biopsies, ring fibers are a pathologic criterion of myotonic disorders. The ring is formed by a bundle of peripheral myofibrils that are circumferentially oriented such that they encircle the internal portion of the sarcoplasm, which is normal in structure and orientation. In cross sections of muscle, the ring is especially well visualized in PAS stains where the striations of the transversely oriented peripheral myofibrils are seen in contrast to the inner sarcoplasmic contents (Figure 8.25). Rings are also seen to advantage in PTAH stains, resin sections, or under phase contrast microscopy. Under the electron microscope,

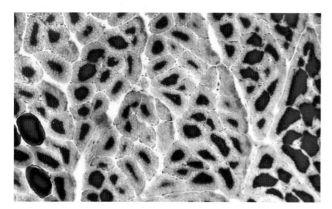

Figure 8.23 Exposure of fresh muscle to water during transport may cause an abnormal staining pattern in RTC, obscuring the detail and granular appearance of mitochondria (RTC).

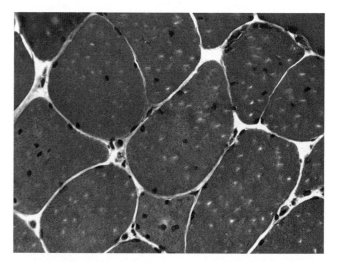

Figure 8.24 Nuclear internalization. Several fibers contain internal pyknotic nuclei, a common nonspecific pathologic change (H&E).

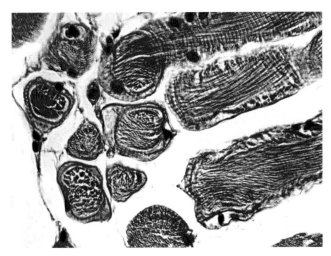

Figure 8.25   Ring fibers. Bundles of myofibrils are circumferentially oriented, forming rings that encircle transversely sectioned fibers. (PAS).

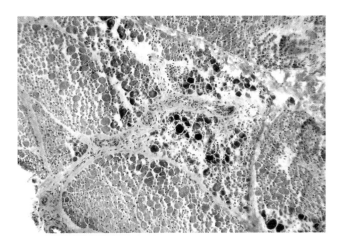

Figure 8.27   Infant muscle. A relative increase in perimysial connective tissue is normal (trichrome).

the pathologically oriented myofibrils are generally normal in structure except for hypercontraction of the sarcomeres (75).

Along with ring fibers, hyalin fibers are evident in specimens damaged by contraction artifact. These fibers are abnormally increased in diameter and rounded in configuration. Their sarcoplasm in both paraffin and frozen sections is smudged or glassy and more deeply stained than in normal fibers (Figure 8.26). The hyalin appearance is the legacy of hypercontraction, as shown in electron microscopic studies. In clamped specimens that are free of excessive contraction, true hyalin fibers are a common feature of Duchenne muscular dystrophy. The pathogenesis of true hyalin fiber formation, which is believed to precede subsequent fiber necrosis (76), is apparently related to excessive irritability secondary to cell membrane instability. It is possible that sarcolemmal damage allows excessive contraction and also

promotes cell necrosis. In serial sections of hyalin fibers, areas of necrosis may be found, indicating the importance of hyalinization as a sign of fiber destruction.

Excessive quantities of endomysial connective tissue usually represent reactive fibrosis accompanying neuromuscular disease. However, as pointed out above, at the interface between muscle and tendons or fascia, abundant connective tissue is normally present and should not be regarded as reactive fibrosis. Although endomysial connective tissue is not prominent in the biopsies of infants, as indicated previously, the perimysial connective tissue far exceeds the amount present in older children and adults (Figure 8.27).

Interstitial and perivascular inflammatory cells almost always reflect clinical disease, most frequently immunologically mediated or idiopathic inflammatory myopathies such as polymyositis or dermatomyositis. However, in the biopsies of infants it is well to remember that small foci of hematopoiesis are normally present and do not represent true inflammatory infiltrates. Muscles subjected to trauma such as EMG needles may harbor foci of inflammation for months following the diagnostic study and are not clinically significant.

One of the most demanding challenges to the diagnostic pathologist is the muscle biopsy characterized by a variation in fiber diameters or by what appears to be atrophy or hypertrophy. The utility of enzyme histochemistry in these situations cannot be overstated. It is important to recall from previous discussions that (a) a normal variation in fiber size occurs at the junctions of muscle fibers and either tendons or fascia and (b) what at first seems to be atrophy may be normal, depending upon the muscle examined and upon the patient's age and sex. Smaller muscles, and especially those devoted to finely coordinated activities, have much smaller diameters than large, bulky muscles. Muscle fibers are expected to be much smaller in infants and children than in mature adults; and, as previously noted, there

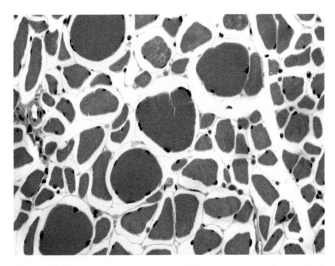

Figure 8.26   Hyalin fibers. Several fibers are enlarged, rounded, with darkly stained sarcoplasm. (H&E).

is an increasing reduction in fiber diameters with advancing age. The significance of fiber hypertrophy should be evaluated in light of the patient's activity and level of regular exercise. In evaluating fiber size, it may be necessary to measure fiber diameters.

Morphometric analysis of the muscle biopsy is imperative when the changes in fiber diameters are minimal and subtle. In order to obtain statically significant morphometric data, the lesser diameter of each muscle fiber should be determined, based upon a minimum number of 200 fibers in the sample (77). The atrophic or hypertrophic process may be selective, affecting only one fiber type, or it may be nonselective (78). True selective atrophy of type 1 fibers is most commonly encountered in myotonic dystrophy. Type 2 fiber atrophy is a common finding in acute denervation, disuse, and myasthenia gravis. True hypertrophy of type 1 fibers is relatively specific for infantile spinal muscular atrophy. True type 2 fiber hypertrophy is generally restricted to congenital fiber-type disproportion. The pattern of atrophy is important in distinguishing between normal and abnormal. Randomly distributed small or large fibers may be normal, depending on other factors discussed above. Grouped atrophy, where five or more small angular fibers cluster together is essentially diagnostic of chronic neurogenic disease. Panfascicular atrophy, in which the majority of fibers in each fascicle are atrophic, is virtually specific for infantile spinal muscle atrophy. Perifascicular atrophy is typical of dermatomyositis.

Ragged red fibers can be observed in elderly people (79). These fibers are recognized in RTC stains performed on frozen sections, where they exhibit an irregular surface and collections of red staining subsarcolemmal material (Figure 8.28). The ragged red areas represent foci of increased, often abnormal mitochondria. Ragged red fibers are generally the hallmark of the mitochondrial myopathies, which are characterized by mitochondrial dysfunction and often mutations of mitochondrial genes (41). It is now known that mitochondrial damage occurs in the aging cell, including skeletal muscle. Ragged red fibers are considered to be a reflection of this damage, which may be associated with clinical disease but frequently is not.

SPECIMEN HANDLING

Muscle biopsies should be performed by physicians with expertise in biopsy technique and a sincere interest in obtaining the best possible specimen. The physician who has direct responsibility for the patient's care needs to be sure that the biopsy comes from an appropriate muscle so that it is representative of the disease process. In some conditions, the disease process is widespread, such as in many metabolic diseases, and virtually any muscle is suitable for biopsy. However, in other disorders where, for example, symptoms are referable to the legs and spare the arms, a biopsy of the deltoid or biceps brachii muscle is unlikely to reflect the disease process accurately and may be normal or nondiagnostic. Moreover, whenever possible, the tissue sample should be obtained from a region in which the disease process remains active rather than quiescent. In a muscle where the disease process has subsided, the biopsy is apt to be unremarkable. In severely involved muscle, particularly if there is marked weakness or wasting, the pathologic findings are likely to be those of end-stage disease which may defy conclusive pathologic interpretation. Muscles subjected to previous traumatic injury, such as needle tracts incurred during EMG or intramuscular injections of medications, and muscles altered by an unrelated disease process should not be biopsied. The pathologic picture in such muscles may simulate that associated with a variety of neuromuscular diseases and will confuse the pathologist.

The special handling of the muscle biopsy precludes submission of the specimen on weekends and holidays or late in the workday afternoon when laboratory personnel are not available to receive and process the tissue. If possible, a technician familiar with the biopsy technique should assist the physician performing the biopsy and collect the specimen properly. Two separate specimens from the same site are routinely required. The first specimen is maintained at isometric length by its insertion in a muscle clamp. This device is designed to minimize contraction artifact, which inevitably results when an incision is made in the muscle, and it is immersed in fixative. Since the muscle is introduced into the instrument lengthwise, the sample is conveniently oriented for further processing. The biopsy must extend entirely across the clamp, thereby ensuring an acceptable specimen size of at least 1 cm in length. The biopsy should be of sufficient size to maximize the opportunity of observing the entire pathologic process. To

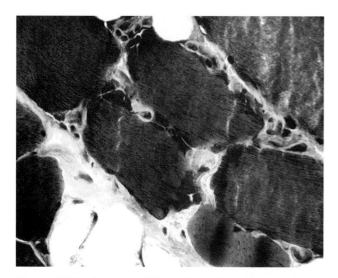

Figure 8.28 Ragged red fibers. Ragged red fibers are recognized in RTC stain as having an irregular sarcolemmal surface with collections of red-staining material (RTC).

attain this goal, some clinicians favor obtaining two biopsies routinely, one from the arm and one from the leg, for example. Thus, the major drawback to needle biopsy, which has certain advantages over open biopsy, is the limited size of the sample.

While there is some disagreement regarding the primary fixative for muscle biopsies, we have elected to use 10% formalin, buffered to a pH of 7.4 in a 0.1 M phosphate buffer. Strips of muscle 1 mm in width are dissected from the edges of the sample and postfixed in phosphate-buffered 2% glutaraldehyde for electron microscopic study. After fixation for a minimum of 24 hours in 10% phosphate-buffered formalin, the remainder of the sampled specimen is used for routine paraffin sections. A second unfixed specimen measuring $1 \times 0.5 \times 0.5$ cm is obtained for the preparation of frozen sections. Although the utilization of a muscle clamp is not mandatory, clamping the specimen will help in its orientation.

Several techniques are described for flash freezing (80), but we prefer freezing the sample in liquid nitrogen after coating the surface of the specimen with talc. Whatever technique is employed, the condition on which the freezing technique is based is that it proceeds with extreme rapidity, within 10 to 15 seconds. Freezing the tissue in a cryostat in a fashion similar to most specimens submitted for frozen section diagnosis from the operating room is contraindicated. The frozen sample should be oriented so that cross sections of muscle are cut. Serial frozen sections in our laboratory are stained with H&E, rapid Gomori's trichrome (RTC), and three standard histochemical reactions: ATPase (pH 9.4 and 4.6) and NADH-TR. Other stains such as periodic acid-Schiff (PAS) for glycogen, phosphorylase, and fat stains are performed when indicated. Frozen tissue may also be used for biochemical analysis, for immunohistochemical preparations, and for immunofluorescence microscopy. Inasmuch as frozen tissue may be needed for future additional studies, muscle biopsies can be sealed in airtight plastic capsules or bags to prevent dessication and freezing artifact while stored in an ultralow freezer at $-70\,^{\circ}$C.

REFERENCES

1. Jacob M, Christ B, Jacob HJ. On the migration of myogenic stem cells into the prospective wing region of chick embryos. A scanning and transmission electron microscope study. *Anat Embryol (Berl)* 1978;153:179–193.
2. Larsen WJ. *Human Embryology.* New York: Churchill Livingstone; 1993:281–307.
3. Okazaki K, Holtzer H. Myogenesis: fusion, myosin synthesis, and the mitotic cycle. *Proc Natl Acad Sci U S A* 1966;56:1484–1490.
4. Yaffe D. Developmental changes preceding cell fusion during muscle differentiation in vitro. *Exp Cell Res* 1971;66:33–48.
5. Wakshull E, Bayne EK, Chiquet M, Fambrough DM. Characterization of a plasma membrane glycoprotein common to myoblasts, skeletal muscle satellite cells, and glia. *Dev Biol* 1983;100: 464–477.
6. Keeter JS, Pappas GD, Model PG. Inter- and intramyotomal gap junctions in the axolotl embryo. *Dev Biol* 1975;45:21–33.
7. Chiquet M, Eppenberger HM, Turner DC. Muscle morphogenesis: evidence for an organizing function of exogenous fibronectin. *Dev Biol* 1981;88:220–235.
8. Kelly AM, Zacks SI. The histogenesis of rat intercostal muscle. *J Cell Biol* 1969;42:135–153.
9. Ishikawa H, Bischoff R, Holtzer H. Mitosis and intermediate-sized filaments in developing skeletal muscle. *J Cell Biol* 1968;38: 538–555.
10. Franklin GI, Yasin R, Hughes BP, Thompson EJ. Acetylcholine receptors in cultured human muscle cells. *J Neurol Sci* 1980;47: 317–327.
11. Martin L, Joris C. Histoenzymological and semiquantitative study of the maturation of the human muscle fiber. In: Walton JN, Canal N, Scarlato G, eds. *Disease of Muscle.* Amsterdam: Excerpta Medica; 1970:657.
12. Wohlfart G. Ueber das vorkommen verschiedener arten von muskelfarsern in der skelettmusculatur der menschen und einiger saugetiere. *Acta Psychiatr Neurol* 1937;12(suppl):119.
13. Fenichel GM. A histochemical study of developing human skeletal muscle. *Neurology* 1966;16:741–745.
14. Carlson BM. *Human Embryology and Developmental Biology.* Philadelphia: Mosby; 2005.
15. Goldspink G. Sarcomere length during post-natal growth of mammalian muscle fibers. *J Cell Sci* 1968;3:539–548.
16. Close RI. Dynamic properties of mammalian skeletal muscles. *Physiol Rev* 1972;52:129–197.
17. Goldspink G. Postembryonic growth and differentiation of striated muscle. In: Bourne GH, ed. *The Structure and Function of Muscle.* Vol. 1. New York: Academic Press; 1972:179–236.
18. Stickland NC. Muscle development in the human fetus as exemplified by m. sartorius. *J Anat* 1981;132(pt 4):557–579.
19. Adams RD, DeReuck J. Metrics of muscle. In: Kakulas BA, ed. *Basic Research in Myology.* Amsterdam: Exerpta Medica; 1972.
20. Kakulas BA, Adams RD. Embryology and histology of skeletal muscle. *Diseases of Muscle. Pathological Foundations of Clinical Myology.* 4th ed. Philadelphia: Harper and Row; 1985:8–9.
21. Adhihetty PJ, Hood DA. Mechanisms of apoptosis in skeletal muscle. *Basic Appl Myol* 2003;13:171–179.
22. Hamburger V. History of the discovery of neuronal death in embryos. *J Neurobiol* 1992; 23:1116–1123.
23. Sohal GS. Sixth Annual Stuart Reiner Memorial Lecture: embryonic development of nerve and muscle. *Muscle Nerve* 1995; 18:2–14.
24. McClearn D, Medville R, Noden D. Muscle cell death during the development of head and neck muscles in the chick embryo. *Dev Dyn* 1995;202:365–377.
25. Abood EA, Jones MM. Macrophages in developing mammalian skeletal muscle: evidence for muscle fiber death as a normal developmental event. *Acta Anat* 1991;140:201–212.
26. Fidzianska A, Goebel HH. Human ontogenesis. 3. Cell death in fetal muscle. *Acta Neuropathol (Berl)* 1991;81:572–577.
27. MacKenzie WC. *The Action of Muscles, Including Muscle Rest and Muscle Re-education.* New York: Hoeber; 1921.
28. Feinstein B, Lindegård B, Nyman E, Wohlfart G. Morphological studies of motor units in normal human muscles. *Acta Anat* 1955;23:127–142.
29. Clemente CD, ed. *Gray's Anatomy.* 30th Amer. ed. Philadelphia: Lea and Febiger; 1985:434–436.
30. Blomfield LB. Intramuscular vascular patterns in man. *Proc Roy Soc Med* 1945;38:617–618.
31. Renkin EM, Hudlicka O, Sheehan RM. Influence of metabolic vasodilatation on blood-tissue diffusion in skeletal muscle. *Am J Physiol* 1966;211:87–98.
32. Emslie-Smith AM, Engel AG. Microvascular changes in early and advanced dermatomyositis: a quantitative study. *Ann Neurol* 1990;27:343–356.
33. Schmalbruch H. Rote muskelfasern. *Z Zellforsch Mikrosk Anat* 1971;119:120–146.
34. Heuser JE, Reese TS, Landis DM. Functional changes in frog neuromuscular junctions studied with freeze-fracture. *J Neurocytol* 1974;3:109–131.

35. Ellisman MH, Rash JE, Staehelin LA, Porter KR. Studies of excitable membranes. II. A comparison of specializations at neuromuscular junctions and nonjunctional sarcolemmas of mammalian fast and slow twitch muscle fibers. *J Cell Biol* 1976;68:752–774.

36. Ross MJ, Klymkowsky MW, Agard DA, Stroud RM. Structural studies of a membrane-bound acetylcholine receptor from Torpedo californica. *J Mol Biol* 1977;116:635–659.

37. Carpenter S, Karpati G. *Pathology of Skeletal Muscle.* New York: Churchill Livingstone; 1984.

38. DeGirolami U, Smith TW. Teaching monograph: pathology of skeletal muscle diseases. *Am J Pathol* 1982;107:231–276.

39. Dubowitz V, Brooke MH. *Muscle Biopsy. A Modern Approach.* Philadelphia: WB Saunders; 1973.

40. Engel AG, Franzini-Armstrong C, eds. *Myology.* 2nd ed. New York: McGraw-Hill; 1994.

41. Heffner RR, ed. *Muscle Pathology.* New York: Churchill Livingstone; 1984.

42. Heffner RR Jr. Muscle biopsy in the diagnosis of neuromuscular disease. *Semin Diagn Pathol* 1984;1:114–151.

43. Heffner RR Jr, Balos LL. *Muscle biopsy in neuromuscular diseases.* In: Mills SE, ed. *Sternberg's Diagnostic Surgical Pathology.* Vol. 1. 4th ed. Philadelphia: Lippincott Williams & Wilkins; 2004:111–135.

44. Kakulas BA, Adams RD. *Diseases of Muscle. Pathological Foundations of Clinical Myology.* 4th ed. Philadelphia: Harper & Row; 1985.

45. Karpati G, ed. *Structural and Molecular Basis of Skeletal Muscle Diseases.* Basel: ISN Neuropathology Press; 2002.

46. Mastaglia FL, Walton JN, eds. *Skeletal Muscle Pathology.* 2nd ed. Edinburg: Churchill Livingstone; 1992.

47. Pearson CM, Mostofi FK, eds. *The Striated Muscle.* Baltimore: Williams & Wilkins; 1973.

48. Swash M, Schwartz MS. *Neuromuscular Diseases. A Practical Approach to Diagnosis and Management.* New York: Springer-Verlag; 1981.

49. Schmalbruch H. Muscle fibers as members of motor units. *Skeletal Muscle.* Berlin: Springer-Verlag; 1985:301.

50. Brooke MH, Engel WK. The histographic analysis of human muscle biopsies with regard to fiber types. 4. Children's biopsies. *Neurology* 1969;19:591–605.

51. Bowden DH, Goyer RA. The size of muscle fibers in infants and children. *Arch Pathol* 1960;69:188–189.

52. Vogler C, Bove KE. Morphology of skeletal muscle in children. An assessment of normal growth and differentiation. *Arch Pathol Lab Med* 1985;109:238–242.

53. Miosge N, Klenczar C, Herken R, Willem M, Mayer U. Organization of the myotendinous junction is dependent on the presence of α7β1 integrin. *Lab Invest* 1999;79:1591–1599.

54. Kolliker A. Mikroskopische Antomie odor Gewebelehre des Menschen. Leipzig: Engelmann; 1850:253–255.

55. Bakker GJ, Richmond FJ. Two types of muscle spindles in cat neck muscles: a histochemical study of intrafusal fiber composition. *J Neurophysiol* 1981;45:973–986.

56. Swash M, Fox KP. Muscle spindle innervation in man. *J Anat* 1972;112(pt 1):61–80.

57. Campion DR. The muscle satellite cell: a review. *Int Rev Cytol* 1984;87:225–251.

58. Hoffman EP, Wang J. Duchenne-Becker muscular dystrophy and the nondystrophic myotonias. Paradigms for loss of function and change of function of gene products. *Arch Neurol* 1993;50:1227–1237.

59. Johns DR. Mitochondrial DNA and disease. *N Engl J Med* 1995;333:638–644.

60. Jay V, Becker LE. Fiber-type differentiation by myosin immunohistochemistry on paraffin-embedded skeletal muscle. A useful adjunct to fiber typing by the adenosine triphosphatase reaction. *Arch Pathol Lab Med* 1994;118:917–918.

61. Ohlendieck K, Matsumura MD, Ionasescu VV, et al. Duchenne muscular dystrophy: deficiency of dystrophin-associated proteins in the sarcolemma. *Neurology* 1993;43:795–800.

62. Coers C, Woolf AL. *The Innervation of Muscle: A Biopsy Study.* Springfield, Il: Charles C Thomas; 1959.

63. Koelle GB, Friedenwald JS. A histochemical method for localizing cholinesterase activity. *Proc Soc Exp Biol Med* 1949;70:617–622.

64. Engel AG, Lindstrom JM, Lambert EH, Lennon VA. Ultrastructural localization of the acetylcholine receptor in myasthenia gravis and in its experimental autoimmune model. *Neurology* 1977;27:307–315.

65. Engel AG, Fukunaga H, Osame M. Stereometric estimation of the area of the freeze-fractured membrane. *Muscle Nerve* 1982;5:682–685.

66. Wray JS, Holmes KC. X-ray diffraction studies of muscle. *Annu Rev Physiol* 1981;43:553–565.

67. Bennington JL, Krupp M. Morphometric analysis of muscle. In: Heffner RR, ed. *Muscle Pathology.* New York: Churchill Livingstone; 1984:43–71.

68. Goodman SR. *Medical Cell Biology.* Philadelphia: Lippincott; 1994;61–100.

69. MacLennan DH, Duff C, Zorzato F, et al. Ryanodine receptor gene is a candidate for predisposition to malignant hyperthermia. *Nature* 1990;343:559–561.

70. Brooke MH, Kaiser KK. Muscle fiber types: how many and what kind? *Arch Neurol* 1970;23:369–379.

71. Gunby P. Runner's ability depends partly on muscle fiber type. *JAMA* 1979;242:1712–1713.

72. Lexell J, Henriksson-Larsen K, Winblad B, Sjostrom M. Distribution of different fiber types in human skeletal muscles: effects of aging studied in whole muscle cross sections. *Muscle Nerve* 1983;6:588–595.

73. Karpati G, Engel WK. "Type grouping" in skeletal muscles after experimental reinnervation. *Neurology* 1968;18:447–455.

74. Engel WK. Muscle target fibres, a newly recognized sign of denervation. *Nature* 1961;191:389–390.

75. Heffner RR Jr. Electron microscopy of disorders of skeletal muscle. *Ann Clin Lab Sci* 1975;5:338–347.

76. Cullen MJ, Fulthorpe JJ. Stages in fibre breakdown in Duchenne muscular dystrophy. *J Neurol Sci* 1975;24:179–200.

77. Dubowitz V, Brooke MH. *Muscle Biopsy. A Modern Approach.* Philadelphia: WB Saunders; 1973.

78. Engel WK. Selective and nonselective susceptibility of muscle fiber types. A new approach to human neuromuscular diseases. *Arch Neurol* 1970;22:97–117.

79. Mendell JR. Mitochondrial myopathy in the elderly: exaggerated aging in the pathogenesis of disease. *Ann Neurol* 1995;37:3–4.

80. Bossen EH. Collection and preparation of the muscle biopsy. In: Heffner RR, ed. *Muscle Pathology.* Vol 3. New York: Churchill Livingstone; 1984:11–14.

Blood Vessels

9

Patrick J. Gallagher   Allard C. van der Wal

GROSS AND LIGHT MICROSCOPIC FEATURES

The normal structure of vessels, particularly the aorta, elastic and muscular arteries, and the larger veins, change progressively throughout life (Table 9.1) (1,2). These aging changes lead to increased arterial stiffness, detected clinically by alterations in pulse wave velocity (3). It is now clear that aging arteries are especially affected by common disorders such as atherosclerosis, hypertension, and diabetes (Table 9.2). Surgical pathologists must be fully aware not only of the nature and extent of these alterations, but also of their variation from site to site.

Aorta

The length and breadth of the aorta increase progressively throughout life. Although there are some variations in the rate of these changes, both between men and women and from decade to decade, the process continues well into a person's seventies and eighties. This enlargement produces the characteristic unfolding of the aorta so often seen in chest radiographs; and, if the aortic valve annulus is also involved, aortic incompetence can result. Some atherosclerosis is almost inevitable in the abdominal aorta in the middle aged and elderly, but aging changes are independent of this.

The principal components of all arteries are elastic and collagen fibers, smooth muscle cells, and a mucopolysaccharide-rich ground substance (4). In the media of the aorta and the carotid, the innominate and proximal axillary arteries elastic fibers predominate. Parallel lamellar units of elastin enclose smooth muscle cells, ground substance, and collagen (Figure 9.1). There are about 40 lamellar units at birth and at least 50 in adult life, each measuring about 11 μm in thickness. Interconnecting bands of collagen and elastin fibers provide strength, whereas the lamellar arrangement distributes stress evenly across the wall, smoothing the cyclical pressure waves of cardiac contraction (5). Elastic fragmentation with associated foci of fibrosis are the most prominent aging changes and account for the weakening that leads to aortic dilatation (Figure 9.2). The changes in the structure of the extracellular matrix are

TABLE 9.1

AGING CHANGES IN BLOOD VESSELS

	Major Macroscopic and Histologic Features
Aorta	Progressive and linear increase in diameter with age. Eccentric or diffuse fibrous intimal thickening. Fragmentation of elastic lamellae with widening of interlamellar spaces. Focal amyloid deposits. Thickening of walls of vasa vasorum.
Muscular arteries	Progressive dilatation and tortuosity. Caliber of vessels usually less in females, especially coronary arteries. Intimal fibrosis, sometimes suggesting reduplication of the internal elastic lamella. Focal fragmentation and calcification of internal elastic lamella. Increased fibrosis and hyalinization of media. No significant inflammation in atheroma-free segments.
Arterioles	Intimal thickening, usually as concentric layers of fibroelastic tissue. Hyalinization of media.
Capillaries	Basement membrane thickening, approximately twofold increase in thickness from puberty to old age.
Venules and veins	Few detailed studies of small veins. Larger veins show intimal fibrosis and hypertrophy of both circular and longitudinal bundles.

thought to be the result of upregulation of genes that mediate matrix metalloproteinase production (6). Apoptosis can be demonstrated in a number of cell types within atheromatous plaques (7) but is unlkely to be a key factor in the aging of the arterial wall (8). Calcification is a common complication; and, although it is most frequent in atheromatous segments, it may occur in areas where the intima is virtually normal. The underlying causes of aortic and coronary arterial calcification remain poorly understood (9,10). Small amounts of amyloid can be detected in aortic atheromatous lesions of middle-aged and elderly subjects and may be derived from serum amyloid A or other apolipoproteins (11,12).

Cystic medial degeneration (CMD), originally called *medionecrosis aortae* by Erdheim, is a difficult concept, and many pathologists are unsure about the exact meaning of the term. Histologically, the condition is characterized by degeneration and fragmentation of the elastic layers of the media and formation of mucoid pools (Figure 9.1B–C). Some areas have few, if any, stainable nuclei, and this is the result of smooth muscle cell death. More recently, areas of smooth muscle cell apoptosis and disorganized proliferation, fibrosis, and angiogenesis have been described, suggesting that CMD is a process of degenerative injury and repair. In 1977, Schlatmann and Becker (13) showed that the histological alterations of CMD showed a striking correlation with age and

may therfore represent the normal aging process of elastic arteries. The same features are seen in hypertensive patients, who have an altered hemodynamic profile, and in genetic disorders of connective tissue, such as Marfan's or some types of the Ehlers-Danlos syndrome. They have also been reported in patients with a history of cocaine abuse (14). In connective tissue disorders, CMD is more pronounced and leads to complications such as intramural hematoma formation or aortic dissection at an earlier age.

Although the exact cause of CMD is unknown, it appears to be related to an imbalance between the mechanical forces imposed on the aortic wall during systole and the

TABLE 9.2

HISTOLOGIC CHANGES IN ARTERIES AND ARTERIOLES

Condition	Major Histologic Features
Normal adults	Minimal intimal thickening, may be eccentric or diffuse. Intact internal elastic lamella, occasional small breaks only. No significant inflammation.
Atherosclerosis	Eccentric fibrous intimal thickening, intimal and medial foam cell and lipid deposition. Neovascularization with intimal and medial hemorrhage. Dystrophic calcification. Adventitial aggregates of plasma cells, lymphocytes, and histiocytes. Intimal and medial aggregates of T lymphocytes, especially at shoulders of lesion. The most important complication is rupture of fibrous cap of the lesion with associated thrombus formation.
Systematic hypertension	Concentric fibrous intimal thickening and medial hypertrophy, especially in arterioles. Changes pronounced in accelerated or malignant phase, with fibrinoid necrosis. Aneurysmal dilation of intracerebral arterioles and capillaries. Increased atherosclerosis.
Diabetes mellitus	Hyalin change in arterioles. Capillary microaneurysms with basement membrane thickening. Loss of pericytes; retinal neovascularization. Increased atherosclerosis in arteries.
Active arteritis	Acute or chronic inflammatory cell inflammation of adventitia and media. Mural edema, reactive intimal thickening, and endothelial necrosis. Fibrinoid necrosis of wall, occasionally aneurysmal dilatation.
Healed arteritis	Bizarre patterns of disordered fibrous intimal thickening. Medial scarring with patchy aggregates of chronic inflammatory cells. Abnormally prominent medial blood vessels.

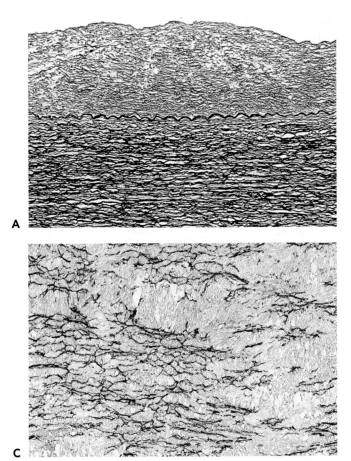

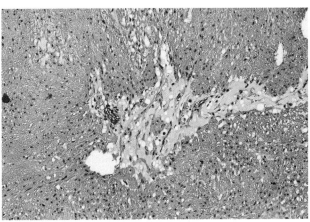

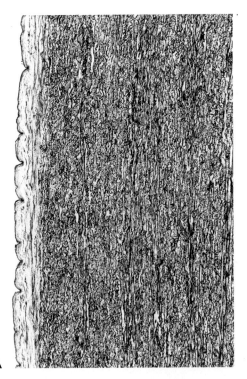

Figure 9.1 **A.** Inner half of the aortic wall of a 62-year-old man. There is a moderate degree of fibrous intimal thickening, which has no immediate clinical relevance but may predispose to atherosclerosis. There was only slight fragmentation of the elastic lamellae; the overall appearance is well within normal limits for a patient of this age (elastic van Gieson). **B.** The typical appearance of cystic medial degeneration in an H&E–stained section. Note the prominent pool of mucoid material. **C.** This shows a corresponding section to B but is stained for elastic tissue. There is extensive loss of the normal elastic framework.

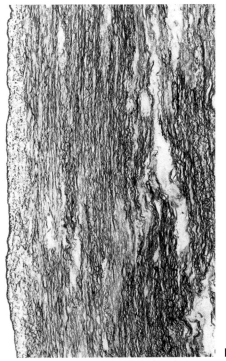

Figure 9.2 **A.** The normal appearance of the aortic media of a 48-year-old man. There are many parallel lamellae of elastic tissue. There is no significant intimal thickening. **B.** The aortic wall of a 31-year-old man with Marfan's syndrome. The medial elastic tissue is extensively fragmented, and there is fibrosis and loose mucopolysaccharide-rich areas. Such extensive changes would be unusual even in an elderly patient. (Elastic van Gieson.)

capacity of the aortic wall to resist these forces. The resulting shear forces may cause alterations in the secretion pattern of smooth muscle cells or their death by apoptosis. More recently, p53 accumulation, *bax* upregulation, and both vascular smooth muscle cell apoptosis and regeneration have been demonstrated in areas of cystic medial necrosis (15). In Marfan's syndrome, the histologic changes suggest exaggerated aging, but there are no features that allow a specific diagnosis to be made (Figure 9.2B). The underlying genetic abnormality involves a glycoprotein, fibrillin, that is closely associated with elastin fibers. The exact functions of fibrillin and other associated glycoproteins are uncertain, but they may act as a "scaffold" on which elastin fibers are laid down. There is a wide spectrum of clinical abnormalities in Marfan's syndrome, and certain clinical features, such as arachnodactyly or aortic dissection, are especially common in some families (16).

Elastic fragmentation and associated medial necrosis are the most common histologic findings in both ascending and thoracic aortic aneurysms. Despite thinning of the wall due to vascular dilatation, the cellular and matrix components in thoracic aneurysms are in fact increased as a result of vascular smooth muscle hyperplasia. In contrast in abdominal aortic aneurysms there is a reduction in smooth muscle density in abdominal aortic aneurysms (17,18). Traditionally, abdominal aortic aneurysms have been considered atheromatous in origin, but this is an oversimplification. Genetic studies have provided compelling evidence for an inherited basis of this disease. Aneurysms have been detected in up to 20% of first degree relatives, especially when the affected subject is female (19). Whether the atherosclerosis is the primary cause or a secondary complication, the inflammation and medial scarring that accompany all but the earliest stages of atheroma further damage a wall already weakened by normal aging or by specific genetically determined alterations in the matrix of the aortic wall. Patchy chronic inflammatory

aggregates, including lymphocytes and plasma cells, are often present in the adventitia of atheromatous segments of the aorta and coronary arteries (Figure 9.3). In biopsies of the ascending aorta during repair of dissecting aneurysms or aortic reconstructions for root dilatation, these chronic adventitial infiltrates must not be mistaken as evidence of aortitis. Small collections of lymphocytes, macrophages, and giant cells are occasionally seen in these biopsies. Although they should be reported, our experience is that they have no clinical significance. In some abdominal aneurysms, the inflammatory infiltrates are especially dense, and surgical repair may be difficult. The inflammation may be a reaction to ceroid pigment, and there can be associated retroperitoneal fibrosis (20).

Cardiac surgeons have several techniques for repairing aortic coarctations and may submit samples of aorta, the narrowed aortic segment, the subclavian artery, or the ductus arteriosus (arterial duct) for histologic identification. The aorta around the coarctation may show reactive intimal thickening, even in neonates, but the underlying elastic structure is usually well preserved. The coarctation itself can have a variety of appearances. In long-standing cases, there may be dense intimal and medial fibrosis. In neonates, the intima may have a distinctly irregular pattern of fibroelastic intimal thickening, resembling some forms of arterial dysplasia (Figure 9.4). The structure of the arterial duct changes progressively during intrauterine growth and in the postnatal period (21) and can be influenced by prostaglandin treatment. Unlike the aorta and the proximal subclavian artery, which are elastic vessels, the arterial duct has a muscular media and a defined internal elastic lamella.

Arteries

It is only in children and young adults that muscular arteries conform to the classical descriptions of textbooks. The

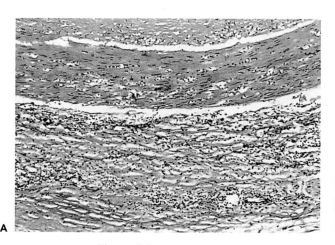
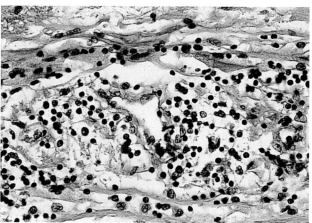

A   B

Figure 9.3 A. and B. Adventitial chronic inflammatory infiltrates in the wall of an atheromatous coronary artery. A few inflammatory cells have infiltrated into the media. The magnified view on the right confirms that most of the inflammatory cells are lymphocytes or plasma cells.

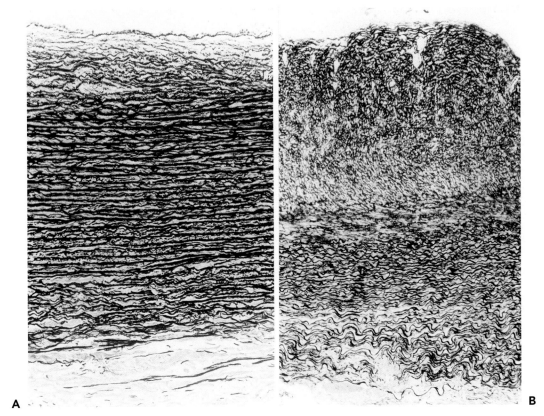

Figure 9.4 Coarctation of the aorta. **A.** The aortic wall distal to a coarctation in a 3-month-old child. There is slight intimal edema only. **B.** The coarctation itself; note the irregular arrangement of the intimal fibroelastic tissue. (Elastic van Gieson.)

intima of arteries is defined as the region from and including the endothelium to the luminal margin of the media (22). At birth, the intima is a virtual space with the endothelium closely opposed to the internal elastic lamella. This layer thickens slowly with age, either (a) eccentrically at branching points or bifurcations or (b) diffusely. Both types occur preferentially at sites of altered blood flow or mechanical stress, suggesting that they are adaptive changes (a response to injury). Vascular smooth muscle cells derived from the underlying media and extracellular matrix proteins accumulate in the thickened intima and may serve as a "soil" for the development of atherosclerotic plaques. For example, in the aorta and coronary arteries, the so-called atherosclerosis prone areas are those that show early diffuse or eccentric thickening.

Progressive intimal fibrosis affects nearly all arteries (Figure 9.5), but in surgical pathology material it is especially noticeable in the spleen, myometrium, and thyroid (Figure 9.6). As in the aorta, fragmentation of the elastic tissue, usually the internal elastic lamella, is common and is of no specific significance (Figure 9.7). In some aging arteries, the internal lamella appears to repeatedly reduplicate, producing a pattern of concentric intimal thickening (Figure 9.5). Small foci of calcification can be identified in

otherwise normal vessels, usually just to the medial aspect of the internal elastic lamella. These aging changes, often loosely termed arteriosclerosis, have been studied most extensively in the coronary arteries, where women generally show substantially less elastic fragmentation and intimal fibrosis than do men of the same age (45). About 75% of the mass of the media is smooth muscle cells. These run in a spiral or circumferential pattern around the wall. As in the intima the small amounts of associated collagen and elastin increase throughout life. Arteries dilate and become more tortuous with increasing age, and this has a fortuitous antiocclusive effect. The caliber of the coronary arteries in middle-aged and elderly women is less than that of men. This may make coronary artery surgery more difficult and contribute to the poorer results recorded in women (23). If arterial dilatation is pronounced and irregular, as in so-called coronary artery ectasia, spontaneous thrombosis may result.

Nutrients reach the media of elastic or muscular arteries by direct diffusion through the intima or via small branches, the vasa vasorum, which reenter the media from the adventitial aspect. Vasa are best seen in biopsy samples taken from the ascending aorta during root repairs and sometimes have remarkably thick muscular walls (Figure 9.8). In

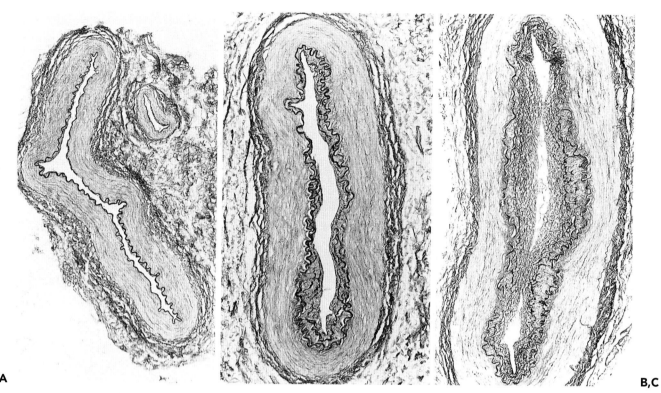

A   B,C

Figure 9.5 Aging changes in muscular arteries. **A.** (left) Normal appearing artery from a 17-year-old girl. **B. and C.** Note the progressive intimal fibrosis in arteries from elderly males. In C there is some reduplication of the internal elastic membrane. (Elastic van Gieson.)

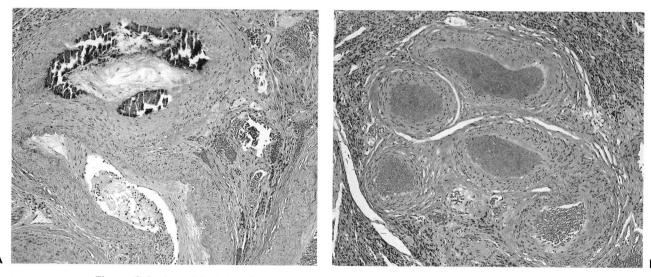

A   B

Figure 9.6 **A. and B.** Aging changes in arteries. These thick-walled vessels were close to the serosa of the myometrium in a 52-year-old woman. Note the prominent calcification in A and the increased tortuosity in B. These changes have no importance. They can be seen in other sites, especially in thyroidectomy specimens.

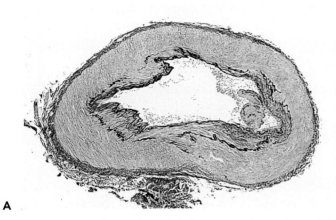
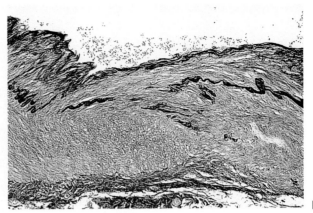

A

B

Figure 9.7   A. and B. Temporal artery from a 72-year-old woman who died suddenly from coronary heart disease. There was no past history of headache or temporal arteritis. Note the fragmentation of the elastic lamella with a little associated fibrosis (red coloration in B). Changes such as these are commonplace in the elderly and must not be interpreted as evidence of previous arteritis (elastic van Gieson).

atheromatous arteries, there is often marked neovascular proliferation. Hemorrhage from these vessels contributes to the growth of lesions and their lipid content (24).

The different stages, or phases, of atherosclerotic plaque development have been categorized in the American Heart Association (AHA) classification into three types of early lesions (plaque types I–III) and three types of mature late lesions (plaque types IV–VI). Early lesions consist of adaptive intimal thickening (type I), fatty streaks (type II) with accumulation of lipid-rich foam cells and T lymphocytes), and pathological intimal thickening (type III, early atheroma). Late stages include fibroatheroma (type IV), fibrotic or calcified plaques (type V), and complicated plaques (type VI) (25,26). Recently, there has been much

interest in the concept of the so-called vulnerable plaque: plaques at high risk for development of superimposed thrombosis or plaque hemorrhage. Several postmortem studies of coronary arteries from patients with myocardial infarction or sudden cardiac death have shown that vulnerable lesions have specific features such as a large lipid core, a thin fibrous cap, and marked inflammatory activity in the plaque tissue (27).

Virmani et al. (28) have modified the AHA classification in order to highlight the variation in plaque morphology in relation to the onset and evolution of atherothrombotic complications. In their classification, the late stages of plaque development are divided into fibrous cap atheroma, thin cap fibroatheroma, healed plaque rupture or erosion, and calcified plaques. This classification emphasizes that complicated (thrombosed) plaques can be the result of rupture of a fibrous cap or erosion of the endothelial lining (Table 9.3).

Inflammatory Infiltrates in Arteries

Apart from a few scattered macrophages or mast cells, the adventitia of arteries is devoid of inflammatory cells. However, for many years it has been known that, in the chronic advanced stages of atherosclerosis, nodular or patchy inflammatory infiltrates can form at the sites of atheromatous lesions, a process that increases with the severity of atherosclerosis (29). These aggregates can resemble the lymphoid follicle-like lesions that form in diseases of disordered immunity, such as rheumatoid disease. Immunohistochemistry has shown that these highly organized structures containing germinal centers surrounded by both T and B cells. Small vessels are lined by plump endothelium, which stains with antibodies that identify high endothelial venules (see Immunohistochemistry section,

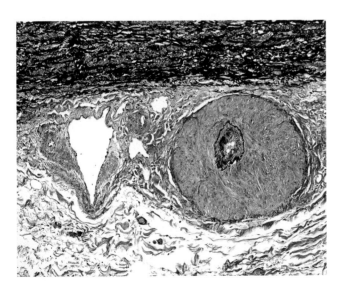

Figure 9.8 The aortic adventitia. The thick-walled vessel is a vasa vasorum. The thin-walled vessel (*left*) is a small vein.

TABLE 9.3

MODIFIED AMERICAN HEART ASSOCIATION CLASSIFICATION OF ATHEROMATOUS LESIONS

Lesion	Histologic Features
Pathologic intimal thickening	Smooth muscle cell proliferation, intimal fibrosis, extracellular lipid but no lipid core or necrosis
Fibrous cap atheroma	Well-formed lipid core with thick fibrous cap, free of inflammatory cells (>80 μm coronary artery >200 μm carotid artery)
Thin fibrous cap atheroma	Thin cap of inflamed fibrous tissue with underlying lipid core
Ruptured plaque	Luminal thrombus communicating with lipid core via a ruptured fibrous cap
Eroded plaque	Luminal thrombus with endothelial ulceration; lipid core may be absent or small and does not communicate with lumen
Calcified lesions	Heavily calcified plaques with or without thrombus or lipid core

This is a simplified version of the classification of Virmani R, Kolodgie FD, Burke AP, et al. Lessons from sudden cardiac death: a comprehensive morphological classification for atherosclerotic lesions. *Arterioscler Thromb Vasc Biol* 2000;20:1262-1275; Virmani R, Farb A, Burke A, et al. Coronary heart disease and its syndromes. In: Virmani R, Farb A, Burke A, et al. *Cardiovascular pathology.* Philadelphia: WB Saunders, 2001:26–53, with permission. Reprinted with permission from: Mills SE, ed. *Sternberg's Diagnostic Surgical Pathology.* 4th ed. Philadelphia: Lippincott Williams & Wilkins; 2004.

below). Arteries in chronically inflamed tissues and within tumors often show pronounced fibrous intimal thickening, sometimes termed endarteritis obliterans (Table 9.2). In the early stages of this process, the fibrous tissue has a loose histologic appearance, and the ground substance may be basophilic. Although inflammatory or tumor cells often closely surround the adventitia, they do not usually penetrate far into the muscular wall.

These changes must be carefully distinguished from those of systemic vasculitis. In general terms, vasculitis tends to affect vessels of a specific size, cause necrosis of vessel walls (Figure 9.9) with associated hemorrhage, and lead to tissue infarction. In healed vasculitis, there is irregular fibrosis of the muscular wall (Figure 9.10).

Arterioles

There are no specific histologic features that accurately distinguish small arteries from larger arterioles; but, for convenience, arterioles are said to have a diameter of less than 100 μm. However, in biopsy material, there is so much variation in the contours of these small vessels that accurate distinction is often impossible and probably unnecessary. Larger arterioles have an obvious media and an adventitial layer of connective tissue. In the smallest (terminal) arterioles, an internal elastic lamella may not be identified. The smooth muscle cells are arranged circumferentially, each cell winding around the wall several times. This is the structural basis of the precapillary sphincter. Small arterioles have a very thin adventitia but are richly supplied by sympathetic nerve fibers.

Hyalinization is a common lesion of arterioles and small arteries and increases with age and in conditions such as hypertension and diabetes. The glassy uniform appearance is the result of accumulation of a variety of plasma proteins and small amounts of lipids. As in arteries, reduplication of elastic tissue and intimal fibrosis are common changes in the aged. In severe longstanding benign hypertension and in the malignant phase, the arteriolar lumen can be substantially narrowed by concentric layers of fibrous tissue and smooth muscle cells, changes that are outside the normal range of aging (Table 9.1). Fibrinoid necrosis of the arteriolar media is the hallmark of malignant hypertension and some forms of acute vasculitis (Figure 9.9). It must always be regarded as pathologic. In the earliest changes of diabetic microangiopathy, arterioles and capillaries often show prominent basement membrane thickening (30). This thickening can be readily identified in renal and peripheral nerve biopsies. Although there is physiologic evidence of small vessel disease in the heart and the peripheral vasculature, characteristic histologic changes of diabetic microangiopathy are seldom seen in these sites. In diabetes the amounts of type IV collagen and laminin are increased, but the proteoglycan component of the basement membrane is reduced. Albumin and immunoglobulins accumulate in these abnormal basement membranes, binding to glycosylated protein residues and contributing to the overall eosinophilic appearance.

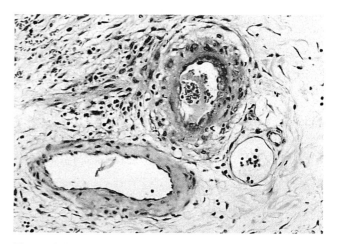

Figure 9.9   Florid fibrinoid necrosis in a small intestinal vessel of a girl with systemic lupus erythematosus. Fibrinoid necrosis is not a feature of normal aging or uncomplicated hypertension. It always should be regarded as pathologic. In this case, the involved vessel is probably an arteriole. Note the small vein (*lower left*) and capillary (*lower right*).

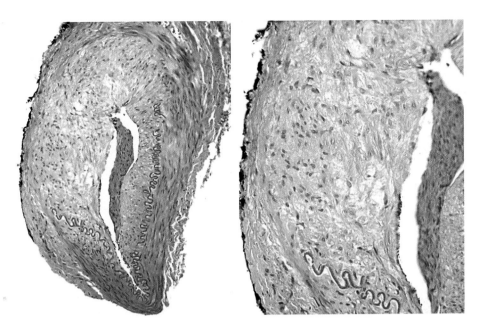

A, B

Figure 9.10 Healed temporal arteritis. This patient had been receiving steroid therapy for two weeks when this biopsy was performed. **A.** The low power view shows irregular thickening of the wall and a loss of about 50% of the internal elastic lamella. **B.** This higher power view shows fresh fibrous scarring of the media. Changes such as these are not part of the normal aging process (see Figure 9.6).

Capillaries

In contrast to arterioles, capillaries have neither a muscular media nor an elastic lamella. A single but complete layer of endothelial cells lies on a basement membrane whose thickness varies from site to site. Basement membrane thickness increases with age, almost doubling in muscle capillaries from 10 to 70 years of age. There is no fibrous tissue support peripheral to this, but pericytes are present in and among the basement membrane. It is difficult to identify pericytes in routine sections, but they are easily seen by electron microscopy and also stain with antismooth muscle actin antibodies. They provide structural support; and, because they contain several forms of myosin, they may be able to regulate blood flow. It is likely that they are involved in the synthesis of vascular basement membrane and are capable of phagocytosis (31). It is generally accepted that the turnover of pericytes is increased in the capillaries of diabetics, and this may contribute to the development of small vessel disease (30).

The endothelium of capillaries may have circular fenestrations that act as pores through the full thickness of the endothelial cell. Fenestrations are especially prominent in renal glomerular endothelial cells and are found in the intestinal mucosa, skin, and endocrine glands. In contrast, fenestrations are poorly developed or absent in brain, muscle, lung, and connective tissue (5).

In certain sites, such as the liver, spleen, pituitary, adrenals, and bone marrow, the vessels that connect arterioles and venules are known as sinusoids rather than capillaries. With diameters of up to 30 to 40 μm, they are generally more distended than capillaries. They have prominent fenestrations, but there are also significant gaps between endothelial cells. In the liver, there is no significant associated basement membrane.

Venules and Veins

The transition from venous capillary to muscular venule and small collecting vein is characterized by the gradual acquisition of a muscular media. Even in medium-sized veins (Figure 9.11), the internal elastic lamella is often incomplete and the muscle fibers are only poorly oriented into circular and longitudinal layers. The paracortical or high endothelial venules of lymph nodes have an important role in T-lymphocyte recirculation (32). The endothelial cells of postcapillary venules have a prominent cuboidal or columnal appearance, usually with an ovoid nucleus and a single central nucleolus. They stain specifically with the HECA-452 antibody (see below).

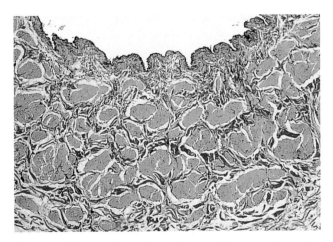

Figure 9.11 A renal vein from a 58-year-old woman, close to the junction with the inferior vena cava. There is no significant intimal thickening, and a thin internal elastic lamella can be identified. Note the thin layer of subendothelial collagen. The muscular wall is composed of coarse fascicles, which are not clearly arranged into circular and longitudinal layers (elastic van Gieson).

Placental, dural, and retinal veins and the veins of erectile tissue have very little muscle. In general, the veins of the lower limb have thicker walls than those of the arm and abdomen. Most veins have valves to prevent the reflux of blood. The increasing use of the saphenous vein as an arterial conduit has led to a greater understanding of the normal structure of larger veins and the changes that occur in them as a result of aging. Large veins have a thin layer of subendothelial connective tissue with one or more incomplete elastic lamellae. Around this, there is an inner longitudinal and outer circular smooth muscle coat. The connective tissue adventitia is often well developed. Saphenous veins in middle-aged and elderly patients show intimal fibrosis and longitudinal and circular muscle hypertrophy with a substantial increase in medial connective tissue. Sometimes a prominent third outer longitudinal muscle layer (Figure 9.12) forms between the circular coat and the adventitia (33). These changes must be distinguished from the form of atherosclerosis that develops in vein bypass grafts.

Lymphatics

At the light microscopic level, small lymphatics closely resemble capillaries. In general terms, lymphatics have a larger diameter and a less regular cross-sectional profile (34). They begin as dilated channels with closed ends and anastomose freely. Although they are present in most

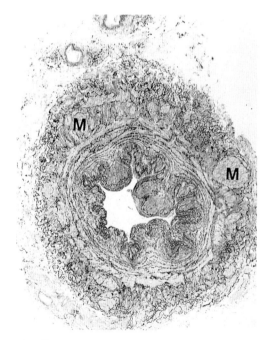

Figure 9.12 A saphenous vein with a prominent third outer longitudinal muscular coat (*M*). Reprinted with permission from: Milroy et al. Histological appearances of the long saphenous vein. *J Pathol* 1989;159:311–316. With permission.

tissues, they are rarely found in the epidermis, nails, cornea, articular cartilage, central nervous system, or bone marrow. Lymphatic channels have numerous valves and are often slightly distended at these sites, producing a slightly beaded appearance. Lymphatics with a diameter of more than 0.2 mm usually have a thin muscular media, with no clear division into circular or longitudinal coats, and a fibrous adventitia. A longitudinal muscular layer is present in the right lymphatic and thoracic ducts. As detailed and illustrated below, lymphatic vessels stain specifically with two antibodies, D2-40 and LYVE-1.

Pulmonary Arteries and Veins

Although the basic histologic structure of pulmonary vessels resembles that of their systemic counterparts, there are differences that reflect the much lower pressure of the pulmonary circuit. The lumina of major pulmonary arteries are widely dilated in comparison with wall thickness. The intima is hardly discernible. In an adult, the pulmonary arterial media is composed of only 10 to 15 parallel elastic lamellae, whereas, even in a young child, 40 aortic lamellae can be identified. The thickness of the pulmonary trunk is about 40 to 80% that of the aorta (Figure 9.13).

In the systemic circulation, the transition from elastic to muscular arteries is abrupt and is usually at the point of a major arterial orifice. In contrast, even pulmonary arteries as small as 0.5 to 1.0 mm in diameter are elastic vessels (35,36). Muscular pulmonary arteries and arterioles also have thin walls in relationship to their luminal diameter, but this may be difficult to appreciate unless special techniques of perfusion or fixation are used. In comparison with systemic arteries, there is usually a prominent internal and external elastic lamella. Arterioles give rise to a rich network of alveolar capillaries. Pericytes are not easily identified, and in places the endothelium and alveolar epithelium appear to share a common basement membrane. The walls of pulmonary veins are less structured than their systemic counterparts. The media is composed of a rather haphazardly arranged but roughly circular layer of connective tissue and muscle. No distinct and continuous elastic lamellae are present, and valves are said to be absent (Figure 9.14).

It can be difficult to distinguish the early vascular changes of pulmonary hypertension from those of normal aging (Table 9.4). The histologic changes have been described and comprehensively illustrated (35,36). The initial changes in both conditions include intimal fibrosis and medial muscular hypertrophy, and each of these features is most prominent in muscular arteries and larger arterioles (37). The absence of significant changes in the larger arteries may be misleading. In long-standing pulmonary hypertension, the complex changes in muscular arteries include florid intimal thickening, marked medial hypertrophy, and prominent dilatation of small branches of parent vessels (Figures 9.13D, 9.15). In the

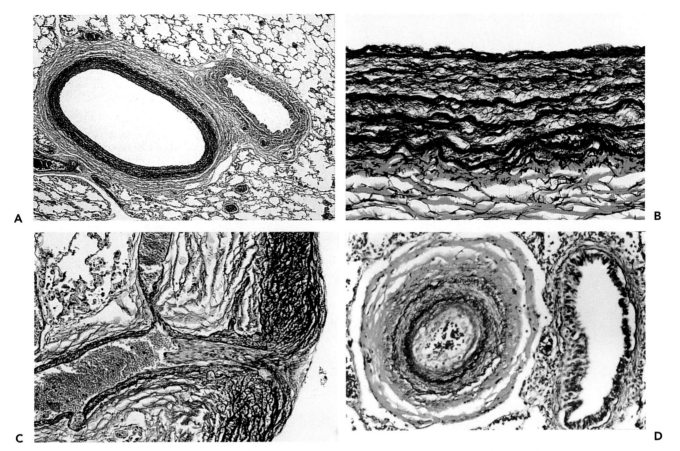

Figure 9.13   A. Elastic pulmonary artery from a 1-year-old child. The lung was inflated via the main pulmonary artery, which therefore appears much larger than the corresponding bronchus. **B.** A magnified view of the elastic wall (Gomori's trichrome). **C.** The transition from elastic to muscular pulmonary arteries in a 73-year-old man. Note the larger number of elastic lamellae. There is slight fibrous intimal thickening only (elastic van Gieson). **D.** A small pulmonary artery from a patient with longstanding pulmonary hypertension and chronic obstructive airways disease. There is hypertrophy of the muscular wall and pronounced fibrous intimal thickening (Gomori's trichrome).

most extreme examples, angiomatoid malformations may develop, and occasionally there is fibrinoid necrosis of the vessel wall (38,39). Lung biopsy is no longer used for the assessment of pulmonary hypertension in children with congenital heart disease nor in adults with primary pulmonary hypertension. However surgical pathologists must make a careful assessment of the pulmonary arteries and veins in lung biopsy specimens and be able to describe and grade these alterations accurately (40).

Aging changes in pulmonary veins are seldom described in detail. In severe, long-standing cardiac failure, intimal fibrosis, medial hypertrophy, and hyalinization are prominent pulmonary venous abnormalities. Marked medial hypertrophy may confer an arterialized appearance to pulmonary veins, and they may appear to have an internal and external elastic lamina. Multiple levels should be taken and stained for elastin and by a trichrome method. The elastic lamellae are seldom complete in these abnormal veins, and there is often more medial fibrosis than in corresponding pulmonary arteries. Even so, accurate distinction of abnormal pulmonary arteries and veins can be difficult.

Anastomoses, Angiodysplasias, and Vascular Malformations

There is potential for anastomoses between many arteries and veins. These are especially developed in the skin, where they contribute to thermoregulation. They vary in size from about 200 to 800 μm and in some sites, such as the nail bed, have a complex structure. There are also anastomoses between pulmonary and bronchial veins and between the portal and systemic circulations. Peripheral glomus tumors almost certainly arise from supporting cells that surround the normal but rather complex anastomosing channels between digital arterioles and venules. Glomus cells do not express endothelial markers but, because they stain with smooth muscle actin and vimentin, may be related to vascular smooth muscle (41). The potential connections

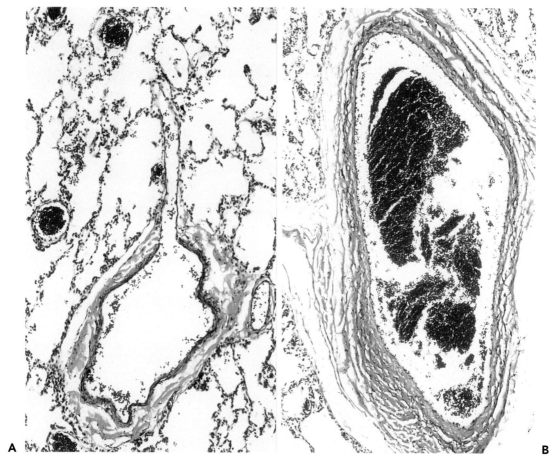

Figure 9.14 Normal pulmonary veins. **A.** A pulmonary venule draining into a small vein. Very little muscle is present in the wall. **B.** A large pulmonary vein close to the hilum of the lung. (Gomori's trichrome)

TABLE 9.4

HISTOLOGIC FEATURES OF PULMONARY VESSELS

Vessel	Normal	Age-Related Changes	Pulmonary Hypertension
Elastic arteries (>500 µm)	Widely patent lumen, media of 10 to 15 parallel lamellae of elastic tissue	Slight intimal fibrosis; increased medial thickness due to collagen deposition; occasional atheromatous plaques	Atherosclerosis and dilation of main pulmonary arteries; medial thickening due to hypertrophy of admixed muscular elements
Muscular arteries or arterioles	Thin muscular wall often with distinct internal and external elastic lamina	Increased muscular media, eccentric intimal fibrosis, especially in vessels less than 300 µm in diameter	Complex changes include florid intimal thickening, medial hypertrophy, dilation of small branches, angiomatoid (plexiform) lesions, and fibrinoid necrosis
Veins	Thin media of irregularly arranged fibrous tissue and muscle. No distinct elastic lamella. No valves.	Few detailed studies. The media may appear hyalinized.	Intimal fibrosis, medial muscular hypertrophy—occasionally sufficient to mimic appearance of arteries

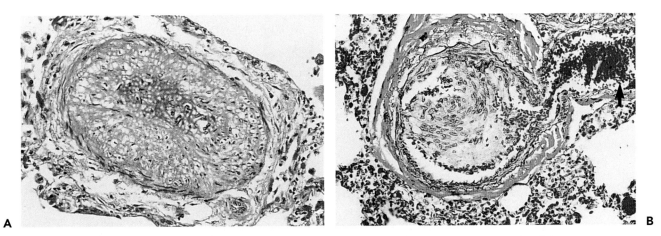

A   B

Figure 9.15 Advanced pulmonary hypertensive changes. **A.** There is marked hypertrophy of the medial muscle in a small pulmonary artery. **B.** An early plexiform lesion with nearby dilated thin-walled branches (*arrow*). (Gomori's trichrome.)

between the portal and systemic circulations, either in the submucosa of the esophagus or rectum or in the periumbilical or diaphragmatic region, may be massively dilated in advanced hepatic disease. Biopsies are seldom performed surgically.

Surgical pathologists must be familiar with the normal vascular patterns of the cerebral meninges and the colonic submucosa if cerebral arteriovenous malformations and large intestinal angiodysplasia are to be accurately assessed. Each of these areas has a rich vascular supply with numerous, sometimes thick-walled, venous channels. Malformations or angiodysplasias must only be diagnosed if there is undoubted evidence of an abnormal vessel wall. Aging changes and atherosclerosis seldom involve the smaller leptomeningeal arteries. In arteries, eccentric fibrous intimal thickening or disruption of the elastic lamellae support a diagnosis of a malformation. Veins in these malformations have irregular contours, the thickness of their muscular wall may vary markedly, and the wall can be uniformly fibrosed.

Angiodysplasia of the colon is a common cause of lower gastrointestinal hemorrhage. The lesions are usually present on the antimesenteric border of the cecum, often close to the ileocecal valve (42). They are not direct arteriovenous anastomoses but rather dilatations of preexisting, and previously normal, capillary rings and veins (Figure 9.16). The dilatation of these vessels may be the result of increased colonic muscular pressure causing intermittent obstruction of draining vessels. Multiple blocks must be examined and the appearances contrasted with a control section of submucosa from a normal colon. Submucosal arteries of the large intestine may show pronounced age-related tortuosity, and this must not be interpreted as an abnormality. A proportion of cases with good clinical or radiologic evidence of angiodysplasia will not be confirmed histologically. Some cases of massive gastrointestinal hemorrhage result from abnormally large submucosal arteries. This is most common

in the stomach but also has been reported in the large and small intestine. Arteries in the submucosa of the proximal portion of the stomach can arise directly from omental vessels and may have a larger caliber than superficial arteries arising from a submucosal plexus, the so-called caliber-persistent artery or Dieulafoy's lesion (43,44).

Vascular malformations are congenital lesions composed of mature but often malformed (dysplastic) blood vessels. They result from dysregulation in the signalling pathways of vasculogenesis in early embryonic life (45) and must be distinguished from true angiomas and reactive hyperplasias. They may be solitary lesions or be part of a dysmorphic syndrome and grow slowly but progressively, usually commensurate with the growth of the patient (46,47).

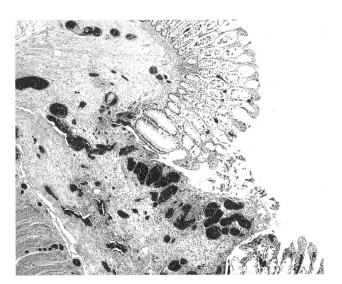

Figure 9.16 Angiodysplasia of the colon. Note the many dilated thin-walled blood vessels in the submucosa. Although these vessels are distended, their basic structure is unaltered.

They are classified according to the size of the predominate type of vessel. Clinically, a distinction is made between low- and high-flow lesions. The latter are usually arteriovenous malformations characterized by connections between feeding arteries and draining veins, without an interconnecting capillary bed, the so-called arteriovenous fistula (48). Fistulae are rarely found in tissue sections; but in these lesions arteries have a tortuous course, and a proportion of veins may show intimal thickening with collagen and elastin deposition in their walls. Pure venous malformations are composed of dilated vascular channels with walls of variable size, showing irregular degrees of attenuation and fibrosis. Complications include thrombosis with organization, papillary endothelial hyperplasia (Masson's pseudotumor), and nodular calcification. In lymphatic malformations, the vascular channels vary considerably in size and may have an incomplete muscular wall. As in other vessels their endothelium stains with CD31 and CD34 antibodies and with factor VIII-related antigen.

Vascular Surgery

The changes commonly seen in vessels after surgical procedures and interventions are summarized in Table 9.5.

Endarterectomy

Patency can be restored to a partially occluded artery by drawing out a proportion of the atherosclerotic intima. The procedure is usually applied to the carotid bifurcation, the iliac, femoral, or, occasionally, coronary arteries. Ideally, the surgeon should establish a plane between the innermost media and the intima, and the atheromatous material should be removed in its entirety. At its bifurcation the carotid artery has an elastic wall, and the material removed will include layers of elastic tissue, atheromatous debris, and thrombus. Acute postoperative thrombus formation is the most important immediate complication of the procedure. Longer term complications are recurrent thrombosis, aneurysmal dilatation, and restenosis due to fibrous intimal proliferation (49).

Bypass Grafts

The pathologic changes that occur in autologous saphenous vein bypass grafts have been described in detail (50). Care must be taken to distinguish these changes from those associated with normal aging. When subjected to arterial pressure, many vein grafts dilate and most develop some fibrous intimal thickening and medial muscular hypertrophy. In time, many develop pronounced fibrous intimal thickening with areas of lipid deposition, intramural hemorrhage, and thrombosis. These appearances closely mimic atherosclerosis and are an important cause of graft failure. In one postmortem study in which saphenous vein conduits were sampled throughout their length, more than 75% narrowing

TABLE 9.5 PATHOLOGIC CHANGES AFTER VASCULAR SURGERY	
Procedure	**Spectrum of Histologic Change**
Endarterectomy	*Acutely:* surface platelet and fibrin deposits on inner face of surgical dissection, occasionally progressing to occlusive thrombosis. *Chronically:* variable degrees of fibrous intimal hyperplasia, occasionally progressing to restenosis. "False" aneurysm formation.
Vein bypass grafting	*Acutely:* thrombosis, dissection at anastomosis site. *Chronically:* dilatation with fibrous intimal thickening and medial muscular hypertrophy (to be contrasted with preimplant state). Occasionally, marked intimal fibrosis with lipid deposition and hemorrhage, leading to occlusion ("vein atherosclerosis").
Internal mammary and radial artery grafting	*Acutely:* thrombosis at anastomoses sites. *Chronically:* occasional grafts become fibrosed. Graft atherosclerosis uncommon.
Angioplasty and stenting	*Acutely:* acute inflammation, dissection, and thrombosis. *Chronically:* restenosis due to reactive fibrous intimal thickening, now reduced by drug eluting stents.
Prosthetic vessels	*Acutely:* thrombotic occlusion. *Chronically:* extensive macrophage and giant cell infiltration of fabric wall. Formation of fibrin-rich pseudointima, occasionally progressing to partial or complete occlusion. Graft failure and thrombosis.

was demonstrated in 11 to 26% of the segments examined (51). Grafts can sometimes be dilated by angioplasty, but redo coronary bypass procedures are now a significant part of the work of all cardiac surgery departments.

In cardiac surgery, coronary artery stenoses are routinely bypassed with the left or right internal mammary artery. The origin of the artery from the subclavian artery is preserved, and it is then dissected away from the chest wall. There is usually a surrounding cuff of soft tissue, but some surgeons dissect this away, producing a so-called "skeletalized" graft. Long-term patency rates are superior to saphenous vein grafts. The caliber of the normal internal mammary artery is similar to that of distal coronary arteries. Preexisting occlusive disease is present in fewer than 5% of patients, and only occasional grafts develop atheromatous obstructions (52). In its proximal portion, the internal mammary is an elastic

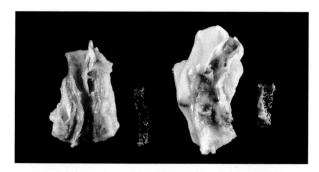

Figure 9.17 Coronary artery stenting. Metallic stents were inserted three weeks before this patient's death. The stent placed in the left anterior descending artery (*left*) is fully patent and an excellent result has been obtained by the angioplasty procedure. In contrast, some reactive fibrosis has formed in the stent that was placed in the right coronary artery (*right*).

artery, but the media is muscular from about the level of the fourth rib.

Segments of the radial artery are also used as free grafts. Like saphenous vein grafts, they are anastomosed proximally to the aortic root and distally to the coronary arteries. The radial artery is muscular and is invariably free of significant atheroma.

Angioplasty

Percutaneous coronary angioplasty (PTCA) with stent emplacement is now the treatment of choice for many proximal coronary stenoses and is increasingly used as a primary intervention to open thrombosed coronary arteries after myocardial infarction (53). The mortality rate in most centers is now less than 1%, and over 90% of procedures are initially successful (52). In order to dilate the vessel, the heavily fibrous and focally calcified atheromatous plaque must be cracked open. Only when this has occurred can the deeper intima and underlying media be distended by the inflated balloon and held open by the expandable metallic stent. Early histologic studies of patients dying soon after angioplasty demonstrated a characteristic pattern of radial tears or splits, sometimes with dissections extending into the underlying media.

Stents minimize the complications of these changes, but stent thrombosis is an occasional complication (54). Restenosis is the result of fibrous intimal proliferation, thrombus formation, and an overall reduction in the size of the vessel lumen, the so-called constrictive remodelling (55,56). Stents coated with immunosuppressant or antineoplastic agents, such as sirolimus or paclitaxel, are now used routinely and have reduced rates of restenosis as compared to bare metal stent (57,58). If death occurs soon after the procedure, the stent can be carefully extracted from the opened artery (Figure 9.17), which is then processed in the usual way. After late closure, stents can be cut with an electric diamond saw and then embedded in hard plastic.

Prosthetic Vessels

Various types of fabric graft are used for the treatment of peripheral vascular disease, for closing cardiac septal defects, or in other more complex procedures in children with congenital heart disease. Acute occlusion of prosthetic vessels is usually the result of surgical technique or poor flow rates. In time, prosthetic grafts develop a pseudointima. This has a jellylike consistency, may develop a partial (though not a complete) endothelial lining, and is composed of fibrin and enmeshed leukocytes (59). However, the most striking feature of these prosthetic vessels is the intense mononuclear and giant cell reaction that develops around the woven fibers of the graft. There is usually a moderate degree of adventitial fibrosis that binds the prosthesis to the surrounding tissues and reduces its elasticity. Long-term complications include thrombosis, particularly at flexures or surgical anastomoses, infection, and deterioration of the fibers of the graft.

ELECTRON MICROSCOPY

Ultrastructural studies have made enormous contributions to our understanding of vascular biology. However, even surgical pathologists with a specific interest in vascular pathology have only limited experience and expertise in electron microscopy. Some of the most important ultrastructural features of vessels are summarized in Table 9.6.

TABLE 9.6

ULTRASTRUCTURAL FEATURES OF VASCULAR TISSUES

Endothelial cells are joined by tight, adherans or gap junctions.
Transendothelial channels characterize fenestrated endothelium, as in hepatic sinusoids, glomeruli, and endocrine organs.
Cytoplasmic inclusions of endothelium include lysosomes, plasmalemmal vesicles, and Weibel-Palade bodies (see Figure 9.19).
Capillary endothelium is surrounded by basement membrane in which pericytes are embedded. There is very little basement membrane around lymphatic vessels. There are direct appositions between processes of pericytes and endothelium through gaps in the basement membrane.
Smooth muscle cells are invested in basement membrane and are linked by communicating (gap) junctions. Elastin and collagen fibers may be closely opposed to the surfaces of smooth muscle cells.
No significant media in small arterioles, capillaries, or lymphatics.
The adventitia is composed of collagen and some elastin fibers. It has a well-developed structure in large veins but is very thin in some arteries.

Endothelial Cells

The entire vascular system is lined internally by a single layer of rather spindle-shaped endothelial cells. Small fingerlike microvilli, 200 to 400 nm long, may be seen on the surface of endothelial cells (Figure 9.18). A thin polysaccharide layer, the glycocalyx, coats the luminal surface of the endothelium. This is up to 100 nm in thickness, but its exact function is uncertain. Although endothelial cells have relatively sparse endoplasmic reticulum, a small number of free ribosomes, and an inconspicuous Golgi apparatus they produce a variety of molecules that are important in blood coagulation and the regulation of vascular tone.

Junctional complexes between endothelial cells are tight, adherens, or gap junctions (60). Tight junctions have a barrier function and help to maintain cell polarity. Molecules of the claudin family create the barrier and regulate electrical resistance between cells (61,62). Loss of this barrier function may be important in disorders such as diabetic retinopathy (63,64). Adherens junctions regulate permeability to white cells and soluble molecules and have a role in contact inhibition. Gap junctions are assembled from proteins known as connexins and form channels between adjacent cells (65). Alterations in gap junction proteins have been documented in human heart disease, including atrial and ventricular arrhythmias (66).

Inclusions of Endothelial Cells

Lysosomes are readily identified in most endothelial cells and are involved in intracytoplasmic digestion of foreign

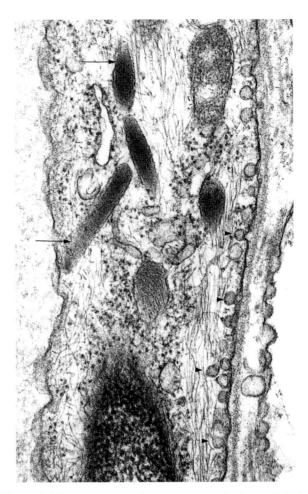

Figure 9.19   Transmission electron micrograph of an endothelial cell from a small subcutaneous capillary. Plasmalemmal vesicles are present on the abluminal surface (*arrowheads*). There are conspicuous Weibel-Palade bodies (*arrows*). Only part of the endothelial cell nucleus is included (*bottom*) (original magnification ×15,000).

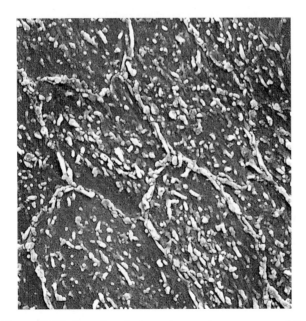

Figure 9.18   Scanning electron microscopic appearances of the endothelium from an experimental animal perfused under pressure with fixative. The junctions between individual endothelial cells are clearly seen; and, in this preparation, microvilli are particularly prominent (original magnification ×1,200).

debris and products of metabolism. In many areas of the vascular system, membrane-bound vesicles measuring up to 80 to 90 nm can be identified (Figure 9.19). They are most prominent on the abluminal surface of the endothelial cell. They were originally known as plasmalemmal vesicles but are now usually termed caveolae. Their functions include the sequestration and concentration of small molecules, and they contribute to the endothelial barrier function, regulation of nitric oxide synthesis, and cholesterol metabolism (67). Weibel-Palade bodies are characteristic inclusions of endothelium and measure up to 3 μm in maximum dimension. These membrane-bound structures contain up to 25 parallel tubular arrays. Immunologic studies have shown that Weibel-Palade bodies are sites of storage of von Willebrand factor. They are a useful marker of endothelial cells but are seldom as conspicuous as in Figure 9.19.

The permeability of capillaries varies considerably from organ to organ. In some sites, such as the renal glomerulus, the hepatic sinusoids, the small intestine, and some endocrine glands, there is a rapid interchange between blood and the surrounding tissue. Some of these permeability differences are related to the exact nature of the junctions between endothelial cells, but endothelial fenestrae also have an important role in this respect. These fenestrations are in fact the openings of irregular, and sometimes incomplete, transendothelial channels that allow the rapid interchange of fluid between the blood vessel lumen and the interstitium.

Media

In the human aorta, homogeneous parallel elastic lamellae alternate with layers containing smooth muscle cells and a variety of extracellular components. Smooth muscle predominates in muscular arteries. The power of contraction of smooth muscle is as great as skeletal muscle and can be maintained for longer periods with greater shortening. The structure of smooth muscle cells is maintained by the intermediate filaments vimentin and desmin, and the contractile forces are generated by actin and myosin filaments. Smooth muscle cells are arranged in parallel longitudinal bundles with the wide part of one cell opposed to the tapering part of another. Each smooth muscle cell is covered by a basal lamina which merges with fine collagen and elastin fibers (5).

Individual smooth muscle cells are often linked by communicating (gap) junctions, but tight junctions are not generally seen. In the microcirculation and in some larger arteries and arterioles, there are gap junctions between the smooth muscle cells and the overlying endothelium (68). These myoendothelial junctions could have an important role in relaying physiologic or pharmacologic stimuli between the blood vessel lumen and the media.

Adventitia and Supporting Cells

The adventitial layer consists almost entirely of collagen and elastic fibers. The thickness of this layer varies with the size of the vessel, and it may be continuous with the surrounding connective tissue. In some medium-sized veins, it is particularly well developed but in cerebral arteries may be as thin as 80 μm. A layer of elastic tissue, the external elastic lamella, is present at the junction of the media and adventitia. In human material, it is seldom as pronounced as the internal elastic lamella but is prominent in many other mammalian arteries. The pericytes that are present in and among the basement membrane of capillaries and small venules superficially resemble fibroblasts. The ultrastructural appearance of their cytoplasmic filaments suggests that they are contractile, and this is further evidence that they are of mesenchymal origin (31).

Lymphatics and Veins

The smallest lymphatic vessels have wider lumina than blood capillaries and a discontinuous basement membrane. A variety of anchoring filaments bind the lymphatic endothelium to the surrounding collagenous tissues, perhaps providing the sort of support normally produced by basement membrane and enmeshed pericytes in capillaries. The ultrastructural appearances of venous capillaries, venules, and small veins mirror those seen at the light microscopic level.

ANTIGEN EXPRESSION OF NORMAL AND NEOPLASTIC VASCULAR TISSUE

Endothelium

Endothelial cells cover the inner surface of the entire vascular tree, arterial, venous, capillary, and lymphatic. The most widely used antibodies are directed against von Willebrand factor (factor VIII), CD31, and CD34 (Figure 9.20). Because these antigens are present in all types of endothelial cells, they are considered to be panendothelial markers. The lectin Ulex europaeus 1 agglutinin binds to some α-L-fructose containing glycocompounds and therefore to virtually all human endothelia (69). The staining pattern is sometimes more intense than with factor VIII antibodies, especially in immature vessels (70). However, all endothelial markers cross-react to some extent with other cell components. For example, in areas of hemorrhage or thrombosis, CD31 reacts strongly with platelets, macrophages, and lymphocytes, and von Willebrand factor can produce diffuse extracellular staining. Nevertheless these antibodies are indispensable for the identification of vascular tumors such as angiomas, hemangioendotheliomas, and angiosarcomas and can be helpful in the identification of tumor emboli in vascular or lymphatic channels, rather than in artifactual tissue spaces.

Antibodies that recognize proteins involved in the early steps in angiogenesis include antiendoglin (CD105) and anti-VEGF (71). In different sites in the vascular system, the endothelium may show marked heterogeneity in morphology, gene expression patterns, and related differences in functional status. However, there are only limited variations in the immunophenotypic profile of endothelial cells. Antibodies to glucose transporter protein–1 (GLUT-1 antibodies) react with the endothelium of cerebral capillaries, the placental vasculature, and one specific type of angioma—the juvenile capillary angioma (Figure 9.21) (72). Another site specific antibody is anti-HECA 452, which reacts specifically with the plump endothelial cells of high endothelial venules in lymphoid tissue and postcapillary venules in chronically inflamed tissues (Figure 9.22). In inflamed tissues and in atheromatous lesions, endothelial cells undergo profound functional alterations (endothelial activation) associated with upregulation of antigens such

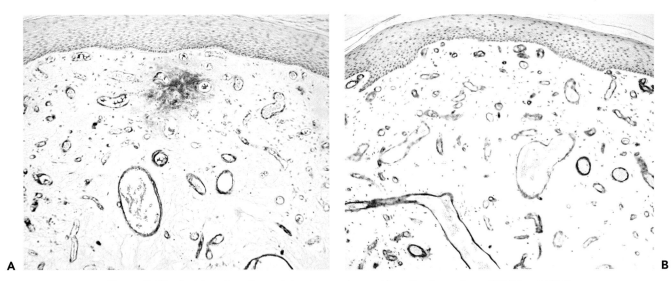

Figure 9.20 Staining of small vessels in a hemangioma with antibodies to factor VIII (**A**) and CD34 (**B**). As in these illustrations, the staining with CD34 is usually sharper than with factor VIII. Some non-specific extravascular staining is often seen with factor VIII but has no significance.

as ICAM-1, VCAM-1, and CD31 or with de novo expression of leukocyte adhesion molecules such as E-selectin. Until recently, there were no specific markers of lymphatic endothelium. Both D2-40 and LYVE-1 stain lymphatic endothelium specifically (Figure 9.22) (73), and D2-40 staining has confirmed the lymphatic origin of Kaposi's sarcoma (74) (Figure 9.23).

Smooth Muscle

Biochemical and immunohistologic studies have demonstrated that vascular smooth muscle has a distinctive component of contractile and intermediate filament proteins (75). In most smooth muscle, γ-smooth muscle actin and desmin predominate. In contrast, in vascular tissue there is abundant α-smooth muscle actin, and vimentin exceeds desmin. Antibodies directed against smooth muscle actin (SMA-1) are excellent markers of medial muscle; SMA-1 recognizes the full spectrum of proliferating (or synthetic) and mature (or contractile) smooth muscle phenotypes. As SMA-1 reacts with pericytes, it clearly outlines capillaries in reactive microvascular proliferations and in pyogenic granulomas and juvenile angiomas during their growth phase. Generally all benign vascular proliferations, including glomus tumors, stain strongly with SMA-1 antibodies (Figure 9.24). In contrast, this staining is often incomplete or even

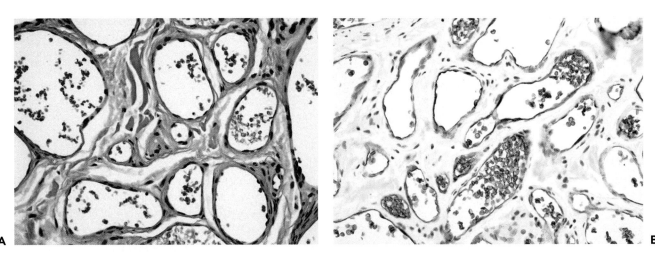

Figure 9.21 Site-specific staining of vascular endothelium. The vascular endothelium in this juvenile capillary hemangioma from a 3-year-old male (**A**) is specifically stained with the GLUT-1 antibody (**B**). This antibody also stains the endothelium of cerebral capillaries and the placenta. In contrast, the more commonly used endothelial antibodies such as factor VIII, CD31, and CD34 stain most types of normal and neoplastic endothelia.

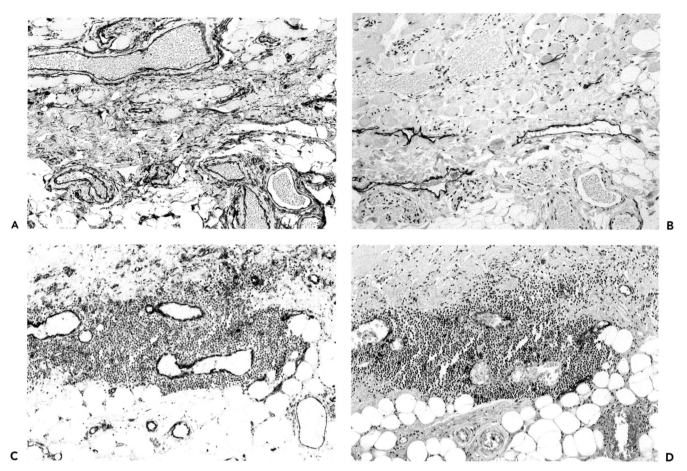

Figure 9.22   Immunohistochemical staining of vessels. **A. and B.** show a mixture of vessels from the subcutaneous tissues of a 68-year-old female from close to a leg ulcer: CD31 antibody staining identifies many vascular spaces (A), and a similar section is stained with the antibody D2-40, which recognizes lymphatic endothelium only (B). **C. and D.** are from a nodular inflammatory infiltrate in the aortic adventitia adjacent to a large atheromatous plaque: C has been stained with CD31, which recognizes most vessels, and D was stained with HECA-452, which recognizes high endothelial venules.

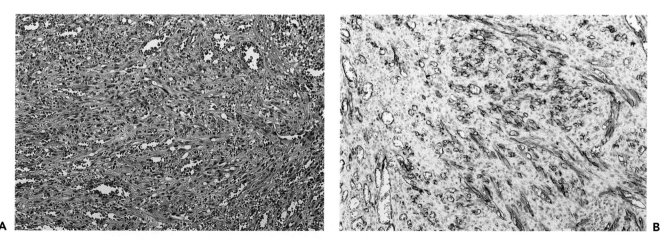

Figure 9.23   Kaposi's sarcoma. **A.** has been stained with H&E. **B.** was immunostained with the D2-40 antibody, a specific marker of lymphatic endothelium. Note the strong positive staining; LYVE-1 is another antibody that specifically stains lymphatic endothelium.

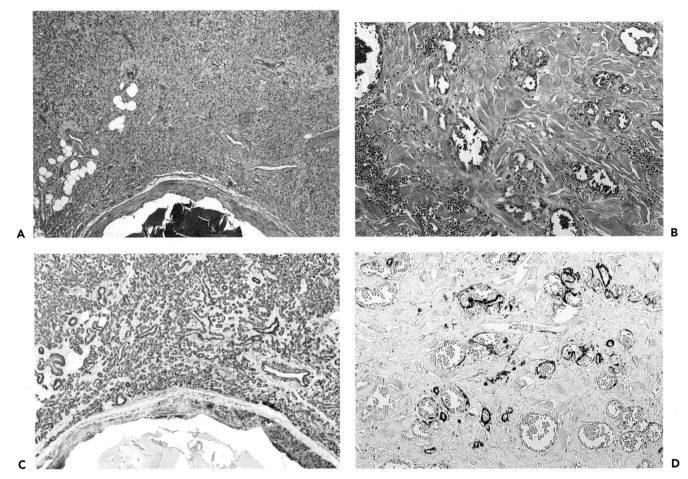

Figure 9.24 Patterns of staining with smooth muscle actin antibody. **A. and C.** are from a benign vascular proliferation. Note the intense staining of the walls of these small vessels. **B. and D.** are from an angiosarcoma. Only small amounts of actin are present in the walls of the malignant blood vessels (D).

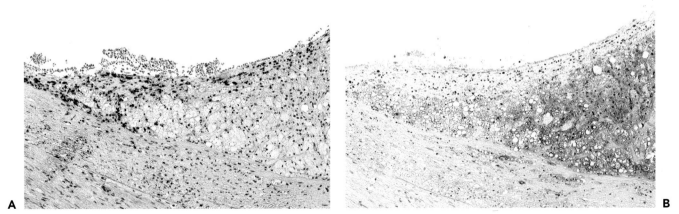

Figure 9.25 Immunohistochemical staining in atherosclerosis. **A.** CD3 positive lymphocytes are present at the edge of a lesion. **B.** Macrophages react for CD68.

absent in angiosarcoma, hemangiopericytoma, or Kaposi's sarcoma (Figure 9.23).

Other Useful Antibodies for Diagnostic Vascular Pathology

Immunohistochemical studies of the inflammatory infiltrates in atheromatous lesions (Figure 9.25) have contributed greatly to our understanding of the pathogenesis of atherosclerosis (76) but, as yet, have no value in everyday surgical pathology. T-lymphocyte markers, such as CD3 and CD4, may be of use in the diagnosis of vasculitis, especially temporal arteritis with minimal inflammatory activity (77). In transplant arteriosclerosis, there is a high relative proportion of CD8+ T lymphocytes, which also express granzyme B. In addition to von Willebrand factor (factor VIII), antifibrinogen antibodies are excellent for the demonstration of vascular leakiness and tissue damage (24,78); CD61 stains platelet aggregates in microvessels [for example in small vessel vasculitis (78)], angiolipomas, and coagulopathies [such as in the antiphospholipid syndrome]. Glycophorin A is a specific marker of erythrocytes and their precursors in the bone marrow. The epitopes are preserved in tissues for long periods, and the antibody is valuable in the detection of old hemorrhage; for example, in completely organized pulmonary thromboemboli (79) and in atherosclerotic plaques (80).

Antiamyloid antibodies (antiamyloid A, anti-immunoglobulin antibodies) are used to differentiate the nature of amyloid depositions, which have a preferential distribution in vessel walls. Cerebral vascular amyloid deposits usually do not stain with these antibodies. In pathologic conditions, such as cerebral amyloid angiopathy or amyloid found occasionally in cerebral vascular malformations, the depositions show positive staining with anti-β-amyloid antibody.

REFERENCES

1. Ferrari AU, Radaelli A, Centola M. Invited review: aging and the cardiovascular system. *J Appl Physiol* 2003;95:2591–2597.
2. Plante GE. Impact of aging on the body's vascular system. *Metabolism* 2003;52(suppl 2):31–35.
3. Lakatta EG, Levy D. Arterial and cardiac aging: major shareholders in cardiovascular disease enterprises: Part I: aging arteries: a 'set up' for vascular disease. *Circulation* 2003;107:139–146.
4. Robins SP, Farquharson C. Connective tissue components of the blood vessel wall in health and disease. In: Stehbens WE, Lie JT, eds. *Vascular Pathology*. London: Chapman & Hall; 1995:89–127.
5. Wigley C. Smooth muscle and the cardiovascular and lymphatic systems. In: Standring S, ed. *Gray's Anatomy: The Anatomical Basis of Clinical Practice*. 39th edition Philadelphia: Elsevier; 2005: 137–156.
6. Jacob MP. Extracellular matrix remodeling and matrix metalloproteinases in the vascular wall during aging and in pathological conditions *Biomed Pharmacother* 2003;57:195–202.
7. Kavurma MM, Bhindi R, Lowe HC, Chesterman C, Khachigian LM. Vessel wall apoptosis and atherosclerotic plaque instability *J Thromb Haemostasis* 2005;3:465–472.
8. Boddaert J, Mallat Z, Fornes P, et al. Age and gender effects on apoptosis in the human coronary arterial wall. *Mech Ageing Dev* 2005;126:678–684.
9. Doherty TM, Detrano RC. Coronary arterial calcification as an active process: a new perspective on an old problem. *Calcif Tissue Int* 1994;54:224–230.
10. Elliott RJ, McGrath LT. Calcification of the human thoracic aorta during aging. *Calcif Tissue Int* 1994;54:268–273.
11. Maier W, Altwegg LA, Corti R, et al. Inflammatory markers at the site of ruptured plaque in acute myocardial infarction: locally increased interleukin-6 and serum amyloid A but decreased C-rective protein. *Circulation* 2005;111:1355–1361.
12. Mucchiano GI, Häggqvist B, Sletten K, Westermark P. Apolipoprotein A-1-derived amyloid in atherosclerotic plaques of the human aorta. *J Pathol* 2001;193:270–275.
13. Schlatmann TJ, Becker AE. Histologic changes in the normal aging aorta: implications for dissecting aortic aneurysm. *Am J Cardiol* 1977;39:13–20.
14. Hsue PY, Salinas CL, Bolger AF, Benowitz NL, Waters DD. Acute aortic dissection related to crack cocaine. *Circulation* 2002;105: 1592–1595.
15. Ihling C, Szombathy T, Nampoothiri K, et al. Cystic medial degeneration of the aorta is associated with p53 accumulation, Bax upregulation, apoptotic cell death, and cell proliferation. *Heart* 1999;82:286–293.
16. Judge DP, Dietz HC. Marfan's syndrome. *Lancet* 2005;366: 1965–1976.
17. Ghorpade A, Baxter BT. Biochemistry and molecular regulation of matrix macromolecules in abdominal aortic aneurysms. *Ann N Y Acad Sci* 1996;800:138–150.
18. Lopez-Candales A, Holmes DR, Liao S, Scott MJ, Wickline SA, Thompson RW. Decreased vascular smooth muscle cell density in medial degeneration of human abdominal aortic aneurysms. *Am J Pathol* 1997;150:993–1007.
19. Alexander JJ. The pathobiology of aortic aneurysms. *J Surg Res* 2004;117:163–175.
20. Ramshaw AL, Parums DV. The distribution of adhesion molecules in chronic periaortitis. *Histopathology* 1994;24:23–32.
21. Szyszka-Mroz J, Wozniak W. A histological study of human ductus arteriosus during the last embryonic week. *Folia Morphol (Warsz)* 2003;62:365–367.
22. Stary HC, Blankenhorn DH, Chandler AB, et al. A definition of the intima of human arteries and of its atherosclerosis-prone regions. A report from the Committee on Vascular Lesions of the Council on Arteriosclerosis, American Heart Association. *Circulation* 1992;85:391–405.
23. Farrer M, Skinner JS, Albers CJ, Alberti KG, Adams PC. Outcome after coronary artery surgery in women and men in the north of England. *QJM* 1997;90:203–211.
24. Kolodgie FD, Gold HK, Burke AP, et al. Intraplaque hemorrhage and progression of coronary atheroma. *N Engl J Med* 2003;349: 2316–2325.
25. Stary HC, Chandler AB, Glagov S, et al. A definition of initial, fatty streak, and intermediate lesions of atherosclerosis. A report from the Committee on Vascular Lesions of the Council on Arteriosclerosis, American Heart Association. *Arterioscler Thromb* 1994;14: 840–856.
26. Stary HC, Chandler AB, Dinsmore RE, et al. A definition of advanced types of atherosclerotic lesions and a histological classification of atherosclerosis. A report from the Committee on Vascular Lesions of the Council on Arteriosclerosis, American Heart Association. *Arterioscler Thromb Vasc Biol* 1995;15: 1512–1531.
27. van der Wal AC, Becker AE. Atherosclerotic plaque rupture—pathologic basis of plaque stability and instability. *Cardiovasc Res* 1999;41:334–344.
28. Virmani R, Kolodgie FD, Burke AP, Farb A, Schwartz SM. Lessons from sudden coronary death: a comprehensive morphological classification scheme for atherosclerotic lesions. *Arterioscler Thromb Vasc Biol* 2000;20:1262–1275.
29. Schwartz CJ, Mitchel JR. Cellular infiltration of the human arterial adventitia associated with atheromatous plaques. *Circulation* 1962;26:73–78.

30. Hammes HP. Pericytes and the pathogenesis of diabetic retinopathy. *Horm Metab Res* 2005;37(suppl 1):39–43.
31. Allt G, Lawrenson JG. Pericytes: cell biology and pathology. *Cells Tissues Organs* 2001;169:1–11.
32. Azzali G. Structure, lymphatic vascularization and lymphocyte migration in mucosa-associated lymphoid tissue. *Immunol Rev* 2003;195:178–189.
33. Langes K, Hort W. Intimal fibrosis (phlebosclerosis) in the saphenous vein of the lower limb: a quantitative analysis. *Virchows Arch A Pathol Anat Histopathol* 1992;421:127–131.
34. O'Morchoe CC, O'Morchoe PJ. Differences in lymphatic and blood capillary permeability: ultrastructural–functional correlations. *Lymphology* 1987;20:205–209.
35. Wagenvoort CA, Mooi WJ. *Biopsy Pathology of the Pulmonary Vasculature.* London: Chapman & Hall; 1989.
36. Edwards WD. Pulmonary hypertension and related vascular diseases. In: Stehbens WE, Lie JT, eds. *Vascular Pathology.* London: Chapman & Hall; 1995:585–621.
37. Warnock ML, Kunzmann A. Changes with age in muscular pulmonary arteries. *Arch Pathol Lab Med* 1977;101:175–179.
38. Rubin LJ. Primary pulmonary hypertension. *N Engl J Med* 1997;336:111–117.
39. Farber HW, Loscalzo J. Pulmonary arterial hypertension. *N Engl J Med* 2004;351:1655–1665.
40. Patchefsky AS. Nonneoplastic pulmonary disease. In: Mills SE, ed. *Sternberg's Diagnostic Surgical Pathology.* 4th ed. Vol 1. Philadelphia: Lippincott Williams & Wilkins; 2004:1111–1172.
41. Weiss SW, Goldblum JR. Perivascular tumors. In: Weiss SW, Goldblum JR, eds. *Enzinger and Weiss's Soft Tissue Tumors.* 4th ed. St. Louis: Mosby; 2001:985–1035.
42. Warkentin TE, Moore JC, Anand SS, Lonn EM, Morgan DG. Gastrointestinal bleeding, angiodysplasia, cardiovascular disease, and acquired von Willebrand syndrome. *Transfus Med Rev* 2003;17:272–286.
43. Veldhuyzen van Zanten SJ, Bartelsman JF, Schipper ME, Tytgat GN. Recurrent massive haematemesis from Dieulafoy vascular malformations—a review of 101 cases. *Gut* 1986;27:213–222.
44. Sone Y, Kumada T, Toyoda H, et al. Endoscopic management and follow up of Dieulafoy lesion in the upper gastrointestinal tract. *Endoscopy* 2005;37:449–453.
45. Vikkula M, Boon LM, Mulliken JB. Molecular genetics of vascular malformations. *Matrix Biol* 2001;20:327–335.
46. Mulliken JB, Glowacki J. Hemangiomas and vascular malformations in infants and children: a classification based on endothelial characteristics. *Plast Reconstr Surg* 1982;69:412–422.
47. Requena L, Sangueza OP. Cutaneous vascular anomalies. Part I. Hamartomas, malformations, and dilation of preexisting vessels. *J Am Acad Dermatol* 1997;37:523–552.
48. Calonje E. Haemangiomas. In: Fletcher CDM, Unni KK, Mertens F, eds. *World Health Organisation Classification of Tumours: Pathology and Genetics of Tumours of Soft Tissue and Bone.* Lyon, France: IARC Press; 2002:156–158.
49. Clagett GP. Cerebrovascular disease. In: Harris JW, Beauchamp RD, Evers BM, Mattox KL, Townsend CM. *Sabiston Textbook of Surgery.* 17th ed. Philadelphia: WB Saunders; 2004:1939–1963.
50. Garratt KN, Edwards WD, Kaufmann UP, Vlietstra RE, Holmes DR Jr. Differential histopathology of primary atherosclerotic and restenotic lesions in coronary arteries and saphenous vein bypass grafts: analysis of tissue obtained from 73 patients by directional atherectomy. *J Am Coll Cardiol* 1991;17:442–448.
51. Kalan JM, Roberts WC. Morphologic findings in saphenous veins used as coronary arterial bypass conduits for longer than 1 year: necropsy analysis of 53 patients, 123 saphenous veins, and 1865 five-millimetre segments of veins. *Am Heart J* 1990;119:1164–1184.
52. Popma JJ, Kuntz RE, Baim DS. Percutaneous coronary and valvular intervention. In: Braunwald E, Zipes DP, Peter L, Bonow R, eds. *Braunwald's Heart Disease.* 7th ed. Philadelphia: WB Saunders; 2005:1367–1369.
53. Keeley EC, Boura JA, Grines CL. Primary angioplasty versus intravenous thrombolytic therapy for acute myocardial infarction: a quantitative review of 23 randomised trials. *Lancet* 2003;361:13–20.
54. Wenaweser P, Rey C, Eberli FR, et al. Stent thrombosis following bare-metal stent implantation: success of emergency percutaneous coronary intervention and predictors of adverse outcome. *Eur Heart J* 2005;26:1180–1187.
55. Kearney M, Pieczek A, Haley L, et al. Histopathology of in-stent restenosis in patients with peripheral artery disease. *Circulation* 1997;95:1998–2002.
56. Sangiorgi G, Taylor AJ, Farb A, et al. Histopathology of postpercutaneous transluminal coronary angioplasty remodeling in human coronary arteries. *Am Heart J* 1999;138(pt 1):681–687.
57. Windecker S, Remondino A, Eberli FR, et al. Sirolimus-eluting and paclitaxel-eluting stents for coronary revascularization. *N Engl J Med* 2005;353:653–662.
58. Dibra A, Kastrati A, Mehilli J, et al. Paclitaxel-eluting or sirolimus-eluting stents to prevent restenosis in diabetic patients. *N Engl J Med* 2005;353:663–670.
59. Clowes AW, Kirkman TR, Reidy MA. Mechanisms of arterial graft healing. Rapid transmural capillary ingrowth provides a source of intimal endothelium and smooth muscle in porous PTFE prostheses. *Am J Pathol* 1986;123:220–230.
60. Bazzoni G, Dejana E. Endothelial cell-to-cell junctions: molecular organization and role in vascular homeostasis. *Physiol Rev* 2004;84:869–901.
61. Van Itallie CM, Anderson JM. The molecular physiology of tight junction pores. *Physiology (Bethesda)* 2004;19:331–338.
62. Sawada N, Murata M, Kikuchi K, et al. Tight junctions and human diseases. *Med Electron Microsc* 2003;36:147–156.
63. Harhaj NS, Antonetti DA. Regulation of tight junctions and loss of barrier function in pathophysiology. *Int J Biochem Cell Biol* 2004;36:1206–1237.
64. Hsueh WA, Quinones MJ. Role of endothelial dysfunction in insulin resistance. *Am J Cardiol* 2003;92:10J–17J.
65. Sohl G, Willecke K. Gap junctions and the connexin protein family. *Cardiovasc Res* 2004;62:228–232.
67. Gratton JP, Bernatchez P, Sessa WC. Caveolae and caveolins in the cardiovascular system. *Circ Res* 2004;94:1408–1417.
68. Giepmans BN. Gap junctions and connexin-interacting proteins. *Cardiovasc Res* 2004;62:233–245.
69. Holthofer H, Virtanen I, Kariniemi AL, Hormia M, Linder E, Miettinen A. Ulex europaeus I lectin as a marker for vascular endothelium in human tissues. *Lab Invest* 1982;47:60–66.
70. Ordonez NG, Batsakis JG. Comparison of Ulex europaeus I lectin and factor VIII-related antigen in vascular lesions. *Arch Pathol Lab Med* 1984;108:129–132.
71. Dales JP, Garcia S, Carpentier S, et al. Prediction of metastasis risk (11 year follow-up) using VEGF-R1, VEGF-R2, Tie-2/Tek and CD105 expression in breast cancer (n=905). *Br J Cancer* 2004;90:1216–1221.
72. North PE, Waner M, Mizeracki A, Mihm MC Jr. GLUT1: a newly discovered immunohistochemical marker for juvenile hemangiomas. *Hum Pathol* 2000;31:11–22.
73. Jackson DG. Biology of the lymphatic marker LYVE-1 and applications in research into lymphatic trafficking and lymphangiogenesis. *APMIS* 2004;112:526–538.
74. Kahn HJ, Bailey D, Marks A. Monoclonal antibody D2-40, a new marker of lymphatic endothelium, reacts with Kaposi's sarcoma and a subset of angiosarcomas. *Mod Pathol* 2002;15:434–440.
75. Desmouliere A, Chaponnier C, Gabbiani G. Tissue repair, contraction, and the myofibroblast. *Wound Repair Regen* 2005;13:7–12.
76. Hansson GK. Inflammation, atherosclerosis and coronary artery disease. *N Engl J Med* 2005;352:1685–1695.
77. Weyand CM, Goronzy JJ. Medium- and large-vessel vasculitis. *N Engl J Med* 2003;349:160–169.
78. Meijer-Jorna LB, Mekkes JR, van der Wal AC. Platelet involvement in cutaneous small vessel vasculitis. *J Cutan Pathol* 2002;29:176–180.
79. Arbustini E, Morbini P, D'Armini AM, et al. Plaque composition in plexogenic and thromboembolic pulmonary hypertension: the critical role of thrombotic material in pultaceous core formation. *Heart* 2002;88:177–182.
80. Virmani R, Kolodgie FD, Burke AP, et al. Atherosclerotic plaque progression and vulnerability to rupture. Angiogenesis as a source of intraplaque hemorrhage. *Arterioscler Thromb Vasc Biol* 2005;25:2054–2061.

NERVOUS SYSTEM

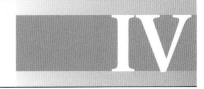

Peripheral Nervous System

Carlos Ortiz-Hidalgo   Roy O. Weller

INTRODUCTION

From a practical point of view, the pathology of peripheral nerves falls into two main categories: (a) peripheral neuropathies, which are diagnosed and treated by physicians and for which an elective nerve or muscle biopsy may be performed as a diagnostic procedure rather than as a therapeutic exercise, and (b) tumors and traumatic lesions, which are removed surgically mainly as a therapeutic measure to alleviate symptoms.

For the diagnosis of peripheral neuropathies, a detailed knowledge of the structure, immunohistochemistry and ultrastructure of peripheral nerves, and clinicopathological correlations is essential. The diagnosis of tumors and traumatic lesions, conversely, relies more on identifying the cellular components within the lesion and their interrelationships. This chapter, therefore, concentrates first on how to identify different cellular components in normal peripheral nerves and, second, on how knowledge of the normal structure of peripheral nerves can be used to identify and assess pathological lesions.

DEVELOPMENT OF THE PERIPHERAL NERVOUS SYSTEM

The first anatomical evidence of nervous system differentiation is the neural plate, which develops as a thickened specialized area in the middorsal ectoderm of the late gastrula stage of the developing embryo. This zone later becomes depressed along the axial midline to form a neural groove that folds inward to form the neural tube (1). Before fusion is completed, groups of cells become detached from the lateral folds of the neural plate to form the neural crests. Anteriorly, neural crests are located at the level of the presumptive diencephalon and extend backward along the whole neural tube (2).

The neural crest yields pluripotent cells endowed with migratory properties (1). In the peripheral nervous system, the neural crest is the source of neurons and satellite cells in the autonomic and sensory ganglia; ectodermal placodes may also give rise to ganglion cells in the cranial region. Schwann cells are also derived from the neural crest. Migrating pluripotent neural crest cells and their subsequent development is determined and progressively limited, perhaps by the inductive effect of neuregulins and their receptors erbB2 and erbB3, by environmental factors, and by relations with other cell types (1,3). The transcription factor Sox-10, that is initially expressed in the earliest migrating neural crest cells, appears to be intimately involved in the development of Schwann cells from the neural crest. Interestingly, the major myelin protein, P0, is also a transcriptional target for Sox-10 (3).

Many of the events that occur during the later stages of development of peripheral nerves are recapitulated during the regeneration that follows nerve damage in postnatal life. Developing neuroblasts of the dorsal root ganglia (posterior sensory root ganglia) extend neurites both centrally into the neural tube and toward the periphery. Developing motor neurons in the anterior lateral parts of the neural tube extend their neurites toward the periphery. Schwann cells derived from the neural crest become associated with the developing peripheral nerves and eventually form myelin around many of the axons. The proximal portions of the anterior horn cell axons and the central axons of the sensory ganglion cells are myelinated within the neural tube by oligodendrocytes (Figure 10.1).

Growth of Axons

One of the major questions that has been raised is how neuronal processes grow over long distances and arrive at specific terminal regions. Genetic determinants, growth factors, and the extracellular matrix appear to play important roles in the appropriate guidance of neuronal processes (4,5). In 1909, Santiago Ramón y Cajal proposed the concept of neurotrophic substances to explain the directionality and specificity of axonal growth in the developing nervous system, but it was not until the 1960s that nerve growth factor (NGF) was discovered by Rita Levi-Montalcini and Stanley Cohen, as a target-derived neurotrophic factor that supports the survival and differentiation of sensory and autonomic ganglia in the peripheral nervous system (6).

Nerve growth factor is a protein composed of three subunits—alpha (α), beta (β), and gamma (γ)—but only the β-NGF has nerve growth–promoting activity. Beta-NGF in humans is a 14.5 KDa polypeptide, γ-NGF is an arginyl esterase, whereas the function of the α subunit is not known (6,7). Other substances that participate in axon growth are members of the NGF family [such as brain-derived neurotrophic factor (BDNF)]; neurotrophins 3 (NT-3), 4/5 (NT-4/5), and 6 (NT-6); semaphoring-3A, neuropilin-1, and ephrin (8). The tips of growing axons possess multiple surface receptors for soluble and bound molecules that provide information for the axons' growth course (8). Nerve growth factor interacts with the NGF receptor on the surface of the axon and promotes motility of the growing tip of the axon by interaction with the cytoskeleton of the cell. Mitochondria, neurotubules, neurofilaments, actin filaments, and some cisternae of smooth endoplasmic

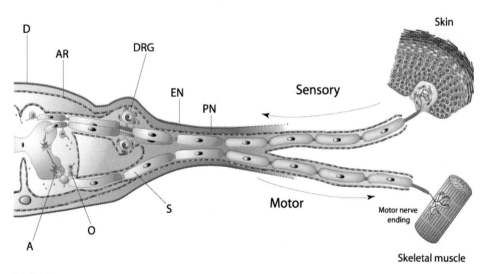

Sergio Piña-Oviedo

Figure 10.1 Anatomy of spinal nerve roots. Motor axons arising from the anterior horn cell (*A*) are initially myelinated by oligodendrocytes (*O*) and then pass into the anterior root to be myelinated by Schwann cells (*S*). Sensory nerve axons pass into the dorsal root ganglion (*DRG*), and the central extension of the sensory neuron passes via the dorsal root into the spinal cord. Arachnoid (*AR*) appears to be continuous with the perineurium of the peripheral nerve (*PN*). Dura (*D*) extends from the spinal cord to coat the roots within the intervertebral foramen and is continuous with the epineurium (*EN*).

reticulum are incorporated into the axonal growth cone by axoplasmic flow. In addition to its growth promoting properties, NGF also promotes the early synthesis of neurotransmitters.

Schwann cells in the developing nerve produce NGF and possess NGF receptors on their surface membranes, but expression of these receptors diminishes markedly as the peripheral nerve matures. As NGF binds to Schwann cell receptors and becomes concentrated on the surface of the primitive Schwann cell, it provides a chemotactic stimulus for growing axons (9). Failure of trophic interactions between the target organ and its innervation may result in nerve dysfunction. Indeed, cases of human neuropathies have been attributed to deficiency of neurotrophic factors; important data that provides a rational basis for the clinical use of neurotrophic agents in peripheral neuropathies (7).

The extracellular matrix also plays an important role in axonal growth and guidance. The tip of the growing axon has receptors for adhesion to extracellular substances such as collagen, fibronectin, laminin, and entactin; binding of extracellular components to these receptors promotes elongation of axons and stimulates cytoskeletal protein synthesis—and therefore cell movement and axon growth. Some of these extracellular components are found within or near basement membranes surrounding Schwann cells (10,11).

Schwann Cells and Myelination

Schwann cells move freely between and around developing peripheral nerve axons, forming primitive sheaths around the neurites and growing in parallel with them. Contact with axons stimulates Schwann cell division in vitro (12). In vivo Schwann cell multiplication virtually ceases in the normal adult animal, but mitotic activity is induced by peripheral nerve damage. It is thought that exposure of the axon to the Schwann cell following loss of myelin sheaths (demyelination) or during axonal regeneration following axonal degeneration (wallerian degeneration) promotes Schwann cell division and that the relationship between Schwann cells and axons in the normal nerve induces some sort of contact inhibition in the Schwann cells. If axon regeneration does not occur following axon damage, Schwann cells gradually decrease in number, suggesting that Schwann cell growth and survival depend on contact with axons (12). Experimental evidence also suggests that continued axon regeneration depends on the presence of Schwann cells (13).

By the ninth week of gestation, fascicles of the human sural nerve are identifiable and contain large axon bundles surrounded by Schwann cell processes (14). Between weeks 10 and 15, Schwann cells extend several long flattened processes that wrap around large clusters of fine axons. At this stage, two to four Schwann cells are located within a common basement membrane and form Schwann "families" (15).

Myelination of peripheral nerves in humans commences between the twelfth and eighteenth week of gestation (16). Initiation of myelination depends on the diameter of the axon and its association with Schwann cells. By the time that axons have increased in diameter to between 1.0 and 3.2 μm, they are in a 1:1 relationship with Schwann cells and have either formed mesaxons or membrane spirals with compact sheaths of 3 to 15 layers (12,15). The reason why some nerves become myelinated and others do not is not clear. Schwann cells around myelinated fibers and around unmyelinated fibers are both able to produce myelin, but the factors that determine whether myelination occurs are unknown. Certain transcription factors, such as Krox-20 and Oct-6, are known to be involved in the myelination program (3,4). In Oct-6 null mice, for instance, myelination is severely delayed, while in Krox-20 null mice myelination fails completely (3). Schwann cells in developing and regenerating peripheral nerves also express high levels of the neurotrophin receptor p75NTR. Neurotrophins are a family of proteins that play a variety of functions in the development and maintenance of the peripheral nervous system (17). Certain glycoproteins, such as myelin-associated glycoproteins, are believed to participate in establishing specific Schwann cell–axon interactions in the developing peripheral nervous system (18).

Experimental studies have shown that axons may induce the formation of myelin if the unmyelinated sympathetic chain is grafted onto a myelinated nerve such as the saphenous nerve. Schwann cells that had not previously formed myelin will do so if they come into contact with large, regenerating axons that were previously myelinated (3). It appears also that Schwann cells may influence the caliber of axons since axonal diameter may be decreased markedly in some hereditary demyelinating neuropathies in which there is a genetic defect in Schwann cells and in myelination (12,13). It has been demonstrated that myelinating Schwann cells control the number and phosphorylation state of neurofilaments in the axon, leading to enlargement of the axon itself. Conversely, absence of myelin results in fewer neurofilaments, reduced phosphorylation levels, and therefore smaller axon diameters (18). Myelin-associated glycoprotein (MAG) acts as a myelin signal that modulates the caliber of myelinated axons (19). Maintenance of an axon therefore appears to depend not only on influences from the neuron cell body but also on interactions of the axon with the accompanying Schwann cells (12).

Some 70% of axons within a mixed sensory nerve, such as the sural nerve, are very small and will become segregated into groups of 8 to 15 axons lying in longitudinal grooves within one Schwann cell; these will form the unmyelinated fibers within the peripheral nerve. Thus, all axons in the peripheral nervous system are invaginated into the surfaces of Schwann cells, but myelin sheaths only form around the larger axons, which represent only a small proportion of peripheral nerve fibers.

ANATOMY OF PERIPHERAL NERVES

An understanding of the anatomy of peripheral nerves is essential for the interpretation of clinical signs and symptoms and for planning an autopsy to investigate a patient with a peripheral neuropathy (14,15,19,20).

Major nerves, such as the sciatic and median nerves, contain motor, sensory, and autonomic nerve fibers; they are thus compound nerve trunks. It was Sir Charles Bell, the Scottish physician, who first demonstrated that motor function lay in the anterior roots; François Magendie, the French physiologist, showed that the sensory function lay in the posterior roots. This (anterior-motor; posterior-sensory) is known as the Bell-Magendie law. Motor nerves are derived from anterior horn cells in the spinal cord or from defined nuclei in the brainstem. The initial segment of the axon lies within the central nervous system and is ensheathed by myelin formed by oligodendrocytes (Figure 10.1). As the axons pass out of the brainstem or spinal cord they become myelinated by Schwann cells. Anterior spinal roots join the posterior roots as they pass through the intervertebral foramina to form peripheral nerve trunks. Cranial nerves leave the skull through a number of different foramina. The junction point between oligodendrocytes and the Schwann sheath of the cranial nerves, known as Obersteiner-Redlich zone (O-Rz), has some clinical significance. For example, the pulsatile compression of the O-Rz by a vessel in some exit foramina may be responsible for the clinical symptoms of trigeminal and glossopharyngeal neuralgia, hemifacial spasm, torticollis spasmodicus, or even symptoms of essential hypertension when a vascular cross-compression of the left vagus nerve occurs (21)

Motor nerves end peripherally at muscle endplates and many of the sensory nerves are associated with peripheral sensory endings. The cell bodies of sensory nerves lie outside the central nervous system in the dorsal root ganglia or in cranial nerve ganglia (15). Each ganglion contains numerous, almost spherical neurons (ganglion cells) with their surrounding satellite cells. Such satellite cells are derived from the neural crest and have an origin similar to that of Schwann cells (22). Satellite cells have been referred to in the past by a large variety of names such as amphicyte, capsular cells, perisomatic gliocyte, or perineuronal satellite Schwann cells.

Dorsal root ganglion cells were first described by the Swiss anatomist Albert von Kolliker in 1844. They are examples of pseudounipolar cells, which means that a single, highly coiled axon, or stem process, arises from each perikaryon; but, at varying distances from the neuron, there is a T- or Y-shaped bifurcation, always at a node of Ranvier, with the formation of central and peripheral axons. Thus, the initial segment of axon gives the impression that the cell is a unipolar neuron when it actually has two axons (Figure 10.1). The central axon passes into the spinal cord, either to synapse in the posterior sensory horn of gray matter or to pass directly into the dorsal columns. Peripheral axons pass into the peripheral nerves (15).

Autonomic nerves are either parasympathetic or sympathetic. Preganglionic parasympathetic fibers pass out of the brainstem in the cranial nerves III, VII, IX, and X and from the sacral cord in the second and third sacral nerves. Postganglionic neurons are situated near or within the structures being innervated. Sympathetic preganglionic fibers arise from neurons in the intermediolateral cell columns of gray matter in the thoracic spinal cord and pass out in thoracic anterior roots (15). These preganglionic fibers are myelinated and reach the sympathetic trunk through the corresponding anterior spinal roots; they synapse with the sympathetic ganglion cells in paravertebral or prevertebral locations. The autonomic nervous system innervates viscera, blood vessels, and smooth muscle of the eye and skin (15).

HISTOLOGY, IMMUNOCYTOCHEMISTRY, AND ULTRASTRUCTURE OF PERIPHERAL NERVES

Components of the Nerve Sheath

Macroscopic inspection of a normal peripheral nerve reveals glistening white bundles of fascicles bound together by connective tissue. The intraneural arrangement of fascicles is variable and changes continuously throughout the length of every nerve. Damaged peripheral nerves are often gray and shrunken due to the loss of myelin. Microscopically, transverse sections of a peripheral nerve (Figure 10.2) show how endoneurial compartments containing axons and Schwann cells are surrounded by perineurium to form individual fascicles embedded in epineurial fibrous tissue.

Epineurium

The epineurium consists of moderately dense connective tissue binding nerve fascicles together. It merges with the adipose tissue that surrounds peripheral nerves (Figure 10.2A), particularly in the subcutaneous tissue. In addition to fibroblasts, the epineurium contains mast cells. Although mostly composed of collagen, there are elastic fibers in the epineurium so that, when a specimen of unfixed nerve is removed from the body, there is some elastic recoil of the epineurium (20,23). The amount of epineurial tissue varies and is more abundant in nerves adjacent to joints. As nerve branches become smaller to consist of only one fascicle, epineurium is no longer present. In nerves that consist of several fascicles, one or more arteries, veins, and lymphatics run longitudinally in the epineurium parallel to the nerve fascicles (the vasa nervorum) (15,20,25) (Figure 10.2). Inflammation and occlusion of such arteries is an important cause of nerve damage in vasculitic diseases (25). The overgrowth of epineurial adipose tissue produces

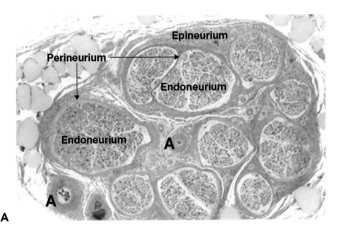 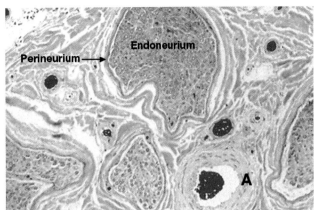

A

B

Figure 10.2 Peripheral nerve sheaths and compartments. **A.** A low-power view of a transverse section of a normal sural nerve. The nerve fascicles with roughly circular outlines are surrounded by perineurium and embedded in the connective tissue of the epineurium. Epineurial blood vessels (*arrow*) are also cut in cross section, and there is adherent adipose tissue (*upper left*) (1-μm resin section, toluidine blue, ×16). **B.** The endoneurial compartment containing myelinated and nonmyelinated nerve fibers and their accompanying Schwann cells is surrounded by perineurium. A large epineurial artery (*arrow*) is seen at the lower right (paraffin section, H&E, ×45).

the so-called lipofibromatous hamartoma, which classically affects the hands and is associated with enlargement of the affected digit (26).

Perineurium

Originally described by Friedrich G.J. Henle in the nineteenth century, the perineurium has, in the past, been known by a variety of different terms, such as mesothelium, perilemma, neurothelium, perineurothelium, and, more recently, perineurial epithelium (15,20).

Based on the pioneer work of the 1995 Nobel Prize winners Christiane Nüsslein-Volhard and Wieschaus, an intercellular signaling molecule secreted by Schwann cells known as Desert Hedgehog, was described, that functions as an important molecule in the formation of the perineurium. Apparently this molecule signals to the surrounding connective tissue cells to organize the perineurium (3).

The perineurium consists of concentric layers of flattened cells separated by layers of collagen (Figures 10.2–10.4). The number of cell layers varies from nerve to nerve and depends on the size of the nerve fascicle. In the sural nerve, for example, there are 8 to 12 layers of perineurial cells, but the number of layers decreases progressively so that a single layer of perineurial cells surrounds fine distal nerve branches (20). Perineurial cells eventually fuse to form the outer-core of the terminal sensory endings in pacinian corpuscles and muscle spindles (20,24,27). In motor nerves, the perineurial cells form an open funnel as the nerve ends at the motor endplate. Paraganglia of the vagus nerve may lie just underneath the perineurium (28).

By electron microscopy, perineurial cells are seen as thin sheets of cytoplasm containing small amounts of endoplasmic reticulum, filaments, and numerous pinocytotic vesicles that open on to the external and internal

surfaces of the cell. Basement membrane is usually seen on both sides of each perineurial lamina (29,30). Numerous cell junctions, including well-formed tight junctions (zonulae occludentes), are present between adjacent perineurial cells and appear to be critical for the formation of

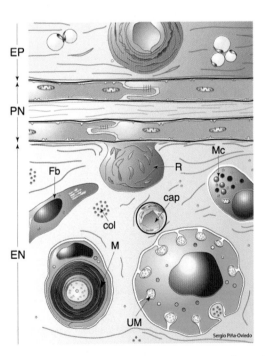

Figure 10.3 Diagram to show the major elements of peripheral nerve compartments. The epineurium (*EP*) contains collagen, blood vessels, and some adherent adipose tissue. The flattened cells of the perineurium (*PN*) are joined by tight junctions and form flattened layers separated by collagen fibers. Renaut bodies (*R*) project into the endoneurium (*EN*). Schwann cells forming lamellated myelin (*M*) (drawn uncompacted in this diagram) surround the larger axons. Multiple unmyelinated axons (*UM*) are invaginated into the surface of Schwann cells. Other elements include fibroblasts (*Fb*), mast cells (*Mc*), capillaries (*cap*), and collagen (*col*).

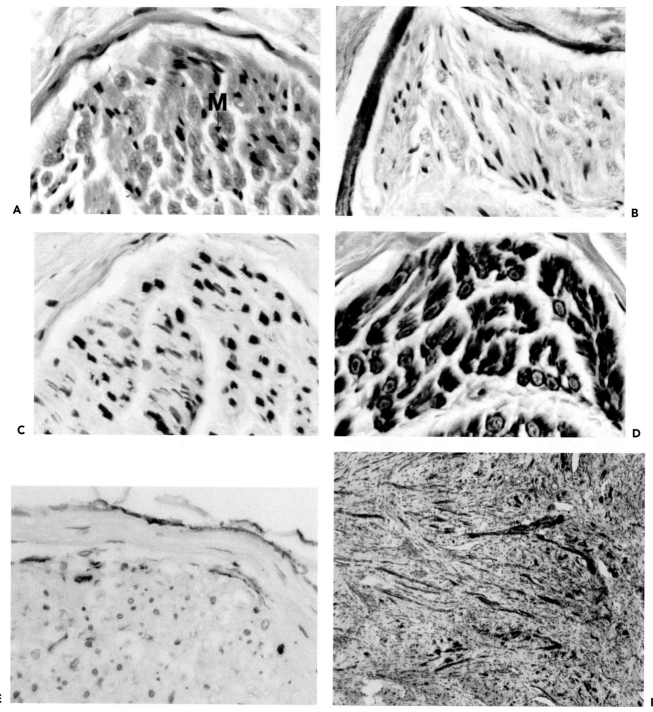

Figure 10.4 Immunocytochemistry of a normal peripheral nerve. **A.** Part of single nerve fascicle, cut in transverse section. Perineurium (*top*) surrounds the endoneurium containing myelinated nerve fibers (*M*). The nuclei are mainly those of Schwann cells (paraffin section, H&E, ×160). **B.** Similar field to (A) stained for epithelial membrane antigen. The perineurium (*top*) is densely stained [immunoperoxidase technique (ABC) with antiepithelial membrane antigen (anti-EMA) antibody, ×160]. **C.** Part of a nerve fascicle stained for neurofilament protein. Large myelinated axons are well stained, but unmyelinated axons are much smaller and more difficult to detect [immunoperoxidase technique (ABC) using an antibody against the 80 KDa neurofilament protein, ×160]. **D.** Part of a nerve fascicle stained for S-100 protein showing densely stained Schwann cells [immunoperoxidase (ABC) using anti-S-100 protein antibody, ×160]. **E.** Part of a nerve showing CD34+ endoneurial cells. These cells are clearly distinct from the Schwann cells that comprise the bulk of the cell in the nerve [immunoperoxidase technique (ABC) using anti-CD34 (QBend10) antibody, ×160]. **F.** A traumatized nerve cut in longitudinal section showing regenerating axons (stained brown) (immunohistochemistry for GAP 43, ×40). (Photograph provided by Professor James Nicoll.)

the blood-nerve barrier (15,30). Claudins are integral membrane proteins that play a major role in tight junctions and are present in normal and neoplastic perineurium. Claudins comprise a group of approximately 20 different proteins that are exclusively localized in tight junctions (31). In peripheral nerves, claudin-1 expression is largely limited to perineurial cells but is also present in paranodal regions and in the outer mesaxon along internodes (31,32). When tracer substances such as ferritin and horseradish peroxidase are injected into the blood, they do not enter peripheral nerves. Their entry is prevented by tight junctions in endoneurial capillaries and by the tight junctions in the inner layers of the perineurium. Thus, there is a blood-nerve barrier analogous to the blood-brain barrier (30). The blood-nerve barrier is present soon after birth and may prevent the entry of drugs and other substances into nerves that may otherwise interfere or block nerve conduction (30,33). No such blood-nerve barrier exists in the dorsal root ganglia or in autonomic ganglia; these sites in the peripheral nervous system are vulnerable to certain toxins, such as mercury (34).

If the perineurium is injured, there is breakdown of the blood-nerve barrier and perineurial cells migrate into the endoneurium to surround small fascicles of nerve fibres (35). This is classically seen in amputation neuromas but is also observed in focal compressive lesions of nerve (36). The swelling of the nerve and the concentric arrangement of the perineurial cells in the compressive lesions spawned the term *localized hypertrophic neuropathy*, but it is quite different from hypertrophic neuropathy (36), in which Schwann cells form whorls around individual axons in response to recurrent segmental demyelination (see below).

Whereas the epineurial sheath of the nerve is continuous with the dura mater at the junction of spinal nerves and spinal nerve roots (Figure 10.1), the perineurium blends with the pia-arachnoid. There are some morphological similarities between perineurium and arachnoid cells, although arachnoid cells are not usually coated by basement membrane. Immunocytochemically, perineurial cells and pia-arachnoid cells are positive for epithelial membrane antigen (EMA) (Figure 10.4) and vimentin but are negative for S-100 protein and CD57 (37,38). Perineurial cells also express insulin-dependent glucose transporter protein I (Glut-1) (32,39).

Epithelial membrane antigen belongs to a heterogenous family of highly glycosylated transmembrane proteins found originally on the surface of mammary epithelial cells (40) but which are also present in the cells of virtually all epithelial tumors (40). However, EMA is not restricted to epithelial structures and has been identified on plasma cells and on cells in certain lymphomas and soft tissue tumors (20,40). Perineurial cells, arachnoid, and pia share certain ultrastructural characteristics and express EMA and vimentin in their cytoplasm. Immunohistochemistry has demonstrated that perineurial cells proliferate in some conditions, such as traumatic neuroma, Morton's neuroma, neurofibroma, solitary circumscribed neuroma, neurothekeoma, pacinian neuroma, and in the mucosal neuromas associated with multiple endocrine neoplasia (vide infra) (33,41).

Some tumor cells break through the perineurial sheath to grow along the perineurial space; perineurial invasion has been correlated with decreased survival times in some cancers (42). The problem for the histopathologist, however, is that sometimes perineurial invasion cannot be unequivocally determined on hematoxylin and eosin (H&E)–stained sections. Immunocytochemistry for Glut-1, EMA, and claudin-1 may be used to rapidly and accurately assess the presence of perineurial invasion (38,43). Care must be taken, however, when examining cases of vasitis nodosa, in which benign proliferating ductules may be found within the perineurium and endoneurium (44). Nerve involvement has also been reported in fibrocystic disease of the breast, normal and hyperplastic prostate, and normal pancreas (44).

Endoneurium

The endoneurium is the compartment that contains axons and their surrounding Schwann cells, collagen fibers, fibroblasts, capillaries, and a few mast cells (Figures 10.3–10.5).

In cross sections of peripheral nerves, some 90% of the nuclei belong to Schwann cells, 5% to fibroblasts, and 5% to other cells (such as mast cells and capillary endothelial cells). Within the endoneurium, CD34+ bipolar cells with delicate dendritic processes have been identified and are distinct from Schwann cells (45,46). Similar cells have been identified in peripheral nerve sheath tumors in various proportions (45).

Some investigators have observed endoneurial dendritic cells, distinct from Schwann cells and conventional fibroblasts, that may function as phagocytes under certain conditions (47). In this regard, it has been described within the human endoneurium, an intrinsic population of immunocompetent and potentially phagocytic cells (endoneurial macrophages), that share several lineage-related and functional markers with macrophages and may represent the peripheral counterpart of del-Rio-Hortega cells (microglia) of the CNS (48,49).

Nerve fibers may be myelinated or unmyelinated but not all nerves have the same nerve fiber composition. Most biopsies of peripheral nerves in humans are taken from the sural nerve at the ankle, and it is the composition of this nerve that has been most closely studied (50). Fibroblasts are ultrastructurally identical to fibroblasts elsewhere in the body. Mast cells are a normal constituent of the endoneurium and are also seen in sensory ganglia and in the epineurial sheath of peripheral nerves. There is an increase in the number of mast cells in some pathological conditions such as axonal (wallerian) degeneration

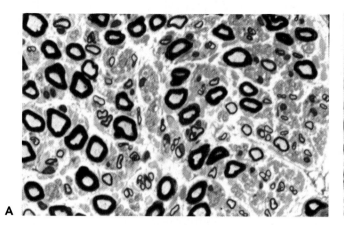
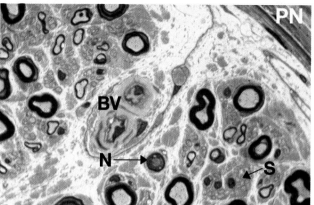

Figure 10.5 High-power histology of human sural nerve in transverse section. **A.** Large- and small-diameter myelinated fibers are seen. In the normal nerve, these fibers are separated from each other, but small numbers of clusters (see Figure 10.12B) are seen in this illustration (1-μm resin section, toluidine blue, ×160). **B.** Part of a sural nerve fascicle cut in transverse section. Perineurium is at the top right (*PN*). Both large and small myelinated fibers vary in cross-sectional outline. Splits within the sheath are Schmidt-Lanterman incisures. Also visible are an endoneurial blood vessel (*BV*) and a section through a fiber near the node of Ranvier (*N*). Unmyelinated axons are seen as unstained circles within Schwann cells (*S*). (1-μm resin section, ×310.)

and in some neoplastic entities such as von Recklinghausen's disease (neurofibromatosis). A characteristically high number of mast cells is seen in neurofibromas, but they are only present in the Antoni B areas of schwannomas (24,51). Mast cells are thought to influence growth of neurofibromas because some of their mediators may also act as growth factors (52). Apparently the inciting factor for mast cell migration into nerve sheath tumors is Kit ligand that is hypersecreted by NF−/− Schwann cell populations (52). Mast cell stabilizers are claimed to reduce proliferation and itching of neurofibromas (52). Following nerve injury, there is breakdown of the blood-nerve barrier as endoneurial vessels become permeable to fluid and protein; this increase in permeability may be related to the release of biogenic amines from mast cells within the endoneurium. Proteases released from mast cells have a high myelinolytic activity and may play a role in the breakdown of myelin in certain demyelinating diseases (52,53).

Collagen within the endoneurial compartment is highly organized and forms two distinct sheaths around myelinated and unmyelinated nerve fibers and their Schwann cells (see Figures 10.8, 10.10). The outer endoneurial sheath (of Key and Retzius) is composed of longitudinally oriented large diameter collagen fibers; the inner endoneurial sheath (of Plenk and Laidlaw) is composed of fine collagen fibers oriented obliquely or circumferentially to the nerve fibers. The term *neurilemma* has been applied to the combined sheath formed by the basement membrane of the Schwann cell and the adjacent inner endoneurial sheath (15,24). Thus the term *neurilemmoma* is inappropriate when used to describe tumors of Schwann cell origin

(schwannomas). The longitudinal orientation of collagen fibers in the outer endoneurial sheath, together with the Schwann cell basement membrane tubes, may play an important role in guiding axons as they regenerate following peripheral nerve damage (3,24).

Renaut bodies (Figures 10.3, 10.6) are seen not infrequently in the endoneurium of human peripheral nerves. Described in the nineteenth century by the French physician Joseph Louis Renaut, they are cylindrical (circular in cross section), hyalin bodies attached to the inner aspect of the perineurium. Composed of randomly oriented collagen fibers, spidery fibroblasts, and perineurial cells, Renaut bodies stain positively with Alcian blue because of the presence of acid glycosaminoglycans. The rest of the endoneurium also contains Alcian blue–positive mucoproteins (24,54). Renaut bodies express vimentin and EMA and produce extracellular matrix highly enriched in elastic fiber components (55). In longitudinal section, they may extend for some distance along the nerve and end in a blunt and abrupt fashion (55). These bodies are more prominent in horses and donkeys than in humans (2). Their precise function is not known, but Renaut himself thought that they may act as protective cushions within the nerve. They increase in number in compressive neuropathies and in a number of other neuropathies, including hypothyroid neuropathy, and may be a reaction to trauma (54,55).

Blood Supply of Peripheral Nerves

Vasa nervorum supplying peripheral nerves are derived from a series of branches from associated regional arteries. Branches from those arteries enter the epineurium (Figures

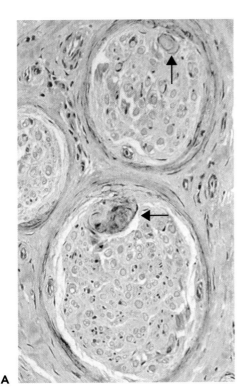
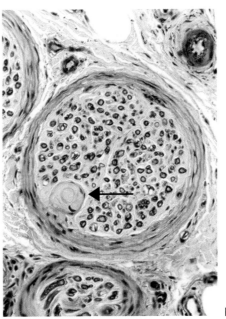

A   **B**

Figure 10.6 Nerve fascicles showing Renaut bodies (*arrows*). **A.** Immunostaining for epithelial membrane antigen (EMA). **B.** Russell-Movat pentachrome, showing the Renaut bodies in blue.

10.2, 10.3) to form an intercommunicating or anastomosing plexus. From that plexus, vessels penetrate the perineurium obliquely and enter the endoneurium as capillaries often surrounded by pericytes (Figure 10.5). Tight junctions between the endothelial cells of the endoneurial capillaries constitute the blood-nerve barrier (30).

Complete infarction of peripheral nerves is very uncommon, probably due to the rich anastomotic connections of epineurial arteries. However, inflammation and thrombotic occlusion of epineurial arteries is seen in vasculitides (56), and occlusion by emboli occurs in patients with atherosclerotic peripheral vascular disease; both these disorders result in ischemic damage to peripheral nerves with axonal degeneration and consequent peripheral neuropathy (50).

Nerve Fibers

Most peripheral nerves contain a mixture of myelinated and unmyelinated nerve fibers. As the axons are oriented longitudinally along the nerve, quantitative estimates of the number of fibers in the nerve and their diameters are only adequately assessed in exact transverse sections. Staining techniques that can be used to identify nerve fibers and other components within peripheral nerves are summarized in Table 10.1. Longitudinal sections of peripheral nerve are less valuable than transverse sections, but teased nerve fibers (see Figure 10.15D) are very valuable for detect-

ing segmental demyelination and remyelination and for assessing past axonal degeneration and regeneration (50).

In a transverse section of a human sural nerve, there are approximately 8,000 myelinated fibers/mm^2, whereas the unmyelinated axons are more numerous at 30,000 myelinated fibers/mm^2. Peripheral nerve fibers are classified as class A, class B, and class C fibers, according to their size, function, and the speed at which they conduct nerve impulses. Class A fibers are myelinated and are further subdivided into six groups covering three size ranges. The largest are 10 to 20 μm diameter myelinated fibers that conduct at 50 to 100 m/sec; myelinated fibers 5 to 15 μm in diameter conduct at 20 to 90 m/sec, and 1 to 7-μm diameter myelinated fibers conduct at 12 to 30 m/sec. Class B fibers are myelinated preganglionic autonomic fibers some 3 μm in diameter and conducting at 3 to 15 m/sec. Unmyelinated fibers are small (0.2 to 1.5 μm in diameter), conduct impulses at 0.3 to 1.6 m/sec, and include postganglionic autonomic and afferent sensory fibers, including pain fibers (57).

Myelinated Axons

Ultrastructure

Although myelinated nerve fibers can be demonstrated in paraffin sections (Figure 10.4), they are best visualized by light microscopy in 0.5- to 1-μm thick toluidine blue–stained resin sections (Figure 10.5). They exhibit a bimodal

TABLE 10.1

HISTOLOGIC TECHNIQUES FOR PERIPHERAL NERVES

Technique	Application
A. General	
1. Hematoxylin and eosin (H&E)	Detection of inflammation, myelin, and axons (Figure 10.2B, 10.4A)
2. Hematoxylin-van Gieson	Collagen stains red; myelin black
3. Reticulin stains	Basement membrane around each Schwann cell in normal (e.g., Gordon-Sweet) nerve and schwannomas (Figure 10.17C)
4. Masson's trichrome	Fibrinoid necrosis in vasculitis
5. Alcian blue	Glycosaminoglycans stain blue
6. Toluidine blue	(a) Mast cells in paraffin section (b) general stain for 1 μm resin sections, (c) metachromatic stain for sulfatide lipid
B. Stains for myelin	
1. Luxol fast blue	Myelin stains blue; can be combined with silver stains for axons
2. Loyez	Myelin stains black
3. Osmium	Myelin stains black
4. Periodic acid-Schiff (PAS)	Myelin stains bright pink (good for detecting small number of nerve fibers in muscle biopsies)
5. Polarized light (frozen section)	Normal myelin, birefingent; degenerating myelin isotropic (nonbirefingent)
6. Marchi's	Degenerating myelin stains black (due to the presence of cholesterol esters); normal myelin is unstained.
7. Oil red O	Degenerating myelin stains bright red; normal myelin, pink
C. Stains for axons	
1. Palmgren's or Bodian's (silver stains)	Axons stain black.
D. 0.5 to 1 μm resin sections	
1. Toluidine blue	Myelin stains black; axons unstained; Schwann cells and other cells, blue; collagen, blue (Figures 10.2A, 10.5, 10.12 and 10.14A,B)
2. Toluidine blue and carbol fuschin.	Myelin stains black; axons, unstained; cells and collagen, pink/blue (Figure 10.14C)
3. Immunohistochemistry can be performed on these sections.	
E. Electron microscopy	(Figures 10.8, 10.9, 10.10, and 10.16)
F. Teased fibers	
1. Osmium tetraoxide stained	Myelin; nodes of Ranvier; demyelination and remyelination (Figure 10.14D)
2. Enzyme histochemistry	
a. Mitochondrial enzymes	Schwann cytoplasm; axoplasm
b. Acid phosphatase	Lysosomal activity associated with degenerating myelin
c. Polarized light	Myelin
3. Lipid histochemistry	
a. Sudan black B	Myelin
b. Oil red O	Normal and degenerating myelin
4. Immunohistochemistry	
a. S-100 protein	
b. CD57 (Leu-7)	Schwann cells (Figure 10.4); schwannomas
c. CD56 (NKH1)	Schwann cells; schwannomas
d. Calretinin	Schwann cells and some schwannomas
e. CD146 (Mel-CAM)	Schwann cells; some schwannomas
f. GFAP (glial fibrillary acidic protein)	Some schwannoma cells; possibly unmyelinated
g. Myelin basic protein	Myelin
h. Neurofilament protein	Axons (Figure 10.4C)
i. Epithelial membrane antigen/Glut-1/claudin-1	Perineurium (Figure 10.4B)
j. CD34 (QBend10)	CD34 positive endonerual fibroblasts
k. CD68 (KP-1/PGM1)	Endoneurial macrophages.
l. GAP 43	Regenerating axons (Figure 10.4F)

distribution of fiber diameter in the normal nerve, with peaks at 5 and 13 μm and a range of 2 to 20 μm. Most axons above 3 μm in diameter are myelinated. Although along much of its length a myelinated nerve fiber has a circular outline in cross section, there is considerable variation in shape within the normal nerve, especially in the perinuclear regions and in the regions around the node of Ranvier (paranodal regions) (Figure 10.7).

The axon itself is limited by a smooth plasma membrane (axolemma), that is separated from the encompassing Schwann cell by a 10 to 20 nm gap (periaxonal space of Klebs) (Figure 10.8). The axonal cytoplasm (axoplasm) contains mitochondria, cisternae of smooth endoplasmic reticulum, occasional ribosomes and glycogen granules, peroxisomes, and vesicles containing neurotransmitters. The most prominent components of the axoplasm, however, are the filamentous and tubular structures. Microfilaments, 5 to 7 μm in diameter, are composed of chains of actin and comprise approximately 10% of the total axonal

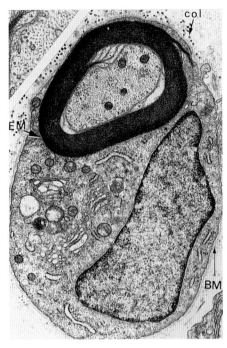

Figure 10.8 Transverse section of a myelinated nerve fiber in the perinuclear region. The axon contains mitochondria, small vesicles, and numerous neurofilaments and neurotubules cut in cross section (**inset**,*top left*). A distinct periaxonal space separates the axon from its encompassing Schwann cell. Myelin is compacted except at the external mesaxon (*EM*) and internally around the internal mesaxon near the axon itself. Part of a Schmidt-Lanterman incisure is seen on the inside of the myelin sheath. Abundant rough and smooth endoplasmic reticulum is seen in the perinuclear cytoplasm of the Schwann cell. A basement membrane (*BM*) surrounds the Schwann cell plasma membrane, and endoneurial collagen fibers are seen cut in cross section (*col*). (Electron micrograph, ×18,400); inset, ×40,000.)

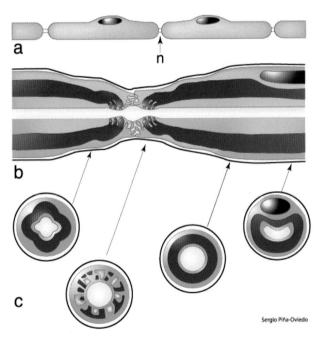

Sergio Piña-Oviedo

Figure 10.7 Diagram to show the relationships between (A) teased fibers, (B) nerve fibers in longitudinal section, and (C) nerve fibers in transverse section. **A.** In teased fibers, nodes of Ranvier (*N*) are separated by internodal portions of the Schwann cell and myelin sheath. The Schwann cell nucleus is roughly in the center of the internode. **B.** Longitudinal section through the node of Ranvier shows how the myelin sheath terminates as a series of end-loops. The axon narrows as it passes through the node of Ranvier. **C.** Transverse sections of peripheral nerve as seen in electron micrographs and 1 μm resin sections are here related to the different portions of the internode and the node of Ranvier. *From left to right*, the paranodal region shows crenation of both axon and myelin sheath in larger fibers. At the node of Ranvier, the axon is small and coated by radially arranged Schwann cell processes and myelin end-loops. Throughout most of the internode, the myelinated fiber is circular. In the region of the nucleus, the axon and the myelin sheath may be ovoid rather than circular in outline.

protein. They are virtually confined to the cortical zone of the axoplasm immediately beneath the axolemma (15). Neurofilaments (Figures 10.4C, 10.8) are 8- to 10-μm diameter intermediate filaments of indeterminant length, and they constitute a major filamentous component in larger axons (58). They were described originally by Ramón y Cajal and Bielschowsky as argentophilic neurofibrillae. In the neuronal perikaryon, neurofilaments tend to appear in multiple whorled bundles with no clear orientation to elements of the cell. In the axons, however, neurofilaments appear in longitudinal, mostly parallel orientation (59). Small arm-like filaments are seen by electron microscopy. They project from the surface of the neurofilaments to form an irregular polygonal lattice. Neurofilaments are composed of protein triplets that are chemically and immunochemically distinct (59). Three major subunits are recognized and are classified according to their molecular weights of 68, 150, and 200 KDa. Within axons, neurofilaments are phosphorylated and are immunocytochemically distinct from the nonphosphorylated filaments within neuron cell bodies. Immunocytochemistry for neurofilament protein (Figure 10.4C) is often valuable for detecting large- or medium-sized axons in normal nerves, in traumatic lesions, in tumors involving peripheral nerves, and occasionally for detecting axonal processes in neuronal tumors (58,59).

The third "filamentous" component in the axoplasm is the microtubule (neurotubule). Microtubules are cylindrical (Figure 10.8), unbranched, longitudinally oriented, hollow tubules 24 nm in diameter and composed of globular subunits of tubulin 4 to 5 nm in diameter. Periodic radial projections of high-molecular weight proteins, which are part of the microtubule-associated proteins (MAPs), arise from the surface of the neurotubules. These armlike projections bind neurofilaments and actin filaments and together form neurotubule-neurofilament-actin filament lattices. The three-dimensional lattices form an ordered structure in the axoplasm that appears to play an important role in axonal transport and contributes directly to the axon's shape (60). Microtubules also direct the transport of vesicular organelles between the cell body and the axon and thereby determine, in part, the composition of the axon (60).

Axoplasmic Flow

In 1906, Scott proposed that neuron cell bodies secreted "growing substances" in order to maintain the function of the axon. He suggested that such substances pass down the axon cytoplasm to the axon terminals. This suggestion was endorsed by Ramón y Cajal when he observed how regeneration occurs from the proximal stump of a damaged axon as long as continuity with the cell body is maintained (15). More definitive evidence of axonal transport was provided later by experimental studies using autoradiography and other techniques. Not only can labeled substances such as tritiated leucine be traced by autoradiography as they are transported along axons from the cell body, but the transport of organelles within the axon can also be directly observed by the use of dark-field microscopy or Nomarski optics (60). The term *axoplasmic flow* was coined by Weiss to describe the movement of different materials along the axoplasm. Axoplasmic flow and transport occur in two directions, away from the cell body (anterograde) and toward the cell body (retrograde) (61).

Anterograde axoplasmic transport occurs at two velocities: fast and slow. Most organelles and large-molecular weight substances within the axon are conveyed by fast axoplasmic transport, up to 400 mm/day. If a ligature is placed around a nerve, transported material accumulates proximal to the ligature and to some degree distal to it, due to interference with anterograde and retrograde transport, which both occur at the same rate and by the same mechanisms. The filamentous lattice component of neurotubules, neurofilaments, and actin filaments is responsible for fast axoplasmic flow, and these three elements probably act as rails along which the various transported organelles and substances move. Fast axoplasmic transport is dependent on oxidative energy mechanisms and adenosine triphosphate (ATP); it also depends on calcium and magnesium ions and is blocked by calcium channel blocking agents. Some substances, such as trifluoperazine, that block calmodulin (calcium-activating protein) also block axoplasmic flow. Neurotubules, as an integral part of the axoplasmic transport mechanism, are depolymerized by cold and by colchicine; vincristine, and vinblastine are known to bind tubulin and prevent the normal assembly of neurotubules. Such substances block fast axoplasmic flow (60).

Retrograde axoplasmic transport may convey information and organelles back to the cell body. In immature nerves, nerve growth factor is taken up by nerve terminals and retrogradely transported to the cell body, where it may play a role in the maturation of neurons (62). It has been suggested that the transport of such growth factors may also influence the metabolism of mature neurons and that the absence of such signals from the distal part of the neuron when the axon is severed may trigger chromatolysis (61). Retrograde transport is also a pathway by which certain toxins (tetanus neurotoxin) and some metals (lead, cadmium, and mercury) may bypass the blood-brain barrier and accumulate in neurons (63). Neurotropic viruses such as herpes, rabies, and poliomyelitis may be transported to the central nervous system by retrograde transport (64,65). In addition to toxic neuropathies, axonal transport is defective in diabetes, peroneal muscular atrophy, and probably in amyotrophic lateral sclerosis. Axoplasmic transport is reduced with age (66).

Slow axoplasmic transport at 1 to 3 mm/day concerns the distal movement of cytoskeletal elements such as neurofilaments, microtubules, and actin. It is a one-way process, and neurofilaments are broken down by calcium-activated proteases at the distal end of the axon. Similarly, microtubules are depolymerized distally (67). Various toxins such as hexocarbons and their derivatives may interfere with slow axoplasmic transport so that neurofilaments accumulate and form large swellings within the axon (34,68). It is thought that neurofilaments within an axon may act primarily to maintain the bulk and the shape of large axons; neurofilaments are less numerous in small axons.

The Periaxonal Space of Klebs

As the Schwann cell enwraps the axon, it leaves a space, 20 nm wide, between the Schwann cell membrane and the axolemma (Figure 10.8); this is the periaxonal space of Klebs (69). This space is in continuity with the extracellular space at the node of Ranvier through a narrow helical channel at the site where the terminal cytoplasmic processes of the Schwann cell approach the axolemma (14) (Figure 10.7). The maintenance of the periaxonal space of Klebs appears to be mediated by an intrinsic 100 KDa myelin-associated glycoprotein (MAG) in the periaxonal membrane of the Schwann cell (70). This protein has a heavily glycosylated domain, with sialic acid and sulfate residues on the external surface of the plasma membrane extending into the periaxonal space; in fact, about half of the peptide of MAG is in the periaxonal space (71). Mutant mice that do not express MAG do not form a periaxonal space, and the Schwann cell membrane fuses with the axolemma. Experimental studies with giant squid axons and mammalian nerve axons show that there is an increase in potassium concentration in the periaxonal space during repetitive conduction of nerve impulses. The full significance of the periaxonal space, however, is not clearly understood.

Schwann Cells

In his book on the microscopic structure of animals and plants published in Berlin in 1839, Theodore von Schwann identified a vague sheath of cells within nerve fibers; these cells have subsequently borne his name as Schwann cells. As described previously in the section on development of peripheral nerves, Schwann cells are derived from the neural crest and migrate with growing axons into the developing peripheral nerves (3,72). Schwann cells produce nerve growth factor both in development and during regeneration; and, as the nerves grow, Schwann cells divide axons into groups and eventually establish 1:1 relationships with the larger fibers that they will ultimately myelinate (15,25,72). Immature proliferating Schwann cells have a relatively large volume of cytoplasm compared with mature Schwann cells. The Schwann cytoplasm is rich in mitochondria, polyribosomes, Golgi cisternae, and rough endoplasmic reticulum (Figure 10.8). The cytoskeleton within the cells includes vimentin intermediate filaments and is particularly obvious during the active proliferative and migrating phases of development and regeneration.

Schwann cells in a normal adult peripheral nerve are associated with both myelinated fibers and unmyelinated fibers. In myelinated fibers the Schwann cytoplasm is divided into two compartments: (a) around the nucleus and on the outside of the myelin sheath, and (b) that thin rim of cytoplasm on the inside of the myelin sheath and around the internal mesaxon (Figure 10.8). Using electron microscopy, Schwann cells within a nerve can be identified by their relationship with myelinated or unmyelinated fibers. In damaged peripheral nerves, however, Schwann cells can be identified most easily by the presence of an investing basement membrane (Figure 10.8). Other cells within the endoneurium, such as fibroblasts, do not have a basement membrane; and, although macrophages may invade the basement membrane tubes, they have a distinct ruffled border that distinguishes them from Schwann cells. Perineurial cells may be found in the endoneurial compartment, particularly in damaged nerves; they possess a basement membrane, but they can be distinguished from Schwann cells by the presence of tight junctions that are not a feature of Schwann cells (3,54,72). With increasing age,

normal Schwann cells accumulate lipofuscin and lamellated structures in the paranuclear cytoplasm in the form of pi (π) granules of Reich. Such granules are composed of wide-spaced lamellated structures and amorphous osmiophilic material; they are rich in acid phosphatase and stain metachromatically with toluidine blue in frozen sections (73). Other inclusions such as the corpuscles of Erzholz are seen in Schwann cytoplasm; these bodies are spherical, 0.5 to 2.0 μm in diameter, and stain intensely with the Marchi method. Few Pi granules remain in Schwann cells following nerve damage in which there has been extensive Schwann cell mitosis and proliferation (73).

In addition to an investing basement membrane, composed of laminin, fibronectin, and entactin/nidogen, Schwann cells also produce heparan sulfate, N-syndecan, glypican, collagens type I, III, IV, and V, β1 and β4 integrin, and the protein BM-40 (74). All these secreted products are incorporated into the basement membrane except type I and type II collagen (3,72). Schwann cells can be identified in paraffin sections by immunocytochemistry and by the presence of close investment by reticulin staining. There is a rich reticulin network investing each cell, not only in the normal peripheral nerve but also in Schwann cell tumors. The S-100 protein in the cytoplasm and nuclei of Schwann cells can be identified by immunocytochemistry (Figure 10.4D). This acidic protein, which is 100% soluble in ammonium sulfate at neutral pH, was described by Blake W. Moore in 1965, is a calcium-binding EF-hand type molecule, and has no known function, but it is present in Schwann cells and not in fibroblasts or perineurial cells (37,75) (Figure 10.4). In vitro studies have reported the presence of Schwann cells that are weakly reactive for S-100 protein and that may correspond to the nonmyelinating (Remak) cell population (76). Schwann cells are also immunolabeled using CD57 and CD56 but perineurial cells are again negative (37,77). Calretinin, the 29-KDa, calcium-binding protein that also belongs to the family of EF-hand proteins, is expressed in Schwann cells but not consistently in schwannomas (78). Normal and some neoplastic Schwann cells also express the cell adhesion molecule CD146 (79). Occasionally, Schwann cells are labeled by anti-GFAP antibodies, but this may depend on the antibody used (37,80). GFAP immunoreativity in the peripheral nervous system has been demonstrated in enteric ganglia, olfactory nerve cells, and in Schwann cells in the sciatic, splenic and vagus nerves (81). Schwann cells also participate in the formation, function, and maintenance of neuromuscular junctions and Meissner corpuscles (82,83). These "terminal Schwann cells" may be identified by their expression of Herp-protein, which is not present in nonterminal myelinating Schwann cells (84). An interesting and peculiar intermediate glial cell type known as the olfactory ensheathing cell (OEC) is associated with neuronal processes of the olfactory bulb; OECs share astrocytic and Schwann cell phenotypes, promote axonal regeneration, and are potentially useful cells for xenotransplantation procedures (85).

Myelin

Myelin sheaths appear as slightly basophilic rings in H&E–stained transverse paraffin sections of nerve (Figure 10.4). They can be more prominently stained by Luxol fast blue or by hematoxylin stains such as Loyez (Table 10.1). In frozen sections, myelin is well depicted by Sudan black staining; and, in unstained frozen sections, myelin can be identified due to its birefringence in polarized light, a technique that is particularly suitable for identifying myelin in enzyme histochemical preparations (57).

Myelin is formed by the fusion of Schwann cell membranes and, by electron microscopy, it is seen as a regularly repeating lamellated structure with a 12 to 18 nm periodicity (86). On the outer and inner aspects of the sheath, external and internal mesaxons can be traced from the cell surface (Figure 10.8). The myelin membrane is divided into two structurally and biochemically distinct domains: the compact and the noncompact myelin, each of which is characterized by a unique set of proteins. Compact myelin, for instance, contains P0, PMP22, and MBP, whereas noncompact myelin contains MAG, Cx32, $\alpha 6\beta 4$ integrin and E-cadherin (3,72).

As the external aspects of the Schwann cell membranes fuse to produce compact myelin, an interrupted interperiod line forms in the myelin. The more densely stained period line is formed by fusion of the cytoplasmic aspects of the cell membrane. A narrow cleft can be resolved between the components of the interperiod line. In myelinating Schwann cells, noncompact myelin is present in paranodal loops, Schmidt-Lanterman incisures, nodal microvilli, and the inner and outer edges of the myelin (87). Several types of cell junction, including tight, gap and adherens junctions, are seen between the myelin lamellae (known as autotypic junctions) (87).

Biochemically, myelin is 75% lipid and 25% protein. The major lipids are cholesterol, sphingomyelin, and galactolipids, which are present in a rather higher proportion than they are in other cell membranes. It is the arrangement of the lipids that produces the liquid crystalline fluid birefringent myelin sheath, and it is esterification of the cholesterol in degenerating myelin that can be detected by Sudan dyes, by oil red O, and by the Marchi technique (Table 10.1). As myelin degenerates and the cholesterol becomes esterified, the ultrastructural lamellated pattern of myelin is lost and replaced by the amorphous osmiophilic globules seen in electron micrographs. More than half the protein in myelin is a transmembrane 28 to 30 KDa glycoprotein, P0 (88); other proteins are P1 and P2. The protein mediates homophilic adhesive interactions between Schwann cell plasma membranes, is a key structural constituent of both the major dense line and interperiod line of compact myelin, and is involved in myelin compaction (88). Numerous mutations in P0 have been described in a variety of demyelinating diseases (see below) (88).

Although the lipid composition of myelin in the peripheral nervous system (PNS) is very similar to that of the central nervous system (CNS), the protein components are markedly different. Central nervous system myelin has no P0 protein but has a proteolipid that is soluble in organic solvents; it also has an 18KDa basic protein that is probably homologous to the P1 protein of peripheral nerve myelin. These biochemical differences may account for differences in the structure between PNS and CNS myelin; for example, the spaces between the dense lines are less for CNS myelin (89). Biochemical differences in the proteins definitely account for the distinct antigenicities of peripheral and central nervous system myelin. Thus, injection of CNS myelin with Freund's adjuvant will produce allergic encephalomyelitis in experimental animals, with destruction of myelin in the brain and spinal cord (90), whereas injection of peripheral nervous system myelin with Freund's adjuvant will produce allergic neuritis with demyelination in the peripheral nervous system.

Myelin sheaths are essential for the normal functioning of the PNS; and, in those hereditary neuropathies in which myelination is defective, severe disability and retardation of development are seen (91). Acting as a biological electrical insulator, myelin allows discontinuous (saltatory) and very rapid conduction of a wave of depolarization along the nerve fiber. It appears that myelination is an evolutionary adaptation that allows increased conduction velocities without excessive increases in axon diameter (72).

Myelination in the PNS in humans occurs well in advance of that of the CNS (89). Although there is little myelin in human cerebral hemispheres at birth, myelin sheaths have already started to form around peripheral nerves at this time. Myelination is initiated by contact between Schwann cells and future myelinated axons. The Schwann cell rotates around the axon and may form 50 or more spirals, resulting in formation of the myelin sheath.

As the Schwann cell differentiates and produces a basement membrane, it acquires polarity via interaction of its cytoskeleton and some basement membrane components (mainly laminin and fibronectin) (3,92). The Schwann cell then begins to extend processes around individual axons. Once the lips of the Schwann cell start to wrap around the axon, they generate traction to pull the whole cell around, and a spiral wrapping made up of many lamellae is formed (18). The importance of basement membrane formation as a prerequisite for the formation of myelin is emphasized by the lack of myelination when the basement membrane is deficient (92,93).

Myelin-associated glycoprotein also plays an important role in myelination (88). It is present in the membranes of Schwann cells around myelinated fibers but not in those cells associated with unmyelinated fibers. Myelin-associated glycoprotein probably functions through its interaction with the Schwann cell cytoskeleton, and this facilitates process lengthening and rotation during myelination (71). Periaxin, a 47 KDa protein constituent of the dystroglycan-dystrophin–related protein-2 complex that links the Schwann cell cytoskeleton to the extracellular matrix, is located in the periaxonal region of Schwann cell plasma membrane that possibly interacts with myelin-associated glycoprotein during myelination (94). Mutations in the periaxin gene result in the autosomal recessive demyelinating Charcot-Marie-Tooth (CMT4F) and Déjérine-Sottas diseases (94) (see below). As myelination proceeds, cytoplasm is expressed from the spiral of Schwann cell processes and membranes compact to form the 12 to 18 nm lamellated structure of myelin.

The length of an embryonic Schwann cell is 30 to 60 μm, and it becomes associated with that length of axon in the developing nerve. As the nerve lengthens with growth of the body and limbs, so does the Schwann cell so that the length of the Schwann cell or internodal distance (Figure 10.7) in myelinated fibers reaches some 190 μm at 18 weeks gestation and 475 μm at birth. In the adult nerve, normal Schwann cells may extend for up to 1 mm in length along myelinated fibers. Schwann cells associated with unmyelinated fibers lengthen to reach approximately 250 μm in the adult sural nerve. Following damage to a peripheral nerve, Schwann cell lengths revert to their embryonic length, and thus give short internodes in regenerating and remyelinating nerve fibers (see Figures 10.12, 10.14).

Schmidt-Lanterman Clefts or Incisures

Once viewed as artifacts, the clefts or incisures described by H.D. Schmidt and A.J. Lanterman (Figure 10.9) are now known to be fixed components of the myelin sheath (24). Each Schmidt-Lanterman incisure (S-L I) consists of a continuous spiral of Schwann cytoplasm that runs from the outer (nuclear) to the inner (paraxonal) Schwann cell compartment in an oblique fashion at about 9 degrees to the long axis of the sheath. The cleft splits the cytoplasmic membranes at the major dense line and forms a route for the passage of substances from the outer cytoplasmic layer through the myelin sheath to the inner cytoplasm. This function was suggested by Ranvier as early as 1897. Near the external surface of the cleft, stacks of desmosome-like structures and gap junctions rich in connexin 32, are sometimes seen, possibly maintaining the integrity of the spiral (95). The cell junction proteins claudin-5, MUPP1, E-cadherin, as well as a 155-KDa isoform of neurofascin, have been selectively detected at the S-L I (31). Cytoplasm in the clefts contains membrane-bound dense bodies, lysosomes, an occasional mitochondrion, and a single microtubule (Figure 10.9) that runs circumferentially around the fiber; this microtubule may be associated with transport and with stabilization of the cytoplasmic spiral (15). The number of S-L Is correlates with the diameter of the axon; the larger the

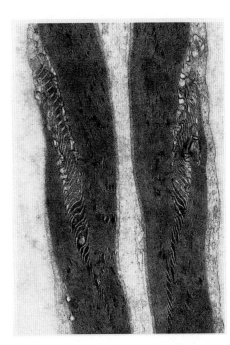

Figure 10.9 Longitudinal section of peripheral nerve: a Schmidt-Lanterman incisure. Blebs of cytoplasm are seen running through the myelin sheath. Densities in the cytoplasm (*top left*) suggest some form of junction between the spiral turns of the incisure. The axon is cut tangentially. (Electron micrograph, ×30,000). (Reprinted from Weller RO, Cervos-Navarro J. *Pathology of Peripheral Nerves: A Practical Approach.* London: Butterworths; 1977 with permission.)

fiber, the more clefts in the myelin sheath per Schwann cell. The presence of these clefts throughout myelogenesis suggests that they are an important functional part of the sheath (24). Balice-Gordon et al. (96) have suggested that the incisures may provide some degree of flexibility and may protect the peripheral nerve from mechanical stress during stretching and recoil. It also seems obvious that they are pathways of communication between the inner and outer Schwann cell cytoplasm, but their full significance remains to be elucidated.

Node of Ranvier

With the introduction of techniques whereby individually separated or teased myelinated nerve fibers could be stained black with osmium tetroxide, a new view of nerve fibers was obtained. In his publication of 1876, Louis-Antoine Ranvier, Professor of Histology in Paris, described and illustrated the constrictions or "étranglements annulaires," that are now known as the nodes of Ranvier (20,24). The functions of the node at that time were not known, but Ranvier did suggest that the constrictions may prevent displacement or flow of the semiliquid myelin along the nerve fibers (20,24). He also suggested that the gap in the myelin sheath at the node of Ranvier might allow diffusion of nutrients into the axon (15).

In teased fibers stained with osmium tetroxide or viewed in polarized light, the nodal gap is readily visible, as is the bulbous swelling of the fiber on either side of the node of Ranvier (see Figure 10.15D). The distance between each node along a myelinated fiber (Figure 10.7) is approximately proportional to the thickness of the myelin sheath. In a normal adult mammalian nerve, internodal segments between the nodes of Ranvier vary from 200 to 1500 μm in length; the Schwann cell nucleus is usually sited around the middle of the internode.

Histological study of 1-μm transverse resin sections of nerve and electron microscopic observations reveal a complex structure at the node of Ranvier and in the paranodal regions. As the axon approaches a node of Ranvier, it may become cruciform in cross section, especially in large fibers (Figure 10.7). Deep furrows develop in the surrounding myelin sheath, and those furrows are filled with cytoplasm that is rich in mitochondria. As the axon passes through the node it is reduced to one-third or one-sixth of its internodal diameter. There may be a slight swelling at the midpoint of the node. Amorphous, osmiophilic material rich in ankyrin, Nr CRM, and neurofascin (97) may be deposited under the axolemma (98). Ankyrin-binding proteins are also localized in the initial segment of the axon, the voltage-dependent sodium channel, the sodium/potassium ATPase, and the sodium/calcium exchanger (97). These specialized areas of axon membrane may reflect the site of high ionic current density during transmission of a nerve impulse. Numerous ion channels are present in this region of the axolemma, and they are responsible for the changes in ionic milieu that occur during the conduction of nerve impulses (98).

There is considerable specialization of the Schwann cell and the myelin sheath at the node of Ranvier. The myelin sheath terminates by forming dilated looplike structures that are closely apposed to the axon surface (Figure 10.7). Occasionally, desmosome-like structures are formed between Schwann cell terminal loops. The tight junction protein claudin-2, and the ERM (ezrin, radizin, moesin) proteins have been identified as a ring that surrounds sodium channels at the node of Ranvier, possibly participating in the junctions formed at the outer collars of two adjacent Schwann cells at the node zone (31). The abundance of mitochondria in the paranodal cytoplasm is an indication of the high energy requirements of the node. Right in the center of the node, the myelin end-loops are replaced by multiple fingerlike Schwann cell processes (nodal villi) that contain f-actin and are 70 to 100 nm in diameter. The villi extend from the Schwann cells into the nodal gaps and interdigitate with processes of adjacent Schwann cells (98). This interlacing pattern of cell processes around the axon at the node of Ranvier is more prominent and complex in larger fibers.

Basement membrane from the two adjacent Schwann cells is continuous over the nodal gap. Around the villous Schwann cell processes, there is an electron-dense polyanionic-rich material that constitutes the extracellular matrix of the node. This gap substance creates a ringlike structure (ring of Nemiloff) and may provide an ion pool necessary for nodal function. It has been demonstrated that the gap substance contains glycosaminoglycans with cation binding substances (95).

The myelin sheath acts as a biological insulator for the internodal portion of the axons. Conduction of impulses along myelinated fibers proceeds in a discontinuous manner from node to node (saltatory conduction). Numerous sodium channels with a suggested density of approximately 100,000/μm^2 are present on the axolemma at the node of Ranvier in contrast to the very low density of sodium channels (less than 25/μm^2) in the internodal axon membrane; the internodal membrane may be regarded as inexcitable (3,98). Potassium channels show a complementary distribution to that of the sodium channels; they are less common than in the nodal membrane but are present in the paranodal and internodal axon membrane. Potassium channels contribute to the stabilization of the axon by preventing repetitive firing responses to a single stimulus and also help to maintain the resting potential of the myelinated fiber (98).

In demyelinating diseases, when the myelin sheath is stripped from the axon, there is gross slowing or cessation of nerve conduction along the affected fibers. Spread of a continuous wave of depolarization along the axon membrane is prevented due to the absence of an adequate density of sodium channels in the internodal axon membrane. Furthermore, the exposure of the internodal axon cell membrane, which is rich in potassium channels, will also interfere with induction of the impulse (15,98).

Unmyelinated Axons

Unmyelinated fibers can be detected as unstained structures by light microscopy in toluidine blue–stained 0.5-μm transverse resin sections of peripheral nerve (Figure 10.5) (99). However, at 1 to 3 μm diameter, they are almost at the limit of resolution and are only seen in good quality sections. Such fibers can be stained by silver techniques, such as Palmgren's or Bodian's, but are poorly visualized in immunocytochemical preparations using antineurofilament antibodies (Figure 10.4), probably because unmyelinated fibers contain few neurofilaments and a high proportion of microtubules.

The structure of unmyelinated fibers and their quantitation are most adequately studied by transmission electron microscopy (Figure 10.10). They are more numerous than myelinated fibers in mixed peripheral nerves by a factor of 3 or 4:1 (25,54) and were first recognized in 1838 by the Polish physician Robert Remak as "fibriae organicae"; the Schwann cells associated with unmyelinated axons are sometimes referred to as Remak cells (54). Schwann cells

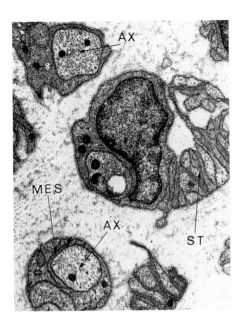

Figure 10.10 Unmyelinated axons (1.3 μm in diameter) cut in transverse section. The axons (AX) are surrounded by Schwann cells, Mesaxons (MES). Stacks of Schwann cell processes (ST) are commonly seen in adult nerves. (Electron micrograph, ×13,000.)

have the potential to differentiate into either a myelinating or nonmyelinating ensheathing cell, depending upon the signals received from the axons that they contact. Schwann cells must form basal laminae in order to myelinate axons (24,54). Schwann cells around myelinated and unmyelinated axons may thus be regarded as originating from the same cell type but developing morphological, biochemical, and physiological differences (106).

The cytoplasm of Schwann cells associated with unmyelinated fibers contains a Golgi apparatus, rough endoplasmic reticulum, mitochondria, microtubules, and microfilaments and may exhibit centrioles near the nucleus. Pi (π) granules, however, are not present, although there are lysosomes containing acid phosphatase present in the cytoplasm (73). The nuclei of these cells are ellipsoid with one or more prominent nucleoli. A continuous basement membrane surrounds each cell (98). Schwann cells associated with unmyelinated fibers express different phenotypic characteristics from Schwann cells around myelinated axons. Although both types of Schwann cell contain immunocytochemically detectable vimentin intermediate filaments and S-100 protein, and almost the same basement membrane components, Schwann cells associated with unmyelinated axons are more likely to express GFAP (101). Such cells also lack MAG, which is apparently necessary for segregation and myelination of axons. *Mycobacterium leprae* (Hansen's bacilli) colonize nonmyelinating Remak cells by attaching to laminin-2 and its receptor α-dystroglycan. Myelin-forming Schwann cells seem to be relatively free from infection by *M. leprae*. There is often a strong cell-mediated immune response with extensive in-

flammation and peripheral nerve damage that causes paralysis and loss of sensation and frequently leads to unintentional mutilation of hands and feet (102).

Electron microscopy of transverse sections of normal peripheral nerve show how numerous unmyelinated axons 0.2 to 3.5 μm in diameter are associated with a single Schwann cell. Short mesaxons extend from the surface of the cell (Figure 10.10), and the Schwann cell is separated from the axon plasma membrane by a space 10 to 15 nm wide that is analogous to the periaxonal space of Klebs seen around myelinated fibers. Although many axons may be gathered close to the cell body in the perinuclear region of the Schwann cell (24,54), away from the nuclear region, single axons become more widely separated and are enclosed by thin Schwann cell processes (Figures 10.3, 10.10). Each Schwann cell associated with unmyelinated axons in the sural nerve is between 200 and 500 μm in length. As axons pass from one Schwann cell to another, they are surrounded by flattened irregular, fingerlike processes that interlock and become telescoped into the adjacent Schwann cell. The surface of the axon is therefore always in contact with the Schwann cell. In young children, only a single thin layer of Schwann cytoplasm surrounds each axon away from the nuclear region; but the picture is more complex in adult nerves, with several Schwann cell processes stacked together and associated with each unmyelinated axon.

Pockets of collagen bundles are frequently invaginated into the surface of Schwann cells associated with unmyelinated fibers (Figure 10.3), particularly in aging nerves and when there is loss of unmyelinated fibers. The pockets of collagen fibers are separated from the surface of the Schwann cell by a layer of basement membrane. The significance of this phenomenon is not fully known.

Endocrine cells have been identified within the perineurium in close contact with unmyelinated nerves in the lamina propria of the appendix (103). These cells were demonstrated in 1924 by Masson, and later Auböck coined the term *endocrine cell–nonmyelinated fiber complex*, emphasizing the association between endocrine cells and unmyelinated fibers (104). These complexes are separated from the interstitial connective tissue by a common continuous basement membrane, leaving the cells in intimate contact with each other. It has been suggested that such endocrine cells could participate in the pathogenesis of the so-called neuromas of the appendix and appendiceal carcinoids (105,106). It is not known whether such endocrine cells exist in nerves other than those located in the wall of the appendix, but there are reports of extraepithelial carcinoid tumors in stomach, small intestine, and bronchus, which suggests that there may also be endocrine cells related to nerves in these regions (107).

Interesting immunological properties have been ascribed to Schwann cells. Numerous in vitro studies have shown that Schwann cells display a large repertoire of properties, ranging from the participation in antigen presentation, to secretion of pro- and anti-inflammatory cytokines, chemokines, and neurotrophic factors (108). Schwann cells express Ia determinants on their membranes and are able to present foreign antigens to specific synergic T cells. When Schwann cells are exposed to inflammatory cytokines they have the capacity of inducing selective damage to T cells and have the potential of regulating the immune response in the peripheral nervous system (109). A role for Schwann cells has been suggested in myasthenia gravis (110).

Schwann cells also express complement receptor CR1 (CD35) and CD59, a 19 to 25 KDa glycoprotein that binds to complement proteins C8 and C9 in the assembling cytolytic membrane attack complex. This may indicate that regulation of complement activation by these proteins is important in neural host defense mechanisms and may be implicated in the complement-mediated damage occurring in inflammatory demyelinating diseases such as Guillain-Barré syndrome (111,112).

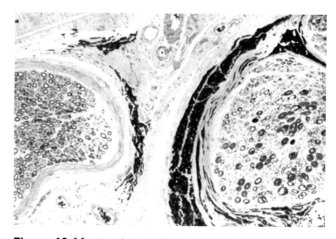

Figure 10.11 Histologic artifact in a peripheral nerve. In this transverse 1-μm resin section, the fascicle to the left of the picture is well-preserved. However, there is extensive recent hemorrhage (*center*) that occurred during the biopsy procedure; the myelinated axons in the nerve fascicle are squeezed and distorted (*right*) (toluidine blue, ×40.)

CORRELATION OF NORMAL HISTOLOGY WITH THE PATHOLOGY OF PERIPHERAL NERVES

Handling and Preparation of Peripheral Nerve Biopsy and Autopsy Specimens

The sural nerve is the nerve that is most commonly biopsied in the investigation of peripheral neuropathies. It is a sensory nerve so that in some motor neuropathies it may be totally normal, in which case examination of small branches of motor nerves within a muscle biopsy may be more fruitful (48,54,54). At autopsy, a wider range of motor and sensory nerves may be sampled, depending on the clinical picture. Whether taken at biopsy or autopsy, peripheral nerves are very easily damaged. The myelin sheaths are semiliquid and may be crushed by indelicate handling (Figure 10.11). The specimen should be gripped at only one end and then gently dissected free before laying it, very gently stretched, on a piece of dry card and placing it in fixative or in liquid nitrogen for snap freezing. Fresh, frozen nerve should be used for enzyme and lipid histochemical studies whereas formalin-fixed nerve can be embedded in paraffin for the application of routine stains and immunocytochemistry (see Table 10.1). Although formalin-fixed material can be used for the preparation of 0.5- to 1-μm resin-embedded sections and for electron microscopy, ideally the tissue should be fixed in glutaraldehyde and postfixed in osmium for ultrastructural studies. Teased fibers can be prepared from either glutaraldehyde- or formalin-fixed material (24,54).

The method of preparation really depends on the information sought. Frozen sections are ideal for detecting abnormal lipids, such as sulfatide in metachromatic leukodystrophy, and for detecting the cholesterol ester droplets of degenerating myelin by staining for Sudan red or oil red O. Increased lysosomal enzyme activity as in Krabbe's leukodystrophy or in human and experimental neuropathies in which axonal degeneration or segmental demyelination is suspected can be detected in frozen sections stained histochemically for acid phosphatase (54). Brief formalin or glutaraldehyde fixation can be used in some cases for electron microscopic enzyme histochemistry (54,113). Frozen sections can also be used for immunofluorescence for the detection of immunoglobulin binding to myelin sheaths in paraproteinemias. Transverse frozen sections of nerve are ideal for these purposes although they are often more difficult to prepare than longitudinal sections.

There is a variety of methods of preparing and examining fixed specimens of peripheral nerve, and each method reveals different information (24,54). Ideally, exact transverse sections should be cut from the peripheral nerve; occasionally, longitudinal sections are also useful, particularly for detacting regenerating axons by immunocytochemistry (Figure 10.4F). Paraffin-embedded sections can be stained for a variety of histological stains and for immunocytochemistry to reveal nerve components (Table 10.1). Blood vessels and inflammatory exudates are ideally studied in paraffin sections, but quantitation of nerve fibers, the detection of axon degeneration and regeneration, and the assessment of segmental demyelination and remyelination are more satisfactory in 0.5- to 1-μm toluidine blue–stained resin sections or by electron microscopy. The presence of amyloid in the endoneurium or giant axons in some hereditary neuropathies and in some toxic neuropathies can be detected both in paraffin- and in resin-embedded sections. Teased preparations are most useful for detecting segmental demyelination and remyelination and for assessing whether axonal degeneration and regeneration have occurred within the nerve in the past (24,56).

Peripheral Neuropathies

The pathological diagnosis of a peripheral neuropathy usually requires close clinicopathologic correlation and knowledge of the electrophysiologic data, such as nerve conduction velocities and electromyography. Moderate slowing of nerve conduction velocities usually indicates loss of large myelinated fibers, whereas excessive slowing of conduction velocity suggests that segmental demyelination has occurred. Although there are a number of specific histopathological features that aid in the diagnosis of peripheral neuropathy [e.g., amyloid, the presence of *M. leprae* bacilli, abnormal lipids such as sulfatide within the nerve, giant axons, and vasculitis (15,56)], for the most part, assessment of peripheral nerve pathology depends on detection and quantitation of general pathological features and good clinicopathological correlation.

General Pathology of Peripheral Nerves

The general pathological reactions of peripheral nerves are, for most practical purposes, limited to (a) axonal degeneration and regeneration and (b) segmental demyelination and remyelination. Hypertrophic changes with onion-bulb formation occur most commonly as a result of recurrent segmental demyelination and are most often seen in hereditary neuropathies.

Axonal Degeneration and Regeneration

If a neuron in the anterior horn of the gray matter of the spinal cord or in a dorsal root ganglion dies, its axon degenerates and no regeneration occurs. Such neuronal destruction is seen in poliomyelitis, motor neuron disease (amyotrophic lateral sclerosis), spinal muscular atrophy, and infarction of the spinal cord. Dorsal root ganglion cells may be lost in viral infections such as varicella zoster or in a variety of hereditary sensory neuropathies. If an axon in a peripheral nerve is injured, for example, by trauma, entrapment, or ischemia, the distal end of the axon degenerates and subsequently regeneration occurs from the proximal stump of the damaged axon (Figure 10.12). The success of the regeneration depends on the distance of the site of damage from the nerve end organ (either motor endplate or sensory nerve ending) and the amount of scarring or other obstruction laid in the path of the regenerating axons.

Axonal degeneration was described by Waller in 1850 in London and the eponym *wallerian degeneration* is still used. Much of the fundamental work on nerve degeneration and regeneration, however, was performed by Ramón y Cajal in

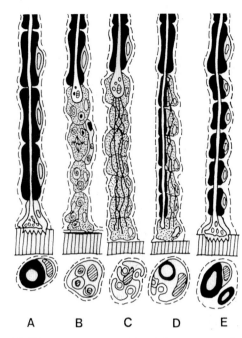

Figure 10.12 Diagram summarizing the events occurring during axonal degeneration and regeneration. **A.** Normal nerve. **B.** By seven days after axonal damage, Schwann cells containing axon and myelin debris have divided to form bands of Büngner. **C.** Axon sprouts grow from the swollen end bulb of the proximal axon. **D.** An axon becomes myelinated. **E.** Connection with the end organ is reestablished; regenerated internodes are short. (Reprinted from: Weller RO, Cervos-Navarro J. *Pathology of Peripheral Nerves: A Practical Approach.* London: Butterworths; 1977 with permission.)

the early part of the twentieth century. Twenty-four hours after nerve injury, most myelinated and nonmyelinated axons start to show degenerative changes. There is retraction of myelin from the nodes of Ranvier and dilatation of Schmidt-Lanterman incisures in the proximal as well as in the distal stump. By 48 hours, myelin and axon changes become more obvious as the axon disintegrates and myelin sheaths become disrupted and form globules (Figure 10.13) in which axon fragments are enclosed. Disintegration of the myelin appears to start with dilatation of the Schmidt-Lanterman incisures during the first day or two after injury (24,54). Myelin debris is initially birefringent and has a lamellated ultrastructure, as does normal myelin. But, as proteins break down and lysosomal enzymes become active around the myelin debris (54,113,114), cholesterol within the myelin is esterified to cholesterol esters, and lipid debris loses its birefringence in polarized light and its lamellated ultrastructure to become amorphous globular lipid, which now stains strongly with Sudan dyes and oil red O. The Marchi technique also differentiates between normal myelin and degenerating myelin (56).

During the second week after nerve injury, much of the myelin debris is removed from the distal part of the nerve, and regenerative features become more prominent. Axon fragments and myelin debris are broken down by both

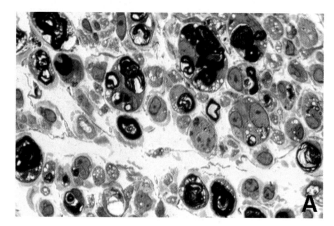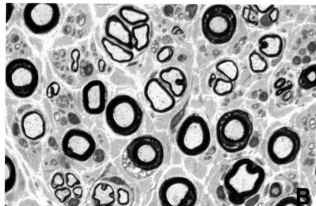

Figure 10.13 Axonal degeneration and regeneration in transverse sections of peripheral nerve. **A.** Axonal degeneration four days after nerve section. Few axons are visible and myelin is forming globules in Schwann cells and macrophages (1-μm section, toluidine blue, ×310). **B.** Axonal regeneration in a human nerve biopsy. Normal myelinated fibers are interspersed with clusters of closely associated thinly myelinated regenerating fibers (*top and bottom right*) (1-μm section, toluidine blue, ×310).

Schwann cells and macrophages (116). Schwann cells directly attract macrophages by secretion of different proteins, probably regulated by autocrine circuits involving the neuropoietic cytokines, IL-6, and leukemia inhibitory factor (113). Macrophages, in addition to their phagocytic function may help to promote nerve repair through the elaboration of Schwann cell mitogens and may also affect neurons and axonal growth directly through the release of neurotrophins (115,117–119).

Although Schwann cell mitoses are seen as early as 24 hours after nerve injury, the peak of proliferation is between 3 and 15 days after nerve damage (120). As Schwann cells proliferate, they form columns (bands of Büngner) surrounded by basement membrane (Figure 10.12); often redundant, old Schwann cell basement membrane is associated with these bands. Regenerating axons grow along the bands of Büngner; and, if regeneration fails, the bands shrink and Schwann cells may disappear and become replaced by fibrous tissue (121).

"Importins" are proteins involved in the retrograde transport of substances collectively known as *injury signals;* such transport is through a complex of proteins acting in association with neurotubules and into the cell nucleus, where gene transcription subsequently occurs (122).

Several easily detectable histological changes occur during axonal regeneration The neuron cell bodies in the anterior horns of the spinal cord or in the dorsal root ganglia show changes of chromatolysis during the first three weeks after axonal injury (120). The nerve cell perikaryon swells by some 20%, and the nucleus becomes eccentric, as does the nucleolus. Nissl substance (a mixture of rough endoplasmic reticulum and polyribosomes) is dispersed so that the cytoplasm becomes pale when stained by H&E or by the Nissl stain (24,54). During this stage of chromatolysis, there is a marked increase in polyribosomal ribonucleic

acid (RNA) with an upregulation of a number of regeneration-associated genes, including those encoding growth-associated protein-43 (GAP 43), cytoskeleton protein-23, and β-tubulin, and in peptides such as galanin and vasoactive intestinal polipeptide (VIP), reflecting the metabolic events involved in axon regeneration (122–124). Regenerative changes in axons are seen within the first few hours after nerve damage but are most easily detected 5 to 20 days after injury. Using immunocytochemistry, GAP 43 can be identified in regenerating axons 4 to 21 days after injury (125) (Figure 10.4F). The proximal stump of the axon swells to create a balloonlike structure, often 50 μm in diameter and 100 μm in length. The balloons are filled with organelles and fibrils, which can be detected by electron microscopy; they can be visualized by light microscopy using immunocytochemical stains for neurofilament protein, GAP 43, or silver stains such as were used by Ramón y Cajal when he first described them. Myelin sheaths become stretched around the swollen axon balloons (114,126).

Starting around the fourth day after injury, multiple nerve sprouts, or neurites, extend from the axon balloon (growth cone) and grow distally at 1 to 2.5 mm/day. As the neurites enter the bands of Büngner, they become invaginated into the surface of the Schwann cell and, if growth continues, they become myelinated. Unmyelinated fibers regenerate in a similar way, but they are smaller and no myelin sheaths form around them. Regenerating neurites can be detected in the classical way by silver staining; but, in cross sections of peripheral nerve, they are best demonstrated in 0.5- to 1-μm resin sections or by electron microscopy. Characteristically, regenerating axons form clusters encircled by a single basement membrane. In the light microscope, these clusters (Figure 10.13) are recognized by the close association of small, thinly myelinated axons within the nerve; myelinated nerve fibers in a normal nerve are well-separated from each other by endoneurial collagen (Figure 10.5).

Axon growth and regeneration are stimulated by nerve growth factor that is synthesized by Schwann cells, fibroblasts, and macrophages and transported back along the axon by retrograde axoplasmic transport to stimulate nerve cell protein synthesis (60,126,127,128). In addition to growth factors, there appears to be topographical affinity between regenerating axons and certain pathways; for example, it appears that regenerating tibial nerve axons grow toward the distal tibial nerve rather than toward the distal peroneal nerves. Connective tissue elements may also play a role in guiding regenerating axons (10). Neurite outgrowth–promoting factors on cell surfaces (cell adhesion molecules) or in the extracellular matrix promote extension of the axon by providing an appropriate "adhesivness" in the substrate (129). Both neurotrophic and neurite outgrowth–promoting factors are essential for axonal growth after injury (129).

The success of regeneration, with axons reaching effective end organs, may be influenced by several factors. If the injury is far proximal from the end organ, few regenerating axons may make effective reconnections. But, regeneration over short distances may be very effective in the peripheral nervous system. The presence of scar tissue or discontinuity of anatomical pathways may also inhibit regeneration. A number of grafting techniques are employed to overcome this problem (13,120). If regeneration to the distal stump of a nerve is blocked by scar tissue, axons may grow outside the original course of the nerve and even back alongside the proximal stump (terminals of Perroncito); thus, small bundles of regenerating neurites, often surrounded by perineurial cells, form amputation neuromas. Microscopically, there are interlacing bundles containing axons surrounded by myelin sheaths and with fine perineurial coverings. Immunocytochemistry for neurofilament proteins (axons), EMA, and Glut-1 (perineurial cells), and S-100 (Schwann cells) may be very useful in establishing the structure and identity of the nerve bundles in an amputation neuroma. Immunohistochemical and radioimmunoassay data have shown a focal accumulation of sodium channels within the tips of injured axons that may be responsible, in part, for the ectopic axonal excitability and the resulting abnormal sensory phenomena (pain and paresthesia) which frequently complicate peripheral nerve injury (130). Macropaghes migrate into the neuroma within the first two weeks after the injury, and later they are seen with numerous large cytoplasmic vacuoles filled with myelin fragments. This suggests that macrophages may also participate in the genesis of chronic pain after the neuroma has formed possibly by: (a) creating demyelinating axonal regions susceptible to external stimuli; (b) by releasing substances that influence regeneration of axons; or (c) by direct action on the denuded remodelling membranes (131).

Axon degeneration, often with regeneration, is a feature of numerous peripheral neuropathies, including those associated with diabetes, amyloidosis, infections (such as leprosy), sarcoidosis, paraneoplastic syndromes, vascular disease, and metabolic diseases (24,54,132,133). Most toxic neuropathies (34,68) result in chronic axonal degeneration at the extreme distal ends of sensory and motor nerves (distal axonopathies). The distal ends of long tracts in the spinal cord (dorsal columns and corticospinal tracts) are often affected as well as the peripheral nerves. Timely withdrawal of the toxin may allow effective regeneration to occur, but only in the peripheral nerves, not in the spinal cord. Many peripheral neuropathies induced by the diseases itemized above are slowly progressive, so that nerve biopsies in these conditions do not usually reveal the early stages of axonal degeneration and regeneration. More frequently, the histological picture is characterized by loss of large myelinated axons and, to a lesser extent, loss of small myelinated and unmyelinated axons. Nerve root or peripheral nerve compression and trauma to peripheral nerve trunks result in axonal degeneration. Regeneration may be recognized in transverse sections of peripheral nerve by the presence of clusters (Figure 10.13). In teased fiber preparations, short internodes in the distal part of the nerve indicate that axonal degeneration and regeneration have occurred in the past (121).

Segmental Demyelination and Remyelination

When demyelination occurs in peripheral nerves, it has a segmental distribution with each segment representing the internodal portion of an axon myelinated by one Schwann cell (Figures 10.7, 10.14). Such segments can be contiguous, and thus demyelination may occur over long lengths of the nerve or in short sporadic segments (55,118). The axon remains intact except in severe demyelinating neuropathies in which secondary axonal degeneration occurs. Remyelination is often rapid and effective, with restoration of nerve function. Demyelination may occur as a result of direct interference with Schwann cell metabolism, as in diphtheria; myelin sheaths are broken down through the lysosomal action of Schwann cells, although macrophages are later involved in the destruction of myelin debris (116,120). Another mechanism that is seen in the commonest acute demyelinating neuropathy, Guillain-Barré syndrome, in which there is an immunological attack on peripheral nerve myelin by lymphocytes and macrophages; segmental demyelination occurs and is followed by remyelination (Figures 10.14, 10.15). Functional recovery occurs following both types of demyelination except in the most severe cases (134).

The first stages of segmental demyelination are seen at the node of Ranvier, where the nodal gap becomes widened; subsequently, the whole internode of myelin may be broken down (135). This destruction results in severe slowing of conduction of nerve impulses across the demyelinated segment and the onset of symptoms for the patient. Preserved axons remain invaginated within Schwann cells as the

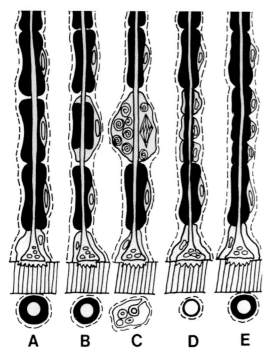

Figure 10.14 Summary of the events occurring in primary segmental demyelination and remyelination. **A.** Normal nerve. **B.** Early segmental demyelination; retraction of paranodal myelin with widening of the nodal gap. **C.** Destruction of myelin sheath and Schwann cell mitosis. **D. and E.** Remyelination; intercalated short segments. (Reprinted from: Weller RO, Cervos-Navarro J. *Pathology of Peripheral Nerves: A Practical Approach.* London: Butterworths; 1977 with permission.)

myelin sheaths are broken down (Figures 10.15 and, 10.16). Schwann cells proliferate and within a few days start to remyelinate the demyelinated axons by a similar mechanism to that seen during myelination in the fetus. Remyelination may be well advanced by two weeks after demyelination as the thickness of myelin sheaths increases and conduction velocities return to normal.

Classically, segmental demyelination can be detected in teased nerve fibers, first by the presence of widening of the gap of the node of Ranvier and then by the presence of axons devoid of myelin sheaths. Intercalated thin myelin sheaths along the axon are seen as remyelination proceeds (Figure 10.15). In electron micrographs or in resin-embedded light microscope sections, naked axons can be recognized in transverse section and remyelinating fibers detected by the presence of inappropriately thin myelin sheaths (Figures 10.12–10.14). Segmental demyelination is a feature of a number of peripheral neuropathies (132,133), particularly mild vascular damage to peripheral nerves as in rheumatoid arthritis (136), diabetes (24), Guillain-Barré syndrome, occasional toxic neuropathies (131), and metabolic neuropathies such as metachromatic leukodystrophy (15,56) (Figure 10.15). Throughout the range of neuropathies, however, segmental demyelination is less common than axonal degeneration.

Hypertrophic Neuropathy

Recurrent segmental demyelination is a feature of a number of chronic hereditary neuropathies, particularly Charcot-Marie-Tooth (CMT) disease, Déjérine-Sottas disease (hereditary motor and sensory neuropathy types I and III), and Refsum's disease (138,139). In such diseases, repeated segmental demyelination appears to be responsible for a florid proliferation of Schwann cells and the formation of onion-bulb whorls (139,140) (Figures 10.14, 10.15), giving a distinctive histological picture of hypertrophic neuropathy to these peripheral neuropathies. So far, at least 16 genetic loci and 9 caustive genes have been identified for primary heritable demyelinating neuropathies (HDN); therefore, although histopathological analysis is still important for the diagnosis of HDN, it is gradually being replaced by molecular diagnosis (139,141).

Traumatic Lesions of Peripheral Nerve

An understanding of the structure and staining reactions of normal peripheral nerve is essential for unraveling the complexities of traumatic lesions of nerve. Identification of cell types, recognition of patterns of organization, and the detection of normal elements within a traumatic lesion allow a more confident diagnosis and description to be formulated.

Amputation neuromas may develop as painful swellings at the distal ends of amputated limbs or at sites of nerve damage without amputation. They consist of disoriented bundles of axons surrounded by Schwann cells and divided into compartments by perineurial cells. In H&E–stained paraffin sections, the tubular formation of the perineurial compartments can be recognized (56). By immunocytochemistry, axons can be stained with antibodies to neurofilament protein and GAP 43; the Schwann cells associated with them contain S-100 protein, and the perineurial cells are EMA-, Glut-1–, and claudin-1–positive but do not contain S-100 protein (142). Silver stains can also be used to identify the twisted and disoriented axons. The histological picture reflects the processes seen in the normal regeneration of peripheral nerve; but in amputation neuromas, appropriate regeneration along the distal part of the nerve is prevented.

In 1876, Thomas G. Morton, from Pennsylvania, described a neuroma that involves the plantar interdigital nerves, almost always between the third and the forth toes (Morton's metatarsalgia), and consists of small painful swellings on the nerves. Histologically, there is fibrosis and edema of the endoneurium and perineurium and the accumulation of mucosubstances similar to endoneurial glycosaminoglycans. The detection of axons and Schwann cells by immunohistochemistry is often a useful adjunct to the diagnosis of this lesion (142).

A pseudocyst or nerve sheath ganglion, containing mucinous material that stains with Alcian blue, may form on a

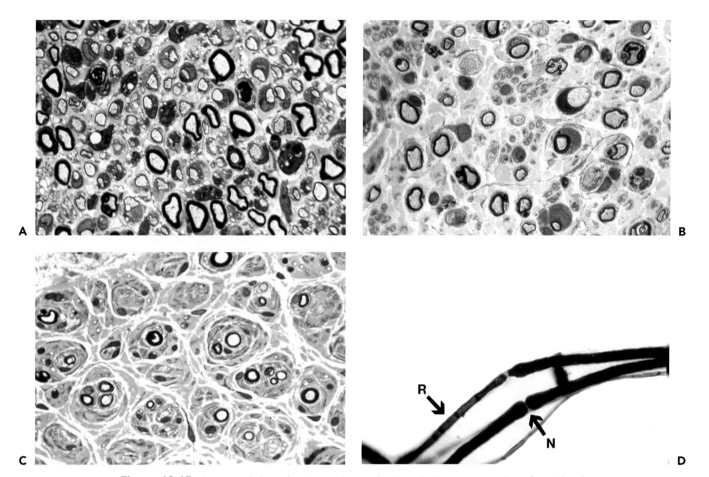

Figure 10.15 Segmental demyelination and remyelination. **A.** Transverse section of peripheral nerve showing early remyelination in an experimental animal. There are normal, large myelinated fibers with axons 8 to 10 μm in diameter and axons 3 to 5 μm in diameter, which have thin myelin sheaths and are remyelinating. Myelin debris is seen in Schwann cells and macrophages (1-μm resin section, toluidine blue, ×310). **B.** Nerve biopsy from a child with metachromatic leukodystrophy (sulfatide lipidosis). Large axons with either thin myelin sheaths (remyelination) or with no myelin sheath at all (demyelinated) (*right of center*) are seen in the biopsy. Unmyelinated fibers (*center*) are unaffected (1-μm resin section, toluidine blue, ×310). (Reprinted from Ahmed AM, Weller RO. The blood-nerve barrier and reconstitution of the perineurium following nerve grafting. *Neuropathol Appl Neurobiol* 1979;5:469–483 with permission.) **C.** Hypertrophic neuropathy (Charcot-Marie-Tooth disease-HSMN type I). Demyelinated and remyelinated axons are seen at the centers of onion-bulb whorls formed by Schwann cell processes; there is abundant endoneurial collagen (pink) (1-um resin section, toluidine blue and carbol fuchsin, ×240). **D.** Teased fibers. Normal fiber (*lower*) with a normal node of Ranvier (*N*). The fiber above has a thin, remyelinating segment (*R*) on one side of the node and a normal segment on the other side (osmium stain, ×200). (Reprinted from: Weller RO. *Colour Atlas of Neuropathology.* Oxford: Oxford University Press and Harvey Miller; 1984 with permission.)

peripheral nerve, generally at a site of repeated trauma. Although the fibrous capsule of the cyst and its mucinous contents may dominate the picture, damaged nerve components can usually be detected adjacent to the cyst (142).

Compressive lesions of peripheral nerves have resulted in some debate regarding their origin. Because of the resemblance of whorls within these lesions to those seen in hypertrophic neuropathies, they have been labeled *localized hypertrophic neuropathy* (36). Such lesions usually occur at sites of compression over the fibula or on the posterior interosseous nerve (137), although some lesions present with

no obvious nerve compression. Although there is well-marked onion-bulb formation, ultrastructural studies have shown that the onion bulbs are formed not by Schwann cells, as in hypertrophic neuropathies, but by perineurial cells (141,143). Such compressive lesions should not be confused with perineuromas in which immunocytochemistry has confirmed that the cell whorls are formed by EMA-, Glut-1-, and claudin-1–positive perineurial cells (40,143), and there are abnormalities of chromosome 22. (143,144).

In 1972, Reed described a small (1–15 mm), typically solitary neuroma that presents in adults and affects the face,

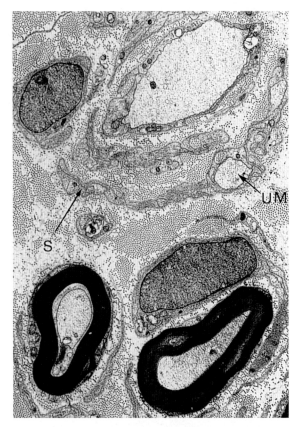

Figure 10.16 Demyelination. A large diameter axon (*top*) is demyelinated and devoid of a myelin sheath. A small onion-bulb whorl has formed around this axon with the encirclement by Schwann cell processes (*S*), one of which contains an unmyelinated fiber (*UM*). Thickly myelinated fibers are seen at the bottom of the picture. (Electron micrograph,×6,600.)

with no clinical manifestations of neurofibromatosis or MEN-IIb (multiple endocrine neoplasia). This lesion is known as solitary circumscribed neuroma (SCN) (palisaded encapsulated neuroma) and is currently viewed as a form of true neuroma. Histologically, SCN appears as one or more circumscribed nodules in the dermis, sometimes partially encapsulated by a delicate compact EMA-positive perineurial layer. The process consists of a solid proliferation of tightly interwoven fascicles of Schwann cells, sometimes separated by narrow gaps that create a characteristic appearance of the lesion at low magnification. The Schwann cells are often arranged as palisades, and there may be numerous axons scattered troughout the lesion, which are best demonstrated with Bodian's silver stain or by immunohistochemistry for neurofilament proteins (145).

Tumors of the Peripheral Nervous System

A variety of cells and structures may be identified in tumors of the peripheral nervous system; they include perineurial cells, Schwann cells, axons, and neurons (142,146,147). The diagnosis frequently depends on the histologic analysis of the tumor and thus the detection of cellular components forming the tumor and their relationship with normal nerve structures (142).

Perineurioma is a rare true perineurial neoplasm (135). Perineuriomas can arise in a wide variety of sites and may exhibit different histological patterns with extra and intraneural forms (29,148). Histologically, *intraneural perineuriomas* affect individual fascicles with concentric proliferation of spindle cells around nerve fibers in the endoneurium; extraneural (soft tissue) perineuriomas show paucicellular to cellular forms (with some cases showing dense collagenization–*sclerosing perineurioma*) with proliferation of spindle cells with extremely thin and elongated profile resembling normal perineurial cells (148). The key diagnostic finding is that the proliferation cells are labeled with EMA, Glut-1 and claudin1 but fail to stain for S-100 protein, neurofilaments, and CD34 (39–41,142). Perineuromas may be closely related to cutaneous meningioma since shared histologic features, and positive staining for vimentin and EMA in both conditions, suggest close similarities between these lesions (41).

Schwannomas are tumors of peripheral nerves composed almost entirely of Schwann cells (28,142,146). Neoplastic Schwann cells may produce and respond to trophic factors, particularly to the growth factor–like polypeptides known as neuregulins, in an autocrine and/or paracrine fashion to promote proliferation. In fact the presence of neuregulins in certain schwannomas has been demonstrated by immunohistochemistry (149).

Histologically, schwannomas show the classical patterns of spindle cells in a compact (Antoni type A) or loose (Antoni type B) arrangement. Neoplastic Schwann cells may exhibit different morphologies (Figure 10.17) (142,146, 150–152). Occasionally, the Schwann cells have an epithelioid appearance (epithelioid schwannomas) (152), are surrounded by an abundant myxoid stroma (nerve sheath myxoma) (153), have a high nuclear-cytoplasmic ratio (cellular schwannoma), exhibit a plexiform pattern (plexiform schwannoma), contain copious melanin (melanotic schwannoma) or exhibit xanthomatous change with many foamy cells containing oil red O–positive neutral lipid (142,146,154). Schwannomas usually grow on the sides of

Figure 10.17 Panel showing the different morphology that the Schwann cells may present in schwannomas. **A.** Benign schwannoma, showing the typical biphasic appearance. **B.** Benign schwannoma with Verocay bodies. **C.** Reticulin (Gordon-Sweet) stain in a benign schwannoma, showing the positive basement membrane. **D.** Cellular schwannoma with uniform fascicular growth pattern. **E.** Granular cell schwannoma. Note the granular cells are originating from a nerve fascicle (*N*) (anti-S-100 protein). (Photograph supplied by Dr. Javier Baquera.) **F.** Melanotic schwannoma. **G.** Nerve sheath myxoma. **H.** Malignant peripheral nerve sheath tumor (malignant triton tumor) with rhabdomyoblastic differentiation (*arrowheads*).

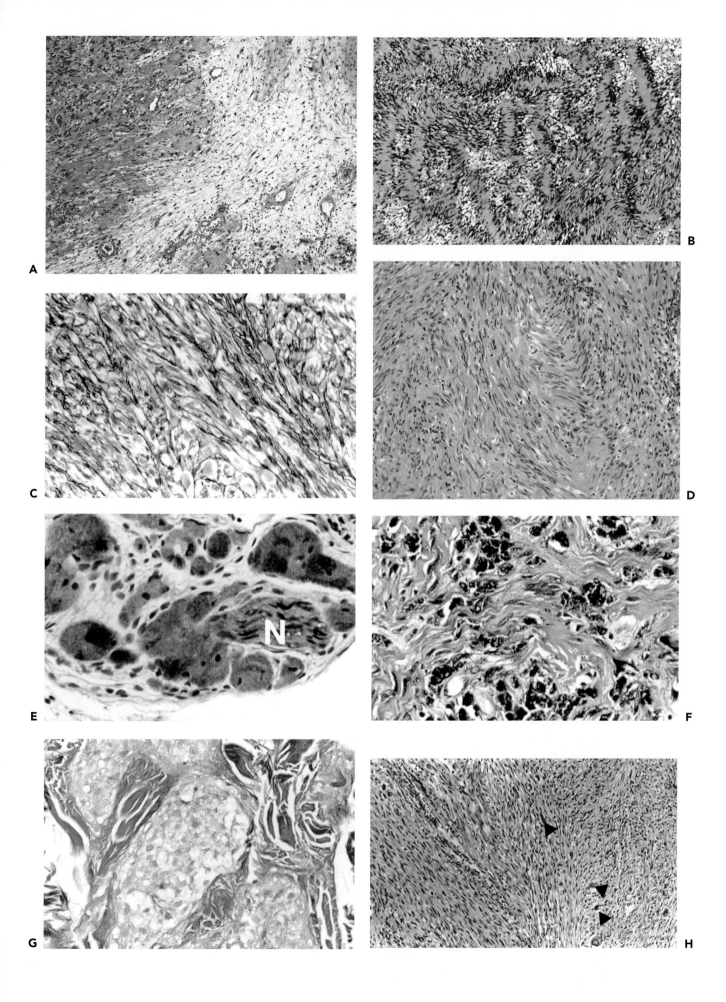

nerves and do not infiltrate nerve bundles (54). Thus, normal nerves may be seen within the fibrous capsule that is usually present around schwannomas.

Histologically, the tumor cells have elongated nuclei and long eosinophilic processes, often forming palisades first described by the Uruguayan-born pathologist José Verocay and known today as Verocay bodies (155). The palisades are parallel arrays of tumor nuclei separated by the eosinophilic, periodic acid-Schiff (PAS)–positive processes of Schwann cells. The basement membrane investing each Schwann cell in the tumor is well-demonstrated by electron microscopy but can also be demonstrated in reticulin stains by light microscopy (54,142). Collagen bundles within schwannomas may have a distinctive long spaced appearance (Luse bodies) (156). Immunocytochemistry shows the presence of S-100 protein, CD57 (Leu-7), CD56, and calretinin in schwannoma cells, but they are negative for EMA (37,38,157). Some schwannomas associated with the spinal cord and those deep in the body or close to major joints stain by immunocytochemistry for GFAP, while the superficial, subcutaneous schwannomas are negative (158). Schwann cells associated with unmyelinated fibers are more likely to express GFAP, and it has been proposed that the GFAP-positive schwannomas may arise from unmyelinated nerves (158).

Melanin may be seen in schwannomas; and, by electron microscopy, premelanosomes and melanosomes may be identified (142,145). Such structures emphasize the common origin of Schwann cells and melanocytes from the neural crest (159,160). There are two types of melanotic schwannomas. The *conventional type* is composed of plump spindle and epithelioid cells arranged in whorls and streaming fascicles containing melanin pigment. *Psammomatous melanotic schwannomas* are mainly in autonomic/visceral locations with the same cell arrangement as melanotic schwannomas but with the additional feature of PAS-positive, von Kossa-positive, mineralized, laminated calcospherites (161). Approximately 50% of patients with psammomatous melanotic schwannomas may have evidence of Carney's syndrome, which includes primary pigmented nodular adrenocortical disease; pituitary-independent, primary adrenal form of hypercortisolism; lentigines; ephelides and blue nevi of the skin and mucosae; and a variety of nonendocrine and endocrine tumors, such as myxomas, pituitary adenomas, testicular Sertoli cell tumor, and other benign and malignant neoplasms (including tumors of thyroid and ductal adenomas of the breast) (161).

Granular cell tumor (GCT, or Abrikosoff tumor) is not a specific entity. Granular cytoplasmic change is the expression of a metabolic alteration occurring often, but not exclusively, in Schwann cells (162). The tumor cells have abundant granular cytoplasm and a small eccentric nucleus; they invade small nerve branches in the skin. Immunocytochemical studies have shown that the tumor cells express S-100 protein, CD57, CD68, neurospecific enolase (NSE),

Protein Gene Product PGP9.5, and also occasionally myelin (P0 and P2) and myelin-associated proteins (28,163). Expression of calretinin has been demonstrated in GCT. As this calcium-binding protein is typically expressed in neurons, ganglion cells, and Schwann cells, GTC expression may further support a neuronal origin or differentiation of these tumors (157). Interestingly, calretinin positivity may be increased in the pseudoepitheliomatous hyperplasia of the squamous epithelium overlying the tumor cells seen in some cases of GCT, which may indicate a role of calretinin in the interaction between GCT cells and hyperplastic epithelium (157). Granular cells have also been described in nerves undergoing wallerian degeneration (162).

Neurofibromas are complex benign lesions frequently associated with neurofibromatosis (147). As distinct from schwannomas, neurofibromas are diffuse lesions in the skin or around peripheral nerves that invade the peripheral nerve endoneurium and enlarge nerve branches (54,142, 147). They also diffusely invade surrounding tissues and may cause bone destruction. Histologically, neurofibromas are as a rule not encapsulated, and they contain a variety of cells that are associated with peripheral nerves; unlike schwannomas, neurofibromas are not predominantly composed of Schwann cells. Mast cells are frequently seen in the stroma and can be identified using toluidine blue or Giemsa or by anti-triptase, CD117, and calretinin immunohistochemistry (51,52,152). Mast cells induce factor XIIIa-positive fibroblast-like cells to synthesize the large amount of extracellular matrix in neurofibromas, and mast cells are one of the inflammatory cell types involved in tumor promotion (52,164–166). It has been hypothesized that when mast cells are lost, as seen in cases of malignant peripheral nerve sheath tumors, there may be a diminution of the anti-cancer effect of mast cells in maintaining the benign nature of some of these proliferations (51,52). By immunocytochemistry, S-100- and CD57 (Leu-7)-positive Schwann cells can be detected within neurofibromas, in addition to EMA-, Glut-1–, and claudin-1–positive perineurial cells and CD34 endoneurial fibroblasts (37,38). Entrapped axons can be seen coursing through neurofibromas in immunocytochemical preparations for neurofilament protein or in silver-stained sections. All of these cellular components are set in a variable fibromyxoid stroma that in some cases may be so prominent (the myxoid part) that it may be mistaken for a myxoma or myxoid liposarcoma. Distorted structures resembling Wagner-Meissner or pacinian corpuscles are sometimes seen (pacinian neurofibromas), and melanin may be found in pigmented neurofibromas (167).

Neurofibromatosis is an autosomal dominant disease that is part of the group of neurocutaneous disorders collectively known as phacomatoses (137,142,168). It presents as two major diseases, peripheral (type 1, or von Recklinghausen's disease; NF1) and central (type 2; NF2) (163). Both type 1 and type 2 are inherited as autosomal dominant traits, but many cases are new mutations. Over 90% of cases of neurofibromatosis are type 1 (peripheral); a gene defect has been located on the long arm of chromosome 17 (17q11.2; *NF1* gene) near the centromere and has been linked to the locus encoding nerve growth factor (147,168). There is an increase in nerve growth factor in the serum of patients with this disorder (169). The *NF1* suppresor gene, which spands over 350 kb of genomic DNA and contains 60 exons, encodes a ubiquitous protein known as neurofibromin. This 2818 amino acid protein has been shown to be associated with cytoplasmic microtubules and functions as a GTPase-activating protein for *ras* (170,171).

A wide variety of disorders occur in patients with NF1, including elephantiasis neuromatosa, in which there are redundant folds of skin associated with plexiform neurofibromas (24,162,168,170,171) and, more commonly, multiple cutaneous neurofibromata. Other tumors, such as gliomas, carcinoid tumors, pheochromocytomas, neuroblastomas, gastrointestinal stromal tumors, Wilms' tumors, and pigmented hamartomas of the iris (Lisch nodules), are also seen in patients with this disorder (142,167).

Central, or type 2, neurofibromatosis is much less common than NF1 and is characterized by bilateral vestibular schwannomas; skin lesions are uncommon. Approximately 40% of the vestibular schwannomas in NF2 tend to have a lobular grapelike pattern, while this arrangement is extremely uncommon in sporadic schwannomas (169,172). A proportion of these patients have multiple tumors, including meningiomas, intramedullary spinal ependymomas, and glial microhamartomas of the cerebral cortex (169,170). A gene deletion on chromosome 22q12 (*NF2* gene) was identified in 1993 in patients with this disorder, and it is associated with abnormalities of glial growth factor and nerve growth factor activity (169). The *NF2* gene spans 110 kb and encodes a membrane-cytoskeleton linking protein that is a member of the protein 4.1 family, known as merlin, (for *m*oezin-*e*zrin-*r*adixin-*li*ke prot*ein*). Merlin, also known as schwannomin, may be detected immunohistochemically in the cytoplasm of many cells, including Schwann cells, and it is believed to act as a tumor suppressor gene, the loss of function of which is a fundamental event in the genesis of schwannomas (172,173,174). Normal Schwann cells express merlin, which is known to play a crucial role in cytoskeleton-associated events. Since merlin is a tumor suppressor gene, and all schwannomas lack merlin, it is proposed that the mutation of *NF2* may cause tumor formation through disruption of cell shape, cell matrix, and cell-cell communication or signaling functions, attributed to actin-cytoskeleton-plasma membrane interaction (173,174). Sporadic schwannomas from non-*NF2* individuals also have *NF2* mutations (175).

Neuronal tumors such as ganglioneuromas occur in association with autonomic ganglia in the peripheral nervous system. Histologically, neurons can be identified within these tumors; axons and Schwann cells may be identified by immunocytochemistry. Electron microscopy reveals the presence of 100-nm dense-core vesicles resembling catecholamine granules in the neurons. In addition to well-differentiated ganglioneuromas, primitive neuroectodermal tumors such as neuroblastoma and ganglioneuroblastomas arise within the abdomen and thorax (172). Cell types within the more primitive tumors may be difficult to identify by immunocytochemistry, but electron microscopy usually reveals the presence of 100-nm dense-core catecholamine vesicles within the tumor cell cytoplasm (142,176).

Malignant peripheral nerve sheath tumors (MPNST, or malignant schwannomas) (142) are derived from specialized cells of the endoneurium and perineurium and show great histological variation and many similarities to other soft tissue tumors (28,142). The term *MPNST* incorporates previously used terms such as neurofibrosarcoma and malignant schwannoma. Mutation in the *NF1* tumor suppressor gene is the most important molecular genetic event in the development of MPNST (177). Malignant change in a benign scwhannoma is an extremely rare event (142); however, two forms of neurofibroma, plexiform and localized intraneural neurofibroma, are significant precursors of MPNST (178). Immunocytochemistry has demonstrated EMA-, S-100–, and CD57-positive cells in MPNST (154,177), and occasional tumors that are EMA-positive and S-100–negative have been described as MPNST with perineurial cell differentiation (179). This suggests that cells of MPNST may produce proteins characteristic of perineurial cells or of both perineurium and Schwann cells. Neurospecific enolase, neurofilament protein, and myelin-basic protein have also been occasionally identified in MPNST (17,180). Heterogeneity is common, and so histological sampling should include wide areas of tumor (142,181). Unusual elements (such as cartilage, bone, squamous elements, and muscle) may be encountered occasionally. Malignant peripheral nerve sheath tumors may also present with malignant glands (glandular malignant schwannoma) or rhabdomyosarcoma, features that may be highlighted by immunocytochemistry for cytokeratins and desmin, respectively. In an attempt to explain the occurrence of malignant muscle differentiation (rhabdomyosarcoma) in malignant schwannomas, Pierre Masson suggested that endoneurial cells might differentiate into muscle cells under the inductive influence of nerve cells, a situation that was thought to be operative in regenerating limbs in triton salamanders, hence the name *triton tumor* (malignant schwannoma with rhabdomyoblastic differentiation) (182).

ACKNOWLEDGMENTS

We thank the staff of the Neuropathology and Cell Pathology laboratories and the Imaging Unit of Southampton University Hospitals NHS Trust, Southampton, England, and the Immunohistochemistry section of the ABC Medical

Center in Mexico City for their generous and expert cooperation. Special thanks are due to Margaret Harris, who typed the original manuscript, to Dr. Sergio Piña-Oviedo, who drew the diagrams, and to Professor James Nicoll and Dr. Javier Baquera, who supplied Figures 10.4F and 10.17E respectively.

REFERENCES

1. Le Douarin NM, Creuzet S, Couly G, Dupin E. Neural crest cell plasticity and its limits. *Development* 2004;131:4637–4650.
2. Gogly B. Embryology of neural crests and their classification [in French]. *Rev Orthop Dento Faciale* 1990;24:401–426.
3. Scherer SS. The biology and pathobiology of Schwann cells. *Curr Opin Neurol* 1997;10:386–397.
4. Jessen KR, Mirsky R. Signals that determine Schwann cell identity. *J Anat* 2002;200:367–376.
5. Young HM, Anderson RB, Anderson CR. Guidance cues involved in the development of the peripheral autonomic nervous system. *Auton Neurosci* 2004 31;112:1–14.
6. Levi-Montalcini R. The nerve growth factor and the neuroscience chess board. *Prog Brain Res* 2004;146:525–527.
7. Anand P. Neurotrophic factors and their receptors in human sensory neuropathies. *Prog Brain Res* 2004;146:477–492.
8. Petruska JC, Mendell LM. The many functions of nerve growth factor: multiple actions on nociceptors. *Neurosci Lett* 2004;361: 168–171.
9. Markus A, Patel TD, Snider WD. Neurotrophic factors and axonal growth. *Curr Opin Neurobiol* 2002;12:523–531.
10. Chernousov MA, Carey DJ. Schwann cell extracellular matrix molecules and their receptors. *Histol Histopathol* 2000;15: 593–601.
11. Letourneau PC, Condic ML, Snow DM. Extracellular matrix and neurite outgrowth. *Curr Opin Genet Dev* 1992;2:625–634.
12. Michailov GV, Sereda MW, Brinkmann BG, et al. Axonal neuregulin-1 regulates myelin sheath thickness. *Science* 2004;304: 700–703.
13. Nadim W, Anderson PN, Turmaine M. The role of Schwann cells and basal lamina tubes in the regeneration of axons through long lengths of freeze-killed nerve grafts. *Neuropathol Appl Neurobiol* 1990;16:411–421.
14. Shield LK, King RHM, Thomas PK. A morphologic study of human fetal sural nerve. *Acta Neuropathol (Berlin)* 1986;70:60–70.
15. Thomas PK, Ochoa J. Microscopic anatomy of peripheral nerve fibers. In: Dyck PJ, Thomas PK, Lambert EH, Bunge R, eds. *Peripheral Neuropathy*. 2nd ed. Vol 1. Philadelphia: WB Saunders; 1984:39–96.
16. Moore JK, Linthicum FH Jr. Myelination of the human auditory nerve: different time courses for Schwann cell and glial myelin. *Ann Otol Rhinol Laryngol* 2001;110(pt 1):655–661.
17. Notterpek L. Neurotrophins in myelination: a new role for a puzzling receptor. *Trends Neurosci* 2003;26:232–234.
18. Martini R. The effect of myelinating Schwann cells on axons. *Muscle Nerve* 2001;24:456–466.
19. Yin X, Crawford TO, Griffin JW, et al. Myelin-associated glycoprotein is a myelin signal that modulates the caliber of myelinated axons. *J Neurosci* 1998;18:1953–1962.
20. Reina MA, López A, Villanueva MC, Andrés JA, León GI. Morfología de los nervios periféricos, de sus cubiertas y de su vascularización. *Rev Esp Anesesiol Reanim* 2000;47:464–475.
21. Sloniewski P, Korejwo G, Zielinski P, Morys J, Krzyzanowski M. Measurements of the Obersteiner-Redlich zone of the vagus nerve and their possible clinical applications. *Folia Morphol (Warsz)* 1999;58:37–41.
22. Lieberman AR. Sensory ganglia. In: Landon DN, ed. *The Peripheral Nerve*. London: Chapman and Hall; 1976:188–278.
23. Tassler PL, Dellon AL, Canoun C. Identification of elastic fibres in the peripheral nerve. *J Hand Surg Br* 1994;19:48–54.
24. Rushing EJ, Bouffard JP. Basic pathology of the peripheral nerve. *Neuroimaging Clin N Am* 2004;14:43–53, vii.
25. Cavanagh JB. Pathology of peripheral nerve diseases. In: Weller RO, ed. *Systemic Pathology*. 3rd ed. Vol. 4: *Nervous System, Muscle and Eyes*. Edinburgh: Churchill Livingstone; 1990:544–578.
26. Kameh DS, Perez-Berenguer JL, Pearl GS. Lipofibromatous hamartoma and related peripheral nerve lesions. *South Med J* 2000;93:800–802.
27. Vega JA, Del Valle ME, Haro JJ, Naves FJ, Calzada B, Uribelarrea R. The inner-core, outer-core and capsule cells of the human Pacinian corpuscles: an immunohistochemical study. *Eur J Morphol* 1994;32:11–18.
28. Enzinger FM, Weiss SW.. *Soft Tissue Tumors*. 4th ed. St Louis: Mosby; 2001.
29. Tsang WYW. Perineuriomas: perineurial cell neoplasms with distinctive extra- and intraneural forms. *Adv Anat Pathol* 1996; 212–222.
30. Reina MA, López A, Villanueva MC, De Andrés JA, Machés F. La barrera hemato-nerviosa en los nervios. *Rev Esp Anesesiol Reanim* 2003;50:80–86.
31. Poliak S, Matlis S, Ullmer C, Scherer SS, Peles E. Distinct claudins and associated PZD proteins form different autotypic tight junctions in myelinating Schwann cells *J Cell Biol* 2002;159:361–372.
32. Folpe AL, Billings SD, McKenney JK, Walsh SV, Nusrat A, Weiss SW. Expression of claudin-1, a recently described tight junction-associated protein, distinguishes soft tissue perineurioma from potential mimics. *Am J Surg Pathol* 2002;26:1620–1626.
33. Erlandson RA. The enigmatic perineurial cell and its participation in tumors and in tumorlike entities. *Ultrastruct Pathol* 1991;15: 335–351.
34. Cavanagh JB. Toxic and deficiency disorders. In: Weller RO, ed. *Systemic Pathology*. 3rd ed. Vol 4. *Nervous System, Muscle and Eyes*. Edinburgh: Churchill Livingstone; 1990:244–308.
35. Ahmed AM, Weller RO. The blood-nerve barrier and reconstitution of the perineurium following nerve grafting. *Neuropathol Appl Neurobiol* 1979;5:469–483.
36. Weller RO. Localized hypertrophic neuropathy and hypertrophic polyneuropathy. *Lancet* 1974;ii:529–593.
37. MacKeever PE. Immunohistochemistry of the nervous system. In: Daabs DJ, ed. *Diagnostic Immunohistochemistry*. Philadelphia: Chirchill Livingstone; 2002:559–624.
38. Hirose T, Tani T, Shimada T, Ishizawa K, Shimada S, Sano T. Immunohistochemical demonstration of EMA/Glut1-positive perineurial cells and CD34-positive fibroblastic cells in peripheral nerve sheath tumors. *Mod Pathol* 2003;16:293–298.
39. Yamaguchi U, Hasegawa T, Hirose T, et al.. Sclerosing perineurioma: a clinicopathological study of five cases and diagnostic utility of immunohistochemical staining for GLUT1. *Virchows Arch* 2003;443:159–163.
40. Wick MR, Cerilli LA. Applications of immunohistochemistry in the diagnosis of undifferentiated tumors. In: Lloyd RV, ed. *Morphology Methods: Cell and Molecular Biology Techniques*. Totowa, NJ: Human Press; 2001:323–360.
41. Zelger B, Weinlich G, Zelger B. Perineurioma. A frequently unrecognized entity with emphasis on a plexiform variant. *Adv Clin Path* 2000;4:25–33.
42. Hirai I, Kimura W, Ozawa K, et al. Perineural invasion in pancreatic cancer. *Pancreas* 2002;24:15–25.
43. Fogt F, Capodieci P, Loda M. Assessment of perineural invasion by GLUT-1 immunohistochemistry. *Appl Immunohistochem* 1995;3: 194–197.
44. Zimmerman KG, Johnson PC, Paplanus SH. Nerve invasion by benign proliferating ductules in vasitis nodosa. *Cancer* 1983;51: 2066–20610.
45. Khalifa MA, Montgomery EA, Ismiil N, Azumi N. What are the CD34+ cells in benign peripheral nerve sheath tumors? Double immunostaining study of CD34 and S-100 protein. *Am J Clin Pathol* 2000;114:123–126.
46. van de Rijn M, Rouse RV. CD34: a review. *Appl Immunohistochem* 1994;2:71–80.
47. Maurer M, Muller M, Kobsar I, Leonhard C, Martini R, Kiefer R. Origin of pathogenic macrophages and endoneurial fibroblast-

like cells in an animal model of inherited neuropathy. *Mol Cell Neurosci* 2003;23:351–3510.

48. Bonetti B, Monaco S, Giannini C, Ferrari S, Zanusso G, Rizzuto N. Human peripheral nerve macrophages in normal and pathological conditions. *J Neurol Sci* 1993;118:158–168.

49. Griffin J, George R. The resident macrophages in the peripheral nervous system are renewed from the bone marrow: new variations on an old theme. *Lab Invest* 1993;3:257–260.

50. Gabriel CM, Howard R, Kinsella N, et al. Prospective study of the usefulness of sural nerve biopsy. *J Neurol Neurosurg Psychiatry* 2000;69:442–446.

51. Zochodne DW, Nguyen C, Sharkey KA. Accumulation and degranulation of mast cells in experimental neuromas. *Neurosci Lett* 1994;182:3–6.

52. Viskochil DH. It takes two to tango: mast cell and Schwann cell interactions in neurofibromas. *J Clin Invest* 2003;112:1791–1793.

53. Esposito B, De Santis A, Monteforte R, Baccari GC. Mast cells in Wallerian degeneration: morphologic and ultrastructural changes. *J Comp Neurol* 2002;445:199–210.

54. Weller RO, Cervos-Navarro J. *Pathology of Peripheral Nerves: A Practical Approach*. London: Butterworths; 1977.

55. Weis J, Alexianu ME, Heide G, Shroder JM. Renaut bodies contain elastic fiber components. *J Neuropathol Exp Neurol* 1993;52:444–451.

56. Weller RO. *Colour Atlas of Neuropathology*. Oxford: Oxford University Press and Harvey Miller; 1984.

57. Baker MD. Electrophysiology of mammalian Schwann cells. *Prog Biophys Mol Biol* 2002;78:83–103.

58. Lariviere RC, Julien JP. Functions of intermediate filaments in neuronal development and disease. *J Neurobiol* 2004;58:131–148.

59. Al-Chalabi A, Miller CC. Neurofilaments and neurological disease. *Bioessays* 2003;25:346–355.

60. Mukhopadhyay R, Kumar S, Hoh JH. Molecular mechanisms for organizing the neuronal cytoskeleton. *Bioessays* 2004;26:1017–1025.

61. von Bartheld CS. Axonal transport and neuronal transcytosis of trophic factors, tracers, and pathogens. *J Neurobiol* 2004;58:295–314.

62. Baas PW, Buster DW. Slow axonal transport and the genesis of neuronal morphology. *J Neurobiol* 2004;58:3–17.

63. Arvidson B. A review of axonal transport of metals. *Toxicology* 1994;88:1–14.

64. Coleman MP, Perry VH. Axon pathology in neurological disease: a neglected therapeutic target. *Trends Neurosci* 2002;25:532–537.

65. Bearer EL, Breakefield XO, Schuback D, Reese TS, LaVail JH. Retrograde axonal transport of herpes simplex virus: evidence for a single mechanism and a role for tegument. *Proc Natl Acad Sci U S A* 2000;97:8146–8150.

66. Peters A. The effects of normal aging on myelin and nerve fibers: a review. *J Neurocytol* 2002;31:581–593.

67. Terada S. Where does slow axonal transport go? *Neurosci Res* 2003;47:367–372.

68. Spencer PS, Schaumburg HH, eds. *Experimental and Clinical Neurotoxicology*. 2nd ed. New York: Oxford University Press; 2000.

69. Katalymov LL, Glukhova NV. Some characteristics of periaxonal space in myelinated nerve fibers. *Dokl Biol Sci* 2003;388:9–11.

70. Trapp B, Quarles R, Suzuki K. Immunocytochemical studies of quaking mice support a role for myelin-associated glycoprotein in forming and maintaining the periaxonal space and periaxonal cytoplasmic collar of myelinating Schwann cells. *J Cell Biol* 1984;99:594–606.

71. Quarles RH. Myelin sheaths: glycoproteins involved in their formation, maintenance and degeneration. *Cell Mol Life Sci* 2002;59:1851–1871.

72. Mirsky R, Jessen KR. The neurobiology of Schwann cells. *Brain Pathol* 1999;293–311.

73. Weller RO, Herzog I. Schwann cell lysosomes in hypertrophic neuropathy and in normal human nerves. *Brain* 1970;93:347–356.

74. Tsiper MV, Yurchenco PD. Laminin assembles into separate basement membrane and fibrillar matrices in Schwann cells. *J Cell Sci* 2002;115(pt 5):1005–1015.

75. Gonzalez-Martinez T, Perez-Pinera P, Diaz-Esnal B, Vega JA. S-100 proteins in the human peripheral nervous system. *Microsc Res Tech* 2003;60:633–638.

76. Garavito ZV, Sutachan JJ, Muneton VC, Hurtado H. Is S-100 protein a suitable marker for adult Schwann cells? *In Vitro Cell Dev Biol Anim* 2000;36:281–283.

77. Le Forestier N, Lescs MC, Gherardi RK. Anti-NKH-1 antibody specifically stains unmyelinated fibres and non-myelinating Schwann cell columns in humans. *Neuropathol Appl Neurobiol* 1993;19:500–506.

78. Fine SW, Li M. Expression of calretinin and the alpha-subunit of inhibin in granular cell tumors. *Am J Clin Pathol* 2003;119:259–264.

79. Shih IM. The role of CD146 (Mel-CAM) in biology and pathology. *J Pathol* 1999;189:4–11.

80. Yasuda T, Sobue G, Ito T, et al.. Human peripheral nerve sheath neoplasm: expression of Schwann cell-related markers and their relation to malignant transformation. *Muscle Nerve* 1991;14:812–8110.

81. Kawahara E, Oda Y, Ooi A, Katsuda S, Nakanishi Y, Umeda S. Expression of glial fibrillary acidic protein (GFAP) in peripheral nerve sheath tumors. A comparative study of immunoreactivity of GFAP, vimentin, S-100 protein, and neurofilament in 38 schwannomas and 18 neurofibromas. *Am J Surg Pathol* 1988;12:115–120.

82. Koirala S, Reddy LV, Ko CP. Roles of glial cells in the formation, function, and maintenance of the neuromuscular junction. *J Neurocytol* 2003;32:987–1002.

83. Paré M, Elde R, Mazurkiewicz JE, Smith AM, Rice FL. The Meissner corpuscle revised: a multiafferented mechanoreceptor with nociceptor immunochemical properties. *J Neurosci* 2001;21:7236–7246.

84. Oda R, Yaoi T, Okajima S, Kobashi H, Kubo T, Fushiki S. A novel marker for terminal Schwann cells, homocysteine-responsive ER-resident protein, as isolated by a single cell PCR-differential display. *Biochem Biophys Res Commun* 2003;308:872–877.

85. Wewetzer K, Verdú E, Angelov DN, Navarro X. Olfactory ensheathing glia and Schwann cells: two of a kind? *Cell Tissue Res* 2002;309:337–345.

86. Ffrench-Constant C, Colognato H, Franklin RJM. The mysteries of myelin unwrapped. *Science* 2004;304:688–6810.

87. Spiegel I, Peles E. Cellular junctions of myelinated nerves (Review). *Mol Membr Biol* 2002;19:95–101.

88. Eichberg J. Myelin PO. New knowledge and new roles. *Neurochem Res* 2002;27:1331–1340.

89. Garbay B, Heape AM, Sargueil F, Cassagne C. Myelin synthesis in the peripheral nervous system. *Prog Neurobiol* 2000;61:267–304.

90. Raine CS. Multiple sclerosis and chronic relapsing EAE: comparative ultrastructural neuropathology. In: Hallpike JF, Adams CWM, Tourtelotte WW, eds. *Multiple Sclerosis. Pathology, Diagnostic and Management*. London: Chapman and Hall; 1983:413–460.

91. Shy ME, Garbern JY, Kamholz J. Hereditary motor and sensory neuropathies: a biological perspective. *Lancet Neurol* 2002;1:110–118.

92. Chen ZL, Strickland S. Laminin gamma1 is critical for Schwann cell differentiation, axon myelination, and regeneration in the peripheral nerve. *J Cell Biol* 2003;163:889–8910.

93. Podratz JL, Rodriguez E, Windebank AJ. Role of the extracellular matrix in myelination of peripheral nerve. *Glia* 2001;35:35–40.

94. Takashima H, Boerkoel CF, De Jonghe P, et al. Periaxin mutations cause a broad spectrum of demyelinating neuropathies. *Ann Neurol* 2002;51:709–715.

95. Meier C, Dermietzel R, Davidson KG, Yasumura T, Rash JE. Connexin32-containing gap junctions in Schwann cells at the internode zone of partial myelin compaction and in Schmidt-Lanterman incisures. *J Neurosci* 2004;24:3186–3198.

96. Balice-Gordon RJ, Bone LJ, Scherer SS. Functional gap junctions in the Schwann cell myelin sheath. *J Cell Biol* 1998;142:1095–1104.

97. Custer AW, Kazarinova-Noyes K, Sakurai T, et al. The role of ankyrin-binding protein NrCAM in node of Ranvier formation. *J Neurosci* 2003;23:10032–10039.

98. Scherer SS. Nodes, paranodes, and incisures: from form to function. *Ann N Y Acad Sci* 1999;883:131–142.

99. Ochoa J. The unmyelinated fibre. In: Landon DN, ed. *The Peripheral Nerve*. London: Chapman and Hall; 1976:106–158.

100. Mirsky R, Jessen KR. The biology of non–myelin-forming Schwann cells. *Ann N Y Acad Sci* 1986;486:132–146.

101. Gray MH, Rosenberg AE, Dickersin GR, Bhan AK. Glial fibrillary acidic protein and keratin expression by benign and malignant nerve sheath tumors. *Hum Pathol* 1989;20:1089–1096.

102. Britton WJ, Lockwood DNJ. Leprosy. *Lancet* 2004;363:1209–12110.

103. Schmidt HG, Schmid A, Domschke W. Nerve-neuroendocrine complexes in stomach mucosa in Zollinger-Ellison syndrome [in German]. *Pathologe* 1995;16:404–407.

104. Auböck L, Hofler H. Extraepithelial intraneural endocrine cells as starting-points for gastrointestinal carcinoids. *Virchows Arch A Pathol Anat Histopathol* 1983;401:17–33.

105. Franke C, Gerharz CD, Bohner H, et al. Neurogenic appendicopathy in children. *Eur J Pediatr Surg* 2002;12:28–31.

106. Ortiz-Hidalgo C, de León-Bojorge B, Torres JE. Neuroma apendicular asociado a microcarcinoide solitario. *Patología* 1995;33:83–85.

107. Schmidt HG, Schmid A, Domschke W. Nerve-neuroendocrine complexes in stomach mucosa in Zollinger-Ellison syndrome [in German]. *Pathologe* 1995;16:404–407.

108. Colomar A, Marty V, Combe C, Medina C, Parnet P, Amedee T. The immune status of Schwann cells: what is the role of the P2X7 receptor? [in French] *J Soc Biol* 2003;197:113–122.

109. Bonetti B, Valdo P, Ossi G, et al. T-cell cytotoxicity of human Schwann cells: TNFalpha promotes fasL-mediated apoptosis and IFN gamma perforin-mediated lysis. *Glia* 2003;43:141–148.

110. Zhang YP, Porter S, Wekerle H. Schwann cells in myasthenia gravis. Preferential uptake of soluble and membrane-bound AChR by normal and immortalized Schwamm cells, and immunogenic presentation to SChR-specific T line lymphocytes. *Am J Pathol* 1990;136:111–112.

111. Vedeler C, Ulvestad E, Borge L, et al. The expression of CD-59 in normal human nervous tissue. *Immunology* 1994;82:542–547.

112. Gold R, Archelos JJ, Hartung HP. Mechanisms of immune regulation in the peripheral nervous system. *Brain Pathol* 1999;9:343–360.

113. Glass JD. Wallerian degeneration as a window to peripheral neuropathy. *J Neurol Sci* 2004;220:123–124.

114. Fu SY, Gordon T. The cellular and molecular basis of peripheral nerve regeneration. *Mol Neurobiol* 1997;14:67–116.

115. Hirata K, Kawabuchi M. Myelin phagocytosis by macrophages and nonmacrophages during Wallerian degeneration. *Microsc Res Tech* 2002;57:541–547.

116. Tofaris GK, Patterson PH, Jessen KR, Mirsky R. Denervated Schwann cells attract macrophages by secretion of leukemia inhibitory factor (LIF) and monocyte chemoattractant protein-1 in a process regulated by interleukin-6 and LIF. *J Neurosci* 2002;22:6696–6703.

117. Shen ZL, Lassner F, Bader A, Becker M, Walter GF, Berger A. Cellular activity of resident macrophages during Wallerian degeneration. *Microsurgery* 2000;20:255–261.

118. Burnett MG, Zager EL. Pathophysiology of peripheral nerve injury: a brief review. *Neurosurg Focus* 2004;16:E1.

119. Horie H, Kadoya T, Hikawa N, et al. Oxidized galectin-1 stimulates macrophages to promote axonal regeneration in peripheral nerves after axotomy. *J Neurosci* 2004;24:1873–1880.

120. Blackemore WK. Myelination, demyelination and remyelination. In: Thomas Smith W, Cavanagh JB, eds. *Recent Advances in Neuropathology*. Vol 2. Edinburgh: Churchill Livingstone; 1982:53–82.

121. Lee SK, Wolfe SW. Peripheral nerve injury and repair. *J Am Acad Orthop Surg* 2000;8:243–252.

122. Blesch A, Tuszynski MH. Nucleus hears axon's pain. *Nat Med* 2004;10:236–237.

123. Boeshore KL, Schreiber RC, Vaccariello SA, et al. Novel changes in gene expression following axotomy of a sympathetic ganglion: a microarray analysis. *J Neurobiol* 2004;59:216–235.

124. Bergner AJ, Murphy SM, Anderson CR. After axotomy, substance P and vasoactive intestinal peptide expression occurs in pilomotor neurons in the rat superior cervical ganglion. *Neuroscience* 2000;96:611–618.

125. Khullar SM, Fristad I, Brodin P, Kvinnsland IH. Upregulation of growth associated protein 43 expression and neuronal co-expression with neuropeptide Y following inferior alveolar nerve axotomy in the rat. *J Peripher Nerv Syst* 1998;3:79–90.

126. Fenrich K, Gordon T. Canadian Association of Neuroscience review: axonal regeneration in the peripheral and central nervous systems: current issues and advances. *Can J Neurol Sci* 2004;31:142–156.

127. Terenghi G. Peripheral nerve regeneration and neurotrophic factors. *J Anat* 1999;194(pt 1):1–14.

128. Welcher AA, Suter U, De Leon M, Bitler CM, Shooter EM. Molecular approaches to nerve regeneration. *Philos Trans R Soc Lond B Biol Sci* 1991;331:295–301.

129. Boyd JG, Gordon T. Neurotrophic factors and their receptors in axonal regeneration and functional recovery after peripheral nerve injury. *Mol Neurobiol* 2003;27:277–324.

130. Craner MJ, Hains BC, Lo AC, Black JA, Waxman SG. Co-localization of sodium channel Nav1.6 and the sodium-calcium exchanger at sites of axonal injury in the spinal cord in EAE. *Brain* 2004;127(pt 2):294–303.

131. Frisen J, Risling M, Fried K. Distribution and axonal relations of macrophages in neuroma. *Neuroscience* 1993;55:1003–1013.

132. King RM. *Atlas of Peripheral Nerve Pathology*. London: Edward Arnold; 19910.

133. Dyck PJ, Dyck PJB, Giannini C, Sahenk Z, Windebank AJ, Engelstad JN. Peripheral nerves. In: Graham DI, Lantos PL, eds. *Greenfield's Neuropathology*. 7th ed. Vol. 2. London: Arnold; 2002:551–676.

134. Kuwabara S. Guillain-Barre syndrome: epidemiology, pathophysiology and management. *Drugs* 2004;64:597–610.

135. Weller RO, Nester B. Early changes at the node of Ranvier in segmental demyelination: histochemical and electron microscopic observations. *Brain* 1972;95:665–674.

136. Weller RO, Bruckner FE, Chamberlain MA. Rheumatoid neuropathy: a histological and electrophysiological study. *J Neurol Neurosurg Psychiatry* 1970;33:592–604.

137. Weller RO, Mitchell J, Daves GD Jr. Buckthorn (Karwinskia humboldtiana) toxins. In: Spencer PS, Schaumburg HH, eds. *Experimental and Clinical Neurology*. Baltimore: Williams & Wilkins; 1980;336–347.

138. Shy ME, Garbern JY, Kamholz J. Hereditary motor and sensory neuropathies: a biological perspective. *Lancet Neurol* 2002;1:110–118.

139. Klein CJ. Pathology and molecular genetics of inherited neuropathy. *J Neurol Sci* 2004;220:141–143.

140. Bertorini T, Narayanaswami P, Rashed H. Charcot-Marie-Tooth disease (hereditary motor sensory neuropathies) and hereditary sensory and autonomic neuropathies. *Neurologist* 2004;10:327–337.

141. Zhou L, Griffin JW. Demyelinating neuropathies. *Curr Opin Neurol* 2003;16:307–313.

142. Ironside JW, Moss TH, Louis DN, Lowe JS, Weller RO. Tumours of peripheral nerves. In: *Diagnostic Pathology of Nervous System Tumors*. Churchill Livingstone; 2002:425–464.

143. Giannini C, Scheithauer BW, Jenkins RB, et al. Soft-tissue perineurioma. Evidence for an abnormality of chromosome 22, criteria for diagnosis, and review of the literature. *Am J Surg Pathol* 1997;21:164–173.

144. Rankine AJ, Filion PR, Platten MA, Spagnolo DV. Perineurioma: a clinicopathological study of eight cases. *Pathology* 2004;36:309–315.

145. Kossard S, Kumar A, Wilkinson B. Neural spectrum: palisaded encapsulated neuroma and verocay body poor dermal schwannoma. *J Cutan Pathol* 1999;26:31–36.

146. Kurtkaya-Yapicier O, Scheithauer B, Woodruff JM. The pathobiologic spectrum of Schwannomas. *Histol Histopathol* 2003;18:925–934.

147. Ferner RE, O'Doherty MJ. Neurofibroma and scwhannoma. *Curr Opin Neurol* 2002;15:679–684.

148. Canales-Ibarra C, Magariños G, Olsoff-Pagovich P, Ortiz-Hidalgo C. Cutaneous sclerosing perineurioma of the digits: an

uncommon soft-tissue neoplasm. Report of two cases with immunohistochemical analysis. *J Cutan Pathol* 2003;30: 577–581.

149. Hansen MR, Linthicum FH Jr. Expression of neuregulin and activation of erbB receptors in vestibular schwannomas: possible autocrine loop stimulation. *Otol Neurotol* 2004;25:155–1510.

150. de Saint Aubain Somerhausen N, Valaeys V, Geerts M, Andre J. Neuroblastoma-like schwannoma: a case report and review of the literature. *Am J Dermatopathol* 2003;25:32–34.

151. Kim YC, Park HJ, Cinn YW, Vandersteen DP. Benign glandular schwannoma. *Br J Dermatol* 2001;145:834–837.

152. Kindblom LG, Meis-Kindblom JM, Havel G, Busch C. Benign epithelioid schwannoma. *Am J Surg Pathol* 1998;22:762–770.

153. Laskin WB, Fetsch JF, Miettinen M. The "neurothekeoma": immunohistochemical analysis distinguishes the true nerve sheath myxoma from its mimics. *Hum Pathol* 2000;31:1230–1241.

154. Scheithauer BW, Woodruff JM, Erlandson RA, eds. Neurofibroma. Tumors of the peripheral nervous system. *Atlas of Tumor Pathology.* Series 3, fascicle 24. Washington, DC: Armed Forces Institute of Pathology; 1999:177–218.

155. Ortiz-Hidalgo C, Verocay J. Verocay neurinomas and bodies and other contributions to medicine. *Rev Neurol* 2004;39:487–491.

156. Dingemans KP, Teeling P. Long-spacing collagen and proteoglycans in pathologic tissues. *Ultrastruct Pathol* 1994;18:539–547.

157. Fine SW, McClain SA, Li M. Immunohistochemical staining for calretinin is useful for differentiating schwannomas from neurofibromas. *Am J Clin Pathol* 2004;122:552–5510.

158. Yen SH, Fields KL. A protein related to glial filaments in Schwann cells. *Ann N Y Acad Sci* 1985;455:538–551.

159. Fullen DR, Reed JA, Finnerty B, McNutt NS. S100A6 preferentially labels type C nevus cells and nevic corpuscles: additional support for Schwannian differentiation of intradermal nevi. *J Cutan Pathol* 2001;28:393–3910.

160. Katati MJ, Martin JM, Massare E, Arjona V. Melanocytic schwannoma. A case report and review of the literature [in Spanish]. *Rev Neurol* 2000;31:427–430.

161. Stratakis CA, Matyakhina L, Courkoutsakis N, et al. Pathology and molecular genetics of the pituitary gland in patients with the "complex of spotty skin pigmentation, myxomas, endocrine overactivity and schwannomas" (Carney complex). *Front Horm Res* 2004;32:253–264.

162. Ordoñez NG. Granular cell tumor: a review and update. *Adv Anat Pathol* 1999;6:186–203.

163. Kurtin PJ, Bonin DM. Immunohistochemical demonstration of the lysosome-associated glycoprotein CD68 (KP-1) in granular cell tumors and schwannomas. *Hum Pathol* 1994;25:1172–1178.

164. Skovronsky DM, Oberholtzer JC. Pathologic classification of peripheral nerve tumors. *Neurosurg Clin N Am* 2004;15:157–166.

165. Zhu Y, Ghosh P, Charnay P, Burns DK, Parada LF. Neurofibromas in NF1: Schwann cell origin and role of tumor environment. *Science* 2002;296:920–922.

166. Takata M, Imai T, Hirone T. Factor-XIIIa-positive cells in normal peripheral nerves and cutaneous neurofibromas of type-1 neurofibromatosis. *Am J Dermatopathol* 1994;16:37–43.

167. Rosai J. Soft tissues. In: *Rosai and Ackerman's Surgical Pathology.* 9th ed. Vol 2. Edinburgh: Mosby; 2004:2266–22610.

168. Arun D, Gutmann DH. Recent advances in neurofibromatosis type 1. *Curr Opin Neurol* 2004;17:101–105.

169. Lim DJ, Rubenstein AE, Evans DG, et al. Advances in neurofibromatosis 2 (NF2): a workshop report. *J Neurogenet* 2000;14: 63–106.

170. Yang FC, Ingram DA, Chen S, et al. Neurofibromin-deficient Schwann cells secrete a potent migratory stimulus for Nf1+/− mast cells. *J Clin Invest* 2003;112:1851–1861.

171. Young H, Hyman S, North K. Neurofibromatosis 1: clinical review and exceptions to the rules. *J Child Neurol* 2002;17:613–621.

172. Baser ME, R Evans DG, Gutmann DH. Neurofibromatosis 2. *Curr Opin Neurol* 2003;16:27–33.

173. Xiao G-H, Chernoff J, Testa JR. NF2: the wizardry of Merlin. *Genes Chromosomes Cancer* 2003;38:389–3910.

174. Bashour AM, Meng JJ, Ip W, MacCollin M, Ratner N. The neurofibromatosis type 2 gene product, merlin, reverses the F-actin cytoskeletal defects in primary human schwannoma cells. *Mol Cell Biol* 2002;22:1150–1157.

175. Pelton PD, Sherman LS, Rizvi TA, et al. Ruffling membrane, stress fiber, cell spreading and proliferation abnormalities in human Schwannoma cells. *Oncogene* 1998;17:2195–2201.

176. Mora J, Gerald WL. Origin of neuroblastic tumors: clues for future therapeutics. *Expert Rev Mol Diagn* 2004;4:293–302.

177. Bilgic B, Ates LE, Demiryont M, Ozger H, Dizdar Y. Malignant peripheral nerve sheath tumors associated with neurofibromatosis type 1. *Pathol Oncol Res* 2003;9:201–205.

178. Woodruff JM. Pathology of tumors of the peripheral nerve sheath in type 1 neurofibromatosis. *Am J Med Genet* 1999;89:23–30.

179. Zamecnik M, Michal M. Malignant peripheral nerve sheath tumor with perineurial cell differentiation (malignant perineurioma). *Pathol Int* 1999;49:69–73.

180. Zamecnik M, Michal M. Perineurial cell differentiation in neurofibromas. Report of eight cases including a case with composite perineurioma-neurofibroma features. *Pathol Res Pract* 2001;197:537–544.

181. Yamaguchi U, Hasegawa T, Hirose T, et al. Low grade malignant peripheral nerve sheath tumour: varied cytological and histological patterns. *J Clin Pathol* 2003;56:826–830.

182. Malerba M, Garofalo A. A rare case of nerve-sheath sarcoma with rhabdomyoblastic differentiation (malignant triton tumor) [in Italian]. *Tumori* 2003;89:246–250.

Central Nervous System

11

Gregory N. Fuller   Peter C. Burger

INTRODUCTION

The central nervous system (CNS) is unparalleled among natural systems in terms of structural and functional complexity. As a consequence of its intricate regional architecture, heterogeneous cellular constituents, and an associated extensive and somewhat arcane lexicon, the nervous system is often viewed as a formidably Byzantine realm by many nonneuropathologists; and yet, a working familiarity with the normal morphology of this complex organ must precede optimal evaluation of the many disease states that afflict it. To this end, this chapter will present the salient features of regional neuroanatomy followed by a description of the essentials of microscopic anatomy of the CNS, with special emphasis on those aspects that constitute potential diagnostic pitfalls, including normal anatomic variations, alterations associated with advancing age, reactive changes, and common artifacts.

REGIONAL NEUROANATOMY

We have limited this discussion of regional neuroanatomy to those principles of structural organization that are of practical value to the diagnostician, emphasizing the rudiments of neuroembryology by which the basic organization of the nervous system is best understood. Further details about topographical neuroanatomy can be found in the list of suggested readings provided at the end of the chapter.

Organization of the Spinal Cord and Brainstem

Embryologically, the nascent CNS is a hollow tube formed by the invagination of the neural plate ectoderm. This primitive cylinder is subdivided functionally into a dorsal sensory (alar) plate and a ventral motor (basal) plate. The two are separated by a lateral groove, termed the sulcus limitans, along which develops the efferent autonomic system (Figure 11.1). This primitive organizational pattern is retained, essentially unaltered, in the mature spinal cord. The central gray matter consists of: (a) dorsal horns that receive sensory input from the dorsal roots; (b) ventral horns that contain motor neurons whose axons are conducted to the somatic periphery by the ventral roots; and (c) the lateral autonomic gray matter. Spinal autonomic neurons are confined to thoracic (sympathetic) and sacral (parasympathetic) levels, forming the intermediolateral cell columns. The axons of these preganglionic neurons exit the spinal cord through the ventral roots, ultimately to synapse on postganglionic neurons in the peripheral autonomic ganglia. The sympathetic intermediolateral cell column produces a third horn of gray matter in the thoracic cord, termed the lateral horn (Figures 11.1–11.2). The parasympathetic intermediolateral cell column occupies a similar lateral position in the sacral cord (at the S2, S3, and S4 levels) but does not form a distinct horn.

Spinal Cord

The anatomy of the spinal cord varies according to the level (Figure 11.2). Two enlargements of the ventral horns, one in the cervical region (Figure 11.2A) and another in the lumbosacral region (Figure 11.2C), provide motor innervation for the upper extremities and lower extremities, respectively. In contrast, the ventral horns of the thoracic cord provide innervation for the more limited axial musculature of the trunk and are, accordingly, much smaller (Figure 11.2B). As mentioned earlier, the lateral horns of the gray matter (sympathetic neurons) are a unique feature of the thoracic cord. The thickness of the surrounding white matter fiber bundles (termed funiculi) also varies with cord level, being greatest in the cervical cord, where the thickness reflects the summated accrual of ascending fiber tracts that have successively entered at lower levels, as well as the maximum content of descending tracts that are en route to lower levels, and thinnest in the lumbosacral cord. The terminus of the spinal cord, the filum terminale, is composed primarily of meningeal connective tissue in the human and is discussed separately with the pia-arachnoid (Figure 11.56).

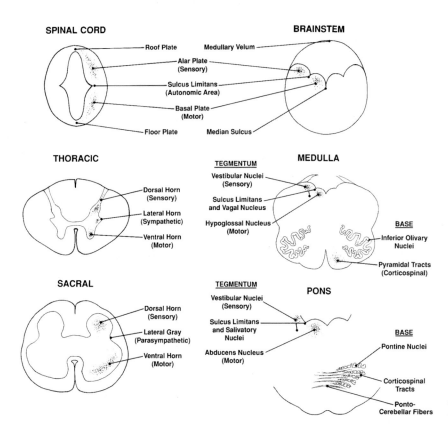

Figure 11.1 Structural organization of the spinal cord and brainstem. (See text for discussion.)

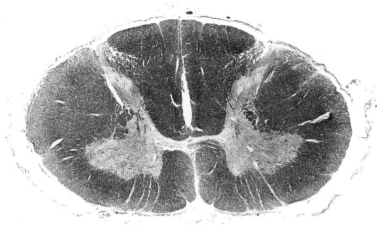

A

Figure 11.2 Spinal cord: regional variation of spinal cord structure is illustrated in these cross sections taken from the cervical enlargement (**A**), midthoracic cord (**B**), and lumbosacral enlargement (**C**). The cervical enlargement (A) is typified by an oval shape with large white matter funiculi and prominent, broad anterior gray horns that contain the motor neurons that innervate the upper extremities. In contrast, sections from thoracic cord (B) have a more rounded profile and exhibit small, slender, peglike anterior gray horns. In addition, lateral horns, which house the intermediolateral cell column neurons of the sympathetic nervous system, are unique to thoracic segments (see Figure 11.1). The lumbosacral cord (C) has very large anterior gray horns (motor supply to the lower extremities) like those of the cervical enlargement but only a very small surrounding mantle of white matter (see Figure 11.1).

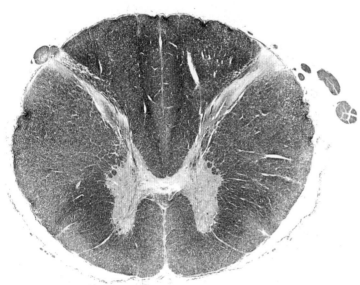

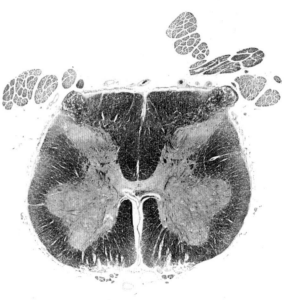

B   **C**

Brainstem

The brainstem is innately more complex than the spinal cord, but its basic organization is readily understood when viewed as a slightly modified version of the basic plan. Thus, the stem is also a neural tube but one that has been stretched dorsally and splayed out laterally so that the ventrally located embryonic motor plate is now medial and the dorsal sensory plate is lateral (Figure 11.1). Therefore, within the brainstem, the cranial nerve motor nuclei are located medially, the sensory nuclei laterally, and the autonomic nuclei are intermediate in position.

The brainstem can be further subcategorized in cross section into tectum, tegmentum, and base. The tectum is the roof of the ventricular system, as exemplified by the superior and inferior colliculi (corpora quadrigemina) of the midbrain and the superior medullary vela of the pons and medulla. The tegmentum forms the floor of the cerebral aqueduct and fourth ventricle and is divisible into the medial motor and lateral sensory areas discussed previously

(Figure 11.1). The "base" is located subjacent to the tegmentum and is the most ventral portion of the stem. It is composed principally of the so-called long tracts—that is, the descending motor pathways and ascending sensory pathways that link the spinal cord with higher neural centers. The combination of long tract signs with dysfunction of specific cranial nerves allows the precise anatomic localization of brainstem lesions by clinical examination.

Cerebellum

Embryologically, the cerebellum arises as a dorsal outgrowth of the fetal brainstem and remains connected to it in the adult by the three pairs of cerebellar peduncles: the superior (brachium conjunctivum), middle (brachium pontis), and inferior (restiform body). They join with the midbrain, pons, and medulla, respectively. The cerebellum is composed of three structural and functional compartments: cortex, medulla, and deep nuclei. The cortex

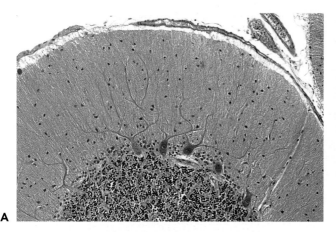

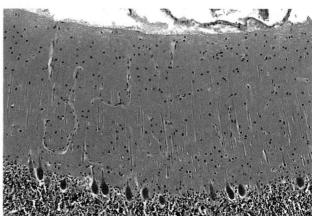

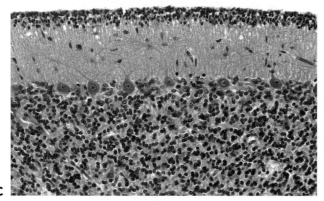

Figure 11.3 Cerebellar cortex. The adult cerebellar cortex is composed of three layers: an outer hypocellular molecular layer, middle Purkinje cell layer, and inner densely populated granular cell layer. Whereas the Purkinje cells are prototypically neuronal in appearance, the small cells of the granular layer are hardly recognizable as neurons by traditional histologic criteria (see Figure 11.7). **A.** A cross section of a cerebellar folium shows the typical broadly branching Purkinje cell dendritic arbor. **B.** However, sections taken parallel to the folia reveal the streamlined "on edge" appearance of the arbor, which should not be interpreted as pathological pruning. **C.** The fetal cerebellum has an additional cortical lamina, the external granular layer, applied to the surface of the cortex. This pool of cells populates the internal granular cell layer during development and is, thereby, depleted by the end of the first year of postnatal life.

plays three distinct laminae: an outer hypocellular molecular layer, an intermediate single-cell thick Purkinje cell layer (described below), and a deep hypercellular granular cell layer (Figure 11.3). Before one year of age, the cerebellar cortex is conspicuous for remnants of a fourth layer of small neurons, the fetal external granular cell layer, which is located immediately subjacent to pia (Figure 11.3C). The external granular cells are gradually depleted during the first year of life as they descend the processes of Bergmann glia to reach their final position in the internal granular cell layer. Embedded within the white matter of the cerebellar medulla are four pairs of nuclei, from medial to lateral: fastigial, globosus, emboliform, and dentate. The dentate is by far the largest and is usually the only deep nucleus seen on routine sections. Its serpiginous profile is strikingly similar to that of the inferior olivary nucleus of the medulla oblongata (illustrated in Figure 11.1) which is a major source of afferent fibers to the cerebellum.

The Purkinje cell dendritic arbor extends into the molecular layer like a hand with outstretched fingers. Its broad, flat palm and radiating fingers are oriented perpendicular to the long axis of the cerebellar convolutions (folia). Thus, routine folia cross sections show the typical, elaborate dendritic branching pattern, whereas longitudinal sections present a dramatically different "on edge" view of the arbor (Figure 11.3). This should not be mistaken for pathologic dendritic tree "pruning" seen in some disease states.

Diencephalon

The diencephalon is interposed between the brainstem (midbrain, pons, and medulla) and the cerebrum. Four major divisions are recognized: epithalamus (pineal gland and habenula), thalamus, subthalamus, and hypothalamus. The medial and lateral geniculate nuclei of the thalamus are sometimes considered together as the metathalamus.

The strategic location of the thalamus is related to its major role in processing and relaying information passing between the cerebral cortex and brainstem and spinal cord. All sensory data (with the exception of olfaction) are processed by specific thalamic nuclei before distribution to the primary sensory cortices.

Of clinical significance to the pathologist, certain portions of the diencephalon immediately subjacent to the third ventricle (in particular, the large dorsomedial nuclei of the thalamus and the mammillary bodies of the hypothalamus) are often prominently involved in Wernicke's encephalopathy. The lesions at these sites are postulated to account for the memory disturbance that accompanies this disorder.

Cerebrum

Supratentorially, the CNS becomes so much more complicated that it is difficult to describe in terms of any general pattern of orientation. It remains a hollow structure, but one that is no longer easy to consider as a tube with fold-ings and regional overgrowths. In light of this complexity, it is appropriate to review only those areas that are of par-ticular diagnostic relevance.

Basal Ganglia

The term *basal ganglia* refers to the deep gray matter masses of the telencephalon and encompasses the caudate nucleus, putamen, globus pallidus, and amygdala (Figure 11.4). The term *ganglion* was formerly used interchangeably with *nucleus,* and *ganglion cell* was synonymous with *neuron* to earlier neuroanatomists. With the exception of the basal ganglia, the current definition of a ganglion is now gener-ally restricted to mean a collection of neuronal cell bodies

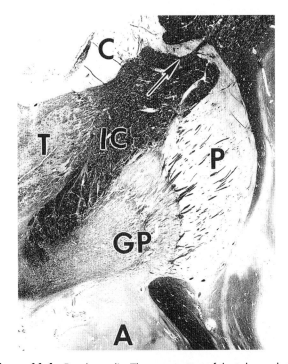

Figure 11.4 Basal ganglia. The gray matter of the telencephalon is broadly divisible into two components—the superficial cortical gray matter mantle and the deep gray nuclei. The latter are known as the basal ganglia and consist of the caudate nucleus (*C*), puta-men (*P*), globus pallidus (*GP*), and amygdala (*A*). The lenticular nu-cleus is composed of the medially situated, diffusely myelinated globus pallidus and the laterally placed putamen, whose myeli-nated fibers are grouped into slender fascicles known as the pencil bundles of Wilson. The internal capsule (*IC*) separates the lenticular nucleus from the caudate and the thalamus (*T*). Gray matter bridges (*arrow*) occasionally span the capsule to connect the cau-date and putamen, a reflection of the close functional relationship between these two nuclei. The lenticular nucleus receives its blood supply from several lenticulostriate arteries, which are direct branches of the middle cerebral artery, and is the most common site of intracerebral hypertensive hemorrhage and lacunar infarc-tion. The large lenticulostriate artery coursing through the lateral putamen was known in former times as Charcot's artery, or, more colorfully, as the artery of internal hemorrhage. The lenticulostriate vessels are often surrounded by dilated perivascular spaces that should not be mistaken for lacunar infarcts.

located outside the CNS, namely, the sensory and auto-nomic ganglia of the peripheral nervous system. Reference to CNS neurons as *ganglion cells* is still occasionally en-countered, and this historical sense of the term is reflected in the names of such neoplastic entities as *ganglioglioma,* *ganglioneuroma,* and *ganglion cell tumor.*

The amygdala (archistriatum) is located in the mesial temporal lobe immediately rostral to the hippocampus and is functionally related to the limbic system. The re-maining nuclei of the basal ganglia play an integral role in the modulation of motor function and probably partici-pate in other higher neural systems as well. The caudate nucleus, as the name implies, has a long tapering tail that intimately follows the curvature of the lateral ventricle. The caudate is morphologically and functionally closely related to the putamen. These two nuclei are appropriately referred to collectively as the neostriatum, or simply the striatum. For descriptive purposes, the putamen and the medially situated globus pallidus (paleostriatum, or pallidum) are collectively referred to as the lenticular (lentiform) nucleus. The putamen and globus pallidus are separated from one another by the external medullary lamina of the globus pallidus, whereas the globus pallidus is itself divided into medial and lateral segments by the internal medullary lamina. The globus pallidus (pale globe) is so named because of its pallor in the fresh state compared to the putamen. This contrast is attributable histologically to the dense meshwork of myelinated fibers in the globus pallidus. In contrast, myelinated axons in the putamen are grouped into slender fascicles (pencil bundles of Wilson) that project medially to the globus pallidus and to the substantia nigra. The histologic ap-pearance of the lentiform nucleus is distinctive and per-mits unambiguous identification of even very limited amounts of tissue from this site.

The basal ganglia are prominently involved in a vari-ety of pathological processes, including kernicterus (lit-erally, nuclear jaundice) in the neonate and lacunar infarction in adults. Carbon monoxide poisoning classi-cally produces selective necrosis of the inner segment of the globus pallidus. A frequent incidental finding of no diagnostic significance on routine sections of the lentiform nucleus is micronodular mineralization of small blood vessels, which is typically most prominent in the globus pallidus. Histologically, similar micronodular mineralization is also commonly seen in the hippocam-pus (Figure 11.5C).

Hippocampal Formation

The hippocampal formation comprises the subiculum, Ammon's horn (hippocampus proper), and dentate gyrus (Figure 11.5). In coronal sections of the medial tem-poral lobe, the subiculum forms the inferior base of the hippocampal formation, joining the parahippocampal

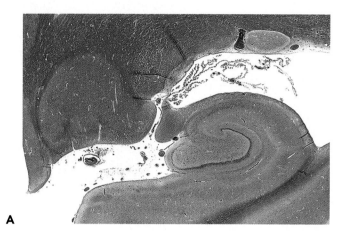

A

Figure 11.5 Hippocampal formation. The hippocampal formation is composed of the subiculum, Ammon's horn (cornu Ammonis, abbreviated CA; divided into regions CA1–CA4), and the dentate gyrus (**A, B**). CA1 is equivalent to Sommer's sector and is the region of the hippocampus that is most sensitive to a variety of insults. In contrast, the adjacent CA2 region is known as the dorsal resistant zone. Two common incidental findings are also illustrated—micronodular mineralization (**B, C**), which is also seen in the globus pallidus, and a residual hippocampal fissure (**B, D**), which should not be misinterpreted as a healed infarct. [*CN,* tail of the caudate nucleus; *HF,* residual hippocampal fissure; *LGN,* lateral geniculate nucleus (note the "Napoleon's hat" profile and distinctive lamination); *MM,* micronodular mineralization.]

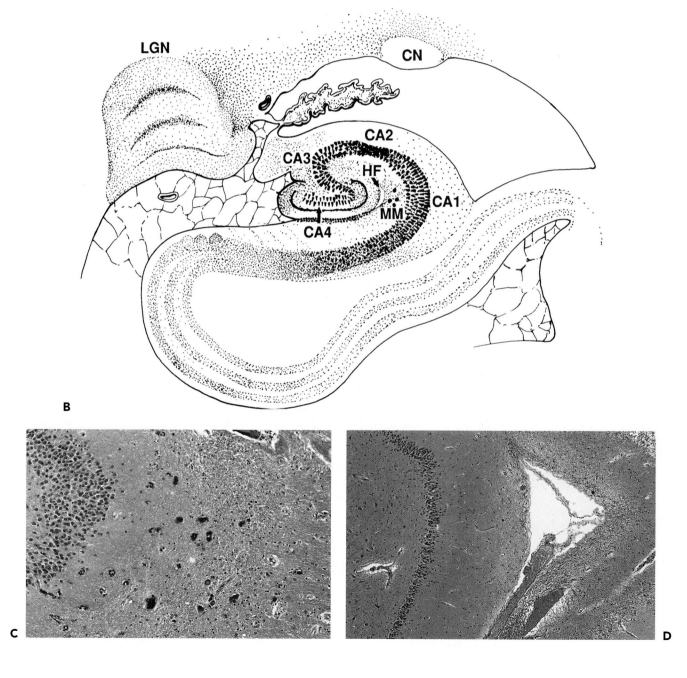

B

C

D

gyrus with Ammon's horn. Ammon's horn, routinely abbreviated CA (for cornu Ammonis), is divided into four regions, CA1 through 4, based on cytological architecture and synaptic connectivity. (This nomenclature was introduced by Lorente de No in 1934.) The superiorly arching CA1 is joined by CA2 to form the medial floor of the temporal horn of the lateral ventricle. The dorsally situated CA2 is usually recognizable by the greater compactness of the pyramidal cell layer, as compared to CA1, and CA3 forms a descending medial arch that terminates in the hilus of the dentate gyrus. The final segment of Ammon's horn, CA4, lies within the hilus of the dentate gyrus and is often referred to as the end-plate. Essentially equivalent to Sommer's sector, CA1 is the zone that is most sensitive to various insults, including seizures, ischemia, and Alzheimer's disease changes. In contrast, the adjacent CA2 segment is known as the dorsal resistant zone, in recognition of its relative sparing compared to the other three sectors. The exquisite sensitivity of CA1 to injury, with sparing of the adjacent CA2, is routinely observed as mesial sclerosis of the hippocampus, which is seen in many temporal lobes resected for intractable epilepsy. The classic histologic description of the pattern of neuronal loss in Ammon's horn was based on observations made on the brains of such epileptic patients by Wilhelm Sommer in 1880; E. Brotz coined the term *Sommer's sector* in 1920.

There are several notable features that are frequently encountered incidentally in the examination of routine hippocampal sections and can be mistakenly interpreted as evidence of disease. One is an asymptomatic micronodular mineralization comparable to that seen in the globus pallidus. In the hippocampal formation, it is most commonly seen just outside the apex of the dentate gyrus (Figure 11.5B, C). A second common finding is a residual hippocampal fissure, which produces a rarefied lamina or cystic cleft that can be mistaken for a healed infarct (Figure 11.5B, D). In addition, pyramidal neurons of the CA are often dark and shrunken in autopsy material, and care must be taken not to overinterpret such changes as evidence of ischemia (Figures 11.16, 11.17).

Cerebral Cortex

From antiquity, neuroscientists have sought to divide the cortical mantle into discrete, functionally significant units. Early efforts yielded fanciful maps akin to those of phrenology and physiognomy. More recently, the application of light microscopy and special staining techniques for cell bodies (Nissl stains), dendritic arbors and unmyelinated axons (Golgi's stains), and the myelin sheaths of myelinated axons (myelin stains such as the Weil's, Weigert's, and Luxol fast blue methods) have permitted a more scientific approach, although the details are beyond the scope of this chapter. In brief, the parcellation of the cortex is based on regional variation in the relative number, composition, and distribution of cortical neurons and their processes (cytoarchitectonics and myeloarchitechtonics). Various neuroanatomists have divided the cortex into a number of regions, varying from 20 to more than 200 and depending on the particular morphologic criteria and degree of subtlety employed. Currently, the most popular cortical map is that devised by Korbinian Brodmann in 1909. Brodmann's map and the classical nomenclature for the gross anatomy of the cerebral sulci and gyri are the two systems most commonly used at present for reference purposes in the neuroanatomic and clinical literature.

Within the context of even the simplest cortical map, it is generally not possible to assign a given histologic section of cortex to a precise anatomic locus without prior knowledge of the section's provenance. However, two cortical areas do exhibit distinctive features: primary motor cortex and primary visual cortex. The motor cortex, located on the precentral gyrus of the frontal lobe, is distinguished by the presence of the giant pyramidal cells of Betz. Pyramidal cells generally range from 10 to 50 mm in soma height from base to origin of the apical dendrite. By comparison, Betz cells may exceed 100 mm in soma height. The primary visual cortex, located on the banks of the calcarine fissure of the medial occipital lobe, is remarkable for the presence of a prominent external band of Baillarger, termed the line (or stria) of Gennari. This myelinated stratum located in lamina IV is usually visible to the naked eye and permits exact delineation of the primary visual cortex (Brodmann area 17) from the adjacent visual association cortex (Brodmann area 18).

CELLULAR CONSTITUENTS OF THE CENTRAL NERVOUS SYSTEM

Gray Matter and White Matter

By volume, most of the central nervous system is composed of gray matter and white matter. Specialized types of CNS tissues include the choroid plexus, pineal gland, circumventricular organs, and the infundibulum and neurohypophysis (discussed later). The hallmark of gray matter (Figure 11.6A) is the presence of neuronal cell bodies embedded within a finely textured eosinophilic background termed neuropil (Figure 11.6B, C). Neuropil (literally, nerve felt) is an interwoven meshwork of neuronal and glial cell processes. The individual neurites that compose the neuropil are not generally distinguishable in routine hematoxylin-eosin (H&E)–stained sections (Figure 11.6B) but are resolvable at the ultrastructural level (Figure 11.6C). White matter, in contrast, is composed primarily of myelinated axons and the supporting cells, oligodendroglia, that produce and maintain the myelin sheaths (Figure 11.6D).

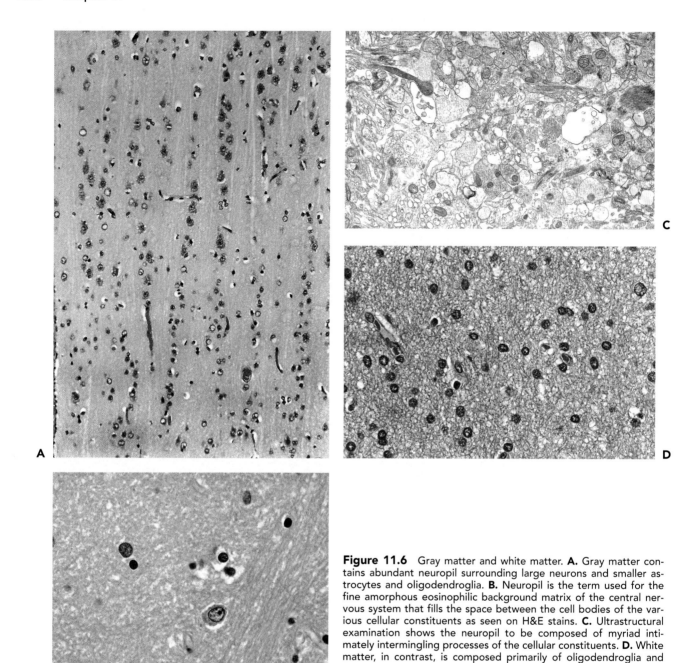

Figure 11.6 Gray matter and white matter. **A.** Gray matter contains abundant neuropil surrounding large neurons and smaller astrocytes and oligodendroglia. **B.** Neuropil is the term used for the fine amorphous eosinophilic background matrix of the central nervous system that fills the space between the cell bodies of the various cellular constituents as seen on H&E stains. **C.** Ultrastructural examination shows the neuropil to be composed of myriad intimately intermingling processes of the cellular constituents. **D.** White matter, in contrast, is composed primarily of oligodendroglia and the axons that they myelinate, and it displays a much more uniform appearance.

Neurons

Normal Microscopic Anatomy

The prototypical neuron is exemplified by the large multipolar Betz cells of the motor cortex, the α motor neurons of the ventral horn of the spinal cord, and the Purkinje cells of the cerebellum. These neurons are characterized by large perikarya (cell bodies or somas) with abundant Nissl substance (rough endoplasmic reticulum), robust dendritic arborizations, and large nuclei with prominent single nucleoli (Figure 11.7A). Such large multipolar forms, however, represent only one type of neuron; the diapason of neuronal morphologies is remarkable. This is readily apparent by comparison of a motor neurons with granular cell neurons (Figure 11.7A, D). These two neuronal populations typify the classical dichotomous subdivision of CNS neurons into large extroverted projection neurons with long axons (Golgi type I neurons) and small introverts that function regionally with restricted connections (Golgi type II

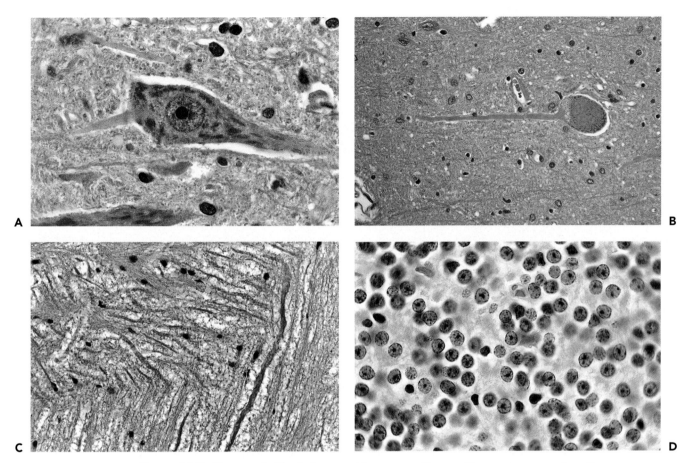

Figure 11.7 Neurons. **A.** Classical neuronal features, as illustrated by a motor neuron from the ventral horn of the spinal cord, include a large cell body (soma, perikaryon) with abundant cytoplasmic Nissl substance (rough endoplasmic reticulum, the "tigroid substance" of early microscopists), cytoplasmic processes, and a large nucleus with a single prominent nucleolus. The large process extending to the right is clearly recognizable as a dendrite by its content of Nissl substance, whereas, in this fortuitous section, the smaller process extending to the left is identified as the neuron's axon by its lack of Nissl substance. **B.** Axons are further distinguished from dendrites by their nontapering profile. **C.** The nontapering profile of axons is easily recognized in white matter. The extremes of neuron size and shape are readily apparent from a comparison of a large motor neuron (A) with the small granular cell neurons of the cerebellar cortex (**D**) that are approximately the same size as a motor neuron's nucleolus!

neurons). Between these two poles is a full spectrum of neuronal sizes and shapes, with an equally impressive variety of dendritic arbor configurations. The details of the latter are generally appreciable only with special stains for neuronal processes. The cell processes of neurons are separated into two categories: axons (Figure 11.7A–C), of which each neuron only has one, and dendrites (Figure 11.7A), which are often multiple.

With respect to morphologic variants, one unique population of CNS neurons merits brief mention. The mesencephalic nucleus of the trigeminal nerve, which is concerned chiefly with the mediation of jaw proprioception, is composed of true primary (first order) sensory neurons that possess only a single process emanating from the cell body (Figure 11.8A). This nucleus constitutes the only intraparenchymal example of this class of neurons; all other primary sensory neuronal perikarya are gathered outside the CNS in the spinal and cranial nerve ganglia (Figure 11.8B–D).

Immunohistochemistry

Antibodies have been raised against a wide variety of the many unique neuronal proteins that are being isolated and characterized at an ever-increasing rate. A majority of these markers are confined to use for research purposes but several have found utility in the diagnostic laboratory. One of the earliest such markers, neuron specific enolase (NSE), has proven notoriously unreliable as a marker of neuronal differentiation. Its use for this purpose in evaluating neoplasms of the central nervous system is not recommended.

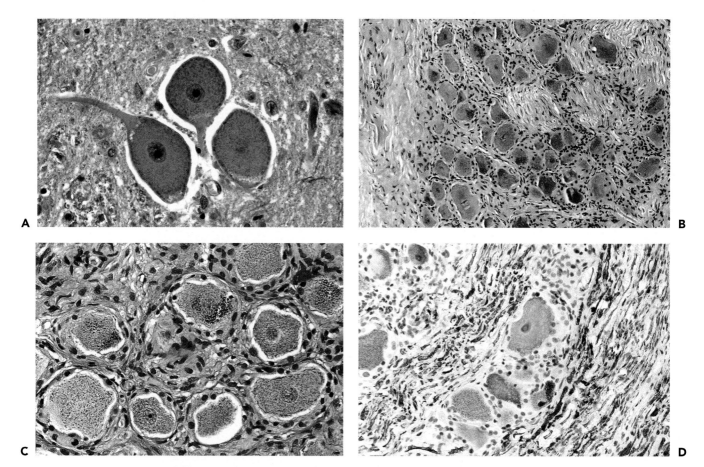

Figure 11.8 Unipolar neurons. Another neuronal morphologic variant is the unipolar (pseudounipolar) neuron. These large neurons possess only a single cell process, an axon, but no dendrites. **A.** Unipolar neurons are primary sensory neurons, and the only example of this class of neuron within the central nervous system is the mesencephalic nucleus of the trigeminal nerve in the upper pons and midbrain lateral to the periaqueductal gray matter. **B.** All other unipolar neurons are located in the peripheral nervous system ganglia. The dorsal root ganglia of the spinal cord provide a good example, with large unipolar neurons surrounded by satellite cells (B). **C.** Ganglionic neurons typically display cytoplasmic pigment. **D.** Their cell bodies and axons are strongly positive for phosphorylated neurofilament proteins.

Antibodies directed against epitopes on the constituent proteins of neurofilaments, which are major cytoskeletal elements of the neuronal perikaryon and cytoplasmic processes, have been used extensively in both experimental and clinical studies (Figure 11.9).

One of the most useful and widely employed neuronal markers is synaptophysin. Synaptophysin is an integral membrane protein of synaptic vesicles. In the normal nervous system, antisynaptophysin antibodies yield a diffuse, finely granular pattern throughout the gray matter neuropil (Figure 11.10A). In addition, punctate granular decoration is seen along the cell bodies and proximal dendrites of several types of large, projection class neurons, including the Purkinje cells of the cerebellum, α motor neurons of the spinal cord, extraocular motor neurons of the brainstem, and Betz cells of the precentral gyrus (Figure 11.10B).

Age-Related Neuronal Inclusions

A variety of inclusions, largely intracytoplasmic, appear with increasing frequency as we age. By far, the most common is lipofuscin (lipochrome, or aging pigment), whose yellow-to-pale-brown color is unaltered by most histologic procedures, including the H&E method (Figure 11.11). Its autofluorescence and partial avidity for the acid-fast stain can be used to visualize differentially this "wear-and-tear" pigment, although little functional significance is generally assigned to lipochrome accumulation in normal aging. In larger neurons, lipofuscin may accumulate to such an extent that it displaces organelles and creates an appearance similar to the cell swelling of central chromatolysis, described below (Figure 11.18). The lateral geniculate body provides an example of a densely populated nucleus whose constituent neuron's prominent accumulation of lipofus-

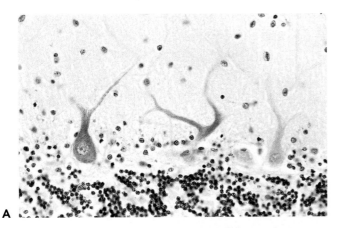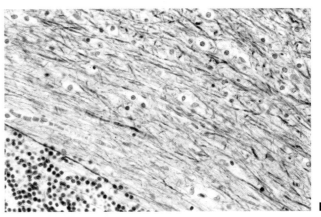

Figure 11.9 Neurofilament proteins (NFPs). Antibodies directed against neurofilament protein epitopes illuminate the cytoskeleton of neurons and their processes. As illustrated in the cerebellar cortex, specific antibodies directed against either nonphosphorylated (**A**) or phosphorylated (**B**) NFPs differentially identify cell bodies and dendrites or axons, respectively.

cin is often discernible macroscopically as a distinctly mahogany hue compared to adjacent cortex. Interestingly, lipofuscin accumulation is not simply a function of cell size because some classes of large neurons appear comparatively immune to significant accrual (e.g., the cerebellar Purkinje cells).

Functionally more significant neuronal inclusions that may be seen in asymptomatic individuals are those associated with Alzheimer's disease. They are neurofibrillary tangles, neuritic plaques, granulovacuolar degeneration, and Hirano bodies. These illustrate the often ill-defined distinction between health and disease, because these changes can be seen in the elderly, albeit in limited numbers, in the absence of antemortem disturbances of mentation.

In some cases, neurofibrillary tangles may be found in asymptomatic individuals in occasional neurons of the subiculum or CA. Although silver stains greatly aid visualization and quantitation, these structures may be identified on routinely stained H&E sections if the observer is familiar with their appearance. In pyramidal cells, they appear as a slightly basophilic wisp of faintly fibrillar material that extends out into cell processes, most notably the apical dendrite, and they are often more prominent on one side of the nucleus (flame-shaped tangle; Figure 11.12A). This morphology reflects the fact that tangles generally conform to the shape of the cell body. For example, in the pigmented neurons of the locus ceruleus, which are multipolar and lack the dominant apical dendrite of pyramidal neurons,

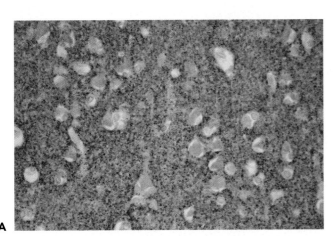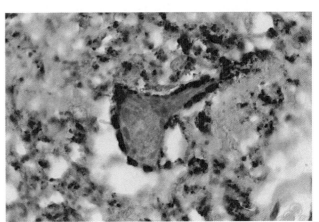

Figure 11.10 Synaptophysin is one of the most useful and widely employed markers of neuronal differentiation. **A.** The neuropil of gray matter, which is rich in synaptic contacts, shows a diffuse, finely granular pattern. **B.** Several specific types of large projection class neurons show prominent punctate decoration of the cell body and proximal dendrites, as illustrated here by a motor neuron in the hypoglossal nucleus of the medulla. Other groups of large neurons exhibiting this pattern of synaptophysin immunopositivity include Purkinje cells of the cerebellum, motor neurons of the ventral horn of the spinal cord, and Betz cells of the precentral gyrus in the cerebral cortex.

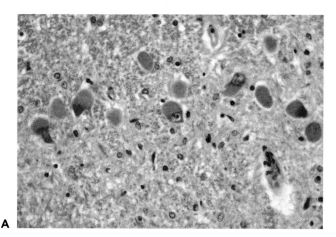
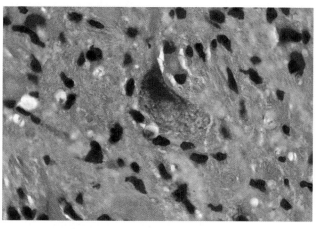

Figure 11.11 Lipofuscin. **A.** Prominent accumulation of lipofuscin pigment in large neurons with increasing age, as seen for example in the lateral geniculate nucleus, can result in peripheral displacement of the nucleus and Nissl substance, mimicking central chromatolysis. **B.** As a practical application of normal neurohistology, the presence of lipofuscin can sometimes aid in the identification of neurons in intraoperative frozen sections. As illustrated here, a neuron, identified by its lipofuscin content, is surrounded by tumor cells, thereby supporting a diagnosis of infiltrating glioma.

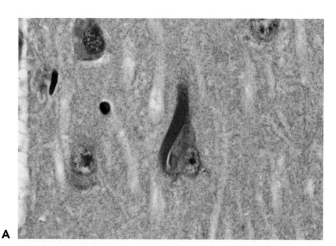
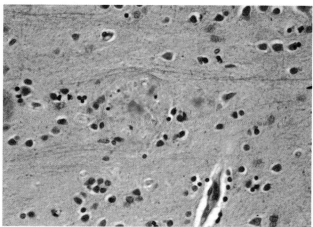
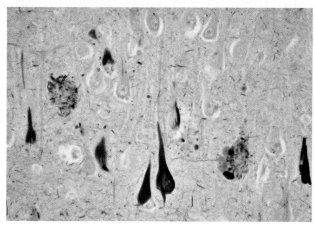

Figure 11.12 Neurofibrillary tangles and neuritic plaques. Neurofibrillary tangles (**A**) may be seen sporadically in the hippocampal formation of aging brains and have a fibrillary texture in H&E-stained sections. Mature senile (neuritic) plaques (**B**) deform the smooth texture of the neuropil and appear in H&E-stained sections as spherical, somewhat granular foci with a central eosinophilic core that is composed of amyloid. Note that adjacent myelinated axons are focally displaced as they pass by the plaque. In earlier stages, the plaques are less well defined and are not identifiable in H&E-stained sections. Although both neurofibrillary tangles and large mature neuritic plaques can be seen in H&E-stained sections, use of special techniques, such as silver stains (**C**), greatly facilitates visualization and quantitation.

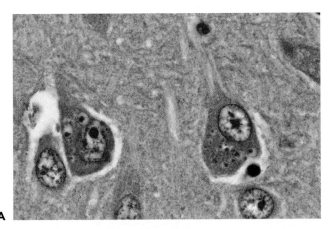

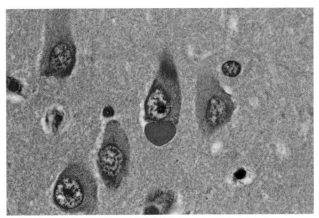

A   B

Figure 11.13 Granulovacuolar degeneration (of Simchowitz) (**A**) and Hirano bodies (**B**). Like neurofibrillary tangles, both of these intracytoplasmic inclusions can occasionally be seen in the hippocampal formation of normal older individuals. However, although these alterations are not pathognomonic for dementing illness, an appreciable number of affected cells should prompt a search for evidence of Alzheimer's disease in the form of a thorough examination for senile (neuritic) plaques and neurofibrillary tangles.

tangles that are globular in shape are occasionally encountered as an incidental finding.

The senile plaque is also a manifestation of cell injury, but one that, like slight atherosclerosis, is not an unexpected finding in the brains of asymptomatic adults. In such individuals, the plaque is usually seen in its primitive form as a somewhat ill-defined, roughly circular region of abnormal argyrophilic neurites that is not visualized in the H&E-stained section. As the plaques mature they become visible in the latter preparation, particularly when a central core of eosinophilic amyloid appears (Figure 11.12B). The latter can be more readily seen by Congo red or periodic acid-Schiff (PAS) staining. As noted earlier, both neurofibrillary tangles and neuritic plaques are more easily identified and quantitated with special techniques such as immunofluorescence or silver stains (Figure 11.12C).

Two additional intraneuronal inclusions that are seen in Alzheimer's disease, but only rarely in nondemented individuals, are granulovacuolar degeneration (GVD) and Hirano bodies (Figure 11.13). As the name implies, the inclusion of GVD consists of a dark, basophilic granule inside a small, clear vacuole. Clusters of these cytoplasmic inclusions may be present within a single neuron (Figure 11.13A). Depending on the plane of section, Hirano bodies appear in H&E-stained sections as brightly eosinophilic oval, elliptical, or elongated rodlike refractile inclusions that are located either in very close apposition to a neuronal perikaryon (Figure 11.13B) or within the neuropil. Ultrastructural examination supports a localization in neuronal cell bodies and processes, and immunohistochemical studies reveal the presence of actin and actin-associated proteins. Unlike neurofibrillary tangles and neuritic plaques, both GVD and Hirano bodies exhibit a very limited neuroanatomic distribution and are, in fact, virtually

confined to the hippocampal formation. Encountering more than one or two cells with these alterations should raise the issue of Alzheimer's disease and prompt a search for other attendant histologic features.

A particularly striking cytoplasmic inclusion occasionally encountered in routine sections of the hypoglossal nuclei of the medulla (less often in the ventral horn motor nuclei of the spinal cord) is the hyalin (colloid) inclusion (Figure 11.14). These inclusions, which consist of ectatic cisternae of endoplasmic reticulum, are rarely seen in the first few decades of life but appear with increasing

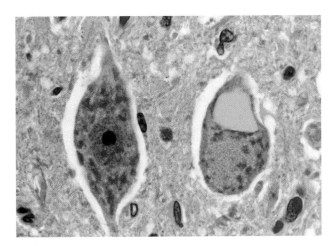

Figure 11.14 Hyalin (colloid) inclusion: these eye-catching inclusions, as seen in the neuron on the right, may be observed sporadically throughout the neuraxis but are most commonly encountered in the large motor neurons of the hypoglossal nuclei in the medulla (as in this micrograph). Less frequently, they may be seen in the motor neurons of the ventral horn of the spinal cord. Electron microscopic examination reveals ectatic cisternae of endoplasmic reticulum.

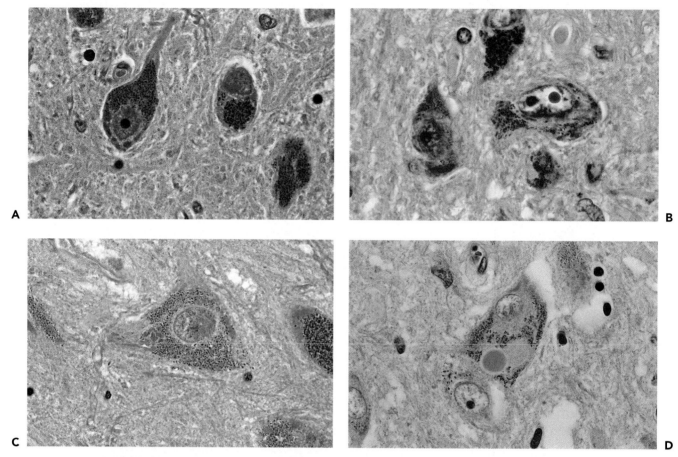

Figure 11.15 Pigmented neurons of the brainstem. **A.** Neuromelanin is a coarse, dark brown cytoplasmic pigment that is formed as a byproduct of catecholamine synthesis and is frequently encountered microscopically in scattered catecholaminergic neurons distributed widely throughout the brainstem. Two large populations are visible grossly: the substantia nigra (black substance) of the midbrain and the locus ceruleus (blue spot) of the pons. **B.** Marinesco bodies are eosinophilic, spheroidal, paranucleolar bodies that are often observed in the nuclei of pigmented neurons, especially those of the substantia nigra. The number of Marinesco bodies increases with advancing age and can be quite striking in some individuals. They should not be mistaken for intranuclear viral inclusions. **C.** Clusters of minute intracytoplasmic eosinophilic granules, seen in this micrograph to the left of the nucleus, may occasionally catch the eye of an obsessive observer. They have no known pathologic significance and are much smaller than Lewy bodies (**D**), which are the characteristic intracytoplasmic inclusions of Parkinson's disease.

frequency thereafter. They are occasionally mistaken by the uninformed for viral inclusions.

Catecholaminergic neurons throughout the brainstem gradually accumulate neuromelanin as a byproduct of neurotransmitter synthesis. The largest and most densely populated of these nuclei is the substantia nigra (black substance), which contains dopaminergic neurons. The locus ceruleus (blue spot), which is also seen by the unaided eye, is a collection of noradrenergic neurons in the rostral pontine tegmentum. It is of practical importance that the Lewy bodies of Parkinson's disease can be found in both of these neuroanatomic locales. Of the smaller and more diffusely distributed pigmented neurons, those in the vicinity of the dorsal motor nucleus of the vagus nerve in the medulla oblongata are most commonly encountered during routine histologic examination. Microscopically, neuromelanin

appears as coarse, dark brown granules (Figure 11.15A) and should not be confused with melanocytic melanin. The latter is also present in the central nervous system but is confined to leptomeningeal melanocytes as discussed below (see Figure 11.57).

Several eosinophilic inclusions may be seen in pigmented brainstem neurons. The most striking of these are the commonly encountered Marinesco bodies (Figure 11.15B). These bright red, hyalin-appearing structures are located within the nucleus, often adjacent to and about the same size as a nucleolus (an alternative designation is paranucleolar body). Multiple Marinesco bodies may occur within a single nucleus, and, in some cases, a large percentage of pigmented neurons exhibit these eye-catching inclusions. In such cases, they may raise concern about a viral infection to the unaccustomed observer but are not

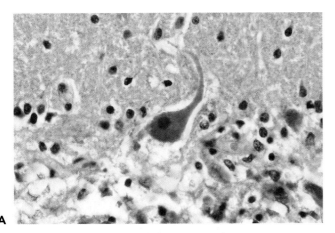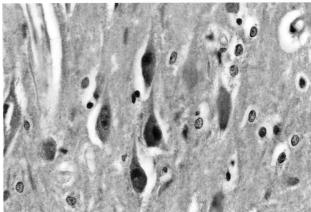

A   B

Figure 11.16 Ischemic injury: the sine qua non of ischemic damage to the nervous system is the so-called red neuron. As illustrated here by a Purkinje cell of the cerebellum (**A**) and pyramidal neurons of the hippocampal CA1 region (**B**), the soma (cell body) is shrunken, the cytoplasm is intensely eosinophilic, and the nucleus is pyknotic with no discernible nucleolus. It is largely the pronounced eosinophilia that distinguishes this cellular alteration from autolytic neuronal condensation, in which the cytoplasm is dark and basophilic (Figure 11.17).

pathologic and have yet to be correlated with any significant process except advancing age. Two types of eosinophilic inclusions may be encountered in the cytoplasm of pigmented neurons. Clusters of diminutive acidophilic granules are occasionally noted (Figure 11.15C) but have no pathologic significance. Lewy bodies, in contrast, are much larger, notably displace the cytoplasmic neuromelanin from which they are separated by a small clear halo, and are associated with Parkinson's disease (Figure 11.15D).

Autolysis and Basic Neuronal Reactions to Injury

As captured in their normal state by perfusion fixation or rapid immersion fixation, neurons are generally rotund with lightly eosinophilic cytoplasm that is stippled with basophilic Nissl substance in the case of the larger neurons. The surrounding glia are inconspicuous, and few clear vacuoles are seen. This perfection in fixation is rarely achieved in human material, however; and, in virtually all autopsy and surgical specimens, autolysis alters this ideal appearance to a greater or lesser extent. Neurons are, thereby, rendered somewhat contracted and basophilic. Nuclei are also somewhat condensed. Simultaneously, the processes of glia that surround neurons and blood vessels imbibe water to produce clear vacuoles (Figure 11.29). The neuronal response to injury overlaps in some cases with these autolytic changes, and it may not be possible to distinguish agonal hypotensive injury from autolysis in autopsy specimens. In the former setting, the neuronal contraction is pronounced, and the perineuronal and perivascular spaces are exceptionally prominent.

There are, however, three neuronal changes that provide unequivocal evidence of antemortem injury. One is the

"red" neuron, which is the sine qua non of ischemic damage. The second is central chromatolysis, and the third is ferruginization. The red neuron is characterized by a shrunken cell body and intense cytoplasmic eosinophilia with complete loss of Nissl basophilia (Figure 11.16). The nucleus is dark and usually lacks a distinguishable nucleolus but may be pale and demonstrate early karyolysis. At times, it has a somewhat fragmented look suggesting karyorrhexis, although clearly defined karyorrhexis is rare. In surgical specimens, tissue-handling artifact ("crush" artifact) also results in dark, shrunken neuronal perikarya; however, as with autolytic autopsy specimens, these cells lack the distinctive cytoplasmic eosinophilia of ischemia (Figure 11.17).

Central chromatolysis, the second unequivocally abnormal finding, consists of a loss of central basophilic staining of the cell body with peripheral margination of the Nissl substance (Figure 11.18). It is seen in a number of pathologic

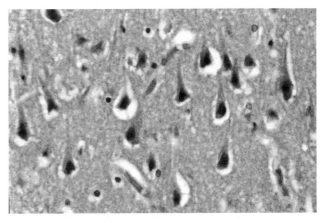

Figure 11.17 Neuronal contraction as a tissue-handling artifact. In contrast to ischemic insult (Figure 11.16), in "crush" artifacts the cytoplasm is dark and basophilic rather than brightly eosinophilic.

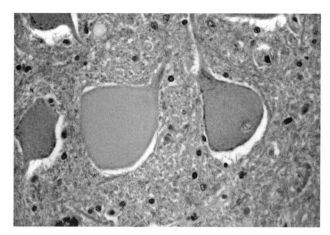

Figure 11.18 Central chromatolysis. Cytoplasmic hyalinization and swelling with peripheral displacement of the nucleus and lipofuscin can be a response to either intrinsic neuronal disease (such as in poliomyelitis or other viral infections) or to interruption of the axon in close proximity to the cell body. In the latter setting, the term *axonal reaction* is applied.

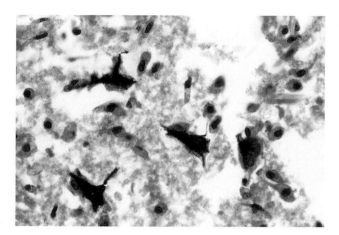

Figure 11.19 Mineralized (ferruginized) neurons. These encrusted relics resembling petrified tree trunks are most commonly encountered around the margins of old infarcts.

states (the ballooned anterior horn cells of poliomyelitis being the classical example). There are numerous mimickers that lie in wait for the unwary. For example, some normal neuronal populations, such as the supraoptic and paraventricular nuclei of the hypothalamus and the dorsal nucleus of Clarke of the thoracic spinal cord, display Nissl substance that is preferentially distributed peripherally in the soma. Other neurons, such as those of the mesencephalic nucleus of the trigeminal nerve discussed previously (Figure 11.8), have large, exquisitely rounded somas and, hence, mimic that aspect of chromatolysis. The giant pyramidal cells of Betz in the motor cortex are so large in comparison to surrounding neurons, that at low magnification they may give an initial impression of chromatolytic swelling. Finally, as discussed earlier, one must be careful not to mistake the accumulation of various substances that displace the Nissl substance peripherally, such as lipofuscin, for central chromatolysis (Figure 11.11).

A striking finding sometimes encountered near old infarcts is the presence of ferruginized or fossilized neurons, in which both perikarya and axons are encrusted by blue-staining minerals (Figure 11.19). This arresting phenomenon is not limited to the vicinal tissue of old infarcts, although this is the most common context, nor is it confined to the adult nervous system, because prenatal insults may result in similar findings. Clusters of axons thus affected can be mistaken for fungal hyphae (Figure 11.20).

A common reaction of axons to injury seen in a wide variety of pathologic states is the formation of localized dilatations known as axonal spheroids or axon "retraction balls" (Figure 11.21A). Ultrastructural examination shows greatly distended axis cylinders filled with bundles of neurofilaments and cellular organelles. A regional variant of this process may be observed in the granular cell layer of the cerebellum where focal dilatations of Purkinje cell axons are

termed *torpedoes*. These structures are seen in a number of cerebellar degenerative diseases, as well as in normal aging. The most common site in the central nervous system where scattered axonal spheroids are routinely encountered as an incidental finding in aged individuals is in the rostral fasciculus gracilis of the medulla (Figure 11.21B). Spheroids in this location are often mineralized.

Astrocytes

Normal Microscopic Anatomy

Like neurons, astrocytes are also heterogeneous. The cells of one class conform to the classic star shape and occur as either the fibrillary or protoplasmic form. Fibrillary astrocytes populate the white matter, whereas the latter inhabit the gray matter. Other important subtypes of astrocytes include the Bergmann astrocytes, which are distributed in a narrow lamina between the cell bodies of Purkinje neurons in the cerebellar cortex, and the "pilocytic" astrocytes of the periventricular region, cerebellum, and spinal cord (Figure 11.22).

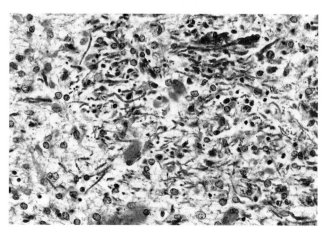

Figure 11.20 Mineralized axons. Clusters of mineralized axons have a superficial resemblance to fungal hyphae.

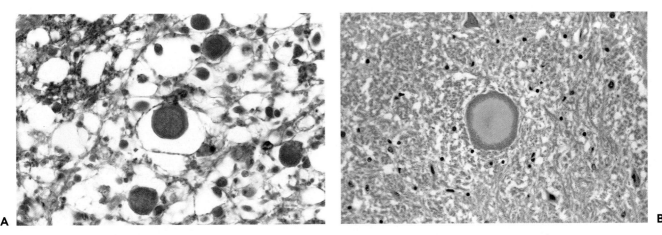

Figure 11.21 Axonal spheroids. **A.** Focal dilatations known as spheroids are a common axonal reaction to injury that are seen in a wide array of pathologic conditions, including radiation damage and posttraumatic diffuse axonal injury. **B.** Axonal spheroids are also frequently encountered incidentally in older individuals in the dorsal medulla oblongata (rostral fasciculus gracilis near the nucleus gracilis), where, as in this example, they are often mineralized.

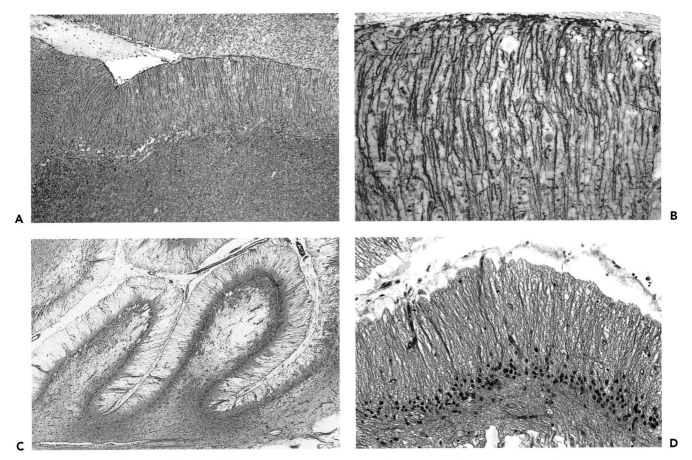

Figure 11.22 Bergmann glia. These astrocytes illustrate the fact that specialization is not confined to neurons. Bergmann astrocytes have cell bodies distributed in a narrow lamina of the cerebellar cortex coextensive with that of the Purkinje cells. Each cell sends an elongated process through the molecular layer to the subpial surface. **A.** and **B.** These processes are not usually well seen in healthy cerebellum with routine H&E staining (Figure 11.3A) but can be exquisitely visualized with immunohistochemistry for glial fibrillary acidic protein (GFAP). **C.** and **D.** An equally striking unmasking of this elegant architecture is often seen without the use of specialized staining techniques in areas of cerebellar cortex adjacent to healed infarcts, in which the degree of ischemia was sufficient to kill the indigenous neuronal populations but spared the more resistant Bergmann glia. Like other astrocytes throughout the central nervous system, Bergmann glia respond to ischemic insult by proliferating, resulting in an increased thickness of the cell body lamina referred to as Bergmann gliosis (D).

In gray matter, nuclei of protoplasmic astrocytes cannot generally be distinguished from those of small neurons because the cytoplasm of both blends imperceptibly into the surrounding neuropil and is not normally discernible as a discrete entity. In white matter, it is usually difficult in H&E-stained sections to distinguish fibrillary astrocytes from the much more numerous oligodendroglia. The nuclei of oligodendrocytes are smaller and more hyperchromatic, but usually these two cell types do not fall into two clearly defined groups. In sections stained for myelin, a very small amount of eosinophilic cytoplasm may occasionally, but not invariably, be seen surrounding normal astrocytic nuclei. This helps distinguish this cell from the oligodendrocyte whose cytoplasm, other than the myelin sheath, is not usually apparent by conventional light microscopy (Figure 11.32). Astrocytic cytoplasm becomes much more prominent when astrocytes respond to CNS injury, culminating in the abundant glassy cytoplasm of the gemistocyte (Figure 11.24).

To appreciate the distinctive morphology of the star cell, one must visualize its radiating processes. These threadlike extensions reach out to define a sphere of influence that is many times greater in extent than one would have suspected by looking at an H&E-stained section alone. Historically, this tinctorial feat was achieved through the technically capricious metallic impregnations but now is accomplished with ease and predictability by the immunohistochemical localization of glial fibrillary acidic protein (GFAP) (Figure 11.24). In the case of the fibrillary astrocyte, processes branch infrequently, whereas those of the protoplasmic astrocyte are more numerous and divide more frequently. They are often less well stained with GFAP than the fibrillary types. Neither type of resting astrocyte is as apparent immunohistochemically as are reactive astrocytes.

The polar forms of astrocytes include the pilocytic and Bergmann types. The pilocytic astrocyte is not conspicuous in its native state but becomes so when responding as gliosis and forming Rosenthal fibers. The latter are hyaline, often corkscrew-shaped, eosinophilic structures that are wedged within one of the cell's bipolar processes (Figure 11.25). These structures are occasionally seen in normal brains in the hypothalamus or pineal gland but become much more prominent in gliosis about such lesions as craniopharyngiomas, pineal cysts, cerebellar hemangioblastomas, and chronic lesions of the spinal cord.

The Bergmann astrocytes are confined to a one-to-two-cell thick lamina. Their polar processes extend to the pial surface of the cerebellum and are only faintly seen with difficulty in standard sections. Yet, they are well visualized with immunohistochemistry for GFAP and at the margins of old cerebellar infarcts (Figure 11.22). The Bergmann glia provide an excellent illustration of astrocytic specialization. Their processes are a form of scaffold and serve as a reminder of the cooperative interplay between astrocytes and neurons during embryological development. At that time, the small neurons of the external granular cell layer spiral down the Bergmann processes to reach their final destination in the internal granular cell layer.

Age-Related Inclusions in Astrocytes: Corpora Amylacea

The ubiquitous corpora amylacea are, by far, the most salient astrocytic inclusions encountered in routine sections. These faintly laminated, slightly basophilic polyglucosan bodies accumulate with age and are observed in greatest numbers where astrocytic foot processes are most numerous, particularly around blood vessels and beneath the pia (Figure 11.23). The olfactory tracts of adults are also typically rich in corpora amylacea (Figure 11.45).

The similarity between corpora amylacea and fungal yeast forms such as cryptococcus is a source of potential diagnostic error since both are strongly positive for methenamine silver, Alcian blue, and PAS (Figure 11.23).

In some individuals, corpora amylacea are strikingly numerous although no pathologic significance has yet been attributed to this abundance.

Astrocytic Reactions to Injury

Although normally among the most morphologically demure of nervous system constituents (only naked nuclei are typically visible on routine H&E histology), astrocytes respond rapidly and dramatically to CNS injury. This response typically consists of two components: hypertrophy and hyperplasia. The initial hypertrophic response, an increase in cell size and cytoplasmic prominence, occurs rapidly following CNS insult. Conspicuous cytoplasm is generally indicative of reactive gliosis and constitutes prima facie evidence of CNS injury. Reactive astrocytes display a broad range of cytoplasmic quantity, from just barely perceptible to robustly embonpoint (Figure 11.24). The latter cells are known as *gemistocytes* (literally stuffed cells). Gliosis may, of course, also present as an increase in the number and density of astrocytic nuclei (hyperplasia) without attendant cytoplasmic prominence. This chronic type of gliosis is frequently subtle and often requires special stains for confirmation and quantitation.

The end result of acute reactive astrogliosis, such as that accompanying cerebral infarction, is frequently a dense fibrillary gliosis (Figure 11.24D). The often-invoked analogy of the astrocyte as the "fibroblast of the CNS" (i.e., a ubiquitously distributed cell with mitotic capability that responds with alacrity to a wide range of deleterious stimuli) is quite apt.

A distinctive cytoplasmic inclusion seen in fibrillary astrogliosis is the Rosenthal fiber (Figure 11.25). These strikingly eosinophilic, elongated, anfractuous structures are observed in a wide variety of reactive states that share in common significant chronicity. Rosenthal fibers are also characteristic of several specific nosologic entities, including

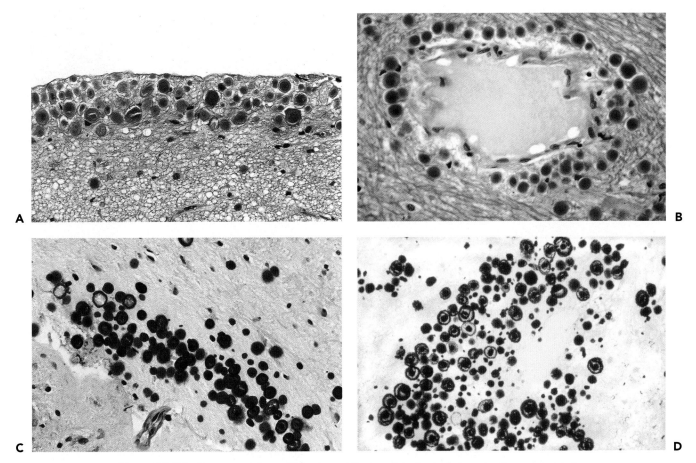

Figure 11.23 Corpora amylacea. These basophilic, lamellated polyglucosan bodies accumulate in astrocytic processes with age, most prominently in subpial (**A**) and perivascular (**B**) locations. Corpora amylacea can resemble fungal yeast forms and show strong positivity for fungal stains such as PAS-fungus (**C**) and Gomori's methenamine silver (GMS) (**D**).

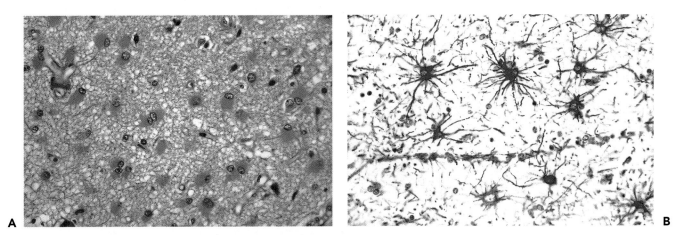

Figure 11.24 Reactive astrocytosis. The plainly visible cytoplasm and processes of the astrocytes (**A**) is proof of an insult to the nervous system. Under normal conditions, only bare nuclei are usually seen. The extensive, radiating cytoplasmic processes for which the astrocyte received its name are most readily appreciated when reactive astrocytes are immunostained for GFAP (**B**). Reactive astrocytes have been descriptively classified according to the amount and configuration of visible cytoplasm, and include the aptly named gemistocytic "laden" or "stuffed" cell (**C**), and pilocytic "hair cell" (**D**) types. Reactive gemistocytes are typical of the acute astrocytic reaction to CNS damage whereas dense fibrillary gliosis is commonly seen in longstanding lesions such as healed infarcts.

(continued)

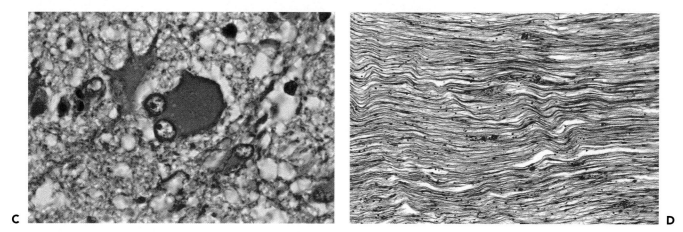

C

D

Figure 11.24 *(continued)*

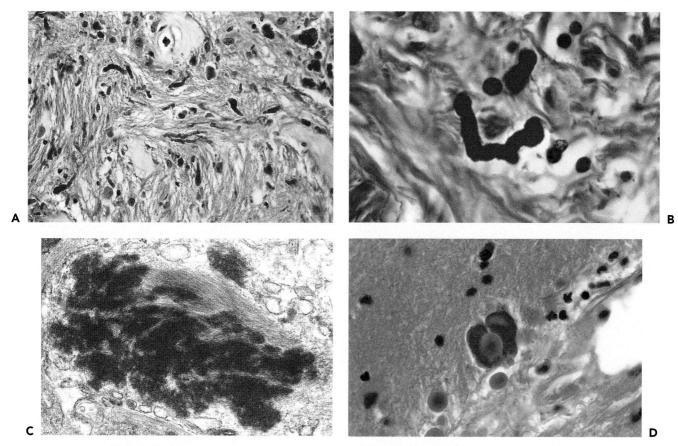

A

B

C

D

Figure 11.25 Rosenthal fibers. Chronic reactive fibrillary astrogliosis is often accompanied by Rosenthal fiber formation (**A**). Rosenthal fibers are brightly eosinophilic, lumpy, elongated structures (**B**) that, by ultrastructural examination, appear as electron-dense amorphous masses surrounded by and merging with dense bundles of glial filaments (**C**). Occasionally, the two most common intracytoplasmic inclusions of astrocytes (corpora amylacea and Rosenthal fibers) may coexist in the same astrocytic process (**D**).

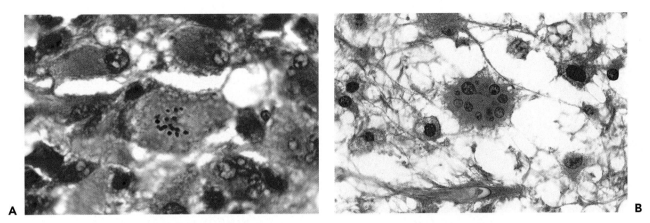

Figure 11.26 Granular mitoses (**A**) and Creutzfeldt astrocytes (**B**) in demyelinating diseases. These distinctive reactive astrocytes occur in a variety of pathologic conditions but are particularly characteristic of demyelinating diseases.

Alexander's disease and, perhaps most widely known, pilocytic astrocytoma. It should be stressed, however, that Rosenthal fibers may be strikingly abundant in the chronically compressed glial stroma surrounding a large number of nonneoplastic conditions (such as syringomyelia) and slowly expanding nonglial tumors (such as craniopharyngioma).

There are several specialized forms of reactive astrogliosis that deserve brief description. Reactive astrocytes with multiple small, variably sized, nuclei (micronuclei), termed Creutzfeldt astrocytes, may be seen in a number of reactive states but are especially typical of demyelinative processes (Figure 11.26). A specific type of astrocytic reaction to injury

is seen in a variety of hepatic diseases that produce hyperammonemia. The reaction consists of nuclear changes exclusively: swelling with contortion of the nuclear membrane, chromatin clearing, and development of one or two prominent nucleoli (Figure 11.27). In sharp contrast to all of the other types of reactive astrocytes, these Alzheimer type II astrocytes fail to exhibit prominent (or even subtle!) cytoplasm by routine H&E microscopy. Alzheimer type II astrocytes may be seen throughout the neuraxis but are particularly prominent in certain locations, most notably the globus pallidus. Alzheimer type I astrocytes differ from type II astrocytes in displaying abundant eosinophilic cytoplasm (Figure 11.27) and are only seen with frequency in

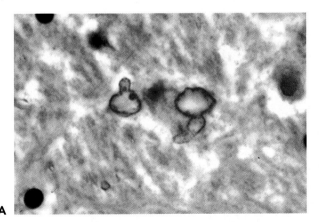
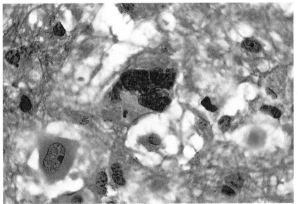

Figure 11.27 Alzheimer astrocytes in hyperammonemia. Two types of reactive astrocytic morphologies, termed Alzheimer type II and Alzheimer type I astrocytes, are associated with hyperammonemic conditions. They were described by Alois Alzheimer and bear his name but have nothing to do with the dementing disease that was also a subject of the famous neurologist's investigations. By far, the most frequently encountered are Alzheimer type II astrocytes (**A**). Typical features include an enlarged pale nucleus with an irregular contour and one or more small nucleoli. In marked contrast to other types of reactive astrocytes, visible cytoplasm is lacking. Alzheimer type II astrocytes are commonly seen in a wide variety of diseases that result in increased blood ammonia. In contrast, Alzheimer type I astrocytes (**B**) have large, irregularly lobulated or multiple nuclei and clearly discernible eosinophilic cytoplasm. These cells are not seen in most hyperammonemic diseases, with the exception of hepatolenticular degeneration (Wilson's disease).

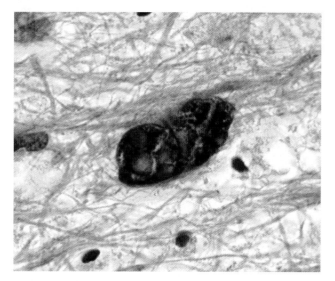

Figure 11.28 Bizarre reactive astrocytes of progressive multifocal leukoencephalopathy (PML). Atypical-appearing reactive astrocytes are sometimes the most striking finding in a PML biopsy and can be mistaken for neoplasia by the unprepared.

Wilson's disease (hepatolenticular degeneration). As the eponyms imply, both types of reactive astrocytic morphologies were described by Alois Alzheimer and have no relationship to the dementing disease of the same ilk.

Among astrocytic reactions to injury, none is more striking than that observed in some cases of progressive multifocal leukoencephalopathy (PML). Not infrequently, the most eye-catching aspect of a PML biopsy is an alarming nuclear hyperchromatism and pleomorphism exhibited by scattered astrocytes—a vignette that has on more than one occasion elicited a mental frisson from even the most experienced observer (Figure 11.28).

Perivascular clearing is a routinely observed artifact of autolysis (Figure 11.29). By electron microscopy, these clear spaces are revealed to be greatly dilated astrocytic perivascular foot processes. This phenomenon of water imbibition by astrocytes is seen both as an autolytic change in virtually all autopsy specimens and, when extreme, as a marker of antemortem hypoxic/ischemic injury.

Oligodendroglia

The oligodendroglia ("few branch" glia) are small cells that are active in the formation and maintenance of myelin and in the, as yet, poorly understood capacity of attending to neuronal cell bodies (satellitosis). In white matter, the oligodendrocytes' obligatory orientation to fiber pathways is occasionally made apparent by a fortuitous plane of section wherein the fascicular distribution of these cells is seen (Figure 11.30). In gray matter, oligodendrocytes are encountered as two to three small, dark nuclei that are pressed against the cell membrane of larger neurons (Figure 11.31). In surgical specimens obtained from infiltrating gliomas, these normal satellite oligodendroglia must be distinguished from infiltrating neoplastic cells that, like their nontransformed counterparts, are attracted to the immediate perineuronal region. Both astrocytomas and oligoden-

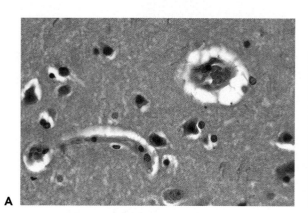

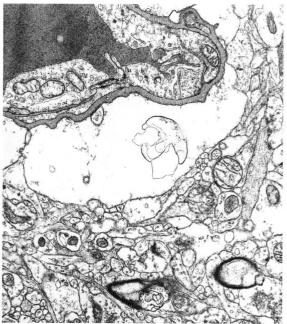

Figure 11.29 Perivascular astrocytic foot process swelling in autolysis. **A.** This common artifact of routine tissue processing is observed by light microscopy as apparent perivascular clearing of the neuropil. **B.** As seen by electron microscopy, the clearing is due to dilated astrocyte foot processes.

Figure 11.30 Oligodendroglia. As seen here in a white matter tract (the corpus callosum) cut in longitudinal section, these glia may be identified, even at low power, as rows of nuclei that queue up between fascicles of myelinated axons.

drogliomas may exhibit such satellitosis, but it is most prominent in the latter neoplasm. Generally, the nuclei of the neoplastic satellites are larger, more pleomorphic, and more coarsely constructed than the normal orbiting cortical oligodendrocytes.

Identification of normal oligodendroglia in both gray and white matter is greatly facilitated by these cells' perinuclear halo (the so-called fried egg appearance), which results from swelling and vacuolation of the cytoplasm (Figure 11.32A). This is analogous to the perivascular swelling and vacuolation of astrocytic foot processes. In oligodendroglial neoplasms (oligodendrogliomas), the perinuclear halo is a well-known, distinctive, and diagnostically useful feature (Figure 11.32B). Oligodendroglia and their neoplastic counterparts exhibit strong immunopositivity for S-100 protein (Figure 11.32C).

Ependyma

This cuboidal-to-columnar epithelium provides a lining for the CNS ventricular system (Figure 11.33) and specializes focally as a covering for the choroid plexus (Figure 11.47). The ciliated nature of the ependyma is readily appreciable in the child but is generally less so thereafter. Tanycytes (literally, stretched cells) are specialized constituents of the ependyma, the elongated abluminal processes of which reach the subependymal vasculature. Thus, these cells provide a physical link between the ventricular, vascular, and intraparenchymal compartments of the CNS. Tanycytes are

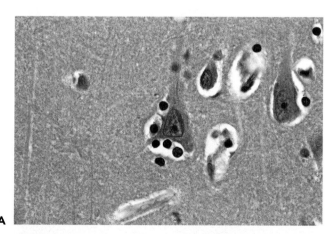

A

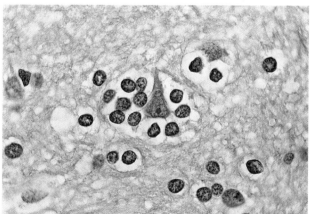

B

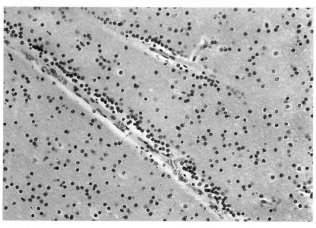

C

Figure 11.31 Perineuronal satellitosis. **A.** Normal perineuronal glia consist primarily of oligodendroglial satellite cells, together with occasional astrocytes and microglia. **B.** This affinity of normal oligodendroglia for neuronal perikarya is often retained by their neoplastic counterparts, oligodendrogliomas, in the form of neoplastic satellitosis. **C.** Nonneoplastic oligodendroglial hyperplasia can also be seen, as for example in some cases of longstanding epilepsy.

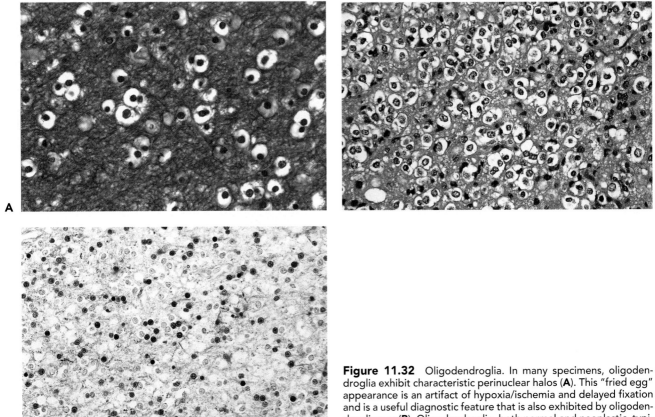

Figure 11.32 Oligodendroglia. In many specimens, oligodendroglia exhibit characteristic perinuclear halos (**A**). This "fried egg" appearance is an artifact of hypoxia/ischemia and delayed fixation and is a useful diagnostic feature that is also exhibited by oligodendrogliomas (**B**). Oligodendroglia, both normal and neoplastic, typically show strong nuclear immunopositivity for S-100 protein (**C**).

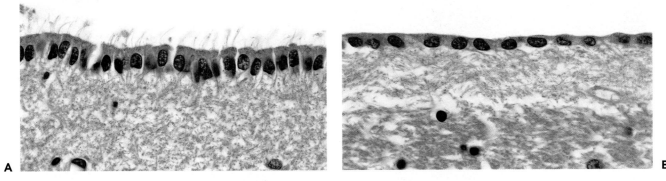

Figure 11.33 Ependyma and the subependymal plate. The lining of the ventricular system varies from a robust ciliated-columnar epithelium (**A**) to nearly squamous flattened cuboidal (**B**). The relative abundance of cilia and the height of the ependyma vary with anatomic location, and both decrease with age. The hypocellular fibrillary zone located immediately subjacent to the ependyma is known as the subependymal plate and contains scattered glia as single cells and in small clusters (Figure 11.36B). Glia of the subependymal plate respond to ependymal injury with a proliferative response termed granular ependymitis (Figure 11.36A). Subependymomas originate from the glia of the ependyma and subependymal plate.

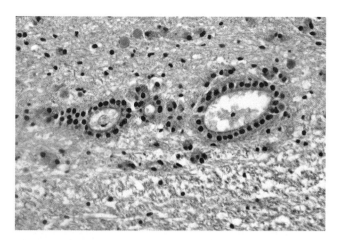

Figure 11.34 Ependymal rosettes. Clusters of ependymal rosettes may be found subjacent to the ependymal lining of the ventricular system throughout the neuraxis. They are particularly common in areas where opposed ventricular surfaces fuse during development, such as at the tips of the lateral ventriculur horns, especially the occipital horns (as illustrated here), and at the lateral angles of the fourth ventricle. These normal rosette clusters are occasionally sampled in surgical specimens and should not be misinterpreted as evidence of disease.

most numerous in the modified ependyma covering many of the circumventricular organs (discussed below). Visualization of these cells is best effected through use of the Golgi's stain.

The closely apposed ependymal surfaces of the tips of the lateral ventriculur horns frequently fuse during development, resulting in cords of ependymal cell nests and rosettes. This is especially typical of the distal portions of the posterior horns in the occipital lobes (Figure 11.34). The white matter in such areas appears pale and can simulate the rarefaction seen after ischemic insult.

Detached ependymal rosettes may be encountered subjacent to the ventricular lining at any location throughout the neuraxis.

The ependyma-lined central canal of the spinal cord is patent in the child (Figure 11.35) but generally becomes obliterated about the time of puberty unless obstructive hydrocephalus is present. In the latter case, the canal may remain patent and even become dilated (hydromyelia). In the normal adult, however, the spinal ependymal cells have completed their role as a generative epithelium and remain as scattered clumps and rosettes (Figure 11.35). Occasional sections of adult spinal cord may exhibit a focally patent central canal.

The primary ependymal response to injury is loss. The resultant focal denudation of the ventricular wall is often accompanied by a proliferation of local cells, the subependymal glia. This nonspecific reaction, termed *granular ependymitis* (Figure 11.36A), is the potential product of a broad range of disparate etiologies, from viral infection to hydrocephalus. It is seen frequently at autopsy as a very focal, limited response and has, in this setting, little diagnostic significance. The normal ependyma is commonly thrown into folds, termed *plicae*, in many parts of the ventricular system (Figure 11.36B). These normal undulations should not be confused with granular ependymitis.

Microglia and the Monocyte—Macrophage System

Normal Microscopic Anatomy

The small, dark, elongated nuclei of microglia are ubiquitous in the normal brain. They are so small and inconspicuous

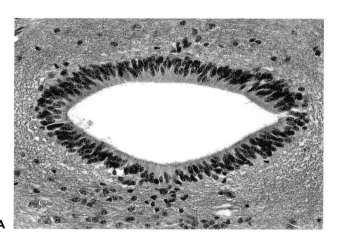

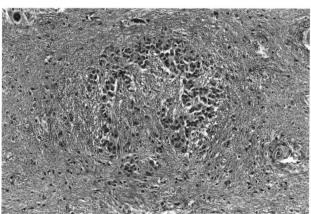

Figure 11.35 Central canal of the spinal cord. **A.** In the child, the central canal is widely patent and exhibits the ciliated columnar ependymal lining expected in a young individual. **B.** In contrast, the central canal of adults is typically obliterated over much of its length, with only residual small nests and occasional rosettes of ependymal cells.

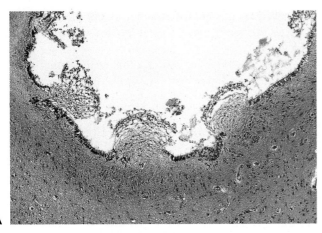
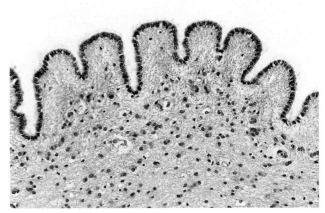

Figure 11.36 Granular ependymitis. **A.** The combination of focal denudation of the ependyma, coupled with an exophytic fusiform proliferation of the subependymal glia constitutes granular ependymitis. Despite the implication of an inflammatory etiology inherent in the name, this common alteration can result from many diverse insults, ranging from hydrocephalus to viral infections. **B.** Normal undulations of the ependyma, termed plicae, should not be confused with granular ependymitis.

uous in H&E-stained sections, however, that they are rarely noticed (Figure 11.37A). They must be distinguished from the commonly encountered tangential or *en face* sections of endothelial cells, which possess similarly elongated, albeit somewhat larger and plumper, nuclei. Special staining techniques such as the classic silver carbonate method, the more predictable lectin histochemistry (Figure 11.37B), and immunohistochemical markers such as HAM-56 uncloak the dendritic processes of microglia and permit unambiguous visualization. By these techniques, microglia are seen to be strikingly pervasive throughout the CNS parenchyma.

Response to Injury

In contrast to the relative passivity and anonymity of microglia in healthy nervous tissue, their activity is by no means subtle when called to action by parenchymal injury. Two variants are seen: microglial nodules and diffuse microgliosis. Microglial nodules (also called microglial stars) are frequent concomitants of viral or rickettsial infection, and they are generally acknowledged to consist of both astrocytes and microglia (Figure 11.38A). The microglia have an elongated shape and are known as rod cells. A form of glial nodule is also seen about degenerating neurons, as in amy-

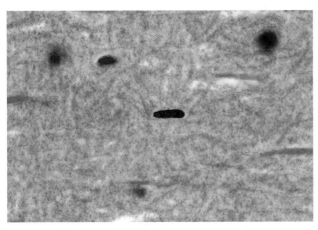
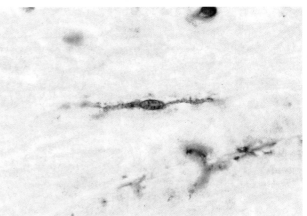

Figure 11.37 Microglia. **A.** These normally inconspicuous residents of the CNS parenchyma are identifiable by their classical rod-shaped nuclei on routine H&E staining. **B.** Dendritic processes, often bipolar, are vividly demonstrated by lectin staining.

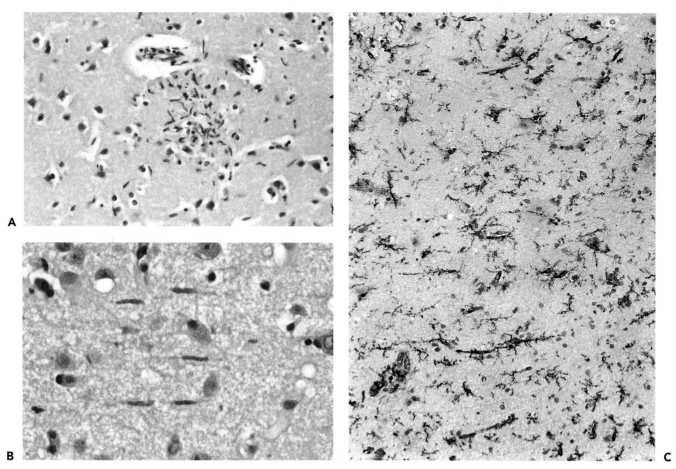

Figure 11.38 Microglia. Reactive microglia may assume several forms. Microglial nodules (**A**) are focal hypercellular collections of microglia together with reactive astrocytes that commonly form as a response to viral and rickettsial infections. In diffuse microgliosis (**B**), seen in a variety of conditions, including ischemia, the characteristic elongated rod-shaped nuclei can be identified on H&E-stained sections; however, the true extent of their presence is more accurately visualized through immuno-histochemistry, as seen here with HAM-56 (**C**).

otrophic lateral sclerosis. Diffuse microgliosis is equally distinctive. In this context, the rod-shaped nuclei of microglia may be present in such numbers as to be easily identified (Figure 11.38B); however, the full extent of microgliosis is often best appreciated through immunohistochemistry for markers such as CD68 or HAM-56 (Figure 11.38C).

Destruction of nervous tissue, by whatever mechanism, generally elicits a macrophage response that serves to clear nonviable debris (Figure 11.39A). Both the activation of autochthonous tissue microglia and the diapedesis of blood monocytes are sources for these scavengers. The weight of evidence suggests that the recruitment of blood monocytes plays a predominant role in large lesions such as infarcts but that the supply of indigenous cells is sufficient for lesser insults.

Macrophages are proliferative cells (Figure 11.39A, B). Mitotic figures will, therefore, usually be present in disease processes that elicit a macrophage response, such as infarction and demyelination. They should not be interpreted as suggestive of a neoplastic process. Macrophages often contribute substantially to the cellularity of tissue samples and, depending on preservation and fixation conditions, their identity may not always be obvious. For example, in some specimens, clearing of the macrophage cytoplasm lends an appearance similar to that of oligo-dendroglial cells, to the extent that, together with the attendant hypercellularity, an infiltrating glioma might be suspected. In such instances a number of antibodies, such as CD68 or HAM-56, can be used to identify the macrophage component (Figure 11.39C, D).

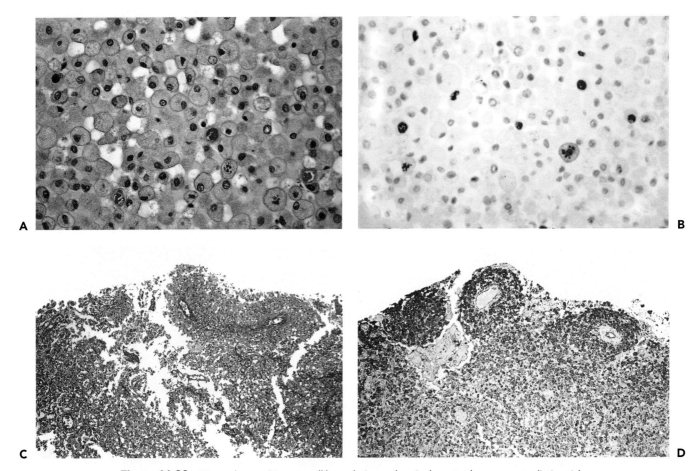

Figure 11.39   Macrophages. Discrete cell boundaries and vesicular cytoplasm serve to distinguish macrophages from other cellular constituents of the nervous system (**A**). Cognoscenti will be familiar with the colorful appellations given these cells in former times, including gitter cells (lattice cells) and compound granular corpuscles. Macrophages are mitotically active cells, and populations responding to CNS injury are readily labeled with proliferation markers such as the monoclonal antibody MIB-1 (**B**). Mitotic figures are, thus, to be expected in tissue samples from a wide range of nonneoplastic conditions that elicit a macrophage response, including infarcts and demyelinative diseases. In hypercellular biopsies (**C**), macrophages can be distinguished from other cellular constituents by a number of commercially available antibodies such as HAM-56 (**D**).

SPECIALIZED ORGANS OF THE CENTRAL NERVOUS SYSTEM

Pineal Gland

The pineal body (epiphysis, or conarium) presents a singular histologic appearance among CNS tissues with a prominently lobulated architecture (Figures 11.40–11.41). This glandular appearance might be mistaken for carcinoma by the unwary, and it can be difficult to distinguish the normal pineal gland from a well-differentiated pineocytoma in small surgical specimens.

Generally present in the pineal gland after puberty are corpora arenacea (acervuli cerebri, or brain sand). These mineralized concretions accrue with age and confer the radiologic hyperdensity that, before the era of computerized tomography and magnetic resonance imaging, made the normal midline position of the pineal gland a useful radiologic landmark (Figure 11.40).

The increase in corpora arenacea with senescence is accompanied by gradual gliosis and cystic change, with attendant effacement of the lush glandular appearance of the pineal gland seen in the earlier decades of life. The ubiquitous incidental pineal cysts typically have densely gliotic walls with scattered Rosenthal fiber formation (Figure 11.41C). The investing leptomeninges of the pineal contain arachnoid cell nests that occasionally give rise to meningiomas of the pineal region (Figure 11.41D).

Pineocytes express strong immunopositivity for the neuronal marker synaptophysin (Figure 11.42A). This useful phenotypic marker is retained by most pineal parenchymal neoplasms. In addition to pineocytes, the pineal gland also

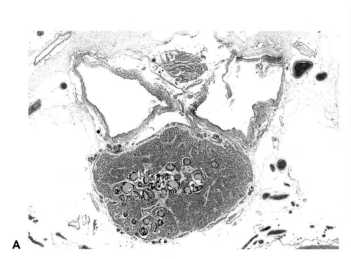

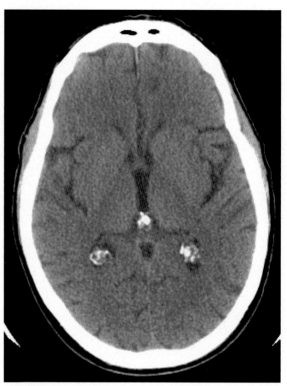

Figure 11.40 Pineal gland (epiphysis). **A.** Whole mount of a cross section of the pineal gland and its environs in situ reveals the typical mineralized concretions variously referred to as corpora arenacea (sand bodies), acervuli cerebri (little heaps), or simply brain sand. Superior to the pineal gland are the paired internal cerebral veins, and between them is the suprapineal recess of the third ventricle, which is lined with ependyma and often contains a tuft of choroid plexus. The loose connective tissue (redundant leptomeninges), in which all of these structures are located, is called the velum interpositum. **B.** The calcification of the pineal gland increases with age and was, thereby, quite useful as a radiographic midline marker prior to the advent of contemporary high resolution neuroimaging modalities. Also seen in this CT scan of a normal adult brain are prominently calcified tufts of choroid plexus (glomera choroidea; also Figure 11.47) in the atria of both lateral ventricles.

contains an indigenous population of astrocytes whose distribution is revealed by immunostaining for GFAP (Figure 11.42B).

Median Eminence and Infundibulum

The median eminence, infundibulum, and neurohypophysis display a unique constellation of morphologic features that reflect their specialized neuroendocrine functions. The background stroma is highly spindled (Figure 11.43A) and contains nodular microvascular tangles termed gomitoli (Figure 11.43B), spherical granular bodies called Herring bodies (Figure 11.43C; Table 11.1), which are storage sites for oxytocin and vasopressin, and scattered cells bearing lipofuscin-like brown pigment (Figure 11.43D). The constellation of features comprising a highly spindled background, vascular tangles, and granular bodies gives this region of the CNS more than a passing resemblance to pilocytic astrocytoma. An additional incidental finding,

particularly in tissue sections of the infundibulum, is the presence of small clusters of granular cells, termed granular cell tumorlets (Figure 11.43E).

Olfactory Bulbs and Tracts

The intracranial components of the olfactory apparatus (the olfactory bulbs and tracts) have a very distinctive histologic appearance. Familiarity with these structures is useful, not only for the neuropathologist, but also for the general surgical pathologist who may encounter them in resections performed as part of the surgical treatment for regionally invasive entities of the nasal and paranasal sinuses. In such situations, the surgical pathologist may be called upon to render an intraoperative frozen-section assessment of tissue resected superior to the cribriform plate. The ability to recognize the normal histologic features of olfactory bulb tissue is, thus, of more than pedantic importance.

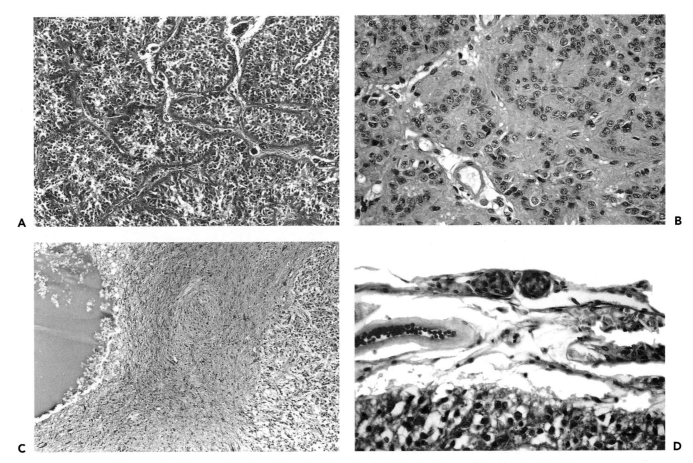

Figure 11.41   Pineal histology. The pineal gland has a richly glandular architecture that is totally unlike any other region of the central nervous system. Salient features include a prominent lobular organization with connective tissue septa (**A**) and pineocytic rosettes (**B**). The latter impart a distinctly neuroendocrine character. Two additional histologic features of note are the ubiquitous incidental pineal cysts, whose walls (**C**) typically exhibit astrogliosis with scattered Rosenthal fibers, and arachnoid cell nests of the investing velum interpositum (**D**) that occasionally provide a source for meningiomas arising in this region.

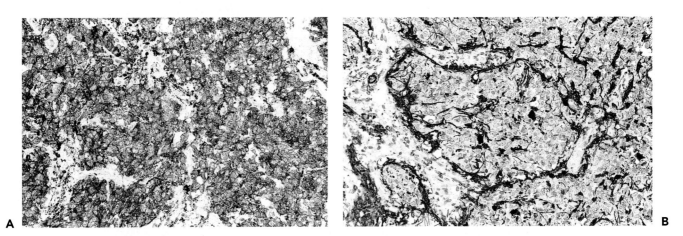

Figure 11.42   Pineal immunohistochemistry. **A.** Pineocytes (and their neoplastic progeny, the pineal parenchymal tumors) are strongly immunopositive for the neuronal marker synaptophysin. **B.** As expected, the indigenous population of pineal astrocytes are well visualized with antibodies directed against GFAP.

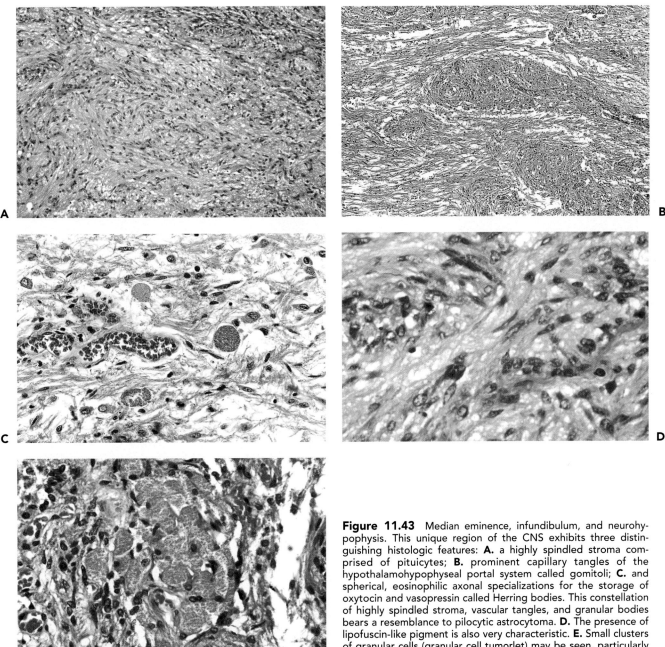

Figure 11.43 Median eminence, infundibulum, and neurohypophysis. This unique region of the CNS exhibits three distinguishing histologic features: **A.** a highly spindled stroma comprised of pituicytes; **B.** prominent capillary tangles of the hypothalamohypophyseal portal system called gomitoli; **C.** and spherical, eosinophilic axonal specializations for the storage of oxytocin and vasopressin called Herring bodies. This constellation of highly spindled stroma, vascular tangles, and granular bodies bears a resemblance to pilocytic astrocytoma. **D.** The presence of lipofuscin-like pigment is also very characteristic. **E.** Small clusters of granular cells (granular cell tumorlet) may be seen, particularly in the infundibulum, as an incidental finding but occasionally reach a sufficient size to produce compression of the infundibulum and subsequent clinical presentation with mildly elevated serum prolactin (stalk effect).

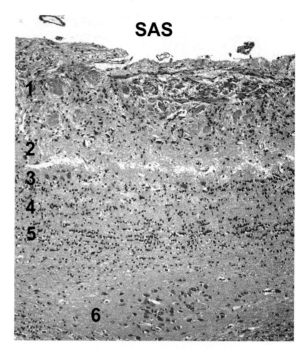

Figure 11.44 Olfactory bulb. The olfactory bulbs have a very distinctive laminar organization. The most superficial layer, termed the glomerular layer (*1*) is covered by the leptomeninges (pia-arachnoid) and the subarachnoid space (*SAS*). The glomerular layer displays a unique architecture, with spindled olfactory nerve fascicles intermixing with spherical hypocellular synaptic zones called glomeruli (*1*). Deeper layers include the external plexiform (*2*), mitral cell (*3*), internal plexiform (*4*), and granular cell layer (*5*). Deeper still is the anterior olfactory nucleus (*6*). A working familiarity with olfactory bulb histology is essential for the surgical pathologist because this structure is frequently seen in the frozen section laboratory during resection of superior nasal cavity tumors that may invade the cribriform plate and overlying olfactory bulbs.

TABLE 11.1

GRANULAR BODIES IN THE CNS: THREE ETIOLOGIC CLASSES

Normal
Herring bodies of the neurohypophysis
Reactive
Granular bodies adjacent to vascular malformations and conditions with iron deposition
Neoplastic
Pilocytic astrocytoma
Pleomorphic xanthoastrocytoma
Ganglioglioma

The olfactory bulb has a laminar organization (Figure 11.44). The outer layer is composed of spindled bundles of entering olfactory nerve fascicles intermixed with distinctive spherical, anuclear areas (termed glomeruli) that constitute specialized zones of synaptic contact between olfactory nerve collaterals and the dendrites of intrinsic olfactory bulb neurons. Mitral cells are large neurons, so-named for a resemblance of the perikaryon shape to a bishop's mitre. Their cell bodies are located in a lamina deep to that of the glomeruli (Figure 11.44). The deepest layer consists of a thick lamina of granular cell neurons that are comparable in size to those of the cerebellum and dentate gyrus.

The olfactory tracts (sometimes incorrectly referred to as olfactory nerves) extend posteriorly from the olfactory bulbs. They are triangular in cross section and, in adults, are notable for their profuse numbers of corpora amylacea (Figure 11.45).

Choroid Plexus

The choroid plexus is a specialized organ of the CNS that is responsible for the production of cerebrospinal fluid. It is found in the body, atrium, and temporal horns of the lateral ventricles, in the interventricular foramina of Monro, in the roof of the third ventricle, and in the roof and lateral recesses of the fourth ventricle. The frontal and occipital horns of the lateral ventricles and the aqueduct of Sylvius

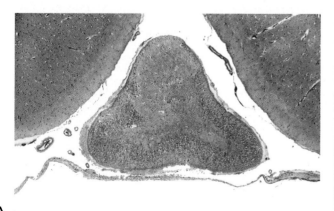
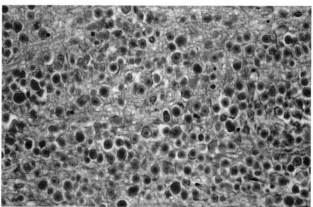

A   B

Figure 11.45 Olfactory tracts. **A.** The olfactory tracts contain myelinated fiber bundles and are roughly triangular in cross section. **B.** A distinctive feature of the tracts frequently observed in adults is their remarkable content of corpora amylacea.

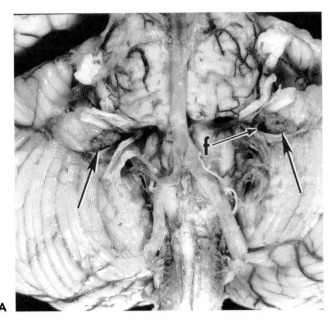

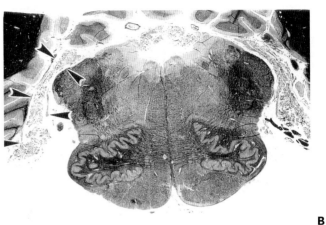

Figure 11.46 Choroid plexus. **A.** Small tufts of choroid plexus are normally visible on the basal surface of the brainstem in the cerebellopontine angle (*arrows*), and indicate the location of the lateral foramina of Luschka (*f*) from which they protrude. The dusty discoloration of the inferior medulla is due to the presence of leptomeningeal melanocytes (Figure 11.57). **B:** The ependyma-lined sleeve of the lateral recess of the fourth ventricle (*arrowheads*), together with the protruding tuft of choroid plexus, is referred to in the older literature as the "flower basket of Bochdalek" or "cornucopia." Pieces of the ependymal cuff are often seen adherent to the lateral aspect of the medulla in autopsy brainstem sections and should be recognized as a normal finding.

are devoid of choroid plexus. The plexus is most obvious in the atria of the lateral ventricles (Figures 11.40B, 11.47), where prominent bilateral tufts (glomera choroidea) are formed. Cystic xanthomatous change is a common incidental finding in these botryoid structures. The plexus is also a normal resident in the subarachnoid space of the cerebellopontine angle (CPA) cisterns, which it reaches from the lateral recesses of the fourth ventricle by protruding through the foramina of Luschka (Figure 11.46). The paired foramina of Luschka (lateral), which open laterally into the ventral basilar CPA cisterns, are to be distinguished from the single foramen of Magendie (median), which opens in the dorsal midline into the cisterna magna.

Microscopically, choroid plexus consists of invaginated fronds of vascular leptomeninges covered by an ependyma that is modified to become a highly secretory epithelium (Figure 11.47). The cells are larger and more cobblestoned than those of the adjacent ependyma (Figure 11.33). In addition to collagen and blood vessels, small nests of meningothelial (arachnoid) cells are common normal habitués of the choroid plexus; whorls of these cells frequently give rise to psammoma bodies (Figure 11.47G). Nonspecific deposition of mineral salts also occurs commonly throughout the connective tissue core with increasing age and accounts for most of the plexuses' radiodensity. An additional aging change of no specific pathological significance is cytoplasmic vacuolization of the ependyma-derived lining cells (Figure 11.47E).

Circumventricular Organs

The circumventricular organs (CVOs) comprise a diverse group of specialized CNS centers that share two morphologic features: a periventricular location and vasculature that lacks the characteristic blood-brain barrier properties found throughout the rest of the brain and spinal cord. There are six CVOs: the pineal gland, subfornical organ, organum vasculosum of the lamina terminalis, area postrema, subcommissural organ, and the median eminence-infundibulum-neurohypophysis (Figures 11.48–11.49). Of these, all except the subcommissural organ are fully developed in the adult human (Figure 11.49). The subcommissural organ, which is located on the ventral surface of the posterior commissure just caudal to the pineal gland, is a very prominent CVO in most vertebrates (Figure 11.49B); although it generally regresses near the end of gestation in humans, vestigial remnants may be present (Figure 11.49C).

INTRADURAL ELEMENTS OF THE PERIPHERAL NERVOUS SYSTEM

The major intradural representatives of the peripheral nervous system are the cranial and spinal nerves and small autonomic fibers in the adventitia of blood vessels. In all of the cranial nerves except cranial nerve VIII, the transition from central to peripheral nervous system occurs within 2

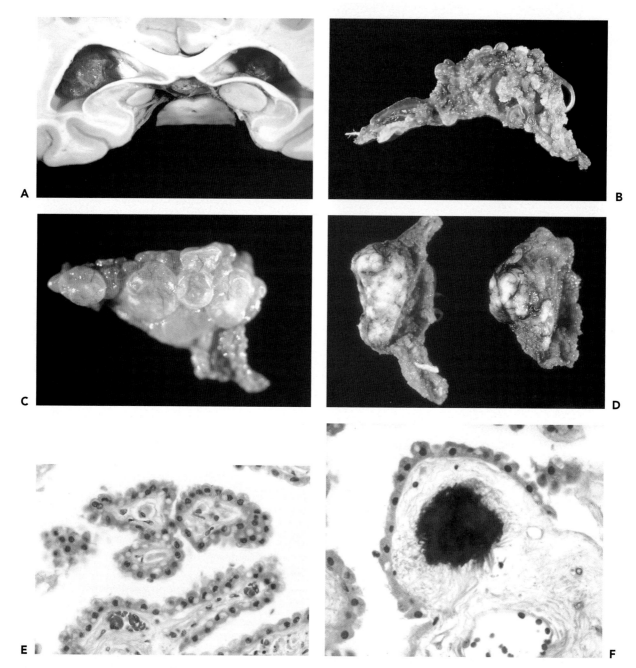

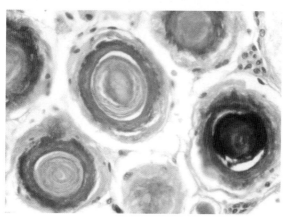

Figure 11.47 Choroid plexus. Choroid plexus produces the cerebrospinal fluid and is found in the lateral ventricles, foramen of Monro, roof of the third ventricle, and fourth ventricle. The largest tufts are called the glomera choroidea and are located in the atria of the lateral ventricles (**A**). Choroid plexus consists of a botryoid, finely tufted tangle of epithelium-covered fibrovascular tissue (**B**) that is formed during embryonic development through an invagination of the vascular pia-arachnoid into the ventricular system, whereby it acquires its covering of modified ependyma. Two common incidental findings on MRI scans and in autopsy specimens are cystic change (**C**) and xanthogranulomas (**D**), both of which may be bilateral. Histologically, choroid plexus is seen to be covered by simple cuboidal epithelium (modified ependyma); in adults, each choroid epithelial cell bears a single prominent paranuclear cytoplasmic vacuole (**E**). An additional aging change seen in normal choroid plexus is calcification, which occurs in two forms: nonspecific deposition of calcium salts in the collagenous stroma (**F**) and as psammoma bodies (**G**). The latter arise from meningothelial cell nests that normally are present in the choroid plexus as a result of the stroma's embryologic derivation from the leptomeninges.

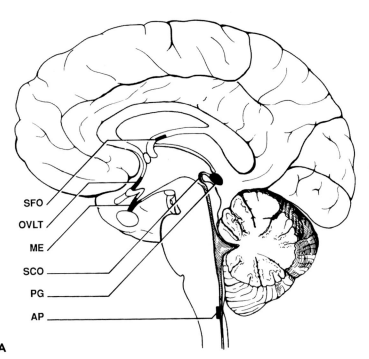
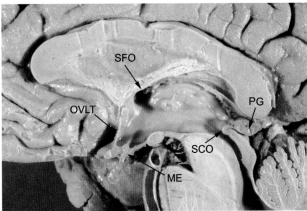

A
B

Figure 11.48 Circumventricular organs. The circumventricular organs share a midline or paramidline position, proximity to the ventricular system, and lack of the usual blood-brain barrier. The subcommissural organ is present in the developing fetus but is vestigial in the adult. (*AP*, area postrema; *ME*, median eminence and infundibulum; *OVLT*, organum vasculosum of the lamina terminalis; *PG*, pineal gland; *SCO*, subcommissural organ; *SFO*, subfornical organ)

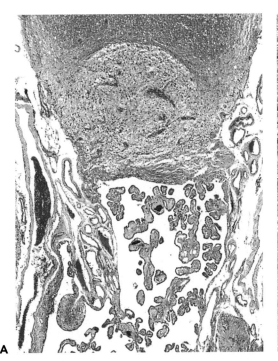
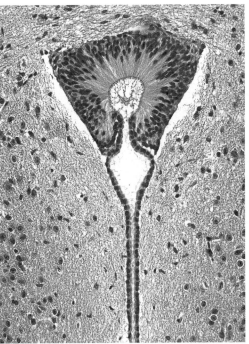

A
B

Figure 11.49 Circumventricular organs (CVOs). Histologically, all of the CVOs except for the subcommissural organ are very similar, with a loose neuropil that is highly vascular and lacks a blood-brain barrier as illustrated by the subfornical organ (**A**). The subcommissural organ is located in the region of the pineal gland just beneath the posterior commissure in the posterior dorsal third ventricle and is highly developed in most mammalian species, as illustrated by the mouse (**B**).

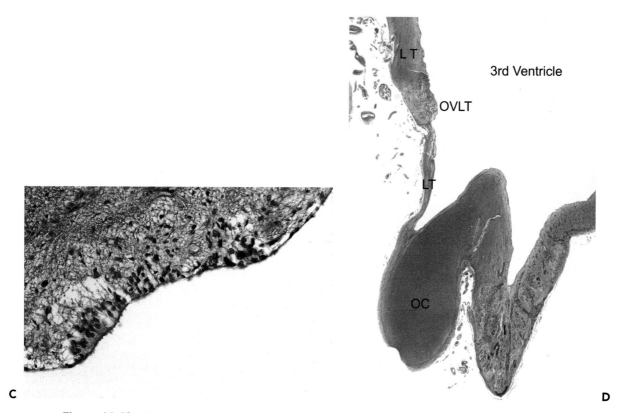

C

D

Figure 11.49 *(continued)* In humans, the subcommissural organ is vestigial, but remnants are occasionally encountered (**C**). The organum vasculosum of the lamina terminalis (*OVLT*) and the median eminence-infundibulum-neurohypophysis are two additional CVOs that are in contact with the third ventricle (**D**). (*I*, infundibulum; *LT*, lamina terminalis; *OC*, optic chiasm)

mm of the pial surface. In the eighth cranial nerve, the central nervous system extends out along the nerve for a centimeter or so to the level of the internal auditory meatus. At this point, the transition occurs between the medial central nervous system segment and the lateral peripheral segment that emerges from the apparatus for hearing and balance (Figure 11.50). The myelin of the central nervous system is formed by oligodendrocytes, whereas that of the peripheral nervous system is formed by Schwann cells. Peripheral nerve is noted for its content of interstitial collagen and the elongated nuclei of Schwann cells.

Two additional intrathecal components of the peripheral nervous system may pique interest on fortuitous encounter. The first is the so-called microneuroma, which is usually found in the parenchyma of the spinal cord or, more rarely, the medulla (Figure 11.51). These structures consist of a Gordian knot of unmyelinated axons that have been hypothesized to arise secondary to traumatic injury of peripheral nerve roots whose regenerating axons follow penetrating spinal or medullary arteries into the CNS parenchyma along the Virchow-Robin spaces. According to the hypothesis, the tapering perivascular spaces ultimately block further advance of the regenerating axons and, thereby, result in the observed neuroma.

An additional component of the peripheral nervous system that occasionally arouses interest is the unmyelinated terminal nerve (variously termed *nervus terminalis*, *cranial nerve zero*, and *terminal nerve*), which courses in the subarachnoid space covering the gyri recti of the orbital

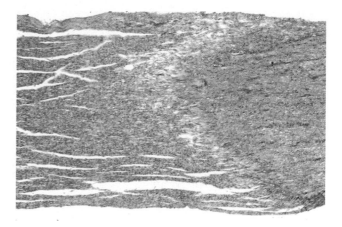

Figure 11.50 Transition zone from central to peripheral nervous system myelin. For cranial nerve VIII (vestibulocochlear), this transition occurs in the vicinity of the internal acoustic meatus.

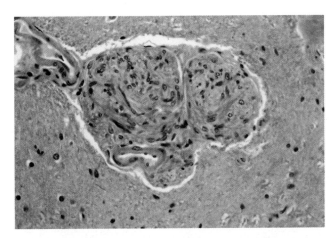

Figure 11.51 Microneuroma. These tangled balls of unmyelinated axons are most often encountered in the spinal cord, less often in the medulla, as an incidental finding in an otherwise unremarkable specimen.

surface of the frontal lobes (Figure 11.52). Although usually composed of multiple small anastomosing fascicles, it occurs as a single trunk in some specimens and can be quite striking. Rarely, intrafascicular ganglion cells may be observed.

MENINGES

Dura Mater (Pachymeninx)

The dura mater is composed of two tightly annealed layers of fibrous connective tissue. The outer layer functions as the periosteum of the cranium, whereas the inner meningeal layer is joined to the arachnoid membrane by weak intercellular junctions and focally forms the four dural reduplications that compartmentalize the cranial cavity: the falx cerebri, falx cerebelli, tentorium cerebelli, and diaphragma sellae. The two layers of the dura separate to accommodate the dural venous sinuses; the inner meningeal layer is pierced by draining veins and by arachnoid villi. The latter conduct cerebrospinal fluid back into the venous circulation and are obvious over the superior parasagittal convexities of the cerebral hemispheres, where they project into the superior sagittal sinus (Figure 11.53). They are present in all other major venous sinuses, as well. They are often observed along the posterior margin of the cerebellar hemispheres in relation to the sinus confluens and the transverse venous sinuses. Small villi are also present intraspinally.

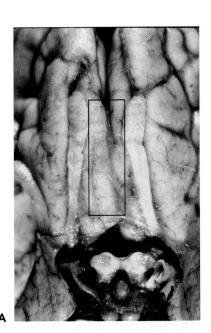

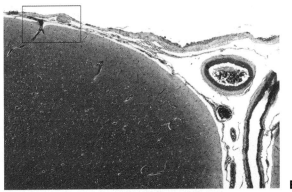

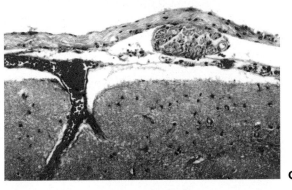

Figure 11.52 Cranial nerve zero. Cranial nerve zero (CN0), also known as the terminal nerve or nervus terminalis, is present in humans as a plexus of small peripheral nerve fascicles found in the subarachnoid space that covers the gyri recti that lie between the olfactory bulbs and tracts (**A**). Tissue sections taken through the gyri recti that include the overlying leptomeninges (**B**) will often include a terminal nerve fascicle cut in cross section (**C**). The small peripheral nerve fascicles of cranial nerve zero are one potential source of subfrontal schwannomas.

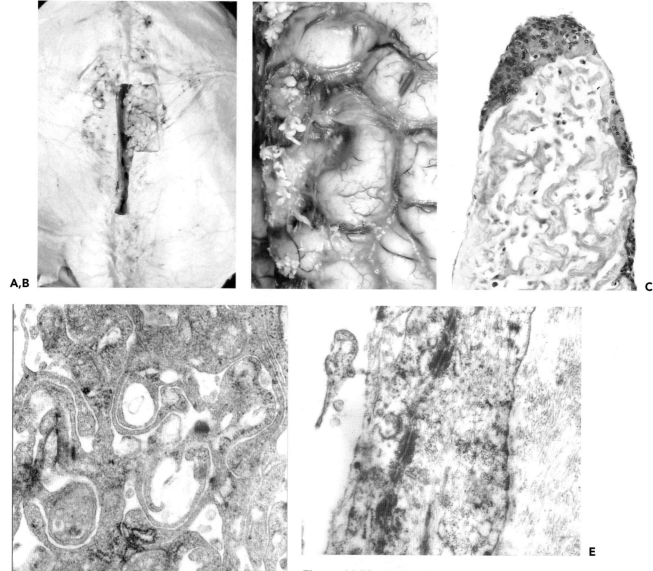

A,B

C

D

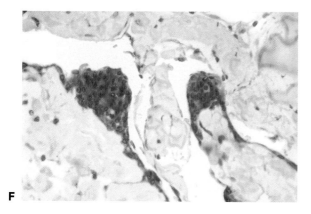

E

F

Figure 11.53 Arachnoid granulations (villi). Specialized structures of the arachnoid membrane serve to return cerebrospinal fluid from the subarachnoid space to the venous circulation and are accordingly found in relation to all major dural venous sinuses. The villi are most prominent in the superior sagittal (**A, B**) and transverse sinuses. With advancing age, they undergo collagenous hypertrophy, as seen in these micrographs, and may then be referred to as pacchionian bodies. The enlarged villi remodel the overlying bone of the inner table of the calvarium to produce small pits termed pacchionian foveolae, or foveolae granulares. Nests of meningothelial cells may be seen anywhere along the arachnoid membrane but are especially prominent in the apical regions of arachnoid granulations, where they are termed arachnoid cap cells (**C**), and in the arachnoid covering the orbitofrontal cortex. Normal meningothelial cells are innately inclined to form whorls and psammoma bodies, two features that are often retained by their neoplastic counterparts, meningiomas. The meningothelial cells of the arachnoid membrane, including the cap cells, serve an epithelial function. Accordingly, they possess elongated, intertwined cell processes (**D**) that are tightly spot welded together by numerous desmosomes (**E**) and exhibit strong immunopositivity for epithelial membrane antigen (EMA) (**F**). Like the tendency to form whorls and psammoma bodies, these epithelial phenotypic traits are retained by neoplastically transformed meningothelial cells and serve as useful diagnostic features of the vast majority of meningiomas, which otherwise exhibit a very broad range of light microscopic morphologies.

The epithelial properties of arachnoid granulations are reflected ultrastructurally in elongated, interdigitating cell processes bonded together with desmosomes and immunohistochemically, by positivity for epithelial membrane antigen (Figure 11.53). These features are also characteristic of meningiomas.

With age, the deposition of collagen enlarges the arachnoid villi, which are then referred to as pacchionian bodies (Figure 11.53). Such large granulations frequently press through the overlying roof of the superior sagittal sinus and its lateral lacunae to produce small pits or depressions in the inner table of the calvarium. These are known as the *foveolae granulares* or *pacchionian foveolae*. Portions of the dura, particularly the falx cerebri and parasagittal dura associated with the superior sagittal sinus, often calcify nonspecifically with age. Calcification may also be seen in association with chronic renal failure. Focal ossification is sometimes encountered as an incidental finding.

Pia-Arachnoid (Leptomeninges)

The arachnoid forms a continuous sheet immediately subjacent to the dura. Based on descriptive and experimental ultrastructural observations, it is now generally accepted that the dura and arachnoid exist in vivo as a physically continuous tissue, with sparse but unequivocal intercellular junctions linking these two historically discrete membranes. The storied subdural space has, thus, taken its rightful place in the pantheon of neuromythology, alongside brain lymphatics and the syncytial theory of the neural net. It has been proposed that the term *spatium subdurale* be eliminated from the standardized nomenclature of Nomina Anatomica. Nevertheless, there is no disputing the fact that the interface between dura and arachnoid constitutes the weak link or path of least resistance for pathologic processes that tend to disrupt the meninges. It seems unlikely

that such venerable terms as *subdural hematoma* will soon be cashiered.

The pia mater and arachnoid are often considered as a single delicate covering of the brain and spinal cord (the pia-arachnoid, or leptomeninges). The arachnoid is connected to the pia by delicate strands termed *arachnoid trabeculae* (Figure 11.54A). In the young, the arachnoid is crystal clear, but with age it becomes gradually thickened. The extent of this change varies considerably. In some cases, it is severe enough to raise concern about a pathologic process—meningitis and meningeal carcinomatosis being the two usual suspects. This normal age-related arachnoid thickening is typically most pronounced over the dorsal parasagittal cerebral convexities. Microscopically, it results from the deposition of dense bundles of collagen (Figure 11.54B), analogous to the collagenous hypertrophy of arachnoid villi that occurs prominently in the same vicinity.

Focal nests of arachnoid cells (also called meningothelial cells) may be seen throughout the arachnoid membrane but are concentrated over the arachnoid villi (arachnoid cap cells) (Figure 11.53C). These distinctive elements become more obvious and more clustered with advancing age and, in the adult, often form whorls with centrally placed psammoma bodies. At this point, the resemblance of these nests to those of the meningioma is inescapable. As mentioned previously, small nests of arachnoid cells are also present intraventricularly in the vascular connective tissue core of the choroid plexus (Figure 11.47G). Both normal and neoplastic meningothelial cells are immunoreactive for epithelial membrane antigen—an understandable property considering the epithelial phenotype of the desmosome-containing meningothelial cell (Figure 11.53).

The dorsal leptomeninges of the thoracic and lumbosacral spinal cord occasionally contain white waferlike

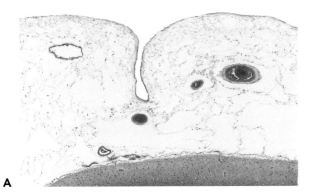
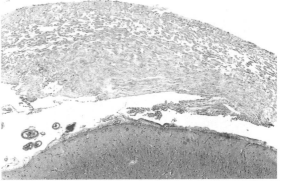

A   **B**

Figure 11.54 Subarachnoid space. **A.** The subarachnoid space is delimited by the arachnoid membrane externally and by the pia mater internally. Delicate arachnoid trabeculae course between these two membranes. **B.** In adults, gradual collagen deposition in the subarachnoid space results in grossly appreciable "clouding" of the leptomeninges. This aging fibrosis appears grossly as diffuse opacification with focal plaques and small punctate nodules. It is characteristically most prominent along the dorsal cerebral convexities adjacent to the superior sagittal sinus.

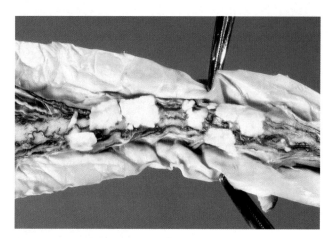

Figure 11.55 Hyaline plaques of the spinal leptomeninges. These plaques are common incidental findings at autopsy and occur most frequently in the dorsal spinal arachnoid, although they may occasionally be seen in the cerebral leptomeninges as well.

plaques (Figure 11.55), a finding that is often termed *arachnoiditis ossificans*. In fact, in the majority (but not all) of cases, these brittle lesions are roentgenographically and histologically devoid of bone or mineral. Rather, they most often consist of laminated, hyalinized fibrous tissue. True arachnoiditis ossificans generally occur in the context of prior symptomatic inflammation or trauma to the leptomeninges. Hyalin plaques, in contrast, are typically discovered as an incidental finding at autopsy in the absence of any relevant clinical history.

Like the dura, the pia is traditionally divided into two layers: the epipia, which covers the surface of the CNS parenchyma and surrounds the vasculature, and the intima pia, which extends into the CNS parenchyma as the posterior median and intermediate septa of the spinal cord. Classically, three specialized structures of the epipia are recognized: the denticulate ligaments on either side of the spinal cord, the linea splendens adjacent to the anterior spinal artery, and the filum terminale. All three structures are composed primarily of dense bundles of collagen.

The filum terminale, which forms the terminus of the spinal cord, warrants additional brief description. As noted earlier, it is composed largely of leptomeningeal collagen but also contains small blood vessels and occasional small nerve fascicles; it may harbor focal collections of adiposites in a minority of normal individuals. Most importantly, however, is an ependymal remnant of the central canal (Figure 11.56). This structure is the source of origin for a unique neoplasm of the conus medullaris and filum terminale: the myxopapillary ependymoma.

Leptomeningeal Melanocytes

True melanocytes like those found in the skin are normal cellular constituents of the meninges. They are typically most concentrated in the leptomeninges of the ventral aspect of the upper cervical spinal cord and medulla oblongata (Figure 11.57). In individuals with an abundant melanocytic presence, the distribution territory extends upward through the pontine cistern and mesencephalic interpeduncular fossa, lateral to the inferior cerebellar hemispheres and mesial aspects of the temporal lobes, and as far rostrally as the gyri recti of the orbitofrontal cortex. It is not unusual for melanocytes to follow the investing leptomeninges of the perivascular Virchow-Robin spaces around large penetrating arteries for short distances into the CNS parenchyma.

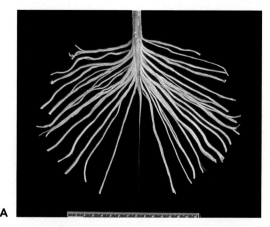

A

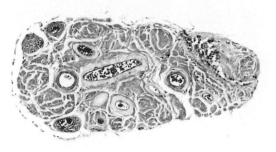

B

Figure 11.56 Filum terminale. **A.** The filum terminale is the terminus of the spinal cord and extends downward from the conus medullaris surrounded by the nerve roots of the cauda equina. **B.** As seen in cross section, the filum is composed primarily of dense collagenous tissue and contains blood vessels, small peripheral nerve fascicles, and, of significant clinical importance, a small, often eccentrically located, ependymal remnant of the central canal (*upper right*). The latter structure, shown at higher magnification in **C**, is the origin of myxopapillary ependymoma. **D.** A remnant of the embryonic terminal ventricle of Krause (ventriculus terminalis), which consists of a focal dilatation of the central canal located in the region of the junction of the conus medullaris with the filum, may be encountered in sections from this vicinity.

(continued)

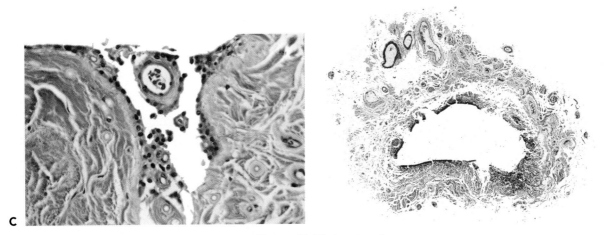

Figure 11.56 (continued)

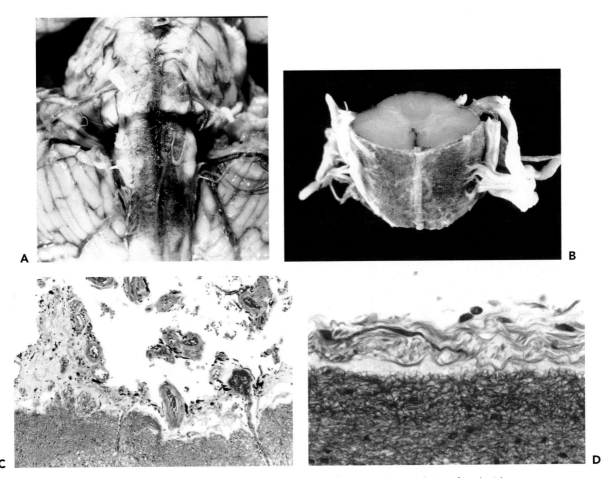

Figure 11.57 Leptomeningeal melanocytes. True melanocytes (not to be confused with neuromelanin-containing catecholaminergic neurons) are normal constituents of the pia-arachnoid and are often grossly visible as a dusky brown discoloration of the leptomeninges overlying the ventral aspect of the brainstem (**A**) and cervical spinal cord (**B**). On cross section their rounded profiles might be confused with hemosiderin-laden macrophages; but on longitudinal section their elongated, dendritic quality is evident (**C, D**).

TABLE 11.2

"BROWN PIGMENT" IN THE CENTRAL NERVOUS SYSTEM (CNS)

Normal
  Lipofuscin in large neurons
  Lipofuscin-like pigment in the infundibulum and
    neurohypophysis
  Neuromelanin (catecholaminergic neurons)
  Melanocytic melanin (leptomeningeal melanocytes)
  Melanin in fetal pineal gland
Abnormal
  Hemosiderin from hemorrhage
  Melanin of metastatic melanoma
  Melanin of pigmented primary CNS tumors
  Lipochrome-like pigment in many "melanotic" CNS tumors
  Pigmented fungi
  Malaria pigment
Artifact
  "Formalin pigment"

Intrinsic melanocytes of the leptomeninges may be involved in a spectrum of proliferative conditions ranging from benign melanocytoma to primary CNS melanoma, with all of these entities being exceptionally rare. In contrast, the normal presence of melanocytes in the leptomeninges must always be borne in mind when examining surgical biopsies from CNS sites known to harbor these distinctive elements; one must avoid misinterpreting them as evidence of a melanocytic neoplasm or as hemosiderin-laden macrophages (Table 11.2). With regard to the latter, the long dendritic processes of the melanocytes are generally quite distinctive (Figure 11.57).

OPTIC NERVE

The optic nerves (as well as the optic tracts and optic chiasm) are direct extensions of the CNS and not peripheral nerves. The significance of this fact is that the myelin of the optic nerves is of the central type and is produced by oligodendroglia, not Schwann cells. Thus, the optic nerves are susceptible to diseases of CNS white matter, such as multiple sclerosis. Being extensions of the CNS, the optic nerves are surrounded by the three meninges, pia mater, arachnoid, and dura mater, with the enclosed subarachnoid space (Figure 11.58). The presence of an arachnoid layer surrounding the optic nerve explains the occurrence of optic sheath meningiomas.

FETAL BRAIN

The two most distinctive histologic features of fetal brain compared to adult brain are active neurogenesis and paucity of myelin. The former is observed as a prominent, dense aggregation of neuroblasts and immature neurons in the periventricular and subpial zones. A similarly transient layer of migrating neurons in the fetal and infant

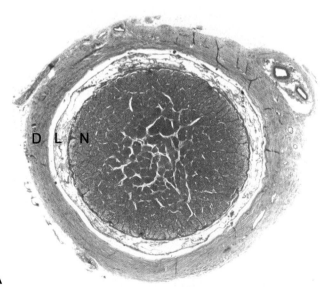

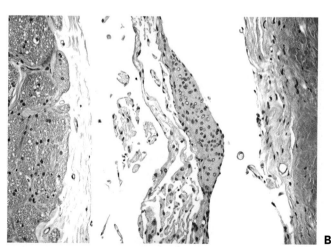

A

B

Figure 11.58 Optic nerve. **A.** A whole-mount cross section reveals that the optic nerve (*N*) is surrounded by leptomeninges (*L*), which include the pia mater and arachnoid together with the enclosed cerebrospinal fluid-containing subarachnoid space. The leptomeninges and subarachnoid space are in turn covered by the densely fibrous dura mater (*D*), which, in this location, is often referred to as the optic nerve sheath. **B.** At higher magnification, leptomeningeal arachnoid cell clusters are clearly seen. The presence of arachnoid cell nests around the optic nerve must be borne in mind when examining intraoperative frozen tissue sections from this neuroanatomic vicinity.

TABLE 11.3
ARTIFACTS

Postal service artifacts
  Crush (glass slides)
  Paraffin pox (paraffin blocks melted into bubble-wrap during
    shipping in hot weather)
Cautery artifact
  Tissue
  Blood vessels
Freeze artifact
Crush artifact
  Embedding sponge
  Surgical or histology forceps
Cavitron ultrasonic surgical aspirator (CUSA) artifacts
  Pseudonecrosis
  Admixed exogenous constituents
  Cranial bone fragments ("bone dust")
  Hemostatic agents
Pseudomineralization
  Bone dust
  Laminar pseudomineralization

Delayed fixation artifact
  Perinuclear halos—oligodendroglial (useful)
  Perinuclear halos—neurons (mimics oligodendroglioma)
  Pseudohypercellularity on smear preparations (uneven
    thickness mimics glioma)
Air-drying artifact on touch/smear/drag preps
**Collapsed leptomeningeal vessels (mimics vascular
  malformation)**
Formalin pigment
Extraneous contaminants
  Iatrogenic foreign material
  Tissue fragments ("floaters")
  Microtome waterbath fungi and bacteria
  Airborne plant pollen spores
Autopsy artifacts
  Cerebellar conglutination
  Mechanical herniation ("toothpaste") artifact of spinal cord
  Macroscopic gas-forming bacteria vacuolation ("Swiss
    cheese brain")

cerebellum (the external granular layer) has been discussed. These generative laminae begin involuting during the latter part of gestation; remnants are present during the first year of postnatal life (Figure 11.3C).

ARTIFACTS

A variety of gross and macroscopic artifacts may complicate evaluation of the CNS. Many of these are seen frequently in surgical neuropathology practice, while a few are limited primarily to autopsy neuropathology (Table 11.3). Artifacts can be broadly separated into those that hinder diagnostic evaluation versus those that mimic histopathologic lesions. Among the former are artifacts of the crush-burn-freeze-suck-soak group (Figure 11.59). The cavitron ultrasonic surgical aspirator (CUSA) is widely employed by neurosurgeons for the safe removal of diseased CNS tissue, particularly soft tumors, and a trap can be used to collect the aspirated tissue and saline irrigation solution for submission for histologic evaluation. Although microscopic examination of CUSA material can be very informative, the

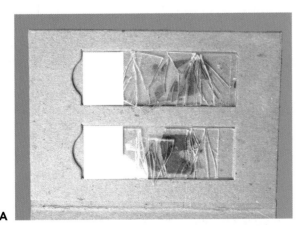
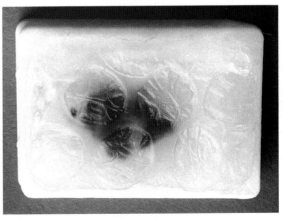

Figure 11.59 Artifacts. Many artifacts encountered in surgical pathology of the central nervous system prevent or severely hinder interpretation of the specimen. Among these, some are unique to the consultation service, such as postal service crush artifact (**A**) and hot weather bubble-wrap "paraffin pox" (**B**), while others are secondary to surgical and laboratory tissue insults, such as severe freeze artifact (**C**), cautery artifact (**D**), and ultrasonic aspiration of brain tissue (**E**).

(continued)

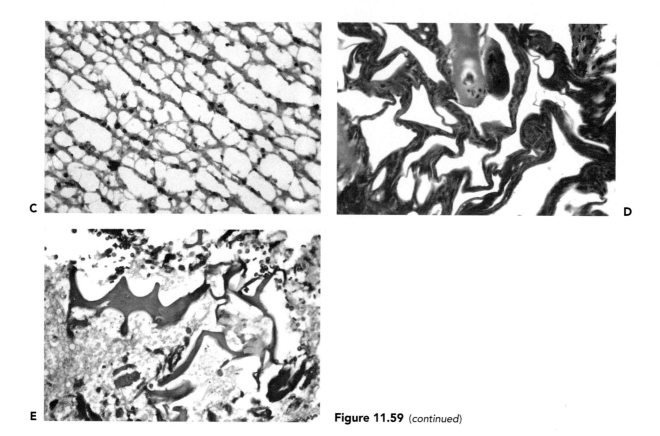

Figure 11.59 (*continued*)

pathologist must be aware of the artifacts that frequently accompany such specimens, including artificial distortion and smearing, and the introduction of extraneous material (bone dust, hemostatic agent); CUSA artifact is one cause of pseudonecrosis in CNS tissue samples (Table 11.4). Among artifacts that mimic lesions, the most common are perinuclear halo artifact, collapsed leptomeningeal vessels, and "bone dust" (Figure 11.60).

Iatrogenically introduced foreign material is also encountered with regularity by pathologists who examine

CNS specimens and warrants brief mention (Table 11.5; Figure 11.61). A variety of foreign agents are used to control bleeding during surgery and may be introduced preoperatively by the interventional radiologist for embolization of vascular lesions or intraoperatively by the surgeon to control hemorrhage during and after surgery. All of these agents periodically appear in tissue sections. Because they are designed to be resorbable and can therefore be left in place, the morphologic appearance will vary depending on the time interval from placement at the initial surgery and subsequent resection during a second surgery (as, for example, resection of recurrent tumor). Resorbable hemostatic agents elicit a chronic inflammatory reaction of variable intensity, which occasionally may be severe enough to create mass effect and clinical symptoms (textiloma, gossypiboma).

There are a few artifacts with which the pathologist who examines postmortem CNS specimens should be familiar (Figure 11.62), the most common being autolysis of the cerebellar granular cell layer (cerebellar conglutination), mechanical distortion of the spinal cord produced by forceps pressure during removal ("toothpaste" artifact), and the production of cystic cavities of varying size in the brain by the postmortem proliferation of gas-forming bacteria ("Swiss cheese brain").

TABLE 11.4
PSEUDONECROSIS ETIOLOGIES

Artifact
  CUSA*/saline solution artifact
  Hematoxylin absence artifact
Normal regional histology
  Cerebellar cortex on smear preparation (hypocellular
    eosinophilic molecular layer mimics necrosis)
Iatrogenic
  Degenerating microfibrillar collagen (Avitene) textiloma
    (gossypiboma)

*Cavitron ultrasonic surgical aspirator (CUSA).

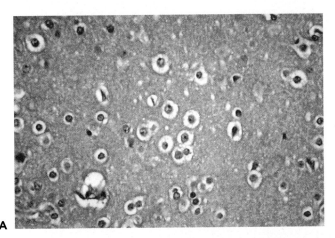

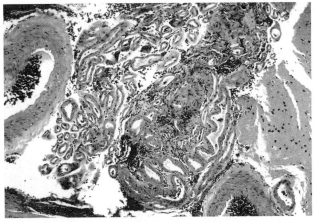

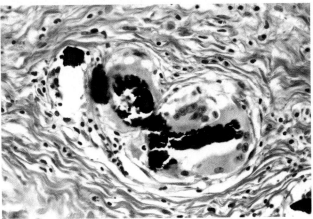

Figure 11.60 Artifacts. Several types of artifacts may not be recognized as artifactual in nature to the unaware and so may be particularly misleading. For example, one of the most characteristic morphologic features of normal oligodendrocytes and their derivative tumors, oligodendrogliomas, in formalin-fixed paraffin-embedded tissue sections is the presence of perinuclear halos. However, depending on fixation conditions and other factors, prominent halos may sometimes be seen around other cell types, including neurons (**A**); care must be exercised in such situations to avoid misdiagnosis. Another example of misleading artifact is the tangle of normal blood vessels that results from collapsed vascular leptomeninges (**B**). The result can mimic vascular malformation. Before rendering a diagnosis of vascular abnormality in such circumstances, the adjacent brain or spinal cord tissue should be examined for evidence of associated features, such as gliosis, hemosiderin deposition, and granular bodies. Finally, also under the category of misleading artifact is "bone dust," which consists of microscopic fragments of cranial bone produced by the surgeon's drill that become intermixed with the tissue sample and can mimic calcification or ossification. In repeat operations, such bone dust fragments left in situ at the previous operation can be seen accompanied by a foreign body–type giant cell reaction (**C**).

TABLE 11.5
IATROGENICALLY-INTRODUCED FOREIGN MATERIAL

Preoperative embolic agents
   Gelatin foam (Gelfoam)
   Polyvinyl alcohol particles
   Acrylic microspheres (Embospheres)

Intraoperative hemostatic agents
   Resorbable hemostatic agents
      Gelatin foam (Gelfoam)
      Oxidized cellulose (Surgicel, Oxycel)
      Microfibrillar bovine collagen (Avitene)
   Nonresorbable hemostatic agents
      "Retained" cotton ball/pledgers
      Cottonoids and kites (synthetic)

Surgically introduced therapeutic materials
   Gliadel wafers (chemotherapy delivery)
   Muslin (cotton) fabric (aneurysm wrapping)

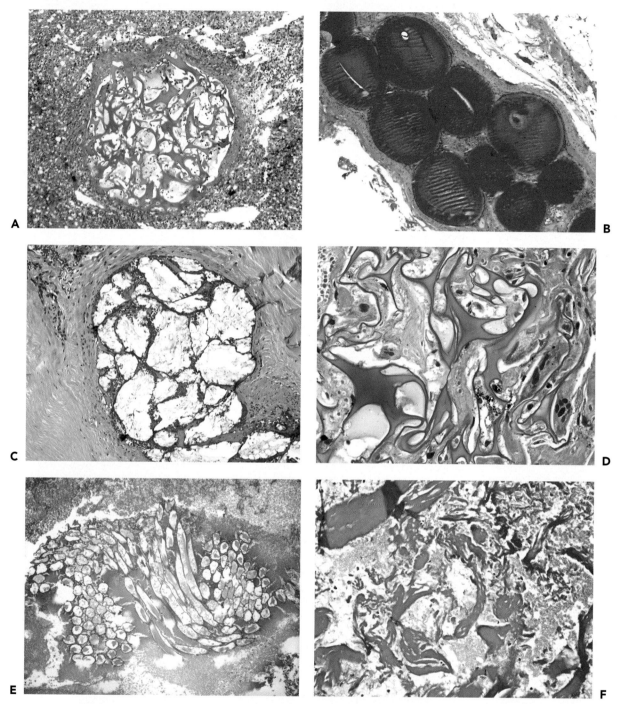

Figure 11.61 Artifacts. An additional category of artifacts seen in surgical neuropathology consists of foreign material placed by the interventional radiologist or neurosurgeon and subsequently encountered by the pathologist upon tissue resection. The most common examples of this are embolic and hemostatic agents. Embolic materials are introduced by catheter prior to surgery for highly vascular lesions to reduce intraoperative bleeding; the most common are gelatin foam (**A**), acrylic resin spheres (**B**), and polyvinyl alcohol particles (**C**). Hemostatic agents, in contrast, are placed in the surgical site to stop bleeding during the operation and often are left in place after closing to prevent postoperative bleeding. The most commonly employed agents are gelatin foam (**D**), oxidized cellulose (**E**), and microfibrillar bovine collagen (**F**).

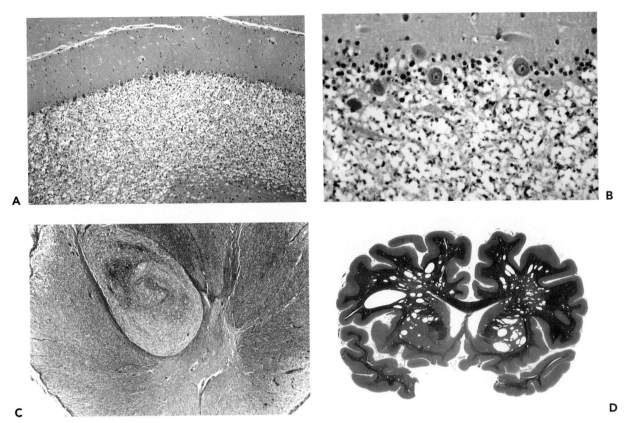

Figure 11.62 Artifacts. There are a number of gross and histologic artifacts that are usually encountered only in autopsy specimens of the central nervous system. The most common of these are cerebellar conglutination (**A, B**), also known as "etat glace," which consists of autolytic dissolution of the granular cell layer of the cerebellum; "toothpaste" or "squeeze" artifact of the spinal cord (**C**), which results from focal crushing of the cord by forceps during removal at autopsy and resultant internal herniation of the central gray matter, mimicking malformation or heterotopia; and "Swiss cheese brain" (**D**), which is a striking macroscopic vacuolization of the brain resulting from postmortem proliferation of gas-forming bacteria.

SUGGESTED READINGS

Neuropathology Textbooks

Burger PC, Scheithauer BW. Tumors of the central nervous system. In: *Atlas of Tumor Pathology*, series 4. Washington, DC: Armed Forces Institute of Pathology; 2006.

McLendon RE, Rosenblum M, Bigner DD. *Russell & Rubinstein's Pathology of Tumors of the Nervous System*. 7th ed. London: Arnold; 2006.

Prayson RA, ed. *Neuropathology*. Philadelphia: Elsevier; 2005.

Love S, Louis D, Ellison D, eds. *Greenfield's Neuropathology*. 8th ed. London: Arnold; 2006.

Burger PC, Scheithauer BW, Vogel FS. *Surgical Pathology of the Nervous System and Its Coverings*. 4th ed. New York: Churchill Livingstone; 2002.

Ironside JW, Moss TH, Louis DN, Lowe JS, Weller RO. *Diagnostic Pathology of Nervous System Tumours*. New York: Churchill Livingstone; 2002.

Neuropathology Review Books

Gray F, De Girolami U, Poirer J, eds. *Escourolle and Poirier's Manual of Basic Neuropathology*. 4th ed. Boston: Butterworth-Heinemann; 2004.

Nelson JS, Mena H, Parisi JE, Schochet SS, eds. *Principles and Practice of Neuropathology*, 2nd ed. New York: Oxford University Press; 2003.

Citow JS, Wollmann RL, Macdonald RL. *Neuropathology and Neuroradiology: A Review*. New York: Thieme; 2001.

Fuller GN, Goodman JC. *Practical Review of Neuropathology*. Philadelphia: Lippincott Williams & Wilkins; 2001.

Prayson RA. *Neuropathology Review*. Totowa, NJ: Humana Press; 2001.

Neuropathology Atlases

Ellison D, Love S, Chimelli L, Harding B, Lowe JS, Vinters H. *Neuropathology: A Reference Text of CNS Pathology*. 2nd ed. London: Mosby; 2004.

Hirano A. *Color Atlas of Pathology of the Nervous System*. 2nd ed. New York: Igaku-Shoin; 1988.

Okazaki H, Scheithauer BW. *Atlas of Neuropathology*. New York: Gower Medical; 1988.

Schochet SS, Nelson J. *Atlas of Clinical Neuropathology*. East Norwalk, CT: Appleton & Lange; 1989.

Weller RO. *Color Atlas of Neuropathology*. London: Oxford University Press; 1984.

Veterinary Neuropathology

Summers BA, Cummings JF, de Lahunta A, eds. *Veterinary Neuropathology*. St. Louis: Mosby; 1995.

Pituitary and Sellar Region

M. Beatriz S. Lopes   Peter J. Pernicone

Bernd W. Scheithauer   Eva Horvath   Kalman Kovacs

12

EMBRYOLOGY

To fully appreciate the anatomy of the pituitary (hypophysis), an understanding of its embryogenesis is essential. The gland consists of an anterior lobe (adenohypophysis), a posterior lobe (neurohypophysis), and an intermediate zone (Figure 12.1). The development of each differs significantly.

The adenohypophysis has its origin in a thickening of oral ectoderm (1–4). During the third week of gestation, this thickened plate invaginates in a cephalad direction to form the Rathke's pouch, which retains its connection to the stomodeum via a narrow stalk. In the sixth week, the stalk becomes so attenuated that the pouch loses its stomodeal attachment as it comes into contact with the infundibulum. Cellular proliferation in the anterior wall of Rathke's pouch gives rise to the pars distalis, the principal portion of the anterior lobe. In addition, a "tonguelike" extension of the pars distalis, the pars tuberalis, grows upward to partially surround the anterior surface of the infundibulum. The posterior portion of Rathke's pouch gives rise to what in humans is a thin segment of pituitary, the pars intermedia or intermediate lobe. In this zone, microcystic remnants of

Rathke's pouch containing colloidlike material are commonly seen (Figure 12.1). Gross cystic dilatation of such remnants is common but infrequently produces clinically significant intermediate lobe or Rathke's cleft cysts.

A remnant of the pharyngohypophysial stalk, demonstrable in fetuses and occasionally encountered in adults, comprises the pharyngeal pituitary (5,6). Located in the midline, beneath the muco-periosteum of the nasopharynx, it extends from the posterior border of the vomer along the sphenoid bone. Although the full spectrum of anterior pituitary hormone-producing cells may be demonstrated in pharyngeal pituitaries, they are rarely the seat of medical or surgical disease.

The neurohypophysis develops from a neuroectodermal bud first noticeable in the floor of the diencephalon at 4 weeks' gestation (1,3). Two weeks later, the outgrowth grows ventrally to abut the posterior portion of Rathke's pouch. This specialized portion of the nervous system comprises magnocellular nuclei, their axons within the median eminence and infundibular stalk, and their terminations in the pars nervosa (posterior lobe). Oxytocin and vasopressin, as well as their carrier proteins, the neurophysins,

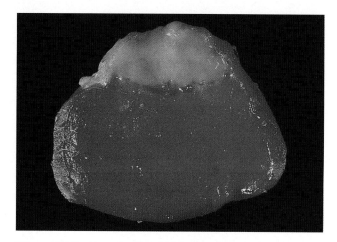

Figure 12.1 Normal unfixed adult pituitary gland cut in the horizontal plane. The posterior lobe is located at the top of the field. A few intermediate lobe cysts are present. The deep red color of the anterior lobe is a reflection of its extensive vascularity.

are detectable in supraoptic and paraventricular nuclei at 19 weeks and in the posterior lobe at 23 weeks (7).

As early as 7 to 8 weeks' gestation, the portal system begins to develop. Although by 12 weeks both the median eminence and the anterior lobe are vascularized, the circulation of the hypothalamic–pituitary portal system is not completed until 18 to 20 weeks (7).

The hypothalamus develops from a swelling in the diencephalon. Although the hypothalamic nuclei as well as the supraopticohypophysial tract are demonstrable at 8 weeks' gestation, unmyelinated axons, growing ventrally from the magnocellular (supraoptic and paraventricular) nuclei, do not reach the posterior lobe until 6 months.

By 12 weeks, a number of cartilaginous plates have fused to form the cartilaginous neurocranium (1). The body of the sphenoid bone and the sella turcica result from fusion of hypophysial cartilaginous plates located on either side of the developing pituitary. The sella is well formed by 7 weeks and matures through a process of enchondral ossification.

Rare developmental malformations of the pituitary gland, including ectopic pituitary gland and pituitary dystopia, have been reported (8,9).

The understanding of pituitary development has recently expanded as a result of the identification of molecular mechanisms that may specify cell determination and differentiation. Recent advances in pituitary development in mammals have suggested that pituitary organogenesis is controlled by a combination of sequential exogenous and endogenous signals (10–12). These signals induce the expression of interacting transcriptional regulators in temporal and spatial patterns. Pituitary cell types appear to emerge from a common stem cell under the response of transcription regulators critical for determination and differentiation of specific cell type. Briefly, the transcription factor pituitary homeobox 1 (*Ptx1*) appears in early

development of the pituitary and cooperates with more functionally oriented transcription factors. *Pit-1* is a transcription factor that regulates the functional differentiation of the somatotrophs, lactotrophs, and thyrotrophs. A family of basic helix-loop-helix transcription factors, *Neuro D1*, and a novel T box factor, *Tpit*, appear to synergistically play a role in the functional differentiation for pituitary pro-opiomelanocortin (POMC) cell lineage and corticotroph cells. The nuclear receptor steroidogenic factor-1, *SF-1*, is a key factor for differentiation of LH and FSH cells.

On the other hand, the time period of recognition of the various human pituitary hormone–producing cells during embryonal development have been well determined by immunohistochemical stains. Corticotrophs are the first cells to differentiate in the human fetal pituitary (at around 5 weeks gestational age). Somatotrophs appear around 8 to 9 weeks, followed by thyrotrophs and gonadotrophs at 12 to 15 weeks. Lactotrophs, although seen in small numbers as early as 12 weeks, are only fully recognizable at 23 weeks (7,13,14).

GROSS ANATOMY

Bony Sella

The pituitary gland is centrally situated at the base of the brain, where it lies safely nestled in the sella turcica, a saddle-shaped concavity within the sphenoid bone (Figures 12.2–12.4). It is attached to the hypothalamus by both the pituitary stalk and a tenuous vascular network (Figures 12.5–12.7). By virtue of its location, the pituitary

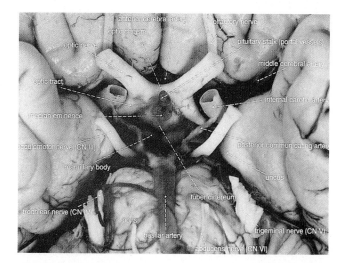

Figure 12.2 Ventral surface of normal brain showing the pituitary stalk and surrounding structures. The pituitary gland has been removed. The proximity of the optic chiasm to the pituitary is the basis for the visual field deficits accompanying suprasellar extension of pituitary adenomas. Visible along the posterior aspect of the stalk are tributaries of the portal system.

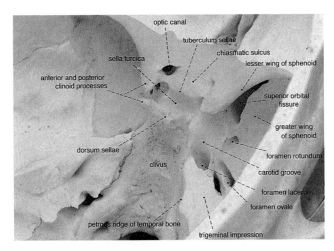

Figure 12.3 Oblique view of the normal skull base; the various skull bones are indicated in color. The sella turcica is centrally located with several foramina nearby. The foramen spinosum is not visible in this view. Yellow, sphenoid; pink, occipital; light blue, temporal; green, parietal; white, frontal.

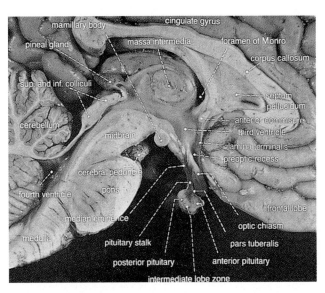

Figure 12.5 Midline sagittal section through the brain at the level of the pituitary stalk and pituitary gland, showing the pituitary gland with surrounding structures including hypothalamus, third ventricle, optic chiasm, and sphenoid sinus.

gland has many important anatomic relations (15–17). Anterior to the sella, the sphenoid bone forms a midline slope, the tuberculum sella, as well as a transverse indentation, the chiasmal sulcus, so named for the overlying optic chiasm (see Figures 12.3–12.4). The optic canals, which transmit the optic nerves, lie anterolateral to the sulcus, whereas the optic tracts are posterolateral. In view of the pituitary's proximity to the optic apparatus, pituitary lesions that extend superiorly may cause significant visual field deficits (Figures 12.2, 12.5–12.11). Specifically, compression of decussating fibers in the chiasm produces bitemporal hemianopsia, whereas compromise of an optic tract leads to homonymous hemianopsia. Further suprasellar extension may cause hypothalamic dysfunction and hydrocephalus.

The floor of the sella forms a portion of the roof of the sphenoid air sinus, a fortuitous relationship that permits ready surgical access (18) (Figures 12.4, 12.6–12.12). Indeed, the transsphenoidal approach to the pituitary initially involves mobilization of the nasal septal cartilage followed by resection of a portion of the ethmoid plate. A sublabial incision is then made, and the sphenoid

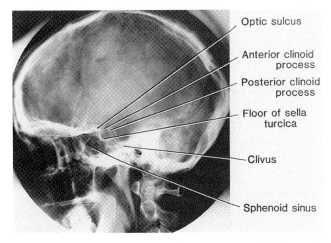

Figure 12.4 This normal lateral skull radiograph shows the central location of the sella turcica and surrounding bony anatomy.

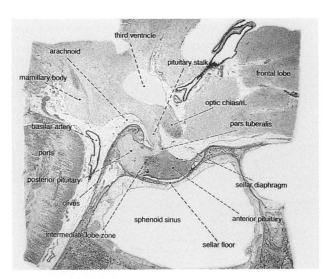

Figure 12.6 Sagittal whole-mount section of normal pituitary gland and surrounding structures. The anterior (*at right*) and posterior (*at left*) lobes are clearly delineated. The pars tuberalis is the thin tongue-shaped portion of anterior lobe that extends for a short distance up the stalk. This diagram illustrates the proximity of the optic chiasm to the pituitary. Superior extension of a pituitary tumor may compress the optic chiasm with resultant visual field deficits, whereas downward extension may fill the sphenoid sinus (Luxol-Fast Blue–PAS).

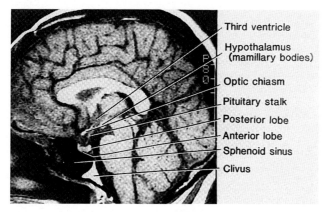

Figure 12.7 Magnetic resonance imaging (MRI): sagittal view of the brain at the level of the pituitary stalk and gland. The clarity of the pituitary gland, stalk, hypothalamus, and optic chiasm is remarkable, making MRI an excellent imaging modality for the assessment of pituitary lesions. One advantage of MRI over computed tomography (CT) is the absence of bony artifact with MRI.

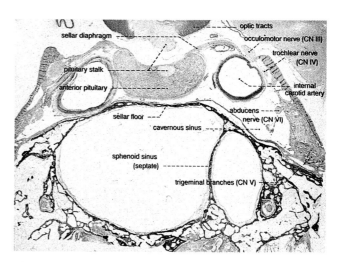

Figure 12.9 Coronal whole-mount view of the normal pituitary gland and surrounding structures. Note the location of cranial nerves III, IV, VI, and branches of cranial nerve V within the cavernous sinuses, a relationship explaining the occurrence of cranial nerve palsy in association with invasive pituitary adenomas. This section also illustrates the proximity of the internal carotid arteries to the pituitary gland (Luxol-Fast Blue–PAS).

speculum is placed in the septal space, permitting direct visualization of the anterior wall of the sphenoid sinus. Upon breaking through the anterior sphenoid wall, the sella may be seen bulging into the roof of the sinus. A septated sphenoid sinus may affect the surgeon's orientation at surgery (Figures 12.8–12.9). The pituitary is then exposed by traversing the bony sellar floor and incising the dural investment around the gland.

The sloping anterior sellar wall terminates in posterolateral projections, the anterior clinoid processes (Figures 12.3–12.4). Posterior to the sella, the sphenoid bone continues as the dorsum sellae, anterolateral portions of which form the posterior clinoid processes (see Figures 12.3–12.4). Posterior to the dorsum sellae lies the downward-sloping clivus, notorious as the site of predilection of chordomas (Figures 12.3, 12.4, 12.6–12.7). A number of neurovascular foramina are situated in the sellar region; by name and contents from anterior to posterior, they include the foramen rotundum (maxillary nerves), ovale (mandibular nerves), spinosum (middle meningeal arteries), and lacerum (internal carotid arteries) (Figure 12.3).

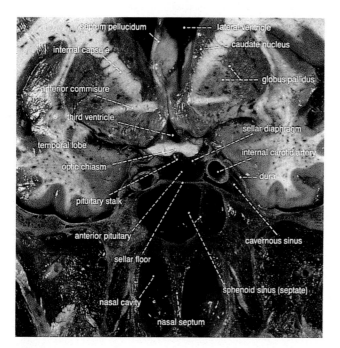

Figure 12.8 Coronal section of the head at the level of the pituitary stalk and gland. This photograph clearly illustrates the intimate relationships between the cavernous sinuses, the sphenoid sinus, and the pituitary gland. Invasive adenomas may extend laterally into one or both cavernous sinuses or inferiorly into the sphenoid sinus. Note the proximity of the optic chiasm to the pituitary.

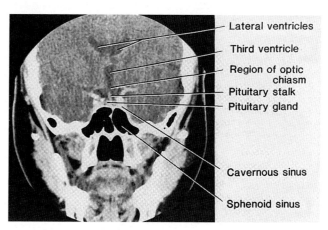

Figure 12.10 A computed tomographic (CT) coronal view of the normal skull and brain at the level of the pituitary stalk and gland. The CT scan is a good imaging modality for assessing the pituitary gland; however, radiologists often encounter problems with bony artifact. For this reason, MRI is superior.

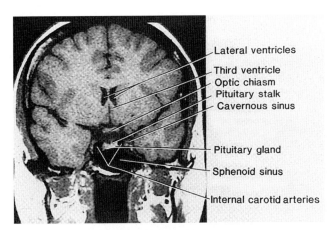

Figure 12.11 Coronal MRI of the skull and brain at the level of the pituitary stalk and gland.

Meninges

The physical relationship of the meninges to the pituitary and sella is unusual in that the pituitary lacks a leptomeningeal investment. Periosteal dura lines the sella turcica, whereas the dura proper covers the lateral aspects of the cavernous sinuses and forms the sellar diaphragm. The diaphragm is usually thin at the center and thick at its periphery and possesses a variably sized central aperture through which the pituitary stalk passes (15). Leptomeninges do encircle the stalk; however, below the level of the sellar diaphragm, they reflect back upon themselves to form a circumferential channel, the infradiaphragmatic hypophysial cistern. This arrangement explains the higher incidence of development of meningiomas in the suprasellar surface of the diaphragm rather than in the intrasellar compartment.

In some individuals, the leptomeninges exhibit an important anatomic variation. It consists of extension or

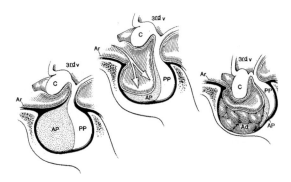

Figure 12.13 Illustration of normal as well as variants of the empty sella. **A.** The normal pituitary-sellar relationships. The leptomeninges cover the stalk and sellar diaphragm but do not extend into the sella. **B.** In primary empty sella syndrome, an excessively large diaphragmatic orifice permits herniation of leptomeninges into the sella. Prolonged CSF pressure compresses the gland against the sellar floor. **C.** Secondary empty sella may result from infarction of a pituitary adenoma, infarction of the pituitary gland, and surgical or radioablation of the gland. (Ar, arachnoid; AP, anterior pituitary; PP, posterior pituitary; C, optic chiasm; 3rd v, third ventricle)

herniation of the arachnoid through an inordinately large diaphragmatic opening. In one study, the incidence of an intrasellar arachnoidocele was found to exceed 20% (19). In such cases, transsphenoidal surgery may result in persistent cerebrospinal fluid (CSF) rhinorrhea because of inadvertent violation of the subarachnoid space. With prolonged exertion of even normal CSF pressure, enlargement of such arachnoidoceles may produce sellar enlargement and pituitary compression, the gland being reduced to a thin crescent on the posterior sellar floor (Figures 12.13). The so-called empty sella syndrome, shows a distinct predilection for obese, multiparous females (Figure 12.14). Its anatomic manifestations are fully expressed in as many as 5.5% of autopsies (20–21). Compression of the gland

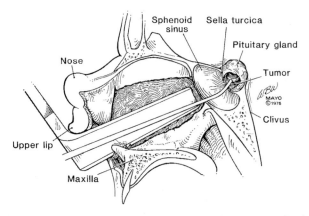

Figure 12.12 Transsphenoidal approach to the pituitary gland. After mobilizing the nasal septal cartilage and resecting a portion of ethmoid plate, a sublabial incision is made, and a sphenoid speculum is placed. Next, the floor of the sphenoid sinus and the floor of the sella turcica are traversed. Finally, the dural investment of the pituitary gland is incised, and the gland is exposed. This diagram illustrates a curette in place for removal of a pituitary adenoma.

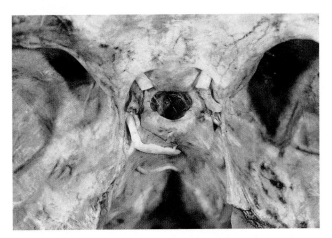

Figure 12.14 Superior view of the skull base, demonstrating an incidentally encountered primary empty sella. Normally in this view the upper surface of the pituitary gland would be visible through the diaphragmatic aperture, but here the sella appears empty. Only rarely is primary empty sella syndrome symptomatic. This specimen is from a 57-year-old obese diabetic woman.

and traction deformation of the pituitary stalk may cause mild to moderate hypopituitarism and hyperprolactinemia, respectively.

Vasculature

Vascular structures of major surgical significance abound in the sellar region. The paired cavernous sinuses are situated on either side of the sella and, in part, lie lateral and superior to the sphenoid sinuses (Figures 12.8–12.11). Each cavernous sinus is partially invested by dura of the middle fossa, as well as by thin bony walls of the sphenoid sinus. Venous drainage to the sinuses comes from a number of sources, including the eye (superior ophthalmic vein), brain (inferior and middle cerebral veins), and sphenoparietal sinus. Communication between right and left cavernous sinuses takes place through intercavernous sinuses bordering the anterior and posterior aspects of the sella (22). The complex thus forms a venous ring around the sella and its contents. Additional intercavernous sinuses are located along the ventral surface of the pituitary. The cavernous sinuses proper contain, in addition to their content of venous sinuses, a number of vital neurovascular structures (23,24). These include the cavernous segments of the internal carotid arteries and segments of cranial nerves III (oculomotor), IV (trochlear), V (trigeminal), and VI (abducens) (Figures 12.8–12.9). Delicate areolar tissue fills the interstices between venous channels, arteries, and nerves. The location of the horizontal portions of the internal carotid arteries within the cavernous sinuses varies, not only from person to person but from left to right. As a result, the carotids may lie immediately adjacent to the sella, in which case they may create a surgical risk (19) (Figures 12.8–12.9). Furthermore, the anterior portions of the carotids may indent the sphenoid bone and thus be separated from the cavity itself by as little as 1 mm of bone (15). Several branches of the internal carotid artery arise within the cavernous sinus, including the meningohypophysial trunk (the largest intracavernous branch), the artery of the inferior cavernous sinus, and small capsular branches (23,24). The meningohypophysial trunk gives rise to several vessels, one of which, the inferior hypophysial artery, supplies the posterior or neural lobe and the pituitary capsule.

Given their location, the cavernous sinuses may be directly involved by pituitary tumors. For example, extension of an invasive adenoma into the cavernous sinuses may produce neuropathies of cranial nerves III through VI (Figure 12.9), including ptosis, facial pain, or diplopia.

The principal arterial supply of the pituitary originates in two branches of the internal carotids: the superior and inferior hypophysial arteries (25,26) (Figure 12.15). A single superior hypophysial artery springs from each carotid shortly after its entry into the cranial cavity and promptly divides into posterior and anterior branches, each of which anastomoses with the corresponding branch from the

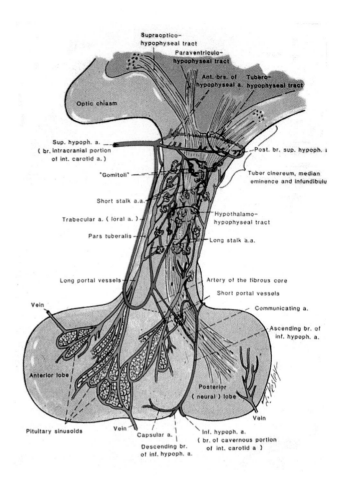

Figure 12.15 Diagrammatic representation of the vasculature of the pituitary gland. The superior and inferior hypophysial arteries and branches of the internal carotid arteries comprise the major blood supply of the gland. Small terminal branches of the superior and inferior hypophysial arteries give rise to tangled capillary loops termed gomitoli, which drain into portal vessels. The latter traverse the length of the stalk and terminate as a capillary bed in the anteior lobe. The anterior pituitary thus receives the majority of its blood supply not from arteries but from the portal system. The portal system forms a vital link between the hypothalamus and the pituitary gland.

opposite side to form an arterial ring around the upper pituitary stalk. The anterior branches give rise to trabecular or loral arteries, which descend on the upper surface of the anterior lobe, course toward the pituitary stalk, and terminate in long stalk arteries along the pars tuberalis. In their brief course along the anterior lobe, trabecular arteries each give rise to a small artery of the fibrous core (25). The posterior and anterior branches of the superior hypophysial arteries are also the source of short stalk arteries, which penetrate the superior aspect of the pituitary stalk to run upward or downward within it. In contrast to the superior hypophysial arteries, the inferior branches originate from the meningohypophysial trunks within the cavernous sinuses. They contact the inferolateral portions of the gland and bifurcate into medial and lateral branches that anastomose with their opposite counterparts to form an

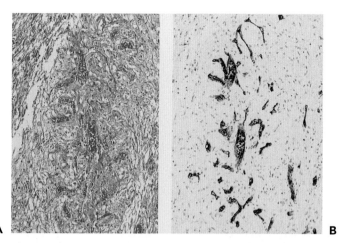

Figure 12.16 Gomitoli, tortuous capillary loops surrounding a central arteriole in the upper portion of the pituitary stalk (**A**) (H&E, original magnification ×100). The complex vascularity of the gomitoli is highlighted by staining with *Ulex europeus* lectin (**B**) (immunostain, original magnification ×100).

arterial circle about the posterior lobe. Thus, branches of the inferior hypophysial arteries supply primarily the posterior lobe and lower portion of the stalk, contributing only small capsular branches to the periphery of the anterior lobe (27). Although many of the arterial branches in the pituitary stalk and infundibulum form arterioles and capillaries, some give rise to unique vascular complexes termed gomitoli (Figures 12.15–12.16). These "balls of thread" consist of a central artery surrounded by a glomeruloid tangle of capillaries. The transition from central arteries to the capillaries is via short specialized arterioles endowed with thick smooth muscle sphincters that serve to regulate blood flow. The mixture of periarteriolar capillaries drains into an extensive pampiniform network, the portal system, which envelopes the stalk (Figures 12.2, 12.15).

The hypophysial portal system, the critical link between hypothalamus and pituitary, takes its origin from the capillary plexus of the median eminence and stalk, which itself is derived from terminal ramifications of the superior and inferior hypophysial arteries (22). The capillary plexus in the median eminence and superior stalk, the site of uptake of hypophysiotrophic factors, drains into the long portal vessels that course along the surface of the stalk to supply the majority (90%) of the anterior lobe, whereas the smaller capillary plexus in the lower stalk gives rise to the short portal vessels that descend into its central portion, including that bordering the posterior lobe (27,28). Distally, the portal system communicates with a delicate capillary network in the anterior lobe, which carries hypophysiotrophic factors into the pituitary and conveys anterior lobe hormones to the general circulation (Figure 12.17).

Venous outflow of the pituitary is via collecting vessels that drain into the subhypophysial sinus, cavernous sinus, and superior circular sinus (26).

There is considerable variability in the vascular anatomy of the pituitary. Aside from a minor direct arterial supply via capsular branches of the inferior hypophysial arteries, the majority of the anterior lobe's circulation is venous, originating from the portal vessels (25,26). In contrast to that of the anterior lobe, the blood supply of the posterior lobe is direct and arterial, a characteristic that explains the predilection of metastatic carcinomas for the neural lobe.

PHYSIOLOGY AND HISTOLOGY

Hypothalamus

The pituitary is known to be under significant hypothalamic control. In fact, the pituitary and the hypothalamus form a complex neurohormonal circuit, a vital element for maintainance of a normal endocrine status. Weighing approximately 5 g and forming the walls and floor of the inferior third ventricle, the hypothalamus lies above the

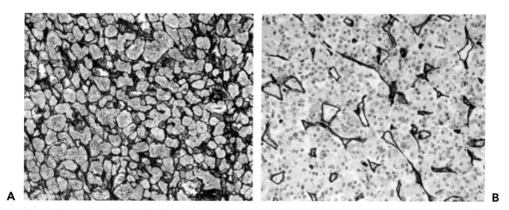

Figure 12.17 Adenohypophysis. **A.** The intricate capillary and connective tissue network outlined in reticulin stain. The reticulin stain is invaluable in the evaluation of pituitary adenomas, which are largely devoid of reticulin, whereas the surrounding normal gland retains it (Wilder reticulin, original magnification ×40). **B.** The capillary endothelium of the anterior lobe capillary network stains strongly for CD31 (immunostain ×100).

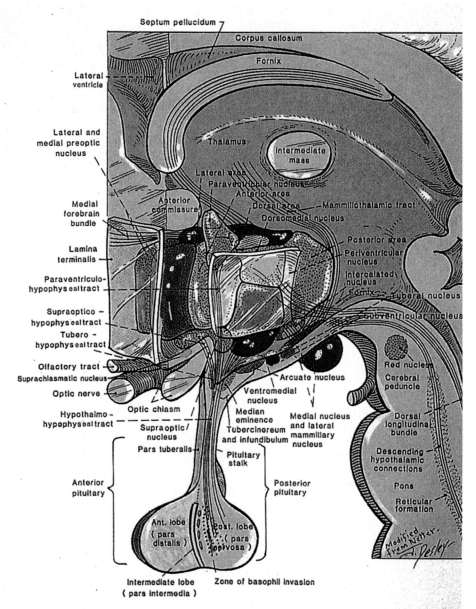

Septum pellucidum

Corpus callosum

Fornix

Lateral ventricle

Lateral and medial preoptic nucleus

Thalamus

Intermediate mass

Medial forebrain bundle

Lateral area
Paraventricular nucleus
Anterior area
Anterior commissure
Dorsal area
Dorsomedial nucleus

Mammillothalamic tract

Lamina terminalis

Posterior area
Periventricular nucleus
Intercalated nucleus
Fornix
Tuberal nucleus

Paraventriculo-hypophyseal tract

Supraoptico-hypophyseal tract
Tubero-hypophyseal tract

Subventricular nucleus

Olfactory tract
Suprachiasmatic nucleus
Optic nerve

Arcuate nucleus

Red nuclei
Cerebral peduncle

Ventromedial nucleus

Hypothalmo-hypophyseal tract
Optic chiasm
Supraoptic nucleus
Pars tuberalis

Median eminence
Tubercinereum and infundibulum

Medial nucleus and lateral mammillary nucleus

Dorsal longitudinal bundle

Pituitary stalk

Descending hypothalamic connections

Pons

Anterior pituitary

Posterior pituitary

Reticular formation

Ant. lobe (pars distalis)
Post. lobe (pars optvosa)

Modified from Netter.

Intermediate lobe (pars intermedia)
Zone of basophil invasion

Figure 12.18 A diagrammatic representation of the hypothalamic nuclei, showing the supraoptico-hypophysial and paraventriculohypophysial tracts, as well as the tuberohypophysial tract. The former carry vasopressin and oxytocin along axons to the posterior lobe, whereas the latter carries hypothalamic releasing and inhibiting hormones to the median eminence, where they enter the portal system for transport to the anterior lobe.

pituitary to which it is connected by the pituitary stalk (Figures 12.5–12.7, 12.18–12.19). As the name suggests, the hypothalamus lies inferior to the thalamus. Although at first glance it appears poorly demarcated, the hypothalamus is bordered anteriorly by the anterior commissure, lamina terminalis, and optic chiasm; posteriorly and superiorly by the midbrain tegmentum and mamillary bodies; dorsally by the hypothalamic sulcus; and laterally by subthalamic nuclei (29,30). The region consists of several ill-defined but functionally related neuronal nuclei (Figures 12.18–12.21). Afferent and efferent connections bring these nuclei into contact with nearby as well as remote portions of the central nervous system, including other diencephalic structures, the cerebrum, brain stem, and spinal cord. Two major and

distinct hypothalamohypophysial secretory systems are recognized. One consists of the supraoptic and paraventricular nuclei and their projections to the posterior lobe (supraopticohypophysial and paraventriculohypophysial tracts); the other is composed mainly of nuclei of the tuberal region, the funnel-shaped floor of the third ventricle, and their processes terminating in the median eminence (tuberohypophysial tract) (Figure 12.18).

The supraoptic nuclei are located superior to the optic tracts, whereas the wedge-shaped paraventricular nuclei lie ventromedial to the fornix and abut the walls of the third ventricle (Figure 12.19). Due to their predominant composition of large neurons measuring up to 25 μm, these are termed magnocellular nuclei (Figure 12.20). Each contains

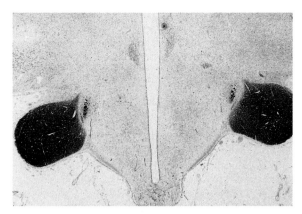

Figure 12.19 Coronal whole-mount section through the hypothalamus and third ventricle. The paraventricular nuclei are visible as darkly staining areas beneath the ependyma of the third ventricle (*upper field*), whereas the supraoptic nuclei lie above the heavily myelinated optic tracts. The arcuate nucleus lies inferior to the base of the third ventricle (cresyl violet).

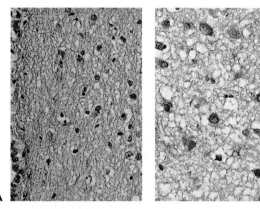

Figure 12.21 Periventricular nucleus. **A.** Lying beneath the ependyma of the third ventricle (bottom left), this ill-defined nucleus is composed of small nerve cell bodies (H&E, original magnification ×63). **B.** Its constituent neurons stain for CRH, a tropic hormone that exerts its effect on corticotrophs in the anterior lobe (immunostain, original magnification ×100).

vasopressin- and oxytocin-producing neurons, but only one hormone is produced by a given neuron. Their axons form the supraopticohypophysial and paraventriculohypophysial tracts, which carry vasopressin and oxytocin (the two so-called neurohypophysial hormones), as well as their respective carrier proteins, the neurophysins, to the posterior lobe of the pituitary gland. Oxytocin and vasopressin, both nonapeptides, are synthesized as 20-kDa prohormones, which include in their structure the cysteine-rich neurophysin carrier proteins, neurophysin I and neurophysin II, respectively. The precursor molecules are packaged into secretory granules within the Golgi apparatus and transported by axoplasmic flow within unmyelinated axons to nerve terminals in the posterior pituitary lobe, where they are released into the circulation by a calcium-dependent exocytosis (31). Large intra-axonal accumulations of these hormones, named Herring bodies, are often

visible by light microscopy as round, granular structures that appear eosinophilic on hematoxylin and eosin (H&E) sections (Figure 12.22). In transit from the hypothalamus to the posterior lobe, prohormones undergo extensive processing and cleavage to form the final products, vasopressin and oxytocin. Although these hormones differ by only two amino acids, oxytocin exhibits virtually no antidiuretic activity, and vasopressin has negligible oxytocic effect. Oxytocin mediates the "milk let-down reflex" by stimulating contraction of myoepithelial cells surrounding terminal mammary lobules. In addition, it serves a role in parturition, binding, and facilitating contraction in the final stages of parturition. The major physiologic role of vasopressin, also called antidiuretic hormone (ADH), is the formation of hypertonic urine. Acting via cyclic adenosine

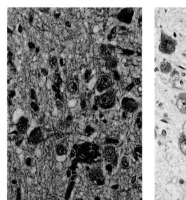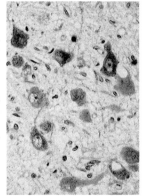

Figure 12.20 Paraventricular nucleus of the hypothalamus. **A.** Its high degree of vascularity is a characteristic of magnocellular nuclei (H&E, original magnification ×100). **B.** The nerve cell bodies stain positively for vasopressin (immunostain, original magnification ×100).

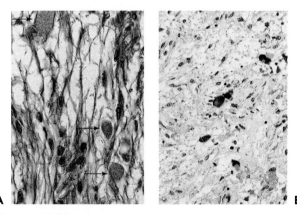

Figure 12.22 Pituitary stalk. Axonal swellings termed Herring bodies characterize its axons. **A.** They are distinguished by their ovoid shape and granular character on H&E [*upper left and lower right; arrows*]. Herring bodies represent intra-axonal accumulations of oxytocin- and vasopressin-containing granules en route to the posterior lobe (H&E, original magnification ×100). **B.** Herring bodies staining for vasopressin (immunostain, original magnification ×100).

monophosphate, vasopressin increases the water permeability of renal collecting ducts, allowing the hypotonic intraductal fluid to equilibrate with the hypertonic fluid in the medullary interstitium. The results are concentrated urine and conservation of body water. Damage to the neurohypophysis from head trauma, surgery, inflammatory processes, or neoplasms may destroy vasopressin-producing neurons and cause diabetes insipidus.

The second component of the hypothalamohypophysial system is the tuberoinfundibular tract. Its fibers originate in a number of hypothalamic nuclei lying within the walls of the inferior third ventricle and tuberal region (29) (Figures 12.18–12.19, 12.21). Products of these nuclei, targeted for the anterior pituitary, consist of releasing and inhibiting hormones. Unlike the magnocellular neurons of the supraoptic and paraventricular nuclei, these are small neurons and for this reason are termed parvicellular neurons (Figure 12.21). Their processes project to the median eminence, a highly vascular zone, located in the posterior proximal portion of the pituitary stalk. Here, the hypothalamic hormones are released into the first portion of the portal system for transport to the anterior lobe. Ultrastructurally, the median eminence consists of closely packed nerve terminals containing membrane-bound neurosecretory granules. Because the terminals lie in close proximity to the fenestrated capillaries that form the origin of the portal system, the overall anatomic arrangement permits ready entry of hypothalamic releasing and inhibiting hormones and perhaps other modulators into the portal system and consequently the anterior lobe. The hypothalamic hormones include five peptide hormones: corticotropin-releasing hormone (CRH), growth hormone-releasing hormone (GHRH), somatostatin, gonadotropin-releasing hormone (GnRH or LHRH), and thyrotropin-releasing hormone (TRH). The sites of synthesis of the various hypothalamic hormones,

their characteristics, and target cells are summarized in Tables 12.1 and 12.2. In addition to these hormones, several bioactive substances produced in the hypothalamus participate in the regulation of anterior pituitary hormone secretion. The most significant one is dopamine, which has a tonic inhibitory control of pituitary lactotrophs (32).

Adenohypophysis

The pituitary is a tan to brown, bean-shaped structure varying in weight from 500 to 700 mg (Figure 12.1). An average-sized gland of 600 mg measures about $13 \times 10 \times 6$ mm. Generally, the weight of the female pituitary is greater than that of the male (33). Among females, the gland is smaller in nulliparas than in multiparas. In pregnancy the gland enlarges significantly (up to 30%) primarily as a result of lactotroph cell hyperplasia (33,34). The anterior lobe comprises 80% of the pituitary and includes the pars distalis, intermedia, and tuberalis. The body and stalk of the gland are surrounded by a delicate capsule derived from the meninges (35). Staining characteristics roughly divide the pars distalis into a central mucoid wedge and two lateral wings, zones best visualized in coronal and horizontal sections.

By light microscopy, the cells of the anterior lobe show variation, not only in size and shape but also in their histochemical staining characteristics (Figure 12.23–12.24). They are arranged in nests, cords, and small acini bounded by an interlacing capillary network that is best seen on reticulin stain (see Figure 12.17). This architectural pattern, altered in hyperplasia and conspicuously absent in adenomas, is of considerable diagnostic significance. The pars intermedia, poorly developed in humans, consists in large part of epithelium-lined spaces containing periodic acid-Schiff (PAS)-positive colloid; the constituent cells are ciliated, goblet, and endocrine; the last show variable immunoreactivity

---

TABLE 12.1

PITUITARY HORMONES AND HYPOTHALAMIC STIMULATORY AND INHIBITORY HORMONES

	Hypothalamic Hormone	
Affected Pituitary Hormone	**Stimulatory**	**Inhibitory**
Growth hormone (GH)	Growth hormone-releasing hormone (GHRH)	Somatostatin
Prolactin (PRL)	Thyrotropin-releasing hormone (TRH) Vasoactive intestinal peptide (VIP)	Dopamine
Adrenocorticotropin (ACTH)	Corticotropin-releasing hormone (CRH) Arginine vasopressin (AVP)	?
Follicle-stimulating hormone (FSH) Luteinizing hormone (LH)	Gonadotropin-releasing hormone (GnRH)	?
Thyroid-stimulating hormone (TSH)	Thyrotropin-releasing hormone (TRH)	Somatostatin

TABLE 12.2

MAJOR HYPOTHALAMIC HORMONES: THEIR COMPOSITION AND LOCALIZATION

Hormone	Abbreviations	Hypothalamic Sites	Extrahypothalamic Sites
Growth hormone-releasing hormone	GHRH	Arcuate nucleus	?
Thyrotopin-releasing hormone	TRH	Widely distributed in CNS with concentration in ventromedial, dorsal, and paraventricular nuclei, particularly on left	Brain and spinal cord, fetal pancreatic islet cells, intestine neuroendocrine cells
Gonadotropin-releasing hormone or luteinizing hormone-releasing hormone	GnRH or LHRH	Widespread distribution with concentration in the arcuate, ventromedial, dorsal, and paraventricular nuclei	Brain (limbic system), breast (lactation), placenta
Corticotropin-releasing hormone	CRH	Periventricular, medial paraventricular nuclei; co-localized with arginine vasopressin	Brain (cerebral cortex, limbic system, brain stem, spinal cord)
Somatostatin or Growth hormone-release inhibiting hormone		Periventricular nucleus, paraventricular (parvocellular neurons), arcuate nuclei	Brain, retina, peripheral nervous system, pancreatic islet cells, intestinal neuroendocrine cells, thyroid, placenta
Dopamine		Arcuate nucleus	Brain, GI tract
Arginine vasopressin	AVP	Paraventricular, supraoptic nuclei	Brain
Oxytocin	OT	Paraventricular, supraoptic nuclei	Brain

for pituitary hormones (36) (Figure 12.25). Incidental Rathke's cleft remnants, the vast majority of which are microscopic in size, are present in 30% of pituitaries; the majority of them are located in the intermediate lobe (37).

In H&E-stained sections, three principal cell types are identified in the normal anterior lobe: acidophils (40%), basophils (10%), and chromophobes (50%) (Figures 12.23–12.24). The designations reflect their staining affinities for acidic and basic dyes, with the chromophobic cells lacking affinity for either. These reactivities form the basis of an outdated classification of pituitary adenomas that offers little in specifying their hormone content or endocrine function. On the other hand, advances in immunohistochemistry permit morphologic and functional correlation (Figure 12.26). Numerous cells in the central or mucoid wedge are basophilic and stain strongly via the PAS method. Such cells produce adrenocorticotropin (ACTH) and glycoprotein hormones (LH, FSH, TSH). In contrast, most cells in the lateral wings are acidophilic and are engaged either in growth hormone (GH) or, less frequently, in prolactin (PRL) production. The essential morphologic features of the five principal cell types and the biochemical characteristics of the six hormones of the anterior pituitary are summarized in Table 12.3. Their ultrastructural features are presented in Table 12.4.

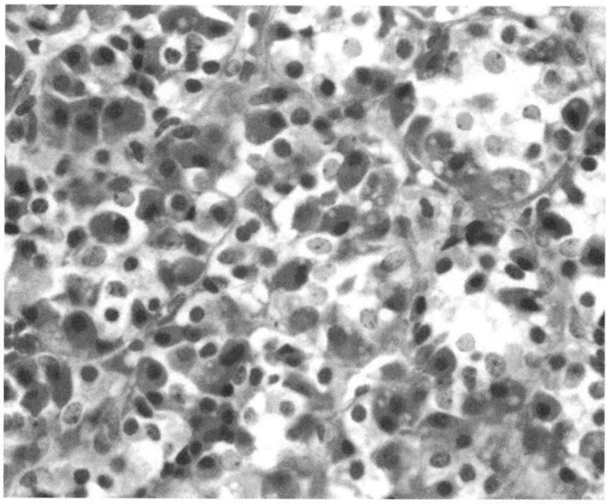

Figure 12.23 Anterior lobe. An H&E-stained section shows chromophobic, acidophilic, and basophilic cells. Acidophils are most numerous in the lateral wings, whereas basophils are found in greatest number in the central or mucoid wedge. The different cell types are arranged in acinar formations that can be highlighted by reticulin stain (see Figure 12.17) (original magnification ×200).

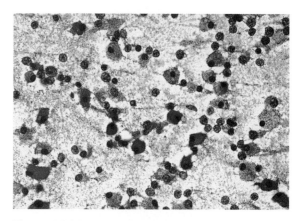

Figure 12.24 H&E-stained cytologic smear of the normal anterior lobe, demonstrating acidophils, chromophobes, and basophils. Delicate nuclei, inconspicuous nucleoli, and variable cytoplasmic staining characterize normal cells and permit their distinction from adenoma cells (original magnification ×100).

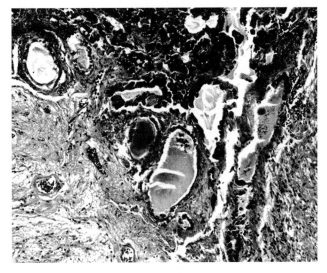

Figure 12.25 Intermediate lobe remnant. Such cysts are lined by a single layer of cuboidal to columnar epithelium that may be nonciliated, ciliated, mucin-producing, or granulated. The cyst contains an eosinophilic colloid (H&E, original magnification ×100).

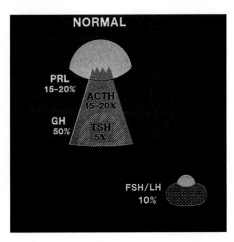

Figure 12.26 Preferential localization and relative frequency of functional anterior lobe cell types in the normal pituitary gland. Note that gonadotrophs (LH/FSH cells), represented in the small gland (*lower right*), are distributed diffusely and show no preferential localization.

TABLE 12.3

THE NORMAL ANTERIOR PITUITARY: MORPHOLOGIC AND FUNCTIONAL FEATURES OF SECRETORY CELLS

Cell Type	Product	Location	Percentage of Cells	Histochemical Staining[a]	Immunoperoxidase Staining
Somatotroph[b]	Growth hormone (GH); 21,000 dalton polypeptide	Lateral wings	50	Acidophilic; PAS (−)	GH
Lactotroph[b]	Prolactin (PRL); 23,500 dalton polypeptide	Resting cells— generalized; Secreting cells— postero-lateral wings	15 to 20	Acidophilic; PAS (−)	PRL
Corticotroph	Adrenocorticotrophic hormone (ACTH); 4,507 dalton polypeptide	Mucoid wedge	15 to 20	Basophilic; PAS and lead hematoxylin (+)	ACTH, β-LPH, MSH, endorphin, enkephalin
Gonadotroph	Follicle stimulating & luteinizing hormone (FSH & LH); 35,100 and 28,260 dalton glycoprotein	Generalized	10	Basophilic; PAS, lead hematoxylin, aldehyde fuchsin, and aldehyde thionine (+)	FSH and LH[c]
Thyrotroph	Thyrotrophic hormone (TSH); 28,000 dalton glycoprotein	Anterior mucoid wedge	< 5	Same as for gonadotroph	TSH

[a] The tinctorial characteristics of normal pituitary cells depend on adequate cytoplasmic granulae storage. If sparsely granulated, cells that are otherwise functional may appear nonreactive or "chromophobic."
[b] Rare acidophillic stem cells (presumed somatotroph and lactotroph precursor cells producing both GH and PRL) are present in the normal pituitary.
[c] Many gonadotrophs are capable of producing both FSH and LH, although immunohistochemical and ultrastructural evidence suggests that some gonadotrophs may produce only one hormone.

TABLE 12.4
THE NORMAL PITUITARY: ULTRASTRUCTURAL FEATURES

Cell Type	Granularity	Cell Size and Shape	Nucleus	Cytoplasm	Golgi Complex	Rough Endoplasmic Reticulum	Granules
Somatotroph Densely granulated (resting phase)	+++, ++++	Medium, spherical oval	Spherical and central, with prominent nucleoli	Lucent	+	+	Abundant; dense, spherical; closely apposed limiting membrane; no exocytosis; 350 to 600 nm (range 250 to 600 nm)
Somatotroph Sparsely granulated (secretory phase)	+, ++	Medium, spherical oval	Irregular	Lucent	+++	+++ Peripherally disposed	Sparse; dense, spherical; closely apposed limiting membrane; no exocytosis; 350 to 600 nm (range 250 to 600 nm)
Lactotroph Densely granulated (resting phase)	+++, ++++	Large, polyhedral-elongate	Oval-elongate	Lucent	+	++	Abundant, dense, spherical-oval, irregular; occasional exocytosis; 500 to 800 nm
Lactotroph Sparsely granulated (secretory phase)	+, ++	Medium, polyhedral-elongate	Oval	Lucent	+++, ++++ Juxtanuclear	++++ "Nebenkern" formation	Sparse; dense, irregular; frequent normal and misplaced exocytosis 200 to 350 nm
Corticotroph	++, +++	Medium, oval-polygonal	Spherical, eccentric	Electron-dense; cytoplasmic type I microfilaments; large lysosomes	++	++, +++ Dispersed, slightly dilated	Variable density, spherical-irregular; frequently peripheral; no exocytosis; 300 to 350 nm (range 250 to 700 nm, rarely 1,000 nm)
Gonadotroph	++	Medium, oval	Spherical, eccentric	Lucent	++, +++ Prominent, globular	++, +++ Stacked or dispersed and slightly dilated	Dense, spherical; no exocytosis; 250 to 400 nm;
Thyrotroph	+, ++	Medium, polygonal	Spherical, eccentric	Lucent; scattered lysosomes	++, +++ Globular, with numerous vesicles	+++ Short dispersed profiles	Dense, spherical; frequently peripheral; no exocytosis; 150 nm

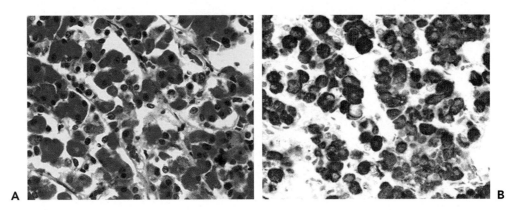

Figure 12.27 Somatotrophs. **A.** By H&E stain, somatotrophs are medium-sized cells with abundant, eosinophilic and granular cytoplasm GH. Somatotrophs comprise 50% of anterior lobe cells (original magnification ×200). **B.** The strong staining reaction is a reflection of the numerous secretory granules present at the ultrastructural level (see Figure 12.28) (immunostain, original magnification ×200).

Somatotroph cells. Somatotrophs, or GH cells, occur in greatest density in the lateral wings and comprise approximately 50% of all adenohypophysial cells. A minority of somatotroph cells are scattered throughout the median portion of the gland. They are medium-sized, ovoid cells with round, centrally located nuclei, relatively prominent nucleoli, and with abundant acidophilic granules (Figure 12.27). Immunohistochemical stains for GH shows strong and diffuse cytoplasm staining, consistent with the numerous secretory granules present at the ultrastructural level (Figures 12.27–12.28).Somatotroph cells are rather stable during life, and their number, morphology, and immunoreactivity are unchanged by age.

The product of GH cells has extensive effects by direct action of GH and actions through mediators of hepatic origin called somatomedins (insulin-like growth factor-I, or IGF-1) (32). Growth hormone functions as the major promotor of growth but also in several other metabolic pathways, including glucose, insulin, and fatty acid. The pulsatile secretion of GH from the anterior lobe is under the control of the two hypothalamic regulatory hormones: growth hormone releasing hormone (GHRH) and somatostatin

(growth hormone-release inhibiting hormone). The GHRH controls GH synthesis by regulating transcription of GH mRNA via control of cAMP levels. Somatostatin appears to determine the timing and amplitude of GH pulses but has no effect on GH synthesis. Hypersecretion of GH in children causes gigantism, whereas its overproduction in adults leads to acromegaly.

Lactotroph cells. Lactotrophs, or PRL cells, comprise approximately 20% of anterior pituitary cells and are concentrated in the posterior portions of the lateral wings. Histologically, they appear either acidophilic (densely granulated) or chromophobic (sparsely granulated). Chromophobic cells are more numerous, are located predominantly in the posterior lateral wings, possess elongate processes, and, despite an abundance of endoplasmic reticulum and well-developed Golgi complexes, contain relatively few cytoplasmic granules (Figures 12.29–12.30, and Table 12.4). Densely granulated lactotrophs are thought to represent a storage phase, whereas sparsely granulated cells are engaged in active secretion. A characteristic pattern of PRL staining of lactotrophs by immunohistochemistry, the so-called "Golgi pattern," is the presence of paranuclear staining corresponding to PRL in the Golgi apparatus (Figure 12.29).

With the exception of pregnancy and lactation, there is no significant difference in PRL cell number between males and females. The doubling in volume of the pituitary during pregnancy is due to striking hyperplasia as well as hypertrophy of chromophobic lactotrophs, termed pregnancy cells. They persist until shortly after delivery or the termination of lactation (33,34). Prolactin cell hyperplasia also may accompany estrogen administration and hypothyroidism (32). The existence of mammosomatotrophs, cells engaged in PRL and GH production and possessing unique ultrastructural features, attests to the existence of a histogenetic relationship between PRL and GH cells (38).

Prolactin secretion is unique among the anterior pituitary hormones in that it is under tonic hypothalamic

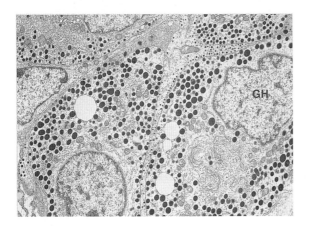

Figure 12.28 Densely granulated somatotrophs (GH cells) showing prominent Golgi and numerous 200- to 500-nm secretory granules (original magnification ×11,700).

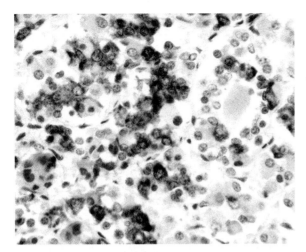

Figure 12.29 Lactotrophs. Lactotrophs comprise 15% to 20% of anterior lobe cells. The majority are sparsely granulated, angular cells with processes that may wrap around adjacent cells. Many lactotrophs in this field show paranuclear staining, a pattern corresponding to PRL in the Golgi apparatus (PRL immunostain, original magnification ×100).

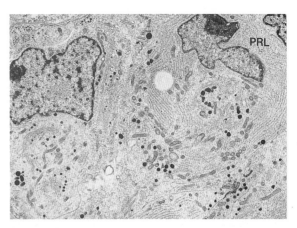

Figure 12.30 Sparsely granulated PRL cell. Note the abundant cisternae of rough endoplasmic reticulum and the prominent Golgi complex containing pleomorphic developing granules. Mature PRL granules range in size from 200 to 350 nm (original magnification ×8,700).

inhibition by dopamine (hypothalamic PRL-inhibitory factor, or PIF) produced by tuberoinfundibular dopamine neurons. Several prolactin-releasing factors participate in PRL secretion, including TRH and vasoactive intestinal peptide (VIP). A fragment of GnRH also has been shown to inhibit PRL release. Prolactin synthesis is also regulated by effects of estrogen on PRL gene expression. Disruption of the hypothalamus or the hypothalamic–hypophysial stalk may impede dopamine delivery to the anterior lobe, causing hyperprolactinemia, a phenomenon termed "stalk effect." Common situations are any space-occupying sellar or parasellar mass (e.g., pituitary macroadenoma, Rathke's cleft cyst, craniopharyngioma, or glioma) that compresses the pituitary stalk. The most striking example of stalk effect is the hyperprolactinemia that follows surgical transection of the stalk, a practice now obsolete but once used in the past for the treatment of metastatic breast cancer (39).

Prolactin acts through specific prolactin receptors in multiple tissues, including breast, liver, ovary, testis, and prostate. The main site of PRL action is in the breast, where it stimulates the formation of casein, lactalbumin, lipids, and carbohydrates, all essential components of breast milk. During pregnancy, high levels of estrogen, progesterone, placental lactogen, and PRL induce acinar development and promote milk formation. As previously noted, milk secretion is under the control of oxytocin, a potent stimulator of myoepithelial cell contraction in breast tissue.

Corticotroph cells. Corticotrophs, or ACTH cells, comprise 15% to 20% of adenohypophysial cells and are most numerous in the mid- and posterior portions of the mucoid wedge (Figure 12.26). Histologically, corticotroph cells are polygonal, medium- to large-sized, and basophilic (Figure 12.31). A paranuclear vacuole that corresponds to one or several lysosomal structures at the ultrastructural level is

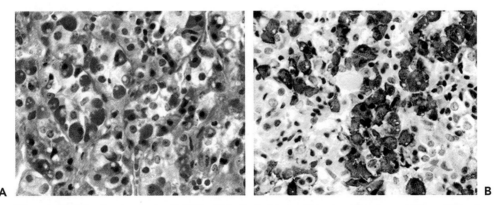

Figure 12.31 Corticotrophs (ACTH cells). **A.** Corticotrophs comprise about 15% to 20% of anterior lobe cells and are mainly located in the mucoid wedge. By H&E stain, corticotrophs are basophilic cells with ovoid to polyhedral shape and central nucleus. Many have a small vacuole near the nucleus, representing a massive lysosome (original magnification ×200). **B.** Note the clustering of cells, a characteristic feature of corticotrophs (ACTH immunostain, original magnification ×200).

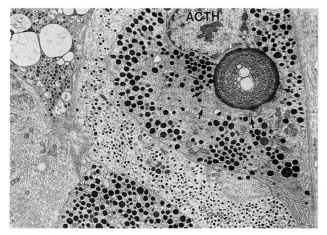

Figure 12.32 Corticotroph (ACTH cell). The cell contains the typical large lysosome and spherical to slightly pleomorphic and variably electron-dense secretory granules measuring 150 to 450 nm. Bundles of intermediate filaments (*arrows*) are a regular feature of corticotrophs. The adjacent cells with small granules are likely TSH cells (original magnification ×8,250).

typically seen in the cytoplasm (Figure 12.32) (36,40). Corticotroph cells are strong PAS positive due to a carbohydrate moiety contained in proopiomelanocortin (POMC), the precursor molecule of ACTH. In immunostained preparations, corticotrophs may be shown to contain not only ACTH (Figure 12.31) but also other POMC derivatives, including β-lipotropin (β-LPH), melanocyte-stimulating hormone (MSH), endorphin, and enkephalin. Perinuclear bundles of cytokeratin filaments are also a characteristic feature of ACTH cells (Table 12.4). Under conditions of glucocorticoid excess, either exogenous or endogenous, corticotrophs accumulate cytokeratin as a manifestation of Crooke's hyaline change (Figures 12.33–12.34).

Adrenocorticotropin (ACTH), the principal product of corticotrophs, stimulates the adrenal cortex to secrete glucocorticoids, mineralocorticoids, and androgens (32). It plays a critical role in both the transport of amino acids and glucose into muscle, as well as the stimulation of insulin release from the pancreas. Pituitary ACTH secretion is

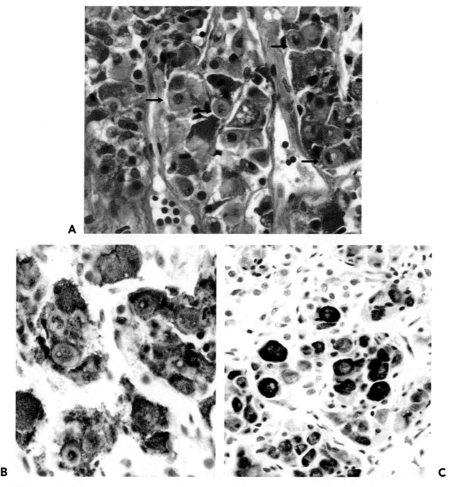

Figure 12.33 Crooke's hyaline change. **A.** Crooke's cells (*arrows*) are characterized by a conspicuous eosinophilic perinuclear ring consisting of cytokeratin (H&E, original magnification ×100). **B.** ACTH stains show central displacement of the nucleus and organelles by filament accumulation (ACTH immunostain, original magnification ×100). **C.** Staining for cytokeratin show strong reactivity of the Crooke's cells (CC immunostain, original magnification ×100).

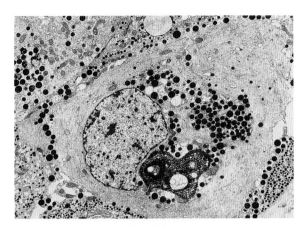

Figure 12.34 Crooke's cell. This electron micrograph of the pituitary adjacent to a corticotroph cell adenoma displays massive accumulation of cytokeratin filament. Secretory granules are displaced to the perinuclear zone or to the periphery of the cytoplasm. Note the large lysosome in the lower portion of the field (original magnification ×6,720).

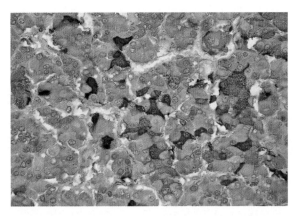

Figure 12.35 Thyrotroph (TSH cell). Thyrotrophs are medium-sized angulated cells with some demonstrating elongate processes. They comprise only about 5% of anterior lobe secretory cells and show strong TSH immunoreactivity (TSH immunostain, original magnification ×100).

regulated by hypothalamic corticotropin-releasing hormone (CRH) and arginine vasopressin (AVP). Adrenocorticotropin is part of a larger precursor molecule, proopiomelanocortin (POMC), which is enzymatically cleaved in the anterior pituitary into β-LPH and ACTH. In the intermediate lobe, ACTH is cleaved into melanocyte-stimulating hormone (MSH) and other ACTH-like peptides. Excess secretion of ACTH, such as occurs in Cushing's disease, leads to stereotypic abnormalities such as truncal obesity, hypertension, diabetes mellitus, amenorrhea, hirsutism, muscle atrophy, striae, impaired wound healing, and mental status changes. Hyperpigmentation also may occur in this setting and is due to the effects of MSH.

Thyrotroph cells. Thyrotrophs, or TSH cells, are located primarily in the anterior part of the mucoid wedge and comprise only 5% of adenohypophysial cells (41). They are medium sized and angular or elongate (Figures 12.35–12.36). Like corticotrophs, normal TSH cells are basophilic and are PAS positive (see Table 12.4 for ultrastructural features).

Thyroid-stimulating hormone (TSH, a glycoprotein hormone) binds to thyroid cells, inducing RNA and protein synthesis and thereby the production of thyroglobulin and thyroid hormones. Like the other two glycoprotein hormones of the pituitary [luteinizing hormone (LH) and follicle-stimulating hormone (FSH)], TSH consists of two noncovalently bound subunits, alpha (α) and beta (β). The α-subunit is common to all three glycoprotein hormones; the β-subunit is specific for each hormone and confers biological specificity. Secretion of TSH is regulated by both hypothalamic hormones and circulating thyroid hormones. Thyrotropin-releasing hormone (TRH) stimulates TSH release, while somatostatin and dopamine can inhibit TSH secretion. In the setting of primary hypothyroidism,

thyrotrophs undergo hypertrophy and hyperplasia. When excessive, the response may produce sufficient hypertrophy of the pituitary gland to mimic adenoma. Pituitary adenomas that elaborate TSH are rare; most occur in the setting of hypothyroidism (36), although a minority result in hyperthyroidism.

Gonadotroph cells. Gonadotrophs, or FSH and LH cells, comprise 10% of the adenohypophysis, show a strong affinity for both basic and PAS stains, and generally are evenly distributed throughout the anterior lobe. Immunohistochemical and ultrastructural studies have shown that FSH and LH may be produced in isolation or by the same cell (42) (Figures 12.37–12.38) (see Table 12.4 for ultrastructural features). In the daily practice of surgical pathology, monoclonal antibodies against the specific β-subunits of LH and FSH are universally applied. In addition, antibodies

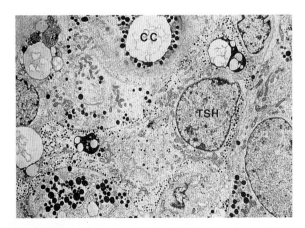

Figure 12.36 Thyrotroph (TSH cell). This micrograph of the normal anterior pituitary shows the characteristic elongate thyrotrophs, the large lysosomes frequently observed in cells of this type, and small (150-nm) peripherally located secretory granules. Part of a Crooke's cell (CC) is also shown (original magnification ×5,300).

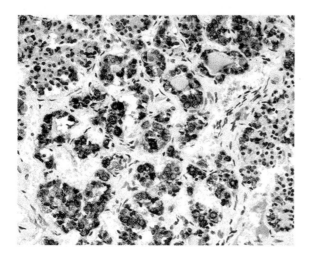

Figure 12.37 Gonadotroph (FSH/LH cell). Gonadotroph cells manufacture both LH and FSH. The paucity of strongly staining cells in this field reflects the fact that only 10% of anterior lobe secretory cells are gonadotrophs (FSH immunostain, original magnification ×100).

against the α-subunit of the glycoprotein pituitary hormones (LH, FSH, and TSH) is useful for determination of abnormal production and/or secretion of this subunit hormone.

Both LH and FSH play distinct but essential roles in the reproductive physiology of males and females. Secretion of these hormones from the gonadotroph cells is regulated by integration of the GnRH (LHRH) signal and feedback effects of gonadal steroids and the peptides inhibin, follistatin and activin (43). GnRH (LHRH) interacts with a membrane receptor to regulate both LH and FSH release and synthesis, and it is necessary for gonadotroph cells' function; gonadal steroids and peptides are ineffective alone in stimulating release. In the female, LH is required for ovulation and follicular luteinization. In males, it stimulates interstitial Leydig cells to produce testosterone.

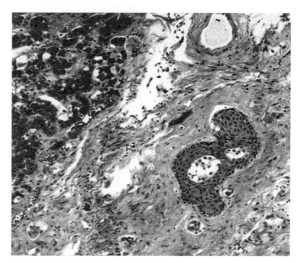

Figure 12.39 Anterior pituitary, pars tuberalis. Squamous metaplasia of secretory cells is a common feature of this portion of the gland.

Follicle-stimulating hormone promotes follicular development in the female, whereas in the male it induces Sertoli cells to produce an androgen-binding protein.

Par Tuberalis. The pars tuberalis, an upward extension of the anterior lobe along the pituitary stalk, is composed of normal acini of pituitary cells scattered among surface portal vessels. These cells often show immunoreactivity for ACTH, FSH, LH, and α-subunit. Although in functional terms they may or may not differ from similar cells in the pars distalis, these cells do show a distinct tendency to undergo squamous metaplasia (Figure 12.39) (44).

Follicles are not an uncommon feature of the normal anterior pituitary. Their functional constituent cells, termed follicular cells, appear to be derived in large part from various secretory cells (Figure 12.40). Ultrastructurally, they are

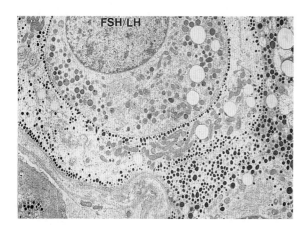

Figure 12.38 Gonadotroph (FSH/LH cell). The dull, low-contrast appearance of the cell is typical of gonadotrophs. Their spherical and slightly irregular secretory granules are characteristic; they have variable electron density and measure 250 to 400 nm. The cell process surrounding the gonadotroph likely belongs to a thyrotroph (original magnification ×8,250).

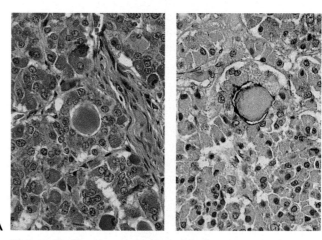

A   **B**

Figure 12.40 Anterior pituitary, follicle formation. **A.** Follicles, some containing a small quantity of colloid-like material, are commonly found in the anterior lobe (H&E, original magnification ×100). **B.** Follicles show prominent apical staining for epithelial membrane antigen (EMA) (EMA immunostain, original magnification ×100).

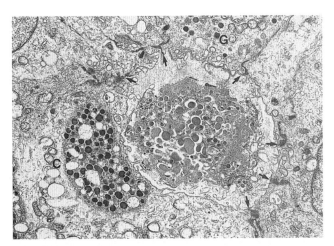

Figure 12.41 Electron micrograph of a pituitary follicle. This young follicle contains cell debris within its lumen. The gonadotroph (G), but not the corticotroph (C), is part of this follicle. Follicles are composed of granulated adenohypophysial cells that, through the formation of junctional complexes *(arrows)*, surround damaged adenohypophysial cells (original magnification ×12,600).

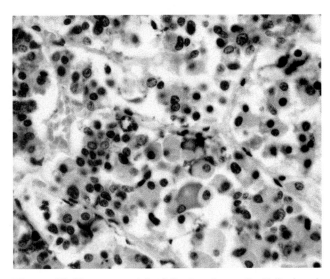

Figure 12.42 Anterior lobe folliculostellate cells. Folliculostellate cells comprise less than 5% of anterior lobe cells and are scattered throughout the pituitary, including the intermediate lobe zone. Folliculostellate cells staining for S-100 protein, GFAP, and vimentin (S-100 immunostain, original magnification ×100).

often poorly granulated or agranular and linked by apical junctional complexes. Within follicular lumina, one often finds cellular debris (Figure 12.41). The stimulus for follicle formation is therefore thought to be damage or rupture of anterior lobe secretory cells (45).

Folliculostellate cells. The folliculostellate cell is the sixth cellular element of the adenophypophysis, a specialized sustentacular-like cell that appears to have multiple functions related to phagocytosis and secretion of growth-factors (46,48). They comprise less than 5% of the anterior lobe cells, are scattered about the anterior lobe, and contribute to the formation of anterior lobe follicles and cysts of the intermediate lobe. They are readily identified by their reactivity for S-100 protein (Figure 12.42), and can also be identified by glial fibrillary acidic protein (GFAP) and vimentin. They participate in regulating the activity of anterior pituitary endocrine cells through the production of cytokines (such as interleukin-6, and leukemia inhibitory factor) and growth factors (including basic fibroblast growth factor and vascular endothelial growth factor) (48). Additionally, ultrastructural and immunohistochemical studies on human adenomatous and nonneoplastic pituitary folliculostellate cells suggest that they may represent an adult stem cell progenitor population (47,48).

Variation in Normal Morphology of the Adenohypophysis

A number of normal histologic variations in the pituitary gland may mimic clinically significant lesions. Examples include squamous cell nests in the pars tuberalis, basophil invasion of the posterior lobe, granular cell clusters and tumorlets of the stalk and neurohypophysis, and salivary gland rests.

Squamous cell nests show a definite predilection for the pars tuberalis; they have been found in up to 24% of autopsy cases, occur more commonly in elderly patients, and show no sex predilection (49). They arise through a process of metaplastic transformation from adenohypophysial cells, as evidenced by simultaneous expression of keratin and pituitary hormones, most often FSH, LH, or ACTH (44) (Figure 12.39). Because squamous metaplasia also may accompany foci of ischemic infarction in the anterior lobe, it appears to be an inherent property of pituitary secretory cells.

Basophil invasion, a finding more common in males and the elderly, may at first glance mimic an adenoma. It consists of corticotrophic basophils extending from the pars intermedia into the neurohypophysis (Figures 12.43–12.44). Similar to ordinary corticotrophs, these basophilic cells are immunoreactive for ACTH, β-LPH, endorphins, and other POMC derivatives; however, they contain few cytokeratin filaments and are less susceptible to Crooke's hyalinization in response to hypercortisolism (36).

Salivary gland rests appear as tubular glands upon the surface or in the substance of the neurohypophysis, often just posterior to the pars intermedia (Figure 12.45). They are composed of a single layer of cuboidal to columnar epithelium with basally oriented nuclei and finely granular, strongly PAS-positive cytoplasm. Salivary gland rests are often oncocytic. Their ultrastructural features include well-developed rough endoplasmic reticulum, secretory droplets, microvilli, and desmosomes, all of which support the contention that they are indeed salivary glands (50).

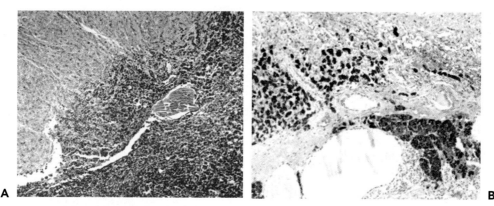

Figure 12.43   Basophil invasion. **A.** This subpopulation of corticotroph cells appears to infiltrate the substance of the posterior lobe (H&E, original magnification ×4). **B.** The invading cells are strongly immunoreactive for ACTH and other POMC derivate hormones (ACTH immunostain, original magnification ×40).]

Age-Related Changes of the Adenohypophysis

The cytology of the anterior pituitary varies with age. For instance, the late fetal or term pituitary gland shows PRL cell hyperplasia, a reflection of high maternal estrogen levels. Also, when compared with the adult pituitary, the prepubertal gland shows gonadotrophic cells to be poorly developed. In adults the pituitary undergoes several changes with increasing age (51,52).

With few exceptions, the main one being pregnancy, the gland weight remains stable throughout life, decreasing only slightly in the elderly due to anterior lobe atrophy. Pregnancy results in a doubling of the size of the pituitary due to gradual increase in large chromophobic PRL cells ("pregnancy cells") (53,54) (Figure 12.46). The increase in PRL-producing cells during pregnancy appears to result not only from proliferation of PRL cells but also from recruitment of GH cells to PRL production (55). This increase in PRL-producing cells, in large part a hyperplasia, gradually disappears within months after delivery or abortion. The process is often incomplete; hence, the pituitaries of

multiparas are larger than those of women who were never pregnant. Pregnancy also results in a significant decrease of gonadotropin immunoreactivity, a reflection of the production of gonadotropic hormones by the placenta.

The effects of age on the cellular contents of several pituitary hormones has been studied. Specifically, GH and PRL cells have been shown to undergo no significant decrease in number, granularity, distribution, or immunoreactivity with increasing age (56,57). Both ACTH and TSH cells also appear to be unaffected by age, but no data are available regarding the effects of senescence on FSH and LH cells. Small foci of lymphocytes, usually in the intermediate lobe, are present in about 40% of adult pituitaries but are conspicuously absent in newborns and very young children (51).

Fibrosis is the most frequent age-related change in elderly patients. It is generally perivascular in distribution

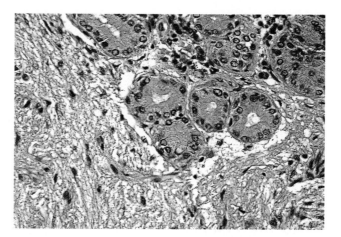

Figure 12.45   Salivary gland rest in the posterior lobe. The glands are composed of a single layer of cuboidal to columnar epithelium with basally oriented nuclei and granular PAS-positive cytoplasm. Salivary gland rests are encountered both on the surface of or within the posterior lobe, where it abuts the intermediate lobe zone (H&E, original magnification ×63).

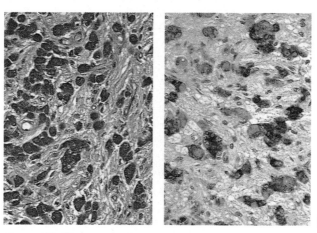

Figure 12.44   Basophil invasion. **A.** PAS staining (original magnification ×63). **B.** ACTH immunostain (original magnification ×63).

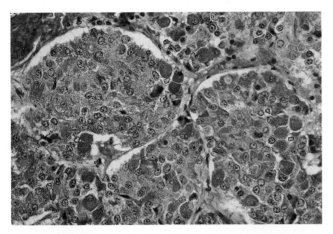

Figure 12.46 The pituitary in pregnancy features abundant pale chromophobic PRL cells (pregnancy cells) (H&E, original magnification ×100).

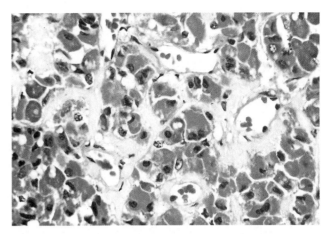

Figure 12.47 Perivascular fibrosis is a common feature of the aging pituitary (H&E, original magnification ×100).

(Figure 12.47) but is on occasion patchy, suggesting a remote microinfarct. Interstitial and intracellular deposits of amyloid have been demonstrated in the majority of autopsy-derived anterior pituitaries (58). Immunohistochemically, these reacted for antiamyloid lambda (λ) light chain and amyloid P component. The mean volume percentage of such deposits is approximately 0.5% of the anterior lobe. The occurrence of amyloid and its degree of deposition was related not only to patient age but also to the prevalence of chronic obstructive pulmonary disease and to non–insulin-dependent diabetes mellitus.

Neurohypophysis

As a functional unit, the neurohypophysis consists of the infundibulum, pituitary stalk, and posterior lobe. The posterior lobe, a ventral extension of the central nervous system, is the site of release of the hypothalamic hormones oxytocin and vasopressin. Its cellular elements consist of unmyelinated axons originating from the supraoptic and paraventricular nuclei and, to a lesser extent, from cholinergic neurons of the hypothalamus, an extensive vascular network, and specialized glial cells termed pituicytes (Figure 12.48).

Pituicytes, the most numerous cells of the neurohypophysis, are morphologically elongated, uni- or bipolar cells that display the prolongation of the cytoplasm into one or more processes. Pituicytes are strongly positive for glial fibrillary acidic protein (GFAP) (Figure 12.48), as well as S-100 protein and vimentin. Similar to glial cells of other areas of the central nervous system, pituicytes expand processes to adjacent connective tissue or to a blood vessel wall. Pituicytes appear to exist in five principal forms: major, dark, ependymal, oncocytic, and granular (59). Their morphologic diversity, ranging from astrocytic to ependymal, is thought to be a reflection of their physiologic role, which as yet is unclear (60).

Histologically, the axons of the posterior lobe are readily identified using silver stains and/or immunostains for

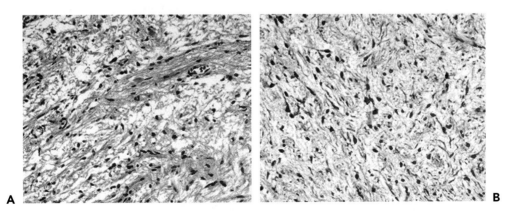

Figure 12.48 Posterior lobe. **A.** Pituicytes have elongated nuclei dispersed within the neuropil of the neurohypophysis (H&E, original magnification ×100). **B.** These cells stain positively for glial fibrillary acid protein (GFAP) (GFAP immunostain, original magnification ×100).

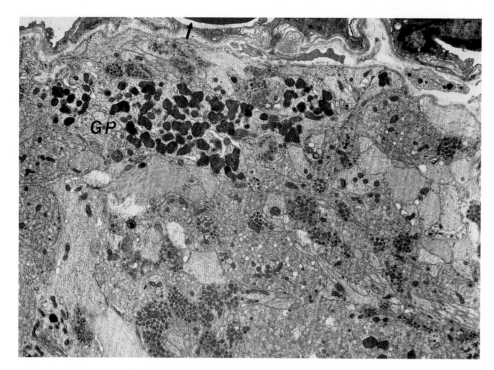

Figure 12.49 Pituitary, posterior lobe. This electron micrograph shows axonal processes containing neurosecretory granules of varying electron density. A granular pituicyte (GP) containing numerous prominent lysosomes lies in close proximity to the intravascular space (*arrow*). The intravascular space is bounded by fenestrated endothelial cells as seen here. Outside the endothelium lies the perivascular space, a region containing a variety of cell types (not shown here), including pericytes, histiocytes, fibroblasts, and mast cells (original magnification ×6,200).

neuronal markers. Focal axonal dilatations, known as Herring bodies, represent intra-axonal accumulations of posterior lobe hormones (Figure 12.22). At the ultrastructural level, the unmyelinated axons appear as delicate fibers, measuring 0.05 to 1.0 μm in diameter, which contain longitudinal arrays of microtubules and neurofilaments. Two types of neurosecretory axon, A and B, have been described based on the morphology of their neurosecretory granules. Type A fibers, far more numerous than type B, contain 100- to 300-nm oxytocin and vasopressin granules, whereas type B fibers, likely aminergic in nature, contain granules ranging from 50 to 100 nm (61). Neurosecretory fibers are closely associated with pituicytes, their axons often being ensheathed by them (Figure 12.49).

The most important function of the neurohypophysis is the transfer of hormonal substances from neurosecretory granules to the intravascular space. The complex anatomy of the neuronal, vascular, and perivascular compartments forms the basis for this elaborate process. Beginning at the neuronal side, neurohormonal factors appear to be released into minute channels that traverse the outermost, or abluminal, basement membrane of vessels to communicate with the perivascular space. They then traverse the inner, or luminal, basement membrane and endothelium in order to gain access to the vascular space (62) (Figure 12.49).

Variation in Normal Morphology of the Neurohypophysis

Granular cell nests or tumorlets, most located in the stalk or posterior lobe, are found in about 6% of autopsy pituitaries and are more common among the elderly (63). Vary-

ing from scattered cells to compact tumorlike nodules, they are composed of plump cells with granular acidophilic and strongly PAS-positive cytoplasm and relatively small nuclei (Figure 12.50). Only rarely do granular cells form clinically significant tumors (64). The origin of granular cell tumorlets and tumors of the neurohypophysis is uncertain. In rare cases, GFAP immunoreactivity has been shown, providing some evidence of the hypothesis that these granular cell nests may originate from pituicytes (65).

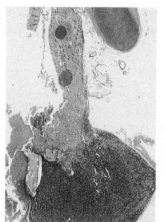 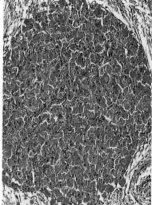

A   B

Figure 12.50 Pituitary stalk, granular cell tumorlets. **A.** Low-power view of the stalk shows two tumorlets. The optic chiasm is at the upper portion of the field; the anterior lobe is at the lower portion of the field (H&E, original magnification ×20). **B.** High-power view of a granular cell tumorlet. Such nodules are composed of pituicytes, modified glial cells, with abundant lysosome-rich eosinophilic cytoplasm. Tumorlets, as well as individual granular cells, are of no clinical significance (H&E, original magnification ×100).

DIFFERENTIAL DIAGNOSIS

The principal consideration in differential diagnosis of pituitary lesions is the distinction of normal pituitary tissue from adenoma. The most conspicuous architectural feature of the adenohypophysis is the arrangement of its cells in acini that, depending on orientation of section, vary from round to oval or somewhat elongate. The acini are surrounded by a delicate reticulin- or PAS-positive capillary network (Figure 12.17). In contrast, pituitary adenomas lack this uniform acinar architecture, showing only scant reticulin that is limited to scattered vessels (Figure 12.51). Although most normal pituitary acini are heterogeneous in their cellular content, thus permitting the distinction of normal from adenomatous tissue on H&E sections alone, some parts of the pituitary contain largely a single cell type and appear fairly monomorphous. For instance, eosinophilic GH cells are present in large numbers in the lateral wings. On the other hand, occasional adenomas composed of mixed cell populations (often ones associated with acromegaly) superficially resemble normal adenohypophysis. As a result, the distinction of normal from adenomatous tissue may be more easily achieved by PAS and reticulin staining than by immunohistochemistry alone. Small biopsies of the intermediate lobe may include the so-called basophilic infiltration normally seen in the posterior pituitary (Figures 12.43–12.44). Since these basophilic cells are arranged diffusely or in clusters, and lack the typical acinar formation seen in the anterior pituitary, they may be mistaken for ACTH-microadenomas.

A limited biopsy of the pituitary may occasionally include intermediate zone cysts, which are normal derivatives of Rathke's cleft. Correlation with radiologic and operative data usually obviates confusion with Rathke's cleft cyst. Clinically significant cysts are readily evident on neuroimaging and are identified as sizable cysts by the experienced surgeon.

As previously noted above, adenohypophysial cells may undergo squamous metaplasia, particularly in the pars tuberalis. This location is only occasionally sampled in surgical specimens. Scant in extent, intimately associated with adenohypophysial cells, and cytologically benign, they are unlikely to be confused with either cysts (epidermoid or dermoid cysts) or with neoplasms (craniopharyngiomas). In very small numbers, cytologic benign lymphocytes are seen in the intermediate zone of the normal pituitary in 10% of autopsied subjects (66). Unassociated with endocrine disease, such cells are readily distinguished from the far more widespread and dense infiltrates of lymphocytic hypophysitis or abscess.

A limited biopsy of the neurohypophysis can readily be mistaken for glioma in that the vast majority of its nucleated cells are specialized astrocytes (pituicytes). Unlike pilocytic astrocytomas, the tumor most closely mimicked by posterior pituitary tissue, the neurohypophysis contains large numbers of axons terminating on vessels. Of these axons, some possess PAS-positive swellings (Herring bodies). Secondary involvement of the pituitary by more ordinary diffuse astrocytomas is exceedingly rare.

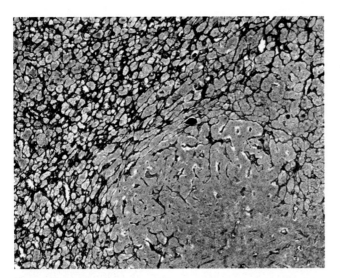

Figure 12.51 Disruption of the reticulin network in a pituitary adenoma. Compare the acinar pattern of the normal adenophypophysis (*upper left*) with the adenoma (*bottom right*) (Wilder reticulin, original magnification ×100).

REFERENCES

1. Moore KL. The Developing Human: Clinically Oriented Embryology. Philadelphia: WB Saunders; 1988:170–205.
2. Conklin JL. The development of the human fetal adenohypophysis. *Anat Rec* 1968;160:79–91.
3. Sabshin JK. The pituitary gland—anatomy and embryology. In: Goodrich I, Lee KJ, eds. *The Pituitary: Clinical Aspects of Normal and Abnormal Function.* Amsterdam: Elsevier Science; 1987:19–27.
4. Falin LI. The development of human hypophysis and differentiation of cells of its anterior lobe during embryonic life. *Acta Anat (Basel)* 1961;44:188–205.
5. Boyd JD. Observations on the human pharyngeal hypophysis. *J Endocrinol* 1956;14:66–77.
6. McGrath P. Aspects of the human pharyngeal hypophysis in normal and anencephalic fetuses and neonates and their possible significance in the mechanism of its control. *J Anat* 1978;127:65–81.
7. Asa SL, Kovacs K. Functional morphology of the human fetal pituitary. *Pathol Annu* 1984;19:275–315.
8. Colohan AR, Grady MS, Bonnin JM, Thorner MO, Kovacs K, Jane JA. Ectopic pituitary gland simulating a suprasellar tumor. *Neurosurgery* 1987;20:43–48.
9. Lennox B, Russell DS. Dystopia of the neurohypophysis: two cases. *J Pathol Bacteriol* 1951;63:485–490.
10. Scully KM, Rosenfeld MG. Pituitary development: regulatory codes in mammalian organogenesis. *Science* 2002;295:2231–2235.
11. Osamura RY, Egashira N. Recent developments in molecular embryogenesis and molecular biology of the pituitary. In: Lloyd RV, ed. *Endocrine Pathology: Differential Diagnosis and Molecular Advances.* Totowa, NJ: Humana Press, Inc; 2004:75–86.
12. Asa SL, Ezzat S. Molecular basis of pituitary development and cytogenesis. In: Kontogeorgos G, Kovacs K, eds. *Molecular Pathology of the Pituitary. Frontiers of Hormone Research.* Vol 32. Basel, Switzerland: Karger; 2004:1–19.
13. Dubois PM, Begeot M, Dubois MP, Herbert DC. Immunocytological localization of LH, FSH, TSH and their subunits in the pituitary of normal and anencephalic human fetuses. *Cell Tissue Res* 1978;191:249–265.

14. Begeot M, Dubois MP, Dubois, PM. Growth hormone and ACTH in the pituitary of normal and anencephalic human fetuses: immunocytochemical evidence for hypothalamic influences during development. *Neuroendocrinology* 1977;24:208–220.
15. Renn WH, Rhoton AL Jr. Microsurgical anatomy of the sellar region. *J Neurosurg* 1975;43:288–298.
16. Lang J. Anatomy of the midline. *Acta Neurochir Suppl (Wien)* 1985;35:6–22.
17. Osteology. In: Williams PL, Warwick R, eds. *Gray's anatomy*. 36th ed. Philadelphia: WB Saunders; 1980:230–418.
18. Kern EB, Laws ER Jr. The rationale and techniques of selective transsphenoidal microsurgery for the removal of pituitary tumors. In: Laws ER Jr, Randall RV, Kern EB, Abboud CF, eds. *Management of Pituitary Adenomas and Related Lesions with Emphasis on Transsphenoidal Microsurgery*. New York: Appleton-Century-Crofts; 1982:219–233.
19. Bergland RM, Ray BS, Torack RM. Anatomical variations in the pituitary gland and adjacent structures in 225 human autopsy cases. *J Neurosurg* 1968;28:93–99.
20. Berke JP, Buxton LF, Kokmen E. The empty sella. *Neurology* 1975;25:1137–1143.
21. Kaufman B, Chamberlain WB Jr. The ubiquitous empty sella turcica. *Acta Radiol* 1972;13:413–425.
22. Kaplan HA, Browder J, Krieger AJ. Intercavernous connections of the cavernous sinuses. The superior and inferior circular sinuses. *J Neurosurg* 1976;45:166–168.
23. McGrath P. The cavernous sinus: an anatomical survey. *Aust N Z J Surg* 1977;47:601–613.
24. Harris FS, Rhoton AL. Anatomy of the cavernous sinus. A microsurgical study. *J Neurosurg* 1976;45:169–180.
25. Stanfield JP. The blood supply of the human pituitary gland. *J Anat* 1960;94:257–273.
26. Xuereb GP, Prichard MM, Daniel PM. The arterial supply and venous drainage of the human hypophysis cerebri. *Q J Exp Physiol Cogn Med Sci* 1954;39:199–217.
27. Gorczyca W, Hardy J. Arterial supply of the human anterior pituitary gland. *Neurosurgery* 1987;20:369–378.
28. Xuereb GP, Prichard MM, Daniel PM. The hypophyseal portal system of vessels in man. *Q J Exp Physiol* 1954;39:219–230.
29. Scheithauer BW. The hypothalamus and neurohypophysis. In: Kovacs K, Asa SL (eds). *Functional Endocrine Pathology*. Boston: Blackwell; 1991:170–224.
30. Pansky B, Allen DJ. *Review of Neuroscience*. New York: Macmillan; 1980.
31. Brownstein MJ, Russell JT, Gainer H. Synthesis, transport, and release of posterior pituitary hormones. *Science* 1980;207:373–378.
32. Thorner MO, Vance ML, Laws ER Jr, Horvath E, Kovacs K. The anterior pituitary. In: Wilson JD, Foster DW, Kronenberg HM, Larsen PR, eds. *Williams Textbook of Endocrinology*. 9th ed. Philadelphia: WB Saunders; 1998:249–340.
33. Scheithauer BW, Sano T, Kovacs KT, Young WF Jr, Ryan N, Randall RV. The pituitary gland in pregnancy: a clinicopathologic and immunohistochemical study of 69 cases. *Mayo Clin Proc* 1990;65:461–474.
34. Goluboff LG, Ezrin C. Effect of pregnancy on the somatotroph and the prolactin cell of the human adenohypophysis. *J Clin Endocrinol Metab* 1969;29:1533–1538.
35. Ciric I. On the origin and nature of the pituitary gland capsule. *J Neurosurg* 1977;46:596–600.
36. Kovacs K, Horvath E. *Tumors of the Pituitary Gland*. Washington, DC: Armed Forces Institute of Pathology; 1986.
37. McGrath P. Cysts of sellar and pharyngeal hypophyses. *Pathology* 1971;3:123–131.
38. Mulchahey JJ, Jaffe RB. Detection of a potential progenitor cell in the human fetal pituitary that secretes both growth hormone and prolactin. *J Clin Endocrinol Metab* 1988;66:24–32.
39. Turkington RW, Underwood LE, Van Wyk JJ. Elevated serum prolactin levels after pituitary-stalk section in man. *N Engl J Med* 1971;285:707–710.
40. Horvath E, Ilse G, Kovacs K. Enigmatic bodies in human corticotroph cells. *Acta Anat (Basel)* 1977;98:427–433.
41. Phifer RF, Spicer SS. Immunohistochemical and histologic demonstration of thyrotropic cells of the human adenohypophysis. *J Clin Endocrinol Metab* 1973;36:1210–1221.
42. Phifer RF, Midgley AR, Spicer SS. Immunohistologic and histologic evidence that FSH and LH are present in the same cell type in the human pars tuberalis. *J Clin Endocrinol Metab* 1973;36:125–141.
43. Muttukrishna S, Tannetta D, Groome N, Sargent I. Activin and follistatin in female reproduction. *Mol Cell Endocrinol* 2004;225:45–56.
44. Asa SL, Kovacs K, Bilbao JM. The pars tuberalis of the human pituitary. A histologic, immunohistochemical, ultrastructural and immunoelectron microscopic analysis. *Virchows Arch A Pathol Anat Histopathol* 1983;399:49–59.
45. Horvath E, Kovacs K, Penz G, Ezrin C. Origin, possible function and fate of "follicular cells" in the anterior lobe of the human pituitary. *Am J Pathol* 1974;77:199–212.
46. Marin F, Stefaneanu L, Kovacs K. Folliculo-stellate cells of the pituitary. *Endocr Pathol* 1991;2:180–192.
47. Horvath E, Kovacs K. Folliculo-stellate cells of the human pituitary: a type of adult stem cell? *Ultrastruct Pathol* 2002;26:219–28.
48. Inoue K, Mogi C, Ogawa S, Tomida M, Miyai S. Are folliculostellate cells in the anterior pituitary gland supportive cells or organ-specific stem cells? *Arch Physiol Biochem* 2002;110:50–53.
49. Luse SA, Kernohan JW. Squamous-cell nests of the pituitary gland. *Cancer* 1955;8:623–628.
50. Schochet SS Jr, McCormick WF, Halmi NS. Salivary gland rests in the human pituitary. Light and electron microscopical study. *Arch Pathol* 1974;98:193–200.
51. Shanklin WM. Age changes in the histology of the human pituitary. *Acta Anat (Basel)* 1953;19:290–304.
52. Sano T, Kovacs KT, Scheithauer BW, Young WF Jr. Aging and the human pituitary gland. *Mayo Clin Proc* 1993; 68:971–977.
53. Scheithauer BW, Sano T, Kovacs KT, Young WF Jr, Ryan N, Randall RV. The pituitary gland in pregnancy: a clinicopathologic and immunohistochemical study of 69 cases. *Mayo Clin Proc* 1990;65:461–474.
54. Stefaneanu L, Kovacs K, Lloyd RV, et al. Pituitary lactotrophs and somatotrophs in pregnancy: a correlative in situ hybridization and immunocytochemical study. *Virchows Arch B Cell Pathol Incl Mol Pathol* 1992;62:291–296.
55. Frawley LS, Boockfor FR. Mammosomatotropes: presence and functions in normal and neoplastic pituitary tissue. *Endocr Rev* 1991;12:337–355.
56. Calderon L, Ryan N, Kovacs K. Human pituitary growth hormone cells in old age. *Gerontology* 1978;24:441–447.
57. Kovacs K, Ryan N, Horvath E, Penz G, Ezrin C. Prolactin cells of the human pituitary gland in old age. *J Gerontol* 1977;32:534–540.
58. Röcken C, Saeger W, Fleege JC, Linke RP. Interstitial amyloid deposits in the pituitary gland. Morphometry, immunohistology, and correlation to diseases. *Arch Pathol Lab Med* 1995;119:1055–1060.
59. Takei Y, Seyama S, Pearl GS, Tindall GT. Ultrastructural study of the human neurohypophysis. II. Cellular elements of neural parenchyma, the pituicytes. *Cell Tissue Res* 1980;205:273–287.
60. Hatton GI. Pituicytes, glia, and control of terminal secretion. *J Exp Biol* 1988;139:67–79.
61. Seyama S, Pearl GS, Takei Y. Ultrastructural study of the human neurohypophysis. I. Neurosecretory axons and their dilatations in the pars nervosa. *Cell Tissue Res* 1980;205:253–271.
62. Seyama S, Pearl GS, Takei Y. Ultrastructural study of the human neurohypophysis. III. Vascular and perivascular structures. *Cell Tissue Res* 1980;206:291–302.
63. Luse SA, Kernohan JW. Granular-cell tumors of the stalk and posterior lobe of the pituitary gland. *Cancer* 1955;8:616–622.
64. Lopes MBS, Scheithauer BW, Saeger W. Granular cell tumour. In: DeLellis RA, Lloyd RV, Heitz PU, Eng C, eds. *World Health Organization Classification of Tumours, Pathology and Genetics of Tumours of Endocrine Organs*. Lyon: IARC Press; 2004:44–45.
65. Nishioka H. Immunohistochemical study of granular cell tumors and granular pituicytes of the neurohypophysis. *Endocr Pathol* 1993;4:140–145.
66. Shanklin WM. Lymphocytes and lymphoid tissue in the human pituitary. *Anat Rec* 1951;111:177–191.

HEAD AND NECK

Normal Eye and Ocular Adnexa

13

Gordon K. Klintworth   *Thomas J. Cummings*

INTRODUCTION

The eye and surrounding tissues are subject to a wide variety of primary ocular and systemic disease processes. An understanding of ocular anatomy will enable the general surgical pathologist to appreciate morphologic abnormalities and will facilitate the diagnosis of many of the pathologic conditions affecting those structures. Similar to other specimens received by the surgical pathologist, in some cases a discussion with the ophthalmologist who is submitting the tissue is important for proper handling, sectioning, and processing of the tissue. Proper handling of the tissue is required so as to not artifactually mask the diagnostic histologic features, such as the common age-related arcus lipoides.

This chapter presents an overview of the normal histology of the eye and ocular adnexa. Several excellent texts are available for more detailed information on ocular anatomy and development (1–5).

The eye is roughly spherical in shape and external measurements are routinely obtained in three dimensions. In the adult, the anteri_oposterior plane of the eye measures approximately 24 mm, whereas the vertical and the horizontal dimensions are both about 23 to 23.5 mm. Located midway between the anterior and posterior poles of the eye is the equator of the globe.

Several external landmarks allow the pathologist to orient the globe and to determine whether an eye is from the right or the left side (Figure 13.1). By establishing the nasal (medial) and temporal (lateral) sides of the globe and the superior surface of the eye, the side of the eye can easily be deduced. The six extraocular muscles (four rectus and two oblique muscles) that arise in the posterior orbit and run forward to insert upon the sclera are important in this regard. The rectus muscles arise from a fibrous ring at the apex of the orbit, the annulus of Zinn, and are enveloped by a fascial membrane that creates a cone-shaped structure posterior to the globe. The levator palpebrae superioris also arises at the orbital apex and extends anteriorly to the eyelids. Of the extraocular muscles, only the inferior oblique has a muscular insertion upon the sclera; the other muscles have tendinous insertions. The extraocular muscle insertions are usually removed by the surgeon when the globe is excised (enucleated), but they are frequently present on eyes obtained postmortem. The superior and inferior oblique muscles are most useful in orientating the globe. The tendinous insertion of the superior oblique muscle behind the superior rectus muscle insertion indicates the top of the eye. The inferior oblique muscle inserts on the sclera temporally in the horizontal meridian, and its fibers run inferiorly toward the back of the orbit. The optic nerve is also useful in assessing orientation because it exits the globe slightly nasal to the posterior pole of the eye. Adjacent to the optic nerve, the prominent long posterior ciliary arteries course through the superficial sclera in opposite directions in a horizontal plane. Anteriorly, the dimensions of the cornea may be helpful in topographic orientation. In the adult, the cornea is elliptical in shape with its horizontal diameter being slightly greater than its vertical breadth. In young children, this difference is less apparent.

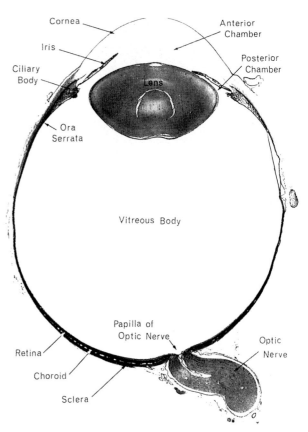

Figure 13.2 This photomicrograph of a histologic section of an eye from a rhesus monkey illustrates the major tissue layers of the eye, the lens, the vitreous humor body, and the spaces of the anterior and posterior chambers. (Reproduced with permission from: Bloom W, Fawcett DW. *A Textbook of Histology*. 12th ed. New York: Chapman and Hall; 1994.)

The eye is traditionally described as having three tissue layers that surround the vitreous humor, the lens, and the spaces of the anterior and posterior chambers (Figure 13.2). The outermost part of the eye is composed of the transparent cornea and the opaque sclera. The ocular middle layer is made up of the iris, ciliary body, and the choroid. The innermost retina is in direct contact with the vitreous humor body.

CORNEA

The transparent cornea occupies one-sixth of the anterior surface of the globe and refracts the entering light. Although individual variation is common, the cornea measures approximately 11.7 mm in the horizontal plane and 10.6 mm in the vertical plane. Centrally, the cornea is about 0.5 mm thick, but peripherally it thickens to about 0.67 mm. Histologically, the cornea consists of six distinct layers: (a) the epithelium; (b) the basal lamina of the epithelium; (c) Bowman's layer; (d) the stroma; (e) Descemet's membrane; and (f) the endothelium (Figure 13.3).

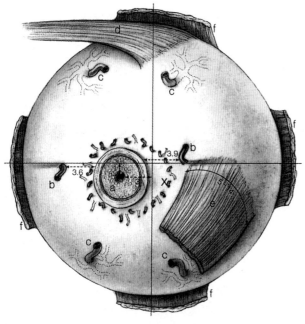

Figure 13.1 This drawing depicts the right eye as seen from behind. Several external landmarks are useful in determining orientation of the globe. The optic nerve (*a*) is located approximately 1 mm inferior to and 3 mm nasal to the posterior pole of the eye. The long posterior ciliary arteries (*b*) are located in the horizontal plane, and four vortex veins (*c*) exit the sclera posteriorly. The superior oblique muscle (*d*) inserts on the top of the globe, whereas the inferior oblique muscle (*e*) inserts temporally, and its fibers run posteriorly and nasally. The rectus muscles (*f*) insert horizontally, inferiorly, and superiorly. The approximate location of the macula (*x*), the part of the retina responsible for the most distinct vision, is slightly temporal to the optic nerve. (Reproduced with permission from: Hogan MJ, Alvarado JA, Weddell JE. *Histology of the Human Eye: An Atlas and Text*. Philadelphia: WB Saunders; 1971.)

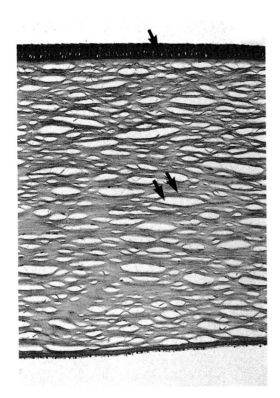

Figure 13.3 The stratified squamous epithelium of the cornea (*arrow*) overlies the basal lamina and Bowman's layer. The clefts within the collagenous stroma (*double arrows*) represent artifacts of tissue processing. No blood vessels or lymphatics are normally present within the cornea. Descemet's membrane and the corneal endothelium are located just posterior to the stroma. (H&E, ×33.)

The corneal epithelium, which is composed of stratified nonkeratinized squamous cells, is about five cell layers thick centrally. The peripheral cornea is often twice as thick. The basilar epithelial cells are polygonal in shape; and, as they become displaced to the corneal surface during differentiation, a more flattened appearance is acquired. In the normal cornea, even the most superficial epithelial cells retain their nuclei. Mitotic figures are uncommon in the epithelium but are observed in the basal cells occasionally. Some Langerhans cells are present within the corneal epithelium, especially peripherally (6). Apoptosis is also uncommonly seen in the epithelium of the normal cornea. Langerhans cells are most readily identified by special histochemical and immunohistochemical methods and are not normally recognizable in routinely stained tissue sections.

The corneal epithelium rests upon a basal lamina, which is difficult to see in hematoxylin and eosin (H&E)–stained tissue sections. Staining with the periodic acid-Schiff (PAS) reaction makes this layer apparent (Figure 13.4). In certain pathologic conditions, the epithelial basal lamina assumes an intraepithelial location.

Bowman's layer is an acellular structure located just posterior to the epithelial basal lamina (Figure 13.4). It is

approximately 8 to 14 μm thick. As shown by transmission electron microscopy, Bowman's layer is not a true basement membrane but is composed of randomly oriented delicate collagen fibers. The anterior face of Bowman's layer ends distinctly at its junction with the epithelial basal lamina. Posteriorly, Bowman's layer merges inconspicuously with the underlying corneal stroma. Unmyelinated sensory nerves reach the epithelium from the stroma after crossing Bowman's layer. However, nerve processes are difficult to detect in the cornea in standard tissue sections, even with the use of special histologic techniques.

The stroma accounts for approximately 90% of the cornea's thickness. It is composed of numerous layers of collagen fibers embedded in a proteoglycan-rich extracellular matrix, and the anterior and posterior portions of the cornea have several differences. The stroma contains keratan sulfate proteoglycans (lumican, keratocan, mimecan), as well as a galactosaminoglycan-rich proteoglycan (decorin). Transmission electron microscopy has disclosed that the corneal collagen fibers are regularly spaced and of a uniform diameter; this arrangement contributes to the transparency of the cornea. The corneal fibroblasts (keratocytes) are surrounded by the stromal collagen lamellae. Other cell types are seldom identified in tissue sections of the normal corneal stroma, but rarely an occasional mononuclear leukocyte or granulocyte may be present. The normal cornea lacks blood vessels, and its nutrition is obtained from an arterial plexus at the junction of the cornea and sclera and from direct contact with the aqueous humor of the anterior chamber. In tissue sections of routinely processed formalin-fixed corneas, clefts are almost invariably present between the collagen lamellae. Initially interpreted as lymphatic channels by early histologists, these clefts are artifacts of tissue processing. Lymphatic vessels are not present in the normal cornea.

Descemet's membrane, a true basal lamina elaborated by the underlying corneal endothelial cells, begins to form

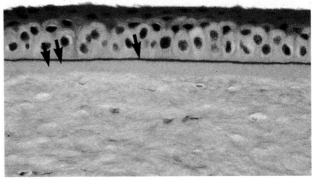

Figure 13.4 The corneal epithelium rests upon a thin basal lamina (*arrow*), which is prominent in this section following periodic acid-Schiff staining. The acellular band directly underneath the basal lamina is Bowman's layer (*double arrows*) (PAS, ×132).

during fetal life. At birth, it is approximately 3 to 4 μm thick (Figure 13.5). Basal laminar material is continuously added to the posterior part of Descemet's membrane throughout life so that by adulthood, this structure attains a thickness of approximately 10 to 12 μm. The fetal and postnatal regions of Descemet's membrane differ ultrastructurally. This difference is occasionally discernible by light microscopy.

The corneal endothelium (Figure 13.5) is directly exposed to the aqueous humor in the anterior chamber. Although this cell layer does not line blood vessels or lymphatic spaces, the term *endothelium* is firmly entrenched in the literature. These cells function as an osmotic pump to regulate a necessary state of stromal dehydration that preserves corneal clarity. Endothelial decompensation results in corneal edema and diminished optical transparency. The corneal endothelium has been shown by immunohistochemistry to be S-100 protein–positive, a finding supportive of other evidence suggesting a neural crest origin (7). They react with the monoclonal antibody 2B4.14.1, which recognizes the renal Tamm-Horsfall glycoprotein (THGP) antigen, raising the possibility that the cornea expresses a molecule with homeostatic properties similar to that ascribed to THGP (8). The endothelial cells of the cornea normally form a single flattened layer and, virtually, never regenerate by mitosis in human eyes. Under pathologic conditions (epithelial ingrowth and posterior polymorphous corneal dystrophy), cytokeratin-containing squamous cells replace the endothelium and form a layer that is more than one cell thick.

After the second decade of life, age-related focal excrescences (Hassall-Henle warts) commonly form on the peripheral part of Descemet's membrane (Figure 13.6). Virtually identical focal thickenings occur on the central part of Descemet's membrane (corneal guttae) under pathologic circumstances and most notably in Fuchs's corneal dystrophy. The presence of excrescences on Descemet's membrane in tissue sections of corneal buttons removed at penetrating

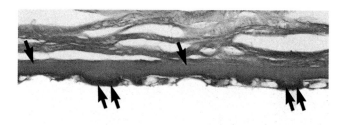

Figure 13.6 Descemet's membrane *(single arrows)* is located immediately posterior to the corneal stroma. The excrescences on the peripheral portion of Descemet's membrane (Hassall-Henle warts) *(double arrows)* represent an aging change. Descemet's membrane also thickens with age. (H&E, ×132.)

keratoplasty (full-thickness corneal transplant) is always abnormal. Hassall-Henle warts are too peripheral in location to be present in a surgically excised corneal button.

Corneal epithelium and endothelium are prone to being artifactitiously "rubbed-off" during prosection of the tissue, and it is important to distinguish this artifact from the true loss of corneal epithelium and endothelium.

SCLERA

The sclera, which accounts for approximately five-sixths of the surface area of the eye, begins at the periphery of the cornea and extends posteriorly to the optic nerve. The sclera's relatively rigid nature protects the eye from trauma and helps maintain intraocular pressure. Anteriorly, the sclera is visible underneath the transparent conjunctiva and is normally white in adults. The sclera varies in thickness, being about 0.8 mm thick near its junction with the cornea. At the insertions of the four rectus muscles (approximately 5 to 8 mm posterior to the corneoscleral junction), the sclera is at its thinnest, measuring approximately 0.3 mm. From this point posteriorly, the sclera gradually thickens and attains its maximal width of about 1.0 mm adjacent to the optic nerve.

The sclera has three components: the episclera, the stroma, and the lamina fusca. The episclera, its most superficial part, is located between the fibrous structure that envelops the globe (Tenon's capsule) and the underlying scleral stroma with which it merges. The episclera is composed of loosely arranged collagen fibers and fibroblasts embedded in an extracellular matrix. Occasional melanocytes and mononuclear leukocytes are also present. Anteriorly, the episclera is richly vascularized.

The largest component of the sclera is its stroma, which consists of fibrous bands of collagen, occasional elastic fibers, and scattered fibroblasts (Figure 13.7). The corneal

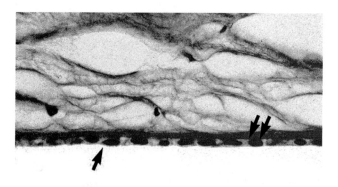

Figure 13.5 A thin monolayer of corneal endothelial cells *(arrow)* is adjacent to Descemet's membrane *(double arrows)*. These cells are in direct contact with the aqueous humor of the anterior chamber (H&E, ×132).

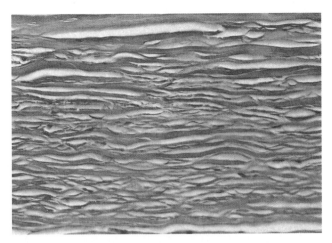

Figure 13.7 The scleral stroma is predominantly composed of collagen fibers that vary in diameter and are in haphazard array. Scattered fibroblasts occur between the collagen bundles. (H&E, ×100.)

and scleral stroma appear similar at the light microscopic level; but, when viewed by transmission electron microscopy, the individual collagen fibers within the sclera vary in diameter and are randomly arranged, in contrast to the orderly packed corneal collagen fibers of uniform diameter. This largely accounts for the opaque nature of the sclera.

Although the scleral stroma is relatively avascular, blood vessels, as well as accompanying nerves and scattered melanocytes, are present in perforating emissarial canals (Figure 13.8). The anterior ciliary arteries perforate the sclera near the insertion of the rectus muscles. Venous channels draining the iris, ciliary body, and choroid (vortex veins) exit the sclera several millimeters posterior to the equator of the eye. The posterior ciliary arteries pass through the sclera near the optic nerve. In some individuals, a nerve

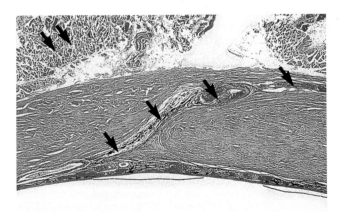

Figure 13.8 This figure illustrates a blood vessel that penetrates the sclera and extends to the prominently vascularized choroid through an emissarial canal (*single arrows*). Pigmented melanocytes are also present. The fibers of the inferior oblique muscle are present at the site of insertion upon the outer sclera (*double arrows*). (H&E, ×50.)

in an emissarial canal near the corneoscleral junction may be prominent and attain a diameter of 1 to 2 mm. The nodular appearance of this so-called *nerve loop of Axenfeld* may mimic a neoplasm or conjunctival cyst clinically (9). To the unwary surgical pathologist, this totally normal nerve bundle may be mistaken for a neurofibroma (10).

The innermost layer of the sclera, the lamina fusca, contains loose collagen fibers, fibroblasts, and scattered melanocytes. It represents a region of transition between the sclera and the underlying choroid. The sclera is weakly attached to the choroid below by thin fibers of collagen.

With increasing age, several histologic changes occur in the sclera. Calcium may deposit diffusely between the individual collagen fibers throughout the entire scleral stroma. Localized abnormalities, known as senile scleral plaques, may occur just anterior to the insertion of the lateral or horizontal rectus muscles. These lesions are characterized by decreased stromal cellularity, abnormal collagen, and, in advanced cases, calcification (11).

CORNEOSCLERAL LIMBUS

The corneoscleral limbus, or junction, is not a distinct anatomic site but is a significant landmark clinically. Most surgical procedures on the anterior part of the eye are accomplished after access via an incision in the limbal area. For purposes of discussion, the trabecular meshwork and Schlemm's canal will be considered as part of the corneoscleral limbus.

The limbus is approximately 1.5 to 2.0 mm wide, and separate layers of the cornea merge with components of the sclera or conjunctiva in this area (Figure 13.9). The squamous epithelium of the cornea extends centrifugally beyond the limbus until it meets the epithelium of the bulbar conjunctiva. At the limbus, Bowman's layer of the cornea blends into the subepithelial tissues of the conjunctiva, and the corneal and scleral stroma become continuous with each other. Descemet's membrane abruptly terminates in the limbal region and gives rise to the clinically significant landmark known as Schwalbe's ring. In about 15% of eyes, a prominent area of thickening is identified histologically at this site (Figure 13.10) (2). Immediately adjacent to Schwalbe's ring is the most anterior aspect of the trabecular meshwork. Both the trabecular meshwork and Schlemm's canal constitute the apparatus responsible for the removal of aqueous humor from the eye (Figure 13.11). Aqueous humor drainage occurs in the angle between the anterior surface of the iris and the sclera. Histologically, the meshwork appears as a collection of finely branching and delicately pigmented connective tissue bands. The cells, which line the trabecular meshwork, are continuous with the corneal endothelium. Posteriorly, the trabecular meshwork extends to a roughly triangular-shaped projection of scleral connective tissue, known as the scleral spur.

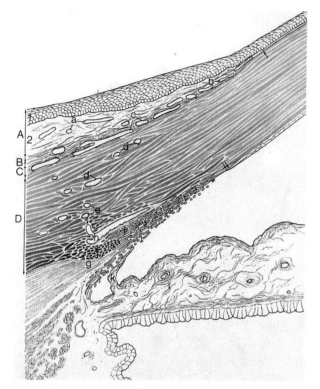

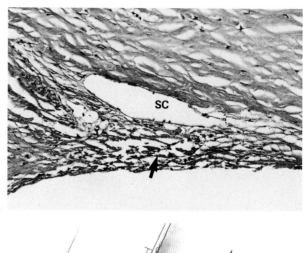

Figure 13.9   The corneoscleral limbus represents the junction of the peripheral cornea with the anterior sclera and is not a distinct anatomic site. Clinically, the limbus is an important landmark. The conjunctiva of the limbus (*A*) is composed of epithelium (*1*) and stroma (*2*). The thin connective tissue layer of Tenon's capsule (*B*) overlies the episclera (*C*). The corneal and scleral stroma merge gradually in the area marked *D*. Vessels of the conjunctival stroma (*a, b*), episclera (*c*), and limbal plexus (*d, e*) are illustrated. The projection of collagen fibers known as the scleral spur (*f*) merges with the smooth muscle fibers of the ciliary body (*g*). Schlemm's canal (*h*) and the trabecular meshwork (*i, j*) are responsible for removal of aqueous humor from the eye. Occasionally, processes from the iris (*k*) insert upon the trabecular meshwork. Bowman's layer (*arrow*) and Descemet's membrane (*double arrows*) both terminate in the area of the limbus. (Reproduced with permission from: Hogan MJ, Alvarado JA, Weddell JE. *Histology of the Human Eye: An Atlas and Text.* Philadelphia: WB Saunders; 1971.)

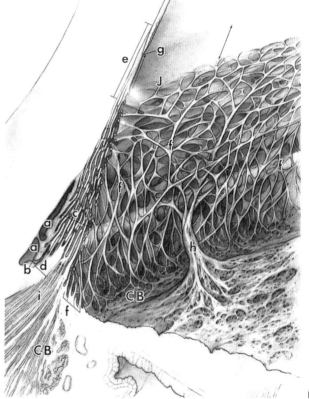

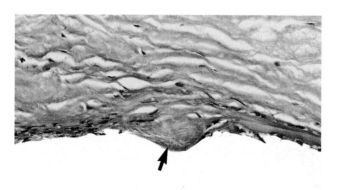

Figure 13.10   Schwalbe's ring is a significant clinical landmark in the limbal area and represents the peripheral termination of Descemet's membrane. Prominent Schwalbe's rings (*arrow*) are identified histologically in about 15% of eyes. (H&E, ×80.)

Figure 13.11   **A.** Located in the angle of the anterior chamber is Schlemm's canal (*SC*) and the trabecular meshwork (*arrow*). Schlemm's canal is an endothelial channel that enables aqueous humor to drain from the eye. Aqueous humor reaches Schlemm's canal after percolating through the connective tissue strands of the trabecular meshwork. (H&E, ×66.) **B.** Structures within and near the angle of the anterior chamber are depicted in this drawing. In this illustration, Schlemm's canal (*a*) has two channels, one of which is in communication with a small collecting channel (*b*). The collecting channel is intimately associated with the limbal part of the trabecular meshwork (*c*). The scleral spur (*d*) is closely associated with the trabecular meshwork. Descemet's membrane terminates peripherally in the area denoted *e* and *g*. Some components (*f*) of the trabecular meshwork arise at the ciliary body (*CB*). Isolated strands of meshwork merge with a nearby process (*h*) from the anterior surface of the iris. A muscle of the ciliary body (*i*) attaches to the trabecular meshwork (*arrows*). The corneal endothelium merges with endothelial cells of the meshwork (*j*). (Reproduced with permission from: Hogan MJ, Alvarado JA, Weddell JE. *Histology of the Human Eye: An Atlas and Text.* Philadelphia: WB Saunders; 1971.)

Located slightly anterior and superficial to the trabecular meshwork is Schlemm's canal, an endothelial-lined venous channel that completely encircles the limbus. Because Schlemm's canal sometimes gives off smaller branches, two lumens are occasionally seen on histologic sections of the anterior chamber angle. Although the trabecular meshwork and Schlemm's canal appear to be in intimate contact in tissue sections, they are separated from each other by a thin layer of connective tissue and separate endothelial linings. Aqueous humor percolates among the delicate beams of the trabecular meshwork before becoming transported to Schlemm's canal. Ultrastructural examination of this region discloses giant cytoplasmic vacuoles in the endothelial lining of Schlemm's canal, adjacent to the trabecular meshwork. These vacuoles are thought by some to contain fluid in the process of being transported from the trabecular meshwork into the lumen of Schlemm's canal (12). Once in Schlemm's canal, aqueous humor drains into the episcleral venous plexus by way of numerous small collector channels. Prolonged obstruction to the outflow of aqueous humor results in increased intraocular pressure and glaucoma.

CONJUNCTIVA, CARUNCLE, AND PLICA SEMILUNARIS

The conjunctiva is a thin continuous mucous membrane lining the inner surface of the eyelids and much of the anterior surface of the eye. In addition to its protective function, the conjunctiva allows the eyelids to move smoothly over the globe. The conjunctival epithelium is composed of two to five layers of columnar cells and rests upon a basal lamina. Within the conjunctival epithelium are goblet cells that secrete mucoid material that becomes incorporated into the tear film (Figure 13.12). Melanocytes are present in the basal epithelial layers and, like melanocytes in the skin, transfer melanosomes into adjacent epithelial cells. These pigmented epithelial cells are numerous in dark-skinned individuals (Figure 13.13). The loose, fibrovascular subepithelial connective tissue of the conjunctival stroma normally contains nerve cells, melanocytes, and accessory lacrimal glands. Lymphoid follicles with germinal centers reside in the conjunctiva (Figure 13.14), particularly in areas where the conjunctiva lining the inner surface of the eyelid merges with the portion covering the eyeball (superior and inferior fornices); scattered lymphocytes are not unusual within the conjunctiva. Hence, their presence is not indicative of chronic conjunctivitis unless both plasma cells and significant numbers of lymphocytes are present. Three distinct areas of the conjunctiva are recognized (Figure 13.15): the palpebral conjunctiva, the bulbar conjunctiva, and the conjunctiva lining the fornices.

The morphologic attributes of the conjunctiva vary in different parts of this tissue. Although goblet cells exist throughout the epithelium of the bulbar conjunctiva, they

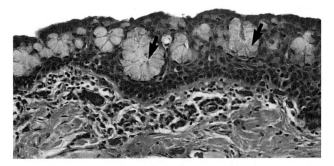

Figure 13.12 Goblet cells (*arrows*) are prominent in this section of conjunctival epithelium. Scattered mononuclear cells are often present in apparently healthy individuals in the underlying conjunctival stroma. (H&E, ×66.)

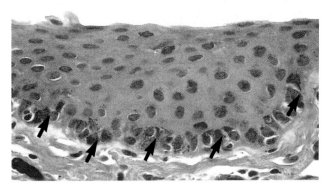

Figure 13.13 In dark-skinned individuals, the basal layers of the conjunctival epithelium are pigmented (*arrows*) (H&E, ×160).

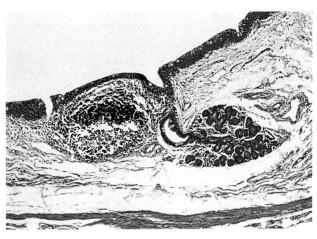

Figure 13.14 A small lymphoid follicle and island of accessory lacrimal tissue are present in the stroma of the palpebral conjunctiva (H&E, ×25).

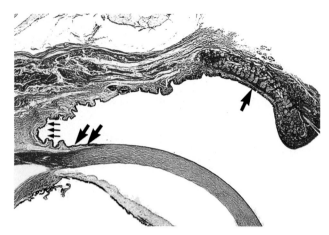

Figure 13.15 The conjunctiva can be divided into three parts. The palpebral conjunctiva (*arrow*) lines the posterior surface of the eyelid. The bulbar conjunctiva (*double arrows*) extends from the limbus over the anterior sclera. The bulbar and palpebral conjunctiva converge upon the conjunctiva of the superior and inferior fornices (*triple arrows*). (H&E,×2.5.)

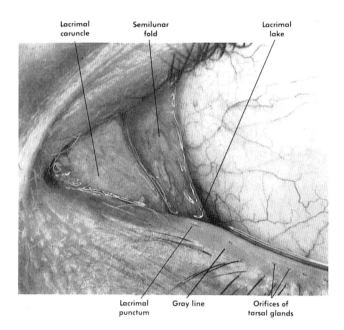

Figure 13.16 The caruncle and semilunar fold are specialized portions of the conjunctiva and are located in the medial interpalpebral angle of the eye. Before tears enter the lacrimal drainage apparatus through the lacrimal punctum, they accumulate at the medial canthus (lacrimal lake). The demarcation between the conjunctival and cutaneous portions of the eyelid is discernible clinically at the so-called *gray line*. The secretions of the meibomian glands (tarsal glands) reach the surface of the eyelids at small orifices. (Reproduced with permission from: Newell FW. *Ophthalmology: Principles and Concepts*. 6th ed. St. Louis: CV Mosby; 1986.)

are more common in the inferior and nasal parts. Goblet cells are particularly abundant in the forniceal regions. The conjunctival stroma is thickest in the fornices and bulbar areas and thinnest in the palpebral conjunctiva and at the corneoscleral limbus, where small conjunctival papillae, known as the pallisades of Vogt, are evident. The palpebral conjunctiva is firmly attached to the inner surface of the eyelids, but the bulbar conjunctiva is loosely adherent to the underlying sclera by thin connective tissue strands.

The palpebral conjunctiva, which lines the posterior surface of the eyelids, extends from the fornices to the mucocutaneous junction at the eyelid margins, where the epithelium of the conjunctiva merges abruptly with the epidermis of the anterior surface of the eyelids. The palpebral conjunctiva contains several infoldings of epithelium (crypts of Henle). Islands of accessory lacrimal glands that are morphologically identical to the main tear-producing gland within the orbit occur within the palpebral conjunctiva. The subconjunctival tissue of the upper fornix may contain over 40 such glands, but fewer than 10 accessory lacrimal glands are present in the lower fornix (glands of Krause). The upper eyelids have approximately two to five accessory lacrimal glands (glands of Wolfring) located at the superior aspect of the tarsus. The bulbar conjunctiva begins at the limbus, at which point the corneal epithelium gradually becomes replaced by conjunctival epithelium and continues over the sclera to the superior and inferior fornices. There, the conjunctiva is thrown into small folds before becoming the palpebral conjunctiva.

Both the caruncle and plica semilunaris (semilunar fold) represent specialized segments of the conjunctiva (Figure 13.16). The caruncle is the nodular mass of fleshy tissue located in the medial interpalpebral angle of the eye. Its surface is covered by a stratified nonkeratinized squamous epithelium. The subepithelial stroma of the

caruncle contains hair follicles, smooth muscle, sebaceous glands, adipose connective tissue, and, occasionally, accessory lacrimal glands and sweat glands. The plica semilunaris, an arc-shaped fold of conjunctiva located immediately lateral to the caruncle, is thought to be a vestigial remnant of the nictitating membrane of lower species. The histologic features of the plica semilunaris are similar to those in other areas of the conjunctiva, except that the epithelium contains abundant goblet cells and, rarely, cartilage is present within the stroma.

THE UVEAL TRACT

Located between the outer scleral covering and the inner retina is the uveal tract, which begins anteriorly as the iris, extends to the ciliary body, and then to the choroid posteriorly. The designated term *uvea* is derived from the Latin word *uva* (grape) because this portion of the eye was thought to somewhat resemble the dark color of a grape after the sclera and cornea are stripped from the globe.

The Iris

The iris is a thin diaphragm of tissue with a central opening, the pupil, which functions to regulate the amount of

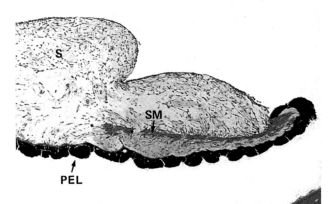

Figure 13.17 The iris is composed of stroma (*S*) and a posterior epithelial lining (*PEL*). The sphincter muscle (*SM*) of the iris is evident within the stroma. The pigmented posterior epithelial lining normally extends around the lip of the pupil anteriorly for a short distance. (H&E, ×25.)

light reaching the retina (Figure 13.17). Muscles within the iris dilate or constrict the pupil in response to sympathetic or parasympathetic nerve impulses. The diameter of the iris is approximately 21 mm, whereas the diameter of the pupil ranges from 1 to 8 mm. The iris is thinnest at its point of attachment with the ciliary body peripherally, the iris root. Normally, the iris rests gently upon the crystalline lens and, therefore, bulges slightly forward. Structurally and developmentally, the iris consists of two main parts: the stroma and the posterior epithelial lining.

Numerous ridges and depressions may be identified in tissue sections of the anterior iris stroma. These correspond to the contraction folds and furrows seen on clinical examination. The anterior surface of the iris lacks a cellular

lining. The stroma contains melanocytes, nerve cells, blood vessels, and smooth muscle in a loose connective tissue background. The color of the iris is due to the number of stromal melanocytes present. Lightly pigmented individuals with blue irises have relatively few stromal melanocytes. In contrast, darkly pigmented individuals with brown irises have numerous melanocytes within the iris stroma (Figure 13.18). In addition to melanocytes, melanosome-containing macrophages are also scattered within the iris stroma, particularly at the iris root. A thick collar of collagen fibers normally surrounds the blood vessels within the iris stroma. To the inexperienced observer, these normal vessels may appear to have arteriolosclerosis. In the pathologic process of iris neovascularization, thin-walled blood vessels, which lack such a collagenous coat, cover the anterior surface of the iris.

The sphincter muscle (sphincter pupillae), a bundle of circularly arranged smooth muscle innervated by parasympathetic nerves, acts to constrict the pupil. Located within the posterior stroma of the pupillary zone, the sphincter pupillae is nearly 1 mm wide. Radially oriented smooth muscle fibers with scattered cytoplasmic melanosomes are also located within the stroma of the iris (dilator pupillae). Innervated by sympathetic nerves, this muscle is active in pupil dilatation.

Posteriorly, the iris is lined by two separate but closely apposed epithelial layers derived from neuroectoderm. The cells of the anterior epithelial layer, which are in direct contact with the posterior aspect of the stroma, are continuous with smooth muscle fibers of the dilator pupillae; the sphincter pupillae are of similar developmental origin. The posterior iris pigment epithelial layer is in direct contact

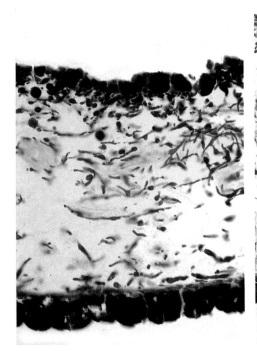
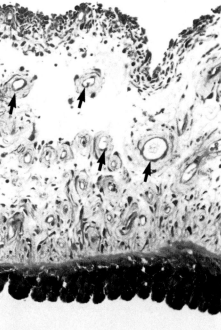

Figure 13.18 The color of the iris is due to the number of stromal melanocytes, which are more abundant in the stroma of an individual with a brown iris (*left*) than with a blue iris (*right*). The amount of pigment in the posterior epithelial lining is similar in irises of different color. Blood vessels in the iris stroma are normally surrounded by a thick collar of collagen fibers (*arrows*); this should not be confused as arteriolosclerosis. In contrast to the posterior surface of the iris, the anterior iris lacks a cellular lining. (Left, H&E, ×66; right, H&E, ×66.)

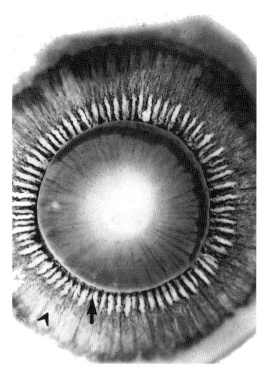

Figure 13.19 The lens and ciliary body are viewed from behind in this photograph. The ciliary body has two components: the pars plicata and the pars plana. The pars plicata contains about 70 sagitally oriented folds, or ciliary processes (*arrow*). The pars plicata gradually merges with the flat pars plana (*arrowhead*). (Reproduced with permission from: Klintworth GK, Landers MB III. *The Eye: Structure and Function.* Baltimore: Williams & Wilkins; 1976.)

layers does not vary significantly between lightly and darkly pigmented individuals. In persons with ocular and oculocutaneous albinism, the pigmented epithelia, as well as the stromal melanocytes, contain fewer melanin granules than in normal individuals. The pigmented epithelia of the iris normally extend around the lip of the pupil anteriorly for a short distance. In certain pathologic conditions, fibrovascular tissue on the anterior surface of the iris everts the pupillary margin and pulls the pigmented epithelia onto the anterior surface of the iris. This displaced pigmented epithelium may be apparent clinically and is known as ectropion uveae.

The Ciliary Body

The middle segment of the uveal tract, the ciliary body, is located between the iris and the choroid. Situated interior to the anterior sclera, it is made up of two ring-shaped components: the pars plicata and the pars plana (Figure 13.19). The anteriormost aspect of the ciliary body, the pars plicata begins at the scleral spur and contains approximately 70 sagitally oriented folds (approximately 2 mm long and 0.8 mm high). Continuous with these folds, the flat pars plana, which is approximately 4 mm wide, merges posteriorly with the serrated anterior border of the retina (ora serrata). Both portions of the ciliary body consist of epithelium, stroma, and smooth muscle.

The ciliary epithelium embraces two distinct layers, both of which share a similar development derivation from neural ectoderm (Figure 13.20). The inner epithelial layer is virtually nonpigmented and is contiguous with the aqueous humor of the posterior chamber. At the ora serrata, the sensory retina converges into the nonpigmented ciliary epithelial monolayer, which extends anteriorly until it

with the aqueous humor of the posterior chamber. The cytoplasm of both epithelial layers contains numerous melanosomes (approximately 1 μm in diameter), which are larger than those of the iris stroma (diameter of about 0.5 μm). The number of melanosomes in the iris epithelial

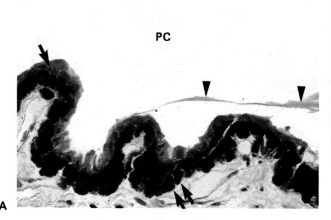

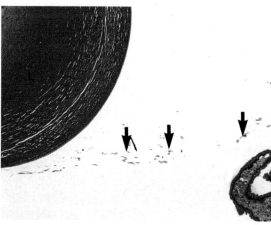

Figure 13.20 **A.** The epithelium of the ciliary body has two distinct layers. The inner nonpigmented layer (*arrow*) is in direct contact with the aqueous humor of the posterior chamber (*PC*). The outer pigmented epithelial layer (*double arrows*) is adjacent to the underlying stroma. Acellular eosinophilic fibers attach to the crests of the nonpigmented epithelium of the pars plicata (zonules) (*arrowheads*). Zonules do not originate in the valleys between the ciliary processes (H&E, ×132). **B.** Zonular fibers (*arrows*) span between the pars plicata of the ciliary body (right) and the lens (*L*) and hold the lens in place (H&E, ×25).

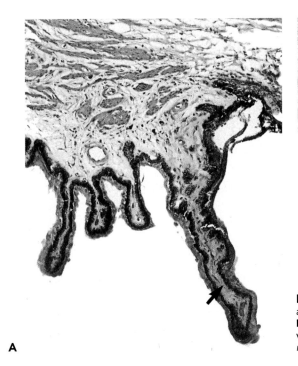

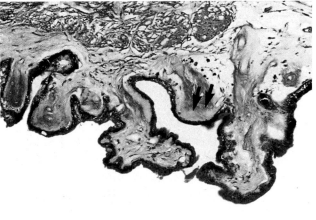

B

A

Figure 13.21 The pars plicata of the ciliary body changes with age. **A.** In infancy the stroma of the ciliary processes is sparse (*arrow*). **B.** The stroma continues to expand until adulthood; and, with advancing age, the ciliary processes become hyalinized (*double arrows*). (**A,** H&E, ×40; **B,** H&E, ×40.)

becomes the posterior epithelial layer of the iris. In contrast, the outer ciliary epithelial layer is pigmented and unites with the retinal pigment epithelium at the ora serrata. The pigmented epithelium of the ciliary body overlies a periodic acid-Schiff (PAS)– positive basal lamina that is closely adherent to the adjacent stroma. The basal lamina of the pigmented epithelium can become conspicuously thickened in diabetes mellitus. Acellular fibers, known as zonules (Figure 13.20), attach the crests of the nonpigmented ciliary epithelium in the pars plicata to the capsule of the crystalline lens.

The stroma of the ciliary body, composed of fibroblasts, blood vessels, nerve cells, and melanocytes, is most abundant in the ciliary processes of the pars plicata and least plentiful in the valleys between these processes and in the pars plana. During infancy, the stroma of the ciliary body is sparse (Figure 13.21, *left*), but it expands until adulthood. With advanced age, the ciliary body stroma becomes hyalinized (Figure 13.21, *right*) and frequently calcifies.

The smooth muscle of the ciliary body (Figure 13.22) forms three distinct bundles. The outermost muscle runs in a longitudinal, or meridonal, direction, whereas the middle layer contains radially oriented fibers and the innermost muscle cells are aligned in a circular fashion. In routinely processed globes, histologic differentiation of these three muscular layers is difficult. Muscles of the ciliary body attach in large part to the scleral spur. The ciliary muscle assists in accommodation. As it contracts, the ciliary body extends forward, reducing pressure on the zonules and enabling the lens to become less concave—and thereby increasing its refractive power.

Choroid

The richly vascularized choroid (Figure 13.23) extends from the ciliary body to the optic nerve. Its inner aspect is firmly adherent to the retinal pigment epithelium. The outer surface of the choroid is loosely attached to the overlying sclera. Bruch's membrane delineates the choroid from the overlying retinal pigment epithelium and is approximately 2 to 4 μm thick. Although Bruch's membrane appears as a thin eosinophilic layer in tissue sections, ultrastructural analysis has disclosed it to be composed of five distinct layers: the basal lamina of the overlying retinal pigment epithelium, a collagenous layer, an elastic fiber-rich component, another collagenous portion, and the

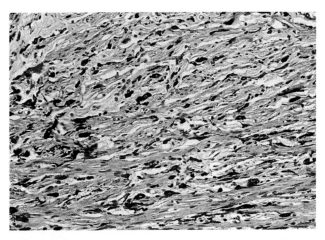

Figure 13.22 Smooth muscle constitutes a large portion of the ciliary body. Pigmented melanocytes are often present in between the smooth muscle bundles (H&E, ×66.)

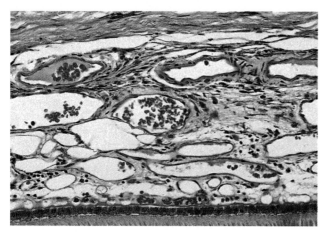

Figure 13.23 This photomicrograph illustrates the well-vascularized choroid. At the top of the figure, the choroid abuts the sclera. The single layer of retinal pigment epithelium is present at the bottom of the figure. (H&E, ×66.)

basal lamina of the endothelial cells of the underlying capillary network (choriocapillaris). Located in the innermost choroidal stroma adjacent to Bruch's membrane, the choriocapillaris connects with arterial and venous channels from vessels in the outer choroidal stroma. Its function is to nourish the outer retinal layers. With age, Bruch's membrane thickens and commonly acquires focal excrescences known as drusen (Figure 13.24). Both drusen and Bruch's membrane may calcify.

The choroidal stroma is thinnest anteriorly, near the ciliary body, where it is approximately 0.1 mm thick. Posteriorly, at the optic nerve, the choroidal stroma thickens to nearly 0.22 mm. The tenuous connection between the choroidal stroma and the sclera is responsible for both the pathologic and artifactual separations often seen between these two layers in histologic sections. The stroma contains abundant pigmented melanocytes (Figure 13.25), which are more numerous in heavily pigmented

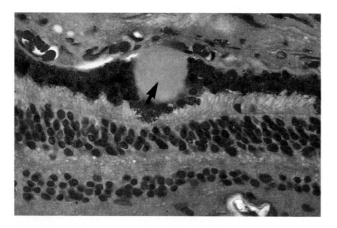

Figure 13.24 An amorphous excrescence (*arrow*) in Bruch's membrane appears to extend into the underlying retina. Such so-called *drusen* are common and occasionally calcify. (H&E, ×160.)

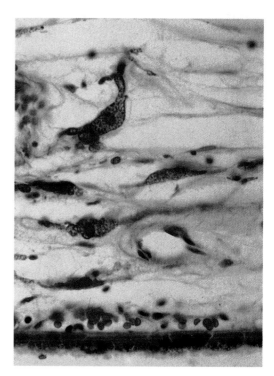

Figure 13.25 Numerous pigmented melanocytes are located within the choroidal stroma (H&E, ×160.)

individuals than in persons with little pigment. Collagen fibers, some smooth muscle, neurons of the autonomic nervous system, and a prominent vascular system are also present. Large- and medium-sized arteries (branches of the posterior ciliary arteries) and veins (vortex veins) are situated in the outermost choroid.

RETINA

The cellular components of the retina include the photoreceptors (rods and cones), a variety of different neurons (ganglion, bipolar, horizontal, and amacrine cells), and neuroglial cells (Müller cells and astrocytes). Many of these special types of cells can only be detected with the aid of specific staining techniques. These constituents of the retina are stratified into several distinct layers (Figure 13.26). The rods and cones comprise the outermost part of the sensory retina and are closely apposed to the retinal pigment epithelium. The retina's anterior boundary has a serrated edge (ora serrata), at which point it is approximately 0.1 mm thick. Cysts develop in the peripheral retina (peripheral cystoid degeneration) in virtually everyone over age 20 (13) (Figures 13.27, 13.28). Here, the retina converges into a single layer of nonpigmented epithelium, which continues anteriorly to where it merges with the nonpigmented epithelium of the ciliary body (Figure 13.28). Posteriorly, the retina extends to the optic nerve, where it is approximately 0.5 to 0.6 mm thick. The sensory retina is in direct

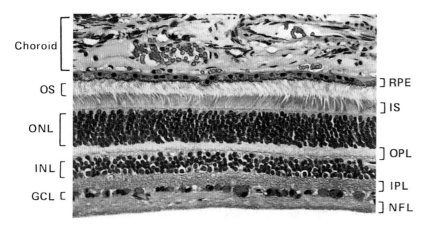

Choroid

OS
ONL
INL
GCL

RPE
IS
OPL
IPL
NFL

Figure 13.26 The cellular components of the retina are organized in well-defined layers. The choroid is directly above the retinal pigment epithelium (*RPE*) in this figure. Specialized extensions of the photoreceptors known as the outer and inner segments (*OS* and *IS*) are located immediately adjacent to the RPE. Cell bodies of the photoreceptors are present in the outer nuclear layer (*ONL*); synapses between the bipolar cells, horizontal cells, and the photoreceptors occur in the outer plexiform layer (*OPL*); the inner nuclear layer (*INL*) embraces nuclei of the amacrine, bipolar, horizontal, and Müller's cells; the inner plexiform (*IPL*) contains axons and dendrites of amacrine, bipolar, and ganglion cells; ganglion cell bodies are located in the ganglion cell layer (*GCL*); the nerve fiber layer (*NFL*) contains ganglion cell axons. (Reproduced with permission from: Klintworth GK, Landers MB III. *The Eye: Structure and Function*. Baltimore: Williams & Wilkins; 1976.)

contact with the vitreous humor and lies interior to the retinal pigment epithelium, which defines the outermost border of the retina.

The retinal pigment epithelium is a monolayer of cells. These epithelial cells contain numerous intracytoplasmic melanosomes; cellular processes envelope part of the overlying rods and cones as shown by transmission electron microscopy. The phagocytic function of the retinal pigment epithelium assists in the turnover of the photoreceptor elements. Undigested products of phagolipsomes culminate in the progressively increasing number of lipofuscin granules that accumulate within the retinal pigment epithelium, with time.

Some photoreceptors are cylindrical in appearance (rods), whereas others are conical-shaped and somewhat longer and thicker (cones). Internal to the photoreceptors is the outer plexiform layer, formed from cell processes of the horizontal and bipolar cells and axonal extensions of the rods and cones. The inner nuclear layer embraces the nuclei of several cell types (the bipolar, Müller, horizontal, and amacrine cells). Constituents of the inner plexiform layer include bipolar and amacrine cell axons and dendrites of the ganglion cells. Near the vitreal aspect of the retina is the ganglion cell layer, composed predominantly of ganglion cell bodies. The axons of these large neurons make up the nerve fiber layer; these processes are usually unmyelinated; but, as an incidental developmental anomaly, bundles of some nerve fibers are occasionally myelinated. In older individuals, basophilic PAS-positive intracellular rounded bodies (corpora amylacea), indistinguishable from similar structures in the brain, often accumulate in the nerve fiber layer of the retina near the optic disc. By light microscopy, two acellular zones can be distinguished within the retina: the external and internal limiting membranes. The so-called *external limiting membrane* is located between the photoreceptors and the outer nuclear layer.

The membrane represents firm junctions between Müller cells and adjacent photoreceptors (zonula adherens). The basal lamina of the Müller cells accounts for the hyalin structure seen on light microscopy and is known as the *internal limiting membrane*. Similar to the neuroglial tissue of the brain, by immunohistochemistry the neuronal cells of the retina show strong immunopositivity to synaptophysin (Figure 13.29) and NeuN (*Neu*ronal *N*uclei) (14) (Figure 13.30). Neurofilament protein highlights the axons of the

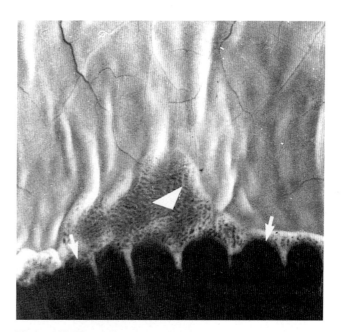

Figure 13.27 The ora serrata marks the anterior boundary of the retina. An almost invariable finding in the retina of all human eyes after the age of 20 is peripheral cystoid degeneration. Macroscopically, the peripheral retina immediately behind the ora serrata (*arrows*) has a focally vacuolated appearance (*arrowhead*). (Reproduced with permission from: Klintworth GK, Landers MB III. *The Eye: Structure and Function*. Baltimore: Williams & Wilkins; 1976.)

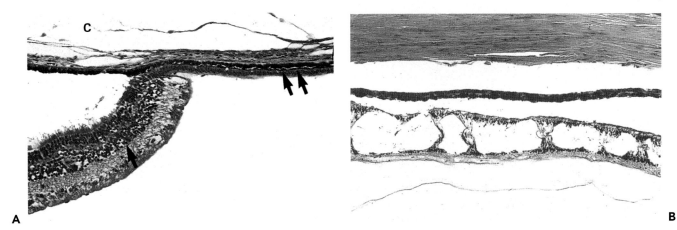

Figure 13.28 **A.** At the ora serrata, the multilayered retina (*arrow*) converges with the single layer of nonpigmented epithelium of the ciliary body (*double arrows*). The retina is loosely attached to the choroid (*C*) in the region of the ora serrata and is artifactually separated from it in this figure (H&E,×50). **B.** Microscopically, peripheral cystoid degeneration is characterized by the presence of numerous cystlike spaces within the retina. (Reproduced with permission from: Klintworth GK, Landers MB III. *The Eye: Structure and Function*. Baltimore; Williams & Wilkins, 1976.)

nerve fiber layer as they continue posteriorly to enter the optic nerve. Glial cells and their processes react with glial fibrillary acidic protein (GFAP) (Figure 13.31).

Light passes through the entire sensory retina before it is converted by the photoreceptor cells into electric impulses. The impulses are eventually transmitted to the visual cortex in the occipital lobe of the brain through a complex series of intercellular connections.

The retina varies in structure in different sites (Figure 13.32). A yellow specialized portion of the retina is located in the posterior pole of the eye (in an area slightly temporal to the optic disc). This is the macula lutea (yellow spot), where the bipolar and ganglion cells contain the pigment xanthophyll. In the macular region of the retina, the ganglion cells are several layers thick. The center of the macula contains a slightly depressed area (the fovea centralis) measuring almost 1.5 mm in diameter; it is responsible for most visual acuity. The walls of the fovea centralis are known as the clivus, and the precise center is designated the foveola. Blood vessels are absent in the foveola, which measures approximately 0.4 mm in diameter. The inner layers of the retina are displaced peripherally in the foveola so that only photoreceptors, the outer nuclear layer, and outer plexiform layer are present. Cones are located within the foveola, but rods are absent.

The microvasculature of the normal retina is composed of branches of the central retinal artery and tributaries of the central retinal vein. It contains arterioles, venules, and intervening capillaries (Figure 13.33). In capillaries from normal individuals, endothelial cells and pericytes are present in a ratio of approximately 1:1. The retinal microvasculature is affected in hypertension, diabetes mellitus, and other conditions. Capillary microaneurysms and the loss of capillary pericytes are characteristics of diabetic retinopathy. These are

best visualized in flat preparations of the retina after trypsin digestion of the retinal cells.

Artifacts of the Retina

It is necessary to distinguish a true detachment of the sensory retina from the retinal pigment epithelium from an artifactitious retinal detachment in the same location. True retinal detachments are characterized by the presence of blood or eosinophilic proteinaceous fluid in the space between the two retinal layers (Figure 13.34), rounded edges at the site of the retinal break, photoreceptor elements of one fold of retina adjacent to the internal

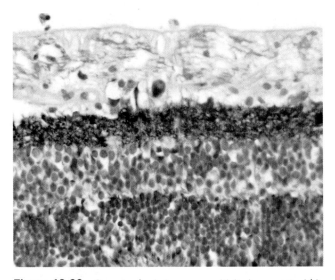

Figure 13.29 Synaptophysin immunopositivity is present within the ganglion cell layer, inner and outer nuclear layers, and inner and outer plexiform layers (×40).

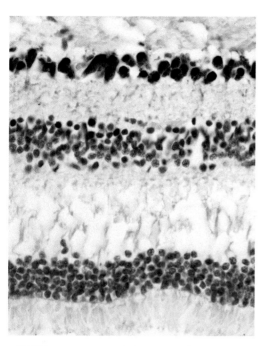

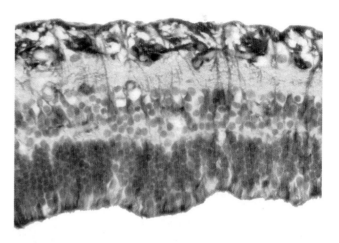

Figure 13.31   Glial fibrillary acidic protein (GFAP) highlights the retinal glia and their processes (×40).

Figure 13.30   Reactivity with the immunohistochemical marker NeuN is restricted to neurons of the ganglion cell layer and a few cells in the inner nuclear layer (×40).

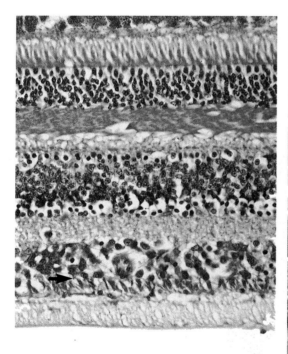

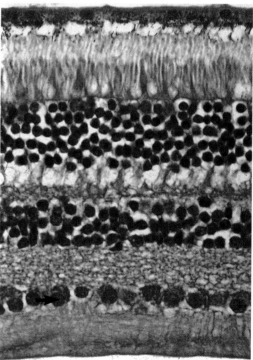

Figure 13.32   The retina has regional histologic variations. In the macular region (*left*), the ganglion cells (*arrow*) are multilayered. In areas outside of the macula (*right*), ganglion cells (*arrow*) form a single layer. (Left, H&E, ×80; right, H&E, ×160.)

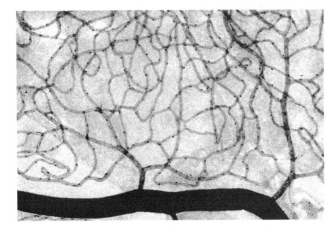

Figure 13.33 This flat preparation of a normal retina following trypsin digestion discloses retinal capillaries adjacent to a retinal arteriole (H&E, ×25).

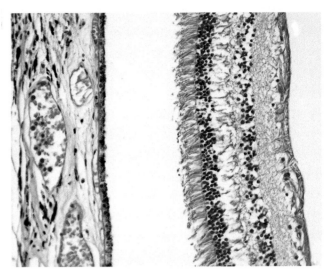

Figure 13.35 Artifactual retinal detachments are characterized by retinal pigment epithelium granules within the tips of the photoreceptors and the absence of subretinal eosinophilic fluid (H&E, ×20).

limiting membrane of another fold (Zimmerman's sign), an absence of photoreceptor outer segments (except in a very acute detachment), and the presence of cyst-like spaces within the detached retina. In contrast, artifactitious retinal detachments typically lack subretinal fluid that is rich in eosinophilic protein or blood, have squared-off edges at the site of the break with intact photoreceptor outer segments, and fragments of pigment epithelium cell debris are adherent to the photoreceptor outer segments (Figure 13.35) (15).

At the ora serrata, the sensory retina of neonates and children folds inwardly upon itself (Lange's fold) in eyes that have been subjected to a fixative such as formalin (Figure 13.36). This artifact of fixation is not observed in the living eye or in unfixed enucleated eyes that have been sectioned to observe the peripheral retina. Lange's fold is thought to result

from traction on the peripheral retina by a shortening of the vitreous humor base and posterior lens zonules caused by tissue fixation. After the age of 20 years, Lange's fold is not observed, presumably because the peripheral retina has become firmly bound to the subjacent retinal pigment epithelium. The convexity of this artifact of fixation is directed anteriorly and axially in neonates; but, in older infants and children, the fold is initiated some distance from the ora serrata, apparently because of a propensity for peripheral retinal adhesions to the subjacent retinal pigment epithelium with increasing age. In contrast to a true retinal

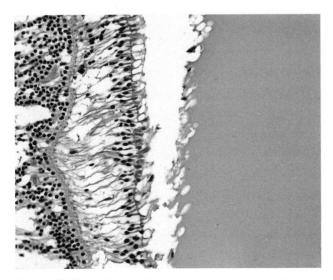

Figure 13.34 A feature of a true retinal detachment is the presence of eosinophilic proteinaceous fluid within the subretinal space (H&E, ×20).

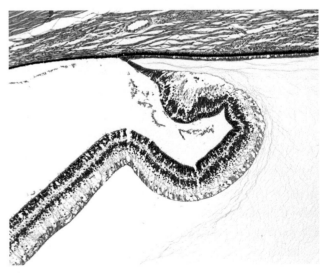

Figure 13.36 Lange's fold is a postmortem artifact usually seen in infant eyes. At the ora serrata, the peripheral retina typically takes on a bowed or concave appearance anteriorly. The absence of subretinal fluid distinguishes this from a true retinal detachment (H&E, ×10).

detachment, subretinal fluid is not present between the layers of the sensory retina in Lange's fold (16).

THE OPTIC NERVE

More than one million axons from the retinal nerve fiber layer converge at the optic nerve head, which accounts for the physiologic blind spot in the normal visual field and represents the beginning of the optic nerve. The central retinal artery and vein traverse the optic nerve; and, within a slight depression at the origin of the nerve, they are surrounded by glial tissue (Figure 13.37). From the optic nerve head, the axons extend for approximately 1 mm to a sievelike partition of connective tissue in the sclera (the lamina cribrosa) through which the nerve fibers pass on their way to the brain. Over one thousand nerve fiber bundles surrounded by astrocytes, oligodendroglia, and collagenous septae (Figure 13.38) can be identified in cross sections of the optic nerve, which is a tract of the central nervous system. Like the brain, the optic nerve is surrounded by dura, arachnoid, and pia mater. Small focal meningothelial proliferations occasionally form within the leptomeninges surrounding the optic nerve. Some orbital meningiomas presumably arise from them. Laminated products of the meningothelial cells (psammoma bodies) sometimes occur in the arachnoid mater (Figure 13.39). Pigmented melanocytes are sometimes encountered within the leptomeninges and optic nerve head.

After leaving the globe, each optic nerve continues posteriorly through the orbit to its respective optic foramen, and then to the optic chiasm before terminating in the lateral geniculate bodies.

At the level of the lamina cribrosa, the axons within the optic nerve become myelinated by concentric membranous processes of the oligodendroglia. The rather abrupt transition between myelinated and nonmyelinated nerve fibers is eminently appreciated in tissue sections stained with Luxol fast blue or other dyes with an affinity for myelin (Figure 13.40). As the axons acquire myelin coats, the diameter of the optic nerve doubles to nearly 3 mm. Located within the central core of the optic nerve, adjacent to the globe, is the central retinal artery and vein. Both of these vascular channels exit the nerve some 8 to 15 mm posterior to the lamina cribrosa; the channels are not evident within tissue sections of the optic nerve closer to the brain. The orbital portion of the optic nerve extends some 25 mm from the lamina cribrosa to the optic foramen at the apex of the orbit. If the optic nerve becomes compressed during enucleation of the globe, some optic nerve tissue may extrude into the eye and become dislodged into the lumen of blood vessels near the optic disc, between the sensory retina and the retinal pigment epithelium, and even into the vitreous humor. Neural tissue within the optic nerve may become displaced in a manner comparable to the "toothpaste" artifact of the

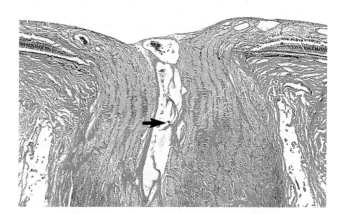

Figure 13.37 The optic nerve penetrates the sclera near the posterior pole of the eye. This histologic section contains the central retinal artery (*arrow*) in the central part of the optic nerve. Both the central retinal artery and the central retinal vein traverse the optic nerve until they exit the nerve about 8 to 15 mm posterior to the eyeball. (Masson's trichrome, ×10.)

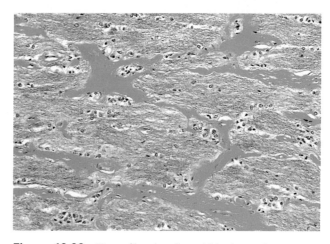

Figure 13.38 Nerve fiber bundles within the optic nerve are surrounded by thin collagenous septae (Masson's trichrome, ×50).

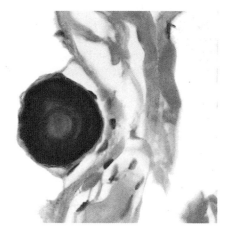

Figure 13.39 Laminated psammoma bodies, such as this one, are often closely associated with the meningothelial cells of optic nerve (H&E, ×160).

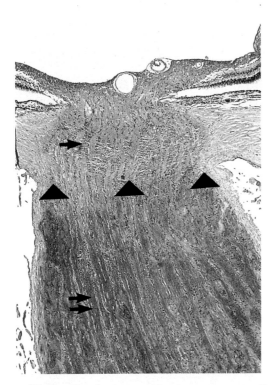

Figure 13.40   The abrupt transition between nonmyelinated (*arrow*) and myelinated (*double arrows*) nerve fibers of the normal optic nerve at the level of the lamina cribrosa (*arrowheads*) is dramatically illustrated in this tissue section stained with a dye that has an affinity for myelin (Luxol fast blue, ×10).

spinal cord that follows a traumatic insinuation of white matter into the grey matter. This artifact should not be mistaken for ectopic intraocular nervous tissue, tumors, giant drusen, vitreous humor worms, or subretinal exudates (17). With age, corpora amylacea, similar to those in the retina and brain, may become evident in the optic nerve.

THE CRYSTALLINE LENS

The biconvex ocular lens (Figure 13.41) is located directly behind the pupil and in front of the anterior face of the vitreous humor. In the adult, it measures approximately 10 mm in diameter and 4 to 5 mm in width. The lens is held in place by zonules that connect it to the pars plicata of the ciliary body. The lens is encircled by a collagen- and carbohydrate-rich capsule that serves as the site of attachment for the zonules. The capsule over the anterior surface of the lens thickens with time. At 2 to 3 years of age, the anterior capsule is almost 8 to 15 μm wide and increases to 14 to 21 μm by 35 years (Figure 13.42). The posterior lens capsule reaches its maximum thickness at about 35 years of age (4–23 μm) and then diminishes to 2 to 9 μm after age 70 years (Figure 13.43) (2). Directly interior to the anterior lens capsule is a

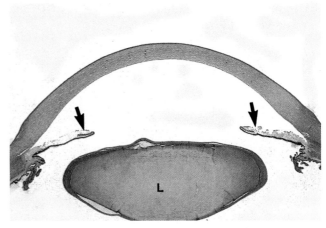

Figure 13.41   The crystalline lens (*L*) is situated just posterior to the pupil and iris (*arrows*) (H&E, ×2.5).

single layer of cuboidal epithelium. These cells extend to about the level of the lens equator; they do not normally exist posterior to this point. Proliferating epithelial cells elongate at the lens equator and become displaced toward the center of the lens, known as the lens nucleus, where they are retained for life. This process continues throughout life, and the long slender cells are designated lens fibers. In the peripheral part of the lens near the equator, the fibers retain their nuclei; but, as the fibers become displaced toward the center of the lens, their nuclei disintegrate so that the center of the lens lacks nuclei. In some cataractous lenses, such as the cataract of rubella, the fibers within the center of the lens retain their nuclei.

The normally transparent lens commonly opacifies with age. Discrete globules of degenerate lens fibers may form. They are frequently accompanied by the presence of an extension of epithelial cells posterior to the equator. The high density of the lens fibers makes it difficult to obtain histologic sections of the lens that are free from artifact.

Infant eyes can demonstrate an artifact of fixation resulting in an umbilicated, dimpled, or concave configuration of the posterior surface of the lens (18) (Figure 13.44).

INTRAOCULAR COMPARTMENTS

The eye accommodates two major fluid-containing intraocular compartments. One is filled with aqueous humor, the other with vitreous humor. The aqueous humor compartment is divided into an anterior and posterior chamber (Figure 13.45). The anterior chamber is delineated in front by the cornea, peripherally by the drainage angle of the eye, and posteriorly by the pupil and the iris. The small posterior chamber is situated between the pigmented epithelia of the iris, the ciliary body, the anterior face of the vitreous humor, and the lens.

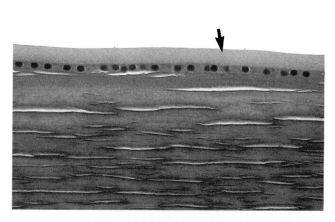
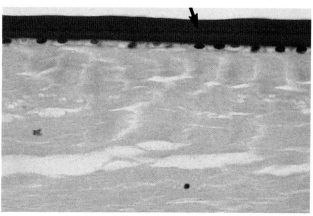

Figure 13.42 The anterior lens capsule (*arrow*) appears as an eosinophilic acellular band overlying a single layer of epithelial cells in hematoxylin and eosin-stained preparations (*left*). The lens capsule is rich in carbohydrate and reacts intensely with the periodic acid-Schiff stain (*arrow*) (*right*). (Left, H&E, ×132; right, PAS, ×160.)

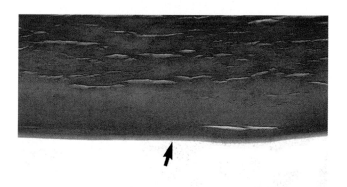

The aqueous humor, a watery solution that does not normally stain with routine histologic techniques, is produced by the ciliary body and flows forward through the aperture of the pupil to the anterior chamber, where it leaves the eye through the trabecular meshwork and Schlemm's canal. The anterior chamber contains approximately 0.25 ml of aqueous humor; the posterior chamber has a volume of only approximately 0.06 ml. Normal human aqueous humor has a density slightly greater than water; and, like plasma, it contains protein, ascorbic acid, electrolytes, and glucose. The major differences between

Figure 13.43 Posteriorly, the lens capsule (*arrow*) is thinner than anteriorly, and epithelial cells are absent (H&E, ×132).

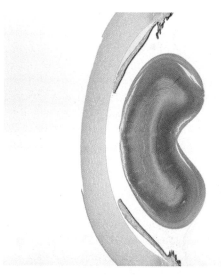

Figure 13.44 Infant eye demonstrating an artifact of fixation resulting in a posterior concave or umbilicated appearance of the lens. This figure also illustrates an artifactual absence of most of the corneal epithelium (H&E, ×1).

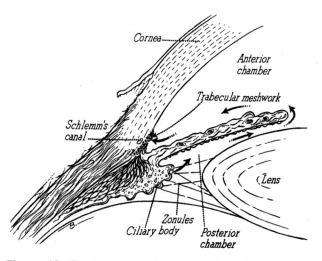

Figure 13.45 The anterior chamber is defined by the cornea, anterior surface of the iris, and pupil. The boundaries of the much smaller posterior chamber include the posterior surface of the iris, the ciliary body, and the anterior face of the vitreous humor. Aqueous humor is produced by the ciliary body and circulates from the posterior chamber through the pupil into the anterior chamber. Aqueous humor drains from the eye by way of the trabecular meshwork and Schlemm's canal. (Reproduced with permission from: Klintworth GK, Landers MB III. *The Eye: Structure and Function.* Baltimore: Williams & Wilkins; 1976.)

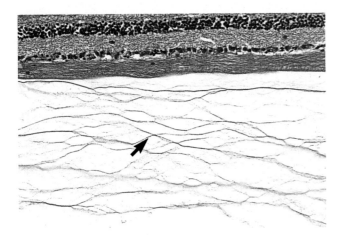

Figure 13.46 The vitreous humor (*arrow*) appears as an amorphous material in standard tissue sections (H&E, ×50).

aqueous humor and plasma are the relatively low-protein and high-ascorbic acid concentration of aqueous humor, relative to plasma.

The vitreous humor extends from the sensory retina to the lens and contains a gel-like material composed of water, protein, hyaluronic acid, and a small population of cells, designated hyalocytes, which are rarely noted in standard tissue sections. These tissue macrophages are thought to synthesize collagen and hyaluronic acid. The gelatinous consistency of the vitreous humor is due to a framework of numerous, randomly oriented collagen fibrils. The concentration of glucose and ascorbic acid is much lower than in the aqueous humor, whereas the concentration of soluble protein is similar to that of the aqueous humor (19). The vitreous humor is attached securely to the retina at the ora serrata and near the optic disc. Occasionally, vitreous humor may be identified as an amorphous acellular material on hematoxylin and eosin-stained sections (Figure 13.46).

THE EYELIDS

The eyelids (Figure 13.47) can be divided into cutaneous and conjunctival portions. The cutaneous segment of the eyelid is composed of a stratified squamous epidermis overlying a loosely arranged dermis, beneath which is muscular tissue. The eyelids contain several types of skin appendages. Sebaceous glands deposit their secretions, together with decomposed whole cells, via ducts into hair follicles of the eyelashes (glands of Zeis) or into ducts that open into the lid margins (meibomian glands) (Figure 13.48). Apocrine glands, whose secretions represent the pinched-off luminal aspect of the lining acinar cells, also open into the follicles of the eyelashes (glands of Moll) (Figure 13.49). In addition, the dermis of the eyelid contains eccrine sweat glands, which discharge secretions

directly onto the skin via a convoluted duct. The subcutaneous portion of the upper and lower eyelids contains concentrically arranged skeletal muscle fibers (orbicularis oculi) but very little adipose connective tissue. Striated muscle of the palpebral portion of the levator palpebrae superioris is also present in the upper eyelid; it terminates in a dense fibrocollagenous aponeurosis. Small bundles of smooth muscle fibers (Müller's muscle) are located within the upper and lower eyelids.

The junction between the cutaneous and conjunctival parts of the eyelid is demarcated clinically by a sulcus (the gray line), located between the ducts of the meibomian glands and the eyelashes. The conjunctival portion of the eyelid is made up of dense connective tissue containing the meibomian glands and the palpebral conjunctiva (Figure 13.50). The tarsus, located immediately posterior to the muscles of the eyelid, accounts for most of the rigidity of the eyelids and is covered posteriorly by conjunctival epithelium and a thin subepithelial stroma. As described earlier, accessory lacrimal glands are present in the palpebral conjunctiva.

The presence of more prominent subcutaneous, suborbicularis, and pretarsal fat tissue in the upper eyelid (the pretarsal fat pad) distinguishes an Asian eyelid from a Caucasian eyelid (20).

THE ORBIT

The posterior and peripheral borders of the orbit are defined by bones of the skull, face, and nose. At the anterior orbital margin, the periosteum of the orbital bones gives rise to a dense connective tissue sheet (the orbital septum) (Figure 13.47A), which extends forward to insert into the eyelids. Tissue posterior to this septum is considered to be within the orbit. In the human adult, the orbit measures approximately 40 mm in height, 45 mm in depth, and has a volume of almost 30 mL. Several bony canals allow for transmission of blood vessels and nerves into and out of the orbit, posteriorly. The contents of the orbit are organized in a complex three-dimensional arrangement (Figure 13.51). Aside from the eye, the optic nerve and its meningeal coverings, Tenon's capsule, the extraocular muscles, the lacrimal gland, blood vessels, and a delicate framework of fibroadipose connective tissue constitute the major components of the orbit.

The only epithelial structure normally present in the orbit is the lacrimal gland (Figure 13.52). Closely apposed to the globe and situated in the superolateral aspect of the orbit, this gland is traditionally divided into two parts: a larger orbital lobe and a smaller palpebral lobe. About a dozen ducts from the lacrimal gland open into the superior conjunctival fornices and transmit their secretions into the tear film. The lacrimal gland is not encapsulated, and thin fibroconnective tissue septae divide the tissue into lobules

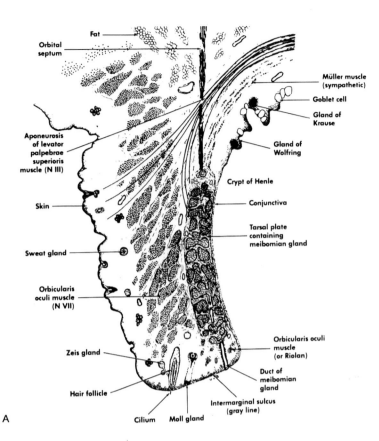

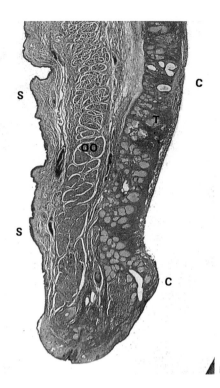

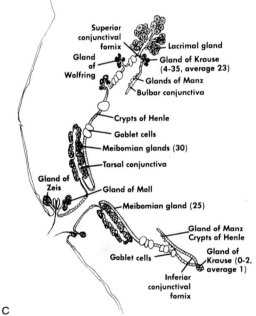

Figure 13.47 **A.** Components of the eyelid as illustrated on this drawing include skin and cutaneous appendages, muscle, connective tissue, and conjunctiva. (Reproduced with permission from FW Newell. *Ophthalmology: Principles and Concepts.* 6th ed. St. Louis: CV Mosby; 1986.) **B.** The skin surface (*S*), the orbicularis oculi muscle (*OO*), the tarsus (*T*), and the conjunctiva (*C*) are evident in this histologic section of an eyelid (H&E, ×3.3). **C.** Multiple foci of accessory lacrimal gland tissue (glands of Krause and Wolfring) are present in the eyelids. (Reproduced with permission from: Newell FW. *Ophthalmology: Principles and Concepts.* 6th ed. St. Louis: CV Mosby; 1986.)

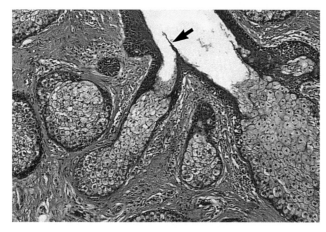

Figure 13.48 Modified sebaceous glands, the meibomian glands, deposit secretions into ducts that open onto the eyelids. A valve is evident (*arrow*) in this duct of a meibomian gland. (H&E, ×33.)

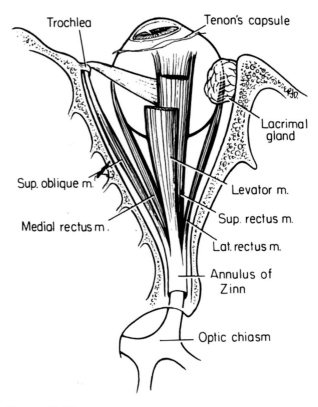

Figure 13.51 The bony cavity of the orbit contains the eyeball and its fibrous covering (Tenon's capsule), the cartilagenous trochlea, the lacrimal gland, and the extraocular muscles. The trochlea and the lacrimal gland are located within the superonasal and superotemporal aspects of the orbit respectively. Some of the extraocular muscles originate from a ring of fibrous tissue in the posterior orbit known as the annulus of Zinn. (Reproduced with permission from: Tasman W, Jaeger EA, eds. *Duane's Clinical Ophthalmology*. Vol. 2. Philadelphia: JB Lippincott; 1989.)

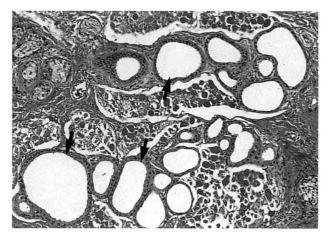

Figure 13.49 Apocrine glands (glands of Moll) (*arrows*) occur in the eyelid and open into the follicles of the eyelashes (H&E, ×33).

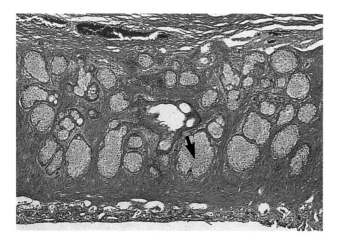

Figure 13.50 The tarsus, composed of dense fibrous tissue, contains the meibomian glands (*arrow*). The palpebral conjunctiva is immediately beneath the tarsus at the bottom of this figure. (H&E, ×13.2.)

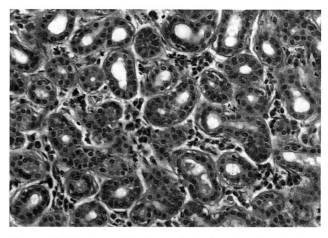

Figure 13.52 Acini of the lacrimal gland are lined by columnar-shaped epithelial cells. Scattered lymphocytes and plasma cells are normally present in the gland. (H&E, ×80.)

composed of acini and lined by columnar-shaped cells. Occasionally, some lobules extend posteriorly behind the globe. Most cells are serous in type and contain scattered intracytoplasmic fat droplets and granules. Mucinous cells similar to those of salivary glands are not usually present in the acini but may be identified in the ducts. In addition to secretory cells, the lining of the larger peripheral ducts within the lacrimal gland contain myoepithelial cells external to the serous cells. Occasional lymphocytes and plasma cells are commonly present between the acini of the lacrimal gland.

The orbit contains the cranial nerves, which innervate the extrinsic muscles of the eye (oculomotor, trochlear, and abducens nerves) and branches of the ophthalmic division of the trigeminal nerve, as well as parasympathetic and sympathetic nerves that innervate the cornea, conjunctiva, and the muscles of the ciliary body and iris. Neurons of the ciliary ganglion, which is located near the optic nerve close to the orbital apex and which measures approximately 2 mm in diameter, receive parasympathetic and sympathetic nerve fibers.

Other constituents of the orbit include smooth muscle (Figure 13.53) (21) and the arc-shaped structure (trochlea), through which the tendon of the superior oblique muscle passes before insertion upon the eyeball (Figure 13.54). The trochlea is the only cartilaginous structure normally present in the orbit. It arises from the superior nasal aspect of the frontal bone.

Lymphatic channels do not exist in the orbit according to traditional teaching; but this point is disputed because lymphangiomas develop in the orbit on rare occasions (22). The orbit normally lacks lymphoid tissue but contains scattered lymphocytes. These cells presumably give rise to the monoclonal and polyclonal lymphoid proliferations that frequently develop within the orbit, creating diagnostic and prognostic difficulty for the pathologist (23).

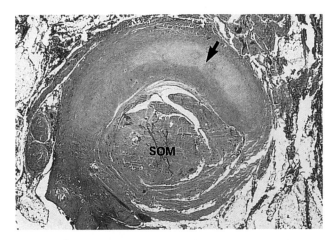

Figure 13.54 The arc-shaped trochlea (*arrow*), the only cartilaginous structure of the normal orbit, envelops the skeletal muscle fibers of the superior oblique muscle (*SOM*) (H&E, ×5).

LACRIMAL DRAINAGE APPARATUS

The lacrimal drainage apparatus (Figure 13.55), composed of the puncta, canaliculi, lacrimal sac, and the nasolacrimal duct, collects the tears and drains them to the nose. Tear fluid drains toward the medial canthus and then passes through an opening in the medial aspect of each eyelid, known as the lacrimal punctum. The puncta drain into the lacrimal canaliculi, tubular structures approximately 0.5 mm in diameter. Initially, The canaliculi are oriented vertically but, within 2 mm of their origin, bend at right angles to become almost horizontal within the eyelids. The distal portions of the canaliculi exit the

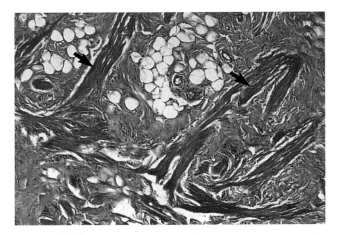

Figure 13.53 Smooth muscle bundles (*arrows*) are present in the soft tissues of the orbit (H&E, ×10).

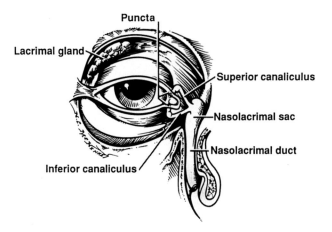

Figure 13.55 The lacrimal gland and drainage apparatus are illustrated here. The lacrimal gland is located in the superotemporal aspect of the orbit and contributes secretions to the tear film. Tears enter the canaliculi through the puncta and drain through the nasolacrimal sac and duct to eventually reach the inferior meatus within the nose.

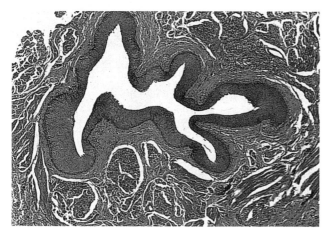

Figure 13.56 The lacrimal canaliculi are lined by nonkeratinizing stratified squamous epithelium and are surrounded by fibrous tissue (H&E, ×13.2).

upper and lower eyelids. They merge to form the lacrimal sac, which is encased by bones located in the inferomedial wall of the orbit. A duct (the nasolacrimal duct) that is nearly 1 cm long drains the lacrimal sac into the inferior nasal meatus of the nose. The epithelium lining the lacrimal drainage apparatus varies in different regions. In the canaliculi, it is a nonkeratinizing stratified squamous epithelium (Figure 13.56), but in the lacrimal sac and duct, the epithelium is stratified columnar in type and contains mucus-secreting goblet cells surrounded by connective tissue (Figure 13.57).

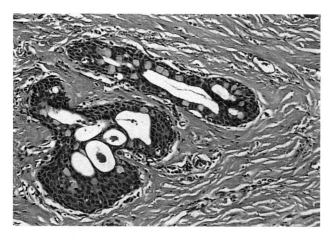

Figure 13.57 The epithelium of the lacrimal sacs and ducts is stratified columnar and contains goblet cells (H&E, ×50).

ACKNOWLEDGMENT

The authors acknowledge the contribution of Mark W. Scroggs to previous editions of this chapter.

REFERENCES

1. Bron AJ, Tripathi RC, Tripathi BJ. *Wolff's Anatomy of the Eye and Orbit.* 8th ed. London: Chapman & Hall Medical; 1997.
2. Hogan MJ, Alvarado JA, Weddell JE. *Histology of the Human Eye: An Atlas and Text.* Philadelphia: WB Saunders; 1971.
3. Fine BS, Yanoff M. *Ocular Histology: A Text and Atlas.* 2nd ed. Hagerstown, Md: Harper & Row; 1979.
4. Jakobiec FA, ed. *Ocular Anatomy, Embryology and Teratology.* Philadelphia: Harper & Row; 1982.
5. Bloom W, Fawcett DW. *A Textbook of Histology.* 12th ed. New York: Chapman and Hall; 1994.
6. Gillette TE, Chandler JW, Greiner JV. Langerhans cells of the ocular surface. *Ophthalmology* 1982;89:700–711.
7. Shamsuddin AK, Nirankari VS, Purnell DM, Chang SH. Is the corneal posterior cell layer truly endothelial? *Ophthalmology* 1986;93:1298–1303.
8. Howell DN, Burchette JL Jr, Paolini JF, Geiser SS, Fuller JA, Sanfilippo F. Characterization of a novel human corneal endothelial antigen. *Invest Ophthalmol Vis Sci* 1991;32:2473–2482.
9. Reese AB. Intrascleral nerve loops. *Arch Ophthalmol* 1931;6:698–703.
10. Spencer WH. Sclera. In: Spencer WH, ed. *Ophthalmic Pathology: An Atlas and Textbook.* 4th ed. Philadelphia: WB Saunders; 1996:337.
11. Scroggs MW, Klintworth GK. Senile scleral plaques: a histopathologic study using energy-dispersive x-ray microanalysis. *Hum Pathol* 1991;22:557–562.
12. Tripathi RC. Aqueous outflow pathway in normal and glaucomatous eyes. *Br J Ophthalmol* 1972;56:157–174.
13. Straatsma BR, Foos RY. Typical and reticular degenerative retinoschisis. *Am J Ophthalmol* 1973;75:551–575.
14. Mullen RJ, Buck CR, Smith AM. NeuN, a neuronal specific nuclear protein in vertebrates. *Development* 1992;116:201–211.
15. Folberg R. The eye. In: Spencer WH, ed. *Ophthalmic Pathology: An Atlas and Textbook.* 4th ed. Philadelphia: WB Saunders; 1996:25–27.
16. Gartner S, Henkind P. Lange's folds: a meaningful ocular artifact. *Ophthalmology* 1981;88:1307–1310.
17. Zimmerman LE, Fine BS. Myelin artifacts in the optic disc and retina. *Arch Ophthalmol* 1965;74:394–398.
18. Eagle RC Jr. *Eye Histology. An Atlas and Basic Text.* Philadelphia: WB Saunders; 1999:101–114.
19. Kaufman PL, Alm A, eds. *Adler's Physiology of the Eye.* 10th ed. St. Louis: CV Mosby; 2003.
20. Jeong S, Lemke BN, Dortzbach RK, Park YG, Kang HK. The Asian upper eyelid. An anatomical study with comparison to the Caucasian eyelid. *Arch Ophthalmol* 1999;117:907–912.
21. Koornneef L. New insights in the human orbital connective tissue. Result of a new anatomical approach. *Arch Ophthalmol* 1977;95:1269–1273.
22. Harris GJ. Orbital vascular malformations: a consensus statement on terminology and its clinical implications. Orbital Society. *Am J Ophthalmol* 1999;127:453–455.
23. Bardenstein DS. Ocular adnexal lymphoma: classification, clinical disease, and molecular biology. *Ophthalmol Clin North Am* 2005; 18:187–197.

The Ear and Temporal Bone

Bruce M. Wenig   Leslie Michaels

INTRODUCTION

The ear can be considered as three distinct regions, or compartments, to include the external ear, the middle ear and temporal bone, and the inner ear (Figure 14.1).

■ The external ear consists of the auricle (pinna), external auditory canal (or meatus), and the tympanic membrane at the medial end of the auditory canal.
■ The middle ear cavity includes the ossicles, auditory (eustachian or pharyngotympanic) tube connecting the middle ear space to the nasopharynx, and expansion of the middle ear cavity in the form of air cells in the temporal bone.
■ The inner ear is embedded in the petrous portion of the temporal bone and consists of a membranous (otic) labyrinth that lies within a dense bone referred to as the otic capsule, which is excavated to form the osseous (periotic) labyrinth (1).

The inner ear is the sense organ for both hearing and balance. The external and middle ears are the sound-conducting apparatus for the auditory part of the inner ear.

EXTERNAL EAR

Embryology

The external ear develops from the first brachial groove. The external auricle (pinna) forms from the fusion of the auricular hillocks or tubercles (a group of mesenchymal tissue swellings from the first and second branchial arches) that lie around the external portion of the first branchial groove (2). The external auditory canal is considered a normal remnant of the first branchial groove. The tympanic membrane forms from the first and second branchial pouches and the first branchial groove (2). The ectoderm of the first

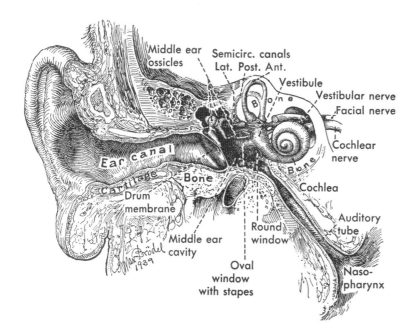

Figure 14.1 Modified coronal section through the ear and temporal bone depicting the anatomic compartments of the ear: the external, middle, and inner ears (Reprinted with permission from: Hollinshead WH. The ear. In: Hollinshead WH, ed. *Anatomy for Surgeons*. 3rd ed. Philadelphia: Harper and Row; 1982:159–221).

branchial groove gives rise to the epithelium on the external side; the endoderm from the first branchial pouch gives rise to the epithelium on the internal side; and the mesoderm of the first and second branchial pouches gives rise to the connective tissue lying between the external and internal epithelia (Figure 14.2) (2).

Anatomy

The anatomy of the external ear is seen in Figure 14.3. The outer portion of the external ear includes the auricle leading into the external auditory canal. The skeleton of the auricle consists of a single plate of elastic cartilage conforming to the shape of the ear. The lobule is the only part of the auricle that is devoid of skeletal support. The cartilage of the auricle is continuous with that of the external auditory canal.

The auricle is attached to the bony skull by three ligaments: anterior, superior, and posterior (1). The anterior ligament attaches the helix and the tragus to the zygomatic process. The superior ligament attaches the spine of the helix to the superior margin of the bony external meatus. The posterior ligament attaches the medial surface (eminence) of the concha to the mastoid process. The auricle is anchored through its continuity with the cartilage of the meatus and through the skin and extrinsic muscles.

The extrinsic muscles of the ear include the anterior, superior, and posterior auricular muscles. These muscles are usually functionless but may be subject to voluntary control (as in ear "wiggling"). There are also small intrinsic muscles in connection with the cartilage of the external ear, but they are of no apparent importance. The extrinsic and intrinsic muscles of the ear are innervated by the facial nerve.

DEVELOPMENT OF THE EPITHELIAL SYSTEMS OF THE EAR

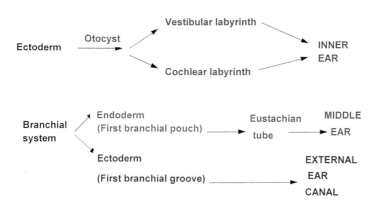

Figure 14.2 Diagrammatic representation of the embryology of the epithelia of the inner, middle, and external ears.

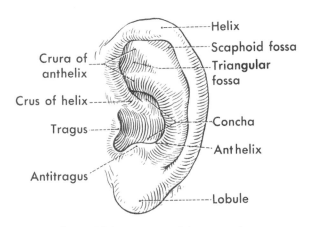

Figure 14.3 Anatomy of the external ear.

The external auditory canal or meatus extends from the concha to its medial limit, which is the external aspect of the tympanic membrane. The lateral portion of its wall consists of cartilage and connective tissue (1); the medial portion of its wall consists of bone. The cartilaginous part of the external auditory canal constitutes slightly less than half its total length. Inconstant fissures, referred to as the fissures of Santorini, occur in the cartilage; these fissures may transmit infection from the canal to the parotid gland and superficial mastoid regions, or vice versa. The bony part of the canal is formed by both the tympanic part and the petrous part of the temporal bone. The anterior, inferior, and lower posterior parts of the bony wall are formed by the C-shaped part of the temporal bone developed from the annulus tympanicus of the fetus. However, the annulus is incomplete in the posterosuperior part of the wall, and this part of the wall in adults is formed by the squamous and petrous parts of the temporal bone. In adults, the anterior and inferior walls of the cartilaginous canal are closely related to the parotid gland. The anterior wall of the bony canal is closely related to the mandibular condyle, the posterior wall to the mastoid air cells, and the medial portion of the superior wall to the epitympanic recess.

The tympanic membrane (eardrum) is situated obliquely at the end of the external auditory canal, sloping medially both from above downward and from behind forward. The tympanic membrane is a fibrous sheet interposed between the external auditory canal and the middle ear cavity (Figure 14.4). The connective tissue interposed between these two layers consists of radiating fibers that are attached to the manubrium of the malleus and are reinforced peripherally by circular fibers. The latter are thickened at the margin of the tympanic membrane to form a fibrocartilaginous ring (annulus fibrocartilagineus membranae tympani), attaching the tympanic membrane to the tympanic sulcus of the tem-

poral bone. In the upper portion of the tympanic membrane, there is a limited area where the connective tissue fibers are lacking; this area is referred to as the pars flaccida, or Schrapnell's membrane. In this area, the tympanic portion of the temporal bone is deficient; this gap is referred to as the tympanic incisure, or the notch of Rivinus. The tympanic membrane attaches to the temporal bone. The remainder of the tympanic membrane, in which there are intact connective tissue fibers, is referred to as the pars tensa.

The outer aspect of the tympanic membrane is concave. The center of the concavity is referred to as the umbo, which is the strong point of attachment of the manubrium of the malleus to the tympanic membrane. In the anteriosuperior portion of the tympanic membrane, the lateral process of the malleus is attached; from this point of attachment, the anterior and posterior mallear folds pass to the cartilaginous annulus and separate the pars flaccida from the pars tensa. In otoscopic examinations of the tympanic membrane, the bright area of light reflection present downward and forward from the umbo is referred to as the "cone of light."

Histology

Histologically, the auricle is essentially a cutaneous structure composed of keratinizing, stratified squamous epithelium with associated cutaneous adnexal structures that include hair follicles, sebaceous glands, and eccrine sweat glands (Figure 14.5). In addition to the hair follicles and sebaceous glands, the outer third of the external auditory canal is noteworthy for the presence of modified apocrine glands (called ceruminal glands) that replace the eccrine glands seen in the auricular dermis (Figure 14.6). Ceruminal glands produce cerumen and are arranged in clusters

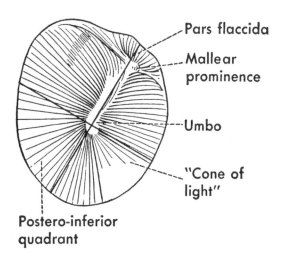

Figure 14.4 External (lateral) view of the tympanic membrane.

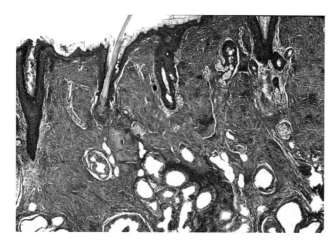

Figure 14.5 The auricle is a cutaneous structure histologically composed of keratinizing stratified squamous epithelium with associated cutaneous adnexal structures that include hair follicles, sebaceous glands, and eccrine sweat glands.

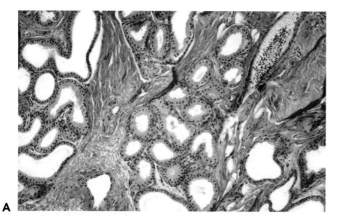

A

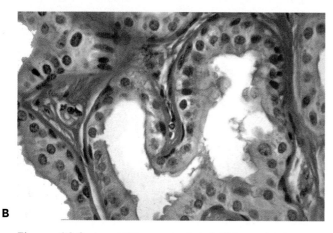

B

Figure 14.6 In addition to the hair follicles and sebaceous glands, the outer third of the external auditory canal is noteworthy for the presence of modified apocrine glands called ceruminal glands that replace the eccrine glands seen in the auricular dermis. **A.** Ceruminal glands are submucosal in location and are arranged in clusters or lobules. **B.** Ceruminal glands are composed of two cell layers, including the inner or secretory cells (containing intracytoplasmic cerumen and appearing as granular, golden-yellow pigmentation) and flattened-appearing myoepithelial cells located peripheral to the secretory cells. Focally, the secretory cells show holocrine (decapitation) type secretion.

composed of cuboidal cells with eosinophilic cytoplasm, often containing a granular, golden-yellow pigment. These cells have secretory droplets along their luminal border. Peripheral to the secretory cells are flattened myoepithelial cells. The ducts of the ceruminal glands terminate in the hair follicle or on the skin. The ducts of ceruminal glands lack apocrine or myoepithelial cells. In the inner portion of the external auditory canal, ceruminal glands and the other adnexal structures are absent.

The subcutaneous tissue is composed of fibroconnective tissue, fat, and elastic-type fibrocartilage, which gives the auricle its structural support (Figure 14.7). The ear lobe is devoid of cartilage and is replaced by a pad of adipose tissue. The perichondrium is composed of loose vascular connective tissue.

Similar to the auricle, the external auditory canal is lined by keratinizing squamous epithelium that extends to include the entire canal and covers the external aspect of the tympanic membrane. The tympanic membrane has a central bilaminated zone, including lateral radially arranged

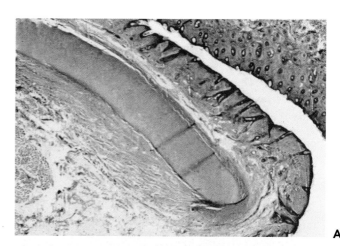

A

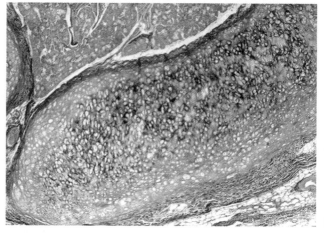

B

Figure 14.7 **A.** The cartilage of the external ear is elastic. **B.** Elastic stains show the abundant amount of elastic fibers (black staining) in the auricular cartilage.

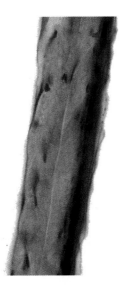

Figure 14.8 Section of pars tensa of tympanic membrane. The following layers may be distinguished from left to right: middle ear epithelium, lamina propria, circular arrangement of collagenous fibers (i.e., at right angles to former layer), radial arrangement of collagenous fibers, lamina propria, and stratified squamous epithelium.

and medial circularly arranged collagenous fibers (Figure 14.8). The inner two-thirds of the external auditory canal contain bone rather than cartilage. Because adnexal structures are absent, there is relatively close apposition of the epithelium to the subjacent bone.

Auditory Epithelial Migration

Auditory epithelial migration represents the mechanism by which keratin is removed from the tympanic membrane. Without such a self-cleaning process, the keratin squames normally produced by the stratified squamous epithelium of the tympanic membrane would continuously build up and interfere with the conduction of sound via the tympanic membrane. The entire epithelium, including keratin, moves from the tympanic membrane onto the deep external auditory canal. From the deep external auditory canal, the epithelium moves laterally to the junction of the deep (osseous) canal and the cartilaginous canal, where it is desquamated (3–5).

Auditory epithelial migration occurs in two separate and discrete pathways (Figure 14.9) (6). In one pathway, the epithelium moves upward over the handle of the malleus and then posterosuperiorly across the pars flaccida, moving laterally over the deep canal (Figure 14.10). The other pathway is radially moving away from the handle of the malleus and pars flaccida to the periphery of the tympanic membrane and then to the deep canal (Figure 14.11). Michaels and Soucek (3–5) have extensively evaluated the process of auditory epithelial migration and correlate the pathways to the development of the epithelia of the tympanic membrane and deep external canal in the embryo and fetus (6). The process of auditory epithelial migration has been felt to represent a possible pathogenesis for the development of cholesteatoma

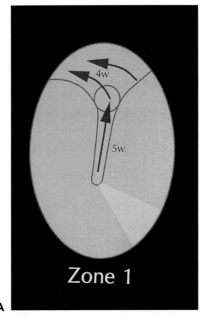

A

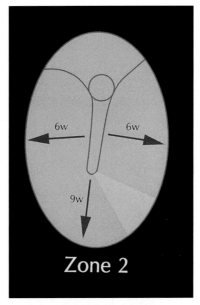

B

Figure 14.9 Summary of pathways of migration on tympanic membrane as determined by serial photography of dye markings. The tympanic membrane and adjacent deep external canal epithelium are depicted as being viewed en face. Two discrete pathways are present: **A.** passing upward along a tongue of epithelium and over the handle of the malleus to join epithelium, moving in a postero-superior direction over the pars flaccida region (*Zone 1*), and **B.** a radial pathway moving centrifugally from the pars flaccida and handle of malleus regions to the periphery (*Zone 2*). The times given for each region are the weeks required for dye to be completely cleared from that region.

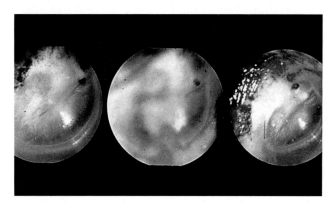

Figure 14.10 Pathway of auditory epithelial migration as shown by movement of blue dye daubed on tympanic membrane. Dye is seen on the day it was daubed, just anterior and inferior to the lateral process of the malleus. In the next photograph, taken 9 days later, it has moved posteriorly and superiorly to lie over that structure. Thirteen days later, in the third photograph, it has crossed the pars flaccida region, moving in the same direction toward the external canal.

(see below). However, there is no definitive evidence linking auditory epithelial migration to the development of cholesteatoma.

MIDDLE EAR

Embryology

The middle ear space develops from invagination of the first branchial pouch (pharyngotympanic tube) from the primitive pharynx. The auditory tube and tympanic cavity develop from the endoderm of the first branchial pouch;

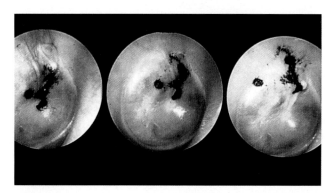

Figure 14.11 In this daubed tympanic membrane, an irregular array of dye is seen on the handle of malleus region on the sixth day after its deposition. By the fifteenth day, in the second photograph, a round dot that was just posterior to the handle of the malleus has separated and is commencing to travel backward; the main mass of dye is moving discretely upward along the handle of the malleus. This process has advanced on the twenty-seventh day in the third photograph, the posterior dye having reached the back edge of the tympanic membrane and the large mass now situated across the pars flaccida at an angle that has now changed to a posterosuperior one.

the malleus and incus develop from the mesoderm of the first branchial arch (Meckel's cartilage), while the stapes develops from the mesoderm of the second branchial arch (Reichert's cartilage) (Figure 14.2) (2).

Anatomy

The middle ear, or tympanic cavity, lies within the temporal bone between the tympanic membrane and the squamous portions of the temporal bone laterally and the petrous portion of the temporal bone surrounding the inner ear medially. The anatomic limits of the tympanic cavity include (1,7,8):

1. lateral or internal aspect made up by the tympanic membrane and squamous portion of the temporal bone
2. medial aspect bordered by the petrous portion of the temporal bone
3. superior (roof) delimited by the tegmen tympani (a thin plate of bone that separates the middle ear space from the cranial cavity)
4. inferior (floor) aspect bordered by a thin plate of bone separating the tympanic cavity from the superior bulb of the internal jugular vein
5. anterior aspect delimited by a thin plate of bone separating the tympanic cavity from the carotid canal (that houses the internal carotid artery)
6. posterior aspect delimited by the petrous portion of the temporal bone, containing the mastoid antrum and mastoid air cells

The tympanic cavity communicates anteriorly with the nasopharynx by way of the auditory tube, and it communicates posteriorly with the mastoid air cells by way of the aditus and mastoid antrum.

The contents of the tympanic cavity include the ossicles (malleus, incus, and stapes), ligaments of the ossicles, tendons of the ossicular muscles, auditory tube, tympanic cavity proper, epitympanic recess, mastoid cavity, and chorda tympani of the facial nerve (cranial nerve VII). The middle and external ears function as conduits for sound conduction for the auditory part of the internal ear.

Lateral Wall

The tympanic cavity extends above the level of the tympanic membrane as the epitympanic recess (attic). In this area lie the head of the malleus and the body of the short process of the incus. The epitympanic recess projects laterally above the external acoustic meatus; it is this portion of the tympanic cavity that has a part of the squamous portion of the temporal bone as its lateral wall.

Roof

The roof of the tympanic cavity is the tegmen tympani, a thin plate of bone separating the middle ear cavity from the cranial cavity. In children, the unossified petrosquamous suture of the tegmen tympani may allow the direct passage of infection from the middle ear to the meninges of the middle cranial fossa (1). In adults, especially in the setting of a long-standing history of chronic otitis media, compromise of the tegmen tympani may result in acquired encephalocele, in which glial-type tissue is present within the middle ear cavity. In adults, veins from the middle ear perforate the petrosquamous suture to end in the petrosquamous and the superior petrosal sinuses and may potentially transmit infection directly to the cranial venous sinuses (1).

Floor

The floor of the tympanic cavity is usually a thin plate of bone separating the cavity from the internal jugular vein. In the presence of a large superior bulb of the internal jugular vein, it may bulge into the middle ear and may present dehiscences (9).

Posterior Wall

The posterior wall of the tympanic cavity opens through the narrow aditus ad antrum in the wider mastoid (tympanic) antrum. Below the aditus is a relatively thin bone separating the tympanic cavity from the antrum, and it is from this posterior wall that the pyramidal eminence projects, with an aperture at its apex from which the tendon of the stapedius muscle is transmitted. Above and behind the pyramidal eminence, the facial nerve curves downward to change its course from horizontal to vertical. The chorda tympani, arising from the facial nerve, then enters the tympanic cavity through the canaliculus of the chorda in the posterior wall.

Anterior Wall

The lower part of the anterior wall is part of the petrous apex. This area consists of a thin plate of bone (which may be incomplete or may contain air cells) that separates the cavity from the carotid canal in which the internal carotid artery is located. The upper part of the anterior wall is deficient since the canal containing the tensor tympani muscle opens in this location, and immediately below this area is the tympanic orifice of the auditory tube.

Medial Wall

The medial wall of the tympanic cavity is the petrous portion of the temporal bone surrounding the internal ear and separating the middle ear cavity from the inner ear cavity.

Several markings of importance are found on its surface, including the broad prominence produced by the anterior end of the lateral semicircular canal and the prominence of the facial (fallopian) canal produced by the horizontal portion of the facial nerve in its course between the inner and middle ears. The cochleariform process transmits the tendon of the tensor tympani muscle. Its apex is the landmark for the position of the turn (geniculum, or external genu) between the anterolaterally and posteriorly directed horizontal portions of the facial nerve. Immediately below the facial canal is the fossula fenestrae vestibuli (the stapes niche); it contains the oval window, which is closed by the base of the stapes. Below the oval window is the promontory formed by the basal turn of the cochlea. The tympanic nerve plexus lies on the promontory. Below the back part of the promontory, the cochlear fossula (the round window niche) leads to the round window or fenestrae cochlea. Behind the promontory is a depression referred to as the sinus tympani, a site that may harbor infections and may transmit infections to the ampullary end of the posterior canal and posterior end of the lateral canal if the infection is deeply situated (1).

Middle Ear Ossicles and Muscles

The middle ear bones, or ossicles, include the malleus, incus, and stapes (Figure 14.12). The parts of the malleus include a head, upper and lower manubrium (handle), lateral process, and anterior process. The malleus is closely attached to the tympanic membrane by its manubrium (handle) and its lateral process, while its head projects above the epitympanic recess to articulate with the body of the incus. The anterior (long) process (processus gracilis) of the malleus extends obliquely downward from the neck toward the tympanosquamous fissure. In infants, the anterior process may reach the tympanosquamous fissure; but, in adults, the distal part is transformed to connective tissue, forming the anterior ligament of the malleus (1). The malleus is also attached to the tympanic wall by superior and lateral mallear ligaments. The lateral ligament attaches the neck of the malleus to the margin of the tympanic notch.

The parts of the incus include its body and the long and short processes. The body of the incus is fitted against the head of the malleus and lies in the epitympanic recess. The short process (crus) rests in a depression referred to as the fossa of the incus, which is situated in the posterior wall of the tympanic cavity below the aditus ad antrum. The long process (crus) of the incus descends parallel and slightly posteromedial to the manubrium of the malleus but at its lower end turns medial to articulate with the stapes (1). The incus is held in place by a posterior ligament that attaches to its short process and by a superior ligament to attach to the body. The knoblike expansion of the long crus of the incus (at the incudomallear joint) is referred to as the lenticular process.

The stapes is formed by its two crura, a head that lies at the junction of the crura and a footplate that lies on the oval window (Figure 14.13). The head of the stapes articulates with the incus. From its articulation with the incus, the

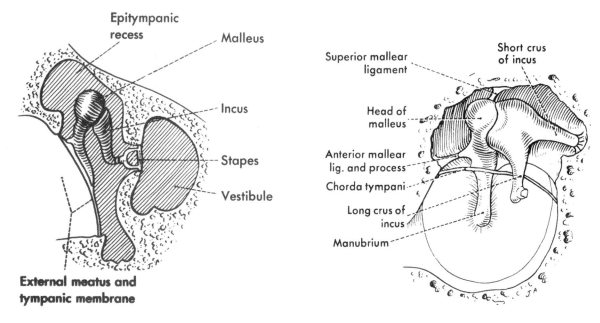

Figure 14.12 Diagrammatic depiction of the anatomy of the middle ear ossicles: **A.** frontal aspect (rotated through approximately 90°), and **B.** medial aspect. (Reprinted with permission from Hollinshead WH. The ear. In: Hollinshead WH, ed. *Anatomy for Surgeons.* 3rd ed. Philadelphia: Harper & Row; 1982:159–122.)

stapes passes almost horizontally to the oval (vestibular) window. The footplate of the stapes is attached to the oval window by the annular ligament. The latter, a ring of elastic fibers, allows movement of the stapes but seals any potential space between its footplate and the edges of the oval window.

The incudomallear and incudostapedial joints are synovial (diarthroidal) (see below). In addition to their ligaments, the stapes and manubrium of the malleus have muscles attached to them. The stapedius muscle diminishes the excursion of the base of the stapes by its reflex contraction. Important functions ascribed to the stapedius muscle are to protect the inner ear from excessive sound and to improve discrimination for higher frequencies in speech. The stapedius muscle is innervated by a branch of the facial nerve.

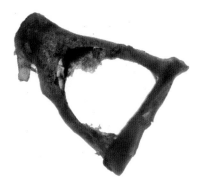

Figure 14.13 Intact resected stapes, showing (from *left* to *right*) its head, two crura, and footplate.

The tensor tympani muscle draws the manubrium medially, thereby tightening the tympanic membrane. The tensor tympani muscle is felt to primarily protect against excessive noise but also functions, in conjunction with the tensor veli palitini muscle, to respond to swallowing and electric stimulation from the tongue. The action of these two muscles pumps air from the tympanic cavity into the auditory tube, forcing air into the nasopharynx and helping to open the isthmus (10). The tensor tympani muscle is innervated by a branch of the mandibular nerve.

Auditory (Eustachian or Pharyngotympanic) Tube

The auditory tube extends from its tympanic ostium high on the anterior wall of the tympanic cavity to a nasopharyngeal ostium situated posterior to the inferior nasal concha (1). The tube is not straight but slightly S-shaped. In the adult, the tympanic ostium is approximately 2 to 2.5 cm higher than is the nasopharyngeal end; the tube runs downward, medially, and anteriorly to the nasopharynx. The length of the tube in adults varies from 31 to 38 mm (11). In infants, the tube is shorter, relatively wider, and more horizontal in its course—and, therefore, an easier pathway for infections ascending from the nasopharynx to the tympanic cavity.

The tube can be divided into an osseous portion and cartilaginous portion. The osseous portion or canal has a bony wall and is the lateral, or tympanic, third of the tube. The anteromedial two-thirds has a cartilaginous and connective tissue wall and is referred to as the cartilaginous portion of the tube. The cartilaginous and osseous tubes meet at an obtuse angle.

Histology

Tympanic Cavity Proper

Histologically, the epithelial lining of the tympanic cavity is a single layer of respiratory epithelium of flattened to cuboidal epithelium (Figure 14.14). Under normal conditions, there are no glandular elements within the middle ear; the presence of glandular epithelium in the middle ear is abnormal (see below under Selective Abnormalities). Further, stratified squamous epithelium is not present in the tympanic cavity under normal conditions nor does squamous metaplasia occur in the middle ear (5). Ciliated pseudostratified columnar epithelium may be found in limited patches among the flattened or cuboidal epithelium.

Auditory Tube

The lining of the auditory tube is a low ciliated epithelium for much of its length except as it approaches its nasopharyngeal end, where it becomes ciliated pseudostratified columnar epithelium containing goblet cells. In its cartilaginous portion, it also contains seromucinous glands (Figure 14.15). The auditory tubes contain a lymphoid component, particularly in children, that is referred to as Gerlach's tubal tonsil (Figure 14.16). Reactive hyperplasia of this lymphoid component, particularly in children, may close off the auditory tube, providing a desirable milieu for otitis media. The mucosa of the osseous portion of the auditory tube is separated from the carotid canal by a thin plate of bone measuring 1 mm in thickness (5). Dehiscence

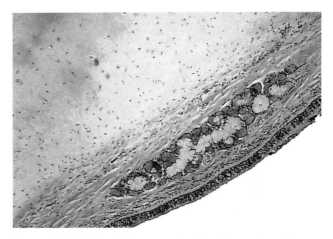

Figure 14.15 Cartilaginous portion of auditory tube with seromucinous glands.

of the carotid canal is fairly frequent (12). Squamous carcinoma of the middle ear or auditory tube, a rare occurrence, may easily penetrate this area and gain access to the carotid artery, with the potential for widespread dissemination (13). The cartilage of the nasopharyngeal portion of the auditory tube is hyalin type.

Mastoid Air Cells

The mastoid air cells represent a network of intercommunicating spaces that emanate from the tympanic cavity (5). Each air cell is lined by flattened to cuboidal epithelium, which rests on periosteum that covers a thin frame of lamellar bone (Figure 14.17).

Pneumatization of the Temporal Bone

In the newborn, the rudimentary mastoid bone contains a single air space, the antrum, surrounded by diploic bone

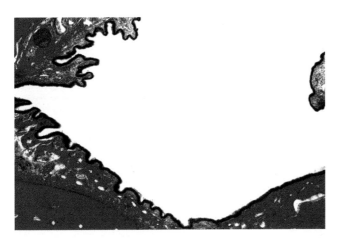

Figure 14.14 The epithelial lining of the tympanic cavity is a single layer of epithelium (cuboidal to respiratory). Under normal conditions, glands are not identified within the tympanic cavity.

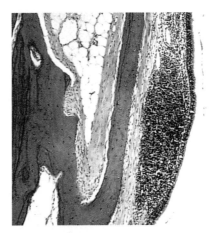

Figure 14.16 Mucosa of auditory tube. The lining is of ciliated columnar epithelium. In the lamina propria beneath, there are numerous lymphocytes that are probably the result of inflammation.

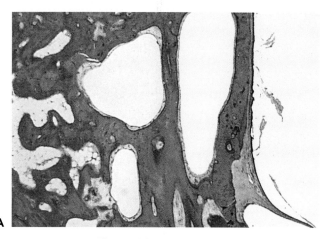

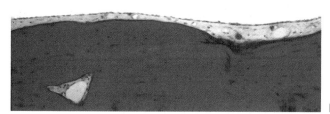

A
B

Figure 14.17 **A.** Mastoid air cells (*center*), tympanic membrane (*lower right*), and squamous epithelium of the osseous portion of the external canal (*right*). Note the thin covering of skin over the external ear canal and the proximity of bone to it. **B.** Higher magnification shows the very thin epithelial layer of the mastoid air cells resting on perisoteum covering lamellar bone.

containing hematopoietic elements (14). As the mastoid process develops, the marrow spaces hollows out. The mesenchymal component occupying the space is resorbed and the developing air-containing cells become lined by the advancing endodermal epithelium. The mastoid process is constantly pneumatized in adults, although not in the infant. The cells grow out from the antrum, as well as from each other, forming complex interlocking chains of thin-walled cavities opening into each other. The antrum apparently always has air cells; the mastoid process is usually one of several types, including pneumatized (containing air cells), diploic (containing marrow), mixed (containing air cells and marrow), or sclerotic. Approximately 80% of mastoid are well pneumatized by the age of 3 or 4 years; but, in approximately 20% of people, normal pneumatization fails to occur (1,15).

Middle Ear Ossicles

The middle ear ossicles develop from cartilage with a single center of ossification for bone; there is no epiphyseal ossification. The persistence of cartilage in each of the ossicles (Figure 14.18) and the bifurcation of the stapes to form the crura with the obturator foramen between them distinguishes the middle ear ossicles from other long bones (5).

The head of the stapes is formed of endochondral bone with a cartilaginous cap at the incudostapedial joint. The crura of the stapes are formed of periosteal bone only. From the middle ear aspect of the stapes footplate to its vestibular surface, the histologic findings include the flattened to cuboidal epithelium of the tympanic cavity, a thin layer of bone, cartilage, and a single flattened (perilymphatic) epithelial cell layer (Figure 14.19).

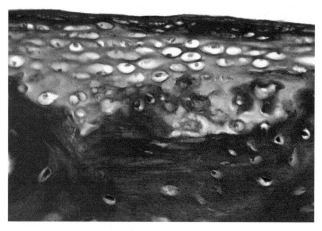

Figure 14.18 Stapes footplate showing persistence of cartilage.

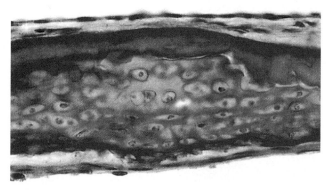

Figure 14.19 Stapes footplate. Beneath the cubical epithelium of the middle ear (*above*), there is a thin layer of bone. Below this, the footplate consists of cartilage, and there is a basal flattened layer of cells comprising the lining of the vestibule.

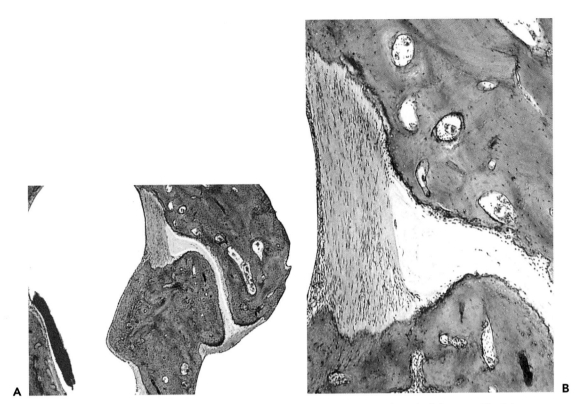

A

B

Figure 14.20 **A.** Incudomalleal joint. Note the joint capsule at each end of the joint. The joint space is occupied by the fibrocartilage of the articular disk. **B.** Higher power view of the incudomalleal joint; note one end of joint capsule and articular disk.

The malleus and incus have an outer covering of periosteal bone layer and an inner core of endochondral bone with well-formed haversian systems. The manubrium (handle) of the malleus is predominantly covered by retained cartilage rather than periosteal bone. The entire inner core of the manubrium, as well as the rest of the malleus, is composed of endochondral bone. The anterior process is formed in membrane early in fetal life and merges with the malleus after its formation (5). At its superior aspect, the manubrium is separated from the tympanic membrane by a ligament covered by the middle ear epithelium. The short process of the incus shows a tip of unossified cartilage.

Middle Ear Joints

Both the incudomalleal and incudostapedial joints are diarthrodial. Middle ear epithelium is present on the outer surface of the joint capsule, and synovial membrane is present on its inner surface. The joint capsule is comprised of fibrous tissue with a high elastic fiber content (5). The articular disk, representing the space in between the articular ends, is comprised predominantly of fibrocartilage (Figure 14.20). The articular processes of both the malleus and the incus are covered by cartilage.

The annular ligament binds the cartilaginous edge of the stapes footplate to the cartilaginous rim of the vestibular window (stapediovestibular joint) (Figure 14.21) and is composed of fibrous tissue, with elastic fibers being prominent near the ligament surfaces (16). Cartilage also covers the articular surfaces of the stapediovestibular joints.

The fissula ante fenestrum is the canal linking the middle ear with the vestibule. It lies in the bone just anterior to the stapediovestibular joint and develops as a slit filled with fibrous tissue that is often with associated cartilage (Figure 14.22).

Middle Ear Muscles

The muscles of the middle ear, including the tensor tympani and stapedius muscles, are composed of a central tendon formed by elastic tissue with muscle fibers radiating from it (Figure 14.23). This configuration has been described as feather-shaped. The tensor tympani muscle has a prominent mature adipose tissue component (Figure 14.24) that is believed to function as insulation for the cochlea against electric effects from its contraction (5).

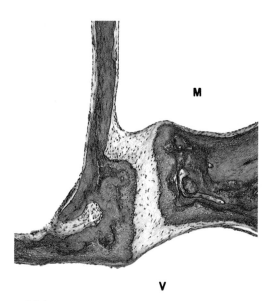

Figure 14.21 Stapediovestibular joint, part of footplate of stapes, adjacent bony labyrinthine wall, and crus of stapes. The footplate shows a lamina of cartilage on its vestibular surface, which is continuous with the cartilage of the stapediovestibular joint. (*M*, middle ear cavity; *V*, cavity of vestibule)

INNER EAR

Embryology

The first division of the ear to develop is the inner ear, which appears toward the end of the first month of gestation (2,17). The membranous labyrinth, including the utricle, saccule, semicircular ducts, cochlear duct, and endolymphatic sac, arises from the placodal thickening of the ectoderm to become a closed otic vesicle (otocyst). The otic vesicle forms from the invagination of the surface ectoderm, located on either side of the neural plate, into the

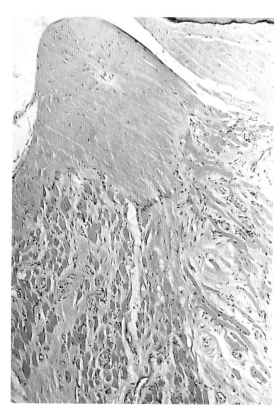

Figure 14.23 Stapedius muscle and tendon. The skeletal muscle fibers and fibrous bands between them radiate to a tendon.

mesenchyme. This invagination eventually loses its connection with the surface ectoderm. The membranous labyrinth, which is essentially tubular and saccular is filled with fluid, the endolymph or endolymphatic fluid. The early development of the membranous labyrinth takes place in mesenchyme and subsequently in the cartilage destined to form the petrous portion of the temporal bone (1). The membranous labyrinth lies in cavities excavated from

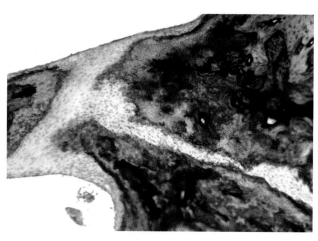

Figure 14.22 Fissula ante fenestrum is the canal within bone that links the middle ear with the vestibule and develops as a slit filled with fibrous tissue.

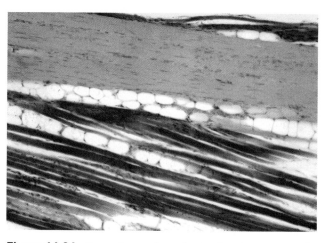

Figure 14.24 Tensor tympani muscle showing the presence of a mature adipose tissue component.

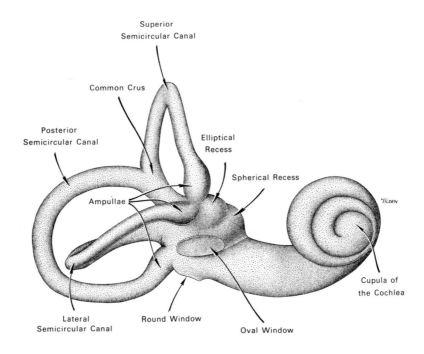

Figure 14.25 Schematic depicting the osseous labyrinth.

this mesenchyme or cartilage. The space lying between the inner surface of the bony wall and the outer surface of the membranous labyrinth is the perilymphatic space. The perilymphatic space develops around the membranous labyrinth by fusion of mesenchymal spaces to form larger ones surrounding the membranous portion. The bony labyrinth, including the vestibule, semicircular canals and cochlea arises from the mesenchyme around the otic vesicle (2,17,18).

Anatomy

The internal (inner) ear, or labyrinth, is embedded within the petrous portion of the temporal bone and comprises the medial portion of the temporal bone adjacent to the cranial cavity. The inner ear contains the membranous labyrinth, which is surrounded by an osseous layer or bony shell termed the osseous (bony) labyrinth (Figure 14.25). The membranous labyrinth contains the cochlea, which is the organ of hearing, and the vestibular system, which is the system of balance (equilibrium).

Osseous Labyrinth (Otic Capsule)

The osseous labyrinth consists of the vestibule and cochlear capsule. The central portion of the osseous labyrinth cavity is the vestibule, a large ovoid perilymphatic space approxi-

mately 4 mm in diameter and containing both the saccule and utricle of the membranous labyrinth. In the floor of the bony vestibule are seen the elliptical recess for the anterior end of the utricle and, anterior and lateral to this, the spherical recess for the saccule. In the lateral wall of the vestibule is the oval window, in which the base of the stapes is situated. Through the stapes, the perilymph of the vestibule receives vibrations from the tympanic membrane and ossicular chain (set up by sound waves reaching the tympanic cavity). Along the medial wall and floor of the vestibule, where it abuts the lateral end of the internal acoustic meatus, are small openings for the entrance of the nerve branches to the vestibular portion of the ear (1).

The bony cochlea, a part of the otic capsule, is a hollowed spiral about two- to three-fourths turns, diminishing from a relatively broad base to a pointed cupula, or apex. It is so named because of its resemblance to a snail shell. The base of the cochlea lies against the anteromedial surface of the vestibule and next to the anterior surface of the lateral (blind) end of the internal auditory canal. A central core of bone called the modiolus runs forward from the cochlea but does not reach the cupula. It is around this central core that the spiral channels of the cochlea (perilymphatic and endolymphatic) are arranged. A layer of bone arranged in a spiral fashion unites the modiolus to the peripheral wall of the bony cochlea and separates successive spiral cavities from each other (1). The modiolus is hollow to accommodate the cochlear nerve. The base of the modiolus lies against the lateral end of the internal auditory canal, to which the cochlear nerve runs.

The vestibular aqueduct extends through the otic capsule from the vestibule to the posterior cranial fossa, transmitting the endolymphatic duct. The terminal end of the vestibular aqueduct is the endolymphatic sac, a dilated area that ends blindly outside the dura (1). The cochlear duct opens at one end into the lower end of the scala tympani and at the other end into the subarachnoid cavity (1). The issue as to whether the cochlear duct represents an open channel between the subarachnoid space and the perilymphatic space at the lower end of the scala tympani remains controversial (1). A possible role ascribed to the cochlear duct is to serve as part of the pressure-adjusting mechanism of the perilymph in conjunction with the round window (19–21).

Membranous Labyrinth

The membranous (otic) labyrinth is the spiral-appearing structure that resembles the shell of a snail. The principle components of the membranous labyrinth are the cochlear duct, utricle, saccule, ductus reuniens, semicircular canals with their ampullae, and the endolymphatic sac and duct.

Cochlear Duct

The membranous cochlea, or cochlear duct, is a cone-shaped spirally oriented membranous tube between the osseous spiral lamina and the outer osseous wall of the cochlea, to which it is attached (7). The cochlear duct, also referred to as the scala media, lies between the scala vestibuli and the scala tympani (Figure 14.26). These three compartments are fluid-filled. The cochlear duct, as well as the entire membranous labyrinth, contains endolymph. The scala vestibuli and the scala tympani contain perilymph. The cerebrospinal fluid communicates directly with the perilymphatic space through the cochlear aqueduct (perilymphatic duct) (Figure 14.27).

The cochlear duct contains the sensory end organ of hearing known as the spiral organ of Corti. The organ of Corti rests on the basilar membrane, which separates the

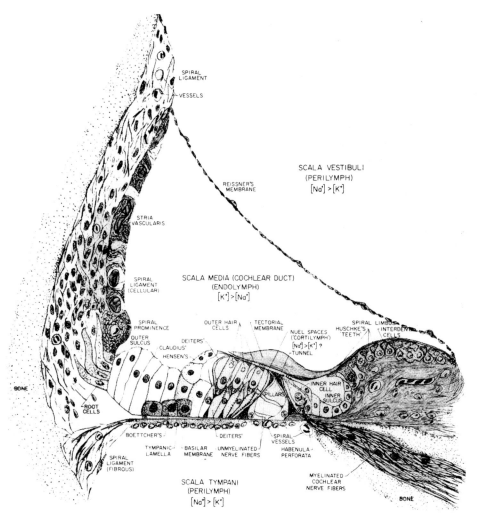

Figure 14.26 Schematic illustration of the membranous labyrinth, containing the cochlea (organ of hearing) and the vestibular (system of balance) systems. The relationship between the endolymph, containing scala media (cochlear duct), and the perilymph, containing scala vestibuli and scala tympani, is shown. (Reprinted with permission from: Nager GT. Anatomy of the membranous cochlea and vestibular labyrinth. In: Nager GT, ed. *Pathology of the Ear and Temporal Bone.* Baltimore: Williams & Wilkins; 1993:3–48.)

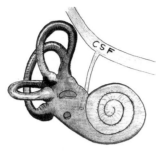

PERILYMPH

Figure 14.27 Schematic depicting the direct communication between the perilymphatic space and cerebrospinal fluid (*CSF*) through the cochlear aqueduct (perilymphatic duct).

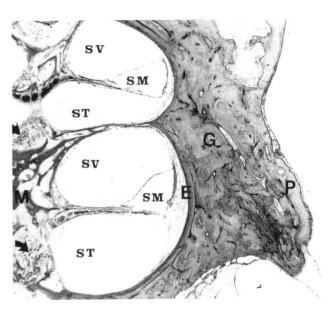

Figure 14.28 Cochlea, bony cochlea, and modiolus. (*Arrows,* spiral ganglion cells of basal and middle coils in modiolus; *E,* endosteal layer of bone; *G,* endochondral layer containing globuli interossei; *M,* modiolus; *P,* periosteal layer; *SM,* scala media; *ST,* scala tympani; *SV,* scala vestibuli)

cochlear duct from the scala tympani (Figure 14.26). Together, the organ of Corti and the basilar membrane form the spiral membrane that is the floor or tympanic wall of the cochlear duct. The spiral ligament is a thickened, modified portion of periosteum of the bony cochlea, forming the outer curved wall of the cochlea duct and adjacent parts of the scalae. The scala tympani lies below the basilar membrane, while the scala vestibuli lies above the cochlear duct and is separated from it by Reissner's membrane. Reissner's membrane forms the roof of the cochlear duct. The scala tympani and scala vestibuli communicate with each other only at the apex, known as the helicotrema. The scala vestibuli winds toward the apex of the cochlea at the helicotrema, becoming the scala tympani—which, in turn, coils back toward the round window (Figure 14.28). The scala vestibuli and the scala tympani communicate with the middle ear via the oval window and round window, respectively. The scala tympani ends blindly at the round window membrane, but the scala vestibuli opens up at that level into the perilymphatic space of the vestibulum. The cochlear duct connects with the vestibular system via ductus reuniens located at the saccule. In this way, the three semicircular canals that comprise the vestibular system are filled with endolymph.

Utricle

The utricle is an elongated to oval-shaped portion of the membranous labyrinth, lying superior to the saccule in the medial wall of the vestibule (Figure 14.29). It is larger in diameter than the semicircular ducts and receives both ends of each semicircular duct (for a total of five, since the anterior and posterior ducts share a common opening). The macule of the utricle, located on the inferior surface of the utricle (utricular recess), is a sensory end organ. The utriculosaccular duct usually arises from the utricle; it communicates with the endolymphatic duct and connects the utricle to the saccule. As previously indicated, the three semicircular canals communicate with the utricle via

openings formed by the union of the nondilated or nonampullary ends of the superior and posterior canals, termed the commun crus.

Saccule

The saccule is located anteromedial to the upper (anterior) end of the utricle (Figure 14.29) and tends to be more round than the utricle. The saccule and utricle are continuous via the utriculosaccular duct and with the cochlear duct by the ductus reuniens (also referred to as the canalis reuniens of Hensen) (1). The macule of the saccule contains

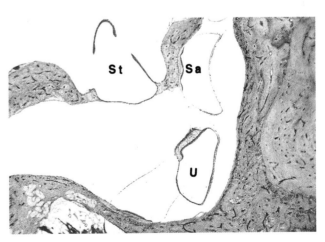

Figure 14.29 Ventricle of cat showing utricle (*U*) and saccule (*Sa*). (*St,* stapes)

the sensory nerve endings of this portion of the inner ear and is an oval thickening on the lateral wall.

Semicircular Canals

The semicircular ducts include the anterior or superior duct, the posterior duct, and the lateral ducts. The end of each semicircular duct is expanded to form the ampulla. The anterior duct is directed anterolaterally, the posterior duct is directed posterolaterally, and the lateral ducts form a laterally directed angle of approximately 90° between themselves. The osseous canals follow a similar direction. The three semicircular canals communicate with the utricle via openings formed by the union of the nondilated or nonampullary ends of the superior and posterior canals (the common crus). From the common crus, the anterior duct curves upward, while the posterior duct curves backward and then downward. The other (membranous) ampullary ends of the semicircular canals contain the sensory endings of the ducts. At the ampullary ends, the anterior and posterior ducts empty into the utricle. The lateral semicircular duct lies in an approximate horizontal plane; both of its ends also connect to the utricle, with the anterior end being the ampulla.

Endolymphatic Duct and Sac

The endolymphatic duct traverses the medial portion of the petrous pyramid in its own bony canal, the vestibular aqueduct (7). The endolymphatic duct can be divided into segments. The first segment is the dilated portion referred to as the sinus, representing the common channel into which the utricular and saccular ducts open. The next segment of the duct is narrow and referred to as the isthmus. After the isthmus, the duct widens again to become the endolymphatic sac. The majority of the endolymphatic sac is located within the funnel-shaped cranial aperture of the cochlear duct, lying within a duplication of the posterior fossa dura and partially covered medially by a thin bony shelf referred to as the operculum. The endolymphatic sac ends in a terminal dilatation or fovea of the sac. Two portions of the endolymphatic sac are recognized: a proximal rugose portion with an irregular lumen caused by numerous folds of the epithelial lining and a distal portion with a smooth epithelial lining.

The membranous vestibular system contains the receptor organs for sense of motion and position. The neural structures of the inner ear, including the vestibulocochlear nerve and the facial nerve, enter the inner ear through the internal auditory canal.

Inner Ear Innervation

The nerve to the inner ear is cranial nerve VIII, variably referred to as the acoustic, auditory, or vestibulocochlear nerve. This nerve functionally consists of vestibular and cochlear divisions. In the internal auditory canal, these two parts are closely associated; but, at the lateral end of the canal, the nerve trunk divides into three parts, including two vestibular and one cochlear.

The vestibular nerve arises from the bipolar cells of the superior and inferior division of the (afferent) vestibular, or Scarpa's, ganglion located at the lateral end of the internal auditory canal. Peripherally, the vestibular nerve divides into two main divisions, the superior and inferior divisions. The superior part of the ganglion gives nerves to the ampullae of the lateral and anterior (superior) canals and to the saccular and utricle maculae. The inferior part of the ganglion gives rise to a posterior ampullary nerve and a nerve to the saccule. The inferior part also gives rise to a branch to the cochlear division.

The cells of origin for the cochlear nerve form the spiral ganglion, which represents the first of four neurons between the auditory end organ and the auditory cortex. The spiral ganglion is located in coils of the modiolus at the base of attachment of the osseous spiral lamina (see Figure 14.28). The osseous spiral lamina is a thin trabecula of bone surrounding afferent nerve fibers that run from the organ of Corti through the habenula perforata to the acoustic nerve and efferent fibers to the outer hair cells that arise from the olivocochlear system of Rasmussen. The efferent fibers make their exit from the brain with the vestibular part of the nerve and join the cochlear branch of cranial nerve VIII via the vestibulocochlear communicating branch, or nerve of Oort through the modiolus (1). Prior to reaching the modiolus, the nerve fibers are unmyelinated but are myelinated upon reaching the cochlear modiolus. The central fibers, or axons, of these bipolar neurons unite to form nerve bundles and pass from the cochlear modiolus through nerve channels in the osseous spiral foraminous tract into the internal auditory canal, where they form the cochlear nerve.

Within the internal auditory canal, the vestibulocochlear nerve is usually connected to the facial nerve. Together, the three nerves enter the posterior cranial fossa, transverse the cerebellopontine angle, and enter the brainstem at the posterior lower lateral aspect of the pons. The central auditory pathways consist of three additional neurons that form numerous connections with nuclei throughout the central nervous system as part of a complex auditory reflex system reaching the auditory cortex in the anterior transverse gyrus of the superior temporal lobe (7,8).

The facial nerve enters the temporal bone through the internal auditory meatus within the petrous portion of the temporal bone in company with (lying above) the vestibulocochlear nerve and the internal auditory artery. The facial nerve then passes Bill's bar, which represents a pointed bony projection separating the facial nerve from the superior division of the vestibular nerve. At the outer end of the canal, the facial nerve pierces arachnoid and dura to enter its own bony canal, the facial canal (fallopian canal, or aqueduct of Fallopius). This canal continues for a short distance, and the facial nerve comes to lie just above the cochlea, where it bears the geniculate ganglion. The greater petrosal nerve comes off the geniculate ganglion and passes anteriorly and medially to enter the middle cranial fossa. Immediately beyond the geniculate ganglion, the facial nerve turns sharply (external genu; geniculum) laterally and posteriorly. As it runs backward in the bone of the lateral wall of the vestibule (which is the medial wall of the tympanic cavity), the facial nerve inclines downward and laterally where the bone surrounding it forms a bulge or projection, referred to as the prominence of the facial canal. This bulge or prominence is a normal finding, and it may be large enough to cover the oval window and base of the stapes. The facial nerve then makes a broad curve downward to run almost vertically through the mastoid process to the stylomastoid foramen, where the facial canal ends and the nerve exits from the skull.

Shortly before leaving the stylomastoid foramen, the facial nerve gives off the chorda tympani, which is composed of sensory and preganglionic motor fibers. Slightly above the stylomastoid foramen, the chorda tympani leaves the facial trunk and takes a recurrent course upward and forward in its canaliculus ("iter chordae posterius") to enter the tympanic cavity through its posterior wall. Within the tympanic cavity, it passes between the malleus and incus and leaves the tympanic membrane through a canal in the pterygotympanic fissure ("iter chordae anterius"), where it joins the lingual nerve to be distributed to the anterior two-thirds of the tongue (taste buds) and to the submandibular ganglion, through which postganglionic fibers reach the submandibular and sublingual salivary glands.

Histology

Osseous Labyrinth

The cavity of osseous labyrinth (otic capsule) surrounds and replicates the outline of the membranous labyrinth lying within it. The osseous labyrinth is extremely dense and includes three layers: an outer periosteal layer; a middle layer in which there is persistence of much of the calcified cartilaginous matrix referred to as globuli interossei or globuli ossei (Figure 14.30); and an inner layer abutting the membranous labyrinth and lined by a thin layer of internal periosteum (also referred to as endosteum) (5). The density of the osseous labyrinth is necessary to insulate and safeguard the delicate vibrations of the fluids contained within it and is necessary in maintaining the integrity and functions of hearing and balance (5). As noted by Michaels (5) the bone of the adult osseous labyrinth is neither lamellar nor woven bone but "somewhere in be-

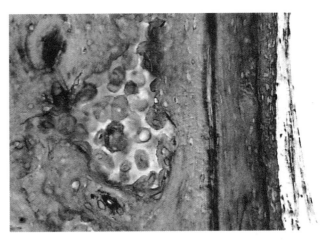

Figure 14.30 Globuli ossei (*left*) and endosteum (*right*) of cochlea.

tween"; in contrast to other adult bone, the osseous labyrinth lacks the normal developmental process of removal and replacement of calcified cartilaginous matrix and of primitive bone (5).

Membranous Labyrinth

The membranous labyrinth consists of epithelium-lined channels surrounded by connective tissue. The three basic divisions of the membranous labyrinth (including the semicircular canals, the utricle and saccule, and the cochlear duct) have similar structure, consisting of a specialized thickened epithelium surrounded by and attached to a fibrogelatinous membrane. The specialized epithelium consists of supporting cells and neuroepithelium or hair cells. The neuroepithelium has processes ("hairs") that project from the free edge of the cells.

Cochlea

The organ of Corti consists of neurotransmitting hair cells that rest on the basilar membrane and is arranged in a spiral like the duct itself (Figure 14.31). The organ of Corti consists of supporting cells and hair cells. The supporting, or pillar, cells are of several different types. Among the more important supporting cells are the phalangeal cells, which are arranged in two groups: an inner or single row of cells and an outer row of cells (cells of Deiters) formed from three to five rows of cells, depending on the level of the cochlea, with more rows of cells toward the apex and fewer rows of cells toward the base.

The inner row of phalangeal cells is associated with a single layer of hair cells; the outer row of phalangeal cells alternate with rows of hair cells. The phalangeal cells get their name from the shape of the stiff processes that project

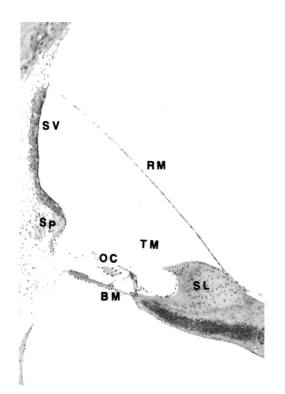

Figure 14.31 Scala media of cat. (*BM*, basilar membrane; *OC*, organ of Corti; *RM*, Reissner's membrane; *SL*, spiral limbus; *SP*, spiral prominence; *SV*, stria vascularis; *TM*, tectorial membrane)

helicotrema. The tectorial membrane is a gelatinous structure with numerous fine fibers. Like the basilar membrane, the tectorial membrane increases in size from the base to the apex of the cochlea and is believed to have a vibratory effect on the hair cells.

Together, the organ of Corti and the basilar membrane form the spiral membrane, which is the floor or tympanic wall of the cochlear duct. The spiral ligament is a thickened, modified portion of periosteum of the osseous cochlea, which forms the outer or curved wall of the cochlear duct and adjacent parts of the scalae. The vestibular, or Reissner's, membrane is thin and consists of two layers of cells: an inner cell layer of ectodermal origin (consisting of epithelial-like clusters) and an outer layer of mesodermal origin (consisting of large, flat, and elongated cells) (5). This membrane forms the roof of the cochlear duct. In Ménière's disease (see below), the vestibular membrane bulges toward the scala vestibuli. In the outer (vertical) wall of the cochlear duct is the stria vascularis, which is supplied by 30 to 35 small arteries that originate from the modiolar region of the scala vestibuli and pass outward to the lateral wall of the osseous labyrinth (Figure 14.31) (22). It is believed to be the source of the endolymph (23). The tissue spaces of the spiral ligament serve as a site of absorption (24). The stria vascularis is altered in ototoxic conditions, as may occur secondary to use of cisplatin, diuretic agents, and other drugs (see below under **Presbycusis and Other Hearing Loss**) (5).

from the cells contributing to the reticular membrane that covers the free surface of the organ (1). The hair cells have numerous (40 to 100 per cell) "hairs" projecting from the reticular (cuticular) surface. The outer hair cells are more sensitive, are short and wedge-shaped between the apices of the phalangeal cells in order to reach the basilar membrane, and are believed to be responsible for the cochlear microphonics (1). The inner hair cells are long, are less susceptible to damage than the outer hair cells, and believed to be less sensitive to sound.

Intercellular spaces among the cells of the organ of Corti are apparently filled with intercellular substance. The largest of these spaces runs the entire length of the organ of Corti between inner and outer rows of phalangeal and hair cells and is referred to as the tunnel, or canal, of Corti (Figure 14.32). The tunnel of Corti is bounded by special supporting cells, the inner and outer pillars (Corti's rods) (Figure 14.32). The tunnel and pillars together form Corti's arch.

The basilar membrane is fibrous tissue that supports the organ of Corti. The basilar membrane has the tectorial membrane attached to it. The basilar membrane has fibers that pass from the bony spiral lamina to the spiral crest of the spiral ligament. The basilar membrane increases in size from the base to the apex of the cochlea and is felt to have resonator action with deformation of the membrane by sound, beginning at its lower end and traveling toward the

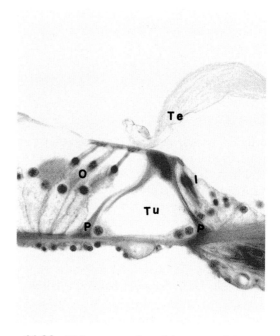

Figure 14.32 Higher power view of the organ of Corti (see Figure 14.31). (*I*, inner hair cells; *O*, outer hair cells; *P*, pillar cells (walls of tunnel); *Te*, tectorial membrane; *Tu*, tunnel of Corti)

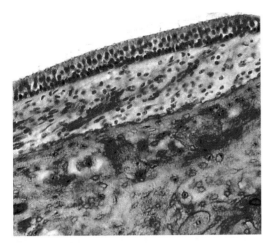

Figure 14.33 Higher power of a part of Figure 14.29, showing macula of the saccule.

Semicircular Canals, Utricle, and Saccule

The end of each semicircular duct is expanded to form an ampulla. The sensory endings in the ampullae of the ducts are the cristae. Each crista consists of thickened epithelium; above each crista rests a gelatinous formation of viscous protein polysaccharide called the cupola. The hairs of the neuroepitheial hair cells project into the base of the cupola. As a result of the gelatinous nature of the cupola, it may be bent by the pressure of the endolymph, which apparently stimulates the hair cells and, therefore, the nerve endings of the cristae.

The utricle and saccule, representing the two main membranous structures of the vestibule, are lined by a sensory epithelium known as the macula (Figure 14.33). The maculae are identical to one another in structure and are similar to the cristae of the semicircular canals. By transmission electron microscopy, these sensory cells are of two types: type I cells are flask-shaped with a swollen basal portion; type II cell is cylindrical. Type I cells are attached to fibers of the sensory nerves by a wide chalicelike terminal, and the terminal of type II cells is connected by buttonlike attachments of the nerve (Figure 14.34) (5). The sensory epithelium consists of hair cells, which in turn have stiff, immotile projections embedded in the gelatinous otolithic membrane. Also embedded in the otolithic membrane are crystalline bodies, referred to as otoliths, that contain calcium carbonate and a protein suspended in a jellylike polysaccharide. It is only in the presence of otoliths that the maculae differ from the other sensory areas of the ear.

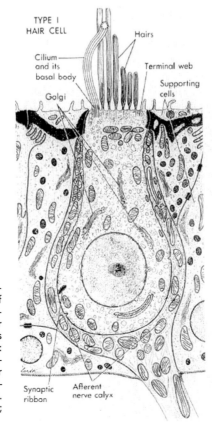

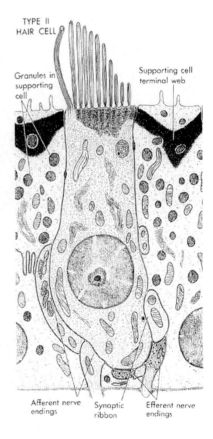

Figure 14.34 Schematic representation of the ultrastructure of vestibular hair cells showing the principal features of type I and type II hair cells and their supporting cells (Reprinted with permission from: Nager GT. Anatomy of the membranous cochlea and vestibular labyrinth. In: Nager GT, ed. *Pathology of the Ear and Temporal Bone.* Baltimore: Williams & Wilkins; 1993:3–48).

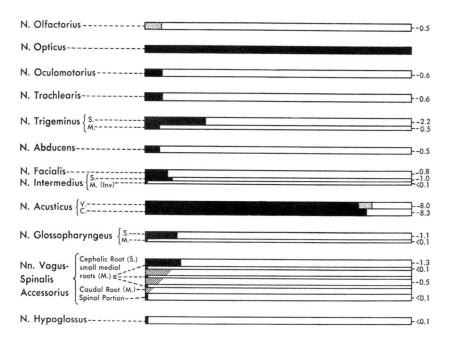

Figure 14.35 Schematic illustration of the cranial and spinal nerves showing that most of the nerves have glia extending for only a fraction of a millimeter beyond their external origins with the exceptions of the optic nerve, which is really a tract of brain (given the presence of neuroglia throughout its length), and the vestibulocochlear nerve (cranial nerve VIII). The vestibulocochlear nerve typically has glia extending from 6 to 8 mm along its course. (From: Tarlov IM. Structure of the nerve root. II. Differentiation of sensory from motor roots: observations on identification of function in roots of mixed cranial nerves. *Arch Neurol Psychiatr* 1937;37:1338–1355).

Nerves and Paraganglia

Most cranial and spinal nerves have glia extending only a fraction of a millimeter beyond their external origins (25,26). The optic nerve contains neuroglia throughout its length and, thereby, really is a tract of brain rather than a true nerve. The exception to the other cranial nerves is the eighth (vestibulocochlear) nerve, which typically has glia extending from 6 to 8 mm along its course (Figure 14.35). This distribution of glia along cranial nerve VIII helps explain the greater occurrence of glial tumors on this nerve as compared to the other cranial nerves (25). The vestibular and cochlear divisions are fused near the entrance to the internal auditory meatus; at this location, the nerve changes in appearance from pale staining proximally to dark staining distally. This change in appearance is the result of the abrupt transition of the coverings of the nerve fibers from the pale staining oligodendroglia to the darker staining Schwann cells (Figure 14.36). This glial-Schwann sheath junction of the cranial nerve VIII is referred to as the Obersteiner-Redlich zone. Acoustic neuromas (also referred to as vestibular neuromas) may arise anywhere between this junction and the cribrosa area at the fundus of the canal (27).

Paraganglia similar in structure to the carotid body are identified in the ear and may give rise to jugulotympanic paragangliomas. The majority of paraganglia are found in relation to the jugular bulb, and a minority are found under the mucosa of the medial side of the middle ear promontory (Figure 14.37).

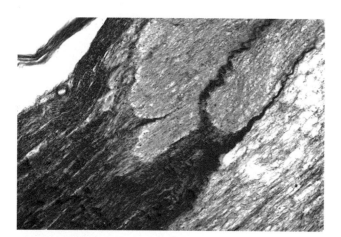

Figure 14.36 The vestibular and cochlear divisions of the vestibulocochlear nerve are fused near the entrance to the internal auditory meatus. At this location is the glial-Schwann sheath junction, also referred to as the Obersteiner-Redlich zone, where the nerve changes in appearance from pale staining proximally to dark staining distally as a result of the abrupt transition of the coverings of the nerve fibers from the pale staining oligodendroglia to the darker staining Schwann cells.

Endolymphatic Sac and Duct

The lining epithelium of the endolymphatic duct is low cuboidal (Figure 14.38), and the epithelium of the endolymphatic sac is taller and has a papillary appearance (Figure 14.39). An aggressive neoplasm, termed the endolymphatic sac papillary tumor, is presumed to originate from the endolymphatic sac epithelium (28). This tumor, initially considered to represent a low-grade malignancy (i.e., adenocarcinoma), is potentially a locally destructive but not metastatic tumor characterized by variably appearing epithelium, including nondescript low-cuboidal to

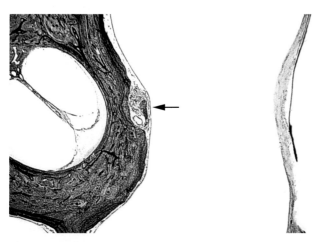

Figure 14.37 Normal tympanic paraganglion (arrow) under mucosa of medial side of middle ear over promontory. The tympanic membrane is on the right (Gomori's reticulin stain).

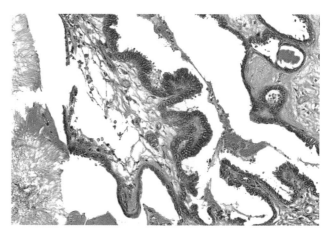

Figure 14.39 Endolymphatic sac, which is lined by tall columnar epithelium arranged on papillae.

papillary and glandular appearing neoplasm (28,29). Patients with this tumor often describe symptoms similar to those occurring in Ménière's disease, including vertigo and spinning of the room. This tumor has been found to be associated with von Hippel-Lindau (VHL) syndrome, including the identification of the VHL gene (30,31).

Composition and Circulation of the Perilymph and Endolymph

Perilymph, which is partly a filtration of cerebrospinal fluid (CSF) and partly a filtration from blood vessels of the ear, has a similar chemical composition as CSF, resembling extracellular fluid with low potassium and high sodium concentrations. The similarities of perilymph and CSF support the concept that perilymph is derived from CSF. The anatomic basis for this concept is based on the consideration that the cochlear aqueduct (perilymphatic duct) opens into both the

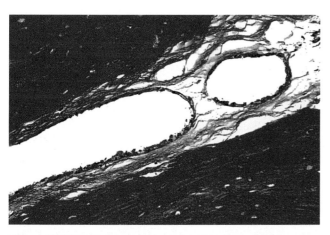

Figure 14.38 Endolymphatic duct within the vestibular aqueduct. The duct is lined by low cuboidal epithelium.

subarachnoid and perilymphatic spaces (1). An increase in CSF pressure results in flow into the labyrinth.

The perilymphatic spaces of each osseous semicircular canal are continuous on both ends with the perilymphatic space of the vestibule, and this space is continuous with the scala vestibuli, which is continuous with the scala tympani at the helicotrema. All perilymphatic spaces open widely into each other. Due to areas of discontinuity or deficiency in the compact bone of the petrous portion of the temporal bone, foci of communication may exist between the perilymphatic space and other cavities. Such areas of potential communication include the middle and inner ear via the round and oval windows. In addition, the vestibular and cochlear aqueducts and the foramina for the nerves and blood vessels of the inner ear serve as potential channels between the inner ear and the cranial cavity.

Endolymph is an intracellular-like fluid containing high potassium and low sodium concentrations. Endolymph contains more than 30 times as much potassium as does perilymph or CSF but about one-tenth as much sodium (32). Endolymph has a low protein content; its protein is entirely globulin instead of an admixture of globulin and albumin (1). It has a viscosity similar to the vitreous of the eye because of its high mucopolysaccharide content. The electrolyte concentration of the endolymph is critical for normal functioning of the sensory organs. It is generally believed that the main sources of endolymph are the stria vascularis, the epithelium of the ampullae of the semicircular ducts, and the epithelium of the maculae of the utricle and saccule.

Endolymph circulates through the cochlear duct (scala media) downward to the base of the cochlea, through the ductus reuniens into the saccule, and then into the endolymphatic sac and duct, where it is reabsorbed. The cochlear duct communicates with the vestibular endolymph-containing sacs through two canals so that the endolymphatic system is, like the perilymphatic system, a continuous one.

Conduction of Sound

Conduction of sound occurs via air and via bone. The pinna and external auditory canal conduct sound waves in air to the tympanic membrane. Conduction of sound by air is less efficient as compared with the ossicular route. The ossicular chain, including the malleus, incus, and stapes, enhances the sound energy transmission by conveying vibrations from the tympanic membrane to the footplate of the stapes and hence through the oval window of the vestibule to the perilymph. From the vestibular perilymph, vibrations derived from sound waves pass directly to the perilymphatic spaces of the cochlea, first via the scala vestibuli (upper compartment) ascending from the oval window, and then to the scala tympani (lower compartment) descending to the round window. The walls of the scala media (i.e., the cochlear duct, which contains endolymph) receive waves of vibrations from the adjacent perilymph (containing the scala vestibuli and scala tympani). Through the endolymph, the waves of vibrations affect the sensory cells of the organ of Corti, the sensory organ of sound reception located in the scala media, from which it passes to the cochlear nerve with transmission via central pathways to the cerebral cortex.

SELECTED ABNORMALITIES AND PATHOLOGY

External Ear

Abnormalities of the external ear include those associated with first and second branchial arch syndromes. First and second branchial arch syndromes include otologic and nonotologic abnormalities. The otologic manifestations or abnormalities include malformed or absent external ears, atretic external auditory canal, and impaired hearing. The nonotologic abnormalities include asymmetric facies, abnormalities of the temporomandibular joint, neuromuscular abnormalities, and associated abnormalities of the cardiovascular, renal, and central nervous systems. Goldenhar's syndrome, also known as oculoauriculovertebral dysplasia, is a first and second branchial arch syndrome characterized by ear tags, preauricular pits and fissures, epidermoids, lipodermoids, and vertebral column abnormalities (33).

Ear abnormalities can also be seen in association with other abnormalities, including Down's syndrome (Figure 14.40). Cryptotia is a rare anomaly in which the superior portion of the auricle is buried in the scalp (Figure 14.41). Microtia represents gross hypoplasia of the pinna with a blind or absent external auditory canal. Microtia is typically bilateral although the degree of hypoplasia may differ on the two sides.

Accessory tragi (also referred to as accessory or supernumerary ears, accessory auricle, or polyotia) appear at birth

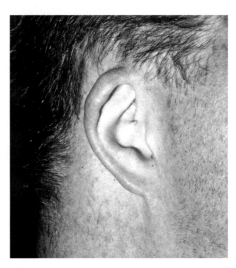

Figure 14.40   Individual with Down's syndrome. In comparison to non-Down's syndrome individuals, patients with Down's syndrome have external ears that are smaller, low set, and have an incompletely developed superior helix.

and may be solitary or multiple, unilateral or bilateral, sessile or pedunculated, and soft or cartilaginous skin-covered nodules or papules. They are located on the skin surface, often anterior to the auricle, and may be mistaken clinically for a papilloma. Histologically, accessory tragi recapitulate the normal external auricle and include skin, cutaneous adnexal structures, and a central core of cartilage. Accessory tragi are thought to be related to second branchial arch anomalies. They may occur independently of other congenital anomalies but also may occur in association with cleft palate or lip, mandibular hypoplasia, or other anomalies such as Goldenhar's syndrome (oculoauriculovertebral dysplasia) (33).

In adults, diagonal earlobe crease has been associated with coronary artery disease and has been referred to as Frank's sign (34). The crease runs diagonally backward and downward across the lateral surface of the earlobe from the external meatus (Figure 14.42). Depending on the extent and depth of the crease, three grades have been assigned, with grade 1 being the least obvious appearing crease, grade 2 including a superficial crease across 100% of the earlobe or a deep crease across 50% of the earlobe, and grade 3 represented by a deep crease along 100% of the earlobe. Bilateral grades 2 and 3 creases are associated with a significantly higher risk of death from atherosclerosis and myocardial infarction (35).

Middle Ear

Otitis Media

Otitis media is either an acute or chronic infectious disease of the middle ear space. Otitis media is predominantly, but not exclusively, a childhood disease. The most common

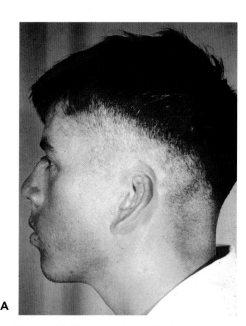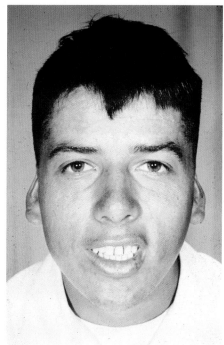

A   B

Figure 14.41   A. and B. Individual with cryptotia, a rare anomaly in which the superior portion of the auricle is buried in the scalp.

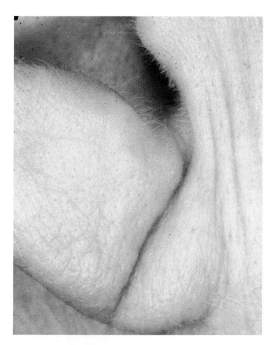

Figure 14.42 Individual with a grade 3 earlobe crease represented by a deep crease along 100% of the earlobe. This person had a similar earlobe crease of the opposite ear. Bilateral grades 2 and 3 creases are associated with a significantly higher risk of death from atherosclerosis and myocardial infarction.

microorganisms implicated in causing disease of the middle ear are *Streptococcus pneumoniae* and *Haemophilus influenzae* (36). Otoscopic examination reveals a hyperemic, opaque, bulging tympanic membrane with limited mobility; purulent otorrhea may be present. Bilateral involvement is not uncommon. The middle ear infection is felt to result from infection via the auditory tube at the time of or following a pharyngitis (bacterial or viral).

In general, otitis media is managed medically. However, at times tissue is removed for histopathologic examination. The pathologic alterations are generally straightforward, but secondary changes such as glandular metaplasia of the surface epithelium (the result of chronic infection) may occur that might be confused with a true gland-forming neoplasm.

The histologic changes in chronic otitis media include a variable amount of chronic inflammatory cells, consisting of lymphocytes, histiocytes, plasma cells, and eosinophils. Multinucleated giant cells and foamy histiocytes may be present. The middle ear low cuboidal epithelium may or may not be seen. However, glandular metaplasia, a response of the middle ear epithelium to the infectious process, may be present (Figure 14.43). The glands tend to be more common in nonsuppurative otitis media than in suppurative otitis media. The metaplastic glands are unevenly distributed in the tissue specimens, are variably shaped, and are separated by abundant stromal tissue. The glands are lined by a columnar to cuboidal epithelium, with or without cilia or goblet cell metaplasia. Glandular secretions may or may not be present so that the glands may appear empty or contain varying

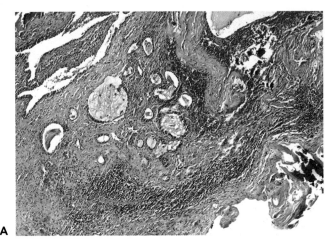
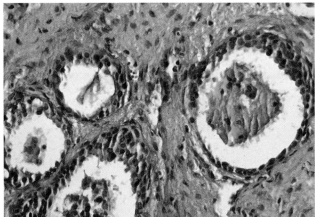

A

B

Figure 14.43 Under normal conditions, glands are not identified in the middle ear space; however, glandular metaplasia can be found in the setting of otitis media. **A.** Otitis media, showing chronic inflammation, fibrosis, glandular metaplasia, and foci of calcifications (*lower right*); residual normal cuboidal epithelium of the middle ear is seen in the upper left. **B.** Higher magnification showing glandular metaplasia is the setting of chronic otitis media.

secretions, including thin (serous) or thick (mucoid) fluid content. The identification of cilia is confirmatory of middle ear glandular metaplasia and is a feature is not found in association with middle ear adenomas (36). Further, the haphazard arrangement of the glands in the background of changes of chronic otitis media should allow for differentiating metaplastic from neoplastic glands. Acute inflammatory cells may be superimposed by chronic otitis media.

In addition to the inflammatory cell infiltrate and glandular metaplasia, other histopathologic findings can be seen in association with chronic otitis media (or represent sequelae of chronic otitis media) and include fibrosis, granulation tissue, tympanosclerosis, cholesterol granulomas, and reactive bone formation. Due to the presence of scar tissue, the middle ear ossicles may be destroyed (partial or total) or may become immobilized. Perforation of the tympanic membrane pars tensa may occur with resulting ingrowth of squamous epithelium, potentially leading to the development of cholesteatoma (see below).

Tympanosclerosis represents dystrophic mineralization (calcification or ossification) of the tympanic membrane or middle ear that is associated with recurrent episodes of otitis media (37). The incidence of tympanosclerosis in otitis media varies from 3 to 33% (37). Tympanosclerosis of the tympanic membrane can be seen in children following myringotomy and tube insertion. In this setting, the tympanosclerotic foci may or may not be permanent. Tympanosclerosis of the middle ear typically affects older patients, represents irreversible accumulation of mineralized material, and is associated with conductive hearing loss (38,39).

On gross examination, tympanosclerotic foci may be localized or diffuse and appear as white nodules or plaques (Figure 14.44). Histologically, dense "clumps" of mineral-

ized, calcified, or ossified material or debris can be seen within the stromal tissues or in the middle (connective tissue) aspect of the tympanic membrane (Figure 14.45). Tympanosclerosis may cause scarring and ossicular fixation.

Cholesterol granuloma is a histologic designation describing the presence of a foreign body granulomatous response to cholesterol crystals derived from the rupture of red blood cells with breakdown of the lipid layer of the erythrocyte cell membrane. Cholesterol granulomas arise in the middle ear and mastoid in any condition in which there is hemorrhage combined with interference in drainage and ventilation of the middle ear space (40). Cholesterol granuloma of the middle ear may present as idiopathic hemotympanum; patients may also complain of hearing loss and tinnitus. The majority of cholesterol

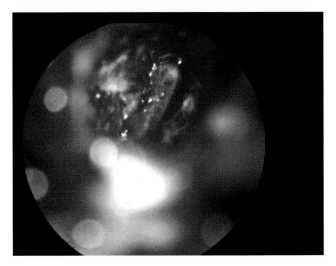

Figure 14.44 Tympanic membrane in tympanosclerosis showing calcified plaque on the tympanic membrane.

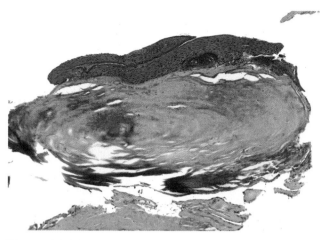

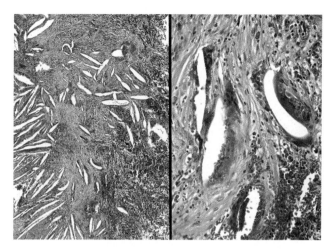

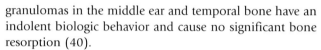

Figure 14.45 Tympanosclerosis. The tympanic membrane is thickened and calcified and is covered on its external (external auditory canal) aspect by keratinizing squamous epithelium (*top*) and on its internal (tympanic cavity) aspect by cuboidal epithelium (*bottom right*).

Figure 14.46 Cholesterol granuloma appears as empty, irregularly shaped clefts or spaces surrounded by histiocytes and multinucleated giant cells. Fresh hemorrhage and hemosiderin pigment are readily apparent.

granulomas in the middle ear and temporal bone have an indolent biologic behavior and cause no significant bone resorption (40).

In contrast to cholesterol granulomas of the middle ear and temporal bone, cholesterol granulomas of the petrous apex may behave aggressively, producing a tumorlike mass with expansion of the cyst and erosion/destruction of adjacent structures. Depending on the direction of expansion, apical cholesterol granulomas may invade into the cochlea, cerebellopontine angle, jugular foramen, cranial nerves V to XI, brain stem, and cerebellum, producing life-threatening symptoms (41). Involvement of the petrous apex is more likely to be associated with sensorineural hearing loss; additional signs and symptoms may include headaches, cranial nerve deficits, and bone erosion with involvement of the posterior or middle cranial fossa (41,42). On axial computed tomography, apical cholesterol granulomas appear as round to ovoid to irregular-shaped cysts with smooth margins and evidence of bone remodeling.

The histology of cholesterol granulomas is the same irrespective of location and includes the presence of irregular-shaped clear-appearing spaces surrounded by histiocytes and/or multinucleated giant cells (foreign body granuloma) (Figure 14.46). Cholesterol granulomas are not related to cholesteatomas but may occur in association with or independent of a cholesteatoma.

Cholesteatoma (Keratoma)

Cholesteatoma is a pseudoneoplastic lesion of the middle ear characterized by the presence of stratified squamous epithelium that forms a saclike accumulation of keratin within the middle ear space (akin to an epidermal inclusion cyst). De-

spite their invasive growth, cholesteatomas are not considered to be true neoplasms. The term *cholesteatoma* is a misnomer in that it is not a neoplasm nor does it contain cholesterol. Perhaps the designation of *keratoma* would be more accurate, but the term cholesteatoma is entrenched in the literature. In the middle ear and inner ear, cholesteatomas take three forms: acquired cholesteatoma, congenital cholesteatoma, and cholesteatoma of the petrous apex. Depending on the site of origin in the tympanic membrane, each of these cholesteatomas may be subdivided into pars flaccida (Schrapnell's membrane) and pars tensa cholesteatomas.

Acquired Cholesteatoma

Acquired cholesteatoma is the most common type of cholesteatoma. It tends to be more common in men than in women and occur in older children and young adults. Acquired cholesteatoma is derived from entry of external ear canal epidermis into the middle ear. The latter may occur in one of several ways: via perforation of the tympanic membrane, following localized retraction of the tympanic membrane with epithelial invagination or ingrowth of a band of stratified squamous epithelium into the middle ear; via entrapment of squamous epithelium following surgery and/or trauma; or via squamous metaplasia of the middle ear mucosa (43). A decrease in middle ear pressure can induce retraction of certain regions of the tympanic membrane in the pars flaccida, pars tensa, or both (43). Retraction pockets are felt to represent the precursors for the development of cholesteatoma (Figure 14.47) (44,45). Dysfunction of the auditory tube leading to chronic (recurrent) otitis media is felt to represent a causative factor (43).

The upper posterior part of the middle ear space is the most common site of acquired cholesteatoma. Initially,

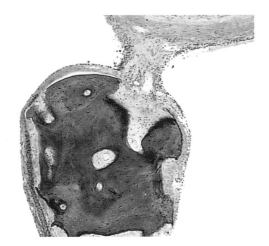

Figure 14.47 Section of malleus from an adult ear with a retraction pocket of the tympanic membrane at autopsy. There is a thin layer of stratified squamous epithelium between the bone and middle ear epithelium. This was found on serial section to be an ingrowth of the stratified squamous epithelium from the outer epithelial covering of the retraction pocket.

cholesteatomas may remain clinically silent until extensive invasion of the middle ear space and mastoid occurs. Symptoms include hearing loss, malodorous discharge, and pain and may be associated with a polyp arising in the attic of the middle ear or perforation of the tympanic membrane. Otoscopic examination may reveal the presence of white debris within the middle ear, which is considered diagnostic.

Congenital Cholesteatoma

Congenital cholesteatoma is a cholesteatoma of the middle ear that exists in the presence of an intact tympanic membrane, presumably occurring in the absence of chronic otitis media that may result in perforation or retraction of the tympanic membrane. Congenital cholesteatomas are found in infants and young children. Small colonies of epidermoid cells, referred to as epidermoid formations, are found on the lateral anterior superior surface of the middle ear in temporal bones after 15 weeks gestation (43). During the first postpartum year, the epidermoid colonies disappear; however, if the epidermoid cells do not disappear but continue to grow, they will become a congenital cholesteatoma. The latter have also been referred to as epidermoid cysts (46). In the majority of cases, congenital cholesteatomas are found in the anterosuperior part of the middle ear. Early lesions show no symptoms and are discovered by otoscopic examination. In later lesions, the signs and symptoms may be the same as acquired cholesteatoma.

Cholesteatoma of the Petrous Apex

Cholesteatoma of the petrous apex is an epidermoid cyst of this location and bears no relation to cholesteatoma of the middle ear. It is likely of congenital origin, but no cell rests have been discovered that may explain the origin of these lesions. Symptoms usually relate to involvement of the cranial nerves VII and VIII in the cerebellopontine angle (46).

Pathology

Cholesteatomas appear as cystic, white to pearly appearing masses of varying size that contain creamy or waxy granular material. The histologic diagnosis of cholesteatoma is made in the presence of a stratified keratinizing squamous epithelium, subepithelial fibroconnective or granulation tissue, and keratin debris (Figure 14.48). The essential diagnostic feature is the keratinizing squamous epithelium, and the presence of keratin debris alone is not diagnostic of a cholesteatoma. The keratinizing squamous epithelium is

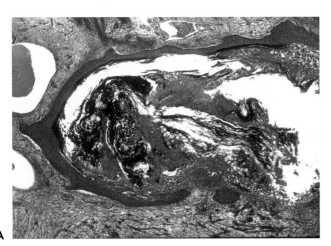

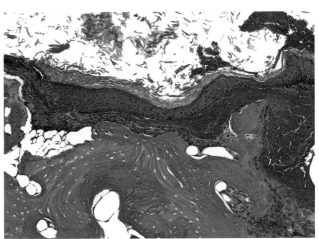

Figure 14.48 Cholesteatoma of the middle ear. **A.** The histologic diagnosis of cholesteatoma is based on the presence of finding keratinizing squamous epithelium within the middle ear space. **B.** Osseous involvement.

cytologically bland and shows cellular maturation without evidence of dysplasia. In spite of its benign histology, cholesteatomas are "invasive" and have widespread destructive capabilities.

The destructive properties of cholesteatomas result from a combination of interrelated reasons, including mass effect with pressure erosion of surrounding structures from the cholesteatoma, the production of collagenase (which has osteodestructive capabilities by its resorption of bony structures), and bone resorption (20). Collagenase is produced by both the squamous epithelial and the fibrous tissue components of the cholesteatoma. This local aggressive behavior is the result of the continuing accumulation of the cholesteatomatous material with progressive erosion of surrounding structures. Depending on the location and extent of the cholesteatoma, erosion may include the lateral wall of the attic, the middle ear ossicles, the tegmental bone over the attic and antrum, and the mastoid cortex (43). Less frequent progression includes erosion of the lateral sinus and jugular bulb, the vestibular and cochlear capsules, the facial canal, the dura of the middle and posterior cranial fossa, the semicircular canals, and the facial nerve (43). Sequelae of such erosions may include semicircular canal fistulas, exposed tympanic facial nerve, or brain herniation through the tegmen.

The histologic diagnosis of cholesteatomas is relatively straightforward in the presence of keratinizing squamous epithelium. In contrast to cholesteatomas, squamous cell carcinoma shows dysplastic or overtly malignant cytologic features with a prominent desmoplastic stromal response to its infiltrative growth. Cholesteatomas do not transform into squamous cell carcinomas. In an attempt to determine whether cholesteatomas were low-grade squamous carcinomas, Desloge et al. (47) performed DNA analysis on human cholesteatomas to determine whether ploidy abnormalities were present. In ten cases with interpretable data, nine were euploid and one was aneuploid. These authors concluded that, due to a lack of overt genetic instability, cholesteatomas could not be considered to be malignant neoplasms. Cholesterol granuloma is not synonymous with cholesteatoma. These entities are distinctly different pathologic entities and should not be confused with one another.

Otosclerosis

Otosclerosis is a disorder of the bony labyrinth and stapedial footplate that exclusively occurs in humans and is of unknown etiology. Otosclerosis means hardening of the ear and is derived from Greek (*ous*, ear; *skleros*, hard; *osis*, condition); osseous ankylosis (from the Greek *ankoulon*, to stiffen); chronic metaplastic ostitis; progressive otospongiosis. Otosclerosis primarily causes conductive hearing loss that usually begins in the second and third decades of life and is slowly progressive. The extent of the hearing loss directly correlates with the degree of stapedial footplate fix-

ation. It is not uncommon for patients with otosclerosis also to have vestibular disturbances (48,49). Otosclerosis usually involves both ears; however, unilateral disease can occur in up to 15% of cases (50).

Although many theories regarding the etiology of otosclerosis appear in the literature, there is no consensus. Hereditary factors are often cited as among the causes. Surgical management of the conductive hearing loss caused by stapes fixation (stapedectomy) is the treatment of choice, with replacement of the fixed stapes by a prosthesis. The resected bone may include the entire stapes (with the footplate) or only the superstructure that includes the head and crura (without the footplate).

Histologically, the initial alterations include resorption of bone around blood vessels. The cellular fibrovascular tissue replaces the resorbed bone, resulting in softening of the bone (otospongiosis). Immature bone is laid down with continuous active resorption and remodeling. The new bone is rich in ground substance and deficient in collagen; but, over time, more mature bone with increased collagen and less ground substance is produced, resulting in densely sclerotic bone. This process most often begins from the adjacent temporal bone (anterior to the oval window) and eventually involves the footplate of the stapes moving across the annulus fibrosus or stapediovestibular joint (Figure 14.49). Stapedial involvement causes fixation of the stapes, with inability to transmit sound waves resulting in conductive hearing loss. While the otosclerotic changes can be seen in the resected stapedial footplate, even when the footplate is removed intact it may be free of otosclerotic changes as fixation results via pressure on the nonotosclerotic footplate from swelling of the otosclerotic process in the adjacent temporal bone (7).

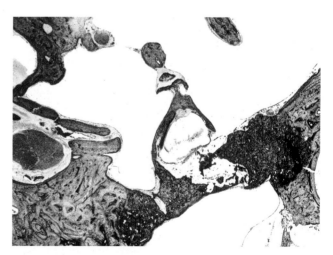

Figure 14.49 Otosclerosis of the temporal bone (anterior to the oval window) involving the footplate of the stapes moving across the annulus fibrosus or stapediovestibular joint. Stapedial involvement causes fixation of the stapes, with inability to transmit sound waves resulting in conductive hearing loss.

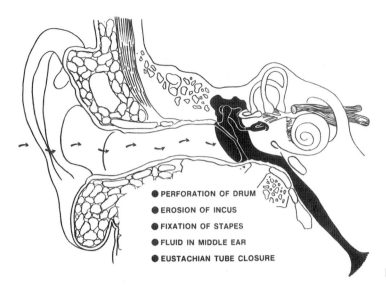

Figure 14.50   Causes of conductive hearing loss.

Inner Ear

Presbycusis and Other Hearing Loss

Hearing loss may include conductive hearing loss and sensorineural hearing loss. There are many causes for conductive and sensorineural hearing loss, respectively (Figures 14.50–14.51). Hearing loss that occurs with increasing age is referred to as presbycusis. There is still controversy as to the underlying electrophysiologic and histopathologic alterations associated with the development of presbycusis. Degenerative alterations within various microanatomic structures of the cochlea, including the hair cells, spiral ganglion cells, stria vascularis, and basilar membrane, have been invoked as the cause of presbycusis (51). Alternatively, damage to the outer hair cells alone has been invoked as the cause of presbycusis (52,53). As Soucek and colleagues have

shown in their studies of aged ears (52,53), the histopathologic changes include scanty to absent outer hair cells of the third row (Figure 14.52), with complete loss of both inner and outer hair cells of all rows at the extreme lower end of the basal coil. In contrast to these aforementioned sites, Soucek and colleagues found that the inner hair cells sustained minimal loss, the first row of outer hair cells had

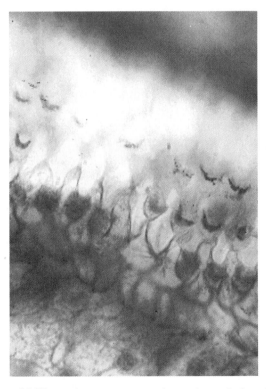

Figure 14.52   Surface preparation of outer hair cells from basal coil of cochlea of an elderly man. There are many gaps among the hair cells of the first two rows. (P, pillar cells) (Osmic acid, Alcian blue, and phloxine eosin, oil immersion.)

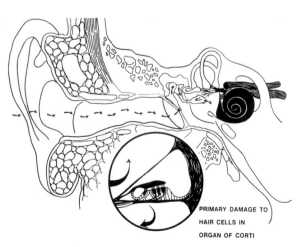

Figure 14.51   Cause of sensorineural hearing loss.

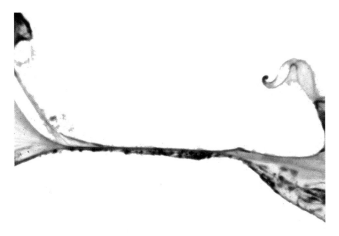

Figure 14.53 Viral labyrinthitis- (end stage) related hearing loss with total degeneration of the organ of Corti.

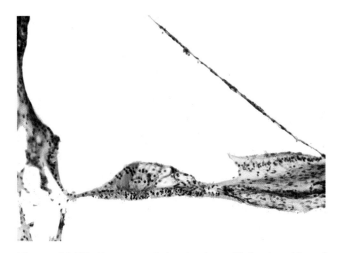

Figure 14.55 Posttraumatic hearing loss with focal avulsion of the organ of Corti.

greater loss, and the second row more loss but not to the extent seen in the third row of outer hair cells or at the extreme lower end of the basal coil (54,55). In addition, these authors also found the presence of enormously lengthened and thickened sterocilia and giant stereocilia, which they felt contributing to the development of presbycusis.

Degenerative alterations within various microanatomic structures of the membranous labyrinth resulting in sensorineural hearing loss may occur secondary to infectious disease (Figure 14.53), metabolic abnormalities (Figure 14.54), trauma (Figure 14.55), sensory presbycusis (Figure 14.56), and use of certain medications, including cisplatin, diuretic agents, and other drugs (Figures 14.57–14.58).

Ménière's Disease

Ménière's disease is an idiopathic disorder of the inner ear associated with a symptom complex of spontaneous,

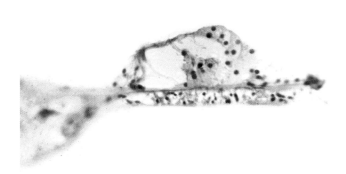

Figure 14.56 Sensory presbycusis characterized by the loss of hair cells in the organ of Corti.

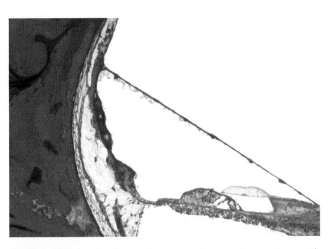

Figure 14.54 Metabolic-related hearing loss in a patient with diabetes is characterized by the presence of hyalinized vasculature structures in the stria vascularis.

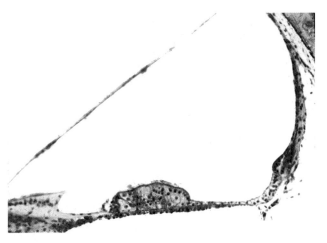

Figure 14.57 Strial presbycusis with atrophy; this is secondary to ototoxic effect caused by cisplatin therapy.

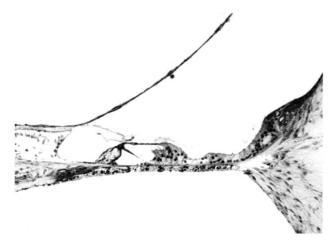

Figure 14.58 Kanamycin ototoxic effects on the organ of Corti, including loss of hair cells.

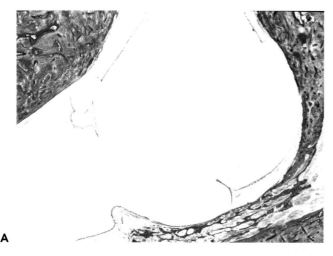

A

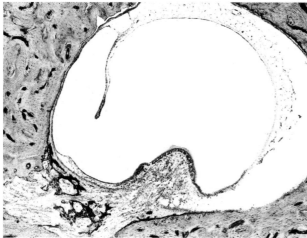

B

Figure 14.59 Ménière's disease showing dilatation (**A**) and rupture of the membranous labyrinth (**B**).

episodic attacks of vertigo, sensorineural hearing loss, tinnitus, and a sensation of aural fullness. The onset of vertigo is frequently sudden, reaching maximum intensity within a few minutes, lasting from an hour or more, and either subsiding completely or continuing as a sensation of unsteadiness for hours to days.

The pathogenesis of Ménière's disease is distortion of the membranous labyrinth, defined as changes in the microanatomy of the membranous labyrinth as a consequence of the over-accumulation of endolymph (endolymphatic hydrops) and at the expense of the perilymphatic space (54,55). Endolymph, which is produced by the stria vascularis in the cochlea and by cells in the vestibular labyrinth, circulates in a radial and longitudinal fashion. In patients with Ménière's disease, it is believed that there is inadequate absorption of endolymph by the endolymphatic sac (55).

In the early stages of the disease, endolymphatic hydrops primarily involves the cochlear duct and saccule, but in the later stages the entire endolymphatic system is involved. Alterations of the membranous labyrinth include dilatation, outpouching, rupture, and collapse (Figure 14.59). Fistulae (unhealed ruptures) may occur. Severe cytoarchitectural and atrophic changes may occur in the sense organs with loss of neurons in the cochlea.

TEMPORAL BONE DISSECTION

For a detailed discussion of proper postmortem removal, sectioning, and processing for microscopic evaluation of the temporal bone, the reader is referred to other texts (7,56).

REFERENCES

1. Hollinshead WH. The ear. In: Hollinshead WH, ed. *Anatomy for Surgeons.* 3rd ed. Philadelphia: Harper & Row; 1982:159–221.
2. Moore KL. The ear. In: Moore KL, ed. *The Developing Human: Clinically Oriented Embryology.* 4th ed. Philadelphia: WB Saunders; 1988:412–420.
3. Michaels L, Soucek S. Development of the stratified squamous epithelium of the human tympanic membrane and external canal: the origin of auditory epithelial migration. *Am J Anat* 1989;184: 334–344.
4. Michaels L, Soucek S. Stratified squamous epithelium in relation to the tympanic membrane: its development and kinetics. Int J Pediatr Otorhinolaryngol 1991;22:135–49.
5. Michaels L. The ear. In: Sternberg SS, ed. *Histology for Pathologists.* 2nd ed. Philadelphia: Lippincott-Raven; 1997:337–366.
6. Michaels L, Soucek S. Auditory epithelial migration on the human tympanic membrane: II. The existence of two discrete migratory pathways and their embryologic correlates. *Am J Anat* 1990;189: 189–200.
7. Nager GT. Anatomy of the membranous cochlea and vestibular labyrinth. In: Nager GT, ed. *Pathology of the Ear and Temporal Bone.* Baltimore: Williams & Wilkins; 1993:3–48.
8. Schuknecht HF. Anatomy. In: Schuknecht HF, ed. *Pathology of the Ear.* 2nd ed. Philadelphia: Lea & Febiger; 1993:31–74.

9. Maybaum JL, Goldman JL. Primary jugular bulb thrombosis. A study of twenty cases. *Arch Otolaryngol* 1933;17:70–84.

10. Kamerer DB. Electromyographic correlation of tensor tympani and tensor veli palatini muscles in man. *Laryngoscope* 1978;88:651–662.

11. Graves GO, Edwards LF. The Eustachian tube: a review of its descriptive, microscopic, topographic and clinical anatomy. *Arch Otolaryngol* 1944;39:359–397.

12. Moreano EH, Paparella MM, Zelterman D, Goycoolea MV. Prevalence of carotid canal dehiscence in the human middle ear: a report of 1000 temporal bones. *Laryngoscope* 1994;104(pt 1): 612–618.

13. Michaels L, Wells M. Squamous cell carcinoma of the middle ear. *Clin Otolaryngol Allied Sci* 1980;5:235–248.

14. Nager GT. Pneumatization of the temporal bone. In: Nager GT, ed. *Pathology of the Ear and Temporal Bone*. Baltimore: Williams & Wilkins; 1993:53–62.

15. Tremble GE. Pneumatization of the temporal bone. *Arch Otolaryngol* 1934;19:172–182.

16. Davies DV. A note on the articulations of the auditory ossicles and related structures. *J Laryngol Otol* 1948;62:533–536.

17. Dayal VS, Farkashidy J, Kokshanian A. Embryology of the ear. *Can J Otolaryngol* 1973;2:136–142.

18. Lysakowski A, McCrea RA, Tomlinson RD. Anatomy of vestibular end organs and neural pathways. In: Cummings CW, Frederickson JM, Harker LA, Krause CJ, Richardson MA, Schuller DE, eds. *Otolaryngology: Head and Neck Surgery*. 3rd ed. St. Louis: Mosby; 1998: 2561–2583.

19. Kobrak HG. Influence of the middle ear on labyrinthine pressure. *Arch Otolaryngol* 1935;21:547–.

20. Lindsey JR, Schuknecht HF, Neff WD, Kimura RS. Obliteration of the endolymphatic sac and the cochlear aqueduct. *Ann Otol Rhinol Laryngol* 1952;61:697–716.

21. Tonndorf J, Tabor JR. Closure of the cochlear windows: its effect upon air- and bone-conduction. *Ann Otol Rhinol Laryngol* 1962;71:5–29.

22. Belemer JJ. The vessels of the stria vascularis: with special reference to their functions. *Arch Otolaryngol* 1936;23:93–97.

23. Guild SR. The circulation of the endolymph. *Am J Anat* 1927;39: 57–81.

24. Altmann F, Waltner JG. New investigations on the physiology of the labyrinthine fluids. *Laryngoscope* 1950;60:727–739.

25. Tarlov IM. Structure of the nerve root. II. Differentiation of sensory from motor roots: observations on identification of function in roots of mixed cranial nerves. *Arch Neurol Psychiatr* 1937;37: 1338–1355.

26. Hollinshead WH. The cranium. In: Hollinshead WH, ed. *Anatomy for Surgeons*. 3rd ed. Philadelphia: Harper & Row; 1982:26–27.

27. Hyams VJ, Batsakis JG, Michaels L. Acoustic neuroma. In: Hartmann WH, Sobin LH, eds. *Atlas of Tumor Pathology. Tumors of the Upper Respiratory Tract and Ear*, Second Series, Fascicle 25. Washington, DC: Armed Forces Institute of Pathology; 1988: 323–326.

28. Heffner DK. Low-grade adenocarcinoma of probable endolymphatic sac origin. A clinicopathologic study of 20 cases. *Cancer* 1989;64:2292–2302.

29. Wenig BM, Heffner DK. Endolymphatic sac tumors: fact or fiction? *Adv Anat Pathol* 1996;3:378–387.

30. Megerian CA, McKenna MJ, Nuss RC, et al. Endolymphatic sac tumors: histopathologic confirmation, clinical characterization, and implication in von Hippel-Lindau disease. *Laryngoscope* 1995; 105(pt 1):801–808.

31. Sgambati MT, Stolle C, Choyke PL, et al. Mosaicism in von Hippel-Lindau disease: lessons from kindreds with germline mutations identified in offspring with mosaic parents. *Am J Hum Genet* 2000; 66:84–91.

32. Smith CA, Lowry OH, Wu ML. The electrolytes of the labyrinthine fluids. *Laryngoscope* 1954;64:141–153.

33. Schuknecht HF. Developmental defects. In: Schuknecht HF, ed. *Pathology of the Ear*. 2nd ed. Philadelphia: Lea & Febiger; 1993: 115–189.

34. Frank ST. Aural sign of coronary heart disease. *N Engl J Med* 1973;289:327–328.

35. Patel V, Champ C, Andrews PS, Gostelow BE, Gunasekara NP, Davidson AR. Diagonal earlobe creases and atheromatous disease: a postmortem study. *Jr Coll Physicians Lond* 1992;26:274–277.

36. Wenig BM. The ear. In: Mills SE, Carter D, Greenson JK, Oberman HA, Reuter VE, Stoler MH, eds. *Sternberg's Diagnostic Surgical Pathology*. 4th ed. Philadelphia: Lippincott Williams & Wilkins; 2004:1033–1072.

37. Bhaya MH, Schachern PA, Morizono T, Paparella MM. Pathogenesis of tympanosclerosis. *Otolaryngol Head Neck Surg* 1993;109(pt 1):413–420.

38. Gibb AG, Pang YT. Current considerations in the etiology and diagnosis of tympanosclerosis. *Eur Arch Otorhinolaryngol* 1994; 251: 439–451.

39. Nager GT, Vanderveen TS. Cholesterol granuloma involving the temporal bone. *Ann Otol Rhinol Laryngol* 1976;85(pt 1):204–209.

40. Nager GT. Cholesterol granulomas. In: Nager GT, ed. *Pathology of the Ear and Temporal Bone*. Baltimore: Williams & Wilkins; 1994: 914–939.

41. Thedinger BA, Nadol JB Jr, Montgomery WW, Thedinger BS, Greenberg JJ. Radiographic diagnosis, surgical treatment, and long-term follow-up of cholesterol granulomas of the petrous apex. *Laryngoscope* 1989;99:896–907.

42. Nager GT. Cholesteatomas of the middle ear. In: Nager GT, ed. *Pathology of the Ear and Temporal Bone*. Baltimore: Williams & Wilkins; 1994:298–350.

43. Michaels L. The biology of cholesteatoma. *Otolaryngol Clin North Am* 1989;22:869–881.

44. Wells MD, Michaels L. Role of retraction pockets in cholesteatoma formation. *Clin Otolaryngol Allied Sci* 1983;8:39–45.

45. Schuknecht HF. Cholesteatoma. In: Schuknecht HF, ed. *Pathology of the Ear*. 2nd ed. Philadelphia: Lea & Febiger; 1993:204–206.

46. de Souza CE, Sperling NM, da Costa SS, Yoon TH, Abdel Hamid M, de Souza RA. Congenital cholesteatomas of the cerebellopontine angle. *Am J Otol* 1989;10:358–363.

47. Desloge RB, Carew JF, Finstad CL, et al. DNA analysis of human cholesteatomas. *Am J Otol* 1997;18:155–159.

48. Cody DT, Baker HL Jr. Otosclerosis: vestibular symptoms and sensorineural hearing loss. *Ann Otol Rhinol Laryngol* 1978;87(pt 1):778–796.

49. Morales-Garcia C. Cochleo-vestibular involvement in otosclerosis. *Acta Otolaryngol* 1972;73:484–492.

50. Schuknecht HF. Otosclerosis. In: Schuknecht HF, ed. *Pathology of the Ear*. 2nd ed. Philadelphia: Lea & Febiger; 1993:365–379.

51. Schuknecht HF. Disorders of aging. In: Schuknecht HF, ed. *Pathology of the Ear*. 2nd ed. Philadelphia: Lea & Febiger; 1993: 415–446.

52. Soucek S, Michaels L, Frohlich A. Pathological changes in the organ of Corti in presbyacusis as revealed in microslicing and staining. *Acta Otolaryngol Suppl* 1987;436:93–102.

53. Soucek S, Michaels L, Frohlich A. Evidence for hair cell degeneration as the primary lesion in hearing loss of the elderly. *J Otolaryngol* 1986;15:175–183.

54. Paparella MM. The cause (multifactorial inheritance) and pathogenesis (endolymphatic malabsorption) of Meniere's disease and its symptoms (mechanical and chemical). *Acta Otolaryngol* 1985;99:445–451.

55. Klis SF, Buijs J, Smoorenburg GF. Quantification of the relation between electrophysiologic and morphologic changes in experimental endolymphatic hydrops. *Ann Otol Rhinol Laryngol* 1990;99(pt 1):566–570.

56. Schuknecht HF. Histologic techniques. In: Schuknecht HF, ed. *Pathology of the Ear*. 2nd ed. Philadelphia: Lea & Febiger; 1993:7–12.

Mouth, Nose, and Paranasal Sinuses

15

Karoly Balogh   Liron Pantanowitz

EMBRYOLOGY AND PRENATAL CHANGES

The development of this highly specialized part of the head is restricted to structures of importance to the surgical pathologist. For details, the reader is referred to other sources (1–2).

The oral region develops from an ectodermal depression, the stomodeum. The deep oral cavity is formed by the forward growth of structures about the margins of the stomodeum, giving rise to superficial parts of the face and jaws, as well as the walls of the oral cavity. The stomodeal prominence is surrounded bilaterally by the maxillary and mandibular processes and rostrally by the unpaired frontal prominence. The upper lip, maxilla, and nose are derived from structures surrounding the stomodeum. The caudal boundary of the oral cavity is formed by the paired mandibular processes, which, during the second year of life, fuse in the midline to form the mandible. The paired maxillary processes likewise meet in the midline, crowding the nasal elevation to ultimately form the maxilla and, by fusion in the midline, the palate. The contours of the face change with the rapid growth of the nose and jaws (2). The nose is formed on either side of the frontonasal elevation by an invagination of ectoderm into the mesoderm to form two nasal pits that gradually converge toward the midline, where they merge with each other. The underlying mesenchyme develops into bone, cartilage, and skeletal muscle.

At the end of the second month of fetal life, the formation of the bony structures begins; the maxilla is one of the first bones to calcify. Simultaneously, the nasal pits become progressively deeper and extend downward toward the oral cavity. Later, elevations appear on the lateral walls of the right and left nasal cavity that will become the scroll-like nasal turbinates (conchae). The nasal cavities communicate with chambers in the adjacent bones known as paranasal sinuses. Named for the bones in which they lie, they comprise the frontal, maxillary, sphenoidal, and ethmoidal sinuses. The paranasal sinuses can be first identified around the fourth month of fetal life, but most of their expansion occurs after birth, and they attain full size many years later. The mucosa lining the nasal cavities invaginates into the surrounding bone, thereby lining the expanding sinus. While the palate has been taking shape from the roof of the mouth, the tongue has been forming in the floor. The posterior part of the tongue (behind the sulcus terminalis) is derived from the midventral areas of branchial arches II, III, and IV.

The tonsils first develop as endodermal epithelial buds that arise from the lining of the primitive oronasal cavity and grow into the subjacent mesenchyme to eventually give rise to the tonsillar crypts. Crypt formation may be simple, as in the lingual tonsil, or more complex, as in the palatine tonsils. Lymphoid tissue begins to accumulate and organize around the crypts at around the time when secondary budding of the crypts takes place. This development occurs in close association with mucous glands, which explains the close anatomic proximity of such glands to the tonsils.

Tooth development (odontogenesis) is of considerable importance to an understanding of the pathogenesis of odontogenic tumors and cysts. Odontogenesis is a highly coordinated and complex process that relies upon several genes, growth factors, structural proteins (e.g., amelogenin, tuftelin, predentin, cementum, enamelin), and extracellular matrix molecules being expressed in temporal- and space-specific patterns (3). The teeth begin to develop inside the gums of the upper and lower jaw (Figure 15.1). Such regulatory interactions occur during the early stages of morphogenesis, particularly when the dental epithelium induces the condensation of mesenchymal cells around the epithelial bud. Teeth pass through three stages of development: growth, mineralization, and eruption. The growth period is further subdivided into the bud, cap, and bell stages.

Initially, the oral epithelium shows definite thickening and begins to grow into the subjacent mesenchyme around the entire arc of each jaw. The free margin of this epithelial band gives rise to two invaginating processes. The outer process (vestibular lamina) will form the vestibule that demarcates the cheeks and lips. From the inner horseshoe-shaped process (dental lamina), tooth buds (bud stage) arise at the site of each future tooth. Thus, the primordia for the temporary deciduous (primary) teeth are formed. Shortly afterward, the primordia of the succedaneous (permanent) teeth develop in the same way. The permanent tooth germs lie in a hollow of the alveolar sockets on the lingual side of the deciduous teeth. The developing enamel organ of each tooth takes the shape of a goblet with the dental lamina as its stem. As the dental lamina disintegrates, the inner lining cells (inner enamel epithelium) of the enamel organ differentiate to become columnar epithelial cells called ameloblasts, whereas the outer layer of cells (outer enamel epithelium) flatten into a layer of closely packed cells. Between the ameloblasts and the outer enamel epithelium is the loosely arranged epithelium of the stellate reticulum. Inside the goblet-shaped enamel organ, the mesenchymal cells proliferate to form a dense aggregate, the dental papilla (cap stage).

The dental papilla will form the dentin, cementum, and pulp. The dentin is the internal layer of the tooth, the cementum is the bony tissue covering the root of the tooth, and the pulp is the soft inner part of the tooth. More peripherally, the condensing mesenchymal cells extend around the enamel organ as the dental follicle. The cells of the dental follicle eventually produce alveolar bone and collagen fibers of the periodontium. In the final

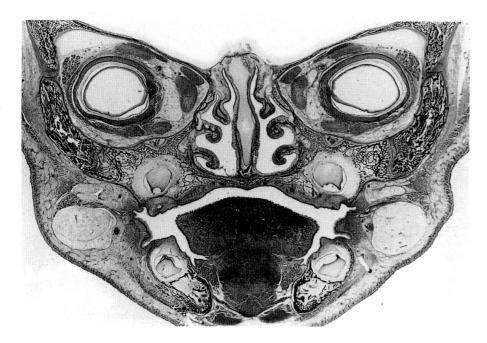

Figure 15.1 Coronal section of head of a human fetus about 30 weeks of age (284 mm crown-rump length). The bell-shaped enamel organs are present in each quadrant. The tongue is relatively large. The paranasal sinuses are not yet discernible at this stage of fetal development.

(bell) stage of growth, the epithelium of the cap will form the enamel. During this stage, the outer and inner enamel epithelium meet at their apical ends, where they proliferate to form Hertwig's epithelial root sheath, which initiates the differentiation of the outermost cells of the papilla to become arranged in a row of single columnar cells to form the odontoblasts (Figures 15.2–15.3). Nerves and blood vessels in the dental papilla begin to form the primitive dental pulp. The dental papilla grows toward the gum, crowding in on the enamel organ, which by then has lost its connection with the oral epithelium. During dentinogenesis nonmineralized predentin is produced by the odontoblasts against the inner surface of the enamel organ. As the odontoblasts produce predentin, their cell bodies recede toward the center of the tooth, so that each odontoblast leaves behind a thin process (Tomes' fiber) that occupies a dentinal tubule. The organic matrix of the predentin eventually mineralizes to become dentin, which is arranged in the shape of tubules running from the pulp chamber toward the periphery. Meanwhile the enamel cap of the tooth is being formed (amelogenesis) by the ameloblasts (4). The formation of dentin and enamel begins at the tip of the crown and progresses toward the root of the tooth (5). As the developing

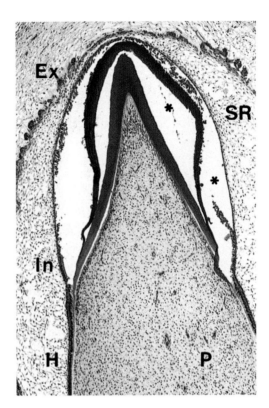

Figure 15.3 Enamel organ. Amelogenesis and dentinogenesis progress from crown to root. Early enamel and dentin appear as black bands, widest at the crown area and become thinner toward the root. [*Ex*, external enamel epithelium; *In*, inner enamel epithelium; *SR*, stellate reticulum; *H*, Hertwig's epithelial root sheath; *P*, dental papilla; *, artifact (separation)]

root increases in length, the previously formed crown moves closer to the surface of the gum. Even when the crown of the tooth begins to erupt, the root is still incomplete and continues growing until the crown has completely emerged (6,7) (Figures 15.4–15.5). The

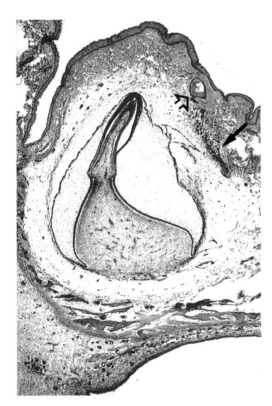

Figure 15.2 Enamel organ of deciduous tooth. Formation of enamel and dentin has begun at the crown area of the tooth. [*Arrow*, remnants of dental lamina; *arrowhead*, a small epithelial cyst (rest of Serres)]

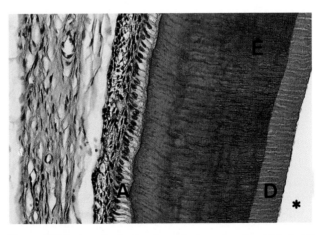

Figure 15.4 Developing tooth, sagittal section. Ameloblasts (*A*) line the surface of the enamel matrix (*E*) which is partly mineralized. Dentin (*D*) is not mineralized (predentin) and has been separated by an artifact (*) from pulp (missing).

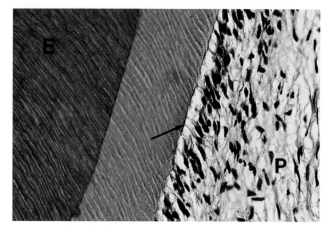

Figure 15.5 Developing tooth. Layer of polarized odontoblasts with Tomes' fibers (*arrow*) extending into tubules of predentin. Fibroblasts of pulp (*P*) are loosely arranged. (*E*, enamel matrix)

enamel is made by differentiated ameloblasts that produce long, thin enamel prisms, or rods; these rods become calcified and are surrounded by a thin organic matrix. Enamel production is completed when the crown is mineralized and its final size attained (8). At this point in time, the flattened ameloblasts and remainder of the cells of the enamel organ form a cuticle on the surface of the enamel; this membrane is then shed (9).

After the root has attained its full length and definitive position in the jaw, a bone-like hard substance, cement, is deposited on it (cementogenesis). Cement is produced by the mesenchymal cells adjacent to the root. These cells become differentiated into a cementoblast layer that resembles the osteogenic (cambial) layer of the periosteum (10,11). Fibers from the rest of the dental sac form the periodontal ligament, which firmly attaches the tooth in the bony alveolar socket (12).

As the jaws approach their adult size, the latent primordia of the permanent teeth follow the same developmental process as did the deciduous teeth (13) (Figure 15.6). When a developing permanent tooth increases in size, the root of the corresponding deciduous tooth is partly resorbed by osteoclastic activity (Figure 15.7). Thus, the anchorage of the deciduous tooth becomes weakened and the tooth is shed, permitting the underlying permanent tooth to erupt.

The minor salivary glands in the mouth develop following a pattern of epithelial-mesenchymal interactions between the outgrowth of an ectodermal bud from the lining of the stomodeum and the underlying mesenchyme. The proliferation, differentiation, and morphogenesis of these glands depend on intrinsic (programmed pattern of cell-specific gene expression) and extrinsic factors. The extrinsic factors include cell-cell and cell-matrix interactions, as well as growth factors (14).

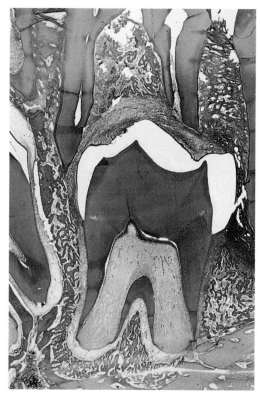

Figure 15.6 Deciduous and unerupted permanent teeth in a 10-year-old child. Perpendicular section through the roots of two deciduous teeth with underlying permanent molar tooth. Empty space was left by enamel that was dissolved by decalcification. Note relationship between teeth and bone, respectively.

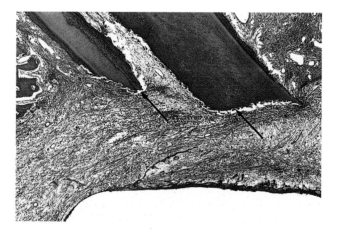

Figure 15.7 Roots of deciduous molar tooth before shedding. Resorption of dentin is indicated by numerous Howship's lacunae and osteoclasts (*arrows*). The thin band (*bottom*) is the reduced internal enamel epithelium that covered the crown of the underlying permanent tooth; the enamel dissolved with decalcification.

GROSS ANATOMY

In this chapter we will consider only those features that are important for the surgical pathologist.

Jawbone

The mandible is a horseshoe-shaped bone; its horizontal part forms the body, which is continuous with the vertical parts of the two sides, the rami. The bone of the body has a thick cortex, and the compact shell contains plates of cancellous bone arranged along the trajectories. The upper part of the body is hollowed into sockets that carry eight teeth on each side. Each ramus is a nearly vertical, flattened, oblong plate of bone surmounted by two processes. The posterior articular process ends in the condyle, articulating with the articular disk of the temporomandibular joint. The anterior (coronoid) process serves for the insertion of the temporal muscle.

The right and left maxillae jointly form the upper jaw; they participate in forming boundaries of four cavities: the roof of the mouth, the floor and lateral wall of the nose, the floor of the maxillary sinus, and the floor of the orbit. The alveolar processes of the maxillae together form the alveolar arch.

Nose

The external nose and nasal septum are partly composed of hyaline cartilage and bone. The two orifices of the external nose, the nares (nostrils), are separated from each other by the median vertical soft tissue columella. The columella is attached posteriorly to the nasal septum, which forms the medial wall of the two approximately symmetrical chambers, the right and left nasal cavities. The nasal cavity extends from the nares anteriorly to the choanae posteriorly. Just behind the nares, the nasal cavity widens to form the vestibule. A ridge (limen nasi) on the lateral nasal wall separates the vestibule from the rest of the nasal cavity proper. In each nasal fossa is an olfactory region that occupies the superior part of the nasal cavity. The rest of the nasal fossa consists of the respiratory region. On the lateral wall of each nasal fossa are the superior, middle, and inferior turbinates. A fourth supreme turbinate may be present at the uppermost portion of the lateral nasal wall. The scroll-shaped turbinates hang over the corresponding funnel-shaped nasal passages, or meatuses, into which the various paranasal sinuses open. The nasal mucosa is in continuity with the mucosa of these sinuses through their corresponding openings. The nasal mucous membrane is most vascular and thickest over the turbinates and is also relatively thick over the nasal septum.

Paranasal Sinuses

The air-filled paranasal cavities (sinuses) are located in the bones around the nasal cavity. The maxillary and frontal sinuses open into the middle meatus of the nose. The sphenoidal sinus opens into the sphenoethmoidal recess above the superior turbinate. There are numerous ethmoidal sinuses that form small communicating cavities, also called ethmoid air cells (or ethmoid labyrinth). The ethmoid air cells have thin bony walls. According to their location, the ethmoidal sinuses can be divided into three groups: the anterior and middle ethmoidal sinuses, which open into the middle meatus, and the posterior ethmoidal sinus, which opens into the superior meatus of the nose. There are many variations in size, shape, and location of all paranasal sinuses. One or more of them may even be underdeveloped or absent.

Blood Vessels

The nasal cavity has an extraordinarily rich blood supply. The anterior and posterior ethmoidal branches of the ophthalmic artery supply the frontal and ethmoidal sinuses, as well as the roof of the nasal cavity. The sphenopalatine branch of the maxillary artery supplies the mucosa of the turbinates, meatuses, and the nasal septum. The mucosa of the maxillary sinus is supplied by branches of the maxillary artery and the sphenoidal sinus by the pharyngeal artery. The branches of all these vessels form a plexiform network in and below the mucous membrane. The veins of the nasal mucosa are well developed, particularly in the inferior turbinate and in the posterior part of the nasal fossa, where they form a cavernous plexus. The veins of the lower jaw drain via the inferior central vein into the pterygoid plexus. Blood from the upper jaw and facial structures drains in two directions: the more anterior parts into the anterior facial vein and the more posterior parts into the pterygoid plexus. The pterygoid plexus drains the teeth, soft palate, fauces, and pharynx. These anatomic relationships are particularly important because infections and tumors of the face, mouth, nose, and paranasal sinuses can reach the intracranial cavernous sinus either via the emissary vein of Vesalius or by way of veins communicating with the inferior or superior ophthalmic veins. The latter veins drain the structures of the anterior face, such as lips, cheek, and external nose, as well as the mucosa of the frontal sinuses, ethmoidal cells, and upper lateral nasal wall. The cavernous sinus also receives venous blood from the mucosa of the sphenoidal sinus.

Nerves

The regions discussed here have a rich and complex innervation, the description of which is beyond the scope of this chapter. However, many nerves of the head lie in close proximity to the mucosa and submucosa of the upper aerodigestive tract and are therefore prone to early invasion by carcinoma.

Lymph Nodes

Lymph nodes of the head and neck are abundant and can be divided into 10 groups: the occipital, mastoid, parotid, facial, sublingual, submaxillary, submental, retropharyngeal, anterior cervical, and lateral cervical nodes. Only those lymph nodes related to the regions covered in this chapter are discussed here. There are three principal parotid lymph node groups: superficial (suprafascial or preauricular) nodes; subfascial (extraglandular) nodes contained in the parotid sheath; and deep intraglandular nodes. The parotid lymph nodes drain the parotid gland, external ear, frontotemporal facial region, eyelids, upper lip, root of the nose, floor of the nasal cavity, soft palate, and buccal mucosa. Their efferents pass into the superior deep cervical nodes.

The small superficial group of facial nodes include, from rostral to caudal, the infraorbital (nasolabial) nodes situated in the nasolabial fold, the buccal nodes placed external to the buccinator muscle and its fascia, and the mandibular nodes located external to the mandible. The facial nodes receive afferent lymphatics from the eyelids, nose, cheek, upper lip, and subjacent nodes, and they empty into the submaxillary nodes. There are also deep facial nodes situated deep to the ramus of the mandible near the maxillary artery. Heterotopic buccal nodes may rarely be encountered immediately beneath the buccal mucosa near the orifice of Stensen's duct, giving the false clinical impression of a neoplasm (15,16). The sublingual (or lingual) nodes are intercalated along the course of the collecting lymph trunks of the tongue. The submaxillary (submandibular) nodes, situated in the space lodging the submaxillary salivary gland, are located around or within the fascial sheath of this gland. They receive lymph vessels from the chin, lips, cheeks, nose (including the anterior nasal cavity), gums, teeth, floor of the mouth, hard palate, tongue, and other nearby nodes. The submental nodes receive lymphatics from similar regions. Their afferent vessels connect partly with the submaxillary and internal jugular nodes. The retropharyngeal nodes, which lie between the posterior wall of the pharynx and prevertebral fascia, may project anteriorly onto the soft palate and therefore may be mistaken for palatine tonsils. The more lateral retropharyngeal nodes atrophy with age. These nodes drain the nasal cavities, palate, middle ear, nasopharynx, and oropharynx. They send efferent vessels to the internal jugular chain of nodes.

Lymphatics

For a detailed description of the lympahtic system draining the head and neck, the reader is referred to the compendium by Tobias, which is a translation of the original work by Rouviére (17). Lymphatics arising from the upper lip terminate in the parotid, submental, and submaxillary lymph nodes. Central lymphatics from the lower lip drain into the submental node, while those originating more laterally empty into the submaxillary nodes. Lymphatics arising from the mucosa of the cheeks traverse the buccinator muscle to eventually terminate in the submaxillary nodes. Their course may be interupted by the buccinator nodes. Cutaneous lymphatics of the cheek end in the submaxillary, submental, and parotid nodes. The lymphatic network of the tongue is divided into a superficial and deep (muscular) set. They drain to the linguinal and submaxillary nodes but end mainly in the deep cervical lymph nodes. The node at the bifurcation of the common carotid artery is considered to be the principal lymph node of the tongue (17). Lymphatics in the region of the tongue may cross the midline to reach nodes of the opposite side. The gingiva contain a similar superficial and deep anastomosing lymphatic network that drains into the sublingual, submental, submaxillary, internal jugular, and occasionally the retropharyngeal nodes. Lymphatic vessels that exit from the dental pulp of the teeth are in direct communication with those of the gingiva. Lymphatics from the floor of the mouth are continuous with those from the tongue and gums. Afferent lymphatics from the floor of the mouth drain into the sublingual, submental, and deep cervical nodes, while those from the posterolateral region terminate in the submaxillary and deep cervical nodes. The draining lymphatics of the palate, which are continuous with those of the gums and palatine tonsils, reach the submaxillary, retropharyngeal, and deep nodes of the neck.

The cutaneous lymphatics of the nose terminate in the submaxillary lymph nodes. Lymph from the nasal vestibule goes to the parotid and submaxillary nodes. Lymphatics originating from the anterior nasal cavities drain to the submental nodes, while those from the posterior cavities pass to the retropharyngeal and deep superior cervical nodes. The lymphatics from the olfactory region do not communicate with those of the respiratory region (17). Lymphatics arising from the olfactory region communicate to the subarachnoid space of the brain via small cannaliculi passing through the foramina of the cribiform plate along with the olfactory nerve filaments. The lower aspect of the inferior turbinate drains to the internal jugular lymph nodes. The upper portion of the inferior turbinate, along with lymphatics from the middle turbinate, drain into the retropharyngeal and internal jugular lymph nodes. The superior turbinates drain to the retropharyngeal and deep cervical nodes. Lymphatics from the frontal and maxillary sinuses, along with the anterior and medial group of ethmoidal sinuses, drain to the submaxillary nodes. The posterior ethmoidal group and sphenoidal sinuses drain lymph into the retropharyngeal nodes.

Tonsils

Nonencapsulated lymphoid tissue present in the oropharynx is normally organized into epithelial-covered lymphoid aggregates termed *tonsils*. Tonsils are typically softer than lymph nodes on palpation because they lack a fibrous capsule or trabeculae. The word *tonsil* has also been used to refer to the palatine tonsils. Waldeyer's ring, described by the nineteenth century anatomist Wilhelm von Waldeyer, refers to the circular collection of submucosal lymphoid tissue that gaurds the opening into the upper aerodigestive tract (18). Waldeyer's ring is comprised of the palatine, pharyngeal, tubal, and lingual tonsils, as well as the lateral pharyngeal lymphoid bands and intervening isolated lymphoid follicles (pharyngeal granulations) (19,20). The pharyngeal bands are located on the posterolateral wall of the oropharynx, just behind the posterior tonsillar pillar. The oval shaped palatine (faucial) tonsils are situated laterally in the oropharynx within the triangular tonsillar fossa, which is bound by the palatoglossal arch anteriorly and palatopharyngeal arch posteriorly. Their tonsillar crypts usually become occupied with desquamated epithelium, debris, and microorganisms that are grossly visible on the surface as white spots (follicles). Such crypt plugs may calcify. The palatine tonsils are the only tonsils with a partial capsule, which is formed by compressed connective tissue on their attached side. This capsule separates the tonsils from the underlying musculature of the pharyngeal wall. The tonsils are largest in early childhood; after about four years of age, they begin to gradually atrophy. Following puberty, the tonsils become increasingly fibrotic. The pharyngeal tonsil (adenoid, or tonsil of Luschka) is a single pyramidal-shaped aggregate of lymphoid tissue located superiorly in the midline of the nasopharyngeal wall. Unlike the other tonsils, the adenoid does not have typical crypts, but rather numerous surface folds extending from the tonsillar base anterolaterally. The surface of the pharyngeal tonsil also forms a median recess known as the pharyngeal bursa. The tubal tonsil (eustachian tonsil or Gerlach's tonsil) is that small portion of the pharyngeal tonsil that is located behind the pharyngeal opening of the eustachian tube. The lingual tonsil is situated on the dorsum of the tongue posteriorly, between the sulcus terminalis and the valleculae. In most individuals the median glossoepiglottic ligament divides the lingual tonsil into bilateral lobes.

Additional tonsillar structures may also be found in the normal human oropharynx. These include the so-called oral tonsils, which are structurally similar to the palatine tonsils (21). Oral tonsils occur chiefly in the palate, floor of the mouth, and on the ventral surface of the tongue. They are small (1–3 mm in diameter), firm, circumscribed, mobile lymphoid aggregates present under intact oral mucosa. Oral tonsils contain a single central crypt. It has been proposed by some authors that intraoral lymphoepithelial cysts originate from occluded crypts of oral tonsils (22,23). Reactive tonsillar tissue has also been noted in the region of the pyriform sinus, palate, and lateral surface of the tongue (24,25).

MICROSCOPY

Mouth

Lips and Vermilion Border

The entrance to the digestive tract is surrounded by two fleshy folds of skin, the lips. They are partly covered by skin that bears hairs, sweat glands, and sebaceous glands and is richly endowed with sensory nerves. The inner surface of the lips is covered by the oral mucosa and forms a part of the wall of the oral cavity. Between the external integument and the oral mucosa are the orbicularis oris muscle, the labial vessels, nerves, and adipose tissue with numerous minor salivary glands. The latter are easily accessible for biopsies to diagnose Sjögren's syndrome. The junction between the skin and oral mucosa is known as the vermilion border, where the keratinized squamous epithelium of the skin changes to the mucous membrane of the oral cavity. The squamous epithelium of the vermilion border is thin, and the tall connective tissue papillae are close to the surface. The blood in the rich capillary network shows through the thin epithelium, accounting for the redness of the lips. The transition zone has no hairs. In adults, ectopic sebaceous glands are commonly observed in the vermilion border, at the corners of the mouth, or in the buccal mucosa; these are termed Fordyce's spots (or Fox-Fordyce granules) and increase with age, so that 70 to 80% of elderly persons have them. These ectopic sebaceous glands are considered normal (Figure 15.8) (26,27). Like the skin, the vermilion border

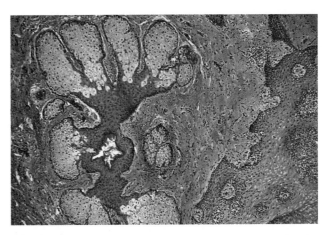

Figure 15.8 Ectopic sebaceous glands in the vermilion border (Fox-Fordyce granule).

is exposed to physical forces and chemical agents. For this reason, actinic keratosis and solar elastosis can be seen on the vermilion border. The squamous epithelium of the transitional zone imperceptibly merges with the stratified squamous epithelium of the oral mucosa.

Oral Mucosa and Submucosa

The oral mucosa consists of an epithelial layer and an underlying layer of connective tissue, the lamina propria (Figure 15.9). The mucosa of the oral cavity shows regional modifications in structure and cytokeratin expression that correspond to functional requirements. The stratified squamous epithelium of the oral mucosa has three functional types: the lining mucosa, masticatory mucosa, and specialized mucosa (28). Most of the oral mucosa is lined by nonkeratinized squamous epithelium, representing the lining mucosa. The palate, gingiva, and dorsum of the tongue are exposed to the forces of mastication and are covered by keratinized epithelium of the masticatory mucosa type. The mucosa of the palate is orthokeratinized, whereas the epithelium of the gingiva is often parakeratinized. Details of the specialized mucosa are described with the tongue. Throughout the oral cavity the epithelium is worn off by mastication and speaking; hence, exfoliated epithelial cells are a normal constituent of the saliva and are frequently encountered by the pathologist in sputum or as "contaminants" in bronchoscopic specimens. Squamous cells of the buccal mucosa have also been a convenient source for the microscopic demonstration of the sex chromosome (Barr body) (Figure 15.10). The shed epithelial cells are replaced by the basal cells, which divide then migrate to the surface and are themselves eventually worn off. The renewal of the oral mucosa takes about 12 days (29). As the name implies, the squamous epithelium of the mucosa is kept moist and glistening by mucus that is secreted by the numerous minor and paired major salivary glands. This thin film of mucus

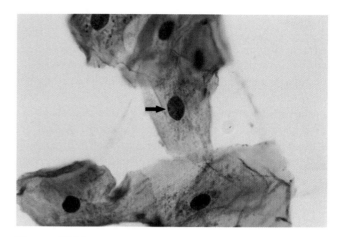

Figure 15.10 Cytologic image of a scraping of the buccal mucosa. Intermediate squamous cell with sex chromatin body (Barr body) (*arrow*) lying against the inner nuclear membrane (Papanicolaou stain).

covers and protects all intraoral structures, including the teeth, which are bathed by saliva. Saliva rinses away bacteria, provides buffering agents (e.g., phosphate and bicarbonate) that neutralize acids created by bacteria that inhabit dental plaque, contains antibacterial agents, and minerals required for tooth remineralization. Hence, xerostomia promotes tooth decay

The interface of the epithelium and lamina propria is delineated by the basal lamina, or basement membrane. In hematoxylin and eosin (H&E)–stained sections, it is sometimes hard to see the basal lamina, but special stains (e.g., reticulin) demonstrate it well (Figure 15.11). The basal lamina is secreted by the epithelial cells and serves supportive and filtering functions. It also regulates differentiation, migration, and polarity of the epithelial cells. The basal lamina is composed of type IV collagen and heparan sulfate, as well

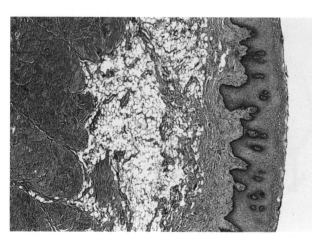

Figure 15.9 Inner aspect of cheek, cross section. *Left* to *right*: cross-striated muscle, adipose tissue, lamina propria, buccal mucosa.

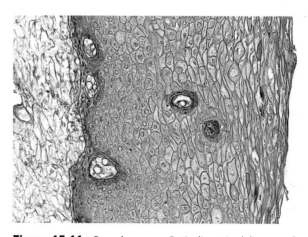

Figure 15.11 Buccal mucosa. Reticulin stain delineates the cell membrane of nonkeratinized squamous epithelial cells and the delicate basement membrane. Papillae of the lamina propria contain blood vessels.

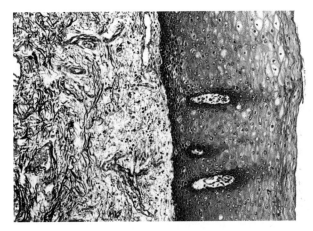

Figure 15.12 Buccal mucosa showing maturation of squamous epithelium: there is a row of small basal cells, larger cells of stratum spinosum, and parallel arranged flat surface cells. No keratinization is seen. Lamina propria shows delicate strands of connective tissue, blood vessels, and a few lymphocytes. (Mallory's trichrome.)

as the two glycoproteins, laminin and entactin, that interact with other components of the extracellular matrix. A single layer of basal cells rests on the basal lamina. The basal cells continuously divide, and the new cells push the overlying ones toward the surface. During this process of differentiation, the small cuboidal basal cells become polyhedral and larger, forming the stratum spinosum. These cells contain abundant intracytoplasmic fibrils (tonofilaments) that attach to desmosomes, connecting the squamous epithelial cells with each other. Toward the superficial layers the cells gradually become flat. The nonkeratinized squamous epithelium lacks a stratum granulosum and stratum corneum. The surface cells may retain their nuclei, and their cytoplasm does not contain keratin filaments (Figure 15.12) (30). In keratinizing epithelium, the cells form a stra-

tum granulosum, which is a prominent layer three to five cells thick. The cells of this layer have numerous intracytoplasmic granules, called keratohyalin granules, which stain with hematoxylin. As the process of keratinization advances, the nucleus and cytoplasmic organelles become disrupted and disappear while the cell becomes filled with an intracellular protein, keratin. Thus, the surface layer, the stratum corneum, is formed.

All oral epithelia show expression of cytokeratin 5 and 14 (CK5 and CK14, respectively), the keratin pair typically expressed by basal cells of stratifying epithelium. The oral mucosa from various sites exhibits striking differences in cytokeratin synthesis (Table 15.1) (31,32). Such differences usually appear in the fetus by 23 weeks. The differences in the distribution of these cytoskeletal proteins reflect the relationship between morphology and function of these epithelia (33). The gingiva expresses a great complexity of cytokeratins, similar to that of the epidermis. For example, gingival epithelia are immunoreactive for CK1 and CK10 (differentiation that is associated with epithelial properties of toughness and rigidity), as well as CK4 and CK13 (differentiation associated with epithelial properties of flexibility and elasticity). In contrast, the lining mucosa shows a paucity of cytokeratins, resembling stratified nonkeratinizing squamous epithelium of the esophagus. Malignant transformation is often associated with alterations in the cytokeratin pattern.

Normal oral mucosal epithelial cells, even in the fetus, express the ABO blood group antigens (34). In fact, the oral mucosa has become a model for studying cellular glycosylation. In general, the blood group antigen expression on epithelial cells follows the general phenotype of the host individual as determined by routine serologic methods. The loss of these antigens on malignant epithelial cells may be a valuable marker for primary carcinoma. All epithelial

TABLE 15.1

CYTOKERATIN EXPRESSION PROFILES OF DIFFERENT ORAL EPITHELIA, AS DETERMINED BY IMMUNOHISTOCHEMICAL AND ELECTROPHORETIC STUDIES.

Cytokeratin Type	CK1	CK4	CK5	CK6	CK7	CK8	CK10	CK13	CK14	CK16	CK18	CK19
Epidermis (for comparison)	++	/	++	+	/	−	++	/	++	+	/	/
Oral lining mucosa	/	++	++	+	/	−	−	++	+	−	−	+
Oral gingival epithelium	++	+	++	+	−	−	++	+	++	++	−	+
Epithelium of oral sulcus	−	++	++	/	−	+	−	++	++	++	+	++
Junctional epithelium	−	−	++	/	−	+	−	++	++	+	+	++
Masticatory mucosa (e.g., hard palate)	++	/	++	/	/	/	/	/	++	++	/	/
Epithelia of enamel organ	/	−	++	/	+	+	−	−	/	/	−	++
Rests of Malassez	/	−	++	/	−	−	−	−	+	−	−	++

+ (weak or occasional expression); ++ (strong expression); − (expression absent); / (no data)
(Modified from: Mackenzie IC, Rittman G, Gao Z, Leigh I, Lane EB. Patterns of cytokeratin expression in human gingival epithelia. *J Periodontal Res* 1991;26:468–478.)

cell layers of the enamel organ, however, are normally devoid of the blood group antigens.

The lamina propria is a delicate layer of connective tissue situated beneath the squamous epithelium. It contains few elastic and collagenous fibers and is rich in blood vessels, lymphatics, and nerves. The nerves belong to the sensory branches of the trigeminal nerve. The lamina propria also contains scattered lymphocytes, which are often found migrating through the epithelium. Consequently, few lymphocytes are a normal constituent of the saliva (salivary corpuscles).

The submucosa under the lining mucosa is composed of fairly loosely arranged connective tissue, which contains larger blood vessels, lymphatics, nerves, adipose tissue, and numerous minor salivary glands. Where the mucosa is in close proximity to the underlying bone (e.g., the hard palate), there is no submucosa and the fibers of the lamina propria are directly and tightly attached to bone. In these areas, the mucosa, lamina propria, and periosteum are joined together as one membrane and are generally referred to as a mucoperiosteum.

Palate and Uvula

The roof of the oral cavity is formed by the palate; the anterior two-thirds consists of the hard palate, and the posterior one-third is comprised of the soft palate. The palate separates the oral and nasal cavities. Anteriorly and laterally, the palate is bounded by the alveolar arches and gums; posteriorly, it is continuous with the soft palate. The hard palate is covered by masticatory mucosa, which has a series of ridges (palatal rugae) running across, but not crossing, the midline. The ridges are easily seen and palpated and can be felt with the tongue. The supporting dense connective tissue fibers of these ridges pass directly from the papillary layer of the lamina propria into the underlying bone. In the anterior lateral regions of the hard palate, the submucosa contains fat tissue, whereas more posteriorly its lateral regions contain minor salivary glands (palatine glands), which are pure mucous glands (Figure 15.13).

The soft palate is the mobile portion. With no bony support, it is suspended from the posterior border of the hard palate like a curtain. Its oral surface is covered by lining mucosa, and its nasal surface, which is continuous with the floor of the nasal cavity, is mostly lined by ciliated respiratory epithelium. The soft palate contains fibers of striated muscle, blood vessels, and nerves (Figure 15.14). Larger mucous glands underlie the oral epithelium of the soft palate, whereas smaller groups of mixed glands are present on the nasal surface under the respiratory epithelium. From the middle of the posterior border of the soft palate hangs a small, conical process of soft tissue, the uvula. The uvula is microscopically similar to the

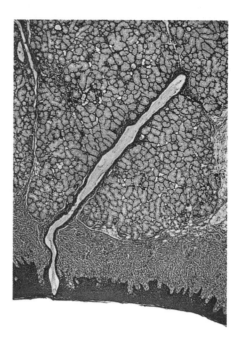

Figure 15.13 Hard palate with pure mucous minor salivary glands and duct. Note dense connective tissue of lamina propria (H&E).

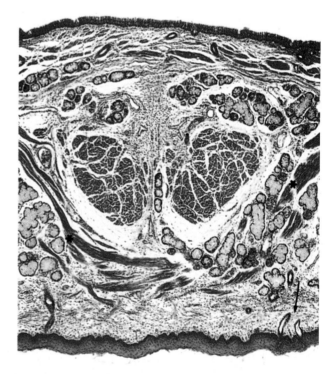

Figure 15.14 Soft palate sectioned in the coronal plane. Nasal respiratory mucosa (*top*), oral squamous mucosa (*bottom*). Fascicles of pharyngopalatine muscle are to the right and left of the midline. Fibers of levator veli palatini muscle (*) are obliquely descending. Ducts of minor salivary glands are near the oral mucosa (*arrow*), respectively.

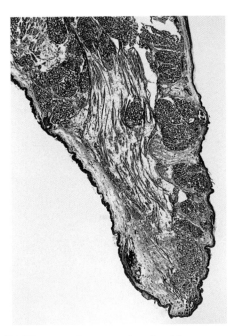

Figure 15.15 Sagittal section of uvula with numerous mucous glands and bundles of cross-striated muscle. More glands are seen near the oral surface (*right*).

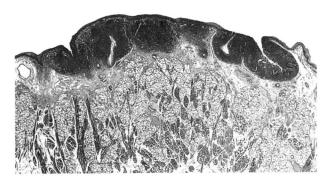

Figure 15.16 Lingual tonsil. Low-power view of lymphoid tissue and underlying mucous glands that appear as pale areas among bundles of skeletal muscle.

soft palate (Figure 15.15). It contains predominantly mucous glands and muscle fibers that become more sparse from the proximal to the distal end. The musculus uvulae muscle inserts into the actual mucosa of the uvula. Mast cells, usually located around blood vessels, are a frequent finding (35).

Floor of the Mouth

The mucous membrane of the floor of the mouth is thin and loosely attached to the underlying structures. The rete ridges are short. The submucosa contains some adipose tissue and numerous minor salivary glands (sublingual mucous glands).

Tonsils

The tonsils are organized aggregates of lymphoid tissue covered on their luminal surface by a mucous membrane. The close proximity of lymphocytes to the surface epithelium facilitates the direct internal transport of foreign material from the exterior. Epithelial-lined crypts and folds further aid in trapping foreign material. Tonsils normally lack a prominent fibrous capsule. This is in contrast to lymph nodes, which have a capsule and subcapsular sinus that reflects the antigenic delivery through afferent lymphatics. The mucosa lining the palatine and lingual tonsils consists of stratified squamous epithelium, whereas the mucosa overlying the pharyngeal tonsil is pseudostratified

ciliated respiratory type epithelium that contains occasional goblet cells. The epithelium lining the crypts or folds represents an extension of the regional surface epithelium. However, the epithelial lining of some crypts in the palatine tonsil may occasionally consist of respiratory mucosa. The palatine tonsil contains 10 to 30 crypts that may extend to the deep juxtacapsular region. In the lingual tonsil (Figure 15.16) and pharyngeal tonsil, the lining epithelium forms only shallow folds 0.5 to 1.0 cm deep. Sulfur granules comprised of *Actinomyces* and other *Actinomyces*-like oral flora are a frequent finding within tonsillar crypts. As in lymph nodes, the lymphoid component may contain lymphoid follicles, some with active germinal centers. Intraepithelial lymphocytes within the surface and crypt-lining epithelium (called lymphoepithelium) is commonly observed (Figures 15.17–15.18) and merely reflects the normal passage of lymphocytes. Sometimes the epithelium is so heavily infiltrated by lymphocytes that it is scarcely

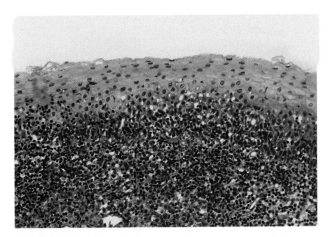

Figure 15.17 Lingual tonsil. The mucosa (nonkeratinized stratified squamous epithelium) is infiltrated with numerous lymphocytes that obscure the basement membrane.

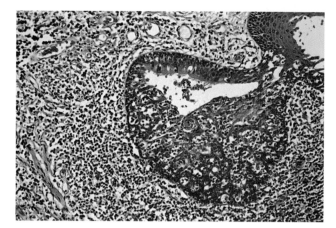

Figure 15.18   Lingual tonsil. Squamous epithelium of crypt is disrupted by lymphocytes that have migrated into it.

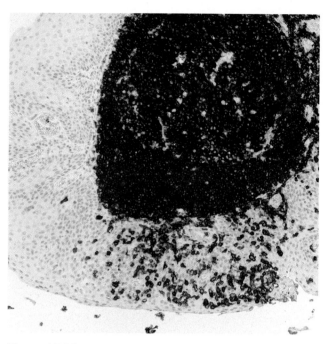

Figure 15.20   Tonsil showing CD20 (B-cell marker) immunoreactive lymphocytes located within a lymphoid follicle. B cells focally pass through the lymphoepithelium. (We acknowledge Christopher N. Otis for his help with this photomicrograph.)

distinguishable. Intraepithelial lymphocyte trafficking primarily overlies subepithelial lymphoid follicles (Figures 15.19–15.20), resembling Peyer's patches of the small intestinal mucosa. Intraepithelial lymphocytes of the surface mucosa are predominantly T cells (CD3+, CD5+, CD7+, and CD8+), whereas those present within the crypt epithelium include both T cells and B cells (36). The epithelial cells of lymphoepithelium (known as M cells) exhibit numerous surface microvilli and microfolds. At the ultrastructural level, intraepithelial lymphocytes have been shown to

be located within intracytoplasmic compartments that communicate with each other to form an intraepithelial network of channels (37).

Tonsils are normally found in close association with minor salivary glands (Figure 15.21). Frequently, the excretory ducts of these mucous glands empty into the tonsillar crypts. The minor salivary glands (Weber's glands) adjacent to the palatine tonsils are thought to be a putative reservoir of pathogenic bacteria and therefore should be removed along with the tonsil during a tonsillectomy. Small foci of elastic cartilage and even bone may be present close to the

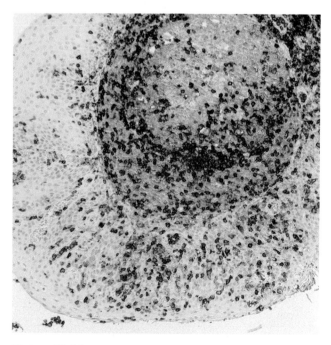

Figure 15.19   Tonsil lymphoepithelium overlying a secondary lymphoid follicle with a germinal center. The CD3 (T-cell marker) immunostain highlights abundant T cells trafficking through the epithelium. (We acknowledge Christopher N. Otis for his help with this photomicrograph.)

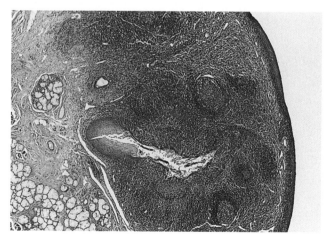

Figure 15.21   Lingual tonsil. Lymphoid tissue with follicles under mucosa and around its infolding (crypt). Note mucous glands and ducts.

TABLE 15.2
MINOR SALIVARY GLANDS OF THE MOUTH, NOSE, AND PARANASAL SINUSES

Name	Location	Type of Acini
Labial (superior and inferior)	Lips	Mixed (predominantly mucous)
Buccal	Cheek	Mixed (predominantly mucous)
Glossopalatine	Anterior faucial pillar Glossopalatine fold	Pure mucous
Palatine	Hard palate Soft palate	Pure mucous (mixed in avula)
	Uvula	Mixed (predominantly mucous)
Palatine tonsil (Weber's glands)	Subjacent to tonsil capsule	Pure mucous
Sublingual	Floor of mouth	Mixed (predominantly mucous)
Lingual (glands of Blandin and Nuhn)	Anterior tongue	Mixed (predominantly mucous)
Tongue (Ebner's glands)	Circumvallate papillae	Pure serous
Lingual tonsil	Base of tongue	Pure mucous
Nasal and paranasal	Nose and sinuses	Mixed

fibrous capsule of the palatine tonsil, which has been proposed by some authors to represent metaplasia or heteretopia (38) but more than likely is an embryological remnant of Reichert's cartilage that originates from the second branchial arch.

Minor Salivary Glands

Numerous small salivary glands are scattered throughout the submucosa of the oral cavity, nose, and paranasal sinuses, as well as adjacent to the palatine and pharyngeal tonsils. These glands are not encapsulated and are named by their location. They can be classified as mucous, serous, and mixed seromucinous types (Table 15.2). These glands produce secretions similar to those of the major salivary glands, which empty onto the mucosal surface through numerous small excretory ducts. The secretory activity of these glands appears to be continuous, although they can respond to specific local chemical or physical stimuli.

Structurally, the minor salivary glands are compound tubular or tubuloacinar glands. Their secretory portions are the acini that are designated according to their secretion as mucous, serous, or mixed. Within mixed acini, the mucous cells are nearest to the excretory duct, whereas the serous cells are at the cul-de-sac of the acini and appear as crescents, called the demilunes of Giannuzzi (Figures 15.22–15.23). The mucous acini are more tubular than those of the serous type. The mucous cells are also larger,

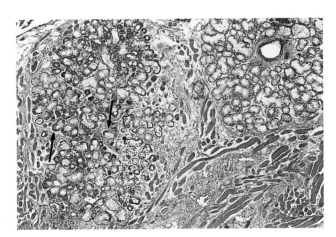

Figure 15.22 Minor salivary glands in the uvula are surrounded by cross-striated muscle. The gland with the distinct duct is of the pure mucous type. The other gland is seromucinous, with the serous cells forming darker staining crescents (*arrows*).

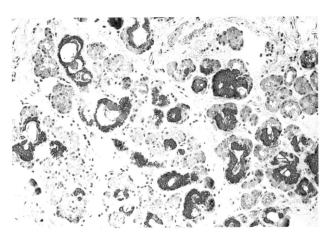

Figure 15.23 Mixed minor salivary gland of the uvula. Acid mucopolysaccharides in mucous cells are stained turquoise (Alcian blue at pH 2.6).

and their flattened nuclei are present at the cell bases. The mucous cells have a pale-appearing cytoplasm in H&E-stained sections (Figure 15.13) and will also stain with Alcian blue, periodic acid-Schiff (PAS), or mucicarmine (39,40). The smaller serous cells have more rounded basal nuclei and have an eosinophilic cytoplasm that contains zymogen granules. Contractile myoepithelial cells are wrapped around the acinus and assist by squeezing the secretion from the acinar cells into the excretory ducts (41). The myoepithelial cells of the minor salivary glands are variably immunoreactive with antibodies to cytokeratin (CK5, CK14, and CK17), to smooth muscle markers (smooth muscle actin, h-caldesmon, calponin), p63 (nuclear immunoreactivity), and, rarely, to S-100 protein (42). It should be noted that melanocytes may be found in a small proportion (<2%) of minor salivary glands (43).

It is important to note that the minor salivary glands, wherever they occur in the mouth, nose, or paranasal sinuses, can become involved by the same pathologic processes as the major salivary glands. This is especially true for neoplasms, which arise from various cellular components of the minor salivary glands.

The surgical pathologist must be well aware of the fact that squamous metaplasia can occur in the excretory ducts and acini of minor salivary glands. For instance, epithelial regeneration after injury of various types may lead to squamous metaplasia that can mimic squamous cell carcinoma. A good example of this is seen in necrotizing sialometaplasia or in irradiated salivary glands. In the latter case, the diagnostic dilemma is usually compounded by the possibility of a recurrence of previous squamous cell carcinoma. Oncocytic cells may be found in minor salivary glands in varying numbers and distribution patterns (Figure 15.24). Oncocytes ("swollen cells") are large, cuboidal, or columnar epithelial cells with a finely granular eosinophilic cytoplasm that have been identified in many exocrine or endocrine glands (44). Up to 60% of their cytoplasm is usually occupied by mitochondria that

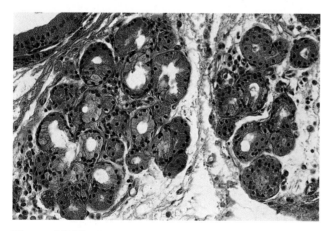

Figure 15.24 Oncocytes in minor salivary gland appear as cuboidal swollen cells with a finely granular oxyphilic cytoplasm.

can be visualized after long-term (48 hours) staining with phosphotungstic acid-hematoxylin on fresh-frozen sections incubated for the histochemical demonstration of mitochondrial enzyme activity, by means of immunohistochemistry (e.g., antimitochondrial antibody), or by electron microscopy. Oncocytes are benign cells that occur with increasing frequency in older persons. They develop due to metaplasia of ductal and acinar epithelium. However, the etiology and functional significance of oncocytic metaplasia is not clear. In the minor salivary glands, oncocytes can be seen in nodular or diffuse oncocytosis, oncocytoma (45,46), and even oncocytic carcinomas (47).

Cheeks

The skin of the cheek is part of the facial skin. The inner surface of the cheeks is covered by squamous lining mucosa. The submucosa contains some fat cells and many minor salivary glands of the mixed type, embedded in loose connective tissue. The mucosa and submucosa are bound to the underlying buccal musculature by connective tissue fibers.

Juxtaoral Organ of Chievitz

Deep in the wall of the cheeks overlying the angle of the mandible sits an anatomically well-defined small fusiform structure, the juxtaoral organ (JOO) of Chievitz, which is normally present in the buccotemporal space (48,49). In adults, it measures 0.7 to 1.7 cm in length and 0.1 to 0.2 cm in diameter and persists throughout life. It is multilobulated, has a dense fibrous capsule, and consists of round or elongate nests of nonkeratinizing squamouslike epithelial cells embedded in an organized connective tissue stroma that is rich in small nerves and sensory receptors innervated by two to four branches of the buccal nerve (50). The connective tissue envelope is divided into a thin inner stratum fibrosum internum, middle stratum nervosum, and outer stratum fibrosum externum. These nests of epithelial cells appear in a cluster on histologic sections, but serial sectioning shows them to be small sprouts and folds in continuity with a mass of epithelium (49). Thus, cross sections through different portions of the JOO can show considerable variation in number and shape of epithelial sprouts (Figure 15.25). The larger nests of epithelium are composed of cells with a clear PAS-positive cytoplasm and round or oval nuclei, forming "light centers." Intercellular bridges can be seen toward the center of the cell nests. The cells in the smaller nests can show a whorl-like or concentric arrangement. Occasionally, a glandlike lumen or a follicle filled with colloidlike mucin-negative material is encountered. Melanin pigmentation has been reported in the JOO (51). The central epithelial cells of the JOO appear to be immunoreactive for cytokeratins, whereas the outer

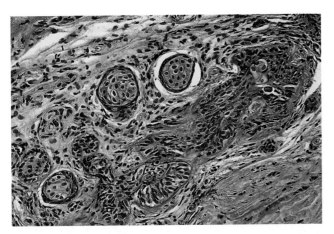

Figure 15.25 Juxtaoral organ of Chievitz. Small nests of nonkeratinized squamous epithelial cells are delineated by basement membrane. The elongated cells outside the epithelial islands are fibroblasts and Schwann cells. Nerve is seen below and to the right.

more basaloid cells are usually keratin negative. The cell nests are also positive for vimentin and epithelial membrane antigen (EMA) but are negative for S-100 protein, glial fibrillary acidic protein (GFAP), neurospecific enolase (NSE), synaptophysin, and chromogranin (52,53).

The seemingly esoteric and minute JOO has considerable importance for the surgical pathologist because the presence of squamous epithelial nests intimately admixed with numerous small nerves may be misinterpreted as perineural invasion by squamous cell carcinoma (54). On the other hand, astute pathologists aware of this pitfall have, in a case of a mucoepidermoid carcinoma with lymphatic spread in the retromolar region, correctly recognized the epithelial nests of the juxtaoral organ (55). Such cases unequivocally demonstrate the importance of awareness of this small organ. Cases of clinically enlarged (56) and hyperplastic JOOs have been described (57), but so far no carcinoma originating from it has been reported. The function of the JOO is unknown. Since Johan Henrik Chievitz, a Danish anatomist, described this structure in 1885 in a 10-week-old human embryo (58), it has been widely believed that the organ of Chievitz is a rudimentary structure, representing an abortive salivary gland anlage. More recently, the possibility of a neurosecretory and receptor function of the organ has been raised (59). The JOO has been shown to contain pacinian corpuscles (60), supporting its mechanosensory function. For a thorough review of the literature, the reader is referred to the small monograph by Zenker (49) or review paper by Pantanowitz and Balogh (59). Finally, we would like to alert our readers to the fact that similar benign epithelial islands may reside within peripheral nerves in the maxilla (61) and mandible (62).

Tongue

Situated in the floor of the mouth, the tongue is an organized mass of cross-striated muscle invested by mucous membrane. Its muscles are partly extrinsic (i.e., have their origins outside the tongue) and partly intrinsic, being contained entirely within it. The bundles of cross-striated muscle are embedded in connective tissue with some adipocytes and are arranged three-dimensionally. The tongue is well-supplied with blood vessels that form numerous anastomoses. The tongue is richly endowed with myelinated and nonmyelinated nerves containing motor, sensory, and vegetative nerve fibers, some with ganglion cells. The ventral (under) surface of the tongue is covered by smooth lining mucosa that has short, blunt rete ridges (Figure 15.26). Its submucosa merges with the connective tissue that intersects with the ventral muscle bundles of the tongue.

The dorsal (upper) surface of the tongue is divided into an anterior and posterior part by a V-shaped shallow groove, the sulcus terminalis. The anterior two-thirds of the dorsum of the tongue is lined by specialized mucosa, which is bound by connective tissue fibers to the underlying skeletal muscle of the tongue. This specialized mucosa is modified keratinized squamous epithelium covered with small projections (papillae) that are visible to the naked eye. The pathologist has to be aware of these papillae so as not to mistake them for papillary epithelial hyperplasia, papillomas, or oral hairy leukoplakia. According to their shape, the papillae can be filiform, fungiform, foliate, or circumvallate. The great majority are filiform papillae, conical projections of the keratinized epithelium (Figure 15.27). Among these are scattered the fungiform papillae, which are rounded elevations above the surface of the tongue; their surface is not keratinized (Figure 15.28). Clinically, fungiform papillae appear as small red nodules because the thin epithelium does not mask the underlying vascular connective tissue. Microscopically, fungiform papillae should not be misinterpreted as denture-induced fibrous hyperplasia or small traumatic fibromas. The foliate papillae are located posteriorly along the sides of the tongue. At

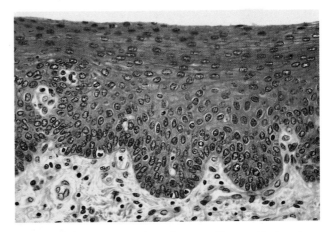

Figure 15.26 Ventral surface of tongue. The stratified nonkeratinized squamous epithelium of the lining mucosa has a slightly wavy interface with the lamina propria. A few scattered lymphocytes are seen in the lamina propria and in the epithelium.

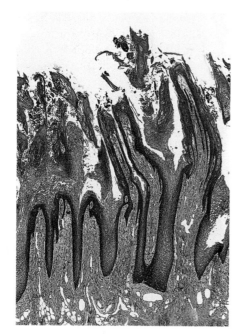

Figure 15.27 Dorsal surface of tongue. Filiform papillae have a connective tissue core beset with secondary papillae with pointed ends. The superficial squamous cells are keratinized. Note the slender, pointed rete ridges.

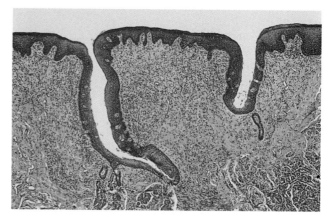

Figure 15.29 Circumvallate papilla. Numerous taste buds are on the lateral walls of the papilla and on the epithelium facing the papilla within the furrow. Ducts of serous glands open into the furrow surrounding the circumvallate papilla.

the junction of the anterior two-thirds and the posterior one-third of the tongue are the circumvallate papillae. These are the largest papillae, measuring 0.1 to 0.2 cm in diameter and are arranged in a V-shape immediately anterior to the sulcus terminalis. The circumvallate papillae number 6 to 12. A small, ring-shaped furrow surrounds each circumvallate papilla and separates it from a circular, palisade-like mucosal elevation (vallum), which is the outer border of the circumvallate papilla (Figure 15.29).

Taste buds are present in large numbers on the side of the circumvallate papillae and in lesser numbers on the fungi-

form and foliate papillae, as well as elsewhere on the dorsal and lateral aspects of the tongue. These small epithelial organs stain lighter than the surrounding epithelium. Like other simple epithelia, taste buds express low-molecular weight keratins such as CK18, and, accordingly, they are immunoreactive with the antibody CAM5.2 (Figure 15.30). Numerous small serous glands (Ebner's glands) are located under the circumvallate papilla. The ducts of these glands empty their secretion into the small furrow around each papilla; this serous secretion flushes out the furrows, thus facilitating perception of new tastes (Figure 15.29). The taste buds are barrel-shaped intramucosal sensory receptors that occupy the full thickness of the mucosa and communicate with the surface through a small opening, the gustatory pore (Figure 15.31). The taste buds are composed of three types of cells: (a) gustatory or taste cells, (b) supporting, or sustentacular, cells, and (c) basal cells. The taste cells are crescent-shaped, have lightly staining cytoplasm, and possess numer-

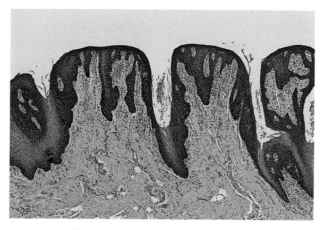

Figure 15.28 Fungiform papillae. Slightly rounded, elevated structures with a larger connective tissue core. Smaller connective tissue papillae project into the base of the surface epithelium.

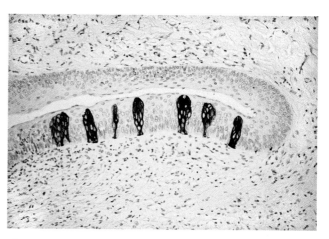

Figure 15.30 Taste buds showing immunoreactivity for CAM 5.2.

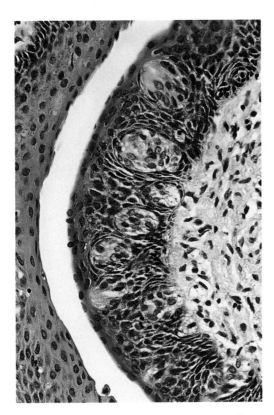

Figure 15.31 Taste buds on the side of a circumvallate papilla. The cells of the intraepithelial taste buds are spindle-shaped and oriented at a right angle to the surface. The cell nuclei are elongated and are situated mainly in the basal half of the buds. Nerve fibers ending on the sensory (gustatory) cells cannot be seen with H&E stain.

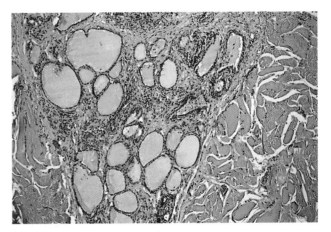

Figure 15.32 Lingual thyroid. The glandular parenchyma is embedded in skeletal muscle. The thyroid tissue is not encapsulated, and care should be taken to avoid mistaking it for invasive growth.

ous fine microvilli that protrude through the taste pore as gustatory hairs. The basal end of the taste cells has intimate contact with many fine nerve terminals that leave through the basement membrane and become myelinated outside the taste bud. The supporting cells are likewise crescentic, extending between the basement membrane and the surface; they form a shell for the taste bud and are also scattered between the gustatory cells. The supporting cells have a dark cytoplasm and possess microvilli that also protrude through the taste pore. The small basal cells, situated between the bases of the other cells, give rise to the other cells of the taste bud (63,64).

The apex of the V-shaped sulcus terminalis projects backward and is marked by a small pit, the foramen cecum, which is an embryologic remnant indicating the upper end of the thyroglossal duct. Correspondingly, ectopic thyroid tissue can occur at the base of the tongue (lingual thyroid) or anywhere along the tract of the thyroglossal duct caudally (Figure 15.32). Microscopically, ectopic thyroid resembles normal thyroid tissue. However, the surgical pathologist should be aware that the presence of thyroid glands within muscle may mimic carcinoma. Ectopic thyroid tissue may undergo all the physiologic and pathologic changes of the thyroid gland proper.

Gingiva

The gingiva (gum) is that portion of the oral mucosa that surrounds the neck of the teeth like a collar. Masticatory mucosa (i.e., parakeratinized or keratinized stratified squamous epithelium) covers the gum. There is no submucosal layer. Instead, the connective tissue of the lamina propria contains collagenous fibers that bind the epithelium tightly to the underlying alveolar periosteum and bone. The gingival epithelium interdigitates with the underlying connective tissue, forming long, interconnected rete ridges that are separated by connective tissue plates and papillae (Figures 15.33–15.34). The gingival epithelium is divided anatomically into oral gingival, oral sulcular, and junctional epithelia. The cytokeratin expression profile of gingival epithelium corresponds to this anatomical division (Table 15.1).

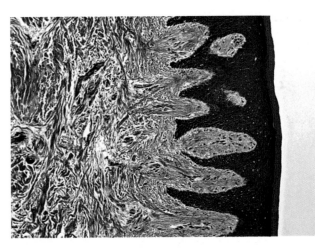

Figure 15.33 Gingiva (gum). The masticatory mucosa has tall rete ridges. A dense network of collagen fibers (blue) tightly anchors the epithelium to the underlying bone (not shown); the keratin layer (orange band) on the surface of the epithelium imparts further strength to it (Mallory's trichrome).

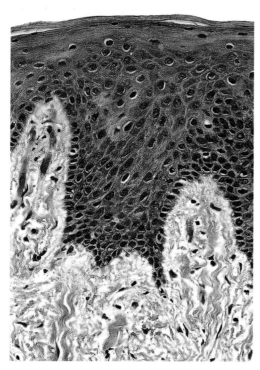

Figure 15.34 Gingiva. Tall rete ridges and dense lamina propria with blood vessels in papillae.

Oral gingival epithelium that extends onto the oral surface of the gum best fits the general pattern of masticatory mucosa. The short portion of gingiva apposed to the tooth (sulcular gingiva) differs from the rest of gingival epithelium in that it is thinner, lacks the characteristic rete ridges, and is not keratinizing (65,66).

The gingiva is highly vascular; its vessels originate in the periodontium and extend into the lamina propria, forming well-organized capillary loops. Occasionally random biopsies of gingiva have been performed to support the diagnosis of systemic diseases (e.g., amyloidosis).

Intraepithelial Nonkeratinocytes

Four different nonepithelial cell types normally occur in the oral mucosa: melanocytes, Merkel cells, Langerhans cells, and lymphocytes.

Melanocytes are found mainly in a basal location in the oral mucosa; they are more common in people with darker complexions (67,68). Small areas of melanin pigmentation, mostly less than 10 mm in diameter, may occur. They are most common on the gingiva but are also seen in the lips, palate, and buccal mucosa and are called mucosal melanosis (melanotic macules) (69) (Figure 15.35). Melanin pigment formed by melanocytes in the basal layer is transferred to adjacent epithelial cells. Such changes can sometimes occur after inflammatory reactions, in smokers,

with Peutz-Jeghers syndrome and Addison's disease, or secondary to drugs and human immunodeficiency virus (HIV) infection. Melanocytic hyperplasia (lentigo) and pigmented nevi may also occur in the oral mucosa but less commonly than on the skin (70–73). Histologically, a lentigo shows increased melanin pigmentation in the basal cell layer without an increase in the number of melanocytes. Intramucosal nevi, similar to intradermal nevi, are the most common type of nevus. Other types of nevi, such as compound nevi, junctional nevi, blue nevi, and combined forms can be observed on the vermilion border, cheek mucosa, gingiva, palate, and tongue. Understandably, primary malignant melanomas can arise anywhere from the oral mucosa (74).

Merkel cells also occur in the basal layer of the oral epithelium, either individually or in clusters (75). Clusters are preferentially located in masticatory mucosa in close contact with the tongue, which supports the notion that they have a mechanoreceptor function. On routine H&E-stained sections, their cytoplasm appears lighter than that of the surrounding basal cells. These neuroendocrine cells are morphologically and functionally identical to those in the skin. They are immunoreactive with antibodies to S-100 protein, chromogranin, CK20, and villin. Their ultrastructure is characterized by many intracytoplasmic dense-core, membrane-bound granules, 80 to 100 μm in diameter (Figure 15.36).

Langerhans cells, mostly located suprabasally, are microscopically similar to melanocytes and cannot be distinguished with certainty in routine H&E-stained sections. In the gingiva, the Langerhans cells are structurally and functionally similar to those in the skin (76,77). Their cytoplasm appears clear, and their small indented ("coffee bean") nucleus stains heavily with hematoxylin. Their dendritic processes, spread among the cells of the stratum spinosum, can be seen well with the immunohistochemical stain for S-100 protein (Figure 15.37), as well as CD1a, the MHC class II

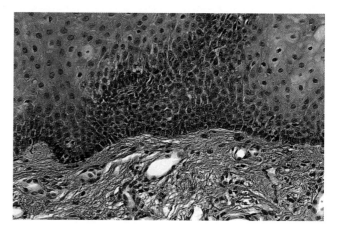

Figure 15.35 Mucosal melanosis of the lip. Numerous melanocytes above the basal lamina appear as a brown ribbon.

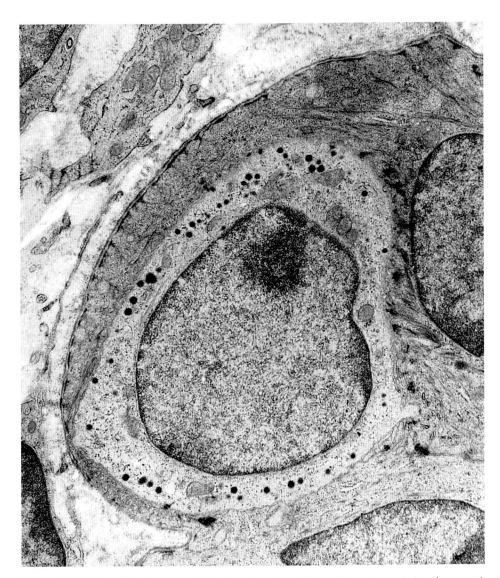

Figure 15.36 Merkel cell surrounded by keratinocytes in the basal layer. Transmission electron micrograph shows the lighter-staining cytoplasm with characteristic and subplasmalemmal, membrane-bound, dense-core granules. The nucleus has no fibrous lamina, unlike melanocytes. The adjacent dermis contains fibroblasts. (Original magnification ×11,500.)

molecules (e.g., HLA-DR), and various adhesion molecules (78). Electron microscopy shows characteristic Birbeck granules in their cytoplasm and a lack of tonofilaments and desmosomes. The frequency of oral mucosal Langerhans cells varies inversely with the degree of keratinization. They are quantitatively lowest in the floor of the mouth and do not occur only around the basal portion of the taste buds and in epithelium lining periodontal pockets.

Langerhans cells play an important role in the immune response, being involved in the processing and presentation of antigens to subjacent lymphocytes. An increased number of Langerhans cells is seen in biopsy samples of the oral mucosa in oral lichen planus, associated with dental caries, with tobacco and alcohol consumption, and in tumor epithelium of invasive oral squamous cell carcinoma.

Teeth and Supporting Structures

The deciduous and permanent teeth have a similar microscopic appearance. The teeth are set in bony sockets on the alveolar processes of the maxillae and the mandible. The part of the tooth that lies within the socket is called the root; there may be multiple roots. The tip of each root is called the apex. The alveolar processes are covered by the gum, and the crowns of the teeth project above the gums. The roots of the teeth are held securely in their sockets by bundles of collagen fibers called the periodontal ligament (periodontal membrane) (12,66). The periodontium includes the tissues investing and supporting the teeth: the cementum, periodontal membrane, alveolar bone, and gingiva (Figures 15.38–15.39). The center of each tooth has a

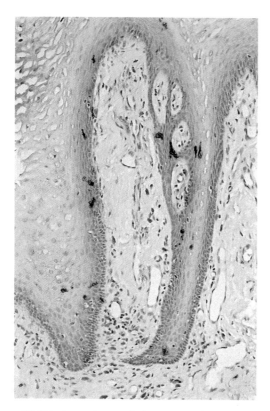

Figure 15.37 Langerhans cells in mucosa of tongue. Dendritic cells in the suprabasal epidermis demonstrate immunoreactivity for S-100 protein.

ologic or pathologic stimuli, odontoblasts can upregulate their protein synthetic activity.

As the dental pulp ages, the number of fibroblasts decreases and, concomitantly, the number and size of collagen fibers increases. Pulp stones (denticles) are commonly observed in the dental pulp of aging individuals. True denticles contain dentinal tubules within a mineralized matrix and are surrounded by odontoblasts. False denticles are composed of a mineralized matrix arranged in concentric lamellae. Most denticles are asymptomatic.

Enamel covers the crown of the tooth. It is the hardest material found in the body and consists of 99.5% apatite crystals (82). Mature enamel is made up of long thin rods that dissolve during decalcification and are therefore not seen on conventional histologic sections. The dentin-enamel junction lies at the former interface between the inner enamel epithelium and dental mesenchyme. Coronal dentin is covered with enamel, and radicular dentin is covered with cementum. Thus, cementum covers the root of the tooth. A slight indentation (cervical line) encircles the tooth and marks the junction of the crown with the root.

pulp chamber, or pulp cavity, that is filled with dental pulp containing loosely arranged fibroblasts, nerves, blood vessels, and lymphatics (79) (Figure 15.40). The pulp chamber narrows toward the root and becomes the root canal. The vessels and postganglionic sympathetic and sensory nerve fibers enter and leave the root canal through a small opening, the apical foramen. The pulp chamber of the growing tooth is lined by a single continuous layer of odontoblasts, which are tall columnar cells with oval nuclei. An elongated cell process, also known as Tomes' fiber, reaches from each odontoblast into the extracellular matrix secreted by them (Figure 15.5). The matrix around the odontoblastic process eventually mineralizes, so that Tomes' fiber comes to lie within a dentinal tubule (80,81). Besides the odontoblastic process, the tubules also contain 200 μm-long unmyelinated nerve fibers, which account for the well-known sensitivity of dentin. Dentin is arranged in the shape of tubules running from the pulp chamber toward the periphery. The dentinal tubules and the meshwork of collagen between them are embedded in hydroxyapatite crystals. On a weight basis, 80% of dentin consists of inorganic calcium salts and 20% of organic material. It is harder than bone but softer than enamel. Dentin makes up most of the wall of the tooth. In the mature tooth, many odontoblasts become inactive, but some continue producing predentin at a reduced rate throughout the life of the tooth. In response to physi-

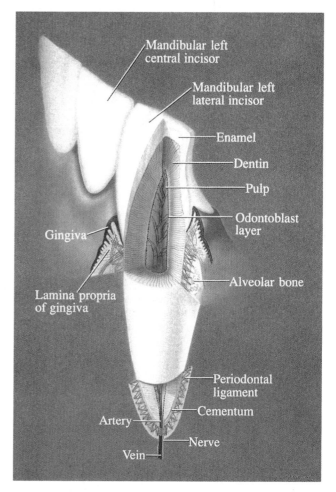

Figure 15.38 Schematic drawing depicts the periodontium including the gingiva, alveolar bone, periodontal ligament, and cementum.

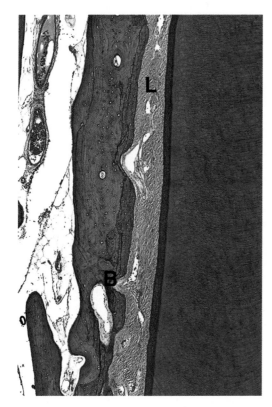

Figure 15.39 Root of tooth and supporting structures, perpendicular section. Dentin is covered by a thin layer of cementum (appearing as a blue band). The periodontal ligament (*L*) holds the tooth in the bony socket of the alveolar process (*B*).

The cementum joins the enamel at this junction (cementoenamel junction). Cementum is similar in structure and composition to bone but has fewer cells, called cementocytes, that occupy lacunae (10,11). It is composed of 55% organic material (mainly calcium) and 45% inorganic material. Cementum is attached by the periodontal ligament to the surrounding bone (Figure 15.39). In older persons, many cementocytes die, and only the surface layer

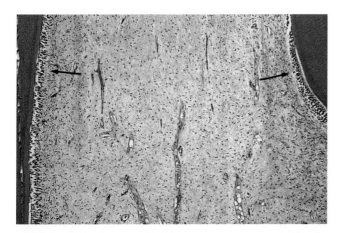

Figure 15.40 Pulp of developing tooth. Odontoblasts (*arrows*) line dentin. The pulp consists mostly of loosely arranged fibroblasts. Note the delicate wall of blood vessels.

appears viable. Another aging phenomenon are cementicles, which are small round calcified bodies on or in the cementum and in the periodontal ligament. Cementicles are of no clinical significance.

From the pathologist's point of view, it is noteworthy that examination of teeth involved in neoplastic growth in most cases shows tumor invading the periodontal ligament and the alveolar bone, destroying these structures. The roots of the teeth may remain intact or may undergo resorption. However, the dental pulp is rarely invaded by neoplasm.

Odontogenic epithelium changes over time. Before tooth eruption, it consists of the external enamel epithelium, inner enamel epithelium, stellate reticulum, Hertwig's epithelial root sheath, and dental lamina; after complete tooth formation, it comprises the epithelial rests of Malassez. Most odontogenic epithelia express cytokeratins 5, 8 and 19 (83). In addition, the external enamel epithelium and stellate reticulum also express cytokeratins 7, 13, 14, 17, and 18; the inner enamel epithelium, cytokeratins 14 and 18; dental lamina, cytokeratins 7, 13, and 14; and epithelial rests of Malassez, cytokeratins 14 and 19. During odontogenesis, CK14 expression in ameloblasts is gradually replaced by CK19. Odontogenic epithelium is the source of odontogenic cysts and some neoplasms, which explains why CK19 is present in almost all epithelial cells of odontogenic cysts.

Pathologic Correlates of the Rests of Serres and Rests of Malassez

Developmental remnants of the dental lamina, called the rests of Serres, commonly occur under the gum as small nests of squamous epithelium (10,14) (Figures 15.2, 15.41). These epithelial islands may proliferate and undergo cystic degeneration, which leads to the formation of gingival cysts. Similarly, epithelial remnants of Hertwig's root sheath, called the rests of Malassez, are universally present in the periodontal membrane and, exceptionally, even in the bone of the alveolar ridge. When dental caries cause a bacterial infection and necrosis of the pulp, the infection usually spreads toward the apical foramen, and a periapical granuloma may develop. As a result of the inflammatory stimulus, the nearby epithelium of the rests of Malassez begins to proliferate and forms an epithelial lining in these apical granulomas (Figure 15.41). It is also assumed that the rests of Serres and the rests of Malassez are potential sources of ameloblastomas and odontogenic cysts.

Nose and Paranasal Sinuses

External Nose and Nasal Vestibule

The external nose is covered by skin that is rich in sebaceous glands, sweat glands, and small hairs. The anterior skin of the nares and widened nasal vestibule, lined by skin that is

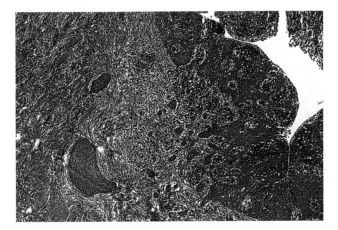

Figure 15.41   Rests of Malassez in periodontium near the apical granuloma.

continuous with the integument of the nose, similarly contains many hair follicles and sebaceous and sweat glands. The squamous epithelium of the vestibule merges with the respiratory mucosa, which covers the respiratory portion of the nasal cavity and all of the paranasal sinuses.

Nasal Mucosa

At the level of the limen nasi, the lining of the nasal cavity gradually changes from squamous epithelium to nonciliated cuboidal or columnar epithelium. Farther into the nasal cavity, this becomes continuous with the pseudostratified ciliated columnar epithelium (respiratory epithelium). The mucosa of the respiratory portion is continuous with that of the ostia and contiguous paranasal sinuses. The mucosal lining contains three main cell types: basal (reserve) cells, goblet cells, and ciliated cells (Figure 15.42). Basal cells, confined to the vicinity of the basal lamina,

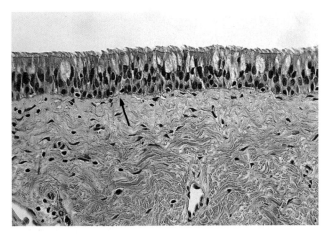

Figure 15.42   Pseudostratified respiratory mucosa of the nose with predominantly ciliated cells. Goblet cells have clear cytoplasm. The basal cells (*arrow*) are lying on thin basal lamina.

divide to produce new daughter cells that differentiate to become mucous or ciliated cells. The mucous cells rest on the basement membrane with a slender stem, and the cytoplasm of their apical portion contains varying amounts of mucus. As these cells fill up with mucus, they resemble a goblet with a foot and a stem. The cells discharge their contents to form a blanket of mucus that covers the surface of the respiratory epithelium. Another source of this mucous coat is the secretion from the seromucinous glands in the lamina propria.

The majority of the cells of the respiratory epithelium are normally made up of ciliated cells bearing small fingerlike cell processes, the cilia, which project into the lumen. Each cell has over 200 cilia, each about 5 μm long. Ultrastructurally, on cross section the ciliary shafts show a highly characteristic circular arrangement of nine pairs of microtubules (doublets), which are arranged symmetrically around two central microtubules (Figure 15.43). Longitudinal sections of the cilia show that the ciliary shaft ends in a basal body (kinetosome), from which it is derived (84). The nasal mucosa is a convenient site to biopsy when ultrastructural abnormalities of cilia are suspected, such as in immotile-cilia syndrome (85,86). The function of the ciliated cells in the nose is to constantly move the protective mucous blanket by the coordinated sweeping motion of the cilia toward the pharynx. In order to perform this function, the cilia beat at 10 to 20 cycles/second. They have an effective whiplike stroke forward and a recovery stroke backward. The propulsive forward phase is much faster and more vigorous than the recovery phase (87). Ciliary activity is optimal at the normal nasal temperature of about 30°C. However, cilia are hardy and persist under unfavorable conditions, including under extreme cold and heat. They will also beat normally and forcefully in a pus-filled cavity. When injured or destroyed by an acute infection, they regenerate rapidly. They do not, however, tolerate excessive drying. Accordingly, they are dependent always upon a coating of moisture for their activity and preservation. The blanket of mucus covering the nasal mucosa and paranasal sinuses forms a conveyor of the bacteria and other foreign matter. The nasal mucociliary layer is the first line of defense against bacterial invasion in this location.

Melanocytes are also present in the normal mucosa of the upper airways. In the nasal cavity they can be seen in the respiratory epithelium and nasal glands. Melanocytes are commonly encountered in the lamina propria of the septum and turbinates, particularly in dark-skinned adults (88). This explains why primary malignant melanomas are well-known to arise in the nose and paranasal sinuses (89).

Intraepithelial lymphocytes are diffusely scattered throughout the nasal mucosa. These are uniformly CD8+ T cells (36). These T cells coexist with a population of dendritic cells that lack CD1a expression. The nasal mucosa and subepithelial tissue contain virtually no B cells. This

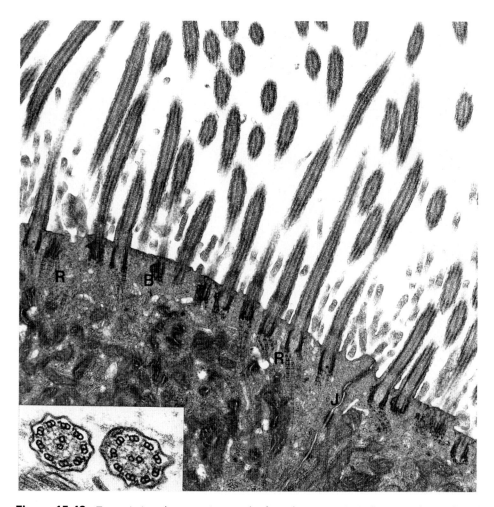

Figure 15.43 Transmission electron micrograph of nasal mucosa. Vertical section shows ciliated epithelial cells extending to the surface. The shafts of the slender long cilia have peripheral and central microtubules that appear as darker linear structures extending from the kinetosome (basal body) (*B*). Cross-banded filamentous rootlets (*R*) are associated with kinetosomes. Note junctional complexes (*J*). Inset: Cross section of the shaft of two cilia. Note the symmetrically arranged nine peripheral doublets and the central pair of single microtubules. (Original magnification ×25,000; inset, original magnification ×87,500.)

finding may explain why most primary nasal lymphomas are of CD8+ T-cell derivation.

Beneath the mucous membrane is the lamina propria, containing numerous small mucous and serous glands that discharge their secretion through lobular ducts onto the surface (Figure 15.44). These glands are embedded in vascular fibroconnective tissue, which is attached to the perichondrium and periosteum of the cartilages and bones forming the nasal cavity (90–92).

The turbinates are somewhat curved structures that are supported by an osseous axis enveloped by relatively thick mucosa (Figures 15.1, 15.45). Their convex surface protrudes toward the nasal cavity. Located beneath their mucosa is a tunica propria or stroma that attaches the mucosa to the underlying structures. Their tunica propria is of variable thickness, being thickest in the areas more exposed to

inhaled and exhaled air (i.e., over the nasal septum and medial aspects of the inferior and middle turbinates). In these areas, the epithelium contains many goblet cells and the basement membrane is prominent (93). These areas also have abundant blood vessels and clusters of mixed seromucinous glands (6–10 glands/mm²) (Figure 15.46). The glands vary from simple straight tubules lined with goblet cells to tubuloalveolar glands. The chief ducts of the latter open onto the mucosal surface by minute orifices. The glands tend to be at a level between the mucosa and the underlying bone.

The turbinates and the lower part of the septum are rich in venous sinuses, which are of variable size and shape, forming a dense network of large veins that resemble erectile tissue (Figure 15.47). These blood vessels are of irregular shape, have muscular walls, and can rapidly dilate and

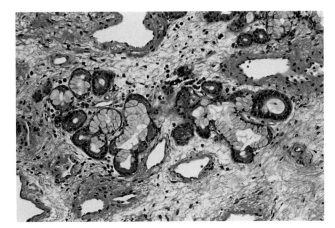

Figure 15.44 Nasal seromucinous gland with duct. Serous cells with darker staining cytoplasm are at the periphery of tubuloacinar glands and form the demilunes of Giannuzzi.

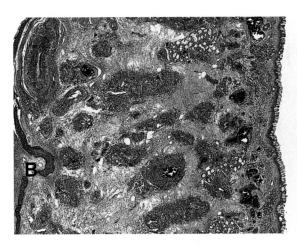

Figure 15.46 Turbinate, coronal section. Mucosal blood vessels are surrounded by a thick sheath of connective tissue (blue); note the large artery near the bone (*B*) (Mallory's trichrome).

constrict, thereby permitting fast adjustments of mucosal temperature and secretion to climatic changes. It is important for the surgical pathologist to know about the normal rich vascular anatomy of the turbinates in order to avoid mistaking them for a hemangioma, angiofibroma, or angioleiomyoma. The stroma of the nasal mucosa also contains lymphatics, small nerves, and a sprinkling of lymphocytes and plasma cells but no lymphoid aggregates. A few mast cells and eosinophils are normally also present.

The osseous portion of the turbinates consists of thin, interconnecting laminae of lamellar bone, forming a continuous shell that is interconnected with bone trabeculae. The interosseous spaces contain numerous large veins, arteries, and some nerves. In contrast to the submucosal veins, the intraosseous veins have a rather large round or oval lumen on cross section and have proportionately thin walls. Occasional adipocytes, but no hematopoietic marrow, are seen in turbinated bone. The presence of prominent hematopoiesis in the facial and nasal bones or the paranasal sinuses is abnormal and may be observed in conditions such as thalassemia major.

The nasal septum consists of a large cartilaginous plate and four small osseous plates, all of which firmly unite with sutures (Figure 15.48). The nasal mucosa is closely apposed to the underlying structures of the nasal septum. The periosteum and perichondrium of the nasal septum attach so closely to the overlying submucosa as to constitute one

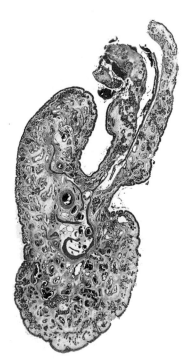

Figure 15.45 Middle turbinate, coronal section. Bone in the axis of the turbinate appears as a delicate, curled structure. The covering mucous membrane and tunica propria are rich in blood vessels and mucous glands, particularly on the convexity and inferior border of the turbinate, areas that are most exposed to the airstream in the nasal cavity. (Low-power view.)

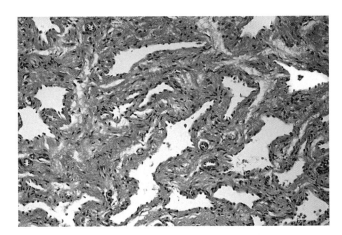

Figure 15.47 Inferior turbinate. Numerous larger blood vessels of variable size and shape are closely packed and form a sponge-like vascular system resembling erectile tissue. The endothelial cells are evenly distributed. Capillaries are lacking.

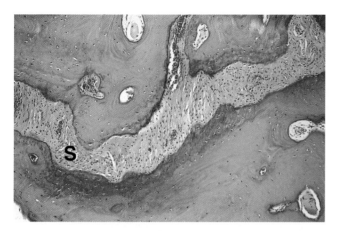

Figure 15.48 Suture (*S*) in the nasal septum. Parallel edges of the vomer (*top*) and maxilla are connected by parallel, densely arranged collagen fibers that are anchored in the bones.

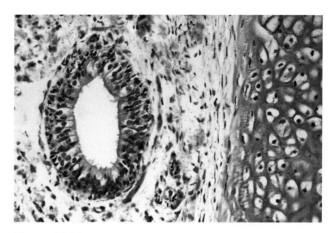

Figure 15.50 Vomeronasal organ of Jacobson in a 22-week-old embryo (180 mm crown-rump length), including a cross section of the tubular structure adjacent to vomeronasal cartilage. In humans the columnar epithelium has microvilli but no sensory epithelium.

membrane, called the mucoperiosteum. A common site of nosebleed is Little's area (or **Kiesselbach's area**) on the anterior part of the cartilaginous nasal septum above the intermaxillary line. The submucosa of this area is richly supplied with thin-walled dilated blood vessels (Figure 15.49). Although rarely seen in surgical specimens, Little's area should not be mistaken for a pyogenic granuloma, which frequently occurs in this location.

Vomeronasal Organ of Jacobson

The vestigial remains of a paired embryonic structure, the vomeronasal organ of Jacobson, are situated under the mucosa of the lower anterior side of the nasal septum covering an area of 0.2 to 0.6 cm. In adults, it consists of a small tubular sac lined by columnar epithelium with microvilli, but it has no sensory cells with cilia and lacks other well-differentiated olfactory structures (Figure 15.50). The organ

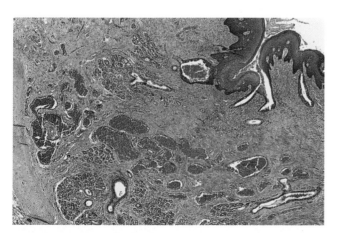

Figure 15.49 Little's area. Teleangiectatic, thin-walled blood vessels are clustered under the epithelium in the anterior portion of the nasal septum. This area is above the level of mucous glands.

is best developed in the twentieth week of embryonic life, after which regressive changes occur and it becomes rudimentary. In humans it has no known function and is of no pathologic significance (94). In many vertebrates, Jacobson's organ is highly developed, particularly in animals of keen olfactory sensibility (95–97).

Olfactory Mucosa

The roof of the nasal cavity and contiguous portions of the nasal septum and superior turbinate form the olfactory region (98). Here, the ciliated columnar epithelium of the nasal mucosa is modified by liberally scattered cells of the sensory organ of smell. The olfactory epithelium consists of three types of cells: (a) olfactory nerve cells, (b) supporting, or sustentacular, cells, and (c) basal cells that lie on the basal lamina (99,100) (Figure 15.51). The olfactory nerve cells are spindle-shaped and have a spherical nucleus. The dendrites of these bipolar cells extend to the surface of the pseudostratified olfactory epithelium and send out a tuft of fine processes known as olfactory cilia (hairs). The cilia, which function as receptors for the detection of odorants, are 2 μm long and lie along the surface of the mucosa embedded in mucus. The deep processes of these bipolar cells form axons that find their way through the basal lamina and join neighboring processes to become bundles of unmyelinated olfactory nerve fibers (100). These fibers collect to form myelinated nerves, which then pass through the cribriform plate of the ethmoid bone to end on the mitral cells in the olfactory bulb. The supporting cells are tall, cylindrical cells that in the elderly contain lipofuscin, giving the yellow hue characteristic of the olfactory mucous membrane. The free surface of these cells possesses many slender microvilli that protrude into the covering mucus. The basal cells are small and conical, lying with their base on the basement membrane. They are believed to represent

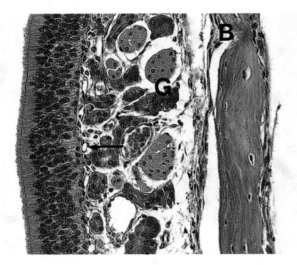

Figure 15.51 Olfactory mucosa. The population of olfactory nerve cells and supporting cells forms a pseudostratified columnar epithelium with distinct microvilli. Basal cells lie on basal lamina (*arrow*). Bowman's glands (*G*) with excretory ducts and nerves are between the epithelium and bone of nasal septum (*B*).

stem cells that can give rise to new supporting and sensory cells. Under the mucosa is the lamina propria, composed of loose connective tissue in which are found the olfactory glands of Bowman (101). The secretion of these tubuloalveolar glands is carried to the surface of the mucosa by narrow ducts.

Paranasal Sinuses

The sinuses are lined with a mucous membrane that is continuous with the nasal mucosa. The mucosa is therefore similar to that of the nasal cavity. However, the epithelium (schneiderian epithelium) and lamina propria are thinner and less vascular. Seromucous glands present in the sinuses are more sparse compared to in the nasal mucosa and are largely concentrated at the ostium of the maxillary sinus. The mucus formed in the sinuses is moved by the action of the cilia through the apertures to the nasal cavities.

REFERENCES

1. Moore KL, Persaud TVN. *The Developing Human: Clinically Oriented Embryology.* 5th ed. Philadelphia: WB Saunders; 1993.
2. Sperber GH. *Craniofacial Embryology.* 4th ed. London: Butterworth-Heinemann; 1989.
3. Thesleff I, Vaahtokari A, Kettunen P, Aberg T. Epithelial-mesenchymal signaling during tooth development. *Connect Tissue Res* 1995;32:9–15.
4. Listgarten MA. Phase-contrast and electron microscopic study of the junction between reduced enamel epithelium and enamel in unerupted human teeth. *Arch Oral Biol* 1966;11:999–1016.
5. Schour I, Massler M. Studies in tooth development: the growth pattern of human teeth. *J Am Dent Assoc* 1940;27:1918–1931.
6. Gorski JP, Marks SC Jr. Current concepts of the biology of tooth eruption. *Crit Rev Oral Biol Med* 1992;3:185–206.
7. Marks SC Jr, Gorski JP, Cahill DR, Wise GG. Tooth eruption—a synthesis of experimental observations. In: Davidovitch Z, ed. *The Biological Mechanisms of Tooth Eruption and Root Resorption.* Birmingham, AL: EBSCO Media; 1988:161–169.
8. Orban B, Sicher H, Weinmann JP. Amelogenesis (a critique and a new concept). *J Am Coll Dent* 1943;10:13–22.
9. Schroeder HE. Development and structure of the tissues of the tooth. In: Schroeder HE. *Oral Structural Biology.* New York: Thieme Medical; 1986:4–184.
10. Bhaskar SN, Orban BJ, eds. *Orban's Oral Histology and Embryology.* 11th ed. St. Louis: CV Mosby Year Book; 1990.
11. Held AJ. Cementogenesis and the normal and pathologic structure of cementum. *Oral Surg Oral Med Oral Pathol* 1951;4:53–67.
12. Smukler H, Dreyer CJ. Principal fibres of the periodontium. *J Periodont Res* 1969;4:19–25.
13. Logan WHG, Kronfeld R. Development of the human jaws and surrounding structures from birth to the age of fifteen years. *J Am Dent Assoc* 1933;20:379–427.
14. Schroeder H. *Oral Structure Biology: Embryology, Structure and Function of Normal Hard and Soft Tissues of the Oral Cavity and the Temporomandibular Joints.* New York: Thieme; 1991.
15. Gorlin RJ. Heterotopic lymphoid tissue: a diagnostic problem. *Oral Surg Oral Med Oral Pathol* 1957;10:87–89.
16. Sadeghi EM, Ashrafi MH. Heterotopic lymph node of the buccal mucosa simulating a tumor: a clinicopathological appraisal. *ASDC J Dent Child* 1982;49:304–306.
17. Tobias MJ. *Anatomy of the Human Lymphatic System.* Ann Arbor, MI: Edwards Brothers, Inc.; 1938.
18. Richtsmeier WJ, Shikhani AH. The physiology and immunology of the pharyngeal lymphoid tissue. *Otolaryngol Clin North Am* 1987;20:219–228.
19. Goeringer GC, Vidic B. The embryogenesis and anatomy of Waldeyer's ring. *Otolaryngol Clin North Am* 1987;20:207–217.
20. Dolen WK, Spofford B, Selner JC. The hidden tonsils of Waldeyer's ring. *Ann Allergy* 1990;65:244–248.
21. Knapp MJ. Oral tonsils: location, distribution, and histology. *Oral Surg Oral Med Oral Pathol* 1970;29:155–161.
22. Knapp MJ. Pathology of oral tonsils. *Oral Surg Oral Med Oral Pathol* 1970;29:295–304.
23. Buchner A, Hansen LS. Lymphoepithelial cysts of the oral cavity. A clinicopathologic study of thirty-eight cases. *Oral Surg Oral Med Oral Pathol* 1980;50:441–449.
24. Napier SS, Newlands C. Benign lymphoid hyperplasia of the palate: report of two cases and immunohistochemical profile. *J Oral Pathol Med* 1990;19:221–225.
25. Simpson HE. Lymphoid hyperplasia in foliate papillitis. *J Oral Surg Anesth Hosp Dent Serv* 1964;22:209–214.
26. Miles AEW. Sebaceous glands in the lip and cheek mucosa of man. *Br Dent J* 1958;105:235–248.
27. Sewerin I. The sebaceous glands in the vermilion border of the lips and in the oral mucosa of man. *Acta Odontol Scand* 1975;33(suppl 68):13–226.
28. Meyer J, Squier CA, Gerson SJ, eds. *The Structure and Function of the Oral Mucosa.* New York: Pergamon Press; 1984.
29. Skougaard MR. Cell renewal, with special reference to the gingival epithelium. *Adv Oral Biol* 1970;4:261–288.
30. Squier CA, Finkelstein MW. Oral mucosa. In: Ten Cate AR, ed. *Oral Histology, Development, Structure and Function.* St. Louis: CV Mosby; 1989:341–382.
31. Mackenzie IC, Rittman G, Gao Z, Leigh I, Lane EB. Patterns of cytokeratin expression in human gingival epithelia. *J Periodontal Res* 1991;26:468–478.
32. Sawaf MH, Ouhayoun JP, Forest N. Cytokeratin profiles in oral epithelial: a review and a new classification. *J Biol Buccale* 1991;19:187–198.
33. Ouhayoun JP, Gosselin F, Forest N, Winter S, Franke WW. Cytokeratin patterns of human oral epithelia: differences in cytokeratin synthesis in gingival epithelium and the adjacent alveolar mucosa. *Differentiation* 1985;30:123–129.
34. Mandel U. Carbohydrates in oral epithelia and secretions: variation with cellular differentiation. *APMIS Suppl* 1992;27:119–129.

35. Olofsson K, Mattsson C, Hammarstrom ML, Hellstrom S. Structure of the human uvula. *Acta Otolaryngol* 1999;119:712–717.
36. Graeme-Cook F, Bhan AK, Harris NL. Immunohistochemical characterization of intraepithelial and subepithelial mononuclear cells of the upper airways. *Am J Pathol* 1993;143:1416–1422.
37. Winther B, Innes DJ. The human adenoid. A morphologic study. *Arch Otolaryngol Head Neck Surg* 1994;120:144–149.
38. Bhargava D, Raman R, Khalfan Al Abri R, Bushnurmath B. Heterotopia of the tonsil. *J Laryngol Otol* 1996;110:611–612.
39. Eversole LR. The histochemistry of mucosubstances in human minor salivary glands. *Arch Oral Biol* 1972;17:1225–1239.
40. Munger BL. Histochemical studies on seromucous- and mucous-secreting cells of human salivary glands. *Am J Anat* 1964;115:411–429.
41. Tandler B, Denning CR, Mandel ID, Kutscher AH. Ultrastructure of human labial salivary glands. III. Myoepithelium and ducts. *J Morphol* 1970;130:227–246.
42. Ogawa Y. Immunocytochemistry of myoepithelial cells in the salivary glands. *Prog Histochem Cytochem* 2003;38:343–426.
43. Takeda Y. Existence and distribution of melanocytes and HMB-45-positive cells in the human minor salivary glands. *Pathol Int* 2000;50:15–19.
44. Hamperl H. Über das vorkommen von onkocyten in verschiedenen organen und ihren geschwülsten: (mundspeicheldrüsen, bauchspeicheldrüse, epithelkörperchen, hypophyse, schilddrüse, eileiter). *Virchows Arch A* 1936;298:327–375.
45. Chang A, Harawi SJ. Oncocytes, oncocytosis and oncocytic tumors. *Pathol Annu* 1992;27:263–304.
46. Balogh K Jr, Roth SI. Histochemical and electron microscopic studies of eosinophilic granular cells (oncocytes) in tumors of the parotid gland. *Lab Invest* 1965;14:310–320.
47. Goode RK, Corio RL. Oncocytic adenocarcinoma of salivary glands. *Oral Surg Oral Med Oral Pathol* 1988;65:61–66.
48. Tschen JA, Fechner RE. The juxtaoral organ of Chievitz. *Am J Surg Pathol* 1979;3:147–150.
49. Zenker W. *Juxtaoral Organ (Chievitz' Organ). Morphology and Clinical Aspects.* Baltimore: Urban & Schwarzenberg; 1982.
50. Pantanowitz L, Tschen JA. Organ of Chievitz. *Ear Nose Throat J* 2004;83:230.
51. Ide F, Mishima K, Saito I. Melanin pigmentation in the juxtaoral organ of Chievitz. *Pathol Int* 2003;53:262–263.
52. Pantanowitz L, Tschen JA, Balogh K. The juxtaoral organ of Chievitz. *Int J Surg Pathol* 2003;11:37.
53. Pantanowitz L. Immunophenotype of the juxtaoral organ. *Int J Oral Maxillofac Surg* 2004;33:113.
54. Lutman GB. Epithelial nests in intraoral sensory nerve endings simulating perineural invasion in patients with oral carcinoma. *Am J Clin Pathol* 1974;61:275–284.
55. Mikó T, Molnár P. The juxtaoral organ—a pitfall for pathologists. *J Pathol* 1981;133:17–23.
56. Soucy P, Cimone G, Carpenter B. An unusual intraoral mass in a child: the organ of Chievitz. *J Pediatr Surg* 1990;25:1200.
57. Leibl W, Pflüger H, Kerjaschki D. A case of nodular hyperplasia of the juxtaoral organ in man. *Virchows Arch A Pathol Anat Histol* 1976;371:389–391.
58. Chievitz JH. Beiträge zur entwicklungsgeschichte der speicheldrüsen. *Arch Anat Physiol* 1885;9:401–436.
59. Pantanowitz L, Balogh K. Significance of the juxtaoral organ (of Chievitz). *Head Neck* 2003;25:400–405.
60. Ide F, Mishima K, Saito I. Pacinian corpuscle in the juxtaoral organ of Chievitz. *J Oral Pathol Med* 2004;33:443–444.
61. Eversole LR, Leider AS. Maxillary intraosseous neuroepithelial structures resembling those seen in the organ of Chievitz. *Oral Surg Oral Med Oral Pathol* 1978;46:555–558.
62. Jensen JL, Wuerker RB, Correll RW, Erickson JO. Epithelial islands associated with mandibular nerves. Report of two cases in the walls of mandibular cysts. *Oral Surg Oral Med Oral Pathol* 1979;48:226–230.
63. Kruger L, Mantyh PW. Gustatory and related chemosensory systems. In: Björklund A, Hökfelt T, Swanson LW, eds. *Handbook of Chemical Neuroanatomy.* Vol. 7. Integrated Systems of the CNS Part II. Amsterdam: Elsevier; 1989:323–411.
64. Oakley B. Neuronal–epithelial interactions in mammalian gustatory epithelium. In: Bock GR, ed. *Regeneration of Vertebrate Sensory Receptor Cells.* Chichester, England: Wiley; 1991:277–287.
65. Ainamo J, Loe H. Anatomical characteristics of gingiva: clinical and microscopic study of the free and attached gingiva. *J Periodontol* 1966;37:5–13.
66. Melcher AH, Bowen WH, eds. *Biology of the Periodontium.* New York: Academic Press; 1969.
67. Squier CA, Waterhouse JP. The ultrastructure of the melanocyte in human gingival epithelium. *Arch Oral Biol* 1967;12:119–129.
68. Schroeder HE. Melanin containing organelles in cells of the human gingiva. I. Epithelial melanocytes. *J Periodont Res* 1969;4:1–18.
69. Kaugars GE, Heise AP, Riley WT, Abbey LM, Svirsky JA. Oral melanotic macules: a review of 353 cases. *Oral Surg Oral Med Oral Pathol* 1993;76:59–61.
70. Buchner A, Merrell PW, Hansen LS, Leider AS. Melanocytic hyperplasia of the oral mucosa. *Oral Surg Oral Med Oral Pathol* 1991;71:58–62.
71. Buchner A, Ledier AS, Merrell PW, Carpenter WM. Melanocytic nevi of oral mucosa: a clinicopathologic study of 130 cases from northern California. *J Oral Pathol Med* 1990;19:197–201.
72. Buchner A, Hansen L. Pigmented nevi of the oral mucosa: a clinicopathologic study of 36 new cases and review of 155 cases from the literature. Part I. A clinicopathologic study of 36 new cases. *Oral Surg Oral Med Oral Pathol* 1987;63:566–572.
73. Buchner A, Hansen L. Pigmented nevi of the oral mucosa: a clinicopathologic study of 36 new cases and review of 155 cases from the literature. Part II. Analysis of 191 cases. *Oral Surg Oral Med Oral Pathol* 1987;63:676–682.
74. Trodahl JN, Sprague WG. Benign and malignant melanocytic lesions of the oral mucosa. An analysis of 135 cases. *Cancer* 1970;25:812–823.
75. Hashimoto K. Fine structure of Merkel cell in human oral mucosa. *J Invest Dermatol* 1972;58:381–387.
76. Waterhouse JP, Squier CA. The Langerhans cell in human gingival epithelium. *Arch Oral Biol* 1967;12:341–348.
77. Chou JM, Daniels TE. Langerhans cells expressing HLA-DQ, HLA-DR and T6 antigens in normal oral mucosa and lichen planus. *J Oral Pathol Med* 1989;18:573–576.
78. Barrett AW, Cruchley AT, Williams DM. Oral mucosal Langerhans' cells. *Crit Rev Oral Biol Med* 1996;7:36–58.
79. Baume LJ. The biology of pulp and dentine. A historic terminologic-taxonomic, histologic-biochemical, embryonic and clinical survey. *Monogr Oral Sci* 1980;8:1–220.
80. Holland GR. The odontoblast process: form and function. *J Dent Res* 1985;64:499–514.
81. Thomas HF. The dentin–predentin complex and its permeability: anatomical review. *J Dent Res* 1985;64:607–612.
82. Nylen UM, Termine JD, eds. Tooth enamel III. Its development, structure, and composition. *J Dent Res* 1979;58:675–1031.
83. Domingues MG, Jaeger MM, Araujo VC, Araujo NS. Expression of cytokeratins in human enamel organ. *Eur J Oral Sci* 2000;108:43–47.
84. Fawcett DW, Porter KR. A study of the fine structure of ciliated epithelium. *J Morphol* 1954;94:221–281.
85. Afzelius BA. The immotile-cilia syndrome and other ciliary disease. *Int Rev Exp Pathol* 1979;19:1–43.
86. Howell JT, Schochet SS Jr, Goldman AS. Ultrastructural defects of respiratory tract cilia associated with chronic infections. *Arch Pathol Lab Med* 1980;104:52–55.
87. Sleigh MA, Blake JR, Liron N. The propulsion of mucus by cilia. *Am Rev Respir Dis* 1988;137:726–741.
88. Zak FG, Lawson W. The presence of melanocytes in the nasal cavity. *Ann Otol Rhinol Laryngol* 1974;83:515–519.
89. Cove H. Melanosis, melanocytic hyperplasia, and primary malignant melanoma of the nasal cavity. *Cancer* 1979;44:1424–1433.
90. Rhys-Evans PH. Anatomy of the nose and paranasal sinuses. In: Kerr AG, Groves J, Scott-Brown WG, eds. *Scott-Brown's Otolaryngology.* 5th ed. Vol I. London: Butterworth; 1987:138–161.

91. Drake-Lee AB. Physiology of the nose and paranasal sinus. In: Kerr AG, Groves J, Scott-Brown WG, eds. *Scott-Brown's Otolaryngology.* 5th ed. Vol I. London: Butterworth; 1987:162–182.

92. Ballenger JJ. The clinical anatomy and physiology of the nose and accessory sinuses. In: Ballenger JJ, ed. *Diseases of the Nose, Throat, Ear, Head and Neck.* 14th ed. Malvern, PA: Lea & Febiger; 1991:3–22.

93. Trotter CM, Hall GH, Salter DM, Wilson JA. Histology of the mucous membrane of the human inferior nasal concha. *Clin Anat* 1990;3:307–316.

94. Zuckerkandl E. Das Jacobsonsche organ. *Erg Anat Entwicklungsgesch* 1910;18:801–843.

95. Pearlman SJ. Jacobson's organ (Organon vomeronasale Jacobsoni): its anatomy, gross, microscopic and comparative, with some observations as well on its function. *Ann Otol Rhinol Laryngol* 1934;43:739–768.

96. Negus VE. The organ of Jacobson. *J Anat* 1956;90:515–519.

97. Seifert K. Licht- und elektronenmikroskopische untersuchungen am Jacobsonschen organ (organon vomero-nasale) der Katze. *Arch Klin Exp Ohr Nas Kehlk Heilk* 1971;200:223–251.

98. Naessen R. The identification and topographical localization of the olfactory epithelium in man and other mammals. *Acta Otolaryngol* 1970;70:51–57.

99. Schneider RA. The sense of smell in man—its physiologic basis. *N Engl J Med* 1967;277:299–303.

100. Palay SL. The general architecture of sensory neuroepithelia. In: Bock GR, ed. *Regeneration of Vertebrate Sensory Receptor Cells.* Chichester, England: Wiley; 1991:3–24.

101. Seifert K. Licht- und elektronenmikroskopische untersuchungen der Bowman-Drüsen in der riechschleimhaut makrosmatischer säuger. *Arch Klin Exp Ohren Nasen Kehlkopfheilkd* 1971;200:252–274.

Larynx and Pharynx

16

Stacey E. Mills

LARYNX

Definition and Boundaries

The larynx is a complex organ with numerous connective tissue elements and a variety of epithelia. The superior border of the larynx is the tip of the epiglottis and the aryepiglottic folds. The inferior limit is the inferior rim of the cricoid cartilage. The anterior boundary is composed of the lingual surface of the epiglottis, the thyroid cartilage, the anterior arch of the cricoid cartilage, the thyrohyoid membrane, and the cricothyroid membrane. The posterior boundary is the cricoid cartilage and the arytenoid region. The piriform fossa is frequently, and erroneously, considered to be a part of the larynx. In reality, it is a pouch of the hypopharynx that passes on each side of the larynx. It is, thus, a conduit for food and water, not air.

Although not part of the larynx per se, the pre-epiglottic space is an important area for the spread of carcinoma. This more or less triangular space is filled with fat and loose connective tissue. It is bounded posteriorly by the epiglottis, anteriorly by the thyroid cartilage and thyrohyoid membrane, and superiorly by the hyoepiglottic ligament.

Embryology

The supraglottic portion of the larynx is derived from the third and fourth branchial arches and is, therefore, related to the development of the oral cavity and oropharynx. The glottis and subglottis arise from the sixth branchial arch, which also give rise to the trachea and lungs. Bocca et al. (1) have demonstrated that the larynx virtually consists of two hemilarynges (superior and inferior), each of them with its own different derivation and its own largely independent lymphatic circulation. These authors also discuss the importance of this embryologic derivation with respect to the origin and spread of laryngeal carcinoma. Each of these hemilarynges may become invaded by cancer independent of one another. The extension of cancer is often limited within the boundaries of this embryologic demarcation (1).

The first embryologic appearance of the respiratory apparatus occurs at approximately 21 days in the 3-mm embryo. At this time, an evagination, or groove, forms adjacent to the superior portion of the foregut, above the fourth branchial arch. The inferior portion of this evagination is the pulmonary anlage. The first portion of the larynx to develop is the epiglottis, but this does not appear as a definitively formed structure until approximately the fifth week of intrauterine development.

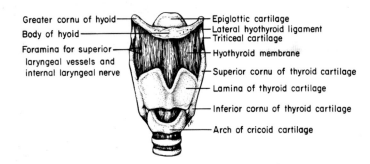

Figure 16.1 Anterior view of an unopened larynx shows the lamina of thyroid cartilage, the arch of the cricoid cartilage, and the hyothyroid membrane as the major structures that define the anterior external surface of the larynx. (From: Mills SE, Fechner RE. Pathology of the larynx. *Atlas of Head and Neck Pathology Series.* Chicago: American Society of Clinical Pathologists Press; 1985.)

The outline of the larynx is recognizable in the 6-mm embryo. At this time, the respiratory groove described previously begins to close; this closure is completed with the formation of the arytenoid cartilages. By 60 to 70 days, at the stage of the 30-mm embryo, the vocal cords begin to differentiate. The embryonic development of the larynx is complex, and it is not surprising that at least 30 different congenital malformations have been described (2).

Gross and Functional Anatomy

The larynx is composed of an elastic cone, cartilages, intrinsic and extrinsic muscles, submucosa, and an overlying mucous membrane (Figures 16.1–16.3). The elastic cone provides most of the structural strength to support the true vocal cords. The elastic tissue is thickened just under the mucosa of the free edge of the cord. This portion of the elastic cone is referred to as the vocal ligament. It is visible grossly as a white band beneath the mucous membrane (Figure 16.3). The vocal ligament inserts on the thyroid cartilage anteriorly and the vocal process of the arytenoid cartilage posteriorly (Figure 16.4).

The major cartilages of the larynx are the cricoid, thyroid, and the paired arytenoid cartilages (Figure 16.5). These major structural cartilages are all of hyalin type. The epiglottis, in contrast, is composed of elastic cartilage containing numerous fenestrations. Calcification of the thyroid and cricoid cartilages begins during the second decade of life in males and somewhat later in females. In older individuals, the thyroid cartilage is frequently ossified, replete with fibrofatty and hematopoietic bone marrow

elements. The ossification of the thyroid cartilage is important in regard to the spread of laryngeal carcinoma. This cartilage is involved by continuous or metastatic carcinoma only when ossified. Hyalin cartilage, perhaps because of its elaboration of angiogenesis inhibiting factors, is remarkably resistant to the spread of neoplasia.

The cricoid and thyroid cartilages articulate with one another, but their motion is limited by several dense ligaments that anchor the cartilages together. The arytenoid cartilages articulate with the cricoid cartilage. Both the cricothyroid and cricoarytenoid joints are diarthrodial and lined by flattened synovial cells. These tiny joints are susceptible to conditions that more commonly affect larger synovial-lined spaces, such as gout and rheumatoid arthritis.

Each arytenoid cartilage attaches to the thyroarytenoid muscle and has a protrusion, the vocal process, that is the posterior point of insertion of the vocal ligament. The position of the arytenoid cartilage determines the tension of the vocal ligament. During adduction of the cords, the arytenoid cartilages move medially along the facets of the cricoid cartilage; they also pivot or rock (Figure 16.4). The rocking motion causes the vocal processes to move downward and toward the midline to complete the adduction of the vocal cords.

The muscles of the larynx can be divided into two groups. The extrinsic muscles originate from neighboring structures outside the larynx and insert on the thyroid, cricoid, or hyoid cartilages. These muscles include the omohyoid, sternohyoid, sternothyroid, and thyrohyoid muscles; they act as a whole upon the larynx during swallowing.

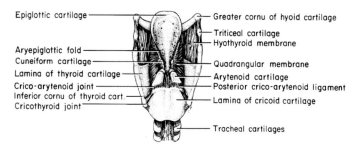

Figure 16.2 Posterior view of an unopened larynx emphasizes the position of the arytenoid cartilages. Major support and posterior definition of the larynx are provided by the lamina of the cricoid cartilage. (From: Mills SE, Fechner RE. Pathology of the larynx. *Atlas of Head and Neck Pathology Series.* Chicago: American Society of Clinical Pathologists Press; 1985.)

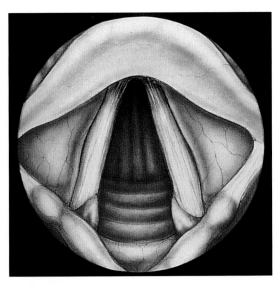

Figure 16.3 Larynx as viewed endoscopically from above. The elastic cone is visible through the mucosa of the true cord as a gray-to-white zone. False cords are loose folds of mucosa without further distinguishing features.

The principle intrinsic muscles of the larynx are the cricothyroid, posterior cricoarytenoid, lateral cricoarytenoid, and thyroarytenoid. There are also small strands of muscle that are in continuity with the thyroarytenoid muscle and insert along the length of the vocal ligaments. This is frequently referred to as the vocalis muscle. It should be remembered that the vocalis muscle is actually a component of the thyroarytenoid muscle, and some authors use these names interchangeably.

The lateral cricoarytenoid muscle adducts the vocal cord, and the posterior cricoarytenoid muscle abducts the cord.

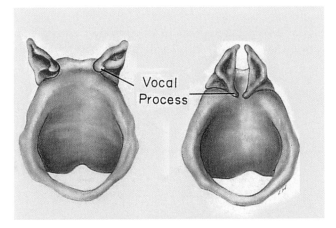

Figure 16.4 The arytenoid cartilage articulates with the posterior lamina of the cricoid cartilage. When the arytenoid cartilages are abducted, they are widely separated and the airway is open (*left*). When adducted, the arytenoid cartilages pivot, as well as move medially, thus bringing the vocal cords together (*right*). (From: Mills SE, Fechner RE. Pathology of the larynx. *Atlas of Head and Neck Pathology Series.* Chicago: American Society of Clinical Pathologists Press; 1985.)

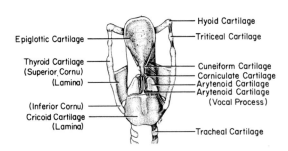

Figure 16.5 The major cartilages of the larynx are better seen in this drawing that deletes the associated soft tissues. (From: Mills SE, Fechner RE. Pathology of the larynx. *Atlas of Head and Neck Pathology Series.* Chicago: American Society of Clinical Pathologists Press; 1985.)

During phonation, the thyroarytenoid muscle slightly moves the thyroid cartilage. The degree of contraction of the thyroarytenoid muscle determines the length and tension of the vocal cord.

The larynx can be divided into three major compartments (supraglottic, glottic, subglottic) for purposes of discussing its submucosal and mucosal components. The supraglottic larynx extends from the tip of the epiglottis to the true cord (3). This portion of the larynx also includes the aryepiglottic (arytenoepiglottic) folds, false vocal cords, and ventricles. The arytenoepiglottic folds run posteriorly from the base of the epiglottis to the region of the arytenoid cartilages. The false vocal cords are soft, rounded protrusions of the mucous membrane that lie superior to the true cords. The ventricles form the lower boundary of the false cords and separate them from the inferiorly located true cords. The ventricles extend upward behind the false cords as elliptical pouches. The greatest extension of the ventricles is slightly forward, where they end as dilated, blind pouches called the saccules. Involvement of the ventricle is a frequent route of superior spread by glottic carcinoma, and this spread may be difficult to detect clinically.

The glottic compartment consists of the true vocal cords and the narrow band of mucous membrane called the anterior commissure, which bridges the vocal cords anteriorly (4,5). The subglottic compartment is the area between the lower border of the true vocal cords, where the squamous epithelium normally ends, and the first tracheal cartilage (6).

Microscopic Anatomy

Studies of larynges from newborns have shown that, except for the true vocal cords, the larynx initially is lined by ciliated epithelium (7) (Figures 16.6–16.7). Squamous epithelium begins to appear on the false vocal cords by about 6 months of age but does not necessarily completely replace the ciliated respiratory mucosa (8,9). The lingual, or anterior, surface of the epiglottis is invariably covered by stratified squamous epithelium. The posterior, or laryngeal, surface of the epiglottis is covered by stratified squamous epithelium in its upper portion, but this merges with

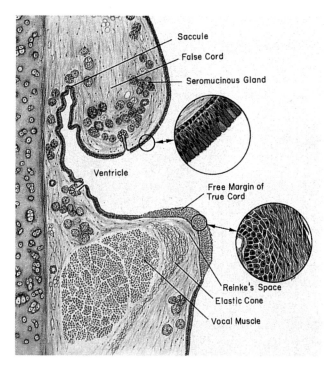

Figure 16.6 Drawing of the normal microscopic anatomy of the larynx. Seromucinous glands are prominent in the false cord, and this cord is lined by ciliated columnar epithelium at birth. The vocalis muscle, elastic cone, and Reinke's space are also visualized in the true cord. (From: Mills SE, Fechner RE. Pathology of the larynx. *Atlas of Head and Neck Pathology Series.* Chicago: American Society of Clinical Pathologists Press; 1985.)

respiratory-type epithelium inferiorly (10). About one-half of nonsmoking adults have patches of squamous epithelium intermixed with ciliated epithelium, both in the supraglottic and infraglottic regions. In smokers, the ciliated, respiratory epithelium of the larynx often is totally replaced by squamous epithelium.

The normal ciliated epithelium of the larynx has an innermost layer of small, round cells—the basal, or reserve, cell layer. This single cell layer of basal cells is overlaid by a

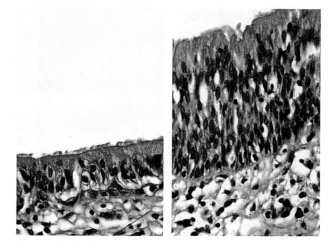

Figure 16.8 The ciliated columnar epithelium of the larynx may be only a few cells in thickness (*left*), or it may form a considerably thicker layer (*right*). (From: Mills SE, Fechner RE. Pathology of the larynx. *Atlas of Head and Neck Pathology Series.* Chicago: American Society of Clinical Pathologists Press; 1985.)

second row of ciliated columnar cells. Variation in the position of the nuclei within the columnar cell layer imparts a pseudostratified appearance to the epithelium. The ciliated layer may vary considerably in thickness (Figure 16.8). Mucus-secreting cells may be numerous or rare. When there is abundant mucin, the cells assume a goblet configuration and may be located either within the middle portion of the epithelium or near the surface (Figure 16.9). Other mucus-secreting cells are barely recognizable and have only a few faintly discernible vacuoles within otherwise eosinophilic columnar cells.

The squamous epithelium of the larynx has a basal layer of small cells with scant cytoplasm and ovoid nuclei that are typically oriented perpendicular to the surface. Mitotic figures are normally confined to this layer. Dendritic melanocytes may be present in the basal layer, especially in African Americans (11,12). The frequency with which this

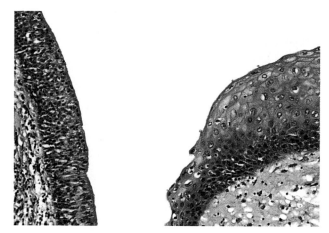

Figure 16.7 Section through ventricle discloses ciliated columnar to intermediate epithelium lining false cord (*right*) and squamous epithelium lining true cord (*left*).

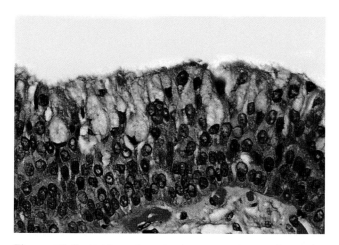

Figure 16.9 Goblet cells and columnar mucinous cells may be present in variable numbers within the nonsquamous epithelium of the larynx.

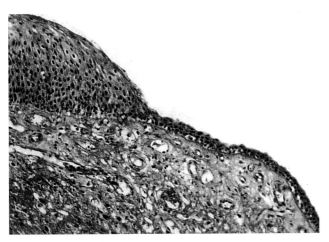

Figure 16.10 The squamous epithelium of the larynx can vary from approximately 5 cells to over 25 cells in total thickness, even within the same larynx.

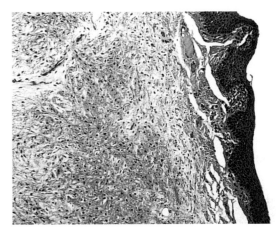

Figure 16.11 The true vocal cord is lined by squamous epithelium. A narrow, sparsely vascular zone (Reinke's space) lies between the squamous epithelium and the underlying vocal ligament.

melanocytic change is observed, and whether it represents a congenital or acquired process, remain unclear. Rare laryngeal malignant melanomas presumably arise in such foci.

As the squamous cells in laryngeal mucosa mature and migrate toward the lumen, the nuclei enlarge, assume a more spherical shape, and have more vesicular chromatin. The eosinophilic cytoplasm becomes abundant, and slight cell shrinkage during fixation produces numerous, thin strands of cytoplasm from adjacent cells that remain attached by desmosomes. Because of these thin cytoplasmic strands between cells, the term *prickle cell layer* (malpighian layer) has been applied to this zone. This is the broadest component of the squamous epithelium. The superficial layer is composed of one to three flattened cells with small, condensed nuclei. The squamous epithelium of the larynx can vary from about 5 cells in total thickness to over 25 cells (Figure 16.10). Normally, the larynx lacks a layer of parakeratotic surface cells. Continued exposure to irritants, such as cigarette smoke, may lead to foci of parakeratosis that may also be associated with orthokeratin formation.

The lamina propria of the true vocal cord is loose or dense connective tissue that lies between the vocal ligament and the squamous epithelium (Reinke's space) (Figure 16.11). Reinke's space contains a few capillaries but lacks lymphatics and only rarely has sparse seromucinous glands. As a result of this limited vascular access, carcinomas confined to the true vocal cords tend to remain localized and are amenable to curative radiation or surgical therapy. The poor lymphatic drainage of Reinke's space also probably contributes to the development of vocal cord nodules and polyps when abnormal amounts of edemalike fluid collect in this region. Likewise, vocal abuse or upper respiratory tract infections frequently produce edema in this region and manifest clinically as hoarseness or dysphonia. The anterior commissure, unlike the true cords, contains more abundant capillaries, lymphatics, and seromucinous glands.

The junction between the ciliated columnar epithelium, inferior and superior to the squamous epithelium of the true vocal cords, may be abrupt, but usually there is a transitional zone that varies from several cells to a width of 1 to 2 mm. The transitional zone consists of columnar cells that are gradually replaced by small, basaloid or immature squamous cells (Figure 16.12). In effect, this is a zone of immature squamous metaplasia in which the cells become progressively larger until they reach the size of the fully mature squamous epithelium that lines the true vocal cord.

The transitional zone often has a microscopically disorganized appearance when compared to the adjacent squamous and ciliated epithelium (Figure 16.12). Furthermore, the epithelium in this zone may be thickened and consist predominantly of basaloid cells. The latter

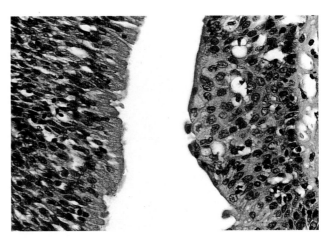

Figure 16.12 Ciliated columnar epithelium lines the false cord (*left*). A transitional zone is seen on the true cord (*right*). This zone of immature squamous metaplasia has a disorganized appearance that should not be confused with dysplasia. (From: Mills SE, Fechner RE. Pathology of the larynx. *Atlas of Head and Neck Pathology Series.* Chicago: American Society of Clinical Pathologists Press; 1985.)

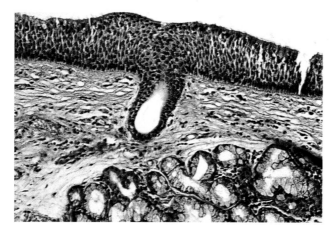

Figure 16.13 Seromucinous glands in the false cord drain into a duct that enters the overlying ciliated columnar epithelium. (From: Mills SE, Fechner RE. Pathology of the larynx. *Atlas of Head and Neck Pathology Series.* Chicago: American Society of Clinical Pathologists Press; 1985.)

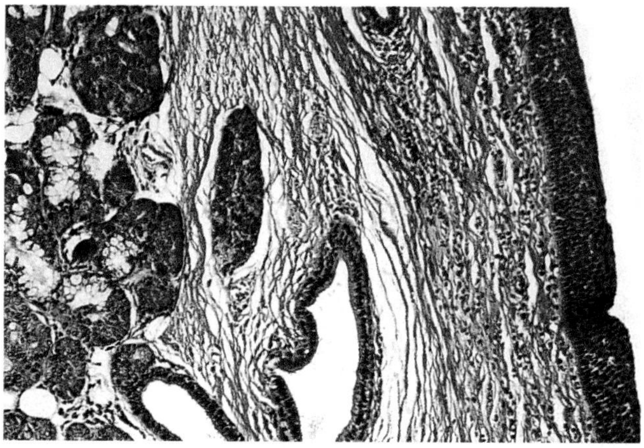

Figure 16.15 Seromucinous glands and their ducts are most prominent in the false cord.

cells have uniform nuclei with mitotic figures confined to the basal-most cell layer. This normal pattern can easily be confused with dysplasia or so-called carcinoma in situ, particularly in frozen sections or otherwise suboptimal preparations. Awareness of this transitional zone and attention to cytologic detail will avoid confusion.

Human papillomavirus (HPV) subtypes have been implicated in the pathogenesis of a variety of squamous proliferations in the larynx and elsewhere in the head and neck. Using sensitive polymerase chain reaction (PCR) techniques, studies are beginning to document some HPV subtypes, such as type 11 in approximately 25% of light microscopically normal laryngeal specimens (13). Thus, the finding of this HPV subtype adjacent to a laryngeal carcinoma cannot be assumed to represent a causative association. HPV subtypes more commonly associated with malignancy (HPV-16, HPV-18) have not yet been demonstrated in light-microscopically normal laryngeal mucosa.

Seromucinous glands are present throughout most of the larynx and communicate with the surface epithelium by ducts that are lined either by squamous cells, columnar epithelium (Figures 16.13 and 16.14), or a mixture of the two (14). The columnar epithelial component may or may not be ciliated. The glands are most abundant in the false cords (Figure 16.15), and there is also an extensive group of seromucinous glands just below the anterior commissure. Just superior to the anterior commissure is a narrow zone that is devoid of glands. In most cases, no glands are found beneath the squamous epithelium lining the free edge of the true vocal cords. Glands are present, however, beginning immediately at the squamocolumnar junction, both above and below the squamous epithelium of the true cords. Occasionally, there are glands in the stroma of the true vocal cord, and glands may be present in the underlying vocalis muscle (Fig-

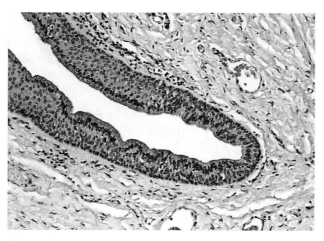

Figure 16.14 Ducts from seromucinous glands may be lined by squamous cells, ciliated columnar epithelium, or a mixture of the two.

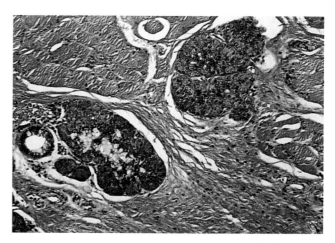

Figure 16.16 Seromucinous glands are occasionally located deep within the vocalis muscle.

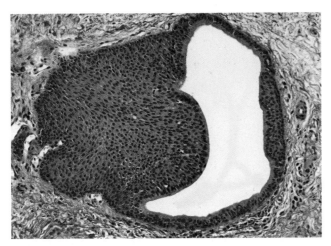

Figure 16.17 This seromucinous gland duct is associated with a large aggregate of metaplastic, nonkeratinizing squamous cells.

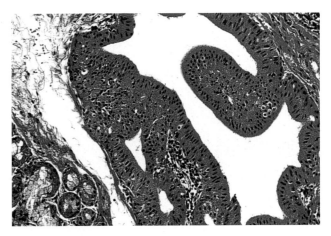

Figure 16.19 Oncocytic transformation of seromucinous epithelium can result in cystic structures.

ure 16.16). The fenestration in the elastic cartilage of the epiglottis are filled with abundant seromucinous glands. These glands penetrate completely through the cartilage and afford a ready path for the spread of supraglottic carcinoma.

Laryngeal biopsies, particularly from the region of the false cords, will often contain seromucinous gland ducts lined by squamous epithelium and located deep beneath the surface mucosa (Figure 16.17). Because of tangential sectioning, these ducts may appear as seemingly isolated squamous nests. Distinction from infiltrating carcinoma should not be a problem in adequately prepared sections. However, changes of basal cell hyperplasia or dysplasia also can involve these ducts. Fortuitous sections of such ducts may then result in seemingly isolated nests of basaloid or overtly dysplastic epithelium that are much more likely to be mistaken for invasive carcinoma (Figure 16.18).

Oncocytic metaplasia of ductal and acinar cells in the seromucinous glands of the larynx is a common, age-

related change. Oncocytes are not seen in the seromucinous glands of individuals younger than 18 years of age, but oncocytes are present in these glands in approximately 80% of people over the age of 50 (15,16). Uncomplicated oncocytic metaplasia is asymptomatic; but, occasionally, oncocytic metaplasia may become cystic (Figure 16.19) and, if sufficiently large, produce symptoms.

The seromucinous glands of the larynx may also undergo infarction and associated squamous metaplasia (Figures 16.20–16.21). The resultant process, termed necrotizing sialometaplasia, is much more common in the oral cavity and probably results from a traumatic or spontaneous ischemic event (17). The islands of metaplastic cells may be mitotically active and exhibit mild-to-moderate nuclear atypia. Confusion with mucoepidermoid or squamous cell carcinoma is common, particularly in frozen section specimens. At low-power magnification, the preservation of the acinar pattern, in association with infarction, inflammation, and extravasation of mucin, will aid in the correct diagnosis.

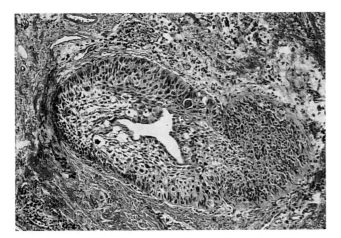

Figure 16.18 When ducts are involved with cytologically atypical squamous epithelium resembling surface dysplastic changes, they should not be misinterpreted as invasive carcinoma. In this example, the inner columnar cell lining is retained.

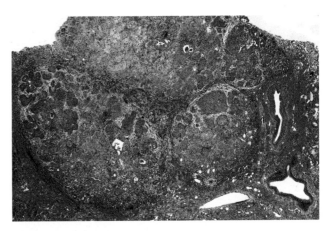

Figure 16.20 This low-power example of necrotizing sialometaplasia shows preservation of the pre-existing lobular architecture of the seromucinous glands.

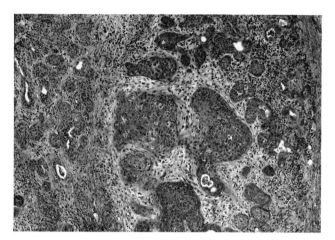

Figure 16.21 Higher magnification of necrotizing sialometaplasia shows replacement of the seromucinous lobules by aggregates of squamous cells with associated inflammation.

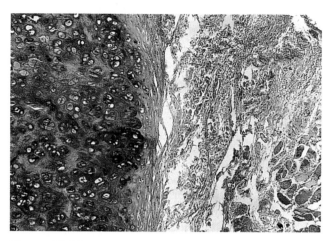

Figure 16.22 The vocal process of the arytenoid cartilage is a sharply circumscribed nodule of elastic-type cartilage. (From: Mills SE, Fechner RE. Pathology of the larynx. *Atlas of Head and Neck Pathology Series.* Chicago: American Society of Clinical Pathologists Press; 1985.)

If the external surface of the larynx is carefully sampled, it is not unusual to find microscopic islands of normal thyroid tissue within the fibrous capsule of the larynx and trachea, just external to the cricothyroid membrane (18). The thyroid follicles are small and appear normal, with well-formed colloid. Continuity with the main thyroid gland is not usually demonstrable (19). Less commonly, microscopic foci of thyroid tissue will be encountered internal to the cartilage of the larynx and trachea, usually at the junction of the cricoid cartilage and the first tracheal ring (18,20). These isolated foci of extrathyroidal thyroid tissue probably lose their connection to the main portion of the thyroid gland during embryologic development (18). Awareness of this phenomenon and attention to the microscopic features will avoid confusion with invasive or metastatic thyroid carcinoma.

The normal larynx contains at least two pairs of paraganglia. The superior, supraglottic paraganglia are sharply localized to the upper, anterior third of the false cords, in close approximation to the margin of the thyroid cartilage and the internal branch of the superior laryngeal nerves (21,22). The paired inferior paraganglia are more variably situated and may be found between the thyroid and cricoid cartilages or just below the cricoid cartilage (21,22). They are closely associated with the inferior laryngeal nerves. Aberrant or ectopic paraganglia have been described in various sites throughout the larynx. Laryngeal paraganglia are minute, neuroendocrine structures (0.1–0.4 mm) of unknown physiologic activity. Their close association with neurovascular bundles suggests chemoreceptor function, but this has not been proved. Laryngeal paraganglia presumably give rise to the rare paragangliomas of the larynx.

The vocal process of the arytenoid cartilage is a normal structure that is occasionally encountered in biopsy specimens from the posterior portion of the true cord. It is

a sharply circumscribed nodule of uniformly mature, elastic-type cartilage (Figure 16.22). Its elastic nature, demonstrable with appropriate elastin stains, allows distinction from cartilaginous neoplasms of the larynx, all of which are composed of hyalin-type cartilage. The sharp circumscription of the cartilaginous arytenoid process allows it to be differentiated from chondroid metaplasia of the vocal ligament. Chondroid metaplasia of the vocal cord is a common, usually asymptomatic, finding that typically affects the mid- and posterior portions of the vocal cord (23,24). The margins of the cartilage are blurred, and there is a peripheral zone of connective tissue that is rich in acid mucopolysaccharides (Figure 16.23) (24). The metaplastic nodules contain dense aggregates of elastic fibers throughout the lesion. The multilobular pattern, typical of cartilaginous neoplasms, is absent. Chondroid metaplasia can occur

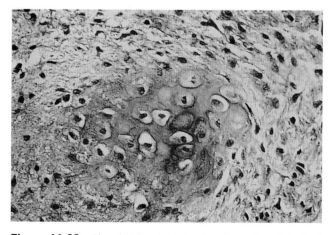

Figure 16.23 Chondroid metaplasia of the larynx has ill-defined margins. (From: Mills SE, Fechner RE. Pathology of the larynx. *Atlas of Head and Neck Pathology Series.* Chicago: American Society of Clinical Pathologists Press; 1985.)

in other soft tissues of the larynx, particularly in the region of the false cord. In one study, foci of chondroid metaplasia were found in 1 to 2% of larynges at autopsy (23).

Neural, Vascular, and Lymphatic Components

The intrinsic laryngeal muscles are innervated by branches of the vagus nerve. The cricothyroid muscle is supplied by the superior laryngeal branch of the vagus, and the remainder of the intrinsic musculature has been conventionally viewed as being innervated by the recurrent laryngeal branch of the vagus nerve. The terminal portion of the recurrent laryngeal nerve is referred to as the inferior laryngeal nerve (25). More recently, it has been shown that branches of the superior and recurrent laryngeal nerves form anastomoses, most commonly within the interarytenoid muscle but less consistently in the piriform sinus. Branches from the superior laryngeal nerve, referred to as the communicating nerve, may pass through the cricothyroid muscle to partially innervate the vocalis muscle (26,27). It has been suggested that the communicating nerve may be the nerve of the elusive fifth branchial arch (27).

The lower portions of the larynx are supplied with blood from the inferior laryngeal artery, a small branch of the inferior thyroid artery that accompanies the inferior laryngeal nerve. The inferior laryngeal artery has anastomoses with the larger superior laryngeal artery, derived from the superior thyroid artery. The laryngeal arteries are accompanied by similarly named veins. The superior laryngeal vein joins the superior thyroid vein and drains into the internal jugular vein (25). The inferior laryngeal vein joins the inferior thyroid vein. Numerous anastomoses across the front of the trachea between the left and right inferior laryngeal veins may lead to contralateral venous return (25).

The lymphatics of the larynx tend to drain along with the vasculature. Therefore, supraglottic lymphatics drain superiorly, and subglottic lymphatics drain inferiorly (1,25). As discussed earlier, lymphatics are scarce in the glottis. Some of the laryngeal lymphatics end in very small lymph nodes on the thyrohyoid membrane, cricotracheal ligament, or superior trachea (25). These nodes, however, drain into the deep cervical nodes (25). Lymphatics in the supraglottic larynx are prominent and, typically, terminate in the anterior jugular chain (28). Subglottic lymphatics terminate in the midline pretracheal nodes or, less commonly, in the lower cervical lymph nodes (28).

PHARYNX

Definition and Boundaries

The pharynx has three functionally and structurally dispersed subparts—the nasopharynx, oropharynx, and hypopharynx (Figure 16.24). The nasopharynx is the portion

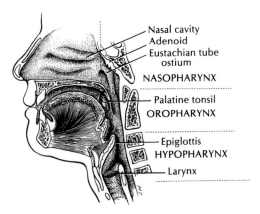

Figure 16.24 This sagittal section delineates the boundaries of the nasopharynx, oropharynx, and hypopharynx.

of the pharynx that lies above the soft palate. It has anterior, posterior, and lateral walls. The anterior wall is perforated by the posterior nares (choanae). The posterior wall is an arch that includes the roof of the nasopharynx, as well as the posterior portion against the base of the skull. The posterior wall extends inferiorly and, at the level of the horizontal projection of the soft palate, continues inferiorly as the posterior wall of the oropharynx. The anterior and posterior walls are connected by the lateral walls into which the eustachian (pharygotympanic, or auditory) tubes empty.

The oropharynx lies between the soft palate and the tip of the epiglottis. By definition, its superior boundary is a horizontal projection of the soft palate. Anteriorly, it is bounded by the fauces or opening from the mouth and, below this, the posterior aspect of the dorsum of the tongue. The inferior margin of the anterior portion of the oropharynx is marked by the opening of the piriform recess at the level of the tip of the epiglottis. A horizontal projection posteriorly from this point, marks the posterior aspect of the inferior margin, which is continuous with the hypopharynx.

The hypopharynx is the portion of the pharynx below the tip of the epiglottis and extending downward to the beginning of the esophagus. The hypopharynx is wide superiorly, but rapidly narrows as it approaches the level of the cricoid cartilage and becomes continuous with the esophagus. The hypopharynx partially surrounds the larynx laterally and is separated from it by the aryepiglottic folds. The latter extend from the upper posterior border of the larynx to the side of the epiglottis. The lateral extensions of the hypopharynx are called the piriform recesses or sinuses (25) (Figure 16.25).

Embryology

The embryologic pharynx is of endodermal derivation and, at its cephalic end, is in direct continuity with the ectoderm forming the stomodeum. Recent observations have

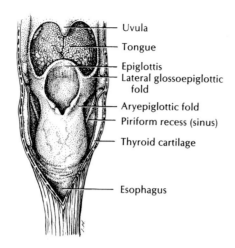

Uvula
Tongue
Epiglottis
Lateral glossoepiglottic fold
Aryepiglottic fold
Piriform recess (sinus)
Thyroid cartilage

Esophagus

Figure 16.25 The piriform sinuses are a conduit between the oropharynx and the opening of the esophagus. They surround the larynx laterally.

suggested that the development of the roof of the pharynx is highly dependent on the closely adjacent notochord (29). The stomodeum and pharynx are separated by the buccopharyngeal membrane, which is lined on its external surface by ectoderm and internally by endoderm. At the end of the third week of embryologic development, the buccopharyngeal membrane ruptures, establishing contact between the stomodeum and the primitive pharyngeal portion of the foregut (29,30). Superiorly, the buccopharyngeal membrane corresponds to approximately the level of the nasal choanae. In the subsequent fifth through seventh weeks of gestation, the primitive nasal cavity forms and enlarges, with formation and later rupture of the bucconasal membrane, establishing the final connection between the nasal cavity and pharynx (29). In the eighth through the tenth gestational weeks, the secondary palate develops behind the primary palate, ending the formation of the basic pharyngeal structures. At this point, however, the pharynx is proportionally quite small; and, after the tenth week of gestation, remarkable growth in this region occurs with enlargement of the pharynx and downward movement of the palate and tongue (29).

Thus, the lining of the nasal cavity and paranasal sinuses is of ectodermal origin and constitutes the so-called schneiderian membrane. The nasopharynx, oropharynx, and hypopharynx are, at least in large part, of endodermal origin. The sharp demarcation between endoderm and ectoderm at the level of the nasal cavity is of considerable practical importance. Certain neoplasms, such as angiofibromas and lymphoepitheliomas, are virtually confined to the endodermally derived nasopharynx. In contrast, schneiderian papillomas and intestinal-type adenocarcinomas arise from the ectodermally derived lining of the nasal cavity and paranasal sinuses; they do not occur in the nasopharynx.

Gross Anatomy

By nature of their boundaries and lack of resectability, the nasopharynx and oropharynx are practically never encountered as gross specimens. The roof of the nasopharynx is composed of mucosa overlying the basal portions of the sphenoid and occipital bones (25). The lateral and posterior walls of the nasopharynx are composed of the superior constrictor muscles and the pharyngobasilar fascia. The soft palate is the floor of the anterior portion of the nasopharynx: the only truly mobile portion of the nasopharynx (25). Although the opening between the nasopharynx and oropharynx is normally patent, the soft palate can be moved posteriorly and superiorly to completely separate the nasal and oral segments. This is important as a component of proper speech and to keep food and water out of the nasal region during eating and drinking.

The most important gross features of the nasopharynx encountered by pathologists are the pharyngeal tonsil, pharyngeal recess, and the eustachian tube openings. The pharyngeal tonsil, or adenoids, is a prominent, convoluted mass in the roof of the nasopharynx in children. (It typically atrophies in adults.) The pharyngeal recess, or Rosenmüller's fossa, is a mucosal-lined depression in the posterolateral portion of the nasopharynx. Just anterior to the recess, located in the lateral wall, is the ostium of the eustachian tube. This opening is surrounded on its superior and posterior aspects by mucosa-covered cartilage, the tubal torus, from the eustachian tube wall (25).

The superior portion of the anterior oropharynx is bounded by the fauces, or opening of the mouth into the oropharynx. The lateral walls of the fauces are composed, on each side, of the two tonsillar pillars, between which lies the palatine tonsil in the tonsillar fossa. The anterior tonsillar pillar is the palatoglossal arch. This structure curves downward and forward, from the soft palate to the tongue. The posterior tonsillar pillar, or palatopharyngeal arch, extends downward from the posterolateral border of the soft palate laterally along the pharyngeal wall. Each of the arches contains a similarly named muscle (25).

The palatine tonsil, more commonly referred to as simply the tonsil, varies tremendously in size, depending on its state of lymphoid reactivity. The surface of the tonsil is covered with epithelial-lined pits, the tonsillar crypts that pass into the underlying lymphoid tissue. Beneath the tonsil is the pharyngobasilar fascia, which sends branches of fibrous tissue into and around the tonsil, forming the so-called tonsillar capsule. Loose connective tissue between this capsule and the deeper superior constrictor muscle forms a plane of cleavage that facilitates surgical removal (25).

The parapharyngeal, or lateral pharyngeal, space is an important zone of loose connective tissue lying deep to the tonsil and lateral to the pharynx (Figure 16.26). This space is roughly pyramidal, with the base of the skull forming the base of the pyramid superiorly (18,25). Inferiorly, the apex

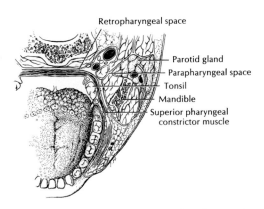

Figure 16.26 The parapharyngeal space lies deep to the tonsil and contains several vital structures. It is in continuity, posteriorly, with the retropharyngeal space.

is formed by the attachment of the cervical fascia to the hyoid bone; medially is the superior constrictor muscle of the pharynx; and, laterally, the pterygoid lamina, inner surface of the mandibular ramus, and the deep lobe of the parotid gland (18). Contained within the parapharyngeal space are the internal carotid artery, internal jugular vein, cranial nerves IX to XII, the cervical sympathetic chain, vagal and carotid bodies, and multiple lymph nodes (18). Mass-producing lesions involving any of these structures may cause medial displacement of the tonsil and lateral pharyngeal wall. Tonsilar abscesses or other sources of infection may also involve and rapidly spread throughout this space. Posteriorly, the parapharyngeal space is in direct continuity with loose connective tissue behind the pharynx and anterior to the prevertebral fascia of the vertebral column (25). This has been referred to as the retropharyngeal space (Figure 16.26).

Inferior to the fauces, the oropharynx is bounded anteriorly by the posterior aspect of the immobile portion of the tongue. The base of the tongue contains abundant submucosal lymphoid tissue that constitutes the lingual tonsil. Along with the palatine and pharyngeal tonsils, this structure forms an oblique wreath of lymphoid tissue that encompasses the oropharynx and nasopharynx and is often referred to as Waldeyer's ring.

The most important structures in the hypopharynx are the piriform sinuses (Figure 16.25). These elongated, pear-shaped gutters extend laterally along both sides of the larynx, and posteriorly from the pharyngoepiglottic fold to the opening of the esophagus (28). Laterally, the piriform sinus lies against the thyroid cartilage. Medially, it is separated from the laryngeal ventricle by a thin layer of muscles derived from the aryepiglottic fold and the opening of the esophagus (28). Just posterior and lateral to the piriform sinus is the common carotid artery. Because of their close association, tumors arising in the hypopharynx often invade the larynx secondarily. These tumors should be distinguished from primary laryngeal neoplasms because of their poorer prognosis.

Microscopic Anatomy

The nasopharyngeal mucosa in the adult has a surface area of about 50 cm^2. Most of it is lined by stratified squamous epithelium, and about 40% is covered by respiratory-type, columnar epithelium (31). Squamous epithelium predominantly lines the lower portion of the anterior and posterior nasopharyngeal walls, as well as the anterior half of the lateral walls. Ciliated respiratory epithelium predominantly carpets the region of the posterior nares (choanae) and the roof of the posterior wall. The remainder of the nasopharynx, including the posterior lateral walls and the middle-third of the posterior wall, has alternating islands of squamous and respiratory epithelium.

The junction between squamous and respiratory epithelium may be sharp, or there may be zones of transitional or intermediate epithelium as previously described in the larynx. We prefer the term *intermediate epithelium*, as opposed to *transitional epithelium*, because these cells lack the ultrastructural features of urinary tract epithelium. Intermediate epithelium primarily forms a wavy ring at the junction of the nasopharynx and oropharynx. The intermediate cells may be basaloid with minimal cytoplasm, and they typically have a cuboidal or round configuration. As discussed under the larynx, biopsy specimens containing intermediate epithelium must not be overly interpreted as areas of dysplasia or carcinoma in situ. This is most likely to be a problem when this zone is encountered in a frozen section.

In addition to the pharyngeal tonsil, less-prominent collections of lymphoid follicles may be present submucosally throughout the nasopharynx (Figure 16.27). These follicles are particularly abundant in the rim of the eustachian tube opening (Gerlach's, or tubal, tonsil), but they are also

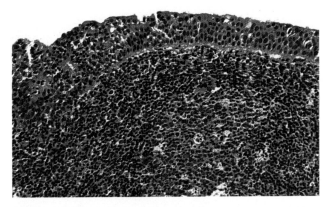

Figure 16.27 Submucosal lymphoid aggregates are present normally throughout the nasopharynx and should not be overly interpreted as severe chronic inflammation.

present under mucosa of the lateral and posterior walls of the nasopharynx, as well as on the nasopharyngeal surface of the soft palate (28). Thus, a submucosal follicular lymphoid infiltrate is normal in nasopharyngeal biopsies and should not be overinterpreted as a pathologic inflammatory process.

Throughout the nasopharynx, there are numerous submucosal seromucinous glands that produce predominantly mucin. These glands are particularly numerous in the region of the eustachian tube opening. As with the laryngeal seromucinous glands, oncocytic metaplasia in the glandular and ductal epithelium becomes increasingly frequent with advancing age (32,33).

The anterior portion of the pituitary gland forms from an intracranial invagination of epithelium in the form of Rathke's pouch. Microscopic remnants of Rathke's pouch epithelium are present in the roof of the nasopharynx in 95 to 100% of individuals (34–36). In most instances, this so-called pharyngeal pituitary is located in the midline, in the region of the vomerosphenoidal articulation. The nests of epithelial cells measure 0.2 mm to approximately 6 mm in greatest dimension. They are located deep in the mucosa or in the underlying periosteum (34). Most of the epithelial cells appear undifferentiated, but occasional basophilic and eosinophilic cells may be present (Figure 16.28). Although it is not entirely clear, the pharyngeal pituitary may not have any physiologic function. Most pituitary adenomas that involve the nasopharynx reach this location by invasion from the pituitary fossa. Occasionally, however, apparently ectopic pituitary adenomas present in the nasopharynx, and it is tempting to speculate that such lesions arise from the pharyngeal pituitary (37,38).

The pharyngeal bursa is a normal embryonic structure situated posterior to Rathke's pouch. Remnants of this bursa may be found in approximately 3% of normal adults (39,40). Cysts derived from this structure may be found in all ages, occasionally as an incidental finding, and occur in the regions of the adenoid (41). The cysts are separated

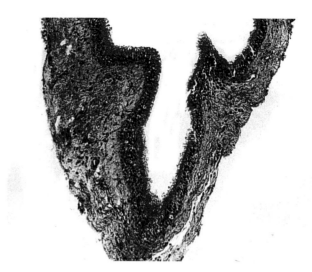

Figure 16.29 Nasopharyngeal cysts are rimmed by fibrous tissue and lined by ciliated columnar epithelium.

from the adenoid by a fibrous membrane and will not be removed with routine adenoidectomy specimens (Figure 16.29) (10). The median pharyngeal recess is a shallow depression formed normally in association with the pharyngeal tonsil. Unlike cysts derived from the pharyngeal bursa, those formed from the median pharyngeal recess are located within the adenoid and will be removed with it (10).

The cranial end of the embryonic notochord is closely associated with the roof of the developing nasopharynx (42). Although most of the notochord degenerates during embryonic and fetal development, notochordal remnants have been demonstrated in the submucosa of the nasopharynx and other closely adjacent locations (10,43). Most chordomas involving the nasopharynx are downgrowths of cranio-occipital tumors, but rare primary nasopharyngeal tumors presumably arise from these nasopharyngeal notochord remnants (42,43).

Both the oropharynx and hypopharynx are lined continuously by stratified squamous epithelium. This mucus is typically nonkeratinizing, although areas of parakeratin or orthokeratin may be seen secondary to chronic irritation. As in the nasopharynx, the submucosa of the oropharynx and hypopharynx contains scattered lymphoid aggregates, as well as prominent submucosal seromucinous glands.

The stratified squamous epithelium covering the tonsils extends into the tonsillar crypts for considerable distances. As these cords of epithelium merge with the underlying lymphoid tissue, the epithelial cells assume a more basaloid appearance and have uniform but vesicular nuclei. The junction between the lymphoid cells and the islands of squamous cells is often blurred (Figure 16.30). Apparently isolated, irregular nests of basaloid, focally keratinized squamous cells, often with vesicular nuclei, are common deep within the tonsil (Figure 16.31), and such nests must not be confused with carcinoma. Attention to the low-power

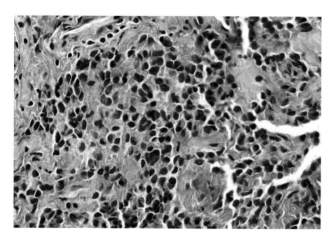

Figure 16.28 Nests of ectopic pituitary cells present in the superior portion of the nasopharynx.

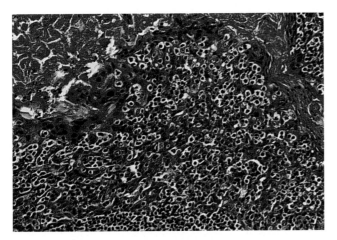

Figure 16.30 The junction between lymphoid tissue and the squamous cells lining the tonsillar crypts is often blurred.

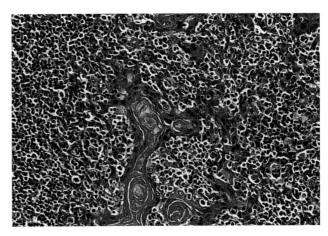

Figure 16.31 Irregular nests of epithelium are frequently present deep within the tonsil. These are closely approximated to tonsillar crypts and are a normal finding not to be misinterpreted as carcinoma.

architecture will confirm that these nests are closely approximated to tonsillar crypts and are a normal finding.

Occasionally, islands of metaplastic cartilage and bone are encountered within or immediately adjacent to the tonsils (18,44). This presumably represents a secondary, reactive change to prior inflammation. Eggston and Wolff (44) described this change in about one-fifth of all resected tonsils. These authors noted that patients with this change had an average age of 24 years and, therefore, were older than most individuals undergoing tonsillectomy (44).

Neural, Vascular, and Lymphatic Components

The nerves supplying the constrictor muscles of the phaynrx, the stylopharyngeus muscle, and the muscles of the soft palate are derived almost entirely from the pharyngeal plexus. The latter structure is formed by the union of the pharyngeal branches of the glossopharyngeal and vagus nerves.

The inferior constrictor muscle may receive a portion of its innervation from the external laryngeal nerve, a separate branch of the vagus that primarily supplies the larynx (25).

The blood supply to the superior portion of the pharynx is from the ascending pharyngeal artery, which runs upward along the posterior lateral wall of the pharynx (25) (Figure 16.32). The inferior portion of the pharynx is supplied by branches from the superior and inferior thyroid arteries. The veins draining the pharynx merge posteriorly to form the pharyngeal plexus, which in turn drains at irregular intervals into the pterygoid plexus and the superior and inferior thyroid veins (25).

The lymphatics from the roof and posterior wall of the nasopharynx join in the midline, and pass through the pharyngeal fascia. They then split to the right or left retropharyngeal lymph nodes. Some of the nasopharyngeal lymphatics terminate in the highest lymph nodes of the internal jugular and spinal chains (28). Most of the

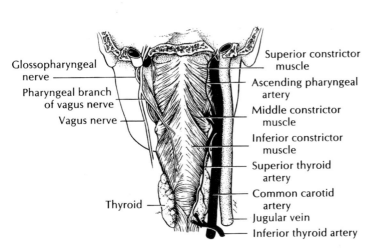

Glossopharyngeal nerve

Pharyngeal branch of vagus nerve

Vagus nerve

Thyroid

Superior constrictor muscle

Ascending pharyngeal artery

Middle constrictor muscle

Inferior constrictor muscle

Superior thyroid artery

Common carotid artery

Jugular vein

Inferior thyroid artery

Figure 16.32 Posterior view of the pharynx with emphasis on vascular and neural components.

lymphatics from the soft palate converge at a group of lymph nodes located below the anterior belly of the digastric muscle, immediately in front of the jugular chain (28). Lymphatics from the tonsil pass through the lateral wall of the pharynx and terminate in subdigastric nodes located anterior to the jugular chain (28). The hypopharynx is rich in lymphatics. These converge at an orifice in the thyrohyoid membrane, through which also passes the superior laryngeal artery. After exiting the thyrohyoid membrane, the lymphatics ramify into several trunks that terminate in lymph nodes of the internal jugular chain (28).

ACKNOWLEDGMENTS

The author thanks Linda Hamme for her expert artistic assistance and Joshua Weikersheimer, director of the American Society of Clinical Pathologists Press, for obtaining and allowing the use of several illustrations from Mills and Fechner (45).

REFERENCES

1. Bocca E, Pignataro O, Mosciaro O. Supraglottic surgery of the larynx. *Ann Otol Rhinol Laryngol* 1968;77:1005–1026.
2. Cotton A, Reilly JS. Congenital malformations of the larynx. In: Bluestone CD, Stool SE, eds. *Pediatric Otolaryngology.* Philadelphia: WB Saunders; 1983:1215–1224.
3. Stell PM, Gudrun R, Watt J. Morphology of the human larynx. III. The supraglottis. *Clin Otolaryngol* 1981;6:389–393.
4. Stell PM, Gregory I, Watt J. Morphometry of the epithelial lining of the human larynx. I. The glottis. *Clin Otolaryngol* 1978;3:13–20.
5. Andrea M, Guerrier Y. The anterior commissure of the larynx. *Clin Pathol* 1981;6:259–264.
6. Stell PM, Gregory I, Watt J. Morphology of the human larynx. II. The subglottis. *Clin Otolaryngol* 1980;5:389–395.
7. Hopp ES. The development of the epithelium of the larynx. *Laryngoscope* 1955;65:475–499.
8. Tucker JA, Vidic B, Tucker GF Jr, Stead J. Survey of the development of laryngeal epithelium. *Ann Otol Rhinol Laryngol* 1976;85(suppl 30, pt 2):1–16.
9. Scott GBD. A quantitative study of microscopical changes in the epithelium and subepithelial tissue of the laryngeal folds, sinus, and saccule. *Clin Otolaryngol* 1976;1:257–264.
10. Hyams VJ, Batsakis JG, Michaels L. Tumors of the upper respiratory tract and ear. *Atlas of Tumor Pathology*, 2nd ser, fasc 25. Washington, DC: Armed Forces Institute of Pathology; 1988.
11. Busuttil A. Dendritic pigmented cells within human laryngeal mucosa. *Arch Otolaryngol Head Neck Surg* 1976;102:43–44.
12. Goldman JL, Lawson W, Zak FG, Roffman JD. The presence of melanocytes in the human larynx. *Laryngoscope* 1972;82:824–835.
13. Nunez DA, Astley SM, Lewis FA, Wells M. Human papilloma viruses: a study of their prevalence in the normal larynx. *J Laryngol Otol* 1994;108:319–320.
14. Nassar VH, Bridger GP. Topography of the laryngeal mucous glands. *Arch Otolaryngol Head Neck Surg* 1971;94:490–498.
15. Lundgren J, Olofsson J, Hellquist H. Oncocytic lesions of the larynx. *Acta Otolaryngol* 1982;94:335–344.
16. Gallagher JC, Puzon BQ. Oncocytic lesions of the larynx. *Ann Otol Rhinol Laryngol* 1969;78:307–318.
17. Wenig BM. Necrotizing sialometaplasia of the larynx. A report of two cases and a review of the literature. *Am J Clin Pathol* 1995;103:609–613.
18. Michaels L. *Ear, Nose, and Throat Histopathology.* New York: Springer–Verlag; 1987.
19. Richardson, GM, Assor D. Thyroid tissue within the larynx. Case report. *Laryngoscope* 1971;81:120–125.
20. Bone RC, Biller HF, Irwin TM. Intralaryngotracheal thyroid. *Ann Otol Rhinol Laryngol* 1972;81:424–428.
21. Lawson W, Zak FG. The glomus bodies ("paraganglia") of the human larynx. *Laryngoscope* 1974;84:98–111.
22. Kleinsasser O. Das Glomus laryngicum inferior. Ein bisher. unnbekanntes, nicht chromaffines Paraganglion vom Bau der sog. Carotisdrüse im menschlichen Kehlkopf. *Arch Ohren Nasen Kehlkopfheilkd* 1964;184:214–224.
23. Hill MJ, Taylor CL, Scott GBD. Chondromatous metaplasia in the human larynx. *Histopathology* 1980;4:205–214.
24. Iyer PV, Rajagopalan PV. Cartilaginous metaplasia of the soft tissues in the larynx. Case report and literature review. *Arch Otolaryngol Head Neck Surg* 1981;107:573–575.
25. Hollingshead WH. *Textbook of Anatomy.* 2nd ed. New York: Harper & Row; 1967.
26. Sanders I, Wu BL, Mu L, Li Y, Biller HF. The innervation of the human larynx. *Arch Otolaryngol Head Neck Surg* 1993;119:934–939.
27. Wu BL, Sanders I, Mu L, Biller HF. The human communicating nerve. An extension of the external superior laryngeal nerve that innervates the vocal cord. *Arch Otolaryngol Head Neck Surg* 1994;120:1321–1328.
28. del Regato JA, Spjut HJ. Ackerman and del Regato's Cancer: *Diagnosis, Treatment, and Prognosis*. 6th ed. St. Louis: Mosby; 1985.
29. Sumida S, Masuda Y, Watanabe S, Nishizaki K, Slipka J. Development of the pharynx in normal and malformed fetuses. *Acta Otolaryngol* 1994;suppl 517:21–26.
30. Langman J. *Medical Embryology.* 2nd ed. Baltimore: Williams & Wilkins; 1969.
31. Ali MY. Histology of the human nasopharyngeal mucosa. *J Anat* 1965;99 (pt 3):657–672.
32. Morin GV, Shank EC, Burgess LPA, Heffner DK. Oncocytic metaplasia of the pharynx. *Otolaryngol Head Neck Surg* 1991;105:86–91.
33. Benke TT, Zitsch RP III, Nashelsky MB. Bilateral oncocytic cysts of the nasopharynx. *Otolaryngol Head Neck Surg* 1995;112:321–324.
34. Melchionna RH, Moore RA. The pharyngeal pituitary gland. *Am J Pathol* 1938;14:763–771.
35. Boyd JD. Observations on the human pharyngeal hypophysis. *J Endocrinol* 1956;14:66–77.
36. McGrath P. Extrasellar adenohypophyseal tissue in the female. *Australas Radiol* 1970;14:241–247.
37. Langford L, Batsakis JG. Pituitary gland involvement of the sinonasal tract. *Ann Otol Rhinol Laryngol* 1995;104:167–169.
38. Kikuchi K, Kowada M, Sasaki J, Sageshima M. Large pituitary adenoma of the sphenoid sinus and the nasopharynx: report of a case with ultrastructural evaluations. *Surg Neurol* 1994;42:330–334.
39. Hollender AR. The nasopharynx. A study of 140 autopsy specimens. *Laryngoscope* 1946;56:282–304.
40. Toomey JM. Cysts and tumors of the pharynx. In: Paparella MM, Shumrick DA, eds. *Otolaryngology.* Philadelphia: WB Saunders; 1980.
41. Nicolai P, Luzzago F, Maroldi R, Falchetti M, Antonelli AR. Nasopharyngeal cysts. Report of seven cases with review of the literature. *Arch Otolaryngol Head Neck Surg* 1989;115:860–864.
42. Binkhorst CD, Schierbeek P, Petten GJW. Neoplasms of the notochord. Report of a case of basilar chordoma with nasal and bilateral orbital involvement. *Acta Otolaryngol (Stockh)* 1957;47:10–20.
43. Batsakis JG. *Tumors of the Head and Neck: Clinical and Pathological Considerations.* 2nd ed. Baltimore: Williams & Wilkins; 1979.
44. Eggston AA, Wolff D. *Histopathology of the Ear, Nose and Throat.* Baltimore: Williams & Wilkins; 1947.
45. Mills SE, Fechner RE. Pathology of the larynx. *Atlas of Head and Neck Pathology Series.* Chicago: American Society of Clinical Pathologists Press; 1985.

Major Salivary Glands

Fernando Martínez-Madrigal   *Jaques Bosq*
Odile Casiraghi

INTRODUCTION

The primary function of the salivary glands is to moisten the mucous membranes of the upper aerodigestive tract. In humans, this function is fulfilled by the continuous exocrine secretion of numerous minor salivary glands. These glands are located in the submucosa throughout the oral cavity, pharynx, and upper airways. In developed species, most of the saliva is elaborated by three pairs of major glands, or salivary glands, named by their location: the parotid, the submaxillary or submandibular, and the sublingual glands. They are connected symmetrically to the oral cavity, where they empty their secretion only under specific stimuli. The saliva produced by these glands (750–1000 mL/24 hours) plays an important role in preparing food for digestion, as well as in controlling the bacterial flora of the mouth. The quality of the saliva produced by the major glands is variable and depends on both the stimuli and the predominant participating gland.

EMBRYOLOGIC AND POSTNATAL DEVELOPMENTAL CHANGES

Parotid Gland

During embryologic life, the parotid is the first of the three major glands to appear and is seen by the sixth week. It derives from the ectoderm as an epithelial bud from the primitive oral epithelium, at the angle between the maxillary process and the mandibular arch (1). As the primordia grow, they ramify into a bushlike system surrounded by mesenchymal tissue. This mesenchyma and, particularly, the basal lamina play an important role in the lobular organization of the gland (2–5), and in vascular and neural development. By the seventh week, the primitive gland moves in a dorsal and lateral direction and reaches the preauricular region. Development of the facial nerve divides the gland by approximately the tenth week into superficial and deep portions (6).

By the third month, the gland has attained its general pattern of organization. The epithelial structures are arranged in lobules, limited by a capsule of loose connective tissue (Figure 17.1A). The mesenchyma is then colonized by numerous lymphocytes that are later disposed in intraglandular and extraglandular lymph nodes. By the sixth month, the epithelial cordons are canalized and exhibit a double-cell ciliated cover. Cell differentiation begins in the excretory ducts with the progressive transformation of ciliated cells by columnar, squamous, and goblet cells (Figure 17.1B) (7). Intralobular duct and acinar differentiation, including myoepithelial cell formation, begins about the eighth month (8) and myoepithelial cell differentiation by the nineteenth- to twenty-fourth–week period. These cells,

arranged in the basal portions of the acini and intercalated ducts, appear as clear cells with electron microscopy. Between 25 and 32 weeks, the myoepithelial cells become flattened and show cytoplasmal prolongations (9–11). Saliva production starts as a mucinous liquid at this time; but several studies in rodents suggest that full maturation is completed only after birth (12–15).

The definitive location of the parotid is behind the inferior facial nerve maxillary branch, below and in front of the external ear. It is enclosed within a fibroadipose capsule in a depression whose anterior limit is the masseter muscle. Its superior limit is the zygomatic arch; the posterior limit is the tragus, and the inferior limit is the anterior border of the sternocleidomastoid muscle (16). The adult parotid is the largest of the three major salivary glands and weighs between 14 and 28 g. The gland is surrounded by a fine capsule and is divided into two portions by the facial nerve. The main portion, or superficial lobe, is flattened and quadrilateral; it is here that the majority of salivary tumors develop. This observation has permitted the development of conservative surgical treatment of many parotid tumors. The rest of the gland, called the deep lobe, is irregularly wedge-shaped in anatomic relationship with the parapharyngeal space (17).

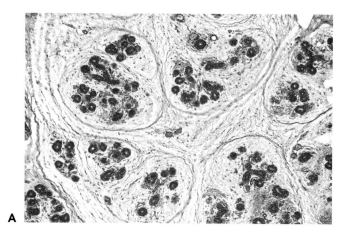

A

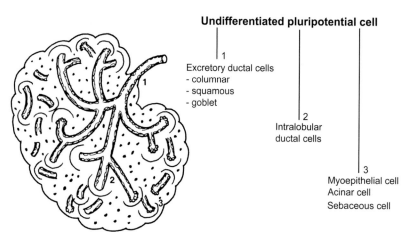

Undifferentiated pluripotential cell

1
Excretory ductal cells
- columnar
- squamous
- goblet

2
Intralobular
ductal cells

3
Myoepithelial cell
Acinar cell
Sebaceous cell

B

Figure 17.1 Development and histogenesis of the epithelial constituents of the salivary gland. **A.** Fetal parotid gland at 4 months; a lobular architecture is present. **B.** Drawing of (A), showing the cellular lines of differentiation for the excretory ducts, (1); excretory ducts, (2); intralobular ducts, (3); and acini.

The surgical anatomic area where the parotid gland is located, is called the parotid region. In this region it is important to keep in mind the anatomical relations between the facial nerve, the gland, and the subcutaneous planes. The facial nerve has four parts, designated as retro-, inter-, intra-, and preglandular. The parotid gland is covered by a superficial musculoaponeurosis and the skin (18). Accessory parotid tissue is found in approximately 20% of cases. Nevertheless, in a recent study, the incidence was found to be 56% with no differences between right and left sides or between sexes (19). This accessory tissue may be found on the anterior surface of the gland, as well as along the parotid duct (20).

Like all the exocrine glands, the parotid is composed of numerous tubuloacinar units connected through the excretory ducts to a main duct (Stensen's duct) located in the anterior portion of the gland. The parotid duct follows a twisted course of 7 cm, crossing the masseter muscle, the corpus adiposum of the cheek, and the buccinator muscle before opening into the oral vestibule. The secretion of the accessory parotid is emptied by an independent duct reaching the parotid duct in the masseter portion.

Blood supply is by arterial branches from the external carotid. The veins are tributaries of the external jugular, and the lymphatics join the superficial and deep cervical lymph nodes. Innervation is derived from the sympathetic and auriculotemporal nerves.

Submaxillary Gland

In the submaxillary gland, the primordia appear at the end of the sixth week and, unlike the parotid, are probably of endodermal derivation (21,22). However, a recent study suggests that the sublingual process of the submandibular gland originates from a lateral ectodermal bud of the anlage of the submandibular gland (23). The epithelial bud appears in the groove between the lower jaw and tongue, at one side of the midplane. Extension of the glandular tissue in the mesenchyma goes backward beneath the lower jaw. Subsequent maturation and cell differentiation are similar to those of the parotid gland except for the lymphoid tissue, which is less obvious than in the parotid. In addition, there is no lymph node formation inside the gland. Recent studies have demonstrated that the extracellular matrix protein fibronectin is essential for cleft formation during the initiation of epithelial branching in submaxillary gland. It has also been demonstrated that inhibition of fibronectin blocks cleft formation and branching (24,25). This mechanism could be applied for other salivary glands and other exocrine glands (such as the mammary glands).

The submaxillary gland is finely encapsulated; it lies inside the submandibular triangle, an osteofibrous cavity from which it takes the form of a triangular prism. This gland weighs approximately 7 to 8 g and, like the other major salivary glands, is organized in lobules connected to a main excretory duct—the submaxillary duct (Wharton's duct)—which measures 5 cm in length and 2 to 3 mm in diameter. The duct originates near the surface; runs between the mylohyoideus, the hyoglossus, and genioglossus muscles; and finally opens through a narrow orifice in a small papilla called the caruncula sublingualis on each side of the frenulum linguae. A submandibular gland having three ducts that open separately into the oral cavity has also been reported (26). The blood supply is from branches of the facial and sublingual arteries. The secretomotor nerves are fibers from the cranial parasympathetic branch of the facial nerve; the vasomotor nerves are derived from the superior cervical ganglion. The lymph nodes are arranged in a row in the spaces between the mandible and the gland and are disposed in anterior, medial, and posterior groups (16,17).

Sublingual Gland

The sublingual glands are the last of the three major salivary glands to appear. Their primordia are located immediately lateral to the submaxillary glands for the greater sublingual glands and in the linguogingival sulcus for the lesser sublingual glands. The epithelial buds grow downward from the groove between the lower jaw and the tongue. Parenchymal organization and differentiation are similar to those of the submaxillary gland and are also probably of endodermal derivation.

The principal sublingual gland weighs 3 g. It lies in the sublingual fossa of the mandible and is surrounded by loose connective tissue. Its secretion is drained through a main duct called the Bartholin's duct, which opens into the submandibular duct, and various small ducts (Rivinus' ducts) that open separately into the mouth in the plica sublingualis or join the submandibular duct (16,17).

Vascular supplies come from the sublingual and submental arteries; the veins are tributaries of the external jugular. Innervation is similar to that of the submaxillary gland.

APOPTOSIS

In the literature, studies concerning apoptosis in salivary glands are not very frequent. Contrary to other glandular tissue, programmed cell death in the salivary glands has been sporadically studied in less-developed and developed species, using experimental animals such as rats or monkeys and, less frequently, humans (27–29).

In normal salivary glands, apoptosis was uncommon when observed in acinar cells and epithelial duct cells and never observed in myoepithelial cells. In specific pathologic contexts, such as duct obstruction or irradiation of the salivary glands, programmed cell death was observed with many significant changes in the structure of the glands (30–31). In some salivary gland diseases, such as Sjögren's syndrome, accelerated apoptosis may explain acinar and ductal cell loss with the typical functional loss of the secretory activity seen in patients with this disease.

In experimental models, apoptosis is regulated by two kinds of protein families, bcl-2-related proteins and the inhibitor of apoptosis proteins (IAP). Activation of caspase-3 is inhibited by bcl-2 or Bcl-XL and accelerated by Bax. In addition, an X chromosome–linked inhibitor of apoptosis called XIAP inhibits caspase-3 activation. Several gene products induce apoptosis in salivary gland diseases (32–34). A particular focus has been put on the expression of Fas (CD95) and its ligand FasL (CD95L), which are members of the TNF (tumor necrosis factor) receptors superfamily. In Sjögren syndrome, contradictory results have been found so the importance of apoptosis in epithelial cell loss in these patients remains speculative (35–37).

Duct obstruction due to calculi or strictures induces salivary gland atrophy. Histologically, the disappearance of acinar cells within the presence of groups of ductlike structures in a fibrous and inflammatory stroma was observed. The acinar cells had disappeared by apoptosis; this acinar cell death was observed a few hours after duct obstruction. In the first cell death, a few days after duct obstruction, the number of intraepithelial macrophages located in the acinar and duct epithelium of a normal salivary gland multiplied. These macrophages removed the dying cells and apoptotic cellular fragments by phagocytosis, and then they migrated to the interstitium. Simultaneous proliferation of duct epithelial cells by an increase in mitosis contributed to the groups of ductlike structures with some features of squamous metaplasia. Myoepithelial cells became more prominent at the periphery of residual ducts. According to many experimental studies, myoepithelial cells become more prominent as the epithelial cell loss increases, and no myoepithelial cell apoptosis has been observed (38–45).

Irradiation of the major salivary glands is unavoidable during radiotherapy for many head and neck cancers. In fact, radiotherapy induced dryness of the oral cavity, contributing to deterioration of oral mucosa and loss of teeth.

The death of salivary gland acinar cells by apoptosis was observed within 24 hours after irradiation. This mode of cell death occurs with relatively low doses of radiation. An acute inflammatory response located among the destroyed acini was observed.

In normal adult salivary glands, cell division is infrequent in the acini. Development and replenishment of acini destroyed by low doses of radiation comes from stem cells that are located in the terminal intralobular ducts. It is possible that radiation-induced apoptosis of acinar cells could be a stimulus for replication of duct stem cells. However, the death of the ductal stem cells by high-dose radiation did not induce complete regeneration of the destroyed acini and resulted in atrophy of the salivary glands (46).

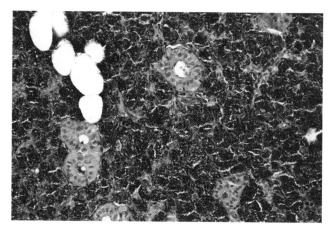

Figure 17.2   Serous-type acini of a parotid gland, with dense secretory granules.

LIGHT MICROSCOPY

The salivary glands are compound exocrine tubuloacinar glands characterized by the aggregation of numerous secretory units. These units consist of acini, where secretion is produced, and a duct system that carries the secretion to the oral cavity and regulates the concentration of water and electrolytes. There are three types of salivary secretory units: the serous ones that contain amylase; the mucous ones that secrete sialomucins; and mixed units made up of mucous and serous cells. According to the predominance of these types of secretory units, the salivary glands may be classified into three categories: serous, mucous, and mixed glands.

With the exception of some mucous units, the parotid gland is of the serous type (Figure 17.2). The submaxillary and the sublingual glands are mixed, with a predominance of serous units in the submaxillary glands (Figure 17.3) and

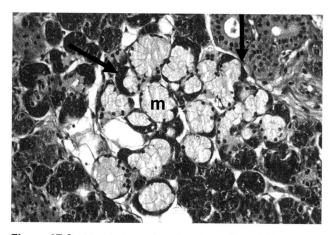

Figure 17.3   Histologic section of a submaxillary gland. In mixed units (*arrows*), serous cells are grouped in a crescent-shaped formation on the periphery of the acini, whereas the mucous cells (*m*) are in direct contact with the duct system.

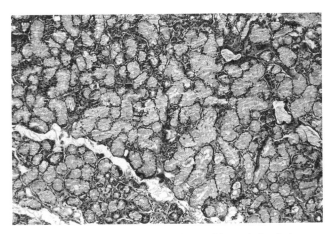

Figure 17.4 Mucous-type acini of the sublingual gland; they are larger and more irregular than the serous and mixed types. Note an inconspicuous duct system.

a mucous predominance in the sublingual glands (Figure 17.4). Mixed secretory units can be found in accessory parotid glands (19).

The lobular architecture of the glands is well defined by the anastomosed connective tissue trabeculae carrying the vascular and neural branches, as well as by the excretory ducts.

SECRETORY UNITS

Acini

Serous acini consist of pear-shaped groups of epithelial cells surrounded by a distinct basement membrane. The epithelial cells have a basal nucleus and dense cytoplasm packed with basophilic [periodic acid-Schiff (PAS)-positive] zymogen granules. They vary in number, depending on the different phases of the secretory cycle (Figure 17.2) (46). The primary enzyme present in the zymogen granules is amylase, or α–amylase, which splits starch into smaller water-soluble carbohydrates. However, there are other proteins in these granules, including agglutinin, proline-rich proteins, and histatins (47). Other enzymes, such as nonspecific antibacterial lysozyme, lactoferrin, trypsin- and chymotrypsin-like proteases, lysine endopeptidase, and histidine peptidase, also have been shown in the cytoplasm of acinar cells (47–51). Each acinus has a central lumen, rarely visible by light microscopy, through which the secretion drains into the intercalated ducts. The excretion seems to be promoted by the contraction of myoepithelial cells that lie between the outer surface of the acinus and the basement membrane. (Given the importance of myoepithelial cells in the pathology of salivary glands, a separate section, below, is devoted to their description.)

Mucous acini are larger than the serous type and have an irregular pattern (Figure 17.4). The secretory cells have abundant cytoplasm filled with clear mucous substance. They contain acid sialomucins (Alcian blue and mucicarmine-positive) and neutral sialmucins (PAS-positive) in different concentrations (52). The characteristics of these sialomucins also differ between submandibular and sublingual glands (53).

Mixed acini (Figure 17.3) are typically found in the submaxillary gland. These structures are characterized by the concentration of mucous cells near the intercalated duct and bordered by a crescent-shaped formation of serous cells. In mixed acini, the serous cells are more or less conspicuous, according to the amount of secretion accumulated in the mucous cells.

Ducts

A peculiar duct system transports the saliva from the gland to the oral cavity and modifies its water and electrolyte concentration. The first two segments, the intercalated and the striated ducts, are intralobular (Figure 17.5). They are also known as secretory ducts because of their metabolic activity (54). The other segments are interlobular and are called excretory ducts (54).

The intercalated duct lies directly in contact with the acinus. It is lined with a single layer of cuboidal epithelium and an irregular layer of myoepithelial cells. The epithelial cells show a progressive transformation between the secretory and ductal cells and a strong cytoplasmic activity of lactoferrin and lysozyme (55). The lengths of the intercalated ducts are variable in the three major glands (Figure 17.6). In the parotid gland, because they are relatively long, they are easy to recognize in the histologic sections (Figure 17.5A). In contrast, they are short in the submaxillary gland and hardly visible in the sublingual gland (Figure 17.4). Some authors have found undifferentiated cells on the basal side of the intercalated and striated ducts (56). These cells are positive for cytokeratins 13 and 16 on immunohistochemical staining (57,58).

The striated ducts are obvious in routine sections, particularly in the submaxillary gland, where they are relatively longer (Figures 17.3, 17.6). The epithelial lining is simple columnar. On the basal side, it has characteristic parallel striations caused by the deep cell membrane invaginations and mitochondria (Figure 17.5B). This structure represents a specialized surface on the epithelia involved in the transport of water and electrolytes. The numerous mitochondria are correlated with the strong eosinophilia of the duct. Various enzymes such as adenosine triphosphatase (ATPase), succinyl dehydrogenase, and carbonic anhydrase (59) are present in the cytoplasm of the striated ducts and provide them with a metabolic and energy system capable of concentrating some of the elements present in the saliva.

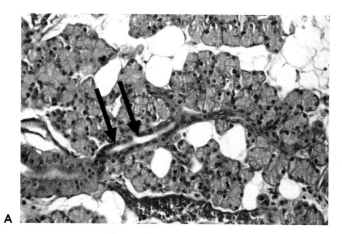
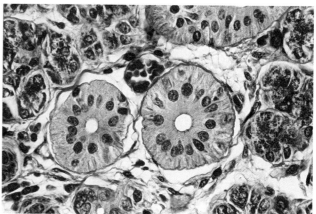

Figure 17.5 Parotid intralobular ducts. **A.** The intercalated ducts (*arrows*) (sectioned longitudinally) lie in contact with the acinus. **B.** The striated ducts (sectioned transversely) are lined with a columnar epithelium of basal-striated appearance.

The striated ducts are connected with the interlobular ducts located in the septal connective tissue. These ducts are lined with a columnar pseudostratified epithelium with sparse goblet cells (Figure 17.7). They become progressively larger before joining the principal duct. The principal function of interlobular ducts is to transport saliva, but their role in regeneration is proposed by means of the hypothetical undifferentiated pluripotential cells. In theory, these cells may follow the same cellular lines as in embryonic development (Figure 17.1B) and are perhaps implicated in the metaplastic and neoplastic alterations of salivary glands (60), which are more frequent in these ducts.

The principal duct consists of a thick external fibrous coat of collagen (similar to dermal collagen) and elastic fiber bundles. The epithelium is pseudostratified columnar and becomes squamous and stratified near the opening in the mucous membrane (Figure 17.8).

ULTRASTRUCTURE

At the electron microscopy level, the serous cells show all the characteristics of a specialized cell for secretion and export of proteins. The cytoplasm possesses abundant endoplasmic reticulum, Golgi vesicles, mitochondria, lipid droplets, and secretory granules (Figure 17.9). The last are more common on the apical side of the cell. They consist of a membrane, which encloses the secretion, and a matrix of low-electron density and homogeneous aspect in immature granules and high-electron density in mature granules (61,62). The electron density of the granules differs according to the package of the different proteins within the same granule (46). All the cytoplasmic organelles increase during protein synthesis and decrease during discharge (59). The basal surface of the cell shows numerous folds of plasma and basal membranes. They cover the entire cell base and

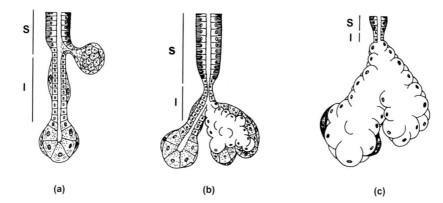

(a)   (b)   (c)

Figure 17.6 The morphology of the major salivary glands is characterized by three types of secretory unit. In the parotid (**A**) the intercalated duct (*I*) is longer than in the submaxillary (**B**) and sublingual glands (**C**). In contrast, the striated duct (*S*) is longer in the submaxillary gland. Sebaceous glands are more frequent in the parotid gland; in the sublingual gland. the intralobular ducts are inconspicuous.

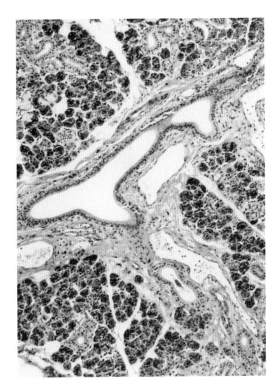

Figure 17.7 Interlobular duct adjacent to vessels in the septal connective tissue.

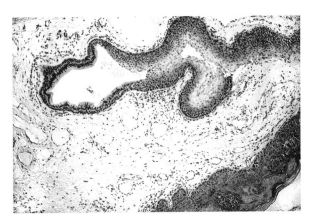

Figure 17.8 Main excretory duct in the caruncula sublingualis. Near the oral surface, the duct is lined with a squamous stratified epithelium.

extend beyond the lateral margins in the manner of foot processes. Therefore, the basal surface of the cell is greatly expanded, facilitating diffusion of materials into the cell (59). Most of the cytoplasm in mucous cells is occupied by mucous vacuoles and Golgi apparatus. Only a small basal and lateral portion of the cytoplasm contains endoplasmic reticulum and mitochondria (63).

At the apical pole, the secretory cells are joined by an adhesive zone, whereas the basal side is adhered by desmosomes (62). Between the junctions, virtual spaces form the secretory capillaries, which are in continuation with the acinar lumen. Numerous microvilli protrude into the capillary lumen (Figure 17.9).

The cytoplasm of myoepithelial cells may be separated into two portions (61): one, in contact with the basal lamina, is occupied by myofilaments and pinocytotic vesicles; the other portion is in contact with the secretory cell and contains mitochondria, endoplasmic reticulum, lysosome-like complexes, and Golgi vesicles. The visualization of myofilaments may vary in different myoepithelial cells; some of them have only focal aggregates of myofilaments, while others show a typical basal distribution resembling

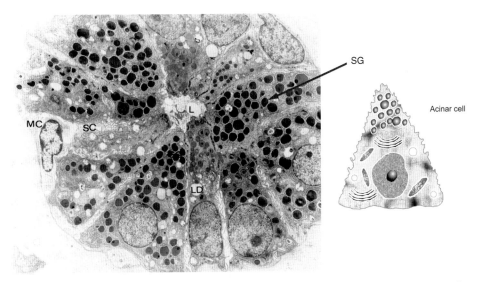

Figure 17.9 **A.** Ultrastructure of a parotid acinus: lumen (*L*), secretory granules (*SG*), lipid droplets (*LD*), secretory capillaries (*SC*), and myoepithelial cell (*MC*) (×6000). **B.** Drawing of an acinar cell.

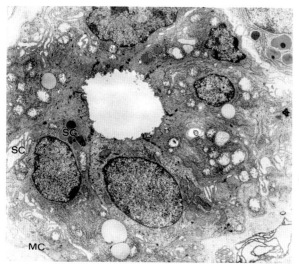

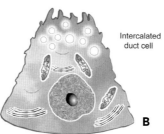

Figure 17.10   A. Intercalated duct of parotid gland. Some secretory granules (*SG*) and secretory capillaries (*SC*) are present on the apical side. On the external surface, myoepithelial cell prolongations (*MC*) are found (×10,300). **B.** Drawing of an intercalated ductal cell.

smooth muscle cells (62). The junction between myoepithelial and secretory cells is ensured by desmosomes.

Transition from acinus to intercalated duct is gradual. In the latter, epithelial cells have relatively large nuclei and few cytoplasmic organelles, consisting principally of mitochondria, some cisternae of endoplasmic reticulum, lipid droplets, and a few apical secretory granules (54,58) (Figure 17.10). Scattered secretory capillaries may be found, as well. On the external surface, myoepithelial cell prolongations are usually present.

The striated ducts (Figure 17.11) are composed of tall cylindrical cells with central nuclei. On the basal side, the cell membrane is extensively folded into fingerlike structures. The space between these folds is occupied by vertically oriented mitochondria. This cytoplasmic organization is specialized in the active transport of water and electrolytes from the vascular system to the lumen of the duct; the rest of the cytoplasm contains mitochondria and scattered endoplasmic reticulum (63–65).

SEBACEOUS GLANDS

In 1931, Hamperl (66) described the presence of sebaceous glands histologically similar to those of the cutaneous adnexa. Other authors have indeed recognized such structures, which appear as isolated cells in the wall of either an intercalated or a striated duct (Figure 17.12A) (67–70). Larger cell accumulations form a sebaceous gland limited by a well-defined basal membrane (Figure 17.12B–C). They vary in size, have a diverticular aspect, and are permanently linked to an interlobular duct. At the periphery of the gland, the cells are flattened with round or oval nuclei. The central cells have an abundant vacuolated cytoplasm rich in lipids, which may be stained, in frozen sections, with fat colorations (Sudan III and IV, oil red O, osmic acid). The nuclei become irregular or pyknotic and finally disappear. When the gland reaches a certain size, the holocrine-type secretion is emptied into the ductal system and is mixed with the saliva (Figure 17.12D).

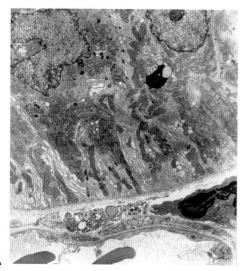

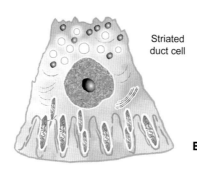

Figure 17.11   A. Striated duct cells possess vertically oriented mitochondria and extensively folded plasma membrane; the basal side is in close relationship to the blood capillary (×7920). **B.** Drawing of a striated duct cell.

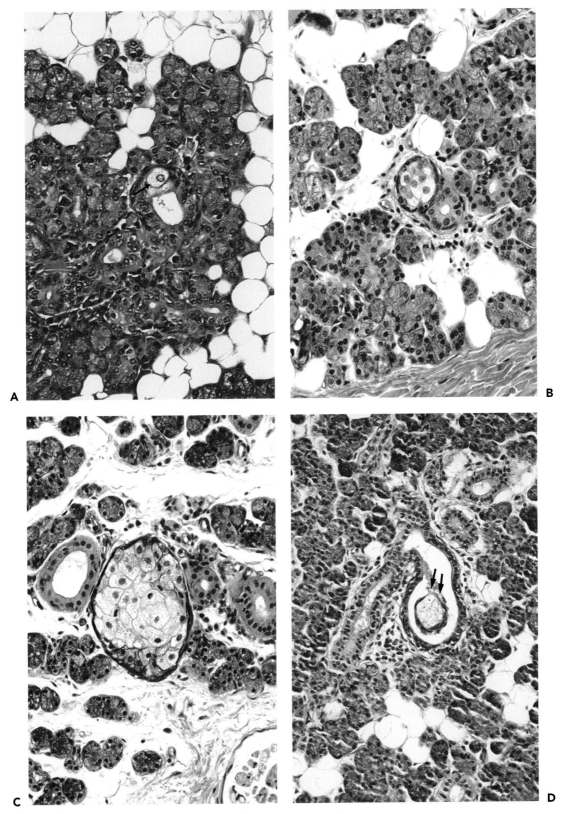

Figure 17.12 Sebaceous elements in a parotid gland. **A.** Isolated sebaceous cells can be seen in the duct wall (*arrow*). They proliferate to form a well-defined gland (**B, C**); secretion is present in the lumen of the duct (**D**) (*arrows*).

(continued)

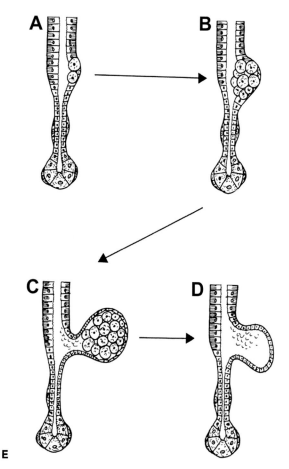

E

Figure 17.12 *(continued)* **E.** Drawing illustrates the previous features.

The number of sebaceous glands in major salivary glands varies; they are common in the parotid gland, rare in the submaxillary gland, and probably absent in the sublingual gland. They are diffusely scattered throughout the parenchyma, where their numbers also vary greatly. Their presence or absence in the different lobules is not related to either age or sex (70).

In a review of 100 parotid glands selected at random from our material, we found sebaceous glands in 42% of cases. They were also found in 5% of 100 submaxillary glands. These findings are in agreement with other authors. Thus, we conclude that their incidence in the parotid gland is more frequent than imagined. The more sections that are examined, the more sebaceous glands are found; it is, therefore, merely a question of looking for them. If the entire parotid gland were examined meticulously, it would be difficult not to find a sebaceous gland (69).

The presence of sebaceous glands in the salivary tissue has not been satisfactorily explained. A heterotopic phenomenon (67,68) similar to the occurrence of sebaceous glands in the oral mucosa (Fordyce's disease) seems

unlikely. In the mouth, this condition may result from aberrant buds along the fetal line of closure (70–72); but in the parotid and submaxillary glands, there are no lines of closure. Metaplasia (66,70) beginning in the ducts does not explain the high frequency of sebaceous glands in parotid parenchyma. Therefore, it seems reasonable to consider the sebaceous glands as a normal holocrine differentiation. Their occurrence in the parotid gland appears to be related to a specific function that is not yet understood. Sebaceous glands analogous to those of the salivary glands have been found in the oral mucosa. In the oral mucosa, androgen receptors participate in the histogenesis of sebaceous glands (73–74). A similar mechanism may be proposed for the histogenesis of sebaceous glands in salivary glands.

The belief that a potential for sebaceous differentiation exists in the salivary parenchyma is further supported by the fact that salivary tumors or tumorlike conditions with a sebaceous character or sebaceous gland participation have been described. These rare lesions include sebaceous adenoma, sebaceous lymphadenoma, sebaceous carcinoma, and parotid cyst. They have also been noted in pleomorphic adenoma and mucoepidermoid carcinoma (69,74–87).

MYOEPITHELIAL CELLS

Myoepithelial cells (basket cells) are derived from early modification and differentiation of primitive pluripotential salivary duct cells by the tenth week of gestation. It has also been suggested that the precursor of myoepithelial cells are the clear cells located in the terminal and striated ducts (63). In regeneration, these cells migrate from the acinar periphery to the duct-acinar region (32).

These cells lie between the epithelial cells and the basal lamina of acini, in the intercalated ducts, and probably also in the union of the striated and intercalated ducts (56,87,88). The cells are flat and have long cytoplasmic processes extending over the epithelial surface (Figure 17.13) in a network that makes it difficult to discern them in routine histologic sections. However, myoepithelial cells may assume morphologic modification at different anatomic locations within the ductal acinar structure (56,64). These cells are best studied by electron microscopy.

The most outstanding characteristic is the presence of cytoplasmic filaments on the basal side. Most of these consist of the myofilaments actin, tropomyosin, and myosin (63,88–90), which are arranged in a pattern similar to that of the smooth muscle. Tonofibril-like bundles of intermediate filaments are attached to the cellular junctions, particularly in desmosomes where the filaments are cytokeratin. Some forms of myoepithelial cells may also show scattered, rather than basal, cytoplasmic distribution of these filaments, which may reflect structural and functional morphology of many salivary neoplasms and in the morphologic variability of some tumors (106).

The Role of Myoepithelial Cells in Salivary Gland Tumors

The presence of myoepithelial cells in different histologic types of salivary gland tumors (Table 17.1) is well documented, as is the role of these cells in the pathogenesis and in its biologic behavior.

The role of myoepithelial cells in the histogenesis of the pleomorphic adenoma has been extensively studied. This tumor, sometimes called a mixed tumor because of the epithelial and mesenchymal mixture of tissues, is the most frequent neoplasm of the major salivary glands (107,108). It is now accepted that myoepithelial cells play a crucial role in the neoplastic process by expressing both epithelial and mesenchymal structures in the majority of pleomorphic adenomas (109–117). The participation of the contractile elements is also accepted in epithelial-myoepithelial carcinoma [clear cell carcinoma, a malignant tumor that mimics the normal structure of the intercalated duct (118–123)] and myoepithelioma [in which the myoepithelial cells are the only tumoral element showing different cellular forms (124–129)]. They also have been demonstrated in terminal duct adenocarcinoma (polymorphous low-grade adenocarcinoma) (130,131); monomorphic adenoma, which includes basaloid monomorphic adenoma (132–134); adenoid cystic carcinoma (96,100,113,135–138); and basaloid adenocarcinoma (139). Myoepithelial cell participation is also present in congenital tumors of salivary gland origin, such as sialoblastoma (140) and the salivary gland anlage tumor (141). Although there are rare reports of myoepithelial cells in mucoepidermoid carcinoma (135,142), it is difficult to fully accept these statements because mucoepidermoid carcinoma arises from a ductal segment that lacks myoepithelial cells.

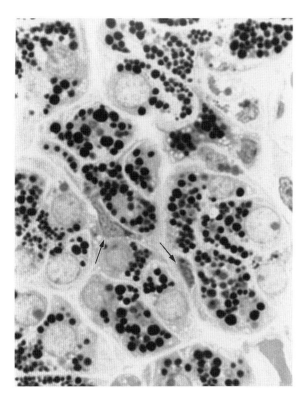

Figure 17.13 Myoepithelial cells (*arrows*) on the acinic surface (semithin section, toluidine blue).

differences (64). The presence of vimentin is not constant, and the filament desmin is absent in normal myoepithelium (91). The cytoplasm shows a strong activity of ATPase and alkaline phosphatase (92,93).

It is generally accepted that myoepithelial cells are contractile. This function speeds up the outflow of the saliva by increasing the pressure on the excretory unit (94). It has been extensively studied in the mammary gland of the rat, where these cells are more frequently found. Oxytocin-induced contraction in the myoepithelial cells is similar to that of true muscle cells (95). The presence of myofilaments in the cytoplasm of these cells correlates strongly with this function. In addition, myoepithelial cells support the underlying parenchyma and participate in the elaboration of the basal lamina. This last function is important in some hyperplastic and neoplastic alterations, where the myoepithelial cells produce fibronectin, laminin, and type III collagen (96–103). All these proteins are constituents of the basal lamina (104). In addition, myoepithelial cells are also involved in the production of tenascin, an extracellular matrix glycoprotein (105,106).

Regardless of endodermal or ectodermal origin, the myoepithelial cells share an epithelial and mesenchymal structure and function. Altered myoepithelial cells may manifest (in neoplastic proliferation) one or both characteristics. These cells are now considered the key factor in the

TABLE 17.1
SALIVARY GLAND TUMORS WITH MYOEPITHELIAL CELL PARTICIPATION

Benign tumors	Myoepitheliomas
	Pleomorphic adenoma
	Basaloid adenomas
Malignant tumors	Epithelial-myoepithelial carcinoma
	Adenoid cystic carcinoma
	Polymorphous low grade adenocarcinoma
	Basaloid carcinoma
Congenital tumors	Sialoblastoma
	Salivary gland anlage tumor

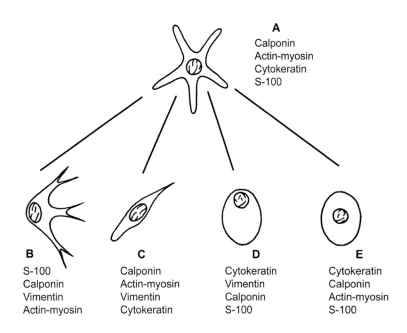

Figure 17.14   Morphology and histologic markers of the normal (**A**) and modified myoepithelial cells (**B–E**). The most constant markers are present in order of frequency: chondromyxoid type (B), spindle-shaped type (C), hyalin or plasmocytoid type (D), and epithelial (clear) type (E).

The principal morphologic types of altered myoepithelial cells are (Figure 17.14):

1. Stellate or myxoid cells, which are typically present in chondromyxoid areas of pleomorphic adenoma.
2. Spindle-shaped or myoid cells, which can be identified in pleomorphic adenoma and some types of myoepithelioma.
3. Hyalin or plasmocytoid cells (143), which can be seen in pleomorphic adenomas and can be present in myoepitheliomas. These cells show abundant cytoplasmic filaments that give a hyalin eosinophilic aspect.
4. Clear or epithelial cells, which are found in many salivary tumors on the external surface of ducts or ductlike structures. This is also characteristic in epithelial-myoepithelial carcinoma.

Bidirectional differentiation of the modified myoepithelium has been well documented. Myoepithelial cells with mesenchymal characteristics secrete mesenchymal mucins such as the acid glycosaminoglycans (hyaluronic acid, heparin sulfate, chondroitin-4-sulfate, and chondroitin-6-sulfate) (144,145), basement membrane constituents, elastin (111,112), and tenascin (105). In addition to contractile filaments (actin and myosin) and related proteins such as calponin, vimentin becomes strongly positive, particularly in spindle-shaped form (138–140,146–148). The S-100 protein, which is a common marker used for the myoepithelium, enhances its positivity in chondroid, myxoid, and stellate cells, particularly if they are associated with a myxoid stroma (104,149–150). Plasmocytoid myoepithelial cells are frequently negative for the muscular markers (151). However, these cells express several ultrastructural and immunomarkers characteristic of myoepithelial cells (127). On the other hand, epithelial differentiation may

take the form of clear or squamous cells, which can contain both vimentin and keratin filaments in the same cell (110). Figure 17.14 illustrates the histologic and immunohistochemical patterns of modified myoepithelium.

Myoepithelial cells are a central element in the histologic formation and organization of different salivary gland tumors. The cytomorphologic features and the variability of the extracellular products account for the morphologic heterogeneity of these lesions. The presence of these cells varies widely, from minimal as in monomorphic adenomas (136), to marked, as in myoepitheliomas. Evidence of the protective effect of myoepithelial cells in malignant tumors is growing. Protease inhibitors like maspin, α1-antitrypsin, TIMP-1, and nexin II are anti-invasive factors produced by the myoepithelial cells in myoepithelial cells rich tumors (152–153). Now it is well accepted that malignant tumors with important myoepithelial cell components behave less aggressively. Myoepithelial carcinoma tends to be lobulated tumors rather than infiltrating, and patients with myoepithelial carcinoma show a better survival when they are compared to carcinomas that do not express myoepithelial cell differentiation. In addition, there is also evidence that myoepithelial cells may inhibit angiogenesis (154).

LYMPHOID TISSUE

The immune system of salivary glands comprises two elements of the mucosa-associated immune system. One is the secretory component, a glycoprotein receptor for dimeric IgA and pentameric IgM that is produced by epithelial cells in the acini, intercalated ducts, and striated ducts (155–156). The other element is lymphoid tissue, which is either distributed diffusely or organized in lymph nodes. Isolated

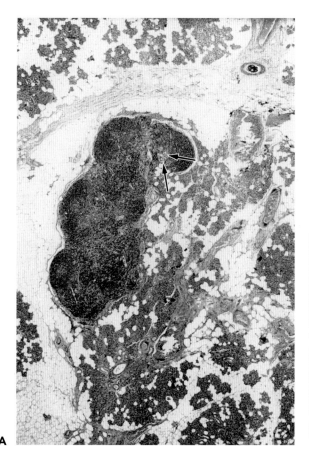

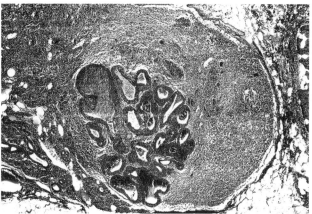

Figure 17.15   Lymph node of the parotid gland. **A.** Presence of glandular ducts in the medullary region (*arrows*). **B.** Duct dilatation and oncocytic transformation in another lymph node of the same patient.

lymphoid cells are present in the connective tissue near the acini and ducts. They are variable in number in the different glands (157) and yield principally IgA (nearly 80% of the immunoglobulins in saliva), along with a lesser quantity of IgG and IgM (159). Small lymph nodes are usually present near the surface of the parotid gland but not in the other salivary glands. Nevertheless, lymphoid cell aggregates are present in fetal submandibular and sublingual glands (158). These nodes usually contain salivary ducts and acini in the medullary region (Figure 17.15A), a phenomenon probably due to the close relationship between developing gland and lymphoid tissue during embryonic life.

Lymph nodes are thought to participate in the histogenesis of Warthin's tumor. Although they have been pinpointed as the origin of the lymphoid tissue that characterizes this neoplasm, the hypothesis is still under debate. Different mechanisms have been proposed, but the most widely accepted one states that the lesion originates from the ducts inside lymph nodes within or adjacent to the parotid gland (85,160–162). According to this concept, the epithelial component of the tumor corresponds to altered ducts inside a lymph node, and the lymphatic component is, in fact, a lymph node. The following arguments support this hypothesis: salivary tissue is frequently present in intraparotid or periparotid lymph nodes (Figure 17.15A); with the exception of a few cases, this tumor

is exclusive to the parotid region; it is common to find early stages of oncocytic and papillary transformation in lymph nodes of the parotid region (Figure 17.15B); and, finally, tumors identical to the epithelial structure of Warthin's tumor occur outside the lymph nodes but without lymphocytic components (160).

The diffuse lymphoid tissue may increase in chronic sialadenitis, particularly in immunologic reactions such as the benign lymphoepithelial lesion associated with Sjögren's syndrome. In these instances, lymphoid tissue may obscure the glandular parenchyma in a diffuse or nodular manner, and epimyoepithelial islands may be formed (91,160). The polyclonal character of the lymphoid cells and the presence of epimyoepithelial islands are useful criteria in the differential diagnosis of malignant lymphoma, which can occur in a preexisting benign lymphoepithelial lesion (162).

THE HETEROTOPIC SALIVARY TISSUE AND ITS SIGNIFICANCE

The presence of salivary tissue outside the major salivary glands and the oral cavity, pharynx, and upper airways is considered heterotopia. This heterotopia may be classified as intranodal and extranodal in a number of locations in the head and neck.

Heterotopia is common in the lymph nodes near the parotid gland but is much less frequent in the submaxillary region and in other upper cervical nodes (163–164). The glandular elements are either normal or atrophic; they consist mainly of ducts, but acini are also found. They are localized in the medullary region and comprise a variable proportion of lymphoid and salivary tissues. Although all types of secretory units are found, serous ones are predominant. The histologic architecture is similar to a normal gland. The lymph nodes exhibit a normal structure or some degree of lymphoreticular hyperplasia.

The incidence of heterotopic salivary tissue in the lymph nodes has been well documented (165). It is typically found in the parotid region of fetuses during various stages of development, usually in more than one lymph node. In adults, although the incidence is not constant, it is nonetheless frequent (166). In most of the reports, the histogenetic mechanisms of this phenomenon have been related to embryonic development. From this point of view, the salivary tissue is trapped during embryologic development. In the fetus, the parotid gland is closely related to lymphoid tissue from the beginning of the second month. Moreover, Bairati (166) found that, at least in the first years of life, this salivary tissue is connected to the parotid gland. Although lymphatic dissemination has been proposed as a mechanism of salivary heterotopia in lymph nodes, in particular when they are located in the lower neck, this hypothesis is only speculative (167).

Extralymphatic heterotopias are rare and often latent but may be responsible for symptomatology. Heterotopic salivary tissue has been described in several sites, including head and neck, thorax, and abdomen (Table 17.2). In the upper neck, heterotopia is limited to the mandible, ear, palatine tonsil, mylohyoid muscle, pituitary gland, and cerebellopontine angle (164,168–169). All these sites, with the exception of the last, may be related to the embryonic migration of the salivary glands. In the lower neck, heterotopias

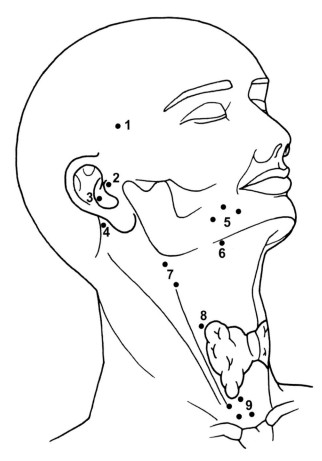

Figure 17.16 Extranodal salivary heterotopias. Pituitary gland (*1*), middle ear (*2*), external auditory canal (*3*), cerebellopontine angle (*4*), mandible (*5*), oropharynx (*6*), cervical superior (*7*), thyroid capsule (*8*), and lower anterolateral neck (*9*).

are localized in the base of the neck, particularly around the sternoclavicular joint and in the thyroid gland and parathyroid glands (Figure 17.16) (167,171).

Most examples of high salivary heterotopia are explained in relation to lines of migration of the parotid and submaxillary glands. In the mandible, the presence of salivary heterotopia may be related to a bone cavity and usually contains submandibular gland tissue. These inclusions are most common in the posterior lower jaw, near the angle. Originally described in 1942 by Stafne, they are often considered as heterotopias (172). This defect may be found in the anterior position (173). A recent study showed the heterotopic salivary tissue is present in 0.3% of maxillofacial marrow samples. The origin of this tissue is a matter of debate, but the most accepted hypothesis is the metaplasia of the odontogenic epithelial lesions (174). In the lower neck, an association with cysts and sinuses is frequent. This condition, along with the topographic presentation, has been related to the branchial apparatus (164,170) and, in particular, to a defective closure of the precervical His's sinus. The different abnormalities related to this defect (175) correspond embryologically to topographic distribution

---

TABLE 17.2

SALIVARY GLAND HETEROTOPIAS

Lacrimal gland
Pituitary gland
External auditory canal
Middle ear
Cerebellopontine angle
Upper neck
Thyroglossal duct
Thyroid gland
Parathyroid gland
Mediastinum
Stomach
Rectum
Prostate gland

through the neck from the ear to the clavicle. When this defect occurs, the salivary tissue is the result of abnormal tissue differentiation (heteroplasia). Willis (176) has argued that this is the mechanism of heterotopia. This mechanism may also account for the salivary tissue in remnants of Rathke's pouch (169) and the thyroglossal duct.

Neoplastic transformation in heterotopic salivary tissue may pose a problem in differential diagnosis of metastasis in a cervical lymph node (163). Pleomorphic adenoma, mucoepidermoid carcinoma, and adenoid cystic carcinoma are the most frequent tumors arising in heterotopic salivary tissue. In fact, heterotopia is an explanation for many aberrant salivary tumors (167,177) and some cervical lymph node metastases that are thought to be metastases of an unknown primary tumor (178). Primary salivary tumors of the mandible may originate in this aberrant tissue (179).

AGING CHANGES

Oncocytes

The oncocyte is an altered swollen epithelial cell characterized by an abundant eosinophilic granular cytoplasm that is rich in altered mitochondria and enzymes (Figure 17.17A) (180). This cell is frequently present in interlobular ducts

and is less frequent in acinar cells. Oncocytes are more common in the parotid gland. They are rare before 50 years of age, increase in frequency with advancing years, and become constant after 70 years (66,181). Oncocytes may be detected by histochemical methods using phosphotungstic-acid hematoxylin or by more specific immunohistochemical methods with antibodies to human mitichondria (182).

The nature and function of oncocytes are unknown. Their proliferative character is a common finding in organs with endocrine function or endocrine dependence (183). Numerous researchers are presently interested in the production of various peptides with endocrine function in the intralobular ducts of rodent salivary glands (184–186). On the other hand, a number of workers are investigating the presence of neuroendocrine peptides such as the substance P–like, β-endorphin–like (187,188), and a calcitonin-related peptide (189). In addition, neuroendocrine regulation of inflammation by the submandibular gland has been explained by an immunoneuroendocrine communication controlled by cervical sympathetic nerves (190).

The proliferation of oncocytes is called oncocytosis or oncocytic metaplasia when it is diffuse and generally without pathologic significance. In other cases, this proliferation presents a nodular pattern known as nodular hyperplasia (191). Histologically, it is easy to distinguish in the

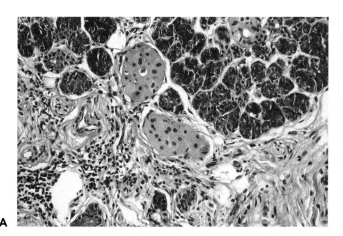

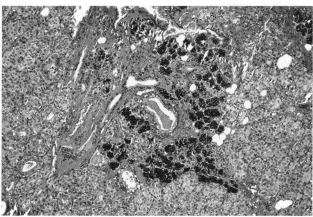

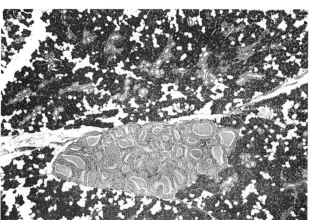

Figure 17.17   A. Oncocytes in intralobular ducts of a normal submaxillary gland. Note the abundant and granulated cytoplasm. **B.** Nodular oncocytic hyperplasia. **C.** Diffuse oncocytosis.

salivary parenchyma as one or several small foci of onco-cytes that are well circumscribed but not encapsulated. The cells may be arranged in solid cords or ductal structures and, in rare cases, may replace most of the gland (Figure 17.17B–C). Oncocytes participate in various salivary gland tumors in approximately 10% of cases (192); the most common is Warthin's tumor, and they are also observed in basal cell adenoma, pleomorphic adenoma, myoepithelioma, polymorphous low-grade adenocarcinoma, mucoepidermoid carcinoma, and acinic cell carcinoma (193–196). The neoplastic proliferation called oncocytoma is rarely found in salivary glands (197).

Fatty Infiltration

Normally, some adipose cells are present in the areolar connective tissue of the salivary glands. This fatty tissue increases in adults; in the elderly, it forms an important proportion of salivary gland tissue. Fatty infiltration may reach huge proportions, especially in alcoholics and the malnourished (198).

REACTIVE CHANGES

Metaplasia

Squamous metaplasia may be present in larger salivary ducts in chronic inflammatory processes, particularly when associated with calculi (Figure 17.18A) (199). (Remember that when the major salivary ducts open into the oral cavity, they are lined with a stratified squamous epithelium). Metaplastic squamous transformation is also present in intralobular ducts and acini in ischemia and radiation injury (200–201).

Mucous metaplasia is found on interlobular ducts and, less frequently, on intralobular ducts in cases of obstructive and postradiotherapy forms of sialadenitis (202). An important proliferation of mucous goblet cells is accompanied by prominent ciliated cells mimicking the respiratory epithelium (Figure 17.18B). Necrotizing sialometaplasia is a type of metaplasia peculiar to salivary tissue, but it is exceptional in major salivary glands (Figure 17.19) (203). It consists of ischemic lobular infarction or necrosis of some acini, accompanied by extensive squamous metaplasia of salivary gland ducts and acini. Severe inflammation and granulation tissue are present. Necrosis of mucous acini is represented by small pools of mucin that, along with the squamous elements, may be mistaken for mucoepidermoid carcinoma (204). The preservation of general lobular morphology and prominent granulation tissue are criteria in favor of benignity. Subacute forms are also described (205).

Hyperplasia

Hyperplasia of mucous acini is an alteration exclusive to the minor salivary glands. In contrast, serous hyperplasia occurs in parotid and, rarely, in submaxillary and sublingual glands; it is called sialadenosis (206). This hyperplasia is associated with a number of metabolic, nutritional, and endocrine conditions or follows the ingestion of chemicals and drugs (207). In most cases, a bilateral swelling of the glands is caused by enlarged acini and an accumulation of secretory granules in the cytoplasm. In other cases, granulation is lost and the cytoplasm looks vacuolated (22). The myoepithelial cells may present nuclear pyknosis or cytoplasmic vacuolation. Adenomatoid salivary gland hyperplasia should be distinguished from true tumors. Recently, adenomatous ductal proliferation in salivary glands has been described; these cases may be misdiagnosed as true adenomas. Adenomatoid hyperplasia contains clusters or lobules of mucous or serous glands with normal or enlarged appearance, whereas adenomatous ductal proliferations show prominent ductal proliferation with some

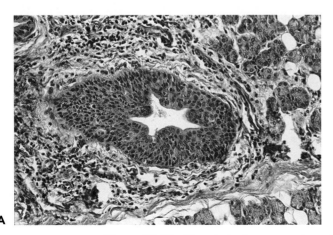
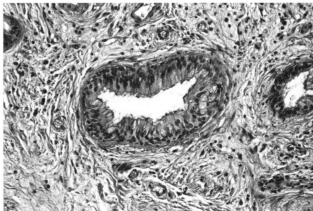

A   **B**

Figure 17.18   Metaplasia of excretory ducts. Squamous (**A**) and mucous metaplasia (**B**) showing cilliated cells simulating respiratory epithelium.

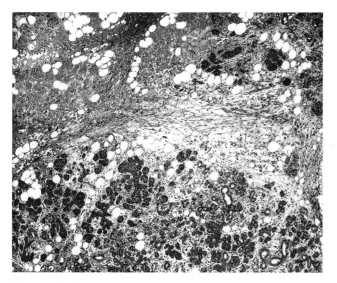

Figure 17.19   Necrotizing sialometaplasia of submaxillary gland.

Atrophy

Atrophy of the salivary tissue is a common finding in surgical specimens of tumoral salivary glands that have one or more atrophied lobules. This atrophy is caused by partial or total obstruction of an excretory duct. Accordingly, secretory units distal to the obstructed duct are dilated, and the acinar lumina become visible. The secretory cells lose their granules and have a similar aspect to that of the intercalated duct. The atrophic lobule has an inflammatory component; the cells gradually disappear, and the parenchyma is replaced by adipose tissue and collagen fibers (Figure 17.20A). The extent of atrophy depends on the size of the affected duct. It is generally greater in lithiasic obstruction. The atrophy present in terminal stage chronic sialadenitis shows a diffuse pattern with prominent periductal sclerosis

and dense inflammatory infiltration (Figure 17.20B) (202). In the submaxillary gland, diffuse atrophy is frequent after radiotherapy, and the gland has a firm consistency (Kuttner's tumor) that may be clinically mistaken for a submaxillary neoplasm. Atypical cells are often found in postradiotherapy atrophy. Dilated ducts lose cell polarity and exhibit hyperchromatic nuclei and prominent myoepithelium. In addition, interlobular ducts lose their continuity, and the interstitium is densely infiltrated with plasma cells (201). In experimental models, atrophy takes place after ligation of main salivary duct. Duct cells persist, in contrast to the disappearance of most acinar cells, which are deleted by apoptosis (210).

Regeneration

The parenchyma of salivary glands have a capacity for regeneration. It is particularly notable in the salivary gland a few weeks after partial resection. In general, regenerating tissue follows an embryonic pattern, showing solid buds and branching columns of undifferentiated cells that eventually form excretory units (22) (Figure 17.21A). In some cases, such regenerating tissue exhibits an atypical appearance. Proliferating solid buds of undifferentiated cells may simulate basal cell adenoma (211) or other undifferentiated cell neoplasms (Figure 17.21B). However, unlike neoplasms, the regenerating tissue preserves the lobular architecture characteristic of the normal salivary gland (Figure 17.21B–C) (22,39). Regeneration after atrophy due to duct obstruction is completed from residual parotid ducts that differentiate into acinar cells (212); this is probably achieved by a stem cell that resides in one of the ducts. The pattern is similar to the high proliferative activity of the terminal tubule, proacinar, and acinar cells during normal embryonic development of the rat submandibular gland (213).

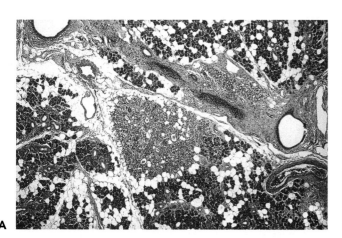
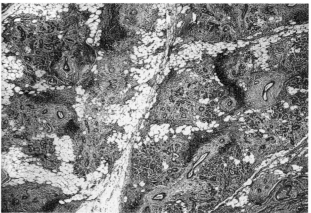

A   **B**

Figure 17.20   Atrophy of the salivary parenchyma. **A.** Focal atrophy in the vicinity of a parotid tumor; note the duct dilatation. **B.** Diffuse atrophy in chronic sialadenitis showing prominent periductal sclerosis.

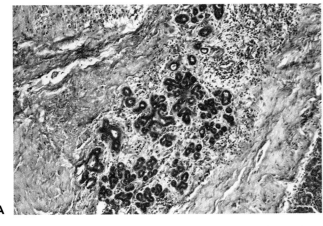

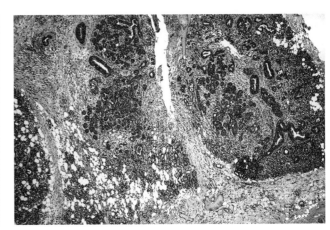

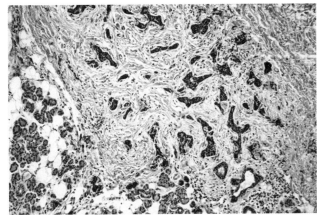

Figure 17.21 Regenerating salivary tissue of parotid gland. **A.** Formation of secretory units with an embryonic pattern. **B.** Atypical regenerating tissue; the lobular pattern is preserved. **C.** Infiltrating residual adenoid cystic carcinoma in a parotid gland. Solid buds consist of undifferentiated cells without lobular arrangement.

CORRELATIVE NORMAL AND NEOPLASTIC HISTOLOGY

A characteristic of salivary glands is the ability to give rise to a large number of histologically distinct tumors (214). The histogenetic origin of these neoplasms is an interesting topic, but the numerous mechanisms that have been proposed remain hypothetical. The most attractive hypotheses attempt to relate this phenomenon to embryonic development and, particularly, to the presence of ductal reserve cells (56,60, 193,214–217). A conjectural role of these reserve cells is the regeneration of salivary parenchyma, as well as the development of metaplastic tissue in reactive conditions. Batsakis (216) hypothesized two stem cells progenitors located at proximal and distal regions of the duct system that are related to tumors mimicking the terminal ductoacinar complex and the excretory ducts system, respectively. Some researchers have demonstrated, by immunohistochemical methods, the presence of basal cells with an undifferentiated aspect in salivary ducts (57,58). However, this does not prove that they act as reserve cells. Conversely, experimental evidence exists of the proliferative capacity of differentiated acinar and myepithelial cells (218–220).

A correlation between the normal structure of the salivary gland and the histologic appearance of salivary tumors can help us to understand morphologic classifications. Nevertheless, we must realize that this histologic similarity does not necessarily imply that a particular tumor arises from the structure that it mimics (217). However, the morphogenetic approach proposed by Dardick relates morphology to cell differentiation derived from different genes' expression of a stem cell (221–222).

The intercalated duct represents the most important segment of the salivary gland in the morphologic organization of many salivary tumors (217). Many distinctive tumors have been related to it, including pleomorphic adenoma, adenoid cystic carcinoma, basal cell adenoma, epithelial-myoepithelial carcinoma, terminal duct carcinoma, basal cell carcinoma, and embryonic tumors (Figure 17.22). These tumors show both epithelial and myoepithelial cell differentiation (93,109,112,113,118,131,132,134,136,139,148,149,217,222, 223), as does the normal intercalated duct. According to Batsakis (216), these tumors develop from "intercalated duct reserve cells" that follow the same direction as the embryonic terminal tubular cell. Statistically, approximately 80% of salivary tumors develop in the parotid gland, where the intercalated ducts are relatively long (Figure 17.6). In contrast, in the sublingual gland, which gives rise to less than 1% of salivary tumors (22), intercalated ducts are hardly visible.

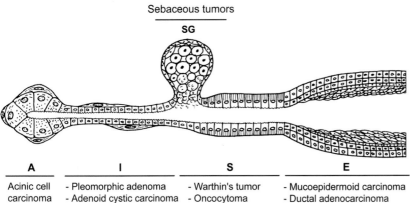

Sebaceous tumors

SG

A	I	S	E
Acinic cell carcinoma	- Pleomorphic adenoma - Adenoid cystic carcinoma - Monomorphic adenoma - Epithelial myoepithelial carcinoma - P L G A	- Warthin's tumor - Oncocytoma	- Mucoepidermoid carcinoma - Ductal adenocarcinoma - Epidermoid carcinoma - Papilloma

Figure 17.22 Morphologic similarity of some salivary tumors and the different epithelial structures of the salivary gland: acinus (*A*), intercalated duct (*I*), striated duct (*S*), sebaceous gland (*SG*), and excretory ducts (*E*). Not necessarily related to histogenesis.

A similar morphologic link exists between the acini, the most differentiated structure of the gland, and the acinic cell tumor, a well-differentiated neoplasm (Figure 17.23A–B) (224); between the mitochondria-rich cells of the striated duct, Warthin's tumor, and oncocytomas (180–181); and between the sebaceous glands and sebaceous tumors (69,76,86). A morphologic analogy also may be found between the larger excretory ducts and mucoepidermoid carcinoma, salivary duct adenocarcinoma, epidermoid carcinoma, adenosquamous carcinoma, and papillary tumors (Figure 17.22) (225–233).

IMMUNOHISTOCHEMISTRY

An important aspect of cytodifferentiation in normal and neoplastic salivary tissue is the expression of different intermediate filaments, enzymes, immunologic components, and other proteins. These proteins may be stained by immunohistochemical methods.

In normal salivary glands, the immunohistochemistry may be summarized as follows (Table 17.3): the expression of cytokeratin varies according to individual cell types of the secretory unit. Acinar cells are stained by several types of lower weight cytokeratins such as CK7, CK8, and CK19. In addition, these cells may be marked by the enzymes usually present in the normal acinus, such as amylase and lysozyme (234). Cytokeratins 6 and 12 are weakly positive in acinar cells but strongly positive in ductal cells, especially in excretory ducts (Figure 17.24) (57). Basal cells are stained with anticytokeratin 19 and 18. Myoepithelial cells may coexpress cytokeratins 14, 17, 19, and vimentin (57,146,148). The most specific markers for myoepithelial cells are S-100 protein, α-smooth muscle actin, calponin, caldesmon, and myosin heavy chain (149,235). In addition, normal myoepithelial cells are

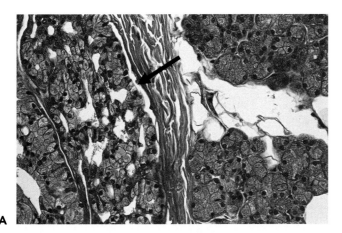

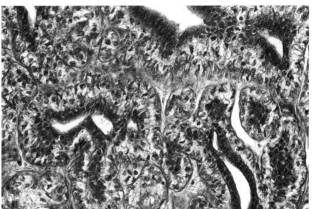

Figure 17.23   A. Acinic cell carcinoma of tha parotid gland (*arrow*), mimicking the normal gland. **B.** Epithelial-myoepithelial carcinoma of parotid gland, showing both epithelial and myoepithelial cells of the intercalated duct.

TABLE 17.3
IMMUNOHISTOCHEMICAL MARKERS OF SALIVARY GLANDS

Structure	LMK	HMK	Vim	A-M	CALP	EMA	S-100	AFP	CEA
Acinus	++	+	−	−	−	−	−	−	+
Intercalated duct	−	++	−	−	−	++	++	++	+
Striated duct	−	++	−	−	−	−	−	++	−
Excretory duct	−	++	−	−	−	++	−	−	−
Myoepithelial cell	+	−	+/−	++	++	−	++	−	−
Basal cell	++	−	−	−	−	−	−	−	−

(*LMK*, low-molecular weight keratin; *HMK*, high-molecular weight keratin; *vim*, vimentin; *A-M*, actin-myosin; *CALP*, calpinin; *EMA*, epithelial membrane antigen; *S-100*, S-100 protein; *AFP*, α-fetoprotein; *CEA*, carcinoembryonic antigen; +, weak positivity; ++, strong positivity; −, negative result)

sometimes stained with glial fibrillary protein (236). The secretory component, except for the mucous units, is present in acinar cells and intercalated and striated ducts (55,237). Carcinoembryonic antigen (CEA) is present in acinar and intercalated duct cells; it is strongly positive in inflamed glands (238). Basal cells are stained with CK14, CK17, and p63 (234). Ductal epithelial cells of intercalated, striated, and interlobular ducts are strongly positive for epithelial membrane antigen (EMA) (239). Recently, the presence of α-fetoprotein in the human submandibular gland has been documented (240). Used as functional markers, the following enzymes may be stained: amylase and lactoferrin in serous acinar cells (241), lysozyme in intercalated ducts (49,50), and alkaline phosphatase and ATPase in myoepithelial cells (92). When used as histologic markers, all these proteins have proven useful in surgical pathology.

SPECIMEN HANDLING

The parotid gland is the most common location of major salivary gland tumors. Because most of them are benign and located on the superficial lobe, partial parotidectomy of the superficial lobe (lateral lobectomy) is the most common treatment. Superficial parotidectomy also suffices for small, well-differentiated, low-grade malignant neoplasms that have not compromised the facial nerve (242). The specimen should be sectioned horizontally, and the relationship between the tumor and the gland should be stated (Figure 17.25). The surgical limits should be described even in benign tumors (Figure 17.26). Total parotidectomy with preservation of the facial nerve is usually indicated in recurrent or multiple benign tumors and large benign tumors of the isthmus and deep lobe.

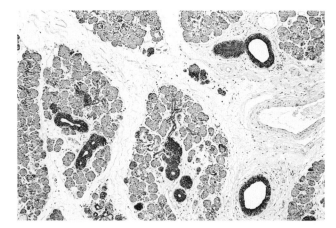

Figure 17.24 Immunostaining for high-molecular weight cytokeratin in a submaxillary gland. The acini are unstained, but intercalated, striated, and excretory ducts show a progressive immunoreaction (peroxidase-antiperoxidase method).

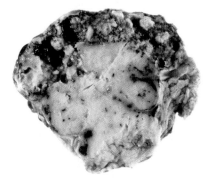

Figure 17.25 Histologic section of a parotid gland showing a pleomorphic adenoma. The tumor is apparently well delimited; tumoral buds may be found separate from the principal tumor.

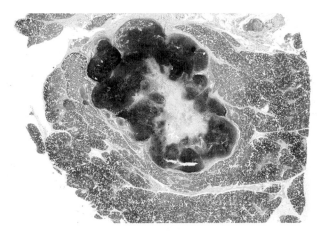

Figure 17.26 Superficial parotidectomy for a pleomorphic adenoma. Note the tumor is well delimited within the normal gland.

Total parotidectomy, including facial nerve resection (radical parotidectomy), is indicated in aggressive malignant tumors, malignant tumors situated in the deep lobe, or those that have compromised the facial nerve. All these specimens should be sectioned on their major axis to evaluate periparotid tissue infiltration (Figure 17.27). Intraparotid and periparotid lymph nodes should be identified; and, when radical parotidectomy includes neck dissection, the lymph nodes should be separated according to the different anatomical regions.

Benign and malignant submandibular gland tumors are rare. Single gland resection is indicated for benign tumors, whereas malignant tumors are treated by a monobloc resection of the gland lesion along with associated muscles, nerves, and mucous membrane.

Sublingual tumors are rare, and most (80%) are malignant. They are also treated by local monobloc resection, including the sublingual compartment and surrounding tissues (243).

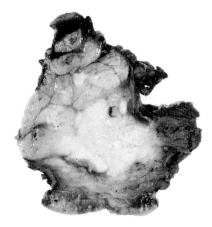

Figure 17.27 Radical parotidectomy for a high-grade mucoepidermoid carcinoma. Note the infiltration of the periparotid tissues.

REFERENCES

1. Arey LB. *Developmental Anatomy*. 7th ed. Philadelphia: WB Saunders; 1974.
2. Cohn RH, Banerjee SD, Bernfield MR. Basal lamina of embryonic salivary epithelia. Nature of glycosaminoglycan and organization of extracellular materials. *J Cell Biol* 1977;73:464–478.
3. Grobstein C. Epithelio-mesenchymal specificity in the morphogenesis of mouse sub-mandibular rudiments in vitro. *J Exp Zool* 1953;124:383–414.
4. Grobstein C. Mechanisms of organogenetic tissue interaction. *Natl Cancer Inst Monogr* 1967;26:279–299.
5. Lawson KA. The role of mesenchyme in the morphogenesis and functional differentiation of rat salivary epithelium. *J Embryol Exp Morphol* 1972;27:497–513.
6. Gasser RF. The early development of the parotid gland around the facial nerve and its branches in man. *Anat Rec* 1970;167:63–77.
7. Azuma M, Sato M. Morphogenesis of normal human salivary gland cells in vitro. *Histol Histopathol* 1994;9:781–790.
8. Donath K, Dietrich H, Seifert G. Enwicklung und ultrastrukturelle cytodifferenzierung der parotis des menschen. *Virchows Arch A Pathol Anat Histopathol* 1978;378:297–314.
9. Lee SK, Hwang Jo, Chi JG, Yamada K, Mori M. Prenatal development of myoepithelial cell of human submandibular gland observed by immunohistochemistry of smooth muscle actin and rhodamine-phalloidin fluorescence. *Pathol Res Pract* 1993;189:332–341.
10. Adi MM, Chisholm DM, Waterhouse JP. Stereological and immunohistochemical study of development of human fetal labial salivary glands and their S-100 protein reactivity. *J Oral Pathol Med* 1994;23:36–40.
11. Lee SK, Kim EC, Chi JG, Hashimura K, Mori M. Immunohistochemical detection of S-100, S-100 alpha, S-100 beta proteins, glial fibrillary acidic protein, and neuron specific enolase in the prenatal and adult human salivary glands. *Pathol Res Pract* 1993;189:1036–1043.
12. Line SE, Archer FL. The postnatal development of myoepithelial cell in the rat submandibular gland. An immunohistochemical study. *Virchows Arch B Cell Pathol* 1972;10:253–262.
13. Gresik EW. Postnatal developmental changes in submandibular glands of rats and mice. *J Histochem Cytochem* 1980;28:860–870.
14. Strum JM. Unusual peroxidase-positive granules in the developing rat submaxillary gland. *J Cell Biol* 1971;51:575–579.
15. Yamashina S, Barka T. Localization of peroxidase activity in the developing submandibular gland of normal and isoproterenol-treated rats. *J Histochem Cytochem* 1972;20:855–872.
16. Testut L. *Traité d'Anatomie Humaine*. Paris: Octave Doin; 1931.
17. Gray H, Gross CM, eds. *Gray's Anatomy of the Human Body*. 29th ed. Philadelphia: Lea & Febiger; 1973.
18. Gola R, Chossegros C, Carreu P. Anatomie chirurgicale de la région parotidienne. Concepts actuels. *Rev Stomatol Chir Maxillofac* 1994;95:395–410.
19. Toh H, Kodama J, Fukuda J, Rittman B, Mackenzie I. Incidence and histology of human accessory parotid glands. *Anat Rec* 1993;236:586–590.
20. Frommer J. The human accessory parotid gland: its incidence, nature, and significance. *Oral Surg Oral Med Oral Pathol* 1977;43:671–676.
21. Hamilton WJ, Boyd JD, Mossman HW. *Human Embryology, Prenatal Development of Form and Function*. London: Williams & Wilkins; 1972.
22. Evans RW, Cruickshank AH. *Epithelial Tumors of the Salivary Glands*. Philadelphia: WB Saunders; 1970.
23. Merida-Velasco JA, Sanchez-Montesinos I, Espin-Ferra J, García-García ID, García-Gomez S, Roldan-Schilling V. Development of the human submandibular salivary gland. *J Dent Res* 1993;73:1227–1232.
24. Sakai T, Larsen M, Yamada KM. Fibronectin requirement in branching morphogenesis. *Nature* 2003;423:876–881.
25. Hu MC, Rosenblum N. Genetic regulation of branching morphogenesis lessons learned from loss-of-function phenotypes. *Pediatr Res* 2003;54:433–438.

26. Gaur V, Choudhry R, Anand C, Choudhry S. Submandibular gland with multiple ducts. *Surg Radiol Anat* 1994;16:439–440.

27. Bowen ID, Morgan SM, Mullarkey K. Cell death in the salivary glands of metamorphosing Calliphora vomitoria. *Cell Biol Int* 1993;17:13–33.

28. Tomei LD, Cope FO, eds. *Apoptosis: The Molecular Basis of Cell Death*. Plainview, NY: Cold Spring Harbor Laboratory Press; 1991.

29. Lu QL, Poulsom R, Wong L, Hanby AM. Bcl-2 expression in adult and embryonic non-haematopoietic tissues. *J Pathol* 1993;169: 431–437.

30. Walker NI, Gobé GC. Cell death and cell proliferation during atrophy of the rat parotid gland induced by duct obstruction. *J Pathol* 1987;153:333–344.

31. Stephens LC, Schultheiss TE, Price RE, Ang KK, Peters LJ. Radiation apoptosis of serous acinar cells of salivary and lacrimal glands. *Cancer* 1991;67:1539–1543.

32. Tamerin A. Submaxillary gland recovery from obstruction II. Electron microscopic alterations of acinar cells. *J Ultrastruct Res* 1971;34:288–302.

33. Burgess KL, Dardick I. Cell population changes during atrophy and regeneration of rat parotid gland. *Oral Surg Oral Med Oral Pathol Oral Radiol and Endod* 1998;85:699–706.

34. Takahashi S, Shinzato K, Domon T, Yamamoto T, Wakita M. Mitotic proliferation on myoepithelial cells during regeneration of atrophied rat submandibular glands after duct ligation. *J Oral Pathol Med* 2004;33:430–434.

35. Kong L, Ogawa N, Nakabayashi T, et al. Fas and Fas ligand expression in the salivary glands of patients with primary Sjögren's syndrome. *Arthritis Rheum* 1997;40:87–97.

36. Bolstand AI, Eiken HG, Rosenlund B, Alarcon-Riquelme M, Jonsson R. Increased salivary gland tissue expression of Fas, Fas ligand, cytotoxic T lymphocyte-associated antigen 4, and programmed cell death 1 in primary Sjögren's syndrome. *Arthritis Rheum* 2003;48:174–185.

37. Hand AR, Ho B. Liquid-diet-induced alterations of rat parotid acinar cells studied by electron microscopy and enzyme cytochemistry. *Arch Oral Biol* 1981;26:369–380.

38. Sharawy M, White SC. Morphometric and fine structural study of experimental autoallergic sialadenitis of rat submandibular glands. *Virchows Arch B Cell Pathol* 1978;28:255–273.

39. Chaudhry AP, Cutler LS, Yamane GM, Satchidanand S, Labay G, Sunderraj M. Light and ultrastructural features of lymphoepithelial lesions of the salivary glands in Mikulicz's disease. *J Pathol* 1986;148:239–250.

40. Fanidi A, Harrington EA, Evan GI. Cooperative interaction between c-myc and bcl-2 proto-oncogenes. *Nature* 1992;359: 554–556.

41. Chen M, Quintans J, Fuks Z, Thompson C, Kufe DW, Weichselbaum RR. Suppression of Bcl-2 messenger RNA production may mediate apoptosis after ionizing radiation, tumor necrosis factor alpha, and ceramide. *Cancer Res* 1995;55:991–994.

42. Tamarin A. Submaxillary gland recovery from obstruction I. overall changes and electron microscopic alterations of glanular duct cells. *J Ultrastruct Res* 1971:34:276–287.

43. Matthews TW, Dardick I. Morphological alterations of salivary gland parenchyma in chronic sialadenitis. *J Otolaryngol* 1988;17: 385–394.

44. Pammer J, Horvat R, Weninger W, Ulrich W. Expression of bcl-2 in salivary glands and salivary adenomas. A contribution to the reserve cell theory. *Pathol Res Pract* 1995;191:35–41.

45. Hockenbery DM, Zutter M, Hickey W, Nahm M, Korsmeyer SJ. BCL2 protein is topographically restricted in tissues characterized by apoptotic cell death. *Proc Natl Acad Sci U S A* 1991;88: 6961–6965.

46. Bloom W, Fawcett DW. *A Textbook of Histology*. 11th ed. Philadelphia: WB Saunders; 1986.

47. Donath K. Die *Sialadenose der Parotis. Ultrastrukturelle, Klinische und Experimentelle Befunde zur Sekretionpathologie*. Stuttgart: Gustav Fischer Verlag; 1976.

48. Takano K, Malamud D, Bennick A, Oppenheim F, Hand AR. Localization of salivary proteins in granules of human parotid and submandibular acinar cells. *Crit Rev Oral Biol Med* 1993;4: 399–405.

49. Caselitz J, Jaup T, Seifert G. Lactoferrin and lysozyme in carcinomas of the parotid gland. A comparative immunocytochemical study with the occurrence in normal and inflamed tissue. *Virchows Arch A Pathol Anat Histol* 1981;394:61–73.

50. Reitamo S, Konttinen YT, Segerberg-Konttinen M. Distribution of lactoferrin in human salivary glands. *Histochemistry* 1980;66: 285–291.

51. Xu L, Lal K, Santarpia RP III, Pollock JJ. Salivary proteolysis of histidine-rich polypeptides and the antifungal activity of peptide degradation products. *Arch Oral Biol* 1993;38:277–283.

52. Quintarelli G. Histochemical identification of salivary mucins. *Ann N Y Acad Sci* 1963;106:339–363.

53. Reddy MS, Bobek LA, Haraszthy GG, Biesbrock AR, Levine MJ. Structural features of the low-molecular-mass human salivary mucin. *Biochem J* 1992;287(pt 2):639–643.

54. Greep RO, Weiss L, eds. *Histology*. New York: McGraw-Hill; 1973.

55. Korsrud FR, Brandtzaeg P. Characterization of epithelial elements in human major salivary glands by functional markers: localization of amylase, lactoferrin, lysozyme, secretory component, and secretory immunoglobulins by paired immunofluorescence staining. *J Histochem Cytochem* 1982;30:657–666.

56. Riva A, Serra GP, Proto E, Faa G, Puxeddu R, Riva FT. The myoepithelial and basal cells of ducts of human major salivary glands: a SEM study. *Arch Histol Cytol* 1992;55(suppl):115–124.

57. Born IA, Schwechheimer K, Maier H, Otto HF. Cytokeratin expression in normal salivary glands and in cystadenolymphomas demonstrated by monoclonal antibodies against selective cytokeratin polypeptides. *Virchows Arch A Pathol Anat Histopathol* 1987;411:583–589.

58. Burns BF, Dardick I, Parks WR. Intermediate filament expression in normal parotid glands and in pleomorphic adenomas. *Virchows Arch A Pathol Anat Histopathol* 1988;413:103–112.

59. Seifert GA, Miehlke A, Haubrich J, Chilla R. *Diseases of the Salivary Glands: Pathology, Diagnosis, Treatment, Facial Nerve Surgery*. Stuttgart: Georg Thieme Verlag; 1986.

60. Regezi JA, Batsakis JG. Histogenesis of salivary gland neoplasms. *Otolaryngol Clin North Am* 1977;10:297–307.

61. Scott BL, Pease DC. Electron microscopy of the salivary and lacrimal glands of the rat. *Am J Anat* 1959;104:115–161.

62. Tandler B. Ultrastructure of the human submaxillary gland. I. Architecture and histological relationships of the secretory cells. *Am J Anat* 1962;111:287–307.

63. Tandler B, Denning CR, Mandel ID, Kutscher AH. Ultrastructure of human labial glands. III. Myoepithelium and ducts. *J Morphol* 1970;130:227–246.

64. Norberg L, Dardick I, Leung R, Burford-Mason AP, Rippstein P. Immunogold localization of actin and cytokeratin filaments in myoepithelium of human parotid salivary gland. *Ultrastruct Pathol* 1992;16:555–568.

65. Sjöstrand FS, Rhodin J. Ultrastructure of the proximal convoluted tubule of the mouse kidney as revealed by high resolution electron microscopy. *Exp Cell Res* 1953;4:426–465.

66. Hamperl H. Beitraäge zur normalen und pathologischen histologic menschlicher speicheldrüsen. *Z Mikorosk Anat Forsch* 1931;27:1–55.

67. Harts PH. Development of sebaceous glands from intralobular ducts of the parotid gland. *Arch Pathol* 1946;41:651–654.

68. Marshall L Jr. Intraparotid sebaceous glands. *Ann Surg* 1949;129: 152–155.

69. Meza-Chavez L. Sebaceous glands in normal and neoplastic parotid glands. *Am J Pathol* 1949;25:627–645.

70. Micheau C. Les glandes dites sébacées de la parotide et de la sous-maxillaires. *Ann Anat Path* 1969;14:119–126.

71. Patey DH, Thackray AC. The treatment of parotid tumours in the light of a pathological study of parotidectomy material. *Br J Surg* 1958;45:477–487.

72. Margolies A, Weidman F. Statistical and histologic studies of Fordyce's disease. *Arch Derm Syph* 1921;3:723–742.

73. Whitaker SB, Vigneswaran N, Singh BB. Androgen receptor status of the oral sebaceous glands. *Am J Dermatopathol* 1997;19:415–418.

74. Laine M, Blauer M, Ylikomi, et al. Immunohistochemical demonstration of androgen receptors in human salivary glands. *Arch Oral Biol* 1993;38:299–302.

75. Brocheriou C. Les tumeurs des glandes salivaires. In: Nezeloff C, ed. *Nouvelles Acquisitions en Pathologie*. Paris: Hermann; 1983:223–268.

76. Albores-Saavedra J, Morris AW. Sebaceous adenoma of the submaxillary salivary gland. Report of a case. *Arch Otolaryngol* 1963;77:500–503.

77. Assor D. Sebaceous lymphadenoma of the parotid gland: a case report. *Am J Clin Pathol* 1970;53:100–103.

78. Cheek R, Pitcock JA. Sebaceous lesions of the parotid. Report of two cases. *Arch Pathol* 1966;82:147–150.

79. Seifert G, Bull HG, Donath K. Histologic subclassification of the cystadenolymphoma of the parotid gland. Analysis of 275 cases. *Virchows Arch A Pathol Anat Histol* 1980;388:13–38.

80. Wasan SM. Sebaceous lymphadenoma of the parotid gland. *Cancer* 1971;28:1019–1022.

81. Kleinsasser O, Hübner G, Klein HJ. Talgzellcarcinom des Parotis. *Arch Klin Exp Ohren Nasen Kehlkopfheilk* 1970;197:59–71.

82. Silver H, Goldstein MA. Sebaceous cell carcinoma of the parotid region. A review of the literature and a case report. *Cancer* 1966; 19:1173–1179.

83. Martínez-Madrigal F, Casiraghi O, Khattech A, Nasr-Khattech RB, Richard JM, Micheau C. Hypopharyngeal sebaceous carcinoma: a case report. *Hum Pathol* 1991;22:929–931.

84. Gnepp DR, Sporck FT. Benign lymphoepithelial parotid cyst with sebaceous differentiation. Cystic sebaceous lymphadenoma. *Am J Clin Pathol* 1980;74:683–687.

85. Peel RL, Gnepp DR. Diseases of the salivary glands. In: Barnes L, ed. *Surgical Pathology of the Head and Neck*. New York: Marcel Dekker; 1985:533–645.

86. Rawson AJ, Horn RC Jr. Sebaceous glands and sebaceous gland-containing tumors of the parotid salivary gland; with a consideration of the histogenesis of papillary cystadenoma lymphomatosum. *Surgery* 1950;27:93–101.

87. Cutler LS, Chaudhry A, Innes DJ Jr. Ultrastructure of the parotid duct. Cytochemical studies of the striated duct and papillary cystadenoma lymphomatosum of the human parotid gland. *Arch Pathol Lab Med* 1977;101:420–424.

88. Archer FL, Kao VC. Immunohistochemical identification of actomyosin in myoepithelium of human tissues. *Lab Invest* 1968;18:669–674.

89. Drenckhahn D, Gröschel-Stewart U, Unsicker K. Immunofluorescence-microscopic demonstration of myosin and actin in salivary glands and exocrine pancreas of the rat. *Cell Tissue Res* 1977;183:273–279.

90. Tandler B. Ultrastructure of the human submaxillary gland. III. Myoepithelium. *Z Zellforsch Mikroskop Anat* 1965;68:852–863.

91. Franke WW, Schmid E, Freudenstein C, et al. Intermediate-sized filaments of the prekeratin type in myoepithelial cells. *J Cell Biol* 1980;84:633–654.

92. Hamperl H. The myoepithelia (myoepithelial cells). *Curr Top Pathol* 1970;53:161–220.

93. Shear M. The structure and function of myoepithelial cells in salivary glands. *Arch Oral Biol* 1966;11:769–780.

94. Garrett JR, Emmelin N. Activities of salivary myoepithelial cells: a review. *Med Biol* 1979;57:1–28.

95. Schroeder BT, Chakraborty J, Soloff MS. Binding of [3H] oxytocin to the cells isolated from the mammary gland of the lactating rat. *J Cell Biol* 1977;74:428–440.

96. Azumi N, Battifora H. The cellular composition of adenoid cystic carcinoma. An immunohistochemical study. *Cancer* 1987;60: 1589–1598.

97. d'Ardenne AJ, Kirkpatrick P, Wells CA, Davies JD. Laminin and fibronectin in adenoid cystic carcinoma. *J Clin Pathol* 1986;39: 138–144.

98. Donath K, Seifert G. Ultrastruktur und pathogenese der myoepithelialen sialadenitis. Über das vorkommen von myoepithelzellen bei der benignen lymphoepithelialen läsion. *Virchows Arch A Pathol Anat Histopathol* 1972;356:315–329.

99. Kallioinen M. Immunoelectron microscope demonstration of the basement membrane components laminin and type IV collagen in the dermal cylindroma. *J Pathol* 1985;147:97–102.

100. Orenstein JM, Dardick I, van Nostrand AW. Ultrastructural similarities of adenoid cystic carcinoma and pleomorphic adenoma. *Histopathology* 1985;9:623–638.

101. Seifert G, Donath K. Classification of the pathology of diseases of the salivary glands. Review of 2,600 cases in the salivary gland register. *Beitr Pathol* 1976;159:1–32.

102. Skalova A, Leivo I. Extracellular collagenous spherules in salivary gland tumors: immunohistochemical analysis of laminin and various types of callagen. *Arch Pathol Lab Med* 1992;116: 649–653.

103. Skalova A, Leivo I. Basement membrane proteins in salivary gland tumors. Distribution of type IV collagen and laminin. *Virchows Arch A Pathol Anat Histopathol* 1992;420:425–431.

104. Laurie GW, Leblond CP, Martin GR. Localization of type IV collagen, laminin, heparan sulfate proteoglycan, and fibronectin to the basal lamina of basement membranes. *J Cell Biol* 1982;95: 340–344.

105. Sunardhi-Widyaputra S, Van Damme B. Immunohistochemical expression of tenascin in normal human salivary glands and in pleomorphic adenomas. *Pathol Res Pract* 1993;189:138–143.

106. Savera AT, Zarbo RJ. Defining the role of myoepithelium in salivary gland neoplasia. *Adv Anat Pathol* 2004;11:69–85.

107. Eneroth CM. Salivary gland tumors in the parotid gland, submandibular gland, and the palate region. *Cancer* 1971;27: 1415–1418.

108. Thackray AC, Sabin LH. Histological typing of salivary gland tumors. In: *International Histological Classification of Tumors*. No. 7. Geneva: World Health Organization; 1972.

109. Dardick I, van Nostrand AW, Jeans MT, Rippstein P, Edwards V. Pleomorphic adenoma. I. Ultrastructural organization of "epithelial" regions. *Hum Pathol* 1983;14:780–797.

110. Dardick I, van Nostrand AW, Phillips MJ. Histogenesis of salivary gland pleomorphic adenoma (mixed tumor) with an evaluation of the role of the myoepithelial cell. *Hum Pathol* 1982;13:62–75.

111. David R, Buchner A. Elastosis in benign and malignant salivary gland tumors. A histochemical and ultrastructural study. *Cancer* 1980;45:2301–2310.

112. Erlandson RA, Cardon-Cardo C, Higgins PJ. Histogenesis of benign pleomorphic adenoma (mixed tumor) of the major salivary glands. An ultrastructural and immunohistochemical study. *Am J Surg Pathol* 1984;8:803–820.

113. Hubner G, Klein HJ, Kleinsasser O, Schiefer HG. Role of myoepithelial cells in the development of salivary gland tumors. *Cancer* 1971;27:1255–1261.

114. Seifert G, Langrock I, Donath K. Pathomorphologische subklassifikation der pleomorphen speicheldrüsen adenomen. Analyse von 310 pleomorphen parotisadenomen. *HNO* 1976;24: 415–426.

115. Shirasuna K, Sato M, Miyazaki T. A myoepithelial cell line established from a human pleomorphic adenoma arising in minor salivary gland. *Cancer* 1980;45:297–305.

116. Yanagawa T, Hayashi Y, Nagamine S, Yoshida H, Yura Y, Sato M. Generation of cells with phenotypes of both intercalated duct-type and myoepithelial cells in human parotid gland adenocarcinoma clonal cells grown in athymic nude mice. *Virchows Arch B Cell Pathol Incl Mol Pathol* 1986;51:187–195.

117. Gallo O, Bani D, Toccafondi G, Almerigogna F, Storchi OF. Characterization of a novel cell line from pleomorphic adenoma of the parotid gland with myoepithelial phenotype and producing interleukin-6 as an autocrine growth factor. *Cancer* 1992;70: 559–568.

118. Corio RL, Sciubba JJ, Brannon RB, Batsakis J. Epithelial-myoepithelial carcinoma of intercalated duct origin. A clinico-pathological and ultrastructural assessment of sixteen cases. *Oral Surg Oral Med Oral Pathol* 1982;53:280–287.

119. Donath K, Seifert G, Schmitz R. Zur diagnose und ultrastruktur des tubulären speichelgangkarzinoms. Epithelial-myoepitheliales schultstückkarzinom. *Virchows Arch A Pathol Anat Histopathol* 1972;356:16–31.

120. Luna MA, Ordonez NG, Mackay B, Batsakis JG, Gillamandegui O. Salivary epithelial-myoepithelial carcinomas of intercalated ducts: a clinical, electron microscopic, and immunocytochemical study. *Oral Surg Oral Med Oral Pathol* 1985;59:482–490.

121. Batsakis JG, el-Naggar AK, Luna MA. Epithelial-myoepithelial carcinoma of salivary glands. *Ann Otol Rhinol Laryngol* 1992;101: 540–542.

122. Nistal M, García-Viera M, Martínez-García C, Paniagua R. Epithelial-myoepithelial tumor of the bronchus. *Am J Surg Pathol* 1994;18:421–425.

123. Palmer RM. Epithelial-myoepithelial carcinoma: an immunocytochemical study. *Oral Surg Oral Med Oral Pathol* 1985;59:511–515.

124. Crissman JD, Wirman JA, Harris A. Malignant myoepithelioma of the parotid gland. *Cancer* 1977;40:3042–3049.

125. Leifer C, Miller AS, Putong PB, Harwick RD. Myoepithelioma of the parotid gland. *Arch Pathol* 1974;98:312–319.

126. Luna MA, Mackay B, Gamez-Araujo J. Myoepithelioma of the palate. Report of a case with histochemical and electron microscopic observations. *Cancer* 1973;32:1429–1435.

127. Sciubba JJ, Brannon RB. Myoepithelioma of the salivary glands: report of 23 cases. *Cancer* 1982;49:562–572.

128. Dardick I, Cavell S, Boivin M, et al. Salivary gland myoepithelioma variants: histological, ultrastructural, and immunocytological features. *Virchows Arch A Pathol Anat Histolpathol* 1989;416:25–42.

129. Martínez-Madrigal F, Santiago Payan H, Meneses A, Domínguez Malagón H, Rojas ME. Plasmacytoid myoepithelioma of the laryngeal region: a case report. *Hum Pathol* 1995;26:802–804.

130. Frierson HR Jr, Mills SE, Garland TA. Terminal duct carcinoma of minor salivary glands. A nonpapillary subtype of polymorphous low-grade adenocarcinoma. *Am J Clin Pathol* 1985;84:8–14.

131. Gnepp DR, Chen JC, Warren C. Polymorphous low-grade adenocarcinoma of minor salivary gland. An immunohistochemical and clinicopathologic study. *Am J Surg Pathol* 1988;12:461–468.

132. Dardick I, Kahn HJ, van Nostrand AW, Baumal R. Salivary gland monomorphic adenoma. Ultrastructural, immunoperoxidase, and histogenetic aspects. *Am J Pathol* 1984;115:334–348.

133. Dardick I, van Nostrand AW. Myoepithelial cells in salivary gland tumors—revisited. *Head Neck Surg* 1985;7:395–408.

134. Hoa W, Kech PC, Swerdlow MA. Ultrastructure of the basal cell adenoma of parotid. *Cancer* 1976;37:1322–1333.

135. Kahn HJ, Baumal R, Marks A, Dardick I, van Nostrand AW. Myoepithelial cells in salivary gland tumors: an immunohistochemical study. *Arch Pathol Lab Med* 1985;109:190–195.

136. Batsakis JG, Luna MA, el-Naggar AK. Basaloid monomorphic adenomas. *Ann Otol Rhinol Laryngol* 1991;100:687–690.

137. Chaudhry AP, Leifer C, Cutler LS, Satchidanand S, Labay GR, Yamane GM. Histogenesis of adenoid cystic carcinoma of the salivary glands. Light and electronmicroscopic study. *Cancer* 1986; 58:72–82.

138. Chen JC, Gnepp DR, Bedrossian CW. Adenoid cystic carcinoma of the salivary glands: an immunohistochemical analysis. *Oral Surg Oral Med Oral Pathol* 1988;65:316–326.

139. Williams SB, Ellis GL, Auclair PL. Immunohistochemical analysis of basal cell adenocarcinoma. *Oral Surg Oral Med Oral Pathol* 1993;75:64–69.

140. Hsueh C, Gonzalez-Crussi F. Sialoblastoma: a case report and review of the literature on congenital epithelial tumors of salivary glands origin. *Pediatr Pathol* 1992;12:205–214.

141. Dehner LP, Valbuena L, Perez-Atayde A, Reddick RL, Askin FB, Rosai J. Salivary gland anlage tumor ("congenital pleomorphic adenoma"). A clinicopathologic, immunohistochemical and ultrastructural study of nine cases. *Am J Surg Pathol* 1994;18:25–36.

142. Dardick I, Daya D, Hardie J, van Nostrand AW. Mucoepidermoid carcinoma: ultrastructural and histogenetic aspects. *J Oral Pathol* 1984;13:342–358.

143. Lomax-Smith JD, Azzopardi JG. The hyaline cell: a distinctive feature of mixed salivary tumors. *Histopathology* 1978;2:77–92.

144. Quintarelli G, Robinson L. The glycosaminoglycans of salivary gland tumors. *Am J Pathol* 1967;51:19–37.

145. Takeuchi J, Sobue M, Yoshida M, Esaki T, Kato Y. Pleomorphic adenoma of the salivary gland. With special reference to histochemical and electron microscopic studies and biochemical analysis of glycosaminoglycans in vivo and in vitro. *Cancer* 1975;36:1771–1789.

146. Caselitz J, Osborn M, Seifert G, Weber K. Intermediate-sized filament proteins (prekeratin, vimentin, desmin) in the normal parotid-gland and parotid-gland tumors. Immunofluorescence study. *Virchows Arch A Pathol Anat Histopathol* 1981;393:273–286.

147. Savera AT, Gown AM, Zarbo RJ. Immunolocalization of three novel smooth muscle-specific proteins in salivary gland pleomorphic adenoma: assessment of the morphogenetic role of myoepithelium. *Mod Pathol* 1997;10:1093–1100.

148. Caselitz J, Osborn M, Wustrow J, Seifert G, Weber K. The expression of different intermediate-sized filaments in human salivary glands and their tumours. *Pathol Res Pract* 1982;175:266–278.

149. Morinaga S, Nakajima T, Shimosato Y. Normal and neoplastic myoepithelial cells in salivary glands. An immunohistochemical study. *Hum Pathol* 1987;18:1218–1226.

150. Markaki S, Bouropoulou V, Milas C. S-100 protein and neuron specific enolase (NSE) immunoreactivity in pleomorphic adenomas of the salivary glands and its relationship to the composition of their extracellular matrix. *Arch Anat Cytol Pathol* 1987;35:211–216.

151. Franquemont DW, Mills SE. Plasmacytoid monomorphic adenoma of salivary glands. Absence of myogenous differentiation and comparison to spindle cell myoepithelioma. *Am J Surg Pathol* 1993;17:146–153.

152. Sternlicht MD, Safarians S, Rivera SP, Barsky SH. Characterizations of the extracellular matrix and proteinase inhibitor content of human myoepithelial tumors. *Lab Invest* 1996;74:781–796.

153. Sternlicht MD, Barsky SH. The myoepithelial defense: a host defense against cancer. *Med Hypotheses* 1997;48:37–46.

154. Savera AT, Sloman A, Huvos AG, Klimtra DS. Myoepithelial carcinoma of the salivary glands. A clinicopathologic study of 25 patients. *Am J Surg Pathol* 2000;24:761–774.

155. Brandtzaeg P. Mucosal and glandular distribution of immunoglobulin components. Immunohistochemistry with a cold ethanol-fixation technique. *Immunology* 1974;26:1101–1114.

156. Brandtzaeg P. Mucosal and glandular distribution of immunoglobulin components: differential localization of free and bound SC in secretory epithelial cells. *J Immunol* 1974;112:1553–1559.

157. Korsrud FR, Brandtzaeg P. Quantitative immunohistochemistry of immunoglobulin- and J-chain-producing cells in human parotid and submandibular salivary glands. *Immunology* 1980;39:129–140.

158. Lee SK, Lim CY, Chi JG, et al. Immunohistochemical study of lymphoid tissue in human fetal salivary gland. *J Oral Pathol Med* 1993;22:23–29.

159. Bernier JL, Bhaskar SN. Lymphoepithelial lesions of salivary glands: histogenesis and classification based on 186 cases. *Cancer* 1958;11:1156–1179.

160. Hsu SM, Hsu PL, Nayak RN. Warthin's tumor: an immunohistochemical study of its lymphoid stroma. *Hum Pathol* 1981;12:251–257.

161. Thompson AS, Bryant HC Jr. Histogenesis of papillary cystadenoma lymphomatosum (Warthin's tumor) of the parotid salivary gland. *Am J Pathol* 1950;26:807–849.

162. Azzopardi JG, Evans DJ. Malignant lymphoma of parotid associated with Mikulicz disease (benign lymphoepithelial lesion). *J Clin Pathol* 1971;24:744–752.

163. Brown RB, Gaillard RA, Turner JA. The significance of aberrant or heterotopic parotid gland tissue in lymph nodes. *Ann Surg* 1953;138:850–856.

164. Micheau C. Les ectopies salivaires. *Arch Anat Cytol Pathol* 1969;17:179–186.

165. Neisse R. Über den einschluss von parotisläppen in lymphknoten. *Anat Hefte* (Wisbaden) 1898;10:289–306.

166. Bairati A. Constate concrescenza fra noduli linfatici ed adenomeri delle ghiandole salivari nellúomo durante lo sviluppo e nell adulto. *Arch Biol (Paris)* 1932;43:415–450.

167. Youngs LA, Scofield HH. Heterotopic salivary gland tissue in the lower neck. *Arch Pathol* 1967;83:550–556.

168. Curry B, Taylor CW, Fisher AW. Salivary gland heterotopia: a unique cerebellopontine angle tumor. *Arch Pathol Lab Med* 1982;106:35–38.

169. Schochet SS Jr, McCormick WF, Halmi NS. Salivary gland rests in the human pituitary: light and electron microscopical study. *Arch Pathol* 1974;98:193–200.

170. Jernstrom P, Prietto C. Accessory parotid gland tissue at base of neck. *Arch Pathol* 1962;73:473–480.

171. Bouquot JE, Gnepp DR, Dardick I, Hietanen JH. Intraosseous salivary tissue: jawbone examples of choristomas, hamartomas, embryonic rests, and inflamatory entrapment: another histogenetic source for intraosseous adenocarcinoma. *Oral Surg Oral Med Oral Pathol Oral Radiol Endod* 2000;90: 205–217.

172. Stafne EC. Bone cavities situated near the angle of the mandible. *J Am Dent Assoc* 1942;29:1969–1972.

173. de Courten A, Küffer R, Samson J, Lombardi T. Anterior lingual mandibular salivary gland defect (Stafne defect) presenting as a residual cyst. *Oral Surg Oral Med Oral Pathol Oral Radiol Endod* 2002;94:460–464.

174. Carney JA. Salivary heterotopia, cysts, and the parathyroid gland: branchial pouch derivatives and remnants. *Am J Surg Pathol* 2000;24:837–845.

175. Willis RA. *The Borderland of Embryology and Pathology.* London: Butterworth; 1962.

176. Willis RA. Some unusual developmental heterotopias. *Br Med J* 1968;3:267–272.

177. Dhawan IK, Bhargava S, Nayak NC, Gupta RK. Central salivary gland tumors of jaws. *Cancer* 1970;26:211–217.

178. Singer MI, Appelbaum EL, Loy KD. Heterotopic salivary tissue in the neck. *Laryngoscope* 1979;89:1772–1778.

179. Martínez-Madrigal F, Pineda-Daboin K, Casiraghi O, Luna MA. Salivary gland tumors of the mandible. *Ann Diag Pathol* 2002;347–353.

180. Micheau C, Riou G. Oncocytes et oncocytomes. Histoenzymologie, ultrastructure et description de l' ADN mitochondrial. *Arch Anat Pathol* 1975;23:123–132.

181. Meza-Chavez L. Oxyphilic granular cell adenoma of the parotid gland (oncocytoma). Report of five cases and study of oxyphilic granular cells (oncocytes) in normal parotid glands. *Am J Pathol* 1949;25:523–538.

182. Shintaku M, Honda T. Identification of oncocytic lesions of salivary glands by anti-mitochondrial immunohistochemistry. *Histopathology* 1997;31:408–411.

183. Hamperl H. Oncocyten und Oncocytome. *Virchows Arch A Pathol Anat Histopathol* 1962;335:452–483.

184. Barka T. Biologically active polypeptides in submandibular glands. *J Histochem Cytochem* 1980;28:836–859.

185. Bing J, Poulsen K, Hackenthal E, Rix E, Taugner R. Renin in the submaxillary gland: a review. *J Histochem Cytochem* 1980;28: 874–880.

186. Murphy RA, Watson AY, Metz J, Forssmann WG. The mouse submandibular gland: an exocrine organ for growth factors. *J Histochem Cytochem* 1980;28:890–902.

187. Whitley BD, Ferguson JW, Harris AJ, Kardos TB. Immunohistochemical localization of substance P in human parotid gland. *Int J Oral Maxillofac Surg* 1992;21:54–58.

188. Pikula DL, Harris EF, Desiderio DM, Fridland GH, Lovelace JL. Methionine enkephalin-like, substance P-like, and beta-endorphin-like immunoreactivity in human parotid saliva. *Arch Oral Biol* 1992;37:705–709.

189. Salo A, Ylikoski J, Uusitalo H. Distribution of calcitonin generelated peptide immunoreactive nerve fibers in the human submandibular gland. *Neurosci Lett* 1993;150:137–140.

190. Mathison R, Davison JS, Befus AD. Neuroendocrine regulation of inflammation and tissue repair by submandibular gland factors. *Immunol Today* 1994;15:527–532.

191. Blanck C, Eneroth CM, Jakobsson PA. Oncocytoma of the parotid gland: neoplasm or nodular hyperplasia? *Cancer* 1970; 25:919–925.

192. Batsakis JG. *Tumors of the Head and Neck.* Baltimore: Williams & Wilkins; 1974.

193. Dardick I, Bireck C, Lingen M, Rowe PE. Differentiation and the cytomorphology of salivary gland tumors with specific reference to oncocytic metaplasia. *Oral Surg Oral Med Oral Pathol Oral Radiol Endod* 1999;88:691–701.

194. Henley JD, Rehan J, Oda D, Gown AM, Gnepp DR. Oncocytic metaplastic tumors of salivary gland origin. *Oral Surg Oral Med Oral Pathol* 1977;84:187.

195. Chang A, Harawi SJ. Oncocytes, oncocytosis, and oncocytic tumors. *Pathol Annu* 1992;27(pt 1):263–304.

196. Palmer TJ, Gleeson MJ, Eveson JW, Cawson RA. Oncocytic adenomas and oncocytic hyperplasia of salivary glands: a clinico-pathological study of 26 cases. *Histopathology* 1990;16:487–493.

197. Gray SR, Cornog JL Jr, Seo IS. Oncocytic neoplasms of salivary glands: a report of fifteen cases including two malignant oncocytomas. *Cancer* 1976;38:1306–1317.

198. Hemenway WG, Allen GW. Chronic enlargement of the parotid gland. Hypertrophy and fatty infiltration. *Laryngoscope* 1959;69: 1508–1523.

199. Isacsson G, Lundquist PG. Salivary calculi as an aetiological factor in chronic sialadenitis of the submandibular gland. *Clin Otolaryngol Allied Sci* 1982;7:231–236.

200. Dardick I, Jeans MT, Sinnott NM, Wittkuhn JF, Kahn HJ, Baumal R. Salivary gland components involved in the formation of squamous metaplasia. *Am J Pathol* 1985;119:33–43.

201. Fajardo LF, Berthrong M. Radiation injury in surgical pathology. Part III. Salivary glands, pancreas and skin. *Am J Surg Pathol* 1981;5:279–296.

202. Seifert G, Donath K. Zur pathoegenese des Küttner-Tumors der submandibularis. *HNO* 1977;25:81–92.

203. Beer GM, Neuwirth A. Nekrotisierende sialometaplasie (speicheldrüseninfarkt) der glandula submandibularis. *Laryngol Rhinol Otol (Stuttg)* 1983;62:468–470.

204. Abrams AM, Melrose RJ, Howell FV. Necrotizing sialometaplasia. A disease simulating malignancy. *Cancer* 1973;32:130–135.

205. Fowler B, Brannon RB. Subacute necrotizing sialadenitis. Report of 7 cases and a review of the literature. *Oral Surg Oral Med Oral Pathol Oral Radiol Endod* 2000;89:600–609.

206. Seifert G, Donath K. Die sialadenose der parotis. *Dtsch Med Wochenschr* 1975;100:1545–1548.

207. Mandel L, Baurmash H. Parotid enlargement due to alcoholism. *J Am Dent Assoc* 1971;82:369–373.

208. Campos LA. Hyperplasia of the sublingual glands in adult patients. *Oral Surg Oral Med Oral Pathol Oral Radiol Endod* 1996;81:584–585.

209. Yu GY, Donath K. Adenomatous ductal proliferation of the salivary gland. *Oral Surg Oral Med Oral Pathol Oral Radiol Endod* 2001;91:215–221.

210. Walker NI, Gobé GC. Cell death and cell proliferation during atrophy of the rat parotid gland induced by duct obstruction. *J Pathol* 1987;153:333–344.

211. Daley TD, Dardick I. An unusual parotid tumor with histogenetic implications for salivary gland neoplasms. *Oral Surg Oral Med Oral Pathol* 1983;55:374–381.

212. Takahashi S, Schoch E, Walker N. Origin of acinar cell regeneration after atrophy of the rat parotid induced by duct obstruction. *Int J Exp Pathol* 1998;79:293–301.

213. Alavres EP, Sesso A. Cell proliferation, differentiation and transformation in the rat submandibular gland during early postnatal growth. A quantitative and morphological study. *Arch Histol Jpn* 1975;38:177–208.

214. Thackray AC, Lucas RB. Tumors of the major salivary glands. In: *Atlas of Tumor Pathology*, Series 2, Fascicle 10. Washington DC: Armed Forces Institute of Pathology; 1974:11–14

215. Eversole LR. Histogenetic classification of salivary tumors. *Arch Pathol* 1971;92:433–443.

216. Batsakis JG. Salivary gland neoplasia: an outcome of modified morphogenesis and cytodifferentiation. *Oral Surg Oral Med Oral Pathol* 1980;49:229–232.

217. Dardick I, van Nostrand AW. Morphogenesis of salivary gland tumors. A prerequisite to improving classification. *Pathol Annu* 1987;22(pt 1):1–53.

218. Barka T. Induced cell proliferation: the effect of isoproterenol. *Exp Cell Res* 1965;37:662–679.

219. Dardick I, Dardick AM, MacKay AJ, Pastolero GC, Guillane PJ, Burford-Mason AP. Pathobiology of salivary glands. IV. Histogenetic concepts and cycling cells in human parotid and submandibular glands cultured in floating collagen gels. *Oral Surg Oral Med Oral Pathol* 1993;76:307–318.

220. Burgess KL, Dardick I, Cummins MM, Burford-Mason AP, Bassett R, Brown DH. Myoepithelial cells actively proliferate during atrophy of the rat parotid gland. *Oral Surg Oral Med Oral Pathol Oral Radiol Endod* 1996;82:674–680.

221. Zarbo RJ. Salivary gland neoplasia: a review for the practicing pathologist. *Mod Pathol* 2002;15:298–323.

222. Dardick I, Burford-Mason AP. Current status of the histogenetic and morphogenetic concepts of salivary gland tumorigenesis. *Crit Rev Oral Biol Med* 1993;4:639–677.

223. Dardick I, van Nostrand AW, Jeans MT, Rippstein P, Edwards V. Pleomorphic adenoma. II. Ultrastructural organization of "stromal" regions. *Hum Pathol* 1983;14:798–809.

224. Micheau C, Lacour J. Epithelioma acineux de la parotide. *Ann Anat Pathol* 1971;16:173–188.

225. Mills SE, Garland TA, Allen MS Jr. Low-grade papillary adenocarcinoma of palatal salivary gland origin. *Am J Surg Pathol* 1984;8:367–374.

226. Garland TA, Innes DJ Jr, Fechner RE. Salivary duct carcinoma: an analysis of four cases with review of literature. *Am J Clin Pathol* 1984;81:436–441.

227. Chen KT, Hafez GR. Infiltrating salivary duct carcinoma. A clinicopathologic study of five cases. *Arch Otolaryngal* 1981;107:37–39.

228. Allen MS Jr, Fitz-Hugh GS, Marsh WL Jr. Low-grade papillary adenocarcinoma of the palate. *Cancer* 1974;33:153–158.

229. Batsakis JG, McClatchey KD, Johns M, Regezi JA. Primary squamous cell carcinoma of the parotid gland. *Arch Otolaryngol* 1976;102:355–357.

230. Martínez-Madrigal F, Baden E, Casiraghi O, Micheau C. Oral and pharyngeal adenosquamous carcinoma. A report of four cases with immunohistochemical studies. *Eur Arch Otorhinolaryngol* 1991;248:255–258.

231. Luna MA, Batsakis JG, Ordonez NG, Mackay B, Tortoledo ME. Salivary gland adenocarcinomas: a clinicopathologic analysis of three distinctive types. *Semin Diagn Pathol* 1987;4:117–135.

232. Micheau C, Lacour J, Genin J, Brugère J. Tumeurs mucoépidermoïdes de la parotide et de la cavité buccale. *Ann Anat Pathol* 1972;17:59–71.

233. White DK, Miller AS, McDaniel RK, Rothman BN. Inverted ductal papilloma: a distinctive lesion of minor salivary gland. *Cancer* 1982;49:519–524.

234. Foschini MP, Eusebi V. Value of immunohistochemistry in the diagnosis of salivary gland tumors. *Pathol Case Rev* 2004;9:270–275.

235. Foschini MP, Scarpellini F, Gown AM, Eusebi V. Differential expression of myoepithelial markers in salivary, sweat and mammary glands. *Int J Surg Pathol* 2000;8:29–37.

236. Zarbo RJ, Hatfield JS, Trojanowski JQ, et al. Immunoreactive glial fibrillary acidic protein in normal and neoplastic salivary glands: a combined immunohistochemical and immunoblot study. *Surg Pathol* 1988;1:55–63.

237. Fantasia JE, Lally ET. Localization of free secretory component in pleomorphic adenomas of minor salivary gland origin. *Cancer* 1984;53:1786–1789.

238. Caselitz J, Jaup T, Seifert G. Immunohistochemical detection of carcinoembryonic antigen (CEA) in parotid gland carcinomas. Analysis of 52 cases. *Virchows Arch A Pathol Anat Histol* 1981;394:49–60.

239. Gusterson BA, Lucas RB, Ormerod MG. Distribution of epithelial membrane antigen in benign and malignant lesions of the salivary glands. *Virchows Arch A Pathol Anat Histol* 1982;397:227–233.

240. Tsuji T, Nagai N. Production of alpha-fetoprotein by human submandibular gland. *Int J Dev Biol* 1993;37:497–498.

241. Caselitz J, Seifert G, Grenner G, Schmidtberger R. Amylase as an additional marker of salivary gland neoplasms. An immunoperoxidase study. *Pathol Res Pract* 1983;176:276–283.

242. Cenley J, Baker DC. Cancer of the salivary glands. In: Suen JY, Myers EN, eds. *Cancer of the Head and Neck.* New York: Churchill Livingstone; 1981.

243. Rankow RM, Mignogna F. Cancer of the sublingual salivary gland. *Am J Surg* 1969;118:790–795.

THORAX AND SEROUS MEMBRANES

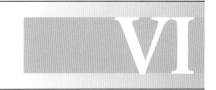

VI

Lungs

Thomas V. Colby   Kevin O. Leslie
Samuel A. Yousem

NORMAL STRUCTURE AND HISTOLOGY

The following review is based on several standard references on the topic (1–16).

General

The lungs are paired intrathoracic organs that are divided into lobes (three on the right—right upper lobe, right middle lobe, right lower lobe; two on the left—left upper lobe, left lower lobe). The lingula is a rudimentary appendage arising from the left upper lobe and is analogous to the middle lobe on the right. The lobes are further divided into bronchopulmonary segments (Table 18.1).

The segmental anatomy of the lung is important for radiologists, bronchoscopists, and pathologists in defining the location of lesions. The lobes are divided by fissures

and have their own pleural investments. The segments are not separated by fissures and do not normally have separate pleural investments, although they are recognizable on the basis of their supplying bronchi (segmental bronchi).

The primordial lungs arise as ventral buds of the foregut extending into the primitive thoracic mesenchyme. Bronchial cartilages, smooth muscle, and other connective tissues are derived from the mesenchyme that surrounds these dichotomatously branching buds. The phases of airway and lung parenchymal development are summarized in Table 18.2.

As the lung progresses through these phases of development, there is a complex series of epithelial-mesenchymal reactions modified by physiologic mechanical forces and humoral factors. These events are overseen by master genes (such as homeobox genes), nuclear transcription factors, hormones, and other soluble mediators such as growth

TABLE 18.1
BRONCHOPULMONARY SEGMENTS*

Right upper lobe	Left upper lobe
1. Apical	1,2. Apical posterior
2. Posterior	3. Anterior
3. Anterior	Lingula
Right middle lobe	4. Superior
4. Lateral	5. Inferior
5. Medial	Left lower lobe
Right lower lobe	6. Superior
6. Superior	7. Anterior-medial basal
7. Medial basal	8. Lateral basal
8. Anterior basal	9. Posterior basal
9. Lateral basal	
10. Posterior basal	

*Modified from: Kuhn C III. Normal anatomy and histology. In: Thurlbeck WM, Churg AM, eds. *Pathology of the Lung.* 2nd ed. New York: Thieme Medical Publishers; 1995:1–36.

TABLE 18.2
PHASES OF LUNG DEVELOPMENT

Phase	Gestation (approx. weeks)	Major Events
Embryonic	3 ½–6 weeks	Development of major airways
Pseudoglandular	6–16	Development of airways to terminal bronchioles
Canalicular	16–28	Development of the acinus and its vascularization
Saccular	28–36	Subdivision of saccules by secondary crests
Alveolar	36 weeks to term (and up to 4 years of age)	Acquisition of alveoli

factors (17,18). Some of these mediators and their relationship to lung development are shown in Table 18.3.

Airways

The airways serve as conduits for air traveling to and from alveoli; for evacuation of material along the mucociliary escalator; and for immunologic, protective, air-moisturizing, and warming functions.

The airways arise by unequal dichotomous branching of the bronchial buds. In a normal individual, there are approximately 20 generations (range: approximately 10–30

divisions, depending on the location in and distance from the trachea) extending from the trachea to the respiratory bronchioles. In histologic sections from normal lungs, the diameter of an airway is approximately the same as its accompanying artery (and vice versa) (19). Disparities in size (of either airway or artery) suggest a pathologic condition. Airways are defined as follows:

- *Bronchi* are cartilaginous airways and are usually more than 1 mm in diameter (Figure 18.1). They are conducting airways, and the cartilage plates in their walls prevent their collapse. The posterior wall is smooth muscle. The cartilage may calcify.

TABLE 18.3
LUNG DEVELOPMENT AND REGULATORY FACTORS*

Phase of Lung Development	Events	Major Molecular Mediators
Embryonic	Outgrowth of trachea, right and left main bronchi, and major airways	HNF-3β, TTF-1, RA, RAR, Shh, Ptch, Gli2, Gli3, FGF-8, FGF-10, NHF-4, N-cadherin, activin-β-r, IIa, lefty-1/2, nodal, Pitx-2
Pseudoglandular	Formation of bronchial tree up to a preacinar level.	GATA-6, N-myc, PDGF, PDGF-R, EGF, EGF-R, FGF, TGF-β, Shh, Ptch, VEGF, BMP-4, RA, RAR
Canalicular	Formation of the pulmonary acinus and of the future air-blood barrier; increase of capillary bed; epithelial differentiation; first appearance of surfactant	GATA-6, TTF-1, HNF-3β, Mash-1, VEGF
Saccular	Formation of transitory air spaces	HNF-3β, TTF-1, NF1, VEGF, VEGF-R
Alveolar	Alveolarization by forming of secondary septa	PDGF, PDGF-R, FGF, FGF-R, VEGF, VEGF-R, angiopoietins, ephrins, RA, RAR
Microvascular maturation (birth–3 years)	Thinning of interalveolar walls; fusion of the capillary bilayer to a single layered network	VEGF, VEGF-R, PDGF, PDGF-R, angiopoietins, ephrins

*Modified from: Roth-Kleiner M, Post M. Genetic control of lung development. *Biol Neonate* 2003;84:83–88.

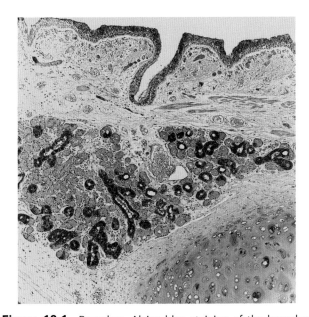

Figure 18.1 Bronchus. Alcian blue staining of the bronchus highlights the presence of goblet cells in the mucosa (slightly increased in this case), as well as the bronchial submucosalglands. Beneath the epithelial basement membrane, there is a vascularized layer of connective tissue with wisps of smooth muscle above the submucosal glands.

■ *Bronchioles* are airways that are usually less than 1 mm in diameter; they lack cartilage (Figure 18.2).
■ *Nonrespiratory bronchioles* represent all bronchioles proximal to respiratory bronchioles.
■ *Terminal bronchioles* are nonrespiratory bronchioles just proximal to respiratory bronchioles.
■ *Respiratory bronchioles* are airways that have alveoli budding from their walls.

In the large bronchi, the surface epithelium rests on a basement membrane, below which there is an elastin-rich layer of connective tissue; together these elements comprise the *bronchial mucosa*. Beneath the bronchial mucosa lies the *submucosa,* in which submucosal glands, cartilage, nerves, ganglia, and branches of the bronchial artery may be found. There is no clear histologic boundary between mucosa and submucosa. Outside the submucosa, there is a peribronchial sheath of loose connective tissue, which is continuous with that of the accompanying artery. The bronchial epithelium is a pseudostratified columnar epithelium composed primarily of ciliated columnar cells with interspersed mucous (goblet) cells. Lesser numbers of neuroendocrine cells, basal cells, brush cells, and migratory inflammatory cells are also normally present (see below).

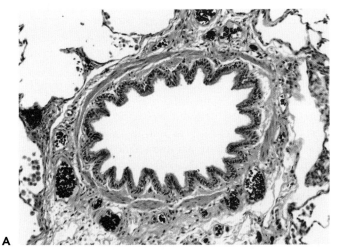

A

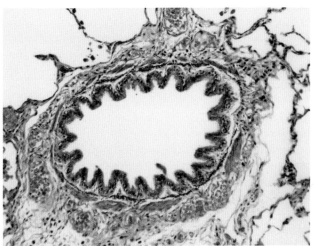

B

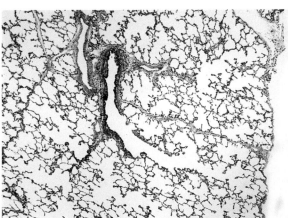

C

Figure 18.2 Bronchioles. Hematoxylin and eosin (**A**) and elastic tissue stains (**B**) illustrate normal bronchioles with a thin layer of connective tissue just beneath the epithelium overlying the elastica (B) and the smooth muscle investiture. The mucosa is low columnar, and there is no thickening of the subepithelial region. The smooth muscle is circumferential and is surrounded by an adventitial layer. **C.** A terminal bronchiole is continuous with the respiratory bronchiole, which extends into the alveolar ducts and ultimately the alveoli.

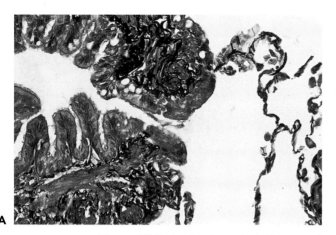

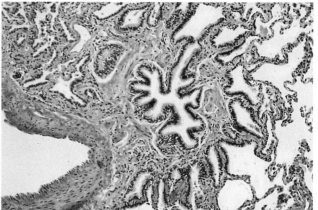

Figure 18.3   Lambert's canals. **A.** These canals represent communications between nonrespiratory bronchioles and adjacent alveoli and are only rarely observed in histologic sections. **B.** It is these canals that are thought to be the origin of peribronchiolar metaplasia, which is seen as a repair phenomenon involving peribronchiolar alveoli after bronchiolar injury.

The height of the pseudostratified columnar epithelium decreases progressively toward the periphery of the lung.

The walls of bronchioles are normally much thinner than those of the bronchi. The surface epithelium rests on a basement membrane, which overlies a thin layer of loose elastin-rich connective tissue. This is surrounded by a muscle layer (muscularis), which is in turn invested by a peribronchiolar connective tissue sheath continuous with that of the adjacent artery. The distinction of mucosa from submucosa in bronchioles is arbitrary, and sometimes the tissue beneath the basement membrane is referred to as submucosal or submembranous connective tissue.

The airway basement membrane region consists of three layers: lamina lucida, lamina densa, and lamina reticularis. The last of these consists of very fine fibrillary collagen and is only found in adults. It is not technically part of the basement membrane, and it is this zone that is thickened in asthma and other inflammatory airway conditions. The basement membrane stains with digested PAS stains and immunostains for type IV collagen and laminin.

Direct communications between nonrespiratory bronchioles and alveoli have been identified and termed Lambert's canals (20). These are thought to be involved in collateral ventilation. Lambert's canals are rarely visible in histologic sections (20). Lambert's canals may be conspicuous in scarred airways surrounded by metaplastic bronchiolar epithelium, which is seen to be continuous with the bronchiolar surface epithelium through Lambert's canals. This has been termed "Lambertosis," bronchiolarization, and peribronchiolar metaplasia (Figure 18.3). Sometimes the marked peribronchiolar metaplasia is the most prominent pathologic finding in a surgical biopsy. Peribronchiolar metaplasia is a not uncommon incidental finding in a variety of diffuse lung diseases. It may also be the sole or predominant change and the cause of the diffuse lung disease as described in some recent studies (21–23).

Cell types lining the airways include basal cells, Kulchitsky cells, ciliated cells, Clara cells, goblet cells, intermediate cells, and brush cells. Ultrastructural abnormalities in the ciliated cells of the respiratory tract are known to be associated with pathologic conditions (e.g., primary ciliary dyskinesia). Goblet cells and ciliated cells decrease in number as the terminal bronchioles are approached; there is a concomitant increase in Clara cells, and the mucosa becomes less columnar and more cuboidal in appearance. Clara cells have secretory functions (e.g., surfactant-like material) and also act as progenitor cells after bronchiolar injury. Clara cell differentiation in tumors of the lung may be appreciated by the presence of apical periodic acid-Schiff (PAS)-positive, diastase-resistant granules, as well as by their electron microscopic apical-dense granules. Kulchitsky cells contain dense core granules and are part of the diffuse neuroendocrine system. Aggregates of neuroepithelial cells are called neuroepithelial bodies; they tend to occur at airway bifurcations. The finding of goblet cells in bronchioles usually signifies chronic airway injury. The cell types in the airways and parenchyma are summarized in Table 18.4 and illustrated in Figures 18.4, 18.5, and 18.6.

Smooth muscle of the airways plays an important functional role in regulating airflow and is arranged in a complex spiral pattern that becomes progressively less prominent in the distal conducting airways. This muscle receives nutrition from the bronchial arteries. At the level of the alveolar ducts, bundles of airway smooth muscle can be seen, interrupted by alveolar openings; in cross section, these may appear as isolated round or oblong aggregates.

Submucosal salivary-type glands containing both serous and mucous cells are found in the larger bronchi. In older individuals, oncocytic metaplasia can be seen in these glands (Figure 18.7). Within the walls of the large airways, ganglia, nerves, and bronchial arteries are found.

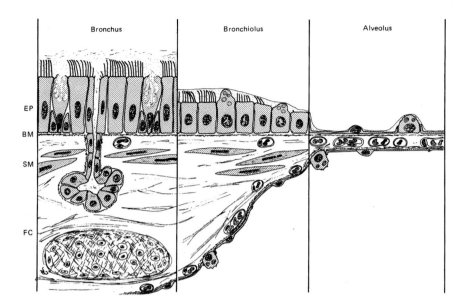

Figure 18.4 Respiratory tract epithelia. There is a progression of pseudostratified columnar epithelium in the large airways, to a more cuboidal epithelium in the small airways, to squamous type epithelial cells (type I pneumocytes) in the alveoli. The epithelium in the large airways is designed for maintaining and moving the mucous stream, whereas the squamous pneumocytes in the airspaces facilitate gas transfer. (Reprinted with permission from: Weibel ER, Taylor CR. Design and structure of the human lung. In: Fishman AP, ed. *Pulmonary Diseases and Disorders*. Vol 1. 2nd ed. New York: McGraw-Hill; 1988:14.)

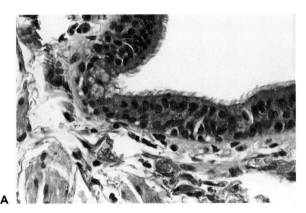

A

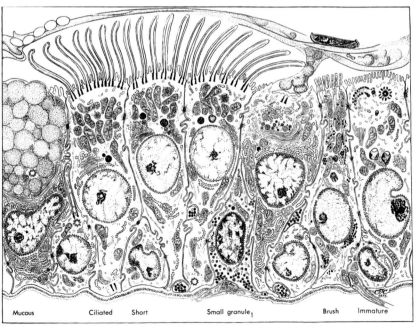

B

Figure 18.5 Bronchial epithelium. **A.** Normal bronchial epithelium is pseudostratified and columnar, with numerous ciliated cells and scattered basophilic and flocculent-appearing goblet cells. **B.** This ultrastructural schematic of bronchial epithelium shows the various cell types present. (Figure 18.5B reprinted with permission from: Sorokin SP. The respiratory system. In: Weiss L, ed. *Cell and Tissue Biology: A Textbook of Histology*. 6th ed. Baltimore: Williams & Wilkins; 1988:769.)

TABLE 18.4
MAJOR CELL TYPES OF THE LOWER RESPIRATORY TRACT*

Cell Type	Features	Function(s)	Location	Histochemical and/or Immunohisto-chemical Staining
Ciliated	Columnar, cuboidal, ciliated bronchial lining cells; each cell has approximately 250 cilia at the apical surface, and each cilium is approximately 6 μm long	Proximal transport of mucous stream (mucociliary escalator)	Bronchi and bronchioles	Epithelial markers[2]
Goblet	Columnar mucus-secreting cells; contain mucous glycoprotein, which discharges apically	Contribute to airway mucus	Bronchi (more numerous proximally); small numbers in bronchioles	Epithelial markers[2], histochemical mucin stains, MUC5
Basal	Short cells with relatively little cytoplasm; oriented along the basement membrane; do not reach the luminal surface of the epithelium	Precursor cell of ciliated and goblet cells	Bronchi; rare in bronchioles	Epithelial markers[2]
Neuroendocrine (Kulchitsky or K cells)	Basal-oriented cells with numerous dense-core (neurosecretory) granules; single or in groups (neuroepithelial bodies), the latter near sites of airway bifurcation	Specific functions not known; considered part of the diffuse neuroendocrine system	Bronchi; rare in bronchioles	Chromogranin-A, synaptophysin, NCAM
Brush	Found infrequently at all levels of the airways; some have termed these type III pneumo-cytes; they are named for a brush border of microvilli approximately 2 μm in length	Thought to be involved in fluid absorption or chemoreceptor function	All airways	Ultrastructurally identified
Serous	Identical to serous cells in the minor salivary gland tissues	Produce secretion of lower viscosity than that from mucous cells	Primarily bronchioles	Lysozyme
Neuroendocrine bodies	Clusters of 4–10 neuroendocrine cells adjacent to the subepithelial basement membrane	Unknown; hypotheses include chemoreceptor, tactile receptor, vasoconstrictive functions	Bronchi, bronchioles, and alveoli	Chromogranin-A, synaptophysin
Oncocytic	Eosinophilic mitochondrial-rich cells in submucosal gland ducts	Ion secretory functions	Submucosal glands	Epithelial markers[2]
Squamous	Stratified squamous epithelium is an abnormal metaplastic replacement of normal pseudostratified respiratory epithelium	Protective, reparative	Bronchi, bronchioles, and occasionally alveoli	Epithelial markers[2], cytokeratin 5/6
Clara	Columnar nonciliated bronchiolar cells; protuberant apical cytoplasm with large, ovoid electron-dense granules; comprise the majority of nonciliated bronchiolar cells	Secretory functions contributing to the mucous pool and maintaining extracellular lining fluid; progenitor for other bronchiolar cells; role in surfactant	Predominantly in bronchioles	CC10, diastase-resistant PAS-positive apical granules

TABLE 18.4
(continued)

Cell Type	Features	Function(s)	Location	Histochemical and/or Immunohisto-chemical Staining
Type I alveolar pneumocyte	Large, flat, squamous alveolar lining cells; cover some 93% of alveolar surface area; incapable of division	Provide a thin air-blood interface for gas transfer	Alveoli	Epithelial markers[2], caveolin, and aquaporin
Type II alveolar pneumocyte	Columnar alveolar lining cells; microvillous surface; synthesize and secrete surfactant (lamellar ultrastructural inclusions); capable of division	Maintain alveolar stability; progenitor for type I pneumocytes	Alveoli	Epithelial markers[2], surfactant protein C
Minor salivary tissue: Serous, Mucous, Ductal Cells	Submucosal minor salivary glands identical to other sites with serous and mucinous acinar cells that secrete into the ducts, which empty at the mucosal surface	Secretion and contribution to airway mucous stream	Bronchial submucosa	Epithelial markers[2], histochemical stains for mucin, Alcian blue/PAS
Smooth muscle	Bundled smooth muscle surrounds the conducting airways to the level of the alveolar ducts	Contraction of the airway	Peripheral in the airway and external to the cartilage in bronchi	Muscle specific actin, smooth muscle actin, desmin, vimentin
Other cells[1]				

[1] Endothelial cells and pericytes; interstitial fibrocytes, fibroblasts, and myofibroblasts; macrophages; lymphoid cells, including Langerhans cells; mast cells; mesothelial pleural lining; cartilage and bone; smooth muscle; peripheral nerves; and myoepithelial cells.

[2] For example, AE1/AE3 and EMA.

*Table is modified from:

Castranova V, Rabovsky J, Tucker JH, Miles PR. The alveolar type II epithelial cell: a multifunctional pneumocyte. *Toxicol Appl Pharmacol* 1988;93:472–483.

Colby TV, Koss MN, Travis WD. Tumors of the lower respiratory tract. In: Rosai J, ed. *Atlas of Tumor Pathology*. 3rd series, fascicle 13. Washington DC: Armed Forced Institute of Pathology: 1995:465–471.

Corrin B. *Pathology of the Lungs*. London: Churchill Livingstone; 2000.

Kasper M, Reimann T, Hempel U, et al. Loss of caveolin expression in type I pneumocyte as an indicator of subcellular alterations during lung fibrogenesis. *Histochem Cell Biol* 1998;109:41–48.

Kreda SM, Gynn MC, Fenstermacher DA, Boucher RC, Gabriel SE. Expression and localization of epithelial aquaporins in the adult human lung. *Am J Respir Cell Mol Biol* 2001;24:224–234.

Lou YP, Takeyama K, Grattan KM, et al. Platelet-activating factor induces goblet cell hyperplasia and mucin gene expression in airways. *Am J Respir Crit Care Med* 1998;157(pt 1):1927–1934.

Rogers AV, Dewar A, Corrin B, Jeffrey PK. Identification of serous-like cells in the surface epithelium of human bronchioles. *Eur Respir J* 1995;6:498–504.

Ryerse JS, Hoffmann JW, Mahmoud S, Nagel BA, deMello DE. Immunolocalization of CC10 in Clara cells in mouse and human lung. *Histochem Cell Biol* 2001;115:325–332.

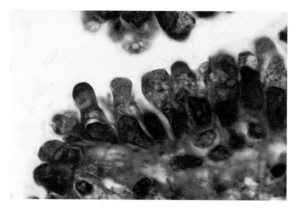

Figure 18.6 Clara cells. Although Clara cells sometimes can be identified in bronchioles, these are seen to best advantage in neoplasms such as this nonmucinous bronchioloalveolar carcinoma. The apical snouting and increased cytoplasmic density are apparent.

Lobule and Acinus

The lung lobule is grossly visible and represents the smallest anatomic subunit of the lung that is bounded by connective tissue (interlobular) septa, which may appear to invaginate from the visceral pleura (Figure 18.8). Lobules are 1 to 2 cm in diameter and are visible to the naked eye on

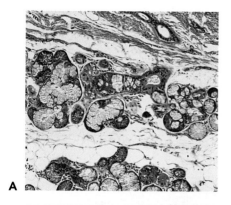

A

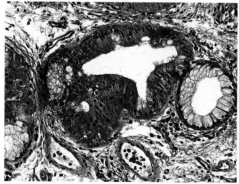

B

Figure 18.7 Bronchial submucosal glands. **A.** The bronchial submucosal glands are normally located in the submucosa above the bronchial cartilage and contain mixed seromucous glands with a duct leading to the bronchial mucosa (also Figure 18.1). **B.** Oncocytic metaplasia involving bronchial submucosal glands is relatively common.

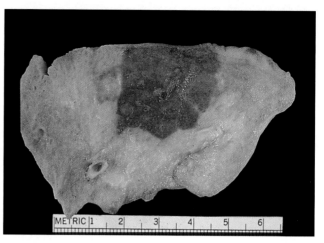

Figure 18.8 Pulmonary lobule. This cut section of normal lung tissue (from an explant that could not be used for technical reasons) shows focal hemorrhage highlighting a pulmonary lobule. The hemorrhage stops abruptly at the interlobular septa and, centrally, a bronchovascular bundle can be appreciated. The lobule is approximately 2.0 cm in diameter.

both the pleural surface of the lung and on cut surfaces of the parenchyma by their septal demarcations. Lobules are accentuated in fibrotic conditions in which the septa contract (e.g., honeycombing, healed infectious pneumonia, chronic pleural inflammation). Pulmonary lobules are identifiable with high-resolution computed tomography (CT) scanning of the lung. The term *lobule* as used here has also been referred to as the secondary lobule of Miller (12). The use of the term *secondary lobule* is discouraged because it implies that there is a primary lobule, and the latter term is not in current use.

The functional unit of the lung is the acinus, where gas transfer takes place (Figure 18.9). The precise definition of the acinus has varied. Some define it as the lung tissue supplied by a single terminal bronchiole (12,15). According to this definition, each pulmonary lobule comprises some 3 to 10 acini. The acinus has also been defined as a respiratory bronchiole and its supplied alveolar ducts and sacs (10,13); using this definition, each lobule comprises some 20 to 30 acini and the acini are 1 to 2 mm in diameter.

Squamous (type I pneumocytes) and cuboidal (type II, or granular, pneumocytes) epithelial cells line the alveoli (Table 18.4). Gas exchange takes place across the cytoplasm of type I cells. Type II cells are the progenitors for type I cells, produce surfactant, and proliferate after injury to restore alveolar epithelial integrity. Type II cell hyperplasia represents a nonspecific marker of alveolar injury and repair (Fig 18.10). Macrophages are a normal finding in the lung, scattered over the surfaces of the alveoli and percolating into the interstitium; a number of subpopulations of pulmonary macrophages are definable, based on their anatomic locations and their role in host defense clearance functions (31). Pulmonary macrophages are greatly increased in cigarette smokers; increased Langerhans cells are also found in the

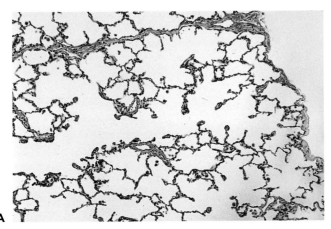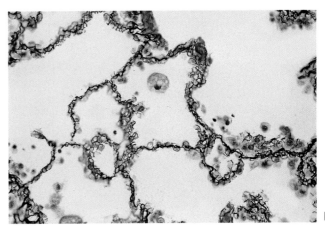

A   B

Figure 18.9 Distal lung parenchyma. The acinus is the functional unit of the lung where a gas transfer takes place. **A.** An alveolar duct extends from the left to right and communicates directly with alveolar spaces; a small interlobular septum (*top*) and the pleura (*right*) are present. (From the case illustrated in Figure 18.2C.) **B.** Reticulin stain highlights the vasculature of the alveolar septum, showing pulmonary capillaries winding around the access of the alveolar wall to maximize gas transfer surface area. A foamy macrophage is present (*upper center*), a normal finding in lung parenchyma.

bronchiolar epithelium of smokers, but their recognition requires special stains (e.g., CD1a) and quantitative studies.

The epithelial and capillary basement membranes in the alveolar septum are irregularly fused. Gas transfer takes place across the alveolar-capillary membrane, which includes the attenuated cytoplasm of the type I cell, the endothelial cell cytoplasm, and their fused basement membranes. Pores of Kohn represent direct communications between adjacent alveoli via a "pore" in the alveolar wall. They are thought to be involved in collateral ventilation. Pores of Kohn are rarely visible with the light microscope.

The lung is invested with a rich framework of connective tissue coursing throughout the interstitium. It is well developed and easily visible along bronchovascular sheaths and in the septa that delimit lobules. This framework is continuous from the hilum to the pleura and encompasses the interstitial compartment of the lung down to the level of the alveolar wall and perivascular areas. Within the alveolar walls, collagen, elastic fibers, mesenchymal cells, and a few inflammatory cells can be identified ultrastructurally. This alveolar interstitial space is normally inconspicuous by light microscopy in adults. In children (up to approximately age 4), some interstitial widening and increased cellularity are a normal histologic finding.

Given the concentration of nuclei of the various cell types comprising the alveolar wall, it may be difficult to decide when some degree of cellularity is pathologic. Although one may attempt to count nuclei in a single alveolar wall, it is more practical to assess inflammatory cell infiltrates in the perivenular regions and to compare various foci in the biopsy since interstitial infiltrates are rarely perfectly uniform in distribution.

Vasculature

The lungs have vascular systems: bronchial (systemic) arteries and veins and pulmonary arteries and veins. The alveolar microvasculature is designed for oxygenation of venous blood derived from the pulmonary arteries. Large (elastic) pulmonary arteries in infants are similar to the aorta in structure; the elastic fiber lamellae become more irregular, fragmented, and less compact in adulthood. Elastic tissue remains relatively prominent in the pulmonary arterial tree to approximately the point where bronchi become bronchioles. At this juncture, the pulmonary arteries become primarily muscular arteries. The muscular pulmonary arteries and arterioles have an internal and external elastic

Figure 18.10 Alveolar cell hyperplasia. A reactive proliferation of type II cells (alveolar cell hyperplasia) is common after injury. This case illustrates how this appears as a single row of cells protruding from the alveolar surface. Cytologic atypia is lacking. The interstitium shows edema, inflammatory cells, and some fibrinous exudate consistent with recent lung injury.

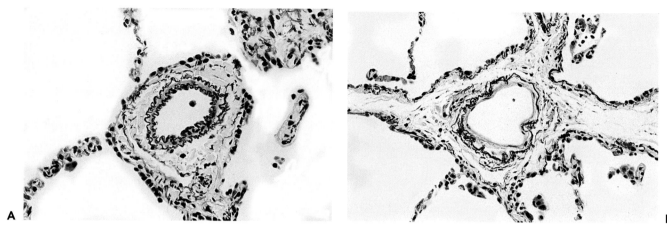

Figure 18.11 Pulmonary vasculature (elastic stains). Normal pulmonary arteries contain two elastic lamina (**A**), whereas veins have a single elastic lamina (**B**). The location of a vein within a septum (**B**) is also very helpful in identifying it as a vein.

membrane (Fig. 18.11A); pulmonary veins have only a lamellated single (outer) elastica (Fig. 18.11B). Small intra-acinar pulmonary veins merge into larger veins in the interlobular septa. The bronchial arteries in the walls of bronchi are part of the systemic circulation and have pressures similar to systemic arterial pressures. The pulmonary circulation is a low pressure system with a normal mean pressure of approximately 10 mmHg (it is somewhat higher at higher elevations).

It may be difficult to separate small pulmonary arterioles from venules, especially since a single elastic lamina forms as arterioles get smaller. In pathologic states, the veins may develop muscular hypertrophy and increased mural thickness (arterialization), making the distinction of arteries from veins difficult. The location of the vessel, particularly if it is in a septum or accompanied by an airway, is extremely helpful (and sometimes the only way) when separating pulmonary veins from pulmonary arteries. In mild pulmonary hypertension, the pulmonary arteries may appear histologically normal; in general, pressure measurements taken at catheterization are more reliable than histologic subtleties in determining the pressure and degree of pulmonary hypertension. Only plexiform lesions and dilatation lesions connote unequivocal pulmonary hypertension. Conversely, the presence of some degree of diffuse interstitial fibrosis or localized pulmonary scars is commonly associated with mural thickening of pulmonary vessels in the absence of pulmonary hypertension.

Lymphatics and Lymphoid Tissue

The lung is invested with a rich supply of lymphatics and lymphoid tissue. Lymphatic drainage is toward the hilum of the lung. Lymph fluid from the lower lobes tends to drain to infratracheal lymph nodes, with lymph fluid from the remaining portions of the lung draining to tracheobronchial lymph nodes. On the left side, the lymph fluid drains into

the thoracic duct; and, on the right side, it drains into the right bronchomediastinal trunk. Both of these ultimately drain into the left and right subclavian veins, respectively. Lymphatic channels are found along bronchovascular structures and pulmonary veins and in the septa and pleura. Valves may be apparent in some sections. Lymphatics do not extend into alveolar walls. The lymphatics vessels are inconspicuous except in pathologic states, such as pulmonary edema or lymphangitic carcinoma. Lymphoreticular infiltrates and some pneumoconioses tend to be distributed along the lymphatic routes, but the lymphatic vessels themselves may not be prominent.

Lymphoid tissue may be seen as small collections of lymphocytes along the lymphatic routes, especially branch points of the bronchovascular bundles; lymphoid tissue is generally absent or inconspicuous except in pathologic states. Lymphoid tissue along the airways is part of the diffuse mucosa-associated lymphoid tissue (MALT) and in the lung is referred to as bronchus-associated lymphoid tissue (BALT). Submucosal lymphoid tissue in the intermediate and small airways is associated with flattening and attenuation of the overlying respiratory mucosa (lymphoepithelium), which has increased HLA class II antigens. At these sites, B lymphocyte emperipolesis is common and is thought to reflect active antigen processing by the BALT. Bronchus-associated lymphoid tissue displays the same reactions observed in lymphoid tissue at other sites; for example, reactive hyperplasia and immunoblastic proliferation, which can be confused with lymphoreticular malignancies.

Immunophenotypically the lymphoid tissue of BALT has an immunoarchitecture with four identifiable compartments, including B-cell–rich follicles, B-cell follicular mantle and marginal zones, and T-cell–rich interfollicular regions. A follicular dendritic cell network is present. Polyclonal plasma cells are identified in the perifollicular tissue. The finer details of the immunoarchitecture and the immunophenotypic characterization of these cells are beyond the scope of this review. The follicles tend to be polarized into a darker side and a paler side, with the latter oriented toward the epithelial surface; BALT also shares features of MALT as seen at other sites. In normal adult lungs, BALT is rarely present, and its presence correlates with some form of chronic antigenic stimulation (32–34). According to Tschernig et al. (34), BALT is not present at birth but is found normally with increasing age, probably as a result of exposure to environmental antigens. After the individual has been exposed to most of the common antigens, the BALT regresses and dendritic cells in the airways assume the role of antigen uptake and presentation. Its reappearance in adults follows chronic antigen stimuli, such as chronic infection.

As currently defined, BALT refers only to lymphoid tissue along the airways (35) and not to the lymphoid tissue that may be seen in the pleura and septa as part of diffuse lymphoid hyperplasia in the lung. Hyperplasia of BALT is frequently accompanied by lymphoid hyperplasia at these other sites.

Intrapulmonary peribronchial lymph nodes are a normal finding, but peripheral intraparenchymal lymph nodes are less common; however, in smokers and others with high dust exposure, they are increasingly recognized (and biopsied) with current imaging techniques (36). Intrapulmonary lymph nodes are usually septal or subpleural in location (see below). Anthracosis and small amounts of silica and silicates in these nodes is common and nonspecific.

Pleura

The visceral pleura is composed of connective tissue, elastic tissue, and an outer mesothelial layer (Figure 18.12). The elastic tissue is often not a single layer, and several layers may be apparent. In pathologic conditions the elastic tissue may greatly increase. Elastic tissue stains are useful in assessing whether a given pathologic process, such as carcinoma, has transgressed the visceral pleura (37), but interpretation is difficult when the pleura is fibrotic and the elastic tissue is increased. Pleural assessment is important in separating T1 carcinomas from T2 carcinomas; the latter invade the visceral pleura (21). Lymphatic vessels that are continuous with those in the interlobular septa are also identifiable in the pleura. When the pleura is fibrotic and in foci of pleural adhesions, vessels may be thick and sclerotic or even pseudoangiomatous in appearance. Fatty metaplasia is often striking in foci of pleural and subpleural scarring. The visceral pleura often remains viable over pulmonary infarcts because it has a separate vascular supply. Submesothelial fibroblasts may undergo mesothelial metaplasia (and become cytokeratin-positive) in inflammatory conditions of the pleura.

SPECIAL STAINS AND THE EVALUATION OF LUNG HISTOLOGY

While most diagnostic work in lung histology and pathology can be performed with routine *hematoxylin-eosin (H&E) staining*, there are a number of special stains that aid interpretation and or highlight findings. *Elastic tissue staining* is helpful in evaluating the pulmonary vasculature, airways, and pleura. Sometimes arteries and veins can be distinguished from each other with elastic tissue staining. Elastic tissue staining highlights damage to the intima and media that might not be apparent on H&E staining. Elastic

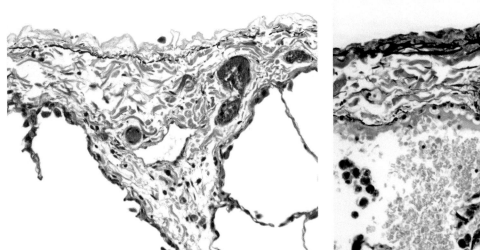

A   B

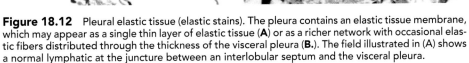

Figure 18.12 Pleural elastic tissue (elastic stains). The pleura contains an elastic tissue membrane, which may appear as a single thin layer of elastic tissue (**A**) or as a richer network with occasional elastic fibers distributed through the thickness of the visceral pleura (**B.**). The field illustrated in (A) shows a normal lymphatic at the juncture between an interlobular septum and the visceral pleura.

tissue stains are also useful in highlighting abnormalities of bronchioles and may confirm the bronchiolar or alveolar duct origin of small scars in cases of complete obliteration of the small airways. Elastic tissue staining is helpful in highlighting the pleural elastica and its relationship to tumors.

Trichrome staining (or other stains highlighting connective tissues) may also be useful in highlighting normal and pathologic findings in the lung, but they do not provide quite as much information as elastic tissue stains. Trichrome staining may be useful in assessing the distribution and extent of fibrosis in fibrosing diseases. *Reticulin stains* and stains for *collagen type IV* may be used to highlight the reticulin network of the lung. This staining may be useful in research studies and in highlighting normal histology but is not generally useful in diagnostic surgical pathology of the lung.

Immunostains for epithelial markers (such as EMA and cytokeratin stains) may be beneficial in atelectatic or fibrotic lung when it is difficult to appreciate the architectural features on H&E staining. Comparing these stains with stains for endothelial cells (such as CD31 or CD34) may provide an additional aid in assessing lung architecture and structural relationships. Use of CD31 may be somewhat confusing since alveolar macrophages frequently show prominent staining. Lymphoid tissue in the lung is assessed with the panoply of lymphoid markers used at other sites. Both CD3 and CD20 are often useful to check the proportion and distribution of T and B cells, respectively. In general, most inflammatory conditions have a preponderance of T cells as the diffuse component of the infiltrates, with scattered B-cell follicles. In lymphoproliferative conditions, cytokeratin staining highlights lymphoepithelial lesions. Both S-100 and CD1a are useful in identifying Langerhans cells; the latter stain is much more specific.

Mesothelial cells lining the pleura typically stain with calretinin, cytokeratin 5/6, and WT-1 (nuclear positivity).

PATTERN RECOGNITION BASED ON NORMAL ANATOMIC LANDMARKS

It is useful to define pathologic conditions in the lung in relation to normal anatomic landmarks (Figure 18.13). This can usually be done with diffuse diseases and often with localized processes. Such an exercise in diffuse lung disease is extremely useful in correlation with gross findings, as well as with high-resolution computed tomography (HRCT) scanning (38). Histologic patterns and their corresponding HRCT patterns can be recognized and are shown in Table 18.5.

It is apparent that there is close correlation (but not a 1:1 relationship) between histology and HRCT. With some communication between the pathologist and the radiologist, there is a significant mutual appreciation for the similarity of the abnormalities seen. In this regard, the pathologist may be significantly aided by HRCT findings, which may suggest distributions that might not be apparent in biopsy material because of such things as the size of the biopsy (e.g., transbronchial biopsy) or sampling issues (nonrepresentative biopsies).

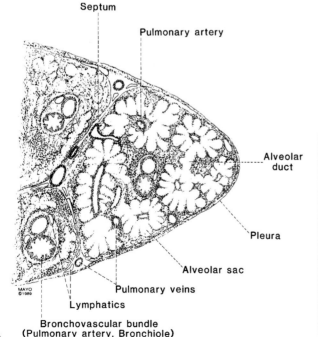

Septum

Pulmonary artery

Alveolar duct

Pleura

Alveolar sac

Pulmonary veins

Lymphatics

Bronchovascular bundle
(Pulmonary artery, Bronchiole)

A

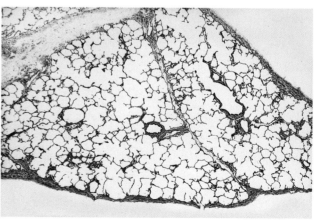

B

Figure 18.13 Wedge lung biopsy. **A.** This stylized diagram is used to depict anatomic landmarks. Structures depicted in (A) can be appreciated in an actual wedge biopsy specimen (**B**).

TABLE 18.5*

CORRESPONDING HISTOLOGIC AND RADIOLOGIC PATTERNS

Histologic	Radiologic (HRCT)
Broncho/bronchiolocentric	Centrilobular
	Bronchovascular
	Nodular
Angiocentric	Bronchovascular (arterial)
	Interlobular septal (venous)
Pleural/subpleural	Pleural/subpleural
Lymphatic	Bronchovascular
	Interlobular septal
	Pleural
Peripheral acinar	Subpleural peripheral distribution (paraseptal)
Septal	Septal
Random nodular	Random nodular
Parenchymal consolidation	Consolidation, ground glass
Diffuse interstitial	Diffuse interstitial, ground glass
Mixed and unclassified	Mixed/unclassifiable

*Modified from: Colby TV, Swensen SJ. Anatomic distribution at histopathologic pattern in diffuse lung disease: correlation with HRCT. *J Thorac Imaging* 1996;11:1–26.

SITE-RELATED CHANGES COMMONLY SEEN IN SURGICAL PATHOLOGY MATERIAL

Site specific changes that may be primary lesions or incidental findings in surgical material are shown in Table 18.6.

Biopsies from lobar tips, particularly from the lingula or right middle lobe, may show incidental inflammatory and fibrotic changes (39), including interstitial fibrosis, epithelial metaplasia, and even focal honeycombing—all of which may not be representative of a diffuse process. Myointimal proliferation is common in the arteries and veins of these biopsies. The airspaces may contain aggregates of macrophages and neutrophils. Because of their accessibility, these sites are often biopsied. Incidental changes in lobar tips are usually obvious as such, since the more proximal lung tissue is either not affected or significantly

TABLE 18.6

SITE-SPECIFIC CHANGES IN LUNG TISSUE

- Inflammatory changes at lobar tips, especially lingula and right middle lobe
- Apical caps: pleural and subpleural fibrosis in the apex and the upper lobes and superior segments of the lower lobes
- Upper lobe centriacinar emphysema
- Visceral pleural/subpleural fibrosis ("subpleural blebs")

less affected. Thus, in evaluation of lobar tip wedge biopsies, the findings of greatest significance are often in the more proximal portions of the specimen. Nonspecific inflammatory changes in lobar tips become a problem in small wedge biopsies, particularly those that are 2 cm or less in greatest dimension. Since lobar tips are so readily accessible to the surgeon, it is difficult to discourage surgeons from biopsying them. If possible, such biopsies should be at least 3.0 cm in greatest dimension. The possibility of middle lobe syndrome (which may affect the lingula, the right middle lobe, or both) (40,41) should be considered for persistent infiltrates in these sites.

Apical caps (Figure 18.14) were once thought to be the result of healed tuberculosis, but they are common in patients who have never had tuberculosis; they are now thought to be an ischemic alteration related to their apical position (42,43). Apical caps are best known in the apex of the upper lobe, but they are also encountered in the upper regions of the lower lobe (44). Apical caps are regions of fibrosis in the pleura and subpleural lung parenchyma that

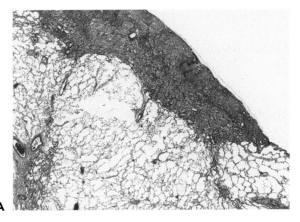

A

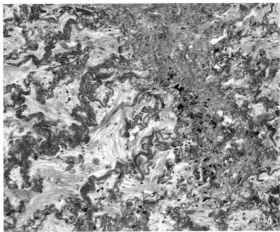

B

Figure 18.14 Apical cap. **A.** Apical caps are found at the apex of the upper lobe, as well as the apex of the lower lobe. They represent regions of pleural and subpleural thickening by elastotic fibrous tissue that may be grayish or eosinophilic in appearance. **B.** Higher power sometimes shows a rich elastic tissue network that appears to highlight alveolar wall structure; some anthracotic pigmented is also noted.

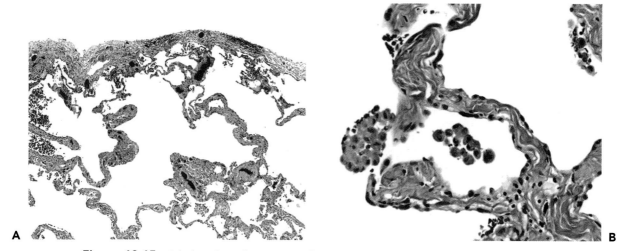

Figure 18.15 Subpleural emphysematous change in smoking. **A.** There is simplification of airspaces. **B.** Some of the alveolar walls show mild fibrosis with hyaline appearing collagen. Occasional clusters of pigmented alveolar macrophages are also noted.

are rich in thickened elastic fibers; the background structure of collapsed alveolar walls and interposed eosinophilic collagen can often be discerned in the tissue; elastic tissue stains enhance these features. Ossification and nests of metaplastic pneumocytes may be present. The changes are sufficiently distinctive that apical caps can often be suspected histologically, even when one does not know the site of origin; even so, any ancient lung scar may sometimes show a similar elastotic appearance. Apical caps in older individuals are sometimes biopsied or resected to exclude a carcinoma or a visceral pleural tumor (44).

Centriacinar (centrilobular) emphysema is a pathologic abnormality that is more common and more severe in the upper lobes (45); it is found predominantly in cigarette smokers and is a common finding in lobes resected for bronchogenic carcinoma. Emphysematous changes are frequently accompanied by some degree of fibrosis, particularly

when bullous change is present. The fibrosis tends to appear as strands of dense, hypocellular, brightly eosinophilic collagenous septa traversing the emphysematous spaces. Anthracosis is also a common finding in smokers and urban dwellers. Focal pleural and subpleural fibrosis (Figure 18.15) is extremely common, especially as an incidental microscopic finding in lobar resections from smokers (46); abnormal airspaces formed by irregular fibrous septa are accompanied by smooth muscle hyperplasia, mucostasis, and bronchiolar metaplasia.

Subpleural blebs (Figure 18.16) are often the only pathologic change found in patients with recurrent pneumothoraces and who don't have diffuse lung disease (47). These are typically evident in the upper lobes. By convention, *blebs* are defined as being less than 1.0 cm in diameter and some are derived from air dissection into the visceral pleura; *bullae* are 1.0 cm or greater in diameter (48).

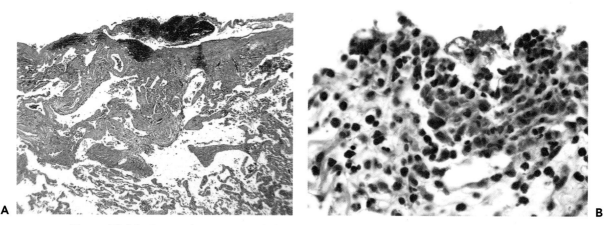

Figure 18.16 Pneumothorax. **A.** So-called "subpleural blebs" are thought to predispose to pneumothorax. These are regions of pleural and subpleural scarring with abnormal airspaces somewhat reminiscent to smoking-related changes (also Figure 18.15). **B.** Pneumothorax is often associated with a pleural reaction (*top*), which has been labeled eosinophilic pleuritis because of the association of eosinophil infiltrate and mesothelial and macrophage reaction on the pleural surface.

Their rupture introduces air into the pleural space, inciting a mesothelial proliferation with numerous macrophages, giant cells, and eosinophils (referred to as eosinophilic pleuritis), and this reaction may accompany any condition that is associated with pneumothorax (49). Collections of interstitial air in the lung tissue, with or without giant cell and/or eosinophilic reaction, may be an accompanying finding. Focal subpleural scarring can usually be distinguished from chronic fibrosing interstitial pneumonias by its restriction to the subpleural region, lack of active fibroblastic proliferation, and the relative abrupt transition to normal alveolar walls. Clinical history and radiographic findings may also be supportive. When an interstitial lung disease such as pulmonary Langerhans cell histiocytosis (eosinophilic granuloma) or lymphangioleiomyomatosis has resulted in pneumothorax, both the primary process and the secondary eosinophilic pleuritis may be recognizable on the biopsy.

Adhesions between the pleura and chest wall are composed of fibrovascular tissue with pockets of bland mesothelial cells and are identical to their peritoneal counterparts. The adhesions identified in surgical specimens and even autopsy tissue often have no obvious cause and represent an incidental finding. Dense, hyalinized fibrotic pleural (visceral or parietal) plaques (50–52) are the consequence of a variety of prior inflammatory events. Their presence bilaterally often is an incidental finding; and, if there is no obvious inflammatory cause, prior asbestos exposure is likely (53).

ARTIFACTS SEEN IN LUNG BIOPSY AND RESECTION MATERIAL

Artifacts related to lung biopsy of prior procedures are described in Table 18.7.

Knowledge of the clinical course of events prior to lung biopsy usually allows the pathologist to avoid

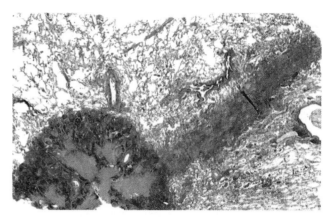

Figure 18.17 Needle tract to a small peripheral adenocarcinoma. The biopsy had been performed a week earlier, and the needle tract shows evidence of hemorrhage, necrosis, organization, and epithelial regeneration.

misinterpreting changes of prior instrumentation. Previous bronchial biopsies may cause hemorrhage, airway inflammation, ulceration, and a granulation tissue reaction. Strips of epithelium may be dislodged by mechanical trauma and embedded in inspissated mucus; residual basal cells may be all that is left adhering to the basement membrane. Bronchoalveolar lavage can produce vacuolation of alveolar pneumocytes and macrophages. Previous needle biopsies may induce necrosis and hemorrhage in the parenchyma, followed by organization and reactive epithelial atypia (Figure 18.17). Patients who have been on positive-pressure ventilation (Figure 18.18) may have disproportional bronchiolar and alveolar duct distension, especially when high inspiratory pressures are used in the adult respiratory distress syndrome (ARDS). Some associated acute inflammatory exudate in the lumen is common, often with relative absence of associated inflammation in the airway wall or surrounding alveolar spaces.

TABLE 18.7
ARTIFACTS SEEN IN LUNG BIOPSIES AND RESECTIONS

- Changes related to prior instrumentation including bronchoscopy, bronchoalveolar lavage, needle aspiration, and ventilatory assistance
- Compression/atelectasis; pseudolipoid change ("bubble artifact")
- Hemorrhage/inflammatory changes
- Septal edema; lymphatic dilatation
- Material from surgical gloves (e.g., talc and starch)
- Inflation-induced alveolar distension resembling emphysema and patchy atelectasis in underinflated zones
- Sponge artifact

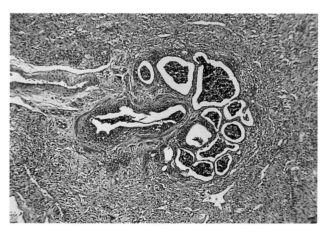

Figure 18.18 Ventilator-associated changes. Common changes in the setting of positive-pressure ventilator therapy include distension of bronchioles, flattening of their epithelium, and an acute inflammatory exudate in the lumen with minimal change in the surrounding alveolar wall.

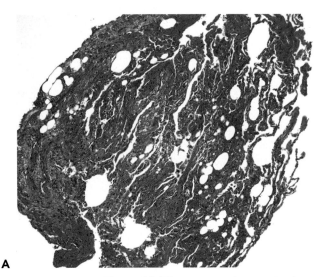

A

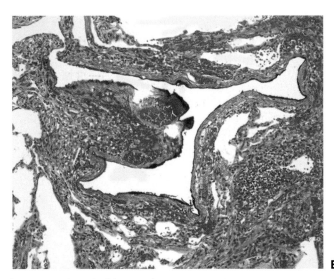

B

Figure 18.19 Bubble artifact. **A.** This fragment from a transbronchial biopsy shows compression and atelectasis (*left*) with some recognizable alveolar walls (*right*). The rounded spaces represent bubble artifact, which is common in such compressed biopsies. **B.** Sponge artifact is illustrated. Note the marked irregularity of the space corresponding to the irregular surface of sponges used in cassettes.

Compression of the lung tissue, particularly in transbronchial biopsies, may produce rounded spaces in alveoli that resemble fat vacuoles and can easily be mistaken for exogenous lipoid pneumonia (Figure 18.19). This artifactual change, often called bubble artifact (54,55), can be recognized because there are no macrophages or giant cells with small intracytoplasmic lipid vacuoles (all the vacuoles are extracellular), and there is usually little fibrosis, which is a constant feature of chronic exogenous lipoid pneumonia.

Compression of airways produces crinkling and telescoping of the epithelium, similar to that seen in endometrial biopsies. Sometimes entire strips of mucosa are displaced into the bronchiolar or alveolar spaces.

Compression-induced nuclear smearing artifact can be produced in any cellular tumor and even in reactive lymphoid tissue in the bronchial mucosa or biopsies of hilar or mediastinal nodes. The resulting changes may suggest small cell carcinoma. Reactive lymphoid follicles, lymphomas, and carcinoid tumors may be extremely difficult to distinguish from small cell carcinoma when this phenomenon is present. Recognition of these diagnostic pitfalls, examining multiple levels (especially at the periphery), and enlisting the aid of concomitant cytology specimens and immunohistochemistry allows resolution of most cases. In rare instances, rebiopsy may be necessary.

Atelectasis may be encountered in all types of lung biopsies since lung tissue is soft and readily compressible (54,55). It is particularly common in video-assisted thoracic surgical wedge biopsies because this procedure requires that the lung be collapsed and samples may become further compressed during retrieval through a small hole in the chest wall (56). Atelectasis may also be encountered in biopsies inflated by the pathologist when not all lobules

uniformly inflate. This phenomenon may be misinterpreted as interstitial pneumonia or interstitial fibrosis because the apposition of alveolar walls produces apparent scarring and hypercellularity (Figure 18.20). With experience, this change can be recognized on routine H&E sections; connective tissue stains show an absence of scarring and a normal background of supporting fibrous tissue along vessels and in septa. In atelectatic lung, the vessels and septa may appear to have more collagen than normal and to be thickened because they are contracted and shortened. Careful assessment of the nuclei in atelectatic lung shows that most

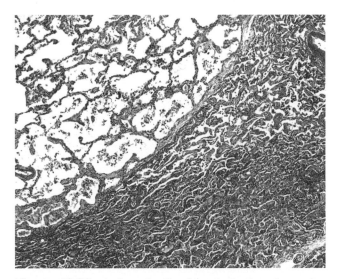

Figure 18.20 Atelectasis. Careful examination shows that recognizable alveolar walls can be traced into the region of atelectasis (*lower right*) and that the process stops somewhat abruptly at an interlobular septum that courses diagonally across the field (*lower left to upper right*).

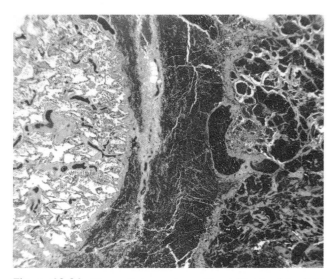

Figure 18.21 Traumatic hemorrhage. The right side of the field shows extensive hemorrhage into alveolar spaces, whereas the tissue on the left shows a complete absence of hemorrhage. There is also dissection of red blood cells into the interlobular septal region (*center*). Such a well-demarcated focus of hemorrhage and dissection of red blood cells into connective tissue would be very unusual in a diffuse alveolar hemorrhage syndrome. The findings are typical of traumatic hemorrhage.

are endothelial or epithelial in origin, rather than inflammatory. Leukocyte common antigen immunostaining and immunohistochemical stains for other lymphoid markers may be useful in this setting. It is also unusual in open biopsies (and larger specimens) for the entire specimen to be uniformly atelectatic; and, therefore, a low-power survey of the entire pattern generally helps one appreciate atelectasis merging with more normal lung. In fact, when significant fibrosis is present (usually associated with foci of honeycombing), atelectasis is rarely a problem because the more rigid fibrotic lung tissue tends to retain its configuration.

Fresh intra-alveolar hemorrhage due to the trauma of surgery is extremely common in biopsy material and should not be overinterpreted as pathologic (Figure 18.21). In fact, hemorrhage related to the trauma of the procedure is the most common cause of fresh blood in alveolar spaces. One can approach this problem from three points of view: the statistical, the histologic, and the clinical. Statistically, the vast majority of cases of fresh alveolar hemorrhage are traumatic since pathologic alveolar hemorrhage is relatively uncommon; thus, in any given case, acute hemorrhage is unlikely to be significant. When pathologic hemorrhage is present, there is usually (but not always) an associated fibrinous exudate or hyalin membranes, obvious distention of alveoli with blood, and evidence of prior hemorrhage manifested by hemosiderin-filled macrophages in the interstitium or airspaces. This last finding is not a reliable histologic criterion in patients who have been smokers and those with venous obstruction or chronic passive congestion.

The most common cause of macrophages staining positively with iron stains is respiratory bronchiolitis in smokers (Figure 18.22). The hemosiderin in smoker's macrophages is finely granular, in contrast to the coarse, dark blue staining in chronic hemorrhage as highlighted by the Prussian blue histochemical stain for iron. Nevertheless, it is surprising how many darkly staining Prussian blue–positive cells can be seen in smokers.

Finally, the clinician can usually confirm whether an alveolar hemorrhage syndrome or alveolar hemorrhage due to some other cause (e.g., cardiac) is in the realm of possibility in any given patient.

Prolonged surgical manipulation of the lung, and even multiple transbronchial biopsies, can lead to margination of neutrophils in capillaries (especially those in the pleura), which mimics capillaritis (56). Capillaritis is usually associated with some evidence of an alveolar hemorrhage syndrome or other clinical or histologic features of a vasculitic syndrome (such as vascular necrosis, karyorrhexis, and fibrin thrombi). It is distributed throughout a biopsy and is not limited to those regions manipulated during surgery. Clamping of the biopsy specimen prior to removal can result in lymphatic obstruction, dilatation, and septal edema.

Lung pathologists are divided on the issue of inflation fixation of biopsy specimens. This can be easily accomplished with a syringe filled with formalin and a fine gauge needle. Careful inflation of a lung biopsy specimen (57) may be helpful diagnostically and is aesthetically pleasing since the lung architecture is more easily appreciated (and particularly amenable to photography). A heavy hand can create overdistension of the alveoli and an emphysematous appearance. If this occurs, clinical correlation may be required to assess whether emphysema is actually a clinical consideration. Patchy atelectatic (uninflated) portions of lung tissue are common in biopsies that have been nonuniformly inflated. One problem that may be encountered in inflated biopsies is that cells and fluid may be "washed out" of the airspaces. This is especially true of smoker's (respiratory) bronchiolitis, which may be quite subtle in inflated specimens. A practical compromise to the issue of whether or not to inflate wedge biopsies was proposed by Dr. Lewis Woolner at the Mayo Clinic several decades ago (personal communication). One takes a wedge biopsy (even specimens from which tissue has been taken for studies such as frozen section) and simply places it in a closed container of formalin and shakes it up for a few seconds. This simple procedure allows the tissue to inflate somewhat on its own and the resultant histologic sections are remarkably good.

Video-assisted thoracic surgical (VATS) lung biopsies (thoracoscopic biopsies) have largely replaced traditional open lung biopsy as the diagnostic procedure for obtaining wedge biopsies of lung tissue for histologic evaluation. Although there are minor disadvantages in comparison to traditional open lung biopsy, diagnostic accuracy does not appear to be compromised (56,58–60). Allowing for the

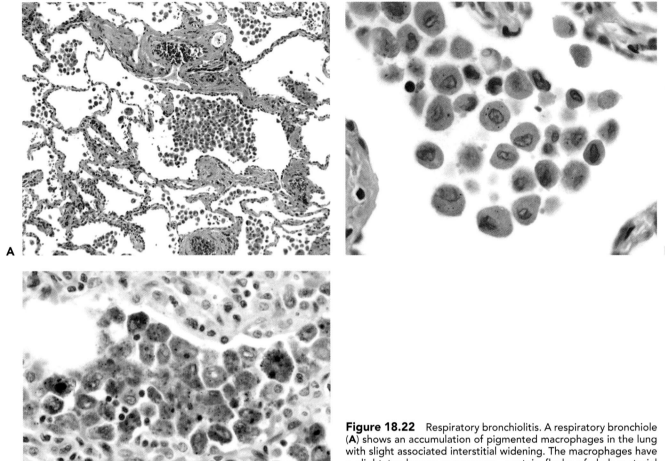

Figure 18.22   Respiratory bronchiolitis. A respiratory bronchiole (**A**) shows an accumulation of pigmented macrophages in the lung with slight associated interstitial widening. The macrophages have a slight tan-brown appearance, contain flecks of dark material (**B**), and are positive with Prussian blue staining (**C**) with a fine granularity.

fact that bimanual palpation is not as feasible with VATS biopsies, and that the tissue is forcibly pulled through a small hole in the chest wall, it is remarkable that sampling error and specimen artifacts are only a minor problem. The specimen size approaches that achieved with traditional open lung biopsy, and the minor degrees of hemorrhage, atelectasis/overinflation, and neutrophil margination represent artifactual changes that do not compromise diagnostic accuracy (56,58–60).

Plastic sponges are often put in cassettes to ensure that small specimens are not lost during processing. Sponge artifact, with triangular "holes" in the tissue, is a well-known artifact in any tissue that is processed this way, particularly if it is placed on the sponges prior to complete formalin fixation (55).

INCIDENTAL FINDINGS IN LUNG BIOPSY AND RESECTION TISSUE

There are a number of incidental findings in lung tissue that may not be related to the primary process that prompted the biopsy or resection (Table 18.8). Sometimes these "incidental" findings are of clinical and pathologic significance, and other times they are of no significance. Correlation of the individual finding(s) with the clinical and radiologic presentation helps to determine their significance.

Findings related to smoking and emphysema are extremely common, especially in lungs resected for bronchogenic carcinoma (46). They may be divided into three broad groups: large airway changes, small airway lesions, and abnormalities of the alveolar parenchyma.

In the large airways, one sees goblet cell hyperplasia, squamous metaplasia (with or without dysplasia), basement membrane thickening, hypertrophy and hyperplasia of bronchial glands with dilated ducts and mucostasis, and, often, a mild submucosal chronic inflammatory infiltrate (45,48).

The changes in the small airways may be quite dramatic and may mimic or even produce an interstitial lung disease (46,61,62). Smoking-induced respiratory bronchiolitis (Figure 18.22) includes goblet cell metaplasia, a mild inflammatory infiltrate in the airway walls, metaplasia of type II cells in the surrounding alveoli, mild peribronchiolar

TABLE 18.8
INCIDENTAL FINDINGS IN LUNG TISSUE

Effects of smoking: emphysema, chronic bronchitis, respiratory (smoker's bronchiolitis, intraparenchymal lymph nodes)

Changes of asthma

Ossification and marrow formation in bronchial cartilages, bronchial submucosal fatty infiltration, and elastotic change

Parenchymal nodules

   Carcinoid tumorlets; DIPNECH (see text)

   Minute (meningothelial-like nodules) pulmonary chemodectomas

   Atypical adenomatous hyperplasia (AAH)

   Healed granulomatous disease, infarcts, etc.

   Hamartomas

   Focal scars

   Occasional (anthraco-) silicotic nodules (in the absence of clinical/radiologic pneumoconiosis)

   Metaplastic bone

   Intrapulmonary lymph nodes

   Small carcinomas (and other tumors)

   Multifocal micronodular pneumocyte hyperplasia (MMPH)

Intracellular/intra-alveolar/interstitial structures

   Macrophages

   Corpora amylacea

   Blue bodies

   Schaumann bodies

   Asteroid bodies

   Calcium oxalate crystals

   Mallory's hyalin-like material in type II cells

   Ferruginous bodies

   Anthracotic pigment/birefringent material (including silica and silicates)

   Metaplastic bone

Epithelioid and/or cholesterol granulomas, giant cells, lipogranulomas

Intravascular/vascular

   Megakaryocytes

   Thrombi (mimic emboli)

   Bone marrow emboli

   Calcification and iron encrustation of the elastic tissue

   Senile amyloid

   Foreign material

Interstitial air in the lung parenchyma

Hilar/peribronchial lymph nodes

   Sinus and paracortical histiocytes (may simulate granulomas)

   Occasional silicotic or anthracosilicotic nodules

   Anthracosis/birefringent material

   Hamazaki-Wesenberg bodies

Pleural adhesions; hyalin pleural plaques

fibrosis, and prominent accumulations of pigmented macrophages in adjacent airspace and the bronchiolar lumen. The pigmented macrophages (smokers' macrophages) contain phagocytosed debris from inhaled cigarette smoke and have prominent secondary lysosomes in their cytoplasm. This results in a dirty granular-tan or brown appearance to the cytoplasm. They contain PAS-positive (lysosomes) and finely granular Prussian blue–positive (hemosiderin) material, as well as tiny, irregular flecks of brown-black material.

The smoking-related changes in the most distal pulmonary parenchyma usually manifest as centriacinar emphysema with airspace enlargement and loss of alveolar walls (45,48). Histologic quantification of emphysema on biopsy material is difficult, although one can often determine whether it is present and subjectively quantify it. Bullous emphysema (with abnormal airspaces greater than 1 cm in diameter) is more common in the upper lobes and is usually associated with some fibrosis in the septa of the bullae and adjacent alveolar walls. The fibrosis is relatively acellular, noninflammatory, eosinophilic, and poorly vascularized. Metaplasia or ulceration of the epithelium and interstitial dissection of air occur in bullae and may induce a giant cell response analogous to that seen in persistent interstitial emphysema.

Asthmatics are predisposed to a number of lung conditions that may lead to lung biopsy, although the asthmatic changes themselves may not be the dominant lesion. These airway changes include goblet cell metaplasia in the airway epithelium, thickening of the basement membrane and submembranous region, smooth muscle hypertrophy and hyperplasia, lymphoid hyperplasia, and a variable infiltrate of eosinophils, lymphocytes, and a few neutrophils, and fibrous tissue in the wall (45,48). Mucostasis (including Curschmann's spirals) may be an accompanying feature; but, when mucostasis is extensive and is associated with sloughing of epithelial fragments into the airways (creola bodies), one should suspect that the asthma itself is the main lesion. Such an appearance is typical of status asthmaticus. Some distal atelectasis with a few airspace macrophages and eosinophils may also be seen. In patients with quiescent asthma or past history of asthma, the airways may be entirely normal or show only minor inflammatory or fibrotic changes.

Metaplastic bone, including bone marrow and calcification, is an aging change that is occasionally seen in bronchial cartilages (63). Metaplastic bone may also be seen in regions of scarring (dystrophic ossification), particularly in apical caps. Small bony nodules may also be seen with no apparent associated pathologic changes. In some older individuals with chronic bronchitis, the bronchial submucosa may have a gray elastotic appearance, particularly in bronchoscopic biopsies.

Carcinoid tumorlets (64–67), now referred to simply as tumorlets, and minute pulmonary meningothelial-like nodules (67–69) are nodular proliferations that are quite common. They may be mistaken for each other, other lesions, or even metastases. Tumorlets (Figure 18.23) represent well-circumscribed proliferations of neuroendocrine cells that usually occur around and within the walls of small airways, particularly in scarred or bronchiectatic airways, and in a small number of patients with airflow destruction. They lack mitotic figures and necrosis; and, while there is a superficial resemblance to small cell carcinoma, they are actually more similar to spindle cell carcinoid tumors. In frozen sections,

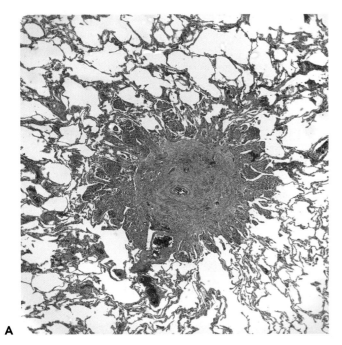

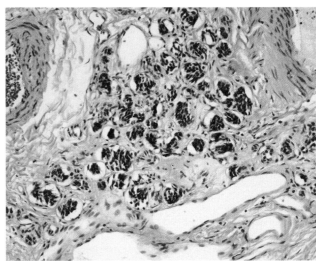

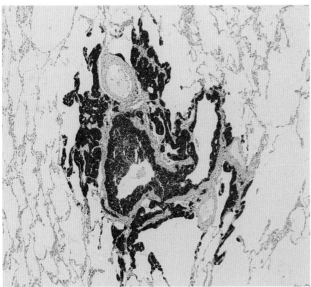

Figure 18.23 Tumorlet. **A.** Tumorlets are typically discrete nodules that are bronchiolocentric. The bronchiole is not apparent in A because it has been overrun by the proliferation, but the adjacent pulmonary artery is identifiable. **B.** Cytologically, tumorlets have a neuroendocrine appearance with nests of cells with granular chromatin and absence of necrosis and significant mitotic activity. The nests are often embedded in a fibrous stroma, and some of them may appear to float freely in airspaces or spaces that resemble lymphatics. **C.** Neuroendocrine markers, such as chromogranin, are strongly positive.

tumorlets may be mistaken for other lesions, particularly metastases. This confusion is compounded by the fact that sometimes tumorlets have cellular clusters at the periphery that retract from the surrounding stroma, simulating lymphatic or airspace invasion.

Tumorlets are often multiple; some may become large enough to be recognized radiographically and to be removed to exclude carcinoma. Exactly where one draws the line between a carcinoid tumorlet and a carcinoid tumor, particularly in cases with multiple lesions, is quite arbitrary, although a cutoff point of 0.5 cm diameter or larger for carcinoid tumor is reasonable (41).

Diffuse intrapulmonary neuroendocrine cell hyperplasia (DIPNECH) is closely related to tumorlets, and the two often

coexist (67). Arbitrarily, DIPNECH is defined as a proliferation of neuroendocrine cells limited to the bronchiolar epithelium. According to the World Health Organization (WHO), DIPNECH is defined as "a generalized proliferation of scattered single cells, small nodules (neuroendocrine bodies), or linear proliferations of pulmonary neuroendocrine cells (PNCs) that may be confined to the bronchiole and bronchiolar epithelium, include local extraluminal proliferation in the form of tumorlets, or extend to the development of carcinoid tumors" (67). When this proliferation expands and goes beyond the bounds of bronchioles, the designation of tumorlet is appropriate. Tumorlets are most frequently encountered as isolated or occasionally multiple nodules. When DIPNECH is encountered, usually multiple airways

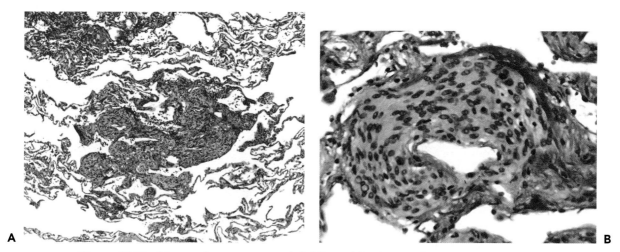

Figure 18.24 Minute pulmonary meningothelial-like nodule. These small parenchymal nodules are sometimes associated with pulmonary veins. **A.** They are associated with syncytial appearing cells in a collagenous stroma. **B.** Cytologically, they bear a distinct resemblance to meningothelial cells.

are involved, and the patients may have evidence of airflow obstruction (67). Similarly, the presence of multiple tumorlets (and multiple carcinoid tumors) should prompt one to search for evidence of DIPNECH and to consider the possibility of clinical evidence of airflow obstruction (70).

Minute pulmonary meningothelial-like nodules (formerly called minute pulmonary chemodectomas) (Figure 18.24) were originally thought to represent an intrapulmonary proliferation of perivenular chemoreceptor cells (67–69). However, the accumulated evidence suggests that the cellular constituents are more closely related to meningothelial cells (67–69). A study by Ionescu et al. (71) showed that meningothelial-like nodules were almost uniformly positive for vimentin, about one-third stain for EMA, and they are negative with cytokeratin and synaptophysin by immunohistochemistry. In a genotypic study, some loss of heterozygosity was demonstrated by the same authors, and this was more common and affected more loci in cases of multiple meningothelial-like nodules in comparison to cases with solitary meningothelial-like nodules (71). The authors concluded that isolated meningothelial-like nodules were probably reactive, that cases of multiple meningothelial-like nodules might represent a transition from a reactive to a neoplastic proliferation, and that meningothelial-like nodules were different from meningiomas based on the major molecular events and their formation and progression (71). Minute pulmonary meningothelial-like nodules are composed of interstitial clusters of fusiform cells with pale eosinophilic cytoplasm, forming small stellate nodules (occasionally grossly appreciable) near small veins. Their location and characteristic bland cytology resembling meningothelial cells are very distinctive.

Atypical adenomatous hyperplasia (AAH) is a proliferative epithelial process occurring as small nodular lesions in the lung parenchyma (Figure 18.25). These were first recognized in resection specimens for carcinoma and named

bronchioloalveolar cell adenomas (72). Miller found these lesions in 23 (10.74%) of 247 consecutive resection specimens for carcinoma (72). They are most easily recognized grossly in cases that are inflated with Bouin's fixative. The WHO defines AAH as "a localized proliferation of mild to moderately atypical cells lining involved alveoli and, sometimes, respiratory bronchioles, resulting in focal lesions in peripheral alveolated lung, usually less than 5 mm in diameter and generally in the absence of underlying interstitial inflammation and fibrosis" (67). The lesions are considered a precursor to some nonmucinous bronchioloalveolar carcinomas and mixed-type adenocarcinomas; and the evidence supporting this is epidemiologic, morphologic, morphometric, cytofluorometric, and genetic. Atypical adenomatous hyperplasia generally represents an incidental histologic finding (rare cases have been identified radiologically) and is found in 2 to 4% of routine autopsies of noncancer–bearing patients and up to 35% of lobectomies for adenocarcinoma of the lung. In general, we advocate a conservative approach to these lesions, since: (a) there are many causes of type II cell proliferation, and many of them are reactive; (b) there are no studies documenting the pathologic progression of AAH to bronchioloalvoelar carcinoma (BAC)—or studies that document how long such a progression takes); and (c) no studies exist showing what percent of lesions of AAH progress to carcinoma.

Focal scars (see following), healed granulomatous disease, and organized infarcts are among other incidental nodular lesions occasionally encountered in the lung. Early infarcts have a wedge shape with hemorrhagic necrosis, and the overlying pleura is viable with a fibrinous pleuritis. They often also have a rim of granulation tissue. Older infarcts are often rounded and have a rim of fibrous tissue; they can even be mistaken for healed granulomas. Necrotic tumor nodules sometimes mimic infarcts. Squamous metaplasia is

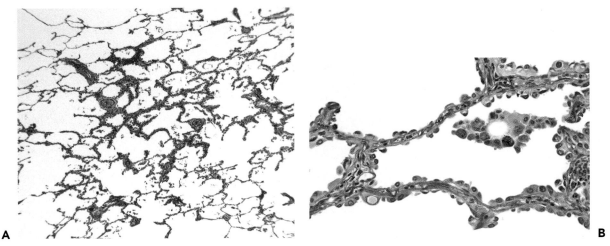

Figure 18.25   Atypical adenomatous hyperplasia (AAH). **A.** In this well-inflated specimen, a 2 to 3 mm diameter lesion is apparent as slight alveolar septal thickening and a proliferation of knob-shaped cells along alveolar walls. **B.** Cytologically, the cells lining the alveoli have mild to moderate atypia but lack the crowding and marked atypia associated with bronchioloalveolar carcinoma. Some nuclear inclusions characteristic of type II cells are also apparent (*lower left*).

common in the airspaces adjacent to organizing infarcts and around bronchioles in organizing diffuse alveolar damage; it may be sufficiently exuberant to be mistaken for a neoplastic process. A single anthracosilicotic nodule is an occasional finding that may be accepted as incidental and insignificant if there is no clinical or radiologic evidence of pneumoconiosis. When silicotic nodules are multiple, the occupational history and the possibility of pneumoconiosis should be explored.

Although extensive parenchymal scarring is usually a pathological process, focal scars a few millimeters in diameter are a common incidental finding in biopsy material. One distinctive form of scar that is frequently observed (and may be identifiable as 2–3 mm centrilobular nodules in CT scans) consists of scars centered on alveolar ducts in the periphery of the lung, particularly common in (ex-) smokers (Figure

18.26). They are round or somewhat stellate in character and have numerous fascicles of smooth muscle—and thus sometimes have been confused with primary muscle proliferations such as lymphangioleiomyomatosis. There are a number of histologic changes that accompany pulmonary scarring, regardless of cause. These include vascular intimal and medial thickening, sometimes to the point of luminal occlusion (endarteritis obliterans); smooth muscle and myofibroblastic hyperplasia in the interstitium; metaplasia and hyperplasia of type II cells or bronchiolar-type epithelium (peribronchiolar metaplasia); accumulations of intra-alveolar macrophages and mucostasis; carcinoid tumorlets (particularly along scarred small airways); dystrophic calcification or ossification; microscopic pericicatricial emphysema; and metaplastic adipose tissue in the pleural and peribronchial regions. The proliferation of type II cells associated with scars may be

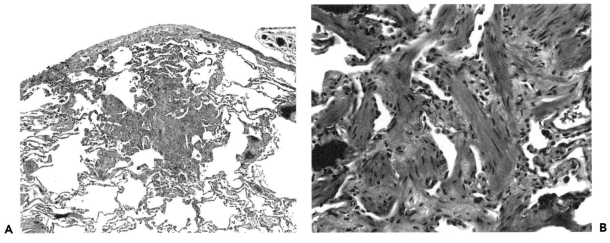

Figure 18.26   Incidental parenchymal scar. These are typically subpleural and appear to center on alveolar ducts (**A**) and commonly have fascicles of normal appearing smooth muscle (**B**).

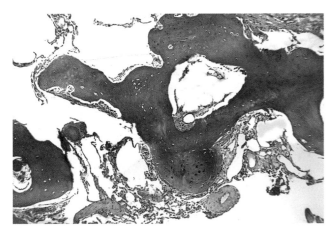

Figure 18.27 Ossification. An incidental focus of pulmonary ossification is noted; tissue is from a patient with usual interstitial pneumonia.

confused with bronchioloalveolar carcinoma. Bronchioloalveolar carcinoma generally has uniform dense cellularity and cellular crowding with abrupt transition to normal alveolar walls, significant cytologic atypia, and lack of ciliated cells. Although AAH tends to have relatively little interstitial widening and fibrosis, AAH enters into the differential diagnosis in this situation.

In rare instances, mature bone is observed in normal alveoli; it may represent the residue of an organized airspace exudate from chronic passive congestion of mitral stenosis or an ancient organized pneumonia (73). Extensive dystrophic ossification (and rarely calcification) occasionally accompanies lesions with diffuse pulmonary fibrosis (Figure 18.27) (74). Focal dystrophic ossification is a common finding in focal lung scar, regardless of cause.

Intrapulmonary lymph nodes (Figure 18.28) are not uncommonly encountered in wedge biopsies. They vary from loosely organized microscopic foci of lymphoid tissue to fully developed lymph nodes identified grossly or radiologically.

Micronodular pneumocyte hyperplasia (MNPH) is defined by the WHO (1999) as "a multifocal micronodular proliferation of type II cells with mild thickening of the interstitium" (Figure 18.29) (67,75). This condition is rare and generally an incidental finding in a biopsy taken for another lesion (usually lymphangioleiomyomatosis). Rarely, MNPH is the sole lesion present, and the lesions may be sufficiently large to be identifiable on CT scans as multiple small nodules. The lesions are typically less than 5 mm in size. They can usually be distinguished from AAH and other causes of alveolar cell hyperplasia by their distinct rounded nodular character at scanning microscopy, the large plump eosinophilic type II cells lacking significant atypia, the slight interstitial collagen deposition within the lesions, and the presence of airspace histiocytes in the regions of the nodules.

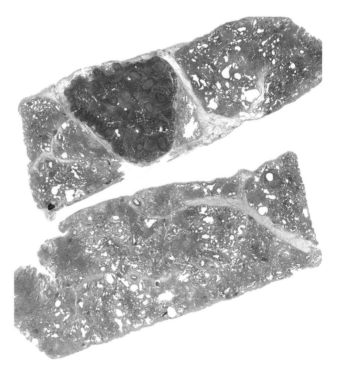

Figure 18.28 Intrapulmonary lymph node. There is a relatively large lymph node that appears to be within or adjacent to an interlobular septum in a wedge biopsy from peripheral lung. Reactive follicles are apparent even at scanning power microscopy.

A number of intra-alveolar and intracellular structures are seen in the lung. Small numbers of intra-alveolar macrophages are a normal finding, and an increase in their numbers is nonspecific and a common reaction in smokers (43). Focal desquamative interstitial pneumonia-like reactions are seen in many pathologic conditions, especially in smokers and in conditions with fibrosis and architectural disorganization (46,76). When hemosiderin is present, causes for alveolar hemorrhage (both primary and secondary) should be excluded.

Corpora amylacea (77,78) are eosinophilic, rounded, slightly lamellated proteinaceous bodies (Figure 18.30) that stain positively with PAS stains and faintly with Congo red stain; they are more common in the lungs of older individuals. Sometimes there is a blue-gray, calcified, or polarizable crystalline particulate body in the center and a macrophage or giant cell response around them. The exact nature and cause of corpora are unclear, but they are of no clinical significance.

Blue bodies (Figure 18.31) are intra-alveolar, lamellated, basophilic, calcified structures found in airspaces associated with alveolar macrophages and giant cells (78). They are a nonspecific finding in a number of diffuse lung diseases related to accumulation of macrophages and are of no diagnostic significance. They are thought to be related to macrophage catabolism; they are composed primarily of calcium carbonate.

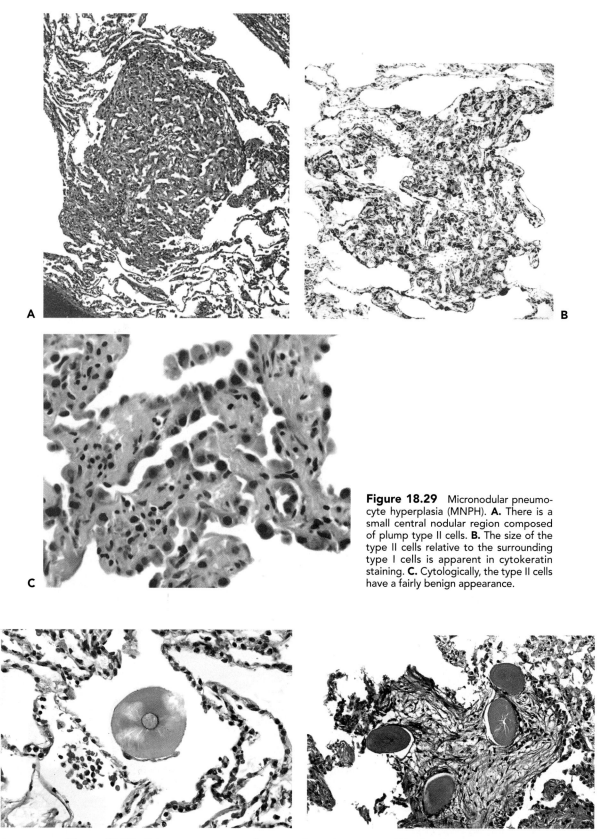

Figure 18.29 Micronodular pneumocyte hyperplasia (MNPH). **A.** There is a small central nodular region composed of plump type II cells. **B.** The size of the type II cells relative to the surrounding type I cells is apparent in cytokeratin staining. **C.** Cytologically, the type II cells have a fairly benign appearance.

Figure 18.30 Pulmonary corpora amylacea. **A.** These show a central bluish nidus and a giant cell or macrophage reaction around them. Others may have radiating proteinaceous arrays and show cracking in histologic sections. They are often Congo red–positive. **B.** Multiple corpora amylacea are seen as an incidental finding associated with organizing pneumonia.

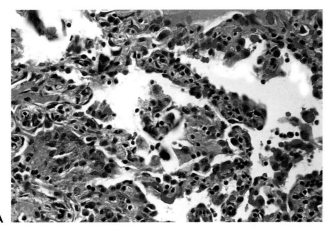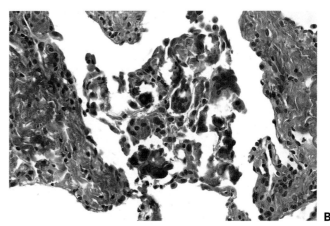

Figure 18.31 Blue bodies. **A. and B.** Blue bodies are gray or blue, intra-alveolar, calcified, lamellated structures often associated with clusters of macrophages, including giant cells.

Schaumann bodies (Figure 18.32) are similar lamellated, calcified bodies seen in giant cells and associated with granulomas (78–80). They are also of no diagnostic significance and may be found in granulomas from diverse causes. Schaumann bodies are endogenously derived and may be mistaken for exogenous material since they may be partially birefringent, due to concomitant presence of oxalate crystals (see following).

Asteroid bodies (Figure 18.33) represent a starlike array of crystallized intracellular protein and are seen in giant cells of many granulomatous conditions; other than being aesthetically pleasing, they are nonspecific.

Calcium oxalate crystals are lucent, birefringent, plate-like crystals, often in giant cells, that may be mistaken for exogenous material (78,79) (Figure 18.34). Accumulation of oxalate crystals around aspergillomas and in patients with forms of invasive aspergillosis is also common.

Material similar to Mallory's hyalin (Figure 18.35) may be found in the reactive type II cells of a number of interstitial diseases. It is distinctive, but nonspecific. It may stain for keratin and ubiquitin (81).

Ferruginous bodies, many of which are asbestos bodies, are indicative of significant inhalational exposure to the ferruginated material, but their presence does not necessarily correspond to clinically significant lung disease. Recent studies with electron-probe analysis have helped elucidate the variety of materials that may become iron encrusted, of which asbestos fibers comprise only a portion (82).

In virtually any urban adult, one may find short, needle-like, birefringent material (usually silica or silicates) in association with anthracotic pigment (Figure 18.36), either along lymphatic routes in the lung or in regional lymph nodes. Silicates are more brightly birefringent than silica.

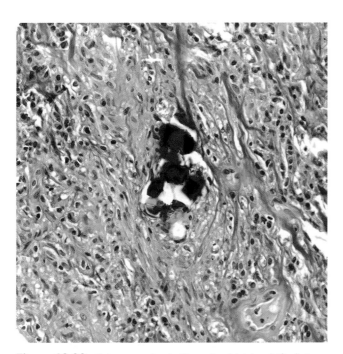

Figure 18.32 Schaumann body. There is a bluish calcified structure associated with surrounding granulomatous inflammation. A lamellated appearance similar to a psammoma body is focally apparent. The pale zones in this case represent loosened oxalate crystals that would be birefringent (see Figure 18.34).

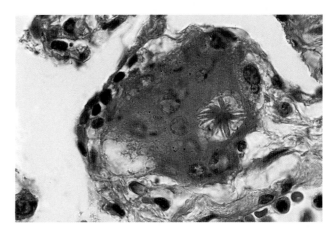

Figure 18.33 Asteroid body. An asteroid body in a giant cell is illustrated from a case of asbestosis.

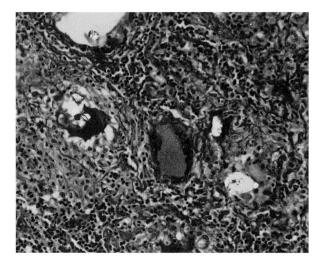

Figure 18.34 Calcium oxalate crystals. Calcium oxalate crystals are commonly associated with Schaumann bodies and granulomatous inflammation and show bright birefringence, as noted in this partially polarized photomicrograph. The association with giant cells is characteristic.

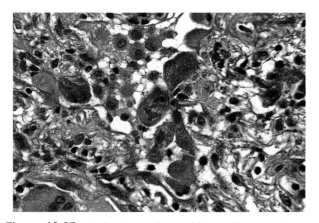

Figure 18.35 Hyalin. Material resembling Mallory's hyalin may be seen in reactive type II cells in a number of acute and chronic conditions.

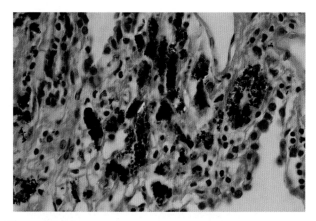

Figure 18.36 Silica and silicates in normal lung. Birefringent silica and silicate particles are a common nonspecific finding in and around the anthracotic pigment that is so commonly seen in urban adults and smokers.

The amount of birefringent material may be quite impressive in individuals (particularly smokers) who have no significant occupational exposure. This material should be distinguished from formalin pigment, as well as from surgical glove talc or starch; the latter are limited to handled surfaces and often demonstrate a Maltese-cross configuration with polarization. The diagnosis of silicosis (and silicatosis) is not based solely on the presence of birefringent material; it requires clinicopathologic correlations: appropriate chest radiograph findings, and parenchymal silicotic nodules or masses of histiocytes (within which early fibrotic nodules may be seen to form) along lymphatic routes. Precise characterization of any material identified requires special techniques such as electron-probe analysis.

An occasional nonnecrotizing epithelioid granuloma may be found in the lungs of patients who have no evidence of granulomatous disease; they are analogous to the occasional granuloma seen at many sites in the body. Likewise, cholesterol granulomas or single giant cells containing cholesterol clefts may also be an occasional incidental finding (Figure 18.37). In some instances, the presence of cholesterol granulomas has been linked to prior alveolar hemorrhage, mucostasis, or pulmonary hypertension (83), but usually no significance can be ascribed to them. Lipogranulomas are an occasional nonspecific finding, said to be more common in diabetics (84).

An interesting finding is the presence of scattered megakaryocytes in alveolar walls (Figure 18.38), predominantly within alveolar capillaries. Large numbers can be seen, particularly during sepsis. They are of no diagnostic significance but should not be overinterpreted as malignant or virally infected cells. Along with the bone marrow and spleen, the lung acts as a major reservoir for megakaryocytes.

Bone marrow emboli, common in autopsy material, are also seen in biopsy specimens (Figure 18.39). Rarely correlated with any clinically significant process, they may be a consequence of bony trauma or excision of ribs. In some cases, however, such as thoracoscopic biopsies, bony

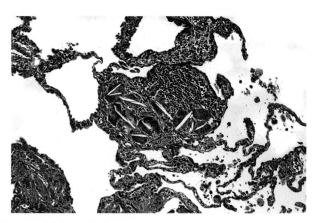

Figure 18.37 Cholesterol granulomas. Granulomas and clusters of giant cells containing cholesterol clefts are a frequent nonspecific finding in interstitial lung disease.

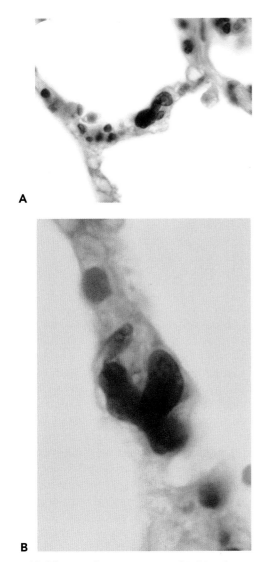

A

B

Figure 18.38 Megakaryocytes. **A. and B.** Megakaryocytes are a common finding in normal lung, often present within alveolar capillaries.

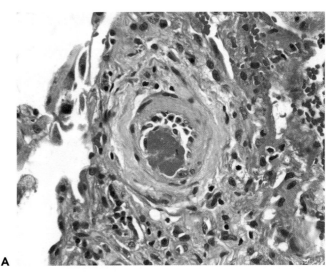

A

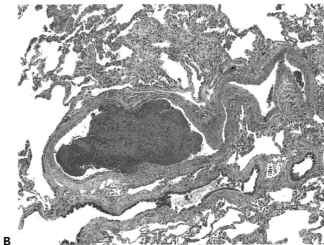

B

Figure 18.40 Thromboemboli in acute lung injury. Small (**A**) or even somewhat large (**B**) fibrin thrombi are commonly present in biopsies showing extensive acute lung injury (A,B). Hyalin membranes are apparent adjacent to the artery in A, and organization is apparent at the top of the field in B.

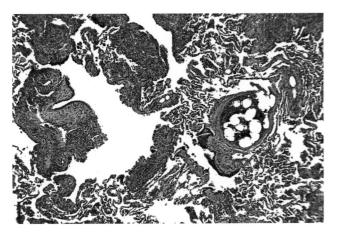

Figure 18.39 Bone marrow embolus. An incidental bone marrow embolus (*right center*) identified in a pulmonary artery in a biopsy from a patient with lymphangioleiomyomatosis (*left*).

trauma cannot be implicated, and the marrow emboli are an unexplained incidental finding.

Recent intravascular thrombi (probably formed in situ) are a relatively common accompanying finding in any severe acute inflammatory lung disease (Figure 18.40), and they should not be considered evidence of pulmonary emboli without corroborating clinical information.

In patients with chronic hemorrhagic, chronic pulmonary congestion, or metabolic abnormalities, calcification and iron encrustation of the pulmonary elastic tissue may occur and even elicit a giant cell reaction (Figure 18.41). This phenomenon has been inappropriately labeled endogenous pneumoconiosis (85).

Intravascular foreign material is usually birefringent and may have a giant cell reaction. While it usually occurs in intravenous drug abuse (IV talcosis), occasional fragments of

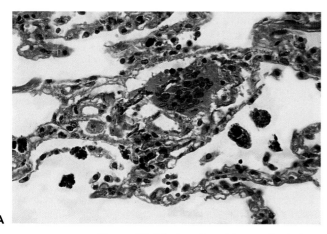 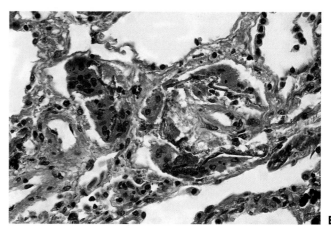

Figure 18.41 Iron deposition on elastic tissue (**A, B**). Chronic hemorrhage, in this case due to severe chronic passive congestion, may result in encrustation of interstitial and vascular elastic fibers by hemosiderin. A giant cell reaction is a frequent accompanying finding (A).

foreign material are seen in patients without a history of drug abuse, perhaps related to intravenous lines during hospitalization or surgery.

The finding of interstitial air, either localized or diffuse, is well known to pediatric lung pathologists and may be an incidental finding in adults who have been on ventilators. Interstitial air can occur as an incidental finding in a region of subpleural fibrosis but also be a significant pathologic finding in its own right (86) (Figure 18.42). The abnormal air-filled spaces resemble honeycombing; however, they lack the expected metaplastic epithelial lining and careful inspection shows either a complete lack of a cellular lining or a histiocytic and giant cell reaction lining the spaces. Interstitial air presenting in this way may be encountered in patients with interstitial lung disease, in patients with a history of pneumothorax, and in and around bullae and blebs.

As in ventilated children, interstitial air may be encountered in adults on assisted ventilation and sometimes may be completely missed, being interpreted as tissue tearing.

Hilar and peribronchial lymph nodes are rarely carefully examined beyond the evaluation for metastatic carcinoma. Nevertheless, they frequently exhibit a number of characteristic changes. Clusters of dust-filled macrophages in the sinuses and paracortical areas may resemble small granulomas (Figure 18.43). Silicotic or anthracosilicotic nodules, old healed infectious granulomas, and sinus histiocytosis are also common. When sarcoidosis is a consideration, one may have difficulty distinguishing the normal histiocytosis of hilar nodes from the granulomas of sarcoidosis. Generally, this problem can be approached by maintaining a high threshold for granulomas, requiring well-formed, rounded granulomatous masses (particularly with accumulations of

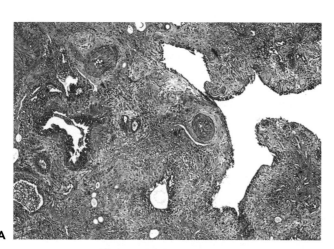 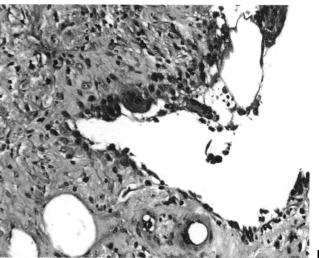

Figure 18.42 Incidental interstitial air. Peculiarly shaped airspaces (**A**) lined by giant cells (**B**) represent interstitial air, which is an occasional incidental finding in patients with interstitial lung disease, including those who have been on positive-pressure ventilation. The case illustrated in A represents an example of nonspecific interstitial pneumonia.

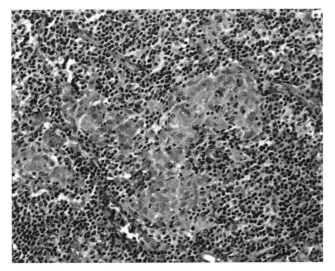

Figure 18.43 Histiocyte clusters in hilar nodes. Normal hilar and mediastinal lymph nodes commonly have clusters of histiocytes with variable amounts of dust particles in them. Sometimes they may appear somewhat granulomatous and may be difficult to distinguish from a true granulomatous reaction.

intergranulomatous fibrinoid or hyalinized material), giant cells, and careful clinicopathologic correlation.

Although multiple intraparenchymal silicotic nodules should make one suspect the possibility of silicosis, anthracosilicotic nodules in hilar nodes are quite common in the absence of silicosis. The nodules are composed of concentric whorled and layered hyalinized collagen and are usually surrounded by a nonpalisaded rim of dust-filled macrophages that contain birefringent material when examined with polarized light. Central degenerative changes may be evident. Silicotic nodules should be distinguished from old/healed granulomatous disease.

Hamazaki-Wesenberg bodies (87) are small (average: 5 μm in length), yellow-brown intracellular or extracellular structures associated with sinus histiocytes in lymph nodes, especially lung hilar nodes (Figure 18.44). The cause of these bodies is unknown, but they resemble lipofuscin. Positive staining with methenamine silver and PAS stains may lead to their confusion with yeast forms, but their H&E appearance, lack of associated necrosis or inflammation, and positive reaction with Fontana-Masson stain should facilitate their recognition and distinction from fungi.

Changes in the pleura in wedge biopsies may be incidental or part of the underlying pathologic process, and their significance needs to be assessed on an individual case basis.

INCIDENTAL FINDINGS IN TRANSBRONCHIAL BIOPSIES

The major artifacts or incidental findings in transbronchial biopsies that lead to misinterpretation include atelectasis

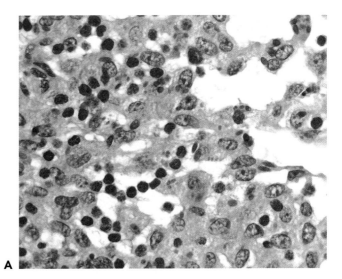

A

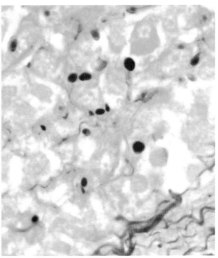

B

Figure 18.44 Hamazaki-Wesenberg bodies. **A.** Hamazaki-Wesenberg bodies represent yellow-brown oval structures associated with histiocytes, occasionally encountered in hilar and mediastinal lymph nodes. **B.** Their positive staining with silver stains sometimes leads to confusion with fungi.

(misinterpreted as interstitial pneumonia), bubble artifact (misinterpreted as lipoid pneumonia), and portions of the pleura (either entirely missed or misinterpreted as neoplastic or suspicious for being neoplastic) (54,55). Such portions of pleura may even include some pleural fat, a particularly common finding in fibrosing interstitial pneumonias. The finding of pleural tissue in transbronchial biopsies (Figure 18.45) is not uncommon but also is not well recognized among most pathologists. Strips of reactive mesothelial cells in such specimens may be confused with carcinoma.

As in wedge biopsies, the most common cause of red blood cells in airspaces in transbronchial biopsies is trauma related to the procedure of the biopsy rather than an alveolar hemorrhage syndrome.

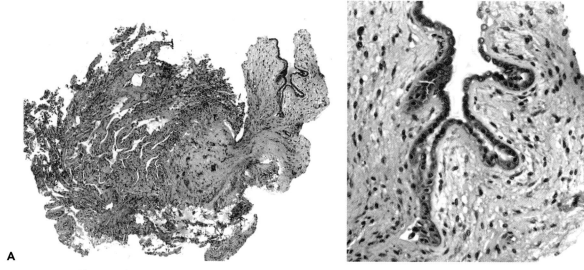

Figure 18.45 Visceral pleura in transbronchial biopsies. Transbronchial biopsies directed toward the periphery of the lung may not uncommonly sample portions of the visceral pleura (**A**, *right*; and **B**). These may lead to misdiagnosis, particularly if there is an associated reactive pleuritis.

EFFECTS OF AGING

Some of the effects of aging on the lung are shown in Table 18.9. Calcification and ossification of cartilages in the large airways may be seen. Intimal thickening is an age-related change in pulmonary arteries and veins (Figure 18.46), and apical pulmonary arteries are affected more often (2). Intimal thickening of veins is often hyalin and sclerotic in character, and should be distinguished from the more cellular intimal and muscular proliferation seen in pulmonary veno-occlusive disease and chronic passive congestion. Mural hyalinization of small arterioles is also an aging change (as well as being common in emphysematous lungs). Some degree of alveolar enlargement accompanies aging (88) and is called senile emphysema. Longitudinal elastic tissue fibers are a normal finding immediately beneath the surface epithelium in the large airways. These may take on an elastotic appearance in the lungs of older individuals. Senile amyloid is usually an incidental finding, is perivascular, and increases in incidence with age (89).

TABLE 18.9
EFFECTS OF AGING SEEN IN LUNG BIOPSIES

- Tracheobronchial cartilage ossification, submucosal fatty metaplasia, oncocytic metaplasia and/or hyperplasia in bronchial glands, and elastotic appearance of the submucosa
- Pulmonary arterial and venous intimal thickening and hyalinization of arterioles
- Alveolar enlargement (rarely appreciated in biopsy material)
- Medial calcification in bronchial arteries
- Senile vascular amyloidosis
- Anthracosis (urban dwellers)

THE BIOPSY THAT LOOKS NORMAL AT FIRST GLANCE

When a lung biopsy for presumed diffuse lung disease initially appears normal, a number of possibilities should be considered (Table 18.10), especially pulmonary edema (Figure 18.47).

Although one can argue that interstitial infiltrates that are so subtle as to be overlooked are probably not clinically significant, their recognition is necessary. This situation can arise, for example, with biopsy material from the less severely affected portions of lungs in patients with interstitial pneumonias, in cases in which the inflammatory infiltrate has

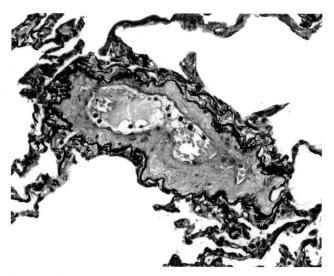

Figure 18.46 Aging change in vessels. In elderly individuals, a hyalin thickening of the intima may be encountered as an incidental finding. Clinical correlation is suggested, since this feature may also be encountered in the setting of pulmonary hypertension.

TABLE 18.10

SITUATIONS IN WHICH A LUNG BIOPSY MAY APPEAR NORMAL

- Sampling error
- Pulmonary vascular disease
- Small airway (bronchiolar) disease
- Pulmonary edema and early diffuse alveolar damage
- Emboli, including fat emboli
- A very subtle interstitial infiltrate
- Cardiac disease with secondary pulmonary abnormalities

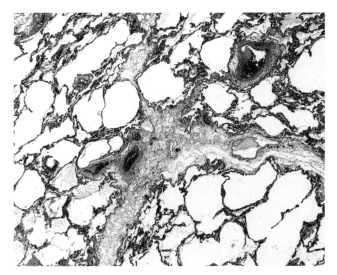

Figure 18.47 Pulmonary edema. Pulmonary edema may produce a deceptively normal appearance in a biopsy. Attention to septal widening, as noted in the accompanying text, and faint flocculent material in airspaces may be a clue to the diagnosis.

been suppressed by steroids or immunosuppressive therapy, and in pathologic entities characterized by patchy inflammation. The presence of inflammatory cells in the perivenular regions and alveolar wall with reactive type II cells is usually indicative of an interstitial pneumonia.

REFERENCES

1. Nagaishi C. *Functional Anatomy and Histology of the Lung.* Baltimore: University Park Press; 1972.
2. Wagenvoort CA, Wagenvoort N. *Pathology of Pulmonary Hypertension.* New York: John Wiley; 1977.
3. Kuhn C III. Ultrastructure and cellular function in the distal lung. In: Thurlbeck WM, Abell MR, eds. *The Lung.* Baltimore: Williams & Wilkins; 1978.
4. Scadding JG, Cumming G, eds. *Scientific Foundations of Respiratory Medicine.* Philadelphia: WB Saunders; 1981.
5. Gail DB, Lenfant CJ. Cells of the lung: biology and clinical implications. *Am Rev Respir Dis* 1983;127:366–387.
6. Bienenstock J, Befus AD. Gut-and-bronchus-associated lymphoid tissue. *Am J Anat* 1984;170:437–445.
7. Langston C, Kida K, Reed M, Thurlbeck WM. Human lung growth in late gestation and in the neonate. *Am Rev Respir Dis* 1984; 129:607–613.
8. Murray JF. *The Normal Lung.* 2nd ed. Philadelphia: WB Saunders; 1986.
9. Fawcett DW. *Bloom and Fawcett: A Textbook of Histology.* 12th ed. New York: Chapman and Hall; 1994.
10. Coalson JJ. The adult lung: structure and function. In: Saldana MJ, ed. *Pathology of Pulmonary Disease.* Philadelphia: JB Lippincott: 1994:3–14.
11. Wang NS. Anatomy. In: Dail DH, Hammar SP, eds. *Pulmonary Pathology.* 2nd ed. New York: Springer-Berlag; 1994:21–44.
12. Kuhn C III. Normal anatomy and histology. In: Thurlbeck WM, Churg AM, eds. *Pathology of the Lung.* 2nd ed. New York: Thieme Medical Publishers; 1995:1–36.
13. Weibel ER, Taylor CR. Functional design of the human lung for gas exchange. In: Fishman AP, ed. *Pulmonary Diseases and Disorders.* Vol 1. 3rd ed. New York: McGraw-Hill; 1998:21–61.
14. Albertine KH, Williams MC, Hyde DM. Anatomy of the lungs. In: Murray JF, Nadel JA, eds. *Textbook of Respiratory Medicine.* 3rd ed. Philadelphia: WB Saunders; 2000:3–33.
15. Corrin B. *Pathology of the Lungs.* London: Churchill Livingstone; 2000.
16. Leslie KO, Wick MR. Lung anatomy. In: Leslie KO, Wick MR, eds. *Practical Pulmonary Pathology.* Philadelphia: Churchill Livingstone; 2005:1–18.
17. Chinoy MR. Lung growth and development. frontiers. *Bioscience* 2003;8:392–415.
18. Roth-Kleiner M, Post M. Genetic control of lung development. *Biol Neonate* 2003;84:83–88.
19. Yaegashi H, Takahashi T. The airway dimension in ordinary human lung. A standardized morphometry of lung sections. *Arch Pathol Lab Med* 1994;118:969–974.
20. Lambert MW. Accessory bronchiolealveolar communications. *J Pathol Bacteriol* 1955;70:311–314.21.
21. Yousem SA, Dacic S. Idiopathic bronchiolocentric interstitial pneumonia. *Mod Pathol* 2002;15:1148–1153.
22. Churg A, Meyers J, Suarez T, et al. Airway-centered interstitial fibrosis: a distinct form of aggressive diffuse lung disease. *Am J Surg Pathol* 2004;28:62–68.
23. Fukuoka J, Franks TJ, Colby TV, et al. Peribronchiolar metaplasia: a common histologic lesion in diffuse lung disease and a rare cause of interstitial lung disease; clinicopathologic features of 15 cases. *Mod Pathol* 2003;17:336a.
24. Colby TV, Koss MN, Travis WD. Tumors of the lower respiratory tract. In: Rosai J, ed. *Atlas of Tumor Pathology.* 3rd series, fascicle 13. Washington DC: Armed Forced Institute of Pathology; 1995: 465–471.
25. Rogers AV, Dewar A, Corrin B, Jeffery PK. Identification of serous-like cells in the surface epithelium of human bronchioles. *Eur Respir J* 1995;6:498–504.
26. Castranova V, Rabovsky J, Tucker JH, Miles PR. The alveolar type II epithelial cell: a multifunctional pneumocyte. *Toxicol Appl Pharmacol* 1988;93:472–483.
27. Kasper M, Reimann T, Hempel U, et al. Loss of caveolin expression in type I pneumocyte as an indicator of subcellular alterations during lung fibrogenesis. *Histochem Cell Biol* 1998;109:41–48.
28. Lou YP, Takeyama K, Grattan KM, et al. Platelet-activating factor induces goblet cell hyperplasia and mucin gene expression in airways. *Am J Respir Crit Care Med* 1998; 157(pt 1):1927–1934.
29. Kreda SM, Gynn MC, Fenstermacher DA, Boucher RC, Gabriel SE. Expression and localization of epithelial aquaporins in the adult human lung. *Am J Respir Cell Mol Biol* 2001;24:224–234.
30. Ryerse JS, Hoffmann JW, Mahmoud S, Nagel BA, deMello DE. Immunolocalization of CC10 in Clara cells in mouse and human lung. *Histochem Cell Biol* 2001;115:325–332.
31. Lehnert BE. Pulmonary and thoracic macrophage subpopulations and clearance of particles from the lung. *Environ Health Perspect* 1992;97:17–46.
32. Gould SJ, Isaacson PG. Bronchus-associated lymphoid tissue (BALT) in human fetal and infant lung. *J Pathol* 1993;169: 229–234.

33. Richmond J, Pritchard GE, Ashcroft T, Avery A, Corris PA, Walters EH. Bronchus associated lymphoid tissue (BALT) in human lung: its distribution in smokers and non-smokers. *Thorax* 1993;48:1130–1134.

34. Tschernig T, Kleemann WJ, Pabst R. Bronchus-associated lymphoid tissue (BALT) in the lungs of children who had died from sudden infant death syndrome and other causes. *Thorax* 1995;50:658–660.

35. Bienenstock J. Bronchus-associated lymphoid tissue. *Int Arch Allergy Appl Immunol* 1985;76(suppl 1):62–69.

36. Kradin RL, Spirn PW, Mark EJ. Intrapulmonary lymph nodes. Clinical, radiologic, and pathologic features. *Chest* 1985;87:662–667.

37. Gallagher B, Urbanski SJ. The significance of pleural elastica invasion by lung carcinomas. *Hum Pathol* 1990;21:512–517.

38. Colby TV, Swensen SJ. Anatomic distribution and histopathologic pattern in diffuse lung disease: correlation with HRCT. *J Thorac Imaging* 1996;11:1–26.

39. Newman SL, Michael RP, Wang NS. Lingular lung biopsy: is it representative? *Am Rev Respir Dis* 1985;132:1084–1086.

40. Albo RJ, Grimes OF. The middle lobe syndrome: a clinical study. *Dis Chest* 1966;50:509–518.

41. Kwon KY, Myers JL, Swensen SJ, Colby TV. Middle lobe syndrome: a clinicopathological study of 21 patients. *Hum Pathol* 1995;26:302–307.

42. Renner RR, Markarian B, Pernice NJ, Heitzman ER. The apical cap. *Radiology* 1974;110:569–573.

43. McCloud TC, Isler RJ, Novelline RA, Putman CE, Simeone J, Stark P. The apical cap. *AJR* 1981;137:299–306.

44. Yousem SA. Pulmonary apical cap: a distinctive but poorly recognized lesion in pulmonary surgical pathology. *Am J Surg Pathol* 2001;25:679–683.

45. Thurlbeck WM, Wright JL. *Thurlbeck's Chronic Airflow Obstruction.* 2nd ed. Hamilton, Ontario: BC Decker; 1999.

46. Fraig M, Shreesa U, Savici D, Katzenstein AL. Respiratory bronchiolitis: a clinicopathologic study in current smokers, ex-smokers and never-smokers. *Am J Surg Pathol* 2002;26:647–653.

47. Lichter I, Gwynne JF. Spontaneous pneumothorax in young subjects: a clinical and pathological study. *Thorax* 1971;26:409–417.

48. Thurlbeck WM. *Chronic Airflow Obstruction in Lung Disease.* Philadelphia: WB Saunders; 1976.

49. Askin FB, McCann BG, Kuhn C. Reactive eosinophilic pleuritis: a lesion to be distinguished from pulmonary eosinophilic granuloma. *Arch Pathol Lab Med.* 1977;101:187–191.

50. Churg A. Asbestos fibers and pleural plaques in a general autopsy population. *Am J Pathol* 1982;109:88–96.

51. Meurman L. Asbestos bodies and pleural plaques in a Finnish series of autopsy cases. *Acta Pathol Microbiol Immunol Scand* 1966;181:1–107.

52. Roberts GH. The pathology of parietal pleural plaques. *J Clin Pathol* 1971;24:348–353.

53. Hillerdal G. Pleural plaques and risk for bronchial carcinoma and mesothelioma. A prospective study. *Chest* 1994;105:144–150.

54. Katzenstein ALA. Katzenstein and Askin's Surgical Pathology of Non-neoplastic Lung Disease. 3rd ed. Philadelphia: WB Saunders; 1997.

55. Kendall DM, Gal AA. Interpretation of tissue artifacts in transbronchial lung biopsy specimens. *Ann Diagn Pathol* 2003;7:20–24.

56. Kadokura M, Colby TV, Myers JL, et al. Pathologic comparison of video-assisted thoracic surgical lung biopsy with traditional open lung biopsy. *J Thorac Cardiovasc Surg* 1995;109:494–498.

57. Churg A. An inflation procedure for open lung biopsies. *Am J Surg Pathol* 1983;7:69–71.

58. Bensard DD, McIntyre RC Jr, Waring BJ, Simon JS. Comparison of video thoracoscopic lung biopsy to open lung biopsy in the diagnosis of interstitial lung disease. *Chest* 1993; 103:765–770.

59. Ferson PF, Landreneau RJ, Dowling RD, et al. Comparison of open versus thoracoscopic lung biopsy for diffuse infiltrative pulmonary disease. *J Thorac Cardiovasc Surg* 1993;106:194–199.

60. Carnochan FM, Walker WS, Cameron EW. Efficacy of video assisted thoracoscopic lung biopsy: an historical comparison with open lung biopsy. *Thorax* 1994;49:361–363.

61. Niewoehner DE, Kleinerman J, Rice DB. Pathologic changes in the peripheral airways of young cigarette smokers. *N Engl J Med* 1974;291:755–758.

62. Myers JL, Veal CF Jr, Shin MS, Katzenstein AL. Respiratory bronchiolitis causing interstitial lung disease. A clinicopathologic study of six cases. *Am Rev Respir Dis* 1987;135:880–884.

63. Ashley DJ. Bony metaplasia in trachea and bronchi. *J Pathol* 1970;102:186–188.

64. Churg A, Warnock ML. Pulmonary tumorlet. A form of peripheral carcinoid. *Cancer* 1976;37:1469–1477.

65. Gould VE, Linnoila RI, Memoli VA, Warren WH. Neuroendocrine components of the bronchopulmonary tract: hyperplasias, dysplasias, and neoplasms. *Lab Invest* 1983;49:519–537.

66. Ranchod M. The histogenesis and development of pulmonary tumorlets. *Cancer* 1977;39:1135–1145.

67. Travis W, Brambilla E, Harris C, Muller-Hermelink K, eds. *World Health Organization Classification of Tumours.* Vol 5. *Pathology and Genetics: Tumors of the Lung, Pleura, Thymus and Heart.* Lyon, France: IARC Press; 2004.

68. Kuhn C III, Askin FB. The fine structure of so-called minute pulmonary chemodectomas. *Hum Pathol* 1975;6:681–691.

69. Gaffey MJ, Mills SE, Askin FB. Minute pulmonary meningothelial-like nodules. A clinicopathologic study of so-called minute pulmonary chemodectoma. *Am J Surg Pathol* 1988;12:167–175.

70. Miller RR, Muller NL. Neuroendocrine cell hyperplasia and obliterative bronchiolitis in patients with peripheral carcinoid tumors. *Am J Surg Pathol* 1995;19:653–658.

71. Ionescu DN, Sasatomi E, Aldeeb D, et al. Pulmonary meningothelial-like nodules: a genotypic comparison with meningiomas. *Am J Surg Pathol* 2004;28:207–214.

72. Miller RR. Bronchioloalveolar cell adenomas. *Am J Surg Pathol* 1990;14:904–912.

73. Elkeles A, Glynn LE. Disseminated parenchymatous ossification in the lungs in association with mitral stenosis. *J Pathol Bacteriol* 1946;58:517–522.

74. Green JD, Harle TS, Greenberg SD, Weg JG, Nevin H, Jenkins DE. Disseminated pulmonary ossification. A case report with demonstration of electron-microscopic features. *Am Rev Respir Dis* 1970;101:293–298.

75. Muir TE, Leslie KO, Popper H, et al. Micronodular pneumocyte hyperplasia. *Am J Surg Pathol* 1998;22:465–472.

76. Bedrossian CW, Kuhn C III, Luna MA, Conklin RH, Byrd RB, Kaplan PD. Desquamative interstitial pneumonia-like reaction accompanying pulmonary lesions. *Chest* 1977;72:166–169.

77. Hollander DH, Hutchins GM. Central spherules in pulmonary corpora amylacea. *Arch Pathol Lab Med* 1978;102:629–630.

78. Koss MN, Johnson FB, Hochholzer L. Pulmonary blue bodies. *Hum Pathol* 1981;12:258–266.

79. Visscher D, Churg A, Katzenstein AL. Significance of crystalline inclusions in lung granulomas. *Mod Pathol* 1988;1:415–419.

80. Schaumann J. On the nature of certain peculiar corpuscles present in the tissue of lymphogranulomatosis benigna. *Acta Med Scand* 1941;106:239–253.

81. Warnock ML, Press M, Churg A. Further observations on cytoplasmic hyaline in the lung. *Hum Pathol* 1980;11:59–65.

82. Churg A, Warnock ML. Asbestos and other ferruginous bodies: their formation and clinical significance. *Am J Pathol* 1981; 102:447–456.

83. Glancy DL, Frazier PD, Roberts WC. Pulmonary parenchymal cholesterol-ester granulomas in patients with pulmonary hypertension. *Am J Med* 1968;45:198–210.

84. Reinila A. Perivascular xanthogranulomatosis in the lungs of diabetic patients. *Arch Pathol Lab Med* 1976;100:542–543.

85. Walford RL, Kaplan L. Pulmonary fibrosis and giant-cell reaction with altered elastic tissue: endogenous pneumoconiosis. *AMA Arch Pathol* 1957;63:75–90.

86. Unger JM, England DM, Bogust GA. Interstitial emphysema in adults: recognition and prognostic implications. *J Thorac Imaging* 1989;4:86–94.

87. Ro JY, Luna MA, Mackay B, Ramos O. Yellow-brown (Hamazaki-Wesenberg) bodies mimicking fungal yeasts. *Arch Pathol Lab Med* 1987;111:555–559.

88. Gillooly M, Lamb D. Airspace size in lungs of lifelong non-smokers: effect of age and sex. *Thorax* 1993;48:39–43.

89. Kunze WP. Senile pulmonary amyloidosis. *Pathol Res Pract* 1979;164:413–422.

Thymus

Saul Suster   Juan Rosai

INTRODUCTION

The thymus is a prototypical lymphoepithelial organ. As such, it is composed of intimately admixed epithelial and lymphoid elements that act in concert to perform their assigned roles. In addition, the thymus harbors other cellular constituents, such as a variety of mesenchymal-derived elements, scattered neuroendocrine cells, and presumably germ cells, all of which may take part in the development of neoplastic and nonneoplastic processes of this organ. Although much progress has been made in the immunohistochemical characterization of the cellular components of the thymus, the diagnosis of thymic lesions still remains largely dependent on the light microscopic interpretation of the findings by the pathologist.

EMBRYOLOGY

The thymus is derived from the third and, to a lesser extent, the fourth pharyngeal pouches, which contain elements derived from all three germinal layers. During the sixth week of gestation, the endodermal lining of the ventral wing of the third pharyngeal pouch forms a pronounced sacculation, which subsequently detaches from the pharyngeal wall, giving rise to the thymic primordia (1,2). It is postulated that, at approximately the same time, the cervical sinus (an ectodermal structure that results from the fusion of the second, third, and fourth branchial clefts) attaches to the thymic primordia, investing them with a layer of ectodermal cells (1,3). As development continues, the thymic primordia migrate in a caudal and medial direction along with the lower parathyroid glands. During the eighth week, these primordia enlarge toward their lower ends, forming two epithelial bars that fuse along the midline to occupy their definitive position within the anterosuperior mediastinum. During this descent, the tail portion of the organ becomes thin and elongated and breaks up into small fragments that usually disappear but that may persist in the soft tissues of the neck, often in intimate connection with the lower parathyroid gland and sometimes embedded within the thyroid gland (see section on Developmental Abnormalities) (1,4).

After migration has been completed, the thymic endodermal-derived epithelial cells develop into stellate elements, forming a reticular meshwork. The surrounding mesenchymal elements form a capsule around it; and, as a result of ingrowth of the capsule, trabeculae form that divide the organ into numerous lobules. By the tenth week, small lymphoid cells originating in the fetal liver and bone marrow populate the thymus, and the organ differentiates into a cortex and a medulla (5). Small, tubular structures composed of epithelial cells (sometimes referred to as medullary duct epithelium) also make their appearance at this time and later give rise to Hassall's corpuscles (6). The thymus progressively enlarges until puberty and from then on begins to involute, although persisting in an atrophic state into old age.

DEVELOPMENTAL ABNORMALITIES

Disturbances in the embryologic development of the thymus may give rise to a series of congenital anomalies. One of the anomalies most frequently encountered is the presence of parathyroid gland tissue within the thymus (7) (Figure 19.1). Such ectopically located tissue is most frequently encountered within the thymic capsule or in close proximity to it (8). This abnormality is easily explained by the close developmental relationship that exists between the two organs, as described in the section on embryology. The thymus itself also may be found in ectopic locations; this usually results from failure of the organ to migrate to its final destination during embryonic development. Undescended thymuses most often are located in the lateral neck, in close association with or even buried within the parathyroid or thyroid glands (9). These rests have a tendency to undergo cystic changes (9). They also may give rise to thymomas, ectopic examples of which have been described in submandibular (10), paratracheal (11,12), and intratracheal locations (13), as well as within the thyroid gland (14,15). A

morphologically distinctive lesion of the thymus displaying combined features of neoplasia and hamartoma occurring in the lower neck has also been recognized (16). Ectopic nodules composed of thymic tissue have been reported in several other locations, including the base of the skull (17) and the pulmonary hilus at the root of the bronchus (18).

Ectopic sebaceous glands have been reported in the thymus (19) and are felt to be related to the contribution of the ectodermally derived cervical sinus to the developing thymus. Mature-appearing salivary gland tissue also may be present in the thymus (Figure 19.2) and has been reported as a component of an intrathoracic cyst that contained normal thymus and parathyroid tissue within its walls (20). It was postulated that this finding could be related to a developmental malformation whereby salivary gland anlagen had been incorporated into the uppermost portion of the third pharyngeal pouch during embryogenesis.

Morphologic abnormalities of the thymus characterized by an embryonal appearance, with a predominance of small spindle epithelial cells adopting a lobular configuration and lacking small lymphocytes and Hassall's corpuscles, have been observed in association with combined immunodeficiency syndromes and T-cell defects (21). Such morphologic alterations have been termed thymic dysplasias and are believed to represent disturbances of normal development. In conditions such as reticular dysgenesis, Swiss-type hypogammaglobulinemia, thymic alymphoplasia, and ataxia-telangiectasia, the immune deficit is accompanied by aplasia or hypoplasia of the thymus (22–24). In DiGeorge syndrome, which is believed to result from an arrest in development of the third and possibly fourth branchial arches, there is a vestigial but normal thymus associated with absence or hypoplasia of the parathyroid glands (25). In Nezelof syndrome (26), the thymic abnormality is similar to that of DiGeorge syndrome except that the parathyroids are normal. The failure of development is thus thought to involve only that part of the branchial endoderm that will

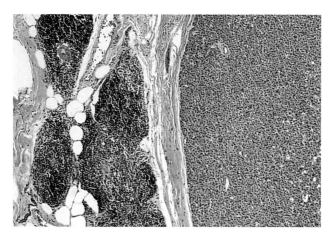

Figure 19.1 Ectopic parathyroid tissue adjacent to normal thymus.

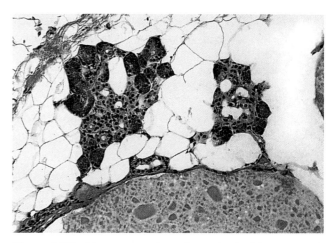

Figure 19.2 Mature-appearing salivary gland acini are seen adjacent to cystically dilated Hassall's corpuscle.

differentiate into thymic epithelium. Histologic changes in the thymus similar to those of thymic dysplasia of primary immunodeficiency disease have been observed in infants as a consequence of graft-versus-host disease after blood transfusions (27). A case of congenital aplasia of the parathyroid glands and thymus in the newborn also has been described (28). The term *thymic dysplasia* in the setting of immunodeficiency conditions may be misleading because of its currently accepted connotation as a preneoplastic cellular status. The alterations in such conditions are unrelated to a neoplastic etiology.

APOPTOSIS

Apoptosis is the name that has been given to the process of physiologic (programmed) cell death. Most thymic lymphocytes die in situ by such a process. During T-cell ontogeny in the thymus, the T cells (T lymphocytes) may undergo a process of positive or negative selection. The accumulated evidence appears to support that apoptosis plays a major role in the process of negative selection and that the vast majority of cortical thymocytes die by this mechanism. Autoreactive thymocytes or harmful cells in the thymus with injured DNA or alterations of their metabolism are also thought to be eliminated by the process of apoptosis at a specific stage of their differentiation (29,30). Therefore, it is believed that disturbances of the apoptotic process within the thymus can be responsible for the appearance of autoreactive cells in the circulation that may give rise to the development of autoimmune disease. In addition, failure of apoptosis also may play a role in carcinogenesis. On the other hand, massive induction of apoptosis within the thymus may lead to immunodeficiency as a result of a decrease in the number of lymphocytes. Thus, thymocyte apoptosis plays an integral role in the pathophysiology of the immune system.

The exact biochemical mechanism involved in thymocyte apoptosis has not yet been completely elucidated; however, it is known that various complex physiologic and nonphysiologic mechanisms can induce it (31). This has led many investigators to seek the genes and their products that are necessary for apoptosis. Several groups have noted that messenger RNA (mRNA) levels for various proteins are increased early in thymocytes after treatment with glucocorticoids or radiation, two agents known to induce massive apoptosis of cortical thymocytes (32,33). A number of genes also have been identified whose expression is increased in cells undergoing apoptosis. Among them, three proto-oncogene products have been shown to act as important regulators of the apoptotic process in mammals: c-myc, bcl-2, and p53. In thymocytes, bcl-2 mRNA is present in the surviving mature thymocytes of the medulla and also in most immature (CD4$^+$/CD8$^+$) thymocytes, although the majority of cortical thymocytes (most of which die by apoptosis) display no bcl-

2, suggesting that this oncogene may be involved in the preservation of T cells (34). Alterations of the *p53* gene also have been shown to play a role in the process of thymocyte apoptosis. Malfunction of the tumor suppressor gene *p53* may promote carcinogenesis by permitting mutated cells to duplicate their DNA before it is repaired. In mice, *p53*-deficient thymocytes have been shown to display drastic resistance to the apoptotic effects of radiation (35). The latter observation suggests that the integrity of the *p53* gene, whose product is known to arrest cell proliferation, may be necessary for the normal apoptotic process in the thymus.

Another pathway of thymocyte apoptosis that has been the object of close scrutiny is the role of the T-cell receptor (TCR)/CD3 complex in this process. During thymocyte development, rearrangement of TCR genes leads to expression of unique, clonally expressed TCRs. Potentially autoreactive thymocytes bearing TCRs with high avidity for self undergo TCR-mediated, activation-induced apoptosis (negative selection), whereas thymocytes with TCRs of low avidity survive (positive selection) (36,37). Recent experiments have demonstrated that the activation of the TCR/CD3 complex leads to the preferential elimination of immature (CD4$^+$/CD8$^+$) thymocytes (38). These and other studies have demonstrated that TCR-mediated signals are involved in apoptosis, and this phenomenon is strongly related to the mechanism of negative selection, although the precise in situ mechanism of apoptosis has not yet been elucidated (39,40).

ANATOMY

The fully mature human thymus is an encapsulated midline structure predominantly located in the anterosuperior mediastinum and composed of two lobules joined in the midline by loose connective tissue and thymic parenchyma. The base of the organ lies on the pericardium and great vessels. The upper poles of each lobe extend into the lower neck and are closely applied to the trachea. The lower poles extend down over the pericardium for a variable distance, generally up to the level of the fourth costal cartilage. The anterior border of the gland is made up by the cervical fascia, strap muscles of the neck, sternum, costal cartilages, and intercostal muscles, and the lateral borders are covered by reflections of the parietal pleura.

The size and weight of the gland may vary considerably depending on the age of the person, although wide variations among individuals in the same age group have been observed (41). The mean weight at birth is about 20 g. The organ exhibits a continuous growth in size until puberty, when it reaches a mean weight of approximately 35 to 50 g; thereafter, it undergoes atrophy, as manifested by a decrease in weight and volume and progressive fatty replacement of the parenchyma.

The blood supply of the organ is derived from the internal mammary, superior and inferior thyroid arteries, and, to a lesser degree, the pericardiophrenic arteries. The arterial branches course along fibrous septa to the region near the corticomedullary junction, where they branch into the cortex and the medulla. The capillaries descend from the outer cortex toward the medulla to form postcapillary venules, and they exit the thymus through the septa as interlobular veins. The venous system drains into the left brachiocephalic, internal thoracic, and inferior thyroid veins. There are no true thymic intraparenchymatous afferent lymphatics. Lymph vessels arise in the interstitium of the lobular septa and merge to form large lymph vessels that course alongside the arteries in the septa. The innervation of the organ is derived from branches of the vagus nerve and the cervical sympathetic nerves.

HISTOLOGY

The basic structural unit of the thymus is the lobule. Each lobule is composed of two morphologically distinctive areas, the cortex and the medulla, both of which are largely composed of varying proportions of epithelial cells and thymic lymphocytes (thymocytes) (Figure 19.3). In the cortex, the sparse epithelial cells present are overshadowed by the numerous, closely packed small lymphocytes. The medulla, in contrast, contains a larger number of epithelial cells and fewer lymphocytes. The cortex and the medulla combined correspond to the thymic epithelial compartment, which is the site of T-cell maturation within this organ. Another important anatomic compartment of the thymus is the perivascular space. In the mature infant thymus, the perivascular space represents a virtual space containing thymic blood vessels and corresponding to a portion of tissue that is contained within the capsule but outside of the thymic epithelial network (42). The perivascular space becomes more prominent with aging and in pathologic processes such as thymoma, and eventually it is replaced with fat and lymphocytes in the involuted thymus of the adult (43). In

addition to the epithelial and perivascular space compartments, there is also a stromal compartment that harbors a variety of other cell types. A thin fibrous capsule is generally present surrounding the entire gland. The interplay of these various cellular elements and compartments contributes to define the various organotypical features of the normal thymus.

One of the problems involved in defining the "normal" thymus is that the histologic appearance of the organ shows progressive changes over time, depending on its stage of maturation or involution. Thus, the "normal" thymus of the adult will look quite different from the "normal" thymus in a child or adolescent. Studies by Hale (43) have shown that the thymus gland does not actually decrease in size or alter its shape over time with the normal process of involution. While the overall size and shape of the gland is retained throughout adulthood into old age, the various cellular constituents are replaced as the normal process of functional involution takes place. Thus, in the thymus of the adult and old age, the normal thymopoietic elements represented by the epithelial compartment become reduced and progressively disappear, being gradually replaced by mature adipose tissue. Residual epithelial elements, however, always remain and generally undergo a process of atrophy that results in a change in the shape of the cells from large, round cells with vesicular nuclei and abundant cytoplasm to small, oval to spindle-shaped cells with hyperchromatic nuclei and scant cytoplasm (44). Small, microscopic, thymopoietic remnants of thymic epithelium can also be found, which usually retain the normal architecture and appearance of the mature cortex in childhood. Other involutional changes include the formation of cystic structures, usually resulting from dilatation of residual Hassall's corpuscles, and the formation of small, abortive glandular or epithelial rosette-like structures within the lymphopoietic islands.

The most distinctive organotypical features of the mature thymus of childhood and adolescence thus include a fibrous capsule, a lobular architecture with sharp separation between the cortex and the medulla, a dual cell population characterized by an admixture of large, round thymic epithelial cells with immature T-cells, and perivascular spaces. The organotypical features of the "normal" involuted thymus of the adult, on the other hand, include the presence of small, spindle-shaped thymic epithelial cells, abundant cystic structures and rosette-like epithelial structures, and the paucity of immature T-cells. Needless to say, these features represent a continuum that will be manifested in various proportions depending on the age, functional status of the organ, various physiologic conditions, and disease states affecting the thymus.

Epithelial Cells

The epithelial cells of the thymus have traditionally been divided into cortical and medullary; some of the latter are arranged in round keratinized structures known as Hassall's

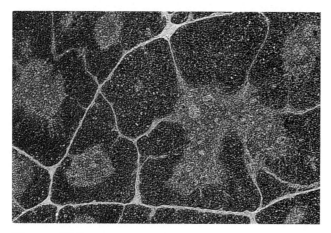

Figure 19.3 Normal lobular architecture of the thymus demonstrating clear separation between cortex and medulla.

corpuscles. In the active thymus of infancy, most epithelial cells are plump, with round or oval nuclei. Their cytoplasm (particularly in the case of the cortical cells) is endowed with numerous prolongations that join with those of adjacent cells to form a veritable network or reticulum. This feature (rather than the relationship with reticulin fibers or presumptive embryologic origin) has led to the previous designation of reticuloepithelial cells. These various epithelial elements play an active role in promoting T-cell maturation in the thymus, either through the action of their humoral substances or through direct contact with thymocytes (45).

A subset of thymic epithelial cells that have predominantly localized to the cortex has been designated as nurse cells. They are characterized by having an abundant cytoplasm within which are engulfed numerous mature thymic T cells. A ringlike staining pattern has been observed in these cells with antiepithelial cell antibodies by immunohistochemistry on sections of human thymus (46). It has been postulated that nurse cells may provide a specialized microenvironment for T-cell maturation, differentiation, and selection in the thymus (46,47).

Hassall's Corpuscles

Hassall's corpuscles constitute the most readily identifiable feature of the thymus at the light microscopic level.

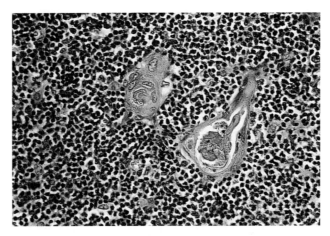

Figure 19.4 Normal Hassall's corpuscles showing characteristic concentric arrangement of keratinizing epithelial cells.

They are restricted to the medulla and are characterized by a concentric pattern of keratinization, the keratin formed being of high-molecular weight (epidermal) type (Figure 19.4). These structures may show much variation in their morphologic appearance, mainly as a result of reactive changes secondary to inflammation. This includes cystic degeneration with accumulation of cellular debris, dystrophic calcification, and infiltration by lymphocytes, foamy macrophages, and eosinophils (Figure 19.5). The

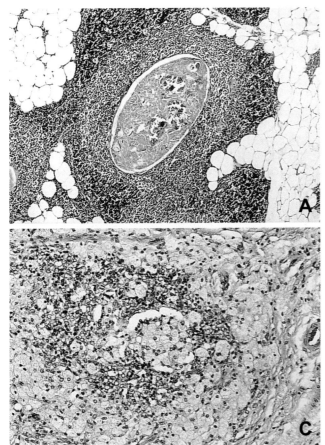

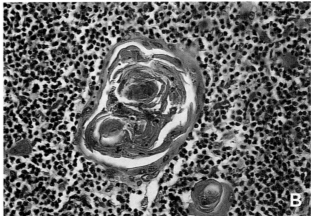

Figure 19.5 Hassall's corpuscles showing (**A**) cystic dilatation with accumulation of cellular debris, (**B**) dystrophic calcification, and (**C**) accumulation of foamy macrophages.

thymic lesions known as Dubois's microabscesses and tra- ditionally ascribed to congenital syphilis (48) represent an exaggeration of the cystic changes in Hassall's corpuscles as a result of infection. We believe that most so-called multilocular thymic cysts are not congenital abnormalities but rather the result of cystic enlargement of Hassall's cor- puscles on the basis of acquired inflammatory changes in this organ (49). An additional change that can be seen in relation to cystic Hassall's corpuscles is the presence of glandular elements, as manifested by the appearance of columnar epithelium (sometimes ciliated- or of goblet- cell type) and the secretion of sulfated acid mucopolysac- charides in the lumen (50). It is likely that these glandu- lar changes are related to the embryologic origin of Hassall's corpuscles (6).

Thymic Lymphocytes (Thymocytes)

The predominant cell population of the thymic cortex is made up of lymphocytes that may be large, medium, or small. Large, mitotically active lymphoblasts comprise about 15% of the lymphoid cells and are found predomi- nantly in the subcapsular portion of the outer cortex (51). These lymphocytes have a round or oval (occasionally con- voluted) nucleus, one or two prominent nucleoli, and rela- tively abundant, strongly basophilic cytoplasm. A gradient of smaller, less mitotically active cells occurs from the outer cortex to the corticomedullary junction and to a lesser de- gree into the medulla of the normal thymus (Figure 19.6). In the capsular region and deep cortex, the vast majority of thymic lymphocytes are short-lived and die in situ (52). This results in lympholysis and active phagocytosis, fea- tures that impart these areas with a prominent "starry sky" appearance and that become particularly prominent in ac- cidental (stress) thymic involution (see section on Thymic Involution) (Figure 19.7).

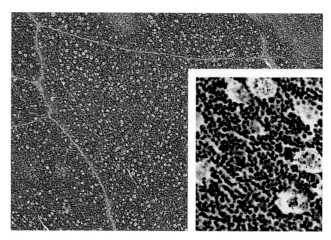

Figure 19.7 Prominent starry sky appearance in the deep cortex of patient with accidental thymic involution. Note abundance of tin- gible-body macrophages (*inset*).

Other Cell Types

In addition to epithelial cells and lymphocytes of T-cell lin- eage, the thymus contains an array of additional cell types. The first of these, B cells (B lymphocytes), can be found ag- gregated as lymphoid follicles or scattered as individual cells. Lymphoid follicles with active germinal centers may be found in otherwise normal thymuses, especially in chil- dren and adolescents (Figure 19.8) (52,53). The presence of such B-cell structures would seem difficult to reconcile with the fact that the thymus constitutes a predominantly T-cell organ. However, ultrastructural studies have indicated that germinal centers in the thymus arise within perivascular spaces, the latter being clearly separated from the thymic parenchyma by a basal lamina (54). This observation led to the proposal that the thymus may be divided into two ma- jor functional compartments: (a) the cortex and medulla (which constitute the true thymic parenchyma) and (b) the

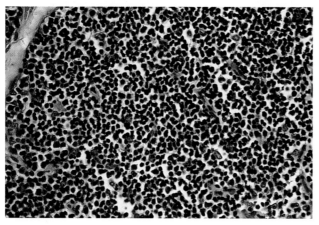

Figure 19.6 Normal thymic cortex. There are numerous cortical thymocytes, most of which have small nuclei with densely packed chromatin.

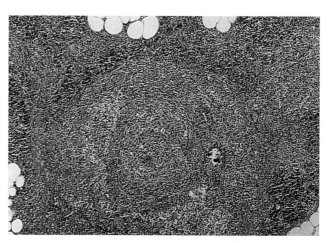

Figure 19.8 Lymphoid follicle with germinal center in normal thymus.

extraparenchymal compartment composed of the perivascular spaces (55). Germinal centers in the thymus could thus be explained as being derived from preexisting perivascular B cells in the extraparenchymal compartment. Germinal centers are well known to be prominent in patients with myasthenia gravis and other immune-mediated diseases (see section on Thymic Hyperplasia) (9), but their presence in an otherwise normal thymus should not necessarily be taken as an indicator of an underlying immune disorder. The incidence of germinal centers in the thymus of normal individuals without septicemia or disease of a presumed autoimmune cause has varied in published studies from 2.1% (53) to 40% (54). This wide variation may be related to a sampling factor or to the age of the patients; germinal centers would be expected to be less frequent in the older age groups. Also, stress has been shown to be a factor responsible for the decrease in the number of these structures (56). Determination of the incidence and number of germinal centers in normal human thymus glands still remains an unsettled issue.

Isolated B cells are found in both fetal and normal adult thymuses distributed along the septa, in close proximity to small vessels at the corticomedullary junction and in the medulla (57). Intrathymic B cells have been found to be significantly increased in patients with myasthenia gravis, a finding that some investigators consider to be a more specific change for this disorder than the presence of germinal centers (57,58). More recently, a population of intramedullary B cells with a tendency to cluster around Hassall's corpuscles has been identified in the thymus gland from fetuses, newborn babies, children, and adults; these lymphocytes show evidence of activation and bear a distinctive immunophenotype (59). Unlike B cells of germinal centers and surrounding mantle zones, the medullary B cells are negative for CD21 and do not express surface/cytoplasmic immunoglobulins. It has been proposed that a significant proportion of non-Hodgkin's lymphomas of the B-cell type located in the anterior mediastinum arise from this intrathymic B-cell population. Additionally, a newly described type of mucosa-associated lymphoid tissue (MALT) lymphoma composed of monocytoid B cells recently was identified as arising from the thymus (60); this finding raises the possibility that monocytoid B cells may be another as yet unidentified cellular constituent of the normal thymus (61).

Several other types of hematolymphoid cells are present in small number but constant fashion in the normal thymus (62–64). Macrophages are mainly located in the cortex, show phagocytic activity, are markedly α-naphthyl acetate esterase positive, acid phosphatase positive, and HLA-DR negative, and are antigenically indistinguishable from macrophages of other organs (45,64). Interdigitating dendritic cells are mainly located in the medulla, are markedly HLA-DR positive, have little lysosomal enzyme activity, and show S-100 protein reactivity (65). Both of

these cell types are thought to be involved in lymphocyte and epithelial cell interaction.

Langerhans cells also have been identified in the thymic medulla; both interdigitating dendritic cells and Langerhans cells are said to be increased in the thymuses of patients with myasthenia gravis (66). The latter cells provide the anatomic substrate for the development of Langerhans cell granulomatosis (histiocytosis X) within the thymus (67). Eosinophils are usually present in the thymus of children, sometimes in large numbers (68). They appear in fetal life and persist until puberty, after which they become infrequent. They are found mainly in the connective tissue septa or within the medulla and occasionally may be present within Hassall's corpuscles.

Mast cells are also normally present in human thymuses. They are usually found within and scattered parallel to the connective tissue septa, often in a perivascular location. The presence of mast cells can be a source of confusion in the course of immunohistochemical and other special stains of the thymus gland because of their propensity to react with a wide variety of reagents; they are easily identified by the use of metachromatic stains. Increased numbers of mast cells in the thymus have been observed in patients with severe combined immunodeficiency and thymic alymphoplasia (69), but the significance of this finding is not understood. Plasma cells are rare in the normal thymus; they are usually located in the connective tissue septa or, more rarely, in the medulla (70). Plasma cells may be numerous in the involuting thymus and also may be present in increased numbers in the thymus of patients with myasthenia gravis (71).

Neuroendocrine cells are now accepted as being a minor but constant component of the normal thymus (72). Peptide- and amine-producing neuroendocrine cells have been identified in the thymus glands of reptiles and birds (73–75) and, to a lesser degree, in mammalian (including human) thymuses. It has been postulated that some of these cells may be embryologically and functionally analogous to C cells of thyroid (76). The physiologic role of these various neuroendocrine elements in the thymus is not yet understood, but their presence has been offered as the probable substrate for the development of carcinoid tumors and other neuroendocrine neoplasms in this organ, including calcitonin-positive medullary carcinomas (77,78).

Myoid cells are located in the thymic medulla. They are common in reptilian and avian thymuses but also can be found (albeit with some difficulty) in human thymuses, particularly in infants. They have microscopic, immunohistochemical, and ultrastructural features of striated muscle cells (79,80). Their histogenesis remains a subject of debate, some studies pointing toward a derivation from the neural crest (81) and others showing the existence of shared epitopes with thymic epithelial cells (82). Myoid cells have been said to be increased in the thymus of patients with myasthenia gravis (57,83) and in patients with true thymic hyperplasia (84), suggesting that these cells may play a role in immunoregulatory mechanisms. Thymic neoplasms thought to represent the neoplastic counterpart of myoid cells also have been described (85).

Germ cells are another cellular element thought to be normally present in the thymus. It has been proposed that scattered germ cells reach the thymus during ontogenesis and that some of them persist into adult life. However, direct evidence of their presence in the normal thymus gland has never been demonstrated, and the only presumptive evidence of their occurrence is the fact that nearly all mediastinal germ cell tumors arise within the thymus (9). Rosai et al. (86) have recently proposed that germ cells in the thymus may develop into somatic cells, thus making their detection and identification difficult by conventional means. They further hypothesized that thymic myoid cells may be of germ cell origin and thus provide indirect evidence for the existence of the latter in this organ (86).

Connective tissue elements of the thymus include vessels, fibrous tissue, nerves, and fat. The vasculature of the thymus arises from arteries that enter the organ via fibrous trabeculae from the capsule. In contrast to other major lymphoid organs, the thymus lacks a hilus. The thymic vessels are ensheathed by a layer of thymic epithelial cells. This anatomic configuration, plus the failure of the thymus to produce antibodies against circulating antigen, led to the concept of the blood-thymus barrier (87). Raviola and Karnovsky (88), in an elaborate study using electron-opaque tracers of different molecular dimensions, demonstrated convincingly that, although some blood-borne macromolecules do penetrate the thymus, their distribution was limited to the medulla, thus pointing to the existence of a blood-thymus barrier operating at the level of the cortex. However, more recent studies have challenged the concept of the blood-thymus barrier by showing that the thymic cortex also may be permeable to immunoglobulin molecules present in the extravascular compartment (89).

The presence of a distinct anatomic compartment bound by the vessel wall and the sheath of epithelial cells has been postulated. It has further been suggested that it is through these perivascular spaces that the mature T-cells exit the thymus to colonize peripheral lymphoid organs once their maturation process is complete. The spaces are inconspicuous in the normal thymus; they may appear dilated in atrophic and involuting organs, but they acquire their greatest prominence in some thymomas (9).

ULTRASTRUCTURE

Ultrastructurally, very elongated cytoplasmic processes can be appreciated in the epithelial cells of the thymic cortex, which are also covered by basal lamina material (Figure 19.9) (90–92). Medullary epithelial cells are more densely packed and have blunted cytoplasmic projections (Figure 19.10). A consistent feature of medullary epithelial cells is the greater frequency of desmosomes and the presence of dense tonofilaments that often insert into desmosomes. This feature is particularly obvious in Hassall's corpuscles. Cortical epithelial cells may display a range of ultrastructural appearances depending on the electron density of their cytoplasm, including pale cells with electron-lucent cytoplasm, intermediate cells with variable electron density, and dark cells with electron-dense cytoplasm. The same range may be observed in medullary epithelial cells; in addition, the medulla contains undifferentiated epithelial cells with sparse cytoplasm (93).

Thymic myoid cells display ultrastructural features of skeletal muscle, including myofilaments with dense

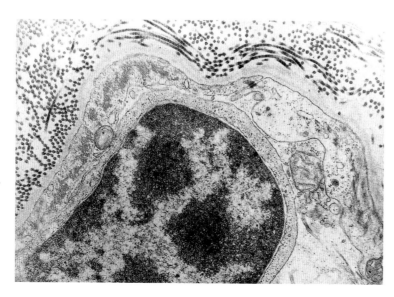

Figure 19.9 Ultrastructural detail of normal cortical epithelial cells showing large cytoplasmic processes joined by a desmosome and wrapped around a small lymphocyte. A thick basal lamina separates the epithelial cells from the surrounding collagen. (Reprinted with permission from: Rosai J, Levine GD. Tumors of the thymus. In: *Atlas of Tumor Pathology.* 2nd series, fascicle 13. Washington, DC: Armed Forces Institute of Pathology; 1976.)

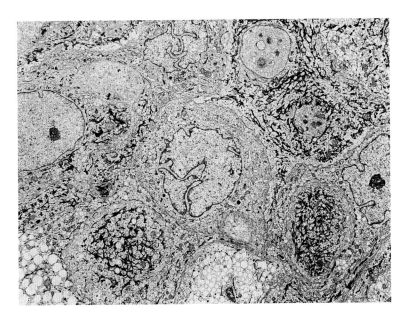

Figure 19.10 Ultrastructural detail of medullary epithelial cells showing compact arrangement and blunted cytoplasmic projections. (Reprinted with permission from: Rosai J, Levine GD. Tumors of the thymus. In: *Atlas of Tumor Pathology*. 2nd series, fascicle 13. Washington, DC: Armed Forces Institute of Pathology; 1976.)

patches (Figure 19.11). Some investigators have identified cells displaying both tonofilaments and myofilaments by electron microscopy, and in some instances myoid cells have been observed to display desmosomal connections with epithelial cells (94).

IMMUNOHISTOCHEMISTRY

Thymic Epithelial Cells

Immunohistochemical studies have demonstrated that thymic epithelial cells may express a variety of distinctive differentiation antigens. Currently, at least four antigeni-

cally distinctive types of epithelial cell are recognized in the normal thymus: subcapsular cortical, inner cortical, medullary, and the cells of Hassall's corpuscles (Table 19.1) (95–98). Inner cortical epithelium, in addition to exhibiting keratin positivity, strongly reacts with TE-3, a murine monoclonal antibody raised against human thymic stroma (99). Subcapsular cortical epithelial cells and medullary epithelial cells react strongly with TE-4 monoclonal antibody. Both of these cells also label with A2B5, a monoclonal antibody directed against a complex neuronal ganglioside found on the cell surface of neurons and neuroendocrine cells (100).

Another marker of subcapsular cortical epithelium and medullary epithelium in normal thymus is that detected

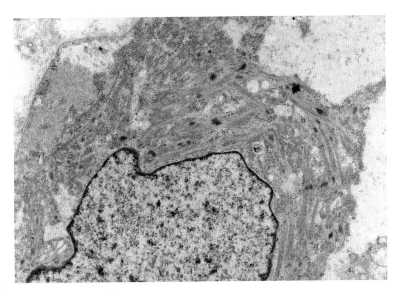

Figure 19.11 Ultrastructural appearance of myoid cell in the thymus. Note bundles of actin and myosin myofilaments with clearly discernible Z lines in the cytoplasm.

TABLE 19.1

SUMMARY OF MAIN ANTIGENIC DETERMINANTS FOUND IN EPITHELIAL CELLS OF THE NORMAL THYMUS

Cells	Keratin	TE-3	TE-4	A2B5	Anti-p19	Antithymosin α1	Antithymopoietin	HLA/Ia
Inner cortical epithelium	+	+	−	−	−	−	−	+
Subcapsular cortical epithelium	+	−	+	+	+	+	+	+
Medullary epithelium	+	−	+	+	+	+	−	−
Hassall's corpuscles	++	−	−	−	−	−	−	−

with anti-p19, an antibody that defines the structural core protein of the human T-cell lymphoma virus and that is believed to be acquired during normal thymic ontogeny. In the normal human thymus, the antigen defined by anti-p19 is found to parallel the reactivity of A2B5 antibody in epithelial cells (101). Interestingly, a recent study on thymomas has demonstrated that the expression of the p19 antigen is lost with malignant transformation (102).

Subcapsular cortical, inner cortical, and medullary epithelial cells also have been found to express class I and class II major histocompatibility antigens (97,103). However, recent studies using double immunolabeling have shown that HLA-DR expression is absent in medullary epithelial cells and that the positivity reported in previous studies may have been the result of diffusion of the stain from surrounding interdigitating dendritic cells (104). A recent study has demonstrated that the epithelial cells in the normal thymus and in thymomas also express epithelium-associated glycoprotein H (tissue blood group O antigen), peanut agglutinin receptor antigen (PNA-r), and Saphora Japonica agglutinin receptor antigen (SJA-r), which are detectable by lectin binding (105). Recent studies also have demonstrated expression of the epidermal growth factor receptor and transforming growth factor alpha in subcapsular, cortical, and medullary epithelial cells, suggesting that this substance plays a role in the growth and differentiation of these cells (106). Subcortical epithelial cells lining the boundaries between the thymic parenchyma and its surrounding fibrous tissue also demonstrate positivity for Leu-7, a differentiation antigen found in human null/killer cells and neuroendocrine cells (107). The cells of Hassall's corpuscles show the strongest keratin positivity of all thymic epithelial cells and react particularly strongly with the high-molecular weight keratin AE2 antibody, which is considered a marker of terminal epithelial maturation (108). Conversely, they are unreactive for the other antigens mentioned above.

Thymic Lymphocytes

The normal lymphoid population of the thymus has been shown to exhibit marked immunophenotypic heterogeneity, reflective of their functional status. The very term *thymocyte*, which was originally introduced to designate all thymic lymphocytes, has acquired a more specific immunologic meaning and is now restricted to immature thymic lymphocytes of T-cell lineage (with the exclusion of pre–T-cell lymphocytes). Thymocytes can be divided into three types in accordance with their different stages of intrathymic maturation (19,109–111) (Table 19.2). The earliest stage of differentiation is found in subcapsular thymocytes, which are characterized by a Leu-1$^+$ (T1), Leu-2a$^+$ (T8), Leu-3a$^+$ (T4), Leu-4$^+$ (T3), Leu-5$^+$ (T11), Leu-6$^+$ (T6), Leu-9$^+$ (T2), Tdt$^+$, and T200$^+$ phenotype (Figure 19.12A). The next stage in maturation is seen in cortical thymocytes, which comprise the majority of thymic lymphocytes (60–70%) and are characterized by a Leu-1$^+$ (T1), Leu-2a$^+$ (T8), Leu-3a$^+$ (T4), Leu-4$^+$ (T3), Leu-5$^+$ (T11), Leu6$^+$ (T6), Leu-9$^+$ (T2), Leu-M3, OKT-10 (T10), Tdt$^+$, and T200$^+$ phenotype. The last stage of intrathymic maturation is seen in medullary thymocytes, which show a Leu-1$^+$ (T1), Leu-4$^+$ (T3), Leu-5$^+$ (T11), Leu -9$^+$ (T2), and T200$^+$ phenotype (Figure 19.12B).

Antigens Leu-2a and Leu-3a are present in only one third to two thirds of these cells, respectively (57,109). Of the above markers, the ones that may distinguish specifically between cortical and medullary thymocytes are CD1, CD14, CD38, and Tdt. Recent studies on thymomas have attempted to correlate the degree of T-cell maturation with the morphologic appearance of the tumor (107,112–114). It has been well established that the lymphoid cell population in thymomas is made up of immature T cells (113,115,116). In lymphocyte-rich thymomas, the lymphocytes have the phenotypic markers of cortical thymocytes; it has, therefore, been proposed that these tumors are attempting to recapitulate the structure and function of the cortical compartment of the normal thymus (114,117,118). In the better-differentiated examples, the analogy with the normal thymus is accentuated by the presence of foci of medullary differentiation. These findings support the originally proposed theory that, in thymomas, prothymocytes from the stem cell compartment undergo a series of maturational events induced by the neoplastic thymic epithelial cells analogous to those that take place in the normal thymus, the lymphoid elements in these tumors thus being an environmental rather

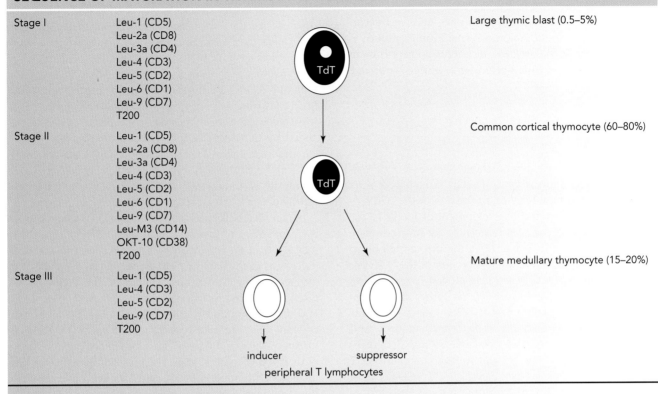

TABLE 19.2		
SEQUENCE OF MATURATION IN THYMIC LYMPHOCYTES		

Stage I	Leu-1 (CD5)	Large thymic blast (0.5–5%)
	Leu-2a (CD8)	
	Leu-3a (CD4)	
	Leu-4 (CD3)	
	Leu-5 (CD2)	
	Leu-6 (CD1)	
	Leu-9 (CD7)	
	T200	
Stage II	Leu-1 (CD5)	Common cortical thymocyte (60–80%)
	Leu-2a (CD8)	
	Leu-3a (CD4)	
	Leu-4 (CD3)	
	Leu-5 (CD2)	
	Leu-6 (CD1)	
	Leu-9 (CD7)	
	Leu-M3 (CD14)	
	OKT-10 (CD38)	
	T200	Mature medullary thymocyte (15–20%)
Stage III	Leu-1 (CD5)	
	Leu-4 (CD3)	
	Leu-5 (CD2)	
	Leu-9 (CD7)	
	T200	

inducer   suppressor

peripheral T lymphocytes

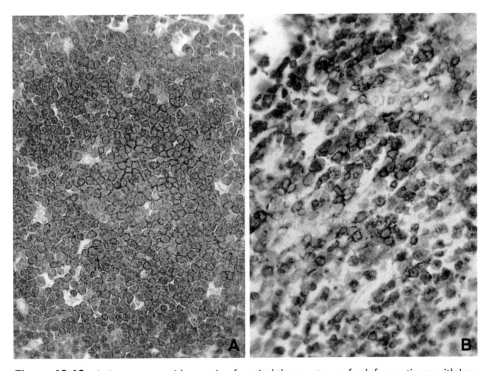

Figure 19.12 **A.** Immunoperoxidase stain of cortical thymocytes on fresh frozen tissue with Leu-1 (CD5) antibody. **B.** Medullary thymocytes showing focal Leu-3a (CD4) positivity on fresh frozen tissue.

than a neoplastic component (9). This contention, which was initially based solely on light microscopic observations of thymomas, has recently gained support from studies with DNA hybridization for T-cell receptor genes that showed that the lymphoid elements in thymomas lacked gene rearrangements that would denote a clonal proliferation of T-cells (119). As already indicated, such interaction is thought to be mediated by thymic hormones produced by thymic epithelial cells.

MOLECULAR BIOLOGY

Molecular studies have demonstrated the presence of rearrangement and expression of T-cell antigen receptors (TCRs) in thymic lymphocytes. Expression of the TCR represents a critical step in the development of T cells in the thymus (120,121). The TCR molecules are heterodimeric proteins analogous in structure to the immunoglobulin molecules. Rearrangement and expression of the TCRs are needed for the T cell to recognize antigen in association with self–major histocompatibility complex (MHC) antigens. There are two major types of TCRs: one type contains α-and β-polypeptide chains, and the other contains γ- and δ-chains. The α-β-TCR is expressed in nearly all T cells, whereas the γ-δ-TCR is expressed in only about 2% of T cells. Immature thymic lymphocytes (CD4$^-$/CD8$^-$) have been shown to contain mRNA only for the β-chain of the TCR. Mature thymic lymphocytes (CD4/CD8$^+$), on the other hand, contain mRNA for both β- and α-chains (122).

As immature thymocytes begin to undergo T-cell receptor gene rearrangements, they first acquire cytoplasmic then cell surface expression of CD3, CD4, and CD8. The CD4$^+$/CD8$^+$ (i.e., "double positive") lymphocytes are located within the thymic cortex and also express CD1a surface marker, as well as strong positivity for the Ki-67 nuclear proliferation antigen (43). As double-positive thymocytes complete their T-cell receptor gene rearrangement and undergo positive and negative selection, they progressively lose their expression of CD1a, Ki-67, and either CD4 or CD8. The resulting "single positive" thymocytes (either CD4$^+$/CD8$^-$ or CD4$^-$/CD8$^+$) migrate into the thymic medulla, where they complete their maturation before they are released into the circulation.

The genetic mechanisms that promote lineage commitment in the thymus are not well understood. Recent studies have suggested that there are at least 25 genes involved in the segregation of the different T-cell lineages. Commitment to the CD4 lineage appears to be controlled by upregulation of genes associated with increased survival followed by expression of genes that regulate nucleosome remodeling and T-cell receptor signaling. Commitment to the CD8 lineage appears to be influenced by upregulation of genes that regulate lymphocyte homing followed by suppression of genes that inhibit apoptosis (123).

FUNCTION

The thymus plays a central role in cell-mediated immunity. In early embryonic development, prothymocytes enter the thymus from the bone marrow and migrate to the outer cortex, where they undergo a process of maturation. Mature thymocytes move from the outer cortex to the medulla then migrate into the peripheral circulation, where they function as mature T cells. During their sojourn in the thymus, T cells learn to distinguish self from nonself and acquire the ability to recognize antigens bound to cell surface molecules encoded by the major histocompatibility complex (MHC). Circulating helper (CD4$^+$) and suppressor (CD8$^+$) thymus-derived T cells play a variety of roles in cell-mediated immunity, including the induction of cytotoxicity, delayed-type hypersensitivity reactions, and transplant rejection.

A controversial aspect of thymic function is that related to the production of thymic hormones, which are thought to play a role in the induction of differentiation of early T-cell precursors in the thymus. Four distinct types of thymic hormones have been identified: thymopoietin, thymosin α1, thymulin (formerly known as facteur thymique serique), and thymic humoral factor (122,124,125). Thymopoietin and thymulin are said to be produced only by thymic epithelium, whereas thymosins are a family of peptides that are synthesized in many organs. The production of thymic hormones by thymic epithelial cells has been an extremely interesting but highly contested subject. At the immunohistochemical level, studies using polyclonal and monoclonal antibodies claim to have demonstrated the presence of thymulin, thymosin α1, and thymopoietin in the cytoplasm of murine and human thymic epithelial cells (125–128). In some studies, the hormone localization has been found to be restricted to A2B5$^+$ cells, that is, subcapsular cortical and medullary epithelial cells (129). This finding has led to the suggestion that these two cell subtypes represent the functional (secretory or endocrine) portion of the thymus, as contrasted with the nonsecretory epithelium of the inner cortical region and of Hassall's corpuscles. In a murine system, thymic hormones also have been described in a subtype of medullary epithelial cell characterized ultrastructurally by numerous cytoplasmic membrane–bound vacuoles containing amorphous material (130). A study by Hirokawa et al. (131), using rabbit antisera against synthetic thymosin α1 and bovine thymosin β3 in 45 cases of human thymomas and normal thymus of newborns, described reactivity of the tumor cells and normal thymic epithelial cells with these antibodies in 80 and 89% of cases, respectively. The thymosin-containing cells were said to be predominantly localized to the medulla and the subcapsular cortex, and the reaction was most intense in the lymphocyte-rich thymomas. These reactions appeared to be specific for thymic tumors because neither thymosin α1 nor thymosin β3 could be detected in other epithelial malignancies tested, including gastric, pulmonary, and hepatic carcinomas. So far, however, sufficiently reliable specific antibodies have not become available for routine use in diagnostic pathology.

In addition to thymic hormones, thymic epithelial cells may contain a wide variety of neuropeptides such as oxytocin, vasopressin, β-endorphin, somatostatin, and other anterior pituitary hormones (132–134), as well as produce various cytokines and growth factors, including interleukin (IL)-1, IL-6, and granulocyte-monocyte colony-stimulating factor (135,136).

The spectrum of biological effects of cytokines in the thymus is determined by the expression of cytokine receptors on the thymic cell surface. Thymic cytokines may act by autocrine or paracrine mechanisms. Examples of paracrine thymic cytokines are IL-7, which induces thymocyte growth and differentiation, and interferon (INF)-γ (produced by thymocytes), which induces thymic epithelial cell activation. An example of an autocrine factor is IL-2, for which the producers and targets are thymocytes. The ability of thymocytes to produce cytokines and express cytokine receptors is gradually reduced as they mature from the stage of precursor cells to cortical thymocytes. After the completion of the selection process of maturation, the ability of thymocytes to produce cytokines and respond to their action is restored (137). The role and function of cytokines in the thymus is different from that of cytokines in the peripheral compartments of the immune system; in the thymus they are involved with the migration and development of thymocytes and autoregulation of thymocytes cell numbers, while in the periphery they are mainly involved in the regulation of inducible processes such as inflammation, immune response, etc.

AGE-RELATED AND OTHER TROPHIC CHANGES

Thymic Involution

The thymus undergoes a slow physiologic process of involution with age. This process starts at puberty, at which time the organ reaches its maximum absolute weight. From then on, it undergoes gradual and progressive atrophic changes (138–140). This process of aging, also known as physiologic involution, is accompanied by gradual changes in thymocyte populations relative to different rates of involution of the cortical and medullary epithelium. In its early stages, the changes consist primarily of a decrease in the number of cortical thymocytes with relative sparing of the epithelial elements (141). In the more advanced stages, the parenchyma of the thymus reverts to a more primitive appearance and is replaced by islands of epithelial cells depleted of lymphocytes, with partly cystic, closely aggregated Hassall's corpuscles and abundant intervening adipose tissue (142). It should be realized that, whereas thymic involution can proceed to a point where no thymic tissue can be appreciated grossly, microscopic thymic remnants are probably always present. The best way to locate them is to examine microscopically the preepicardial fat in a subserial fashion. Recent studies have suggested that the process of involution in the thymus may be quantitative rather than qualitative. It has been demonstrated that thymopoiesis continues to occur in the thymus of adult humans late into life and that thymic activity and function appear to be well maintained into old age and may be indispensable for T-cell reconstitution in different immunological settings (143–145).

A type of change not related to senescence that must be distinguished from the normal physiologic type of involution is accidental or stress involution. This condition results from the dramatic response of the thymus gland to episodes of severe stress, in which the sudden release of corticosteroids from the adrenal cortex leads to rapid depletion of thymic cortical lymphocytes (146). Microscopically, there is prominent karyorrhexis of lymphocytes with active phagocytosis by macrophages, which creates a prominent starry sky appearance characteristically confined to the cortex. If the stimulus persists, a loss of corticomedullary distinction ensues, with accentuation of the epithelial elements, cystic dilatation of Hassall's corpuscles, and the emergence of elongated, epithelium-lined cystic spaces that recapitulate the early stages of Hassall's corpuscle formation. With further loss of thymocytes, the lobular architecture collapses and fibrosis ensues. The thymus is thus transformed into a mass of adipose tissue containing scattered islands of parenchyma with a few lymphocytes.

Acute thymic involution in infancy and childhood has been observed to significantly correlate with the duration of acute illness. It has been proposed that morphologic parameters such as the presence of abundant macrophages in the cortex, increase of interlobular fibrous tissue, and lymphoid depletion of the cortex may enable the pathologist to estimate the duration of acute disease before death (147). A precocious type of thymic involution manifested by epithelial injury also has been observed in both children and adult patients with acquired immunodeficiency syndrome (AIDS) (148,149). These changes have been interpreted by some as an indication that the thymus may constitute a primary target organ in human immunodeficiency virus infection (150), whereas others have considered these changes as an expression of stress involution (149,151).

Thymic Hyperplasia

True thymic hyperplasia is defined as an enlargement of the thymus gland (as determined by weight or volume) beyond that considered as the upper limit of normal for that particular age group (152). The existence of true thymic hyperplasia has been questioned in the past, largely because of the diagnostic excesses committed with the much-abused concept of status thymicolymphaticus. The latter is probably a myth, but true thymic hyperplasia is currently accepted as a distinct entity (153–155).

To establish a diagnosis of true thymic hyperplasia, reference must be made to standard weight charts of normal thymus glands for comparison. Hammar, in 1906 (156), made the first extensive studies on the normal weights of the thymus in fresh autopsy specimens; these studies have remained for many years as the standard. More recently, several workers have updated these studies; the most comprehensive of these is that of Steinman (140), who examined the weight and volume of human thymuses in 136 healthy individuals (Table 19.3). He concluded that determination of the volume of the gland, as measured by the displacement of a physiologic saline solution, was more reliable than weighing the gland and constitutes the optimal parameter for this type of evaluation.

Thymic hyperplasia has been recognized as a complication of chemotherapy for Hodgkin's disease in children (157,158) and germ cell tumors in adults (159,160) and has been interpreted as the expression of an immunologic rebound phenomenon. A similar enlargement of the thymus also has been observed in children recovering from thermal burns (161) and after cessation of administration of corticosteroids in infants (162). Marked enlargement of the thymus has also been observed in the setting of thymic reconstitution after chemotherapy (163) or after the institution of antiretroviral therapy in HIV-infected patients (164).

True thymic hyperplasia must be distinguished from lymphoid hyperplasia. In the latter condition, the term *hyperplasia* refers to an increased number of lymphoid follicles in the medullary region of the gland. This is the result of increased migration of mature T and B cells into the perivascular space, adjacent to but outside of the thymic epithelial meshwork. The problem in establishing the presence of lymphoid hyperplasia vis-à-vis the occurrence of lymphoid follicles in the normal thymus has already been discussed. Lymphoid hyperplasia of the thymus most commonly has been associated with myasthenia gravis but also has been observed in several other immune-mediated disorders, including systemic lupus erythematosus, rheumatoid arthritis, scleroderma, allergic vasculitis, and thyrotoxicosis.

ARTIFACTS AND OTHER POTENTIAL PITFALLS IN DIFFERENTIAL DIAGNOSIS

Microscopic changes related to involution may be a source of considerable confusion in the interpretation of thymic biopsies. Such changes are primarily related to the distribution, architectural arrangement, and cytologic appearance of the epithelial cells (Figure 19.13). Some of these cells may acquire a spindle, mesenchyma-like appearance, whereas others can arrange themselves in rosettelike formations devoid of central lumina (Figure 19.14). The fact that both of these appearances also are found with some frequency in thymic dysplasia and thymoma (but not in the normal active gland of infancy) suggests that they represent regressive and functionally inactive states of the epithelial cells (9).

Sometimes thymic remnants are almost exclusively formed of epithelial elements, arranged in well-defined round nests that may simulate neuroendocrine growths (165) (Figure 19.15). A particularly distinctive appearance is that of thin, elongated strands of thymic epithelium composed of a single or double cell layer, surrounded by or circumscribing dense connective tissue in a fibroepitheliomatous fashion. These thin, elongated epithelial strands may often be flanked by small lymphocytes and may occasionally exhibit an antlerlike, branching configuration (Figure 19.16A). They may be seen by themselves or at the periphery of thymic cysts, thymomas, thymic lymphomas, and other thymic neoplasms. In the case of thymic lymphomas and seminomas, these strands can be present not only around but also within the tumor, surrounded and infiltrated by the neoplastic elements. Their presence, whether detected at the hematoxylin and eosin (H&E) level or with the more sensitive techniques of ultrastructure and immunohistochemistry, can be interpreted erroneously as evidence supporting an epithelial nature for the lesion (Figure 19.16B). As a matter of fact, in our experience these formations constitute the single most important cause of misdiagnosis in cases of large cell lymphoma of the thymus. Conversely, some thymic remnants (perhaps the majority) are made up almost exclusively of lymphocytes,

TABLE 19.3
WEIGHT AND VOLUME OF NORMAL HUMAN THYMUSES

n	Age (years)	Weight (g)[a]	Volume (cm³)[a]
6	0–1	27.3 ± 16.4	26.8 ± 16.1
4	1–4	28.0 ± 19.3	27.9 ± 10.4
7	5–9	22.1 ± 9.2	21.5 ± 8.8
5	10–14	21.5 ± 6.1	21.1 ± 6.4
9	15–19	20.2 ± 10.3	19.3 ± 10.1
18	20–24	21.6 ± 9.5	23.0 ± 10.6
9	25–29	23.1 ± 11.8	23.7 ± 11.9
5	30–34	25.5 ± 9.9	27.6 ± 11.2
17	35–44	21.9 ± 9.2	22.2 ± 10.5
14	45–54	24.8 ± 12.8	26.5 ± 12.4
15	55–64	21.3 ± 9.5	23.5 ± 10.4
17	65–84	23.8 ± 16.1	25.6 ± 17.0
5	85–90	18.2 ± 5.4	20.4 ± 6.8
5	91–107	12.4 ± 6.9	13.4 ± 7.2
136	Total	22.8 ± 12.5	23.4 ± 11.9

[a] Values are means ± SD.
Reprinted from: Le PT, Lazorick S, Whichard LP, et al. Human thymic epithelial cells produce IL-6, granulocyte-monocyte-CSF, and leukemia inhibitory factor. *J. Immunol* 1990; 145: 3310–3315.

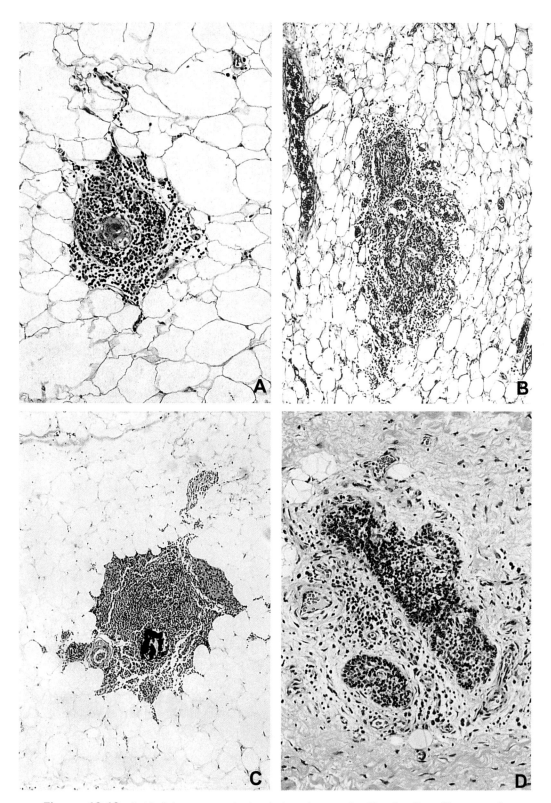

Figure 19.13 Epithelial remnants in involuting thymus. **A.** Abortive Hassall's corpuscle surrounded by small lymphocytes and scattered epithelial cells. **B.** Anastomosing strands of epithelial cells surrounded by small lymphocytes embedded within the preepicardial fat. **C.** Residual thymic island with predominance of lymphocytes, small solid epithelial cell clusters at the periphery, and calcified Hassall's corpuscle. **D.** Anastomosing strands of epithelial cells admixed with small lymphocytes embedded within a collagenized stroma.

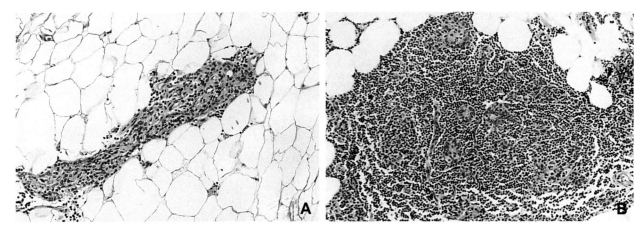

Figure 19.14 **A.** Thymic remnant showing elongated configuration with prominent spindling of the cells. **B.** Involuting thymus with epithelial rosettes.

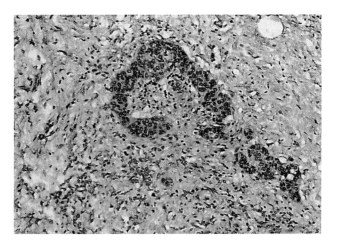

Figure 19.15 Strands of residual thymic epithelium arranged in small nests resembling neuroendocrine growths.

lating lymph nodes. A clue to their real nature should be sought at the very periphery, in which epithelial cells can sometimes be identified encircling the nests, perhaps representing the residual coat of subcapsular cortical cells of the normal organ (Figure 19.17).

Certain patterns of tissue response to injury in the thymus may also constitute a major source of confusion in the interpretation of biopsies of this organ (166). A common form of response of this organ to injury, particularly in cases associated with inflammation, is cystic degeneration of thymic epithelium. The cystic degeneration in such cases is thought to be the result of an acquired process, which in its fullest expression will lead to the formation of a multilocular thymic cyst (167). The main histologic features of such cysts include the formation of large cavities lined by squamous, columnar, or cuboidal epithelium, often in continuity with remnants of normal thymic epithelium within

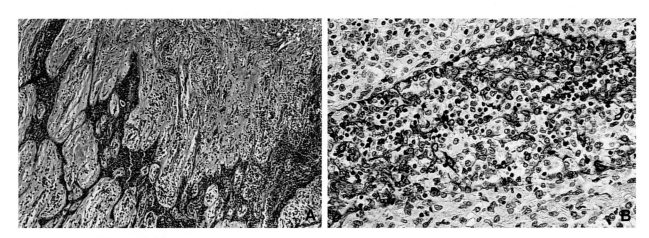

Figure 19.16 **A.** Wall of thymic cyst showing branching strands of thymic epithelial cells surrounded by a fibrous stroma. **B.** Entrapped thymic epithelial elements within anterior mediastinal malignant lymphoma. The strong keratin positivity seen in these cells may lead to an erroneous diagnosis of thymic carcinoma.

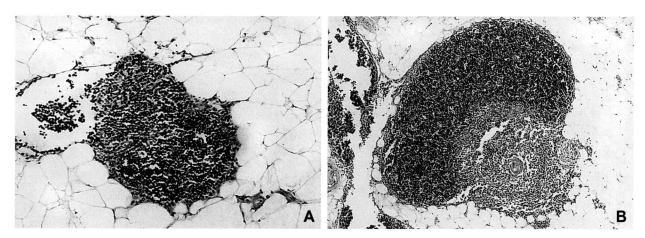

Figure 19.17 **A.** Thymic remnant composed predominantly of small lymphocytes simulating a lymphoid nodule. Note the single row of flattened epithelial cells at the periphery. **B.** Thymic remnant composed of cortical and medullary portion, the latter containing a small Hassall's corpuscle (*bottom half*).

the cyst walls; severe acute and chronic inflammation accompanied by fibrovascular proliferation, necrosis, hemorrhage, and cholesterol granuloma formation; and reactive lymphoid hyperplasia with the formation of prominent germinal centers. In some instances, the cyst lining may show a moderate degree of cytologic atypia with features of pseudoepitheliomatous hyperplasia that can be easily misinterpreted for malignancy (168). In the majority of cases the cystic structures are closely associated with Hassall's corpuscles, many of which show marked dilatation and may be found to be in continuity with the lining of the cystic cavities (Figure 19.18). We believe that this type of reaction is the result of an exaggerated response of medullary duct epithelium–derived structures of the thymus to an underlying inflammatory process (167). However, it is important to point out that seemingly identical changes may take place in uninvolved thymic parenchyma in cases of

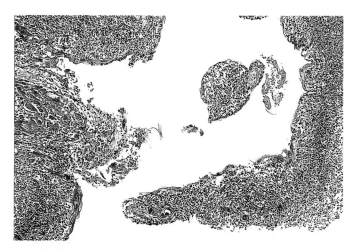

Figure 19.18 Cystic dilatation of Hassall's corpuscle. Notice dense inflammatory infiltrate within the wall of the cyst.

Hodgkin's disease, mediastinal seminoma, and (less commonly) thymoma, to the extent that the neoplastic elements may be overshadowed by the cystic/inflammatory process (169,170). Other primary thymic neoplasms, which also may be closely associated with prominent cystic changes, although to a lesser extent, include basaloid carcinoma and mucoepidermoid carcinoma (171,172). Careful search and extensive sampling must therefore be undertaken in cystic mediastinal lesions for proper identification of the diagnostic neoplastic areas.

Another form of tissue response to injury of the thymus that may introduce difficulties for diagnosis is that of stromal fibrosis. Fibrous overgrowth of the stroma may be the result of various mechanisms in a variety of nonneoplastic conditions [including a specific stimulus such as ionizing radiation or fungal infection (173,174)] or of undetermined etiology [such as in idiopathic sclerosing mediastinitis (175,176). In addition, a variety of malignant conditions of this organ also may be accompanied by prominent fibrous changes of the stroma, including primary diffuse large cell lymphoma of the mediastinum, Hodgkin's disease, and thymic seminoma (166). In many such instances, the gland may show extensive sclerosis with entrapment of a few scattered foci harboring the diagnostic atypical cells. Such cases may prove literally impossible to diagnose in small mediastinoscopic biopsies and will require extensive sampling of the mass to identify the diagnostic areas. The surgeon must be informed of the need for obtaining additional tissue for diagnosis at the time of frozen section examination.

Another potential pitfall for diagnosis is given by the high cellularity, immaturity, and mitotic activity of the normal thymic cortex, which can pose great diagnostic difficulties in mediastinoscopic biopsies and result in a mistaken diagnosis of malignant lymphoma, particularly of the

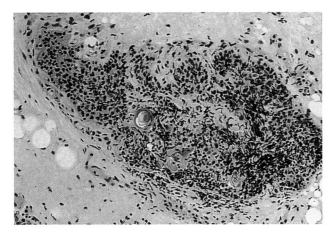

Figure 19.19 Extensive crush artifact is seen in this thymic remnant obtained through mediastinoscopic biopsy.

lymphoblastic type. The paucity or absence of cells with convoluted nuclei and the identification (morphologically or immunohistochemically) of epithelial cells regularly scattered throughout the lymphoid population should point toward the correct interpretation. Finally, an additional source of difficulty for diagnosis lies in the presence of biopsy-induced artifacts, one of the most common being the crush artifact, leading to marked nuclear elongation reminiscent of that seen in small cell carcinoma (Figure 19.19).

REFERENCES

1. Norris EH. The morphogenesis and histogenesis of the thymus gland in man: in which the origin of the Hassall's corpuscles of the human thymus is discovered. *Contrib Embryol Carnegie Inst* 1938;27:193–207.
2. Weller GL Jr. Development of the thyroid, parathyroid and thymus glands in man. *Contrib Embryol Carnegie Inst* 1933;24:93–139.
3. Cordier AC, Haumont SM. Development of thymus, parathyroids and ultimo-branchial bodies in NMRI and nude mice. *Am J Anat* 1980;157:227–263.
4. Gilmour JR. The embryology of parathyroid glands: the thymus and certain associated rudiments. *J Pathol Bacteriol* 1937;45:507–522.
5. Jotereau FV, Houssaint E, Le Douarin NM. Lymphoid stem cell homing to the early thymic primordium of the avian embryo. *Eur J Immunol* 1980;10:620–627.
6. Shier KJ. The thymus according to Schambacher: medullary ducts and reticular epithelium of the thymus and thymomas. *Cancer* 1981;48:1183–1199.
7. Gilmour JR. Some developmental abnormalities of the thymus and parathyroids. *J Pathol Bacteriol* 1941;52:213–218.
8. Nathaniels EK, Nathaniels AM, Wang CA. Mediastinal parathyroid tumors: a clinical and pathological study of 84 cases. *Ann Surg* 1970;171:165–170.
9. Rosai J, Levine GD. Tumors of the thymus. In: *Atlas of Tumor Pathology*. 2nd series, fascicle 13. Washington, DC: Armed Forces Institute of Pathology; 1976.
10. Domaniewski J, Ukleja Z, Rejmanowski T. Problemy immunologiczne I kliniczne w grasiczakach ektopicznych. *Otolaringol Pol* 1975;29:579–585.
11. Martin JME, Rundhawa G, Temple WJ. Cervical thymoma. *Arch Pathol Lab Med* 1986;110:345–357.
12. Yamashita H, Murakami N, Noguchi S, et al. Cervical thymoma and incidence of cervical thymus. *Acta Pathol Jpn* 1983;33:189–194.
13. Wadon A. Thymoma intratracheale. *Zentralbl Allg Pathol Anat* 1934;60:308–312.
14. Harach RR, Day ES, Fransilla KG. Thyroid spindle-cell tumor with mucous cysts. An intrathyroid thymoma? *Am J Surg Pathol* 1985;9:525–530.
15. Miyauchi A, Kuma K, Matsuzuka F, Matsubayashi A, Tamai H, Katayama S. Intrathyroid epithelial thymoma: an entity distinct from squamous cell carcinoma of the thyroid. *World J Surg* 1985; 9:128–135.
16. Rosai J, Limas C, Husband EM. Ectopic hamartomatous thymoma: a distinctive benign lesion of the lower neck. *Am J Surg Pathol* 1984;8:501–513.
17. Gagens EW. Malformation of the auditory apparatus in the newborn associated with ectopic thymus. *Arch Otolaryngol* 1932;15:671–680.
18. Castleman B. Tumors of the thymus gland. In: *Atlas of Tumor Pathology*. 1st series, fascicle 19. Washington, DC: Armed Forces Institute of Pathology; 1955.
19. Wolff M, Rosai J, Wright DH. Sebaceous glands within the thymus. Report of 3 cases. *Hum Pathol* 1984;15:341–343.
20. Breckler IA, Johnston DG. Choristoma of the thymus. *AMA J Dis Child* 1956;92:175–178.
21. Landing B, Yutuc I, Swanson V. Clinicopathologic correlation in immunologic deficiency diseases of children, with emphasis on thymic histologic patterns. In: *Proceedings of the International Symposium on Immunodeficiency*. Tokyo: Tokyo University Press; 1976: 3–33.
22. Blackburn WR, Gordon DS. The thymic remnant in thymic alymphoplasia. Light and electron microscopic studies. *Arch Pathol* 1967;84:363–375.
23. Hoyer JR, Cooper MD, Gabrielsen AE, Good RA. Lymphopenic forms of congenital immunologic deficiency diseases. *Medicine (Baltimore)* 1968;47:201–226.
24. Peterson RD, Kelly WD, Good RA. Ataxia-telangiectasia. Its association with a defective thymus, immunological-deficiency disease, and malignancy. *Lancet* 1964;1:1189–1193.
25. Cooper MD, Petersen RD, Good RA. A new concept of the cellular basis of immunity. *J Pediatr* 1965;67:907–908.
26. Nezelof C, Jammet M-L, Lortholary P, Labrune B, Lamy M. L'hypoplasie hereditaire du thymus: sa place et sa responsabilite dans une observation d'aplasie lymphocytaire, normoplasmocytaire et normoglobulinemique du nourrisson. *Arch Fr Pediatr* 1964;21:897–920.
27. Seemayer TA, Bolande RP. Thymus involution mimicking thymic dysplasia: a consequence of transfusion-induced graft versus host disease in a premature infant. *Arch Pathol Lab Med* 1980;104:141–144.
28. Huber J, Cholnoky P, Zoethout HE. Congenital aplasia of parathyroid glands and thymus. *Arch Dis Child* 1967;42:190–192.
29. Fowlkes BJ, Pardoll DM. Molecular and cellular events of T cell development. *Adv Immunol* 1989;44:207–264.
30. MacDonald HR, Lees RK. Programmed death of autoreactive thymocytes. *Nature* 1990;343:642–644.
31. Kizaki H, Tadakuma T. Thymocyte apoptosis. *Microbiol Immunol* 1993;37:917–925.
32. Colbert RA, Young DA. Glucocorticoid-induced messenger ribonucleic acids in rat thymic lymphocytes: rapid primary effects specific for glucocorticoids. *Endocrinology* 1986;119:2598–2605.
33. Domashenko AD, Nazarova LF, Umansky SR. Comparison of the spectra of proteins synthesized in mouse thymocytes after irradiation or hydrocortisone treatment. *Int J Radiat Biol* 1990;57:315–329.
34. Korsmeyer SJ. Bcl-2: a repressor of lymphocyte death. *Immunol Today* 1992;13:285–288.
35. Lowe SW, Schmitt EM, Smith SW, Osborne BA, Jacks T. p53 is required for radiation-induced apoptosis in mouse thymocytes. *Nature* 1993;362:847–849.
36. Smith CA, Williams GT, Kinsgton R, Jenkins EJ, Owen JJ. Antibodies to CD3/T-cell receptor complex induce death by apoptosis in immature T cells in thymic cultures. *Nature* 1989;337:181–184.

37. von Boehmer H. Positive selection of lymphocytes. *Cell* 1994;76:219–228.
38. Shi Y, Bissonnette RP, Parfrey N, Szalay M, Kubo RT, Green DR. In vivo administration of monoclonal antibodies to the CD3 T cell receptor complex induces cell death (apoptosis) in immature thymocytes. *J Immunol* 1991;146:3340–3346.
39. Blackman M, Kappler J, Marrack P. The role of the T cell receptor in positive and negative selection of developing T cells. *Science* 1990;248:1335–1341.
40. Mountz JD, Zhou T, Wu J, Wang W, Su X, Cheng J. Regulation of apoptosis in immune cells. *J Clin Immunol* 1995;15:1–16.
41. Hammar JA. Die Menschenthymus in Gesundheit und krankheit. *Z Mikrosk Anat Forsch* 1926;6(suppl):107–208.
42. Flores KG, Li J, Sempowski GD, Haynes BF, Hale LP. Analysis of the human thymic perivascular space during aging. *J Clin Invest* 1999;104:1031–1039.
43. Hale LP. Histologic and molecular assessment of human thymus. *Ann Diagn Pathol* 2004;8:50–60.
44. Suster S, Moran CA. Thymoma, atypical thymoma, and thymic carcinoma. A novel conceptual approach to the classification of thymic epithelial neoplasms. *Am J Clin Pathol* 1999;111:826–833.
45. Lobach DF, Haynes BF. Ontogeny of the human thymus during fetal development. *J Clin Immunol* 1987;7:81–97.
46. Dipasquale B, Tridente G. Immunohistochemical characterization of nurse cells in normal human thymus. *Histochemistry* 1991;96:499–503.
47. von Gaudecker B. Functional histology of the human thymus. *Anat Embryol (Berl)* 1991;183:1–15.
48. Rippert H. Die Entwicklungsstörung der Thymusdrüse bei kongenitaler Lues. *Frankfurt Z Pathol* 1912;11:209–218.
49. Suster S, Rosai J. Multilocular thymic cyst: an acquired reactive process. Study of 18 cases. *Am J Surg Pathol* 1991;15:388–398.
50. Henry K. Mucin secretion and striated muscle in the human thymus. *Lancet* 1966;1:183–185.
51. Cantor H, Weissman I. Development and function of subpopulations of thymocytes and T lymphocytes. *Prog Allergy* 1976;20:1–64.
52. Everett NB, Tyler RW. Lymphopoiesis in the thymus and other tissues: functional implications. *Int Rev Cytol* 1967;22:205–237.
53. Middleton G. The incidence of follicular structures in the human thymus at autopsy. *Aust J Exp Biol Med Sci* 1967;45:189–199.
54. Vetters JM, Barclay RS. The incidence of germinal centres in thymus glands of patients with congenital heart disease. *J Clin Pathol* 1973;26:583–591.
55. Levine GD, Rosai J. Light and electron microscopy of the human fetal thymus. In: Johannessen JV, ed. *Electron Microscopy in Human Medicine.* Vol 5. New York: McGraw-Hill; 1980.
56. Goldstein G, Mackay IR. The thymus in systemic lupus erythematosus: a quantitative histopathological analysis and comparison with stress involution. *Br Med J* 1967;2:475–478.
57. Palestro G, Tridente G, Botto Micca F, Novero D, Valente G, Godia L. Immunohistochemical and enzyme histochemical contributions to the problem concerning the role of the thymus in the pathogenesis of myasthenia gravis. *Virchows Arch B Cell Pathol Incl Mol Pathol* 1983;44:173–186.
58. Shirai T, Miyata M, Nakase A, Itoh T. Lymphocyte subpopulation in neoplastic and non-neoplastic thymus and in blood of patients with myasthenia gravis. *Clin Exp Immunol* 1976;26:118–123.
59. Isaacson PG, Norton AJ, Addis BJ. The human thymus contains a novel population of B lymphocytes. *Lancet* 1987;2:1488–1491.
60. Isaacson PG, Chan JK, Tang C, Addis BJ. Low-grade B-cell lymphoma of mucosa-associated lymphoid tissue arising in the thymus: a thymic lymphoma mimicking myoepithelial sialadenitis. *Am J Surg Pathol* 1990;14:342–351.
61. Cardoso De Almeida P, Harris NH, Bhan AK. Characterization of immature sinus histiocytes (monocytoid cells) in reactive lymph nodes by use of monoclonal antibodies. *Hum Pathol* 1984;15:330–335.
62. Duijvestijn AM, Schutte R, Kohler YG, Korn C, Hoefsmit EC. Characterization of the population of phagocytic cells in thymic cell suspensions. A morphological and cytochemical study. *Cell Tissue Res* 1983;231:313–323.
63. Kaiserling E, Stein H, Muller-Hermelink HK. Interdigitating reticulum cells in the human thymus. *Cell Tissue Res* 1974;155:47–55.
64. Ruco LP, Rosati S, Monardo F, Pescarmona E, Rendina EA, Baroni CD. Macrophages and interdigitating reticulum cells in normal thymus and in thymoma: an immunohistochemical study. *Histopathology* 1989;14:37–45.
65. Lauriola L, Michetti F, Stolfi VM, Tallini G, Cocchia D. Detection by S-100 immunolabelling of interdigitating reticulum cells in human thymomas. *Virchows Arch B Cell Pathol Incl Mol Pathol* 1984;45:187–195.
66. Bofill M, Janossy G, Willcox N, Chilosi M, Trejdosiewicz LK, Newsom-Davis J. Microenvironments in the normal thymus and the thymus in myasthenia gravis. *Am J Pathol* 1985;119:462–473.
67. Siegal GP, Dehner LP, Rosai J. Histiocytosis X (Langerhans' cell granulomatosis) of the thymus: a clinicopathologic study of four childhood cases. *Am J Surg Pathol* 1985;9:117–124.
68. Bhathal PS, Campbell PE. Eosinophil leucocytes in the child's thymus. *Australas Ann Med* 1965;14:210–213.
69. Wise WS, Still WJ, Joshi VV. Severe combined immunodeficiency with thymic mast cell hyperplasia. *Arch Pathol Lab Med* 1976;100:283–286.
70. Goldstein G. Plasma cells in the human thymus. *Aust J Exp Biol Med Sci* 1966;44:695–699.
71. Henry K. The human thymus in disease with particular emphasis on thymitis and thymoma. In: Kendall MD, ed. *The Thymus Gland.* London: Academic Press; 1981:85–111.
72. Moll UM, Lane BL, Robert F, Greenen V, Legros JJ. The neuroendocrine thymus. Abundant occurrence of oxytocin-, vasopressin-, and neurophysin-like peptides in epithelial cells. *Histochemistry* 1988;89:385–390.
73. Ciaccio C. Contributo all'istochimica delle cellule cromaffini. II. Cellule cromaffini del timo di gallum domesticus. *Bull Soc Ital Biol Sper* 1942;17:619–620.
74. Hakanson R, Larsson LI, Sundler F. Peptide and amine producing endocrine-like cells in the chicken thymus. A chemical, histochemical and electron microscopic study. *Histochemistry* 1974;39:25–34.
75. Vialli M, Casati C. Sulla presenza di cellule enterocromaffini nel timo dei rettili. *Riv Istochim Norm Patol* 1958;4:343.
76. Vialli M. Elementi del sistema delle cellule enterocromaffinie cellule C nel timo. *Ann Histochem* 1973;18:3–7.
77. Rosai J, Higa E. Mediastinal endocrine neoplasm, of probable thymic origin, related to carcinoid tumor: clinicopathologic study of 8 cases. *Cancer* 1972;29:1061–1074.
78. Wick MR, Rosai J. Neuroendocrine neoplasms of the thymus. *Pathol Res Pract* 1988;183:188–199.
79. Drenckhahn D, von Gaudecker B, Muller-Hermelink HK, Unsicker K, Groschel-Stewart U. Myosin and actin containing cells in the human postnatal thymus: ultrastructural and immunohistochemical findings in normal thymus and in myasthenia gravis. *Virchows Arch B Cell Pathol Incl Mol Pathol* 1979;32:33–45.
80. Hayward AR. Myoid cells in the human fetal thymus. *J Pathol* 1972;106:45–48.
81. Nakamura H, Ayer-Le Lievre C. Neural crest and thymic myoid cells. *Curr Top Dev Biol* 1986;20:111–115.
82. Dardenne M, Savino W, Bach JF. Thymomatous epithelial cells and skeletal muscle share a common epitope defined by a monoclonal antibody. *Am J Pathol* 1987;126:194–198.
83. Van de Velde RL, Friedman NB. Thymic myoid cells and myasthenia gravis. *Am J Pathol* 1970;59:347–368.
84. Judd RL, Welch SL. Myoid cell differentiation in true thymic hyperplasia and lymphoid hyperplasia. *Arch Pathol Lab Med* 1988;112:1140–1144.
85. Murakami S, Shamoto M, Miura K, Takeuchi J. A thymic tumor with massive proliferation of myoid cells. *Acta Pathol Jpn* 1984;34:1375–1383.
86. Rosai J, Parkash V, Reuter VE. On the origin of mediastinal germ cell tumors in men. *Int J Surg Pathol* 1995;2:73–78.
87. Marshall AHE, White RG. The immunological reactivity of the thymus. *Br J Exp Pathol* 1961;42:379–385.
88. Raviola E, Karnovsky MJ. Evidence for a blood–thymus barrier using electron-opaque tracers. *J Exp Med* 1972;136:466–498.

89. Stet RJ, Wagenaar-Hilbers JP, Nieuwenhuis P. Thymus localization of monoclonal antibodies circumventing the blood-thymus barrier. *Scand J Immunol* 1987;25:441–446.

90. Bearman RM, Levine GD, Bensch KG. The ultrastructure of the normal human thymus. A study of 36 cases. *Anat Rec* 1978;190:755–781.

91. Hirokawa K. Electron microscopic observation of the human thymus of the fetus and the newborn. *Acta Pathol Jpn* 1969;19:1–13.

92. Pinkel D. Ultrastructure of the human fetal thymus. *Am J Dis Child* 1968;115:222–238.

93. van de Wijngaert FP, Kendall MD, Schuurman HJ, Rademakers LH, Kater L. Heterogeneity of epithelial cells in human thymus. An ultrastructural study. *Cell Tissue Res* 1984;237:227–237.

94. Henry K. The human thymus in disease with particular emphasis on thymitis and thymoma. In: Kendall MD, ed. *The Thymus Gland.* London: Academic Press; 1981:85–111.

95. de Maagd RA, MacKenzie WA, Schuurman HJ, et al. The human thymus microenvironment: heterogeneity detected by monoclonal anti-epithelial cell antibodies. *Immunology* 1985;54:745–754.

96. Haynes BF. The human thymic microenvironment. *Adv Immunol* 1984;36:87–142.

97. Janossy G, Thomas JA, Bollum FJ, et al. The human thymic microenvironment. An immunohistologic study. *J Immunol* 1980;125:202–212.

98. Van Ewijk W. Immunohistology of lymphoid and non-lymphoid cells in the thymus in relation to T lymphocyte differentiation. *Am J Anat* 1984;170:330–331.

99. McFarland EJ, Scearce RM, Haynes BF. The human thymic microenvironment: cortical thymic epithelium is an antigenically distinct region of the thymic microenvironment. *J Immunol* 1984;133:1241–1249.

100. Eisenbarth GS, Shimizu K, Bowring MA, Wells S. Expression of receptors for tetanus toxin and monoclonal antibody A2B5 by pancreatic islet cells. *Proc Natl Acad Sci U S A* 1982;79:5066–5070.

101. Haynes BF, Robert-Guroff M, Metzgar RS, et al. Monoclonal antibodies against human T cell leukemia virus p19 defines a human thymic epithelial antigen acquired during ontogeny. *J Exp Med* 1983;157:907–920.

102. Savino W, Berrih S, Dardenne M. Thymic epithelial antigen, acquired during ontogeny and defined by the anti-p19 monoclonal antibody, is lost in thymomas. *Lab Invest* 1984;51:292–296.

103. Bhan AK, Reinherz EL, Poppema S, McCluskey RT, Schlossman JF. Location of T cell and major histocompatibility complex antigens in the human thymus. *J Exp Med* 1980;152:771–782.

104. Bofill M, Janossy G, Willcox N, Chilosi M, Trejdosiewicz LK, Newsom-Davis J. Microenvironments in the normal thymus and the thymus in myasthenia gravis. *Am J Pathol* 1985;119:462–473.

105. Wiley EL, Nosal JM, Freeman RG. Immunohistochemical demonstration of H antigen, peanut agglutinin receptor, and Saphora japonica receptor expression in infant thymuses and thymic neoplasias. *Am J Clin Pathol* 1990;93:44–48.

106. Le PT, Lazorick S, Whichard LP, Haynes BF, Singer KH. Regulation of cytokine production in the human thymus: epidermal growth factor and transforming growth factor alpha regulate mRNA levels of interleukin 1 alpha (IL-1 alpha), IL-1 beta, and IL-6 in human thymic epithelial cells at a post-transcriptional level. *J Exp Med* 1991;174:1147–1157.

107. Chan WC, Zaatari GS, Tabei S, Bibb M, Byrnes RK. Thymoma: an immunohistochemical study. *Am J Clin Pathol* 1984;82:160–166.

108. Lobach DF, Scearce RM, Haynes BF. The human thymic microenvironment. Phenotypic characterization of Hassall's bodies with the use of monoclonal antibodies. *J Immunol* 1985;134:250–257.

109. Hsu SM, Jaffe ES. Phenotypic expression of T lymphocytes in thymus and peripheral lymphoid tissues. *Am J Pathol* 1985;121:69–78.

110. Janossy G, Bofill M, Trejdosiewicz LK, Willcox HN, Chilosi M. Cellular differentiation of lymphoid subpopulations and their microenvironments in the human thymus. In: Muller-Hermelink HK, ed. *The Human Thymus: Histophysiology and Pathology.* Berlin: Springer-Verlag; 1986:89–125.

111. Tidman N, Janossy C, Bodger M, Granger S, Kung PC, Goldstein G. Delineation of human thymocyte differentiation pathways utilizing double-staining techniques with monoclonal antibodies. *Clin Exp Immunol* 1981;45:457–467.

112. Chilosi M, Iannucci AM, Pizzolo G, Menestrina F, Fiore-Donati L, Janossy G. Immunohistochemical analysis of thymoma. Evidence of medullary origin of epithelial cells. *Am J Surg Pathol* 1984;8:309–318.

113. Mokhtar N, Hsu SM, Lad RP, Haynes BF, Jaffe ES. Thymoma: lymphoid and epithelial components mirror the phenotype of normal thymus. *Hum Pathol* 1984;15:378–384.

114. Sato Y, Watanabe S, Mukai K, et al. An immunohistochemical study of thymic epithelial tumors. II. Lymphoid component. *Am J Surg Pathol* 1986;10:862–870.

115. Lauriola L, Maggiano N, Marino M, Carbone A, Piantelli M, Musiani P. Human thymoma: immunologic characteristics of the lymphocytic component. *Cancer* 1981;48:1992–1995.

116. van der Kwast TH, van Vliet E, Cristen E, van Ewijk W, van der Heul RO. An immunohistologic study of the epithelial and lymphoid components of six thymomas. *Hum Pathol* 1985;16:1001–1008.

117. Eimoto T, Teshima K, Shirakusa T, et al. Heterogeneity of epithelial cells and reactive components in thymomas: an ultrastructural and immunohistochemical study. *Ultrastruct Pathol* 1986;10:157–173.

118. Shirai T, Miyata M, Nakase A, Itoh T. Lymphocyte subpopulation in neoplastic and non-neoplastic thymus and in blood of patients with myasthenia gravis. *Clin Exp Immunol* 1976;26:118–123.

119. Katzin WE, Fishleder AJ, Linden MD, Tubbs RR. Immunoglobulin and T-cell receptor genes in thymomas: genotypic evidence supporting the nonneoplastic nature of the lymphocytic component. *Hum Pathol* 1988;19:323–328.

120. Swerdlow SH, Angermeier PA, Hartman AL. Intrathymic ontogeny of the T cell receptor associated CD3 (T3) antigen. *Lab Invest* 1988;58:421–427.

121. Nikolic-Zugic J. Phenotypic and functional stages in the intrathymic development of alpha beta T cells. *Immunol Today* 1991;12:65–70.

122. Bach JF, Dardenne M, Pleau JM, Rosa J. Biochemical characteristics of a serum thymic factor. *Nature* 1976;266:55–56.

123. McCarty N, Shinohara ML, Lu L, Cantor H. Detailed analysis of gene expression during development of T cell lineages in the thymus. *Proc Natl Acad Sci U S A* 2004;101:9339–9344.

124. Goldstein AL, Low TLK, McAdoo M, et al. Thymosin alpha 1. Isolation and sequential analysis of an immunologically active thymic polypeptide. *Proc Natl Acad Sci U S A* 1977;74:725–729.

125. Goldstein G. The isolation of thymopoietin (thymin). *Ann NY Acad Sci* 1975;249:177–185.

126. Fabien N, Auger C, Monier JC. Immunolocalization of thymosin alpha 1, thymopoietin and thymulin in mouse thymic epithelial cells at different stages of culture: a light and electron microscopic study. *Immunology* 1988;63:721–727.

127. Jambon B, Montague P, Bene MC, Brayer MP, Faure G, Duheille J. Immunohistologic localization of "facteur thymique serique" (FTS) in human thymic epithelium. *J Immunol* 1981;127:2055–2059.

128. Savino W, Dardenne M. Thymic hormone-containing cells. VI. Immunohistologic evidence for the simultaneous presence of thymulin, thymopoietin and thymosin alpha 1 in normal and pathological human thymuses. *Eur J Immunol* 1984;14:987–991.

129. Haynes BF, Warren RW, Buckley RH, et al. Demonstration of abnormalities in expression of thymic epithelial surface antigens in severe cellular immunodeficiency diseases. *J Immunol* 1983;130:1182–1188.

130. Clark SL Jr. The thymus in mice of strain 129/J, studied with the electron microscope. *Am J Anat* 1963;112:1–33.

131. Hirokawa K, Utsuyama M, Moriizumi E, Hashimoto T, Masaoka A, Goldstein AL. Immunohistochemical studies in human thymomas. Localization of thymosin and various cell markers. *Virchows Arch B Cell Pathol Incl Mol Pathol* 1988;55:371–380.

132. Geenen V, Robert F, Defresne MP, Boniver J, Legros JJ, Franchimont P. Neuroendocrinology of the thymus. *Horm Res* 1989;31:81–84.

133. Jevremovic M, Terzic M, Kartaljevic G, Popovic V, Rosic B, Filipovic S. The determination of immunoreactive beta-endorphin concentration in the human fetal and neonatal thymus. *Horm Metab Res* 1991;23:623–624.

134. Batanero E, de Leeuw FE, Jansen GH, van Wichen DF, Huber J, Schuurman HJ. The neural and neuroendocrine components of the human thymus. II. Hormone immunoreactivity. *Brain Behav Immun* 1992;6:249–264.

135. Le PT, Lazorick S, Whichard LP, et al. Human thymic epithelial cells produce IL-6, granulocyte-monocyte-CSF, and leukemia inhibitory factor. *J Immunol* 1990;145:3310–3315.

136. Wainberg MA, Numazaki K, Destephano L, Wong I, Goldman H. Infection of human thymic epithelial cells by human cytomegalovirus and other viruses: effect on secretion of interleukin 1–like activity. *Clin Exp Immunol* 1988;72:415–421.

137. Yarilin AA, Belyakov IM. Cytokines in the thymus: production and biological effects. *Curr Med Chem* 2004;11:447–464.

138. Hirokawa K. Age-related changes of thymus. Morphological and functional aspects. *Acta Pathol Jpn* 1978;28:843–857.

139. Simpson JG, Gray ES, Beck JS. Age involution in the normal adult thymus. *Clin Exp Immunol* 1975;19:261–265.

140. Steinman GG. Changes in the human thymus during aging. In: Muller-Hermelink HK, ed. *The Human Thymus. Histophysiology and Pathology.* Berlin: Springer-Verlag; 1986:43–88.

141. Steinmann GG, Klaus B, Muller-Hermelink HK. The involution of the aging human thymic epithelium is independent of puberty. A morphometric study. *Scand J Immunol* 1985;22:563–575.

142. Smith SM, Ossa-Gomez LJ. A quantitative histologic comparison of the thymus in 100 healthy and diseased adults. *Am J Clin Pathol* 1981;76:657–665.

143. Jamieson BD, Douek DC, Killian S, et al. Generation of functional thymocytes in the human adult. *Immunity* 1999;10:569–575.

144. Bertho JM, Demarquay C, Moulian N, Van Der Meeren A, Berrih-Aknin S, Gourmelon P. Phenotypic and immunohistological analyses of the human adult thymus: evidence for an active thymus during adult life. *Cell Immunol* 1997;179:30–40.

145. Shanker A. Is thymus redundant after adulthood? *Immunol Lett* 2004;15:79–86.

146. Selye H. Thymus and adrenals in the response of the organism to injuries and intoxications. *Br J Exp Pathol* 1936;17:234–248.

147. van Baarlen J, Schuurman HJ, Huber J. Acute thymus involution in infancy and childhood: a reliable marker for duration of acute illness. *Hum Pathol* 1988;19:1155–1160.

148. Joshi VV, Oleske JM, Saad S, et al. Thymus biopsy in children with acquired immunodeficiency syndrome. *Arch Pathol Lab Med* 1986;110:837–842.

149. Seemayer TA, Laroche AC, Russo P, et al. Precocious thymic involution manifest by epithelial injury in the acquired immune deficiency syndrome. *Hum Pathol* 1984;15:469–474.

150. Grody WW, Fligiel S, Naeim F. Thymus involution in the acquired immunodeficiency syndrome. *Am J Clin Pathol* 1985;84:85–95.

151. Schuurman HJ, Krone WJA, Broekhuizen R, et al. The thymus in acquired immune deficiency syndrome. Comparison with other types of immunodeficiency diseases, and presence of components of human immunodeficiency virus type 1. *Am J Pathol* 1989;134:1329–1338.

152. Kendall MD, Johnson HR, Singh J. The weight of the human thymus gland at necropsy. *J Anat* 1980;131(pt 3):485–497.

153. Lack EE. Thymic hyperplasia with massive enlargement. Report of two cases with review of diagnostic criteria. *J Thorac Cardiovasc Surg* 1981;81:741–746.

154. Katz SM, Chatten J, Bishop HD, Rosenblum H. Massive thymic enlargement. Report of a case of gross thymic hyperplasia in a child. *Am J Clin Pathol* 1977;68:786–790.

155. Judd RL. Massive thymic hyperplasia with myoid cell differentiation. *Hum Pathol* 1987;18:1180–1183.

156. Hammar JA. Uber Gewicht Involution und Persistenz der Thymus im Postfotalleben der Menschen. *Arch Anat Physiol Anat Abt* 1906;(suppl):91–182.

157. Durkin W, Durant J. Benign mass lesions after therapy for Hodgkin's disease. *Arch Intern Med* 1979;139:333–336.

158. Shin M, Ho K. Diffuse thymic hyperplasia following chemotherapy for nodular sclerosing Hodgkin's disease. *Cancer* 1983;51:30–33.

159. Carmosino L, DiBenedetto A, Feffer S. Thymic hyperplasia following successful chemotherapy. A report of two cases and review of the literature. *Cancer* 1985;56:1526–1528.

160. Due W, Dieckmann KP, Stein H. Thymic hyperplasia following chemotherapy of a testicular germ cell tumor. Immunohistological evidence for a simple rebound phenomenon. *Cancer* 1989;63:446–449.

161. Gelfand DW, Goldman AS, Law AJ. Thymic hyperplasia in children recovering from thermal burns. *J Trauma* 1972;12:813–817.

162. Caffey J, Silbey R. Regrowth and overgrowth of the thymus after atrophy induced by the oral administration of adrenocorticosteroids to human infants. *Pediatrics* 1960;26:762–770.

163. Mackall CL, Fleisher TA, Brown MR, et al. Age, thymopoiesis, and CD4$^+$ T-lymphocyte regeneration after intensive chemotherapy. *N Engl J Med* 1995;332:143–149.

164. Markert ML, Alvarez-McLeod AP, Sempowski GD, et al. Thymopoiesis in HIV-infected adults after highly active antiretroviral therapy. *AIDS Res Hum Retroviruses* 2001;17:1635–1643.

165. Croxatto OC. Cordones epiteliales con aspecto endocrino observado en restos timicos del adulto. *Medicina (B Aires)* 1972;32:203–208.

166. Suster S, Moran CA. Malignant thymic neoplasms that may mimic benign conditions. *Semin Diagn Pathol* 1995;12:98–104.

167. Suster S, Rosai J. Multilocular thymic cyst: an acquired reactive process. Study of 18 cases. *Am J Surg Pathol* 1991;15:388–398.

168. Suster S, Barbuto D, Carlson G, Rosai J. Multilocular thymic cysts with pseudoepitheliomatous hyperplasia. *Hum Pathol* 1991;22:455–460.

169. Suster S, Rosai J. Cystic thymomas. A clinicopathologic study of 10 cases. *Cancer* 1992;69:92–97.

170. Moran CA, Suster S. Mediastinal seminomas with prominent cystic changes. A clinicopathologic study of 10 cases. *Am J Surg Pathol* 1995;19:1047–1053.

171. Suster S, Rosai J. Thymic carcinoma. A clinicopathologic study of 60 cases. *Cancer* 1991;67:1025–1032.

172. Moran CA, Suster S. Mucoepidermoid carcinomas of the thymus. A clinicopathologic study of six cases. *Am J Surg Pathol* 1995;19:826–834.

173. Penn CR, Hope-Stone HF. The role of radiotherapy in the management of malignant thymoma. *Br J Surg* 1972;59:533–539.

174. Goodwin RA, Nickell JA, Des Prez RM. Mediastinal fibrosis complicating healed primary histoplasmosis and tuberculosis. *Medicine (Baltimore)* 1972;51:227–246.

175. Light AM. Idiopathic fibrosis of the mediastinum: a discussion of three cases and review of the literature. *J Clin Pathol* 1978;31:78–88.

176. Sobrinho-Simoes MA, Vaz Saleiro JV, Wagenvoort CA. Mediastinal and hilar fibrosis. *Histopathology* 1981;5:53–60.

Normal Heart

20

Gerald J. Berry   Margaret E. Billingham

INTRODUCTION

With the introduction of the cardiopulmonary bypass technique into clinical practice a half-century ago, pathologists found themselves dealing more frequently with cardiac specimens in the surgical pathology laboratory. For many years this consisted of explanted valves, pericardiectomy specimens, ventricular aneurysectomy excisions, and interventricular myomectomy specimens. It was not until cardiac transplantation began in 1968 that the surgical pathologist began handling entire heart specimens. Currently, more than 73,000 heart and combined heart-lung transplant procedures have been recorded in the registry of the International Society of Heart and Lung Transplantation (1). Thoracic transplantation in the pediatric age group ranging from neonates to adolescents is now commonly performed (2). The explanted hearts from infants and children often have complicated congenital heart lesions that have undergone one or more corrective surgical interventions. Surgical pathologists need to have some expertise in the morphologic evaluation of end-stage heart disease of all types. Since the early 1970s, endomyocardial biopsies for the assessment of allograft rejection, infiltrative lesions, and inflammatory disorders are performed routinely. Today many institutions have initiated ventricular assist device (VAD) programs, and ventricular apical specimens are routinely submitted. Like other biopsy specimens, these fall under the auspices of the surgical pathologist. Further, the introduction of complex electrophysiologic mapping techniques and imaging modalities such as transesophageal echocardiography, intravascular ultrasound, cardiac gated spiral-computed tomography (CT) angiography, and magnetic resonance imaging (MRI) have renewed interest in structural-functional correlations. Pathologists have assumed a central role in the clinical evaluation and application of these technologies.

The purpose of this chapter is to review normal cardiac anatomy and histology. The histology of the great vessels is described elsewhere in this book. For the most part, adult histology is described; but, where important differences exist, the histology in infants and children is also addressed. Furthermore, the purpose is not to be encyclopedic. Rather, we will highlight those areas that are of practical importance to the surgical pathologist to enable the distinction between normal and subtle cardiac pathology. As each of the major anatomic divisions of the heart is described, relevant aspects of aging, gender changes, and/or applied anatomy are mentioned. We have also included recommendations for handling endomyocardial biopsy specimens and common artifactual alterations in this discussion.

HEART WEIGHTS

The weight of the normal adult heart is generally achieved by the end of the second decade of life. Heart weight in infants and children is related to age and body size, and tables are readily available in published works (3,4). A variety of approaches to estimating the weight of the adult heart have been used in clinical practice. These differ in complexity and accuracy; for example, the practical guidelines for unfixed adult heart weights published by Hudson in 1965 (5) indicate the male heart weighs 0.45% of the body weight (325 $\pm$ 75 g; average 300 g) and the female heart weighs 0.40% of the body weight (275 $\pm$ 75g; average 250 g). Heart weight varies with age, sex, and body height and weight. Using this type of approach, the heart weight in young athletic adults may approach or exceed the upper limits of normal by up to 25%, whereas in the elderly it may approach or be slightly below the lower limits of normal.

Kitzman and colleagues from the Mayo Clinic (6) proposed a more comprehensive approach that predicts the normal heart weight of a formalin-fixed specimen based on body weight. In their study, body height as a predictor

proved less accurate than body weight. The impact of formalin fixation on the weight of the heart has been addressed with conflicting findings. In one study, the overall finding was that heart weight increased by 5% after fixation, although considerable individual variation—ranging from weight loss to weight gain—was reported (7). Descriptive tables of normal ventricular wall thickness, chamber size, and valvular orifice measurements are available in textbooks and postmortem dissection manuals (4,8–10).

PRENATAL FETAL CIRCULATION

It is beyond the scope of this chapter to discuss cardiac embryology. Developmental molecular biology has provided many new insights in cardiogenesis, some of which have radically altered previously held tenets (11–14). Currently it is thought that the human heart begins to beat around day 17. Well-oxygenated blood leaves the placenta via the umbilical vein, a portion of which passes through the hepatic sinusoids, and the remainder bypasses the liver by way of the ductus venosus to enter the inferior vena cava (IVC). Caval blood enters the right atrium together with an admixture of deoxygenated blood from the lower body. Approximately one-third of this blood is diverted through the interatrial septum (ostium secundum) into the left atrium, where it mixes with the small amount of deoxygenated blood returning from the lungs. The blood then passes into the left ventricle and exits into the ascending aorta to supply the coronary arteries, brain, and upper limbs. Approximately 50% of the blood is returned to the placenta for reoxygenation via the umbilical arteries. The remainder of the blood supplies the lower half of the body. Blood returning to the heart from the upper body reaches the right atrium through the superior vena cava (SCV). It mixes with the residual two-thirds of the blood from the IVC and enters the right ventricle. A small portion is distributed to the lungs, but the majority is diverted across the ductus arteriosus to the descending aorta. Blood is returned to the placenta with only a small amount reaching the lower body of the fetus.

POSTNATAL CIRCULATION

At birth, a series of anatomic and physiologic changes occur, beginning with the infant's first respiratory efforts. The circulation of fetal blood through the placenta ceases, and the infant's lungs expand. As alveoli become aerated, the pulmonary vascular bed dilates, causing increases in pulmonary blood flow and abrupt decline in pulmonary vascular resistance. Additionally, active remodeling of the pulmonary vasculature begins and continues over a period of a few weeks. This consists primarily in the reduction of the muscular medial layer of arterioles and small arteries. Increased blood return to the left atrium by way of the pulmonary veins results in slightly higher left atrial pressures compared to the right atrium. This causes the flap covering the foramen ovale to seal, leaving the indentation called the fossa ovale. By the end of the first month after birth, the significant differences in ventricular hemodynamic load result in thickening of the left ventricular wall and thinning of the right ventricular wall. The ductus arteriosus, located between the left pulmonary artery and aortic arch, functionally closes within 15 hours after birth, and the umbilical veins begin to constrict.

PERICARDIUM

The pericardium surrounds the heart and consists of a fibrous and a serous sac. The fibrous, or parietal, pericardium envelops the heart and is reflected off the ascending aorta, the pulmonary trunk, and the terminal 2 to 4 cm of the SVC, the distal segment of the IVC, and the pulmonary veins. In the normal state, the fibrous pericardium surrounding the heart remains unattached to the serous (visceral) pericardium except at the pericardial reflections. The parietal pericardium is composed of collagenous fibrous tissue (Figure 20.1). Its inelastic tendencies account for the development of cardiac tamponade when it is acutely stretched with more than 250 ml of fluid. It may contain variable amounts of adipose tissue, particularly toward the apex of the heart. A thin layer of mesothelial cells on its inner surface lines the parietal pericardium. It is normally less than 1 mm in thickness. Heterotopic tissues within this layer include thyroid and thymic elements. Neoplastic and hyperplastic alterations have been described, including intracardiac thyroid in the right ventricular outflow tract (15).

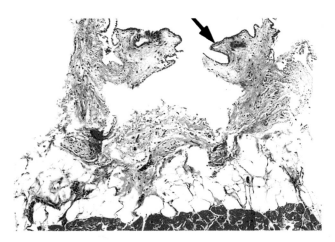

Figure 20.2 Section showing the epicardium lined by mesothelial cells (*arrow*) and covering the subepicardial adipose tissue and myocardium (H&E).

The serous, or visceral, pericardium is also called the epicardium of the heart. It is a single layer of mesothelium that envelops the heart and is in continuity with the fibrous pericardium at the pericardial reflections at the great vessels (Figure 20.2). This delicate membrane covering the heart contains variable amounts of adipose tissue within which are embedded the coronary arteries and veins, lymphatic vessels, nerves, fibroblasts, and macrophages (Figure 20.3). The normal epicardium often has small aggregates of lymphocytes that are present from birth.

Between the two mesothelial layers of the parietal and visceral pericardium is a potential space containing up to 50 mL of straw-colored fluid that allows the surfaces to glide over one another in the normal state. The histologic composition of the two layers of the pericardium does not alter with age and is similar in infants, children, and adults.

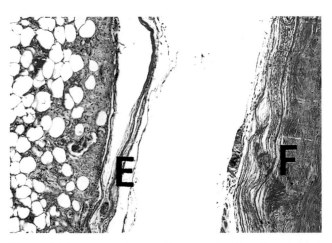

Figure 20.1 Section showing fibrous pericardium (*F*) separated from the thinner epicardium (*E*) (elastic van Giesen).

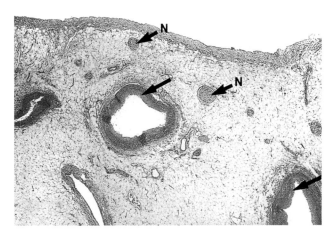

Figure 20.3 Section of the epicardium showing the relationship of coronary vessels (*arrows*) and nerves (*N*) to the epicardium (H&E).

Applied Anatomy

Surgical pathologists may receive pericardiectomy specimens in cases of constrictive pericarditis or recurrent tamponade. Nonspecific fibrosis and chronic inflammation are observed, but granulomatous infection and neoplastic infiltrates should be excluded. In explanted hearts, the pericardial surfaces are often thickened by previous disease states or surgical interventions, in which case the epicardium and parietal pericardium are adherent. Occasionally nodular collections of epicardial fat may be misinterpreted grossly as metastases. Congenital cysts of the pericardium are rare. Heterotopic thyroid and thymic tissue should be distinguished from cardiac involvement by contiguous spread or metastasis. In obese subjects, there may be excessive epicardial deposits of adipose tissue, and the measurement of ventricular thickness should be carefully evaluated. In conditions of cachexia, epicardial fat may undergo serous atrophy, resulting in small gelatinous tissue tags (10).

CARDIAC SKELETON

The cardiac skeleton at the base of the heart is the central supporting structure to which most of the fibers of the myocardium are attached and to which the atrioventricular and aortic valves are anchored. A separate mass of fibrous tissue (the conus ligament) joins the pulmonary ring to the aortic ring. It also serves to separate the atrial and ventricular chambers. It is composed of the right and left fibrous trigones, membranous septum of the interventricular septum, and the fibrous annuli of the atrioventricular foramina (16). The fibrous skeleton is composed of layers of dense collagenous connective tissue admixed with small numbers of elastic fibers and, on occasion, small aggregates of adipose tissue. The fibrous tissue of the mitral and aortic valve rings is more substantial than the right-sided valves, and the right and left trigone create the direct mitral-aortic continuity (17). The right trigone and membranous septum form the central fibrous body within which the atrioventricular bundle is embedded. Bone or cartilage is not normally found in the fibrous skeleton of human hearts, although they have been described in some animal species.

Applied Anatomy

Portions of the cardiac skeleton may be seen in explanted valves. The close proximity of the fibrous skeleton to the conduction system and valvular leaflets is an important consideration for surgeons. Alterations can significantly affect the functional outcomes of all these components.

INTERNAL STRUCTURE OF THE HEART WALL

The wall of the heart in all chambers consists of three main layers: (a) the endocardium, (b) the intermediate muscular portion of the myocardium, and (c) the external portion, or epicardium. Most investigators believe that the endocardium is homologous with the tunica intima of blood vessels, the myocardium with the smooth muscle media, and the external epicardium with the adventitial layer. The endocardium consists of a single layer of endothelial cells (Figures 20.4–20.5) with a subendothelial portion containing a loose elastic framework and collagen bundles, as well as nerves and delicate blood vessels (Figure 20.6).

While the chambers of the heart are composed of these three layers, there can be variation in the thickness of one or more components. A rudimentary layer of smooth muscle is often found in the endocardium of both atria and the

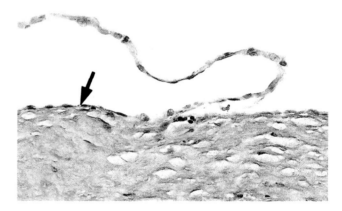

Figure 20.4 Section showing a single layer of endothelial cells covering the myocardium (*arrow*) (H&E).

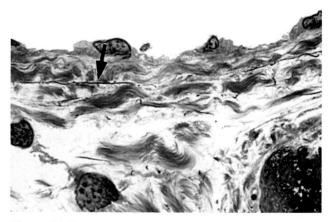

Figure 20.5 One-μm thick section (plastic embedded) of the endothelium covering the fenestrated elastic fibers (*arrow*) and collagen fibers of the subendocardium (toluidine blue).

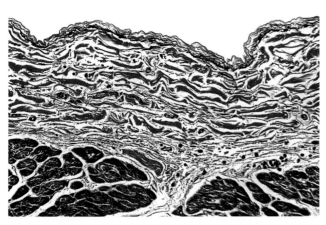

Figure 20.6 Section of the endocardium showing the distribution of the elastic fibers (*black*) and the collagen bundles (*red*), as well as vessels and nerves in the subendocardial layer.

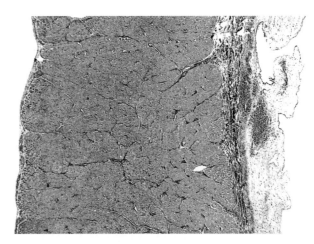

Figure 20.8 Section through the right ventricular wall showing the distribution of collagen from the endocardium (left) through the myocardium and to the epicardium (right) in the normal heart (Masson's trichrome).

ventricles (Figure 20.7). The endocardium of the atria is thicker than the ventricles. Small bundles of smooth muscle are often found but are of questionable functional significance. The myocardium is composed of bundles of myocytes separated by fibrous bands (Figure 20.8). The individual myocytes form a syncytium with end-to-end junctions (called intercalated disks) and sometimes side-to-side junctions. Individual myocytes contain a central ovoid nucleus with a clear zone at the poles (Figure 20.9). The normal cardiac myocyte contains small amounts of lipofuscin granules (lysosomes), which increase in quantity with age. The myocytes are filled with contractile myofibrils (actin and myosin). In addition, atrial myocytes contain atrial dense-core bodies that are demonstrable by electron microscopy (Figure 20.10). The epicardial portion of the chambers was described earlier.

INTERATRIAL SEPTUM

The interatrial septum separates the right and left atrial chambers. In the normal state this separation is complete, although the foramen ovale may retain a small communication at its floor where the septum has not fused (the so-called patent foramen ovale). This is reported in up to 30% of adults and is usually without clinical complications (18). The foramen ovale is closed by the septum to form the circular, dime-sized oval fossa. This represents the true interatrial septum, with the remainder of the anatomic structure being comprised of caval or pulmonary venous infoldings and the muscular and membranous components of the atrioventricular region (17). The membrane covering the oval fossa is a paper-thin, translucent layer early in life that becomes fibrotic and thickened with age, measuring up to

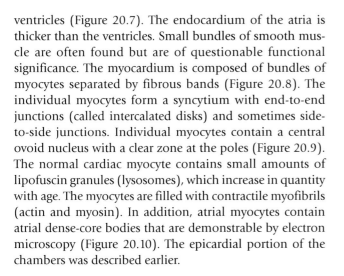

Figure 20.7 Section of endocardium showing smooth muscle bundle (*arrow*) (Masson's trichrome).

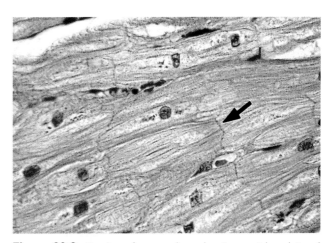

Figure 20.9 Section of myocardium showing ovoid nuclei and intercalated disks (*arrow*) (H&E).

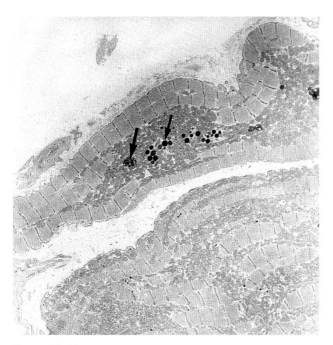

Figure 20.10 Electron micrograph of atrial dense-core granules (*small arrow*) that can be differentiated from the lipofuscin granules (*large arrow*).

2 mm in thickness. The histology of the septum displays variable amounts of atrial muscle, fibrous tissue, mature adipose tissue, and, on occasion, brown fat (Figure 20.11). The thickness of the atrial septum varies considerably.

Applied Anatomy

Lipomatous hypertrophy of the interatrial septum is characterized by accumulations of adipose tissue within the U-shaped lip, or limbus, of the oval fossa and may produce bulging of the interatrial septum. In some patients, the patent foramen ovale can be the site of interatrial shunting or paradoxical embolism.

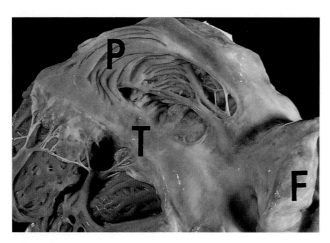

Figure 20.11 The right atrium showing the pectinate muscles (*P*), the crista terminalis (*T*), and the interatrial septal fat (*F*).

RIGHT ATRIUM

Venous return to the heart occurs via the IVC and SCV into the right atrium. The right atrium forms the right lateral cardiac border and is located anterior to the left atrium and to the right of it. Anteromedially, the right atrial appendage protrudes from the right atrium and overlaps the aortic root (17). The atrium is composed of an auricular appendage, a smooth-walled venous sinus that contains the openings of the cavae and coronary sinus, a septal component, and a portion near the opening of the tricuspid valve (19). Extending between the right sides of the openings of both cavae is a prominent muscular ridge called the terminal crest, which underlies the sulcus terminalis. The wide-based triangular appendage defines the anatomic right atrium. The interior surface of this appendage is trabeculated by muscular bands called pectinate muscles. The portion of the right atrium lateral to the terminal crest is smooth-walled and is derived embryologically from the sinus venosus (Figure 20.11). The right atrial wall measures 2 mm in thickness.

The orifice of the SVC is valveless. The opening of the IVC has an inconstant, rudimentary valve called the eustachean valve. It forms a crescentic fold over the orifice and directed blood toward the foramen ovale and into the left atrium during fetal life. The opening of the coronary sinus has a rudimentary flap of tissue called the thebesian valve; these valves vary greatly in size and may be fenestrated or absent. A Chiari's network, usually appearing as a lacelike veil of tissue, represents the remnant of the right sinus venosus valve and is occasionally found in normal hearts (Figure 20.12). The right atrial chamber is covered by endocardium. In the subendocardium, elastic fibers pass into a typical fenestrated elastic membrane that contains blood vessels, nerves, and branches of the conducting system. In the spaces between the muscle bundles of the atria, the wall is so thin that the connective tissue of the endocardium blends with the epicardium. The epicardial surface of the atrium is rich in nerves and ganglia (Figure 20.13).

LEFT ATRIUM

Like the right atrium, this chamber consists of an appendage, a venous component containing the ostia of the four pulmonary veins, a septal component, and a region near the mitral valve orifice. On average, the wall of the left atrium is 3 mm in thickness. The septal surface is smooth. The four pulmonary veins open into the left atrium in the posterior wall. The atrial appendage has a narrow, angulated tubular shape resembling a hockey stick and is lined by pectinate muscles. At its interface with the venous portion of the atrium, it lacks a terminal crest. The endocardial layer is thicker and more opaque than on the right side, due in part to the higher pressures of the pulmonary veins emptying into the atrium. Sometimes a patch of thickened rough

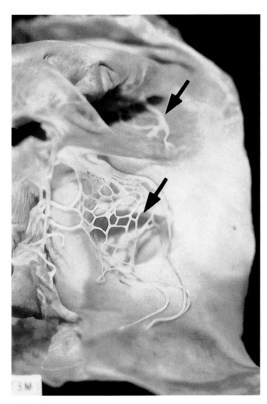

Figure 20.12 Picture of the Chiari's network (arrows), or lacelike pattern of the remnants of the thebesian valve, in the inferior vena cava opening into the right atrium.

endocardium is seen on the posterior wall above the mitral valve as a result of mitral regurgitation. This is called MacCallum's patch but is not usually seen in the normal heart. The two left pulmonary veins enter on the posterolateral surface, and the right veins enter on the posteromedial side; there are no true valves at the venous-atrial junction. Small collections of atrial muscle can be found within the walls of the pulmonary veins at this junction and may act as

physiologic valves. On occasion, this is the source of isolated or left-sided atrial fibrillation and is treated by ablation techniques.

The atrial septum is smooth on the left side but has a central shallow depression corresponding to the oval fossa. The endocardium of the left atrium is thicker as a result of increased collagen layers, particularly near the openings of the pulmonary veins. Otherwise the histology is similar to the right atrium.

RIGHT VENTRICLE

The morphologic right ventricle lies anterior to the other heart chambers. It has an inflow portion (sinus), an apical trabecular component, and an outflow portion (infundibulum conus) (20). The outflow tract is separated anatomically from the inflow tract by a muscular arch called the crista superventricularis. The endocardial surface is coarsely trabeculated, particularly in the apica region.

On sectioning, the trabeculations form the inner two-thirds of the ventricular wall. The septal surface is deeply trabeculated with coarse trabeculae carneae and a thick muscular column called the moderator band (Figure 20.14). This moderator band is found in most hearts and connects the distal portion of the septum to the free wall. It terminates in the region of the anterior papillary muscle. Myocyte disarray is a common finding within trabecular muscles and should not be confused with hypertrophic cardiomyopathy. The right bundle branch travels through the muscular ventricular septum and courses down to end in the moderator muscle. The papillary muscles of the right ventricle are relatively constant, with an anterior papillary muscle located on the anterior wall near its junction with the septum and a small posterior papillary muscle arising under the crista superventricularis at the inferior border of the right ventricular outflow tract. In addition, there is an

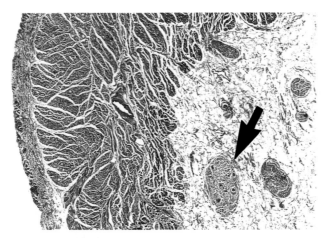

Figure 20.13 Section through the right atrium showing the nerves and ganglion cells (*arrow*) in the overlying subepicardial adipose tissue (elastic van Giesen).

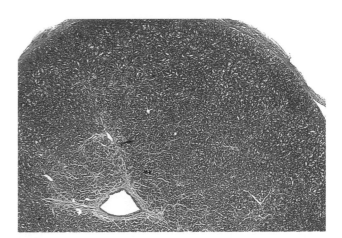

Figure 20.14 A section of trabeculae carneae from the normal right ventricle.

inconstant group of posterior papillary muscles that can arise from the diaphragmatic wall of the right ventricle.

The histology of the right ventricle consists of a thin endocardial layer. The thickness of myocardial wall in normal human adults is about one-third that of the left ventricle and measures up to 5 mm. The endocardium is similar to the other chambers except it has more variability from region to region, with the thickest area found in the septum. The subendocardial space includes a fenestrated elastic membrane and, on occasion, bundles of smooth muscle, particularly in the interventricular septum (Figure 20.7). The interventricular septum also contains blood vessels, nerves, and the left bundle branch of the conduction system. The ventricular free wall has numerous vascular channels consisting of intertrabecular channels that lead into myocardial sinusoids and thebesian veins. Myocardial sinusoids are also found within the trabeculae. Arterioluminal vessels, leading directly from the systemic coronary circulation into the capillary beds, empty into the myocardial sinusoids. The myocardium is richly supplied with small vascular channels that form an intramural circulation (21). There is an extensive web of capillaries that course among the cardiac muscle fibers, are fed by branches of the coronary arteries, and are drained, in part, by the coronary veins. They are also directed to the intramyocardial sinusoids and thence into the lumen of the heart. Deep within the myocardial musculature is found, in addition to the capillary bed, a richly anastomosing network of irregular channels that have been called myocardial sinusoids. These sinusoids receive vessels from the coronary arteries and the capillaries and communicate with coronary veins. The connections between the coronary arteries and the cardiac chambers are called arterioluminal vessels (Figure 20.15). Within the myocardium, variable amounts of adipose tissue can be found,

particularly in the free wall portions. When extensive, it is called fatty infiltration of the right ventricle and represents a metaplastic change. It should not be confused with arrhythmogenic right ventricular dysplasia/cardiomyopathy.

Applied Anatomy

The importance of recognizing the presence of myocyte disarray and adipose tissue as common findings within the trabeculated musculature of the right ventricle of the normal adult heart has been discussed. The apical trabecular region is also the site of pacemaker wire placement and endomyocardial biopsy sampling.

LEFT VENTRICLE

The left ventricle receives blood from the left atrium during ventricular diastole and ejects blood into the systemic arterial circulation across the aortic valve during ventricular systole. The left ventricle is somewhat bullet-shaped, with the blunt tip directed anteriorly and inferiorly and to the left (22). Like the right ventricle, it is composed of inflow, septal, and outflow components. It lacks the moderator band and septomarginal trabeculations of the right ventricle (19). The left ventricular chamber is surrounded by a thick muscular wall measuring up to 15 mm in thickness (note: the papillary muscles are not included in the measurement). The medial wall of the left ventricle is the interventricular septum, which is shared with the right ventricle. The septum is roughly triangular in shape, with the base of the triangle at the level of the aortic cusps; it is entirely muscular, except for the small membranous septum located just below the right coronary and posterior cusps. The upper third of the septum, or outflow tract, is lined by smooth endocardium. The inferior two-thirds of the septum and the remaining ventricular walls are composed of the trabeculae carneae, which are thinner and less prominent than in the right ventricle. The free wall of the left ventricle is that portion that is exclusive of the septum.

The histology of the left ventricle is similar to that of the right side, although the endocardium is slightly thicker as a result of higher hemodynamic pressures. The small arterioles subadjacent to the endocardium have slightly thicker walls than those of the right ventricle, most likely due to the higher pressure in the left ventricle. The myocardium of the left ventricle is arranged in such a way that it appears to spiral inward from the superficial layers. The superficial layers run at right angles to the layers deeper within the wall. These layers are intimately interdigitated to prevent dissection into lamina structures. The attachment of the muscular layers is from the fibrous skeleton at the base of the heart. The deeper muscle layers of the interventricular septum are composed of the deep bulbospiral muscle in the center of the septum originating from the septal portion

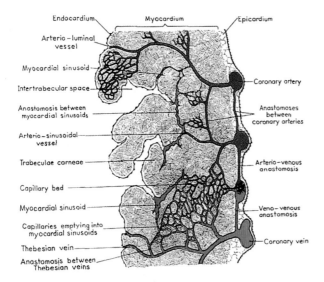

Figure 20.15 Diagrammatic representation of the various intramural vascular channels. Reprinted with permission from: Gittenberger-de Groot AC, Bartelings MM, Deruiter MC, Poelmann RE. Basics of cardiac development for the understanding of congenital heart malformations. *Pediatr Res* 2005;57:169–176.

of the atrioventricular annulus. The fascicles of the deep bulbospiral and sinospiral muscles interdigitate within the muscular interventricular septum. The spiral muscle pulls the base of the ventricle toward the apex during systolic contraction. The blood supply is similar to that of the right ventricle.

Applied Anatomy

Portions of the left ventricular subaortic outflow tract may be submitted as myomectomy specimens in patients with asymmetric hypertrophic cardiomyopathy. Portions of the left ventricular free wall may be removed as aneurysectomy specimens or during VAD placement. The intermediate bulbospiral muscle of the interventricular septum is primarily involved in idiopathic hypertrophic subaortic stenosis (IHSS). Because it lies deep within the septum, the disarray associated with IHSS may not always be seen in the superficial myomectomy specimen.

CARDIAC VALVES

Semilunar Valves

The semilunar valves consist of the pulmonic and aortic valves. The normal valve circumference for the aortic valve is 5.7 to 7.9 cm for women and 6.0 to 8.5 cm for men (23). The normal pulmonic valve circumference is 5.7 to 7.4 cm for women and 9.2 to 9.9 cm for men (23). Interestingly, when adjusted for body surface area, the valves in women are slightly larger than in men (6). Each semilunar valve consists of three semicircular cusps (24), each of which is attached by its semicircular border, or annulus, to the aortic or pulmonic ring. The three points of lateral attachment of adjacent cusps are the commissures (Figure 20.16). The lines of cusp apposition are not at the free margin but are angulated lines extending from well below the point of attachment in the commissure to just below the midpoint of the free edge. In the aortic valve, these lines (the linea alba) and the central nodules (the noduli arenti) can be seen (24). In the pulmonic valve, these landmarks are less obvious because of the lower right-sided pressures. The lunulae are thin, delicate areas of cusp between the linear alba and the free edge.

The semilunar aortic and pulmonic valves are similar in configuration, except that the aortic cusps are slightly thicker and contain coronary ostia. They are situated at the summit at the outflow tract of their corresponding ventricle, the pulmonic valve being anterior, superior, and slightly to the left of the aortic valve in the normal heart. The cusps, which are often slightly unequal in width, circle the inside of the respective vessel root (e.g., pulmonary artery trunk or aortic root). Behind each cusp, the vessel wall bulges outward, creating a pouchlike dilatation known as the sinus of Valsalva. The portion of the cusp adjacent to the rim is thin and may contain small perforations in the normal situation. The noduli arenti meet in the center and contribute to the support of the leaflets. Because the plane of the aortic valve is oblique with the right posterior side lower than the left anterior side, the origin of the left coronary artery is slightly superior to that of the right coronary artery. The ostia of coronary arteries are located in the upper third of their respective sinuses. The right coronary artery passes anteriorly and to the left. In some hearts, there is a separate ostium in the right coronary sinus for the conus artery, sometimes called the third coronary artery (22).

The histology of the semilunar valves is that of a well-defined multilayered structure. Three distinct layers are recognizable: the fibrosa, the spongiosa, and the ventricularis. The fibrosa is a layer of dense collagen that constitutes the major structural component of the cusp and extends to its free edge (25). The densely packed collagen bundles blend into the collagen of the valvular ring in the region of the commissures. Some fibroblasts are present in this layer, as are some very fine elastic fibers. The spongiosa is subadjacent to the fibrosa and occupies a central position in the thickness of the cusp (Figure 20.17). It is best developed in the basal third of the cusp. It does not extend to the free edge, which is composed only of fibrosa and ventricularis layers. The spongiosa is composed of large amounts of proteoglycans, such as glycoaminoglycans, loosely arranged collagen fibrils, scattered fibroblasts, and mesenchymal cells (25). The ventricularis is subadjacent to the spongiosa and is in direct contact with the endothelial layer of the inflow surface of the cusp (i.e., closest to the ventricular surface). It is distinguished from the fibrosa by its abundance of elastic fibers. This feature is often helpful in orienting and identifying the layers of excised aortic valvular cusps. The surface lining of the cusps consists of a single layer of endothelial cells. The surface topography of the aortic cusp varies according to its state of stress. The bundles are wavy and the inflow surface is smoother in the stressed state and rougher in the relaxed state (25).

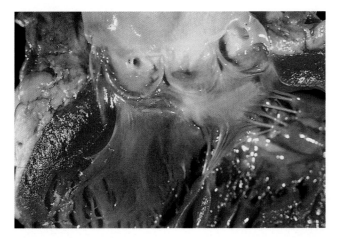

Figure 20.16 Aortic valve from normal heart showing the cusps and the coronary ostia.

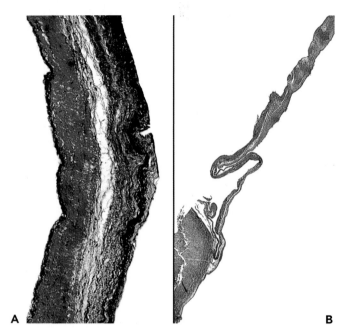

A   **B**

Figure 20.17 High- (**A**) and low-power (**B**) views of a section of the aortic cusp showing the three distinct layers as described in the text.

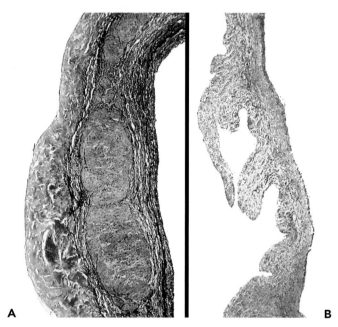

A   **B**

Figure 20.18 High- (**A**) and low-power (**B**) views of a section of the mitral leaflet showing the three distinct layers with muscle in the central portion near the base of the valve.

Atrioventricular Valves

The atrioventricular valves consist of the mitral valve and the tricuspid valve. The normal circumference of the tricuspid valve is 10 to 11.1 cm in women and 11.2 to 11.8 cm in men (23). The normal circumference of the mitral valve is 8.2 to 9.1 cm in women and 9.2 to 9.9 cm in men (23). The valvular apparatus is made up of the annulus, commissures, leaflets, chordae tendineae, and papillary muscles. The annulus is composed of a ring of circumferentially oriented collagen and elastic fibers with extensions into the ventricle and atrium.

The atrioventricular valves have four histologic layers (Figure 20.18). The collagen bundles of the annulus spread down into the cusp of the mitral valve and are known as the fibrosa. They continue into the chordae tendineae and finally spread out into a network that covers the tip of the papillary muscles (Figure 20.19). Adjacent to the fibrosa layer on the ventricular side of the valve is the ventricularis. The ventricularis contains many elastic fibers and is covered by endothelium. Some of the elastic fibers extend into the chordae tendineae; but, in general, this layer is incomplete, as it does not extend to the free edge of the leaflet. The spongiosa is situated on the atrial side of the fibrosa layer. Like the semilunar valves, it has a rich abundance of glycosaminoglycans and a few elastic fibers, collagen fibrils, and connective tissue cells (25). This layer, along with the fibrosa layer, extends through the entire length of the

leaflet. The spongiosa in the anterior and posterior mitral leaflets may contain cardiac myocytes that are a direct extension of the left atrial myocardium (Figure 20.18). In the anterior mitral leaflet, this layer extends into the middle third, whereas in the posterior leaflet it only extends into its proximal third. Neural elements and lymphatics can be found in the leaflets. The atrial aspect of the spongiosa (i.e., layer closest to the atrium) is covered by the auricularis,

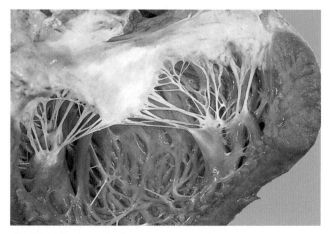

Figure 20.19 A normal mitral valve with chordae tendineae inserting into the papillary muscles.

which in turn has an endothelial lining. The auricularis contains collagen and elastic fibers and smooth muscle cells. It is prominent near the annulus but thins out in the distal third of the leaflet such that the most distal aspect of the valves is composed only of spongiosa and fibrosa. The endothelial cells on the atrial aspect of the atrioventricular valves are plump and have irregular nuclei compared to the flatter endothelial cells on the ventricular aspect.

The architecture of the tricuspid valve apparatus and the layered arrangements of its leaflets are similar to those in the mitral valve; however, the individual layers are thinner in the tricuspid valve. Cardiac muscle bundles insert fairly low into the base of the tricuspid leaflets but do not extend into the leaflet substance. In the posterior and septal leaflets, the auricularis is thicker and contains more abundant smooth muscle cells.

Chordae Tendineae

The chordae tendineae in the normal state are thin fibrous cords that emanate in a fanlike manner from the broad leaflets of the atrioventricular valves and insert into the papillary muscles (Figure 20.19). The central cores of the chordae are composed of longitudinally oriented collagen fibrils. The core is surrounded more peripherally by loosely arranged collagen fibrils and elastic fibers and is embedded in proteoglycan-rich matrix (25) (Figure 20.20). Some chordae contain a small central core of muscle known as chordae muscularis (Figure 20.21), although others contain blood vessels and collagen in variable amounts and appear fleshier in color (Figure 20.22). The endothelial cells on the chordae resemble the flattened ovoid nuclei of the ventricular surface of the leaflets.

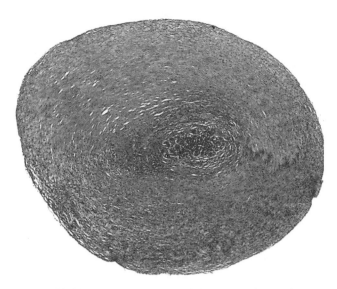

Figure 20.21 Transverse section of chordae tendineae showing central core of muscle (H&E).

Applied Anatomy of Intracardiac Valves

Semilunar and atrioventricular valves are frequently encountered in the surgical pathology laboratory. Indications for valvular replacement or repair include a variety of congenital, infectious, inflammatory, degenerative, and paraneoplastic causes. In many cases, the chordae and portions of papillary muscle may be attached. In the set-

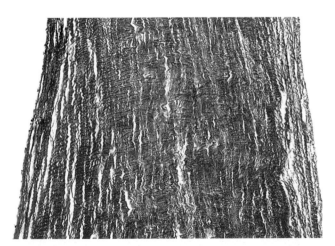

Figure 20.20 Longitudinal section of chordae tendineae showing the relationships of elastic fibers on the surface and collagen in the center (elastic van Giesen).

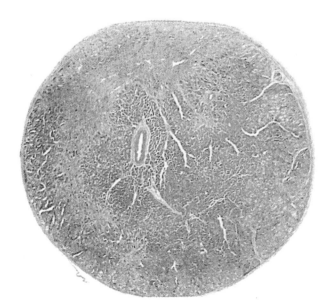

Figure 20.22 Transverse section of a muscular chorda showing fibrous tissue, muscle, and small vessel within the chorda (Masson's trichrome).

ting of myocardial infarction, infection, or valvular prolapse, ruptured papillary muscles may become surgical specimens. Lambl's excrescences and fibrous nodules are papillary projections along the lines of closure or free edge of the valve, respectively.

Aging Changes of Intracardiac Valves

With age, all the cardiac valves become thicker, more opaque, and less pliable. The increase in collagen content may account for the loss of plasticity, and calcifications may occur. The posterior leaflet of the mitral valve often shows yellow atheromatous alteration. The mitral valve annulus may become calcified with age. The valvular circumferences increase with age (6).

PAPILLARY MUSCLES

The two papillary muscles of the right ventricle (anterior and conal) are relatively constant. There is also a group of inconstant posterior papillary muscles on the inferior wall. In the left ventricle there are two constant papillary muscles: the anterior and posterior. The papillary muscles receive the chordae. They are variable in shape and width and on occasion may have multiple heads (Figure 20.19).

The histology of the papillary muscles includes the fibrous cap, into which the chordae insert (Figure 20.23). The small arteries and arterioles in the papillary muscle are notable for their wall thickness and irregularity in comparison to other intracardiac small vessels (Figure 20.24). The myocardium and the endocardial covering are similar to their counterparts described elsewhere. In marked ventricular dilatation, the papillary muscles may become thinned and flattened.

CONDUCTION SYSTEM

Myocardial fibers are delineated along two functional pathways in humans: (a) contractile fibers and (b) myocardial fibers specialized for the initiation and propagation of an impulse for contraction. The conduction system is recognized to be myogenic in origin, with nerves playing only a subsidiary controlling function.

For most pathologists, examining the conduction system is often regarded as a daunting exercise. This is due in large part to the fact that the number of cases requiring detailed morphologic analysis is infrequent and is often limited to specific requests from clinicians. In addition to detailing the microscopic features of the sinoatrial and atrioventricular nodes, we will present our practical approach to the dissection of these structures. We recommend careful

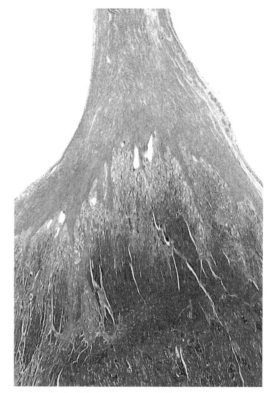

Figure 20.23 Longitudinal section of papillary muscle showing the fibrous cap of the insertion of the chordae tendineae (Masson's trichrome).

attention to key anatomic landmarks to ensure successful retrieval of these structures.

Sinoatrial Node

The sinoatrial (SA) node has the highest intrinsic rate and is recognized as the primary pacemaker of the heart. This node

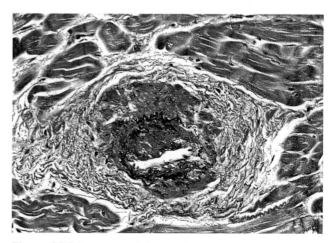

Figure 20.24 Section of abnormally thickened arteriole within a papillary muscle (elastic van Giesen).

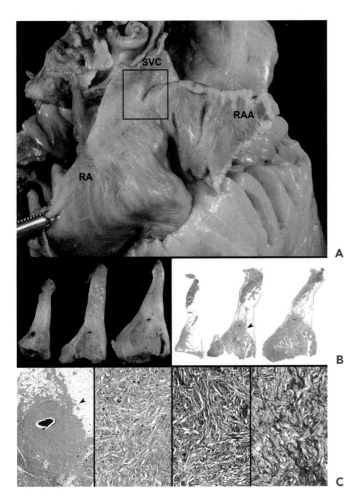

Figure 20.25 The sinoatrial node. **A.** The location of the sinoatrial node within the terminal groove at the junction of the superior vena cava (SVC) and crest of the atrial appendage (*box*). **B.** Macroscopic and low-power magnification of serial sections of nodal tissue. Note the nodal artery that is adjacent to the sinoatrial node. **C.** High-power magnification of the sinoatrial node showing the specialized fibers embedded within collagen and elastic tissue (H&E, trichrome, and elastic van Giesen stains).

of dense connective tissue within which the small muscle fibers are embedded. The muscle fibers contain sparse myofibrils, the striations are not prominent, and the whole mass has a pseudosyncytial appearance. Connective tissue stains such as Masson's trichrome and elastic van Gieson stains highlight the abundant collagen and elastic fibers, respectively (Figure 20.25). Abundant nerve fibers run into the node. The exact pathway(s) carrying the electrical impulse from the SA node to the atrioventricular node remains controversial. Some investigators think that several specialized bundles of conducting system cells (e.g., anterior, middle and posterior internodal tracts) conduct the impulse around the atrium. Others argue that the arrangement of myocardial fibers within the atrium and interatrial septum serves to propagate the impulse (16).

Atrioventricular Node

In our experience a heart opened along the lines of flow provides the optimum exposure for dissecting the atrioventricular (AV) node. From a right-sided approach the interventricular septum is oriented with the tip of the apex pointing downward. The important landmarks include the oval fossa, ostium of the coronary sinus, and tricuspid valve annulus and leaflets. The AV node lies within the subendocardial tissues on the right side of the interatrial septum just anterior to the opening of the coronary sinus, posterior to the membranous interventricular septum, and above the tricuspid valve annulus within the triangle of Koch (26) (Figure 20.26). A rectangular block of tissue, beginning with a vertical incision adjacent to the ostium of the coronary sinus and extending 1 to 2 cm below the annulus, is removed. After careful trimming of valvular structures, the block will contain components of the tricuspid valve (septal leaflet) and mitral and aortic valves (Figure 20.26). Serial sectioning at 2 to 3 mm intervals and sequential placement in tissue cassettes yields a total of 8 to 10 cassettes.

In histologic sections, the AV node is flattened against the central fibrous body and is composed of a network of muscle fibers, with the superficial zone having fibers arranged in a parallel manner. These specialized fibers retain their intercalated disks and striations but are characterized by their pale eosinophilic appearance (Figure 20.26). A small AV nodal artery is often identified adjacent to the AV node. At the anterior end of the AV node, the muscle fibers become arranged in parallel lines to form the main bundle of His or penetrating AV bundle. To reach the ventricle, the AV bundle pierces the central fibrous body and runs forward on the upper margin of the muscular ventricular septum. This penetrating portion of the main bundle is surrounded by dense connective tissue and anatomically is closely related to the aortic and mitral valve rings (Figure 20.26). Connective tissue stains can aid in the localization of the nodal tissue. The

is situated within the terminal groove at the junction of the SVC and the lateral border of the right atrium (Figure 20.25). Its position is constant and is marked by the apex of the crest of the atrial appendage. It is ovoid or cigar-shaped in most hearts, but rare cases of horseshoe-shaped SA nodes are reported. Removal of a rectangular block of tissue that includes the distal SVC and atrium on either side of the terminal groove is recommended. Serial sectioning in a longitudinal plane parallel to the terminal groove at 2 mm intervals is recommended, and all the tissue slices can be accommodated in 2 tissue cassettes. Grossly identifying the SA nodal artery is also helpful in procuring the node (Figure 20.25). This is a branch of the right coronary artery that is found in slightly more than half of the general population. Microscopically, the node is arranged around a central artery adjacent to epicardial adipose tissue. The node is composed

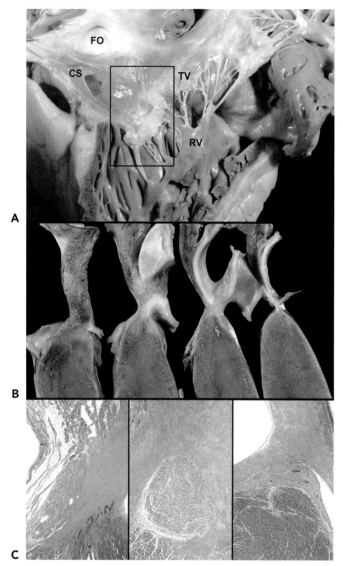

A

B

C

Figure 20.26 The atrioventricular nodal apparatus. **A.** The location of the AV node (*box*) viewed from the right ventricle. Important landmarks include the coronary sinus (*CS*), tricuspid valve annulus and leaflet (*TV*), and fossa ovale (*FO*). **B.** Serial sections of the rectangular block of tissue show the relationship of the nodal tissue to the tricuspid valve, mitral valve, atrioventricular valve, and fibrous skeleton of the heart. **C.** The atrioventricular (AV) node (*left*), AV penetrating bundle (*middle*) and AV bundle with fascicle (*right*) are shown.

fibers of the main bundle are arranged in parallel. The penetrating AV bundle terminates as the left and right bundle branches. The left fascicle runs downward over the endocardial surface of the interventricular septum to the base of the anterior papillary muscle, and the right fascicle ends in the moderator band of the right ventricle. Direct connection of both bundle branches to a complex ramifying system of subendocardial conduction fibers can be demonstrated in mammalian hearts. Light microscopy shows the fibers in the bundle of His and the conduction bundles to be small and contain few myofibrils (Figure 20.27).

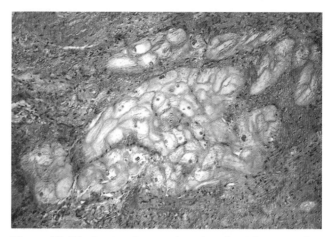

Figure 20.27 Section showing the pale cells of the mammalian conducting system. These cells contain glycogen and only sparse myofibrils (Masson's trichrome).

Aging Changes in the Human Conduction System

With advancing age, the SA node displays progressive increase in fibrous tissue while the AV node remains relatively unchanged. Similarly, fibrous tissue increases in the upper portion of the interventricular septum. These changes are associated with a loss of conduction fibers in the region of the left bundle branch. Up to 50% of the left bundle origin may be lost in people over 60 years of age (27).

CARDIAC INNERVATION

The nerve supply of the heart is autonomic, including both the sympathetic and parasympathetic supply via both the efferent and afferent fibers. Histologically, large nerves can be seen in the epicardium and adjacent to the coronary blood vessels. Small nerves within the myocardium are hard to identify unless special stains are used. Myocardial nerves are best viewed using electron microscopic examination, by which the autonomic nerves can be distinguished. Cardiac ganglia (parasympathetic) can be found over the surface of the atria and in the AV groove (Figure 20.13).

Autonomic Nerves

Axonal varicosities occur at irregular intervals along autonomic fibers, and their morphology is considered useful in determining whether the nerve is adrenergic or cholinergic (25). In cholinergic nerves, the varicosities contain accumulations of agranular vesicles and a few mitochondria. In adrenergic nerves, the varicosities contain vesicles rich in electron-dense cores. Each of these cores is separated from the limiting membrane of the vesicle by an electron-lucent zone (Figure 20.28). Presumptive sensory nerve terminals

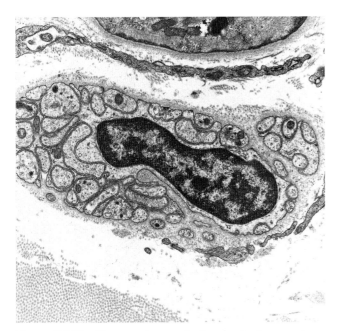

Figure 20.28 Electron micrograph of sympathetic nerve showing dense-core granules in the myocardium (original magnification ×22,500).

have large diameters and contain numerous mitochondria. They are located in perivascular regions and are surrounded by Schwann cells. A given Schwann cell may enclose adrenergic and cholinergic axons together with sensory axons (25). Autonomic ganglia are found in the subepicardial tissue of the atria and atria appendages and at the root of the great vessels, along the interatrial and AV grooves in the atrial septum and in the vicinity of the SA and AV nodes. Large nerves can be seen in the subepicardial layer adjacent to the epicardial coronary arteries.

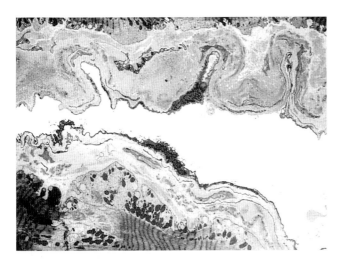

Figure 20.29 Electron micrograph showing an intramyocardial lymphatic with thin walls and no basement membrane (original magnification ×20,000).

LYMPHATICS

There are two networks of lymphatics in the heart: (a) in the endocardium and (b) in the epicardium. The route of drainage of the endocardial network is through channels in the myocardium into the epicardial lymphatics. The epicardial meshwork of channels, containing many valves, drains toward the AV sulcus by means of several longitudinal channels that run for the most part parallel to the coronary veins in the anterior and posterior longitudinal sulci of the ventricles (25). Lymphatics leave the pericardial cavity to empty into one of the pulmonary hilar lymph nodes and join the lymphatic drainage system of the mediastinum or into the thoracic duct. Lymphatics are also found in the myocardial valves and lie within the grooves of the coronary blood vessels.

The lymph capillaries and larger lymphatic vessels accompany blood vessels in the myocardial interstitium. The walls of the myocardial lymphatics consist of extremely thin endothelial cells, the nuclei of which bulge into the lumen (Figure 20.29). In contrast to endothelial cells of blood capillaries, those of the lymphatic capillaries do not have a well-defined external basal lamina. The endothelial cells of lymphatic capillaries may have Weibel-Palade bodies and transplant vesicles (25). The larger lymphatics are confined to the outer third of the myocardial wall and occasionally contain valves. These flaplike structures contain a core of collagen embedded in microfibrils and are covered by endothelium.

SMALL INTRAMURAL CORONARY ARTERIES

The structure of the intramural coronary arteries and the larger coronary arteries is similar and consists of the endothelium, smooth muscle, and adventitia (Figure 20.30).

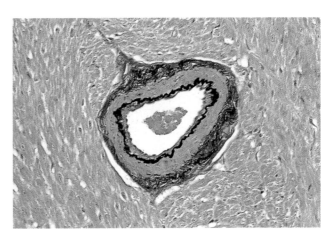

Figure 20.30 Transverse section of intramyocardial arteriole (elastic van Giesen).

These smallest muscular arteries contain three or four layers of smooth muscle. Arterioles have flat, elongated endothelial cells that do not protrude into the lumen. Their internal elastic lamina is discontinuous. Metarterioles are also known as precapillary sphincters. The endothelial cells in metarterioles have numerous surface projections that bulge into the lumen (25). Although the medial smooth muscles form a single discontinuous layer, it gradually disappears as capillaries begin. Capillaries are distinguished by the fact that their walls are composed of only a single layer of endothelial cells. They do not have smooth muscle cells but may have closely associated pericytes (25). Capillary endothelial cells may have microvilli and cytoplasmic processes (filopodia). The myocardium has a rich network of capillaries. These branches undergo anastomosis and eventually become thin-walled venules measuring up to 100 μm in diameter.

VEINS AND VENULES

Venules have thin, flat endothelial cells and characteristically contain a large amount of connective tissue in the vicinity of their external surface; they contain collagen fibrils that approach the endothelial layer and are anchored on its outer surface (25). Venules gradually increase in size to become veins. Veins have larger lumens but thinner walls than their arterial counterparts.

Veins have three layers: the intima, media, and adventitia. The intima is thin, lacks smooth muscle cells and has a poorly defined internal elastic lamina. The media is also thin and contains few smooth muscle cells and elastic fibers. The adventitia is thick with abundant collagen and elastic fibers. Cardiac veins drain blood into either the coronary sinus or directly into the chambers (thebesian veins).

THE ENDOMYOCARDIAL BIOPSY

The transvenous endomyocardial biopsy is currently utilized for the diagnosis of allograft rejection and a variety of inflammatory, metabolic, and neoplastic conditions that affect the heart. Originally introduced in the early 1960s, the bioptome and the technique have undergone modifications that now permit clinicians the opportunity to obtain cardiac tissue in a safe outpatient setting (28). The right internal jugular vein or femoral vein approaches are commonly used. Complications are uncommon and include local problems (such as hematomas and nerve injury) and cardiac problems (such as arrhythmias, tricuspid valve apparatus damage, and ventricular perforation).

Tissue Handling and Processing

Proper tissue procurement and handling are essential for optimal diagnostic evaluation (29). Biopsy specimens should

be gently extracted from the bioptome with a needle tip to limit crush artifactual distortion. The clinical indications for the biopsy determine, in large part, the method of tissue handling. For example, for standard light microscopy, the tissue should immediately be placed in a standard fixative such as 10% neutral buffered formalin. To demonstrate the type of amyloid fibril in cardiac amyloidosis by immunofluorescence (e.g., AL, AA, or transthyretin), one or two pieces should be received in saline or Zeus medium and then snap frozen in a plastic Beem capsule containing an embedding medium. The diagnosis of chronic anthracycline cardiotoxicity requires that *all* the biopsy pieces (minimum of 3–5 pieces) be submitted in fixative for transmission electron microscopy (e.g., 2.5% glutaraldehyde with 2% paraformaldehyde in 0.1M sodium cacodylate buffer, pH 7.2).

For routine diagnostic evaluation, overnight processing and paraffin embedding are sufficient. For emergent cases, a 90-minute rapid ("ultra") processing cycle is available, and microscopic slides can be prepared within three to four hours. All the biopsy pieces should be embedded in the same block. We recommend that a minimum of three slides are prepared, with each sectioned at 4 to 5 μm thickness from various depths within the paraffin block. Multiple fragments, or "ribbons," are placed on each slide.

We routinely stain with hematoxylin and eosin (H&E) and use stains such as Masson's trichrome to confirm the presence of myocyte damage or fibrosis, Congo red stain for amyloid fibrils, and the Prussian blue stain for iron deposition. Immunohistochemical, immunofluorescent, and molecular studies are utilized for specific indications. Paraffin section immunohistochemistry is used to evaluate for the presence of infectious myocarditis (e.g., cytomegalovirus (CMV) or toxoplasmic myocarditis), posttransplant lymphoproliferative disorders (PTLD) [B-cell clonality, Epstein-Barr virus (EBV) latent membrane proteins, anomalous coexpression of B-cell and T-cell antigens] or acute antibody mediated rejection (intravascular collections of CD68+ histiocytes and deposition of C4d on the microvasculature). In situ hybridization is helpful to demonstrate the presence of EBV or other viral genome or light chain restriction in PTLD.

Biopsy Limitations and Tissue Artifacts

Sampling error in the diagnosis of rejection, myocarditis, and infection remains a major consideration in the clinical management of patients and the evaluation of new noninvasive diagnostic modalities. In general, the false-negative rate is low, particularly when four or more pieces of tissue are submitted. The issue of how many lymphocytes are normally found in the myocardium has been addressed. In an endomyocardial biopsy study, the mean number of lymphocytes is fewer than 5.0 per high-power field (30).

A variety of artifacts occur in endomyocardial biopsy specimens that may mimic pathologic lesions. The surgical pathologist must be aware of these patterns to avoid a

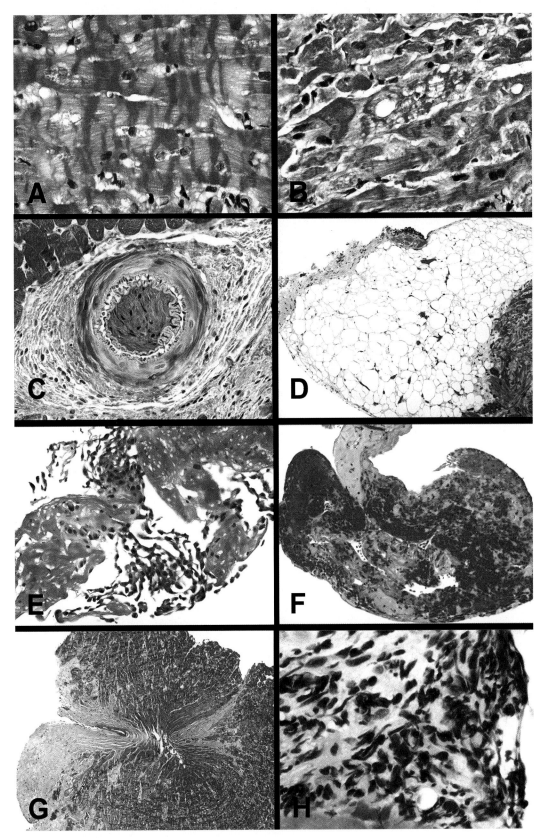

Figure 20.31 Artifacts of endomyocardial biopsy specimens: **A.** Contraction band artifact (H&E); note the normal appearance of myocyte nuclei. **B.** Contraction band necrosis with hyperchromatic py-knotic nuclei and eosinophilic cytoplasm. The changes are contrasted with the common contraction band artifact in A. **C.** Telescoping of intramyocardial is highlighted by a trichrome stain. **D.** Intramyocardial adi-pose tissue. The presence of fat does not imply epicardial localization or perforation. **E.** Mesothelial cells admixed with fibrin indicative of ventricular perforation. **F.** Thrombus without attached myocardial tis-sue. **G.** Bioptome-induced "Victorian waistband" artifact. **H.** Crush artifactual distortion of cells.

misdiagnosis that could lead to unnecessary therapeutic interventions. These have been reviewed in detail in a recent publication and only selected topics will be briefly reviewed (31). The most common biopsy artifact is the presence of contraction bands in myocytes (Figure 20.31A). They are identical to the linear bands observed in acute ischemic necrosis and catecholamine ("pressor") effect. These changes are induced by the biopsy procedure itself and can be diminished by using fixatives stored at room temperature. In ischemic injury, the nuclei of surrounding myocytes are usually pyknotic (Figure 20.31B), while in artifactually induced contraction bands, the nuclei remain normal in appearance.

Another frequent artifact is intussusception, or "telescoping," of small arteries that has been confused with luminal occlusion by thrombus and transplant-related arteriosclerosis. Connective tissue stains such as Masson's trichrome or elastic van Gieson highlight the internal elastic membranes of both vessel segments (Figure 20.31C). Intramyocardial accumulations of mature adipose tissue can simulate epicardial tissue, especially if associated with vessels of relatively large caliber (Figure 20.31D). Both can be found in the right ventricular apical region, and adipose tissue is found not uncommonly in woman and elderly patients. This should not be confused with arrhythmogenic right ventricular cardiomyopathy/dysplasia; clinical-pathologic correlation is essential for this purpose.

Ventricular perforation is identified by the presence of mesothelial cells (Figure 20.31E). Accumulations of fresh platelet- and fibrin-rich thrombus may be identified along the endocardial surface of biopsy fragments (Figure 20.31F). These form as a result of the repetitive placement of the bioptome along the endocardial surface and do not indicate chronic mural thrombi. A number of patterns of bioptome-induced tissue distortion or crush artifact can be observed in biopsy samples. The "hour-glass" or "Victorian waistband" effect is caused by central constriction of the tissue by the bioptome mechanism (Figure 20.31G). A more problematic artifact is the smearing of cytoplasmic and nuclear components of cells that yields strands of basophilic material (Figure 20.31H). In this setting, it may not be possible to distinguish the cell types (lymphocytes, endothelial cells, histiocytes, myocytes), and we do not attempt to evaluate these foci for allograft rejection or myocarditis. In some cases, procurement of additional leveled H&E-stained sections can provide less distorted foci in the deeper aspects of the biopsy sample. In our experience, immunohistochemical stains have not been consistent or helpful.

SUMMARY

Because of the structural-functional nature of cardiac disease, the surgical pathologist should have a working knowledge of both anatomy and histology. Moreover, the alterations produced by the endomyocardial biopsy and the bioptome require familiarity with the myriad of tissue artifacts. With a practical understanding of these points, the evaluation of specimens ranging from endomyocardial samples to explanted hearts will be enhanced and the diagnostic information to clinicians more precise.

REFERENCES

1. Hertz MI, Boucek, MM, Deng MC, et al. Scientific Registry of the International Society for Heart and Lung Transplantation: introduction to the 2005 annual reports. *J Heart Lung Transplant* 2005; 24:939–944.
2. Boucek MM, Edwards LB, Keck BM, Trulock EP, Taylor DO, Hertz MI. Registry of the International Society for Heart and Lung Transplantation: eighth official pediatric report—2005. *J Heart Lung Transplant* 2005;24:968–982.
3. Scholz DG, Kitzman DW, Hagen PT, Ilstrup DM, Edwards WD. Age-related changes in normal human hearts during the first 10 decades of life. Part I. (Growth): a quantitative anatomic study of 200 specimens from subjects from birth to 19 years old. *Mayo Clin Proc* 1988;63:126–136.
4. Ludwig J, ed. *Handbook of Autopsy Practice.* 3rd ed. Totowa, NJ: Humana Press; 2002.
5. Hudson R. Structure and function of the heart. In: Hudson R, ed. *Cardiovascular Pathology.* Vol 1. London: Edward Arnold; 1965: 12–23.
6. Kitzman DW, Scholz DG, Hagen PT, Ilstrup DM, Edwards WD. Age-related changes in normal human hearts during the first 10 decades of life. Part II. (Maturity): a quantitative anatomic study of 765 specimens from subjects 20 to 99 years old. *Mayo Clin Proc* 1988;63:137–146.
7. Hutchins GM, Anaya OA. Measurements of cardiac size, chamber volumes and valve orifices at autopsy. *Johns Hopkins Med J* 1973; 133:96–106.
8. Sheaff MT, Hopster DJ. Organ dissection—cardiovascular system. In: Sheaff MT, Hopster DJ. *Post Mortem Technique Handbook.* London: Springer; 2001.
9. Silver MM, Silver MD. Examination of the heart and of cardiovascular specimens in surgical pathology. In: Silver MD, Gotlieb AI, Schoen FJ, eds. *Cardiovascular Pathology.* New York: Churchill Livingstone; 2001:1–29.
10. Edwards WD. Applied anatomy of the heart. In: Brandenberg RO, Fuster V, Guiliani ER, McGoon ER eds. *Cardiology: Fundamentals and Practice.* Chicago: Year Book Medical; 1987:47–112.
11. Cook AC, Yates RW, Anderson RH. Normal and abnormal fetal cardiac anatomy. *Prenat Diagn* 2004;24:1032–1048.
12. Foley A, Mercola M. Heart induction: embryology to cardiomyocyte regeneration. *Trends Cardiovasc Med* 2004;14:121–125.
13. Gittenberger-de Groot AC, Bartelings MM, Deruiter MC, Poelmann RE. Basics of cardiac development for the understanding of congenital heart malformations. *Pediatr Res* 2005;57:169–176.
14. Pandur P. What does it take to make a heart? *Biol Cell* 2005;97: 197–210.
15. Burke A, Virmani R. Tumors of the heart and great vessels. In: *Atlas of Tumor Pathology.* 3rd series, fascicle 16. Washington, DC: Armed Forces Institute of Pathology; 1995:127–170.
16. Anderson RH, Becker AE. *The Heart: Structure in Health and Disease.* London: Gower Medical Publishing; 1992.
17. Malouf JF, Edwards WD, Tajik AJ, Seward JB. Functional anatomy of the heart. In: Fuster V, Alexander RW, O'Rouke RA, eds. *Hurst's the Heart.* 11th ed. New York: McGraw-Hill; 2004:45–86.
18. Sweeney LJ, Rosenquist GC. The normal anatomy of the atrial septum in the human heart. *Am Heart J* 1979;98:194–199.
19. Sheppard M, Davies MJ. *Practical Cardiovascular Pathology.* London: Arnold Publishers; 1998.
20. Davies MJ. Introduction to normal cardiac anatomy. In: Davies MJ, Mann JM. *The Cardiovascular System. Part B: Acquired Diseases of the Heart.* New York: Churchill Livingstone; 1995:1–6.

21. Barry A, Patten B. The structure of the adult heart. In: Gould SE, ed. *Pathology of the Heart and Blood Vessels.* Springfield, IL: Charles C Thomas; 1968:104-105.

22. James TN, Sherf L, Schlant RC, Silverman ME. Anatomy of the heart. In: Hurst JW, Logue RB, Rackley CE, et al., eds. *The Heart.* 5th ed. New York: McGraw-Hill; 1982:22–74.

23. Silver MM, Freedom RM. Gross examination and structure of the heart. In: Silver MD, ed. *Cardiovascular Pathology.* 2nd ed. Vol 1. New York: Churchill Livingstone; 1991:1–42.

24. Davies MJ, Pomerance A, Lamb D. Techniques in examination and anatomy of the heart. In: Pomerance A, Davies MJ, eds. *Pathology of the Heart.* Oxford: Blackwell Scientific; 1975:1–48.

25. Ferrans VJ, Rodríguez ER. Ultrastructure of the normal heart. In: Silver MD, ed. *Cardiovascular Pathology.* 2nd ed. New York: Churchill Livingstone; 1991:43-101.

26. Edwards WD. Cardiovascular system. In: Ludwig J, ed. *Handbook of Autopsy Practice.* 3rd ed. Totowa, NJ: Humana Press; 2002:21-44.

27. Davies MJ, Anderson RH. The pathology of the conduction system. In: Pomerance A, Davies MJ, eds. *The Pathology of the Heart.* Oxford: Blackwell Scientific; 1975:367–412.

28. Baughman KL. History and current techniques of endomyocardial biopsy. In: Baumgartner WA, Reitz B, Kasper E, Theodore J, eds. *Heart and Lung Transplantation.* 2nd ed. Philadelphia: WB Saunders; 2002:267-281.

29. Berry GJ, Billingham ME. The pathology of human cardiac transplantation. In: Baumgartner WA, Reitz B, Kasper E, Theodore J, eds. *Heart and Lung Transplantation.* Philadelphia: WB Saunders; 2002:286-306.

30. Edwards WD, Holmes DR Jr, Reeder GS. Diagnosis of active lymphocytic myocarditis by endomyocardial biopsy: quantitative criteria for light microscopy. *Mayo Clin Proc* 1982;57:419– 425.

31. Hauck AJ, Edwards WD. Histopathologic examination of tissues obtained by endomyocardial biopsy. In: Fowles RE, ed. *Cardiac Biopsy.* Mount Kisco, NY: Futura Publishing; 1992:95–153.

Serous Membranes

Darryl Carter   Lawrence True   Christopher N. Otis

ANATOMY

The mesothelium lines the pleural, pericardial, and peritoneal cavities. Mesothelial cells on the serous surfaces appear as a simple or cuboidal epithelium, although they are of mesodermal origin. They are supported by a fibrous submesothelial layer, which becomes continuous with the outer layer of invested viscera. The serous membranes show functional differentiation according to their derivation from visceral or parietal mesoderm.

Because of space limitations, description of the gross anatomy of the mesothelium must be somewhat truncated, but some areas have functional differentiation that is reflected by their histologic features. The pleura is a continuous membrane that covers the chest wall and the lungs. The visceral pleura coats the entire pulmonary surface, including the major and minor fissures that divide the lung into lobes, whereas the parietal pleura extends over the ribs, sternum, and supporting structures and is reflected over the mediastinal structures on either side. Posteriorly in the mediastinum, the two layers of parietal pleura are separated by a thin band of fibrovascular connective tissue. Superiorly, the cervical pleura is reflected into the retroclavicular area over the apex of the lung and is coated by a thickened layer of fibrous tissue and skeletal muscle; inferiorly, the diaphragmatic pleura represents its caudal extent. Anteriorly, the pleura is reflected over

part of the pericardium. The posterior visceral pleura becomes continuous with the diaphragmatic pleura over the pulmonary ligament. The heart and great vessels lie in the pericardium, which is lined by a continuous layer of mesothelium. The visceral (epicardial) side is connected to the myocardium, and the parietal (pericardial) layer rests on a dense fibrous tissue layer containing branches of the internal mammary and musculophrenic vessels, descending aorta, and branches of the vagus, phrenic, and sympathetic nerves. The thoracic surface of the pericardium is coated with parietal pleura.

The peritoneum is a nearly continuous membrane lining the potential space between the intra-abdominal viscera and the abdominal wall. In the female, it is normally interrupted by the lumina of the fallopian tubes. Anatomically, it is more complex than either the pleura or pericardium. The parietal layer covers the abdominal wall, diaphragm, anterior surfaces of the retroperitoneal viscera, and the pelvis. The visceral peritoneum invests the intestines and other intra-abdominal viscera. The elongated structures in which the parietal and visceral layers come together are the mesentery, which contains blood vessels, lymphatics, lymph nodes, and nerves.

The greater omentum is a double sheet with four layers of mesothelium between which there are numerous blood vessels and adipose tissue, which may be abundant; lymphatics and lymph nodes are less prominent than in the mesentery. The peritoneal cavity is grossly divided into the greater sac over the intestines, the retrogastric lesser sac, right and left retrocolic areas, and the pelvis. Several out-pouchings of peritoneum are often seen in pathology laboratories. Inguinal hernia sacs are pouches of parietal peritoneum, often invested with fibrous tissue and occasionally with skeletal muscle, which have been pushed through the abdominal musculature into the inguinal canal. Umbilical or ventral hernias are also outpouchings of peritoneum, but the specimens received by pathologists after surgery for their repair are usually preperitoneal fibroadipose tissue pushed ahead of the parietal peritoneum rather than mesothelium itself.

The scrotum acquires a lining of parietal mesothelium, the processus vaginalis, into which the testes descend during the seventh month of gestation. A mesothelial layer forms the surface of the tunica vaginalis. Distention of this mesothelial sac on the tunica vaginalis results in a hydro-cele—communicating with the peritoneal cavity when congenital but noncommunicating in acquired hydroceles. The sac of an inguinal hernia communicates with the peritoneal cavity and not with the mesothelium-lined space of the scrotum. Both hernia and hydrocele sacs are capable of a wide range of reactive changes.

FUNCTIONAL ANATOMY

The functional anatomy of the pleura has been described by Sahn (1) and Pistolesi et al. (2). The pleura is a continuous membrane surrounding a space that normally contains approximately 10 mL of clear colorless fluid. The surface is lined by a single layer of mesothelial cells anchored to a basement membrane that lies on layers of collagen and elastic tissue containing vascular and lymphatic vessels. The lining mesothelial cells are 16 to 40 μm in diameter, have rounded nuclei, usually containing a nucleolus, and a relatively large amount of cytoplasm. Although the visceral and parietal pleurae are opposing parts of the same continuous membrane, there are major functional differences between them.

The human visceral pleura is thick relative to that seen in some other mammals (3) and is similar to that of horses, cattle, sheep, and pigs (4). It has an arterial blood supply from the bronchial arteries, with a venous return that passes first into the pulmonary veins and then into the left atrium except for certain hilar regions that are drained by bronchial veins into the right atrium. The lymphatics that pass through the visceral pleura are the superficial layer of pulmonary lymphatics with extensive connections to the peribronchial, perivascular, and interlobular lymphatic spaces and lymphoid tissue (5). Blood and lymphatic vessels are invested by collagen and elastic fibers, which are divided into two layers: an external elastic lamina supporting

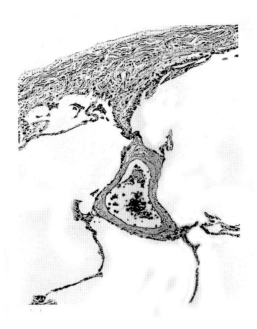

Figure 21.1 Visceral pleura. The mesothelial cells on the surface are thin, in profile, and not apparent. The dense submesothelial layer from the posterior surface of the left lower lobe is composed of collagen and elastin. It extends into adjacent pulmonary interstitium and around pulmonary vessels.

the mesothelial cells and an internal layer investing the vessels and becoming continuous with the pulmonary interstitium (Figures 21.1–21.2). Histologic identification of the layer of elastin has been considered clinically important in determining pleural invasion, which is significant for staging of primary lung cancer (6), but elastin may also be interrupted in nonneoplastic conditions that scar the pleura. In sheep, and probably in humans, the thickness of the external layer increases in both craniocaudal and ventrodorsal directions (7). The visceral pleura is innervated by branches of the vagus nerves and sympathetic nerve trunks.

The parietal pleura is anatomically, histologically, and functionally different. Although the single layer of mesothelial cells that lie on the surface of the parietal pleura are cytologically similar to those that form the continuous membrane over the visceral pleura, they are interrupted by stomata which range in size from 2 to 12 μm in diameter (8–12). The stomata communicate directly with lymphatic lacunae that are surrounded by bundles of collagen and drain directly into intercostal lymphatics and then into the mediastinum, where they are particularly dense along the retrocardiac surface (13–16). Fluid and particulate matter extravasated from the lung are collected in these lymphatics and passed into the mediastinum, where the mesothelium covers collections of macrophages called Kampmeier foci (17,18). The arterial and venous blood supply to the parietal pleura is from the intercostal through mesothelium and submesothelial stroma. Another level of control results in the relatively low protein content (1.0 to 1.5 g/dL) of pleural fluid. The point of protein regulation is unknown, although speculation is that it is at the level of mesothelial microvilli (21). In the thoracic cavity, the direction of flow appears to be via diffusion from capillaries of both visceral and parietal pleurae, with resorption primarily through parietal pleural capillaries. Turnover is estimated at 0.7 mL/hr (21) (Figure 21.3). Small molecules (less than 4 nm in diameter) diffuse through the intercellular spaces and junctions between mesothelial cells. Loss of control results in serous effusions such as those seen in congestive heart failure.

Larger molecules, up to 50 nm in diameter, are transferred across the mesothelium by pinocytotic uptake and transcellular transport. Larger structures, such as cells in bloody effusions, are transported via the stomata and "crevices." Loss of control of these mechanisms results in accumulations of exudative pleural fluid. Mesothelial cells express the secretory component of IgA, which is otherwise limited to surfaces with direct environmental contact (22). The glycoprotein-rich pleural fluid acts as a lubricant to minimize friction between visceral and parietal pleurae. The site of synthesis and mechanisms of control of the carbohydrate-rich fractions of the pleural fluid are unknown. The submesothelial connective tissue distributes mechanical

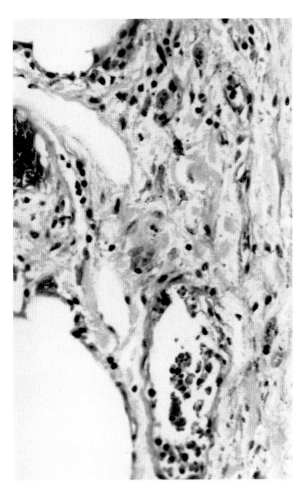

Figure 21.2 Visceral pleura. Capillaries are prominent. The lymphatics are dilated but deeply placed and entirely invested by the submesothelial layer.

vessels. The thickness of the fibroelastic layer investing the parietal pleural lymphatics is relatively constant and considerably less than that of most of the visceral pleura, suggesting that it serves as a membrane across which fluid may diffuse. The parietal pleura is innervated by branches of the intercostal nerves, which are activated in pleurisy. The structures of the peritoneum are similar to those of the pleura (19,20).

FUNCTIONS OF SEROUS MEMBRANES

The serous membranes serve as selective barrier for fluid and cells. A small volume of fluid is required for capillary action to facilitate adherence of visceral and parietal pleurae as the lungs and chest wall expand and contract. Elements of the serous membranes regulate fluid interchange to keep this fluid at a minimal level to prevent compromise of the lung volumes. Control appears to be at the capillary level because fluid is freely diffusible

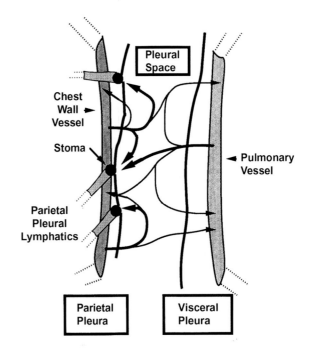

Figure 21.3 Model of the dynamics of pleural fluid formation. A transudate from capillaries in visceral and parietal pleura is partly reabsorbed by those capillaries and the rest diffuses into the pleural space, where it is resorbed via stomata into parietal pleural lymphatics.

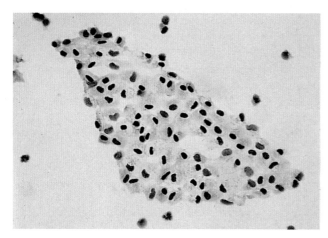

Figure 21.4 In this peritoneal wash specimen, a sheet of normal mesothelial cells has been detached.

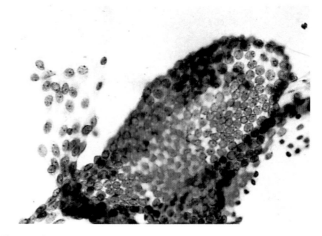

Figure 21.6 This detached fragment of reactive mesothelium shows an intact mesothelial layer with cells in two phases of the reactive process shown in Figures 21.7 and 21.8.

forces from the pleura uniformly throughout the lungs. Such a redistribution of forces is not required of the abdominal serosa. Both mesothelial cells and fibroblasts contribute to collagen synthesis.

Mesothelial Cells

Morphology

Normal mesothelial cells are rarely seen in histologic sections but may be evident in cytologic preparations of peritoneal washes taken during a laparotomy (Figure 21.4). When thus visualized, they have abundant clear cytoplasm with crisply defined cell borders, small and centrally placed nuclei with a homogeneous chromatin pattern, and usually without a nucleolus (Figure 21.5).

In a variety of reactive processes, the mesothelial cells undergo markedly proliferative and hyperplastic changes. A relatively abundant cytoplasm is maintained, but the cell borders are less sharply defined. The nuclei are larger, both absolutely and relatively, the chromatin pattern is more hyperchromatic, and nucleoli are often present and prominent (Figures 21.6–21.9).

As the hyperplastic changes in the reactive mesothelial cells progress, cell groups become smaller, and individual cells predominate. When clustered, reactive mesothelial cells present an irregular outside border. The nucleus, and especially the nucleolus, may enlarge dramatically, but the nuclei are similar in size, shape, and pattern from cell to cell. Mitotic figures may be seen. The cytoplasm may become multivacuolated as the cells degenerate and imbibe fluid (Figures 21.10–21.18).

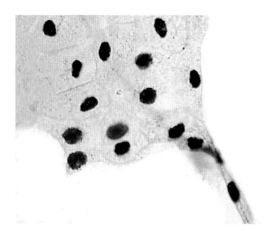

Figure 21.5 At higher magnification, a sheet of relatively normal mesothelial cells with abundant, clear cytoplasm and crisply defined cell borders. The centrally placed nuclei are small and have a homogenous chromatin.

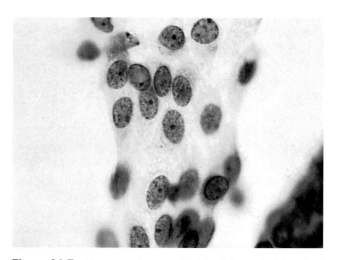

Figure 21.7 These reactive mesothelial cells from the left side of Figure 21.6 have abundant cytoplasm, and the nuclei are larger with a more vesicular chromatin pattern. Nucleoli are present but not prominent.

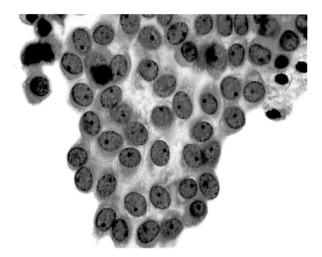

Figure 21.8 The more reactive mesothelial cells from the right side of Figure 21.6 have larger nuclei, a more vesicular chromatin pattern, and more prominently featured nucleoli. Less cytoplasm is present.

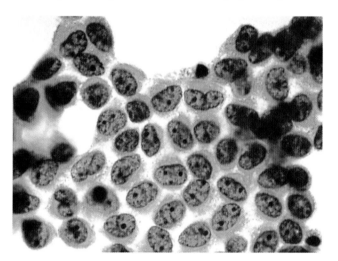

Figure 21.9 In this more reactive sheet of mesothelial cells, the cytoplasm has grown smaller and the nuclei relatively larger. Irregularity of the chromatin pattern is more prominent.

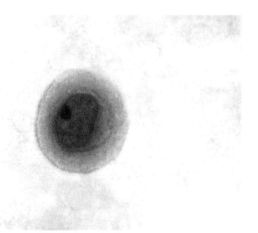

Figure 21.10 This individual reactive mesothelial cell has a restricted amount of cytoplasm and a relatively large nucleus with a nucleolus. The cell border is highly irregular and quezzy, suggesting the presence of the numerous elongated microvilli, which are evident on electron microscopy (see Figure 21.24). The cytoplasm is divided into an inner denser layer and an outer less dense layer. Ultrastructurally, the inner more dense layer corresponds to the presence of intermediate filaments with the characteristics of keratin (see Figure 21.25).

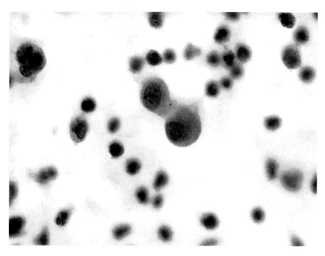

Figure 21.11 Mesothelial reaction is frequently associated with inflammatory cells. These reactive mesothelial cells are joined in pairs. Each is several times the size of either neutrophils or lymphocytes.

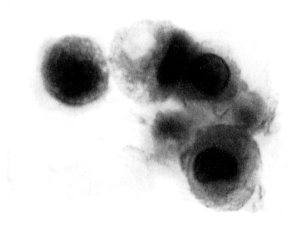

Figure 21.12 These reactive mesothelial cells are loosely joined together. The uppermost cell has a vacuole in the cytoplasm, which could be either a vesicle or an intracytoplasmic lumen.

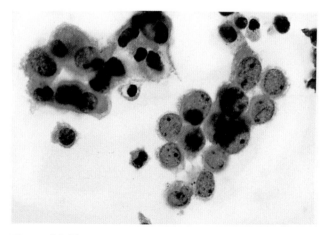

Figure 21.13 When reactive mesothelial cells are in groups, an irregular or "knobby" outside border is formed. Acini form a smooth outer border.

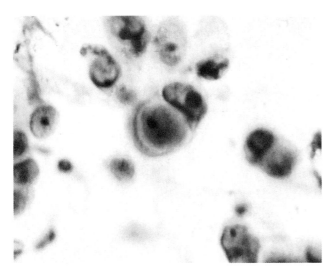

Figure 21.14 Occasionally, very reactive mesothelial cells may show cellular interactions similar to that of a keratin pearl.

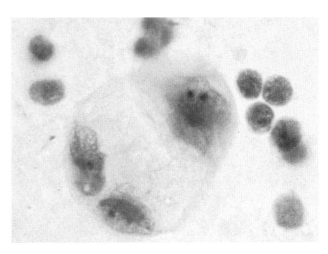

Figure 21.17 Reactive mesothelial cells may degenerate and swell. These three cells have abundant multivacuolated cytoplasm and the large nuclei of the reactive mesothelial cells.

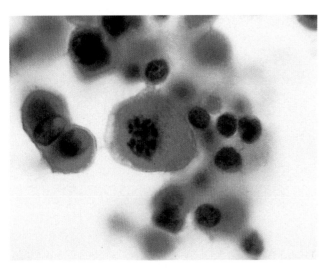

Figure 21.15 Mitotic figures may be seen in the proliferating cells of reactive mesothelium.

Histochemistry

Histochemical stains have provided information about mucoprotein content of the mesothelium. Negativity for the periodic acid-Schiff (PAS) reaction is evidence that mesothelial cells lack significant quantities of neutral mucoproteins. In contrast, positivity for histochemical stains that detect negative groups, such as the positively charged dye Alcian blue, is evidence of acid mucoproteins. That the intensity of staining reactions for acid mucosubstances is diminished by preincubating the tissue sections in hyaluronidase is evidence that at least some of the terminal hexose groups of the mucosubstances are either hyaluronic acid or chondroitin sulfate (Figure 21.19). Furthermore, the fact that histochemical mucin is decreased, but not abolished, by incubating cells in neuraminidase prior to histo-

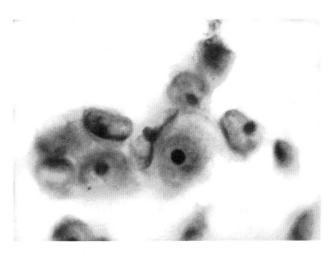

Figure 21.16 Markedly reactive mesothelial cells have large vesicular nuclei with a prominent nucleoli.

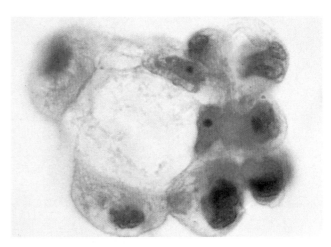

Figure 21.18 When markedly reactive mesothelial cells form irregular groups and combine with degenerating forms, they may mimic the appearance of a mucin-producing adenocarcinoma.

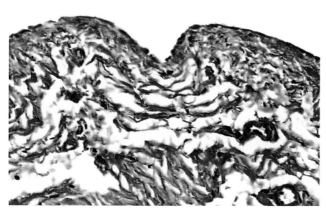

Figure 21.19 Alcian blue stain of serosal membrane. Note staining of both mesothelium and of the matrix proteins, which contain abundant acid mucoproteins.

chemical staining is evidence that some of the terminal carbohydrate groups are sialated (23). MacDougall et al. (24) have documented that neoplastic mesothelial cells may stain with mucicarmine.

The types of terminal carbohydrate groups of membrane proteins and lipids can also be characterized with lectins, which have specific and discrete ranges of sugar group affinities. Concanavalin A mesothelial cell reactivity indicates the presence of terminal groups that are either α-mannose or α-glucose.

Immunohistochemistry

Immunohistochemistry is the most commonly employed method for demonstrating mesothelial differentiation. Mesothelial cells preferentially express a group of so-called mesothelial markers (calretinin, cytokeratin 5/6, WT-1, HBME-1, thrombomodulin, and D2-40) relative to so-called epithelial markers (CEA, CD15, MOC-31, BER-EP4, B72.3, and TTF-1). However, overlap in the expression of any single marker has led to the use of a panel of antibodies to distinguish epithelium and, hence metastatic carcinoma, from reactive mesothelium.

Calretinin, a calcium-binding protein of 29 kDa with similarity to S-100 protein, is found in both the nucleus and cytoplasm of reactive and neoplastic mesothelium but is also found in some adenocarcinomas (25–28) (Figure 21.20). Cytokeratin 5 is found in the cytoplasm of most mesothelial cells and squamous cell carcinomas, but few adenocarcinomas (29); WT-1, a product of the Wilms' tumor gene, is found in the nucleus of reactive and neoplastic mesothelium and in ovarian surface epithelium and tumors derived therefrom (30). Thrombomodulin, a transmembrane glycoprotein, gives a membranous stain in about half the mesotheliomas but also in some adenocarcinomas. Mesothelial cells also express mesothelin, epithe-

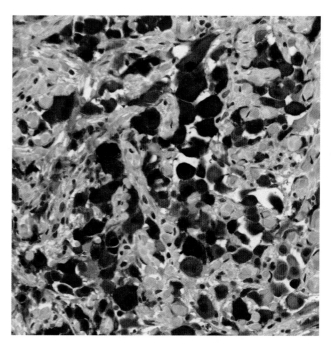

Figure 21.20 Immunohistochemical staining of mesothelial cells for calretinin. Note the nuclear and cytoplasmic staining.

lial membrane antigen (EMA), N-cadherin, E-cadherin, and vimentin (31). Recently, D2-40 (a marker of lymphatic epithelium) has been reported to identify mesothelial cells with a high sensitivity, but it also marks ovarian serous carcinoma (32).

Mesothelial cells usually lack the glycoproteins detected by antibodies to CEA, MOC-31 and BER-EP4 and the determinant detected by Leu-M1 (CD15) (33–36). Latza et al. (37) and Sheibani et al. (38) reported that BER-EP4 was used to distinguish malignant epithelium (adenocarcinoma) from malignant mesothelioma, but Gaffey et al. (39) and Otis (40) reported BER-EP4 immunoreactivity in high proportions of both benign and malignant mesothelial tumors, as well as adenocarcinomas. The tissue specific nuclear transcription protein TTF-1 is important in embryogenesis of thyroid and lung and is found in nuclei of pneumocytes and many adenocarcinomas of the lung but not in mesothelium (41).

Overlap between reactive and neoplastic mesothelium in the expression of even a panel of antibodies leaves only the demonstration of invasion of parietes or organs to confirm the diagnosis of malignant mesothelioma in most cases. The diagnosis of mesothelioma-in-situ requires demonstration of invasive mesothelioma elsewhere in the same specimen or in a subsequent specimen.

Nonproliferating mesothelial cells express both vimentin and a variety of keratins (K7 of 55 kDa, K8 of 53 kDa, K18 of 44 kDa, and K19 of 40 kDa) that can be detected with monoclonal antibodies immunoreactive with the small, acidic, type I keratins (42) (Figures 21.21–21.22).

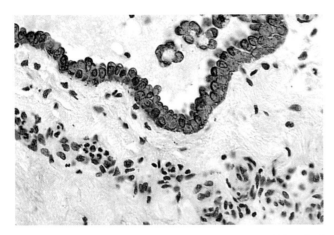

Figure 21.21 Keratin expression by mesothelium and detached mesothelial cells, demonstrated by a mixture of monoclonal anti-keratin antibodies (AE1/AE3). Note that the immunohistochemical pattern of staining is similar to the distribution of intermediate filaments seen at the ultrastructural level.

Mesothelium does not express cytokeratin 20, using monoclonal antibodies (43). These keratins are distinct from those of epithelia, including the epidermis, glandular epithelia, and transitional epithelium (44). Ovarian epithelial tumors express a spectrum of keratins similar to that of mesothelium (44).

The plasticity of the immunophenotype of mesothelial cells is demonstrable in abnormal states. Although mesothelium normally lacks sex steroid receptors, reactive mesothelium adjacent to endometriosis expresses focal immunoreactivity for estrogen and progesterone receptors (45). Furthermore, reactive mesothelial cells can express the muscle cell cytoskeleton proteins desmin and muscle-specific actin (46). There is experimental evidence that the pattern of intermediate filament expression by mesothelial cells is dependent on shape and cell-cell interaction. Induction of a spindle morphology inhibits keratin synthesis.

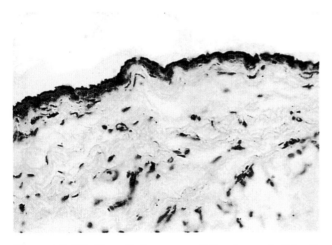

Figure 21.22 Vimentin immunoreactivity of mesothelial cells and fibroblasts.

In contrast, induction of an epithelioid morphology (for example, with retinoids) stimulates keratin synthesis and inhibits vimentin synthesis; the ability of cells to respond in this manner also depends on the presence of cell-cell interactions (47). The pattern of intermediate filament expression by intact mesothelium has not been analyzed in such detail (Figures 21.20–21.21).

Ultrastructure

Numerous long microvilli (Figures 21.23–21.24), measuring up to 3 μm in length and 0.1 μm in diameter, are present and are more numerous in caudal portions of the parietal pleura and in the visceral pleura. The other organelles found in mesothelial cells are not specific for them. Junctions of all types are found—tight junctions that serve as a barrier to certain molecules, gap junctions for cell-cell transport, and desmosomes for cell-cell adherence. Intermediate filaments are somewhat prominent; although they do not aggregate into bundles, they are often arranged in a perinuclear, circumferential distribution (Figures 21.25–21.26).

Submesothelial Layer

Normally, the submesothelial layer contains few cells, and most of these are fibroblasts. Much of the submesothelial layer is composed of collagen, elastin, and other extracellular proteins. During reactive processes, the submesothelial layer may become much more prominent as cells proliferate there.

Histochemistry

The main constituents of the submesothelial tissue are glycosylated proteins, including glycosaminoglycans. Because the majority of carbohydrate groups are negatively charged (as a result of an abundance of hyaluronic acid and other acidic groups), this extracellular matrix stains in a manner characteristic of acidic mucoproteins; that is, it is Alcian blue–positive (Figure 21.19). That staining intensity can be diminished by treating the section with hyaluronidase before histochemical staining is evidence that hyaluronic acid groups are responsible, in large part, for the intensity of staining (21).

Immunohistochemistry

The antigens of the submesothelial layer can be categorized into matrix constituents and antigens of the mesenchymal cells. The extracellular matrix materials are those typical of most connective tissue. Types I and III collagen and fibronectin are abundant. Elastin fibers are plentiful and basement membrane proteins, including type IV collagen and laminin, are found at the mesothelial cell-stromal interface.

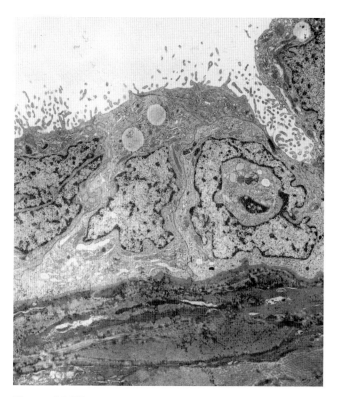

Figure 21.23 Mesothelial cells with their elongated microvilli, cover the surface of the serosa. The subjacent stroma is composed of collagen and fibroblasts.

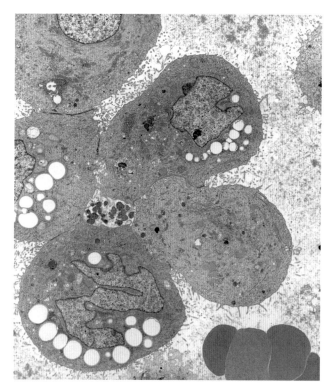

Figure 21.24 EM of a cluster of detached mesothelial cells within a pleural effusion. Cytoplasmic lipid droplets impart a vacuolated appearance to some cells. Note the long microvilli, which impart the "fuzzy" appearance to these cells at the light microscopic level.

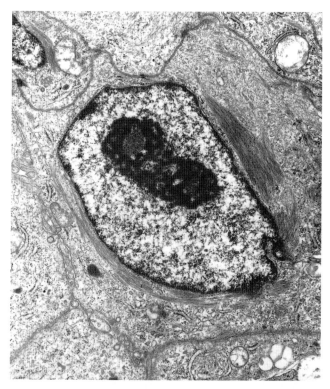

Figure 21.25 Ultrastructure of a mesothelial cell. Intermediate filaments are arranged in a perinuclear distribution.

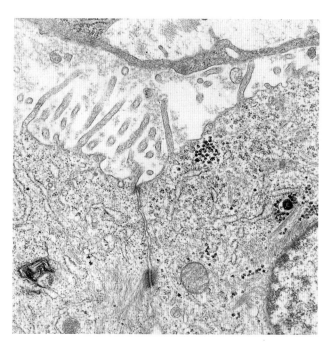

Figure 21.26 High magnification of the luminal aspect of two mesothelial cells. Note the small tight junction, subjacent desmosome, and the cytoskeletal filaments within the microvilli.

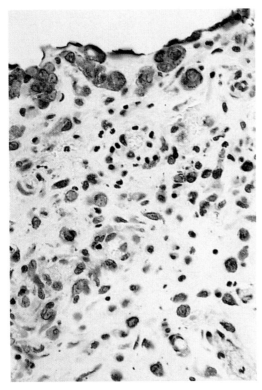

Figure 21.27   Keratin (AE1/AE3) immunoreactivity of proliferating submesothelial spindle cells.

Proteoglycans are plentiful. The pattern of intermediate filament expression by the submesothelial stromal cells varies with their state of "excitation." Quiescent cells contain only vimentin, but stromal cells in regions of injury or inflammation also synthesize keratin detectable with antibodies to type I keratins (47) (Figure 21.27).

RELATIONSHIP OF MESOTHELIAL AND SUBMESOTHELIAL CELLS

The submesothelial mesenchymal cell population serves as the anchoring substratum for the mesothelium. Both mesothelial and submesothelial cells contribute to the extracellular proteins that comprise the matrix. Up to 3% of the total protein synthesized by mesothelial cells are collagens and laminin.

A controversial topic is whether submesothelial cells serve as a source of mesothelial cell renewal, either in normal development, which is the basis for regarding mesothelial cells as mesodermal in origin, or in conditions of rapid mesothelial cell turnover. Earlier ultrastructural and kinetics studies, using thymidine incorporation, suggested that the stromal cells contribute to the repopulation of denuded mesothelium (48,49). Consistent with this scheme is the observation that submesothelial cells, when stimulated to proliferate, synthesize keratin and assume a

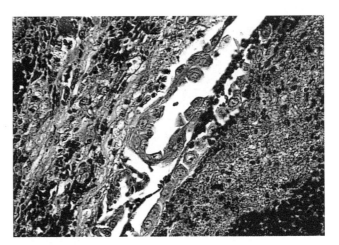

Figure 21.28   In a variety of reactive processes, the mesothelial cells lining serosal surfaces undergo markedly proliferative and hyperplastic changes. This is a section through the pleura of a patient with severe active rheumatoid arthritis.

more epithelioid morphology. However, later studies have demonstrated that healing of injured serosa progresses by multiplication and migration of mesothelial cells at the edges of the wounded area (50).

Reactive Mesothelium

The capacity for mesothelial and submesothelial cellular elements of serous membranes to react and proliferate to produce morphologic patterns mimicking neoplasia is well known and frequently a source of diagnostic confusion (51,52). The process may be diffuse or localized (Figure 21.28). Mesothelial hyperplasia in herniorrhaphy specimens is well described (53) and may be nodular, demonstrate nuclear atypia and frequent mitotic figures, and be accompanied by spindle cell elements (Figures 21.29–21.30).

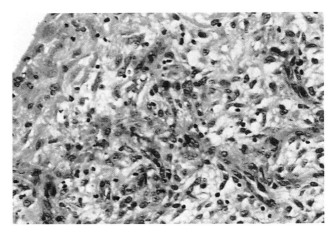

Figure 21.29   This photomicrograph is from a hernia sac of an 18-month-old boy. The reactive mesothelium is composed of proliferative epithelioid cells on the surface and subjacent spindle-shaped cells that give the impression of proliferating fibroblasts.

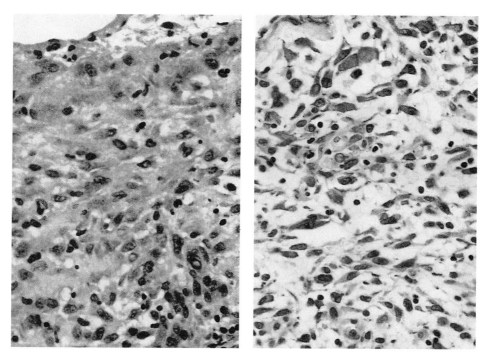

Figure 21.30 The reactive peritoneum in the hernia sac shown in Figure 21.29 (**A**). The immuno-histochemical stain for keratin (AE1/AE3) (**B**) illustrates that both the surface lining mesothelial cells and the subjacent spindle-shaped cells are heavily decorated.

Reactive mesothelial cells in mediastinal lymph nodes have been reported by Brooks et al. (54) and Parkash et al. (55), although the mechanisms by which they enter lymphatics and survive in the sinuses of nodes are not known. This rare event may produce a difficult differential diagnosis. Clear demonstration of the mesothelial nature of these cells is necessary to exclude metastatic carcinoma. If the cells are shown to be mesothelial by electron microscopy or immunohistochemistry, it should be noted that Sussman and Rosai (56) reported that mesothelioma may present as a

lymph node metastasis. Therefore, follow-up may be required to make the distinction between reactive benign mesothelial cells and metastatic malignant ones (Figures 21.31–21.32).

An uncommon manifestation of mesothelial proliferation is the psammoma body—a laminated calcific structure that most likely arises through concentric calcification following cell death. Psammoma bodies are usually nonspecific because they may be observed in inflammatory processes accompanied by mesothelial hyperplasia, malignant mesothelial neoplasia, or epithelial neoplasia (Figure 21.33).

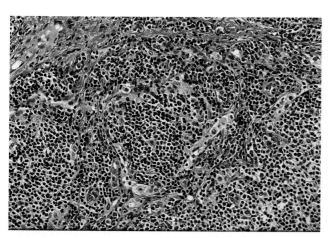

Figure 21.31 Internal mammary lymph node with large epithelioid cells in the sinuses found during coronary artery bypass graft surgery in a 61-year-old man. No pleural lesion was present.

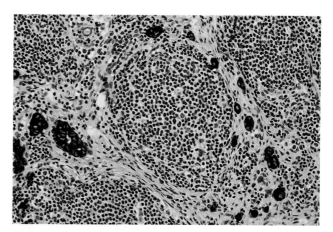

Figure 21.32 Immunohistochemical stain for keratin AE1/AE3 demonstrates the epithelioid cells that were negative for CEA, Leu-M1, BER-EP4, and B72.3 and hence are considered reactive mesothelial cells.

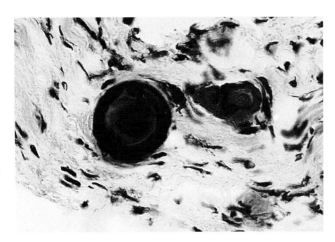

Figure 21.33 Psammoma bodies in the left pelvic peritoneum of a 58-year-old female.

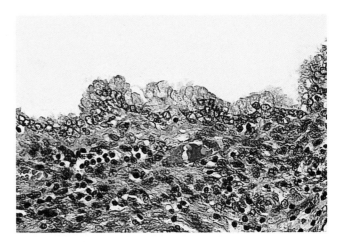

Figure 21.35 Endosalpingiosis involving the omentum contains cystic glands lined by mucinous epithelium with basally oriented nuclei and apical cytoplasm. Periglandular stroma contains mononuclear inflammatory cells.

Endosalpingiosis and Endometriosis

Epithelial elements may be observed in glandular arrangements throughout the peritoneum, omentum, and within lymph nodes. Such glandular structures were recognized in the early 1900s and misinterpreted by some as metastatic carcinoma, a mistake that is unfortunately still committed today. Endometriosis and endosalpingiosis were expounded upon by Sampson (57–59) earlier in this century, with reference to mechanisms of pathogenesis that are still debatable.

Endosalpingiosis refers to glandular spaces lined by epithelium similar to uterine tube epithelium, with three cell types (ciliated, secretory, and intercalated cells) (60) (Figure 21.34). On occasion, psammoma bodies are present. Periglandular stroma containing chronic inflammatory cells is separated from epithelium by PAS-positive basement membrane. Endosalpingiosis may be differentiated from endometriosis by the lack of endometrial stroma or evidence of stromal hemorrhage associated with endometriosis (57,60–63). This condition is seen exclusively in women and has been reported in 12.5% of omenta removed at surgery in females. A large proportion of these

women have coexisting benign disease of the uterine tube (60). The origin of the glandular inclusions is debated but is most likely either related to the influence of müllerian development on the peritoneal mesothelium (coelomic lining) or is a sequela of disease within the uterine tube resulting in extratubal growth of displaced tubal epithelium (60,62). Although definitive evidence of neoplasia arising in endosalpingiosis has not been documented (64), considerable difficulty may be encountered when differentiating extraovarian tumor implants removed in the setting of common epithelial ovarian tumors from endosalpingiosis with cellular atypia. Evaluation of the severity of epithelial atypia, mitotic activity, the presence of ciliated cells, and the presence of invasive characteristics may aid in establishing malignancy in this setting (60). Metaplasia in endosalpingiosis may also be a source of diagnostic difficulty—particularly mucinous metaplasia, which may be mistaken for metastatic mucinous adenocarcinoma (Figures 21.35–21.36).

Endometriosis may be defined by the presence of glands lined by endometrial-type epithelium surrounded by endometrial stroma, outside the uterine endometrial mucosa

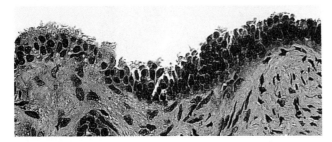

Figure 21.34 Endosalpingiosis involving the serosa of the uterus of a 56-year-old woman. Serous, intercalated, and occasional ciliated cells are present, but endometrial stroma is not.

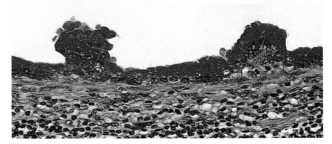

Figure 21.36 Mucicarmine stain of mucinous change in endosalpingiosis demonstrates intracytoplasmic mucin in apical cytoplasm.

and myometrium (64). The condition occurs most frequently in women of childbearing age. It may occur in a variety of body sites, ranging from the pelvic peritoneum to distant organs such as lung, kidney, and skin, but the most frequent site is the peritoneal lining of the pelvic organs (Figure 21.37). Although the histogenesis of endometriosis remains unclear, two general theories have been proposed. The ectopic growth of endometrial elements may result from displacement of endometrial tissue, whether through local means (such as entry of endometrium into the pelvis through the uterine tubes) or via vascular routes to distant organs (57,58). Another possibility includes metaplastic change of the pelvic peritoneum along müllerian lines of differentiation (65,66). Each mechanism may play a role in the histogenesis of endometriosis.

Endometriosis may appear as brown-maroon foci on the peritoneal surfaces and be accompanied by fibrosis or adhesions. Microscopically, endometrial stroma surrounding endometrial epithelium is present (67). Response to hormonal influences is often seen and may be synchronous with intrauterine endometrium. Metaplasia occurs in both epithelial and stromal elements, similar to metaplasias encountered in the endometrium of the uterus. The presence of hemosiderin-laden macrophages and fibrosis may be the only evidence that endometriosis had once been present. However, a definitive diagnosis of endometriosis may not be rendered unless both endometrial glands and stroma are seen.

Another common type of metaplasia, more frequently observed in pregnant than in nonpregnant women, is decidual change. Although usually encountered in the submesothelial layer of pelvic peritoneal surfaces, decidual change may be seen in distant sites including the serosal surfaces of the liver, spleen, diaphragm, and within lymph nodes. In these locations, decidual change may be mistaken for metastatic carcinoma or malignant mesothelioma (Figure 21.38) (66).

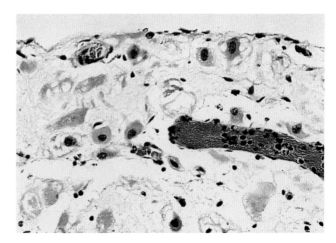

Figure 21.38 Decidual change in the pelvis during pregnancy is seen in subserosal tissue. Loosely cohesive cells with abundant eosinophilic cytoplasm are present.

Fibrous Pleurisy

Fibrous pleurisy is a benign reactive process that usually occurs in the setting of organizing pleural effusions. The differential diagnosis of fibrous pleurisy and desmoplastic mesothelioma may be extremely difficult: both may have regions of increased cellularity in a predominantly fibrous background containing spindle cells that are immunoreactive to keratin antibodies. Fibrous pleurisy tends to have a higher cellularity immediately beneath the fibrinous exudative surface of the pleura and demonstrates a "layering" of spindle cells parallel to the fibrosis with intervening fibrinous exudate. This organization imparts a histologic sense of order to the reactive process that may assist in its recognition. Invasion, bland necrosis, and sarcomatous foci are not seen in fibrous pleurisy (67,68) (Figure 21.39).

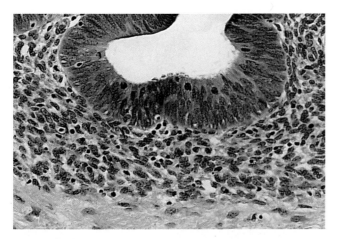

Figure 21.37 Endometriosis involving the peritoneum with extension into the soft tissue of the anterior abdominal wall of a 23-year-old woman. Endometrial glands and stroma are present.

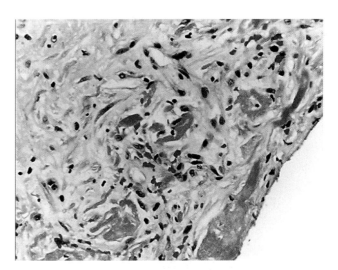

Figure 21.39 The histologic appearance of fibrous pleurisy reflects its inflammatory nature, with granulation tissue, fibrin, and a zonal pattern ranging from active inflammation to quiescent dense fibrosis.

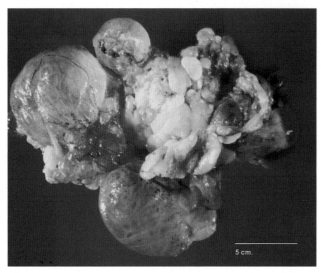

Figure 21.40 Multilocular peritoneal inclusion cyst in the omentum of a 73-year-old patient discovered incidentally at surgery for urogynecologic repair procedure. The cysts vary in size, some being translucent while others are fibrotic, particularly toward the center of the mass.

Multilocular Peritoneal Inclusions Cyst

Multilocular peritoneal inclusions cyst (MPIC) is a mesothelial-lined multilocular lesion that occurs almost exclusively in women. The lesion usually involves the pelvis, although it may occur in other abdominal locations,

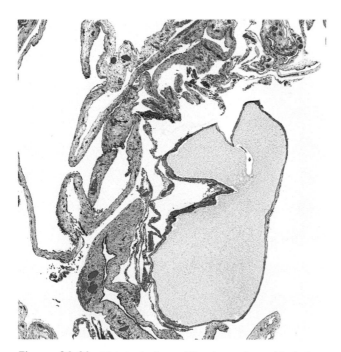

Figure 21.41 Histologically, multilocular peritoneal inclusions cysts (MPIC) reflect the gross features, with septae that vary in thickness and cysts that vary in size.

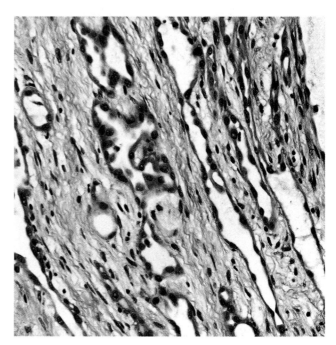

Figure 21.42 Some regions in multilocular peritoneal inclusions cysts may contain mesothelial proliferations that closely resemble an adenomatoid tumor.

including the omentum and mesentery. Usually MPIC is mass forming and may attain diameters up to 20 cm. Grossly, it is composed of multiple cysts, some of which may be thinwalled and translucent (Figure 21.40). Histologically, the septa range from thin and delicate to thickened and inflamed. The mesothelial lining ranges from single flattened cells to hobnail-type cells. Squamous metaplasia of the lining mesothelium may be present. Some regions may resemble the cellular pattern of an adenomatoid tumor (Figures 21.41–21.42) (69).

The true nature of MPIC remains somewhat controversial, with some authors maintaining that it is a neoplasm while others assert it is a reactive lesion that develops in response to injury or even endometriosis. The original designation of *multicystic mesothelioma* reflects the notion that the lesion is neoplastic. Recurrences are frequent, although MPIC-related deaths probably do not occur (70).

REFERENCES

1. Sahn SA. State of the art: the pleura. *Am Rev Respir Dis* 1988;138:184–234.
2. Pistolesi M, Miniati M, Giuntini C. Pleural liquid and solute exchanges. *Am Rev Respir Dis* 1989;140:825–847.
3. Courtice FC, Simmonds WJ. Absorption of fluids from the pleural cavities of rabbits and cats. *J Physiol* 1949;109:117–130.
4. Albertine KH, Wiener-Kronish JP, Roos PJ, Staub NC. Structure, blood supply, and lymphatic vessels of the sheep's visceral pleura. *Am J Anat* 1982;:165:227–294.
5. Grant T, Levin B. Lymphangiographic visualization of pleural and pulmonary lymphatics in a patient without a chylothorax. *Radiology* 1974;113:49–50.

6. Gallagher B, Urbanski SJ. The significance of pleural elastica invasion by lung carcinomas. *Hum Pathol* 1990;21:512–517.

7. Mariassy AT, Wheeldon EB. The pleura: a combined light microscopic, scanning, and transmission electron microscopic study in the sheep. I. Normal pleura. *Exp Lung Res* 1983;4:293–314.

8. Albertine KM, Wiener-Kronish JP, Staub NC. The structure of the parietal pleura and its relationship to pleural liquid dynamics in sheep. *Anat Rec* 1984;208:401–409.

9. Leak LV. Gross and ultrastructural morphologic features of the diaphragm. *Am Rev Respir Dis* 1979;119(pt 2):3–21.

10. Wang NS. The preformed stomas connecting the pleural cavity and the lymphatics in the parietal pleura. *Am Rev Respir Dis* 1975;111:12–20.

11. Wang NS. Morphological data of pleura. Normal conditions. In: Chretien J, Hirsch A, eds. *Diseases of the Pleura.* New York: Masson; 1983:10–24.

12. Wang NS. Anatomy and physiology of the pleural space. *Clin Chest Med* 1985;6:3–16.

13. Bernaudin JF, Fleury J. Anatomy of the blood and lymphatic circulation of the pleural serosa. In: Chretien J, Bignon J, Hirsch A, eds. *The Pleura in Health and Disease.* Vol. 30. New York: Marcel Dekker; 1985:101–124.

14. Cooray GH. Defense mechanism in the mediastinum with special reference to the mechanism of pleural absorptions. *J Pathol Bacteriol* 1949;6:551–567.

15. Courtice FC, Simmonds WJ. Physiological significance of lymph drainage of the serous cavities and lungs. *Physiol Rev* 1954;34:419–448.

16. Staub NC, Wiener-Kronish JP, Albertine KH. Transport through the pleura. Physiology of normal liquid and solute exchange in the pleural space. In: Chretien J, Bignon J, Hirsch A, eds. *The Pleura in Health and Disease.* New York: Marcel Dekker; 1985:169–193.

17. Kampmeier OF. Concerning certain mesothelial thickenings and vascular plexuses of the mediastinal pleura associated with histiocyte and fat-cell production, in the human newborn. *Anat Rec* 1928;39:201–208.

18. Mixter RL. On macrophagal foci ("milky spots") in the pleura of different mammals, including man. *Am J Anat* 1941;69:159–186.

19. Nagel W, Kuschinsky W. Study of the permeability of the isolated dog mesentery. *Eur J Clin Invest* 1970;1:149–154.

20. Tslibari E, Wissig SL. Lymphatic absorption from the peritoneal cavity: regulation of patency of mesothelioma stomata. *Microvasc Res* 1983;25:220–239.

21. Chretien J, Bignon J, Hirsch A, eds. *The Pleura in Health and Disease.* Vol 30. New York: Marcel Dekker; 1985.

22. Ernst CS, Brooks JJ. Immunoperoxidase localization of secretory component in reactive mesothelium and mesotheliomas. *J Histochem Cytochem* 1981;29:1102–1104.

23. Roth J. Ultrahistochemical demonstration of saccharide components of complex carbohydrates at the alveolar cell surface and at the mesothelial cell surface of the pleura visceralis of mice by means of concanavalin A. *Exp Pathol (Jena)* 1973;8:157–167.

24. MacDougall DB, Wang SE, Zidar BL. Mucin-positive epithelial mesothelioma. *Arch Pathol Lab Med* 1992;116:874–880.

25. Doglioni C, Tos AP, Laurino L, et al. Calretinin: a novel immunocytochemical marker for mesothelioma. *Am J Surg Path* 1996;20:1037–1046.

26. Nagel H, Hemmerlein B, Ruschenburg I, Huppe K, Droese M. The value of anti-calretinin antibody in the differential diagnosis of normal and reactive mesothelia versus metastatic tumors in effusion cytology. *Pathol Res Pract* 1998;194:759–764.

27. Oates J, Edwards C. HBME-1, MOC-31, WT1 and calretinin: an assessment of recently described markers for mesothelioma and adenocarcinoma. *Histopathology* 2000;36:341–347.

28. Fetsch PA, Simsir A, Abati A. Comparison of antibodies to HBME-1 and calretinin for the detection of mesothelial cells in effusion cytology. *Diagn Cytopathol* 2001;25:158–161.

29. Chu PG, Weiss LM. Expression of cytokeratin 5/6 in epithelial neoplasms: an immunohistochemical study of 509 cases. *Mod Pathol* 2002;15:6–10.

30. Hecht JL, Lee BH, Pinkus JL, Pinkus GS. The value of Wilms tumor susceptibility gene 1 in cytologic preparations as a marker for malignant mesothelioma. *Cancer* 2002;96:105–109.

31. Ordonez NG. The immunohistochemical diagnosis of mesothelioma: a comparative study of epithelioid mesothelioma and lung adenocarcinoma. *Am J Surg Pathol* 2003;27:1031–1051.

32. Chu AY, Litzky LA, Pasha TL, Acs G, Zhang PJ. Utility of D2-40, a novel mesothelial marker, in the diagnosis of malignant mesothelioma. *Mod Pathol* 2005;18:105–110.

33. Otis CN, Carter D, Cole S, Battifora H. Immunohistochemical evaluation of pleural mesothelioma and pulmonary adenocarcinoma. A bi-institutional study of 47 cases. *Am J Surg Pathol* 1987;11:445–456.

34. Sheibani K, Battifora H, Burke JS, Rappaport H. Leu-M1 antigen in human neoplasms: an immunohistologic study of 400 cases. *Am J Surg Pathol* 1986;10:227–236.

35. Sheibani K, Esteban JM, Bailey A, Battifora H, Weiss LM. Immunopathologic and molecular studies as an aid to the diagnosis of malignant mesothelioma. *Hum Pathol* 1992;23:107–116.

36. Sheibani K. Immunopathology of malignant mesothelioma. *Hum Pathol* 1994;25:219–220.

37. Latza U, Niedobitek G, Schwarting R, Nekarda H, Stein H. Ber-EP4: new monoclonal antibody which distinguishes epithelia from mesothelia. *J Clin Pathol* 1990;43:213–219.

38. Sheibani K, Shin SS, Kezirian J, Weiss LM. Ber-EP4 antibody as a discriminant in the differential diagnosis of malignant mesothelioma versus adenocarcinoma. *Am J Surg Pathol* 1991;15:779–784.

39. Gaffey MJ, Mills SE, Swanson PE, Zarbo RJ, Shah AR, Wick MR. Immunoreactivity for Ber-EP4 in adenocarcinomas, adenomatoid tumors, and malignant mesotheliomas. *Am J Surg Pathol* 1992;16:593–599.

40. Otis CN. Uterine adenomatoid tumors: immunohistochemical characteristics with emphasis on Ber-EP4 immunoreactivity and distinction from adenocarcinoma. *Int J Gynecol Pathol* 1996;15:146–151.

41. Ordonez NG. Value of thyroid transcription factor-1, E-cadherin, BG8, WT1 and CD44S immunostaining in distinguishing epithelial pleural mesothelioma from pulmonary and nonpulmonary adenocarcinoma. *Am J Surg Pathol* 2000;24:598–606.

42. Wu YJ, Parker LM, Binder NE, et al. The mesothelial keratins: a new family of cytoskeletal proteins identified in cultured mesothelial cells and nonkeratinizing epithelia. *Cell* 1982;31(pt 2):693–703.

43. Moll R, Lowe A, Laufer J, Franke WW. Cytokeratin 20 in human carcinomas. A new histodiagnostic marker detected by monoclonal antibodies. *Am J Pathol* 1992;140:427–447.

44. Moll R, Franke WW, Schiller DL, Geiger B, Krepler R. The catalog of human cytokeratins: patterns of expression in normal epithelia, tumors and cultured cells. *Cell* 1982;31:11–24.

45. Nakayama K, Masuzawa H, Li S, et al. Immunohistochemical analysis of the peritoneum adjacent to endometriotic lesions using antibodies for Ber-EP4 antigen, estrogen receptors, and progesterone receptors: implication of peritoneal metaplasia in the pathogenesis of endometriosis. *Int J Gynecol Pathol* 1994;13:348–358.

46. Pitt MA, Haboubi NY. Serosal reaction in chronic gastric ulcers: an immunohistochemical and ultrastructural study. *J Clin Pathol* 1995;48:226–228.

47. Bolen JW, Hammer SP, McNutt MA. Reactive and neoplastic serosal tissue. A light-microscopic, ultrastructural and immunocytochemical study. *Am J Surg Path* 1986;10:34–47.

48. Raftery AT. Regeneration of parietal and visceral peritoneum in the immature animal: a light and electron microscopical study. *Br J Surg* 1973;60:969–975.

49. Raftery AT. Regeneration of parietal and visceral peritoneum: an electron microscopical study. *J Anat* 1984;115(pt 3):375–392.

50. Whitaker D, Papadimitriou JM. Mesothelial healing: morphological and kinetic investigations. *J Pathol* 1985;145:159–175.

51. Ackerman LV. Tumors of the retroperitoneum, mesentery, and peritoneum. In: *Atlas of Tumor Pathology.* 6th series, fascicle 23, 24. Washington, DC; Armed Forces Institute of Pathology; 1954.

52. McCaughey WTE, Kannerstein M, Churg J. Tumors and pseudotumors of the serous membranes. In: *Atlas of Tumor Pathology.* 2nd series, fascicle 20. Washington, DC: Armed Forces Institute of Pathology; 1983.

53. Rosai J, Dehner LP. Nodular mesothelial hyperplasia in hernia sacs: a benign reactive condition simulating a neoplastic process. *Cancer* 1975;35:165–175.

54. Brooks JS, LiVolsi VA, Pietra GG. Mesothelial cell inclusions in mediastinal lymph nodes mimicking metastatic carcinoma. *Am J Clin Pathol* 1990;93:741–748.

55. Parkash V, Vidwans M, Carter D. Benign mesothelial cells in mediastinal lymph nodes. *Am J Surg Pathol* 1999;23:1264–1269.

56. Sussman J, Rosai J. Lymph node metastasis as the initial manifestation of malignant mesothelioma: report of six cases. *Am J Surg Path* 1990;14:819–828.

57. Sampson JA. Heterotopic or misplaced endometrial tissue. *Am J Obstet Gynecol* 1925;10:649–664.

58. Sampson JA. Postsalpingectomy endometriosis (endosalpingiosis). *Am J Obstet Gynecol* 1930;20:443–480.

59. Sampson JA. The pathogenesis of postsalpingectomy endometriosis in laparotomy scars. *Am J Obstet Gynecol* 1946;50:597–620.

60. Zinsser KR, Wheeler JE. Endosalpingiosis in the omentum: a study of autopsy and surgical material. *Am J Surg Pathol* 1982;6:109–117.

61. Hsu YK, Parmley TH, Rosenshein NB, Bhagavan BS, Woodruff JD. Neoplastic and non-neoplastic mesothelial proliferations in pelvic lymph nodes. *Obstet Gynecol* 1980;55:83–88.

62. Horn LC, Bilek K. Frequency and histogenesis of pelvic retroperitoneal lymph node inclusions of the female genital tract. An immunohistochemical study of 34 cases. *Pathol Res Pract* 1995;191:991–996.

63. Schnurr RC, Delgado G, Chun B. Benign glandular inclusions in para-aortic lymph nodes in women undergoing lymphadenectomies. *Am J Obstet Gynecol* 1978;130:813–816.

64. Clement PB. Endometriosis, lesions of the secondary müllerian system, and pelvic mesothelial proliferations. In: Kurman RJ, ed. *Blaustein's Pathology of the Female Genital Tract.* 3rd ed. New York: Springer-Verlag;1987:517–559.

65. Ferguson BR, Bennington JL, Haber SL. Histochemistry of mucosubstances and histology of mixed müllerian pelvic lymph node glandular inclusions: evidence for histogenesis by müllerian metaplasia on coelomic epithelium. *Obstet Gynecol* 1969;33:617–625.

66. Lauchlan SC. The secondary müllerian system. *Obstet Gynecol Surv* 1972;27:133–146.

67. Churg A, Colby TV, Cagle P, et al. The separation of benign and malignant mesothelial proliferations. *Am J Surg Pathol* 2000;24:1183–1200.

68. Mangano WE, Cagle PT, Churg A, Vollmer RT, Roggli VL. The diagnosis of desmoplastic malignant mesothelioma and its distinction from fibrous pleurisy: a histologic and immunohistochemical analysis of 31 cases including p53 immunostaining. *Am J Clin Pathol* 1998;110:191–199.

69. Clement PB. Reactive tumor-like lesions of the peritoneum. *Am J Clin Pathol* 1995;103:673–676.

70. Weiss SW, Tavassoli FA. Multicystic mesothelioma. An analysis of pathologic findings and biologic behavior in 37 cases. *Am J Surg Pathol* 1988;12:737–746.

ALIMENTARY TRACT

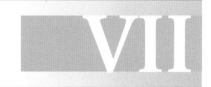

Esophagus

Franco G. DeNardi   Robert H. Riddell

EMBRYOLOGY

In the early stages of development, the notochord induces the formation of the foregut from endoderm (1). At about 21 days' gestation, septa arise from the lateral walls of the foregut, fuse, and divide the foregut into the esophagus and trachea. This process of septation begins at the carina and extends cephalad, being completed by five to six weeks' gestation (Figure 22.1).

The esophagus is initially lined by a thin layer of stratified columnar epithelium, which proliferates to almost occlude the lumen (2). At six to seven weeks, the lumen is reformed as a result of epithelial vacuolization (2) (Figure 22.2). As early as eight weeks' gestation and beginning in the middle one-third of the esophagus, ciliated cells appear and extend cephalad and caudally to almost cover the entire stratified columnar epithelium (2–4). At approximately 10 weeks a single layer of columnar cells populates the proximal and distal ends of the esophagus (2). At approximately four months' gestation, the esophageal cardiac-type glands form

as a result of the downward growth of these columnar cells into the lamina propria, with subsequent proliferation and differentiation (3,5). They go distally as far as the oxyntic mucosa, so that similar glands can be found in the cardia. Some have used this to argue that the cardia is therefore intrinsically part of the esophagus (6), although it could just as easily be interpreted that they are just present in all mucosae proximl to oxyntic mucosa.

At approximately five months' gestation, stratified squamous epithelium initially appears in the middle one-third of the esophagus and extends cephalad and caudally, replacing the ciliated epithelium (3,4). The upper esophagus is the last area to be replaced by squamous epithelium; and, if this process of squamous replacement is not completed at birth, there may be persistence of ciliated cells in the upper esophagus (2,4) (Figure 22.3). These residual cells are usually short lived, being replaced by squamous epithelium within two to three days postpartum (4,7). However, in some patients they either persist into adult life or there is metaplasia back to ciliated cells (8). The single layer of

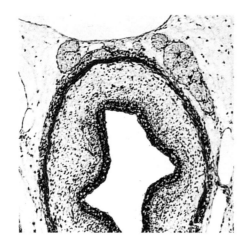

Figure 22.1 Fetal esophagus (late first trimester). Transverse section overview of the esophagus demonstrating inner mucosal layer, middle submucosal layer, and thin outer muscle layer. Note the vagus nerves lying over the esophagus.

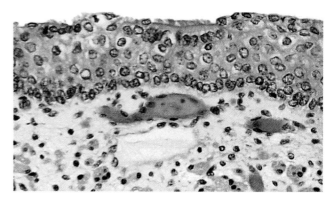

Figure 22.3 Fetal esophagus (third trimester). The epithelial layer at this stage consists of stratified squamous epithelium with occasional ciliated cells on the surface. Note the individual smooth muscle cells of developing muscularis mucosae.

columnar cells is also replaced by squamous epithelium, although some cells may persist at birth, usually located over the esophageal cardiac glands. The submucosal glands develop after the appearance of the squamous epithelium and are likely derived from this squamous epithelial layer (4,7).

Development of the gastrointestinal neuromuscular system begins at four weeks with neural crest cells entering the foregut and migrating rostrocaudally. The myenteric plexus develops first, followed by formation of the submucosal plexus two to three weeks later. At about six weeks' gestation, the circular muscle layer develops, followed by the development of the longitudinal layer at approximately nine weeks' gestation. Initially, the muscularis propria consists entirely of smooth muscle, after which striated muscle gradually develops in the upper esophagus so that by five months the normal ratio and arrangement of both muscle types are established (4). Interstitial cells of Cajal appear at week nine and become closely associated with the myenteric plexus (9). By week 14 the fetal gut has a mature appearance (9).

Developmental defects of the esophagus can be attributed to errors in this morphogenetic sequence. The notochord can induce the formation of the neural tube, gastrointestinal tract, and other organ systems. It has been shown experimentally that a split notochord can result in the duplication of any region of the gastrointestinal tract (1), which may include duplications of the esophagus ranging from the more common cysts to esophagus segments of variable length (1,10,11). As a consequence of this ability to induce development of more than one organ system, any patient presenting with duplications, segmental or cystic, should undergo radiologic evaluation that specifically explores for axial skeletal defects. Occurence of abnormalities during the phase of foregut septation is one proposed mechanism for the formation of tracheoesophageal fistulas (with or without atresia) or of mediastinal cysts of bronchogenic or esophageal origin (12,13). It has been suggested that esophageal duplications also may occur as a result of segments of fused vacuoles formed during the vacuolization phase persisting and differentiating toward esophageal structures (1).

TOPOGRAPHY AND RELATIONS

The esophagus begins in the neck at the cricoid cartilage, passes through the thorax within the posterior mediastinum, and extends for several centimeters past the diaphragm to its junction with the stomach. The overall length varies with trunk length, but in the adult the average length is approximately 23 to 25 cm. In practice, endoscopic distances are measured from the incisor teeth; and, in the average male, the junction of the esophagus and stomach is generally considered to be approximately 40 cm from the incisors. This length may vary from approximately 38 to 43 cm. Although convenient and commonly used in practice, the use of this distance is a crude and unreliable measurement for locating the gastroesophageal junction. It

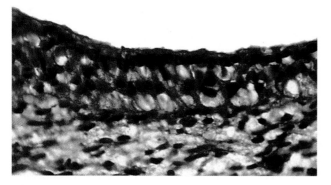

Figure 22.2 Fetal esophagus (late first trimester). The epithelial layer is composed of stratified columnar epithelium. Note the lack of muscularis mucosae.

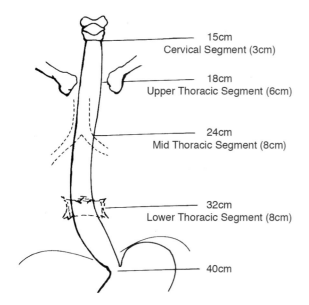

Figure 22.4 Esophageal segments with approximate lengths and distances from the incisors.

esophagus extends from the cricoid cartilage (roughly 15 cm) to the level of the thoracic inlet (approximately 18 cm). The upper thoracic segment extends from the thoracic inlet to the tracheal bifurcation (around 24 cm). The midthoracic segment extends to the level of the eighth thoracic vertebra (approximately 32 cm), and the lower thoracic segment extends to the junction with the stomach (40 cm).

Along its course, the normal esophagus has several points of constriction (Figure 22.5). These occur at the cricoid origin of the esophagus, along the left side of the esophagus at the aortic arch, at the crossing of the left main bronchus and left atrium, and where the esophagus passes through the diaphragm. These constrictions may become clinically significant if food or pills become lodged at these sites of luminal narrowing, with the possibility of contact mucosal injury. The most common sites for lodgement are at the level of the aortic arch and left atrium, where, especially in patients with left atrial enlargement, compression may become significant (16–18).

Knowledge of the relationships of the esophagus with other anatomic structures is important because these relationships may be directly affected by esophageal diseases such as carcinoma or diverticula. Disease of adjacent structures may cause local compression of the esophagus, resulting in dysphagia or lodgement of food or pills. The cervical esophagus is posterior to the trachea and bounded on both sides by the recurrent laryngeal nerve and the carotid sheath and its structures. The thyroid gland overlaps the esophagus in its cervical segment. In the thoracic segment,

has been found that the esophageal length correlates with height in children (14).

For the purpose of classification, staging, and reporting of esophageal malignancy, the International Union Against Cancer suggests division into four segments, with distances measured from the incisors (15) (Figure 22.4). The cervical

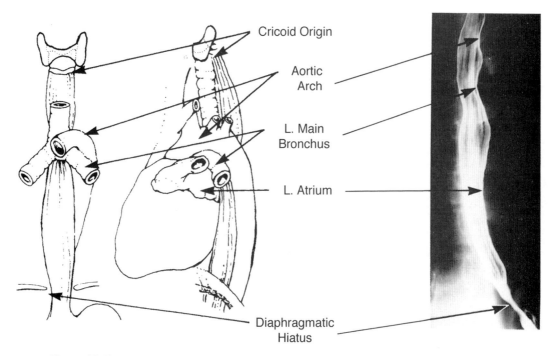

Figure 22.5 Relationship of the esophagus with normal esophageal constrictions. Barium swallow of the normal esophagus (*right*) demonstrates narrowing of the lumen at the sites of constriction.

the esophagus continues posterior to the trachea to the level of bifurcation, a site for the formation of the rare midesophageal diverticula secondary to traction from inflamed mediastinal lymph nodes (19). The esophagus courses posterior to the left atrium. The azygous veins ascend on either side of the thoracic segment.

Initially, the right and left vagus nerves run lateral to the esophagus, giving branches that form plexi on the posterior and anterior esophageal surfaces. At variable sites in the lower thoracic segment, the left and right nerves course onto the anterior and posterior surfaces of the esophagus, respectively, divide to form the anterior and posterior plexuses, and then reunite to form the anterior and posterior vagal trunks that course down to the stomach. An awareness that variations of this pattern exist is most important for the surgeon performing vagotomies. In the abdomen, the liver forms an impression on the anterior aspect of the esophagus. On the right side the junction with the stomach is smooth, whereas on the left the junction forms a sharp angle known as the incisura or angle of His.

The esophagus enters the abdomen by passing through the esophageal hiatus, which is formed by muscles of the diaphragm and contains the phrenoesophageal ligament. In most cases, the muscle sling encircling the esophagus is formed entirely from the right diaphragmatic crus (20), although variations of this pattern do occur. The phrenoesophageal ligament arises from the fascia of the abdominal diaphragm and divides into an ascending and descending leaf. The former passes up through the hiatus to insert approximately 2 to 3 cm above the hiatus, whereas the descending leaf has a variable insertion at or below the gastroesophageal junction or even into the gastric fundus (21). Proposed functions of the phrenoesophageal ligament include (a) assisting in maintaining the pressure differential between the thorax and abdomen, (b) providing fixation mechanisms with maintenance of the gastroesophageal junction within the abdomen during episodes of increased intra-abdominal pressure, and (c) contributing to the competence of the lower esophageal sphincter (LES), thus representing a possible mechanism for the absence of reflux in some patients with hiatal hernias (21–23).

MACROSCOPIC/ENDOSCOPIC FEATURES

In the empty state, the esophagus has an irregular outline as a result of the mucosa and submucosa being thrown into longitudinal folds. During endoscopy, insufflation causes distension so that these folds may not be appreciated, and the mucosa is seen to be a uniform white-pink.

Glycogenic Acanthosis

Glycogenic acanthosis can be seen in up to 25% of the population with the combined use of endoscopy and

barium studies (24–26). Macroscopically, glycogenic acanthosis interrupts the uniformity of the mucosa and presents as white nodules or small plaques on the mucosal folds, primarily in the distal one-third of the esophagus. These lesions vary in size, may be up to 1 cm in diameter, and, if extensive, may coalesce to larger plaques. Microscopically, glycogenic acanthosis consists of hyperplasia of the cells of the prickle layer containing abundant glycogen. Glycogenic acanthosis may resemble, and thus may be confused macroscopically with, monilial plaques or leukoplakia. Glycogenic acanthosis should be considered a variant of normal with as yet no defined relationship to infection or malignancy.

Heterotopias

Heterotopias are defined as normal tissue occurring in sites not expected for that tissue. In the literature, structures accepted as esophageal heterotopias are inconsistently defined. Esophageal cardiac-type glands and ciliated epithelium have been considered as heterotopias (7,8,27, 28) or as embryologic remnants (4) by some investigators. The categorization of melanocytes and argyrophilic cells, including Merkel cells and endocrine cells, presents a similar problem because these cells have not been regularly found in the esophagus (29,30). Melanosis has also been described (31-33).

Gastric body–type mucosa has been described occurring in the upper one-third of the esophagus, usually within 3.0 cm of the upper esophageal sphincter (4,7,27), hence the designation "inlet patch" (Figure 22.6). These heterotopias have been found in approximately 2 to 4% of esophagi and can be found at all ages. Macroscopically, they have a deep pink, velvety appearance, and the junction with squamous epithelium is similar in appearance to the

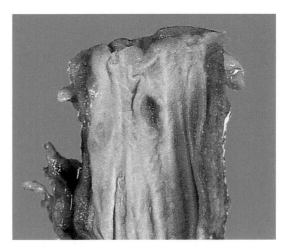

Figure 22.6 Proximal esophagus. Gastric body heterotopia situated slightly distal from the esophageal origin.

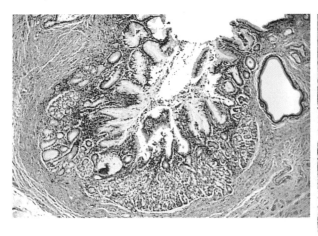

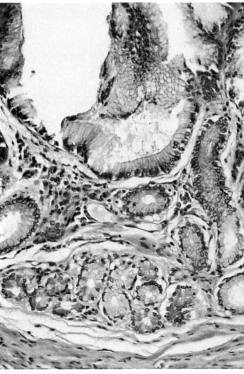

Figure 22.7 Proximal esophagus. Gastric body heterotopia composed of cardiac-type mucosa with scattered chief cells and a mild chronic inflammatory cell infiltrate.

mucosal gastroesophageal junction (27). Associated small peptic erosions or ulcers occasionally are identified nearby.

Microscopically, the heterotopic mucosa contains a variable number of parietal and chief cells with a variable chronic inflammatory cell infiltrate usually related to *Helicobacter* infection (27) (Figure 22.7). Acid production and symptoms have been attributed to heterotopias of larger size. These heterotopias along with the esophageal cardiac-type glands have been implicated as possible origins for the rare occurrence of adenocarcinoma of the upper esophagus (34,35). Theories for the origin of these heterotopias include a metaplastic change in preexisting cardiac-type glands, cell arrest where cells destined to become body mucosa remain in the esophagus rather than descend to the site of the future stomach, or otherwise unexplained heterotopia (4,27).

Sebaceous glands are occasionally found in the esophagus (Figure 22.8) and have been accepted as heterotopias without controversy (36,37). Thyroid tissue also has been described as heterotopic tissue in the esophagus (38). Pancreatic metaplasia is probably the most common form of metaplasia in the cardia, usually close to the Z line, although it also may be found in Barrett's esophagus and in an inlet patch (39–41) (Figure 22.9). While it has no known significance, if it secretes activated pancreatic juice, then it may well potentiate Barrett's esophagus, as it is a normal consituent of duodenal juice, the regurgitation

of which into the esophagus is involved in its pathogenesis. Indeed, it is also possible that an alkaline pH or bile in the esophagus stimulates its formation. Endocrine tissue can be observed (personal observation) but is vanishingly rare.

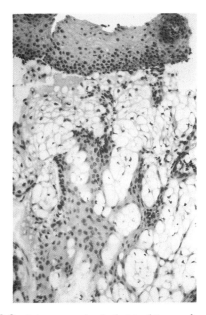

Figure 22.8 Sebaceous glands that in this case formed a nodule that was examined via biopsy.

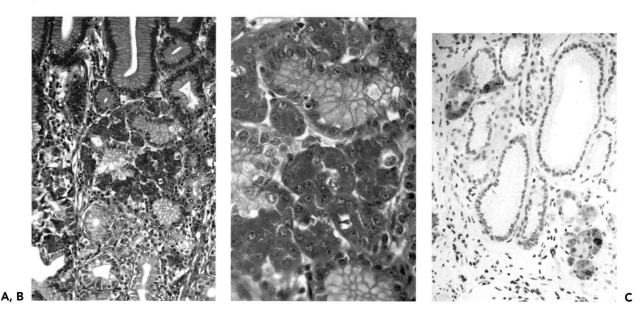

A, B   **C**

Figure 22.9 Pancreatic metaplasia in a biopsy from the cardiac side of the Z line. **A. and B.** Glands are an admixture of mucus glands and eosinophilic granular cells superficially resembling a cross between gastric chief cells and Paneth's cells. **C.** Immunocytochemical reactivity is found to pancreatic exocrine hormones, amylase in this case.

Esophageal Musculature

The muscular coat of the esophagus consists of an outer longitudinal and inner circular layer. The esophageal entrance is bounded superiorly by the cricopharyngeal and inferior pharyngeal constrictor muscles, both of which contribute muscle fibers to the esophageal musculature (22,23). Horizontal fibers from both these muscles form the upper esophageal sphincter, which manometrically is a localized zone of increased pressure measuring 2 to 4.5 cm in length (20,42,43). Together these muscle groups act in tandem to control the act of swallowing.

The longitudinal layer originates as two bands from its origin at the cricoid cartilage. The muscles sweep dorsally where they incompletely interdigitate, leaving a bare V-shaped area (area of Laimer) exposing the underlying circular layer. This area represents an area of potential weakness where a posterior pulsion diverticulum (Zenker's) may form. Theories regarding Zenker's diverticulum center upon a structural or physiologic abnormality of the cricopharyngeus muscle (44). The circular layer of the esophagus is slightly thinner than the longitudinal layer, a pattern that is reversed from the remainder of the gastrointestinal tract (22,23).

At the gastroesophageal junction, the esophageal longitudinal layer is continuous with the outer longitudinal layer of the stomach. The circular layer continues over the stomach, dividing in the region of the cardia to form the middle circular and inner oblique muscle layers of the stomach. The fibers of the inner oblique layer pass in a slinglike manner at the incisura and cross at right angles with the more horizontally oriented fibers of the middle layer, forming a muscular ring (collare Helvetti) to which a possible sphincter function has been ascribed (22,23).

Lower Esophageal Sphincter

The LES is best defined manometrically, where it presents as a 2- to 4-cm zone of pressure that is higher than intragastric or intraesophageal pressure. The distalmost end of the LES defines the muscular component of the gastroesophageal junction (42). At rest, the sphincter maintains an average pressure of 20 mm Hg (range: 10–26) (20). The function of the LES is to keep the lumen closed during rest, thus preventing reflux, and to relax during swallowing, thereby allowing food to pass through. Physiologically, a competent sphincter exists, and various changes in the musculature of the distal esophagus, thought to represent such a sphincter, have been described (43,45–47).

Gastroesophageal Junction

The gastroesophageal junction can be defined physiologically, anatomically, microscopically, or endoscopically and can be considered as being either muscular or mucosal in nature. The muscular gastroesophageal junction is most accurately defined physiologically by manometric studies in which the distalmost segment of the LES defines the junction (42). Unfortunately, in disease states such as severe gastroesophageal reflux disease (GERD) or Barrett's esophagus, the pressure may be so low as to not allow for localization by these means.

Anatomic landmarks that can be used to define the gastroesophageal junction include the peritoneal reflection from the stomach onto the diaphragm or the incisura (angle of His) (22,23); however, their use is limited to the resected surgical specimen.

Endoscopically, there are several landmarks that can be used, the most common of which is the mucosal squamocolumnar junction, or Z line. Sometimes this is accompanied by a ring (Shatzki's ring) that has squamous mucosa above and glandular mucosa distally (48,49), which is sometimes associated with dysphagia. The mucosal squamocolumnar junction is seen macroscopically and endoscopically as a serrated line of contrast known as the Z line or ora serrata (Figure 22.10). The Z line consists of small projections of red gastric epithelium, up to 5 mm long and 3 mm wide, extending upward into the squamous epithelium. Although extension of this gastric mucosa may be circumferentially symmetric, it often is asymmetric. The mucosal gastroesophageal junction may be straight rather than serrated, this occurring most often in the presence of a lower mucosal (Schatzki's) ring.

The mucosal gastroesophageal junction does not correspond to the muscular gastroesophageal junction as defined above; and, particularly if the mucosa is red and inflamed, it may not correspond to the supposed endoscopic junction either. The mucosal junction normally lies within the LES and is therefore found usually within 2 cm of the muscular junction as defined by the proximal edge of the gastric folds (50); thus, the distal 2 cm of the esophagus may be lined by columnar cells of the gastric cardia (it was this fact that led to Barrett's esophagus originally being defined as 3 cm or more of glandular mucosa within the tubular esophagus, as it ensured at least 1 cm of what should be Barrett's mucosa). Irregularities and proximal extensions of the Z line may extend 3 cm into the esophagus and thus endoscopically resemble early Barrett's esophagus. Indeed it is quite possible that some of these are tongues of Barrett's esophagus in which sampling fails to reveal goblet cells, or they may be absent. In one study, 23% of these patients had goblet cells in these tongues if rebiopsied (51).

The upper margin of the diaphragmatic indentation has been used as a guide to define the gastroesophageal junction; however, in the presence of a hiatal hernia, this demonstrates variable movement (22,23).

The proximal margin of the gastric folds has been shown to closely approximate the muscular gastroesophageal junction and thus may provide a fixed and reproducible anatomic landmark for the muscular gastroesophageal junction (50).

In the lower esophagus, the submucosal vessels of the distal esophagus are connected to the gastric submucosal vessels at the first gastric folds by a series of vessels referred to as longitudinal (vertical) vessels. These vessels, present in the lamina propria, are about 2 to 4 cm in length and can be often seen through the squamous or columnar mucosa (52,53). Their lower visible limit is also supposed to mark the original site of the gastroesophageal junction so that "shifts" in this caudally should be apparent. However, in some patients these are quite difficult to visualize, while in others they clearly extend into the gastric rugae. They may therefore be a less sensitive or specific marker of Barrett's esophagus than originally thought, so great care should be taken in making an endoscopic diagnosis of Barrett's esophagus without the usual biopsy confirmation. Even in the studies cited, the endoscopic diagnosis was not confirmed histologically so that the sensitivity and other characteristics of this technique are still unclear.

The longheld view that the distal 2 to 3 cm of the esophagus is normally lined by cardiac-type mucosa has been challenged. In both autopsy and endoscopic based studies (27,40,54–56) that included pediatric aged patients, columnar/cardiac mucosa was either not identified in up to 65% of cases, present as a short segment of less than 1.0 cm., combined with oxyntic (oxyntocardiac) mucosa, or demonstrated considerable circumferential variation within individuals. The authors suggest either that (a) cardiac mucosa of the gastroesophageal junction is not normal (but rather acquired) and that only squamous (esophagus) and oxyntic (stomach) mucosa are normal for this region or (b) it is a physiologic response to gastroesophageal reflux; but, either way it develops in response to a stimulus that includes some degree of acid reflux. To some extent it becomes a matter of semantics as to whether one regards

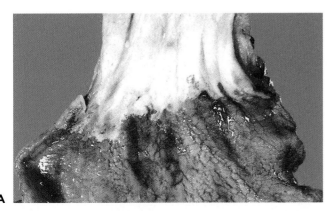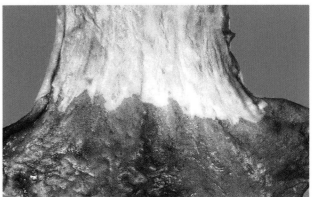

Figure 22.10 Gastroesophageal region. Formalin-fixed specimen demonstrates the variation of the normal squamocolumnar junction (Z line).

reflux as pathologic or physiologic. One could also argue that the normal physiologic position of the anal sphincter is to be closed, but it would cause all sorts of problems if it remained that way permanently! Conversely, it is difficult to see what useful function permitting gastroesophageal reflux serves except that other sphincters (e.g., pylorus) also reflux with some degree of frequency, which may have a physiologic benefit in aiding digestion as well as predisposing to Barrett's esophagus. Furthermore, studies have demonstrated that the length of cardiac or oxyntocardiac mucosa was shown to correlate with the severity of acid reflux suggesting that this metaplastic epithelium results from acid reflux (reflux carditis) (56,57).

Lower Esophageal Rings

Two (possibly three) thin, annular structures known as the lower muscular ring (type A) and lower mucosal ring (Schatzki's, type B) (Figure 22.11) may be identified in at least 10% and 5% of normal esophagi, respectively (48,49,58). A third ring (type C) rarely exists distal to either of these.

The lower muscular ring is the most proximal and is situated slightly more proximal than the Schatzki's ring, often by a centimeter or two. Some have equated the lower muscular ring with the lower esophageal sphincter (43,58). Microscopically, this ring is composed of a thickened circular smooth muscle with overlying squamous mucosa.

The lower mucosal ring (Schatzki's ring) is thought to mark the mucosal gastroesophageal junction. Histologically, the upper surface of the lower mucosal ring is lined by stratified squamous epithelium, whereas the undersurface is lined by columnar-type epithelium with the junction of both usually, but not invariably, being found at the apex of the ring. The core of the ring consists of connective tissue plus fibers of the muscularis mucosae without contribution from the muscularis propria. These rings are usually

asymptomatic but may be associated with intermittent dysphagia, sometimes becoming progressive or associated with attacks of sudden dysphagia (20). A "C ring" is rare, the most distal, and is said to consist of the diaphragmatic pinch, in which case it can be enhanced by sniffing.

HISTOLOGY

The four layers that characterize the gastrointestinal tract—mucosa, submucosa, muscularis propria, and serosa—form the wall of the esophagus.

Mucosa

The mucosa consists of a nonkeratinizing, stratified squamous epithelium, lamina propria, and muscularis mucosae (Figure 22.12).

Epithelium

The squamous epithelium can be divided into the basal, prickle, and functional cell layers. In addition, argyrophilic positive endocrine cells, melanocytes, Merkel cells, intraepithelial antigen-presenting cells and intraepithelial lymphocytes that are virtually impossible to distinguish in routine sections (and therefore perhaps best called collectively intraepithelial mononuclear cells) can be found in the epithelium of the normal esophagus. The basal layer occupies approximately 10 to 15% of the epithelium, being one to three cells thick; however, in the distal 3 cm, approximately 60% of normal individuals (without objective or subjective evidence of gastroesophageal reflux) may show basal cell hyperplasia of greater than 15% (59,60). The upper extent of the basal zone has been arbitrarily defined as the level where the nuclei are separated by a distance equal to their diameter (61). Periodic acid-Schiff (PAS) stain may be used to demonstrate the upper extent of the glycogen-poor basal cells (Figure 22.13). Above the basal cell layer, the

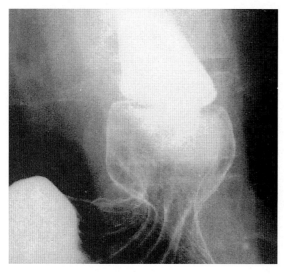

Figure 22.11 Lower esophageal mucosal ring (Schatzki's ring). The mucosal ring is outlined by the column of barium.

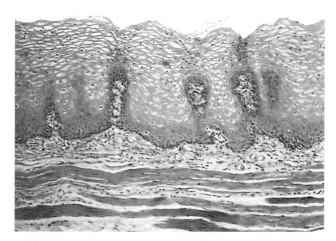

Figure 22.12 Midesophagus. The esophageal mucosa consists of a surface epithelial layer, middle lamina propria, and lower muscularis mucosae, which consists of longitudinally oriented smooth muscle bundles.

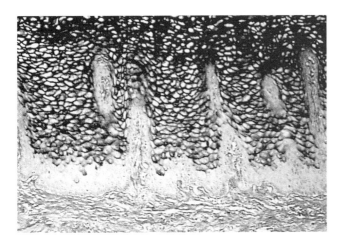

Figure 22.13 Midesophagus. The basal cell layer of the esophageal epithelium shows lack of glycogen, allowing for ready distinction from the overlying glycogen-rich cells (PAS-D).

prickle and functional cell layers consist of glycogen-rich cells that become progressively flatter toward the surface. Glandular mucosa of the distal esophagus is typical cardiac mucosa with variable numbers of specialized gastric cells and cardiac glands as described in the following chapter.

Argyrophilic positive endocrine cells and melanocytes have been found scattered among the basal cells in approximately 25% (62) and 4 to 8% of normal individuals, respectively, while Merkel cells are also described (29–30). The presence of melanocytes, referred to as melanosis (31,32,63), accounts for the occurrence of primary melanoma of the esophagus (64,65) and rare blue nevi (66), whereas the presence of argyrophilic positive cells accounts for the rare occurrence of pure small cell carcinoma (67).

Occasional lymphocytes are a normal finding in the epithelium and usually are located in a suprabasal location (68–70). As they interdigitate between the epithelial cells,

their nuclei become convoluted and may be confused with the nuclei of neutrophils. The term *squiggle cell*, or *intraepithelial cells with irregular nuclear contours*, is used to describe this appearance (Figure 22.14). As in the rest of the gastrointestinal tract, intraepithelial lymphocytes are CD3+/CD8+, indicating suppressor/cytotoxic function. Langerhans cells, which are S-100+, CD6+, and CDla+, also are located in a suprabasal location (Figure 22.15); they function as antigen-presenting cells, similar to Langerhans cells of the skin (68,69).

The cytology of the esophagus is represented by stratified squamous epithelium, gastric-type epithelium representing the distal 1 to 2 cm, and contaminants from the oropharynx, respiratory tract, and foreign material such as food particles. The squamous epithelium in cytologic material consists predominantly of superficial and intermediate squamous cells, with the deeper parabasal cells or squamous "pearls" occasionally observed. The gastric-type epithelium from the lower 1 to 2 cm of the esophagus is brushed as cohesive fragments of uniform cells displaying a honeycomb arrangement. The peripheral cells of the cluster are flattened. The nuclei are regular and paracentrally situated and contain a few granules of chromatin and occasionally a small nucleolus.

The electron microscopic appearance of the epithelial layer demonstrates similarities to nonkeratinizing squamous epithelium elsewhere (Figure 22.16). The cuboidal basal cells are attached to the basement membrane by hemidesmosomes. Progressing superficially, the epithelial cells become more flattened and the nuclei more pyknotic (68). Cell processes and desmosomes are most extensive in the prickle cell layer, becoming fewer and more simplified superficially (71). Membrane-bound, acid phosphatase–containing structures measuring 200 to 300 nm in diameter are identified within the epithelial cells and are

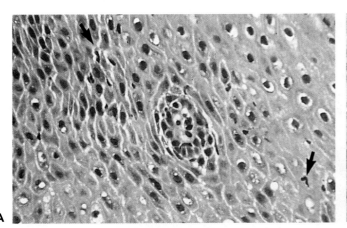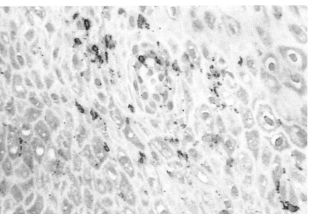

A B

Figure 22.14 A. Numerous lymphocytes within the esophageal epithelium, some of which have a "squiggle" appearance (*arrows*). In addition, the intercellular spaces are dilated causing very prominent prickles, while some of these have formed small "bubbles" primarily at the junction between epithelial cells (best seen in the upper right quadrant). Care needs to be taken not to include perinuclear vacuolization/cytoplasmic retraction or paranuclear vacuoles as dilated intercellular spaces. **B.** Intraepithelial lymphocytes are of T-cell origin, as demonstrated using the T-cell marker UCHL-1, and are primarily suppressor (CD8+) cells.

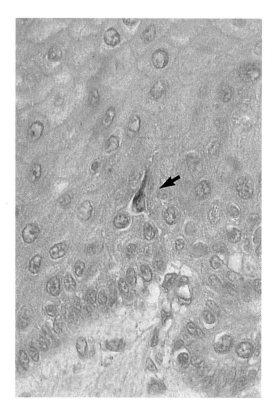

Figure 22.15 Langerhans cell (*arrow*) in a suprabasal position (S-100).

postulated to have a lysosomal function, possibly involved in the digestion of cell junctions necessary for epithelial sloughing (71,72).

Cell kinetics of the human esophagus have not been studied extensively. The basal cells are responsible for epithelial regeneration; and, although data on human esophageal mucosal renewal are not available, epithelial turnover in the esophagus is slower than in the small bowel (73). In the mouse, basal cell proliferation has been shown to have a circadian rhythm (74), and the epithelial turnover

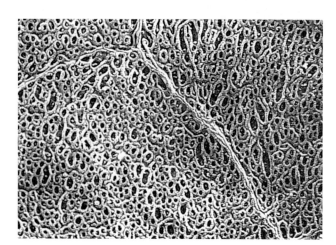

Figure 22.16 Scanning electron micrograph of the surface esophageal mucosa in which intercellular junctions are readily appreciated.

time in the normal rat esophagus is approximately seven days (75). In patients with GERD, there is an increased proliferative activity of the basal cells, resulting in basal cell hyperplasia (76).

Stem cells in the esophagus consist of a single layer of cells attached to the basement membrane that lie between the papillae (interpapillary basal cells) and have a low proliferative activity, being almost entirely Ki-67– (Figure 22.17). In animal models, when these cells divide, one remains attached to the basement membrane, while the

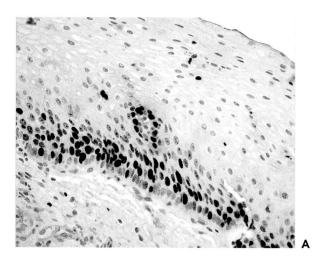

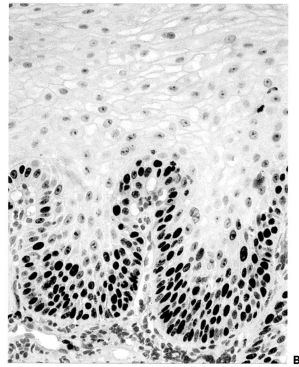

Figure 22.17 Basal layer of esophagus immunostained with MIB-1. **A.** The basal cell layer is relatively thin and unstimulated, consisting of only about 3 cell layers. Many of the cells in the basal layer are completely unstained, therefore representing likely stem cells, while the proliferating cells with black nuclei are in the cell layer immediately above. **B.** In this biopsy, the basal layer is much thicker and therefore more proliferative, and there are fewer non-cycling stem cells in the basal layer.

other migrates and differentiates. They therefore have a high proliferative capacity, divide relatively infrequently in vivo, and are phenotypically "primitive." Under experimental conditions, such stem cells "home" to damaged esophagus, while it can also be shown that bone marrow–derived cells can also home to the esophagus and differentiate into esophageal stem cells, including squamous epithelium (77). As such, basally situated stem cells do not show differentiation characteristics, possessing a different immunophenotype from the more differentiated cells in being CK13 immunoreactive; CK13 is expressed at high levels in the cells of both the papillary basal layer (PBL) and epibasal layers but is absent from the keratinocytes of the interpapillary basal layer (IBL). In addition, CK14 and CK15 are patchy in the IBL, which contrasts with the high levels of expression in the PBL and epibasal layers. Also, mRNA for the differentiation marker CK4 is detectable in the papillary region from the second epibasal layer onwards but does not appear in the interpapillary region until the third epibasal layer (78,79). Therefore, IBL cells appear to be the least differentiated cell type in the tissue (79). Suprabasal integrin expression is a consistent finding at the tips of the esophageal papillae, so PBL cells probably migrate to this site (80). This concept is illustrated in Figure 22.18.

Lamina Propria

The lamina propria is the nonepithelial portion of the mucosa above the muscularis mucosae; it consists of areolar connective tissue and contains vascular structures, scattered inflammatory cells, and mucus-secreting glands. In adults,

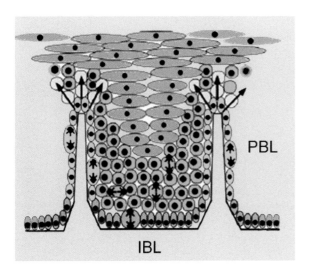

Figure 22.18 A model of the cellular organization in the esophageal epithelium. The interpapillary basal layer (*IBL*) cells (blue-grey) constitute the epithelial stem cell compartment. IBL cells proliferate infrequently and asymmetrically. Proliferating cells reside in the epibasal (suprabasal) layers (blue). Papillary basal cells (*PBL*) (green) are proliferative and intermediate in behavior between IBL and epibasal cells (see text). Differentiated squamous cells are shown in orange. Modified with permission from: Seery JP, Watt FM. Asymmetric stem-cell divisions define the architecture of human oesophageal epithelium. *Curr Biol* 2000;10:1447–1450.

the presence of scattered inflammatory cells, including lymphocytes and plasma cells, is considered a normal finding and does not correlate with acid reflux (61). Lymphocytes identified in the lamina propria are both CD4+ and CD8+, with the T4 population predominating (68). Immunoglobulin (Ig)A-producing B cells (plasma cells) predominate, with a smaller population of IgG- and IgM-producing B cells (plasma cells) (68). Fingerlike extensions of lamina propria, termed papillae, extend into the epithelium, with the maximum depth of extension allowable in the normal esophagus varying from 50% (81) to 75% (81,82). Practically it is easy to use the "rule of thirds" when examining biopsies, in which papillae should not extend into the upper one-third, and basal cells should not get higher than halfway up the basal one-third (adapted from: Ismail-Beigi F, Horton PF, Pope CE II. Histological consequences of gastroesophageal reflux in man. *Gastroenterology* 1970;58:163–174). In the distal 3 cm of the esophagus, up to 60% of individuals without objective evidence of reflux demonstrate papillary lengths that may exceed these values (59). Conversely increasing basal cell hyperplasia and papillary height does correlate with increasing severity of reflux (83).

Esophageal cardiac-type glands are diffusely scattered in the lamina propria through all levels of the esophagus, predominating in the distal and proximal regions (4,27). While they have been variably considered as heterotopias (7,27), normal constituents, or embryologic remnants, there is little doubt that they perform a lubricating function and are physiologically necessary to facilitate bolus passage. However their number is highly variable, and they are not always identified in the esophagus, having been found in 1 to 16% of esophagi in various studies (7,27,62). Histologically, these glands are located within the lamina propria, resemble the cardiac glands of the stomach, and are composed of cells secreting neutral mucins (Figure 22.19). They resemble pyloric glands, even to the extent that they are MUC6 immunoreactive, and may contain variable numbers of both parietal and chief cells and Paneth-like granules. Their ducts are lined by simple mucus-producing cells, in contrast to the submucosal gland ducts, that are frequently squamous-lined. These duct-lining cells may also extend onto the surface for a variable distance, even producing small islands of simple mucus-producing islands with an abrupt junction with squamous mucosa (H. Watanabe, personal communication).

Muscularis Mucosae

The muscularis mucosae is composed of smooth muscle bundles oriented longitudinally (42), rather than having both a circular and longitudinal arrangement as in the stomach and intestines. The muscularis mucosae begins at the cricoid cartilage of the pharynx and become thicker distally. At the gastroesophageal junction, the esophageal muscularis mucosae is thicker than that of the stomach and

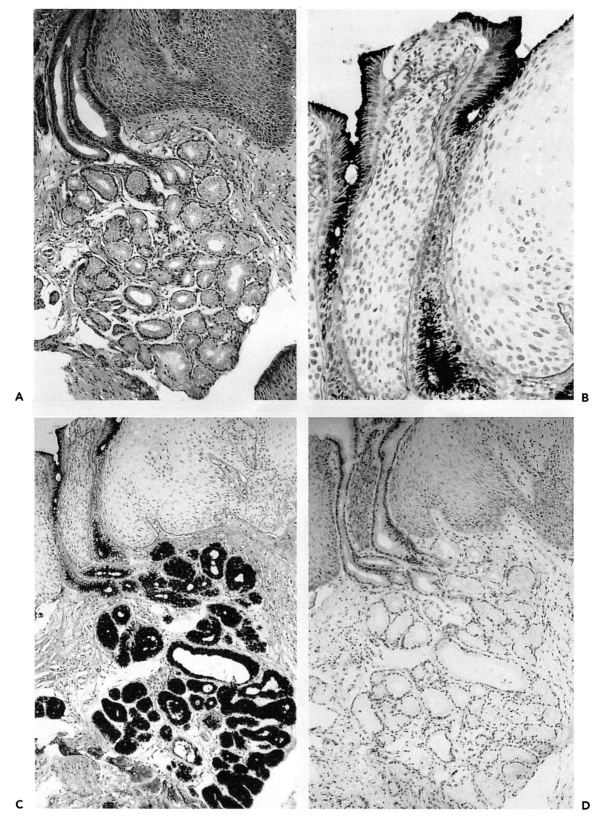

Figure 22.19 Midesophagus. **A.** Esophageal cardiac-type glands are located within the lamina propria. The ducts are lined by gastric foveolar–like cells. **B.** The duct-lining cells may extend over the stratified squamous epithelium for variable distances (PASD). **C, D.** The glands stained PASD positive and alcian blue at pH 2.5 negative, characteristic of neutral mucins.

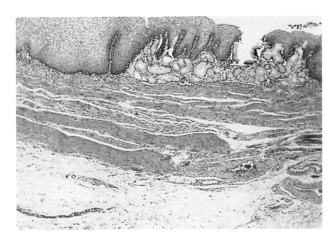

Figure 22.20 Distal esophagus. The mucosal layer at the gastroesophageal junction is characterized by muscularis mucosae that is thicker than the muscularis mucosae of the more proximal esophagus (compare with Figure 22.12). Note the esophageal cardiac-type gland situated above the muscularis mucosae.

may be so thick as to be mistaken for muscularis propria on biopsy (Figure 22.20). This thicker appearance, along with the longitudinal arrangement, is used sometimes to indicate an esophageal origin for the biopsy, and the differences between the muscularis mucosae of the stomach and esophagus can be used to identify the muscular gastroesophageal junction.

Submucosa

The submucosa consists of loose connective tissue containing vessels, nerve fibers (including Meissner's plexus), lymphatics, and submucosal glands (Figure 22.21). The submucosal glands are considered to be a continuation of

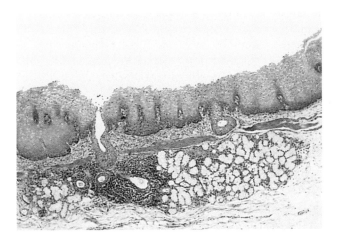

Figure 22.21 Midesophagus. Submucosal glands of the esophagus are located within the submucosa just beneath the muscularis mucosae. Periductal and periglandular chronic inflammation can be a normal finding. Note that in contrast to the columnar-lined glands of the lamina propria, the ducts of the submucosal glands are lined by squamous epithelium.

the minor salivary glands of the oropharynx and are scattered throughout the entire esophagus, but they are more concentrated in the upper and lower regions (4). The glands consist of mucinous cells, with or without a minor serous component, and produce acid mucins (Figure 22.22)

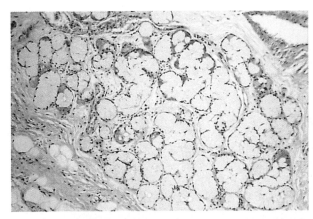

A

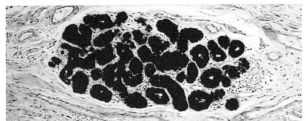

B

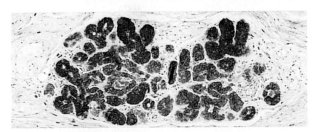

C

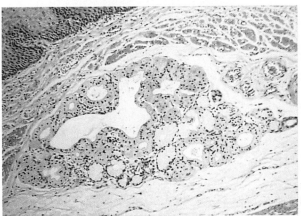

D

Figure 22.22 Midesophagus. **A.** The submucosal glands are composed predominantly of mucus-secreting cells with a variable serous component. **B. and C.** The submucosal glands stained positive with PAS-D and Alcian blue at pH 2.5, a characteristic of acid mucins. **D.** Submucosal glands may demonstrate oncocytic metaplasia.

as well as bicarbonate, which may have a local protective effect. The glands are drained by ducts, initially lined by a single layer of cuboidal epithelium, becoming stratified squamous in type, which penetrate the muscularis mucosae and epithelium to open into the esophageal lumen. This duct epithelium has been immunohistochemically shown to be CK14+/CK19+/CK7+/CK8/18+/variable CK20+ (84). This profile is similar to normal esophageal squamous epithelium and multilayered epithelium (ME), the latter representing a possible intermediate or early stage of Barrett's esophagus (84). Microscopic periductal aggregates of chronic inflammatory cells and duct dilatation are not uncommon findings in the normal esophagus (85). The presence of submucosal glands is indicative of an esophageal origin because these glands are not present in the stomach; unfortunately, submucosal glands are almost never present in mucosal biopsy specimens. However the ducts of the glands may be seen in the lamina propria of mucosal biopsies but are still only demonstrable in up to 14% of biopsies from the lower esophagus (86,87). Esophageal intramucosal pseudodiverticulosis is said to arise from postinflammatory obstruction of the ducts with subsequent duct dilatation (85,88).

Muscularis Propria

It is generally stated that as much as the upper quarter to upper one-third of the proximal muscularis propria is composed of striated muscle (22,23); however, only a short length (approximately 5%) of the proximal muscularis propria is composed of striated muscle (89). Immediately distal to this, smooth and striated muscle intermix, with smooth muscle predominating, whereas slightly more than 50% of the distal muscularis propria is composed solely of smooth muscle (89) (Figure 22.23). Despite the presence of these two different muscle types, they can function as a unit. Auerbach's plexus is found between the two muscle layers. Disease processes may preferentially involve only one of the muscular layers, as in scleroderma (in which atrophy predominantly involves the circular layer) or in achalasia (in which the circular layer may become hypertrophied) (4).

Serosa

Only short segments of the thoracic and intra-abdominal esophagus are lined by serosa derived from the pleura and peritoneum, respectively (4). The majority of the esophagus is surrounded by fascia, which condenses around the esophagus, forming a sheathlike structure. In the upper mediastinum, the esophagus is given support as this fascial tissue extends out to surround and form a similar sheathlike arrangement around adjacent structures (22,23).

ARTERIAL SUPPLY

The cervical portion of the esophagus is supplied by branches of the inferior thyroid artery with contribution from various intercostal arteries. Branches of the bronchial arteries, intercostal arteries, and aorta supply the thoracic segment, whereas the abdominal segment is supplied by branches of the left gastric and inferior phrenic artery (4,22,23,90). Branches from these arteries run within the muscular layer, giving rise to branches that course within the submucosa. Anastomoses are extensive, explaining the rarity of esophageal infarction (4,90).

VENOUS DRAINAGE

The venous return from the upper two-thirds of the esophagus drains into the inferior thyroid vein and azygous system, eventually reaching the superior vena cava. The lower esophageal segment drains into the systemic system through branches of the azygous vein and left inferior phrenic vein. The lower esophageal segment also drains into the portal system from branches of the left gastric vein and through the short gastric veins that empty into the splenic vein (4,22,23,90).

The anatomy of the lower esophageal system has been shown to consist of four layers (91). Radially arranged intraepithelial channels drain into the superficial venous plexus, which is found in the upper submucosa. This superficial venous plexus, consisting of three to five main trunks located in the lower submucosa, communicates with the deep intrinsic veins. Perforating veins connect this layer with the adventitial layer of veins located on the esophageal surface. The venous system appears to be mainly distributed within the esophageal mucosal folds (92).

The portal and caval systems communicate through the esophageal and gastric submucosal veins; and, with increased blood flow, as occurs in portal hypertension, all the venous channels of the normal esophagus dilate and are referred to as varices. In portal hypertension, varices are complicated by ulceration and rupture with hemorrhage. It has been suggested that a major variceal hemorrhage occurs as a result of rupture of a varix of the deep intrinsic veins, whereas minor variceal hemorrhages occur as a result of rupture of a varix in the superficial venous plexus or even from the intraepithelial channels (91).

LYMPHATIC DRAINAGE

A rich network of lymphatics in the lamina propria and submucosa connect with lymphatics in the muscular and adventitial layers. Lymphatics in the muscular layer are predominantly oriented in a longitudinal direction (4). In

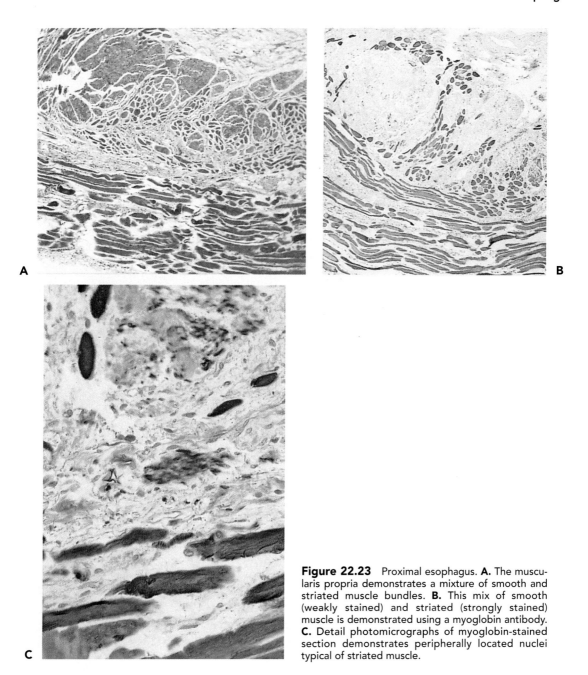

Figure 22.23 Proximal esophagus. **A.** The muscularis propria demonstrates a mixture of smooth and striated muscle bundles. **B.** This mix of smooth (weakly stained) and striated (strongly stained) muscle is demonstrated using a myoglobin antibody. **C.** Detail photomicrographs of myoglobin-stained section demonstrates peripherally located nuclei typical of striated muscle.

view of this longitudinal arrangement, extensive intramucosal and submucosal spread beyond a grossly visible tumor is not uncommon. This becomes an important consideration when assessing resection margins at frozen section.

In general, the cervical esophagus drains into the internal jugular and upper tracheal lymph node groups. The thoracic esophagus drains into the superior, middle, and lower mediastinal lymph node groups, whereas the abdominal segment drains into superior gastric, celiac axis, common hepatic artery, and splenic artery lymph nodes (93). Despite this drainage pattern, in practice the extensive communication of lymphatics results in a varied and unpredictable metastatic pattern (93).

INNERVATION (NERVES AND INTERSTITIAL CELLS OF CAJAL)

The esophagus receives both parasympathetic and sympathetic nerve supplies containing afferent and efferent fibers that innervate glands, blood vessels, and muscles of the esophagus. The vagus nerve carries both parasympathetic and some sympathetic fibers. Sympathetic fibers originating in cervical and paravertebral chains run with vascular structures and end at the esophagus.

As in the rest of the gastrointestinal tract, the esophagus has an intrinsic innervation system. This consists of ganglion cells in the submucosa (Meissner's plexus) and between the circular and longitudinal muscle layers (Auerbach's plexus). These plexuses are less well developed in the esophagus when compared with the remainder of the gastrointestinal tract, and the density of neurons increases as one proceeds toward the stomach (22,23). The submucosal plexus is less well developed than the myenteric nerve plexus.

The plexuses of the esophagus receive input from postganglionic sympathetic and preganglionic and postganglionic parasympathetic fibers, as well as from other intrinsic ganglion cells (20). Three cell types are described in the plexuses (89). Type I neurons are multipolar and confined to Auerbach's plexus, and their axons establish synapses with type II cells. Type II neurons are more numerous, are multipolar, and are found in both Auerbach's and Meissner's plexuses. These cells supply the muscularis propria and muscularis mucosae and stimulate secretory activity.

Interstitial cells of Cajal (ICC) are widely distributed within the submucosal, intramuscular, and intermuscular layers associated with the terminal networks of sympathetic nerves. In the few studies that have examined the distribution of ICCs in the esophagus, they have been identified in the distal one-third of the esophagus in close association with smooth muscle, as well as in the middle one-third associated with both smooth and striated muscle (94). Gastrointestinal stromal tumors (GISTs), including those of esophageal origin, originate from these ICCs. Peculiar to the esophagus, when compared to the rest of the gastrointestinal tract, is that tumors of stromal origin are more frequently benign leiomyomas rather than GISTs (95).

Regulatory peptides identified within nerve fibers and around smooth muscle bundles include vasoactive intestinal peptide (VIP), substance P, enkephalin, and neuropeptide Y (NPY) (96,97). Nerve fibers containing VIP and NPY are the most abundant types present in the esophagus, and the pattern of innervation by these peptide-containing neurons differs from that in the stomach and small intestine (98). Cholecystokinin (CCK) receptors are found in both the mucosa and nerves of the cardia (99).

DIAGNOSTIC CONSIDERATIONS

Commonly received biopsy specimens from the esophagus are for the diagnosis of reflux esophagitis or Barrett's esophagus. The problems of interpretation present in these cases involve the mucosal changes occurring primarily within the confines of the LES.

Barrett's Esophagus

Barrett's esophagus can be defined as the replacement of the esophageal squamous epithelium by metaplastic specialized (ideally intestinalized) columnar epithelium (100) (Figure 22.24). Both macroscopic and microscopic definitions exist, each proposed in an effort to address diagnostic problems encountered in this disease. That most accepted is the presence of an appropriate endoscopic

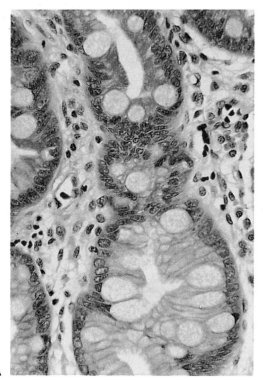

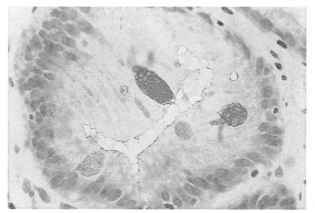

Figure 22.24 Barrett's esophagus. **A.** Intestinal metaplasia is recognized by the presence of goblet cells. Incomplete intestinal metaplasia (lower half of gland) is characterized by goblet cells associated with gastric foveolar–like columnar cells, whereas complete intestinal metaplasia (upper half of gland) is characterized by goblet cells associated with small intestinal, absorptive-like columnar cells. **B.** Goblet cells in intestinal metaplasia stain positive with Alcian blue at pH 2.5.

abnormality that is accompanied by intestinal metaplasia on biopsy (100). This works well except (a) in patients with a highly irregular Z line or very small tongues in whom the endoscopic interpretation of what is within normal limits (or not) may vary considerably; (b) in children, in whom it is rarely found in the first decade of life; and (c) tongues may also fail to yield goblet cells, especially in patients who have been on long-term proton pump inhibitors (PPIs). Indeed, fully 20% of patients rebiopsied for tongues yield goblet cells at the repeat endoscopy (51), a figure virtually identical to that described in long-segment disease (101). Little is known about the dynamics of goblet cells in Barrett's and, if the stimulus for their formation is removed (duodenogastroesophageal reflux) or the amount of gastric secretion reduced (e.g., by use of PPIs), whether their number may diminish or even disappear.

Macroscopically, Barrett's esophagus demonstrates a red velvety mucosa corresponding to the columnar epithelium, with an apparent focal or diffuse cephalad migration of the Z line relative to the previous normal mucosal gastroesophageal junction (Figure 22.25). Barrett's mucosa merges imperceptibly with the gastric mucosa distally. The junction with the esophageal squamous epithelium may appear as a symmetric or asymmetric Z line (as at the normal gastroesophageal junction) or as islands of columnar mucosa alternating with the squamous epithelium ("island pattern"). Foci of squamous epithelium occasionally are identified within Barrett's mucosa. Inflamed squamous mucosa may be indistinguishable from Barrett's mucosa endoscopically, and therefore also the squamo-Barrett junction, when both are present.

The diagnosis of Barrett's esophagus should always be confirmed histologically. If potential Barrett's mucosa is identified endoscopically, it should be examined via biopsy (as outlined below) to confirm the presence of specialized

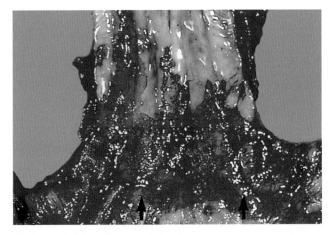

Figure 22.25 Gastroesophageal region. Barrett's esophagus, demonstrating proximal extension of columnar-lined mucosa well into the tubular esophagus. This columnar-lined mucosa extends more than 2 cm from the proximal gastric folds (*arrows*).

epithelium, as well as to exclude dysplasia or carcinoma, both of which may be inapparent endoscopically. Histologic confirmation is also important in cases of short-segment Barrett's esophagus (in which the short tongues of mucosa present may endoscopically resemble hiatal hernias, which are lined by gastric mucosa), inflammatory changes at the gastroesophageal junction, or an exaggerated and asymmetric yet normal mucosal gastroesophageal junction (102–104). Histologic confirmation is also necessary in cases of suspected childhood Barrett's esophagus, where Barrett's mucosa may be indistinguishable from the normal squamous epithelium (105–107). While the term *ultra-short Barrett's esophagus* has been used, primarily for lesions less that 1 cm (108), the interobserver variability of when an irregular Z line stops and Barrett's starts is problematic, rendering the term relatively useless. There also seems little sense in using it for patients with just intestinal metaplasia in an apparently normal cardia.

In adults, specialized epithelium is by far the most frequent epithelial type identified, so much so that the presence of this epithelium is increasingly being used as the sole criterion for the diagnosis of Barrett's esophagus (100). Other epithelial types are of much less value diagnostically and include fundic, junctional, metaplastic pancreatic acinar, and multilayered epithelium. Superimposed dysplasia, primarily of intestinalized epithelium, also may be present.

Specialized-type epithelium is characterized by the presence of goblet and columnar cells (Figure 22.24). The goblet cells contain acid mucins, predominantly sialomucins, thus staining positive with Alcian blue at pH 2.5, MUC2, or CD10 if there is complete intestinal metaplasia. The nongoblet cell population may also show an intestinal phenotype, showing expression of the intestinal markers sucrase-isomaltase and dipeptidilpeptidase IV immunoexpression in the majority of patients examined (109). Similarly goblet cells in Barrett's associated intestinal metaplasia are much more likely to express the mucin antigens MUC1 and MUC6 (110). The columnar epithelial cells may therefore resemble either small intestinal absorptive cells (complete intestinal metaplasia) or gastric foveolar cells, which frequently show evidence of an intestinal phenotype (incomplete intestinal metaplasia); however, these metaplastic cells demonstrate abnormal features that distinguish them from their normal counterparts (Figure 22.24). In the case of complete intestinal metaplasia, the small intestinal-like columnar cells may demonstrate a brush border, but it is not well developed and lacks the uniform enzymatic activity normally found in the brush border of the small intestine (111). Ultrastructurally, these metaplastic cells have been shown to contain mucin granules, which are not present in the absorptive cells of the small intestine, while the gastric foveolar-like columnar cells frequently contain Alcian blue–positive acid mucin, in contrast to those that normally populate the stomach, which contain Alcian blue–negative neutral mucins (111).

Other types of gastric mucosa may be present in Barrett's esophagus but cannot easily be distinguished from mucosa arising from the "normal" gastric cardiac mucosa; their definitive presence in Barrett's esophagus can be accepted only in resections or other circumstances under which specialized mucosa has been identified above the gastroesophageal junction. In the adult, fundic-type mucosa is uncommon and, if present, resembles the transitional epithelium seen at the junction of the gastric body with the antrum or cardia, with only a scattering of parietal and chief cells. Fundic-type mucosa without intestinalization and resembling normal gastric fundus mucosa can be seen in childhood Barrett's esophagus; otherwise, it is rare, and if present one must consider the possibility that the invariably present hiatal hernia has been examined via biopsy. The lack of intestinalized mucosa is a feature usually confined to children; it is likely that specialization occurs later in early adult life. Similarly, junctional-type mucosa that histologically is indistinguishable from normal gastric cardiac mucosa may be present—so much so that, if seen as the only mucosal type in a case of suspected short-segment Barrett's esophagus, a normal exaggerated Z line cannot be excluded.

Multilayered epithelium is a distinctive type of epithelium, histologically characterized by multiple layers of basaloid cells with an overlying layer of columnar epithelium (Figure 22.26). This epithelium has been shown to have mucin and immunohistochemical qualities similar to normal squamous epithelium, duct gland epithelium, and Barrett's epithelium (84); and it is associated with reflux-induced injury (112) and intestinal metaplasia in patients with Barrett's disease (113). As such, it is postulated that

multilayered epithelium may represent an early/transitional phase of columnar metaplasia in Barrett's esophagus, although some believe that this is ciliated ultrastructurally and therefore represents simple metaplasia (8,28).

The diagnosis of Barrett's esophagus is best established by taking biopsy samples from various levels of the gastroesophageal region (114), beginning in the stomach just distal to the upper end of the gastric folds, ideally along the lesser curve, and then every 1 to 2 cm, up into the tongues of mucosa or the most irregular portion of the squamocolumnar junction until squamous epithelium is reached. Obvious islands of columnar-lined epithelium also should be examined via biopsy. This series of biopsy samples yields tissue that initially originates in a site that is clearly of gastric origin (thereby excluding gastric intestinal metaplasia as a cause of proximal intestinalized epithelium), continues through mucosa in which intestinalized epithelium is present (thereby confirming the diagnosis of Barrett's esophagus), and finishes in squamous mucosa. Intestinal metaplasia may be focal and thus may be missed on biopsy. In such cases, if the diagnosis of Barrett's esophagus is suspected, follow-up with repeat biopsy is necessary.

Although there is uncertainty as to the cell of origin for Barrett's esophagus, the cells lining the gland duct may be considered as a possible source (115). Conversely, re-epithelialization of the esophagus following ablation may well be from the squamous-lined submucosal gland ducts.

Intestinal Metaplasia Limited to the Cardiac Region

Intestinal metaplasia (IM) is common and found in up to one-third of patients (116); but, it also depends to some extent on how many biopsies are taken and where a highly irregular but normal Z line stops and short-segment Barrett's esophagus (defined as less than 3 cm of columnar-lined esophagus with goblet cells) begins, a feature with quite marked interobserver variability. In one study, a total of 811 (84.6%) patients had 0 to 0.9 cm of questionably abnormal columnar epithelium between normal oxyntic mucosa and squamous epithelium. Of these, 161 (19.9%) patients had no abnormal epithelium, 158 (19.4%) patients had oxyntocardiac mucosa, 372 (45.9%) patients had cardiac mucosa, and 120 (14.8%) patients had intestinal metaplasia. The prevalence of intestinal epithelium increased progressively with increasing length of abnormal columnar epithelium, being present in 70.4% in the 1- to 2-cm group, 89.5% in the 3- to 4-cm group, and 100% within the greater than or equal to 5 cm group (117).

This raises several issues. First, metaplasia has several causes, although the principle two are GERD and *Helicobacter*. Second, because the diagnosis of Barrett's esophagus requires both intestinal metaplasia and an appropriate endoscopic appearance, the identification becomes key, especially in defining what is unequivocally

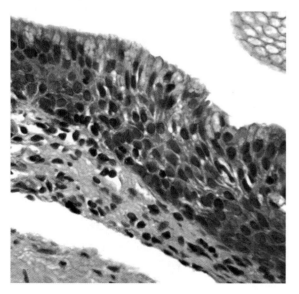

Figure 22.26 Multilayered epithelium, in which there is apical mucin production at the luminal surface (*top*), but the remainder of the epithelium appears squamous with intercellular bridges.

abnormal and where an irregular but normal Z line stops and Barrett's begins (118,119). Clearly, Barrett's esophagus has to begin somewhere, but this distinction is currently impossible to determine because, although some differences between metaplasia in native cardiac mucosa and metaplasia in what was formerly squamous mucosa exist (9), it is unclear how reliable these are. The third issue regarding the type of epithelium in which intestinal metaplasia is occurring is in part the pathogenesis issue but also its implication. Does intestinal metaplasia in what is believed to be the native cardiac side of the Z line have the same malignant potential as recognized Barrett's mucosa? If it does not, then it becomes critical to attempt to separate the two; but, if it does, then the exercise is futile because both diseases are premalignant and the issue becomes the extent of the risk and whether this justifies surveillance. Because metaplasia at the cardia in *Helicobacter* gastritis tends to be complete, while that in Barrett's is often both complete and incomplete, it is likely that Barrett's esophagus is at increased risk of developing carcinoma. This is also supported by mucin immunohistochemistry using MUC1 and MUC6 (110).

Gastroesophageal Reflux Disease (GERD)

The problems encountered in GERD are related to squamous epithelial changes in the distal 3 cm of the esophagus and to the significance of intraepithelial inflammatory cells.

Reactive Squamous Changes

Reflux-associated squamous hyperplasia (RASH) consists of basal cell hyperplasia of greater than 15% and extension of the papillae into the upper one-third of the epithelium (60) (Figure 22.27). Practically, in well-oriented biopsy samples, the esophageal mucosa can be divided into thirds;

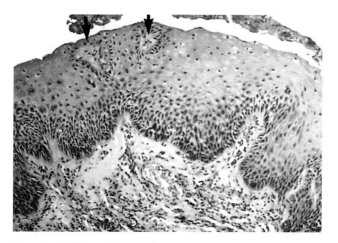

Figure 22.27 Reflux esophagitis. Basal cell hyperplasia and lengthening of the papillae are present. The papillae have extended almost to the surface of the mucosa (arrows).

the papillae should not be seen extending into the upper one-third, and the basal cell layer should not extend more than halfway into the lower one-third. This is operatively a simple and rapid technique for assessing the degree of RASH. However, similar changes have been described in the distal 3 cm of the esophagus in approximately 60% of patients without objective or subjective evidence of acid reflux (59); thus, if present in biopsy samples originating from this zone, such hyperplastic changes should be considered normal, despite the fact that these changes are much more likely to be found in patients with GERD and NERD (nonerosive reflux disease) (83). Changes of RASH are much more likely to be a more specific indicator of reflux if the biopsy samples are taken above the distal 3 cm of the esophagus (59,61). It should be remembered that squamous hyperplasia is a nonspecific reaction to any form of esophageal injury and needs to be interpreted in light of the clinical context.

Dilated Intercellular Spaces

Apart from squamous hyperplasia, dilatation of the intercelluar spaces of the squamous epithelium as a result of gastroesophageal reflux has been demonstrated at both the electron and light microscopic level (120-122) (Figure 22.14). This early epithelial damage is morphologically characterized by irregular dilatation of the intercellular spaces of the basal and prickle cell layers in both erosive and nonerosive esophagitis. Using ultrastructural measurement, it seems that dilatation of more than 2.4 μm is highly suggestive of GERD (123). This is approximately half the diameter of an intaepithelial lymphocyte. Further, patients with NERD have a DIS measurement of approximately half of this at 1.5 μm, which is still about three times the normal value of 0.45 to 0.5 μm (124). Readers will no doubt be pleased to know that these measurements were made ultrastructurally! Treatment with omeprazole results in complete recovery of DIS (125). DIS have also been shown to be one of the histological changes (along with basal cell hyperplasia) seen in biopsies from endoscopic lesions referred to as "red streaks" (86), along with newly re-epithelialized lesions or granulation tissue beneath squamous epithelium. Its utility as a marker of GERD when unaccompanied by other morphological features of reflux disease has yet to be fully determined.

Intraepithelial Inflammatory Cells

Intraepithelial eosinophils (IEEs) and intraepithelial neutrophils (IENs) are generally not considered to be normal constituents of the epithelium throughout its entire length, although rare IEEs in the distal 3 cm of approximately one-third of adult patients is considered normal (61). The presence of IEEs has long been considered a sensitive indicator of reflux esophagitis (61,82,126), although this sensitivity is in question, and not infrequently it is the only pathologic change (Figure 22.28A). Intraepithelial eosinophils are not absolutely specific, having been described in esophagitis due to alkaline reflux, allergic disorders, and infections (82) (Figure 22.28B). In children, although not an absolute criterion, eosinophils within the lamina propria are a significant finding in GERD. However, it is also clear that there is a second syndrome that can be seen in both adults and children in whom the primary symptom may be dysphagia rather than GERD; it tends to occur in younger males, and when fully developed is characterized endoscopically by rings reminiscent of allergic esophagitis. It has therefore been called feline esophagus, ringed esophagus, or trachealization of the esophagus. The esophagus is fragile and can perforate if dilatation of areas of narrowing is attempted. Histologically, the features are massive (usually 20–40/HPF) numbers of eosinophils, that also tend to ex-

tend throughout the esophagus, and also tend to be superficial. Patients often have other evidence of allergies and may respond to steroids or allergen withdrawal, including an elemental diet, rather than to PPIs (127–133).

The presence of IENs obviously implies acute esophagitis and correlates with the presence of erosion or ulceration, albeit of any cause, but is less sensitive for mild GERD. When present, IENs are frequently, but not always, accompanied by the other histologic features of esophagitis. In biopsies, the absence of other features may simply repereresent sampling problems. The use of DIS, IEEs, and IENs as histologic criteria of GERD has the advantage that localization and orientation of the biopsy is not important.

Vascular changes such as dilated capillaries and extravasated red blood cells in the lamina propria should not be considered as criteria for GERD (60,61), although some have been impressed by its usefulness (134). Increased vascularization in the lamina propria, thought of as indicative of RASH is not considered a diagnostic criterion (133). The presence of intraepithelial mononuclear cells (squiggle cells) is associated with GERD but rarely used as the sole criterion (83,135,136).

In the assessment of biopsy tissues for RASH, well-oriented biopsy specimens of full epithelial thickness are necessary. Quite often biopsy samples are taken with small pinch forceps, resulting in a specimen that is small, superficial, and difficult to orient. If endoscopy is being performed to obtain a tissue diagnosis, an appropriate endoscope with large-particle grasp forceps should be used. Changes of GERD may have a patchy distribution; thus, multiple biopsies are recommended. It is important to avoid the use of picric acid containing dyes and fixatives (such as Bouin's solution) because this interferes with the staining of the eosinophil granules, thus preventing their recognition.

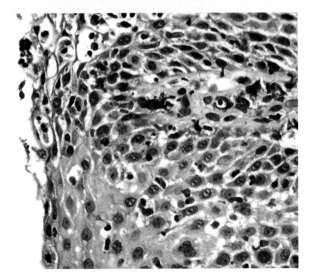

Figure 22.28 Eosinophilic esophagitis. **A.** Reflux esophagitis. Intraepithelial eosinophils are present between the epithelial cells. **B.** Allergic esophagitis (feline esophagus). There is marked basal cell hyperplasia, spongiosis with dilated intercellular spaces, and numerous eosinophils.

Inflammatory Changes on the Cardiac Side of the Z Line

Because of the increasing use of biopsy samples immediately on the squamous side of the Z line to detect inflammatory cells, some biopsy samples inevitably contained cardiac mucosa immediately distal to the Z line. Some of these specimens contained an excess of chronic and sometimes acute inflammatory changes, which were not only unaccompanied by inflammatory changes elsewhere in the stomach, as might be expected with *Helicobacter pylori* gastritis, but inflammation appeared to be completely limited to the gastric cardia and therefore was appropriately termed gastric carditis (114). However, it appears to be a more sensitive marker for GERD than inflammatory changes in the squamous mucosa, as judged by correlation with 24-hour pH studies (57,114,137,138), the proviso being that *Helicobacter* infection (gastritis) is not present as this also causes carditis (139–141).

Adenocarcinomas of the Gastroesophageal Region

Adenocarcinomas arising in the gastroesophageal region may have their origin from the gastric cardia, from Barrett's mucosa, or theoretically from the gastric cardiac-type mucosa present in the distal 2 cm of the esophagus. Gastric cardiac adenocarcinomas can be defined macroscopically as those occurring at or below the gastroesophageal junction, with the bulk of the tumor found in the gastric cardia and not involving the body or distal stomach (142). The presence of premalignant changes in the adjacent cardiac epithelium, such as a villous adenoma or dysplasia, would be confirmatory. Adenocarcinoma arising from Barrett's esophagus are predominantly located in the esophagus and are usually associated with demonstrable Barrett's mucosa histologically. Those arising from the gastric epithelium of the distal 2 cm of the esophagus can be classified with those of the gastric cardia unless associated with Barrett's mucosa. Occasionally, an adenocarcinoma may involve both the lower esophagus and gastric cardia equally, with obliteration of the landmarks of the gastroesophageal junction and any premalignant mucosa. In these cases, identification of the site of origin may be impossible; however, from a practical viewpoint, this distinction may not be important because their clinical behaviors are similar (142–144).

ACKNOWLEDGMENT

We thank Dr. G. W. Stevenson for radiographic material.

REFERENCES

1. Vaage S, Knutrud O. Congenital duplications of the alimentary tract with special regard to their embryogenesis. *Prog Pediatr Surg* 1974;7:103–123.
2. Johns BA. Developmental changes in the oesophageal epithelium in man. *J Anat* 1952;86:431–442.
3. Berardi RS, Devaiah KA. Barrett's esophagus. *Surg Gynecol Obstet* 1983;156:521–538.
4. Enterline H, Thompson J. *Pathology of the Esophagus*. New York: Springer-Verlag; 1984.
5. Borrelli O, Hassall E, D'Armiento F, et al. Inflammation of the gastric cardia in children with symptoms of acid peptic disease. *J Pediatr* 2003;143:520–524.
6. Chandrasoma P, Makarewicz K, Wickramasinghe K, Ma Y, Demeester T. A proposal for a new validated histological definition of the gastroesophageal junction. *Hum Pathol* 2006;37:40–47.
7. Rector LE, Connerley ML. Aberrant mucosa in the esophagus in infants and children. *Arch Pathol* 1941;31:285–294.
8. Takubo K, Vieth M, Honma N, et al. Ciliated surface in the esophagogastric junction zone: a precursor of Barrett's mucosa or ciliated pseudostratified metaplasia? *Am J Surg Pathol* 2005;29:211–217.
9. Wallace AS, Burns AJ. Development of the enteric nervous system, smooth muscle and interstitial cells of Cajal in the human gastrointestinal tract. *Cell Tissue Res* 2005;319:367-82.
10. Le Roux BT. Intrathoracic duplication of the foregut. *Thorax* 1962;17:357–362.
11. Tarnay TJ, Chang CH, Nugent RG, Warden HE. Esophageal duplication (foregut cyst) with spinal malformation. *J Thorac Cardiovasc Surg* 1970;59:293–298.
12. Abell MR. Mediastinal cysts. *AMA Arch Pathol* 1956;61:360–379.
13. Rosenthal AH. Congenital atresia of the esophagus with tracheoesophageal fistula. Report of eight cases. *Arch Pathol* 1931; 12: 756–772.
14. Strobel CT, Byrne WJ, Ament ME, Euler AR. Correlation of esophageal lengths in children with height: application to the Tuttle test without prior esophageal manometry. *J Pediatr* 1979;94: 81–84.
15. Greene FL, Page DL, Fleming ID, et al. Esophagus. In: Greene FL, Page DL, Fleming ID, et al., eds. *AJCC Cancer Staging Manual*. 6th ed. New York: Springer; 2002:91–98.
16. Abid S, Mumtaz K, Jafri W, et al. Pill-induced esophageal injury: endoscopic features and clinical outcomes. *Endoscopy* 2005;37: 740–744.
17. Gulsen MT, Buyukberber NM, Karaca M, Kadayifci A. Cyproterone acetate and ethinylestradiol-induced pill oesophagitis: a case report. *Int J Clin Pract Suppl* 2005;147:79–81.
18. McCullough RW, Afzal ZA, Saifuddin TN, Alba LM, Khan AH. Pill-induced esophagitis complicated by multiple esophageal septa. *Gastrointest Endosc* 2004;59:150–152.
19. Marshall JB, Singh R, Demmy TL, Bickel JT, Everett ED. Mediastinal histoplasmosis presenting with esophageal involvement and dysphagia: case study. *Dysphagia* 1995;10:53–58.
20. Feldman M, Friedman LS, Sleisenger MH. *Sleisenger and Fordtran's Gastrointestinal and Liver Disease: Pathophysiology, Diagnosis and Management*. 7th ed. Philadelphia: WB Saunders; 2002:549–671.
21. Bombeck CT, Dillard DH, Nyhus LM. Muscular anatomy of the gastroesophageal junction and the role of phrenoesophageal ligament. Autopsy study of sphincter mechanism. *Ann Surg* 1966;164:643–654.
22. Netter FH, ed. The CIBA Collection of Medical Illustrations: A Compilation of Pathological and Anatomical Paintings. Vol 3. Digestive System. Part I: Upper Digestive Tract. Summit, NJ: CIBA-Geigy; 1957.
23. Netter FH. Atlas of Human Anatomy. 3rd ed. St. Louis: ICDH Learning/Elsevier; 2003.
24. Katagiri A, Kaneko K, Konishi K, Ito H, Kushima M, Mitamura K. Lugol staining pattern in background epithelium of patients with esophageal squamous cell carcinoma. *Hepatogastroenterology* 2004;51:713–717.
25. McGarrity TJ, Wagner Baker MJ, Ruggiero FM, et al. GI polyposis and glycogenic acanthosis of the esophagus associated with PTEN mutation positive Cowden syndrome in the absence of cutaneous manifestations. *Am J Gastroenterol* 2003;98:1429–1434.
26. Vadva MD, Triadafilopoulos G. Glycogenic acanthosis of the esophagus and gastroesophageal reflux. *J Clin Gastroenterol* 1993;17:79–83.
27. Tang P, McKinley MJ, Sporrer M, Kahn E. Inlet patch: prevalence, histologic type, and association with esophagitis, Barrett esophagus, and antritis. *Arch Pathol Lab Med* 2004;128:444–447.
28. Takubo K, Honma N, Arai T. Multilayered epithelium in Barrett's esophagus. *Am J Surg Pathol* 2001;25:1460–1461.
29. Harmse JL, Carey FA, Baird AR, et al. Merkel cells in the human oesophagus. *J Pathol* 1999;189:176–179.
30. Tateishi R, Taniguchi K, Horai T, Iwanaga T, Taniguchi H. Argyrophil cell carcinoma (apudoma) of the esophagus. A histopathologic entity. *Virchows Arch A Pathol Anat Histol* 1976;371:283–294.
31. Ohashi K, Kato Y, Kanno J, Kasuga T. Melanocytes and melanosis of the oesophagus in Japanese subjects—analysis of factors effecting their increase. *Virchows Arch A Pathol Anat Histopathol* 1990;417:137–143.
32. Bogomoletz WV, Lecat M, Amoros F. Melanosis of the oesophagus in a Western patient. *Histopathology* 1997;30:498–499.
33. Yamazaki K, Ohmori T, Kumagai Y, Makuuchi H, Eyden B. Ultrastructure of oesophageal melanocytosis. *Virchows Arch A Pathol Anat Histopathol* 1991;418:515–522.
34. Abe T, Hosokawa M, Kusumi T, et al. Adenocarcinoma arising from ectopic gastric mucosa in the cervical esophagus. *Am J Clin Oncol* 2004;27:644–645.

35. Hirayama N, Arima M, Miyazaki S, et al. Endoscopic mucosal resection of adenocarcinoma arising in ectopic gastric mucosa in the cervical esophagus: case report. *Gastrointest Endosc* 2003;57:263–266.

36. Nakanishi Y, Ochiai A, Shimoda T, et al. Heterotopic sebaceous glands in the esophagus: histopathological and immunohistochemical study of a resected esophagus. *Pathol Int* 1999;49:364–368.

37. Kushima R, von Hinuber G, Lessel W, Stolte M, Borchard F. Sebaceous gland metaplasia in cardiac-type mucosa of the oesophago-gastric junction. *Virchows Arch* 1996;428:297–299.

38. Postlethwait RW, Detmer DE. Ectopic thyroid nodule in the esophagus. *Ann Thorac Surg* 1975;19:98–100.

39. Polkowski W, van Lanschot JJ, ten Kate FJ, et al. Intestinal and pancreatic metaplasia at the esophagogastric junction in patients without Barrett's esophagus. *Am J Gastroenterol* 2000;95:617–625.

40. Popiolek D, Kahn E, Markowitz J, Daum F. Prevalence and pathogenesis of pancreatic acinar tissue at the gastroesophageal junction in children and young adults. *Arch Pathol Lab Med* 2000;124:1165–1167.

41. Krishnamurthy S, Dayal Y. Pancreatic metaplasia in Barrett's esophagus. An immunohistochemical study. *Am J Surg Pathol* 1995;19:1172–1180.

42. Goyal RK. Columnar cell-lined (Barrett's) esophagus: a historical perspective. In: Spechler SJ, Goyal RK, eds. *Barrett's Esophagus: Pathophysiology, Diagnosis and Management.* New York: Elsevier; 1985:1–18.

43. Goyal RK. The lower esophageal sphincter. *Viewpoints Dig Dis* 1976;8:1–4.

44. van Overbeek JJ. Pathogenesis and methods of treatment of Zenker's diverticulum. *Ann Otol Rhinol Laryngol* 2003;112:583–593.

45. Theisen J, Oberg S, Peters JH, et al. Gastro-esophageal reflux disease confined to the sphincter. *Dis Esophagus* 2001;14:235–238.

46. Wolf C, Timmer R, Breumelhof R, Seldenrijk CA, Smout AJ. Prolonged measurement of lower oesophageal sphincter function in patients with intestinal metaplasia at the oesophagogastric junction. *Gut* 2001;49:354–358.

47. Liebermann-Meffert D, Allgower M, Schmid P, Blum A. Muscular equivalent of the lower esophageal sphincter. *Gastroenterology* 1979;76:31–38.

48. Jamieson J, Hinder RA, DeMeester TR, Litchfield D, Barlow A, Bailey RT Jr. Analysis of thirty-two patients with Schatzki's ring. *Am J Surg* 1989;158:563–566.

49. Mitre MC, Katzka DA, Brensinger CM, Lewis JD, Mitre RJ, Ginsberg GG. Schatzki ring and Barrett's esophagus: do they occur together? *Dig Dis Sci* 2004;49:770–773.

50. McClave SA, Boyce HW Jr, Gottfried MR. Early diagnosis of columnar-lined esophagus: a new endoscopic diagnostic criterion. *Gastrointest Endosc* 1987;33:413–416.

51. Jones TF, Sharma P, Daaboul B, et al. Yield of intestinal metaplasia in patients with suspected short-segment Barrett's esophagus (SSBE) on repeat endoscopy. *Dig Dis Sci* 2002;47:2108–2111.

52. Hoshihara Y, Kogure T, Yamamoto T, Hashimoto M, Hoteya O. Endoscopic diagnosis of Barrett's esophagus [article in Japanese]. *Nippon Rinsho* 2005;63:1394–1398.

53. Choi do W, Oh SN, Baek SJ, et al. Endoscopically observed lower esophageal capillary patterns. *Korean J Intern Med* 2002;17:245–248.

54. Chandrasoma P. Histopathology of the gastroesophageal junction: a study on 36 operation specimens. *Am J Surg Pathol* 2003;27:277–278.

55. Zhou H, Greco MA, Daum F, Kahn E. Origin of cardiac mucosa: ontogenic consideration. *Pediatr Dev Pathol* 2001;4:358–363.

56. Chandrasoma PT, Lokuhetty DM, Demeester TR, et al. Definition of histopathologic changes in gastroesophageal reflux disease. *Am J Surg Pathol* 2000;24:344–351.

57. Der R, Tsao-Wei DD, Demeester T, et al. Carditis: a manifestation of gastroesophageal reflux disease. *Am J Surg Pathol* 2001;25:245–252.

58. Goyal RK, Bauer JL, Spiro HM. The nature and location of lower esophageal ring. *N Engl J Med* 1971;284:1175–1180.

59. Weinstein WM, Bogoch ER, Bowes KL. The normal human esophageal mucosa: a histological reappraisal. *Gastroenterology* 1975;68:40–44.

60. Ismail-Beigi F, Horton PF, Pope CE II. Histological consequences of gastroesophageal reflux in man. *Gastroenterology* 1970;58:163–174.

61. Groben PA, Siegal GP, Shub MD, Ulshen MH, Askin FB. Gastroesophageal reflux and esophagitis in infants and children. *Perspect Pediatr Pathol* 1987;11:124–151.

62. De La Pava S, Nigogosyan G, Pickren JW, Cabrera A. Melanosis of the esophagus. *Cancer* 1963;16:48–50.

63. Sharma SS, Venkateswaran S, Chacko A, Mathan M. Melanosis of the esophagus. An endoscopic, histochemical, and ultrastructural study. *Gastroenterology* 1991;100:13–16.

64. Awsare M, Friedberg JS, Coben R. Primary malignant melanoma of the esophagus. *Clin Gastroenterol Hepatol* 2005;3:xxvii.

65. Suzuki Y, Aoyama N, Minamide J, Takata K, Ogata T. Amelanotic malignant melanoma of the esophagus: report of a patient with recurrence successfully treated with chemoendocrine therapy. *Int J Clin Oncol* 2005;10:204–207.

66. Lam KY, Law S, Chan GS. Esophageal blue nevus: an isolated endoscopic finding. *Head Neck* 2001;23:506–509.

67. Saint Martin MC, Chejfec G. Barrett esophagus-associated small cell carcinoma. *Arch Pathol Lab Med* 1999;123:1123.

68. Seefeld U, Krejs GJ, Siebenmann RE, Blum AL. Esophageal histology in gastroesophageal reflux. Morphometric findings in suction biopsies. *Am J Dig Dis* 1977;22:956–964.

69. Geboes K, De Wolf-Peeters C, Rutgeerts P, Janssens J, Vantrappen G, Desmet V. Lymphocytes and Langerhans cells in the human oesophageal epithelium. *Virchows Arch A Pathol Anat Histopathol* 1983;401:45–55.

70. Geboes K, Haot J, Mebis J, Desmet VJ. The histopathology of reflux esophagitis. *Acta Chir Belg* 1983;83:444–448.

71. Hopwood D, Logan KR, Bouchier IA. The electron microscopy of normal human oesophageal epithelium. *Virchows Arch B Cell Pathol* 1978;26:345–358.

72. Geboes K, Desmet V. Histology of the esophagus. *Front Gastrointest Res* 1978;3:1–17.

73. Bell B, Almy TP, Lipkin M. Cell proliferation kinetics in the gastrointestinal tract of man. 3. Cell renewal in esophagus, stomach, and jejunum of a patient with treated pernicious anemia. *J Natl Cancer Inst* 1967;38:615–628.

74. Burns ER, Scheving LE, Fawcett DF, Gibbs WM, Galatzan RE. Circadian influence on the frequency of labeled mitoses method in the stratified squamous epithelium of the mouse esophagus and tongue. *Anat Rec* 1976;184:265–273.

75. Eastwood GL. Gastrointestinal epithelial renewal. *Gastroenterology* 1977;72(pt 1):962–975.

76. Livstone EM, Sheahan DG, Behar J. Studies of esophageal epithelial cell proliferation in patients with reflux esophagitis. *Gastroenterology* 1977;73:1315–1319.

77. Epperly MW, Guo H, Shen H, et al. Bone marrow origin of cells with capacity for homing and differentiation to esophageal squamous epithelium. *Radiat Res* 2004;162:233–240.

78. Viaene AI, Baert JH. Expression of cytokeratin mRNAs in normal human esophageal epithelium. *Anat Rec* 1995;241:88–98.

79. Seery JP. Stem cells of the oesophageal epithelium. *J Cell Sci* 2002;115(pt 9):1783–1789.

80. Seery JP, Watt FM. Asymmetric stem-cell divisions define the architecture of human oesophageal epithelium. *Curr Biol* 2000;10:1447–1450.

81. Goldman H, Antonioli DA. Mucosal biopsy of the esophagus, stomach, and proximal duodenum. *Hum Pathol* 1982;13:423–448.

82. Brown LF, Goldman H, Antonioli DA. Intraepithelial eosinophils in endoscopic biopsies of adults with reflux esophagitis. *Am J Surg Pathol* 1984;8:899–905.

83. Vieth M, Peitz U, Labenz J, et al. What parameters are relevant for the histological diagnosis of gastroesophageal reflux disease without Barrett's mucosa? *Dig Dis* 2004;22:196–201.

84. Brien TP, Farraye FA, Odze RD. Gastric dysplasia-like epithelial atypia associated with chemoradiotherapy for esophageal cancer: a clinicopathologic and immunohistochemical study of 15 cases. *Mod Pathol* 2001;14:389–396.

85. Muhletaler CA, Lams PM, Johnson AC. Occurrence of oesophageal intramural pseudodiverticulosis in patients with pre-existing benign oesophageal stricture. *Br J Radiol* 1980;53:299–303.

86. Vieth M, Haringsma J, Delarive J, et al. Red streaks in the oesophagus in patients with reflux disease: is there a histomorphological correlate? *Scand J Gastroenterol* 2001;36:1123–1127.

87. Kuramochi H, Vallbohmer D, Uchida K, et al. Quantitative, tissue-specific analysis of cyclooxygenase gene expression in the pathogenesis of Barrett's adenocarcinoma. *J Gastrointest Surg* 2004;8:1007–1017.

88. Medeiros LJ, Doos WG, Balogh K. Esophageal intramural pseudodiverticulosis: a report of two cases with analysis of similar, less extensive changes in "normal" autopsy esophagi. *Hum Pathol* 1988;19:928–931.

89. Meyer GW, Austin RM, Brady CE III, Castell DO. Muscle anatomy of the human esophagus. *J Clin Gastroenterol* 1986;8:131–134.

90. Geboes K, Geboes KP, Maleux G. Vascular anatomy of the gastrointestinal tract. *Best Pract Res Clin Gastroenterol* 2001; 15:1–14.

91. Kitano S, Terblanche J, Kahn D, Bornman PC. Venous anatomy of the lower oesophagus in portal hypertension: practical implications. *Br J Surg* 1986;73:525–531.

92. Vianna A, Hayes PC, Moscoso G, et al. Normal venous circulation of the gastroesophageal junction. A route to understanding varices. *Gastroenterology* 1987;93:876–889.

93. Akiyama H, Tsurumaru M, Kawamura T, Ono Y. Principles of surgical treatment for carcinoma of the esophagus: analysis of lymph node involvement. *Ann Surg* 1981;194:438–446.

94. Faussone-Pellegrini MS, Cortesini C. Ultrastructure of striated muscle fibers in the middle third of the human esophagus. *Histol Histopathol* 1986;1:119–128.

95. Miettinen M, Sarlomo-Rikala M, Sobin LH, Lasota J. Esophageal stromal tumors: a clinicopathologic, immunohistochemical, and molecular genetic study of 17 cases and comparison with esophageal leiomyomas and leiomyosarcomas. *Am J Surg Pathol* 2000;24:211–222.

96. Aggestrup S, Uddman R, Jensen SL, et al. Regulatory peptides in the lower esophageal sphincter of man. *Regul Pept* 1985;10: 167–178.

97. Aggestrup S, Uddman R, Sundler F, et al. Lack of vasoactive intestinal polypeptide nerves in esophageal achalasia. *Gastroenterology* 1983;84(pt 1):924–927.

98. Wattchow DA, Furness JB, Costa M. Distribution and coexistence of peptides in nerve fibers of the external muscle of the human gastrointestinal tract. *Gastroenterology* 1988;95:32–41.

99. Mantyh CR, Pappas TN, Vigna SR. Localization of cholecystokinin A and cholecystokinin B/gastrin receptors in the canine upper gastrointestinal tract. *Gastroenterology* 1994;107:1019–1030.

100. Sharma P, McQuaid K, Dent J, et al. A critical review of the diagnosis and management of Barrett's esophagus: the AGA Chicago Workshop. *Gastroenterology* 2004;127:310–330.

101. Kim SL, Waring JP, Spechler SJ, et al. Diagnostic inconsistencies in Barrett's esophagus. Department of Veterans Affairs Gastroesophageal Reflux Study Group. *Gastroenterology* 1994;107: 945–949.

102. Sharma P. Short segment Barrett esophagus and specialized columnar mucosa at the gastroesophageal junction. *Mayo Clin Proc* 2001;76:331–334.

103. Awad ZT, Filipi CJ. The short esophagus: pathogenesis, diagnosis, and current surgical options. *Arch Surg* 2001;136:113–114.

104. Fletcher J, Wirz A, Henry E, McColl KE. Studies of acid exposure immediately above the gastro-oesophageal squamocolumnar junction: evidence of short segment reflux. *Gut* 2004;53:168–173.

105. Cooper JE, Spitz L, Wilkins BM. Barrett's esophagus in children: a histologic and histochemical study of 11 cases. *J Pediatr Surg* 1987;22:191–196.

106. Hassall E. Columnar-lined esophagus in children. *Gastroenterol Clin North Am* 1997;26:533–548.

107. Hassall E. Childhood Barrett's esophagus under the microscope. *Am J Surg* 1994;167:287–290.

108. Spechler SJ. Short and ultrashort Barrett's esophagus—what does it mean? *Semin Gastrointest Dis* 1997;8:59–67.

109. Chaves P, Cardoso P, de Almeida JC, Pereira AD, Leitao CN, Soares J. Non-goblet cell population of Barrett's esophagus: an immunohistochemical demonstration of intestinal differentiation. *Hum Pathol* 1999;30:1291–1295.

110. Glickman JN, Shahsafaei A, Odze RD. Mucin core peptide expression can help differentiate Barrett's esophagus from intestinal metaplasia of the stomach. *Am J Surg Pathol* 2003;27:1357–1365.

111. Trier JS. Morphology of the columnar-cell-lined (Barrett's) esophagus. In: Spechler SJ, Goyal RK, eds. *Barrett's Esophagus: Pathophysiology, Diagnosis, and Management.* New York: Elsevier; 1985:19–28.

112. Wieczorek TJ, Wang HH, Antonioli DA, Glickman JN, Odze RD. Pathologic features of reflux and Helicobacter pylori-associated carditis: a comparative study. *Am J Surg Pathol* 2003;27:960–968.

113. Shields HM, Rosenberg SJ, Zwas FR, Ransil BJ, Lembo AJ, Odze R. Prospective evaluation of multilayered epithelium in Barrett's esophagus. *Am J Gastroenterol* 2001;96:3268–3273.

114. Riddell RH. The biopsy diagnosis of gastroesophageal reflux disease, "carditis," and Barrett's esophagus, and sequelae of therapy. *Am J Surg Pathol* 1996;20(suppl 1):S31–S50.

115. Takubo K, Vieth M, Aryal G, et al. Islands of squamous epithelium and their surrounding mucosa in columnar-lined esophagus: a pathognomonic feature of Barrett's esophagus? *Hum Pathol* 2005;36:269–274.

116. Odze RD. Unraveling the mysery of the gastroesophageal junction: a pathologist's perspective. *Am J Gastroenterol* 2005;100: 1853–1863.

117. Chandrasoma PT, Der R, Ma Y, Peters J, Demeester T. Histologic classification of patients based on mapping biopsies of the gastroesophageal junction. *Am J Surg Pathol* 2003;27:929–936.

118. Falk GW. Barrett's esophagus. *Gastroenterology* 2002;122: 1569–1591.

119. Sharma P. Recent advances in Barrett's esophagus: short-segment Barrett's esophagus and cardia intestinal metaplasia. *Semin Gastrointest Dis* 1999;10:93–102.

120. Solcia E, Villani L, Luinetti O, et al. Altered intercellular glycoconjugates and dilated intercellular spaces of esophageal epithelium in reflux disease. *Virchows Arch* 2000;436:207–216.

121. Bove M, Vieth M, Dombrowski F, Ny L, Ruth M, Lundell L. Acid challenge to the human esophageal mucosa: effects on epithelial architecture in health and disease. *Dig Dis Sci* 2005;50: 1488–1496.

122. Tobey NA, Hosseini SS, Argote CM, Dobrucali AM, Awayda MS, Orlando RC. Dilated intercellular spaces and shunt permeability in nonerosive acid-damaged esophageal epithelium. *Am J Gastroenterol* 2004;99:13–22.

123. Tobey NA, Carson JL, Alkiek RA, Orlando RC. Dilated intercellular spaces: a morphological feature of acid reflux—damaged human esophageal epithelium. *Gastroenterology* 1996;111:1200–1205.

124. Caviglia R, Ribolsi M, Maggiano N, et al. Dilated intercellular spaces of esophageal epithelium in nonerosive reflux disease patients with physiological esophageal acid exposure. *Am J Gastroenterol* 2005;100:543–548.

125. Calabrese C, Bortolotti M, Fabbri A, et al. Reversibility of GERD ultrastructural alterations and relief of symptoms after omeprazole treatment. *Am J Gastroenterol* 2005;100:537–542.

126. Winter HS, Madara JL, Stafford RJ, Grand RJ, Quinlan JE, Goldman H. Intraepithelial eosinophils: a new diagnostic criterion for reflux esophagitis. *Gastroenterology* 1982;83:818–823.

127. Sant'Anna AM, Rolland S, Fournet JC, Yazbeck S, Drouin E. Eosinophilic esophagitis in children: symptoms, histology and pH probe results. *J Pediatr Gastroenterol Nutr* 2004;39:373–377.

128. Parfitt JR, Gregor JC, Suskin NG, Jawa HA, Driman DK. Eosinophilic esophagitis in adults: distinguishing features from gastroesophageal reflux disease: a study of 41 patients. *Mod Pathol* 2006;19:90–96.

129. Sgouros SN, Bergele C, Mantides A. Eosinophilic esophagitis in adults: a systematic review. *Eur J Gastroenterol Hepatol* 2006;18: 211–217.

130. Onbasi K, Sin AZ, Doganavsargil B, Onder GF, Bor S, Sebik F. Eosinophil infiltration of the oesophageal mucosa in patients with pollen allergy during the season. *Clin Exp Allergy* 2005;35: 1423–1431.

131. Spergel JM, Andrews T, Brown-Whitehorn TF, Beausoleil JL, Liacouras CA. Treatment of eosinophilic esophagitis with specific food elimination diet directed by a combination of skin prick and patch tests. *Ann Allergy Asthma Immunol* 2005;95:336–343.

132. Straumann A, Spichtin HP, Bucher KA, Heer P, Simon HU. Eosinophilic esophagitis: red on microscopy, white on endoscopy. *Digestion* 2004;70:109–116.

133. Straumann A, Rossi L, Simon HU, Heer P, Spichtin HP, Beglinger C. Fragility of the esophageal mucosa: a pathognomonic endoscopic sign of primary eosinophilic esophagitis? *Gastrointest Endosc* 2003;57:407–412.

134. Kobayashi S, Kasugai T. Endoscopic and biopsy criteria for the diagnosis of esophagitis with a fiberoptic esophagoscope. *Am J Dig Dis* 1974;19:345–352.

135. Cucchiara S, D'Armiento F, Alfieri E, et al. Intraepithelial cells with irregular nuclear contours as a marker of esophagitis in children with gastroesophageal reflux disease. *Dig Dis Sci* 1995; 40:2305–2311.

136. Esposito S, Valente G, Zavallone A, Guidali P, Rapa A, Oderda G. Histological score for cells with irregular nuclear contours for the diagnosis of reflux esophagitis in children. *Hum Pathol* 2004;35: 96–101.

137. Csendes A, Smok G, Burdiles P, et al. 'Carditis': an objective histological marker for pathologic gastroesophageal reflux disease. *Dis Esophagus* 1998;11:101–105.

138. Lembo T, Ippoliti AF, Ramers C, Weinstein WM. Inflammation of the gastro-oesophageal junction (carditis) in patients with symptomatic gastro-oesophageal reflux disease: a prospective study. *Gut* 1999;45:484–488.

139. Gulmann C, Rathore O, Grace A, et al. 'Cardiac-type' (mucinous) mucosa and carditis are both associated with Helicobacter pylori-related gastritis. *Eur J Gastroenterol Hepatol* 2004;16:69–74.

140. Voutilainen M, Farkkila M, Mecklin JP, Juhola M, Sipponen P. Chronic inflammation at the gastroesophageal junction (carditis) appears to be a specific finding related to Helicobacter pylori infection and gastroesophageal reflux disease. The Central Finland Endoscopy Study Group. *Am J Gastroenterol* 1999;94:3175–3180.

141. Peitz U, Vieth M, Malfertheiner P. Carditis at the interface between GERD and Helicobacter pylori infection. *Dig Dis* 2004;22: 120–125.

142. Marsman WA, Tytgat GN, ten Kate FJ, van Lanschot JJ. Differences and similarities of adenocarcinomas of the esophagus and esophagogastric junction. *J Surg Oncol* 2005;92:160–168.

143. Sabel MS, Pastore K, Toon H, Smith JL. Adenocarcinoma of the esophagus with and without Barrett mucosa. *Arch Surg* 2000; 135:831–836.

144. Di Martino N, Izzo G, Cosenza A, et al. Adenocarcinoma of gastric cardia in the elderly: surgical problems and prognostic factors. *World J Gastroenterol* 2005;11:5123–5128.

Stomach

23

David A. Owen

EMBRYOLOGY AND POSTNATAL DEVELOPMENT

The stomach develops as a fusiform dilatation of the foregut caudal to the esophagus. This occurs first when the embryo is 7 mm in length. Initially, it is attached to the back of the abdomen by the dorsal mesogastrium and to the septum transversum (diaphragm) by the ventral mesogastrium. As the stomach enlarges, the dorsal mesogastrium becomes the greater omentum and the ventral mesogastrium becomes the lesser omentum.

The stomach is derived from endoderm, and early glandular differentiation of the mucosal lining occurs first at the 80-mm stage of fetal development. Enzyme and acid production first occur at the fourth month of fetal life and are well established by the time of birth. The newborn stomach is fully developed and similar to that of the adult.

GROSS MORPHOLOGIC FEATURES

The stomach is a flattened J-shaped organ located in the left upper quadrant of the abdomen. At its upper end, it joins the esophagus several centimeters below the level of the diaphragm. At its distal end, it merges with the duodenum, just to the right of the midline. The stomach is extremely distensible, and its size varies, depending on the volume of food present.

For the purposes of gross description, the stomach can be divided into four regions: cardia, fundus, corpus (or body), and antrum (1,2) (Figure 23.1). The superomedial margin is termed the lesser curvature, and the inferolateral margin is termed the greater curvature. The cardia is found just distal to the lower end of the esophagus. It is a small and ill-defined area, extending 1 to 3 cm from the gastroesophageal junction. The fundus is that portion of the stomach that lies above the gastroesophageal junction, just below the left

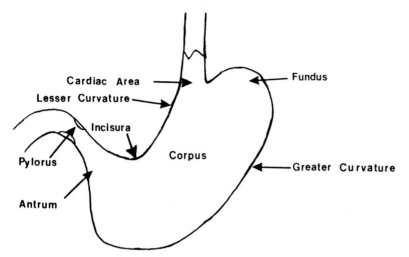

Figure 23.1 Gross anatomical zones of the stomach.

hemidiaphragm. The antrum comprises the distal third of the stomach, proximal to the pyloric sphincter (pylorus), with the remainder of the stomach referred to as the corpus. The junction between the antrum and corpus is poorly demarcated. By external examination, it comprises the portion of stomach distal to the incisura, a notch on the lesser curvature (1). Internally, the gastric mucosa is usually thrown into coarse folds called rugae. These are prominent when the stomach is empty but flattened out when the organ is distended. The rugae are most prominent in the corpus and fundus because this is where the major dilatation to accommodate food occurs. The antrum is characterized by mucosa that is flatter and more firmly anchored to the underlying submucosa (Figure 23.2).

The wall of the stomach has four layers: mucosa, submucosa, muscularis propria, and subserosa. Apart from the mucosa, these layers are structurally similar to the bowel wall elsewhere in the gastrointestinal tract. When viewed close up, the surface of the mucosa is dissected by thin shallow grooves termed areae gastricae (3). These are structurally fixed and do not flatten out when the stomach is distended. They are best seen when the mucosa is viewed *en face* with a hand lens. *Areae gastricae* may be demonstrated radiologically via double-contrast barium examination but also can be recognized on histologic sections—particularly from gastrectomy specimens, where they appear as shallow depressions on an otherwise monotonously smooth surface (Figure 23.3).

Blood Supply

Five arteries supply blood to the stomach. The left gastric artery arises directly from the celiac axis and supplies the cardiac region. The right gastric artery (which supplies the lesser curve) and the right gastroepiploic artery (which supplies the greater curve) arise from the hepatic artery. The left gastroepiploic and the short gastric arteries arise from

the splenic artery and also supply the greater curvature. All these vessels anastomose freely, both on the subserosal layer of the stomach and in the muscularis propria, with extensive true plexus formation present within the submucosa. This richness of blood supply explains why it is so

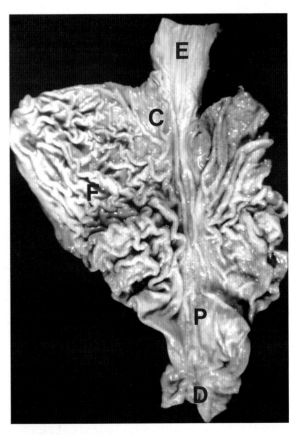

Figure 23.2 Mucosal zones of the stomach. The cardiac mucosa (*C*) is present distal to the lower end of the esophagus (*E*). The pyloric mucosa (*P*) occupies a triangular zone proximal to the duodenum (*D*). Elsewhere, the fundic mucosa (*F*) shows prominent rugal folds.

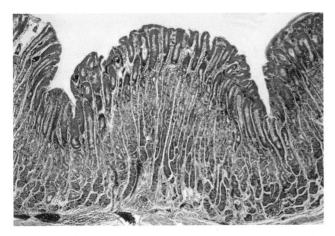

Figure 23.3 Low-power view of the gastric fundal mucosa. The grooves in the mucosa are fixed anatomical features called areae gastricae.

unusual to see gastric infarcts. The mucosal arteries are derived from this submucosal plexus but are end arteries and supply an area of mucosa that is largely independent of the adjacent mucosal arteries (4).

Nerve Supply

The sympathetic nerve supply to the stomach is derived from the celiac plexus via nerves that follow the gastric and gastroepiploic arteries. Branches also are received from the left and right phrenic nerves. The parasympathetic supply is the vagus nerve via the main anterior and posterior trunks that lie adjacent to the esophagogastric junction. Shortly after entering the abdomen, the anterior vagus nerve gives off a hepatic branch, and the posterior vagus nerve gives off a celiac branch. Therefore, truncal vagotomy above these branches results in denervation of not only the stomach but the entire intestinal tract. Sectioning below these nerves results only in gastric denervation. A highly selective vagotomy (gastric corpus denervation) is achieved by sectioning lateral branches as the two main gastric nerves pass along the lesser curvature, with preservation of the terminal portion of the vagi that supply the antrum. No true nerve plexuses occur on either subserosal layer of the stomach but instead are concentrated in Meissner's plexus in the submucosa and Auerbach's plexus between the circular and longitudinal fibers of the muscularis propria.

Lymphatics

Recent studies (5,6) have disproved the former view that lymphatic channels are present at all levels of the lamina propria. By using careful ultrastructural techniques, lymphatics have been demonstrated to be limited to the portion of the lamina propria immediately superficial to the muscularis mucosae. From there, efferents penetrate the

muscle and communicate with larger lymphatic channels running in the submucosa. This arrangement implies that an early gastric cancer may have lymphatic metastases, even though the primary tumor is entirely superficial to the muscularis mucosae.

The lymphatic trunks of the stomach generally follow the main arteries and veins. Four areas of drainage can be identified, each with its own group of nodes. The largest area comprises the lower end of the esophagus and most of the lesser curvature, which drains along the left gastric artery to the left gastric nodes. From the immediate region of the pylorus, on the lesser curvature, drainage is to the right gastric and hepatic nodes. The proximal portion of the greater curvature drains to pancreaticosplenic nodes in the hilum of the spleen, and the distal portion of the greater curvature drains to the right gastroepiploic nodes in the greater omentum and to pyloric nodes at the head of the pancreas. Efferents from all four groups ultimately pass to celiac nodes around the main celiac axis.

GENERAL HISTOLOGIC FEATURES

Histologically, the mucosa has a similar pattern throughout the stomach. It consists of a superficial layer containing foveolae (pits), which represent invaginations of the surface epithelium, and a deep layer consisting of coiled glands that empty into the base of the foveolae (Figure 23.4). The glandular layer differs in structure and function in different zones of the stomach that correspond roughly, but not precisely, to the gross anatomic regions (Figure 23.1).

Adjacent to the gastroesophageal junction is the cardiac mucosa, where the glands are mucus secreting. Extending proximally from the pylorus is the pyloric mucosa (sometimes called the antral mucosa), where the glands are also mucus secreting. This zone is triangular, extending much further (5–7 cm) proximally along the lesser curvature than it does along the greater curvature (3–4 cm). The pyloric mucosal zone is not identical to the antral region, although some accounts use these terms interchangeably. Also, contrary to what is implied in some descriptions, the incisura has no fixed relationship to the proximal margin of the pyloric mucosal zone. Elsewhere within the stomach (corpus and fundus), the mucosa is exclusively fundic in type, where the glands are specialized to secrete acid and pepsin.

Histologic transition between pyloric and fundal mucosa is gradual rather than abrupt, with intervening junctional mucosae (1–2 cm in width) having a mixed histologic appearance. A broad mucosal transition zone is also present at the pylorus, where gastric and duodenal mucosae merge. However, at the lower end of the normal esophagus, the change from nonkeratinizing squamous epithelium to columnar epithelium is abrupt, both grossly and microscopically. The position of this squamocolumnar junction is variable and does not always coincide with the

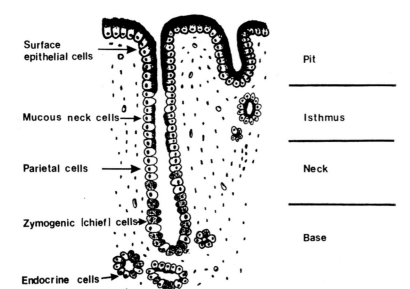

Figure 23.4 Diagrammatic representation of gastric fundal mucosa. Zymogenic (chief) cells are seen mainly in the basal portion of the glands and parietal cells mainly in the isthmic portion. The neck portion contains zymogenic cells, parietal cells, and mucous neck cells. A small number of endocrine cells are present in the basal zone.

strict anatomic esophagogastric junction, that is, the point where the tubular esophagus becomes the saccular stomach. In some individuals the mucosal junction is located 0.5 to 2.5 cm proximal to the anatomic junction and often is serrated, rather than being a regular circumferential line (Z line) (2).

Surface Epithelium

Histologically, the gastric mucosa is covered by tall, columnar, mucus-secreting cells with intervening foveolae that are lined by a similar epithelium (Figure 23.5). The surface and foveolar lining cells are similar throughout all the mucosal zones of the stomach. The gastric glands empty into the base of the foveolae. Separating the foveolae and the

glands is the lamina propria. In the cardiac and pyloric mucosal zones, the foveolae are wider than in other areas, sometimes giving the mucosa a slightly villous appearance (Figure 23.6).

The cells of the surface epithelium and foveolae are tall and columnar with basally situated nuclei and superficial cytoplasm that is almost entirely filled with mucus (Figure 23.7). The nuclei have an even distribution of chromatin, with single inconspicuous nucleoli. On hematoxylin and eosin (H&E)–stained sections, the appearance of the mucus varies, depending on the staining routine and type of stain used. For example, with alcoholic eosin, the mucus appears as a single vacuole that is clear or lightly eosinophilic. With aqueous eosin, the mucus is more heavily eosinophilic and is seen to be present in numerous, small, closely aggre-

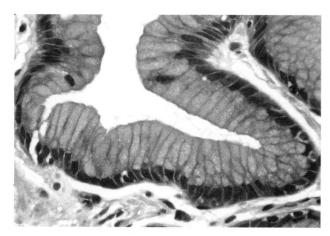

Figure 23.5 Gastric surface epithelium with each cell having a mucous globule in the superficial cytoplasm. Intraepithelial lymphocytes are present. These are surrounded by a clear halo (formalin fixation artifact).

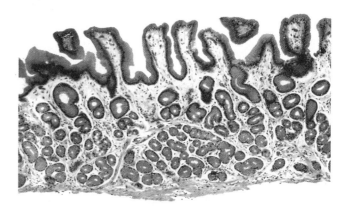

Figure 23.6 Gastric pyloric mucosa. Note that the glands are loosely packed and occupy about half the mucosal thickness. The surface epithelium appears slightly villous.

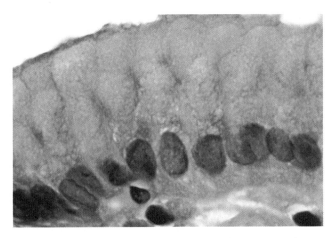

Figure 23.7 Gastric surface epithelium showing cytoplasmic mucus present in multiple small vacuoles.

gated vacuoles. Histochemically, the foveolar mucus is all neutral, periodic acid- Schiff (PAS)–positive, but Alcian blue-negative at pH 2.5 and lower (7).

Cardiac and Pyloric Mucosa

In the cardiac and pyloric zone, the foveolae occupy approximately one-half of the mucosal thickness (Figure 23.6). Both the cardiac and pyloric glands are mucus secreting and are loosely packed with abundant intervening lamina propria (Figure 23.8). Occasional cystic glands may be found in the cardiac mucosa but usually are not encountered in the pyloric mucosa. The cells of the mucus glands have ill-defined borders and a bubbly cytoplasm that is different from the foveolar and surface epithelium. They resemble Brunner's glands of the duodenum. Isolated parietal cells are not infrequently found either singly or in small groups, particularly in the pyloric mucosa and espe-

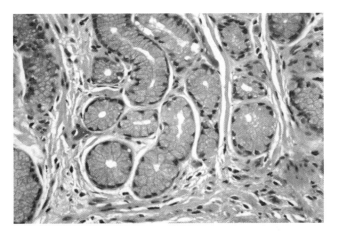

Figure 23.8 Pyloric glands containing cells with a bubbly, foamy appearance.

cially at the junctional zone, where it meets the fundic mucosa (1). However, it is uncommon for zymogenic (chief) cells to be present outside of the fundic mucosa and junctional area. The pyloric glands secrete neutral mucin only. The cardiac glands secrete predominantly neutral mucin with small amounts of sialomucin (7).

The extent of the cardiac mucosa and even its existence as a component of the normal gastroesophageal junction has been disputed. Chandrasoma and his associates (8) studied the gastroesophageal region in unselected adult autopsies. They found that when one histologic section was taken through this region only 27% of cases had a zone of pure cardiac mucosa, 44% of cases had a zone of cardio-fundic mucosa (glands containing a mixture of mucus-secreting cells and parietal cells), and 29% of cases had only pure fundic mucosa. When the entire gastroesophageal junction from a selected group of adult autopsies was examined, all cases had cardiofundic mucosa present, but only 44% had a zone of pure cardiac mucosa. They also found that the zones of pure cardiac mucosa and cardiofundic mucosae were incomplete so that in some sections the esophageal squamous epithelium was present immediately adjacent to pure fundic mucosa. The average length of the cardiac and cardiofundic mucosa was 5 mm, and it never extended beyond 15 mm from the lower margin of the squamous esophageal epithelium. Other investigators have obtained similar results (9). In contrast, Kilgore and associates (10) and Zhou and associates (11) examined autopsy material from fetuses, infants, and young children. They found that pure cardiac mucosa was present in every case and measured 1.0 to 4.0 mm in length (average 1.8 mm). In 38% of cases, there was an abrupt transition from cardiac to fundic glands; and, in the remainder of cases, an additional zone of cardiofundic mucosa was present that generally measured less than 1.0 mm in length. In all instances where cardiofundic mucosa was present, it was in addition to a zone of pure cardiac mucosa. These findings suggest that pure cardiac mucosa and cardiofundic mucosa are normal findings but that the extent of the mucus-secreting mucosa is less than was previously thought. Cardiac mucosal abnormalities may occur when there is gastroesophageal reflux or when the stomach is infected by *Helicobacter pylori*. The changes may include inflammatory nuclear atypia, intestinal metaplasia, and the presence of hybrid mucosa (12). Hybrid mucosa is multilayered, with squamous cells at the base of the mucosa and columnar epithelium on the surface. With the development of these inflammatory changes, it may be difficult or even impossible to distinguish between damaged cardiac mucosa and glandular metaplasia of esophageal squamous epithelium (Barrett's esophagus). Reference to specialized pathology texts is required (13). This distinction has a practical importance because Barrett's esophagus carries a higher potential for malignant change than does metaplastic cardiac mucosa (14).

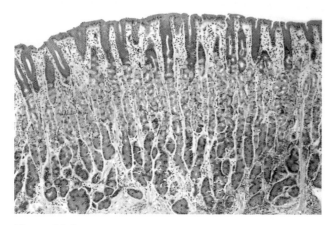

Figure 23.9 Gastric fundic mucosa. Note the short foveolae and the tightly packed glands. Purplish zymogenic cells predominate at the base, and pinkish parietal cells predominate in the upper part of the glands.

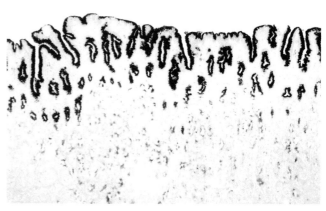

Figure 23.11 Fundic mucosa. The surface and foveolar lining epithelium is intensely positive. Paler staining mucus neck cells are present within the glands (PAS).

Fundic Gland Mucosa

The fundic (or oxyntic) gland mucosa has foveolae that occupy less than one-quarter of the mucosal thickness. In contrast to the cardiac and pyloric mucosa, the glands are tightly packed and are straight rather than coiled (Figure 23.9). For descriptive purposes, they can be divided into three portions: base, neck, and isthmus. The basal portion consists mainly of zymogenic cells (pepsinogen secreting). These are cuboidal and have a basally situated nucleus, which typically contains one or more small nucleoli and cytoplasm that usually stains pale blue-gray with some variation, depending on the type of hematoxylin used (Figure 23.10). The isthmic portion of the glands contains predominantly parietal cells (acid- and intrinsic factor-secreting). These are roughly triangular, with their base along the basement membrane. The nuclei are centrally placed with evenly distributed chromatin, and the cyto-

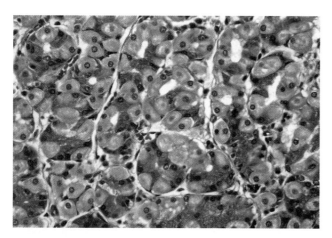

Figure 23.10 Fundic glands, showing parietal cell cytoplasm staining light pink and zymogenic cell cytoplasm staining purplish (H&E).

plasm stains a deep pink on well-differentiated H&E sections (Figure 23.10). The neck portion of the fundic glands contains a mixture of zymogenic and parietal cells, together with a third type, mucous neck cells (Figure 23.11). These are difficult to recognize on an H&E stain but are easily identified using a PAS stain, where they are seen to resemble the mucus-secreting cells of the cardiac and pyloric glands. These cells produce neutral and acidic mucin, especially sialomucin, which stains positively with Alcian blue at pH 2.5 (15). Mucous neck cells are found in lesser numbers in the isthmic portion of the glands, and occasional parietal cells can be encountered in the basal portion of the glands. Mucous neck cells are also present in the pyloric mucosa.

Studies indicate that the mucous neck cells located in glands from all areas of the stomach have proliferation and mucosal regeneration as their major functions. These undifferentiated cells act as stem cells and may migrate upward to renew foveolar and surface epithelium or downward to renew zymogenic, parietal, or neuroendocrine cells (16). It has been estimated that, in humans, the gastric surface epithelium is normally replaced every four to eight days. The parietal and zymogenic cells turn over much more slowly, likely every one to three years.

Endocrine Cells

The stomach contains a wide variety of hormone-producing cells. In the antrum, about 50% of the whole endocrine cell population are G cells (gastrin-producing), 30% are enterochromaffin (EC) cells (serotonin-producing), and 15% are D cells (somatostatin-producing). In the fundic mucosa, however, a major portion of the endocrine cells are enterochromaffin-like (ECL) and secrete histamine. Small numbers of X cells (secretion product unknown) and EC cells are also present. In the fundic mucosa, the cells secreting these

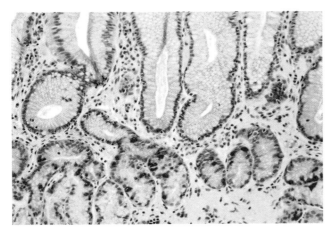

Figure 23.12 Endocrine cells in gastric antral glands. The granules are located between the nucleus and the basement membrane (immunostain for chromogranin).

hormones are mostly located in the glands, particularly toward the base. In the pyloric mucosa, they are most common in the neck region just below the foveolae. Within these neuroendocrine cells, the hormones are present as cytoplasmic granules located between the nucleus and basement membrane; but, because the granules are generally inconspicuous on H&E sections, special techniques are required for their demonstration (Figure 23.12). Hormones from the endocrine cells either enter the blood or modulate other locally situated cells (paracrine effect).

The EC cells and some of the ECL cells have argentaffin granules, which can be stained by Fontana, Masson, or the diazo technique. Other cells are argyrophilic but not argentaffinic and may be stained by the Grimelius technique (17). Silver stains have now been replaced by more sensitive immunologic techniques (synaptophysin and chromogranin) (18). Individual hormones, for example gastrin and somatostatin, may be demonstrated by specific antibodies. In addition to the presence of hormones in epithelial cells, some hormones also are found in neurons and nerve endings present in the stomach wall and mucosa. It is generally believed that vasoactive intestinal peptide is predominant in neural tissue and that catecholamines, bombesin, substance P, enkephalins, and possibly gastrin are also found at these sites. When hyperplasia of G cells occurs, it is generally linear. Overgrowth of ECL cells in the fundic mucosa occurs secondary to hypergastrinemia, arising as a consequence of pernicious anemia. This has been divided into five growth patterns: pseudohyperplasia, hyperplasia, dysplasia, microinfiltration, and neoplasia (19).

Lamina Propria

The epithelial cells of the surface, foveolae, and glands all rest on a basement membrane, which is similar to that seen elsewhere in the intestinal tract. Within the mucosa is a well-developed lamina propria that provides structural support, consisting of a fine meshwork of reticulin with occasional collagen and elastic fibers that are condensed underneath the basement membrane (Figure 23.13). The lamina propria is more abundant in the superficial portion of the mucosa between the pits, especially in the pyloric mucosa. It contains numerous cell types, including fibroblasts, histiocytes, plasma cells, and lymphocytes. It is also normal to find occasional polymorphs and mast cells. As mentioned, the lamina propria also contains capillaries, arterioles, and nonmyelinated nerve fibers. A few fibers of smooth muscle extend upward from the muscularis mucosa into the lamina propria, occasionally reaching the superficial portion of the mucosa, especially in the distal antrum.

The lymphoid tissue of the stomach has not been studied as extensively as that of the small bowel. The isolated lymphocytes and plasma cells in the lamina propria are predominantly of B-cell lineage and IgA secreting. Intraepithelial lymphocytes are present in the stomach but are much less frequent than in the small bowel. They are commonly surrounded by a clear halo, which represents a formalin fixation artifact. These lymphocytes, as well as small numbers of lamina propria lymphocytes, are of T-cell origin.

Recently it has been shown that small numbers of primary lymphoid follicles (aggregates of small lymphocytes) can be found in the normal stomach (20). However, secondary lymphoid follicles (follicles with germinal centers) are found only in gastritis, usually secondary to infection with *Helicobacter pylori*.

Submucosa

The submucosa is located between the muscularis mucosae and the muscularis propria and also forms the cores of the gastric rugae. It consists of loose connective tissue, in which many elastic fibers are found. The autonomic nerve plexus of Meissner is found in the submucosa, as are plexuses of veins, arteries, and lymphatics.

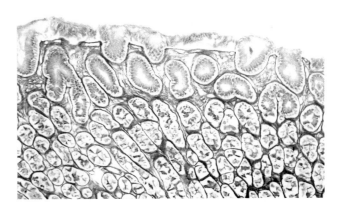

Figure 23.13 Normal gastric fundic mucosa (reticulin).

Muscular Components

In classical anatomy texts (21,22), the main muscle mass of the stomach is referred to as the muscularis externa. In North America, however, the alternative name, muscularis propria, is widely used and preferred. This is because the term *muscularis externa* is ambiguous, and it is sometimes not clear whether it refers to the whole of the main muscle mass or only its external layer.

Three layers of fibers can be recognized in the muscularis propria: outer longitudinal, inner circular, and innermost oblique. The external fibers are continuous with the longitudinal muscle of the esophagus. The inner circular layer is aggregated into a definite sphincter mass at the pylorus, where it is sharply separated from the circular fibers of the duodenum by a connective tissue septum. The oblique muscular fibers are an incomplete layer present interior to the circular fibers and are most obvious in the cardiac area. Evidence for the presence of a circular sphincter at the cardia is controversial (23). Histologic examination is not conclusive; and, although radiologic techniques show arrest of swallowed food at this level, this may be due to external compression from the adjacent crura of the diaphragm.

The muscularis mucosae consist of two layers, the inner circular and outer longitudinal, together with some elastic fibers. Thin bundles of smooth muscle also penetrate into the lamina propria, where they terminate in the basement membrane of the epithelium. This is most obvious in the antral area.

ULTRASTRUCTURE

The surface and foveolar lining epithelial cells are ultrastructurally similar. They are characterized by multiple, rounded, electron-dense mucous vacuoles in the superficial cytoplasm and stubby microvilli projecting from the luminal surface. The basal cytoplasm contains moderate amounts of rough endoplasmic reticulum and some mitochondria. Adjacent epithelial cells are joined by tight junctions (zona occludens) at their luminal aspect and by adherence junctions along the rest of the cell interfaces. These tight junctions are considered to play an important role in maintaining mucosal integrity and the gastric mucosal barrier.

Parietal cells are unique ultrastructurally (Figure 23.14) (24). In the unstimulated state, the cytoplasm contains an apical crescent-shaped canaliculus lined by stubby microvilli (Figure 23.14). Between the microvilli are elongated membrane invaginations termed microtubules. Upon stimulation, the microtubules disappear, to be replaced by a dense meshwork of intracellular canaliculi (25). The canalicular system is considered essential for the formation of hydrochloric acid. This is achieved by active transport of hydrogen ions across the canalicular membrane. Because this process has high energy requirements, most of the remainder of the parietal cell cytoplasm is occupied by mitochondria.

The zymogenic cells are similar to protein-secreting exocrine cells elsewhere in the body. They have rough-

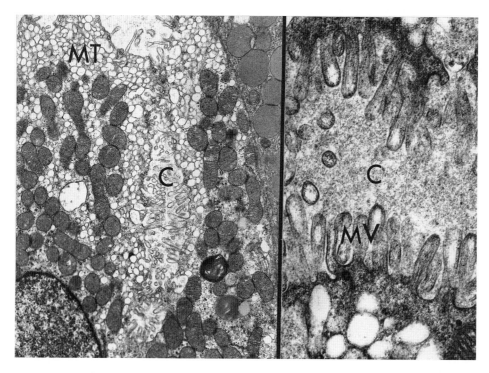

Figure 23.14 Ultrastructural appearances of the parietal cell canaliculus (*C*). Note the fingerlike microvilli (*MV*) and the microtubular invaginations (*MT*). (Original magnifications: *left*, ×9000; *right*, ×41,000.)

surfaced vesicles in the superficial cytoplasm and abundant rough endoplasmic reticulum in the remainder of the cell.

GASTRIC FUNCTION

The function of the stomach is to act as a reservoir and mixer of food and to initiate the digestive process. Gastric secretion of acid, pepsin, and electrolytes is partly under nervous control by the vagus and partly under the control of gastrin, produced by G cells in the antrum. Gastrin release from the G cells may occur either as a result of distention of the antrum or by direct stimulation from ingested food, particularly amino acids and peptides. Hydrochloric acid is produced by the active transport of hydrogen ions across the cell membrane. High concentrations of hydrochloric acid are achieved so that most ingested microorganisms are killed and the contents of the stomach are normally sterile.

Gastric mucus is secreted in two forms: a soluble fraction produced by the gastric glands and an insoluble form produced by the surface and foveolar lining cells. Biochemically, the mucus is a complex glycoprotein consisting of a protein core with branched carbohydrate side chains. Histochemically, gastric mucin is almost entirely neutral, although the mucous neck cells may secrete small amounts of sulfomucin and sialomucin (15). By immunohistochemistry, mucins MUC5AC and MUC6 are detected in the normal stomach (26). The exact physiologic role of gastric mucin is not determined. Clearly, the soluble mucin plays a role in lubrication. The insoluble fraction acts as a surface layer, forming a barrier that, together with bicarbonate secreted by the superficial epithelial cells, prevents back diffusion of acid and gastric autodigestion. The actual structural barrier is formed by the continuous layer of luminal mucosal cells and the tight junctions between adjacent cells. This process is likely modulated by prostaglandins which promote mucosal blood flow.

SPECIAL TECHNIQUES AND PROCEDURES

Relatively few special techniques are applicable to routine diagnosis. Mucin stains are the most widely used, and the combined PAS/Alcian blue is the most versatile. This stains neutral mucin magenta, acid mucin light blue, and combinations purple. The combined stain is preferred over a straight PAS because the mucus in some gastric carcinomas is PAS-negative. A mucicarmine stain is not recommended because it does not permit identification of the mucin type and is also negative with some types of acid mucin. Sialomucin and sulphomucin may be distinguished by a combined high iron diamine and Alcian blue stain, which

stains sulphomucin black and sialomucin light blue. At the present time, however, this distinction is of limited diagnostic utility.

Usually there is no difficulty in distinguishing zymogenic and parietal cells on a good H&E stain (Figure 23.10). If necessary, special stains, such as a Maxwell stain (27), can aid this distinction. Parietal cells can be recognized and quantified by use of a human milk fat globulin antibody (28).

At the present time, the use of cytokeratin 7 and cytokeratin 20 immunostains to distinguish gastric cardiac mucosa from the mucosa of Barrett's esophagus is controversial. Different results have been obtained by different observers, so this methodology cannot be recommended for routine use (13).

AGE CHANGES

Many older adults have a reduced gastric acid output. Histologically, this is characterized by a reduction in the area of fundic mucosa with expansion of the zone of pyloric mucosa. This results in proximal displacement of the pylorofundic junction, a change termed pyloric (or pseudopyloric) metaplasia. Recently it has become recognized that hypochlorhydria of the elderly is not simply the result of aging but is secondary to chronic gastritis (29).

ARTIFACTS

A variety of artifacts may occur in gastric biopsy specimens (Figure 23.15). Most of these artifacts relate to rough handling of the specimen, either at the time the biopsy sample is taken or when it is removed from the forceps. Crushing is common and can result in compression of the lamina propria, leading to a false impression of an inflammatory infiltrate. Crush artifact also produces telescoping of the foveolar lining cells. Stretching of the mucosa results in separation of the pits and glands, leading to the impression of edema. Hemorrhage into the lamina propria is also common in gastric biopsy samples and has to be distinguished from hemorrhagic gastritis. This can be difficult in small biopsy samples, but usually the microscopic appearances of hemorrhagic gastritis are characteristic. They include superficial epithelial damage and erosions.

DIFFERENTIAL DIAGNOSIS

One of the problems for pathologists examining gastric biopsy samples is determining whether the specimen is normal or shows minor degrees of gastritis. It is therefore

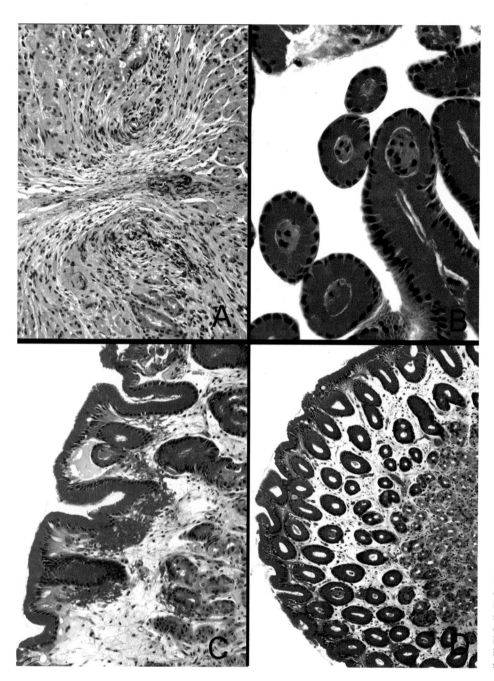

Figure 23.15 Biopsy artifacts: crushing, producing an apparent lamina propria infiltrate (**A**); crushing, resulting in displacement (telescoping) of cells into pit lumen (**B**); biopsy-induced hemorrhage (**C**); and stretching, producing an appearance of superficial edema (**D**).

appropriate to review briefly certain aspects of the classification and diagnosis. Specific types of gastritis, for example, acute hemorrhagic gastritis or granulomatous gastritis, are usually so distinct that confusion with a normal stomach is unlikely (30). On the other hand, *Helicobacter pylori* gastritis may be patchy and may be associated with atrophy. In the early stage of *H. pylori* gastritis (chronic superficial gastritis), an infiltrate of inflammatory cells is observed in the superficial portion of the mucosa, particularly in the lamina propria between the gastric pits (Figure 23.16). Later, the inflammation spreads deeply to involve the whole thickness of the mucosa and is accompanied by atrophy of

gastric glands (chronic atrophic gastritis). Ultimately, the inflammation may burn itself out and all glands are destroyed, leaving only a thinned mucosa containing foveolar structures (gastric atrophy) (30).

The superficial gastric lamina propria normally contains some chronic inflammatory cells. It is often a matter of judgment whether these are considered normal or increased in number because there is no simple satisfactory method of objective measurement. In actual practice, it may be even more difficult to evaluate these cells because the gastric biopsy samples obtained by endoscopists are frequently distorted by crushing or stretching. In assessing possible minor

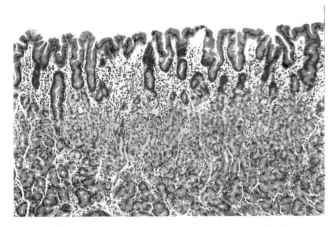

Figure 23.16 Mild chronic superficial gastritis with chronic inflammatory cells present in the superficial lamina propria in excess of normal. This is a borderline biopsy sample and illustrates the least number of cells acceptable for a diagnosis of gastritis.

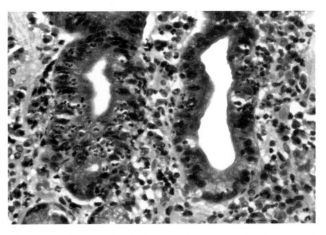

Figure 23.18 Gastric pits infiltrated by neutrophils in a case of *Helicobacter pylori* gastritis.

degrees of inflammation, therefore, study should also be made of the superficial and foveolar lining epithelium, where a number of useful diagnostic features may be identified, depending on the degree of activity of the inflammation. The earliest changes seen are a reduction in the mucin content of the cytoplasm, an increase in nuclear size, and the presence of one or more prominent nucleoli (Figure 23.17). At the base of the foveolae, there may be increased numbers of mitoses, reflecting a more rapid cell turnover. These findings are features of epithelial damage and regeneration and are common to all forms of gastritis and to reactive gastropathy (chemical gastritis). In severe active *H. pylori*-related inflammation, the epithelium and the lamina propria are infiltrated by acute inflammatory cells (Figure 23.18) and organisms may be seen on the mucosal surface (Figure 23.19). Optimum recognition of organisms is enhanced by using special stains (Giemsa, methylene blue, immunohistochemical stains).

Where gastritis has been present for some time, there may be atrophy of the mucosal glands, which can be accompanied by an increase in inflammatory cells in the deeper layers of the mucosa. On an H&E section, this is seen as a separation of the glands with increased intervening lamina propria. However, minor degrees of atrophy may be difficult to distinguish, particularly if there is biopsy artifact. In these instances, a reticulin stain can be useful in confirming atrophy by demonstrating coarse condensation of fibers in the lamina propria (Figure 23.20).

Reactive gastropathy occurs when there is increased exfoliation of cells from the mucosal surface. Chemical agents, especially refluxed bile and nonsteroidal anti-inflammatory drugs, are common causes. The gastric surface and foveolar epitheium show regenerative changes as described above, but the mucosa is not infiltrated by inflammatory cells. The more severe examples of reactive gastropathy may be characterized by a "cork screw" appearance of the foveolae.

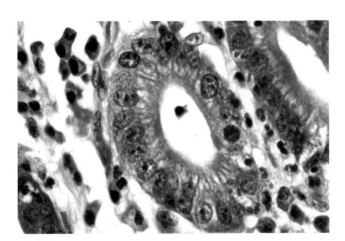

Figure 23.17 Gastritis showing cytoplasmic mucin loss with enlarged nuclei that contain prominent nucleoli.

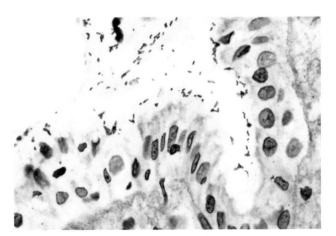

Figure 23.19 *Helicobacter pylori* organisms present in the mucous layer on the gastric mucosal surface.

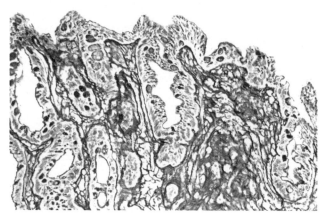

Figure 23.20 Coarse condensation of mucosal fibers in atrophic gastritis (reticulin).

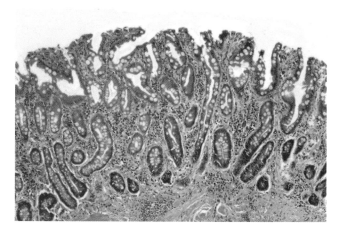

Figure 23.21 Complete intestinal metaplasia (IM).

Metaplasia

There are two major types of metaplasia that are seen in the stomach: intestinal metaplasia (IM) and pyloric (pseudopyloric) metaplasia. Both are thought to be the result of chronic gastritis, and consequently both are more frequently encountered in elderly individuals; neither type is considered symptomatic.

In pyloric metaplasia, there is a replacement of the specialized acid- and enzyme-secreting cells of the fundic glands by mucus-secreting glands of the type present in normal pyloric mucosa. This change occurs in the zone of fundic mucosa adjacent to the histologic fundopyloric junction, and what were typical fundic glands now come to resemble typical pyloric glands. Therefore, in persons with extensive pyloric metaplasia, the fundic gland area of the stomach contracts, the pyloric gland area expands, and the junctional zone is moved proximally toward the cardia (30). Unless the site of biopsy is known with accuracy, pyloric metaplasia cannot be diagnosed on routine H&E sections. However, although the fundic glands lose zymogenic and parietal cells, they still retain pepsinogen I activity. This can be demonstrated by immunohistochemical methods (31).

In IM, there is a change in the cells of the surface and pit epithelium so that morphologically and histochemically they come to resemble the cells of either the small or large bowel; IM may be complete (type I) or incomplete (type II) (32,33). In complete small bowel IM, the gastric mucosa changes to resemble normal small bowel epithelium, characterized by fully developed goblet cells and enterocytes with a brush border (Figure 23.21). In advanced cases, the contour of the mucosa changes with the development of villi and crypts. Paneth's cells may be present in the base of the crypts. In incomplete metaplasia, recognizable absorptive cells are not seen. The epithelium consists of a mixture of intestinal-type goblet cells and columnar mucus-

secreting cells, morphologically resembling those of the normal gastric epithelium.

Histochemical changes detected in the mucus production of the various types of IM are interesting and complex (15,32). In the normal stomach, mucus secreted by the columnar cells is neutral in type, recognized histochemically as PAS-positive and Alcian blue-negative. In complete IM, the enterocyte cytoplasm, apart from the brush border, is mucin-negative, but the goblet cells secrete either sialomucin (an acid mucin that is PAS-positive, Alcian blue-positive at pH 2.5 but Alcian blue-negative at pH 0.5) or sulfomucin (a strongly acidic mucin that is weakly PAS-positive and Alcian blue-positive at pH 2.5 and at pH 0.5) (Figure 23.22). In incomplete small bowel metaplasia, sialomucin is present in the columnar cells; and, in incomplete large bowel metaplasia (also called type III metaplasia) (34), the columnar cells contain sulfomucin (Figure 23.23). Sulfomucin may be recognized separately from sialomucin because it stains positively with high iron diamine (33). The details of

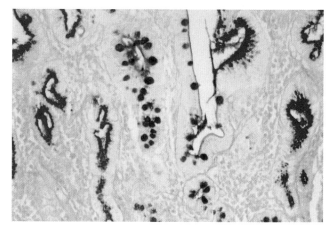

Figure 23.22 Complete intestinal metaplasia (PAS/Alcian blue).

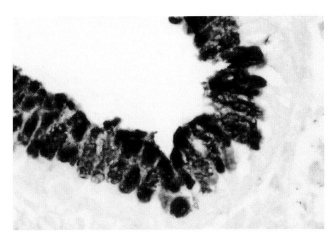

Figure 23.23 Incomplete large bowel metaplasia. The pit contains columnar cells with cytoplasmic sulphomucin (high iron diamine and Alcian blue).

these methods are well described in standard textbooks of histochemistry (34).

Minor degrees of gastric IM are relatively common in persons in North America and elsewhere. The variants described above rarely exist as a pure entity, and mixtures of the various types within the same gastric foveola are encountered frequently. However, IM should never be considered normal and almost always reflects some degree of gastric damage, usually from chronic gastritis.

Less commonly encountered forms of metaplasia include subnuclear vacuolation (35) and ciliated metaplasia (36). These changes all involve the pyloric mucus glands. Subnuclear vacuolation is not strictly a metaplastic change because it does not simulate the appearance of any other type of normal cells and probably represents a degenerative change secondary to gastritis or duodenal reflux. The vacuoles are clear on H&E sections and indent the nucleus. Ultrastructurally, they consist of a membrane-lined space derived either from endoplasmic reticulum or Golgi and probably contain nonglycoconjugated mucus core protein (37). Ciliated cells are found at the base of antral glands where there is superficial IM (36). The cause and significance of this change is not known.

Pancreatic acinar metaplasia (38) may be present in up to 1.2% of gastric biopsy samples or 13% of gastrectomy specimens. The cells, which are indistinguishable from normal acinar cells, also produce lipase and trypsinogen. Seventy-five percent of cases are positive for amylase. Cells are present in nests and variably sized lobules scattered among the cardiac and fundic mucosae.

SPECIMEN HANDLING

Gastric mucosa is delicate and should be handled with care. Tissue should be gently removed from the biopsy forceps and oriented before being placed flat on a supportive mesh, such as filter paper or gelfoam. A variety of fixatives are suitable, depending on personal preferences, although routine formalin is suitable for most purposes. Sections are cut in ribbons, usually at two or three levels.

For the best results, it is suggested that gastrectomy specimens be opened and pinned out on a cork board or wax platform before being immersed in formalin and fixed overnight. If sections are taken directly from a fresh specimen, they almost invariably curl up, resulting in irregular orientation of the final slide.

REFERENCES

1. Lewin KJ, Riddell RH, Weinstein WM. Normal structure of the stomach. In: Lewin KJ, Riddell RH, Weinstein WM, eds. *Gastrointestinal Pathology and its Clinical Implications.* New York: Igaku-Shoin; 1992:496–505.
2. Antonioli DA, Madara JL. Functional anatomy of the gastrointestinal tract. In: Ming SC, Goldman H, eds. *Pathology of the Gastrointestinal Tract.* 2nd ed. Baltimore: Williams & Wilkins; 1998:13–33.
3. Mackintosh CE, Kreel L. Anatomy and radiology of the areae gastricae. *Gut* 1977;18:855–864.
4. Piasecki C. Blood supply to the human gastroduodenal mucosa with special reference to the ulcer-bearing areas. *J Anat* 1974;118 (pt 2):295–335.
5. Lehnert T, Erlandson RA, Decosse JJ. Lymph and blood capillaries in the human gastric mucosa. A morphologic basis for metatasis in early gastric carcinoma. *Gastroenterology* 1985;89:939–950.
6. Listrom MB, Fenoglio-Preiser CM. Lymphatic distribution of the stomach in normal, inflammatory, hyperplastic, and neoplastic tissue. *Gastroenterology* 1987;93:506–514.
7. Filipe MI. Mucins in the human gastrointestinal epithelium: a review. *Invest Cell Pathol* 1979;2:195–216.
8. Chandrasoma PT, Der R, Ma Y, Dalton P, Taira M. Histology of the gastroesophageal junction: an autopsy study. *Am J Surg Pathol* 2000;24:402–409.
9. Sarbia M, Donner A, Gabbert HE. Histopathology of the gastroesophageal junction: a study on 36 operation specimens. *Am J Surg Pathol* 2002;26:1207–1212.
10. Kilgore SP, Ormsby AH, Gramlich TL, et al. The gastric cardia: fact or fiction? *Am J Gastroenterol* 2000;95:921–924.
11. Zhou H, Greco MA, Daum F, Kahn E. Origin of cardiac mucosa: ontogenic consideration. *Pediatr Dev Pathol* 2001;4:358–363.
12. Glickman JN, Chen YY, Wang HH, Antonioli DA, Odze RD. Phenotypic characteristics of a distinctive multilayered epithelium suggests that it is a precursor in the development of Barrett's esophagus. *Am J Surg Pathol* 2001;25:569–578.
13. Genta RM. Inflammatory disorders of the stomach. In: Odze RD, Goldblum JR, Crawford JM. *Surgical Pathology of the GI Tract, Liver, Biliary Tract and Pancreas.* Philadelphia, WB Saunders; 2004: 143–176.
14. Goldblum JR. Inflammation and intestinal metaplasia of the gastric cardia: Helicobacter pylori, gastroesophageal reflux disease or both. *Dig Dis* 2000;18:14–19.
15. Goldman H, Ming SC. Mucins in normal and neoplastic gastrointestinal epithelium. Histochemical distribution. *Arch Pathol* 1968;85:580–586.
16. Matsuyama M, Suzuki H. Differentiation of immature mucous cells into parietal, argyrophil, and chief cells in stomach grafts. *Science* 1970;169:385–387.
17. Grimelius L. A silver stain for alpha-2 cells in human pancreatic islets. *Acta Soc Med Ups* 1968;73:243–270.
18. Rindi G, Buffa R, Sessa F, et al. Chromogranin A, B and C immunoreactivities of mammalian endocrine cells. Distribution,

distinction from costored hormones/prohormones and relationship with the argyrophil component of secretory granules. *Histochemistry* 1986;85:19–28.

19. Solcia E, Fiocca R, Villani L, Luinetti O, Capella C. Hyperplastic, dysplastic, and neoplastic enterochromaffin-like cell proliferations of the gastric mucosa. Classification and histogenesis. *Am J Surg Pathol* 1995;19(suppl1):S1–S7.

20. Genta RM, Hamner HW, Graham DY. Gastric lymphoid follicles in Helicobacter pylori infection: frequency, distribution, and response to triple therapy. *Hum Pathol* 1993;24:577–583.

21. Cormack DH. The digestive system. In: Cormack, DH. *Ham's Histology*. 9th ed. Philadelphia: JB Lippincott; 1987:495–517.

22. Fawcett DW. The esophagus and stomach. In: Fawcett, DW. *Bloom and Fawcett: A Textbook of Histology*. 12th ed. New York: Chapman & Hall; 1994:593–616.

23. Bowden RE, El-Ramli HA. The anatomy of the esophageal hiatus. *Br J Surg* 1967;54:983–989.

24. Rubin W, Ross LL, Sleisenger MH, Jefries GH. The normal human gastric epithelia. A fine structural study. *Lab Invest* 1968;19:598–626.

25. Forte JG, Forte TM, Black JA, Okamoto C, Wolosin JM. Correlation of parietal cell structure and function. *J Clin Gastroenterol* 1983;5(suppl1):17–27.

26. Van Klinken BJ, Dekker J, Buller HA, de Bolos C, Einerhand AW. Biosynthesis of mucins (MUC2-6) along the longitudinal axis of the human gastrointestinal tract. *Am J Physiol* 1997;273(pt 1):G296–G302.

27. Maxwell A. The alcian dyes applied to the gastric mucosa. *Stain Technol* 1963;38:286–287.

28. Walker MM, Smolka A, Waller JM, Evans DJ. Identification of parietal cells in gastric body mucosa with HMFG-2 monoclonal antibody. *J Clin Pathol* 1995;48:832–834.

29. Kekki M, Samloff IM, Ihamaki T, Varis K, Siurala M. Age- and sex-related behaviour of gastric acid secretion at the population level. *Scand J Gastroenterol* 1982;17:737–743.

30. Owen DA. The stomach. In: Mills SE, ed. *Sternberg's Diagnostic Surgical Pathology*. 4th ed. Philadelphia: Lippincott Williams & Wilkins; 2004:1435–1474.

31. Dixon MF, Genta RM, Yardley JH, Correa P. Classification and grading of gastritis. The updated Sydney System. International Workshop on the Histopathology of Gastritis, Houston 1994. *Am J Surg Pathol* 1996;20:1161–1181.

32. Jass JR, Filipe MI. The mucin profiles of normal gastric mucosa, intestinal metaplasia and its variants and gastric carcinoma. *Histochem J* 1981;13:931–939.

33. Filipe MI, Potet F, Bogomoletz WV, et al. Incomplete sulphomucin-secreting intestinal metaplasia for gastric cancer. Preliminary data from a prospective study from three centres. *Gut* 1985;26:1319–1326.

34. Filipe MI, Lake BD. *Histochemistry in Pathology*. Edinburgh: Churchill Livingstone; 1983:310–313.

35. Rubio CA, Slezak P. Foveolar cell vacuolization in operated stomachs. *Am J Surg Pathol* 1988;12:773–776.

36. Rubio C, Hayashi T, Stemmerman G. Ciliated gastric cells: a study of their phenotypic characteristics. *Mod Pathol* 1990;3:720–723.

37. Thompson IW, Day DW, Wright NA. Subnuclear vacuolated mucous cells: a novel abnormality of simple mucin-secreting cells of non-specialized gastric mucosa and Brunner's glands. *Histopathology* 1987;11:1067–1081.

38. Doglioni C, Laurino L, Dei Tos AP, et al. Pancreatic (acinar) metaplasia of the gastric mucosa. Histology, ultrastructure, immunocytochemistry and clinicopathologic correlations of 101 cases. *Am J Surg Pathol* 1993;17:1134–1143.

Small Intestine

24

Terry L. Gramlich   Robert E. Petras

GROSS ANATOMY AND SURGICAL PERSPECTIVE

The small intestine, located within the abdominal cavity, is a multiply coiled tubular organ that extends from the gastric pylorus to the junction of the cecum and ascending colon. Its average length in the human adult is 6 to 7 m (1). Three subdivisions—the duodenum, jejunum, and ileum—are defined and characterized by various anatomic relationships. The duodenum is the most proximal portion of the small intestine; it measures about 12 inches (20–25 cm) in length and extends from the pylorus to the duodenojejunal flexure. The duodenum, excluding the most proximal several centimeters, is a fixed, retroperitoneal structure that forms a C- or U-shape around the head of the pancreas (2). Four subdivisions of the duodenum have been described: (a) the first portion, also known as the duodenal cap or bulb, is the most proximal and superior segment; (b) the descending or second portion, into which the common bile

duct and major and minor pancreatic ducts empty into their respective papillae; (c) the horizontal or third portion; and (d) the ascending or fourth portion, which veers forward at the level of the second lumbar vertebra, just left of midline, to become continuous with the remainder of the small bowel (1,2).

The origin of the jejunum is marked by a strip of fibromuscular tissue, the so-called ligament of Treitz, which anchors the terminal duodenum and duodenojejunal flexure to the posterior abdominal wall (3). Distal to the ligament of Treitz, the remainder of the small bowel is arbitrarily subdivided into the jejunum (the proximal two-fifths) and the ileum (the distal three-fifths, terminating at the ileocecal junction within the right iliac fossa) (1).

Although a discrete point demarcating jejunum from ileum does not exist, several relatively distinctive features become gradually more apparent from proximal to distal; these features help surgeons isolate specific segments of the small bowel. For example, the proximal jejunum has a thicker wall and is about twice the diameter of distal ileum. In addition, jejunal segments have more prominent permanent circular folds (plicae circulares) that can be palpated externally at surgery (1,4). The quantity of mesenteric adipose tissue is greater in the ileum, thus imparting a dense opaque appearance that contrasts with the less fatty, translucent mesentery of the jejunum (4). Finally, most of the jejunum lies within the upper abdominal cavity, whereas most of the ileum lies within the lower abdominal cavity and pelvis.

The arterial vascular supply of the small bowel originates from two major aortic axes: the celiac and superior mesenteric trunks (5). The duodenum is supplied by branches and interanastomosing arcades of both trunks, and its blood supply is intimately associated with that of the pancreatic head (1). The jejunum and ileum receive their blood from more distal branches of the superior mesenteric artery (5). The lymphatic and venous drainage systems follow the arterial supply and flow into regional lymphatics and lymph nodes or the portal venous system, respectively.

Sympathetic neural input to the small bowel is carried by the celiac and superior mesenteric plexuses, whereas the parasympathetic supply is derived from distal branches of the vagus nerve; these both closely follow the arterial paths into the bowel wall.

PHYSIOLOGY

The small intestine has several functional roles, the most important of which is the processing and absorption of ingested nutrients. Pancreatic enzymes act on the larger ingested carbohydrates and proteins to produce more appropriately sized molecules for further digestion. The brush border created by the numerous apical microvilli on absorptive epithelial cells offers an array of peptidases and carbohydrases, which act as key enzymes in additional nutrient breakdown and processing (6). The resulting smaller molecules are subsequently absorbed across the epithelial layer, and most pass into the portal venous system for eventual systemic distribution.

Fat digestion differs somewhat in that pancreatic lipase and bile act intraluminally to create free fatty acids and monoglycerides that migrate via direct diffusion through the lipid-soluble plasma membrane of enterocytes without surface processing or active transport (7). Most undergo intracytoplasmic resynthesis with directed packaging into chylomicrons and are released into regional lymphatic vessels. Water and electrolytes, vitamins, minerals, and various drugs also are absorbed at points along the mucosa of the small bowel. Therefore, the structural integrity of this viscus is critical to the maintenance of nutritional status, as well as in appropriate drug handling.

The small intestine also functions to propel and segmentally mix both newly accepted gastric contents and the residual material left after initial digestive efforts. Although

a number of factors influence gut motility, the most basic contractile activity is initiated at the level of the individual smooth muscle cells within the wall (8). Important functional differences exist, based on whether an individual is feeding or fasting. With feeding, a distended bowel segment initiates peristalsis, a forward propulsive motion that is mediated through the enteric nervous system; the intrinsic neurons of the myenteric plexus of Auerbach are most important in this regard (8,9). In contrast, during fasting or between meals, a slow yet continually recurring set of contractions attempts to clear the enteric lumen of any residual debris. The hormone motilin is believed to be important in the generation of these migratory motor complexes (9). Other endocrine influences, as well as the autonomic and central nervous systems, play a modulatory role in these intrinsic activities.

Advances in the burgeoning field of endocrine gut physiology and immunohistology have disclosed a variety of hormones within individual cells lining the small intestinal mucosa (10). Although the precise physiologic role of most of these cells and their secretory products remains to be determined, some are thought to exert a modulatory effect on gut motility or to influence the function of nearby epithelial cells (9,11).

The gut in general and the small bowel in particular have a crucial function in mucosal immunity. The mucosa/gut-associated lymphoid tissues, which are discussed in detail later in this chapter, are important in the local defense against mucosally encountered microorganisms and generate the initial immunologic responses to these various agents (12). Additionally, these tissues are the breeding ground for various reactive and neoplastic pathologic conditions.

HISTOLOGY

Although regional histologic differences exist within the small intestine, the general microscopic structure is similar throughout its length. The wall of the small bowel can be divided into four basic layers: mucosa, submucosa, muscularis externa or propria, and serosa.

Mucosa

Mucosal Architecture and Design

Because the principal function of the small intestine is absorption of ingested nutrients, the mucosa, which is the layer in contact with luminal contents, is specifically designed for this purpose. Several architectural adaptations augment the otherwise limited surface area of the small intestine (13). One of these, the grossly evident permanent circular folds (plicae circulares), courses perpendicular to the longitudinal axis of the bowel (13,14) (Figure 24.1). These mucosa-covered folds contain submucosal cores and

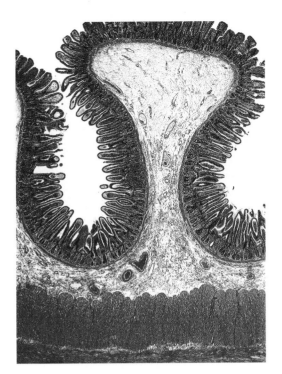

Figure 24.1 A single plica, or permanent circular fold, with its submucosal core and mucosal surface. The absorptive surface area is further augmented by intraluminal mucosal projections (villi).

epithelium and lamina propria form intraluminal projections called villi. These microscopic fingerlike and leaflike projections cover the entire luminal surface of the small bowel and are the most important morphologic modification responsible for enhancing surface area (13,15,16) (Figures 24.2–24.3). Each villous surface is covered by a single layer of epithelium consisting of various cell types. Beneath this epithelial layer lies a core of lamina propria that contains a centrally located, blind-ended lymphatic channel (lacteal), an arteriovenous capillary network, and an abundant migratory cell population (17–19) (Figure 24.4).

In the intervening regions and beneath the villi lie the crypts of Lieberkühn. These tubular intestinal glands open between the villi and extend down to the muscularis mucosae (Figure 24.3). The crypts are depressions of the surface epithelium, whereas the villi are extensions above it. However, these mucosal compartments are contiguous in that the lamina propria forming the villous cores also surrounds the crypts. The ratio of villous length to crypt length in normal small bowel varies from about 3:1 to 5:1 (13) (Figure 24.3). The crypts and surrounding lamina propria lie upon the muscularis mucosae, a thin fibromuscular layer that separates the mucosa from the underlying submucosa.

Mucosal Components and Their Composition

Epithelium

The mucosal epithelium is divided into the villous and crypt compartments. Although similar in appearance, the cell types differ somewhat, and their basic functions are distinct. Common to both, however, is a basic polarity of cellular organization, with nuclei aligned side by side, typically in a basal location within each cell.

traverse nearly the entire circumference of the bowel lumen before overlapping with adjacent permanent folds. In addition to enhancing surface area, they act as partial barriers that attenuate the forward flow of intraluminal contents, thus increasing the time of contact with absorptive surfaces.

The mucosa is composed of an epithelial component, a lamina propria, and a muscularis mucosae. The surface

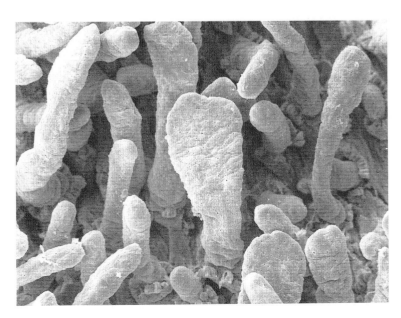

Figure 24.2 Scanning electron micrograph of small intestinal mucosa discloses the fingerlike and leaflike appearance of villi. Fingerlike villi predominate in the more distal segments of small bowel (jejunum and ileum), whereas leaflike villi are more common in the duodenum. Mixed populations, as in this micrograph, are considered normal.

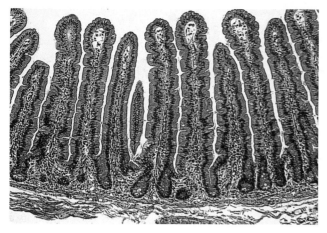

Figure 24.3 Normal jejunal villi. These villi are long and slender mucosal projections with a core of lamina propria covered by a luminal epithelial layer. A single row of intestinal glands (crypts) is found at the base of the mucosa. These crypts lie between adjacent villi and are surrounded by the same lamina propria that forms the villous cores.

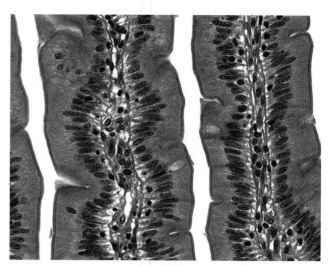

Figure 24.5 High-magnification view of a jejunal villi disclosing the general features of villous morphology. Both columnar absorptive cells and goblet cells (with apical clear vacuole) cover the villous surfaces; each cell type has a basally situated oval-to-round nucleus. Microvilli (brush border) are seen extending from the columnar absorptive cell surface. Note the intraepithelial lymphocytes scattered among and between the epithelial cells.

Villous Epithelium. The absorptive cell is the major villous epithelial cell type encountered. It is tall, columnar, with a basally situated round-to-oval nucleus and an eosinophilic cytoplasm (Figure 24.5). The apical surface contains a brush border that appears densely eosinophilic, stains positive with periodic acid-Schiff (PAS), and is composed of microvilli and the glycocalyx, or fuzzy coat (Figures 24.5–24.6). Microvilli, which are best seen on ultrastructural examination, are evenly spaced surface

projections that also augment the mucosal surface area of the small intestine (20) (Figure 24.7). Multiple filamentous structures emanating from and contiguous with their surface comprise the glycocalyx (17). The microvillous membrane–glycocalyx complex houses important enzymes—peptidases and disaccharidases—that function in terminal digestive processes. This layer probably also acts as a barrier to microorganisms and other foreign matter (21). Components forming the glycocalyx are continu-

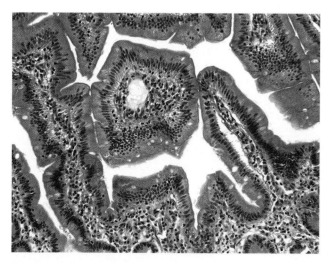

Figure 24.4 The duodenal villous surface is covered by a single layer of tall columnar epithelial cells. The underlying lamina propria core contains lymphoid and plasma cells and a connective tissue framework, including a lymphatic vessel (lacteal) and a subepithelial capillary network.

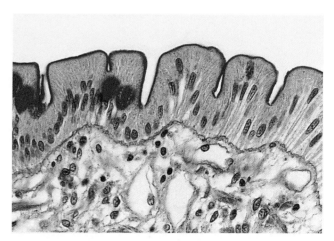

Figure 24.6 Periodic acid-Schiff (PAS) stain highlights the microvillous membrane–glycocalyx complex along the apical surface of the absorptive cells. The thin subepithelial basement membrane that separates the lamina propria from the epithelial compartment also stains with PAS but to a lesser degree. The neutral subgroup of mucins contained within the goblet cells are PAS-positive as well.

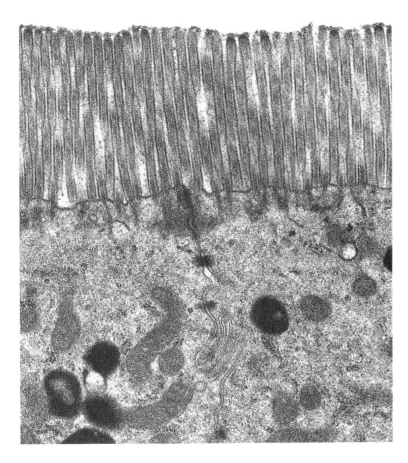

Figure 24.7 Transmission electron micrograph of microvilli emanating from the absorptive columnar cell surfaces. The glycocalyx component is the filamentous layer overlying the microvilli, but most of this has been artifactually removed during processing.

ally synthesized within the absorptive cell and transported to the surface to replace the preexisting coat in a dynamic fashion (17,21,22). Although its functional capacities are uncertain, absence of the glycocalyx of the small bowel mucosa was the sole detectable histologic abnormality found in some children with allergic enteropathy (i.e., cow's milk allergy) (21).

Interspersed among the absorptive cells are goblet cells, which have a characteristic apical mucin droplet and an attenuated, basally situated, bland nucleus (Figure 24.5). They contain both neutral and acid mucin and function as secretory cells, sustaining a moist viscid environment within the lumen (20). In a combined Alcian blue/PAS stain, the droplets appear blue-purple (Figure 24.8). The acid mucins of the small intestine are primarily sialomucins, in contrast to the colonic goblet cell, which contains predominantly acid sulfomucins (23,24). The number of goblet cells increases with distal progression along the small bowel (20).

Scattered endocrine cells are present within the villous epithelium, but they are more abundant within the crypts. Intraepithelial lymphocytes are scattered among and lie between individual epithelial cells, usually just above the basement membrane; normally there is about one lymphocyte for every five epithelial cells (25,26) (Figure 24.5). Intraepithelial lymphocytes mark as T cells (Figure 24.9),

and most are of the T-suppressor/cytotoxic (CD8-positive) variety (27–29). An increase in the number of intraepithelial lymphocytes is characteristic of several disorders, including gluten-sensitive enteropathy (celiac sprue), tropical sprue, and giardiasis (30,31).

Crypt Epithelium. The crypt epithelium primarily functions in epithelial cell renewal (20); and, as a consequence of this regenerative function, mitoses are seen frequently within the crypts (normal range: 1–12 mitoses/crypt) (32). Goblet cells and columnar cells, some of which are undifferentiated or stem cells, are conspicuous. The four major epithelial cell types of the mucosa (absorptive, goblet, endocrine, and Paneth's cells) arise from this stem cell (33). Differentiation and maturation occur in about five to six days as the cells migrate from the crypt depths to the villous tips, where they are subsequently sloughed into the lumen (20,33); however, the Paneth's cell remains within the crypt base (34). It is thought that apoptosis probably functions as a regulator of cell migration toward the villous surface; however, it is not certain whether this form of programmed cell death is responsible for epithelial cell sloughing from the villous tip (35). Morphologically, cells undergoing apoptosis show nuclear condensation and cell shrinkage with subsequent detachment from adjacent epithelium. In addition,

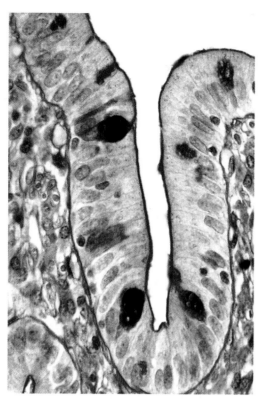

Figure 24.8 Alcian blue/PAS combination stain showing characteristic blue-purple apical mucin droplet of intestinal goblet cells. The heterogeneous composition (neutral and acid mucins) allows both stains to be incorporated into the droplet, imparting this distinctive color.

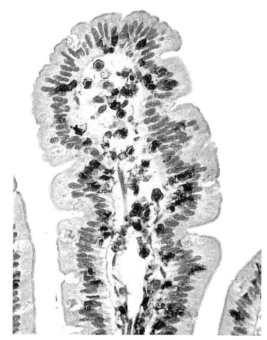

Figure 24.9 Small intestinal mucosa immunostained for UCHL1 (CD45 RO), a pan–T-lymphocyte marker. The positive red-brown reaction highlights both the intraepithelial and lamina propria T cells. Although CD8-positive T-suppressor/cytotoxic lymphocytes predominate within the epithelium, lamina propria T cells usually mark for CD4, the T-helper/inducer subset.

the cell disintegrates into so-called apoptotic bodies and is phagocytosed by local histiocytes (35).

Endocrine cells are relatively abundant in the crypts, occurring as single cells or in discontinuous groupings along the intestinal tract (10). They are of two morphologic types. The "open" type have a pyramidal shape that tapers toward the glandular lumen with which they communicate, whereas "closed" cells are spindle-shaped and have no luminal connection (10). The former are the most frequent type found in the small bowel. Some endocrine cells disclose eosinophilic basal (infranuclear) granules on hematoxylin and eosin (H&E) staining so that they are easily identified on routine preparations (Figure 24.10); however, not all enteroendocrine cells have such a quality, and their identification remains elusive unless special methods are used. Silver (argyrophilic, argentaffinic) preparations or immunocytochemical techniques are useful for visualization in these cases. The disadvantage of silver stains is that no information can be gleaned with respect to endocrine cell type or hormonal composition, and some cells do not reduce silver preparations (10). Immunocytochemistry is, therefore, the best method for definitive evaluation. Antibody preparations to chromogranin and neuron-specific enolase have been shown to be useful nonspecific markers for endocrine cells (36) (Figure 24.11). Precise identifica-

tion of endocrine chemical content requires specific monoclonal or polyclonal antibody preparations. Although most often used in experimental settings, specific hormonal content immunostaining also may have diagnostic value in studying neuroendocrine tumors (37). Electron mi-

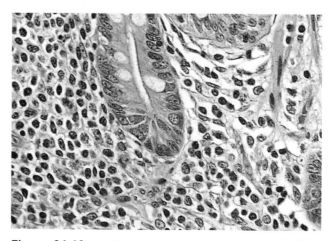

Figure 24.10 A single crypt surrounded by normal cellular lamina propria with abundant migratory cells. Both absorptive columnar and goblet cells are seen lining the crypt. In addition, an endocrine cell (infranuclear eosinophilic granules) and several Paneth's cells (supranuclear granules) are clearly evident.

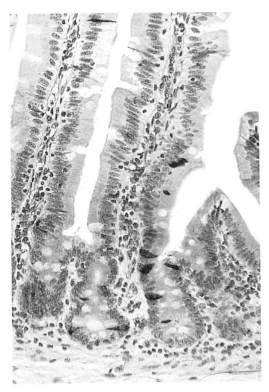

Figure 24.11 Immunostain for chromogranin shows numerous endocrine cells within the crypts and several scattered along the villous surface.

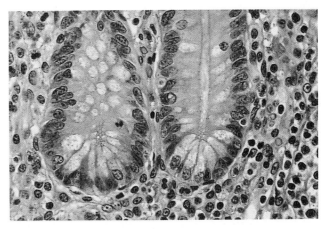

Figure 24.12 Although Hollande's and other picric acid–containing fixatives are superior preservers of cytomorphologic detail, the characteristic supranuclear eosinophilic granules of Paneth's cells are not as easily visualized when compared with the appearance in 4% formaldehyde solution (see Figure 24.10). Clear vacuoles replace the distinct eosinophilic granules within the Paneth's cells (along the crypt bases). Note that the single endocrine cell in this crypt maintains its infranuclear granular staining quality.

croscopy also can be used to identify cytoplasmic neurosecretory granules.

At least 16 distinct types of endocrine cell have been described along the gut (38) and have a characteristic regional distribution and composition. Individual cells containing cholecystokinin, secretin, gastric inhibitory polypeptide, and motilin populate more proximal segments of the small bowel, whereas enteroglucagon-, substance P–, and neurotensin-storing cells are seen in greater frequency in the ileum (38,39). Serotonin- and somatostatin-containing cells are not as regionalized and are found throughout the gastrointestinal tract (38). Some of these endocrine cells are known to play key roles in daily gastrointestinal activity. For example, secretin and cholecystokinin are released in response to various foodstuffs and modulate pancreatic secretion and gallbladder function, respectively (39). Most other gut endocrine cells are still of uncertain or unknown physiologic significance (11,39).

The Paneth's cells, normally found only in the crypt, comprise most of the base of individual crypts throughout the entire small intestine (40). They also are encountered to a lesser degree in the appendix, cecum, and ascending colon (41). Paneth's cells have a pyramidal shape with their apices pointing toward the lumen. Their cytoplasm contains characteristic supranuclear, intensely eosinophilic granules that are easily visualized in H&E–stained sections (Figure 24.10). Interestingly, fixatives containing picric acid

(e.g., Hollande's, Bouin's) mask the eosinophilic staining of these granules, often disclosing only unstained cytoplasmic vacuoles (40) (Figure 24.12). Their round nuclei often contain a prominent nucleolus (20,29). The exact function of Paneth's cells is still uncertain, but they are known to contain lysozyme, defensins (Figure 24.13), and immunoglobulin, and they are capable of phagocytic activity.

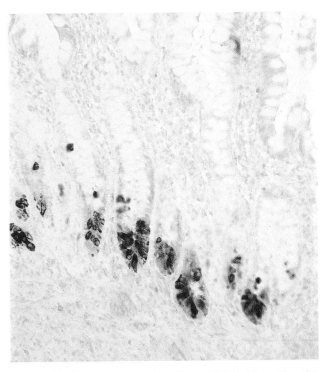

Figure 24.13 Immunostain for defensin HD5 highlights Paneth's cells at the base of the crypts.

These features suggest that they play a role in regulating the intestinal microbial flora (41,42,43).

The crypt epithelium also contains intraepithelial lymphocytes that are predominantly T-suppressor/cytotoxic (CD8-positive) cells (44). Other inflammatory cell types, such as the neutrophil or the plasma cell, are not normally present within either the crypt or villous epithelial compartments; their presence would indicate a pathologic state (31,45).

Immunostaining Patterns of the Epithelium. Carcinoembryonic antigen (CEA) is present on the apical surfaces of cells covering the villi and lining the crypts, and it has been shown to localize to the glycocalyx surface component (46). Additionally, the mucin droplets of goblet cells contain an abundance of CEA and consequently mark intensely with polyclonal anti-CEA. However, no intracytoplasmic immunostaining for CEA is evident in the normal small bowel (46).

Human leukocyte antigen (HLA)-DR–like antigens have been shown to be present in a scattered, focal distribution on the apices of small intestinal columnar-shaped cells (47). Immunostaining with anti–HLA-DR discloses a diminishing intensity of reactivity from the villous surfaces to the crypt bases. Immune-related cells such as lymphocytes (mostly B cells) and macrophages along with the walls of capillaries in the lamina propria also show immunoreactivity for HLA-DR (47).

Lamina Propria

The lamina propria, the intermediate layer of the mucosa, functions both structurally and immunologically. It rests upon the muscularis mucosae, surrounds the crypts, and extends upward as the cores of the intestinal villi. The crypt epithelium and villous epithelium rest upon the lamina propria and are separated from it by a distinct basement membrane recognized as a slender eosinophilic, PAS-positive band at their interface (Figures 24.4–24.6). This subepithelial basement membrane is a continuous structure composed of an ultrastructurally apparent basal lamina and a deeper network of collagenous/reticular fibers and ground substance (17). Interweaving collagen bundles and other connective tissue fibers, fibroblasts, mature fibrocytes, and smooth muscle cells comprise the framework of the lamina propria (45), whereas blood capillaries, lymphatics, and nerves course through this layer on their various routes to and from all portions of the bowel wall.

The most conspicuous feature of the lamina propria is its abundant immunocompetent and migratory cell component (Figures 24.10, 24.12). Five types of immunocompetent or inflammatory cells are normally encountered in the lamina propria: plasma cells, lymphocytes, eosinophils, histiocytes, and mast cells. Neutrophils are not usually encountered in the lamina propria, or for that matter

anywhere in the small bowel wall, with the exception of those confined to vascular lumina.

Plasma cells are the most abundant cellular lamina propria constituent; most contain cytoplasmic immunoglobulin (Ig)A but some contain IgM (Figure 24.14). In contrast to extraintestinal sites (e.g., peripheral lymph nodes) (30,48), IgG-secreting plasma cells are scant. Lymphocytes, both B and T cells, are also common. The predominant subset of T cells within the lamina propria is the T-lymphocytes with the helper/inducer immunophenotype (CD4 positive) (27,48,49) (Figure 24.9). Lymphocytes are found throughout the lamina propria but often form more dense infiltrates just above the muscularis mucosae (45). Moreover, lymphoid aggregates and nodules, many with germinal centers, are scattered along the small bowel and are found in increasing concentration distally. These lymphoid aggregates are based in the lamina propria, but they often extend to some degree into the underlying submucosa.

Histiocytes or macrophages are also seen in the lamina propria but in fewer numbers than lymphocytes or plasma cells. Most are located along the superiormost aspect of the lamina propria near the tips of the villi (28). They function in T-cell regulation as antigen presenters and phagocytes

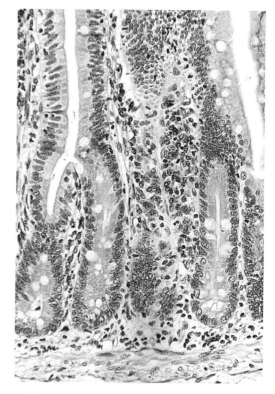

Figure 24.14 Numerous IgA-containing plasma cells (red-brown cytoplasmic staining) within the lamina propria of normal small intestine, immunostained for α-heavy chain. Note that, in contrast to T cells (see Figure 24.9), the plasma cells localize to the lamina propria and are not normally found in the epithelium.

(30). Exaggerated expression of this latter function can be seen pathologically in disseminated *Mycobacterium avium-intracellulare* complex infection and in Whipple's disease, where the lamina propria becomes filled with macrophages engorged with microorganisms (30,50–52).

The only granulocytes normally found in the lamina propria are eosinophils and mast cells. Eosinophilic leukocytes usually are conspicuous, but their role in the normal bowel is uncertain (53). The numbers of eosinophils in the lamina propria increase under various conditions, including those comprising the eosinophilic gastroenteropathies (54–58). Mast cells are relatively abundant in the small intestinal lamina propria, as compared with other body sites (30), but in absolute numbers appear to decrease with distal progression along the small bowel (59). Their function in the gastrointestinal tract in normal and disease states is unknown. Increased numbers of mast cells can be found in inflammatory bowel disease and in the specimens of some individuals with eosinophilic gastroenteropathy (57,60). According to some investigators, a specimen disclosing more than eight mast cells per high-magnification field should suggest the diagnosis of systemic mast cell disease (61). Mast cells can be seen on H&E–stained sections, but they are more easily visualized with special techniques such as toluidine blue, sulfated Alcian blue, or Giemsa stains. Rarely, subepithelial (lamina propria) endocrine cells may be found in the small bowel; however, these are much more prominent in the vermiform appendix (62). Occasionally, in apparently healthy individuals and in certain disease states (e.g., Crohn's disease), ganglion cells are found in the lamina propria of the small bowel. These could potentially be confused with cytomegalovirus infection–induced cellular changes.

Muscularis Mucosae

The muscularis mucosae, which is the outermost layer or limit of the mucosa, is a slender band of tissue composed of elastic fibers and smooth muscle arranged in an outer longitudinal and inner circular layer (Figure 24.15). However, these layers are usually not well delineated on routine light microscopy. Tufts of smooth muscle radiate from the muscularis mucosae into the lamina propria and extend into the villi. The muscularis mucosae provides an important structural foundation for the mucosa, and its absence in some biopsy specimens can cause a loss of villous orientation, an artifact that may interfere with optimal evaluation (53).

Submucosa

Between the muscularis mucosae and muscularis externa is the submucosa, a loose, paucicellular layer composed of a regular, honeycomb-like arrangement (at the ultrastructural level) of collagenous and elastic fibers and related fibroblasts. The submucosa also may contain scattered, rather inconspicuous migratory cells (e.g., histiocytes, lym-

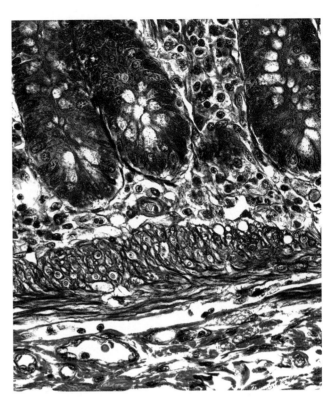

Figure 24.15 High-magnification photomicrograph disclosing inner circular and outer longitudinal smooth muscle bands of the muscularis mucosae; this layering is often inconspicuous on hematoxylin and eosin preparations, where the muscularis mucosae appears as a thin eosinophilic strip between the lamina propria and underlying submucosa (Masson's trichrome).

phoid and plasma cells, and mast cells) and adipose tissue (63). Its histologic appearance and principal role in maintaining the structural integrity of the small bowel are similar throughout the gastrointestinal tract (63). The submucosa is a major focus of vascular routing and related distribution of regional blood and lymphatic flow. Relatively large caliber arterioles, venules, and lymphatic vessels form extensive individual plexuses and networks within this layer (5,19) (Figure 24.16). From this "vascular center," numerous penetrating capillary vessels supply and drain most of the mucosa and muscularis externa (5,19). Lymphatic vessels may be distinguished from blood vessels by the thinner wall of the former and the lack of luminal erythrocytes. However, certain immunohistologic patterns and electron microscopic characteristics are more helpful for definitive identification (18,64,65). Specifically, the endothelial cells of blood capillaries immunostain for PAL-E and factor VIII–related antigen, whereas lymphatic capillary endothelia typically lack these antigenic sites and remain unstained with such antibody preparations (64,65). In addition, blood capillaries as seen by ultrastructural analysis have a continuous basal lamina, endothelial fenestrations, and ensheathing pericytes. However, lymphatic capillaries have a discontinuous basal

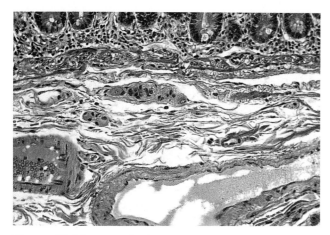

Figure 24.16 Normal submucosa separated from overlying mucosa by the eosinophilic-staining muscularis mucosae. The submucosa is paucicellular, disclosing fibrocollagenous tissue and a prominent vascular component. Note the ganglion cells of Meissner's plexus just beneath the muscularis mucosae.

lamina and lack both fenestrations and surrounding pericytes (17,18). Although small lymphatic vessels are a conspicuous submucosal component, prominent dilated lymphatic structures in this layer, as well as in the mucosa, can be seen in pathologic states such as intestinal lymphangiectasia or Crohn's disease (31,66).

Neural structures are also prominent in the submucosa. The submucosal Meissner's plexus forms one of the two major integrative centers of the enteric nervous system. It consists of a network of ganglia that interconnect through neural processes (67). The ganglia contain compact aggregates of neurons (ganglion cells) routinely identified on

H&E preparations by their characteristic large oval shape, abundant pink cytoplasm, vesicular nucleus, and single prominent, often eosinophilic nucleolus (Figure 24.16). Abundant S-100–positive Schwann cells, glial-like cells, and neural processes are also present in Meissner's plexus. The entire plexus, including the ganglia, contains no connective tissue elements or vascular structures in the normal state (67–70). The plexus is also normally devoid of inflammatory cells; therefore, if these are seen, an injury pattern specific to the neural plexus (such as an inflammatory neuropathy) should be considered, as long as primary inflammatory bowel disease can be excluded (69). Neural interconnections exist between Meissner's plexus and the myenteric plexus of Auerbach (discussed below), as well as with extrinsic (autonomic) neural processes.

Muscularis Externa

The muscularis externa (or muscularis propria) is the thick outer smooth muscle layer that surrounds the submucosa. It is covered externally by subserosal connective tissue and, in most places, by a serosa. Its two distinct muscular layers, oriented perpendicular to each other, are arranged as an outer longitudinally running muscle fiber layer and an inner circular muscle band (Figure 24.17). Blood vessels, lymphatics, and nerves course through the muscularis externa and slender collagenous septa surround groups of smooth muscle cells, creating characteristic bundles and packets of muscle (Figure 24.17). However, fibrous tissue in this layer is minimal in the normal small bowel (69) so even slight fibrous alterations or collagen deposition may be significant. Moreover, the fact that only a few disease entities (including ischemia, irradiation, familial visceral

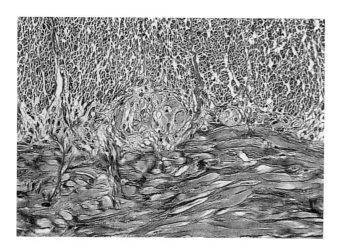

Figure 24.17 Masson's trichrome stain clearly delineates the inner circular (*above*) from the outer longitudinal (*below*) smooth muscle bands of the muscularis externa. The prominent muscular component (*red*) is partitioned into bundles of varying size by delicate collagenous fibers (*blue*). Note the ganglia of the myenteric plexus of Auerbach, characteristically located between the two muscle bands. Fibrous tissue is minimal within the muscularis externa and is also not normally part of the plexus.

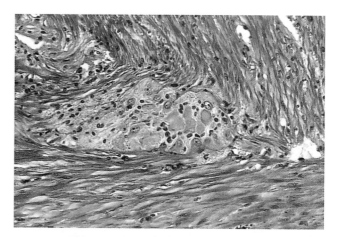

Figure 24.18 A single ganglion of the myenteric plexus of Auerbach located at the interface of the inner (*above*) and outer (*below*) smooth muscle layers of the muscularis externa. Ganglion cells (neuronal cell bodies) are evident and characterized by a polygonal shape, abundant pink cytoplasm, and an eccentric nucleus; spindled neural projections and Schwann cells are also intermixed.

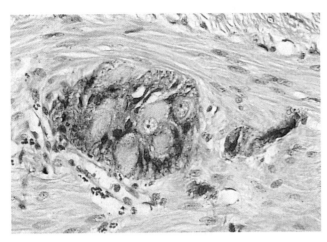

Figure 24.19 This S-100 immunostain highlights the otherwise inconspicuous spindled Schwann cell component of the ganglion. It also marks the Schwann cells accompanying the neural projections that interconnect these ganglia to one another within the plexus system. Note that the ganglion cells show no such immunoreactivity.

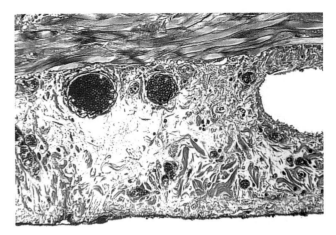

Figure 24.21 The subserosal region contains a delicate fibro-collagenous network, blood vessels, lymphatics, and nerves. The serosa consists of a thin fibrous layer (*blue* and *bottom*) covered by a single layer of mesothelial cells; however, the mesothelium is often denuded in surgical specimens. A portion of the outer layer of the muscularis externa is also present in this field (*top*). (Masson's trichrome.)

myopathy, scleroderma, and mycobacterial infection) are associated with fibrosis of the muscularis propria aids in narrowing a broad differential diagnosis (31).

The myenteric plexus of Auerbach, the other major neural plexus of the enteric nervous system, lies between the outer longitudinal and inner circular muscle layers (Figures 24.17–24.19). Auerbach's plexus is similar in composition to the submucosal plexus, although it typically has larger ganglia, a greater number of neurons, and a more compact plexus network (68,69). As a consequence of these features, it is best to evaluate the myenteric plexus for specific disease processes involving the enteric nervous system, such as the various visceral neuropathies. Because routine processing allows only a small portion of the plexus to be visualized

and because many of these conditions cause no detectable changes on routine H&E-stained sections, special preparations of thicker, larger, and silver-stained sections cut *en face* are currently necessary to diagnose many of these disorders (69). Finally, although of lesser importance, a deep muscular, subserous plexus and several mucosal plexuses are also present within the small bowel (68). Interstitial cells of Cajal (ICC) are located in relation to the myenteric plexus of Auerbach and in septa between circular muscle lamellae (Figure 24.20). These "pacemaker cells" are felt to play a role in intestinal motility (71).

Serosa and Subserosal Region

The serosa is the covering that envelops most of the external surface of the small bowel. Its outermost layer consists of a single row of cuboidal mesothelial cells, under which lies a thin band of loose connective tissue. A subserosal zone of connective tissue lying between this mesothelial covering and the muscularis externa also contains ramifying branches of blood vessels, lymphatics, and nerves (Figure 24.21).

DISTINCTIVE REGIONAL CHARACTERISTICS OF THE SMALL BOWEL

Duodenum

The duodenum exhibits several distinctive histologic features, many related to its proximal location in direct continuity with the pylorus. The gastroduodenal junction,

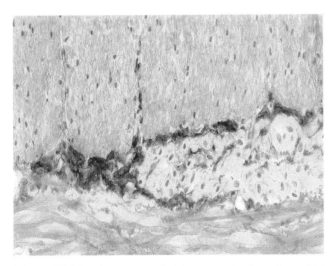

Figure 24.20 The CD117 (c-kit) immunostain shows interstitial cells of Cajal surrounding the myenteric plexus of Auerbach.

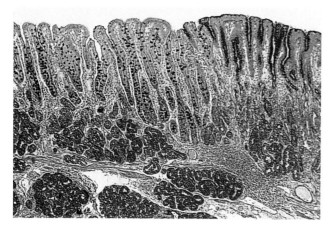

Figure 24.22 Gastroduodenal junction. Note the transition from PAS-positive (*red*) gastric foveolar epithelium and underlying pyloric glands (*right*) to a villous mucosal architecture of the duodenum (*left*) lined predominantly by Alcian blue/PAS-positive (*blue-purple*) goblet cells and absorptive cells. Note that both pyloric (*right*) and Brunner's glands (*left*) are composed predominantly of cells containing only neutral, PAS-positive mucin. Brunner's glands, however, are predominantly submucosal in location, while pyloric glands are an intramucosal structure. (Alcian blue/PAS.)

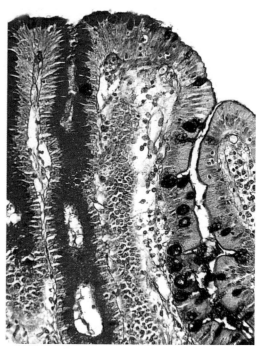

Figure 24.23 Several villi within the confines of the gastroduodenal junction disclosing both "usual small intestinal-type" epithelium and antral-type, PAS-positive, foveolar epithelium. This transitional-type epithelium is a characteristic hybrid found in this region. At more distal small intestinal sites, this transitional type epithelium is termed gastric metaplasia. (Alcian blue/PAS.)

although well-delineated grossly, is poorly demarcated histologically (72) (Figures 24.22–24.23). A gradual transition in epithelial types occurs, with three distinct subtypes in the duodenum (73): (a) an antral-type mucosal epithelium that is identical to the pyloric mucosa; (b) a "usual small intestinal type" (jejunal type) characterized by villi covered by absorptive cells and interspersed goblet cells; and (c) a transitional type (Figure 24.23), in which the same villus is covered by epithelium having features of both antral-type and usual small intestinal-type epithelia. In the region of the gastroduodenal junction, irregular undulating slips of antral-type mucosa extend about 1 to 2 mm into the anatomic duodenum, which then abuts a 2- to 3-mm segment of transitional-type epithelium (73). Distal to this, only the usual small intestinal-type mucosa is found (73). The transitional type epithelium occurring in more distal aspects of the duodenum and in the rest of the small intestine is termed gastric metaplasia (31).

Although the duodenal mucosa may demonstrate long villi with a villous-to-crypt length ratio on the order of 3:1 to 5:1, more commonly, particularly in the first portion (the duodenal cap or bulb), the villi are shorter and broader with occasional branching extensions (74) (Figure 24.24). They often have a leaflike shape with few fingerlike forms when viewed under a scanning electron or dissecting microscope (20,74,75) (Figure 24.25). Also, the number of mononuclear cells within the lamina propria is increased in the duodenum when compared with the rest of the proximal small intestine (74,75). This varied constellation of findings is considered normal and is probably a consequence of the effect of acidic gastric contents on this most proximal intestinal site (40,75).

The submucosa of the gastrointestinal tract lacks glands except at two sites: the esophagus and the duodenum. The submucosal Brunner's glands are the type localized to the duodenum. Indeed, these glands are typically used by the pathologist to identify histologically a segment of small

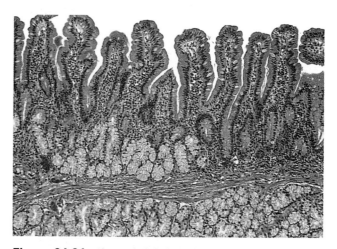

Figure 24.24 Short, slightly broader villi predominate in the duodenum. The underlying submucosal Brunner's glands are a distinctive feature of this portion of small bowel. Note that a fair portion of Brunner's glands normally occurs above the muscularis mucosae.

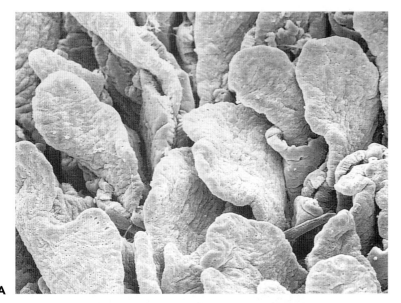

A

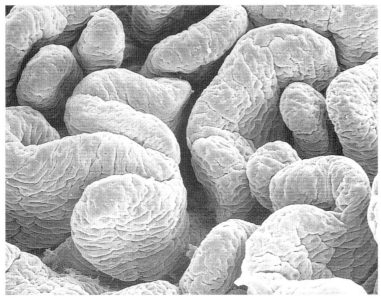

B

Figure 24.25 Two views of duodenal mucosa using scanning electron microscopy: leaflike (**A**) and ridged-shaped (**B**) villi predominate in these normal duodenal specimens.

intestine as duodenum. Brunner's glands, which begin just distal to the gastroduodenal junction, are most concentrated in this region and gradually decrease in quantity along the duodenum (76). Beyond the entrance of the ampulla of Vater, only scattered groups can be found. In rare instances, Brunner's glands extend beyond the duodenojejunal flexure for a short distance (77–79).

Brunner's glands are lobular collections of tubuloalveolar glands predominantly located within the submucosa; however, they often extend through the muscularis mucosae into the deep portions of mucosa beneath the crypts of Lieberkühn (Figures 24.24, 24.26). On average, about one third of the gland population resides within the mucosa (77). Brunner's glands are lined by cuboidal-to-columnar cells with pale, uniform cytoplasm and an oval, basally situated nucleus. Their cytoplasm contains neutral mucins that are PAS positive and diastase resistant (Figure 24.22). Occasionally, mucous cells with apically concentrated mucin and perinuclear vacuolization or clearing are seen. Although opinions vary, these changes are thought to represent the secretory phase of the gland (i.e., recently fed state) (80,81). The glands empty by way of ducts lined by a similar epithelium, which are often seen passing through slips of muscularis mucosae (Figure 24.26). These ducts drain into the crypts at varying levels (79). Brunner's glands and their ducts can be distinguished from surrounding crypts by the absence of goblet cells and by their diffuse cytoplasmic PAS positivity (79).

Although most of the lining epithelial cells of the Brunner's glands are of the mucous type, scattered

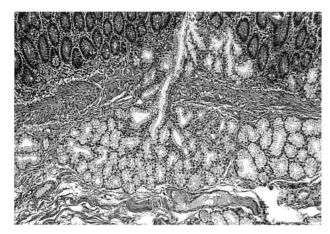

Figure 24.26 Submucosal Brunner's gland lobule with draining duct extending through muscularis mucosae. Note the stark contrast between the crypt epithelium and that of the Brunner's glands and their ducts.

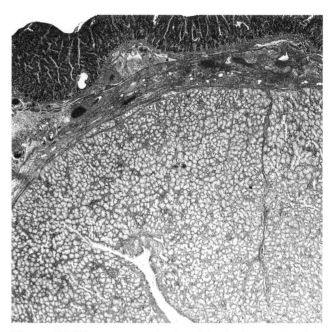

Figure 24.27 Brunner's gland nodule disclosing abundant normal-appearing submucosal glands of Brunner intermixed with smooth muscle, underlying an unremarkable duodenal mucosal villous surface.

endocrine cells are present as well. Many can be detected on routine H&E-stained sections because of their basal eosinophilic granulated cytoplasm (82). By using immunohistologic methods, some have been shown to contain somatostatin, gastrin, and peptide YY (83). However, the ducts that drain Brunner's glands are devoid of endocrine cells (83).

Peptidergic neural fibers, predominantly those with immunoreactivity for vasoactive intestinal peptide and substance P, course within and between individual Brunner's glands. These neuroendocrine substances are probably important in local regulation of acinar secretion, although this function has been verified only for vasoactive intestinal peptide (83). The function of Brunner's glands has not been fully elucidated, but their mucus is felt to be of prime importance for protection of the duodenal mucosa from the potentially damaging effects of the delivered acidic gastric contents (78).

Hyperplasia of Brunner's glands exists in three forms: (a) diffuse glandular proliferation, imparting a coarse nodularity to most of the duodenum; (b) isolated discrete nodules in the proximal duodenum; and (c) a solitary nodule, often designated as an "adenoma" of Brunner's glands (77,84,85). All three types are typically composed of an increased quantity of normal-appearing Brunner's glands, accompanied by variable proportions of smooth muscle (Figure 24.27). The distinction between adenoma and hyperplasia is arbitrary, and no substantial evidence exists to suggest that any of these proliferations are truly neoplastic (84). Moreover, carcinoma arising from a population of Brunner's glands has yet to be convincingly documented (31). Nodules or polypoid structures composed of collections of these submucosal glands in the duodenum are probably best termed Brunner's gland nodules (31).

Pseudomelanosis duodeni, or brown-black pigment, located primarily within lamina propria macrophages, rarely may be observed in the proximal duodenum (86) (Figure 24.28). Lipomelanin, ceroid, iron, sulfide, and hemosiderin have been identified in these deposits. Most reported patients were hypertensive and also suffered from upper gastrointestinal bleeding, chronic renal failure, or diabetes mellitus (86).

Jejunum

The jejunum is the least distinctive segment of the small bowel; and, as such, its histologic features are most similar to those described for the small bowel in general. However, a characteristic feature is the prominent development of the plicae circulares, or permanent circular folds, also termed valves of Kerckring and valvulae conniventes (Figure 24.1). These folds are tallest and most numerous (i.e., closely spaced) in this portion of the small bowel (20). Histologically, the jejunal villi are tall with a villous-to-crypt ratio on the order of 3:1 to 5:1. The vast majority of jejunal villi are slender and fingerlike (Figures 24.2–24.3), in contrast to the slightly shorter villi of the ileum and to the leaflike, occasionally branched and blunted villi of the proximal duodenum (20,40). These morphologic transitions are gradual, particularly in the mobile small intestine, where the separation between jejunum and ileum is arbitrarily defined.

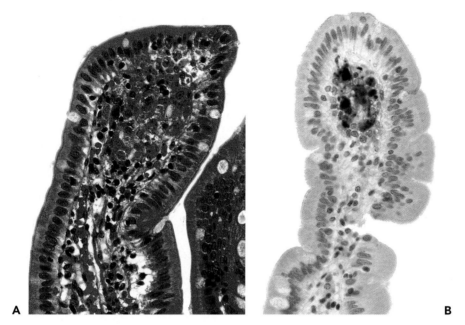

Figure 24.28 **A.** Macrophages containing granular brown-black pigment within the lamina propria of the duodenum, a characteristic of pseudomelanosis duodeni. **B.** Prussian blue stain disclosing the prominent iron content of the pigment.

Ileum

The ileum has a number of distinctive features, including its unique junction with the large intestine. The ileum protrudes approximately 2 to 3 cm into the large intestine at the junction of the cecum and ascending colon. This nipplelike extension of the terminal ileum is encircled by large bowel mucosa and has been likened to the relationship of the uterine cervix with the vagina (87). A muscular sphincter at this site, along with external ligamentous support, is responsible for modifying its function in order to prevent reflux and to allow forward passage of ileal contents (87,88). Histologically, the mucosal transition demonstrates a gradual loss of villi occurring at variable lengths along the short intracecal ileal segment; the ileal mucosa blends rather imperceptibly with the mucosa of the large bowel (Figure 24.29). The ileocecal region normally can contain abundant fat within its submucosa, diffusely distributed and proportional to adipose content in the rest of the abdominal cavity (89) (Figure 24.29). In fact, on rare occasion, a distinct mass of fat is evident. This benign entity, so-called lipohyperplasia of the ileocecal region, reportedly can cause variable symptoms, including abdominal pain and lower gastrointestinal bleeding (89).

The distinctive mucosal characteristics of the ileum, when compared with both jejunum and duodenum, include shorter and fewer plicae circulares and an increased proportion of goblet cells within the epithelium (Figure 24.30). The villi are typically shorter than at more proximal sites and have a predominantly fingerlike shape (20). These features become gradually more apparent along the length of the small intestine and are most evident in the distal ileum. With distal progression, lymphoid nodules that can be found anywhere in the small intestine gradually increase in quantity (20). In addition, specialized clusters of lymphoid aggregates, or Peyer's patches, are most prominent in the ileum.

Peyer's patches are located along the antimesenteric border of the small bowel. They consist of varying numbers of lymphoid follicles, ranging from 5 to over 900, and have been shown to be present during fetal life (90). Until puberty, they increase in size and number and subsequently regress steadily thereafter; nonetheless, Peyer's patches are invariably present even into extreme old age (90). In children, these patches can be grossly visualized near the

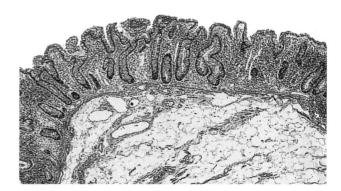

Figure 24.29 Transition from villous mucosal surface of ileum (*left*) to flat mucosa of large intestine (*right*) at the ileocecal junction. Note the prominent submucosal adipose tissue characteristic of this region.

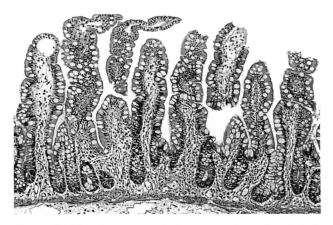

Figure 24.30 Characteristic ileal mucosa with slender relatively short villi (compare with jejunal villi in Figure 24.3) lined by abundant goblet cells with a lesser number of absorptive columnar cells.

ileocecal junction (91); although on the whole, they cannot be seen with the naked eye (92). Moreover, hyperplastic Peyer's patches (or focal lymphoid hyperplasia) may be found in the terminal ileum during childhood and have been linked to more than one-third of the cases of idiopathic intussusception occurring in the ileocecal region in this age group (93–95).

Peyer's patches are basically specialized groups of lymphoid follicles that occupy the mucosa and a variable portion of the submucosa. Structurally, four distinct compartments exist: follicle, dome, follicle-associated epithelium, and interfollicular regions (30,96) (Figure 24.31). Most lymphoid follicles within a Peyer's patch contain a germinal center that is populated by numerous surface IgA-positive B cells, with occasional CD4-positive T cells and macrophages (30,92) (Figures 24.31–24.32). However, the surrounding mantle zone contains a population of small B cells (predominantly surface IgD- and IgM-positive). The dome is the area between the follicle and the overlying surface epithelium; this region contains a heterogeneous population of cells, including B cells of all immunoglobulin isotypes (except IgD), macrophages, and plasma cells (92). The specialized or follicle-associated epithelium overlying lymphoid aggregates is distinct from surrounding villous epithelial surfaces. It characteristically has fewer goblet cells and contains membranous cells, or M cells, interspersed among the usual columnar absorptive cells (30,97) (Figure 24.32). The M cell is a specialized columnar epithelial cell that transports luminal antigens to adjacent extracellular spaces, thus allowing access to immunocompetent cells. These cells play a key role in mucosally based immunity, antigen tolerance, and probably in certain immunopathologic disease states (97). Morphologically, M cells have an attenuated brush border with diminished alkaline phosphatase staining intensity (96,98), a thin strip of apical cytoplasm, and a basally situated round nucleus. The M cell's cytoplasm is often

deformed by several lymphocytes (97). However, definitive M-cell characterization rests upon the identification of specific ultrastructural features (96,97). The follicle-associated epithelium also has a distinctive migratory cell composition because the intraepithelial lymphocyte population is more abundant and has a greater proportion of CD4-positive (T-helper/inducer) cells than does the usual villous epithelium (approximately 40% versus 6%) (96). Last, the fourth component of the Peyer's patch is called the interfollicular region. As in the lymph node, it is predominantly a T-cell zone with CD4-positive T-lymphocytes outnumbering CD8-positive lymphocytes by a 7:1 margin (92).

Plasma cells are a scant component of Peyer's patches, in contrast to the surrounding lamina propria, but they may frequently be found in the dome compartment. Peyer's patches are believed to be important in the generation of the mucosal immune response, in part by supplying the lamina propria with immunocompetent surface IgA-positive B cells

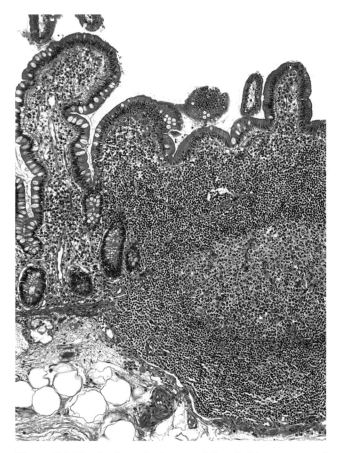

Figure 24.31 Confluent lamina propria lymphoid aggregates of a Peyer's patch. This organized lymphoid tissue typically extends into the underlying submucosa. The four components of the Peyer's patch are seen and include lymphoid nodules with germinal centers, an overlying flattened follicle-associated epithelium, and an intervening pale-staining dome region. The abundant lymphoid population between the follicles is the T-cell–rich interfollicular zone.

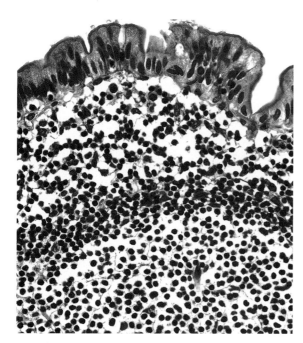

Figure 24.32 High magnification of surface epithelium above a lymphoid nodule within a Peyer's patch. The polymorphous germinal center (*below*) is surrounded by monotonous, small round lymphocytes that comprise the nodule's mantle zone. Above this lies the dome region with lymphocytes, plasma cells, and macrophages. The follicle-associated epithelium characteristically has few, if any, goblet cells; ultrastructurally, most of these cells would be identified as M cells.

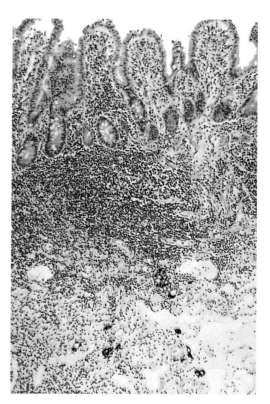

Figure 24.33 Dense brown-black granular pigment within the depths of a Peyer's patch of ileum. The pigment is typically confined to macrophages.

that become functional secretory plasma cells (30,91, 92,97).

Irregularly distributed, granular brown-black pigment can commonly be found in the deep portions of Peyer's patches in adults (99) (Figure 24.33). Although its origin is controversial, atmospheric or dietary sources are most probable (99,100). Accumulating principally within macrophages, this pigment has been shown by x-ray spectroscopy to contain a distinct mineral composition that includes silicates, aluminum, and titanium (99,100). The pigment is inert and has no known clinicopathologic significance.

A final distinctive feature often seen in the ileum is Meckel's diverticulum; it is the most common intestinal congenital anomaly and is found in 1 to 2% of the general population (31). Meckel's diverticulum is an antimesenteric outpouching of the terminal ileum usually located approximately 20 cm from the ileocecal junction. It represents the persistence of the omphalomesenteric duct. Although Meckel's diverticulum is usually an incidental finding, it can cause lower gastrointestinal bleeding or small bowel obstruction (101,102). Histologically, small intestinal mucosa alone lines the diverticulum in about 50 to 70% of cases. Ectopic gastric or pancreatic tissues are found in the remainder, typically encountered at the distal most aspect (102).

SPECIAL CONSIDERATIONS

Geographic, Age-Related, and Dietary Factors

Because geographic and local environmental factors can affect small bowel morphology, historical data about the residence or recent travel of an individual are essential to evaluate histologic material accurately. Specimens from individuals residing in, or visiting at length, certain less developed tropical locations such as Africa, southern India, and Thailand show a distinctly different villous appearance from those of individuals who live in temperate climate zones (45,103–106). The morphologic alterations seen in individuals from such tropical areas include leaflike villi predominating over fingerlike forms in jejunal segments examined via biopsy and an increased number of lamina propria mononuclear cells (107). This difference in the villous population is reflected histologically as stubby villi with a pyramidal shape (i.e., a broader base than apex) and occasional branched and fused villous tips (45,103,104). Interestingly, although the villi are shorter, the villous-to-crypt length ratio usually remains constant in all geographic settings (45,104). Such alterations should probably be considered a normal variant because these individuals are typically asymptomatic and otherwise healthy (103).

The cause of these morphologic changes is uncertain, but environmental factors, particularly regional enteric flora, presumably play a role (103). Similar mucosal changes are seen in normal individuals in temperate environments, but only in proximal portions of the duodenum. Therefore, these particular mucosal alterations must be analyzed in the context of both the patient's residence and the site within the small intestine in order to prevent misinterpretation as a pathologic change, such as tropical sprue.

Aging also modifies small bowel mucosal architecture. Although the literature on humans is limited, it has been shown that specimens from elderly individuals generally have shorter and broader villi than those from younger individuals (108). Moreover, lower animal and human fetuses have been documented as having fingerlike villi exclusively, suggesting that exposure to the environment or aging itself modifies villous architecture (108,109). However, the functional significance of these changes is uncertain (108).

Diet alters villous architecture in laboratory animals. A diet high in fiber results in broad and fused villi, whereas a fiber-free diet seems to prevent the formation of leaflike forms (17). If this finding is valid in humans, it may be one factor related to the presence of stubby, leaflike villi seen in patients in less developed countries where high-fiber diets are common.

Metaplastic and Heterotopic Tissues

Gastric type mucosa is not an unusual finding in the small intestine. A distinction can be made between metaplasia, an acquired alteration, and heterotopia, thought to be congenital in origin. Gastric metaplasia characteristically consists solely of antral-type, PAS-positive, foveolar columnar cells lying along the surface epithelium (Figure 24.23). This change is focal and often in direct continuity with usual columnar absorptive epithelium on the same villus (75). Gastric metaplasia may be encountered in more than 60% of healthy asymptomatic individuals in the duodenal bulb, where it can be regarded as within normal limits (75). More distally, however, it is less commonly seen in the asymptomatic person but rather frequently is associated with duodenitis or mucosal ulceration (75,110). Scattered chief and parietal cells without any organized arrangement are also associated with this type of metaplasia or with reparative processes (110).

In contrast, gastric heterotopia is usually a grossly evident mucosal polyp that contains all cellular elements encountered in the normal gastric fundic mucosa. Characteristically, mucous foveolar epithelium overlies an organized arrangement of glands lined by chief and parietal cells; this is typically well demarcated from the surrounding usual intestinal villous epithelium. Gastric heterotopia is also fairly common, being reported in up to 2% of the population (111); it may be found anywhere along the

gastrointestinal tract (110). Gastric heterotopia is a well-defined entity in the proximal duodenum and usually presents as a mucosal nodule on the anterior wall. Although they are usually of no clinical significance, larger ones may cause obstructive symptoms (111). In contrast, gastric heterotopia distal to the ligament of Treitz is usually symptomatic and often causes intussusception (112). This relationship to clinical symptoms may derive from patient selection bias because asymptomatic gastric heterotopias at a distal site would not be routinely detectable.

Heterotopic pancreas tissue also can be found anywhere along the small intestine but most commonly is found in the duodenum and jejunum (113,114). It can form submucosal, intramural, or serosal nodules and is composed of various admixtures of pancreatic acini, ducts, and islets of Langerhans (113,115) (Figure 24.34). Isolated ductal structures admixed with smooth muscle may be the predominant or exclusive component, and in these instances the alternative term adenomyoma has been used (31,114). Nodules of pancreatic tissue within the small intestine are usually asymptomatic, although larger lesions (greater than 1.5 cm) with prominent mucosal involvement may become clinically significant (114,115). A single case of a combined submucosal pancreatic heterotopia with overlying gastric type mucosa in the duodenal bulb recently was reported (116).

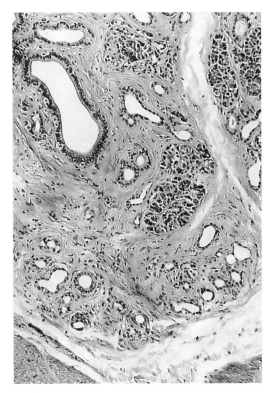

Figure 24.34 Heterotopic pancreas in the duodenum characterized in this instance by variably sized ducts, acini, and abundant smooth muscle.

Lymphoid Proliferations

Lymphoid tissue is a prominent feature of the small bowel. The gut-associated lymphoid system in this region, as in the entire gastrointestinal tract, is compartmentalized into lymphocytes of the epithelium, lamina propria, isolated lymphoid aggregates, and Peyer's patches (117). The normal appearance and immunologic composition of these distinct lymphoid populations have been detailed earlier in the chapter. All these compartments participate at some level in mucosal immune response, but they also provide the milieu for various hyperplastic and neoplastic immunoproliferations, as well as for certain immunodeficiency states. Some of these disorders have histologic features that deviate only slightly from a normal appearance and from one another. Additionally, some are believed to be preneoplastic.

Lymphoid hyperplasias are divided into two broad categories: focal and diffuse forms (118). Focal lymphoid hyperplasia is a localized, well-circumscribed proliferation of benign lymphoid tissue characterized by a polymorphic infiltrate of lymphocytes within which numerous benign follicles with reactive germinal centers are dispersed. These proliferations often involve only the mucosa and submucosa, but they may extend through the entire wall (118). Focal lymphoid hyperplasia is predominantly found in the terminal ileum of children or adolescents who present either with ileocecal intussusception or with a clinical syndrome mimicking appendicitis (93,95,118).

Diffuse or nodular lymphoid hyperplasia is a distinct entity in which multiple nodules composed of aggregates of benign lymphoid follicles disfigure the mucosa and submucosa along extensive lengths of the small intestine, with or without colonic involvement (118–120). It is usually asymptomatic and incidentally encountered (118). However, a distinct clinicopathologic variant exists that is characterized clinically by associated, combined variable immunodeficiency and giardiasis-related diarrhea and histologically by a greatly diminished or absent plasma cell population in the nearby lamina propria (118). Nodular lymphoid hyperplasia, with or without combined variable immunodeficiency, has been associated with an increased risk for the development of various malignancies (e.g., malignant lymphoma, carcinoma) (118–121).

Differentiation of these benign lymphoid lesions from malignant lymphoma can be problematic. However, recognizing the diagnostic morphologic features of malignant lymphoma, such as the usual cytologic monotony of the lymphoid population, the lack of a reactive follicular architecture, and the presence of mucosal ulceration, should resolve most dilemmas (118,122–124). Additionally, because the majority of small bowel malignant lymphomas are of B-cell lineage (124), demonstration of light-chain restriction by immunohistologic techniques or flow cytometric analysis or detection of heavy- or light-chain immunoglobulin gene rearrangements (e.g., monoclonality) by molecular diagnostic methods can aid in certain cases (125–127); T-cell receptor gene rearrangement analysis may be necessary in a minority of cases.

Morphologic Changes Associated with Ileal Diversion and Continence-Restoring Procedures

With the increasing number of diversion and continence-restoring procedures being performed after total colectomy, it has become common to see biopsy and revision specimens after such operations. As a consequence, familiarity with the altered yet "normal" morphology within these ileal creations must be appreciated in order to evaluate them optimally. The expected mucosal changes include villous shortening and crypt lengthening (approximate 1:1 to 2:1 ratio), increased numbers of goblet cells and lymphoid follicles, and a denser mononuclear cell infiltrate within the lamina propria (31,128,129). These alterations are similar after either colectomy with conventional ileostomy or after ileoanal anastomosis with ileal reservoir formation (e.g., pouch) (129–131). However, ileostomy stomas in particular show additional changes of mucosal prolapse exemplified by fibromuscular obliteration of the lamina propria and superficial erosions and microhemorrhages (31). Additionally, goblet cell mucin alterations have been seen in nearly 50% of pouches examined, with conversion to predominantly sulfomucins (i.e., colonic epithelial mucin) (131). However, another group of investigators saw no change in goblet cell mucin from the typical small bowel acid sialomucins in ileal segments after either ileoanal anastomosis with pouch formation or conventional ileostomy (129). Nonetheless, all these changes should be interpreted as "normal" because more definitive and specific criteria need to be met to establish persistent, recurrent, or novel disease in these specimens.

MUCOSAL BIOPSY SPECIMEN EVALUATION IN SUSPECTED MALABSORPTION

Specimen Procurement and Processing

The usefulness of small bowel mucosal biopsy is unquestioned (132), particularly in the evaluation of malabsorptive states. In the past, up to four biopsy samples were usually obtained from the area of the ligament of Treitz via a suction biopsy device attached to a long tube (133). In recent years, the standard upper endoscope has been used, and comparable specimens have been procured (76,134). Because this technique is performed under direct visualization, many more biopsy specimens can be obtained. Regardless of the biopsy technique used, the most critical part of the procedure is proper orientation of the specimen. Ideally, specimens are immediately mounted mucosa side up on a solid substance such as filter paper or plastic mesh and then placed into Hollande's or other fixative. After processing, the histotechnologist embeds the tissue perpendicular to the mounting material. Alternatively, biopsy specimens may be placed unmounted into fixative immediately. The tissue can then be properly oriented after processing at the time of embedding. Because the specimen will naturally curl, some tangential sectioning can be expected. Proper specimen evaluation requires examination of optimally oriented intestinal villi obtained from the central region of the biopsy specimen. Although serial sectioning is advocated by some investigators (107), step-sectioning (three–seven levels) is a reasonable alternative.

Our standard small bowel biopsy procedure consists of obtaining four to six endoscopic biopsy specimens. One can be used to make a touch preparation that is then fixed in alcohol and stained via the Giemsa technique. The other tissue samples are placed in fixative and routinely processed. Step-section slides are obtained: three are stained with H&E and one with alcizn blue/PAS. The PAS stain is a useful screen for Whipple's disease and *Mycobacterium avium-intracellulare* complex infection. Trichrome stain can be used to confirm collagen deposition seen in ischemia or collagenous sprue. In addition, the iron hematoxylin counterstain used in the trichrome technique makes it easier to identify giardiasis.

Specimen Interpretation and Common Artifacts

With appropriate specimen procurement, the mucosa with muscularis mucosae and a small portion of upper submucosa should be available for histologic examination. These specimens should be evaluated in a systematic fashion, including assessment of (a) villous architecture, (b) surface and crypt epithelia, (c) lamina propria constituents, and (d) submucosal structures (53). A well-oriented specimen is essential for optimal evaluation. However, it must be remembered that villi vary in length and shape, particularly in the proximal duodenum, and that villous apices bend and twist in various planes to create unusual forms; these variations should not be misinterpreted as a villous abnormality (40,53). Generally, if four normal villi in a row are observed, the villous architecture of the entire specimen is probably normal (53,107). This does not mean that specimens with fewer than four well-aligned normal villi should be considered inadequate because even one normal intestinal villus in a proximal small bowel biopsy specimen rules out unrelated celiac sprue (31). Conversely, identification of four

normal villi in a row does not necessarily exclude focal lesions, although it almost always does (107). The pathologist must be wary of certain common artifacts that may lead to erroneous interpretations. Careful attention to certain features (described below) within the various mucosal compartments will aid in their recognition.

Tangential Sectioning

Inappropriate orientation of the specimen, occurring at any point during processing, will lead to various tangential cuts or sections. The mucosa must be sectioned perpendicular to its long axis, or a distorted pattern disclosing apparently short and broad villi and an expanded lamina proprial compartment will be observed. However, several features aid in recognizing an oblique cut: (a) numerous elliptically shaped glands, (b) a multilayered arrangement of the crypts (Figure 24.35), or (c) a multilayered surface epithelium (53) (Figure 24.36). If any of these features are present, the villous architecture must be interpreted with caution.

Brunner's Gland–Related Artifact

Brunner's glands have an inconsistent effect on villous architecture (31). Occasionally, normal length villi can be encountered overlying the Brunner's glands (Figure 24.37), but more commonly the villi appear distorted, short, broad, and stubby (31,40) (Figure 24.24). To minimize the potential effects of this artifact on interpretation, biopsy specimens of the small bowel for evaluation of malabsorptive states are routinely obtained as distally as possible in

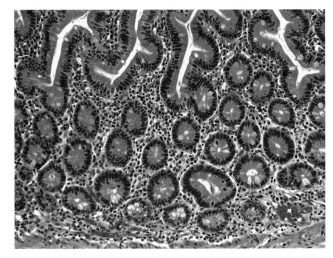

Figure 24.35 Multilayering of crypts indicates a tangential or oblique section of small intestine. The villous architecture overlying the crypts is normal, albeit unusual in appearance; this is also a product of malorientation of the biopsy specimen.

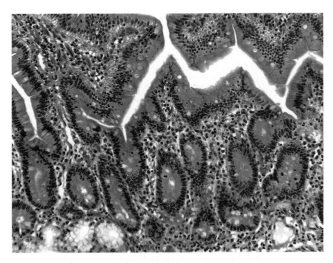

Figure 24.36 Another clue in identifying a tangential cut is multilayering, or "stratification," of the surface epithelium (*left portion of central villus*). The normal surface layer is one-cell thick. This broad and short villous appearance is a consequence of malorientation and should be interpreted accordingly.

the duodenum or from the proximal jejunum (i.e., near the ligament of Treitz) (76,134). Occasionally, however, more proximal small bowel biopsies are necessary for evaluation of duodenitis or ulcer disease.

Lymphoid Aggregate–Related Artifact

Mucosal lymphoid aggregates, or nodules, are scattered along the small bowel and often distort the villous architecture. Villi are usually absent over lymphoid aggregates, and nearby villous forms may be distorted, short, and

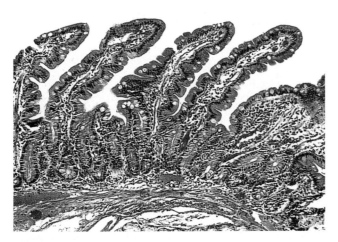

Figure 24.37 Occasionally, long slender villi, similar to those seen in the jejunum, are found overlying Brunner's glands. However, villi associated with Brunner's glands are more commonly shorter and broader (see Figure 24.24).

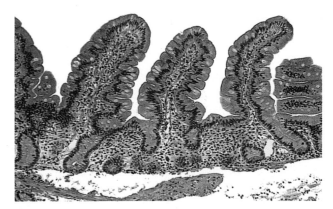

Figure 24.38 Absence of muscularis mucosae in a small bowel biopsy specimen, resulting in shorter- and broader-appearing villi that are widely spaced.

stubby (53) (Figure 24.31). Therefore, when a lymphoid aggregate is seen below an isolated flat portion of the surface epithelium, it should not be misinterpreted as a severe villous abnormality.

Absence of Muscularis Mucosae

As mentioned earlier, the muscularis mucosae is an important structural component of the mucosa. In its absence (for instance, in a very superficial mucosal biopsy specimen), the tissues tend to spread laterally, resulting in villi becoming more widely spaced and appearing short and broad (53,135) (Figure 24.38).

Biopsy Trauma–Related Artifacts

As a direct result of the traumatic pinch or suction biopsy procedures, certain alterations of normal mucosa can be seen. Separation of the villous surface epithelium from the underlying lamina propria or focally denuded epithelium are not unusual (53,135). The lack of acute erosive changes (e.g., neutrophilic infiltrate, cellular necrosis) or chronic evidence of ulceration (e.g., granulation tissue, regenerative epithelium) allow this alteration to be recognized as biopsy related. Additionally, focal hemorrhage and scattered polymorphonuclear leukocytes may be observed in the lamina propria as a consequence of the biopsy procedure. Crush or compression artifact can occur at the site of closure of the endoscopic forceps, resulting in a condensation of the lymphoplasmacytic component that can be misinterpreted as increased chronic inflammation (136). Additionally, the connective tissue may be altered in such a way that it appears more tightly packed, mimicking fibrosis or excessive collagen deposition (136).

Fixative-Related Artifacts

Certain fixatives other than formalin (4% formaldehyde solution) can cause interpretive problems. Although Hollande's fixative better preserves cytologic and nuclear detail, several artifacts may interfere with evaluation. The brightly eosinophilic granules of Paneth's cells and sometimes eosinophilic leukocytes seen readily in formalin-fixed tissue are not as well preserved by Hollande's fixative. Additionally, suboptimal clearing of Hollande's fixative from the specimens before paraffin embedding can result in residual minute, round, basophilic structures that resemble yeast forms or parasites (e.g., cryptosporidium, *Giardia lamblia*) (136)

ACKNOWLEDGMENT

We thank James T. McMahon, Ph.D., for the scanning electron micrographs.

REFERENCES

1. Williams PL, Warwick R, Dyson M, Bannister LH, eds. *Gray's Anatomy*. 37th ed. New York: Churchill Livingstone; 1989.
2. Thorek P. *Anatomy and Surgery*. 3rd ed. New York: Springer-Verlag; 1985.
3. Costacurta L. Anatomical and functional aspects of the human suspensory muscle of the duodenum. *Acta Anat (Basel)* 1972;82:34–46.
4. Trier JS, Winter HS. Anatomy, embryology and developmental abnormalities of the small intestine and colon. In: Sleisenger MH, Fordtran JS, eds. *Gastrointestinal Disease: Pathophysiology, Diagnosis, and Management*. 4th ed. Philadelphia: WB Saunders; 1989:991–1021.
5. Parks DA, Jacobson ED. Physiology of the splanchnic circulation. *Arch Intern Med* 1985;145:1278–1281.
6. Alpers DH. Digestion and absorption of carbohydrates and proteins. In: Johnson LR, ed. *Physiology of the Gastrointestinal Tract*. 2nd ed. New York: Raven Press; 1987:1469–1487.
7. Davenport HW. *Physiology of the Digestive Tract*. 5th ed. Chicago: Year Book Medical; 1982.
8. Quigley EM. Small intestinal motor activity—its role in gut homeostasis and disease. *Q J Med* 1987;65:799–810.
9. Fiorenza V, Yee YS, Zfass AM. Small intestinal motility: normal and abnormal function. *Am J Gastroenterol* 1987;82:1111–1114.
10. Lewin KJ. The endocrine cells of the gastrointestinal tract: the normal endocrine cells and their hyperplasias. In: Sommers SC, Rosen PP, Fechner RE, eds. *Pathology Annual*. Part 1. Norwalk, CT: Appleton-Century-Crofts; 1986:1–27.
11. Solcia E, Capella C, Buffa R, Usellini L, Fiocca R, Sessa F. Endocrine cells of the digestive system. In: Johnson LR, ed. *Physiology of the Gastrointestinal Tract*. 2nd ed. New York: Raven Press; 1987:111–130.
12. Elson CO, Kagnoff MF, Fiocchi C, Befus AD, Targan S. Intestinal immunity and inflammation: recent progress. *Gastroenterology* 1986;91:746–768.
13. Rubin W. The epithelial "membrane" of the small intestine. *Am J Clin Nutr* 1971;24:45–64.
14. Wilson JP. Surface area of the small intestine in man. *Gut* 1967;8:618–621.
15. Holmes R, Hourihane DO, Booth CC. The mucosa of the small intestine. *Postgrad Med J* 1961;37:717–724.
16. Toner PG, Carr KE. The use of scanning electron microscopy in the study of the intestinal villi. *J Pathol* 1969;97:611–617.

17. Trier JS, Madara JL. Functional morphology of the mucosa of the small intestine. In: Johnson LR, ed. *Physiology of the Gastrointestinal Tract*. 2nd ed. New York: Raven Press; 1987:1209–1249.
18. Dobbins WO. The intestinal mucosal lymphatic in man. A light and electron microscopic study. *Gastroenterology* 1966;51:994–1003.
19. Golab B, Szkudlarek R. Lymphatic vessels of the duodenum—deep network. *Folia Morphol (Warsz)* 1981;39:263–270.
20. Neutra MR, Padykula HK. The gastrointestinal tract. In: Weiss L, ed. *Modern Concepts of Gastrointestinal Histology*. New York: Elsevier; 1984:658–706.
21. Poley JR. Loss of the glycocalyx of enterocytes in small intestine: a feature detected by scanning electron microscopy in children with gastrointestinal intolerance to dietary protein. *J Pediatr Gastroenterol Nutr* 1988;7:386–394.
22. Trier JS. The surface coat of gastrointestinal epithelial cells. *Gastroenterology* 1969;56:618–622.
23. Dawson IMP. Atlas of gastrointestinal pathology as seen on biopsy. In: Gresham GA, ed. *Current Histopathology*. Vol 6. Philadelphia: JB Lippincott; 1983:63-67.
24. Filipe MI. Mucins in the human gastrointestinal epithelium: a review. *Invest Cell Pathol* 1979;2:195–216.
25. Dobbins WO III. Human intestinal intraepithelial lymphocytes. *Gut* 1986;27:972–985.
26. Ferguson A, Murray D. Quantitation of intraepithelial lymphocytes in human jejunum. *Gut* 1971;12:988–994.
27. Selby WS, Janossy G, Bofill M, Jewell DP. Lymphocyte subpopulations in the human small intestine: the findings in normal mucosa and in the mucosa of patients with adult coeliac disease. *Clin Exp Immunol* 1983;52:219–228.
28. Cerf-Bensussan N, Schneeberger EE, Bhan AK. Immunohistologic and immunoelectron microscopic characterization of the mucosal lymphocytes of human small intestine by the use of monoclonal antibodies. *J Immunol* 1983;130:2615–2622.
29. Greenwood JH, Austin LL, Dobbins WO III. In vitro characterization of human intestinal intraepithelial lymphocytes. *Gastroenterology* 1983;85:1023–1035.
30. Kagnoff MF. Immunology and disease of the gastrointestinal tract. In: Sleisenger MH, Fordtran JS, eds. *Gastrointestinal Disease*. 4th ed. Philadelphia: WB Saunders; 1989:114–144.
31. Petras RE. Nonneoplastic intestinal disease. In: Sternberg SS, ed. *Diagnostic Surgical Pathology*. Vol 2. Philadelphia: Lippincott Williams & Wilkin; 2004:1475–1542.
32. Ferguson A, Sutherland A, MacDonald TT, Allan F. Technique for microdissection and measurement in biopsies of human small intestine. *J Clin Pathol* 1977;30:1068–1073.
33. Lipkin M. Proliferation and differentiation of normal and diseased gastrointestinal cells. In: Johnson LR, ed. *Physiology of the Gastrointestinal Tract*. 2nd ed. New York: Raven Press; 1987:255–284.
34. Williamson RC. Intestinal adaptation (first of two parts). Structural, functional, and cytokinetic changes. *N Engl J Med* 1978; 298:1393–1402.
35. Watson AJM. Necrosis and apoptosis in the gastrointestinal tract. *Gut* 1995;37:165–167.
36. Facer P, Bishop AE, Lloyd RV, Wilson BS, Hennessy RJ, Polak JM. Chromogranin: a newly recognized marker for endocrine cells of the human gastrointestinal tract. *Gastroenterology* 1985;89:1366–1373.
37. Albrecht S, Gardiner GW, Kovacs K, Ilse G, Kaiser U. Duodenal somatostatinoma with psammoma bodies. *Arch Pathol Lab Med* 1989;113:517–520.
38. Sjolund K, Sanden G, Hakanson R, Sundler F. Endocrine cells in human intestine: an immunocytochemical study. *Gastroenterology* 1983;85:1120–1130.
39. Walsh JH. Gastrointestinal peptide hormones. In: Sleisenger MH, Fordtran JS, eds. *Gastrointestinal Disease*. 4th ed. Philadelphia: WB Saunders; 1989:78–9107.
40. Goldman H, Antonioli DA. Mucosal biopsy of the esophagus, stomach, and proximal duodenum. *Hum Pathol* 1982;13:423–448.
41. Sandow MJ, Whitehead R. The Paneth cell. *Gut* 1979;20:420–431.
42. Geller SA, Thung SN. Morphologic unity of Paneth cells. *Arch Pathol Lab Med* 1983;107:476–479.

43. Shen B, Porter E, Reynoso E, Shen C, Ghosh D, Connor J, Drazba J, Rho H, Gramlich T, Li R, Ormsby A, Sy M, Ganz T, Bevins C. Human defensin -5 expression in intestinal metaplasia of the upper gastrointestinal tract. *J Clin Path*; 2005; 58: 687–694.

44. Jenkins D, Goodall A, Scott BB. T-lymphocyte populations in normal and coeliac small intestinal mucosa defined by monoclonal antibodies. *Gut* 1986;27:1330–1337.

45. Lee FD, Toner PG. *Biopsy Pathology of the Small Intestine.* Philadelphia: JB Lippincott; 1980.

46. Isaacson P, Judd MA. Carcinoembryonic antigen (CEA) in the normal human small intestine: a light and electron microscopic study. *Gut* 1977;18:786–791.

47. Scott H, Solheim BG, Brandtzaeg P, Thorsby E. HLA-DR–like antigens in the epithelium of the human small intestine. *Scand J Immunol* 1980;12:77–82.

48. Chiba M, Ohta H, Nagasaki A, Arakawa H, Masamune O. Lymphoid cell subsets in normal human small intestine. *Gastroenterol Jpn* 1986;21:336–343.

49. Brandtzaeg P, Halstensen TS, Kett K, et al. Immunobiology and immunopathology of human gut mucosa: humoral immunity and intraepithelial lymphocytes. *Gastroenterology* 1989;97: 1562–1584.

50. Comer GM, Brandt LJ, Abissi CJ. Whipple's disease: a review. *Am J Gastroenterol* 1983;78:107–114.

51. Strom RL, Gruninger RP. AIDS with Mycobacterium avium-intracellulare lesions resembling those of Whipple's disease. *N Engl J Med* 1983;309:1323–1325.

52. Roth RI, Owen RL, Keren DF, Volberding PA. Intestinal infection with Mycobacterium avium in acquired immune deficiency syndrome (AIDS). Histological and clinical comparison with Whipple's disease. *Dig Dis Sci* 1985;30:497–504.

53. Perera DR, Weinstein WM, Rubin CE. Symposium on pathology of the gastrointestinal tract. Part II. Small intestinal biopsy. *Hum Pathol* 1975;6:157–217.

54. Klein NC, Hargrove RL, Sleisenger MH, Jeffries GH. Eosinophilic gastroenteritis. *Medicine (Baltimore)* 1970;49:299–319.

55. Johnstone JM, Morson BC. Eosinophilic gastroenteritis. *Histopathology* 1978;2:335–348.

56. Goldman H, Proujansky R. Allergic proctitis and gastroenteritis in children. Clinical and mucosal biopsy features in 53 cases. *Am J Surg Pathol* 1986;10:75–86.

57. DeSchryver-Kecskemeti K, Clouse RE. A previously unrecognized subgroup of "eosinophilic gastroenteritis." Association with connective tissue diseases. *Am J Surg Pathol* 1984;8: 171–180.

58. McNabb PC, Fleming CR, Higgins JA, Davis GL. Transmural eosinophilic gastroenteritis with ascites. *Mayo Clin Proc* 1979;54:119–122.

59. Heatley RV. The gastrointestinal mast cell. *Scand J Gastroenterol* 1983;18:449–453.

60. Befus D, Goodacre R, Dyck N, Bienenstock J. Mast cell heterogeneity in man. I. Histologic studies of the intestine. *Int Arch Allergy Appl Immunol* 1985;76:232–236.

61. Scott BB, Hardy GJ, Losowsky MS. Involvement of the small intestine in systemic mast cell disease. *Gut* 1975;16:918–924.

62. Lundqvist M, Wilander E. Subepithelial neuroendocrine cells and carcinoid tumors of the human small intestine and appendix. A comparative immunohistochemical study with regard to serotonin, neuron-specific enolase and S-100 protein reactivity. *J Pathol* 1986;148:141–147.

63. Lord MG, Valies P, Broughton AC. A morphologic study of the submucosa of the large intestine. *Surg Gynecol Obstet* 1977; 145:55–60.

64. Lee AK, DeLellis RA, Silverman ML, Wolfe HJ. Lymphatic and blood vessel invasion in breast carcinoma: a useful prognostic indicator? *Hum Pathol* 1986;17:984–987.

65. Schlingemann RO, Dingjan GM, Emeis JJ, Blok J, Warnaar SO, Ruiter DJ. Monoclonal antibody PAL-E specific for endothelium. *Lab Invest* 1985;52:71–76.

66. Vardy PA, Lebenthal E, Shwachman H. Intestinal lymphagiectasia: a reappraisal. *Pediatrics* 1975;55:842–851.

67. Gershon MD, Erde SM. The nervous system of the gut. *Gastroenterology* 1981;80:1571–1594.

68. Goyal RK, Crist JR. Neurology of the gut. In: Sleisenger MH, Fordtran JS, eds. *Gastrointestinal Disease.* 4th ed. Philadelphia: WB Saunders; 1989:21–52.

69. Krishnamurthy S, Schuffler MD. Pathology of neuromuscular disorders of the small intestine and colon. *Gastroenterology* 1987;93:610–639.

70. Ferri GL, Probert L, Cocchia D, Michetti F, Marangos PJ, Polak JM. Evidence for the presence of S-100 protein in the glial component of the human enteric nervous system. *Nature* 1982;297:409–410.

71. Romert P, Mikkelsen HB. cC-kit immunoreactive interstitial cells of Cajal in the human small and large intestine. *Histochem Cell Biol* 1998; 109: 195–202.

72. Lawson HH. The duodenal mucosa in health and disease. A clinical and experimental study. *Surg Annu* 1989;21:157–180.

73. Lawson HH. Definition of the gastroduodenal junction in healthy subjects. *J Clin Pathol* 1988;41:393–396.

74. Korn ER, Foroozan P. Endoscopic biopsies of normal duodenal mucosa. *Gastrointest Endosc* 1974;21:51–54.

75. Kreuning J, Bosman FT, Kuiper G, Wal AM, Lindeman J. Gastric and duodenal mucosa in "healthy" individuals. An endoscopic and histopathological study of 50 volunteers. *J Clin Pathol* 1978;31:69–77.

76. Dandalides SM, Carey WD, Petras RE, Achkar E. Endoscopic small bowel mucosal biopsy: a controlled trial evaluating forceps size and biopsy location in the diagnosis of normal and abnormal mucosal architecture. *Gastrointest Endosc* 1989;35:197–200.

77. Robertson HE. The pathology of Brunner's glands. *Arch Pathol* 1941;31:112–130.

78. Lang IM, Tansy MF. Brunner's glands. In: Young JA, ed. *Gastrointestinal Physiology. IV. International Review of Physiology.* Vol 28. Baltimore: University Park Press; 1983:85–102.

79. Treasure T. The ducts of Brunner's glands. *J Anat* 1978;127: 299–304.

80. Leeson TS, Leeson RC. The fine structure of Brunner's glands. *J Anat* 1968;103:263–276.

81. Thompson IW, Day DW, Wright NA. Subnuclear vacuolated mucous cells: a novel abnormality of simple mucin-secreting cells of non-specialized gastric mucosa and Brunner's glands. *Histopathology* 1987;11:1067–1081.

82. Kamiya R. Basal-granulated cells in human Brunner's glands. *Arch Histol Jpn* 1983;46:87–101.

83. Bosshard A, Chery-Croze S, Cuber JC, Dechelette MA, Berger F, Chayvialle JA. Immunocytochemical study of peptidergic structures in Brunner's glands. *Gastroenterology* 1989;97: 1382–1388.

84. Silverman L, Waugh JM, Huizenga KA, Harrison EG Jr. Large adenomatous polyp of Brunner's glands. *Am J Clin Pathol* 1961; 36:438–443.

85. Franzin G, Musola R, Ghidini O, Manfrini C, Fratton A. Nodular hyperplasia of Brunner's glands. *Gastrointest Endosc* 1985;31: 374–378.

86. West B. Pseudomelanosis duodeni. *J Clin Gastroenterol* 1988; 10: 127–129.

87. Rosenberg JC, DiDio LJ. Anatomic and clinical aspects of the junction of the ileum with the large intestine. *Dis Colon Rectum* 1970;13:220–224.

88. Kumar D, Phillips SF. The contribution of external ligamentous attachments to function of the ileocecal junction. *Dis Colon Rectum* 1987;30:410–416.

89. Axelsson C, Andersen JA. Lipohyperplasia of the ileocaecal region. *Acta Chir Scand* 1974;140:649–654.

90. Cornes JS. Number, size, and distribution of Peyer's patches in the human small intestine. Part I. The development of Peyer's patches. Part II. The effect of age on Peyer's patches. *Gut* 1965;6:225–233.

91. MacDonald TT, Spencer J, Viney JL, Williams CB, Walker-Smith JA. Selective biopsy of human Peyer's patches during ileal endoscopy. *Gastroenterology* 1987;93:1356–1362.

92. Spencer J, Finn T, Isaacson PG. Human Peyer's patches: an immunohistochemical study. *Gut* 1986;27:405–410.

93. Pang LC. Intussusception revisited: clinicopathologic analysis of 261 cases with emphasis on pathogenesis. *South Med J* 1989; 82:215–228.

94. Schenken JR, Kruger RL, Schultz L. Papillary lymphoid hyperplasia of the terminal ileum: an unusual cause of intussusception and gastrointestinal bleeding in childhood. *J Pediatr Surg* 1975;10:259–265.

95. Fieber SS, Schaefer HJ. Lymphoid hyperplasia of the terminal ileum—a clinical entity? *Gastroenterology* 1966;50:83–98.

96. Bjerke K, Brandtzaeg P, Fausa O. T cell distribution is different in follicle-associated epithelium of human Peyer's patches and villous epithelium. *Clin Exp Immunol* 1988;74:270–275.

97. Wolf JL, Bye WA. The membranous epithelial (M) cell and the mucosal immune system. *Annu Rev Med* 1984;35:95–112.

98. Owen RL, Jones AL. Epithelial cell specialization within human Peyer's patches: an ultrastructural study of intestinal lymphoid follicles. *Gastroenterology* 1974;66:189–203.

99. Shepherd NA, Crocker PR, Smith AP, Levison DA. Exogenous pigment in Peyer's patches. *Hum Pathol* 1987;18:50–54.

100. Urbanski SJ, Arsenault AL, Green FH, Haber G. Pigment resembling atmospheric dust in Peyer's patches. *Mod Pathol* 1989;2:222–226.

101. Mackey WC, Dineen P. A fifty year experience with Meckel's diverticulum. *Surg Gynecol Obstet* 1983;156:56–64.

102. Artigas V, Calabuig R, Badia F, Rius X, Allende L, Jover J. Meckel's diverticulum: value of ectopic tissue. *Am J Surg* 1986;151:631–634.

103. Bennett MK, Sachdev GK, Jewell DP, Anand BS. Jejunal mucosal morphology in healthy north Indian subjects. *J Clin Pathol* 1985;38:368–371.

104. Cook GC, Kajubi SK, Lee FD. Jejunal morphology of the African in Uganda. *J Pathol* 1969;98:157–169.

105. Lindenbaum J, Gerson CD, Kent TH. Recovery of small-intestinal structure and function after residence in the tropics. I. Studies in Peace Corps volunteers. *Ann Intern Med* 1971;74:218–222.

106. Gerson CD, Kent TH, Saha JR, Siddiqi N, Lindenbaum J. Recovery of small-intestinal structure and function after residence in the tropics. II. Studies in Indians and Pakistanis living in New York City. *Ann Intern Med* 1971;75:41–48.

107. Dobbins WO III. Small bowel biopsy in malabsorptive states. In: Norris HT, ed. *Pathology of the Colon, Small Intestine, and Anus.* New York: Churchill Livingstone; 1983:121–167.

108. Webster SG, Leeming JT. The appearance of the small bowel mucosa in old age. *Age Ageing* 1975;4:168–174.

109. Chacko CJ, Paulson KA, Mathan VI, Baker SJ. The villus architecture of the small intestine in the tropics: a necropsy study. *J Pathol* 1969;98:146–151.

110. Wolff M. Heterotopic gastric epithelium in the rectum: a report of three new cases with a review of 87 cases of gastric heterotopia in the alimentary canal. *Am J Clin Pathol* 1971;55:604–616.

111. Lessells AM, Martin DF. Heterotopic gastric mucosa in the duodenum. *J Clin Pathol* 1982;35:591–595.

112. Tsubone M, Kozuka S, Taki T, Hoshino M, Yasui A, Hachisuka K. Heterotopic gastric mucosa in the small intestine. *Acta Pathol Jpn* 1984;34:1425–1431.

113. Lai EC, Tompkins RK. Heterotopic pancreas. Review of a 26 year experience. *Am J Surg* 1986;151:697–700.

114. Dolan RV, ReMine WH, Dockerty MB. The fate of heterotopic pancreatic tissue. A study of 212 cases. *Arch Surg* 1974;109:762–765.

115. Armstrong CP, King PM, Dixon JM, Macleod IB. The clinical significance of heterotopic pancreas in the gastrointestinal tract. *Br J Surg* 1981;68:384–387.

116. Tanemura H, Uno S, Suzuki M, et al. Heterotopic gastric mucosa accompanied by aberrant pancreas in the duodenum. *Am J Gastroenterol* 1987;82:685–688.

117. Tomasi TB Jr. Mechanisms of immune regulation at mucosal surfaces. *Rev Infect Dis* 1983;5(suppl 4):S784–S792.

118. Ranchod M, Lewin KJ, Dorfman RF. Lymphoid hyperplasia of the gastrointestinal tract: a study of 26 cases and review of the literature. *Am J Surg Pathol* 1978;2:383–400.

119. Rambaud JC, DeSaint-Louvent P, Marti R, et al. Diffuse follicular lymphoid hyperplasia of the small intestine without primary immunoglobulin deficiency. *Am J Med* 1982;73:125–132.

120. Matuchansky C, Touchard G, Lemaire M, et al. Malignant lymphoma of the small bowel associated with diffuse nodular lymphoid hyperplasia. *N Engl J Med* 1985;313:166–171.

121. Hermans PE, Diaz-Buxo JA, Stobo JD. Idiopathic late-onset immunoglobulin deficiency: clinical observations in 50 patients. *Am J Med* 1976;61:221–237.

122. Lewin KJ, Kahn LB, Novis BH. Primary intestinal lymphoma of "Western" and "Mediterranean" type, alpha chain disease and massive plasma cell infiltration: a comparative study of 37 cases. *Cancer* 1976;38:2511–2528.

123. Lewin KJ, Ranchod M, Dorfman RF. Lymphomas of the gastrointestinal tract: a study of 117 cases presenting with gastrointestinal disease. *Cancer* 1978;42:693–707.

124. Grody WW, Magidson JG, Weiss LM, Hu E, Warnke HA, Lewin KJ. Gastrointestinal lymphomas: immunohistochemical studies on the cell of origin. *Am J Surg Pathol* 1985;9:328–337.

125. Tubbs RR, Sheibani K. Immunohistology of lymphoproliferative disorders. *Semin Diagn Pathol* 1984;1:272–284.

126. Little JV, Foucar K, Horvath A, Crago S. Flow cytometric analysis of lymphoma and lymphoma-like disorders. *Semin Diagn Pathol* 1989;6:37–54.

127. Grody WW, Gatti RA, Naiem F. Diagnostic molecular pathology. *Mod Pathol* 1989; 2:553–568.

128. Goldman H, Antonioli DA. Mucosal biopsy of the rectum, colon, and distal ileum. *Hum Pathol* 1982;13:981–1012.

129. Bechi P, Romagnoli P, Cortesini C. Ileal mucosal morphology after total colectomy in man. *Histopathology* 1981;5:667–678.

130. Philipson B, Brandberg A, Jagenburg R, Kock NG, Lager I, Ahren C. Mucosal morphology, bacteriology, and absorption in intra-abdominal ileostomy reservoir. *Scand J Gastroenterol* 1975;10:145–153.

131. Shepherd NA, Jass JR, Duval I, Moskowitz RI, Nicholls RJ, Morson BC. Restorative proctocolectomy with ileal reservoir: pathological and histochemical study of mucosal biopsy specimens. *J Clin Pathol* 1987;40:601–607.

132. Trier JS. Diagnostic value of peroral biopsy of the proximal small intestine. *N Engl J Med* 1971;285:1470–1473.

133. Brandborg LL, Rubin GE, Quinton WE. A multipurpose instrument for suction biopsy of the esophagus, stomach, small bowel, and colon. *Gastroenterology* 1959;37:1–16.

134. Achkar E, Carey WD, Petras R, Sivak MV, Revta R. Comparison of suction capsule and endoscopic biopsy of small bowel mucosa. *Gastrointest Endosc* 1986;32:278–281.

135. Whitehead R. Mucosal biopsy of the gastrointestinal tract. In: Bennington JL, ed. *Major Problems in Pathology.* Vol 3. 3rd ed. Philadelphia: WB Saunders; 1985.

136. Haggitt RC. Handling of gastrointestinal biopsies in the surgical pathology laboratory. *Lab Med* 1982;13:272–278.

Colon

Julia Dahl   *Joel K. Greenson*

EMBRYOLOGY

The gastrointestinal tract is a remarkably complex, three-dimensional, specialized, and vital organ system derived from a simple tubal structure composed of all three germ layers (endoderm, mesoderm, and ectoderm). Early in development, the gut is patterned into four asymmetrical axes—anterior-posterior (AP), dorsoventral (DV), left-right (LR), and radial (RAD), utilizing critical developmental pathways that are directed by reciprocal mesodermal (mesenchymal) to endodermal (epithelial) cell-cell interactions and endodermal to endodermal cell-cell interactions (1–9). Because gut epithelium is a constitutively developing tissue, constantly differentiating from a stem cell in a progenitor pool throughout adult life, these developmental pathways, axes of development, and cell-cell "cross talk" continue to be important in cell differentiation, homeostasis, and apoptosis of the adult intestinal epithelium (8–12).

The adult colon displays a morphologic and functional pattern clearly identifiable in three of the four embryonic axes, and interacts with the gut derivatives (thyroid, lung, liver, and pancreas) produced in the fourth embryonic axis (13,14). Development and differentiation along the AP axis gives rise to the foregut, the midgut, and hindgut, resulting in regionally specific differentiation from mouth to anus. The significant variation in patterns of gene expression, physiologic function, disease distribution, and variations in histologic appearance between the right and left colon reflects the combined midgut and hindgut derivation (8,15–30). The cecum, appendix, ascending, and proximal portion of the transverse colon (right colon) are derived from the midgut while the distal transverse, descending, sigmoid colon, and rectum (left colon) are derived from the hindgut (13,14).

The LR axis is manifested in the colon by characteristic turning and looping of the gut, resulting in portions of colon with varying mesentery and fixation within the abdominal cavity (13).

The fundamental axis maintained in the adult is the radial (crypt to surface) axis. Homeostasis of intestinal epithelium occurs throughout life along this radial axis, with the epithelial and mesenchymal progenitor/proliferative cells being deeper in the radial axis than the differentiated functional cells and the apoptotic cells being luminal (11,31–33).

Abnormalities of any of the developmental pathways or along any axis during organogenesis may result in gross morphologic malformations, including diverticula, rotational malformations, stenoses, atresias, duplications, aganglionic segments, imperforate anus, and others (13,14,34–37). Perturbations of developmental pathways used for organ homeostasis may result in metaplasias, polyposis syndromes, and malignant transformation (10,38–42).

ANATOMIC CONSIDERATIONS

The colon is the terminal 1.0 to 1.5 m segment of the gastrointestinal tract, following the periphery of the peritoneal cavity, with the rectum extending into the pelvis and concluding at the anal canal (Figure 25.1) (43,44). There is considerable anatomic variation in the position of the colon segments, mesenteric coverings, and attachments to the posterior abdominal wall (44,45). Nonetheless, consistency of vascular supply, venous drainage, and innervation distinguishing the two primary (right and left) colon segments along the embryologic AP (midgut/hindgut) axis is maintained. The right colon receives its blood supply from the superior mesenteric artery, parasympathetic nervous innervation from the vagus nerve, and sympathetic innervation from the superior mesenteric ganglia. The left colon receives its blood supply from the inferior mesenteric artery, parasympathetic innervation from sacral nerves S2, S3, and S4 through the nervi erigentes; and sympathetic innervation from the inferior mesenteric ganglia. Venous drainage is predominantly portal. The rectum receives blood from the middle and inferior rectal arteries, parasympathetic innervation from the nervi erigentes, and sympathetic innervation through the hypogastric plexus through lumbar spinal segments L1, L2, and L3 (19,43–45).

Unique external features of the colon include the teniae coli and haustra, visible through the investing serosa and subserosal tissue. The muscular layers of the large intestine are composed of both longitudinally and circularly arranged fibers. The longitudinal fibers are present circumferentially through the length of the colon but are primarily concentrated into three flat bands called the teniae coli (43–45). Convexities of the circular muscular layer, the haustra, are transient and probably the result of structural and functional properties of the colon.

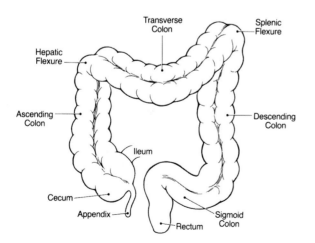

Figure 25.1 Major regions of the colon.

From the luminal perspective, various landmarks are recognized by the endoscopist. The cecum is readily identified by the ileocecal valve, appendiceal orifice, and blind-ended, saclike appearance. The subjacent portal vasculature imparts a blue hue to the mucosa at the hepatic flexure. Orientation of the teniae coli within the transverse colon results in a T-shaped lumen, ending in a slitlike orifice and acute angle of the splenic flexure. Although the descending and sigmoid colon may have thickened mucosal folds and diverticular orifices, calibration marks on the colonoscope are more reliable means of approximating the location within this region.

FUNCTION

The basic function of the large bowel is conservation of salt and water and facilitation of orderly disposal of waste materials (30). Considerable advancements have been made recently in characterizing the vast and interrelated colon functions; these further support the concept of two primary, unique colon segments, the right and left colon (15,19,46). In addition to their distinct embryologic derivation, the right and left colon display segment-specific arrays of physiologic functions, patterns of motility, commensal bacterial populations, and metabolic intermediate and end products; as well as local and systemic immune functions (15,21,23,24,26,29,30,47–51). These varied functions are reflected in differing patterns of gene, lectin and surface marker expression, varying disease distributions, and rates of (and sequences involved in) neoplastic transformation (23,24,28,29,46). Subtle regional variations of the colonic mucosa, reflecting the segmental nature of the right and left colon, have been well recognized by gastrointestinal pathologists (15,20,22) and are described in the following sections.

The most well-recognized function of the colon is absorption of water, desiccation, and transient storage of the feces. The cecum receives 1.3 to 1.8 liters of electrolyte-rich ileal effluent daily and is a high-capacity absorptive surface, effectively absorbing 80% of the chylous water (and sodium ions, Na^+) during the prolonged mucosal exposure created by the retrograde peristalsis unique to the cecum (21,26,27,30). Bulk absorption (of water and sodium) occurs via electroneutral sodium chloride (NaCl) transport at the surface and in the superficial portions of the crypts (21,30,52). Within the left colon, as fecal contents are propagated distally, low-capacity electrogenic absorption via luminal sodium channels, regulated by aldosterone and angiotensin, serve in further absorption of water, as well as preservation of sodium (21,30,53,54), particularly during periods of salt deprivation and/or mucosal injury. An additional mechanism for water absorption unique to the left colon, involving formation of a hyperosmolar (Na^+) compartment between the colonocytes and pericrypt myofibroblasts, has been observed and may be vital in extracting water from the osmotically dense feces, allowing final compaction and storage with a stool output of 200 to 500 g daily (27,55,56).

The colon participates in several diverse and integral metabolic processes through absorption, secretion, fermentation, oxidation, and other processes unique to the colonic epithelium or in concert with the colonic commensal bacteria. Rivaling London's East End or New York City in cultural diversity, there are an estimated 400 to 500 microbial species (bacteria, fungi, and a few protozoa) forming complex ecosystems from the terminal ileum to the rectum (49, 58–60). Bacterial cells outnumber human cells roughly 1000:1, with highest concentration in the cecum and decreasing gradient and varying composition proceeding distally. In the colon of healthy humans, commensal bacteria are required for numerous vital processes: formation of short-chain fatty acids, metabolic intermediates and vitamins; metabolism of proteins and amino acids; detoxification or biotransformation of bile acids, and natural sterols and phytoestrogens, as well as phosphate and oxalate excretion (29,49,50,57,58,60,61). Fermentation of carbohydrates to form short-chain fatty acids, particularly butyrate, serves as a major source of energy for colonocytes, and butyrate plays a crucial role in colonocyte growth and differentiation (51,57,60,62,63). Nearly equal to the activity observed in the liver, colonocytes have the capacity to mediate biotransformation of bile salts, drugs, and xenobiotics (49,50). Many of these processes are segment-specific to either the right or the left colon.

Colonic commensal bacteria are integral to the health and function not only of the large intestine, but to the host at large through activity in local and systemic immune function and regulation. Locally, the colonic epithelium and commensal flora serve as important barriers to infection via tight junctions and secretion of antimicrobial substances, as well as competition for nutrient substrates (64–68).

The intestinal mucosa (terminal ileum through rectum) is the largest immune organ of the body (49,58,59,68,69). Lamina propria and lymphoid aggregate plasma cells represent 80% of the antibody-producing cells within the entire body and produce more antibodies than any other part of the body (49,58,59,69). The process of antigen sampling across specialized regions of the colon results in "gut priming" and routinely confers protection from subsequent infection locally and in other mucosal tissues (systemic immunization) (70–77). At baseline, the gut immune system is highly activated in response to normal flora—so called physiologic inflammation—in which the intestinal microflora and the intestinal immunologic mechanisms influence each other locally and systemically, forming an interdependent mutualistic ecosystem, the balance of which is required for maintenance of health and prevention of disease (71,73,74, 78,79).

LIGHT MICROSCOPY

Although regional histologic differences exist within the right and left colon, the overall microscopic structure is similar throughout its length. The colon contains four histologically distinct compartments: (a) mucosa, (b) submucosa, (c) muscularis externa (or muscularis propria), and (d) serosa. The enteric nervous system spans all four compartments with cell bodies (ganglia and plexi) in both the submucosa and muscularis propria extending processes throughout the lamina propria, submucosa, and muscular layers, while receiving and transmitting information through synapses with the central nervous system via parasympathetic and sympathetic autonomic nervous systems.

Mucosa

The luminal colonic mucosa is the most metabolically and immunologically active compartment of the colon, as reflected in its organization and relative complexity. The luminal surface is covered by glycocalyx (glycans, enzymes, lectins, and mucin), facilitating formation of the commensal microbial ecosystem and serving as an integral barrier function (80–82). Beneath the glycocalyx is polarized columnar epithelium lining millions of regularly spaced crypts that span the depth of the lamina propria. The crypts are aligned perpendicular to and extend to the muscularis mucosae, imparting the well-known "rack of test tubes" appearance (Figure 25.2). Some variation in space between crypts is expected in biopsies of normal individuals; however, irregularly oriented or bifurcated crypts are considered

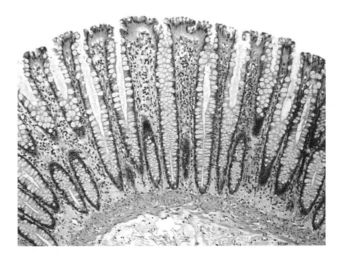

Figure 25.2 Normal colonic mucosa. The histologic section of this endoscopic mucosal biopsy specimen is oriented so the simple columnar surface epithelium facing the lumen is at the top of the figure and the cut surface of the specimen is at the bottom. The mucosal crypts are lined up in parallel, and their mouths are open to the lumen. The lamina propria consists of the stromal elements investing the crypts and extending from the surface epithelium to the smooth muscle cells of the muscularis mucosae at the bottom.

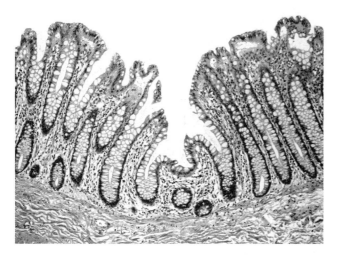

Figure 25.3 Innominate grooves of colonic mucosa. Multiple crypts open in a "mirror image" across a common crypt lumen at the groove, with the common crypt lumen opening to the colonic lumen. This normal finding is not a true branching of the crypts and should not be misinterpreted as architectural distortion indicative of chronic mucosal injury (i.e., inflammatory bowel disease). The innominate groove common lumen is generally within the superficial one-third of the mucosa.

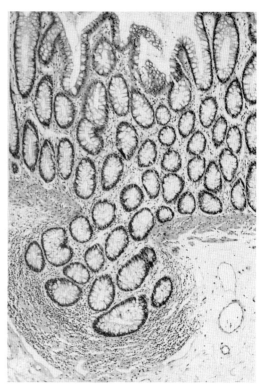

Figure 25.5 Lymphoglandular complex. In this tangential section, crypt epithelium is present within a lymphoid follicle that extends from the mucosa through the muscularis mucosae into the submucosa.

abnormal (see Regional Variation in Histologic Features, below). Variation in the usual pattern of the mucosa is seen at innominate grooves (regularly occurring folds in the mucosa), adjacent to lymphoid follicles, with lymphoglandular complexes and with the normal mucosal folds and ridges created by contraction of the muscularis mucosae (Figures 25.3–25.5). Each of these variations must be distinguished from the histologic changes of chronic mucosal injury (inflammatory bowel disease, or IBD) (Table 25.1).

Advances in immunohistochemistry and development of new antibodies has allowed further classification of cell types, with utility in assessing both normal and pathologic histologic patterns and providing useful adjuncts to standard histochemical stains (Table 25.2) (52,83–123).

Regional Variation in Histologic Features

Although the overall mucosal pattern as described above is maintained, the right and left colon display subtle histologic differences in the ratio of surface epithelial colonocytes to goblet cells, thickness of mucus layer, normal presence of Paneth's cells, crypt length, quantity of surface intraepithelial lymphocytes, lamina propria mononuclear cell distribution, and density, as well as lymphoid aggregate density (Figure 25.6). These subtle, but significant, differences make it essential to dissuade our clinical colleagues from the practice of utilizing pooled biopsies simply labeled *colon*. We encourage gastroenterologists and surgeons to uniformly adopt the practice of separately submitting and appropriately labeling biopsy material from the right and left colon, whether for evaluation of diarrhea or classification of polyps, because the range of normal histologic appearance differs significantly (15,20,22) and neoplastic sequence and progression varies within the right and left colon (19,28,99).

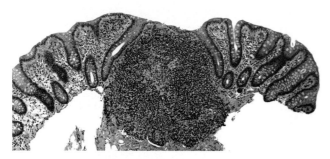

Figure 25.4 Colonic lymphoid aggregate. This lymphoid aggregate splays the adjacent crypts, which appear in a diagonal or near horizontal axis (rather than vertical), and mimics basal lymphoplasmacytosis at the crypt/lymphoid aggregate margin, resembling minor architectural disarray. Goblet cells are absent in the crypt epithelium adjacent to the follicle, while retained on the opposite side of the crypt. These normal features of colonic lymphoid aggregates should not be misinterpreted as architectural distortion indicative of chronic mucosal injury (i.e., inflammatory bowel disease) (see Table 25.2). These aggregates may contain well-formed germinal centers and appear as small polyps endoscopically.

TABLE 25.1
COMMON ARTIFACTS AND VARIANTS: A GUIDE TO EVALUATION AND INTERPRETATION

Histologic Feature:	Common Misinterpretation	Keys to Accurate Interpretation
Mucosa with regular eosinophilic subnuclear material	Collagenous colitis *Accurate Interpretation:* **Normal colon, tangentially sectioned.**	Assess for other features of microscopic colitis.[1] Tangential sectioning of the surface epithelium results in the cytoplasm of adjacent enterocytes appearing below the basally aligned nuclei of "in plane" enterocytes. Levels or a trichrome stain.

Normal colon—histologic features seen in association with adjacent lymphoid aggregates or follicles:

Focally increased surface intraepithelial lymphocytes with otherwise normal architecture.	Lymphocytic colitis *Accurate Interpretation:* **Normal colon**	Assess for other features of the microscopic colitides.[1] Level through the biopsy material to locate the adjacent lymphoid aggregate or lymphoid follicle.
Focal "architectural distortion" in association with numerous lamina propria mononuclear cells. Other biopsy fragments appear normal.	Nonspecific colitis IBD: ulcerative colitis (UC), indeterminate colitis (IDC), Crohn's disease *Accurate Interpretation:* **Normal colon**	Assess for other features of chronic mucosal injury.[2] Level through the biopsy material to locate the adjacent lymphoid aggregate or lymphoid follicle.

Normal colon – histologic features mimicking chronic colitis (IBD).

Biopsy contains horizontal and unusually oriented crypts.	IBD (either UC or IDC). *Accurate Interpretation:* **Normal colon**	Biopsy material evulsed without the muscularis mucosae frequently contains unusually oriented crypts. Assess crypt morphology only in areas in which the muscularis mucosae is present, "tethering" the crypts. Examine other tissue fragments; levels when necessary. Assess for other features of chronic mucosal injury.[2]
Right (or ascending) colon biopsy with numerous lamina propria mononuclear cells	Nonspecific colitis IBD (either UC or IDC) *Accurate Interpretation:* **Normal proximal (right) colon**	Ensure site of biopsy Determine extent of mononuclear expansion, if any. The right colon contains significantly more lamina propria inflammatory cells than the left colon. Assess for other features of chronic mucosal injury.[2]
Deeply eosinophilic granular cells at the base of crypts in the left colon (Paneth cells?) indicating chronic mucosal injury	Nonspecific colitis UC, IDC, or Crohn's *Accurate Interpretation:* **Normal colon**	Assess for other features of chronic mucosal injury.[2] Endocrine cells have apical (luminal) nuclei and fine basal granules and are normal throughout the colon. Paneth cells have basal nuclei; coarse luminal granules are normal in the right colon and pathologic in the left.
Bifurcated crypts in sigmoid colon and/or rectum, without other findings	Inactive IBD *Accurate Interpretation:* **Normal colon or rectum**	One to two bifurcated crypts within the sigmoid colon or rectum is acceptable. Assess for other features of chronic mucosal injury.[2]

Normal colon – histologic features commonly encountered resulting from bowel preparation effects:

Widely spaced crypts, without other findings	Edema Nonspecific colitis *Accurate Interpretation:* **Normal colon**	Water content/edema is not a reproducible finding. Review clinical history for type of bowel preparation, sodium phosphate enemas frequently cause edema. Ensure biopsy fragment contains muscularis mucosa. If other features suggest (i.e., lamina propria pallor [reduced mononuclear cells] and crypt distortion), consider treated IBD.
Basal and/or surface epithelial apoptosis with or without reactive appearing surface enterocytes.	Resolving acute self-limited colitis Antibiotic associated colitis *Accurate Interpretation:* **Normal colon**	Review the clinical history to determine bowel preparation used (oral sodium phosphate frequently causes basal apoptosis, while sodium phosphate enemas may cause surface or basal apoptosis bowel preparation effect). Alert clinical colleagues that sodium phosphate causes bowel preparation effect and is ill advised in the evaluation of diarrhea or GVHD patients.

(*GVHD*, graft-versus-host disease; *IBD*, inflammatory bowel disease; *IDC*, indeterminate colitis; *UC*, ulcerative colitis)

1. Histologic features of microscopic colitis: (a) increased intraepithelial lymphocytes; (b) accompanying damage to surface epithelium (reactive appearance, epithelial sloughing); (c) superficially dense mononuclear inflammatory infiltrate; and with or without (d) thickening or irregularity of the subepithelial basement membrane collagen table (usually entraps superficial capillaries).

2. Histologic features of chronic mucosal injury (chronic colitis, also known as inflammatory bowel disease, or IBD): (a) mononuclear expansion of lamina propria, displacing crypts and resulting in (b) basal plasmacytosis; (c) crypt architectural distortion (bifurcated or irregularly oriented crypts; crypt "dropout"); and (d) Paneth cell (left colon only) or pyloric metaplasia.

TABLE 25.2

PREDOMINANT IMMUNOHISTOCHEMICAL AND HISTOCHEMICAL STAINING PATTERNS OF MANY OF THE NORMAL CELL TYPES PRESENT IN THE HUMAN COLON (51,83–123)

Cell Type	Immunohistochemical Profile		Histochemical Stain
	Positive	**Negative**	
Colonic enterocyte	CK20, pCEA, mCEA, villin, cdx2, AE1/AE3	CK7, EGFR (extremely low expression)	AB2.5–patchy apical blush
Goblet cell (S, surface; C, crypts)	MUC1 (S/C), MUC2 (S/C), MUC3 (S), MUC4 (S/C), MUC5B (C), MUC11 (S/C), MUC12 (S/C)	MUC3 (C) MUC5A (S/C) MUC5B (S)	+AB2.5, mucicarmine, PAS, PAS-D
Enteroendocrine cell	Chromo-A, Chromo-B, synaptophysin, NSE, specific peptides; AE1/AE3	—	Grimelius
Paneth's cell	HL-5, HL-6 (R); AE1/AE3	—	Autofluorescent with eosin
M cell	No known definitive differentiating stains	—	No known definitive differentiating stains
Intraepithelial lymphocytes (surface)	CD3 TCRαβ, CD3 TCRγδ	CD10, CD43, CD138	—
Intraepithelial lymphocytes (M cell)	CD3, CD45 RO, CD45 RA (rare), CD20 (rare)	CD138	—
Lymphoid aggregate (follicle center)	CD 19, CD20, CD10, CD68, occasional CD20, occasional S-100, scattered CD45 RO/CD3	Bcl-2	—
Lymphoid aggregate (periphery/paracortex)	CD3, CD5, CD20 (rare), S-100 (IDC, occasional)	CD138	—
LP plasma cells	CD79a, CD138	CD20, CD3, CD123	—
LP lymphocytes	CD3 (CD4+/CD8+ varying ratio) CD5 (occasional)	Keratin, S100,	—
Eosinophils	CD15	—	Autofluorescent with eosin
Mast cells	Tryptase, CD117 (c-kit)	CD34	Giemsa, toluidine blue
Macrophages	CD68, HAM56, MAC387, lysozyme, α1α-trypsin	LCA, keratin	Iron (hemosiderin and anthracene pigment of melanosis coli)
Dendritic macrophages	CD11b (subepithelial dome), CD123	SMA-α, keratin	
Muciphages	CD68, HAM56	—	AB2.5; PAS-D
Pericrypt myofibroblasts	Vimentin, HHF35, SMMHC, SMA-α	Desmin	MT–mixed blue and red
Subepithelial myofibroblasts	Vimentin, SMA-α	Desmin	MT–mixed blue and red
Basement membrane	Collagen IV, tenascin (minimal)	Tenascin (thick)	MT–blue; saffron–deep red; eosin–autofluorescence
Muscularis mucosa	Vimentin, HHF35, SMA-α, desmin	—	MT–red
Arterioles, capillaries, veins	*Luminal:* CD31, CD34, vimentin, vWF, factor XIII *Wall:* SMA-α	SMA-α, HHF-35	MT–red; elastin
Lymphatic vessels	CD34, vimentin, D2-40 (R)®	vWF	MT–red
Enteric glia and ganglia	Synaptophysin, PDGFR-α(R), NSE	SMA-α	—
Schwann cells	S-100, vimentin	SMA-α	—
Interstitial cells of Cajal	CD34, CD117 (c-kit)	S-100, CD31	—
Submucosal adipose	S-100	—	Oil red O
SM lymphocytes	CD3, scattered CD138 plasma cells	—	—
Muscularis propria	SMA-α, desmin, vimentin	—	MT–deep red
Serosal mesothelium	Calretinin, vimentin, AE1/AE3, CK7	pCEA	—

(—, no information; *AB2.5*, Alcian blue 2.5; *AE1/AE3*, pan-cytokeratin; *C*, crypts; *Chromo-A*, chromogranin A; *Chromo-B*, chromogranin B; *CK20*, cytokeratin 20; *DGFR*, epidermal growth factor; *IDC*, interdigitating dendritic cells; *LCA*, leukocyte common antigen; *LP*, lamina propria; *mCEA*, monoclonal carcinoembryonic antigen; *MT*, Masson's trichrome; *MUC*, mucin gene; *NSE*, neuron specific enolase; *PAS*, periodic acid-Schiff; *PAS-D*, periodic acid-Schiff with diastase digestion; *pCEA*, polyclonal carcinoembryonic antigen; *PDGFRa*, platelet-derived growth factor receptor alpha; *R*, research; *S*, surface; *SM*, submucosa; *SMMHC*, smooth muscle myosin heavy chain; *vWF*, von Willebrand factor)

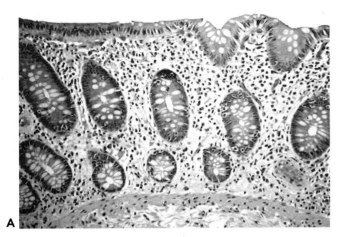
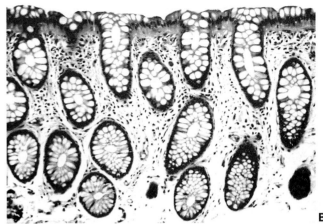

Figure 25.6 Normal mucosa from the cecum (A) and rectum (B). **A.** The mucosa in the cecum has more absorptive cells and fewer goblet cells compared to the rectum. The lamina propria is more cellular, with greater density of plasma cells, eosinophils, and lymphoid aggregates in the cecum as compared to the rectum. Paneth's cells are normally present, residing at the base of the crypts. **B.** The rectal mucosa has a higher ratio of goblet cells to absorptive cells, with a less dense lamina propria and more easily identified muciphages. Paneth's cells are not normally seen within the rectum.

Reflecting a dominant function in absorption and antigen processing, the right colon displays a higher colonocyte (absorptive enterocyte + M cell) to goblet cell (roughly 5:1) ratio as compared to the left colon (Figure 25.6). Proceeding distally, an increase in goblet cells are apparent, with a ratio of 3 or 4:1 (colonocyte:goblet cell), facilitating increased formation of gel-type mucin in the descending and sigmoid colon necessary for consolidation and transit of the increasingly formed fecal matter (15,26,27,124). Paneth cells are normally present at the base of crypts within the midgut-derived right colon but are indicative of metaplasia secondary to chronic mucosal injury after the distal one-third of the transverse colon (Figure 25.6).

Surface intraepithelial lymphocytes are seen in greater concentrations in the right colon than the left and can be marked overlying lymphoid aggregates (20,22,125–127). Similarly, lamina propria mononuclear cell density is also greater in the right colon than the left (descending and sigmoid colon), as are organized lymphoid aggregates, possibly related to the higher concentration of commensal microorganisms and resultant antigen sampling activities (20,22). As goblet cell concentration and mucin increases, lamina propria macrophages, specifically scavenging mucin (muciphages) are observed with an increasing gradient proceeding distally. In the sigmoid colon and rectum, most gastrointestinal pathologists will accept a few bifurcated crypts as being within the range of normal (20), although this has not been systematically studied nor reported.

Epithelium

The colonic mucosa is composed of continuous, polarized surface and crypt epithelium forming millions of crypts (26,128) invested in basement membrane, surrounded by a variably cellular and vascular lamina propria (20,125,127), and with a deep boundary formed by the muscularis mucosae.

The colonic mucosal microarchitecture shows remarkable stability along both the AP and radial axes, despite its high turnover rate and variety of highly specialized cell types (129,130). Albeit based upon circumstantial evidence, it is generally accepted that mucosal renewal is attributed to colonic epithelial stem cells located and maintained within a mesenchymal niche, situated near the base of the intestinal crypts (13,31,32,128,129,131–134). Multipotent stem cells slowly divide, under influence of reciprocal signaling by mesenchymal and other cells, giving rise to a transient population of progenitor cells that rapidly divide and undergo a well-controlled maturation process while migrating toward the lumen (31,128,134). The granule-containing epithelial cell types appear to ignore the rule of luminal progression during maturation, with Paneth's cells (of the right colon) migrating to the crypt base (13,64,135,136) and enteroendocrine cells (throughout the colon) homing to the mid- and deeper regions of the crypts (Figure 25.7) (13,15,137).

During migration, dividing transit cells commit and differentiate to one of five distinct epithelial cell types: absorptive colonocyte, mucus-secreting goblet cell, enteroendocrine cell, Paneth's cell, or M cell. At any given time, 75 to 80% of all colonocytes are associated with the crypts, and only 10 to 15% of colonocytes form the surface epithelium (intercrypt table) (126,130).

Absorptive Colonocytes

Absorptive colonocytes compose the majority of the surface epithelium (80,82,138). The luminal surface is characterized by rigid, tightly packed apical microvilli, (13,130), the tips of which contain integral membrane mucinlike glycoproteins that form a continuous, filamentous brush border glycocalyx (139) that is visible as a striate luminal border. Absorptive

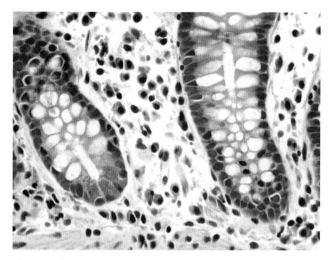

Figure 25.7 Normal right colon with Paneth's cells and an endocrine cell. Within the crypt on the left are three Paneth's cells at the base of the crypt. Note the basal nucleus and coarse, luminal-facing granules that empty into the crypt lumen. Within the crypt on the right is an endocrine cell at the base of the crypt. The endocrine cell is smaller, has a luminal nucleus and fine, basally facing granules, that empty into the pericrypt myofibroblast sheath and adjacent vasculature.

colonocyte cytoplasm is lightly eosinophilic, with small apical vesicles containing mucin (of different composition than goblet cell mucin) positioned for luminal release (21,63, 89,99). The apical poles of columnar cells fan out over goblet cells such that only the small apexes of goblet cells contact the lumen (130). Basally aligned colonocyte nuclei are oval, uniformly sized, and aligned with the long axis parallel to the long axes of the cells, with smooth nuclear contours and frequently observed nucleoli.

Goblet Cells
Goblet cells are dispersed throughout the surface epithelium and crypts and are distinguished by their "wine goblet shape," which results from a large number of mucous granules in the apical pole. Mucin composition varies regionally along the length of the colon due to differential synthesis of the several known secreted and membrane-bound mucins (15). This variation is reflected in the differential histochemical staining patterns commonly observed (99,140,141). Goblet cell cytoplasm is relatively clear with standard hematoxylin and eosin (H&E) stains; however, mucin granules become distinct with mucicarmine, Alcian blue pH 2.5, and periodic acid-Schiff stains (15). Goblet cell nuclei, when compared to adjacent absorptive colonocytes, appear hyperchromatic, dense, and irregular (130).

Endocrine Cells
Endocrine cells within the gut epithelium represent the largest population of hormone-producing cells in the body (128,137,142,143), comprising approximately 1% of the individual cells lining the intestinal lumen, predominantly located in the crypts and, rarely, scattered within the lamina

propria (13,15,28,122,130,142,146–147). More than 30 peptide hormone genes are known to be expressed throughout the digestive tract, in a regionally and spatially distinct pattern (142,148). Enteroendocrine cells contain basally oriented, small, but distinct, deeply eosinophilic granules (137,142). The round, smoothly contoured nuclei of enteroendocrine cells are pushed lumenally, with opposite polarity to the other epithelial cell types (Figure 25.7).

Enteroendocrine cells may be further identified by their histochemical silver staining properties and may also be identified immunohistochemically with varying immunoreactivity to chromogranin A, synaptophysin, neuron-specific enolase, and specific antibodies to the putative peptide hormone of the cell or cell proliferation (i.e., carcinoid tumor) (Table 25.1).

Paneth's Cells
Paneth's cells disregard the rule of luminal migration and are normally encountered at the base of the crypts, within the midgut-derived right colon (13,65,114,128,135). These pyramidal-shaped cells have basally aligned oval nuclei and apical coarse, densely eosinophilic cytoplasmic granules (Figure 25.7) (13,65). Granule and cellular contents include: α-defensins, β-defensins, NOD2, lysozyme, phospholipase A2, secretory leukocyte inhibitor, monomer IgA, TNF-α, heavy metal ions, zinc binding protein, trypsin and trypsinogen, EGF, osteopontin, FAS ligand (CD95L), CD44v6, CD15, REG protein, and numerous others (65,128,135,149,150). The diverse Paneth's cell contents reflect their significant role in innate immunity. Additionally putative roles in regulation of cell matrix interactions, apoptosis, and cellular immunity, as well as stem-cell niche maintenance, have been proposed (65,128,135,149,151).

In addition to characteristic granule staining with H&E stains, granules are conspicuously stained by periodic acid-Schiff, and phloxine-tartrazine (65); and, interestingly, Paneth's cell autofluorescence is elicited by eosin stain (Table 25.2) (114).

M Cells and Follicle-Associated Epithelium
Membranous (M) cells are distinctive epithelial cells that occur in the dome region of organized lymphoid follicles and associated with both the immunologic cells and variants of absorptive colonocytes (the follicle associated epithelium) unique to the dome region (59,126,128,152-154). Estimates of M cells in human colon vary widely, reported from "rare" to approximately 10% of surface epithelial cells (126,153–156). Light microscopy has insufficient magnification to distinguish the unique features of M cells (reduced numbers of an irregular microvilli, apical microfolds, absence of thick filamentous brush border glycocalyx, and the presence of an unusual subdomain of the basolateral membrane that amplifies the cell surface and forms an intraepithelial pocket) visible with electron microscopy. The M cell intraepithelial pocket provides a

docking site for special populations of intraepithelial B and T lymphocytes, along with a small number of macrophages; and immediately overlies the dome region of lymphoid follicles (126,152–154). These unique morphologic features provide local, functional openings in the epithelial barrier through which M cells sample the contents of the lumen and transfer antigents to antigen-presenting cells via a specialized method of transcytosis (67,71,152,155). The follicle associated crypts contains few or no goblet cells, enteroendocrine cells or Paneth cells (153,155). These closely apposed columnar enterocytes may mimic features of low grade cytologic dysplasia (adenoma), particularly with distortion of the crypt architecture generally produced by the adjacent lymphoid aggregate.

Intraepithelial Inflammatory Cells

Intraepithelial lymphocytes (IELs) occur in two compartments: within the paracellular spaces of the absorptive epithelium and in highest density associated with lymphoid aggregates within M-cell pockets (Figure 25.8) (125,127,157–159). The former are predominantly CD3+, CD8+, TCR-$\alpha\beta$+ suppressor T cells, with between 15 and 40% TCR-$\gamma\delta$+ T cells, while the latter are mixture of CD3+/CD45RO+ activated memory, some CD45RA+ naive T cells, and IgM-secreting B cells (86,127,160–162). Intraepithelial lymphocytes are the first members of the immune system to encounter dietary antigens and commensal and pathologic microorganisms, and they likely play an integral role in oral tolerance (58,158,161, 163–165). The IELs home toward their intraepithelial destination, migrating along various chemokine gradients produced by adjacent epithelial, inflammatory, and mesenchymal cells (59,166).

Nuclear molding and indistinct cytoplasmic contours are characteristic of IELs as they extend through the basement membrane to occupy paracellular spaces (Figure 25.8). Retention of the classic lymphocyte round nucleus and thin rim of cytoplasm is more common in IELs overlying aggregates. Normal IEL density ranges from 1 to 5 lymphocytes per 100 colonocytes, except in follicle-associated epithelium, where M-cell associated IELs are abundant (162). The number of IELs decreases from the ascending colon to rectum, with highest concentration in the lymphoid aggregate and commensal bacteria-rich cecum (125,126). It is imperative to ascertain the site of each colon biopsy to avoid misinterpretation of normal IEL density in right colon biopsies as lymphocytic colitis (Table 25.2). Generally, 20 or greater lymphocytes per 100 colonocytes are considered pathologic (59,125,127,168).

Intraepithelial eosinophils may occasionally be seen in the normal colon, although at much lower numbers than lymphocytes (168–170).

Stem and Dividing Transit Cells

It is estimated that between four and six stem cells are present per crypt, with some dividing transit cells apparently able to be "recruited" to serve as stem cells following injury with stem cell loss (31). These proliferative and undifferentiated cells are morphologically indistinct; however, they appear to have a large nucleus with diffuse chromatin and scant cytoplasm with few small organelles (13,128). Mitotic activity is frequently encountered in the basal one-fifth of the crypt, and apoptosis may also be seen (129,131,134).

Apoptosis

The epithelial cells of the colon have remarkably short life spans (Table 25.3), during which they mature, migrate, and function (13,21,33,47,131,134,171). Programmed cell

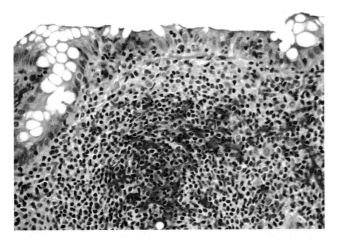

Figure 25.8 Intraepithelial lymphocytes (IELs) overlying a lymphoid follicle. Large numbers of IELs are typically seen overlying lymphoid aggregates. This should not be misinterpreted as lymphocytic colitis.

TABLE 25.3

THE LIFE SPAN OF THE VARIOUS COLON EPITHELIAL CELLS AND NUMBER OF REPLACEMENTS PER AVERAGE HUMAN LIFE SPAN VARY BETWEEN CELL TYPES. DESPITE THE HIGH RATE OF TURNOVER, PRESERVATION OF GENETIC INFORMATION IS THE RULE RATHER THAN THE EXCEPTION

Cell Type	Life Span	Number of Replacements/Life
Absorptive Colonocyte	4–8 days	3285–6570
Goblet Cell	3–4 days	6570–8760
Enteroendocrine Cell	10–15 days	1750–2630
Paneth Cell	20 days	1300
M Cell	Unknown	Unknown
Stem Cell Lineage/Niche	8.2 years	9–10

death (apoptosis), is the conclusion of the normal process of colonocyte turnover, recognizable histologically by identification of apoptotic bodies and debris predominantly in the surface epithelium (Figure 25.9), and less frequently within the colonic crypts. Apoptotic bodies consist of vacuoles containing pyknotic nuclear debris, are surrounded by free space, and generally are at the basal portion of the epithelium or immediately subjacent to the basement membrane (23,132,134,172–180). Lamina propria inflammatory cells similarly undergo apoptosis; however, this is frequently overlooked histologically (174,181,182). Sodium phosphate bowel preparations transiently increase the rate of apoptosis (see Bowel Preparation, below); similar effects are seen with other physical and chemical agents. Increased apoptosis (both surface and/or crypt) may also be seen in several disease states, including graft-versus-host disease, autoimmune enteropathies, systemic autoimmune disorders, and with certain medications (70,183,184). Altered apoptosis (increased, decreased, and abnormal localization) is seen in neoplastic progression (185).

Basement Membrane

The basement membrane complex anchors the various epithelial cells to the underlying myofibroblast network and lamina propria. This fenestrated extracellular support matrix is produced collaboratively by epithelial and mesenchymal cells (98,126,129,186). Basement membrane composition varies, regulated by several factors produced by the epithelium, myofibroblasts, and lamina propria cells (126,129,186,187). In addition to allowing intraepithelial lymphocytes to traverse the basement membrane, the fenestrations allow epithelial, mesenchymal, and dendritic cell processes to sample and/or present antigens and have functional implications in water and ion transport (21,32,129).

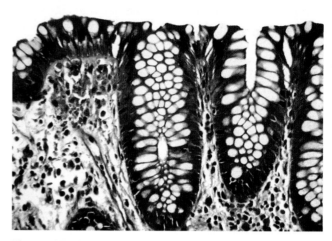

Figure 25.10 Normal basement membrane. The normal basement membrane is 3 to 5 μm thick and has a crisp, delicate, and regular lower border; it blends into the crypt sheath imperceptibly (trichrome stain).

In well-oriented sections, the normal basement membrane is between 3 μm and 5 μm thick, regular, and stains with connective tissue stains (Masson's trichrome, saffron, eosin von Gieson elastin) (Figure 25.10) (187,188). Similar to Paneth's cells, autofluorescence is elicited with eosin stain (115). Basement membrane thickness greater than 10 mm is considered pathologic, as is irregularity of the basement membrane, particularly entrapping superficial lamina propria capillaries (115, 187).

Lamina Propria

The lamina propria invests the colonic crypts, extending from the fenestrated basement membrane complex to the muscularis mucosae. The various lamina propria inflammatory and mesenchymal cells are organized within extracellular matrix, each performing integral immunologic, metabolic, proliferative, and motility functions.

Lamina Propria Inflammatory Cells

As dictated by the wide array of immunologic functions performed by the colonic mucosa, the lamina propria houses localized antigen-sampling and processing factories, with over 30,000 discrete lymphoid aggregates, concentrated within the blind-ended cecum and distributed along the length of the colon (189,190). In addition to lymphoid aggregates, the normal colon contains mature B lymphocytes, plasma cells, T lymphocytes [helper, suppressor, and lymphokine-activated killer (LAK) cells, but unlikely natural killer (NK) cells], eosinophils, mast cells, and macrophages, in combination filling between 30 and 50% of the "free" lamina propria space (22). Normally, there is a decreasing inflammatory cell gradient from lumen to

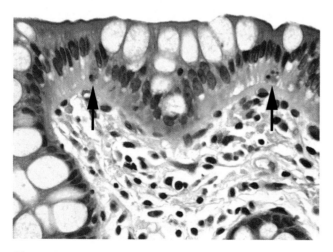

Figure 25.9 Apoptosis. Two apoptotic bodies are seen within the surface epithelium (*arrows*).

muscularis mucosae, in which the lamina propria loose connective tissue is obscured within the superficial aspect of the lamina propria but becomes visible approaching the muscularis mucosa (191). The predominant cell type of the lamina propria is the IgA-secreting plasma cell, with much smaller proportions of IgM-, IgE-, and IgG-secreting plasma cells also present (181,192). Secreted IgA and IgM are transported luminally, providing humoral immune protection (138,181,192). The distinct "cartwheel" nucleus, perinuclear Golgi zone, and amphophilic cytoplasm characteristic of plasma cells observed in other tissues are retained in colonic plasma cells. Of the remaining lamina propria lymphocytes, more than 90% of the lymphocytes were CD3+ T cells, with fewer than 50% also CD8+ (126,127,159). There are also CD 20-positive B lymphocytes present within and adjacent to lymphoid follicles (71,76,78,138,193).

Myeloid cells that normally reside in the lamina propria include eosinophils and mast cells. In the normal colon, the number of eosinophils is highly variable, dependent upon both the region of colon sampled (168–172,194) and the geographic residence of the patient (195). A range of normal eosinophil counts in the lamina propria has been reported as 0 to 8 per high-power field (hpf); however, the eosinophil concentration should be interpreted on the basis of the "company it keeps" (i.e., other features of colitis versus otherwise normal) (Rodger C. Haggitt, MD, personal communication). Higher mean eosinophil concentration is seen in biopsies of patients from the southern United States, compared to the northern United States, with a rather extreme degree of variability (195). Although eosinophils are increased in parasitic and allergic disease, collagenous colitis, ulcerative colitis, Crohn's disease, and other pathologic conditions, consideration of the geographic residence and site of biopsy are integral prior to considering increased eosinophils (as an isolated histologic finding) to be pathologic (170,195). Mast cells, or tissue based basophils, are less numerous than eosinophils, and their density appears to be increased in the ileocecal region compared with other sites of the colon (196,197). Mast cells are difficult to distinguish with routine H&E, but stain well with Giemsa, toluidine blue, tryptase, and CD117 (c-kit) (Figure 25.11, Table 25.2) (194). Neutrophils are not normally seen in any significant number within the lamina propria, although they may be seen in areas of hemorrhage and within blood vessels.

Macrophages are commonly seen scattered throughout the lamina propria and are occasionally concentrated at the basal aspect of the crypts (70,198–201) (Figure 25.12). While macrophages are generally difficult to see with H&E stains, visualization may be enhanced by specific histochemical stains that detect the variety of materials they scavenge and store: apoptotic debris, microbes, lipofuscin, cholesterol esters, gangliosides, mucolipids,

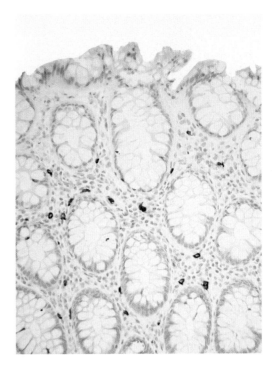

Figure 25.11 Mucosal mast cells. Although difficult to discern on H&E-stained sections, mucosal mast cells are easily identified with CD117. Mucosal mast cells serve well as an internal control when evaluating CD117 stains of gastrointestinal tract mesenchymal tumors. (Anti-CD117 stain.)

glycogen, mucopolysaccharides, and others (Figure 25.12, Table 25.2) (199,200). Muciphages are the most commonly recognized macrophages, ingesting mucin exuded from adjacent goblet cells (and to a lesser extent enterocytes) that crosses the basement membrane. These normal constituents of the lamina propria have increased concentration within the left colon, in keeping with the increased number of goblet cells present in this location. Distention of the lamina propria with the appearance of replacement of other lamina propria inflammatory cells is rarely normal and may indicate bacterial or fungal ingestion/infection (e.g., *Tropheryma whippelii*, *Mycobacterium avium-intracellulare* complex, *Histoplasma capsulatum*, and others) or various metabolic storage disorders, requiring use of histochemical, PCR, or electron microscopic methodologies as well as further laboratory evaluation (97,105,202–205).

Plasmacytoid dendritic cells are scattered throughout the lamina propria, while stellate dendritic cells are concentrated in the subepithelial dome space associated with lymphoid follicles (78,138,206,207). These are histologically indistinct and frequently require immunohistochemistry for definitive identification (Table 25.2) (70,71,76,138). The former have recently been implicated in allergic and autoimmune disorders (88), while the latter are integral in antigen presentation (70,73,208).

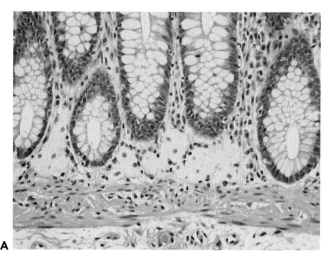
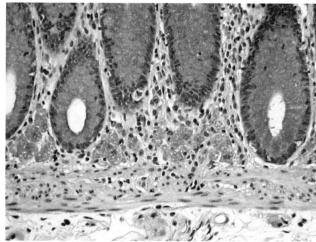

Figure 25.12 Lamina propria muciphages. **A.** These pale macrophages at the base of the mucosa are stuffed with mucins. This finding is not infrequent and does not generally correlate with disease. **B.** The same area stained with Alcian blue pH2.5; the muciphages show strong cytoplasmic staining. Similar findings are seen with PAS with diastase digestion. Of note, bacteria-laden macrophages in Whipple's disease are generally negative when stained with Alcian blue pH 2.5 but densely stain with PAS with diastase.

Myofibroblasts (Pericrypt Myofibroblast Sheath and Lamina Propria Myofibroblasts)

The lamina propria contains two distinct populations of myofibroblasts: the pericrypt myofibroblast sheath and the subepithelial myofibroblast (SEM) syncytia. Interacting closely with the epithelium, lamina propria inflammatory cells, and the muscularis mucosa, myofibroblasts function in absorption, ion and mucin secretion, immune regulation, and differentiation (maintenance of stem cell niche) (521,124,209). The rim of fusiform cells organized in close apposition to each colonic crypt was originally designated the pericryptal fibroblastic sheath (Figure 25.13) (186,209). This specialized population of mesenchymal cells is now known to be a syncytium (both anatomically and functionally) of cells that surrounds the crypts and extends into the lamina propria, forming a reticular network within the extracellular matrix, attaching to one another with both gap and adherens junctions (83,92,186, 209,210), and displaying distinct immunophenotypes (Table 25.2).

In the region of the crypts, the myofibroblasts are oval and scaphoid in appearance and appear to overlap like shingles on a roof. The SEMs exist in two distinct morphological states: (a) the activated myofibroblast and (b) the stellate transformed myofibroblast, similar in appearance to macrophage dendritic cells (186,209). Myofibroblasts often are surrounded by an incomplete basal lamina and embedded in a subepithelial sheet of reticular fibers that also contains fenestrae or foramina through which lymphocytes and macrophages traverse. Gap junctions couple some myofibroblasts to the tissue smooth muscle, and the cells are commonly in close apposition to

varicosities of nerve fibers; however, it is has not been determined whether the interstitial cell of Cajal network is physically connected to the SEM network (186,209,211).

Vasculature and Lymphatics

Vasculature is limited to capillaries and high endothelial venules scattered throughout lamina propria and to

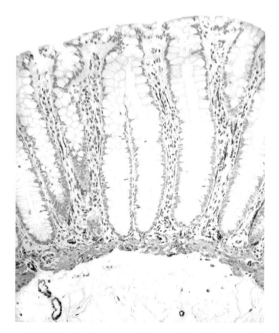

Figure 25.13 Lamina propria myofibroblasts, antimuscle-specific actin (MSA) stain. This stain for muscle-specific actin highlights the pericryptal myofibroblast sheath, muscularis mucosae, and submucosal blood vessels.

lymphatic channels immediately superficial to the muscularis mucosa (212,213). Capillaries are composed of a circumferential endothelial lining and may contain red blood cells as well as inflammatory cells. Irregularly shaped, distorted, and engorged capillaries frequently indicate prolapse of the mucosa. In addition to provision of oxygen and nutrients to mucosal cells, vascular adhesion molecules participate in appropriate "homing" of circulating lymphocytes to their appropriate colonic microenvironment. Lymphatic tributaries rarely initiate within the lamina propria; however, when present, they appear to have thinner walls and cross the muscularis mucosae to join the readily observed submucosal lymphatics (213–215). Definitive differentiation between capillaries and lymphatics requires immunohistochemical analysis (Table 25.2) (84,94,100,216).

Muscularis Mucosae

Forming the deep limiting boundary of the lamina propria is a thin layer of smooth muscle, the muscularis mucosae. This muscle layer is physically tethered to the mucosa, with occasional smooth muscle cells extending into the lamina propria or coalescing with the pericryptal myofibroblast sheath. The muscularis mucosae receives innervation via the submucosal plexus (92,217,218). Because the colonic glands are tethered to the muscularis mucosa, this structure is valuable in evaluating crypt architecture in endoscopic biopsies. Biopsies that do not contain muscularis mucosae may resemble architectural distortion, with glands adopting horizontal or curved configurations. Careful examination of other biopsy fragments with muscularis mucosae, as well as assessment for other features of mucosal injury (Table 25.1), may allow an accurate diagnosis. The muscularis mucosa is normally traversed by lymphoglandular complexes (Figure 25.5), vascular channels, and neural twiglets and participates in absorptive, secretory, proliferative, and possibly motility functions. Isolated thickening may occur with prolapse of the overlying mucosa and adjacent to diverticular orifices. Clear duplication of the muscularis mucosae is generally considered a feature of chronic mucosal injury.

Submucosa

The submucosa is composed of loosely arranged bundles of smooth muscle, fibroelastic tissue, and adipose, in which the local enteric nervous system, vasculature, and lymphatics are embedded. Lymphatic channels may be conspicuous and dilated immediately beneath the submucosa and do not contain cellular elements (213,214,216). Sparse inflammatory cells (relative to the dense "physiologic" inflammation of the mucosa) are scattered throughout, occasionally organized as submucosal lymphoid aggregates. The submucosa provides a flexible matrix—allowing the mucosa to glide and move freely over the rigid muscularis mucosae during peristalsis.

Submucosal smooth muscle consists of loosely woven fascicles of individual smooth muscle cells, forming small bundles. These smooth muscle collections are closely apposed to interstitial cells of Cajal, which in turn are immediately adjacent to nerve varicosities—forming the neuroeffector junctions that receive, transmit, and integrate central, parasympathetic, and sympathetic nervous system commands (211,219,220). The two submucosal neural plexuses are the submucosal plexus of Meissner (located immediately beneath the muscularis mucosae) and Henle's deep submucosal plexus (lying on the inner aspect of the muscularis propria). Neural plexuses are composed of neurons, glial cells, and stromal elements (221–223). Ganglion cells are unique in their histologic appearance with round or oval nuclei, a prominent (often eosinophilic) nucleolus, and ample basophilic cytoplasm stippled with Nissl substance (Figure 25.14). Ganglion cells characteristically cluster together and may mimic giant cells, epithelioid cells, or granulomas. Nerve axons are fibrillar and distinguishing these axons from fibroblasts or their elastofibrotic products may require the use of histochemical or immunohistochemical stains (Figure 25.14B, Table 25.2) (43,112,220,221,223,224).

Interstitial cells of Cajal (ICCs) are modified myofibroblasts. Histologic features evident with routine H&E stain include a fusiform cell body and large oval nucleus; silver stain or immunohistochemical evaluation will reveal two or more dendritic processes, connecting ICCs to one another, to ganglion cells, or to adjacent smooth muscle (210,220,225–227). These intriguing cells are thought to play an important role in the control of gut motor activity (220,228,229). The normal ICC density within the submucosa is substantially less than that seen surrounding the myenteric plexus (see below) (220,228–230). Arterioles (branches from the superior and inferior mesenteric arteries), venules, and lymphatics are present throughout the submucosa (Figure 25.15). These vessels in histologic sections are frequently distended by red blood cells and appear tortuous, with several cross sections of a single arteriole seen adjacent to one another within one field of section.

The amount of adipose within the submucosa varies substantially between the right and left colon and among patients. The ileocecal valve and cecum submucosa may appear particularly expanded by mature adipocytes, resembling a lipoma. However, in the absence of the submucosal adipose forming a discrete, lobulated mass, this may be considered within the range of normal.

Muscularis Externa, Subserosal Zone, and Serosa

The muscularis propria or external smooth muscle layers of the colon consist of an inner circular layer and an outer

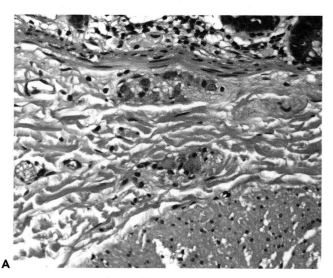

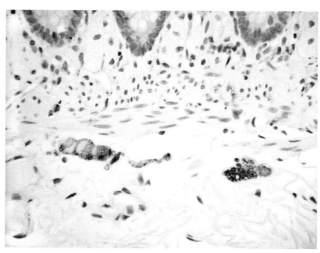

Figure 25.14 Ganglion cells of Meissner's plexus. **A.** Submucosal nerve twigs and clusters of ganglion cells comprising Meissner's plexus. (H&E stain, x20). **B.** Same area stained with S-100 (hematoxylin counter stain), highlighting the Schwann cells. The ganglion cells on the left are conspicuously negative with S-100 (also x20).

longitudinal layer (Figure 25.16) (231,232). Structural variations of the muscularis propria have been identified, which may reflect different motility and storage functions of various regions of the colon (225,226). Auerbach's plexus lies between the two muscle layers and resembles

Meissner's plexus histologically. The interstitial cells of Cajal, the putative pacemaker cells of the gut that drive peristalsis, can be identified throughout the muscularis propria with immunizations for CD117 and CD34 (Figure 25.17) (111,233,234).

Patients with motility disorders may have decreased numbers of these cells within their bowel walls (231,232). The muscularis is perforated by blood and lymphatic vessels and is encased in a subserosal zone of fibroadipose tissue. Strictly speaking, the serosa is limited to the mesothelial lining and immediately adjacent fibroelastic tissue.

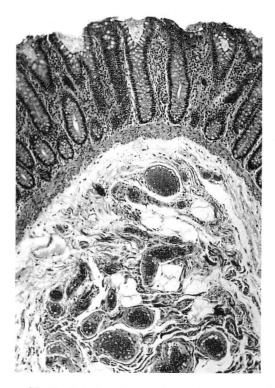

Figure 25.15 Colonic submucosal vasculature. Most of the blood vessels in this section contain erythrocytes.

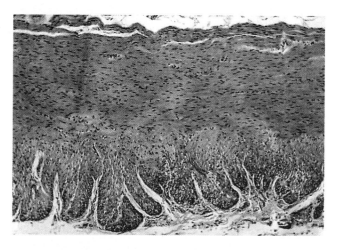

Figure 25.16 Muscularis propria and subserosal tissue. Both layers of the muscularis propria can be seen with the neural tissue of Auerbach's plexus. Below the muscle layers is the fibrovascular adipose tissue of the subserosa.

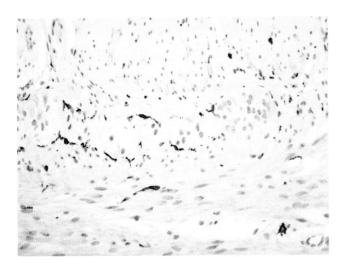

Figure 25.17 Interstitial cells of Cajal (ICC). The CD117 strongly positive, dendritic-appearing cells between the muscle layers and surrounding Auerbach's plexus are the ICCs. These cells are considered to be the pacemaker cell of the gut and perform other functions in gut motility. (Anti-CD117 stain.)

EFFECTS OF PREPARATION AND ARTIFACTS

Bowel Preparation Effects

The most commonly used bowel preparations for colonoscopy and sigmoidoscopy (sodium phosphate enemas, bisacodyl enemas and suppositories, dioctyl sodium sulfosuccinate, soapsuds enemas) can produce abnormalities of the mucosa that may mimic or obscure inflammatory conditions and impart an edematous or hyperemic appearance of the mucosa to the endoscopist (235–237). Histologic features suggesting bowel preparation include: flattening of the absorptive colonocytes to a cuboidal shape, reduction in goblet cell mucus (due to increased mucus secretion), detached surface epithelium leaving an exposed basement membrane, minimal or focal surface epithelial and crypt neutrophilic infiltrate, accentuated extravasation of red blood cells within the lamina propria, and increase in crypt or surface epithelial apoptosis (Figure 25.18). Oral sodium phosphate incites exaggeration of the previously described features of bowel preparation. Endoscopically visible aphthous erosions, erosions, and uncommonly frank ulcers have been reported. Histologically, neutrophilic cryptitis and increased basal apoptosis may be seen in addition to other common features of bowel preparation (Figure 25.19) (235,238,239). This basal apoptosis is histologically identical to low-grade graft-versus-host disease. Hence, oral sodium phosphate bowel preparations should not be used in bone marrow transplant patients. Although bowel preparation histologic changes may not interfere with rendering a polyp diagnosis, subtle inflammatory changes may be overlooked in the midst of

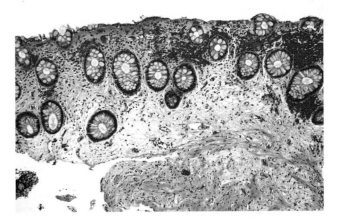

Figure 25.18 Enema effect. There is edema with extravasation and lysis of red blood cells (hemorrhage) within the lamina propria. The surface epithelium is largely denuded. Mucin depletion due to induced goblet cell secretion and increased apoptosis may also be seen.

various bowel preparation changes or alternately misdiagnosed as a pathologic condition. In the evaluation of patients for reasons other than colorectal cancer screening, bowel preparation with polyethylene glycol is suggested, as it appears to incite minimal histologic alterations (240, 241). Nonetheless, polyethylene glycol preparation has also been reported in randomized trials to result in superficial mucus loss, epithelial cell loss, lymphocyte and neutrophil infiltration, and rarely aphthous erosions (242).

Incorrect Tissue Orientation and Tangential Sectioning

Difficulties with proper tissue orientation are most common to endoscopically procured biopsy specimens, owing

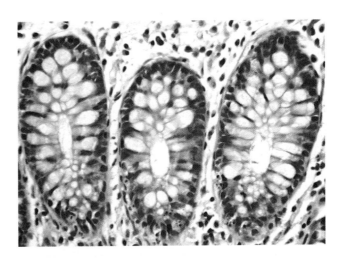

Figure 25.19 Oral sodium phosphate bowel preparation effect. Colonic crypts with apoptotic bodies and neutrophils are secondary to the effects of bowel preparation. Such changes could easily be interpreted as representing infectious colitis or graft-versus-host disease (GVHD) in the right clinical setting.

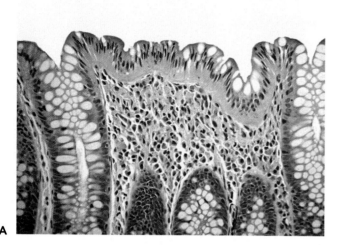
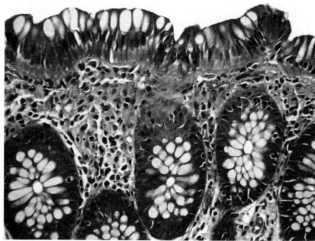

Figure 25.20 Normal colon mimicking collagenous colitis. **A.** This normal mucosa shows blending of the colonocyte cytoplasm with the basement membrane to give the illusion of a thickened subepithelial collagen table. Note that there is no surface damage or colitis present. **B.** This trichrome stained section shows focal thickening in an area where the crypt sheath joins the surface tangentially. Care must be taken when evaluating tangential sections. Again note the lack of colitis or surface damage.

to their small size (sometimes as small as 2 mm). In both endoscopic biopsies and surgical resections, the most accurate interpretation is possible when the tissue is sectioned perpendicular to the plane of the surface epithelium. Evaluation of crypt architecture, inflammatory cell gradient, and thickness and regularity of the subepithelial collagen band may be hindered significantly by tangential sectioning (Table 25.1) (243). The appearance of acini (doughnuts) rather than "test tubes" within the lamina propria is a clear indication of tangential sectioning. Features of chronic mucosal injury may not be sampled in tangential sections that contain only the superficial most aspects of the mucosa. Cytoplasm of adjacent colonocytes in tangentially sectioned tissue may mimic a thickened (but regular) collagen band, risking a misinterpretation of collagenous colitis (Figure 25.20). Tangential sections with exaggerated samples of the basal portions of colonic crypts show cross sections of less mature colonocytes with larger nuclei, less cytoplasm, and without adjacent goblet cells, thus mimicking the features of a tubular adenoma.

Tissue Trauma

Tissue trauma occurs with avulsion of the mucosa during forceps biopsy or in improper handling in the pathology gross room. The former may produce endoscopically visible edema, petechiae, friability, tears, and hemorrhage (241,243), and there may be histologic features of "crush" artifact. Biopsy samples may contain increased cell free space in the lamina propria, resembling edema and extravasation of red blood cells primarily into the luminal portion of the lamina propria. In the absence of other

features of mucosal inflammation (i.e., neutrophilic inflammation), these features should not be considered pathologic. Polyfoam pads may cause triangular artifacts in biopsy material and are not recommended (244). Despite relative fixation, crush artifact may occur with pressure applied to biopsy material with rigid forceps. Use of a plastic pipette with large bore opening (i.e., cutting the tip off of a disposable pipette) to transfer biopsy material to the cassette avoids crush artifact. Crushing of the tissue results in crowding of glands and epithelial cells and is accompanied by stripping of the surface epithelium that then dislodges into the lumen.

Pseudolipomatosis

Pseudolipomatosis is characterized by vacuolated, unlined spaces in the lamina propria and mucosa that resemble loosely arranged adipocytes (Figure 25.21). These lesions are due to air trapping from insufflation of the colon during endoscopy (245).

Electrocautery

Endoscopic removal of polyps with electrocautery ("hot" biopsy, or snare) frequently results in thermodessication of the tissue, compressing crypts together and altering the nuclear features. Characteristically, the crypts are closely apposed, with elongated, pyknotic and distorted nuclei (Figure 25.22). These features may be difficult or impossible to distinguish from a tubular adenoma. Prolonged electrodesiccation may result in loss of both overall architecture and nuclear detail.

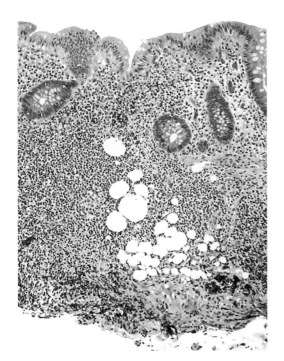

Figure 25.21 Pseudolipomatosis. The clear spaces within this lymphoid aggregate represent air bubbles due to insufflation during endoscopy. This artifact is frequently misinterpreted as adipose tissue/lipoma.

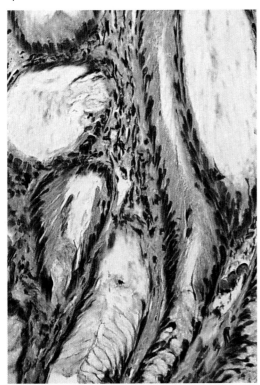

Figure 25.22 Electrodesiccation and compression artifact in the bases of adjacent crypts in normal colonic mucosa produced by an endoscopic electrocautery snare. Affected nuclei are pyknotic and elongated. Colonic crypts distorted by this artifact may be difficult or impossible to differentiate from the tubules of an adenoma.

ACKNOWLEDGMENTS

Dr. Dahl is grateful for the continuing influence of the late Dr. Rodger C. Haggitt in the preparation of this manuscript. Dr. Charles Bevins and Richard Naftalin are thanked for their insight and dialogue.

REFERENCES

1. Batlle E, Henderson JT, Beghtel H, et al. Beta-catenin and TCF mediate cell positioning in the intestinal epithelium by controlling the expression of EphB/ephrinB. *Cell* 2002;111:251–263.
2. Beck F. Homeobox genes in gut development. *Gut* 2002;51: 450–454.
3. Bonhomme C, Duluc I, Martin E, et al. The Cdx2 homeobox gene has a tumour suppressor function in the distal colon in addition to a homeotic role during gut development. *Gut* 2003;52: 1465–1471.
4. Chailler P, Basque JR, Corriveau L, Menard D. Functional characterization of the keratinocyte growth factor system in human fetal gastrointestinal tract. *Pediatr Res* 2000;48:504–510.
5. Haffen K, Kedinger M, Simon-Assmann P. Mesenchyme-dependent differentiation of epithelial progenitor cells in the gut. *J Pediatr Gastroenterol Nutr* 1987;6:14–23.
6. Kedinger M, Simon-Assmann P, Bouziges F, Haffen K. Epithelial-mesenchymal interactions in intestinal epithelial differentiation. *Scand J Gastroenterol Suppl* 1988;23:62–69.
8. Roberts DJ. Molecular mechanisms of development of the gastrointestinal tract. *Dev Dyn* 2000;219:109–120.
9. Stutzmann J, Bellissent-Waydelich A, Fontao L, Launay JF, Simon-Assmann P. Adhesion complexes implicated in intestinal epithelial cell-matrix interactions. *Microsc Res Tech* 2000;51:179–190.
10. Bajaj-Elliott M, Poulsom R, Pender SL, Wathen NC, MacDonald TT. Interactions between stromal cell-derived keratinocyte growth factor and epithelial transforming growth factor in immune-mediated crypt cell hyperplasia. *J Clin Inv* 1998;102:1473–1480.
11. de Santa Barbara P, van den Brink GR, Roberts DJ. Development and differentiation of the intestinal epithelium. *Cell Mol Life Sci* 2003;60:1322–1332.
12. Karam SM. Lineage commitment and maturation of epithelial cells in the gut. *Front Biosci* 1999;4:D286–D298.
13. de Santa Barbara P, van den Brink GR, Roberts DJ. Molecular etiology of gut malformations and diseases. *Am J Med Genet* 2002;115:221–230.
14. Moore KL, Persaud TVN. The digestive system. In: Moore KL, Persaud TVN, eds. *The Developing Human: Clinically Oriented Embryology.* 7th ed. Philadelphia: WB Saunders; 2003:266–284.
15. Arai T, Kino I. Morphometrical and cell kinetic studies of normal human colorectal mucosa. Comparison between the proximal and the distal large intestine. *Acta Pathol Jpn* 1989;39:725–730.
16. Baker K, Zhang Y, Jin C, Jass JR. Proximal versus distal hyperplastic polyps of the colorectum: different lesions or a biological spectrum? *J Clin Pathol* 2004;57:1089–1093.
17. Birkenkam-Demtroder K, Olesen SH, Sorensen FB, et al. Differential gene expression in colon cancer of the cecum versus the sigmoid and rectosigmoid. *Gut* 2005;54:374–384.
18. Calam J, Ghatei MA, Domin J, et al. Regional differences in concentrations of regulatory peptides in human colon mucosal biopsy. *Dig Dis Sci* 1989;34:1193–1198.
19. Gervaz P, Bucher P, Morel P. Two colons-two cancers: paradigm shift and clinical implications. *J Surg Onc* 2004;88:261–266.
20. Greenson JK, Odze RD. Inflammatory bowel disease of the large intestine. In: Odze, RD, Goldblum JR, Crawford JM, eds. *Surgical Pathology of the GI Tract, Liver, Biliary Tract and Pancreas.* Philadelphia: WB Saunders; 2004;213–214.
21. Kunzelmann K, Mall M. Electrolyte transport in the mammalian colon: mechanisms and implications for disease. *Physiol Rev* 2002;82:245–289.

22. Lee E, Schiller LR, Fordtran JS. Quantification of colonic lamina propria cells by means of a morphometric point-counting method. *Gastroenterology* 1988;94:409–418.

23. Liu LU, Holt PR, Krivosheyev V, Moss SF. Human right and left colon differ in epithelial cell apoptosis and in expression of Bak, a pro-apoptotic Bcl-2 homologue. *Gut* 1999;45:45–50.

24. Macfarlane GT, Gibson GR, Cummings JH. Comparison of fermentation reactions in different regions of the human colon. *J Appl Bacteriol* 1992;72:57–64.

25. Moskaluk CA, Zhang H, Powell SM, Cerilli LA, Hampton GM, Frierson HF Jr. Cdx2 protein expression in normal and malignant human tissues: an immunohistochemical survey using tissue microarrays. *Mod Pathol* 2003;16:913–919.

26. Naftalin RJ, Zammit PS, Pedley KC. Regional differences in rat large intestinal crypt function in relation to dehydrating capacity in vivo. *J Physiol* 1999;514(pt 1):201–210.

27. Naftalin RJ. The dehydrating function of the descending colon in relationship to crypt function. *Physiol Res* 1994;43:65–73.

28. Paluszkiewicz P, Berbec H, Pawlowska-Wakowicz B, Cybulski M, Paszkowska A. p53 protein accumulation in colorectal cancer tissue has prognostic value only in left-sided colon tumours. *Cancer Detect Prev* 2004;28:252–259.

29. Priebe MG, Vonk RJ, Sun X, He T, Harmsen HJ, Welling GW. The physiology of colonic metabolism. Possibilities for interventions with pre- and probiotics. *Eur J Nutr* 2002;41(suppl1):I2–I10.

30. Sandle GI. Salt and water absorption in the human colon: a modern appraisal. *Gut* 1998;43:294–299.

31. Booth C, Potten CS. Gut instincts: thoughts on intestinal epithelial stem cells. *J Clin Invest* 2000;105:1493–1499.

32. Marshman E, Booth C, Potten CS. The intestinal epithelial stem cell. *Bioessays* 2002;24:91–98.

33. Seidelin JB. Colonic epithelial cell turnover: possible implications for ulcerative colitis and cancer initiation. *Scand J Gastroenterol* 2004;39:201–211.

34. Bajpai M, Mathur M. Duplications of the alimentary tract: clues to the missing links. *J Pediatr Surg* 1994;29:1361–1365.

35. Bossard P, Zaret KS. Repressive and restrictive mesodermal interactions with gut endoderm: possible relation to Meckel's diverticulum. *Development* 2000;127:4915–4923.

36. Martinez-Frias ML, Bermejo E, Rodrigues-Pinilla E. Anal atresia, vertebral, genital, and urinary tract anomalies: a primary polytopic developmental field defect identified through an epidemiological analysis of associations. *Am J Med Genet* 2000;95:169–173.

37. Robertson K, Mason I, Hall S. Hirschsprung's disease: genetic mutations in mice and men. *Gut* 1997;41:436–441.

38. Houlston R, Bevan S, Williams A, et al. Mutations in DPC4 (SMAD4) cause juvenile polyposis syndrome, but only account for a minority of cases. *Hum Mol Genet* 1998;7:1907–1912.

39. Howe JR, Roth S, Ringold JC, et al. Mutations in the SMAD4/DPC4 gene in juvenile polyposis. *Science* 1998;280:1086–1088.

40. Howe JR, Bair JL, Sayet MG, et al. Germline mutations of the gene encoding bone morphogenetic protein receptor 1A in juvenile polyposis. *Nat Genet* 2001;38:184–187.

41. Roth S, Sistonen P, Salovaara R, et al. SMAD genes in juvenile polyposis. *Genes Chromosomes Cancer* 1999;26:54–61.

42. Ruiz i Altaba A. Gli proteins and Hedgehog signaling: development and cancer. *Trends Genet* 1999;15:418–425.

43. Guyton, AC. The digestive and metabolic systems. In: Guyton AC, ed. *Anatomy and Physiology*. Philadelphia: WB Saunders; 1984:643–700.

44. Smith ME, Morton DG. The colon. In: Smith ME, Morton DG, eds. *The Digestive System* Edinburgh: Churchill Livingstone 2001:175–186.

45. Netter, FH. Abdomen. In: Netter, FH and Colacino S, eds. *Atlas of Human Anatomy*. Summit, NJ: Ciba-Geigy Corp; 1989:251–256, 264–268.

46. Glebov OK, Rodriguez LM, Nakahara K, et al. Distinguishing right from left colon by the pattern of gene expression. *Cancer Epidemiol Biomarkers Prev* 2003;12:755–762.

46. Wood JD, Alpers DH, Andrews PL. Fundamentals of neurogastroenterology. *Gut* 1999;45(suppl2):II6–II16.

47. Howell SJ, Wilk D, Yadav SP, Bevins CL. Antimicrobial polypeptides of the human colonic epithelium. *Peptides* 2003;24:1763–1770.

48. Fihn BM, Jodal M. Permeability of the proximal and distal rat colon crypt and surface epithelium to hydrophilic molecules. *Pflugers Arch* 2001;441:656–662.

49. Mai V, Morris JG Jr. Colonic bacterial flora: changing understandings in the molecular age. *J Nutr* 2004;134:459–464.

50. Roediger WE, Babidge W. Human colonocyte detoxification. *Gut* 1997;41:731–734.

51. Topping DL, Clifton PM. Short-chain fatty acids and human colonic function: roles of resistant starch and nonstarch polysaccharides. *Physiol Rev* 2001;81:1031–1064.

52. Naftalin RJ, Pedley KC. Regional crypt function in rat large intestine in relation to fluid absorption and growth of the pericryptal sheath. *J Physiol* 1999;514(pt 1):211–227.

53. Hirasawa K, Sato Y, Hosoda Y, Yamamoto T, Hanai H. Immunohistochemical localization of angiotensin II receptor and local renin-angiotensin system in human colonic mucosa. *J Histochem Cytochem* 2002;50:275–282.

54. Thiagarajah JR, Griffiths NM, Pedley KC, Naftalin RJ. Evidence for modulation of pericryptal sheath myofibroblasts in rat descending colon by transforming growth factor beta and angiotensin II. *BMC Gastroenterol* 2002;2:4–16.

55. Thiagarajah JR, Pedley KC, Naftalin RJ. Evidence of amiloride-sensitive fluid absorption in rat descending colonic crypts from fluorescence recovery of FITC-labelled dextran after photobleaching. *J Physiol (Lond)* 2001;536:541–553.

56. Hopkins MJ, Sharp R, Macfarlane GT. Age and disease related changes in intestinal bacterial populations assessed by cell culture, 16S rRNA abundance, and community cellular fatty acid profiles. *Gut* 2001;48:198–205.

57. Macfarlane GT, Macfarlane S. Human colonic microbiota: ecology, physiology and metabolic potential of intestinal bacteria. *Scand J Gastroenterol Suppl* 1997;222:3–9.

58. Ouwehand A, Isolauri E, Salminen S. The role of the intestinal microflora for the development of the immune system in early childhood. *Eur J Nutr* 2002;41(suppl1):I32–I37.

59. Pickard KM, Bremner AR, Gordon JN, MacDonald TT. Microbial-gut interactions in health and disease. Immune responses. *Best Pract & Res Clin Gastroenterol* 2004;18:271–285.

60. Pryde SE, Duncan SH, Hold GL, Stewart CS, Flint HJ. The microbiology of butyrate formation in the human colon. *FEMS Microbiol Lett* 2002;217:133–139.

61. Zaharia V, Varzescu M, Djavadi I, et al. Effects of short chain fatty acids on colonic Na+ absorption and enzyme activity. *Comp Biochem Physiol A Mol Integr Phsiol* 2001;128:335–347.

62. Grieg ER, Boot-Handford RP, Mani V, Sandle GI. Decreased expression of apical Na+ channels and basolateral Na+, K+-ATPase in ulcerative colitis. *J Pathol* 2004;204:84–92.

63. Willemsen LEM, Koetsier MA, van Deventer SJH, van Tol EAF. Short chain fatty acids stimulate epithelial mucin 2 expression through differential effects on prostaglandin E_1 and E_2 production by intestinal myofibroblasts. *Gut* 2003;52:1442–1447.

64. Berkes J, Viswanathan VK, Savkovic SD, Hecht G. Intestinal epithelial responses to enteric pathogens: effect on the tight junction barrier, ion transport, and inflammation. *Gut* 2003;52:439–451.

65. Porter EM, Bevins CL, Ghosh D, Ganz, T. The multifaceted Paneth cell. *Cell Mol Life Sci* 2002;59:156–170.

66. Boman HG. Antibacterial peptides: basic facts and emerging concepts. *J Intern Med* 2003;254:197–215.

67. Kohler H, McCormick BA, Walker WA. Bacterial-enterocyte crosstalk: cellular mechanisms in health and disease. *J Pediatr Gastroenterol Nutr* 2003;36:175–185.

68. Lu L, Walker WA. Pathologic and physiologic interactions of bacteria with the gastrointestinal epithelium. *Am J Clin Nutr* 2001;73S:1124S–1130S.

69. Zuercher AW, Jiang HQ, Thurnheer MC, Cuff CF, Cebra JJ. Distinct mechanisms for cross-protection of the upper versus lower respiratory tract through intestinal priming. *J Immunol* 2002;169:3920–3925.

70. Demeter P, De Vos M, Van Huysse JA, et al. Colon mucosa of patients both with spondyloarthritis and Crohn's disease is en-

riched with macrophages expressing the scavenger receptor CD163. *Ann Rheum Dis* 2005;64:321–324.

71. Didierlaurent A, Sirard JC, Kraehenbuhl JP, Neutra MR. How the gut senses its content. *Cell Microbiol* 2002;4:61–72.

72. Girardin SE, Hugot JP, Sansonetti PJ. Lessons from Nod2 studies: towards a link between Crohn's disease and bacterial sensing. *Trends Immunol* 2003;24:652–658.

73. Hershberg RM, Mayer LF. Antigen processing and presentation by intestinal epithelial cells – polarity and complexity. *Immunol Today* 2000;21:123–128.

74. Neutra MR. Current concepts in mucosal immunity. V. Role of M cells in transepithelial transport of antigens and pathogens to the mucosal immune system. *Am J Physiol* 1998;274(pt 1):G785–791.

75. Noverr MC, Huffnagle GB. Does the microbiota regulate immune responses outside the gut? *Trends Microbiol* 2004;12: 562–568.

76. Spahn TW, Kucharzik T. Modulating the intestinal immune system: the role of lymphotoxin and GALT organs. *Gut* 2004;53:456–465.

77. van Niel G, Raposo G, Candalh C, et al. Intestinal epithelial cells secrete exosome-like vesicles. *Gastroenterology* 2001;121: 337–349.

78. Brandtzaeg P, Pabst R. Let's go mucosal: communication on slippery ground. *Trends Immunol* 2004;25:570–577.

79. Rakoff-Nahoum S, Paglino J, Eslami-Varzaneh F, Edberg S, Medzhitov R. Recognition of commensal microflora by toll-like receptors is required for intestinal homeostasis. *Cell* 2004;118: 229–241.

80. Anderson JM, van Itallie CM. Tight junctions and the molecular basis for regulation of paracellular permeability. *Am J Physiol* 1995;269(pt 1):G467–G475.

81. Kucharzik T, Walsh SV, Chen J, Parkos CA, Nusrat A. Neutrophil transmigration in inflammatory bowel disease is associated with differential expression of epithelial intercellular junction proteins. *Am J Pathol* 2001;159:2001–2009.

82. Walsh SV, Hopkins AM, Nusrat A. Modulation of tight junction structure and function by cytokines. *Adv Drug Deliv Rev* 2000; 41:303–313.

83. Adegboyega PA, Mifflin RC, DiMari JF, Saada JI, Powell DW. -Immunohistochemical study of myofibroblasts in normal nic mucosa, hyperplastic polyps, and adenomatous colorectal polyps. *Arch Pathol Lab Med* 2002;126:829–836.

84. Akishima Y, Ito K, Zhang L, et al. Immunohistochemical detection of human small lymphatic vessels under normal and pathological conditions using the LYVE-1 antibody. *Virchows Arch* 2004;444:153–157.

85. Aldenborg F, Enerback L. The immunohistochemical demonstration of chymase and tryptase in human intestinal mast cells. *Histochem J* 1994;26:587–596.

86. Brandtzaeg P, Farstad IN, Helgeland L. Phenotypes of T cells in the gut. *Chem Immunol* 1998;71:1–26.

87. Buffa R, Mare P, Gini A, Salvadore M. Chromogranins A and B and secretogranin II in hormonally identified endocrine cells of the gut and the pancreas. *Basic Appl Histochem* 1988;32:471–484.

88. Castellaneta A, Abe M, Morelli AE, Thomson AW. Identification and characterization of intestinal Peyer's patch interferon-alpha producing (plasmacytoid) dendritic cells. *Hum Immunol* 2004;65:104–113.

89. Corfield AP, Myerscough N, Longman R, Sylvester P, Arul S, Pignatelli M. Mucins and mucosal protection in the gastrointestinal tract: new prospects for mucins in the pathology of gastrointestinal disease. *Gut* 2000;47:589–594.

90. Ferri GL, Probert L, Cocchia D, Michetti F, Marangos PJ, Polak JM. Evidence for the presence of S-100 protein in the glial component of the human enteric nervous system. *Nature* 1982;297: 409–410.

91. Frangsmyr L, Baranov V, Hammarstrom S. Four carcinoembryonic antigen subfamily members, CEA, NCA, BGP and CGM2, selectively expressed in the normal human colonic epithelium are integral components of the fuzzy coat. *Tumour Biol* 1999;20: 277–292.

92. Fulcheri E, Cantino D, Bussolati G. Presence of intra-mucosal smooth muscle cells in normal human and rat colon. *Basic Appl Histochem* 1985;29:337–344.

93. Fujisaki J, Shimoda T. Expression of cytokeratin subtypes in colorectal mucosa, adenoma, and carcinoma. *Gastroenterol Jpn* 1993;28:647–656.

94. Gabbiani G, Schmid E, Winter S, et al. Vascular smooth muscle cells differ from other smooth muscle cells: predominance of vimentin filaments and specific alpha-type actin. *Proc Natl Acad Sci U S A* 1981;78:298–302.

95. Galli SJ, Tsai M, Wershil BK. The c-kit receptor, stem cell factor, and mast cells. What each is teaching us about the others. *Am J Pathol* 1993;142:965–974.

96. Grimelius L. Silver stains demonstrating neuroendocrine cells. *Biotech Histochem* 2004;79:37–44.

97. Hamrock D, Azmi FH, O'Donnell E, Gunning WT, Philips ER, Zaher A. Infection by Rhodococcus equi in a patient with AIDS: histological appearance mimicking Whipple's disease and Mycobacterium avium-intracellulare infection. *J Clin Pathol* 1999;52:68–71.

98. Higaki S, Tada M, Nishiaki M, Mitani M, Yanai H, Okita K. Immunohistological study to determine the presence of pericryptal myofibroblasts and basement membrane in colorectal epithelial tumors. *J Gastroenterol* 1999;34:215–220.

99. Jass JR. Mucin core proteins as differentiation markers in the gastrointestinal tract. *Histopathology* 2000;37:561–564.

100. Jones TR, Kao KJ, Pizzo SV, Bigner DD. Endothelial cell surface expression and binding of factor VIII/von Willebrand factor. *Am J Pathol* 1981;103:304–308.

101. Kato H, Yamamoto T, Yamamoto H, Ohi R, So N, Iwasaki Y. Immunocytochemical characterization of supporting cells in the enteric nervous system in Hirschsprung's disease. *J Pediatr Surg* 1990;25:514–519.

102. Kawana T, Nada O, Ikeda K. An immunohistochemical study of glial fibrillary acidic (GFA) protein and S-100 protein in the colon affected by Hirschsprung's disease. *Acta Neuropathol (Berl)* 1988;76:159–165.

103. Kende AI, Carr NJ, Sobin LH. Expression of cytokeratins 7 and 20 in carcinomas of the gastrointestinal tract. *Histopathology* 2003;42:137–140.

104. Kurki P, Virtanen I. The detection of smooth muscle antibodies reacting with intermediate filaments of desmin type. *J Immunol Methods* 1985;76:329–335.

105. Lamps LW, Molina CP, West AB, Haggitt RC, Scott MA. The pathologic spectrum of gastrointestinal and hepatic histoplasmosis. *Am J Clin Pathol* 2000;113:64–72.

106. Lee MJ, Lee HS, Kim WH, Choi Y, Yang M. Expression of mucins and cytokeratins in primary carcinomas of the digestive system. *Mod Pathol* 2003;16:403–410.

107. Meyer T, Brinck U. Differential distribution of serotonin and tryptophan hydroxylase in the human gastrointestinal tract. *Digestion* 1999;60:63–68.

108. Moll R, Lowe A, Laufer J, Franke WW. Cytokeratin 20 in human carcinomas. A new histodiagnostic marker detected by monoclonal antibodies. *Am J Pathol* 1992;140:427–447.

109. O'Connell FP, Pinkus JL, Pinkus GS. CD138 (syndecan-1), a plasma cell marker immunohistochemical profile in hematopoietic and nonhematopoietic neoplasms. *Am J Clin Pathol* 2004;121:254–263.

110. Ozgul C, Karaoz E, Erdogan D, Dursun A. Expression of epidermal growth factor receptor in normal colonic mucosa and in adenocarcinomas of the colon. *Acta Physiol Hung* 1997–1998; 85:121–128.

111. Park HJ, Kamm MA, Abbasi AM, Talbot IC. Immunohistochemical study of the colonic muscle and innervation in idiopathic chronic constipation. *Dis Colon Rectum* 1995;38:509–513.

112. Petchasuwan C, Pintong J. Immunohistochemistry for intestinal ganglion cells and nerve fibers: aid in the diagnosis of Hirschsprung's disease. *J Med Assoc Thai* 2000;83: 1402–1409.

113. Qualtrough D, Hinoi T, Fearon E, Paraskeva C. Expression of CDX2 in normal and neoplastic human colon tissue and during differentiation of an in vitro model system. *Gut* 2002;51:184–190.

114. Rubio CA, Nesi G. A simple method to demonstrate normal and metaplastic Paneth cells in tissue sections. *In Vivo* 2003;17: 67–71.

115. Rubio CA, Slezak P. The subepithelial band in collagenous colitis is autofluorescent. A study in H&E stained sections. *In Vivo* 2002;16:123–126.

116. Sarsfield P, Rinne A, Jones DB, Johnson P, Wright DH. Accessory cells in physiological lymphoid tissue from the intestine: an immunohistochemical study. *Histopathology* 1996;28:205–211.

117. Sartore S, De Marzo N, Borrione AC, et al. Myosin heavy-chain isoforms in human smooth muscle. *Eur J Biochem* 1989;179:79–85.

118. Smithson JE, Warren BF, Young S, Pigott R, Jewell DP. Heterogeneous expression of carcinoembryonic antigen in the normal colon and upregulation in active ulcerative colitis. *J Pathol* 1996;180:146–151.

119. Truong LD, Rangdaeng S, Cagle P, Ro JY, Hawkins H, Font RL. The diagnostic utility of desmin. A study of 584 cases and review of the literature. *Am J Clin Pathol* 1990;93:305–314.

120. Werling RW, Yaziji H, Bacchi CE, Gown AM. CDX2, a highly sensitive and specific marker of adenocarcinomas of intestinal origin: an immunohistochemical survey of 476 primary and metastatic carcinomas. *Am J Surg Pathol* 2003;27:303–310.

121. West, AB, Isaac CA, Carboni JM, Morrow JS, Mooseker MS, Barwick KW. Localization of villin, a cytoskeletal protein specific to microvilli, in human ileum and colon and in colonic neoplasms. *Gastroenterology* 1988;94:343–352.

122. Wiedenmann B, Waldherr R, Buhr H, Hille A, Roas P, Huttner WB. Identification of gastroenteropancreatic neuroendocrine cells in normal and neoplastic human tissue with antibodies against synaptophysin, chromogranin A, secretogranin I (chromogranin B), and secretogranin II. *Gastroenterology* 1988;95:1364–1374.

123. Wong NA, Herriot M, Rae F. An immunohistochemical study and review of potential markers of human intestinal M cells. *Eur J Histochem* 2003;47:143–150.

124. Thiagarajah JR, Gourmelon P, Griffiths NM, Lebrun F, Naftalin RJ, Pedley KC. Radiation induced cytochrome c release causes loss of rat colonic fluid absorption by damage to crypts and pericryptal myofibroblasts. *Gut* 2000;47:675–684.

125. Kirby JA, Bone M, Robertson H, Hudson, M, Jones DE. The number of intraepithelial T cells decreases from ascending colon to rectum. *J Clin Pathol* 2003;56:158.

126. Kraehenbuhl JP, Neutra MR. Epithelial M cells: differentiation and function. *Annu Rev Cell Dev Biol* 2000;16:301–332.

127. Sapp H, Ithamukkala S, Brien TP, et al. The terminal ileum is affected in patients with lymphocytic or collagenous colitis. *Am J Surg Pathol* 2002;26:1484–1492.

128. Brittan M, Wright NA. The gastrointestinal stem cell. *Cell Prolif* 2004;37:35–53.

129. Bleuming SA, Peppelenbosch MP, Roberts, DJ, van den Brink GR. Homeostasis of the adult colonic epithelium: a role for morphogens. *Scand J Gastroenterol* 2004;2:93–98.

130. Halm DR, Halm ST. Secretagogue response of goblet cells and columnar cells in human colonic crypts. *Am J Physiol Cell Physiol* 2000;278:C212–C233.

131. Kim KM, Shibata D. Methylation reveals a niche: stem cell succession in human colon crypts. *Oncogene* 2002;21:5441–5449.

132. Potten CS. Epithelial cell growth and differentiation. II. Intestinal apoptosis. *Am J Physiol* 1997;273(pt 1):G253–G257.

133. Potten CS, Booth C, Tudor GL, et al. Identification of a putative intestinal stem cell and early lineage marker; musashi-1. *Differentiation* 2003;71:28–41.

134. Sancho E, Batlle E, Clevers H. Live and let die in the intestinal epithelium. *Curr Opin Cell Biol* 2003;15:763–770.

135. Ayabe T, Ashida T, Kohgo Y, Kono T. The role of Paneth cells and their antimicrobial peptides in innate host defense. *Trends Microbiol* 2004;12:394–398.

136. Ouellette AJ. Mucosal immunity and inflammation IV. Paneth cell antimicrobial peptides and the biology of the mucosal barrier. *Am J Physiol Gastrointest Liver Physiol* 1999;277:G257–G261.

137. Schonhoff SE, Giel-Moloney M, Leiter AB. Minireview: development and differentiation of gut endocrine cells. *Endocrinology* 2004;145:2639–2644.

138. Neutra MR, Mantis NJ, Kraehenbuhl JP. Collaboration of epithelial cells with organized mucosal lymphoid tissues. *Nat Immunol* 2001;2:1004–1009.

139. Corfield AP, Wiggins R, Edwards C, et al. A sweet coating—how bacteria deal with sugars. *Adv Exp Med Biol* 2003;535:3–15.

140. Filipe MI. Mucins in the human gastrointestinal epithelium: a review. *Invest Cell Pathol* 1979;2:195–216.

141. Culling CF, Reid PE, Dunn WL, Freeman HJ. The relevance of the histochemistry of colonic mucins based upon their PAS reactivity. *Histochem J* 1981;13:889–903.

142. Rehfeld JF. The new biology of gastrointestinal hormones. *Physiol Rev* 1998;78:1087–1108.

143. Skipper M, Lewis J. Getting to the guts of enteroendocrine differentiation. *Nat Genet* 2000;24:3–4.

144. Cetin Y, Muller-Koppel L, Aunis D, Bader MF, Grube D. Chromogranin A (CgA) in the gastro-entero-pancreatic (GEP) endocrine system. II. CgA in mammalian entero-endocrine cells. *Histochemistry* 1989;92:265–275.

145. Facer, P, Bishop AE, Lloyd RV, Wilson BS,. Chromogranin: a newly recognized marker for endocrine cells of the human gastrointestinal tract. *Gastroenterology* 1985;39:1366–1373.

146. Hirschowitz L, Rode J. Changes in neurons, neuroendocrine cells and nerve fibers in the lamina propria of irradiated bowel. *Virchows Arch A Pathol Anat Histopathol* 1991;418:163–168.

147. Qian J, Hickey WF, Angeletti RH. Neuroendocrine cells in intestinal lamina propria. Detection with antibodies to chromogranin A. *J Neuroimmunol* 1988;17:159–165.

148. Roth KA, Gordon JI. Spatial differentiation of the intestinal epithelium: analysis of enteroendocrine cells containing immunoreactive serotonin, secretin, and substance P in normal and transgenic mice. *Proc Natl Aca Sci U S A* 1990;87:6408–6412.

149. Lala S, Ogura Y, Osborne C, et al. Crohn's disease and the NOD2 gene: a role for Paneth cells. *Gastroenterology* 2003;125:47–57.

150. Ogura Y, Lala S, Xin W, et al. Expression of NOD2 in Paneth cells: a possible link to Crohn's ileitis. *Gut* 2003;52:1591–1597.

151. Lin PW, Simon PO Jr, Gerwitz AT, et al. Paneth cell cryptidins act *in vitro* as apical paracrine regulators of the innate inflammatory response. *J Biol Chem* 2004;279:19902–19907.

152. Baranov V, Hammarstrom S. Carcinoembryonic antigen (CEA) and CEA-related cell adhesion molecule 1 (CEACAM1), apically expressed on human colonic M cells, are potential receptors for microbial adhesion. *Histochem Cell Biol* 2004;121:83–89.

153. Neutra MR, Mantis NJ, Frey A, Giannasca PJ. The composition and function of M cell apical membranes: implications for microbial pathogenesis. *Semin Immunol* 1999;11:171–181.

154. Sierro F, Pringault E, Simon-Assman P, Kraehenbuhl JP, Debard N. Transient expression of M-cell phenotype by enterocyte-like cells of the follicle-associated epithelium of mouse Peyer's patches. *Gastroenterology* 2000;119:734–743.

155. Gebert A, Fassbender S, Werner K, Weissferdt A. The development of M cells in Peyer's patches is restricted to specialized dome-associated crypts. *Am J Pathol* 1999;154:1573–1582.

156. Jepson MA, Clark MA, Hirst BH. M cell targeting by lectins: a strategy for mucosal vaccination and drug delivery. *Adv Drug Deliv Rev* 2004;56:511–525.

157. Farstad IN, Lundin KE. Gastrointestinal intraepithelial lymphocytes and T cell lymphomas. *Gut* 2003;52:163–164.

158. Helgeland L, Dissen E, Dai KZ, Midtvedt T, Brandtzaeg P, Vaage JT. Microbial colonization induces oligoclonal expansions of intraepithelial CD8 T cells in the gut. *Eur J Immunol* 2004;34:3389–3400.

159. MacDonald TT, Bajaj-Elliot M, Pender SL. T cells orchestrate intestinal mucosal shape and integrity. *Immunol Today* 1999;20:505–510.

160. Brandtzaeg P. Development and basic mechanisms of human gut immunity. *Nutr Rev* 1998;56(pt 2):S5–S18.

161. Ebert EC. Interleukin-12 up-regulates perforin- and Fas-mediated lymphokine-activated killer activity by intestinal intraepithelial lymphocytes. *Clin Exp Immunol* 2004;138:259–265.

162. Kagnoff MF. Current concepts in mucosal immunity. III. Ontogeny and function of gamma delta T cells in the intestine. *Am J Physiol* 1998;274:G455–G458.

163. Chen Y, Chou K, Fuchs E, Havran WL, Boismenu R. Protection of the intestinal mucosa by intraepithelial gamma delta T cells. *Proc Nat Acad Sci U S A* 2002;99:14338–14343.

164. Lin T, Yoshida H, Matsuzaki G, et al. Autospecific gamma delta thymocytes that escape negative selection find sanctuary in the intestine. *J Clin Invest* 1999;104:1297–1305.

165. Melgar S, Hammarstrom S, Oberg A, Danielsson A, Hammarstrom ML. Cytolytic capabilities of lamina propria and intraepithelial lymphocytes in normal and chronically inflamed human intestine. *Scan J Immunol* 2004;60:167–177.

166. Shibahara T, Wilcox JN, Couse, T, Madara JL. Characterization of epithelial chemoattractants for human intestinal lymphocytes. *Gastroenterology* 2001;120:60–70.

167. Lamps LW. Lazenby AJ. Colonic epithelial lymphocytosis and lymphocytic colitis: descriptive histopathology versus distinct clinicopathologic entities. *Adv Anat Pathol* 2000;7:210–213.

168. Rothenberg ME, Mishra A, Brandt EB, Hogan SP. Gastrointestinal eosinophils. *Immunol Rev* 2001;179:139–155.

169. Bochner BS, Schleimer RP. Mast cells, basophils, and eosinophils: distinct but overlapping pathways for recruitment. *Immunol Rev* 2001;179:5–15.

170. Levy AM, Yamazaki K, Van Keulen VP, et al. Increased eosinophil infiltration and degranulation in colonic tissue from patients with collagenous colitis. *Am J Gastroenterol* 2001;96:1522–1528.

171. Harnois C, Demers MJ, Bouchard V, et al. Human intestinal epithelial crypt cell survival and death: complex modulations of Bcl-2 homologs by Fak, PI3-K/Akt-1, MEK/Erk, and p38 signaling pathways. *J Cell Physiol* 2004;198:209–222.

172. Barkla DH, Gibson PR. The fate of epithelial cells in the human large intestine. *Pathology* 1999;31:230–238.

173. Debatin KM. Apoptosis pathways in cancer and cancer therapy. *Cancer Immunol Immunother* 2004;53:153–159.

174. Gomez-Angelats M, Bortner CD, Cidlowski JA. Cell volume regulation in immune cell apoptosis. *Cell Tissue Res* 2000;301:33–42.

175. Gupta S. Molecular signaling in death receptor and mitochondrial pathways of apoptosis (Review). *Int J Oncol* 2003; 22:15–20.

176. Huppertz B, Frank HG, Kaufmann P. The apoptosis cascade—morphological and immunohistochemical methods for its visualization. *Anat Embryol (Berl)* 1999;200:1–18.

177. Luciano L, Groos S, Busche R, von Engelhardt W, Reale E. Massive apoptosis of colonocytes induced by butyrate deprivation overloads resident macrophages and promotes the recruitment of circulating monocytes. *Cell Tissue Res* 2002; 309:393–407.

178. Schuster N, Krieglstein K. Mechanisms of TGF-beta-mediated apoptosis. *Cell Tissue Res* 2002;307:1–14.

179. Watson AJM. Apoptosis and colorectal cancer. *Gut* 2004;53: 1701–1709.

180. Xiao ZQ, Moragoda L, Jaszewski R, Hatfield JA, Flifiel SE, Majumdar AP. Aging is associated with increased proliferation and decreased apoptosis in the colonic mucosa. *Mech Ageing Dev* 2001;122:1849–1864.

181. Medina F, Segundo C, Campos-Caro A, Salcedo I, Garcia-Poley A, Brieva JA. Isolation, maturational level, and functional capacity of human colon lamina propria plasma cells. *Gut* 2003;52:383–389.

182. Simon HU. Regulation of eosinophil and neutrophil apoptosis—similarities and differences. *Immunol Rev* 2001;179: 156–162.

183. Iqbal N, Salzman D, Lazenby AJ, Wilcox CM. Diagnosis of gastrointestinal graft-versus-host disease. *Am J Gastroenterol* 2000;95:3034–3038.

184. Iwamoto M, Koji T, Makiyama K, Kobayashi N, Nakane PK. Apoptosis of crypt epithelial cells in ulcerative colitis. *J Pathol* 1996;180:152–159.

185. Backus HH, Van Groeningen CJ, Vos W, et al. Differential expression of cell cycle and apoptosis related proteins in colorectal mucosa, primary colon tumours, and liver metastases. *J Clin Pathol* 2002;55:206–211.

186. Powell DW, Mifflin RC, Valentich JD, Crowe SE, Saada JI, West AB. Myofibroblasts. II. Intestinal subepithelial myofibroblasts. *Am J Physiol* 1999;277(pt 1):C183–C201.

187. Anagnostopoulos I, Schuppan D, Riecken EO, Gross UM, Stein H. Tenascin labelling in colorectal biopsies: a useful marker in the diagnosis of collagenous colitis. *Histopathology* 1999;34:425–431.

188. Gledhill A, Cole FM. Significance of basement membrane thickening in the human colon. *Gut* 1984;25:1085–1088.

189. Azzali G. Structure, lymphatic vascularization and lymphocyte migration in mucosa-associated lymphoid tissue. *Immunol Rev* 2003;195:178–189.

190. Brandtzaeg P, Johansen FE, Baekkevold ES, Carlsen HS, Farstad IN. The traffic of mucosal lymphocytes to extraintestinal sites. *J Pediatr Gastroenterol Nutr* 2004;39(suppl 3):S725–S726.

191. Goldstein NS, Bhanot P. Paucicellular and asymptomatic lymphocytic colitis. Expanding the clinicopathologic spectrum of lymphocytic colitis. *Am J Clin Pathol* 2004;122:405–411.

192. Fischer M, Kuppers R. Human IgA- and IgM-secreting intestinal plasma cells carry heavily mutated VH region genes. *Eur J Immunol* 1998;28:2971–2977.

193. Azzali G. Structure, lymphatic vascularization and lymphocyte migration in mucosa-associated lymphoid tissue. *Immunol Rev* 2003;195:178–189.

194. Nishida Y, Murase K, Isomoto H, et al. Different distribution of mast cells and macrophages in colonic mucosa of patients with collagenous colitis and inflammatory bowel disease. *Hepatogastroenterology* 2002;49:678–682.

195. Pascal RR, Gramlich TL, Parker KM, Gansler TS. Geographic variations in eosinophil concentration in normal colonic mucosa. *Mod Pathol* 1997;10:363–365.

196. Barbara G, Stanghellini V, DeGiorgio R, et al. Activated mast cells in proximity to colonic nerves correlate with abdominal pain in irritable bowel syndrome. *Gastroenterology* 2004; 126:693–702.

197. Rosenwasser LJ, Boyce JA. Mast cells: beyond IgE. *J Allergy Clin Immunol* 2003;111:24–32.

198. Mayer L. Current concepts in mucosal immunity. I. Antigen presentation in the intestine: new rules and regulations. *Am J Physiol* 1998;274(pt 1):G7–G9.

199. Rubio CA. Rectal muciphages are rich in lysozymes: a novel source of antimicrobial mucosal defense? *Scand J Gastroenterol* 2002;37:743–744.

200. Salto-Tellez M, Price AB. What is the significance of muciphages in colorectal biopsies? The significance of muciphages in otherwise normal colorectal biopsies. *Histopathology* 2000;36: 556–569.

201. Schenk M, Bouchon A, Birrer, S, Colonna M, Mueller C. Macrophages expressing triggering receptor expressed on myeloid cells-1 are underrepresented in the human intestine. *J Immunol* 2005;174:517–524.

202. Alkan S, Beals TF, Schnitzer B. Primary diagnosis of Whipple disease manifesting as lymphadenopathy: use of polymerase chain reaction for detection of Tropheryma whippelii. *Am J Clin Pathol* 2001;116:898–904.

203. Dobbins WO III, Weinstein WM. Electron microscopy of the intestine and rectum in acquired immunodeficiency syndrome. *Gastroenterology* 1985;88:738–749.

204. Lee SH, Barnes WG, Hodges GR, Dixon A. Perforated granulomatous colitis caused by Histoplasma capsulatum. *Dis Colon Rectum* 1985;23:171–176.

205. Nguyen HN, Frank D, Handt S, et al. Severe gastrointestinal hemorrhage due to Mycobacterium avium complex in a patient receiving immunosuppressive therapy. *Am J Gastroenterol* 1999;94: 232–235.

206. Hart AL, Lammers K, Brigidi P, et al. Modulation of human dendritic cell phenotype and function by probiotic bacteria. *Gut* 2004;53:1602–1609.

207. Zareie M, Singh PK, Irvine EJ, Sherman PM, McKay DM, Perdue MH. Monocyte/macrophage activation by normal bacteria and bacterial products: implications for altered epithelial function in Crohn's disease. *Am J Pathol* 2001;158: 1101–1109.

208. Bodey, B, Siegel SE, Kaiser HE. Antigen presentation by dendritic cells and their significance in antineoplastic immunotherapy. *In Vivo* 2004;18:81–100.

209. Powell DW, Mifflin RC, Valentich JD, Crowe SE, Saada JI, West AB. Myofibroblasts. I. Paracrine cells important in health and disease. *Am J Physiol* 1999;277(pt 1):C1–C9.

210. Skalli O, Schurch W, Seemayer T, et al. Myofibroblasts from diverse pathologic settings are heterogeneous in their content of

actin isoforms and intermediate filament proteins. *Lab Invest* 1989;60:275–285.

211. Ward SM, Sanders KM, Hirst GD. Role of interstitial cells of Cajal in neural control of gastrointestinal smooth muscles. *Neurogastroenterol Motil* 2004;16(suppl1):112–117.

212. Biberthaler P, Langer S. Comparison of the new OPS imaging technique with intravital microscopy: analysis of the colon microcirculation. *Eur Surg Res* 2002;34:124–128.

213. Fenoglio CM, Kay GI, Lane N. Distribution of human colonic lymphatics in normal, hyperplastic, and adenomatous tissue. Its relationship to metastasis from small carcinomas in pedunculated adenomas, with two case reports. *Gastroenterology* 1973;64:51–66.

214. Dobbins WO III. The intestinal mucosal lymphatics in man. A light and electron microscopic study. *Gastroenterology* 1966;51:994–1003.

215. Fogt F, Zimmerman RL, Ross HM, Daly T, Gausas RE. Identification of lymphatic vessels in malignant, adenomatous and normal colonic mucosa using the novel immunostain D2-40. *Oncol Rep* 2004;11:47–50.

216. Fogt, F, Pascha TL, Zhang PJ, Gausas RE, Rahemtulla A, Simmerman RL. Proliferation of D2-40-expressing intestinal lymphatic vessels in the lamina propria in inflammatory bowel disease. *Int J Mol Med* 2004;13:211–214.

217. Percy WH, Fromm TH, Wangsness CE. Muscularis mucosae contraction evokes colonic secretion via prostaglandin synthesis and nerve stimulation. *Am J Physiol Gastrointest Liver Physiol* 2003; 284:G213–G220.

218. Percy WH, Brunz JT, Burgers RE, Fromm TH, Merkwan CL, van Dis J. Interrelationship between colonic muscularis mucosae activity and changes in transmucosal potential difference. *Am J Physiol Gastrointest Liver Physiol* 2001;281:G479–G489.

219. Daniel EE, Wang YF. Gap junctions in intestinal smooth muscle and interstitial cells of Cajal. *Microsc Res Tech* 1999;47:309–320.

220. Hagger R, Gharaie S, Finlayson C, Kumar D. Regional and transmural density of interstitial cells of Cajal in human colon and rectum. *Am J Physiol* 1998;275(pt 1): G1309–G1316.

221. Coerdt W, Michel JS, Rippin G, et al. Quantitative morphometric analysis of the submucous plexus in age-related control groups. *Virchow Arch* 2004;444:239–246.

222. Wedel T, Spiegler J, Soellner S, et al. Enteric nerves and interstitial cells of Cajal are altered in patients with slow-transit constipation and megacolon. *Gastroenterology* 2002;123:1459–1467.

223. Wilder-Smith CH, Talbot IC, Merki HS, Meier-Ruge WA. Morphometric quantification of normal submucous plexus in the distal rectum of adult healthy volunteers. *Eur J Gastroenterol Hepatol* 2002;14:1339–1342.

224. Eaker EY. Neurofilament and intermediate filament immunoreactivity in human intestinal myenteric neurons. *Dig Dis Sci* 1997;42:1926–1932.

225. Faussone-Pellegrini MS, Pantalone D, Cortesini C. Smooth muscle cells, interstitial cells of Cajal and myenteric plexus interrelationships in the human colon. *Acta Anat (Basel)* 1990;139:31–44.

226. Faussone-Pellegrini MS, Cortesini C, Pantalone D. Neuromuscular structures specific to the submucosal border of the human colonic circular muscle layer. *Can J Physiol Pharmacol* 1990;68:1437–1446.

227. Mazzia C, Porcher C, Jule Y, Christen MO, Henry M. Ultrastructural study of relationships between c-kit immunoreactive interstitial cells and other cellular elements in the human colon. *Histochem Cell Biol* 2000;113:401–411.

228. Rumessen JJ, Peters S, Thuneberg L. Light and electron microscopical studies of interstitial cells of Cajal and muscle cells at the submucosal border of human colon. *Lab Invest* 1993;68:481–495.

229. Ward SM, Sanders KM. Interstitial cells of Cajal: primary targets of enteric motor innervation. *Anat Rec* 2001;262:125–135.

230. Takayama I, Horiguchi K, Daigo Y, Mine T, Fujino MA, Ohno S. The interstitial cells of Cajal and a gastroenteric pacemaker system. *Arch Histol Cytol* 2002;65:1–26.

231. Krishnamurthy S, Schuffler MD. Pathology of neuromuscular disorders of the small intestine and colon. *Gastroenterology* 1987;93:610–639.

232. Fraser ID, Condon RE, Schulte WJ, DeCosse JJ, Cowles VE. Longitudinal muscle of muscularis externa in human and non-human primate colon. *Arch Surg* 1981;116:61–63.

233. Hirota S, Isozaki K, Moriyama Y, et al. Gain-of-function mutations of c-kit in human gastrointestinal stromal tumors. *Science* 1998;279:577–580.

234. Kindblom LG, Remotti HE, Aldenborg F, Meis-Kindblom JM. Gastrointestinal pacemaker cell tumor (GIPACT): gastrointestinal stromal tumors show phenotypic characteristics of the interstitial cells of Cajal. *Am J Pathol* 1998;152:1259–1269.

235. Driman DK, Preiksaitis HG. Colorectal inflammation and increased cell proliferation associated with oral sodium phosphate bowel preparation solution. *Hum Pathol* 1998;29:972–978.

236. Levine DS. Proctitis following colonoscopy. *Gastrointest Endosc* 1988;34:269–272.

237. Pockros PJ, Foroozan P. Golytely lavage versus a standard colonoscopy preparation: effect on normal colonic mucosal histology. *Gastroenterology* 1985;88:545–548.

238. Rejchrt S, Bures J, Siroky M, Kopacova M, Slezak L, Langr F. A prospective, observational study of colonic mucosal abnormalities associated with orally administered sodium phosphate for colon cleansing before colonoscopy. *Gastrointest Endosc* 2004;59:651–654.

239. Wong NA, Penman ID, Campbell S, Lessells AM. Microscopic focal cryptitis associated with sodium phosphate bowel preparation. *Histopathology* 2000;36:476–478.

240. Fa-Si-Oen PR, Penninckx F. The effect of mechanical bowel preparation on human colonic tissue in elective open colon surgery. *Dis Colon Rectum* 2004;47:948–949.

241. Allen TV, Achord JL. The pickle of proper bowel biopsy orientation. *Gastroenterology* 1977;72(pt 1):774–775.

242. Bucher P, Gervaz, P, Egger JF, Soravia C, Morel P. Morphologic alterations associated with mechanical bowel preparation before elective colorectal surgery: a randomized trial. *Dis Colon Rectum* 2005;24:109–112.

243. Haggitt, RC. Handling of gastrointestinal biopsies in the surgical pathology laboratory. *Lab Med* 1982;13:272–278.

244. Carson, FL. Polyfoam pads – a source of artifact. *J Histotechnol* 1981;4:33–34.

245. Snover DC, Sandstad J, Hutton S. Mucosal pseudolipomatosis of the colon. *Am J Clin Pathol* 1985;84:575–580.

Vermiform Appendix

Terry L. Gramlich   Robert E. Petras

GROSS ANATOMY/SURGICAL PERSPECTIVE

The vermiform (wormlike) appendix is a slender tubular extension of the posteromedial aspect of the cecum originating below, and within 1 to 3 cm of, the ileocecal junction. Although the appendix has a relatively constant relationship with the cecum at the appendiceal base, the remainder of its length can be found in a variable number of positions, including retrocecal, subcecal, pelvic, and juxtaileal (1–3). A retrocecal position occurs most commonly, being present in nearly 70% of the population (3,4). Unusual locations, including a vermiform appendix buried within the cecal wall, have been documented (5). Although the appendix itself lacks taeniae, the base of the vermiform appendix lies at the convergence of the three cecal/ascending colon taeniae. These aid in locating the appendix when it is not readily apparent; the prominent anterior taenia is most easily traced for this purpose (1,6).

Vermiform appendices can vary remarkably in length but average 7 to 10 cm (2,4). The peritoneum covers almost all its external surface. The mesoappendix (mesentery of the appendix), a fold of peritoneum contiguous with the mesentery of the terminal ileum, extends along its length, terminating just proximal to the tip (1).

The appendiceal vascular supply courses within the mesoappendix; and, with distal progression, these vessels gradually rest nearer to the appendiceal muscular wall. In the proximity of the tip where there is no mesoappendix, blood vessels lie essentially "unprotected" on its external surface (1). The appendicular artery, a derivative of the inferior branch of the ileocolic artery of the superior mesenteric trunk, provides the majority of blood to the appendix (4,7). However, a variable supply with accessory arterial contributions is not unusual (8). Branches of the ileocolic vein drain the appendiceal venous network into the superior mesenteric vein and eventually into the portal circulation, whereas lymphatic vessels drain into regional (e.g., ileocolic) lymph nodes (6). Innervation is derived from branches of the vagus nerve (parasympathetic) and superior mesenteric plexus (sympathetic). Venous, lymphatic, and neural components closely follow the arterial vasculature (6).

Grossly, the external surface of the vermiform appendix appears smooth, pink-tan or gray, and glistening. The appendiceal diameter typically measures 5 to 8 mm. The wall is tan-white and the mucosal lining is light yellow, often disclosing a nodular appearance imparted by the characteristic and prominent lymphoid component (9). Because of these lymphoid aggregates, the central lumen on cross section is often irregular (stellate) rather than round. The normal luminal diameter measures 1 to 3 mm; however, in one study a luminal diameter of 1.2 cm or more was arbitrarily defined as dilatation (10). Focal occlusions of the appendiceal lumen are not uncommon (9).

Development of the Vermiform Appendix and Congenital Anomalies

The vermiform appendix originates from the primordial structure termed the cecal diverticulum (5,11). First apparent during the sixth week of fetal life, this blind-ended sac progressively develops. Its most proximal portion, in continuity with the remainder of the large bowel, enlarges and expands, forming the cecum proper, whereas its distal aspect or apex simply elongates, remains narrow, and becomes the vermiform appendix (11). Continued growth through infancy and childhood leads to differing cecoappendiceal relationships over this period. For example, the "infantile" cecoappendiceal junction lacks a conspicuous transition; the appendix arises from the inferior aspect of the cecum in this age group. In contrast, an abrupt, easily recognizable junction on the posteromedial cecum is observed in the adult (2).

Abnormal embryologic development can result in agenesis, hypoplasia, and various duplications or even triplication of the appendix (5,9,12–14). Duplication of the appendix can mimic cecal duplication. In general, appendiceal duplication is recognized by the presence of complete and separate inner circular and outer longitudinal muscle bands and the presence of a prominent lymphoid component (12).

Duplications have been well described and categorized and can be associated with other complex and life-threatening congenital anomalies. The classification of appendiceal duplications includes type A, an appendix with a common base, single cecum, and bifurcated distal portion; type B, two separate appendices with distinct bases arising from a single cecum; and type C, two cecal structures, each with its own single appendix (12,13). The type C anomaly is always associated with other organ duplications and often necessitates extensive operative correction in infancy; a type B variant is also associated with other systemic anomalies (12). However, the majority of type B and all type A duplications are found incidentally or during operation for suspected appendicitis in older children and adults.

FUNCTION

The exact role of the appendix is uncertain. However, rather than simply representing a vestigial, functionless structure, the abundant quantity of organized lymphoid tissue suggests involvement in mucosal immunity (15). It has been suggested that B lymphocytes derived from the appendix migrate and populate distant sites of the gastrointestinal tract lamina propria and evolve in these widespread foci into functional immunoglobulin (Ig)A-secreting plasma cells (15,16). In this role, the appendix can both attenuate potentially harmful immunoglobulin responses and enhance regional mucosal immunity (16).

NORMAL HISTOLOGY OF THE APPENDIX

The histologic composition of the appendix is similar to that of the large bowel. The four layers, from its luminal to external surface, include the mucosa, submucosa, muscularis externa (or propria), and serosa. The distinctive features of the appendix are emphasized.

Mucosal Architecture and Design

A single layer of surface epithelium covers the luminal aspect of the appendiceal mucosa. This overlies the lamina propria within which crypts, or intestinal glands, contiguous with the surface epithelial cells are irregularly dispersed (Figure 26.1). The lamina propria is a cellular layer with an abundant migratory cell component and prominent, often

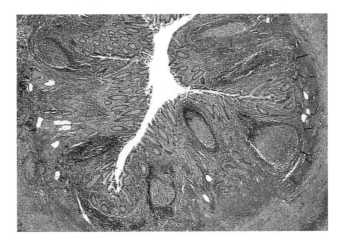

Figure 26.1 Low-magnification view of a cross section of the vermiform appendix. The irregular (stellate) lumen is lined by a single layer of surface epithelium. The remainder of the mucosa (crypts, surrounding lamina propria, and the rather inconspicuous muscularis mucosae) surrounds this surface epithelial layer. Note the characteristic lymphoid nodules within the lamina propria that also extend into the submucosa.

confluent, lymphoid aggregates. In contrast to the scattered lymphoid nodules within the large bowel proper, the appendix, particularly in young individuals, contains abundant and organized lymphoid structures spread around its entire luminal circumference. These lymphoid nodules often distort the luminal contour (9,17). The outermost component and limit of the mucosa is the muscularis mucosae. This slender fibromuscular band is poorly developed in the appendix and often focally deficient.

Surface Epithelium

Several different cell types comprise the surface epithelium. A prominent cell that can be identified at the light microscopic level is tall and columnar with eosinophilic cytoplasm, and it has a round, basally located nucleus (Figure 26.2). These cells represent several distinct cell types that can be differentiated at the ultrastructural level, including "senescent" mucous cells, so-called absorptive cells, and membranous or M cells (18–21). Goblet cells with distinctive apical mucin droplets surrounded by eosinophilic cytoplasm and undermined by an attenuated basal nucleus intermix with the columnar cells (Figure 26.2). The goblet cell apical mucin droplet contains both periodic acid-Schiff (PAS)-positive neutral mucin and Alcian blue–positive acid sulfomucin. This combination results in the formation of a blue-purple color in a mixed Alcian blue/PAS stain (19,22) (Figure 26.3). Overlying lymphoid aggregates, as in other portions of the small

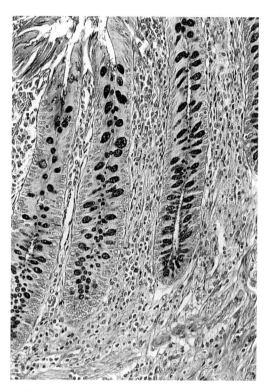

Figure 26.3 Because goblet cells contain both neutral and acid mucopolysaccharides, their apical mucin droplets stain blue-purple with the mixed Alcian blue/PAS preparation.

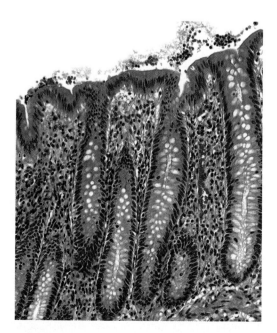

Figure 26.2 The surface epithelium is composed of a single layer of predominantly columnar cells with rare interspersed goblet cells. The crypt linings have a similar cellular composition but contain more goblet cells.

and large bowel, is a specialized or follicle-associated epithelium that is distinct from the surrounding surface epithelium. It characteristically has fewer goblet cells, and many of the columnar cells are of the M-cell type (22) (Figure 26.4). The M cell, a specialized epithelial cell, assists in luminal transport of antigens into the epithelium for appropriate immunologic processing (23,24); M cells are columnar in shape with an attenuated brush border; several lymphocytes are often seen deforming their dependent cytoplasm. Definitive characterization rests on ultrastructural examination, which shows apical cytoplasmic vesicles and shortened microvilli or microfolds (21,23). Because circumferentially distributed organized lymphoid aggregates and lymphoid tissue are prominent in the normal appendix, the specialized follicle-associated epithelium often lines the majority of the appendiceal lumen. Thus, functionally, the surface epithelium is probably primarily involved in antigen processing, as well as in forming a barrier to luminal contents. The luminal surface is also the site where senescent cells are sloughed into the lumen (19,20). Scattered endocrine cells can be seen within the surface epithelium but are more abundant in the underlying crypts. Migratory T and B lymphocytes can be found anywhere within the surface epithelium (25,26) but are more abundant in the follicle-associated epithelium (Figure 26.4).

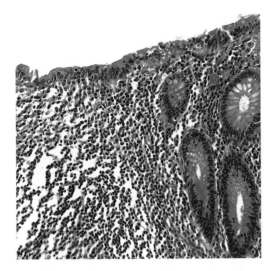

Figure 26.4 Surface epithelium overlying a lymphoid aggregate composed solely of tall columnar cells without intermixed goblet cells. Ultrastructurally, most of these would be classified as membranous or M cells. Note the increased numbers of intraepithelial lymphocytes between the individual columnar cells. Directly beneath the epithelium is the dome region of the lymphoid nodule. The apical portion of the germinal center with surrounding mantle zone is present near the bottom of the micrograph.

Crypt Epithelium

In contrast to the colon, where crypts line up evenly like test tubes in a rack, appendiceal crypts are more irregular in shape, length, and distribution (27). In areas with abundant lymphoid tissue or lymphoid aggregates, crypts are typically absent (28) (Figure 26.5).

Several different cell types line the crypts. The goblet and columnar cell variants discussed above are the most abundant (Figures 26.2, 26.6). Undifferentiated stem cells are scattered about but are inconspicuous. These are typically located at the crypt base, rest on the basement membrane, and do not extend to the crypt lumen; they are best identified by ultrastructural means (19). Isolated or clustered endocrine cells are seen along the crypt epithelium. Their appearance varies from a flask-shaped cell with a narrow strip of apical cytoplasm contiguous with the surface to a spindle-shaped cell with no luminal connection (29,30). Although some endocrine cells can be recognized on hematoxylin and eosin (H&E)–stained sections by their eosinophilic, infranuclear granules (31) (Figure 26.6),

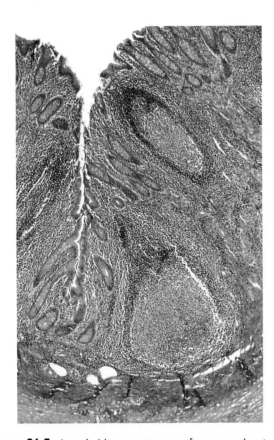

Figure 26.5 Lymphoid aggregates are often a prominent component within the appendiceal mucosa. Note the absence of crypts in the region of the lymphoid nodules and the distortion of surrounding crypts. This is a normal finding in the appendix and is similar to the alteration associated with isolated lymphoid aggregates in the colon.

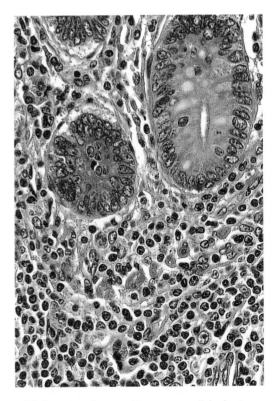

Figure 26.6 Crypts lying within a normocellular lamina propria. The round or ovoid crypts are lined predominantly by eosinophilic columnar cells and goblet cells. A single endocrine cell (containing infranuclear eosinophilic granules) is present at the base of each crypt. The lamina propria contains plasma cells, lymphocytes, and scattered eosinophils. Note the polygonal cells with abundant eosinophilic cytoplasm within the lamina propria. These are the subepithelial (laminal propria) endocrine cells that are often found near the crypt bases.

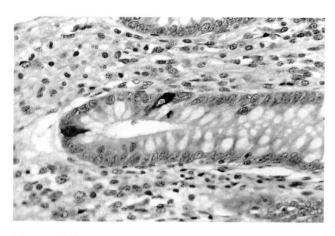

Figure 26.7 Scattered endocrine cells within the epithelium of an appendiceal crypt highlighted with antichromogranin. Intense red-brown cytoplasmic staining is evident in these endocrine cells.

definitive identification rests on immunohistologic analysis for chromogranin (or other pan-reactive neuroendocrine marker) (Figure 26.7) or ultrastructural analysis, which discloses neurosecretory granules within their cytoplasm. More specific immunohistologic methods show that endocrine cells within the appendiceal epithelium contain a variety of amine and polypeptide substances, including serotonin, substance P, somatostatin, and enteroglucagon (32). Paneth's cells also can be found in the crypt bases within the normal appendix in nearly 96% of specimens (33–35). This cell has a basally situated, round nucleus with a conspicuous nucleolus and abundant eosinophilic supranuclear granules (Figure 26.8); their function remains unknown, but they probably play a role in microbial regulation (33).

Intraepithelial lymphocytes occur within the crypt epithelium (36,37), but neutrophils and plasma cells are not normal constituents of either epithelial compartment. Rarely, gastric, ileal, or esophageal squamous-type mucosa can be seen interrupting the normal appendiceal lining; some recognize these as true heterotopias (38–40).

The crypt functions in cell production and renewal because all cells of both epithelial compartments originate from the crypt's stem cells. Most of these cells travel to the surface epithelium, where they are subsequently sloughed intraluminally; the exception (Paneth's cell) remains in the crypt base (36,37). It is believed that apoptosis within the crypt probably functions to regulate cell migration toward the surface; however, it is uncertain whether this type of cell death is responsible for epithelial cell loss into the lumen (41).

Subepithelial Basement Membrane

A slender zone separates the epithelial compartments from the lamina propria and is composed of collagen and other matrix components (42). The subepithelial basement membrane stabilizes the epithelial layers. A PAS stain can be used to highlight this layer, which measures only microns in thickness (20,42) (Figure 26.3).

Lamina Propria

The lamina propria, the central layer of the mucosa, surrounds the crypts and forms a connective tissue framework around them. Its structural components are collagen and elastic fibers and associated fibroblasts intermingled with blood capillaries, lymphatics, and nerve fibers (18–20). As in the large bowel, its migratory cell component consists primarily of plasma cells and T lymphocytes, along with scattered macrophages, eosinophils, B lymphocytes, and mast cells (18,26,43) (Figures 26.6, 26.8). However, depending on an individual's age, a varying number of organized lymphoid nodules distort the lamina proprial architecture. These lymphoid aggregates can extend beneath the muscularis mucosae into the underlying submucosa (Figures 26.1, 26.5), are often confluent, and appear similar in composition and function to the Peyer's patches of the small bowel (21). As in Peyer's patches (see Chapter 24), this lymphoid network of the appendix is compartmentalized into (a) follicle, (b) dome, (c) interfollicular (or parafollicular) region, and (d) follicle-associated epithelium (44–46) (Figure 26.9). The follicle has, in most cases, a germinal center containing a polymorphic cellular population of small and large B lymphocytes in various stages of maturation, occasional CD4+ T-helper cells, and tingible body macrophages; these reactive centers invariably contain mitoses (15,45–47) (Figure 26.10). Immediately surrounding the germinal center is the mantle zone, a darkly staining cuff of small, round B lymphocytes. Overlying the

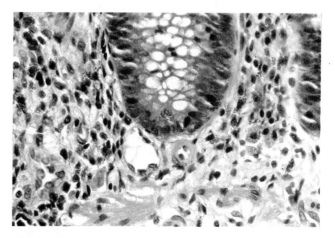

Figure 26.8 Appendiceal crypt disclosing Paneth's cell (at its base) with characteristic supranuclear eosinophilic granules. The surrounding lamina propria has a conspicuous, albeit normal, quantity of eosinophils. Also, note the golden brown, granular pigment within the macrophages, which is characteristic of melanosis.

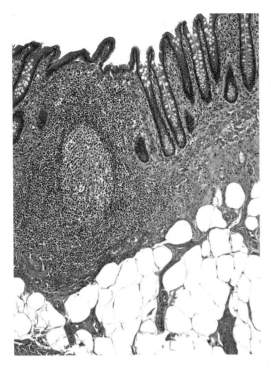

Figure 26.9 Characteristic lymphoid nodule within lamina propria of appendix. A germinal center forms the "core" of the follicle and is surrounded, at least in part, by a mantle zone of small round lymphocytes. Between the overlying epithelium and the mantle is the dome, which contains a mixed cellular population of lymphocytes, plasma cells, and macrophages. A portion of the parafollicular area (T-lymphocyte zone) is seen. Lymphatic and blood vessels are seen beneath the lymphoid nodule in the underlying superficial submucosa.

lymphoid aggregate and beneath the epithelium is the dome region (mixed cell zone), which is composed of a heterogeneous population of cells including B and T lymphocytes, macrophages, and occasional plasma cells (21,46). Both the lymphoid aggregate and the dome region are supported by a structural framework provided by dendritic reticulum cells and their processes (16,47). A prominent collagenous network and closely associated lymphatic vessels surround and define the lymphoid nodule (16). This collagenous/fibrous border is contiguous with the connective tissue framework of the interfollicular zones and adjacent lamina propria (16). The zone surrounding a single lymphoid nodule (parafollicular region) and the area between confluent lymphoid aggregates (the interfollicular region) consist predominantly of T lymphocytes (46) (Figure 26.11). Moreover, the ratio of T-helper/inducer (CD4+) to T-suppressor/cytotoxic (CD8+) lymphocytes is normally about 8:1 in these T-lymphocyte–rich areas (46). Finally, as detailed previously, the overlying epithelium is specialized and distinct from the usual surface epithelium.

The immunophenotypic cellular composition of the appendiceal mucosa is different from the colon. Although the quantity of lymphoid and plasma cells containing IgA and

IgM is similar in both, IgG-containing cells are more abundant in the appendix (15,46) (Figure 26.12). In fact, nearly 50% of the those along the follicle borders, including the dome region, are IgG immunoreactive, whereas IgA-containing cells are more abundant in distant lamina proprial sites (15).

Lymphoid tissue, although a characteristic feature of the appendix, varies in quantity with age. The newborn's appendix contains scant or no lymphoid tissue. With increasing age the lymphoid nodules accumulate, peaking in the first decade (17,48). Lymphoid aggregates then steadily diminish in quantity throughout the remainder of life. However, appendices excised incidentally from middle-aged adults can still occasionally show a prominent organized lymphoid component (10). In contrast, lymphoid nodules and associated lymphocytes can be scant in the central obliterative form of appendiceal neuroma (fibrous obliteration of the appendiceal lumen) and occasionally in appendices removed from normal patients at any age (10). Thus, a great range of normal variation exists in the appendix with respect to its lymphoid content.

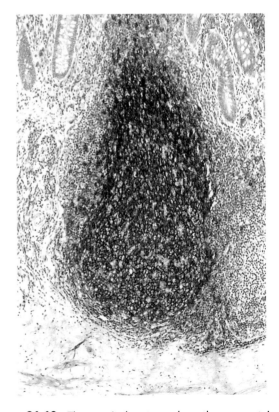

Figure 26.10 The germinal center and mantle zone contain predominantly B-lymphocytes. A pan–B-lymphocyte immunomarker, L26, discloses this characteristic immunophenotype. Scattered macrophages and occasional T lymphocytes (see Figure 26.11) are also normally found within the germinal center. Only scattered B-lymphocytes are present within the interfollicular zone and adjacent lamina propria.

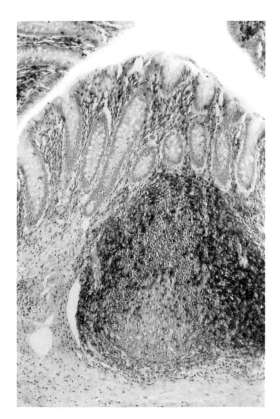

Figure 26.11 A pan–T-cell immunomarker, Leu-22 (CD43), disclosing the characteristic T-lymphocyte distribution within the appendiceal mucosa. The lamina propria and interfollicular regions (between lymphoid follicles) are normally populated by numerous T lymphocytes. There is a sprinkling of T lymphocytes within the germinal center; these are predominantly T-helper/inducer (CD4+) lymphocytes.

Histiocytes with intracellular golden-brown pigment (lipofuscin), not infrequently observed in the colonic mucosa, can also be found in the appendiceal lamina propria; this alteration results from anthracene-containing laxative abuse and has been termed melanosis coli when seen in the colon proper (9,49) (Figure 26.8). Interestingly, this pigmentation is a result of apoptosis induced by anthraquinones (41).

The lamina propria of the appendix contains a well-developed mucosal nervous plexus that is different from the more prominent submucosal and myenteric plexuses. Although all contain neurons (ganglion cells), Schwann cells, and neural processes (axons and neuropil), only the mucosal plexus contains endocrine (neurosecretory) cells. As a consequence, this network has been termed the mucosal neuroendocrine complex (50). These complexes, located just beneath the crypts, are composed of collections of endocrine cells and seen on H&E–stained preparations as polygonal cells with pale granular cytoplasm (Figure 26.6), often intimately associated with spindled Schwann cells, neural processes, and occasional neurons. These

collections, or neuroendocrine ganglia, are interconnected by neural fibers that can be highlighted immunohistologically with antibody preparations to neuron-specific enolase and, in a subset, to substance P (32); anti–S-100 also can outline this network as it marks the accompanying Schwann cells. The mucosal plexus also communicates with other neural networks of the enteric nervous system (50–53). The subepithelial endocrine cells are not always conspicuous but can be highlighted using general neuroendocrine immunomarkers, such as antichromogranin (Figure 26.13) and antineuron-specific enolase, or by using electron microscopy (54,55). Most of these cells have been shown by specific immunohistologic analysis to contain serotonin (51,55). The mucosal neuroendocrine complex is believed to modulate neural communication, through serotonin mediators, between the epithelium and the deeper submucosal and intermuscular plexuses (55). Interestingly, because most appendiceal carcinoids are biphasic, consisting of an admixture of endocrine cells and S-100+ Schwann cells (similar to the architecture of the mucosal neuroendocrine complex), the majority of these appendiceal neoplasms are believed to be derived from these lamina propria endocrine cells rather than from the epithelium-based ones (51).

Muscularis Mucosae

The muscularis mucosae is a thin band of fibromuscular tissue separating the lamina propria and mucosal epithelium from the underlying submucosa. It characteristically forms a continuous layer in the large bowel (18); but, in the appendix, the muscularis mucosae is attenuated, poorly developed, and often focally absent, particularly in the region of penetrating lymphoid aggregates (28,56) (Figure 26.14). In these areas the muscularis mucosae may exist solely as isolated smooth muscle cells in the underlying submucosa (56).

Submucosa

The submucosa separates the mucosa from the muscularis externa. Its loose architectural framework contains a meshwork of collagenous and elastic fibers and associated fibroblasts (Figure 26.15). The submucosa can also contain inconspicuous migratory cells, such as macrophages, lymphoid and plasma cells, and mast cells, along with adipose tissue (17,57) (Figure 26.14). The morphologic appearance of the appendiceal submucosa and its primary role in maintaining structure are similar throughout the gastrointestinal tract (57). Arterioles, venules, blood capillaries, and lymphatic vessels are a prominent component of the submucosa (7,18) (Figure 26.15). Lymphatic vessels (or sinuses) are most prominent just beneath the bases of lymphoid aggregates (16). Neural structures, particularly Meissner's

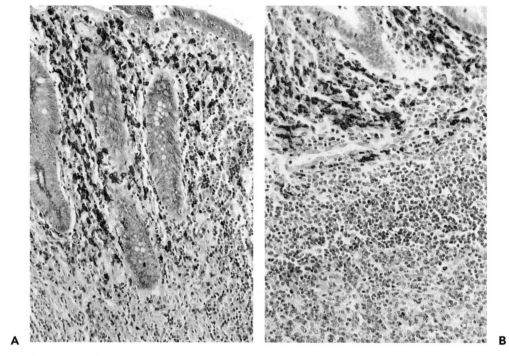

Figure 26.12 A. Immunohistologic preparation showing abundant IgA-containing plasma cells within lamina propria; the epithelial staining is a consequence of the secretory nature of the IgA molecule. **B.** Abundant IgG-bearing cells are characteristically located within the dome region and along the margins of lymphoid nodules in the appendix.

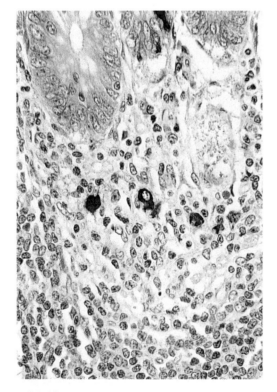

Figure 26.13 Antichromogranin highlights the subepithelial (lamina propria) endocrine cells beneath the crypts. These are more prominent and abundant in the appendix than in any other portion of gastrointestinal tract. Note also the epithelial-based endocrine cell in the overlying crypt.

plexus, are also conspicuous (Figure 26.16). This plexus consists of ganglia, collections of neurons (ganglion cells) with associated neuronal processes, and Schwann cells that interconnect, creating a neural network throughout the submucosal layer (58,59). The ganglion cell is large and oval with abundant eosinophilic cytoplasm; its vesicular nucleus is often eccentrically placed and contains a prominent nucleolus. The surrounding spindle and wavy Schwann cell component of the ganglia is less conspicuous on H&E–stained preparations but can be highlighted with anti–S-100 (Figure 26.16).

Muscularis Externa, Subserosal Region, and the Serosa

The thick smooth muscle layer lying between the submucosa and serosal portions of the appendix is the muscularis externa (or muscularis propria). It is separated into an inner circular layer and an outer longitudinal band (28). The individual smooth muscle cells are oval with blunted ends and form bundles of varying size. Occasionally, granular degeneration (eosinophilic cytoplasmic granularity) of individual or groups of smooth muscle cells is seen, particularly within the inner circular layer (56,60). Between the two muscle bands lies the myenteric (Auerbach's) plexus, which is similar morphologically and functionally to the previously described submucosal plexus of Meissner (59)

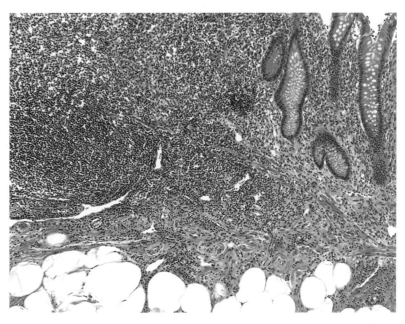

Figure 26.14 Characteristic focal deficiency of muscularis mucosae in region of lymphoid nodule. There is adipose tissue within the submucosa; this is a normal finding.

(Figure 26.17). Additionally, blood and lymphatic vessels and nerve fibers course through this muscular layer (16). Just external to the outer longitudinal smooth muscle layer is the subserosal region, consisting of loose connective tissue and ramifying blood vessels, lymphatics, and nerves. The exteriormost surface, or serosa, is lined by a single layer of cuboidal mesothelial cells that overlies a slender band of fibrous tissue. Only the attachment of the fibrofatty mesoappendix lacks a serosa (1).

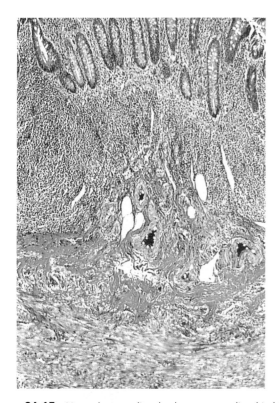

Figure 26.15 Normal appendiceal submucosa outlined in blue, highlighting its prominent collagenous framework. Numerous vascular spaces are also present within this layer. The mucosa (crypts) is *above*, and the inner circular layer of the muscularis externa is *below* (Masson's trichrome).

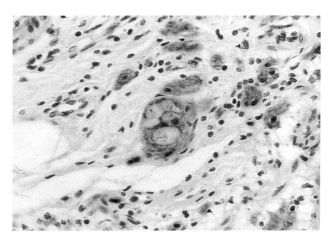

Figure 26.16 Submucosal neural network outlined with anti–S-100. A single ganglion of Meissner's plexus is at the center; the ganglion cells (neurons) have abundant pale cytoplasm, a large eccentric nucleus, and show no immunoreactivity. The Schwann cells of the ganglion and those ensheathing the neuronal processes of the remainder of the plexus are highlighted.

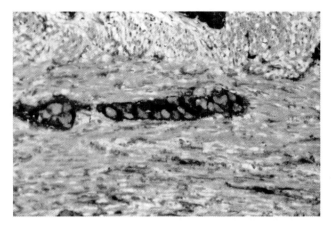

Figure 26.17 Anti–S-100 highlighting Schwann cells of the neural network of the muscularis externa and a ganglion of the myenteric (Auerbach's) plexus.

SPECIAL CONSIDERATIONS

Normal Variation of Mucosal Inflammation Versus Acute Appendicitis

Acute appendicitis is usually characterized by an abundant neutrophilic and eosinophilic infiltrate within the mucosa, submucosa, and often muscularis externa with at least focal mucosal ulceration; frequently suppurative inflammation extends into and through the appendiceal wall (9,10). However, the changes seen in early appendicitis can be quite minimal, and criteria considered sufficient to diagnose early acute appendicitis have varied (9,10,61–66). We agree that "reactive" lymphoid follicles are not a reliable sign of acute appendicitis (9). Focal collections of neutrophils within the lumen and lamina propria have been considered nondiagnostic by some investigators because many "incidental" appendectomy specimens contain these changes (9,10,61,64–66). However, we believe that if care is taken to recognize marginating neutrophils and early mucosal migration of these acute inflammatory cells (i.e., a result of the operative procedure alone), then other collections of neutrophils within the mucosa or intraluminal pus reflect stasis, infection, and changes of early appendicitis (62–64). Whether acute appendicitis becomes chronic or whether it can be recognized in a chronic state has long been debated (63). Fibrous obliteration of the appendiceal lumen is probably not a sequelae of acute appendicitis (53). However, prominent fibrosis, a marked chronic inflammatory cell infiltrate within the wall, and granulation tissue are abnormal and suggest an organizing appendicitis (9). Occasional specimens exhibit infiltration of the appendiceal wall by eosinophilic leukocytes with no other apparent abnormality (10). This change could reflect appendicitis elsewhere in the specimen that was not sampled; however, it remains possible that an infiltrate composed predominantly of eosinophils could represent appendicitis in a resolving phase or be a manifestation of eosinophilic gastroenteritis (62,67,68).

Obliteration of the Appendiceal Lumen (Appendiceal Neuromas)

Obliteration of the appendiceal lumen with absence of the lining mucosa and underlying crypts frequently occurs and has a prevalence in surgical specimens of nearly 30% (9,53). This process usually affects the distal aspect or just the tip, but occasionally the entire lumen is obliterated. This process is often termed fibrous obliteration; however, more recent studies have shown that in some cases the occlusive proliferation appears to be predominantly neurogenic (32,53,69). Other diagnostic terms have been proposed, including neurogenic appendicopathy and appendiceal neuroma. The typical appendiceal neuroma, or the central obliterative form, is composed of a collection of spindle cells in a loose myxoid background with varying amounts of collagen, fat, and chronic inflammatory cells (Figures 26.18–26.19). This typically occludes the lumen and blends imperceptibly with the surrounding submucosa (53). The involved segment usually lacks a mucosa, and lymphoid follicles are typically not seen (20). Immunostaining for neuron-specific enolase and S-100 highlights the spindle cells and identifies their neuronal (axons) and perineuronal (Schwann cell) nature, respectively (32,53) (Figure 26.20). Moreover, endocrine cells visualized with antineuron-specific enolase and antichromogranin (Figure 26.21) occur in many of the cases, usually intermingled with the other elements; serotonin and somatostatin have been identified in some of these endocrine cells by immunohistologic methods (32,53). Ultrastructural analysis discloses neuronal

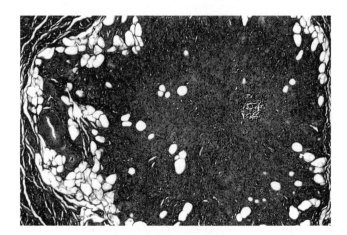

Figure 26.18 Obliteration of appendiceal lumen. The occlusive proliferation is composed of spindled cells within a collagenous and myxoid background, along with scattered adipocytes. A focus of chronic inflammatory cells is also present.

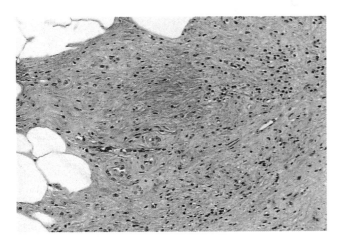

Figure 26.19 High magnification of Figure 26.18 showing spindled cell proliferation in an eosinophilic, fibromyxoid background.

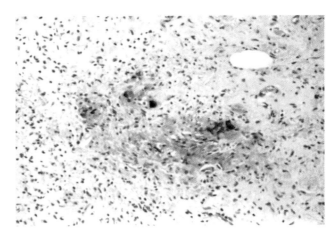

Figure 26.21 Scattered endocrine (neurosecretory) cells are evident within the obliterative luminal proliferation as highlighted by antichromogranin; specific immunomarkers show some of these to contain serotonin or somatostatin.

processes, Schwann cells, and cells with neurosecretory granules (endocrine cells) corroborating the immunostaining results (53).

Another variant of this entity, the intramucosal appendiceal neuroma, primarily affects the mucosa, causing no luminal obliteration. Although morphologically similar to the central obliterative form, this intramucosal variant deceptively expands the lamina propria, separates the crypts, and replaces the usual prominent migratory cell population (53) (Figure 26.22). Immunostaining with S-100 can be helpful in visualizing these more subtle changes.

Both of these entities are believed to be proliferative rather than involutional, progressing through consecutive stages of growth, regression, and finally an end-stage with fibrosis (53,70). Overlapping features are therefore expected with varied admixtures of neurogenic components, collagen, and fat. It is hypothesized that associated endocrine cell hyperplasia, often found in adjacent uninvolved appendiceal

segments, may be responsible for painful stimuli mimicking typical acute appendicitis (53). However, appendiceal neuromas are often found in specimens removed at incidental appendectomy.

Mucocele of the Appendix

The term *mucocele* has been used to describe a dilated appendiceal lumen filled with mucin (71). *Mucocele*, however, should not be used as a specific diagnostic term because the condition is almost always caused by a neoplastic proliferation, either a mucinous cystadenoma or mucinous cystadenocarcinoma (63,71,72). Characteristic architectural and cytologic features should permit identification of these entities.

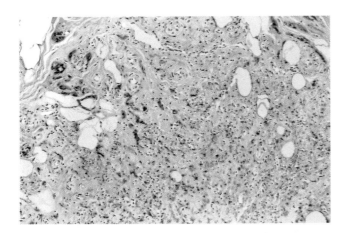

Figure 26.20 Prominent neurogenic (Schwann cell) component highlighted by anti–S-100 within the obliterated lumen.

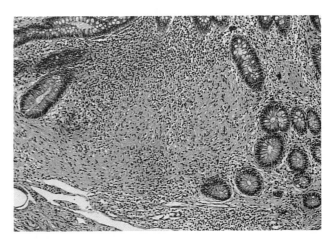

Figure 26.22 Intramucosal variant of appendiceal neuroma. The characteristic subtle spindle cell (schwannian) proliferation expands the lamina propria and separates the crypts. A diminished number of migratory cells is evident in this area.

Dissection and Processing Techniques

Gross dissection and processing of the appendix are generally straightforward. Routine description of size, appearance, and any unusual lesions should be recorded. Luminal patency should be assessed (i.e., obliteration or dilatation) along with the focality and regional distribution of any changes. The tip should be closely inspected for carcinoid tumors because these commonly occur in the distal portion of the appendix (9,73). When grossly evident, they often appear as bulbous, tan-yellow expansions or nodules. However, a routine section of the tip is standard at most institutions and will identify small, grossly unidentifiable tumors (9). The common recommendation of a longitudinal section of the distal several centimeters is often difficult to orient, and we prefer a cross section of the tip. In the usual specimen, 1-cm serial cross-sectioning is performed along the entire length of the appendix. Two cross sections, one from the middle and one of the proximal line of resection, should be submitted for embedding. Because neoplastic proliferations of the appendix (e.g., mucinous cystadenoma/cystadenocarcinoma, carcinoid tumor, and its variants) are not infrequently discovered incidentally during microscopic evaluation of the specimen, we routinely sample the margin of resection. Otherwise, it could be difficult to reconstruct the gross specimen in an attempt to assess the adequacy of excision. The choice of a fixative is not crucial. However, we prefer the superior nuclear detail afforded by Hollande's solution over routine 4% formaldehyde solution. Modifications of dissection and processing may be necessary in certain situations.

REFERENCES

1. Williams PL, Warwick R, Dyson M, Bannister LH, eds. *Gray's Anatomy of the Human Body.* 37th ed. New York: Churchill Livingstone; 1989.
2. Buschard K, Kjaeldgaard A. Investigation and analysis of the position, fixation, length, and embryology of the vermiform appendix. *Acta Chir Scand* 1973;139:293–298.
3. Wakeley CPG. The position of the vermiform appendix as ascertained by an analysis of 10,000 cases. *J Anat* 1933;67:277–283.
4. Thorek P. *Anatomy and Surgery.* 3rd ed. New York: Springer-Verlag; 1985.
5. Abramson DJ. Vermiform appendix located within the cecal wall. Anomalies and bizarre locations. *Dis Colon Rectum* 1983;26: 386–389.
6. Hollinshead WH, Rosse C. *Textbook of Anatomy.* 4th ed. New York: Harper & Row; 1985.
7. Parks DA, Jacobson ED. Physiology of the splanchnic circulation. *Arch Intern Med* 1985;145:1278–1281.
8. Solanke TF. The blood supply of the vermiform appendix in Nigerians. *J Anat* 1968;102(pt 2):353–361.
9. Gray GF Jr, Wackym PA. Surgical pathology of the vermiform appendix. In: Sommers SC, Rosen PP, Fechner RE, eds. *Pathology Annual.* Part 2. Norwalk, CT: Appleton-Century-Croft; 1986:111–144.
10. Butler C. Surgical pathology of acute appendicitis. *Hum Pathol* 1981;12:870–878.
11. Moore KL. The Developing Human: *Clinically Oriented Embryology.* 3rd ed. Philadelphia: WB Saunders; 1982.
12. Bluett MK, Halter SA, Salhany KE, O'Leary JP. Duplication of the appendix mimicking adenocarcinoma of the colon. *Arch Surg* 1987;122:817–820.
13. Wallbridge PH. Double appendix. *Br J Surg* 1962;50:346–347.
14. Tinckler LF. Triple appendix vermiformis—a unique case. *Br J Surg* 1968;55:79–81.
15. Bjerke K, Brandtzaeg P, Rognum TO. Distribution of immunoglobulin producing cells is different in normal human appendix and colon mucosa. *Gut* 1986;27:667–674.
16. Bockman DE. Functional histology of appendix. *Arch Histol Jpn* 1983;46:271–292.
17. Hwang JMS, Krumbhaar EB. The amount of lymphoid tissue of the human appendix and its weight at different age periods. *Am J Med Sci* 1940;199:75–83.
18. Hamilton SR. Structure of the colon. *Scand J Gastroenterol Suppl* 1984;93:13–23.
19. Shamsuddin AM, Phelps PC, Trump BF. Human large intestinal epithelium: light microscopy, histochemistry, and ultrastructure. *Hum Pathol* 1982;13:790–803.
20. Levine DS, Haggitt RC. Normal histology of the colon. *Am J Surg Pathol* 1989;13:966–984.
21. Bockman DE, Cooper MD. Early lymphoepithelial relationships in human appendix: a combined light- and electron-microscopic study. *Gastroenterology* 1975;68(pt 1):1160–1168.
22. Filipe MI. Mucins in the human gastrointestinal epithelium: a review. *Invest Cell Pathol* 1979;2:195–216.
23. Owen RL, Jones AL. Epithelial cell specialization within human Peyer's patches: an ultrastructural study of intestinal lymphoid follicles. *Gastroenterology* 1974;66:189–203.
24. Wolf JL, Bye WA. The membranous epithelial (M) cell and the mucosal immune system. *Annu Rev Med* 1984;35:95–112.
25. Dobbins WO III. Human intestinal intraepithelial lymphocytes. *Gut* 1986;27:972–985.
26. Bartnik W, ReMine SG, Chiba M, Thayer WR, Shorter RG. Isolation and characterization of colonic intraepithelial and lamina proprial lymphocytes. *Gastroenterology* 1980;78(pt 1):976–985.
27. Fawcett DW. *Bloom and Fawcett: A Textbook of Histology.* 11th ed. Philadelphia: WB Saunders; 1986.
28. Neutra MR, Padykula HA. The gastrointestinal tract. In: Weiss L, ed. *Modern Concepts of Gastrointestinal Histology.* New York: Elsevier; 1984:658–706.
29. Lewin KJ. The endocrine cells of the gastrointestinal tract. The normal endocrine cells and their hyperplasias. Part 1. In: Sommers SC, Rosen PP, Fechner RE, eds. *Pathology Annual.* Norwalk, CT: Appleton-Century-Croft; 1986:1–27.
30. Sjolund K, Sanden G, Hakanson R, Sundler F. Endocrine cells in human intestine: an immunocytochemical study. *Gastroenterology* 1983;85:1120–1130.
31. Millikin PD. Eosinophilic argentaffin cells in the human appendix. *Arch Pathol* 1974;98:393–395.
32. Hofler H, Kasper M, Heitz PU. The neuroendocrine system of normal human appendix, ileum and colon, and in neurogenic appendicopathy. *Virchows Arch A Pathol Anat Histopathol* 1983;399: 127–140.
33. Sandow MJ, Whitehead R. The Paneth cell. *Gut* 1979;20:420–431.
34. Geller SA, Thung SN. Morphologic unity of Paneth cells. *Arch Pathol Lab Med* 1983;107:476–479.
35. Vestfrid MA, Suarez JE. Paneth's cells in the human appendix. A statistical study. *Acta Anat (Basel)* 1977;97:347–350.
36. Eastwood GL. Gastrointestinal epithelial renewal. *Gastroenterology* 1977;72(pt 1):962–975.
37. Lipkin M. Proliferation and differentiation of normal and diseased gastrointestinal cells. In: Johnson LR, ed. *Physiology of the Gastrointestinal Tract.* 2nd ed. New York: Raven Press; 1987: 255–284.
38. Aubrey DA. Gastric heterotopia in the vermiform appendix. *Arch Surg* 1970;101:628–629.
39. Ashley DJ. Aberrant mucosa in the vermiform appendix. *Br J Surg* 1958;45:372–373.
40. Droga BW, Levine S, Barber JJ. Heterotopic gastric and esophageal tissue in the vermiform appendix. *Am J Clin Pathol* 1963;40: 190–193.

41. Watson AJ. Necrosis and apoptosis in the gastrointestinal tract. *Gut* 1995;37:165–167.

42. Gledhill A, Cole FM. Significance of basement membrane thickening in the human colon. *Gut* 1984;25:1085–1088.

43. Heatley RV. The gastrointestinal mast cell. *Scand J Gastroenterol* 1983;18:449–453.

44. Tomasi TB Jr. Mechanisms of immune regulation at mucosal surfaces. *Rev Infect Dis* 1983;5(suppl 4):S784–S792.

45. Kagnoff MF. Immunology and disease of the gastrointestinal tract. In: Sleisenger M, Fordtran J, eds. *Gastrointestinal Disease.* 4th ed. Philadelphia: WB Saunders; 1989:114–144.

46. Spencer J, Finn T, Isaacson PG. Gut associated lymphoid tissue: a morphological and immunocytochemical study of the human appendix. *Gut* 1985;26:672–679.

47. van der Valk P, Meijer CJ. The histology of reactive lymph nodes. *Am J Surg Pathol* 1987;11:866–882.

48. Berry RJ, Lack LA. The vermiform appendix of man, and structural changes therein coincident with age. *Anat Physiol* 1906;40:247–256.

49. Walker NI, Bennett RE, Axelsen RA. Melanosis coli: a consequence of anthraquinone-induced apoptosis of colonic epithelial cells. *Am J Pathol* 1988;131:465–476.

50. Papadaki L, Rode J, Dhillon AP, Dische FE. Fine structure of a neuroendocrine complex in the mucosa of the appendix. *Gastroenterology* 1983;84:490–497.

51. Lundqvist M, Wilander E. Subepithelial neuroendocrine cells and carcinoid tumours of the human small intestine and appendix. A comparative immunohistochemical study with regard to serotonin, neuron-specific enolase and S-100 protein reactivity. *J Pathol* 1986;148:141–147.

52. Millikin PD. Extraepithelial enterochromaffin cells and Schwann cells in the human appendix. *Arch Pathol Lab Med* 1983;107:189–194.

53. Stanley MW, Cherwitz D, Hagen K, Snover DC. Neuromas of the appendix. A light-microscopic, immunohistochemical and electron-microscopic study of 20 cases. *Am J Surg Pathol* 1986;10:801–815.

54. Facer P, Bishop AE, Lloyd RV, Wilson BS, Hennessy RJ, Polak JM. Chromogranin: a newly recognized marker of endocrine cells in the human gastrointestinal tract. *Gastroenterology* 1985;89:1366–1373.

55. Rode J, Dhillon AP, Papadaki L. Serotonin-immunoreactive cells in the lamina propria plexus of the appendix. *Hum Pathol* 1983;14:464–469.

56. Sobel HJ, Marquet E, Schwarz R. Granular degeneration of appendiceal smooth muscle. *Arch Pathol* 1971;92:427–432.

57. Lord MG, Valies P, Broughton AC. A morphologic study of the submucosa of the large intestine. *Surg Gynecol Obstet* 1977;145:55–60.

58. Gershon MD, Erde SM. The nervous system of the gut. *Gastroenterology* 1981;80:1571–1594.

59. Krishnamurthy S, Schuffler MD. Pathology of neuromuscular disorders of the small intestine and colon. *Gastroenterology* 1987;93:610–639.

60. Hausman R. Granular cells in musculature of the appendix. *Arch Pathol* 1963;75:360–372.

61. Pieper R, Kager L, Nasman P. Clinical significance of mucosal inflammation of the vermiform appendix. *Ann Surg* 1983;197:368–374.

62. Petras RE. Non-neoplastic intestinal diseases. In: Mills SE, ed. Sternberg's *Diagnostic Surgical Pathology,* 4th ed. Philadelphia: Lippincott Williams & Wilkins; 2004:1475–1541.

63. Morson BC, Dawson IMP, Day DW, Jass JR, Price AB, Williams GT. *Morson and Dawson's Gastrointestinal Pathology.* 3rd ed. Oxford: Blackwell Scientific; 1990.

64. Schenken JR, Anderson TR, Coleman FC. Acute focal appendicitis. *Am J Clin Pathol* 1956;26:352–359.

65. Campbell JS, Fournier P, Da Silva T. When is the appendix normal? A study of acute inflammations of the appendix apparent only upon histologic examination. *Can Med Assoc J* 1961;85:1155–1157.

66. Touloukian RJ, Trainer TD. Significance of focal inflammation of the appendix. *Surgery* 1964;56:942–944.

67. Johnstone JM, Morson BC. Eosinophilic gastroenteritis. *Histopathology* 1978;2:335–348.

68. Klein NC, Hargrove RL, Sleisenger MH, Jeffries GH. Eosinophilic gastroenteritis. *Medicine (Baltimore)* 1970;49:299–319.

69. Aubock L, Ratzenhofer M. "Extraepithelial enterochromaffin cell—nerve-fibre complexes" in the normal human appendix, and in neurogenic appendicopathy. *J Pathol* 1982;136:217–226.

70. Olsen BS, Holck S. Neurogenous hyperplasia leading to appendiceal obliteration: an immunohistochemical study of 237 cases. *Histopathology* 1987;11:843–849.

71. Qizilbash AH. Mucoceles of the appendix: their relationship to hyperplastic polyps, mucinous cystadenomas, and cystadenocarcinomas. *Arch Pathol* 1975;99:548–555.

72. Higa E, Rosai J, Pizzimbono CA, Wise L. Mucosal hyperplasia, mucinous cystadenoma, and mucinous cystadenocarcinoma of the appendix: a re-evaluation of appendiceal "mucocele." *Cancer* 1973;32:1525–1541.

73. Glasser CM, Bhagavan BS. Carcinoid tumors of the appendix. *Arch Pathol Lab Med* 1980;104:272–275.

Anal Canal

27

Claus Fenger

INTRODUCTION

The anal canal has a complex anatomy and histology, and new information still turns up with regard to its embryology, structure, function, and pathology. Unfortunately, much confusion continues about definitions and nomenclature. This chapter therefore includes a historical review and a discussion of the terms used for the different structures (1).

HISTORICAL REVIEW

Anal diseases and their treatment are mentioned as far back as the Egyptian papyri (2). Nevertheless, there are few early descriptions of anal anatomy. Of note is Galenos (130–200 AD), who compared the anus to a laced-up purse (3). The

first observations on the anal canal mucosa were published by Glisson (1597–1677) (4), who noted the anal valves. In 1717, Morgagni (5) mentioned the anal columns and included the now famous drawing in the *Adversaria* (Figure 27.1); in addition, it shows pronounced papillae. In 1727, Heister (6) described the smooth zone between the anal valves and the perianal skin; and, in 1732, Winslöw (7) described the semilunar lacunae between the valves and the bases of the anal columns.

The first exact microscopic description of the different epithelial zones in the anal canal was given by Robin and Cadiat in 1874 (8). The perianal apocrine glands were found by Gay in 1871 (9), and in 1878 Chiari introduced the theory of the anal sinus infection in the pathogenesis of anal fistulas (10). Hermann and Desfosses' (11) microscopic description of anal glands followed shortly afterward.

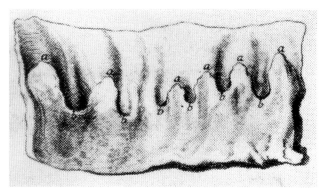

Figure 27.1 The anal canal as seen by Morgagni. Reprinted from: Morgagni GB. Adversaria anatomica omnia. Advers III Animadv. VI. Patavii, Italy: Josephus Cominus; 1717: 10–11.

In 1877 Hilton (12) introduced the term *white line* for the junction between the skin and the mucous membrane and corresponding to the linear interval between the internal and external sphincter muscle. In 1896, Stroud (13) introduced the term *pecten* for the smooth area between the anal valves and Hilton's white line. However, later investigators recommended that use of the term *Hilton's white line* should be discontinued because no anatomic feature identified it (14,15). Detailed macroscopic and stereomicroscopic investigations of surgical specimens of the anal canal have not shown any such structure (16,17).

The term *anal canal* was proposed by Symington in 1888 (18) for what had earlier been described as the third or perineal part of the rectum, that is, the part extending from the level of the pelvic floor backward and downward to the anal opening. This definition corresponds to the *surgical anal canal*, whereas the term *anatomic anal canal* has been used for the area between the line of anal valves and sinuses [dentate line (DL)] and the anal verge alone (Figure 27.2). The anal verge can be defined as the point (line) where the walls of the anal canal come in contact in their normal resting state (19).

As to embryology, Tourneux in 1888 (20) and Retterer in 1890 (21) wrote that the cloacal membrane was divided into anal and urogenital membranes by a descending septum, thus giving basis for the often quoted but never illustrated delusion that the DL is the site of a former anal membrane.

EMBRYOLOGY

In the early embryo (Carnegie stage 13, crown-rump length 5 mm), the primitive urogenital sinus and anorectal canal are separated by the urorectal septum and open into a common cloaca, which is closed at its ventral surface by the cloacal plate. As the embryo grows and its caudal curvature decreases, the distance between the urorectal septum and the cloacal plate decreases, but these two structures never fuse.

Due to apoptosis, the dorsal part of the cloacal plate gradually becomes more like a membrane, which ruptures about 49 days postfertilization (Carnegie stage 19, crown-rump length 16–18 mm). Soon after, a secondary occlusion of the anorectal canal occurs as a result of cell adhesion and formation of an epithelial "plug" at the level of the anal orifice. Recanalization takes place at 30 to 35 mm crown-rump length, again due to apoptosis. The cloaca itself does not contribute to the formation of the anus or rectum (22,23). The characteristic epithelium of the anal transitional zone is present already in the thirteenth week (Figure 27.3).

The prevalence of anal anomalies in Europe is 4 per 10,000 births, and two-thirds occur together with other anomalies. Most of the isolated anomalies are atresias with or without fistula, and 90% of these are located below the levator ani. The etiology to anal atresia is still under discussion (24).

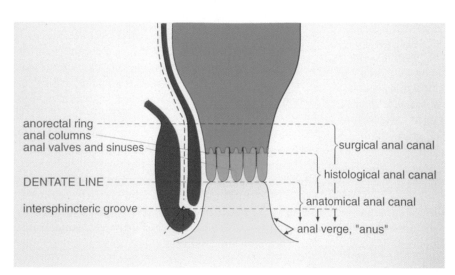

Figure 27.2 Schematic drawing of the anal canal showing the macroscopic landmarks. The "surgical" and "anatomical" anal canals have their lower border at the rather ill-defined anal verge, or anus. This point has sometimes been called the anal margin, whereas other authors have used this term for the same area as the anatomic anal canal. Hilton's "white line" was meant to be located at the intersphincteric groove; Stroud's "pecten" was the area between the dentate line and Hilton's line. The "histologic" anal canal begins at the irregular upper border of the anal transitional zone (compare to Figures 27.9–27.13).

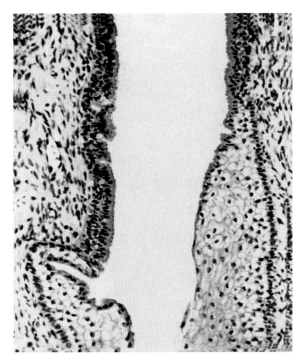

Figure 27.3 Longitudinal section through the middle of an anal canal in a 13-week-old fetus. Squamous epithelium is seen in the lower part; anal transitional zone with the characteristic epithelium is seen in the upper part (H&E).

NOMENCLATURE OF THE ANAL CANAL

It would seem natural to start with a definition of the anal canal; but, because there are several definitions and new terms are still introduced (25,26), a description of the anatomical landmarks and epithelial zones may be the best introduction to this never-ending discussion.

Official Terms

Official terms (27) for the structures seen on the anal canal surface include columnae anales, sinus anales, valvulae anales, linea pectinata, pecten analis, and linea anocutanea. However, the latter three terms are not generally accepted, and many synonyms have been used. Among the epithelial zones, only the anal transition(al) zone has got its own name.

When discussing anal nomenclature, one must always bear in mind that the terms *anal columns, valves,* and *sinuses,* and the line composed by the latter two structures are macroscopic landmarks. However, although they can be visualized by using macroscopic staining (28), the different zones in the anal canal are microscopic structures, and they do not correspond exactly to the macroscopic landmarks (16).

The most important macroscopic landmark is the line composed of the anal valves and sinuses and the bases of the anal columns (Figures 27.4–27.5). A list of names introduced for this line is given in Table 27.1 (1). Among these, the term *dentate line* is chosen by the International

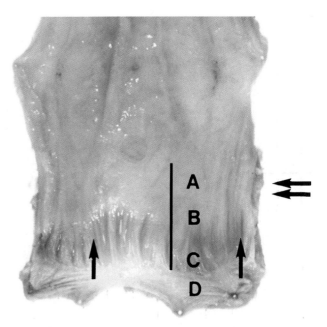

Figure 27.4 Autopsy specimen of the lower rectum and anal canal from an infant. The dentate line is composed of the bases of the well-defined anal columns. Only a narrow rim of perianal skin is at the bottom. The *black vertical line* indicates the extent of the anal canal, the *single arrows* the dentate line, and the *double arrows* the upper border of the anal transitional zone (formalin). (*A*, colorectal zone; *B*, anal transitional zone; *C*, squamous zone; *D*, perianal skin)

Union Against Cancer (UICC) and the World Health Organization (WHO) and is also widely used in textbooks (25,29,30,31,32). Anal valves and papillae are not present as often as reported in anatomy textbooks, and crypts and sinuses may be found over a larger area than compatible

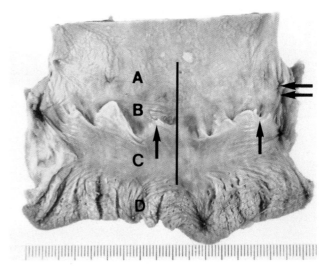

Figure 27.5 Surgical specimen of the lower rectum and anal canal from an adult. Here the dentate line is composed of anal sinuses, valves, and pronounced papillae, whereas the anal columns are nearly invisible. At the bottom, there is a broad rim of wrinkled perianal skin with hairs (formalin). (*Black vertical line*, extent of the anal canal; *single arrows*, the dentate line; *double arrows*, upper border of the anal transitional zone; *A*, colorectal zone; *B*, anal transitional zone; *C*, squamous zone; *D*, perianal skin)

TABLE 27.1

LIST OF TERMS INTRODUCED FOR THE LINE CORRESPONDING TO THE ANAL VALVES, PAPILLAE, AND SINUSES AND THE BASES OF THE ANAL COLUMNSᵃ

Cruveilhier	1843	Ligne sinueuse
Robin and Cadiat	1874	Ligne anale cutanée
Symington	1912	Mucocutaneous junction
		Pectinate line
Abel	1932	Dentate line
Goligher et al.	1955	Valvular line
Parks	1956	Crypt line
Morgan and Thompson	1956	Anorectal line
Walls	1958	Papillary line
Grobler	1977	Hilton's line

ᵃ For references, see Fenger C. The anal transitional zone. *Acta Pathol Microbiol Immunol Scand Suppl* 1987;289:1–42.

with the definition of a line. *Anorectal* and *anocutaneous* refer to special definitions of the anal canal. When no valves, columns, or papillae are present, the line should be defined by the lowest sinuses visible.

Epithelial Zones

Whatever definition of the anal canal is used, the sequence of epithelial zones in this area (i.e., rectum to perianal skin) follows (Figure 27.6):

1. the zone covered with uninterrupted mucosa of colorectal type
2. the zone with epithelial variants [anal transitional zone (ATZ)]
3. the zone covered with uninterrupted squamous epithelium
4. the perianal skin with keratinized squamous epithelium and skin appendages

These zones have been given many different names over the past century (Table 27.2) based on macroscopic, histologic, and embryologic considerations. Among the terms applied to the zone with epithelial variants, situated between the colorectal-type mucosa above and the squamous epithelium below, the most widely accepted term is now the *anal transition(al) zone* (28). The term *zona columnaris* refers to a macroscopic observation; the names *membranous*, *cloacogenic*, and *junctional zones* all indicate the site of the cloacal membrane in early fetal life and the meeting point of endoderm and ectoderm, a theory that was rejected decades ago. The terms *intermediate* or *middle zone* could be used, but neither gives any information about the character of the epithelial lining. *Hemorrhoidal zone* is misleading because hemorrhoids are not confined to this area.

The definition of the anal transitional zone is as follows. The ATZ is the zone interposed between uninterrupted colorectal mucosa above and uninterrupted squamous epithelium below, irrespective of the type of epithelium present in the zone itself (28).

From this it follows that names related to the histologic appearance also would be appropriate for the other zones. One can therefore use the term *colorectal zone* for the mucosa above the ATZ and *squamous zone* for the area below, which gradually merges into the perianal skin (Figure 27.6).

These zones are not always clearly visible to the clinician, and biopsy specimens should therefore be forwarded to the pathologist with an explanation of their location in relation to the DL. Biopsy samples from the lower part of the anal canal can be guided using a colposcope (Figure 27.7) (33,34).

Extent of the Zones

The colorectal zone, ATZ, and the area covered by squamous epithelium can easily be distinguished on longitudinal histologic sections (Figure 27.8). However, this method gives only limited information regarding the extent of the zones because the outlines are highly irregular. A better

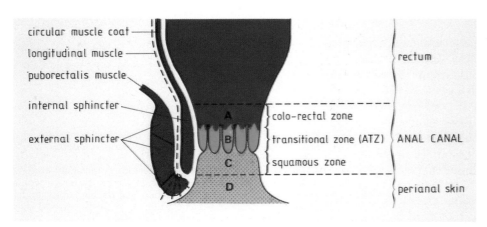

Figure 27.6 Schematic drawing of the anal canal showing the different zones and the proposed nomenclature. Colorectal zone (of anal canal) above (*A*). The extent of the anal transitional zone (*B*) is highly variable. The squamous zone (*C*) gradually merges into the perianal skin (*D*).

TABLE 27.2

LIST OF TERMS FOR THE VARIOUS ZONES IN THE ANAL CANAL AND PERIANAL SKIN[a]

Reference		A	B	C	D
Robin and Cadiat	1874		Zone muqueuse	Zone cutanée lisse	
Duret	1879	Zone muqueuse	Zone moyenne		
			Zone fibroide		
Hermann	1880		Muqueuse anale		
Hermann and Desfosses	1880		Region cloacale		
Stroud	1896			Pecten	
Waldeyer	1899		Zona columnaries	Zona intermedia	Zona cutanea
Szent-Györgyi	1913	Zona intestinalis			
Tucker and Helwig	1935		Intermediate zone		
Tucker and Helwig	1938	Upper zone	Middle zone	Cutaneous zone	Cutaneous zone
Parks	1956		Zone of stratified columnar epithelium		
Grinvalsky and Helwig	1956		Membraneous zone		
Walls	1958		Junctional zone		
Duthie and Gairns	1960		Transitional zone		
Spanner	1970			Zona haemorrhoidalis	
Hollinshead	1974		Zona haemorrhoidalis		
Ferner and Staubesand	1975			Zona alba	
Williams and Warwick	1980			Transitional zone	
Singh	1981		Zone III	Zone II	Zone I
Haas, Fox, and Haas	1984			Anoderm	
Wendell-Smith	2000	Suprazonal part	Transitional zone	Infradentate part	

[a] For detailed references, see Fenger C. The anal transitional zone. *Acta Pathol Microbiol Immunol Scand Suppl* 1987;289:1–42.
(*A*, zone covered with uninterrupted mucosa of colorectal type; *B*, zone with epithelial variants; *C*, zone covered with uninterrupted squamous epithelium; *D*, perianal skin with keratinized squamous epithelium)

impression is provided by staining the whole anal canal with Alcian dye. This method results in dark staining of the abundant mucus in the colorectal zone and an absence of staining in the squamous zone. The interposed ATZ is turquoise, due to sparse mucin production in the surface epithelium and scattered crypts (16). Subsequent serial sectioning of the whole specimen and comparison with the macroscopic picture gives a reliable measurement of the extent of the zones in the whole circumference of the anal canal (28).

By using this method on a consecutive series of 113 anal canals, four main variants could be visualized. In most cases (88%), the ATZ started at the DL and extended on average 9 mm cranially (range: 3–20 mm) (Figure 27.9). In a few cases (7%), the ATZ started below the DL (Figure 27.10) or above the DL (4%) (Figure 27.11). In one case, the ATZ was totally absent (Figure 27.12). In addition, the method clearly demonstrated the highly irregular outlines of the ATZ, especially at the upper border, as visualized by stereomicroscopy (Figure 27.13) (17). Others, using slightly different techniques on 28 anal canals, have found the median length of the ATZ to be about 5 mm (35).

The squamous zone normally extends downward from the DL, but squamous epithelium is often found covering parts of the anal columns (17). The lower border of the squamous zone is difficult to determine because the squamous zone gradually merges into the perianal skin. If the transition is defined by the occurrence of skin appendages, the lower border of the squamous zone is located outside the anal canal. This is particularly the case when hemorrhoids or prolapse is present. From this it follows that the histologic transition to perianal skin does not necessarily correspond to the definitions of the lower border of the anal canal.

The perianal region is not well defined; but, for the purpose of tumor classification, a boundary located 5 to 6 cm from the transition to squamous mucosa is recommended by the American Joint Committee on Cancer (AJCC) (36). This might be inappropriate as the region thus includes the most posterior parts of the vulva or scrotum.

Definitions of the Anal Canal

Various definitions of the anal canal have been suggested through the ages. Some are based on macroscopic landmarks (Figure 27.2), others on the extent of the epithelial zones (Figures 27.2, 27.6). Of the two based on macroscopy, the anatomic anal canal, which extends from the DL down

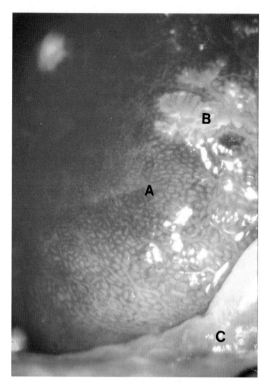

Figure 27.7 Colposcopy of the anal canal at the level of the dentate line. Compare the irregular outlines of the anal transitional zone with Figure 27.13. (*A*, colorectal zone; *B*, anal transitional zone; *C*, squamous zone)

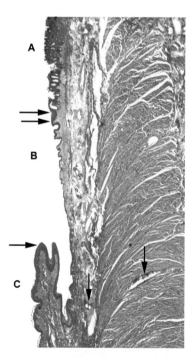

Figure 27.8 Longitudinal section of the anal canal showing the anal transitional zone (ATZ) and parts of the neighboring zones. At the upper border of the ATZ, a little island of squamous epithelium can be seen. The ATZ extends down into an anal sinus. The *vertical arrows* indicate anal glands in the submucosa and internal sphincter (H&E). The double horizontal arrows indicate the upper border of the AZT; the single horizontal arrow, the dentate line. (*A*, colorectal zone; *B*, anal transitional zone; *C*, squamous zone)

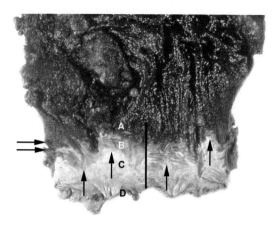

Figure 27.9 Surgical specimen of adult anal canal: normal location of anal transitional zone (Alcian green for 15 min).(*Black vertical line*, extent of the anal canal; *single arrows*, dentate line; *double arrows*, upper border of the anal transitional zone; *A*, colorectal zone; *B*, anal transitional zone; *C*, squamous zone; *D*, perianal skin)

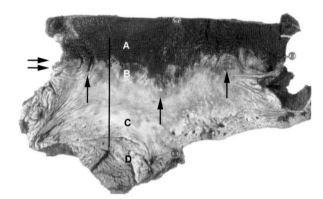

Figure 27.10 Surgical specimen of adult anal canal: low location of anal transitional zone (Alcian green for 15 min). (*Black vertical line*, extent of the anal canal; *single arrows*, dentate line; *double arrows*, upper border of the anal transitional zone; *A*, colorectal zone; *B*, anal transitional zone; *C*, squamous zone; *D*, perianal skin)

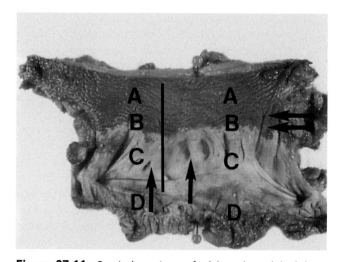

Figure 27.11 Surgical specimen of adult anal canal: high location of anal transitional zone, which here is very narrow (Alcian green for 15 min). (*Black vertical line*, extent of the anal canal; *single arrows*, dentate line; *double arrows*, upper border of the anal transitional zone; *A*, colorectal zone; *B*, anal transitional zone; *C*, squamous zone; *D*, perianal skin)

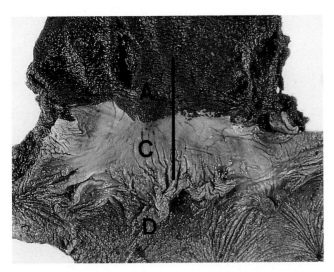

Figure 27.12 Surgical specimen of adult anal canal: no anal transitional zone (Alcian green for 15 min). (*Black vertical line*, extent of the anal canal; *single arrows*, dentate line; *double arrows*, upper border of the anal transitional zone; *A*, colorectal zone; *C*, squamous zone; *D*, perianal skin)

to the anal verge, has been abandoned by most investigators because the definition leaves the ATZ and the characteristic tumors in this area outside the anal canal. The question is, therefore, to choose between the definitions of the *surgical anal canal* and *histologic anal canal*, and there are advantages and drawbacks to both.

The histologic anal canal is defined by the extent of the special mucosa in this area (i.e., the ATZ and the squamous epithelium down to the perianal skin). Using this definition, microscopic identification of the canal is reasonably easy, and all the special tumors in this area have their origin in the canal. The drawback is that the extent of the anal

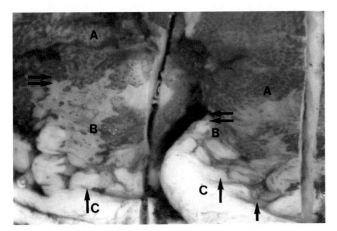

Figure 27.13 Close-up of the anal canal mucosa at the level of the dentate line. The highly irregular outlines of the anal transitional zone (*B*) contrasts to the heavily stained colorectal-type mucosa above (*A*) and the unstained squamous zone below (*C*). The vertical line is for later histologic control of the macroscopic staining (Alcian blue for 15 minutes).

canal cannot be estimated by the clinicians and that colorectal neoplasias can have their origin inside the histologic anal canal because it also harbors colorectal-type epithelium scattered in the ATZ.

The surgical anal canal can be identified easily by the clinician and described in the surgical report, thus making communication between surgeon and pathologist easier. The surgical anal canal is also regarded as a functional unit. However, with regard to the mucosal lining, the surgical anal canal most often includes a ring of more or less normal appearing colorectal mucosa at its upper border.

The lack of agreement between macroscopic and microscopic definitions is well known from other areas (i.e., the cervical transformation zone and the esophagogastric junction) and must be accepted. The essential point is that when the clinician describes the location of a process or a biopsy, the position in relation to the DL is the important message. The pathologist will then report what epithelial types are present in the material and, considering the above-mentioned variations, decide whether it is normal.

As the anal canal is described using the definition of the surgical anal canal by the WHO (31), as well as in the tumor-node-metastasis (TNM) system (32), this definition will also be used in the following text.

ANATOMY

Mucosal Surface

Following the definition of the surgical anal canal (18), the structure extends from the level of the pelvic floor (pelvic visceral aperture, anorectal ring) to the anal opening (anal verge) (Figure 27.2) and in a living person has an average length of 4.2 cm (37). Histologically, the anal canal extends from the upper to the lower border of the internal anal sphincter and has, on formalin-fixed specimens, an average length of 3 cm (16). This slight difference in definitions and measurements must be accepted because the curved appearance of the anal verge cannot be evaluated histologically and because loss of tonus and the fixation procedures may influence the appearance of the specimens.

The anal lumen often forms a more or less triradiate slit when seen at anoscopy. The stem of the Y so formed approaches the midline posteriorly, and the arms embrace a pad of tissue anteriorly. Thus, three folds are seen, named the anal cushions (38). According to some investigators, the Y is asymmetric and usually embraces a pad of tissue to the right anteriorly (38,39). The anal cushions are present already in fetal life. In an opened surgical specimen from adults, these cushions are often inconspicuous.

The surface relief of the anal canal varies with age. The characteristic relief described in all anatomy textbooks is most distinct in children (Figure 27.4). Here the mucosa shows six to ten vertical mucosal folds (the anal columns) that extend from a little below the middle of the anal canal and gradually disappear near the upper end. The anal columns are connected at their bases by small semilunar valves, which occasionally take the form of small papillae. Small pockets, the anal sinuses or crypts, are found behind the valves.

In adults (Figures 27.5, 27.9–27.12), the mucosa often shows less pronounced valves and columns and may exhibit a smooth surface with or without scattered anal sinuses and papillae (16).

The three epithelial zones are faintly visible to the naked eye on unstained, formalin-fixed specimens (Figure 27.5). The upper third shows the same relief as the mucosa of the rectum above. The area immediately above the anal valves and sinuses usually appears more smooth and gray-blue. This is the ATZ. Distal to the sinuses, the squamous epithelium appears as a smooth gray-brown area (Stroud's pecten). At the lower border of the anal canal, the dull, wrinkled perianal skin with hair follicles is obvious.

Musculature

The exact arrangement of the anal musculature is still a subject of debate, and new information is still being added using anal endosonography, magnetic resonance imaging, and manometry (40,41). The muscles here are described from the inside out (Figure 27.6).

Musculus Submucosae Ani

The musculus submucosae ani, originally described by Treitz (42), also have been called musculus sustentator tunicae mucosae, musculus mucosus ani, and musculus canalis ani (43). They consist of fibers from the intersphincteric longitudinal muscle, which pass through the internal sphincter, and from the internal sphincter itself. In the submucosa, they form a network around the vascular plexus (Figure 27.14) and are sometimes connected to the muscularis mucosae upward. Caudally, they rejoin the muscles from which they came. Some fibers fan out in the perianal skin, where they may join fibers from the corrugator cutis ani muscle (38,43).

Internal Anal Sphincter

The internal anal sphincter is a continuation of the circular muscle coat of the rectum but is considerably thicker. In histologic sections it measures 5 to 8 mm in thickness and ends 5 to 19 mm (average: 11.4) below the DL (16). Using anal endosonography, the thickness is maximally 4 to 5 mm (41). The muscle receives sympathetic (motor) fibers and parasympathetic (inhibitory) fibers from the inferior

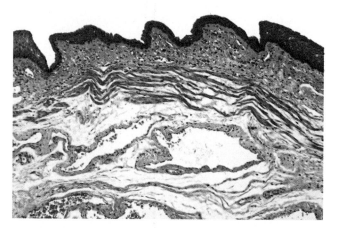

Figure 27.14 Anal transitional zone with columnar surface cells (*central*) and squamous epithelium (*left* and *right*). Vascular spaces located below fibers from the muscularis mucosae (H&E).

hypogastric plexus. In contrast to the adjacent rectum, the internal sphincter contains no enkephalin-immunoreactive fibers, few substance P–reactive fibers, but moderate numbers of fibers reactive for neuropeptide Y and vasoactive intestinal peptide (44). Collagen fiber deposition increases with age (45) and is higher in patients with neurogenic fecal incontinence (46). Pelvic irradiation may result in increased fibrosis and nerve density (47).

Intersphincteric Longitudinal Muscle

The intersphincteric longitudinal muscle is situated between the internal and external sphincters (Figure 27.6). Its thickness varies, and its exact function is unknown (40,48). It contains unstriped fibers from the longitudinal muscle coat of the rectum and striped fibers from the levator ani muscles. At the lower end of the internal sphincter, it breaks up into a number of septae, which diverge fanwise through the subcutaneous part of the external sphincter to end in the corium, thus forming the characteristic corrugation of the perianal skin. These bands are, therefore, referred to as the corrugator cutis ani muscle.

External Sphincter

The striated anal sphincter is traditionally described as a circular muscle, which can be divided into a deep part and a superficial part that surround the internal sphincter and a subcutaneous part below these muscles (Figure 27.6). Most investigators have been unable to find a clear separation between these three parts (40). The puborectalis muscle is situated above the external sphincter. There are two prevailing theories about the arrangement of these muscles.

Shafik (49) has described three U-shaped loops, with their convexity directed backward, forward, and backward, respectively. The top loop comprises the deep part and the puborectalis muscle, which is attached to the lower part of the symphysis; the intermediate loop is formed by the superficial part and is attached by a fibrous tendon to the dorsal part of the tip of the coccyx; the base loop is formed by the subcutaneous part, which is attached anteriorly to the perianal skin and is split from the longitudinal muscle by the above-mentioned fibers. Oh and Kark (50) described a double-loop theory according to which the puborectalis is directed anteriorly and most of the external sphincter posteriorly. This is in better accordance with recent endosonographical studies (40,41).

The superficial and subcutaneous parts differ from normal striated musculature. They consist of relatively small muscle fibers, in the adult predominantly of the slow switch type (type 1), separated by delicate strands of connective tissue (51,52).

Blood Supply

The arterial supply to the anal canal is considerably greater than would be necessary for metabolism alone. Branches from the superior rectal artery reach the ATZ in nearly all cases, but the middle and inferior rectal arteries often also make substantial contributions (38).

The terminal branches of the arteries split up into small tortuous vessels, some of which form tiny arteriovenous anastomoses with the submucosal venous plexus. This plexus consists of small convoluted vessels with discrete dilatations, which may be fusiform, saccular, or serpentine. Connective tissue fibers and fibers from the musculus submucosae ani are situated between the vessels, thus anchoring them to the internal sphincter. The picture is more complex above the DL, whereas the dilatations are fewer and often larger below it. The drainage is mainly cranial to the superior rectal vein, but branches of the superior, middle, and inferior veins communicate freely below as well as through the internal sphincter (38).

Some investigators have described so-called anal glomeruli, in which groups of small convoluted vessels were surrounded by connective tissue, which separated them from the surrounding loose tissue (Figure 27.15). Such structures probably represent thrombosed vessels with recanalization. The whole system has been referred to as the corpus cavernosum recti (although it is situated in the anal canal) and is more pronounced in the areas corresponding to the anal cushions (39) (Figure 27.16).

Hemorrhoids

According to this new understanding of anal vasculature, hemorrhoids or hemorrhoidal disease should be defined as enlargement or prolapse of the anal cushions, in some cases followed by bleeding and thrombosis (53,54,55).

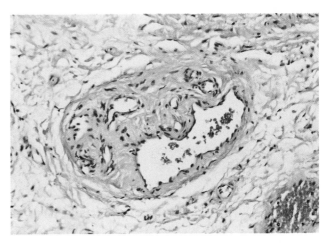

Figure 27.15   So-called anal glomerulus (H&E).

However, it is still debated whether the term *hemorrhoid* or *hemorrhoidal tissue* also should be used to describe the normal anatomical structure or asymptomatic enlargement of the anal cushions (56,57).

The pathogenesis of symptomatic hemorrhoids has been debated for many years, and a low-fiber diet, constipation and prolonged straining, abnormal anal pressure, hypertension in the anal cushions, and hereditary and hormonal factors may be involved. Others have found hemorrhoids associated with diarrhea and obesity but not with age, constipation, cirrhosis, or varicose veins (58).

Deterioration of the supporting and anchoring connective tissue and degenerative changes of the collagen fibers, together with replacement of muscle tissue by collagen, which begins in the third decade, make the structures less stable. The result is venous stasis and dilatation and sliding down of the anal cushions, sometimes followed by prolapse. Damage to the surface may lead to bleeding of arteriolar origin. Inflammation and focal pressure may be

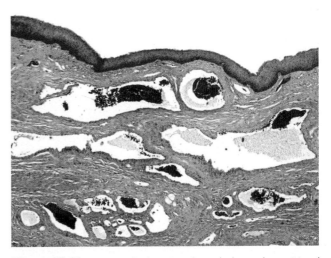

Figure 27.16   Longitudinal section through the anal transitional zone showing an anal cushion (H&E).

followed by further stasis, edema, thrombosis, and neovascularization (59).

This new understanding harmonizes well with the histologic picture of tissue from hemorrhoidectomies. The specimens most often consist of connective tissue stroma with scattered fibers of smooth muscle. The stroma may contain many blood vessels and larger vascular spaces that vary in size and configuration and are often less than 2 to 3 mm in diameter. Inflammatory changes and signs of recent or past thrombosis may be present, as may stromal fibromuscular hyperplasia and elastic fiber proliferation. In some cases the removed hemorrhoid more resembles a fibroepithelial polyp (54). Neuronal hyperplasia is common (60). The surface lining depends on the degree of descent of the cushion and of course the extent of the surgical excision. It therefore may show colorectal, ATZ, or squamous epithelium, as well as perianal skin. The mucosa may show inflammatory reaction or frank erosion or may be the site of regenerative, metaplastic, or keratotic reactions due to recurrent or permanent prolapse. The so-called fibrous anal polyp is assumed to represent an end stage of a prolapsed cushion (61).

Other Vascular Changes

There are a few differential diagnoses to chronic hemorrhoidal disease. Perianal thrombosis, formerly referred to as perianal hematoma, is an acute dark hard lesion arising under the squamous zone of the anal canal or the perianal skin. It represents a thrombus lying in the larger venous dilatations (61,62). Rectal varices are a result of portal hypertension and represent dilated submucosal veins formed when the communicating veins that connect the superior with the middle and inferior hemorrhoidal veins become enlarged. They extend above the level of hemorrhoids and occasionally downward to reach the buttock, perineum, or upper thigh (63,64). Diffuse cavernous hemangioma of the rectosigmoid is a vascular malformation consisting of vascular channels of variable size and thickness, which may involve the whole bowel wall and mesentery or perirectal tissue and may extend down to the DL (65). Recently, two cases of Dieulafoy's lesion in the anal canal have been described (66).

The vast majority of anal fissures occur in the posterior midline. A variant of the course of the inferior rectal artery has been blamed for a reduced perfusion of the posterior commissure and thereby of significance in the pathogenesis (67). Using Doppler laser flow cytometry, it has been shown that the blood flow in the posterior quadrant of the anal canal and perianal skin is significantly lower than in the anterior left and right quadrant and that the higher the anal pressure, the lower the perfusion (68). In addition, histologic studies have shown a lesser arteriolar density in the posterior quadrant throughout the anal canal (69).

These observations have led to the hypothesis that anal fissures are ischemic ulcers.

Nerves

Ganglion cells in the rectum are found in three separate plexuses: the superficial and deep submucous and the myenteric. In the anal canal, ganglion cells belonging to these plexuses are absent or sparse in the first centimeter above the DL (70). The diagnosis of ultrashort Hirschsprung's disease can be made by finding increased acetylcholinesterase reaction in muscularis mucosae and submucosa immediately above the DL (71). The density of interstitial cells of Cajal is significantly lower in the internal sphincter than in the circular muscle layer of the rectum (72).

The sensory innervation (73) of the lower part of the anal canal is accomplished by the inferior rectal nerves. The lining contains free nerve endings as well as organized endings (Meissner's corpuscles, Krause's end bulbs, Golgi-Mazzoni bodies, and genital corpuscles). It is sensitive to touch, pain, heat, and cold.

Sensitivity also can be demonstrated just above the DL in the ATZ, where the same endings can be found just above the anal valves. Thus, pain occasionally can be felt from injections given just above the DL. The ATZ is well supplied with intraepithelial nerve fibers and endings (74). Both types of nerve endings cease abruptly at the transition to the colorectal zone, where only a poorly defined dull sensation is present. However, discrimination seems not to be impaired by excision of the ATZ after restorative proctocolectomy (75).

Patients with hemorrhoids have a mild anal sensory deficit, probably due to the mucosal descent (76). Surgical specimens of hemorrhoids and their end stage, the fibrous polyp, may show proliferation of peripheral nerves without increased terminal density (60) (Figure 27.17).

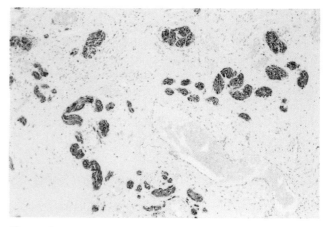

Figure 27.17 Neuromatous hyperplasia in the anal canal (S-100 protein).

Lymphatics

Lymphoid follicles are present in the anal canal from the DL and upward in approximately the same number as in the rectum (about 25/cm^2) (77).

The lower part of the anal canal (below the DL) and the perianal skin are drained to the superficial inguinal nodes. The drainage of the upper part is more complex, and varying results have been obtained from injection studies. Most investigators agree that an indirect or intramural system connects lymphatics in the anal canal to the lymphatic plexuses of the rectum (78). Other more direct lymphatics follow the inferior or medial rectal vessels to end in the hypogastric, obturator, and internal iliac nodes, or they follow the superior rectal vessels to end in nodes in the sigmoid mesocolon and near the origin of the inferior mesenteric artery. Occasional connections also have been demonstrated to the common iliac, middle and lateral sacral, lower gluteal, external iliac, and deep inguinal nodes (79).

Lymphatic metastases from carcinoma of the anal canal are most often found in the inguinal, femoral, pararectal, and iliac nodes, and eventually in the mesenteric or para-aortical nodes. Hematogenous metastases are most often located in the liver and lungs (31,36). Studies on sentinel nodes in anal cancer are ongoing (80).

HISTOLOGY

Colorectal Zone

The mucosa of the upper, colorectal zone is a continuation of the rectal mucosa, and no line of demarcation marks the transition to the anal canal. However, some shortening and irregularity of the crypts often are found in the area closest to the ATZ (Figure 27.18).

Anal Transitional Zone and Anal Glands

As stated above, the upper border of the ATZ is defined by the appearance of other epithelial types. In one-third of cases, the upper part of the ATZ consists of a small rim of mature squamous epithelium (Figures 27.8, 27.18) (16). Many epithelial variants can be found in the ATZ, the most prominent being the so-called ATZ epithelium.

The term *ATZ epithelium* (81) is not generally accepted but can be used until an exact classification is established. It consists of four to nine cell layers. The basal cells are small, and their nuclei are arranged perpendicular to the basement membrane. The surface cells can be columnar (Figure 27.19), cuboidal or polygonal (Figure 27.20), or flattened (Figure 27.21). Small areas can show umbrella-shaped surface cells and more distinct cell borders (Figure 27.22). Other epithelial types are often present in the ATZ. Small areas of mature squamous epithelium may be present, especially at the upper

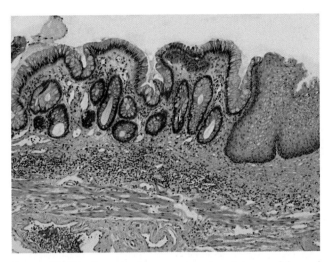

Figure 27.18 Transition between the colorectal zone of the anal canal and the anal transitional zone. Short, slightly irregular crypts. Muscularis mucosae still present (H&E).

border. Scattered crypts of colorectal type and small areas of simple columnar epithelium also may be found.

The anal (intramuscular) glands open in the ATZ (Figure 27.8). These glands seem to be present in all anal canals and the median number is six, with a range of three to ten. Four of five are only present in the submucosa, but the rest extend into the internal sphincter and a few percent reach the intersphincteric space or even penetrate the external sphincter (82,83). The epithelial lining and mucin production are similar to the ATZ epithelium (84), and endocrine cells are occasionally present (85). A characteristic feature is the presence of intraepithelial microcysts and occasionally goblet cell metaplasia (Figure 27.23). The epithelium is surrounded by one or two cell layers of myoepithelial cells that stain positive for smooth muscle actin (83). The glands are often surrounded by groups of lymphocytes. It is

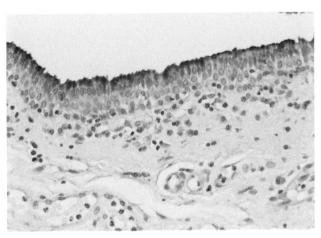

Figure 27.19 Anal transitional zone (ATZ): ATZ epithelium with columnar surface cells and scanty mucin production [Alcian blue pH 2.7, periodic acid-Schiff (PAS)].

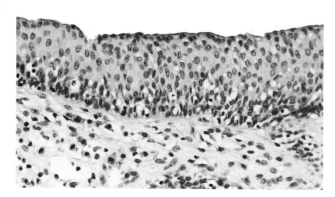

Figure 27.20 Anal transitional zone: ATZ epithelium with cuboidal or polygonal surface cells (H&E).

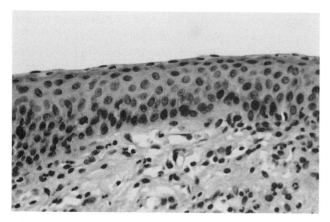

Figure 27.21 Anal transitional zone: ATZ epithelium with flattened surface cells and resemblance to squamous epithelium (H&E).

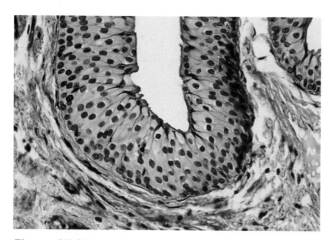

Figure 27.22 Anal transitional zone: ATZ epithelium with umbrella-shaped surface cells resembling urothelium. The surface cells are small (H&E).

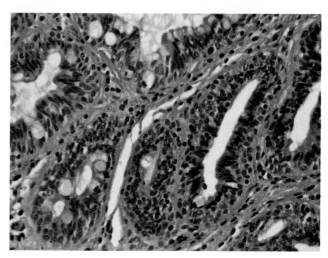

Figure 27.23 Anal gland in the submucosa of the anal transitional zone (ATZ). Epithelium is as in ATZ with scattered goblet cells (H&E).

believed that the anal glands may take part in the formation of fistulas. Cysts are usually due to trauma and inflammation. Well-documented cases of anal gland carcinoma are rare (84,86).

Squamous Zone

The transition to uninterrupted squamous epithelium usually takes place at the level of the DL. The squamous epithelium is unkeratinized with short or no papillae. Melanocytes increase in number as the perianal skin is approached, and the epithelium contains dendritic (Langerhans) cells (60) (Figure 27.24), T lymphocytes (87), and Merkel cells (88) (Figure 27.25). These cells also may be present in squamous metaplasia covering hemorrhoids. The number of dendritic cells is increased in cases of condylomata but decreased in case of concomitant HIV infection (89). Glands or skin appendages are never present in the squamous zone.

Perianal Skin and Glands

Keratinization becomes apparent at the lower end of the anal canal, and the squamous zone gradually merges into the perianal skin with sweat glands, hairs, and sebaceous glands. A characteristic finding is the presence of apocrine glands in the subcutaneous tissue (Figure 27.26). An additional type of glands, the so-called anogenital sweat glands, are lined by a simple columnar epithelium with cytoplasmic "snouts" protruding into the lumen and resting on a layer of flat myoepithelium (90) (Figure 27.27). These glands are probably the point of origin for papillary hidradenoma (91).

Lamina Propria and Muscularis Mucosae

The lamina propria consists of loose connective tissue which in the squamous zone often contains a variable number of

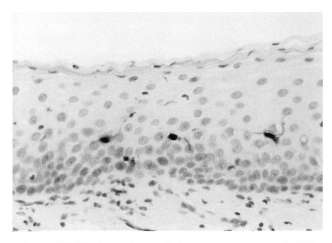

Figure 27.24 Langerhans cells in the squamous zone (S-100).

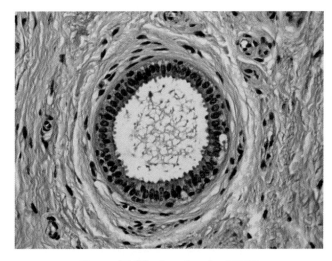

Figure 27.26 Apocrine gland (H&E).

mast cells and small mononuclear or multinucleated CD34+ stromal cells probably of fibroblastic origin (Figure 27.28). It has been suggested that these cells are involved in the formation of fibroepithelial polyps (92,93,94). Fibroepithelial polyps occasionally also show neuronal hyperplasia and hyaline vascular changes (60,94).

The well-defined muscularis mucosae of the rectum continue in the colorectal zone of the anal canal (Figure 27.18) and can be found in the upper part af the ATZ (Figure 27.14). Fibers extending up between colorectal crypts indicate mucosal prolapse, and most fibroepithelial polyps also contain fibers from the muscularis mucosae (92,94).

SPECIAL TECHNIQUES

Mucin Histochemistry

The columnar variant of the ATZ epithelium produces small amounts of a mixture of sulfomucins and sialo-

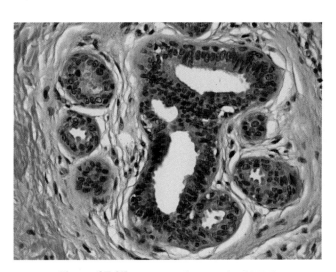

Figure 27.27 Anogenital sweat gland (H&E).

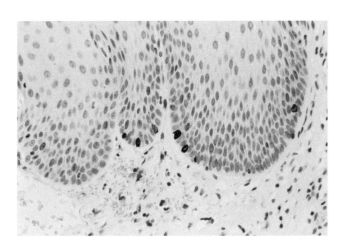

Figure 27.25 Merkel cells in the squamous zone (CK20).

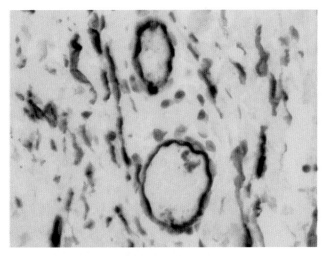

Figure 27.28 Stromal cells (CD34).

mucins, characterized by a scarcity of O-acylated sialic acids, in contrast to the colorectal type mucosa above (95).

Cytokeratins

The keratin expression of the various epithelial types in the anal canal is complex (96). Briefly, the typical reactions in colorectal type epithelium are CK20+/CK7– and in ATZ epithelium and anal glands CK7+/CK20–, and this pattern is also found in tumors originating in the respective epithelia (86,97,98).

The reaction for CK7 varies in the ATZ epithelium, sometimes being very strong throughout all layers, sometimes being absent in the basal layer or the whole epithelium (Figure 27.29). In addition, the ATZ and anal glands are usually positive for cytokeratins 4, 8, 13, 16, 17, 18, and 19. The coexpression of CK4 and CK13 has also been observed in the transitional epithelium of the urinary bladder.

Proliferation Markers

The proliferative marker MIB-1 for Ki-67 is positive in a layer of cells immediately above the basal layer and may be quite pronounced, especially in cases of hemorrhoids and prolapse (Figure 27.30). However, the reaction still differs from that seen in anal intraepithelial neoplasia (Figure 27.31).

Hormone Receptors

Androgen, estrogen, and, to a lesser degree, progesterone receptors have been demonstrated in the squamous epithelium, as well as in the underlying stroma and in the smooth muscle cells of the internal sphincter in most individuals and at all ages, indicating that the organ is a target for sex steroid hormones (99). The anogenital sweat glands and the corresponding papillary hidradenoma show positive re-

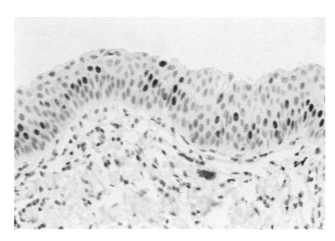

Figure 27.30 ATZ epithelium: proliferative activity (MIB-1).

action for estrogen and progesterone receptors, in contrast to conventional sweat glands (91) (Figure 27.32).

Neuroendocrine Markers

The characteristic epithelia of the ATZ and anal glands contain a heterogeneous population of endocrine cells (81,85), which all show positive reaction for synaptophysin and chromogranin A (Figure 27.33). The cells have slender processes that approximate the surface and a fine granular cytoplasm. The number varies, and the largest population also reacts for serotonin and pancreastatin, but cells positive for somatostatin, peptide tyrosine tyrosine, glucagon-like peptide 1, calcitonin gene–related peptide, protein gene product 9.5, and neurotensin are occasionally present. The pattern is a mixture of products typical for colorectal epithelium and for Merkel cells in the squamous epithelium (88,100).

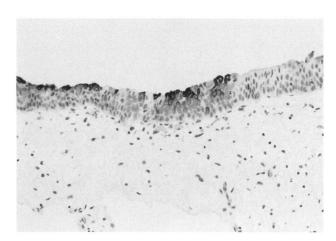

Figure 27.29 ATZ epithelium with varying cytokeratin expression (CK7).

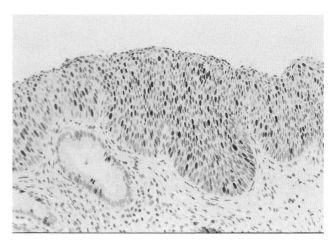

Figure 27.31 Anal intraepithelial neoplasia (AIN): proliferative activity (MIB-1).

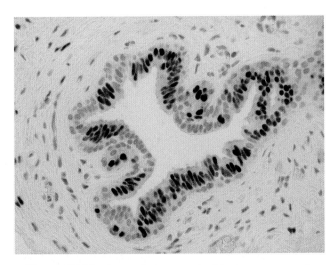

Figure 27.32 Anogenital sweat gland (estrogen receptor).

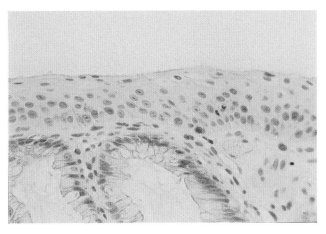

Figure 27.34 Anal transitional zone: three melanin-containing cells in the surface epithelium (HMB-45).

Melanin-Containing Cells

A few melanocytes are also occasionally present in the ATZ (85,101,102). These are CK7–/CK20– and positive for S-100 protein, Melan A, and HMB-45 (Figure 27.34). The corresponding malignant melanoma may be amelanotic and positive for polyclonal but not monoclonal carcinoembryonic antigen (CEA) (103).

Flow Cytometric Microscopy and Electron Microscopy

Flow cytometric DNA analyses of the ATZ epithelium have shown a dominating diploid population with a small hyperdiploid peak, resembling the picture of metaplastic epithelium (104). Transmission electron microscopy has not shown asymmetric unit membranes. In scanning electron microscopy, the surface cells show distinct cell borders and short microvilli (Figure 27.35) (81).

METAPLASIA AND HETEROTOPIA

Other epithelial types may be present and sometimes indicate pathologic conditions. Occasionally, colorectal-type crypts in the ATZ may contain Paneth's cells (Figure 27.36) or show pyloric metaplasia (Figure 27.37), probably as a result of mucosal damage (as in longstanding colitis). Squamous metaplasia in the ATZ and even in the colorectal zone is seen in cases of prolapse, and keratinization may be present (Figure 27.38).

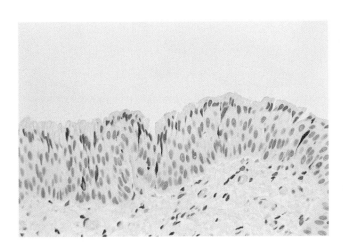

Figure 27.33 Anal transitional zone epithelium: endocrine cells (chromogranin).

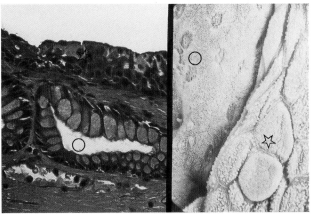

Figure 27.35 Anal transitional zone: **A.** colorectal crypt (*open circle*) and ATZ epithelium (*open star*); **B.** same area in H&E and SEM (original magnification ×1500). Reprinted with permission from: Fenger C, Knoth M. The anal transitional zone: a scanning and transmission electron microscopic investigation of the surface epithelum. *Ultrastruct Pathol* 1981;163–173.

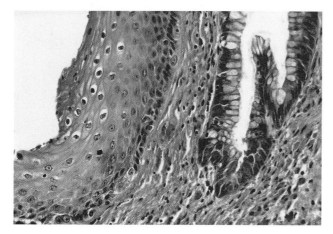

Figure 27.36 Anal transitional zone: area with squamous epithelium covering a colorectal-type crypt with Paneth's cell metaplasia (H&E).

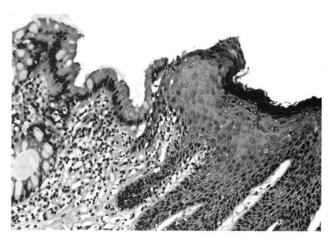

Figure 27.38 Anal transitional zone: keratinizing squamous epithelium extending up to the colorectal zone, as is typical in cases of prolapse (H&E).

I have seen a single example of fundic gastric mucosa in the anal canal. Such areas, rarely found in the rectum, are histochemically almost identical to their orthotopic counterpart (105). Probably *Helicobacter pylori* can turn up in the anal canal as it has done in body-type gastric epithelium in the rectum (106). A unique case has been reported showing ectopic prostatic tissue in the lower anal canal (107).

VIRAL AND NEOPLASTIC CHANGES

Cytomegalovirus, which occasionally infects the rectum, is rarely seem in the anal canal histiocytes (108). Herpesvirus-induced changes are more commonly found in the squamous epithelium (Figure 27.39), and koilocytotic changes due to human papillomavirus (HPV) can be found as high up as in the ATZ (Figure 27.40).

Anal intraepithelial neoplasia (AIN), also referred to as dysplasia or anal squamous intraepithelial lesion (ASIL), is not uncommon. It may be present in the squamous zone as well as in the ATZ and in minor surgical as well as in resection specimens (Figures 27.31, 27.41) (109,110). Squamous carcinoma and AIN are particularly common among men who have sex with men, patients with HIV/AIDS, and transplant recipients and in the rare syndromes Wiskott-Aldrich and epidermodysplasia verruciformis, indicating an attenuated immune response is of importance (111). High-risk HPV is found in most lesions, in particular those located high in the anal canal (112). Exact and reproducible grading of AIN is difficult in biopsies, as well as in cytologic specimens (113,114,115). Follow-up studies have shown that many cases of AIN I–II will regress but that a considerable number of AIN III will recur, even aften highly active antiviral therapy. There are however only few documented cases of transition to

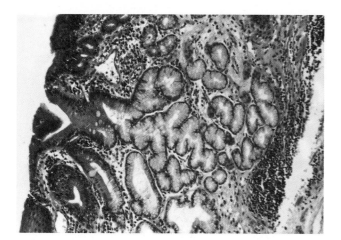

Figure 27.37 Anal transitional zone: area with group of pyloric-type glands (H&E).

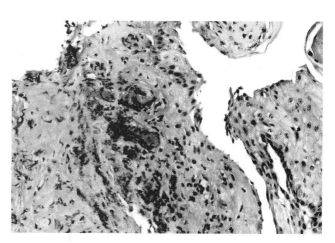

Figure 27.39 Herpes-induced epithelial changes in the squamous zone below the dentate line (H&E).

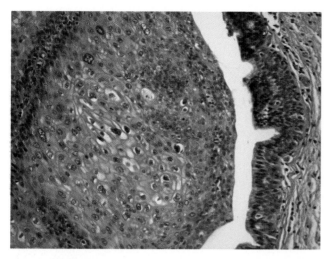

Figure 27.40 Anal transitional zone: area with squamous epithelium showing koilocytotic changes. Normal ATZ epithelium to the *right* (H&E).

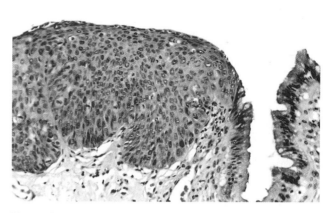

Figure 27.41 Anal transitional zone: area with severe dysplasia (AIN III) (H&E).

squamous carcinoma, and the real risk is unknown (33,116,117).

Squamous carcinoma of the anal canal may have different appearances (i.e., basaloid or keratinizing), but there is substantial overlap of the histologic features found in these tumors (112,118), and the reproducibility of the older WHO classification is rather low (119). In the recent WHO classification, it is therefore recommended that the generic term *squamous carcinoma* be used for these tumors (31). Prognostic

markers have not yet been identified (120). A summary of tumors originating in the different zones is listed in Table 27.3.

Finally, it should be remembered that the anal area is a common site of extramammary Paget's disease and that many of these patients have a synchronous or metachronous malignant tumor. Paget's cells must be distinguished from artifactual clear cells, glycogen-rich cells, koilocytes, and clear cells in pagetoid dyskeratosis, pagetoid Bowen's disease and pagetoid melanoma (121)

TABLE 27.3

ANAL CANAL MUCOSAL ZONES: CELL TYPES AND NEOPLASTIC COUNTERPARTS

Zone*	Cell Type	Neoplasia
A. Colorectal	Colorectal	As in colon and rectum
B. ATZ	ATZ epithelium	Squamous carcinoma variants
		Adenocarcinoma as from anal glands?**
	Squamous	Ordinary squamous carcinoma
	Colorectal type	Adenocarcinoma, colorectal type
	Endocrine cells	Endocrine tumor
	Melanocytes	Malignant melanoma
	Anal glands	Adenocarcinoma, anal gland type
C. Squamous zone	Squamous	Ordinary squamous carcinoma
	Melanocytes	Malignant melanoma
D. Perianal skin	Squamous	Ordinary squamous carcinoma
		Basal cell carcinoma
	Melanocytes	Malignant melanoma
	Apocrine glands	Apocrine tumors
	Anogenital sweat gland	Papillary hidradenoma
	Other appendages	As in skin

*A–D as in Figures 27.5 and 27.6.
** Adenocarcinoma of anal gland type is commonly supposed to originate in anal glands, but the epithelia in the ATZ and anal glands are more or less of the same type. (*ATZ*, anal transitional zone)

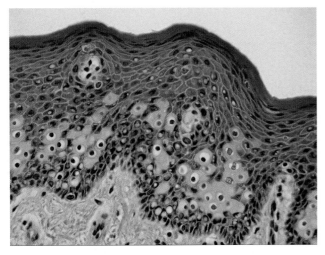

Figure 27.42 Squamous zone: clear cells in pagetoid dyskeratosis (H&E).

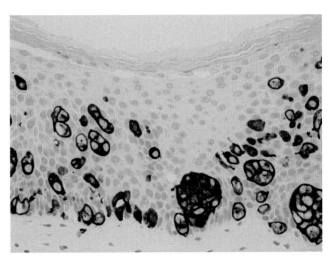

Figure 27.43 Squamous zone: Paget's cells (CK7).

(Figure 27.42). True Paget's cells nearly always show positive reactions for mucin, CEA, and CK7 (Figure 27.43) (122). Primary Paget's is usually positive for gross cystic disease fluid protein and negative for CK20, while the opposite pattern is found in Paget's secondary to colorectal adenocarcinoma (98).

FUNCTION

The normal function of the rectum and anal canal is the result of a combination of factors, including not only the puborectalis and sphincter muscles, but also stool volume and consistency, rectal storage capacity, sensation, and delivery, as well as cognitive and behavioral influences. The functional disorders, the various techniques for investigation of anorectal dysfunction, and the diagnosis and treatment have been extensively reviewed recently (123,124,125). The significance of the ATZ for normal anal function is still a subject of debate (126).

GENDER AND AGING

There is little information on differences in the anal canal between the two sexes and as a result of aging. The surgical anal canal is a few millimeters shorter in females (4.4 cm

TABLE 27.4		
TYPICAL IMMUNOHISTOCHEMISTRY OF NORMAL AND NEOPLASTIC ANAL CANAL		
	Cytokeratins	**Others**
Normal ATZ and anal glands	+7, +19, −20	
AIN and anal canal SCC	+7, +19	+MIB-1, p16, HPV
Anogenital sweat glands	+14	+GCDFP, ER
Anal gland carcinoma	+7, −20	
Rectal adenocarcinoma	−7, +20	
Prostatic adenocarcinoma	−7, −20	+PSA
Primary Paget	+7, −20	+GCDFP
Secondary Paget (CRC)	+7, +20	−GCDFP
Secondary Paget (urotel)	+7, (−20)	−GCDFP
Melanocytic lesions	−7, −20	+HMB45, Melan A

(*CRC*, colorectal type adenocarcinoma; *ER*, estrogen receptor; *GCDFP*, gross cystic disease fluid protein; *HPV*, human papillomavirus; *PSA*, prostate-specific antigen; SCC, squamous cell carcinoma)

vs. 4.0 cm in males) (37), and the external sphincter is also shorter, particularly its anterior part (40,41). With aging, the collagen fiber deposition increases in the internal sphincter (45).

The mucosal surface is often more smooth in the elderly, and the papillae may be more pronounced (Figure 27.5). The underlying connective tissue becomes less stable, which may result in descent of the anal cushions and subsequent squamous metaplasia of the ATZ (54). The number of lymphoid follicles does not change with age (77).

SPECIMEN HANDLING

In minor surgical specimens it is often possible to identify the smooth gray-brown squamous zone from the gray-blue, more glistening anal mucosa. The tissue always should be cut and embedded along the longitudinal axis in order to describe the lesions (i.e., AIN) in relation to the different epithelial zones.

Local excisions should be provided by the surgeon with a suture at the proximal end, pinned up on a plate and sectioned in the same way with special attention to resection lines. Larger surgical specimens are rare nowadays where anal carcinoma most often is treated nonsurgically. They should also be pinned up, and multiple sections may be necessary to find or exclude residual tumor tissue. Information on previous radiation therapy should be provided.

Normally most diagnoses can be established without the use of special stains, but occasionally a panel of immunohistochemical reactions is useful (Table 27.4).

REFERENCES

1. Fenger C. The anal transitional zone. *Acta Pathol Microbiol Immunol Scand Suppl* 1987;289:1–42.
2. Parks AG. De haemorrhois. A study in surgical history. *Guys Hosp Rep* 1955;104:135–156.
3. Braun WO. *Untersuchungen über das Tegument der Analöffnung* [inaugural dissertation]. Königsberg, Germany: R Leopold; 1901.
4. Glisson F. Tractatus de ventriculo et intestinis. In: Clerici D, Mangeti JJ, eds. *Bibliotheca anatomica sive thesaurus.* 2nd ed. Vol 1. Geneva: Chouët et Ritter; 1699. (Quoted in Braun, ref. 3.)
5. Morgagni GB. Adversaria anatomica omnia. Advers III, Animadv. VI. Patavii, Italy: Josephus Cominus; 1717:10–11.
6. Heister L. *Compendium Anatomicum.* 3rd ed. Altorf et Norimbergae; 1727:344.
7. Winslöw JB. *Exposition Anatomique de la Structure de Corps Humain.* Nouvelle édition, Tome III. Amsterdam: Tourneisen; 1732: 346, 351.
8. Robin C, Cadiat A. Sur la structure et les rapports des teguments au niveau de leur jonction dans les regions anale, vulvaire, et du col utérin. *J l'Anat Physiol Pario;*1874;10:589–620.
9. Gay A. Die Circumanaldrüsen des Menschen. *S K Akad Wiss Wien* 1871;43:329–333.
10. Chiari H. Über die nalen Divertikel der Rectumschleimhaut und ihre Beziehung zu den Analisteln. *Med Jahrbücher Wien.* 1878;8: 419–427.
11. Hermann G, Desfosses L. Sur la muquese de la region cloacale du rectum. *C R Acad Sci* 1880;90:1301–1302.
12. Hilton J. In: Jacobsen WHA, ed. *Rest and pain.* 3rd ed. London: Bell & Sons; 1880:288.
13. Stroud BB. The anatomy of the anus. *Ann Surg* 1896;24:1–15.
14. Ewing MR. The white line of Hilton. *Proc R Soc Med* 1954;47: 525–530.
15. Parks AG. Modern concepts of the anatomy of the anorectal region. *Postgrad Med J* 1958;34:360–366.
16. Fenger C. The anal transitional zone. Location and extent. *Acta Pathol Microbiol Scand A* 1979;87:379–386.
17. Fenger C, Nielsen K. Stereomicroscopic investigation of the anal canal epithelium. *Scand J Gastroenterol* 1982;17:571–575.
18. Symington J. The rectum and anus. *J Anat Physiol* 1888;23: 106–115.
19. Buie LA. *Practical Proctology.* Philadelphia: WB Saunders; 1937: 40–50.
20. Tourneux F. Sur le premiers développements du cloaques du tubercule genitale et de l'anus chez l'embryon de mouton. *J Anat (Paris)* 1888;24:503–517.
21. Retterer E. Sur l'origin et l'evolution de la région ano-génitale des mammifères. *J Anat Physiol (Paris)* 1890;26:126–210.
22. Nievelstein RA, van der Werff JF, Verbeek FJ, Valk J, Vermeij-Keers C. Normal and abnormal embryonic development of the anorectum in human embryos. *Teratology* 1998;57:70–78.
23. Rogers DS, Paidas CN, Morreale RF, Hutchins GM. Septation of the anorectal and genitourinary tracts in the human embryo: crucial role of the catenoidal shape of the urorectal sulcus. *Teratology* 2002;66:144–152.
24. Cuschieri A, EUROCAT Working Group. Descriptive epidemiology of isolated anal anomalies: a survey of 4.6 million births in Europe. *Am J Med Genet* 2001;103:207–215.
25. Lewin KJ, Riddell RH, Weinstein WM. The anal canal. In: Lewin KJ, Riddell RH, Weinstein WM, eds. *Gastrointestinal Pathology and Its Clinical Implications.* New York: Igaku-Shoin; 1992:1318–1359.
26. Wendell-Smith CP. Anorectal nomenclature: fundamental terminology. *Dis Colon Rectum* 2000;43:1349–1358.
27. Federative Committee on Anatomical Terminology. *Terminologia Anatomica: International Anatomical Terminology.* Stuttgart: Thieme; 1998.
28. Fenger C. The anal transitional zone. A method for macroscopic demonstration. *Acta Pathol Microbiol Scand A* 1978;86:225–230.
29. Fenoglio-Preiser CM, Noffsinger AE, Stemmermann GN, et al. *Gastrointestinal Pathology. An Atlas and Text.* 2nd ed. Philadelphia: Lippincott-Raven; 1999.
30. Day DD, Jass JR, Price AB, Shepherd NA, Sloan JM, Talbot IC, Warren BF, Williams GT. *Morson and Dawson's Gastrointestinal Pathology.* 4th ed. Oxford: Blackwell Science; 2003;643–646.
31. Fenger C, Frisch M, Marti MC, Parc R. Tumours of the anal canal. In: Hamilton SR, Aaltonen LA, eds. *World Health Organization Classification of Tumours: Pathology and Genetics of Tumours of the Digestive System.* Lyon, France: IARC Press; 2000:145–155.
32. Wittekind C, Greene FL, Hutter RVP, Klimpfinger M, Sobin LH, eds. *UICC TNM Atlas.* 5th ed. Berlin: Springer; 2005.
33. Fenger C, Nielsen VT. Intraepithelial neoplasia in the anal canal. The appearance and relation to genital neoplasia. *Acta Pathol Microbiol Immunol Scand A* 1986;94:343–349.
34. Jay N, Berry JM, Hogeboom CJ, Holly EA, Darragh TM, Palefsky JM. Colposcopic appearance of anal squamous intraepithelial lesions: relationship to histopathology. *Dis Colon Rectum* 1997;40: 919–928.
35. Thompson-Fawcett MW, Warren BF, Mortensen NJ. A new look at the anal transitional zone with reference to restorative proctocolectomy and the columnar cuff. *Br J Surg* 1998;85:1517–1521.
36. Greene FL, Page DL, Fleming ID, et al., eds. *AJCC Cancer Staging Manual.* 6th ed. New York: Springer; 2002.
37. Nivatvongs S, Stern HS, Fryd DS. The length of the anal canal. *Dis Colon Rectum* 1981;24:600–601.
38. Thomson WHF. The nature of haemorrhoids. *Br J Surg* 1975;62: 542–552.
39. Stelzner F, Staubesand J, Machleidt H. Das Corpus cavernosum recti—die Grundlage der inneren Hämorrhoiden. *Langenbecks Arch Klin Chir* 1962;299:302–312.

40. Sultan AH, Kamm MA, Hudson CN, Nicholls JR, Bartram CI. Endosonography of the anal sphincters: normal anatomy and comparison with manometry. *Clin Radiol* 1994;49:368–374.

41. Williams AB, Bartram CI, Halligan S, Marshall MM, Nicholls RJ, Kmiot WA. Multiplanar anal endosonography—normal anal canal anatomy. *Colorectal Dis* 2001;3:169–174.

42. Treitz W. Über einen neuen Muskel am Duodenum des Menschen, über elastische Sehnen, und einige andere anatomische Verhältnisse. *Vierteljahrschrift für die Praktische Heilkunde* 1853;37:113–144.

43. Hansen HH. Die Bedeutung des Musculus canalis ani für die Kontinenz und anorectale Erkrankungen. *Langenbecks Arch Chir* 1976;341:23–37.

44. Wattchow DA, Furness JB, Costa M. Distribution and coexistence of peptides in nerve fibers of the external muscle of the human gastrointestinal tract. *Gastroenterology* 1988;95:32–41.

45. Klosterhalfen B, Offner F, Topf N, Vogel P, Mittermayer C. Sclerosis of the internal anal sphincter—a process of aging. *Dis Colon Rectum* 1990;33:606–609.

46. Speakman CT, Hoyle CH, Kamm MA, et al. Abnormal internal anal sphincter fibrosis and elasticity in fecal incontinence. *Dis Colon Rectum* 1995;38:407–410.

47. Da Silva GM, Berho M, Wexner SD, et al. Histologic analysis of the irradiated anal sphincter. *Dis Colon Rectum* 2003;46:1492–1497.

48. Lunniss PJ, Phillips RK. Anatomy and function of the anal longitudinal muscle. *Br J Surg* 1992;79:882–884.

49. Shafik A. A concept of the anatomy of the anal sphincter mechanism and the physiology of defecation. *Dis Colon Rectum* 1987;30:970–982.

50. Oh C, Kark AE. Anatomy of the external anal sphincter. *Br J Surg* 1972;59:717–723.

51. Lierse W, Holschneider AM, Steinfeld J. The relative proportions of type I and type II muscle fibers in the external sphincter ani muscle at different ages and stages of development—observations on the development of continence. *Eur J Pediatr Surg* 1993;3:28–32.

52. Schröder HD, Reske-Nielsen E. Fiber types in the striated urethral and anal sphincters. *Acta Neuropathol (Berl)* 1983;60:278–282.

53. Johanson JF, Sonnenberg A. Constipation is not a risk factor for hemorrhoids: a case-control study of potential etiological agents. *Am J Gastroenterol* 1994;89:1981–1986.

54. Kaftan SM, Haboubi NY. Histopathological changes in haemorrhoid associated mucosa and submucosa. *Int J Colorectal Dis* 1995;10:15–18.

55. Lunniss PJ, Mann CV. Classification of internal haemorrhoids: a discussion paper. *Colorect Dis* 2004;6:226–232.

56. Haas PA, Haas GP, Schmaltz S, Fox TA Jr. The prevalence of hemorrhoids. *Dis Colon Rectum* 1983;26:435–439.

57. Haas PA. The prevalence of confusion in the definition of hemorrhoids. *Dis Colon Rectum* 1992;35:290–291.

58. Johanson JF, Sonnenberg A. Constipation is not a risk factor for hemorrhoids: a case-control study of potential etiological agents. *Am J Gastroenterol* 1994;89:1981–1986.

59. Chung YC, Hou YC, Pan AC. Endoglin (CD105) expression in the development of haemorrhoids. *Eur J Clin Invest* 2004;34:107–112.

60. Fenger C, Schröder HD. Neuronal hyperplasia in the anal canal. *Histopathology* 1990;16:481–485.

61. Thomson H. The anal cushions—a fresh concept in diagnosis. *Postgrad Med J* 1979;55:403–405.

62. Brearley S, Brearley R. Perianal thrombosis. *Dis Colon Rectum* 1988;31:403–404.

63. Johansen K, Bardin J, Orloff MJ. Massive bleeding from hemorrhoidal varices in portal hypertension. *JAMA* 1980;244:2084–2085.

64. McCormack TT, Bailey HR, Simms JM, Johnson AG. Rectal varices are not piles. *Br J Surg* 1984;71:163.

65. Aylward CA, Orangio GR, Lucas GW, Fazio VW. Diffuse cavernous hemangioma of the rectosigmoid—CT scan, a new diagnostic modality, and surgical management using sphincter-saving procedures. Report of three cases. *Dis Colon Rectum* 1988;31:797–802.

66. Azimuddin K, Stasik JJ, Rosen L, Riether RD, Khubchandani IT. Dieulafoy's lesion of the anal canal: a new clinical entity. Report of two cases. *Dis Colon Rectum* 2000;43:423–426.

67. Klosterhalfen B, Vogel P, Rixen H, Mittermayer C. Topography of the inferior rectal artery: a possible cause of chronic, primary anal fissure. *Dis Colon Rectum* 1989;32:43–52.

68. Schouten WR, Briel JW, Auwerda JJ. Relationship between anal pressure and anodermal blood flow. The vascular pathogenesis of anal fissures. *Dis Colon Rectum* 1994;37:664–669.

69. Lund JN, Binch C, McGrath J, Sparrow RA, Scholefield JH. Topographical distribution of blood supply to the anal canal. *Br J Surg* 1999;86:496–498.

70. Aldridge RT, Campbell PE. Ganglion cell distribution in the normal rectum and anal canal. A basis for the diagnosis of Hirschsprung's disease by anorectal biopsy. *J Pediatr Surg* 1968;3:475–490.

71. Meier-Ruge WA, Bruder E, Holschneider AM, et al. Diagnosis and therapy of ultrashort Hirschsprung's disease. *Eur J Pediatr Surg* 2004;14:392–397.

72. Hagger R, Gharaie S, Finlayson C, Kumar D. Distribution of the interstitial cells of Cajal in the human anorectum. *J Auton Nerv Syst* 1998;73:75–79.

73. Duthie HL, Gairns FW. Sensory nerve-endings and sensation in the anal region of man. *Br J Surg* 1960;47:585–595.

74. Lassmann G. Histologie und Innervation der analen Ductus und Glandulae. *Coloproctology* 1983;5:232–235.

75. Keighley MR, Winslet MC, Yoshioka K, Lightwood R. Discrimination is not impaired by excision of the anal transition zone after restorative proctocolectomy. *Br J Surg* 1987;74:1118–1121.

76. Miller R, Bartolo DC, Roe A, Cervero F, Mortensen NJ. Anal sensation and the continence mechanism. *Dis Colon Rectum* 1988;31:433–438.

77. Langman JM, Rowland R. Density of lymphoid follicles in the rectum and at the anorectal junction. *J Clin Gastroenterol* 1992;14:81–84.

78. Blair JB, Holyoke EA, Best RR. A note on the lymphatics of the middle and lower rectum and anus. *Anat Rec* 1950;108:635–644.

79. Caplan I. The lymphatic vessels of the anal region—a study and investigation of about 50 cases. *Folia Angiol* 1976;24:260–264.

80. Damin DC, Rosito MA, Schwartsmann G. Sentinel node in carcinoma of the anal canal: a review. *EJSO* 2006;32:247–252.

81. Fenger C, Knoth M. The anal transitional zone: a scanning and transmission electron microscopic investigation of the surface epithelium. *Ultrastruct Pathol* 1981;2:163–173.

82. McColl I. The comparative anatomy and pathology of anal glands. Arris and Gale lecture delivered at the Royal College of Surgeons of England on 25th February 1965. *Ann R Coll Surg Engl* 1967;40:36–67.

83. Seow-Choen F, Ho JM. Histoanatomy of anal glands. *Dis Colon Rectum* 1994;37:1215–1218.

84. Fenger C, Filipe MI. Pathology of the anal glands with special reference to their mucin histochemistry. *Acta Pathol Microbiol Scand A* 1977;85:273–285.

85. Fenger C, Lyon H. Endocrine cells and melanin-containing cells in the anal canal epithelium. *Histochem J* 1982;14:631–639.

86. Hobbs CM, Lowry MA, Owen D, Sobin LH. Anal gland carcinoma. *Cancer* 2001;92:2045–2049.

87. Gervaz E, Dauge-Geffroy MD, Sobhani I, et al. Quantitative analysis of the immune cells in the anal mucosa. *Pathol Res Pract.* 1995;191:1067–1071.

88. Hörsch D, Fink T, Göke B, Arnold R, Büchler M, Weihe E. Distribution and chemical phenotypes of neuroendocrine cells in the human anal canal. *Regul Pept* 1994;54:527–542.

89. Sobhani I, Walker F, Aparicio T, et al. Effect of anal epidermoid cancer-related viruses on the dendritic (Langerhans') cells of the human anal mucosa. *Clin Cancer Res* 2002;8:2862–2869.

90. van der Putte SCJ. Anogenital "sweat" glands. Histology and pathology of a gland that may mimic mammary glands. *Am J Dermatopathol* 1991;13:557–567.

91. Offidani A, Campanati A. Papillary hidradenoma: immunohistochemical analysis of steroid receptor profile with a focus on apocrine differentiation. *J Clin Pathol* 1999;52:829–832.

92. Groisman GM, Polak-Charcon S. Fibroepithelial polyps of the anus: a histologic, immunohistochemical, and ultrastructural study, including comparison with the normal anal subepithelial layer. *Am J Surg Pathol* 1998;22:70–76.

93. Groisman GM, Amar M, Polak-Charcon S. Multinucleated stromal cells of the anal mucosa: a common finding. *Histopathology* 2000;36:224–228.

94. Sakai Y, Matsukuma S. CD34+ stromal cells and hyalinized vascular changes in the anal fibroepithelial polyps. *Histopathology* 2002;41:230–235.

95. Fenger C, Filipe MI. Mucin histochemistry of the anal canal epithelium. Studies of normal mucosa and mucosa adjacent to carcinoma. *Histochem J* 1981;13:921–930.

96. Williams GR, Talbot IC, Northover JM, Leigh IM. Keratin expression in the normal anal canal. *Histopathology* 1995;26:39–44.

97. Williams GR, Talbot IC, Leigh IM. Keratin expression in anal carcinoma: an immunohistochemical study. *Histopathology* 1997;30:443–450.

98. Ramalingam P, Hart WR, Goldblum JR. Cytokeratin subset immunostaining in rectal adenocarcinoma and normal anal glands. Implications for the pathogenesis of perianal Paget disease associated with rectal adenocarcinoma. *Arch Pathol Lab Med* 2001;125:1074–1077.

99. Oettling G, Franz HB. Mapping of androgen, estrogen and progesterone receptors in the anal continence organ. *Eur J Obstet Gynecol Reprod Biol* 1998;77:211–216.

100. Hörsch D, Fink T, Büchler M, Weihe E. Regional specificities in the distribution, chemical phenotypes, and coexistence patterns of neuropeptide containing nerve fibres in the human anal canal. *J Comp Neurol* 1993;335:381–401.

101. Fetissof F, Dubois MP, Assan R, et al. Endocrine cells in the anal canal. *Virchows Arch A Pathol Anat Histopathol* 1984;404:39–47.

102. Clemmensen OJ, Fenger C. Melanocytes in the anal canal epithelium. *Histopathology* 1991;18:237–241.

103. Fenger C. CEA reactivity in amelanotic malignant melanoma of the anal canal—critical commentary. *Pathol Res Pract* 1993;189:1077–1078.

104. Fenger C, Bichel P. Flow cytometric DNA analysis of anal canal epithelium and ano-rectal tumours. *Acta Pathol Microbiol Immunol Scand A* 1981;89:351–355.

105. Carlei F, Pietroletti R, Lomanto D, et al. Heterotopic gastric mucosa of the rectum—characterization of endocrine and mucin-producing cells by immunocytochemistry and lectin histochemistry. Report of a case. *Dis Colon Rectum* 1989;32:159–164.

106. Dye KR, Marshall BJ, Frierson HF Jr, Pambianco DJ, McCallum RW. Campylobacter pylori colonizing heterotopic gastric tissue in the rectum. *Am J Clin Pathol* 1990;93:144–147.

107. Morgan MB. Ectopic prostatic tissue of the anal canal. *J Urol* 1992;147:165–166.

108. Blackman E, Vimadalal S, Nash G. Significance of gastrointestinal cytomegalovirus infection in homosexual males. *Am J Gastroenterol* 1984;79:935–940.

109. Fenger C, Nielsen VT. Dysplastic changes in the anal canal epithelium in minor surgical specimens. *Acta Pathol Microbiol Scand A* 1981;89:463–465.

110. Fenger C, Nielsen VT. Precancerous changes in the anal canal epithelium in resection specimens. *Acta Pathol Microbiol Immunol Scand A* 1986;94:63–69.

111. Zbar AP, Fenger C, Efron J, Beer-Gabel M, Wexner SD. The pathology and molecular biology of anal intraepithelial neoplasia: comparisons with cervical and vulvar intraepithelial carcinoma. *Int J Colorectal Dis* 2002;17:203–215.

112. Frisch M, Fenger C, van den Brule AJ, et al. Variants of squamous cell carcinoma of the anal canal and perianal skin and their relation to human papillomaviruses. *Cancer Res* 1999;59:753–757.

113. Lytwyn A, Salit IE, Raboud J, Chapman W, Darragh T, Winkler B, Tinmouth J, Mahony JB, Sano M. Interobserver agreement in the interpretation of anal intraepithelial neoplasia. *Cancer* 2005;103:1447–1456

114. Colquhoun P, Nogueras J, Dipasquale B, Petras R, Wexner SD, Woodhouse S. Interobserver and intraobserver bias exists in the interpretation of anal dysplasia. *Dis Colon Rectum* 2003;46:1332–1338.

115. Friedlander MA, Stier E, Lin O. Anorectal cytology as a screening tool for anal squamous lesions: cytologic, anoscopic, and histologic correlation. *Cancer* 2004;102:19–26.

116. Chang GJ, Berry JM, Jay N, Palefsky JM, Welton ML. Surgical treatment of high-grade anal squamous intraepithelial lesions: a prospective study. *Dis Colon Rectum* 2002;45:453–458.

117. Piketty C, Darragh TM, Heard I, et al. High prevalence of anal squamous intraepithelial lesions in HIV-positive men despite the use of highly active antiretroviral therapy. *Sex Transm Dis* 2004;31:96–99.

118. Williams GR, Talbot IC. Anal carcinoma—a histological review. *Histopathology* 1994;25:507–516.

119. Fenger C, Frisch M, Jass JJ, Williams GT, Hilden J. Anal cancer subtype reproducibility study. *Virchows Arch* 2000;436:229–233.

120. Fenger C. Prognostic factors in anal carcinoma. *Pathology* 2002;34:573–578.

121. Val-Bernal JF, Pinto J. Pagetoid dyskeratosis is a frequent incidental finding in hemorrhoidal disease. *Arch Pathol Lab Med* 2001;125:1058–1062.

122. Helm KF, Goellner JR, Peters MS. Immunohistochemical stains in extramammary Paget's disease. *Am J Dermatopathol* 1992;14:402–407.

123. Diamant NE, Kamm MA, Wald A, Whitehead WE. AGA technical review on anorectal testing techniques. *Gastroenterology* 1999;116:735–760.

124. Cheung O, Wald A. Review article: the management of pelvic floor disorders. *Aliment Pharmacol Ther* 2004;19:481–495.

125. Billingham RP, Isler JT, Kimmins MH, Nelson JM, Schweitzer J, Murphy MM. The diagnosis and management of common anorectal disorders. *Curr Probl Surg* 2004;41:586–645.

126. Choi HJ, Saigusa N, Choi JS, et al. How consistent is the anal transitional zone in the double-stapled ileoanal reservoir? *Int J Colorectal Dis* 2003;18:116–120.

Liver

28

Arief A. Suriawinata   *Swan N. Thung*

INTRODUCTION

The embryology, gross morphology, and histology of the normal human liver—the single largest organ in the human body—are described in this chapter. It is emphasized that liver biopsy specimens must be processed with special care in order to obtain optimal sections for diagnostic histologic evaluation. In many instances, immunohistologic studies of liver tissue have the potential to yield more information than electron microscopy. In surgical and autopsy liver specimens, nonspecific histologic alterations may be prominent, but they often have little significance. On the other hand, some morphologic changes, particularly in needle biopsy specimens, are frequently subtle but may be of diagnostic importance. The pathologist must be familiar with these histologic variations of and from the normal liver.

EMBRYOLOGY

The liver arises as the hepatic diverticulum from the endodermal lining of the most distal portion of the foregut during the third to fourth week of gestation (1–3). In embryos 4 to 5 mm in length, the hepatic diverticulum differentiates cranially into proliferating hepatic cords and caudally into the gallbladder and extrahepatic bile ducts. The anastomosing cords of hepatic epithelial cells grow into the mesenchyme of the septum transversum. As the hepatic cords extend outward during the fifth week of gestation, they are interpenetrated by the inwardly growing capillary plexus, which arises from the vitelline veins in the outer margins of the septum transversum and forms the primitive hepatic sinusoids.

Scattered mesenchymal cells derived from the septum transversum lie between the endothelial wall of the sinusoids and the hepatic cords and form the connective tissue elements of the hepatic stroma, as well as the capsule, which is covered by a mesothelial layer. Hematopoietic tissue and Kupffer cells also derive from splanchnic mesenchyme of the septum transversum. Once these structures are established, the liver grows rapidly to fill most of the embryonal abdominal cavity and by nine weeks' gestation accounts for approximately 10% of the total weight of the embryo (4). The bile canaliculi appear in the 10-mm embryo as intercellular spaces between immature hepatocytes (hepatoblasts).

The epithelium of the intrahepatic bile ducts arises from the proximal part of the primitive hepatic cords. This process is largely determined by the progressive development and branching of the portal vein with its surrounding mesenchyme. First, the epithelial layer in direct contact with the mesenchyme around the portal vein transforms into bile duct–type cells. Then a second layer transforms into bile duct epithelial cells, resulting in a circular cleft in the shape of a cylinder around the portal vein and its enveloping mesenchyme (Figure 28.1). This primitive channel duct in the 8-mm embryo (five to six weeks of gestation) is termed the ductal plate (5), which then undergoes gradual remodeling to form the normal anastomosing system of bile ducts in the portal tracts (6,7). The differentiation of intrahepatic ducts is recognized in embryos of 22 to 30 mm. Despite the common ancestry of hepatic parenchymal cells and ductal epithelium, each cell type is structurally and functionally distinct. The walls of the terminal twigs of the biliary tree, the canals of Hering, which connect bile canaliculi to bile ducts, include both typical hepatocytes and bile duct cells, without intermediate forms.

Functionally, intrahepatic hematopoiesis begins during the sixth week, hepatocyte bile formation by the twelfth week, and excretion of bile into the duodenum by the sixteenth week. The third trimester marks the cessation of hematopoiesis with a concomitant decrease in liver growth so that the liver accounts for approximately 5% of the newborn's body weight.

APOPTOSIS

Apoptosis occurs at all stages during fetal growth and development of ductal plates and hepatoblasts. There is a good correlation between the proliferative and the apoptotic activities in the ductal plate, depending on the remodeling process (8). Involution of liver hyperplasia and neoplasia (9–12) also is controlled by apoptosis, which is induced by transforming growth factor-β1 (11–13). In these regressing livers or tumors, scattered apoptotic bodies, rather than massive lytic necrosis, are observed. In viral infections, such as cytomegalovirus and herpes hepatitis, apoptosis has been proposed as a mechanism of cell death. In viral hepatitis B, however, it is not clear if cell death is mediated directly by the virus or by the host immune system through the release of cytokines such as tumor necrosis factor-a to the infected cells (14). In normal liver tissue, although rare, individual apoptotic bodies may be seen, which suggests that apoptosis is a physiological process in the liver (15) (Figure 28.2).

GROSS MORPHOLOGY

The liver of an adult weighs 1400 to 1600 g, comprising 2% of the body weight (3,16). It is relatively larger in infancy, representing one-eighteenth of the birth weight, mainly

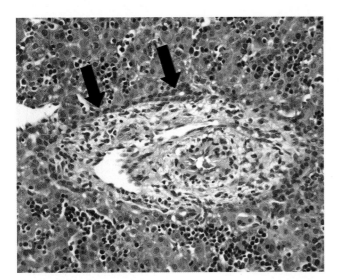

Figure 28.1 Ductal plate (*arrows*) developing around the portal vein mesenchyme in the liver of a 10-week-old embryo. There is extramedullary hematopoiesis in the sinusoids.

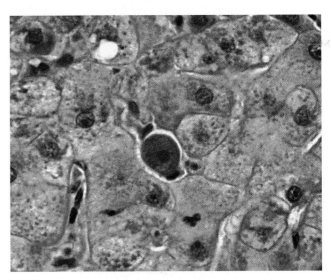

Figure 28.2 An hepatocyte undergoing apoptosis.

due to a large left lobe. The liver resides predominantly in the abdominal right upper quadrant and is completely protected by the rib cage. It extends from the right fifth intercostal space in the midclavicular line down to the right costal margin and to the left as far as the left midclavicular line. It has the appearance of a wedge with the base to the right and measures about 10 cm in vertical span, 12 to 15 cm in thickness, and 15 to 20 cm in its greatest transverse diameter.

It is divided by deep grooves into two large lobes—the right (lateral to falciform ligament) and left (medial to falciform ligament)—and two smaller lobes—the caudate and quadrate lobes. This traditional division is only of topographical significance. Functionally, the division into eight segments, which do not correspond to the anatomical division into lobes (17), is more important. Each segment is served by its own vascular pedicle of arterial and portal venous blood supply and branch of the biliary tree. This segmental division is of critical importance, particularly when dissecting small space-occupying lesions from these areas or when removing segments of liver for transplantation. The superior, anterior, and lateral surfaces of the liver are smooth and almost completely covered by peritoneum, except for a small triangular area—the "bare area" below the diaphragm—which is surrounded by the reflections of the peritoneum forming the coronary ligaments. A thin layer of fibrous connective tissue, the Glisson's capsule, surrounds the liver and extends into the parenchyma to form extensions that support arterial and biliary structures. Anteriorly, the falciform and round ligaments, which during fetal life conducted the left umbilical vein, connect the liver to the abdominal wall. Through the posterior surface of the liver at the base of the bare area runs the inferior vena cava, to which two to four hepatic veins connect. The fossa of the gallbladder and the round ligament separate the quadrate lobe from the right and left liver lobes, respectively. The fossa of the ductus venosus (i.e., the connection of the left umbilical vein to the vena cava inferior) and the inferior vena cava separate the caudate lobe from the left and right lobes of the liver. The horizontal portal fissure (or porta hepatis), which joins the upper ends of the gallbladder fossa and the groove of the round ligament, contains the branches of the hepatic artery, the portal vein, the hepatic nerve plexus, the hepatic ducts, and lymph vessels.

ANATOMY

Blood Supply and Drainage

The liver is nourished by a dual blood supply, approximately three-fourths via the portal vein and the remainder via the hepatic arteries. The portal vein carries venous blood from the alimentary tract, including the pancreas, which is rich in nutrients; whereas the hepatic artery supplies arterial blood from the celiac axis that is rich in oxygen for liver survival.

Venous outflow is provided by the right, middle, and left hepatic veins. The right hepatic vein drains the right lobe, the middle hepatic vein drains primarily the middle portion of the left lobe and a variable portion of the right, and the left hepatic vein provides the principal drainage of the left lateral lobe. The middle and the left hepatic veins often join together to form a common trunk before entering the vena cava. In addition, there are short venous segments that drain the posterior surface of the liver directly into the inferior vena cava (18).

Bile Ducts

Bile ducts accompany the hepatic artery and portal vein while coursing through the liver. They are nourished by the hepatic arteries via a complex peribiliary plexus of capillaries, which supplies all structures within the portal tracts. Bile is formed in hepatocytes, steadily secreted into bile canaliculi, canals of Hering, and then to the intra- and extrahepatic bile ducts. The extrahepatic biliary tract consists of a gallbladder that ends in the cystic duct. The cystic duct joins the hepatic duct to form the common bile duct, which enters the second portion of the duodenum through its muscular structure, the sphincter of Oddi (19).

Lymphatics

The capsule and the stroma of the liver is rich in lymphatic structures. The lymphatic plexus found in the capsule forms significant anastomoses with the intrahepatic lymphatics. The importance of these anastomoses is evident when hepatic venous pressure is increased; exudation of excess lymph from the capsular plexus forms protein-rich ascitic fluid. The intrahepatic lymphatic system exists as a fine, valved plexus associated with branches of hepatic artery in portal tracts. Hepatic lymph is most likely formed in the interstitial space of Disse. Lymphatic capillaries are not observed within the acini (20,21). Most of the hepatic lymphatics leave the liver at the porta hepatis and drain into hepatic nodes along the hepatic artery and into the celiac nodes. Other important efferent routes are via the falciform ligament and the superior epigastric vessels to the parasternal nodes, from the bare area to posterior mediastinal nodes, and from the visceral surface to the left gastric nodes.

The liver represents the largest single source of lymph in the body, producing 15 to 20% of the overall total volume (22) and 25 to 50% of the thoracic duct flow (21). Furthermore, hepatic lymph has an unusually high protein content, about 85 to 95% of that in plasma, and a high content of lymphocytes.

Nerve Supply and Innervation

The liver is innervated by two separate but intercommunicating plexuses around the hepatic artery and portal vein and are distributed with their branches (23). They include parasympathetic fibers from both vagi and sympathetic fibers, which receive their preganglionic connections from spinal segments T7 to T10 (24). The hilar plexuses also include afferent visceral and phrenic fibers. Besides their presence around vascular structures in portal tracts, nerve fibers (mostly sympathetic) are present in the parenchyma along the sinusoids. Release of neurotransmitters from the intrasinusoidal fibers modulate hepatocyte and perisinusoidal cell function. It controls in part carbohydrate and lipid metabolism and induces contraction of perisinusoidal cells, thereby regulating intrasinusoidal blood flow (25). However, neural mechanisms may have only a minor regulatory role because limited reinnervation in liver allografts does not seem to impair their function. Denervation probably explains the impaired normal response of the liver to ischemia, sinusoidal dilatation seen in liver allografts, and impaired metabolic function in cirrhosis (26,27).

HISTOLOGY

The structural organization (16,28–31) of the liver into parenchymal, interstitial, vascular, and ductal elements is based on its many functions and its position between the digestive tract and the rest of the body. The functional unit of the liver is represented by the hepatic lobule or rather, as defined by Rappaport (3,32), the hepatic acinus (Figure 28.3). The latter is a regular, three-dimensional structure in which blood flows from a central axis, formed by the terminal portal venule and terminal hepatic arteriole in the

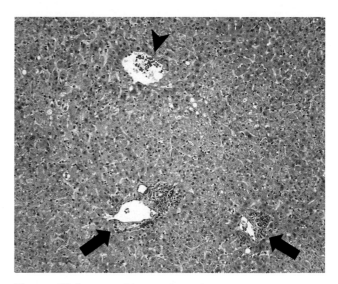

Figure 28.4 Normal human liver showing two portal tracts (*arrows*) and one terminal hepatic venule (*arrowhead*).

portal tract, into the acinar sinusoids and empties into several terminal hepatic venules at the periphery of the acinus (Figure 28.4).

In contrast, the hepatic lobule consists of an efferent central vein with cords of hepatocytes radiating to several peripheral portal tracts (33). Therefore, in a two-dimensional view, the acinus occupies parts of several adjacent lobules. The acini measure 560 to 1050 μm in length and 300 to 600 μm in width. The division of the hepatic parenchyma into the classic lobules, with changes described as being centrilobular, midzonal, and peripheral or periportal, is still used as a convenient landmark. However, Rappaport acinus has now come to be more generally accepted. The acinus is subdivided into zones 1, 2, and 3 with decreasing oxygenation (34). The hepatocytes in zone 1 are nearest to portal tracts and correspond to the peripheral area of the classic lobule. Zone 2 corresponds roughly to the midzonal area of a classic lobule, and zone 3 corresponds to parts of several centrilobular areas.

The terminal vascular branches, which bring substances for nutrition and metabolism into the acinus, run along the terminal bile ducts that drain the secretory products of the same acinus. The vessels form a vascular plexus around the bile ducts (35). Thus, as a result of the sinusoidal blood flow, structural, secretory, and functional unity is established in the acinus. The oxygen gradient, metabolic heterogeneity, and differential distribution of enzymes across the three zones of the acini (14) explain the zonal distribution of liver damage due to ischemia and toxic substances.

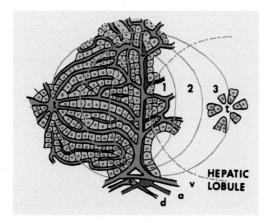

Figure 28.3 Diagram comparing the hepatic acinus with zones 1, 2, and 3 to the hepatic lobule (*dotted line*). Portal tract contains portal venule (*v*), hepatic arteriole (*a*), and hepatic duct (*d*). (*t*, terminal hepatic venule)

Hepatocytes and Bile Canaliculi

The hepatocytes are arranged in spongelike plates that in the adult are normally one-cell layer thick and are separated

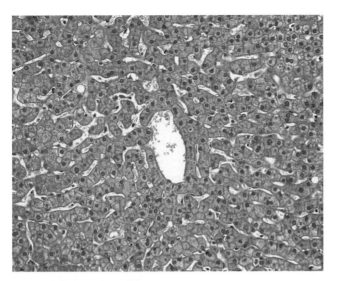

Figure 28.5 Terminal hepatic venule surrounded by converging hepatocyte plates and sinusoids.

by sinusoids along which blood flows from portal tracts to terminal hepatic venules (Figure 28.5). Surrounding the terminal hepatic venules, the hepatocytes exhibit a more regular radial pattern. Away from the perivenular area, the liver cell plates are arranged less regularly without distinct radial arrangement. In children up to 5 or 6 years of age, the liver cells are arranged in two-cell thick plates (Figure 28.6). In adults, the presence of two-cell thick plates and the formation of rosettes indicates regeneration.

The individual hepatocyte is a polygonal epithelial cell approximately 25 μm in diameter with a well-defined plasma membrane that is differentiated into three specialized regions or domains: basolateral (70% of total surface area), which faces the sinusoid; bile canalicular (15%), bounding that part of the intercellular space that constitutes the bile canaliculi; and lateral (15%), facing the rest of the intercellular space. Each domain has different molecular, chemical, and antigenic compositions and functions.

The nucleus is centrally located, round, and contains one or more nucleoli. At birth, all but a few hepatocytes are mononuclear. In adults, although binucleate forms are not uncommon (up to 25% of cells), mitotic activity is rare. Nuclei vary in size in the adult, and the great majority are diploid (36). Some nuclei are larger than others, indicating polyploidy, particularly in persons over 60 years of age (37) (Figure 28.7). The significance of polyploidy is unknown and is usually more marked in the midzonal area. Since cell size is proportional to cell ploidy, polyploidy does not provide an increased quantity of genetic material per unit volume of cytoplasm. The hepatocytes in the portal limiting plates are smaller than other parenchymal cells with more intense nuclear staining and more basophilic cytoplasm. Nuclear displacement to the sinusoidal pole with hyperchromasia is a cytological indication of regenerative activity.

The abundant cytoplasm is eosinophilic and contains fine basophilic granules representing rough endoplasmic reticulum. Cytoplasmic glycogen is present and after proper fixation is stainable with periodic acid-Schiff (PAS) reagent. On hematoxylin and eosin (H&E) preparations, glycogen gives a fine, reticulated, foamy appearance to the cytoplasm. The quantity and distribution of glycogen show diurnal and diet-related variations. An irregular distribution pattern may sometimes be found in biopsies and is not of diagnostic significance (Figure 28.8). Glycogen accumulation in hepatocyte nuclei around portal tracts produces a vacuolated appearance (Figure 28.9) and is common in adolescents. In adults, such an appearance may be conspicuous in

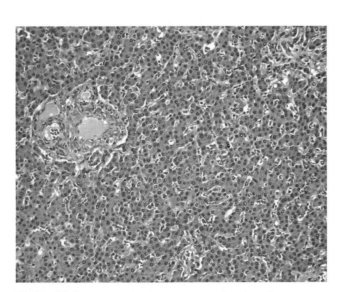

Figure 28.6 Liver of a child showing small uniform hepatocytes that are arranged in two-cell thick plates.

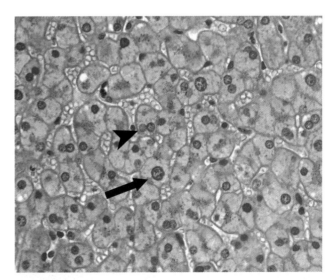

Figure 28.7 Liver of a 65-year-old patient showing significant polyploidy of hepatocyte nuclei (*arrow*) and binucleate forms (*arrowhead*).

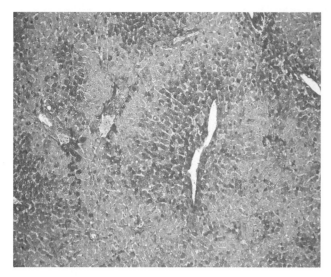

Figure 28.8 Periodic acid-Schiff reaction shows irregular distribution of glycogen (darker color) in the hepatocytes.

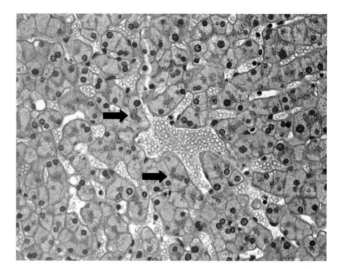

Figure 28.10 Lipofuscin in hepatocytes of zone 3 of the acinus. The finely granular pigment accumulates along the bile canaliculi (*arrows*).

conditions such as diabetes mellitus, pancreatic carcinoma, and chronic heart failure but is usually of no diagnostic significance.

A few vacuoles and small quantities of stainable iron are common in normal hepatocytes, particularly in older individuals. Hemosiderin and copper are abundant in the cytoplasm of hepatocytes during the first week of life, then gradually disappear and should be absent at the age of 6 to 9 months.

Lipofuscin, the "wear and tear" pigment, is seen in varying quantities as fine, well-delineated, light brown, PAS-positive diastase-resistant, partly acid-fast–positive granules in the cytoplasm of hepatocytes in zone 3, particularly at the canalicular pole (Figure 28.10). There is a

progressive increase of its amount in individual hepatocytes and in the number of cells involved in older individuals. It is rich in oxidized lipids accumulating in secondary lysosomes as a result of autophagy and uptake of exogenous substances. It is not found in recently regenerated hepatocytes. It may be difficult to distinguish lipofuscin from the pigment that accumulates in hepatocytes in large amounts in Dubin-Johnson syndrome.

In contrast to lipofuscin, iron and copper are coarser, birefringent, and usually deposited in periportal hepatocytes. Intracellular bile is poorly defined and less granular than the other pigments and often forms thrombi in bile canaliculi in zone 3 (38) (Figure 28.11). Isolated eosinophilic bodies as a result of coagulative necrosis, rare

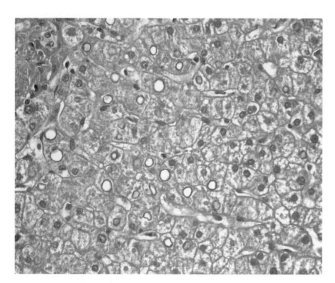

Figure 28.9 Glycogen accumulation in hepatocyte nuclei resulting in clear, empty appearance.

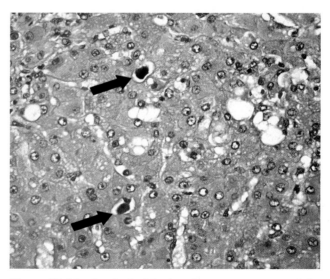

Figure 28.11 Canalicular bile thrombi (*arrows*) in zone 3 of the acinus.

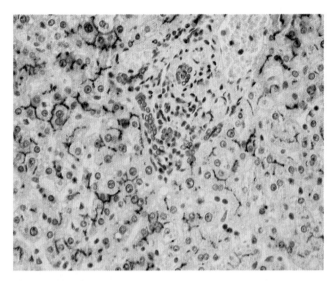

Figure 28.12 CD10 immunostaining delineates the twig-like structures of bile canaliculi, as well as the lumen of bile ducts and ductules.

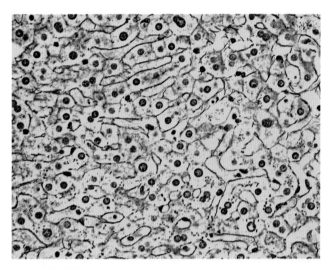

Figure 28.13 Hepatic sinusoids lined by reticulin fibers in a normal liver (reticulin stain).

apoptotic bodies representing normal turnover of hepatocytes (15), and an occasional focal necrosis where chronic inflammatory cells replace a few necrotic hepatocytes are not unusual in otherwise apparently normal livers.

The bile canaliculus is an intercellular space with a diameter of approximately 1 μm, formed by the apposition of the edges of gutterlike hemicanals on adjacent surfaces of two or three neighboring hepatocytes. Bile canaliculi are not readily recognized under the light microscope unless distended in conditions with parenchymal cholestasis, which is accompanied by hepatocyte rosetting. Bile canaliculi form a chicken wire–like network in the center of the hepatic plates, which can be demonstrated immunohistochemically with polyclonal anticarcinoembryonic antigen (pCEA) or CD10 (Figure 28.12). Bile canaliculi connect to bile ductules via canals of Hering.

Sinusoidal Lining Cells

In normal liver biopsy specimens, sinusoids are slitlike spaces that contain a few blood cells. The periportal sinusoids are more tortuous than the perivenular ones.

Hepatic sinusoids separate cords of hepatocytes and are lined by sinusoidal lining cells supported by reticulin fibers (Figure 28.13). These cells, which include endothelial and Kupffer cells, constitute a coordinated defense system. They are not conspicuous in normal biopsy specimens. The endothelial cells have thin, indistinct cytoplasm and small, elongated, darkly stained nuclei without nucleoli. The sievelike plates of the endothelial cytoplasm and the absence of a structurally defined basement membrane (in contrast to capillaries) facilitate exchange between blood and hepatocytes (20,39,40).

The Kupffer cells have a bean-shaped nucleus and plump cytoplasm with star-shaped extensions (41). They are more numerous near the portal tracts. They belong to the mononuclear-phagocytic system and are derived in part from the bone marrow. They contain vacuoles and, particularly in the diseased liver, many diastase-resistant PAS (PAS-D)–positive lysosomes and phagosomes, as well as acid-fast granular aggregates of ceroid pigment. These cells respond actively to many types of injury by proliferation and enlargement.

Between the endothelial cells and the hepatocytes lies the space of Disse, a zone of rapid intercellular exchange. It contains plasma, scanty connective tissue that constitutes the normal framework of the liver, and perisinusoidal cells such as hepatic stellate cells (Ito cells, interstitial fat-storing cells, or hepatic lipocytes) and pit cells. The connective tissue fibers along the sinusoids represent predominantly collagen type III, which stains black in silver impregnations (reticulin) and forms a regular network radiating from the center of the lobules. Elastic fibers and basement membranes are absent from normal sinusoids (42,43). The space of Disse is not discernible in well-fixed, normal liver biopsy material; but in postmortem liver, the hepatocytes shrink, pericellular edema develops, and the space becomes more conspicuous (Figure 28.14).

On light microscopy, hepatic stellate cells (44) are difficult to differentiate from sinusoidal lining cells. They are modified resting fibroblasts that can store fat and vitamin A and produce hepatocyte growth factor (45) and collagen. They play a significant role in hepatic fibrogenesis. When loaded with fat, such as in hypervitaminosis A, they may be recognized due to cytoplasmic fat droplets of rather uniform size with scalloping of the elongated nucleus (Figure 28.15). When activated, these cells contain stainable desmin and actin in their cytoplasm (46), justifying their designation as myofibroblasts.

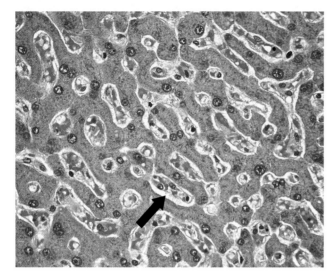

Figure 28.14 Autopsy liver specimen exhibiting dilatation of sinusoids and Disse's space (*arrow*) with prominent sinusoidal lining cells including endothelial and Kupffer cells.

Pit cells (47,48) have not been characterized by light microscopy. Under the electron microscope, they have neurosecretory-like electron-dense granules and rod-cored vesicles. Recent evidence indicates that pit cells are not endocrine cells but correspond to the large granular lymphocytes and have natural killer cell activity (49). Occasional inflammatory cells, lymphocytes, or polymorphonuclear leukocytes may be present in the sinusoids. During the first few weeks after birth, the presence of foci of extramedullary hematopoietic cells in the sinusoids and wall of terminal hepatic venules is a normal feature.

Hepatic Veins

The intrahepatic course of the valveless hepatic veins, which are embedded in a thin sheath of connective tissue, is straight to the inferior vena cava. The smaller branches (or sublobular veins) and the smallest efferent veins (or terminal hepatic venules) are in direct contact with the hepatic parenchyma. There is a defined spatial relationship between the terminal hepatic venules and the branches of the portal vein and hepatic artery in the portal tracts, which interdigitate but do not directly connect in the three-dimensional space.

The distance between two terminal hepatic venules represents the size of an acinus. The terminal hepatic venules have a very thin wall (Figure 28.5) lined by endothelial cells, which is readily demonstrable after staining with trichrome for collagen or Victoria blue for elastic fibers, but they do not have an adventitia around their wall (50).

It has been suggested that perivenular sclerosis in alcoholic patients may be an index of progressive liver injury (50), although this has been disputed subsequently (51). Thickening of the wall of terminal hepatic venules is often part of pericellular fibrosis and central hyalin sclerosis in alcoholic liver disease (51). It may be seen focally in apparently normal individuals, as well as in children up to 2 years of age.

Portal Tracts

Each portal tract contains a bile duct and several bile ductules, a hepatic artery branch, a portal vein branch, and lymphatic channels embedded in connective tissue (Figure 28.16). The amount of connective tissue and the size of the intraportal structures depend on the size of the portal tract.

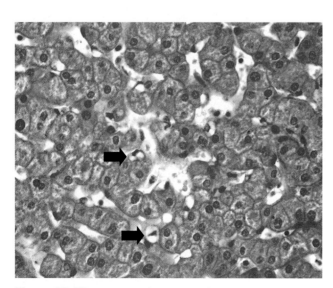

Figure 28.15 Prominent lipocytes in liver biopsy specimen of patient with hypervitaminosis A. The nuclei of the lipocytes are scalloped (*arrows*) due to fat droplets in cytoplasm.

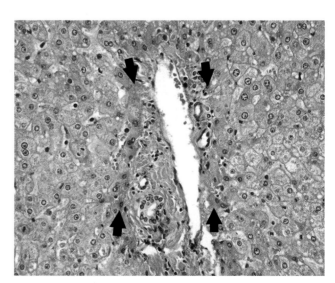

Figure 28.16 Normal portal tract with bile duct, hepatic arteriole, portal venule, and clearly defined limiting plate (*arrows*).

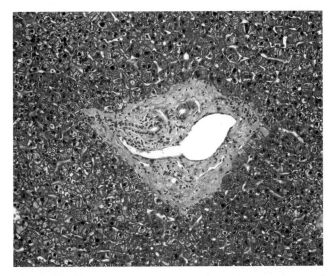

Figure 28.17 The connective tissue of portal tracts consists of mainly collagen type I, which appears as thick, deep blue fibers on trichrome stain.

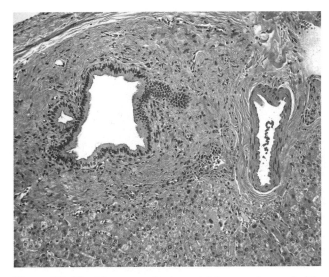

Figure 28.18 A large portal tract containing an artery and a bile duct lined by columnar epithelial cells.

Nerve fibers, both sympathetic and parasympathetic for innervation of blood vessels and bile ducts, can be seen in large portal tracts. The largest portal tracts are round or triangular, the smaller ones are triangular or branching, and the smallest terminal divisions are round or oval. The size of a portal tract is approximately three to four times the diameter of the hepatic artery branch. They normally contain a few lymphocytes, macrophages, and mast cells, but no polymorphonuclear leukocytes or plasma cells. The number of inflammatory cells increases with age. However, their density varies from one portal tract to the next. The connective tissue consists mainly of collagen type I, which is seen as thick, deep blue fibers on the trichrome stain (Figure 28.17). Newly formed collagen type III appears as fine, light blue fibers. In the subcapsular region of the liver, the portal tracts contain more and denser connective tissue. Irregular extensions of fibrous tissue from Glisson's capsule into the parenchyma, sometimes connecting adjacent portal tracts, must not be interpreted as cirrhosis in wedge or superficial biopsy specimens of subcapsular parenchyma (52).

Bile Ducts

The larger intrahepatic or septal bile ducts are lined by tall columnar epithelial cells measuring about 10 mm in diameter with basally situated, pale, oval nuclei and light eosinophilic cytoplasm (53,54) (Figure 28.18). They have an internal diameter greater than 100 μm and a distinct basement membrane stainable with PAS-D. Lymphocytes may occasionally be present within the lining epithelium. The larger bile ducts are located in the central part of the portal tracts and have more periductal fibrous tissue than the smaller ones. The collagen fibers are arranged in an irregular

and circumferential—but not concentric—manner, as may be seen in chronic biliary tract diseases such as primary sclerosing cholangitis and as a sequela of chronic cholecystitis.

The smaller or interlobular bile ducts are lined by cuboidal or low columnar epithelium. They have a basement membrane and a small amount of periductal connective tissue. One or more interlobular ducts may be present in a portal tract. Bile ducts are always accompanied by a portal vein and a hepatic artery, the latter having approximately the same diameter as the bile duct (external caliber ratio of bile duct to artery is 0.7:0.8) (54) (Figure 28.19). The bile ducts are connected to the bile canaliculi by bile ductules and canals of Hering.

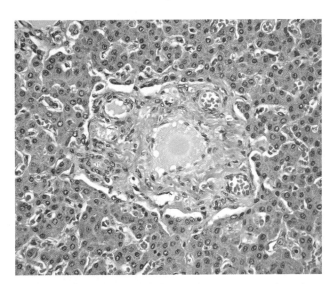

Figure 28.19 Normal portal tract in a newborn, with bile ducts and their corresponding hepatic arterioles of approximately the same diameter.

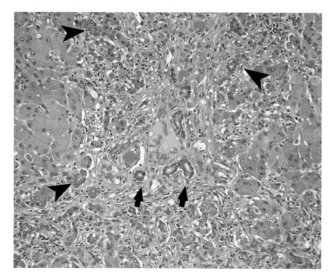

Figure 28.20 Bile ductules (*arrowheads*) are located in the peripheral zone of the portal tract and are smaller than the bile ducts (*arrows*).

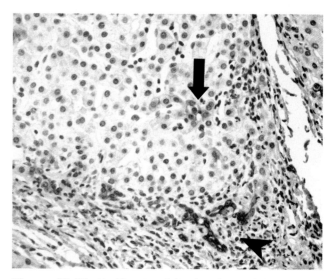

Figure 28.21 Proliferating bile ductules and hepatocytes undergoing ductular metaplasia *(arrow)* in chronic cholestasis are stained brown with anti-CK7.

Bile ductules are located in the peripheral zone of the portal tracts and are smaller (lumen of less than 20 μm) than the interlobular bile ducts (Figure 28.20). They have a basement membrane, are lined by cuboidal cholangiocytes, and are accompanied by a portal vein but not by a hepatic artery branch. Bile ductules may be observed at the edge of the portal tract stroma or may transverse the limiting plate, in which case it will have an "intralobular" as well as an "intraportal" segment. Ductular reaction, or proliferation of bile ductules, occurs in a variety of chronic liver diseases and can be so extensive as to raise the question of adenocarcinoma (55). Proliferating bile ductules should be differentiated from ductular hepatocytes, which are seen in zone 1 of the liver acini in massive hepatic necrosis (56). Canals of Hering, which are the physiologic link between hepatocyte canaliculi and the biliary tree, are not discernible on routine sections of normal liver. They are lined partly by cholangiocytes and partly by hepatocytes—not by cells of intermediate morphology, which are not identified in normal livers (57). They can be demonstrated by staining for high-molecular weight cytokeratin polypeptides (CK7, CK19), which are prominent in all cells of ductal origin (Figure 28.21).

Portal Vein and Hepatic Artery

The lymphatic vessels in portal tracts drain the spaces of Disse. The lymph flows in the same direction as the bile, opposite to that of the blood. The hepatic artery branches are intimately related to the corresponding portal veins. They may show thickening and hyalinization of the wall in older persons, although these changes are usually milder than in other organs. The terminal hepatic arterioles regulate the parenchymal blood supply with their muscular

sphincter (58), whereas the portal venous supply is controlled by mesenteric venous blood flow.

The portal veins are the largest vessels in the portal tracts and produce venules that empty into periportal sinusoids. In contrast to hepatocytes around the terminal hepatic venules, the hepatocytes bordering the portal tracts are joined together and form a distinct row called the limiting plate (59). Destruction of this limiting plate by necroinflammation and/or apoptosis is a hallmark of chronic hepatitis (piecemeal necrosis/interface hepatitis) (Figure 28.22).

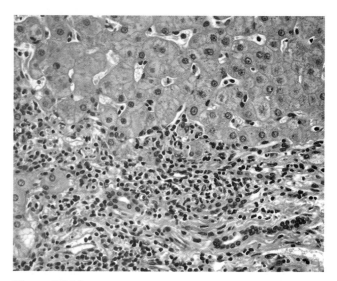

Figure 28.22 Liver from a patient with chronic hepatitis showing destruction of the limiting plate by extension of inflammatory cells from the portal tract into the periportal parenchyma with necrosis/apoptosis of hepatocytes (piecemeal necrosis/interface hepatitis).

EXTRACELLULAR MATRIX

Both interstitial and basement membrane collagens are present in the liver and play an important role, not only as structural elements but also in hepatic function (60). Collagen I—the main component of the dense, birefringent connective tissue fibers—is seen mainly in portal tracts and walls of hepatic veins and rarely in the normal parenchyma, whereas collagen III and IV are present along the sinusoids (5). Collagen I can be demonstrated with connective tissue stains; collagen III can be seen with silver impregnation for reticulin. Collagen II, characteristic of cartilage, is absent from the liver. Collagens IV and V, the basement membrane collagens, and laminin are seen in the basement membrane of vessels, bile ducts, and bile ductules but (except for some collagen IV) not along the sinusoids of normal human liver (42,60). Distribution of elastic fibers in the liver, as demonstrated by orcein, resorcin, or Victoria blue stains, seems to follow that of collagen I (43). Fibronectin, an extracellular matrix glycoprotein, is present diffusely along the sinusoidal surface of hepatocytes and in portal tracts together with the other collagens (61). All components of the extracellular matrix are visualized best by immunohistochemical staining using specific antibodies.

METHODOLOGY

Specimen Handling

At the time of the biopsy procedure, the needle liver biopsy specimen is immediately examined for adequacy. It should be at least 1.5 cm in total length; otherwise, another pass is recommended. Adequate size of the specimen minimizes sampling error.

After the biopsy procedure (62,63), the liver specimen should be handled as little as possible and with utmost care to avoid squeezing and drying artifacts. If the case so indicates, small pieces of liver tissue may be frozen for histochemistry, immunohistochemistry, chemical analysis or fixed in glutaraldehyde for electron microscopy. If required, cultures should be taken. Then the tissue should be transferred quickly into the appropriate fixative solution, usually 10% buffered formalin. Needle biopsy specimens may be arranged on a piece of card to prevent distortion and fragmentation. At this stage, the gross appearance of the liver specimen is noted. Particular attention should be paid to fragmentation, which suggests cirrhosis, and to the number, size, shape, and color of the fragments. Tumors or granulomas, for example, can be recognized as white areas in an otherwise reddish brown tissue. Gray-black discoloration is seen in Dubin-Johnson syndrome, rusty brown in hemochromatosis, green in cholestasis, and yellow in steatosis or in older individuals from the lipofuscin deposition.

Needle biopsy specimens are fixed for at least three hours at room temperature, whereas wedge biopsy specimens, after sectioning into 2-mm thick slices, need longer fixation. Formalin penetrates most tissues at about 0.5 mm per hour at room temperature. In order to avoid shrinkage and hardening of the tissue, it is important to process liver specimens separately from other tissues and on a more rapid schedule in the automated tissue processor. Rush liver biopsy specimens are manually processed to shorten the time schedule to meet the needs of critically ill patients. More than 10 consecutive sections, 3 to 5 μm in thickness, can be cut without artifact from well-embedded specimens. Usually paraffin is used for embedding, but plastic embedding may be used to obtain thinner sections.

Special Stains

The tissue is routinely stained with H&E. Masson's trichrome, Sirius red, or chromotrope-aniline blue stains are used for fibrous tissue; Victoria blue or orcein is used for hepatitis B surface antigen (HBsAg), elastic fibers, lipofuscin, ceroid, and copper-binding protein; PAS with diastase (PAS-D) is used for glycoproteins, including α1-antitrypsin inclusions (Figure 28.23), ceroid in macrophages (Figure 28.24), basement membranes of bile ducts, cytoplasmic inclusions of cytomegalovirus, and *Mycobacterium avium-intracellulare*. Stains for reticulin and iron are also important. If it is not possible to perform all these stains, at a minimum a special stain for connective tissue, such as Masson's trichrome, and/or reticulin should be obtained in order to assess the lobular architecture and to facilitate the diagnosis of cirrhosis.

It should be emphasized that an adequate and properly processed liver specimen without artifacts is an important

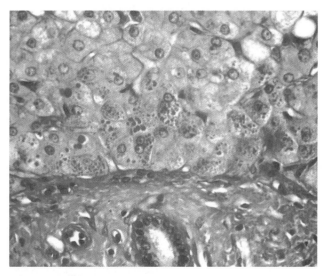

Figure 28.23 Alpha-1-antitrypsin granules and globules in periportal hepatocytes (PAS-D).

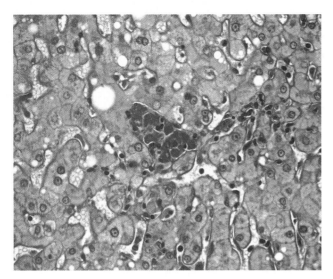

Figure 28.24 Ceroid pigment in macrophages as an indicator of previous hepatocyte injury/necrosis (PAS-D).

prerequisite for the accurate evaluation by an experienced histopathologist, who should be supplied with all relevant clinical and laboratory data.

Microscopic examination should conform to a routine and include all tissue fragments and all structures of the liver (architecture, portal triads, limiting plate, hepatocytes, sinusoidal cells, and terminal hepatic venules). We usually start with careful examination of zone 3 of the acinus because many changes are found here (congestion, fat, necrosis, cholestasis, pigments, endophlebitis) and then move to the remainder of the parenchyma and portal tracts. Sampling error, particularly in focally or irregularly distributed disease processes, always must be taken into consideration. Squeezing of tissue during the biopsy procedure results in distortion of cells and elongation of nuclei, which makes cytologic evaluation of the specimen difficult (for other artifacts, see section In the Liver at Autopsy below).

Immunohistologic Studies

Recent progress in immunology, particularly the development of monoclonal antibodies and of highly sensitive immunohistochemical staining procedures (peroxidase-antiperoxidase and avidin-biotin-peroxidase complex methods), has made it possible to demonstrate many antigens in routinely processed (i.e., formalin-fixed and paraffin-embedded) tissue sections. Blocking of biotin is often required prior to the application of primary antibodies because hepatocytes contain large amount of endogenous biotin, which can give a false positive reaction; such a false positive is even more pronounced with the use of antigen retrievals (64,65).

Cytokeratins (CK) are the intermediate filaments of epithelial cells and are present in hepatocytes and, in greater amounts, in the bile duct epithelium. Different as well as similar cytokeratins are expressed by hepatocytes and bile ducts. Embryonal hepatocytes contain CK8, CK18, and CK19. The expression of CK19 in hepatocytes dissappears by the tenth week of gestation (66). Mature hepatocytes in the normal liver contain only CK8 and CK18 and thus stain diffusely with keratin CAM 5.2. Cytokeratin staining of hepatocytes is usually more intense in the acinar zone 1. Most hepatocytes also stain with keratin 35βH11, which reacts with CK8 only (67). Hepatocytes do not stain with vimentin, epithelial membrane antigen, CK7, and CK19. HepPar1 stains hepatocytes in a diffuse, granular, cytoplasmic pattern (68,69) (Figure 28.25). Normal hepatocytes do not stain with AFP, but hepatocytes in cirrhotic nodules may occasionally show focal positive staining (70).

Cytokeratin polypeptides may be altered in specific liver diseases such as alcoholic hepatitis with formation of Mallory hyalins (67). Mallory hyalins are composed of heterogenous cytokeratin filament and usually react strongly with antibody to CK18, 34βE12, and CAM 5.2 antibodies and with antibody to ubiquitin (71,72). They also react occasionally with CK7 and CK19.

Bile canaliculi can be demonstrated using pCEA and CD10 (73) (Figure 28.12).

Sinusoidal endothelial cells show phenotypic differences with vascular endothelium. Normally, they do not bind the lectin ulex europaeus; they do not express factor VIII–related antigen or contain other molecules found in vascular endothelium, such as CD34 and CD31. They, however, assume these phenotypic properties in chronic liver diseases and in hepatocellular carcinoma (74–76).

Several markers of neural/neuroectodermal differentiation have been found in hepatic stellate cells. These are

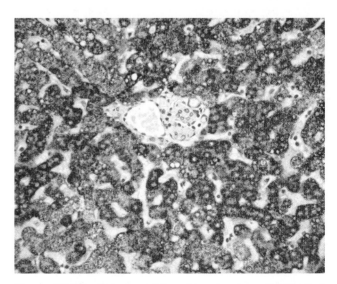

Figure 28.25 Granular staining of hepatocytes using HepPar1 antibody excludes other cells and all structures in the portal tract.

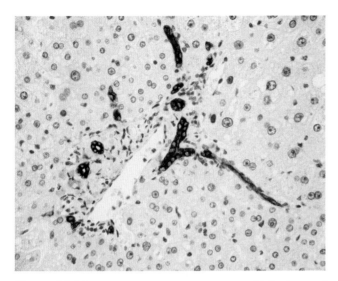

Figure 28.26 Cytokeratin 7 immunostaining of bile duct and bile ductules.

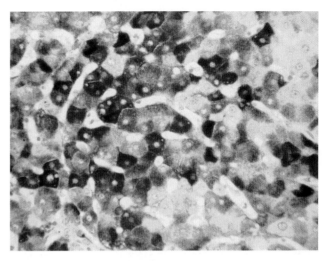

Figure 28.27 Immunostaining of hepatitis B surface antigen (HBsAg) in cytoplasm of ground-glass hepatocytes in an asymptomatic HBV carrier.

synaptophysin, glial fibrillary acidic protein (GFAP), and neural cell adhesion molecule (N-CAM), which can be used to identify resting stellate cells (77–79). When activated, these cells show expression of vimentin, desmin, and smooth muscle actin, which suggests myofibroblastic differentiation (46).

Bile ducts and ductules are readily revealed by immunostaining for bile duct–type CK7 and CK19 (80) (Figure 28.26). Cytokeratin 7 immunostaining is useful to evaluate the presence or loss of bile ducts, such as in cholestatic liver diseases and chronic rejection in liver transplantation. Bile ducts also stain with CK8, CK18, AE1/AE3, 35βH11, and 34βE12 antibodies (67). Some hepatocytes in the periphery of cirrhotic nodules may react with keratin AE1/AE3, CK7, and CK19 antibodies, thus suggesting biliary differentiation (81,82) (Figure 28.21).

Detection of the following antigens is useful in the diagnostic evaluation of liver diseases: α1-antitrypsin in PAS-D–positive intracytoplasmic globules in periportal hepatocytes of patients with α1-antitrypsin deficiency (Figure 28.18); α-fetoprotein in hepatocellular carcinoma; and CEA, CK7, and Lewis blood group antigens in bile duct carcinoma, although CEA is also expressed in some hepatocellular and many other metastatic carcinomas (83,84).

The presence or absence and distribution pattern of viral antigens are helpful in the diagnostic and prognostic evaluation of viral hepatitis, particularly hepatitis B surface (Figure 28.27) and core antigens (Figure 28.28) in hepatitis B virus (HBV) or in dual HBV and HCV (hepatitis C virus) infection. The detection of hepatitis A, C, and delta (D) antigens and of herpesvirus antigens (cytomegalovirus, herpes simplex virus, and Epstein-Barr virus) confirms the cause of acute or chronic hepatitis (85). Since the cloning and sequencing of the HCV genome in 1989, there have

been a number of studies for the detection of HCV antigens in the liver. However, the reports are conflicting (86–88). The detection rate of positive cases varied, which may be related to tissue sampling and differences in sensitivity of various methods and specificity and/or to avidity of the antibodies. Immunohistochemical studies on frozen sections appeared to demonstrate HCV antigens more reliably than on formalin-fixed, paraffin-embedded sections.

The expression of the various components of extracellular matrix in the diseased liver is currently under intensive investigation. It is clear that development of additional monoclonal antibodies to other antigens will further expand the usefulness of immunohistologic stainings to the diagnostic hepatopathologist.

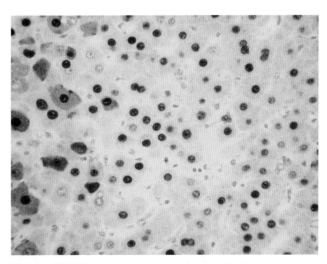

Figure 28.28 Immunostaining of hepatitis B core antigen (HBcAg) in numerous nuclei and cytoplasm of hepatocytes of an immunosuppressed patient with high viral replication.

Molecular Studies

In situ hybridization for the detection of DNA or RNA may be performed on formalin-fixed, paraffin-embedded tissue sections. In situ hybridization for albumin mRNA is highly specific for normal hepatocytes and hepatocellular tumors (69).

The detection of viral sequences such as those of Epstein-Barr virus and more recently of HCV by in situ hybridization appear to be more sensitive than by immunohistochemical methods (89–91). The sensitivity, especially in HCV infection, in which the number of virus in the liver is low, can be further increased by in situ polymerase chain reaction (92).

AGING CHANGES

There are several changes in the liver related to aging. These are commonly seen in individuals 60 years of age and older. There is more variation in the size of the hepatocytes and their nuclei, similar to that seen in patients on methotrexate, due to increased polyploid cells (93). With aging and atrophy of liver cell cords there may be apparent dilatation of sinusoids. More abundant lipofuscin deposition is present in the centrilobular hepatocytes, and sometimes there are some iron pigments in the periportal hepatocytes. The portal tracts contain denser collagen and may exhibit a higher number of mononuclear inflammatory cells than in younger subjects. The arteries may have thickened walls (Figure 28.29), even in normotensive individuals. These histologic changes of aging need to be kept in mind because they are often present in viable donors for which frozen sections are requested and should not be interpreted as pathologic. These aging-related findings are accompanied by alteration in the metabolic function of the liver, including the metabolism of toxins and drugs (94), and therefore may increase the susceptibility of the liver to hypovolemia and decrease its capacity for regeneration.

FREQUENT HISTOLOGIC CHANGES OF LITTLE SIGNIFICANCE

In the Liver at Autopsy

Liver tissue obtained at autopsy often shows changes that are not usually seen in liver biopsy specimens and therefore may cause difficulties in the evaluation. Agonal loss of glycogen from hepatocytes causes increased density and eosinophilia of the cytoplasm. Poor fixation results in irregular staining of hepatocytes, particularly in the center of the specimen. This may result in striking differences in the appearance of liver cells in the peripheral versus the central part of the tissue.

Agonal necrosis, particularly of hepatocytes in zone 3 in patients with shock or heart failure, may not be reflected in elevated aminotransferase levels (Figure 28.30). Its terminal nature is recognized from the lack of any inflammatory response. Autolysis of hepatocytes, particularly in hepatitis and cholestasis resulting in loss of cellular detail and prominent sinusoidal lining cells, is often more pronounced than in other tissues because the liver is rich in proteolytic enzymes. Loss of inflammatory cells by autolysis may make the diagnosis of hepatitis in postmortem specimens difficult (95). Trichrome stain assists greatly in the identification of portal tracts and central venules (and thus the lobular architecture) and, by demonstrating the fibrous septa, the chronicity of the condition.

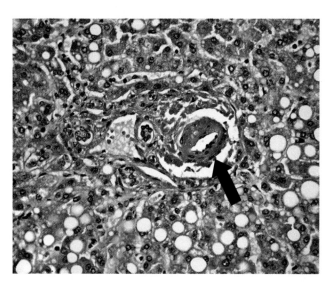

Figure 28.29   Thickened hepatic arteriole in an older individual (*arrow*).

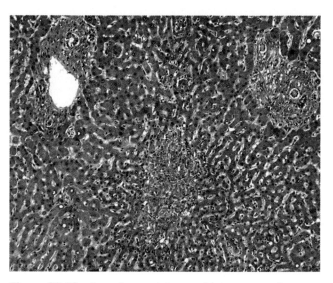

Figure 28.30   Agonal necrosis in zone 3 hepatocytes of autopsy liver without inflammatory cells.

Dilatation of the sinusoidal and perisinusoidal spaces is of little significance in postmortem liver tissues (Figure 28.14) as opposed to similar changes in well-preserved biopsy specimens. Focal accumulation of lymphocytes in scattered portal tracts is frequently seen in autopsy livers and does not justify the diagnosis of chronic hepatitis. Large tissue sections obtained at autopsy often include many large triangular portal tracts with abundant connective tissue that can be distinguished from true portal fibrosis by evaluation of the size of the intraportal structures. Increased fibrous tissue in portal tracts and parenchyma is a normal phenomenon in older individuals.

In Surgical Liver Biopsy Specimens

Surgical biopsy specimens may have several features not seen in needle biopsy specimens that may cause diagnostic difficulties. If the surgeon removes a small, superficial wedge of liver tissue from the inferior margin, the triangular tissue fragment is covered on two sides by the Glisson's capsule. The fibrous connections between the superficial portal tracts and the capsule may imitate cirrhosis (31) (Figure 28.31). However, these changes usually do not extend more than 2 mm into the liver parenchyma.

In biopsy specimens removed at the end of a long surgical procedure, clusters of polymorphonuclear neutrophils are seen in or under the capsule, in sinusoids, around terminal hepatic venules, in portal tracts, and in areas of small focal necroses resembling microabscesses, probably as a result of minor trauma (96) (Figure 28.32). This characteristic lesion must be distinguished from inflammatory liver diseases such as cholangitis. Other "innocent" hepatic lesions include focal steatosis involving small groups of hepatocytes, fat granulomas from mineral oil deposition in

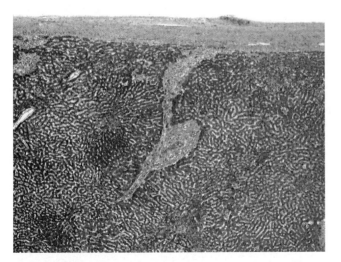

Figure 28.31 Surgical liver biopsy specimen showing fibrous connections between the capsule and superficial portal tracts, imitating the picture of cirrhosis (trichrome stain).

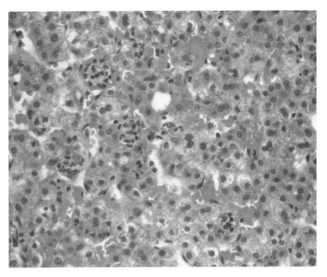

Figure 28.32 Surgical liver biopsy specimen showing clusters of polymorphonuclear neutrophils in sinusoids resembling microabscesses (surgical hepatitis).

perivenular areas and in portal tracts; undefined pigmentation, and unexplained mitoses of hepatocytes that normally have a life span of many years.

MINOR BUT SIGNIFICANT HEPATIC ALTERATIONS

Nonspecific Reactive Hepatitis

This poorly defined histologic change represents a reaction of the liver to a variety of extrahepatic, particularly febrile, and gastrointestinal diseases. Nonspecific reactive hepatitis must be differentiated from primary liver diseases such as mild chronic hepatitis and residual stages of acute viral hepatitis. The alterations consist of activation of sinusoidal lining cells with prominent Kupffer cells, foci of isolated hepatocyte necrosis with accumulation of macrophages and other inflammatory cells, and mild infiltration of some portal tracts by mononuclear cells, without piecemeal necrosis or interface hepatitis (Figures 28.33–28.34). Scattered hepatocytes also may contain microvesicular or macrovesicular fat droplets.

Nonspecific reactive hepatitis with steatosis, increased variation in size and staining quality of hepatocyte nuclei, sinusoidal dilatation, and poorly developed granulomas are seen in livers of patients with acquired immunodeficiency syndrome (AIDS) (97,98). The granulomas are poorly formed and may be difficult to recognize, but special stains may show the a large number of microorganisms such as *M. avium-intracellulare*. Although patients with AIDS are often infected with cytomegalovirus, the characteristic intranuclear and cytoplasmic inclusions are

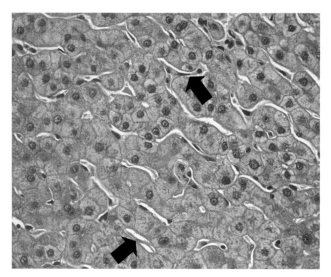

Figure 28.33 Nonspecific reactive hepatitis characterized by activation of sinusoidal lining cells (*arrows*).

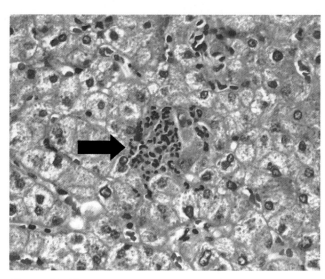

Figure 28.35 Aggregates of polymorphonuclear leukocytes in sinusoid adjacent to a cytomegalovirus-infected cell (*arrow*).

sometimes not detected in the liver. Instead, focal aggregates of polymorphonuclear leukocytes (so-called microabscesses) may be seen in the lobules at the sites of the degenerated infected hepatocytes or sinusoidal lining cells (98,99) (Figure 28.35).

Vicinity of Space-Occupying Lesions

Nonspecific reactive changes are also seen in patients with space-occupying lesions in the liver (100). Although the biopsy specimen may not include the neoplasm, the abscess, or the cyst, a characteristic histologic triad is often observed in the adjacent liver. These changes consist of

proliferated and distorted bile ductules with irregular and even atypical epithelium accompanied by neutrophils in edematous portal tracts, and focal sinusoidal dilatation and congestion (Figure 28.36). In contrast to large bile duct obstruction and other biliary tract diseases such as primary sclerosing cholangitis, cholestasis is usually absent. In addition, the liver cell plates may be compressed and distorted with atrophy of hepatocytes. These histologic changes are the result of focal obstruction of blood and bile flow by the expanding mass. They may be subtle and are usually focal

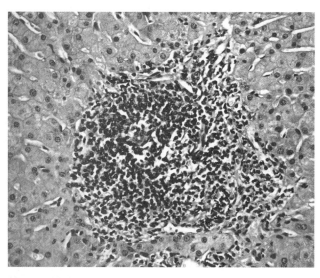

Figure 28.34 Dense lymphocytic aggregate in a portal tract with chronic hepatitis C.

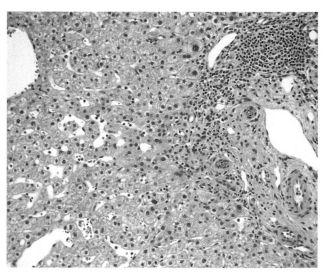

Figure 28.36 Liver biopsy specimen of patient with metastatic carcinoma showing dilatation of sinusoids in zone 2, as well as proliferation of bile ductules and infiltration of portal tract by neutrophils. The specimen did not contain metastatic carcinoma, but the histologic changes are consistent with the vicinity of a space-occupying lesion.

with involvement of small portal tracts. The described triad is characteristic for the vicinity of a space-occupying lesion, and its recognition in a liver specimen should lead to continued search for a neoplasm, cyst, or abscess.

Sinusoidal Dilatation

Acute or chronic venous congestion with dilatation of sinusoids in Rappaport acinus zone 3 and of terminal hepatic venules is frequently seen at autopsy but also in biopsy specimens; it is usually a consequence of right-sided congestive heart failure, whereas irregular necrosis of hepatocytes in zone 3 is often caused by left-sided heart failure or shock (101). In more severe and chronic cases, there is also atrophy of hepatocytes with increased lipofuscin accumulation and scattered small droplet fat vacuoles, enlargement of Kupffer cells containing ceroid pigment, focal cholestasis, and progressive fibrosis in the periphery of the acinus (rather than concentric around the central venules). Engorgement of sinusoids around terminal hepatic venules is also observed in patients with Budd-Chiari syndrome, veno-occlusive disease, sepsis, malignant tumors, so-called collagen diseases, granulomatous diseases, Crohn's disease, and in patients with AIDS (97,102–104).

In contrast, dilatation of sinusoids in Rappaport acinus zone 1 has been observed in pregnancy, in renal transplant patients, after exposure to anabolic/androgenic or contraceptive steroids (105–107), and near space-occupying lesions (100). After exposure to vinyl chloride, thorotrast, arsenicals, and oral contraceptives, sinusoidal dilatation may be accompanied by hepatocellular and sinusoidal cell hypertrophy, hyperplasia, and dysplasia, increased reticulin fibers along sinusoids, and portal fibrosis (106–108).

ACKNOWLEDGMENTS

The late Dr. Hans Popper reviewed the manuscript and offered invaluable constructive criticism. The late Dr. Michael Gerber was the senior author of this chapter in the earlier editions. The authors thank Pamela Ramali for revising illustrations in this chapter.

REFERENCES

1. Desmet VJ, Van Eyken P. Embryology, malformations and malpositions of the liver. In: Haubrich WS, Schaffner F, Berk JE, eds. *Bockus Gastroenterology.* 5th ed. Philadelphia: WB Saunders; 1995: 1849–1857.
2. MacSween RNM, Desmet VJ, Roskams T, Scothorne RJ. Developmental anatomy and normal structure. In: MacSween RNM, Burt AD, Portmann BC, Ishak KG, Scheuer PJ, Anthony PP, eds. *Pathology of the Liver.* 4th ed. London: Churchill Livingstone; 2002:1–66.
3. Wanless IR. Physioanatomic considerations. In: Schiff ER, Sorrell MF, Maddrey WC, eds. *Schiff's Diseases of the Liver.* 9th ed. Philadelphia: Lippincott Williams & Wilkins; 2002:1–57.
4. Moore KL, Persaud TVN. *The Developing Human: Clinically Oriented Embryology.* 7th ed. Philadelphia: WB Saunders; 2003.
5. Hammar JA. Ueber die erste Entstehung der nicht kapillaren intrahepatischen Gallengange beim Menschen. *Z Mikrosk Anat Forsch* 1926;5:59–89.
6. Desmet VJ. Intrahepatic bile ducts under the lens. *J Hepatol* 1985; 1:545–559.
7. Jorgensen MJ. The ductal plate malformation. *Acta Pathol Microbiol Scand Suppl* 1977;257:1–88.
8. Terada T, Nakanuma Y. Detection of apoptosis and expression of apoptosis-related proteins during human intrahepatic bile duct development. *Am J Pathol* 1995;146:67–74.
9. Columbano A, Ledda-Columbano GM, Coni PP, et al. Occurrence of cell death (apoptosis) during the involution of liver hyperplasia. *Lab Invest* 1985;52:670–675.
10. Columbano A, Ledda-Columbano GM, Rao PM, Rajalakshmi S, Sarma DS. Occurrence of cell death (apoptosis) in preneoplastic and neoplastic liver cells. A sequential study. *Am J Pathol* 1984; 116:441–446.
11. Fukuda K, Kojiro M, Chiu JF. Induction of apoptosis by transforming growth factor-β1 in the rat hepatoma cell line McA-RH7777: a possible association with tissue transglutaminase expression. *Hepatology* 1993;10:945–953.
12. Oberhammer F, Bursch W, Tiefenbacher R, et al. Apoptosis is induced by transforming growth factor-β1 within 5 hours in regressing liver without significant fragmentation of the DNA. *Hepatology* 1993;18:1238–1246.
13. Ohno K, Ammann P, Fasciati R, Maier P. Transforming growth factor-β1 preferentially induces apoptotic cell death in rat hepatocytes cultured under pericentral-equivalent conditions. *Toxicol Appl Pharmacol* 1995;132:227–236.
14. Desmet VJ. Liver lesions in hepatitis B viral infection. *Yale J Biol Med* 1988;61:61–83.
15. Wyllie AH. Apoptosis: cell death in tissue regulation. *J Pathol* 1987;153:313–316.
16. Jones AL, Aggeler J. Structure of the liver. In: Haubrich W, Schaffner F, Berk JE, eds. *Bockus Gastroenterology.* 5th ed. Philadelphia: WB Saunders; 1995:1813–1831.
17. Bismuth H. Surgical anatomy and anatomical surgery of the liver. *World J Surg* 1982;6:3–9.
18. Emond JC, Renz JF. Surgical anatomy of the liver and its application to hepatobiliary surgery and transplantation. *Semin Liver Dis* 1994;14:158–168.
19. Behar J. Anatomy and anomalies of the biliary tract. In: Haubrich WS, Schaffner F, Berk JE, eds. *Bockus Gastroenterology.* 5th ed. Philadelphia: WB Saunders; 1995:2547–2553.
20. Henricksen JH, Horn T, Christoffersen P. The blood-lymph barrier in the liver. A review based on morphological and functional concepts of normal and cirrhotic liver. *Liver* 1984; 4:221–232.
21. Barrowman JA. Hepatic lymph and lymphatics. In: McIntyre N, Benhamou JP, Bircher J, Rizetto M, Rodes J, eds. *Oxford Textbook of Clinical Hepatology.* Oxford: Oxford University Press; 1991: 37–40.
22. Witte MH, Witte CL. Lymphatic system in the liver. In: Abramson DI, Dobrin PB, eds. *Blood Vessels and Lymphatics in Organ Systems.* New York: Academic Press; 1984.
23. Tiniakos DG, Lee JA, Burt AD. Innervation of the liver: morphology and function. *Liver* 1996;16:151–160.
24. Friedman JM. Hepatic nerve function. In: Arias IM, Popper H, Jakoby W, Schachter D, Schafritz DA, eds. *The Liver, Biology and Pathobiology.* New York: Raven Press; 1988:948–959.
25. Dhillon AP, Sankey EA, Wang JH, et al. Immunohistochemical studies on the innervation of human transplanted liver. *J Pathol* 1992;167:211–216.
26. Henderson JM, Mackay GJ, Lumsden AB, Atta HM, Brouillard H, Kutner MH. The effect of liver denervation on hepatic haemodynamics during hypovolemic shock in swine. *Hepatology* 1992;15: 130–133.
27. Lee JA, Ahmed Q, Hines JE, Burt AD. Disappearance of hepatic parenchymal nerves in human liver cirrhosis. *Gut* 1992;33: 87–91.
28. Hilden M, Christoffersen P, Juhl E, Dalgaard JB. Liver histology in a "normal" population—examinations of 503 consecutive fatal traffic casualties. *Scand J Gastroenterol* 1977;12:593–597.

29. Millward-Sadler GH, Jezequel AM. Normal histology and ultrastructure. In: Wright R, Millward-Sadler GH, Alberti KGMM KS, eds. *Liver and Biliary Disease*. 2nd ed. London: Bailliere Tindall; 1985:13–44.

30. Patrick RS, McGee JO. Normal liver pathology. In: Patrick RS, McGee JO. *Biopsy Pathology of the Liver*. Philadelphia: JB Lippincott; 1980:4–14.

31. Scheuer P, Lefkowitch JH. The normal liver. In: Scheuer P, Lefkowitch JH, eds. *Liver Biopsy Interpretation*. 6th ed. London: WB Saunders; 2000:36–50.

32. Rappaport AM. The structural and functional unit in the human liver (liver acinus). *Anat Rec* 1958;130:673–689.

33. Elias H. A re-examination of the structure of the mammalian liver. I. Parenchymal architecture. *Am J Anat* 1949;84:311–333.

34. Gumucio JJ, Miller DL. Functional implications of liver cell heterogeneity. *Gastroenterology* 1981;80:393–403.

35. Terada T, Ishida F, Nakanuma Y. Vascular plexus around intrahepatic bile ducts in normal livers and portal hypertension. *J Hepatol* 1989;8:139–149.

36. Ranek L, Keiding N, Jensen ST. A morphometric study of normal human liver cell nuclei. *Acta Pathol Microbiol Scand A* 1975;83: 467–476.

37. Findor J, Perez V, Igartua EB, Giovanetti M, Fioravantti N. Structure and ultrastructure of the liver in aged persons. *Acta Hepatogastroenterol (Stuttg)* 1973;20:200–204.

38. Thung SN, Gerber AM. Differentiation of brown pigments in the liver. In: Thung SN, Gerber MA, eds. *Differential Diagnosis in Pathology. Liver Disease*. New York: Igaku-Shoin; 1995:66.

39. Jones EA. Hepatic sinusoidal cells: new insights and controversies. *Hepatology* 1983;3:259–266.

40. Wisse E, De Zanger RB, Charels K, Van Der Smissen, McCuskey RS. The liver sieve: considerations concerning the structure and function of endothelial fenestrae, the sinusoidal wall and the space of Disse. *Hepatology* 1985;5:683–692.

41. Wisse E, Knook DL. *Kupffer Cells and Other Liver Sinusoidal Cells*. Amsterdam: Elsevier; 1977.

42. Bianchi FB, Biagini G, Ballardini G, et al. Basement membrane production by hepatocytes in chronic liver disease. *Hepatology* 1984;4:1167–1172.

43. Thung SN, Gerber MA. The formation of elastic fibers in livers with massive hepatic necrosis. *Arch Pathol Lab Med* 1982;106: 468–469.

44. Kent G, Gay S, Inouye T, Bahu R, Minick OT, Popper H. Vitamin A-containing lipocytes and formation of type III collagen in liver injury. *Proc Natl Acad Sci U S A* 1976;73:3719–3722.

45. Schirmacher P, Geerts A, Pietrangelo A, Dienes HP, Rogler CE. Hepatocyte growth factor/hepatopoietin A is expressed in fat-storing cells from rat liver but not myofibroblast-like cells derived from fat-storing cells. *Hepatology* 1992;15:5–11.

46. Ogawa K, Suzuki J, Mukai H, Mori M. Sequential changes of extracellular matrix and proliferation of Ito cells with enhanced expression of desmin and actin in focal hepatic injury. *Am J Pathol* 1986;125:611–619.

47. Kaneda K, Kurioka N, Seki S, Wake K, Yamamoto S. Pit cell-hepatocyte contact in autoimmune hepatitis. *Hepatology* 1984;4: 955–958.

48. Wisse E, van't Noordende JM, van der Meulen J, Daems WT. The pit cell: description of a new type of cell occurring in rat liver sinusoids and peripheral blood. *Cell Tissue Res* 1976;173:423–435.

49. Bouwens L, Wisse E. Tissue localization and kinetics of pit cells or large granular lymphocytes in the liver of rats treated with biological response modifiers. *Hepatology* 1988;8:46–52.

50. Van Waes L, Lieber CS. Early perivenular sclerosis in alcoholic fatty liver: an index of progressive liver injury. *Gastroenterology* 1977;73(pt 1):646–650.

51. Nasrallah SM, Nassar VH, Galambos JT. Importance of terminal hepatic venule thickening. *Arch Pathol Lab Med* 1980;104:84–86.

52. Petrelli M, Scheuer PJ. Variation in subcapsular liver structure and its significance in the interpretation of wedge biopsies. *J Clin Pathol* 1967;20:743–748.

53. International Group. Histopathology of the intrahepatic biliary tree. *Liver* 1983;3:161–175.

54. Nakanuma Y, Ohta G. Histometric and serial section observations of the intrahepatic bile ducts in primary biliary cirrhosis. *Gastroenterology* 1979;76:1326–1332.

55. Thung SN, Gerber MA. Adenocarcinoma vs. proliferating bile ductules vs. ductular hepatocytes. In: Thung SN, Gerber MA, eds. *Differential Diagnosis in Pathology. Liver Disorders*. New York: Igaku-Shoin; 1995:128–129.

56. Rubin EM, Martin AA, Thung SN, Gerber MA. Morphometric and immunohistochemical characterization of human liver regeneration. *Am J Pathol* 1995;147:397–404.

57. Roskams TA, Theise ND, Balabaud C, et al. Nomenclature of the finer branches of the biliary tree: canals, ductules, and ductular reactions in human livers. *Hepatology* 2004;39:1739–1745.

58. Yamamoto K, Sherman I, Phillips MJ, Fisher MM. Three-dimensional observations of the hepatic arterial terminations in rat, hamster and human liver by scanning electron microscopy of microvascular casts. *Hepatology* 1985;5:452–456.

59. Elias H. Anatomy of the liver. In: Rouler C, ed. *The Liver: Morphology, Biochemistry, Physiology*. Vol 1. New York: Academic Press; 1963:41–52.

60. Popper H, Martin GR. Fibrosis of the liver: the role of the ectoskeleton. In: Popper H, Schaffner F, eds. *Progress in Liver Disease*. Vol 7. New York: Grune & Stratton; 1982:133–156.

61. Hahn E, Wick G, Pencev D, Timpl R. Distribution of basement membrane proteins in normal and fibrotic human liver: collagen type IV, laminin and fibronectin. *Gut* 1980;21:63–71.

62. Thung SN, Schaffner F. Liver biopsy. In: MacSween RNM, Anthony PP, Scheuer PJ, Burt AP, Portmann BC, eds. *Pathology of the Liver*. 3rd ed. London: Churchill Livingstone; 1994: 787–796.

63. Antonio LB, Suriawinata A, Thung SN. Liver tissue processing techniques. In: Odze RD, Goldblum JR, Crawford JM, eds. *Surgical Pathology of the Gastrointestinal Tract, Liver, Biliary Tract, and Pancreas*. Philadelphia: WB Saunders; 2003:739–756.

64. Bussolati G, Gugliotta P, Volante M, Pace M, Papotti M. Retrieved endogenous biotin: a novel marker and a potential pitfall in diagnostic immunohistochemistry. *Histopathology* 1997;31: 400–407.

65. Dodson A, Campbell F. Biotin inclusions: a potential pitfall in immunohistochemistry avoided. *Histopathology* 1999;34:178–179.

66. Desmet VJ, Van Eyken P, Sciot R. Cytokeratins for probing cell lineage relationships in developing liver. *Hepatology* 1990;12: 1249–1251.

67. Lai YS, Thung SN, Gerber MA, Chen ML, Schaffner F. Expression of cytokeratins in normal and diseased livers and in primary liver carcinomas. *Arch Pathol Lab Med* 1989;113:134–138.

68. Wennerberg AE, Nalesnik MA, Coleman WB. Hepatocyte paraffin 1: a monoclonal antibody that reacts with hepatocytes and can be used for differential diagnosis of hepatic tumors. *Am J Pathol* 1993;143:1050–1054.

69. Kakar S, Muir T, Murphy LM, Lloyd RV, Burgart LJ. Immunoreactivity of Hep Par 1 in hepatic and extrahepatic tumors and its correlation with albumin in situ hybridization in hepatocellular carcinoma. *Am J Clin Pathol* 2003;119:361–366.

70. Theise ND, Fiel IM, Hytiroglou P, et al. Macroregenerative nodules in cirrhosis are not associated with elevated serum or stainable tissue alpha-fetoprotein. *Liver* 1995;15:30–34.

71. Van Eyken P, Sciot R, Desmet VJ. A cytokeratin immunohistochemical study of alcoholic liver disease: evidence that hepatocytes can express 'bile duct-type' cytokeratins. *Histopathology* 1988;13:605–617.

72. Hazan R, Denk H, Franke WW, Lackinger E, Schiller DL. Change of cytokeratin organization during development of Mallory bodies as revealed by a monoclonal antibody. *Lab Invest* 1986;54: 543–553.

73. Borscheri N, Roessner A, Rocken C. Canalicular immunostaining of neprilysin (CD10) as a diagnostic marker for hepatocellular carcinomas. *Am J Surg Pathol* 2001;25:1297–1303.

74. Terayama N, Terada T, Nakanuma Y. An immunohistochemical study of tumour vessels in metastatic liver cancers and the surrounding liver tissue. *Histopathology* 1996;29:37–43.

75. Ruck P, Xiao JC, Kaiserling E. Immunoreactivity of sinusoids in hepatocellular carcinoma. An immunohistochemical study

using lectin UEA-1 and antibodies against endothelial markers, including CD34. *Arch Pathol Lab Med* 1995;119:173–178.

76. Haratake J, Scheuer PJ. An immunohistochemical and ultrastructural study of the sinusoids of hepatocellular carcinoma. *Cancer* 1990;65:1985–1993.

77. Neubauer K, Knittel T, Aurisch S, Fellmer P, Ramadori G. Glial fibrillary acidic protein—a cell type specific marker for Ito cells in vivo and in vitro. *J Hepatol* 1996;24:719–730.

78. Cassiman D, van Pelt J, De Vos R, et al. Synaptophysin: a novel marker for human and rat hepatic stellate cells. *Am J Pathol* 1999; 155:1831–1839.

79. Knittel T, Aurisch S, Neubauer K, Eichhorst S, Ramadori G. Cell-type-specific expression of neural cell adhesion molecule (N-CAM) in Ito cells of rat liver. Up-regulation during in vitro activation and in hepatic tissue repair. *Am J Pathol* 1996;149:449–462.

80. Rubio CA. The detection of bile ducts in liver biopsies by cytokeratin 7. *In Vivo* 1998;12:183–186.

81. Hurlimann J, Gardiol D. Immunohistochemistry in the differential diagnosis of liver carcinomas. *Am J Surg Pathol* 1991;15:280–288.

82. Van Eyken P, Sciot R, Desmet VJ. A cytokeratin immunohistochemical study of cholestatic liver disease: evidence that hepatocytes can express 'bile duct-type' cytokeratins. *Histopathology* 1989;15:125–135.

83. Thung SN, Gerber MA, Sarno E, Popper H. Distribution of five antigens in hepatocellular carcinoma. *Lab Invest* 1979;41:101–105.

84. Gerber MA, Thung SN, Shen SC, Stromeyer FW, Ishak KG. Phenotypic characterization of proliferation: antigenic expression by proliferating epithelial cells in fetal liver, massive hepatic necrosis, and nodular transformation of the liver. *Am J Pathol* 1983; 110:70–74.

85. Gerber MA, Thung SN. The diagnostic value of immunohistochemical demonstration of hepatitis viral antigens in the liver. *Hum Pathol* 1987;18:771–774.

86. Blight K, Lesniewski RR, LaBrooy JT, Gowans EJ. Detection and distribution of hepatitis C-specific antigens in naturally infected livers. *Hepatology* 1994;20:553–557.

87. Krawczynski K, Beach MJ, Bradley DW, et al. Hepatitis C virus antigen in hepatocytes: immunomorphologic detection and identification. *Gastroenterology* 1992;103:622–629.

88. Tsutsumi M, Urashima S, Takada A, Date T, Tanaka Y. Detection of antigens related to hepatitis C virus RNA encoding the NS5 region in the livers of patients with chronic type C hepatitis. *Hepatology* 1994;19:265–272.

89. Negro F, Pacchioni D, Shimizu Y, et al. Detection of intrahepatic replication of hepatitis C virus RNA by in situ hybridization and comparison with histopathology. *Proc Natl Acad Sci U S A* 1992; 89:2247–2251.

90. Tanaka Y, Enomoto N, Kojima S, et al. Detection of hepatitis C virus RNA in the liver by in situ hybridization. *Liver* 1993;13: 203–208.

91. Lones MA, Shintaku IP, Weiss LM, Thung SN, Nichols WS, Geller SA. Posttransplant lymphoproliferative disorder in liver allograft biopsies: a comparison of three methods for the demonstration of Epstein-Barr virus. *Hum Pathol* 1997;28:533–539.

92. Nuovo GJ, Lidonnici K, MacConnell P, Lane B. Intracellular localization of polymerase chain reaction (PCR)-amplified hepatitis C cDNA. *Am J Surg Pathol* 1993;17:683–690.

93. Watanabe T, Tanaka Y. Age-related alterations in the size of human hepatocytes. A study of mononuclear and binucleate cells. *Virchows Arch B Cell Pathol Incl Mol Pathol* 1982;39:9–20.

94. Popper H. Aging and the liver. In: Popper H, Schaffer F, eds. *Progress in Liver Diseases.* Vol 8. Orlando: Grune & Stratton; 1986: 659–683.

95. Gerber MA. Viral hepatitis in the autopsy specimen. *Virchows Arch A Pathol Anat* 1971;354:285–292.

96. Christoffersen P, Poulsen H, Skeie E. Focal liver cell necroses accompanied by infiltration of granulocytes arising during operation. *Acta Hepatosplenol* 1970;17:240–245.

97. Lebovics E, Thung SN, Schaffner F, Radensky PW. The liver in the acquired immunodeficiency syndrome: a clinical and histologic study. *Hepatology* 1985;5:293–298.

98. Sieratzki J, Thung SN, Gerber MA, Ferrone S, Schaffner F. Major histocompatibility antigen expression in the liver in acquired immunodeficiency syndrome. *Arch Pathol Lab Med* 1987;111:1045–1049.

99. Bach N, Thung SN, Berk PD. The liver in acquired immunodeficiency syndrome (AIDS). In: Bianchi L, Gerok W, Maier KP, Deinhard FJ, eds. *Infectious Diseases of the Liver.* Boston: Kluwer Academic; 1990:333–351.

100. Gerber MA, Thung SN, Bodenheimer HC Jr, Kapelman B, Schaffner F. Characteristic histologic triad in liver adjacent to metastatic neoplasm. *Liver* 1986;6:85–88.

101. Arcidi JM Jr, Moore GW, Hutchins GM. Hepatic morphology in cardiac dysfunction. A clinicopathologic study of 1,000 subjects at autopsy. *Am J Pathol* 1981;104:159–166.

102. Banks JG, Foulis AK, Ledingham I, MacSween RN. Liver function in septic shock. *J Clin Pathol* 1982;35:1249–1252.

103. Bruguera M, Aranguibel F, Ros E, Rodes J. Incidence and clinical significance of sinusoidal dilatation in liver biopsies. *Gastroenterology* 1978;75:474–478.

104. Camilleri M, Schafler K, Chadwick VS, Hodgson HJ, Weinbren K. Periportal sinusoidal dilatation, inflammatory bowel disease, and the contraceptive pill. *Gastroenterology* 1981;80:810–815.

105. Ishak KG. Hepatic lesions caused by anabolic and contraceptive steroids. *Semin Liver Dis* 1981;1:116–128.

106. Thung SN, Gerber MA. Precursor stage of hepatocellular neoplasm following long exposure to orally administered contraceptives. *Hum Pathol* 1981;12:472–474.

107. Winkler K, Poulsen H. Liver disease with periportal sinusoidal dilatation: a possible complication to contraceptive steroids. *Scand J Gastroenterol* 1975;10:699–704.

108. Popper H, Maltoni C, Selikoff IJ. Vinyl chloride-induced hepatic lesions in man and rodents. A comparison. *Liver* 1981; 1:7–20.

Gallbladder and Extrahepatic Biliary System

29

Edward B. Stelow   Seung-Mo Hong   Henry F. Frierson, Jr.

INTRODUCTION

The gallbladder is one of the most common surgical pathology specimens. It is most often resected because of stones or inflammatory disease and is only rarely resected because of neoplasia. Somewhat uncommonly, grossly and microscopically "normal" gallbladders are removed incidentally during surgery for other reasons (e.g., liver transplantation). At most institutions, these specimens are rarely seen. The situation is quite different with the extrahepatic bile ducts and ampullae of Vater. These sites are infrequently sampled by biopsy only when neoplasia is suspected, especially cholangiocarcinoma or ampullary adenocarcinoma. The distal common bile duct and ampulla can be studied in the occasional pancreatoduodenectomy specimen but will often be abnormal due to the effects of an ampullary or periampullary neoplasm. The remaining extrahepatic bile duct is rarely resected. The complete biliary system and ampulla can be only studied with autopsy material; however, due in some part to the toxicity of bile, significant autolysis is usually present in these specimens.

This chapter discusses the gross anatomy, physiology, histology, immunohistochemistry, and ultrastructure of the normal gallbladder, extrahepatic bile ducts, ampulla of Vater, and minor papilla.

GALLBLADDER

Gross Anatomy

The gallbladder is a piriform bladder that is attached to the extrahepatic biliary system via the cystic duct and rests in a shallow depression located on the inferior surface of the posterior right lobe of the liver. It measures up to 10 cm long and 3 to 4 cm wide in normal adults, and its wall is approximately 1 to 2 mm thick, varying due to the degree of muscular contraction. The serosal surface of the liver extends to cover the gallbladder, while interlobular connective tissue of the liver merges with the subserosal connective tissue of the gallbladder. The gallbladder is anatomically divided into a blindly ending fundus, a large central body, and a narrow neck that joins the cystic duct. The tapered area of the body that joins the neck is considered the infundibulum. It is here that a peritoneal fold, the cholecystoduodenal ligament, attaches the gallbladder to the first portion of the duodenum. Hartmann's pouch, a small bulge at the infundibulum, is probably not normal and may result from chronic inflammation or stone impaction (1). The neck is somewhat serpentine, measures 5 to 7 mm long, and narrows as it connects with the cystic duct (2).

Physiology

The gallbladder concentrates, stores, and releases bile. Approximately 800 to 1000 mL of bile flow daily into the gallbladder from the liver (3). Its filling results from complex neural and hormonal stimulations that result in its relaxation and the contraction and closing of the sphincter of Oddi. When the sphincter is closed, the intraluminal pressure of the bile ducts will increase as bile is continuously produced by the liver; bile will then flow into the gallbladder. When relaxed the gallbladder can store only 40 to 70 mL of bile and retains a constant intraluminal pressure (3). A much larger volume, however, is handled as the gallbladder concentrates bile via a sodium-coupled transport of chloride, mediated by sodium potassium-ATPase (NaK-ATPase) (4). The active transport of electrolyte into the lateral intercellular space creates an osmotic gradient, and water ultimately flows through the basement membrane into the capillaries of the lamina propria. The gallbladder also has a secretory role, liberating mucosubstances from the surface epithelial cells and neck mucous glands.

Contraction of the gallbladder is also mediated by complex neural and humoral mechanisms and occurs both after and between meals (5). Cholecystokinin, released from the mucosa of the proximal duodenum after fatty meals, is the most important hormone that promotes gallbladder contraction (6). Motilin aids in interdigestive gallbladder contraction, which occurs in tandem with giant migratory complexes of the intestines every two hours or so (5,7). Other peptides including pancreatic polypeptide and somatostatin may affect gallbladder motility (5,7-9). The vagal system may also play a role both directly and indirectly in gallbladder contraction (10). The complicated balance of humoral and neural mechanisms involved in the working of the gallbladder is sometimes disrupted and many disease states have been implicated in the development of gallbladder dysmotility. Dysmotility may, in turn, result in gallbladder pathology (11).

Blood Supply and Lymphatic Drainage

The arterial supply of the gallbladder varies both in its anatomy and in its relationship to the extrahepatic biliary system. The cystic artery supplies the gallbladder and usually arises from the proximal portion of the right hepatic artery. Indeed, 72% of all cystic arteries in a study by Moosman and Collier (12) arose from the right hepatic artery, whereas 13% arose from the superior mesenteric artery; the remainder originated from the common hepatic artery, left hepatic artery, gastroduodenal artery, celiac artery, or aorta. Most commonly, the artery is located superior to the cystic duct (Figure 29.1). In Moosman and Collier's study, 70% of all cystic arteries coursed to the right of the common hepatic duct, and 17% traveled anterior to the common hepatic duct; the remainder of the cystic arteries passed posterior to

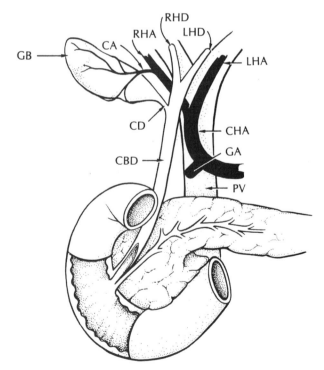

Figure 29.1 Although variations are common, this diagram depicts the "usual" relationships of the extrahepatic bile ducts, portal vein, and branches of the common hepatic artery. (*PV,* portal vein; *GA,* gastroduodenal artery; *CHA,* common hepatic artery; *LHA,* left hepatic artery; *LHD,* left hepatic duct; *RHD,* right hepatic duct; *RHA,* right hepatic artery; *GB,* gallbladder; *CA,* cystic artery; *CD,* cystic duct; *CBD,* common bile duct)

the common hepatic duct, anterior or posterior to the common bile duct, to the right and inferior to the cystic duct, or posterior to both hepatic ducts. The cystic artery branches to form superficial channels that lie over the gallbladder serosa and deep channels that lie between the gallbladder and its hepatic bed (2). One of the more common anatomic variations noted is the double cystic artery. In their study of the extrahepatic biliary tree in 250 cadavers, Moosman and Collier noted a double cystic artery in 14% of their cases. Michels found double cystic arteries in one-quarter of 200 cadavers (13).

A single large cystic vein does not exist (2). The venous drainage consists, in part, of small venous channels on the hepatic side of the gallbladder that lead directly into the liver. Other small veins flow toward the cystic duct and merge with channels from the common bile duct before terminating in the portal venous system.

The lymphatic system of the gallbladder has been investigated by anatomic and physiologic studies and by studies of gallbladder malignancy (14,15). The lymphatics of the gallbladder drain first into lymph nodes at the gallbladder neck or cystic duct. Following this, drainage may proceed to retropancreatic, celiac, or mesenteric lymph nodes. These pathways appear to all converge at abdominal aortic lymph nodes located at the superior mesenteric artery (14). In a study in which dye was injected directly into lymphatic vessels of the gallbladder, the dye flowed initially into the cystic node and pericholedochal nodes, then into lymph nodes posterior to the pancreas, portal vein, and common hepatic artery, and finally into interaortocaval nodes near the left renal vein (15). Ascending lymph flow to the hepatic hilum does not usually occur; however, retrograde flow to the hepatic hilum may occur when there is blockage of lymphatic channels by cancer, inflammation, or surgical ligation (15).

Nerve Supply

Nerve branches from the left trunk of the vagus join the hepatic plexus. The hepatic plexus then supplies the gallbladder with sympathetic, parasympathetic, and possibly afferent nerve fibers (2). Vagal stimulation, both directly and indirectly, may then stimulate interdigestive periodic contractions of gallbladder smooth muscle (10). Neuropeptide Y nerve fibers, which may also participate in gallbladder smooth muscle contraction, are found in all layers of the gallbladder. They form a particularly dense network in the lamina propria, running near the epithelium and paralleling the muscle bundles (16).

Histology

The layers of the gallbladder include the mucosa (surface epithelium and lamina propria), smooth muscle, perimuscular subserosal connective tissue, and serosa. A muscularis mucosae and submucosa are not present. The luminal folds

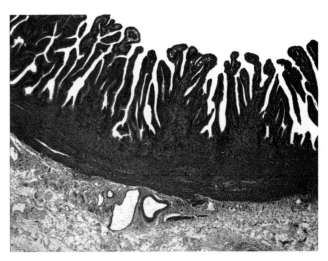

Figure 29.2 The luminal folds of the gallbladder vary in height and contain a delicate core of lamina propria above the bundles of smooth muscle.

are lined by a single layer of columnar epithelium and have cores of lamina propria. The height and width of the folds are variable, and branching is characteristic (Figure 29.2). The columnar epithelial cells have lightly eosinophilic cytoplasm with occasional small apical vacuoles (Figure 29.3). Nuclei are aligned at the cell base or slightly more centrally. They are oval and uniform and have fine chromatin and smooth membranes. Nucleoli are absent or very small and inconspicuous. Occasional columnar cells are

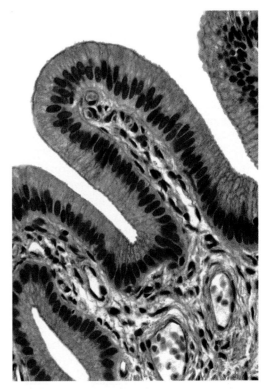

Figure 29.3 The gallbladder is lined by a single layer of tall columnar cells with basally oriented nuclei.

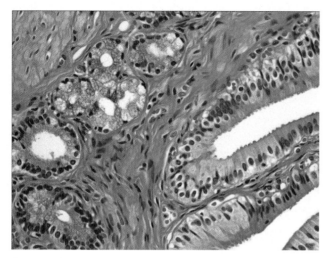

Figure 29.4 Mucous glands are present only in the neck of the normal gallbladder.

narrow with dark eosinophilic cytoplasm (1). These cells, dignified with the appellation "pencil-like" cells, appear to be little more than contracted columnar cells, although they reportedly have a few ultrastructural and enzymatic properties that differ from those of the usual columnar cells. Basal cells are inconspicuous and have nuclei that lie just above and parallel to the basement membrane.

Tubuloalveolar mucous glands are located only in the neck of the gallbladder (17). They have cuboid or low columnar cells with abundant clear to lightly basophilic cytoplasm and round, basally oriented nuclei (Figure 29.4). Their lectin-binding profile is dissimilar to that of the surface epithelial cells (18). The neck mucous glands also differ morphologically and histochemically from the antral-type metaplastic glands found in the fundus, body, or neck of chronically inflamed gallbladders or those that contain gallstones (17). Rare endocrine cells can be found here but are otherwise absent in the normal gallbladder (19,20). Gastric metaplasia (foveolar-type epithelium or antral-type glands) and "intestinal" metaplasia (absorptive cells with prominent brush borders, endocrine cells, goblet cells, and Paneth's cells) are not observed in the normal gallbladder but commonly occur in chronic cholecystitis and cholelithiasis (1,17,21–25). Squamous metaplasia, rarely found in diseased gallbladders, is also absent in normal gallbladders (1). Melanocytes are not found in the normal epithelial lining. However, a few small lymphocytes often are seen between the surface columnar cells.

Gallbladder epithelial cells contain chiefly sulfated acid mucin with very small quantities of nonsulfated acid mucin (17). In contrast, metaplastic cells (goblet cells, superficial gastric-type cells, antral-type glands) contain nonsulfated acid mucin and neutral mucin but little sulfated acid mucin. By immunohistochemistry, the epithelial cells express MUC5AC and MUC6, akin to gastric epithelium; however, pepsinogens I and II, present in pyloric gland metaplasia, are not seen in normal gallblad-

der epithelium (24,26). Lysozyme is also absent in the normal columnar cells but may be found in metaplastic glands (27). Alpha-1-antitrypsin and α1-antichymotrypsin are present in both normal and metaplastic epithelia (27).

Immunohistochemical staining for carcinoembryonic antigen (CEA) (polyclonal; unabsorbed) of normal gallbladders shows focal weak staining along the apices of some lining cells (28). In contrast to the results using monoclonal antibodies to CEA, inflamed epithelium usually shows immunostaining with polyclonal antisera (29). Absorption of at least one polyclonal antibody with human liver powder abolishes the immunoreactivity because there is removal of the CEA-related glycoproteins nonspecific cross-reacting antigen (NCA) and biliary glycoprotein (BGP) (29). The surface epithelium and neck mucous glands are strongly immunoreactive for epithelial membrane antigen and low-molecular weight keratin (CAM 5.2 antibody). The CAM 5.2 antibody also stains some smooth muscle fibers in the gallbladder wall. Normal gallbladder epithelium also reacts with antibody directed against cytokeratin (CK)7 and does not react with antibody directed against CK20 (Figure 29.5) (30). Because endocrine cells are not found in the normal epithelium of the fundus or body, immunohistochemical staining for neuron-specific enolase and chromogranin A is absent (19). A few argentaffin (enterochromaffin) cells are present in the mucous glands of the neck; these cells are readily detected by an antibody to chromogranin A (19). Normal gallbladder mucosa lacks immunoreactivity for estrogen receptor, whereas in 6 of 31 cases of cholelithiasis, a few immunoreactive cells were observed chiefly in metaplastic mucous glands (pseudopyloric glands) (31). Adhesion molecules expressed by normal gallbladder epithelial cells include α-catenin, β-catenin, γ-catenin, CD44, CD99, and E-cadherin (32).

The lamina propria contains loose connective tissue, elastic fibers, nerve fibers, small blood vessels, and lym-

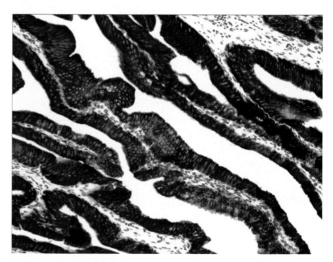

Figure 29.5 The epithelial lining of the gallbladder reacts strongly with antibodies directed against cytokeratin 7 (immunoperoxidase technique).

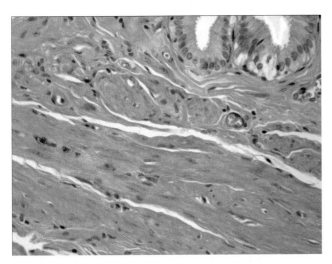

Figure 29.6 Occasional mast cells are identified within the gallbladder by kit-immunostaining. No interstitial cells of Cajal were identified (immunoperoxidase technique).

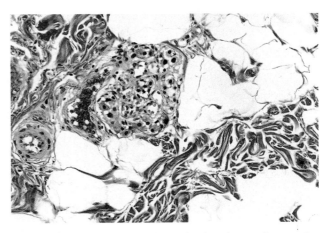

Figure 29.8 Paraganglia are located in the subserosal connective tissue of the normal gallbladder.

phatic channels. Mast cells and macrophages may be seen in small numbers, and it has been noted that these cells are more numerous in normal or minimally inflamed gallbladders than in those with overt chronic cholecystitis (Figure 29.6) (33). Polymorphonuclear leukocytes normally are not present in the lamina propria, but small numbers of lymphocytes and plasma cells are usual. Plasma cells that contain immunoglobulin (Ig)A occur chiefly in the lamina propria, whereas IgM-containing cells are more frequent in the smooth muscle layer (34). A few IgG-containing plasma cells also may be present.

The smooth muscle consists of loosely arranged bundles of circular, longitudinal, and oblique fibers that do not form well-developed layers like they do in the luminal gut. Fibrovascular connective tissue focally separates the muscle bundles. The muscle fibers sometimes extend high into the lamina propria to just beneath the epithelial basement membrane. The thickness of the muscle layer is quite variable, which may simply reflect variable contractile states of

the specimen. Ganglion cells are found in the lamina propria, between smooth muscle bundles, and in the subserosal connective tissue (Figure 29.7). We have been unable to identify interstitial cells of Cajal, although they have been rarely noted by other authors, and rare gastrointestinal stromal tumors of the gallbladder have been reported (1,35).

The subserosal tissue contains loose collagen fibers, fibroblasts, elastic fibers, adipocytes, blood vessels, nerves, and lymphatics. Small aggregates of lymphocytes may occur around vessels. Uncommonly, a lymph node is found in the subserosal connective tissue (36). Paraganglia, infrequently seen in routine sections, are found adjacent to blood vessels and small nerves (Figure 29.8). Examining serial blocks and subserial sections of gallbladders, the investigators of one study found one to five paraganglia in the subserosal tissue of nine of ten cholecystectomy specimens (37).

Rokitansky-Aschoff sinuses represent herniations of epithelium into the lamina propria, smooth muscle, or subserosal connective tissue (Figure 29.9). Although these

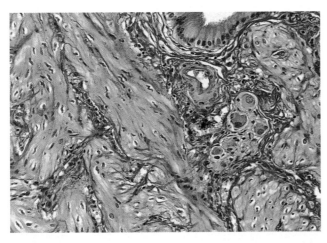

Figure 29.7 Ganglion cells are readily seen in the connective tissue layers of the gallbladder.

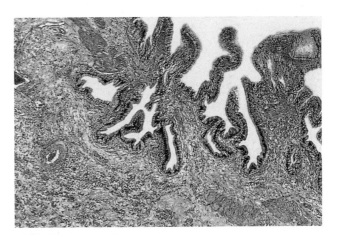

Figure 29.9 Rokitansky-Aschoff sinuses occur in the normal gallbladder but uncommonly penetrate through the smooth muscle bundles.

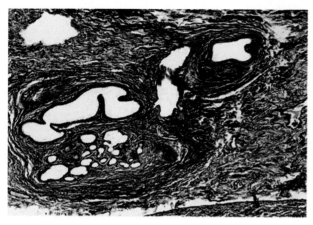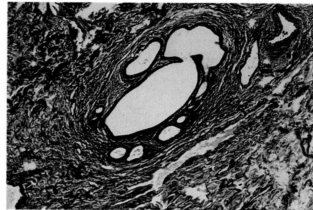

Figure 29.10 Luschka's ducts consist of groups of small ducts having lumina of various caliber. They are surrounded by condensed connective tissue.

are commonly considered a feature of chronic cholecystitis, they are often present in histologically normal gallbladders, albeit more superficially. In a series of 125 cholecystectomy specimens that were inflamed or contained gallstones, 86% had Rokitansky-Aschoff sinuses, almost 90% of which penetrated into or through the smooth muscle (38). The sinuses were also observed in 42% of 112 normal gallbladders examined at autopsy (39). When present in normal gallbladders, they were generally confined to the lamina propria, with infrequent penetration of the smooth muscle. The sinuses are not found in gallbladders from fetuses, but a few superficial outpouchings may be observed in organs from infants (40). The diameters of the sinuses are variable, and flask-shaped formations are usual. Although the exact mechanism for their formation is unknown, herniation of the epithelium may result from overdistension (with increased intraluminal pressure) and extreme contractions of the gallbladder, with subsequent weakening of its wall (40).

Luschka's ducts are small, usually microscopic, bile ducts that lie in the subserosal connective tissue, most commonly on the hepatic side of the gallbladder (Figure 29.10). Occasionally, a few ducts are present in the subserosal connective tissue on the peritoneal side. The ducts have been found in 10 to 12% of routine sections from cholecystectomy specimens, occurring in both normal and diseased organs (39,40). They have been observed in gallbladders from infants, adolescents, and adults and may represent embryonic remnants. Reports of their drainage site are varied. Most have argued that they communicate with intrahepatic bile ducts; however, some have argued that those beneath the serosa possibly drain into the peritoneal cavity, and others, rarely, have suggested that they may drain into the gallbladder lumen, especially within its neck (38,40,41).

The ducts are solitary or multiple but are usually present in small groups surrounded by a distinctive ring of connective tissue and may be adjacent to blood vessels. In serial sections, they sometimes are seen as a system of anastomosing channels. The diameters of their lumina vary from several microns up to a few millimeters. The ducts are lined by cells similar to those of the intrahepatic bile ducts. In some instances, small foci of hepatic parenchyma are located adjacent to the ducts (40). Luschka's ducts are distinct from Rokitansky-Aschoff sinuses, and the two should not communicate. It should be noted that the term *Luschka's duct* has been used somewhat indiscriminately and has been used to refer to entities ranging from Rokitansky-Aschoff sinuses to true accessory ducts.

At surgery and by cholangiography, larger accessory ducts (up to several millimeters long) sometimes are seen in the gallbladder bed. They may be mistaken grossly for small veins or thin strands of fibrous tissue (42). If these ducts are not ligated during surgery, a bile leak may develop, which typically ceases spontaneously. In one study, 9% of 204 patients with randomly selected cholecystectomies had bile leaks from the drain tube; some of these were considered to be due to a divided subvesical duct (43). Although these ducts lie in the gallbladder wall, they usually do not drain into the lumen of the fundus but communicate with the cystic or hepatic ducts (44,45). In a study of 20 autopsy dissections from patients without biliary disease, six subvesical ducts were found, five of which were placed centrally in the gallbladder bed and one in the lateral peritoneal reflection (43). Five led to the right hepatic duct, and one entered the common hepatic duct.

Ectopic hepatic, pancreatic, adrenal, gastric, and thyroid tissues have been reported in the gallbladder (46–49). Ectopic hepatic and adrenal tissues are typically incidental findings, whereas ectopic pancreatic or gastric tissues may lead to symptoms related to their secretions (46).

Ultrastructure

The surface columnar cells measure 15 to 25 μm in height and 2.5 to 7.0 μm in width and rest on a basement membrane (50). These cells have numerous apical microvilli with filamentous glycocalyx and core rootlets (Figure 29.11). The microvilli are shorter and more variable in size and density than those of the intestinal epithelium. Pinocytotic vesicles are formed from the intervillous portions of the cell membrane. The lateral cell membranes are straight at the apex and connected by junctional complexes. Below this boundary, the cell membranes have complex interdigitations that surround lateral intercellular spaces (Figure 29.11). The diameter of the intercellular space varies, depending on the state of fluid transport (51). It is collapsed when there is no water transport but is distended during influx of electrolytes and water. The nuclei are oval, have prominent euchromatin, and occasional small nucleoli. The cytoplasm contains rough endoplasmic reticulum, mitochondria, glycogen, filaments, Golgi apparatus, mucous granules, vesicles, and lysosomes.

Pencil cells have slender outlines, narrow nuclei, and dense cytoplasm that is packed with organelles. At the base of the pencil cell, cytoplasmic extensions project into the basement membrane, unlike that for the typical columnar cell (52). However, microvilli and lateral membrane interdigitations are similar for the pencil cell.

The basal cell measures 10 to 15 μm in diameter, has an irregular nucleus, and has cytoplasmic organelles that

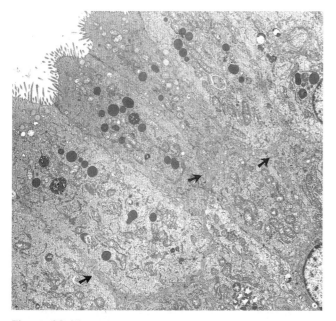

Figure 29.11 Ultrastructurally, the apical portion of the columnar cells of the gallbladder contains abundant microvilli with core rootlets, mitochondria, Golgi apparatus, mucous granules, lysosomes, and a few strands of rough endoplasmic reticulum. The lateral cell membranes form complex interdigitations (*arrows*).

include rough and smooth endoplasmic reticulum, mitochondria, vacuoles, and ring-shaped osmiophilic inclusions (50,52). They have a cytoplasmic extension that runs parallel to the basement membrane, changes direction to run perpendicularly, and then branches toward the lumen (50). The branches are variable in length, delicate, and complex. Throughout the lining epithelium, there are intraepithelial nerve endings that originate from the nerve submucosal plexus and are associated with the small basal cells (50).

Capillaries are found just below the epithelial basement membrane, and their lumina change in size according to the state of fluid transport. The epithelial cells of the glands in the gallbladder neck have a few short microvilli, relatively even lateral membranes, rare secretory granules, and round nuclei (53).

CYSTIC DUCT

The cystic duct is located at the right free edge of the lesser omentum and usually joins the right lateral portion of the common hepatic duct approximately 2 cm distal to the union of the right and left hepatic ducts. In one study, the mean length of the cystic duct was 30 mm and ranged in size from 4 to 65 mm (12). The mean collapsed diameter was 4 mm. Connection and drainage into the common hepatic duct varies. Anatomic studies have found that most cystic ducts drain laterally at an acute angle into the common bile duct (12). In some cases, it may form an angular junction with either the anterior or posterior aspect of the common hepatic duct. A short cystic duct parallel to the common hepatic duct may be present, and a long cystic duct has been rarely noted. Rarely, the cystic duct may spiral and join the common hepatic duct anteriorly or posteriorly. In a cholangiographic study involving large numbers of patients, however, the cystic duct drained laterally at an acute angle into the common bile duct in only 17% of the cases, whereas in 35% it drained in a spiral form, in 41% posteriorly, and in 7% it first ran parallel to the common hepatic duct (54). In rare instances, the cystic duct may join the right and left hepatic ducts, forming a trifurcation. The cystic duct usually passes inferiorly to the cystic artery and to the right of the right hepatic artery.

The lining of the cystic duct is pleated, and in some areas there are short folds of varying width and height. The surface cells are identical microscopically and immunohistochemically to those of the gallbladder (55). Groups of mucous glands are embedded in the dense, collagenous lamina propria. Lectin-binding patterns of the lining cells are similar to those for the surface epithelial cells of the gallbladder body and neck, and the lectin-binding profiles for the mucous glands of the cystic duct are indistinguishable from those of the glands at the gallbladder neck (18). Enterochromaffin

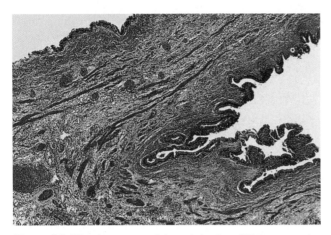

Figure 29.12   The stroma of the spiral valve of Heister contains thin strands of smooth muscle fibers.

cells containing serotonin have been described in cystic ducts from patients with pancreaticobiliary disease (56). In this same group of patients, a few intramural gland cells have shown immunoreactivity for somatostatin.

The connective tissue of the large, oblique folds, grossly visible in the cystic duct at the junction with the gallbladder neck, contains thin groups of smooth muscle fibers (spiral valve of Heister) (Figure 29.12). The smooth muscle is believed to prevent both overdistention and collapse of the cystic duct when it is subjected to changes in pressure (2). Abundant collagen and some elastic fibers, nerve fibers, and ganglion cells are intermixed with the smooth muscle. Nerve fibers showing immunoreactivity for vasoactive intestinal peptide (VIP) and other peptides have been described in the wall (9,56). The loose subserosal connective tissue contains adipose tissue, nerves with occasional ganglion cells, large blood vessels, and lymphatic channels. Lymphocytes and plasma cells are sparse or absent.

RIGHT AND LEFT HEPATIC DUCTS, COMMON HEPATIC DUCT, AND COMMON BILE DUCT

Gross Anatomy

The right and left hepatic ducts, common hepatic duct, and common bile duct are embedded between the serous layers of the hepatoduodenal ligament (the right free border of the lesser omentum). The hepatic ducts emerge from the liver and, in most instances, unite in the hilum approximately 1 cm from the liver to form the common hepatic duct. In 10 to 30% of cases, two large segmental ducts drain the right hepatic lobe and join separately with the left hepatic duct, common hepatic duct, or cystic duct; it is incorrect to label one of these ducts the right hepatic duct and the other as "accessory" (57). In a dissection of 100 au-

topsy specimens, the mean length of the right hepatic duct was 0.8 cm (range: 0.2–2.5 cm) and that of the left hepatic duct 1.0 cm (range: 0.2–3.5 cm) (58). The usual diameter of each hepatic duct was 3 to 4 mm, and the length of the common hepatic duct ranged from 0.8 to 5.2 cm (mean: 2.0 cm) (58). Its diameter ranged from 0.4 to 2.5 cm (59). The diameter of the common hepatic duct and its number of elastic fibers increase with age (59). The common bile duct, resulting from the union of the cystic duct and common hepatic duct, can be divided into supraduodenal, retroduodenal, pancreatic, and intraduodenal segments. It is usually about 1 mm thick and 5 cm long, but its length is quite variable (range: 1.5–9.0 cm) (58). The diameter at its midpoint ranges from 0.4 to 1.3 cm (mean: 0.66 cm), and its lumen narrows approximately 50% after entering the duodenal window (58,60). In an autopsy study of 100 selected subjects who ranged in age from 15 to 102 years, lacked a history of biliary tract disease, and had completely intact biliary tracts, the outer diameters of the upper portions of the common bile ducts ranged from 0.4 to 1.2 cm (mean: 0.74 cm) (61). The outer diameters increased with age but were not related to body weight or length (61). The pits in the surface epithelium (sacculi of Beale) are conspicuous in the extraduodenal portion of the common bile duct and the hepatic ducts. At approximately 2 mm from the duodenal wall, the wall of the common bile duct thickens (due to an increase in muscle), resulting in the abrupt narrowing of the duct's lumen.

Arterial Supply, Venous Drainage, and Relationship to Bile Ducts

The common hepatic artery arises from the celiac trunk and divides into right and left hepatic branches (Figure 29.1). Variations in the origins of the right and left hepatic arteries and their relationships to the extrahepatic bile ducts are typical (62). In one study, almost 42% of 200 cadavers had "aberrant" hepatic arteries (13). Most often, the right hepatic artery is dorsal to the common hepatic duct and right hepatic duct. The common hepatic and left hepatic arteries lie to the left of the extrahepatic bile ducts and ventral to the portal vein. The gastroduodenal artery lies to the left of the common bile duct, and a branch, the superior pancreaticoduodenal, traverses the duct either dorsally or ventrally (2).

The extrahepatic bile ducts are supplied by numerous arteries. The major arteries that supply branches to the common hepatic duct and the common bile duct include the retroduodenal, right and left hepatic, posterior superior and anterior superior pancreaticoduodenal, common hepatic, cystic, gastroduodenal, and retroportal arteries (63). The most important branches travel along the lateral borders of the common bile duct (64).

The portal vein, formed by the union of the splenic and superior mesenteric veins, lies dorsal to the bile ducts

(Figure 29.1). The mean length is 6.4 cm (range: 4.8–8.8 cm) and its mean diameter is 0.9 cm (range: 0.64–1.21 cm) (65). Venous channels that drain the superior portion of the common bile duct enter the liver directly, and those from the inferior portion lead to the portal vein.

Lymphatic Drainage

Lymphatic channels from the common bile duct drain into lymph nodes located along the hepatoduodenal ligament or within the posterior pancreaticoduodenal area. Drainage then proceeds to lymph nodes at the superior mesenteric artery, aorta, and common hepatic duct (66,67).

Nerve Supply

The nerve supply to the cystic and hepatic ducts derives from the anterior portion of the hepatic plexus, whereas nerves that supply the common bile duct arise from the posterior segment of the hepatic plexus. The nerve of the common bile duct, lying dorsally, is the right portion of the posterior hepatic plexus. Smaller branches from the posterior hepatic plexus travel inferiorly along the common bile duct and accompany the duct to the major duodenal papilla (2). Neuropeptide Y–containing nerve fibers have the same pattern of distribution in the common bile duct as in the gallbladder (16).

Histology

The extrahepatic bile ducts, serving as conduits for the flow of bile, are lined by a single layer of tall columnar cells surrounded by a dense connective tissue layer (Figure 29.13). The surface of the epithelium is relatively flat or pleated.

The columnar cells have basally oriented nuclei that are oval and uniform. Nucleoli are absent or very small. Goblet cells are absent in normal epithelium. The epithelium dips into the stroma to form shallow depressions or deeper pits—the sacculi of Beale. In some sections, the deeper sacculi appear isolated from the surface epithelium, but deeper sections will often show their connections. Surrounding the sacculi are unevenly distributed lobules of glands that empty into the sacculi (Figure 29.14). These glands have been termed diverticula, crypts, parietal sacculi, deep glands, biliary glands, periductal glands, and extrahepatic peribiliary glands (68). When located in the more peripheral connective tissue, the glands are encircled by condensed stroma. The peribiliary tubular glands are branched or, occasionally, simple (68). Although they are found in all parts of the extrahepatic bile duct system, they are less frequent in the central portion of the common bile duct and in the intrapancreatic portion than around the bile duct at the ampulla. They are lined by low-columnar or cuboid cells, many of which are filled with mucin (Figure 29.14). With inflammation and fibrosis, the sacculi and glands may be distorted, mimicking well-differentiated

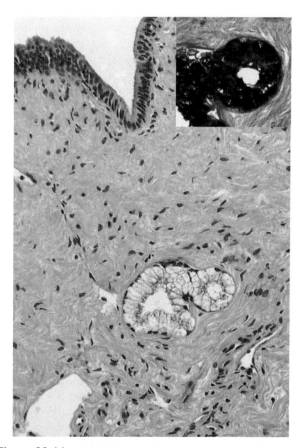

Figure 29.14 Glands embedded in the subepithelial collagenous stroma of the extrahepatic bile ducts typically contain cells with mucin-filled cytoplasm. (Inset: Alcian blue–periodic acid-Schiff (PAS) stain from the same field).

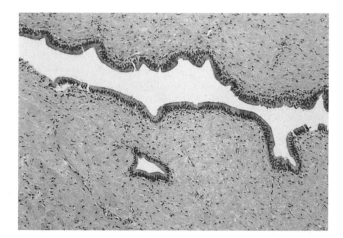

Figure 29.13 Intrapancreatic segment of common bile duct. The extrahepatic bile ducts are lined by a single layer of tall columnar cells overlying dense, collagenous connective tissue. In segments of the common bile duct away from the duodenum, a few small groups of smooth muscle fibers are sometimes found in the outer half of the wall.

adenocarcinoma with desmoplastic stroma. In small biopsy specimens and especially frozen sections, the distinction between adenocarcinoma and distorted benign glands may be impossible. The lack of a lobular arrangement and the presence of marked nuclear atypia and perineural invasion are diagnostic of adenocarcinoma (69). Hence, a haphazard growth pattern and cells whose nuclei vary in size and have irregular nuclear membranes are characteristic of adenocarcinoma. Benign glands of the extrahepatic bile ducts have not been reported to invade nerves.

The surface epithelial cells contain smaller quantities of mucin than the cells that line the gallbladder (70). The former also contain sulfated acid mucin, whereas metaplastic and dysplastic cells primarily contain nonsulfated acid mucin and smaller quantities of sulfated and neutral mucins. The normal lining epithelium stains similarly to that of the gallbladder for epithelial membrane antigen and low-molecular weight keratin (CAM 5.2 antibody). Cytokeratin 7 is consistently expressed in normal epithelium, while CK20 expression depends on the condition of the epithelial cells. In normal cells, expression of CK20 is usually absent; however, it may be expressed when metaplasia, hyperplasia, or carcinoma are present (30,71). Carcinoembryonic antigen immunoreactivity may be absent (using absorbed polyclonal antibody) or appear as focal weak staining along the apices of some cells (using unabsorbed polyclonal antibody) (72). Cytoplasmic staining using either polyclonal or monoclonal anti-CEA antibodies is typically absent (73). Immunoreactivity for lysozyme has been found in the cytoplasm of the cells in the glands, whereas staining of the surface epithelial cells is absent or very weak (72). In addition, cells of the peribiliary glands are usually immunoreactive for pancreatic and salivary α-amylase, trypsin, and lipase (68). The surface epithelium of the common bile duct also shows immunoreactivity for these enzymes.

Gastric metaplasia and intestinal metaplasia are sometimes found in inflamed and fibrotic extrahepatic bile ducts that may also harbor carcinoma (23,70,74). Scattered endocrine cells, including cells immunoreactive for chromogranin and somatostatin, can be observed between mucin-containing cells in normal as well as diseased biliary epithelium (56,74–76).

The stroma directly beneath the surface epithelium is dense and contains abundant collagen and elastic fibers and some small vessels (Figure 29.13). Lymphocytes are sparse. Pancreatic acini and ducts may be seen in the wall of the intrapancreatic portion of the common bile duct (77). Small pancreatic ducts sometimes empty into this segment of the duct. The peripheral stroma of the common bile duct is less dense than the inner connective tissue and contains large blood vessels, lymphatics, nerves and ganglion cells, elastic fibers, and smooth muscle fibers. This stroma merges with the connective tissue of the hepatoduodenal ligament. The distribution of smooth muscle fibers varies

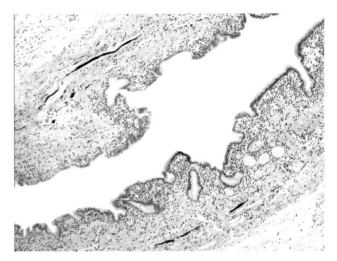

Figure 29.15   Occasional strands of smooth muscle are demonstrated in the upper portion of the common bile duct reacting with antibodies directed against desmin (immunoperoxidase technique).

throughout the bile duct. Scattered muscle fibers or no muscle fibers are present of the upper one-third of the bile duct, whereas a continuous or interrupted pattern of thick smooth muscle bundles is present throughout the lower one-third of the bile duct (Figure 29.15) (78). The muscle fibers are more frequently longitudinal and are intermixed with collagen and elastic fibers. Nerve fibers showing immunoreactivity for VIP are present beneath the epithelium and in muscle fibers (76).

VATERIAN SYSTEM AND MINOR PAPILLA

Gross Anatomy

The Vaterian system is composed of the segments of the common bile duct and major pancreatic duct (occurring either separately or as a common channel) at the duodenum, major papilla, and the sphincteric musculature. It also includes the extraduodenal portion of the common bile duct and major pancreatic duct that join to form a common channel outside the duodenal wall (58). It is a complex structural unit composed of a highly developed mucosa, musculature, and nerve supply that regulates the flow of bile and pancreatic secretions. Its sphincteric function (sphincter of Oddi) is a part of the overall gastrointestinal motility system and is subject to regulation by myogenic, neural, and gastrointestinal hormonal elements (9,79).

The major pancreatic duct of Wirsung drains many small channels in its course from the tail of the pancreas to the duodenal ostium. It typically inserts into the duodenal window caudal or a little lateral to the common bile duct. Its lumen narrows at the duodenal wall. The minor duct of Santorini, usually present, joins the major pancreatic duct at a variety of angles and locations within the pancreas. Uncommonly, the duct of Wirsung is smaller than the duct of Santorini, and the latter may be the chief conduit for drainage of the pancreas (80). The duct of Santorini leads into the minor papilla but also may end blindly in 10 to 20% of cases (80,81). The luminal pressure of the major pancreatic duct is nearly always higher than that for the common bile duct except when the gallbladder empties (82).

The relationship of the common bile duct and duct of Wirsung at the papilla is complex and variable. The ducts may have separate openings into the duodenum, an interposed septum, or a common channel (sometimes forming an ampulla) (Figure 29.16). The ampulla, defined strictly, is a dilated, juglike conduit resulting from the union of the common bile duct and major pancreatic duct. In various studies of the pancreaticoduodenal junction, the frequency for separate openings into the duodenal lumen ranged from 12 to 54% and for a common channel from 46 to 88% (57,80,81,83–87). In most studies, more than two-thirds of the patients had a common channel. In a detailed gross and radiographic study, DiMagno et al. (83) examined 390 pancreaticoduodenal specimens at autopsy and found that 74% of the patients had a common channel, 19% had separate openings for the pancreatic duct and common bile duct, and 7% had an interposed septum. Twenty-five percent of their specimens had a well-defined ampulla, 18% had a long common channel (defined as a channel greater than 3 mm long in the absence of an ampulla), and 31% had a short common channel (defined as a channel less than 3 mm in length) (83). For those specimens with an interposed septum, the two ducts emptied together at the ostium of the papilla. For the ducts that opened separately into the duodenal lumen, their ostia were located from 1 mm to several centimeters apart. On occasion, the ducts will unite before the duodenal wall is breached, forming an extended common channel. In one study, the length of the extended common channel ranged from 0.9 to 3.3 cm (mean: 2.2 cm) (88). This lengthy common channel occurred in 13.8% of patients with carcinoma of the biliary tract (18 of 130 cases) and in those with congenital biliary dilatation (four of four cases) but was

absent in a control group of 30 cases (88). This confluence of the pancreatic and bile ducts outside of the duodenal wall has been increasingly described in association with congenital dilatation of the bile duct, choledochal cyst, and cholangiocarcinoma (89,90).

The major papilla, a cylindrical protuberance housing the terminations of the common bile duct and major pancreatic duct or a common channel, is situated medially at the midportion of the second part of the duodenum. It is usually completely or partially covered by a triangular fold of duodenal mucosa; a longitudinal mucosal fold projects from the caudal portion of its base, forming a frenulum, which was absent in about one-quarter of the cases in one study (91). In one series, the papilla had a mean length of 11.7 mm and a mean width of 5.2 mm (85). Rarely, the major papilla is located at or just below the level of the duodenal mucosa or is absent. Mucosal reduplications (valves of Santorini) at the ostium of the major papilla consist of columnar-shaped protrusions and traverse leaflike flaps of ductal mucosa (92,93). In one study, the columnar-shaped projections that arose from the terminal common bile duct numbered one to four per specimen and ranged from 1 to 5 mm in length (93). They were found in approximately one-third of adults but were not observed in fetuses. Leaflike flaps were present in the caudal wall of the common channel in over 90% of fetuses and adults and were separated by small cul-de-sacs of varying size and depth. The flaps sometimes extended into the major pancreatic duct. In cases in which a common channel was absent, the leaflike flaps were found only at the orifice of the duct of Wirsung. It was postulated by the authors that the flaps may flatten during the flow of pancreatic juice into the duodenum; when the cul-de-sacs are filled, the ostium is blocked and regurgitation is prevented (93).

The sphincter of Oddi consists of the intrinsic circular and longitudinal musculature of the Vaterian system. It is embryologically and functionally distinct from the musculature of the duodenal wall. However, the muscle fibers from the duodenal wall aid in anchoring the Vaterian system in place in the duodenal window. In a study of the structure of the dense connective tissue around the major duodenal

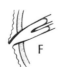

Figure 29.16 Relationship of the common bile duct and duct of Wirsung at the major papilla. (*A*, ampulla; *B*, interposed septum; *C*, separate openings; *D*, short common channel; *E*, long common channel; *F*, extended common channel)

papilla, the papilla and duodenal wall were noted to form both a morphologic and a functional unit (94). Connective tissue fibers spread from the papilla orifice to the circular duodenal musculature and cross at different angles from the orifice to the distal common bile duct. The arrangement and amount of muscle bundles that form the sphincter are highly complex and variable. Important fibers are those around the intrapancreatic (near the duodenal wall) and intraduodenal portions of the common bile duct (sphincter choledochus) (95). In one study, accumulation of circular muscle fibers extended up the common bile duct to a mean distance of 13.6 mm from the pore of the papilla (91). Smooth muscle fibers are also present in the wall of the common channel, around the duct of Wirsung, and near the ostium of the papilla. It is controversial whether the smooth muscle bundles around the pancreatic duct above the common channel have important sphincteric function, but the finding of a sustained pancreatic duct high-pressure zone with phasic contractions after sphincterotomy may be evidence that the sphincter of Oddi extends above the common channel to include portions of the pancreatic duct (95–97). Muscle fibers have been found to extend up the pancreatic duct a mean of 7.3 mm from the papillary pore (91). The tunica muscularis of the duodenum may not have a primary role in managing the flow of bile and pancreatic juice at the choledochoduodenal junction.

The sphincter of Oddi serves to inhibit the flow of bile into the duodenum, pumps bile into the duodenum when necessary, and likely precludes the entry of duodenal contents into the common bile duct or major pancreatic duct (79). Manometric studies have shown that the control of the flow of bile during fasting results from the phasic contractions of the sphincter of Oddi (98). These contractions result in the liberation of small volumes of bile. The flow of pancreatic juice is also regulated. The contractions are in addition to the steady basal pressure of the sphincter of Oddi, which is several mm Hg higher than that for the common bile and pancreatic ducts (99). The high-pressure zone measures 4 to 6 mm long, and the phasic contractions may be antegrade, retrograde, or simultaneous (97). Cholecystokinin has been found to inhibit the phasic contractions of the sphincter and decrease the basal pressure, allowing the flow of large quantities of bile into the duodenum (98). Manometric and contractility studies of the effects of various hormones on the sphincter of Oddi in humans and animals have been summarized (79,97). Glucagon-like cholecystokinin decreases sphincteric pressure, whereas gastrin and secretin elevate basal pressure (97). The phasic contractions and basal tone of the sphincter can be increased or decreased by exogenous drugs. For instance, most narcotics increase sphincteric pressure, whereas atropine decreases it (97).

The minor papilla is nearly always present but may be difficult to locate grossly (81). Its size is variable. It is usually situated 2 cm proximal to the major papilla (81,100).

Vascular and Nerve Supply and Lymphatic Drainage

The intraduodenal portion of the common bile duct is supplied by vessels from the anterior and posterior superior pancreaticoduodenal arteries (2). Venous drainage occurs via small veins that lead to the portal vein. The fine venous architecture of the major papilla has been described in detail (101). Lymphatic drainage is variable, but generally lymphatics from the pancreaticoduodenal junction drain into the anterior and posterior pancreaticoduodenal lymph nodes and then to the nodes at the inferior pancreaticoduodenal artery (102). The Vaterian system is innervated extrinsically by parasympathetic nerve fibers in the vagal nerve and by sympathetic nerve fibers in the splanchnic nerves (9,79). Although little is known regarding the role of these nerve fibers in regulating the motility of the sphincter of Oddi, some evidence indicates that its motility is inhibited by vagal activation (79,103). Three separate ganglia cell groups provide intrinsic innervation. These are found at the base of the papilla in the duodenal wall, within the musculature of the papilla, and within the submucosa (79). This intrinsic innervation appears to provide tonic inhibition and is similar to that for other gastrointestinal sphincters, including the lower esophageal, pyloric, and internal anal sphincters.

Histology

The epithelial lining of the duct of Wirsung is identical to that of the common bile duct. The cytoplasm of the columnar cells also contains sulfated acid mucin (104). The epithelium may undergo hyperplastic, metaplastic, or dysplastic changes. Surrounding the normal epithelium is a dense fibrous layer with abundant collagen and elastic fibers. A few ganglion cells may be seen in the outer half of the fibrous wall. Small pancreatic ducts draining acini traverse the dense fibrous layer. At the orifice of the papilla, the epithelium of Wirsung's duct is thrown into folds (mucosal reduplications) that have cores of fibrovascular stroma. Goblet cells are found interspersed between the columnar lining cells within the papilla. Numerous small accessory pancreatic ducts drain into the ductal lumen near the ostium, and pancreatic acini are sometimes present just beneath the lining of the duct (Figure 29.17). A few lymphocytes may be seen within the ductal epithelium, and lymphocytes, plasma cells, and mast cells sparsely populate the fibrovascular cores. Circular smooth muscle bundles are present around the duct as it penetrates the duodenal wall (100).

The epithelium of the terminal portion of the common bile duct and common channel (if present) covers long, slender papillary fronds, or valvules, that in some respects resemble the fimbriae of the fallopian tube (Figure 29.18). They correspond to the mucosal reduplications seen

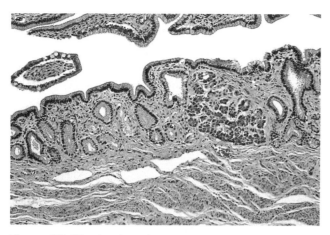

Figure 29.17 The duct of Wirsung at the papilla of Vater is lined by a single layer of tall columnar cells with occasional interspersed goblet cells. Accessory pancreatic ducts and acini are also observed.

grossly. These papillary formations are considerably larger than the duodenal villi, which are few or absent at the surface of the papilla. The valvules may branch and sometimes project beyond the ostium of the papilla, with shorter fronds at the periphery and longer ones centrally (60,105,106). The columnar lining cells have eosinophilic cytoplasm and basal nuclei. Interspersed goblet cells are more numerous near the ostium. The stroma forming the cores of the fronds contains a few lymphocytes, mast cells, and plasma cells. Muscle fibers, present at the base of the fronds, are occasionally found in the stroma of the fronds. The smooth muscle, forming the sphincter choledochus, becomes apparent in the wall of the duct several millimeters before the duct enters the duodenal window. About 5 mm from the duodenal wall, longitudinal muscle fibers are present around two-thirds of the common bile duct; at 2 mm from the duodenal musculature, circular muscle

fibers increase and completely surround the duct (100). These intrinsic muscle fibers are separated from the muscularis propria of the duodenum by connective tissue and, at times, pancreatic tissue (100). Variable amounts of circular and longitudinal muscle fibers also surround the common channel. Before forming a common channel, the common bile duct is set apart from the pancreatic duct by a septum that eventually loses its muscle fibers, becoming a thin connective tissue membrane (100). Interspersed between areas of smooth muscle around the common bile duct or common channel are collagen, elastic fibers, small nerves, and ganglion cells. When the common bile duct and duct of Wirsung are separate within the papilla, they are distinguishable by light microscopy because the common bile duct is larger, has more prominent fronds, a greater amount of enveloping smooth muscle, and bile in its lumen.

A bewildering assortment of glands and ducts of various caliber surround the common bile duct at the papilla. Frequently, it is only possible to distinguish mucous glands from the terminations of accessory pancreatic ducts by studying serial sections (77). Mucous glands drain into the shallow or deep recesses between the papillary fronds (Figure 29.19). The number of these glands and their distribution are variable. Glands near the surface of the papilla may be distended with mucus, and some may even represent dilated accessory pancreatic ducts (105). The number and distribution of accessory pancreatic ducts within the major papilla are also inconstant. These small accessory pancreatic channels, having been studied in serial sections and by camera lucida drawings, empty into the common bile duct (Figure 29.20), duct of Wirsung, common channel, surface of papilla, or through the duodenal mucosa near the papilla (77,107). They are sometimes numerous and may cause obstruction of the common bile duct, duct of Wirsung, or common channel. In such instances, a diagnosis of accessory duct hyperplasia may be

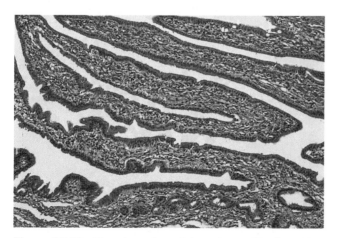

Figure 29.18 Near the ostium of the major papilla, the epithelium of the common bile duct lines prominent papillary fronds (valvules).

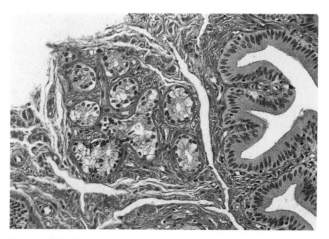

Figure 29.19 Mucous glands are present around the common bile duct at the papilla and drain into recesses between the papillary fronds.

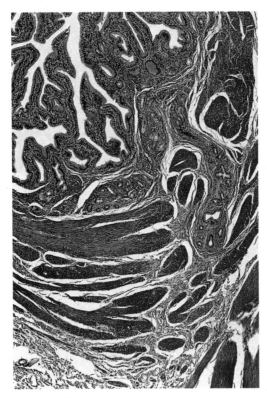

Figure 29.20 Accessory pancreatic ducts pierce the large smooth muscle bundles to empty into the lumen of the common bile duct.

appropriate (105). In an autopsy study, accessory pancreatic ducts were absent in only two of 100 major papillae (107). The ducts drain small lobules of pancreatic acini located within or, more often, near the papilla. In one study, pancreatic acini were found in 8% of 145 major papillae, whereas pancreatic islets were not seen in any of the major papillae (108). The ducts appear as packets of multiple lumens of small caliber encircled by a cellular fibrovascular stroma (Figure 29.21). Within a group of

ducts, the larger central duct is surrounded by smaller branches. Groups of ducts are sometimes seen penetrating the duodenal smooth muscle. Small groups of heterotopic pancreatic acini and ducts also occur in the submucosa of the duodenum away from the major papilla (Figure 29.22).

Immunohistochemically, the cells lining the common bile duct and the duct of Wirsung at the papilla are positive for low-molecular weight keratin (CAM 5.2 antibody), CK7, and epithelial membrane antigen (EMA). There may be linear apical staining for CEA (unabsorbed polyclonal antibody). The adjacent mucous glands and accessory pancreatic ducts have the same immunoreactivity for keratin and EMA. A few scattered cells lining the large ducts within the pancreas are positive for neuron-specific enolase, chromogranin A, insulin, and glucagon (109). Chromogranin-positive cells are sometimes located in the lining epithelium of the duct of Wirsung and common bile duct within the papilla. Mucous glands and accessory pancreatic ducts also contain scattered cells immunoreactive for neuron-specific enolase and chromogranin A (Figure 29.23). In patients with pancreaticobiliary disease, a few cells lining the lumen of the papilla and in adjacent mucous glands have been found to be immunoreactive for somatostatin (56). Although usually absent, endocrine cell micronests may be scattered singly or are grouped in the stroma adjacent to pancreatic ducts, ductules, or accessory

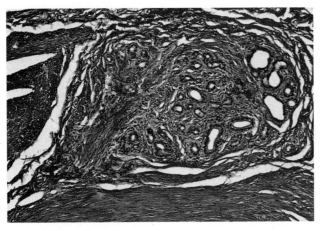

Figure 29.21 Accessory pancreatic ducts that penetrate the smooth muscle bundles at the choledochoduodenal junction are surrounded by a fibrovascular stroma.

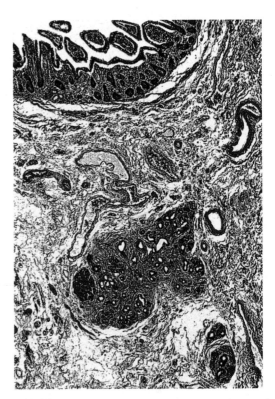

Figure 29.22 Groups of heterotopic pancreatic ducts and acini may be seen in the submucosa of the duodenum away from the papilla of Vater.

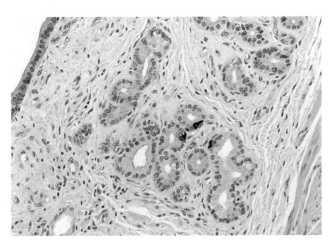

Figure 29.23 Some of the small ducts around the duct of Wirsung at the major papilla contain a few cells that are immunoreactive for chromogranin A (immunoperoxidase technique).

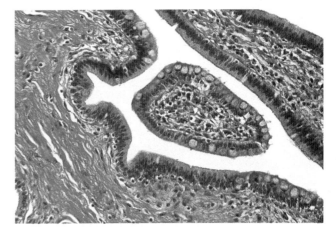

Figure 29.25 The duct of Santorini at the minor papilla is lined by tall columnar cells with interspersed goblet cells.

glands but not around the common bile duct (108). They have been found in about 3% of major papillae. They consist of round, oval, trabecular, or ribbonlike groups of cells that immunohistochemically are distinct from those of pancreatic islets. They are typically scattered, rarely nodular, and immunohistochemically stain for somatostatin and pancreatic polypepide. It is unclear whether they are a normal finding or represent a metaplastic or hyperplastic condition. The functional role of these endocrine cells in the papilla of Vater is unknown.

At the minor papilla, the pancreatic duct of Santorini contains papillary fronds that are lined by simple columnar epithelium with some goblet cells (Figures 29.24–29.25). Small pancreatic ducts open into the lumen of the duct of Santorini at the minor papilla or separately into the duodenum (81). Small lobules of pancreatic acini may be present within the connective tissue of the minor papilla

and were seen in 77% of 167 minor papillae in a study by Noda et al. (108), who noted that 14% of the papillae also contained well-formed pancreatic islets. Atrophic or poorly formed islets are present uncommonly. Smooth muscle bundles separated by collagen, small nerves, and ganglion cells surround the duct. The bundles of muscle occasionally are continuous with those of the muscularis mucosae of the duodenum, but in many instances continuity between the groups of muscle fibers is lacking (81). The lining epithelial cells and those of the small pancreatic ducts stain strongly for low-molecular weight keratin (CAM 5.2 antibody), CK7 and weakly for CEA (unabsorbed polyclonal antibody). A few cells within small ducts and some that line the lumen of the duct of Santorini are flask-shaped and immunoreactive for neuron-specific enolase and chromogranin A (Figure 29.26). Small groups of neuroendocrine cells may extend below the epithelial lining (Figure 29.27). In the above-mentioned study of 167 minor papillae, 16% contained endocrine micronests, which were

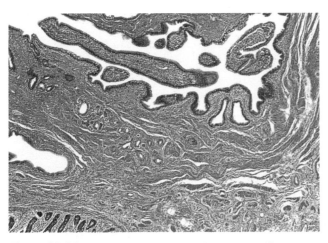

Figure 29.24 The duct of Santorini at the minor papilla contains papillary fronds and is surrounded by muscle bundles.

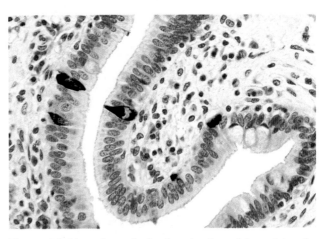

Figure 29.26 A few cells that line the duct of Santorini at the minor papilla are flask-shaped and immunoreactive for chromogranin A (immunoperoxidase technique).

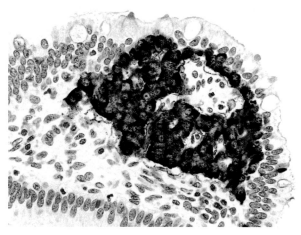

Figure 29.27 A group of cells below the lining epithelium of the duct of Santorini at the minor papilla is immunoreactive for chromogranin A (immunoperoxidase technique).

predominantly scattered and rarely nodular (108). They were usually immunoreactive for somatostatin and pancreatic polypeptide and lacked staining for insulin and glucagon. It is possible that some of these micronests represent metaplasia/hyperplasia or neoplasia.

REFERENCES

1. Albores-Saavedra J, Henson DE, Klimstra. DS. Normal anatomy. In: *Atlas of Tumor Pathology: Tumors of the Gallbladder, Extrahepatic Bile Ducts, and Ampulla of Vater.* 3rd series, fascicle 27. Washington DC: Armed Forces Institute of Pathology; 2000:1–16.
2. Lindner HH. Embryology and anatomy of the biliary tree. In: Way LW PC, ed. *Surgery of the Gallbladder and Bile Ducts.* Philadelphia: WB Saunders; 1987:3–22.
3. Guyton AC. The liver and biliary system. In: Guyton AC. *Textbook of Medical Physiology.* Philadelphia: WB Saunders; 1976:936–944.
4. Frizzell RA, Heintze K. Transport functions of the gallbladder. In: Javitt NB, ed. *International Review of Physiology: Liver and Biliary Tract Physiology.* Vol 21. Baltimore: University Park Press; 1980: 221–247.
5. Shaffer EA. Review article: control of gall-bladder motor function. *Aliment Pharmacol Ther* 2000;14(suppl 2):2–8.
6. Rehfeld JF. Clinical endocrinology and metabolism. Cholecystokinin. *Best Pract Res Clin Endocrinol Metab* 2004;18:569–586.
7. Pomeranz IS, Davison JS, Shaffer EA. In vitro effects of pancreatic polypeptide and motilin on contractility of human gallbladder. *Dig Dis Sci* 1983;28:539–544.
8. Fisher RS, Rock E, Levin G, Malmud L. Effects of somatostatin on gallbladder emptying. *Gastroenterology* 1987;92:885–890.
9. Balemba OB, Salter MJ, Mawe GM. Innervation of the extrahepatic biliary tract. *Anat Rec A Discov Mol Cell Evol Biol* 2004; 280:836–847.
10. Magee DF, Naruse S, Pap A. Vagal control of gall-bladder contraction. *J Physiol* 1984;355:65–70.
11. Colecchia A, Sandri L, Staniscia T, et al. Gallbladder motility and functional gastrointestinal disorders. *Dig Liver Dis* 2003;35(suppl 3):S30–S34.
12. Moosman DA, Collier FA. Prevention of traumatic injury to the bile ducts; a study of the structures of the cystohepatic angle encountered in cholecystectomy and supraduodenal choledochostomy. *Am J Surg* 1951;82:132–143.
13. Michels NA. The hepatic, cystic and retroduodenal arteries and their relations to the biliary ducts with samples of the entire celiacal blood supply. *Ann Surg* 1951;133:503–524.
14. Ito M, Mishima Y, Sato T. An anatomical study of the lymphatic drainage of the gallbladder. *Surg Radiol Anat* 1991;13:89–104.
15. Shirai Y, Yoshida K, Tsukada K, Ohtani T, Muto T. Identification of the regional lymphatic system of the gallbladder by vital staining. *Br J Surg* 1992;79:659–662.
16. Ding WG, Fujimura M, Mori A, Tooyama I, Kimura H. Light and electron microscopy of neuropeptide Y-containing nerves in human liver, gallbladder, and pancreas. *Gastroenterology* 1991;101:1054–1059.
17. Laitio M. Morphology and histochemistry of non-tumorous gallbladder epithelium. A series of 103 cases. *Pathol Res Pract* 1980;167:335–345.
18. Karayannopoulou G, Damjanov I. Lectin binding sites in the human gallbladder and cystic duct. *Histochemistry* 1987;88:75–83.
19. Delaquerriere L, Tremblay G, Riopelle JL. Argentaffine cells in chronic cholecystitis. *Arch Pathol* 1962;74:142–151.
20. Yamamoto M, Nakajo S, Tahara E. Endocrine cells and lysozyme immunoreactivity in the gallbladder. *Arch Pathol Lab Med* 1986;110:920–927.
21. Albores-Saavedra J, Nadji M, Henson DE, Ziegels-Weissman J, Mones JM. Intestinal metaplasia of the gallbladder: a morphologic and immunocytochemical study. *Hum Pathol* 1986; 17:614–620.
22. Kozuka S, Hachisuka K. Incidence by age and sex of intestinal metaplasia in the gallbladder. *Hum Pathol* 1984;15:779–784.
23. Kozuka S, Kurashina M, Tsubone M, Hachisuka K, Yasui A. Significance of intestinal metaplasia for the evolution of cancer in the biliary tract. *Cancer* 1984;54:2277–2285.
24. Tatematsu M, Furihata C, Miki K, et al. Complete and incomplete pyloric gland metaplasia of human gallbladder. *Acta Pathol Jpn* 1987;37:39–46.
25. Tsutsumi Y, Nagura H, Osamura Y, Watanabe K, Yanaihara N. Histochemical studies of metaplastic lesions in the human gallbladder. *Arch Pathol Lab Med* 1984;108:917–921.
26. Chang HJ, Kim SW, Lee BL, Hong EK, Kim WH. Phenotypic alterations of mucins and cytokeratins during gallbladder carcinogenesis. *Pathol Int* 2004;54:576–584.
27. Aroni K, Kittas C, Papadimitriou CS, Papacharalampous NX. An immunocytochemical study of the distribution of lysozyme, a1-antitrypsin and a1-antichymotrypsin in the normal and pathological gall bladder. *Virchows Arch A Pathol Anat Histopathol* 1984;403:281–289.
28. Albores-Saavedra J, Nadji M, Morales AR, Henson DE. Carcinoembryonic antigen in normal, preneoplastic and neoplastic gallbladder epithelium. *Cancer* 1983;52:1069–1072.
29. Maxwell P, Davis RI, Sloan JM. Carcinoembryonic antigen (CEA) in benign and malignant epithelium of the gall bladder, extrahepatic bile ducts, and ampulla of Vater. *J Pathol* 1993;170:73–76.
30. Cabibi D, Licata A, Barresi E, Craxi A, Aragona F. Expression of cytokeratin 7 and 20 in pathological conditions of the bile tract. *Pathol Res Pract* 2003;199:65–70.
31. Yamamoto M, Nakajo S, Tahara E. Immunohistochemical analysis of estrogen receptors in human gallbladder. *Acta Pathol Jpn* 1990;40:14–21.
32. Choi YL, Xuan YH, Shin YK, et al. An immunohistochemical study of the expression of adhesion molecules in gallbladder lesions. *J Histochem Cytochem* 2004;52:591–601.
33. Hudson I, Hopwood D. Macrophages and mast cells in chronic cholecystitis and "normal" gall bladders. *J Clin Pathol* 1986; 39:1082–1087.
34. Green FH, Fox H. An immunofluorescent study of the distribution of immunoglobulin-containing cells in the normal and the inflamed human gall bladder. *Gut* 1972;13:379–384.
35. Mendoza-Marin M, Hoang MP, Albores-Saavedra J. Malignant stromal tumor of the gallbladder with interstitial cells of Cajal phenotype. *Arch Pathol Lab Med* 2002;126:481–483.
36. Weedon D. *Pathology of the Gallbladder.* New York: Masson; 1984.
37. Fine G, Raju UB. Paraganglia in the human gallbladder. *Arch Pathol Lab Med* 1980;104:265–268.
38. Elfving G. Crypts and ducts in the gallbladder wall. *Acta Pathol Microbiol Scand* 1960;49(suppl 135):1–45.
39. Robertson HE, Ferguson WJ. The diverticula (Luschka's crypts) of the gallbladder. *Arch Pathol* 1945;40:312–333.

40. Halpert B. Morphological studies on the gall-bladder. II. The "true Luschka ducts" and the "Rokitansky-Aschoff sinuses" of the human gallbladder. *Bull Johns Hopkins* 1927;41:77–103.

41. Beilby JO. Diverticulosis of the gall bladder. The fundal adenoma. *Br J Exp Pathol* 1967;48:455–461.

42. Moosman DA. Accessory bile ducts: their significance during cholecystectomy. *J Mich State Med Soc* 1964;63:355–358.

43. Foster JH, Wayson EE. Surgical significance of aberrant bile ducts. *Am J Surg* 1962;104:14–19.

44. McQuillan T, Manolas SG, Hayman JA, Kune GA. Surgical significance of the bile duct of Luschka. *Br J Surg* 1989;76:696–698.

45. Goor DA, Ebert PA. Anomalies of the biliary tree. Report of a repair of an accessory bile duct and review of the literature. *Arch Surg* 1972;104:302–309.

46. Tejada E, Danielson C. Ectopic or heterotopic liver (choristoma) associated with the gallbladder. *Arch Pathol Lab Med* 1989;113:950–952.

47. Mutschmann PN. Aberrant pancreatic tissue in the gallbladder wall. *Am J Surg* 1946;72:282–283.

48. Busuttil A. Ectopic adrenal within the gall-bladder wall. *J Pathol* 1974;113:231–233.

49. Curtis LE, Sheahan DG. Heterotopic tissues in the gallbladder. *Arch Pathol* 1969;88:677–683.

50. Gilloteaux J, Pomerants B, Kelly TR. Human gallbladder mucosa ultrastructure: evidence of intraepithelial nerve structures. *Am J Anat* 1989;184:321–333.

51. Kaye GI, Wheeler HO, Whitlock RT, Lane N. Fluid transport in the rabbit gallbladder. A combined physiological and electron microscopic study. *J Cell Biol* 1966;30:237–268.

52. Evett RD, Higgins JA, Brown AL, Jr. The fine structure of normal mucosa in human gall bladder. *Gastroenterology* 1964;47:49–60.

53. Laitio M, Nevalainen T. Gland ultrastructure in human gall bladder. *J Anat* 1975;120(pt 1):105–112.

54. Berci G. Biliary ductal anatomy and anomalies. The role of intraoperative cholangiography during laparoscopic cholecystectomy. *Surg Clin North Am* 1992;72:1069–1075.

55. Repassy G, Schaff Z, Lapis K, Marton T, Jakab F, Sugar I. Mucosa of the Heister valve in cholelithiasis: transmission and scanning electron microscopic study. *Arch Pathol Lab Med* 1978;102:403–405.

56. Dancygier H, Klein U, Leuschner U, Hubner K, Classen M. Somatostatin-containing cells in the extrahepatic biliary tract of humans. *Gastroenterology* 1984;86(pt 1):892–896.

57. Northover JMA, Terblanche. J. Applied surgical anatomy of the biliary tree. In: Blumgart LH, ed. *The Biliary Tract. Clinical Surgery International Series.* Vol 5. Edinburgh: Churchill Livingstone; 1982:1–16.

58. Dowdy GS Jr, Waldron GW, Brown WG. Surgical anatomy of the pancreatobiliary ductal system. Observations. *Arch Surg* 1962;84:229–246.

59. Takahashi Y, Takahashi T, Takahashi W, Sato T. Morphometrical evaluation of extrahepatic bile ducts in reference to their structural changes with aging. *Tohoku J Exp Med* 1985;147:301–309.

60. Baggenstoss AH. Major duodenal papilla. Variations of pathologic interest and lesions of the mucosa. *Arch Pathol* 1938;26:853–868.

61. Mahour GH, Wakim KG, Ferris DO. The common bile duct in man: its diameter and circumference. *Ann Surg* 1967;165:415–419.

62. Benson EA, Page RE. A practical reappraisal of the anatomy of the extrahepatic bile ducts and arteries. *Br J Surg* 1976;63:853–860.

63. Chen WJ, Ying DJ, Liu ZJ, He ZP. Analysis of the arterial supply of the extrahepatic bile ducts and its clinical significance. *Clin Anat* 1999;12:245–249.

64. Northover JM, Terblanche J. A new look at the arterial supply of the bile duct in man and its surgical implications. *Br J Surg* 1979;66:379–384.

65. Douglass BE, Baggenstoss AH, Hollinshead WH. The anatomy of the portal vein and its tributaries. *Surg Gynecol Obstet* 1950;91:562–576.

66. Yoshida T, Shibata K, Yokoyama H, et al. Patterns of lymph node metastasis in carcinoma of the distal bile duct. *Hepatogastroenterology* 1999;46:1595–1598.

67. Yoshida T, Matsumoto T, Sasaki A, et al. Lymphatic spread differs according to tumor location in extrahepatic bile duct cancer. *Hepatogastroenterology* 2003;50:17–20.

68. Terada T, Kida T, Nakanuma Y. Extrahepatic peribiliary glands express alpha-amylase isozymes, trypsin and pancreatic lipase: an immunohistochemical analysis. *Hepatology* 1993;18:803–808.

69. Qualman SJ, Haupt HM, Bauer TW, Taxy JB. Adenocarcinoma of the hepatic duct junction. A reappraisal of the histologic criteria of malignancy. *Cancer* 1984;53:1545–1551.

70. Laitio M. Carcinoma of extrahepatic bile ducts. A histopathologic study. *Pathol Res Pract* 1983;178:67–72.

71. Rullier A, Le Bail B, Fawaz R, Blanc JF, Saric J, Bioulac-Sage P. Cytokeratin 7 and 20 expression in cholangiocarcinomas varies along the biliary tract but still differs from that in colorectal carcinoma metastasis. *Am J Surg Pathol* 2000;24:870–876.

72. Nagura H, Tsutsumi Y, Watanabe K, et al. Immunohistochemistry of carcinoembryonic antigen, secretory component and lysozyme in benign and malignant common bile duct tissues. *Virchows Arch A Pathol Anat Histopathol* 1984;403:271–280.

73. Davis RI, Sloan JM, Hood JM, Maxwell P. Carcinoma of the extrahepatic biliary tract: a clinicopathological and immunohistochemical study. *Histopathology* 1988;12:623–631.

74. Hoang MP, Murakata LA, Padilla-Rodriguez AL, Albores-Saavedra J. Metaplastic lesions of the extrahepatic bile ducts: a morphologic and immunohistochemical study. *Mod Pathol* 2001;14:1119–1125.

75. Yamamoto M, Nakajo S, Tahara E, Miyoshi N. Endocrine cell carcinoma of extrahepatic bile duct. *Acta Pathol Jpn* 1986;36:587–593.

76. Dancygier H. Endoscopic transpapillary biopsy (ETPB) of human extrahepatic bile ducts—light and electron microscopic findings, clinical significance. *Endoscopy* 1989;21(suppl 1):312–320.

77. Cross KR. Accessory pancreatic ducts; special reference to the intrapancreatic portion of the common duct. *AMA Arch Pathol* 1956;61:434–440.

78. Hong SM, Kang GH, Lee HY, Ro JY. Smooth muscle distribution in the extrahepatic bile duct: histologic and immunohistochemical studies of 122 cases. *Am J Surg Pathol* 2000;24:660–667.

79. Allescher HD. Papilla of Vater: structure and function. *Endoscopy* 1989;21(suppl 1):324–329.

80. Millbourn E. On the excretory ducts of the pancreas in man, with special reference to their relations to each other, to the common bile duct and to the duodenum. *Acta Anat (Basel)* 1950;9:1–34.

81. Baldwin WM. The pancreatic ducts in man, together with a study of the microscopical structure of the minor duodenal papilla. *Anat Rec* 1911;5:197–228.

82. Parry EW, Hallenbeck GA, Grindlay JH. Pressures in the pancreatic and common ducts; values during fasting, after various meals, and after sphincterotomy; an experimental study. *AMA Arch Surg* 1955;70:757–765.

83. DiMagno EP, Shorter RG, Taylor WF, Go VL. Relationships between pancreaticobiliary ductal anatomy and pancreatic ductal and parenchymal histology. *Cancer* 1982;49:361–368.

84. Howard J, Jones R. The anatomy of the pancreatic ducts. The etiology of acute pancreatitis. *Am J Med Sci* 1947;214:617–622.

85. Newman HF, Weinberg SB, Newman EB, Northup JD. The papilla of Vater and distal portions of the common bile duct and duct of Wirsung. *Surg Gynecol Obstet* 1958;106:687–694.

86. Stamm BH. Incidence and diagnostic significance of minor pathologic changes in the adult pancreas at autopsy: a systematic study of 112 autopsies in patients without known pancreatic disease. *Hum Pathol* 1984;15:677–683.

87. Sterling JA. The common channel for bile and pancreatic ducts. *Surg Gynecol Obstet* 1954;98:420–424.

88. Suda K, Matsumoto Y, Miyano T. An extended common channel in patients with biliary tract carcinoma and congenital biliary dilatation. *Surg Pathol* 1988;1:65–69.

89. Okada A, Nakamura T, Higaki J, Okumura K, Kamata S, Oguchi Y. Congenital dilatation of the bile duct in 100 instances and its relationship with anomalous junction. *Surg Gynecol Obstet* 1990;171:291–298.

90. Hara H, Morita S, Sako S, et al. Relationship between types of common channel and development of biliary tract cancer in pancreaticobiliary maljunction. *Hepatogastroenterology* 2002;49:322–325.

91. Flati G, Flati D, Porowska B, Ventura T, Catarci M, Carboni M. Surgical anatomy of the papilla of Vater and biliopancreatic ducts. *Am Surg* 1994;60:712–718.

92. Suarez CV. The Santorini valves. *Mt Sinai J Med* 1981;48:149–157.

93. Brown JO, Echenberg RJ. Mucosal reduplications associated with the ampullary portion of the major duodenal papilla in humans. *Anat Rec* 1964;150:293–301.

94. Dziwisch L, Lierse W. Three-dimensional arrangement of dense connective tissue around the human major duodenal papilla. Including the ampullary region and the distal choledochal duct. *Acta Anat (Basel)* 1989;135:231–235.

95. Boyden EA. The anatomy of the choledochoduodenal junction in man. *Surg Gynecol Obstet* 1957;104:641–652.

96. Suarez CV. Structure of the major duodenal papilla. Mt Sinai J Med 1982;49:31–37.

97. Goff JS. The human sphincter of Oddi. Physiology and pathophysiology. *Arch Intern Med* 1988;148:2673–2677.

98. Toouli J, Hogan WJ, Geenen JE, Dodds WJ, Arndorfer RC. Action of cholecystokinin-octapeptide on sphincter of Oddi basal pressure and phasic wave activity in humans. *Surgery* 1982;92:497–503.

99. Coelho JC, Moody FG. Certain aspects of normal and abnormal motility of sphincter of Oddi. *Dig Dis Sci* 1987;32:86–94.

100. Hand BH. An anatomical study of the choledochoduodenal area. *Br J Surg* 1963;50:486–494.

101. Biazotto W. The fine venous architecture of the major duodenal papilla in human beings. *Anat Anz* 1990;171:105–108.

102. Shirai Y, Ohtani T, Tsukada K, Hatakeyama K. Patterns of lymphatic spread of carcinoma of the ampulla of Vater. *Br J Surg* 1997;84:1012–1026.

103. Smirnov VM, Lychkova AE. Mechanism of synergism between sympathetic and parasympathetic autonomic nervous systems in the regulation of motility of the stomach and sphincter of Oddi. *Bull Exp Biol Med* 2003;135:327–329.

104. Kozuka S, Sassa R, Taki T, et al. Relation of pancreatic duct hyperplasia to carcinoma. *Cancer* 1979;43:1418–1428.

105. Edmondson HA. Tumors and tumor-like lesions of the intraduodenal bile duct and papilla of vater. In: *Tumors of the Gallbladder and Extrahepatic Bile Ducts.* 1st series, fascicle 26. Washington DC: Armed Forces Institute of Pathology; 1967:121–167.

106. Suda K, Ootaka M, Yamasaki S, et al. Distended glands or overreplacement of ampullary mucosa at the papilla of Vater. *J Hepatobiliary Pancreat Surg* 2004;11:260–265.

107. Loquvam GS, Russell WO. Accessory pancreatic ducts of the major duodenal papilla. Normal structures to be differentiated from cancer. *Am J Clin Pathol* 1950;20:305–313.

108. Noda Y, Watanabe H, Iwafuchi M, et al. Carcinoids and endocrine cell micronests of the minor and major duodenal papillae. Their incidence and characteristics. *Cancer* 1992;70:1825–1833.

109. Alpert LC, Truong LD, Bossart MI, Spjut HJ. Microcystic adenoma (serous cystadenoma) of the pancreas. A study of 14 cases with immunohistochemical and electron-microscopic correlation. *Am J Surg Pathol* 1988;12:251–263.

Pancreas

David S. Klimstra   Ralph H. Hruban   Martha B. Pitman

INTRODUCTION

The pancreas is an unpaired organ located in the left superior retroperitoneum. It is principally an epithelial organ that includes both exocrine elements (acini and ducts) and endocrine elements (islets of Langerhans). The stroma is sparse in the normal gland, although areas of fibrosis commonly occur as individuals age. There are relatively few opportunities for pathologists to observe the normal histology of the pancreas because (a) the gland quickly autolyzes; (b) normal pancreatic tissue is rarely resected; and (c) when the pancreas is resected for a neoplasm, the adjacent nonneoplastic parenchyma usually has substantial abnormalities. For this reason, minor histologic alterations or even normal structures may not be accurately recognized.

ANATOMIC CONSIDERATIONS

Location and Relationship to Other Structures

Located in the retroperitoneum posterior to the omental bursa at the level of the second and third lumbar verte-

brae, the pancreas extends from the duodenal loop at the right of the midline to the left across the posterior abdominal wall toward the hilum of the spleen (Figure 30.1) (1). The head of the gland is cupped within the C-shaped second and third portions of the duodenum. The distal portion of the common bile duct passes through the posterosuperior head of the pancreas to enter the duodenum at the ampulla of Vater. The left lobe of the liver lies anterior to the head. The neck of the gland is the slender area of the pancreas anterior to the mesenteric vessels and inferior to the pylorus. The body of the pancreas extends from the neck lateral to the left border of the aorta. The posterior wall of the gastric antrum usually overlies the body, and the proximal jejunum immediately distal to the ligament of Treitz passes inferior to the body. The posterior aspect of the body approaches the left adrenal gland and kidney (2). The tail of the pancreas extends from the left border of the aorta laterally and gradually tapers to a blunt end within several centimeters of the hilum of the spleen. In most individuals, the tail is located either centrally (50%) or inferiorly (42%) within the splenic hilum; rarely (8%) it is in the superior hilum (3,4). The anterior aspect of the pancreas, as well as the superior surfaces of

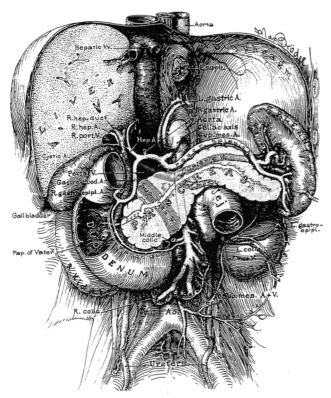

Figure 30.1 Anatomic relationships of the pancreas. The anterior aspect of the upper abdominal viscera is shown after removal of the stomach and omentum. Note the close relationship of the pancreas to the duodenum, jejunum, spleen, and major vessels. Drawing by M. Brödel. Reprinted with permission from: Fawcett DW. *Bloom and Fawcett: A Textbook of Histology*. 12th ed. New York: Chapman & Hall; 1994.

the neck, body, and tail, are covered by the peritoneal surface of the posterior aspect of the lesser sac (5).

Because of the proximity of the pancreas to several organs and other anatomic structures, tumors of these sites may be difficult to distinguish radiographically. Pancreatic masses may be confused with neoplasms of the duodenum, the ampulla of Vater, the distal bile duct, the left adrenal gland, the superior poles of either kidney, the spleen, the left lobe of the liver, the greater curve of the stomach, the root of the mesentery, and the superior retroperitoneum.

A number of major blood vessels are closely related to the pancreas (5,6). The body rests on the aorta. The celiac trunk arises from the aorta superior to the neck of the pancreas and gives off the hepatic artery as well as the tortuous splenic artery, which runs superior to the pancreatic tail. The superior mesenteric artery arises posterior to the junction of the neck and body, and the adjacent superior mesenteric vein passes through a groove between the head and the neck, with a portion of the head (the uncinate process) extending around the superior mesenteric vessels to lie anterior to the aorta. The head of the gland also rests on the inferior vena cava, the right renal vessels, and the left renal vein. These major vessels all lie posterior to the pancreas, allowing for safe surgical access to the gland from the

anterior aspect (7). The splenic vein accompanies the splenic artery along the superior aspect of the tail, joining the superior mesenteric vein to form the portal vein near the posterosuperior border of the head.

The arteries supplying the pancreas are primarily branches of the celiac trunk and the superior mesenteric artery (2,4). The arterial supply has many anastomoses between the different vessels, and numerous anatomic variations exist. The pancreatic head is supplied by the anterior and posterior pancreatoduodenal arteries, which form arcades in the pancreatoduodenal sulcus. The anterior or prepancreatic arcade is formed from the anterior superior pancreatoduodenal artery (a branch of the gastroduodenal artery) and the anterior inferior pancreatoduodenal artery (a branch of the superior mesenteric artery). The posterior arcade is formed from the posterior superior pancreatoduodenal artery (from the gastroduodenal artery) and the posterior inferior pancreatoduodenal artery (from the superior mesenteric artery). Venous drainage is by the pancreaticoduodenal veins, tributaries of the splenic and superior mesenteric vein (7).

The body and tail of the gland are supplied by the dorsal, inferior, and caudal pancreatic arteries and are drained by the inferior and left pancreatic veins. The dorsal pancreatic artery, also know as the superior pancreatic artery, has various origins, including the first 2 cm of the splenic artery, the hepatic artery, the celiac trunk, or the superior mesenteric artery. The right branch of the dorsal pancreatic artery extends across the pancreatic head and supplies the neck of the pancreas, joining the anterior pancreatic arcade. The left branch, known as the inferior pancreatic artery, runs along the inferior body of the pancreas.

Within the pancreas, a large branch of the splenic artery known as the great pancreatic artery, or pancreatica magna, provides left and right branches that course parallel to the main pancreatic duct. The right branch joins the inferior or dorsal pancreatic arteries, and the left branch joins the caudal pancreatic artery. Branches of these pancreatic arteries supply interlobular arteries, and one intralobular artery supplies each lobule.

Major lymphatic vessels follow the course of the blood vessels. Approximately 55% of interlobular lymphatics are closely related to the accompanying artery and vein, 25% are separated from other structures by connective tissue, and 20% are closely related to acinar cells. Only 2% border the ductal system (8). The interlobular lymphatics drain toward the surface of the pancreas and enter a surface network, sometimes referred to as collecting vessels, and converge toward the lymph nodes.

There are two major systems of lymph nodes draining the pancreas: one rings the pancreas and the other surrounds the aorta from the level of the celiac trunk to the origin of the superior mesenteric artery. Lymph nodes may be closely apposed to the periphery of the gland or even embedded within its substance, especially along the inferior and superior borders and in the anterior and posterior pancreatoduodenal regions. Many lymph nodes are also found around the celiac axis, adjacent to the common bile duct, and at the splenic hilus (9). Several classification systems exist for these lymph nodes (9–12), although from the standpoint of involvement by carcinoma, the lymph node classifications appear not to have clinical significance.

Innervation of the pancreas is from the vagus nerve (parasympathetic) and the splanchnic nerves (sympathetic) via the celiac and superior mesenteric plexi (2,5). The course of the nerves accompanies the vasculature (4).

Gross Anatomy

In adults, the pancreas usually measures 15 to 20 cm in length and weighs 85 to 120 g. It is slightly larger in men than in women (6,13). The pancreas weighs 2 to 3 g in the newborn and reaches 7 g at 1 year of age (14). The weight of the gland gradually decreases after 40 years of age to a mean of 70 g in the ninth decade of life (13).

The pancreas is composed of four rather indistinct anatomic regions: the head, neck, body, and tail (Figure 30.2). The bulk of the organ is composed of the head, including the uncinate process, which develops separately and may be anatomically separate in some individuals (see below). The uncinate process (from the Latin *uncus* or "hook") extends inferiorly and posteriorly from the head of the gland and lies behind the pancreatic neck and the superior mesenteric vessels. These vessels frequently indent the uncinate process, producing the hook shape. This vascular sulcus is helpful for orienting the pancreas in pancreatoduodenectomy specimens. The neck of the pancreas is the short constricted area of the pancreas that rests anterior to the mesenteric vessels. The neck and body are somewhat triangular in cross section, whereas the distal-most tail is flat (2).

The normal pancreas is pink-tan to yellow and uniformly lobulated. The anterior surface is smooth and covered by a layer of peritoneum; the remaining surfaces are invested by a thin layer of loose fibroconnective tissue. No discrete capsule is present; and, depending on the amount of parenchymal fat and the extent of any fibrosis, the interface with the surrounding retroperitoneal adipose tissue may be indistinct.

Cut sections of the pancreas reveal arborizing thin-walled white ducts extending into the well-demarcated

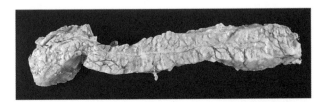

Figure 30.2 Gross appearance of the normal pancreas. The bulbous head (*left*) is connected to the neck, body, and tail, which merge imperceptibly. The parenchyma consists of distinctly lobulated pink-tan fleshy tissue. The pancreatic duct (opened longitudinally) is thin and smooth throughout its course.

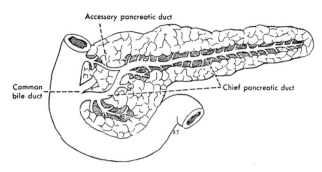

Figure 30.3 Schematic diagram of the pancreas showing the pattern of the major ducts and their tributaries. In this example the accessory duct is patent at the duodenum through the minor papilla. Reprinted with permission from: Cubilla AL, Fitzgerald PJ. *Tumors of the exocrine pancreas.* In: Hartmann WH, Sobin LH, eds. *Atlas of Tumor Pathology.* 2nd series, fascicle 19. Washington, DC: Armed Forces Institute of Pathology; 1984.

lobules. The main pancreatic duct of Wirsung averages 3.0 mm (ranging from 1.8 to 9.0 mm) in diameter (15), gradually enlarging to 4.5 mm near the ampulla of Vater, through which it drains into the duodenum. Main ducts greater than 10 mm in diameter are considered pathologically dilated. Up to 50 secondary or branch ducts drain into the main duct (16,17), entering alternately from either side in a herringbone pattern (Figure 30.3) (6). The course of the major ducts varies depending on the pattern of fusion and atrophy of ducts that occurs during development. In general, the main pancreatic duct of Wirsung begins in the tail, collecting tributaries as it passes through the body and neck toward the head. The duct makes an acute turn inferiorly in the head of the gland, where it is joined by the accessory duct of Santorini from the superior head as well as the major duct from the uncinate process, ultimately exiting through the ampulla at the major papilla. The accessory duct generally does not communicate separately with the duodenum, although retention of embryonic patency through the minor duodenal papilla is not uncommon.

The relationship of the main duct to the distal common bile duct is also highly variable. The prototypical ampulla is a flask-shaped common channel within the wall of the duodenum formed by the fusion of the two ducts. A significant common channel is uncommon, however. In many cases, length of the common channel is less than 3 mm. In others, the two ducts remain separate throughout their course, entering side by side at the major papilla or completely separately (Figure 30.4) (4,13,18). In these individuals, a common channel does not exist or is extremely short. In one study, only 43% of individuals had a common channel greater than 3 mm in length (19). Villiform mucosal projections are present within the distal ducts; these valves of Santorini may prevent the reflux of duodenal secretions (20,21). The intraduodenal portions of the pancreatic and bile ducts are surrounded by thin fascicles of smooth muscle (the sphincter of Oddi), which are continuous with both the muscularis mucosae and the muscularis propria of the surrounding duodenum.

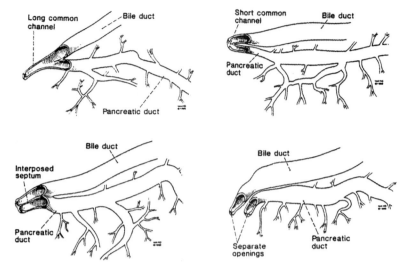

Figure 30.4 Anatomic variations in the paths of the pancreatic and bile ducts at the ampulla. A long common channel (the prototypical ampulla) is only present in some individuals. In others, the ducts fuse within only a few millimeters of the duodenum, resulting in a short common channel, or the two ducts enter separately. Reprinted with permission from: DiMagno EP, Shorter RG, Taylor WF, Go VL. Relationships between pancreaticobiliary ductal anatomy and pancreatic ductal and parenchymal histology. *Cancer* 1982;49:361–368.

DEVELOPMENT

Organogenesis

During the fourth to fifth weeks of gestation, the pancreas forms from the endoderm of the distal embryonic foregut as dorsal and ventral buds (22,23). The dorsal bud forms opposite the hepatic diverticulum, whereas the ventral bud, which may be bilobed, forms adjacent to the hepatic diverticulum (17). Thus, the duct from the ventral pancreas is closely apposed to the common bile duct. With the rotation of the duodenum during the sixth week, the ventral pancreas with the common bile duct migrates circumferentially to the right around the posterior aspect of the duodenum to lie posterior and inferior to the dorsal pancreas (Figure 30.5). The two

portions generally fuse during the seventh week. The dorsal portion makes up the superior head as well as the entire neck, body, and tail of the adult gland, and the ventral portion becomes the remainder of the head, including the uncinate process (23). The ductal systems of the two lobes also normally fuse, with connection of the dorsal duct to the duodenum at the minor papilla being lost and the ventral duct providing the drainage for the exocrine secretions. Thus, the distal two-thirds of the main pancreatic duct (of Wirsung) develop from the embryonic dorsal duct, whereas the proximal one-third forms from the ventral duct. The complicated union of these different ducts accounts for the tortuous nature of the main pancreatic duct in adults. The remaining proximal portion of the dorsal embryonic duct becomes the accessory duct of Santorini. The ampulla of Vater develops during the eighth week.

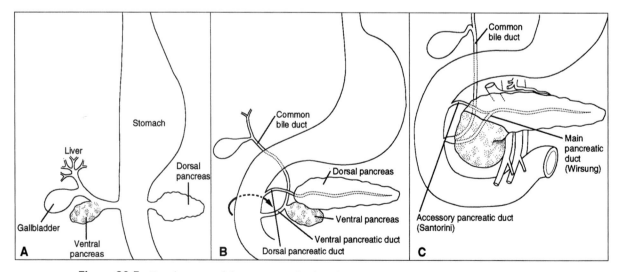

Figure 30.5 Development of the pancreas. The dorsal and ventral buds form on opposite sides of the duodenum (**A**). During the sixth week, the ventral pancreas migrates posteriorly around the duodenum (**B**) to lie inferior to the dorsal pancreas, where it comprises much of the head of the gland (**C**). Reprinted with permission from: Skandalakis LJ, Rowe JS Jr, Gray SW, Skandalakis JE. Surgical embryology and anatomy of the pancreas. *Surg Clin North Am* 1993;73:661–697.

Cytogenesis

The complex events required for normal cellular development of the pancreas have three components (24). First, as described above, the foregut endoderm becomes patterned to form the dorsal and ventral pancreatic buds. Second, the cells undergo lineage commitment to either endocrine or exocrine cell fates. Third, pancreatic morphogenesis occurs by way of extensive growth and branching. Recent studies suggest that distinct signaling pathways control these events, but it is important to note that tissue specification, lineage commitment, and growth are highly interdependent and have considerable spatial and temporal overlap.

Several transcription factors are required for pancreas specification. Prior to and during budding, the pancreatic primordium expresses the homeodomain protein Pdx1 (also known as IPF1) (24), and Pdx1-positive progenitors give rise to all three epithelial cell lines (25). The developing ductal epithelium retains uniform Pdx1 expression, but later Pdx1 expression is lost in the ductal cells, being primarily restricted to the islet cells, with low levels detectable in some acinar cells. Under certain conditions, Pdx1 expression again becomes detectable in individual pancreatic ductal epithelial cells, raising the possibility of multipotential stem cells within the mature ductal epithelium (26).

Among others, additional transcriptional factors involved in pancreatic morphogenesis include Sox17, HLXB9, and PTF1; and many endocrine lineage-specific transcription factors are known, such as Ngn3, NeuroD/Beta2, Nkx2.2, and Nkx6.1 (27–30). However, little information exists regarding similar factors required for exocrine differentiation. The p48 component of the heterotrimeric PTF1 transcription factor complex is required for normal exocrine differentiation (31).

Pancreatic development is also regulated by cell fate determining signals from developmental patterning pathways, such as the *Notch* and *Hedgehog* (*Hh*) signaling pathways. Notch signals are required for epithelial branching and normal exocrine lineage commitment (32). Of the three hedgehog genes essential for mammalian embryogenesis (*sonic hedgehog* [*Shh*], *Indian hedgehog* [*Ihh*], and *desert hedgehog* [*Dhh*]), *Shh* expression in midgestational embryos is critical for proper foregut and gastrointestinal development. In contrast, *Shh* is excluded from the developing pancreas, and repression of *Shh* permits appropriate transcriptional activation of pancreatic genes (33).

The developing ducts form solid cellular cords that proliferate into the surrounding mesenchyme. As the ducts branch progressively, luminal spaces are formed. Both acinar and endocrine cells develop from these primitive ducts (34). The cells at the termini of the branches differentiate into acinar cells during the third month of gestation (34). The pancreatic lobules are formed by the accumulation of acinar units around ductular branches that are separated by layers of mesenchyme. By the fourth

month the acinar cells contain zymogen granules (14). The earliest granules identified in acinar cells are elongated and angular, with a fibrillary internal matrix. These granules, along with small spherical granules, may be detected at 15 to 20 weeks gestation (23,35,36). By 20 weeks, the granules resemble the zymogen granules of the adult pancreas, and the elongate granules disappear. The nature of the elongate granules remains unclear, and enzymes have yet to be detected in them. However, it is interesting that similar "irregular fibrillary granules" have been repeatedly detected in pancreatic neoplasms with acinar differentiation (36–41).

Islet cells also develop from the ducts at 8 to 10 weeks gestation. Most of the islet cells appear to originate from the intralobular and interlobular ducts (16). In the third month, developing endocrine cell clusters bud off from the ducts and surround capillaries to form discrete islets (42,43). In even the earliest developing islets, differentiated α and β cells can be recognized (43–45). At 16 weeks the α and β cells segregate to opposite ends of the islets; these bipolar islets are gradually replaced between 18 and 20 weeks by mantle islets having a central core of β cells surrounded by a rim of α cells (34,43,45). Although the microscopic architecture of the mature adult islets is more complex, the peripheral location of the α cells found in the mantle islets is roughly maintained.

During the third to fourth months, the pancreatic tissue becomes increasingly organized around the branching ductal structures to form lobules (Figure 30.6A–B). The characteristics of the ductal lining cells specific to their level within the ductal system become established during this period. The mesenchymal elements of the early pancreas are prominent. The early periductal stroma is highly cellular (Figure 30.6C), resembling the ovarian-like stroma that characterizes mucinous cystic neoplasms (46,47). As the pancreas develops, the mesenchyme becomes increasingly less abundant and less cellular, ultimately constituting a relatively minimal component of the adult gland.

Developmental Anomalies and Heterotopia

Complete or partial pancreatic agenesis is rare. Complete agenesis is associated with gallbladder agenesis, diaphragmatic hernia, and growth retardation. A homozygous deletion in the *Pdx1* gene was recently identified in a girl born with complete pancreatic agenesis (48), interesting because of the role *Pdx1* plays in pancreatic development. Most patients with partial pancreatic agenesis survive; but, depending upon the amount of pancreatic tissue that develops, they may have diabetes mellitus. More common than pancreatic agenesis is pancreatic hypoplasia, also referred to as congenital short pancreas. This condition may be part of a congenital syndrome or present as an isolated anomaly. The pancreas appears short and stubby but otherwise retains the

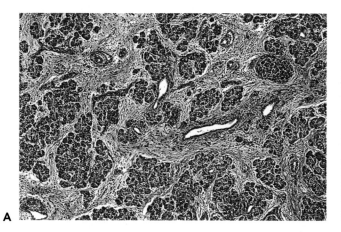

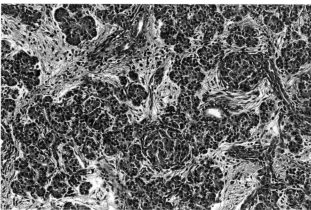

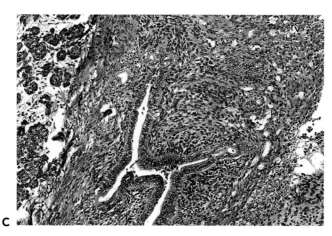

Figure 30.6 **A.** The fetal pancreas at 18 to 20 weeks of gestation exhibits a well-developed lobular architecture. The loose connective tissue between the lobules is relatively abundant. **B.** Both acinar and endocrine elements are well developed and are functioning at this stage. **C.** The mesenchyme surrounding the ducts is highly cellular, resembling the so-called ovarian-like stroma of mucinous cystic neoplasms.

normal appearing lobular architecture. Pancreatic hypoplasia typically is not associated with hypofunction.

Annular or ring pancreas is an extremely rare developmental anomaly in which there is partial or complete encircling of the second part of the duodenum by pancreatic tissue (Figure 30.7) (4,49–51). Pancreas divisum usually accompanies annular pancreas (52), and the condition affects only 0.015% of the population (53). Possibly it is the failure of one of the lobes of the ventral embryonic bud to regress, causing it to encircle the duodenum during the normal rotation of the duodenum. Annular pancreas commonly causes duodenal obstruction, which varies in severity and age of onset, depending on the extent of luminal constriction. Some cases are also associated with duodenal atresia (51). The band of pancreatic tissue partially or completely encircling the duodenum is flattened and may be embedded within the muscularis propria. Histologically it contains all of the normal parenchymal elements. Because the portion of pancreas encircling the duodenum is derived from the ventral pancreas, it is rich in pancreatic polypeptide-containing islets (54).

There are many variations in the paths of the pancreatic ducts and their relationship to the common bile duct (17,51). The communication between the dorsal pancreatic duct and the duodenum fails to obliterate in up to 40% of adults (17,55), resulting in a patent accessory duct (of Santorini) at the minor papilla, proximal to the opening of the

main duct and bile duct at the major papilla. In such instances, the dorsal duct may provide the main route of drainage for the gland and may be much larger in circumference than the ventral duct. This condition appears to be more prevalent in children, suggesting that obliteration of

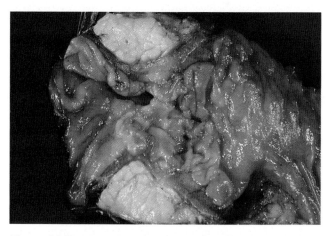

Figure 30.7 Annular pancreas. The pancreatic tissue completely encircles the duodenum, which is opened longitudinally. Reprinted with permission from: Hruban RH, Pitman MB, Klimstra DS. Tumors of the pancreas. In: Silverberg SG, Sobin LH, eds. *Atlas of Tumor Pathology.* 4th series. Washington, DC: Armed Forces Institute of Pathology; 2006.

the accessory duct opening may continue to occur in adulthood (56). Also, the two ducts may fail to fuse entirely, resulting in two separate ductal systems, a condition known as pancreas divisum. This anomaly occurs in 5 to 10% of individuals (17,57). The pancreatic parenchyma of the two lobes is usually fused (23), and the abnormality may not be detected unless a careful study of the ductal system is performed. There are three types of pancreas divisum: type 1, or classical pancreas divisum, involves total failure of duct fusion, causing most of the pancreatic secretions to drain through the duct of Santorini at the diminutive minor papilla, with the duct of Wirsung draining the small ventral pancreas through the major papilla; type 2 involves dominant dorsal drainage in which the ventral duct regresses completely, leaving the single dorsal duct and minor papilla as the only means of egress for exocrine secretions; and type 3 involves incomplete pancreas divisum, where a small communicating branch of the ventral duct remains (58). Patients with pancreas divisum seem to have a higher incidence of pancreatitis, especially when the opening of the dorsal duct at the minor papilla is small (51,57,59).

Anomalous junction of the main pancreatic duct with the distal common bile duct may occur within the head of the pancreas more than 2 cm proximal to the duodenum (17,51). This abnormality may be associated with choledochal cysts and carcinomas of the extrahepatic bile ducts or gallbladder (17,60,61). In a rare abnormality of the pancreatic duct, bifid pancreas, the main pancreatic duct bifurcates within the body of the pancreas (62).

Pancreatic heterotopia is defined as pancreatic tissue located outside of the normal anatomic position of the gland (51). Heterotopic pancreatic tissue is found in portions of the upper gastrointestinal tract and its appendages in up to 15% of individuals at autopsy (63). The surgical incidence, however, is only 0.2% (64). Of the cases detected during life,

25 to 50% are symptomatic (63,65). Although it is presumed to be congenital in origin, most symptomatic cases are detected in adulthood (65). The duodenum and stomach are the most common locations of pancreatic heterotopia (4,66), with most duodenal cases occurring in the second portion several centimeters proximal to the ampulla of Vater. Often the tissue is found in the submucosa beneath the minor duodenal papilla and represents remnants of the embryonic dorsal ductal system. Pancreatic heterotopia also may occur elsewhere in the duodenum and may involve the ampulla of Vater (67,68). Other sites of pancreatic heterotopia include the jejunum, Meckel's diverticulum, the large bowel, and the liver, where it is generally located around the bile ducts (69). In the tubular gastrointestinal tract, heterotopic pancreas appears as lobulated submucosal nodules of yellow to white firm tissue ranging from several millimeters to several centimeters in size. The overlying mucosa may be umbilicated in larger examples (Figure 30.8A). Rarely heterotopic pancreatic tissue is present on the serosal surface. Microscopically, the type and amount of the different pancreatic cell types varies. Most cases have ducts, and they may be the only epithelial component. Such cases have submucosal aggregates of small ducts and lobules of ductules, typically surrounded by interlacing smooth muscle fascicles, resulting in the appearance of so-called adenomyoma. Many cases do show some acinar and endocrine elements, and some resemble normal pancreatic parenchyma (Figure 30.8B). Some duodenal foci of heterotopic pancreas exhibit acini with the features of Brunner's glands, emphasizing the embryologic relationship these glands have with the pancreas (16). One of the important reasons to recognize heterotopic pancreas is to avoid misinterpretation of these ductules as carcinoma; however, cases of adenocarcinoma arising in heterotopic pancreas have been described (70–72), as have pancreatic pseudocysts.

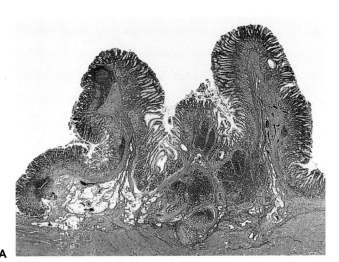

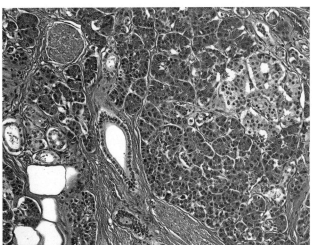

A   B

Figure 30.8 Heterotopic pancreatic tissue in the stomach. **A.** At low power, a submucosal nodule of pancreatic tissue results in an umbilicated appearance. **B.** In this example, lobules of normal-appearing acinar and ductular structures are separated by bands of fibromuscular tissue. Acini, ducts, and islets are arranged in a disorganized pattern, with interspersed bundles of smooth muscle.

Heterotopic tissues also may be found within the pancreas. Accessory splenic tissue may be found in the tail of the pancreas or, more rarely, in the head (73). In most cases, the splenic tissue is small (less than 2 cm), dark red, and spherical. Intrapancreatic adrenal cortical tissue has also been described (74).

MICROSCOPIC FEATURES

Microscopically, the pancreas is arranged in 1- to 10-mm lobules (Figure 30.9). The parenchyma within the lobules consists almost entirely of the epithelial elements of the pancreas, including the acini, the ducts, and the islets of Langerhans. There is minimal intralobular connective tissue, but fibroconnective tissue containing vessels and nerves separates the lobules.

Acini

Acinar cells make up approximately 85% of the mass of the pancreas and constitute the main exocrine secretory component of the gland. The prototypical architecture of the acinus in routine histologic sections appears to be a single layer of polygonal cells surrounding a minute central lumen, suggesting a spherical configuration (Figure 30.10); however, the three-dimensional architecture of the pancreatic acini is much more complex (75). In fact, tubular acini are commonly detected in histologic sections (Figure 30.11). Also, not all acini are located at the terminal end of ductules. Some acini bud from the sides of the ductules or are situated between two ductules. Anastomosing loops of acini also may be found (75). Thus, the secretions of a given acinus may pass through a number of different pathways to reach the ductal system.

Individual acinar cells are polarized, with basally situated round nuclei and apical granular eosinophilic cyto-

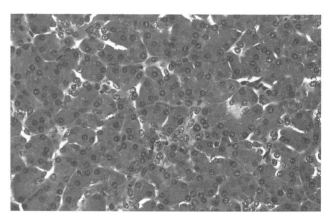

Figure 30.10   Acinar cells contain abundant granular eosinophilic cytoplasm in the apical aspect, with basophilic basal cytoplasm. The nuclei are also basally located. Most acini consist of spherically arranged individual acinar cells.

plasm. The eosinophilia of the apical cytoplasm reflects the accumulation of numerous zymogen granules (Figure 30.10), which contrast with the basophilic zymogen granules of salivary serous acini. The zymogen granule content is highly dynamic, depending on the secretory state of the pancreas, which is largely regulated by digestive hormones (1). The basal cytoplasm of the acinar cells is basophilic due to the high concentration of ribonucleoproteins in the abundant rough endoplasmic reticulum (RER). There may be a clear cytoplasmic zone on the luminal side of the nucleus that contains the Golgi apparatus. The nuclei are uniform and frequently contain distinct central nucleoli; clumps of chromatin are generally present beneath the nuclear membrane. The acinar cells sit directly upon the basement membrane; in contrast to salivary acini, there are no myoepithelial cells surrounding the pancreatic acini.

Although the acinar cells from different regions of the pancreas are all morphologically and functionally similar, there are subtle differences in the size and zymogen granule

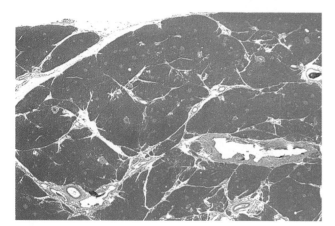

Figure 30.9   At low power, the normal pancreas has a well-developed lobular arrangement of highly cellular glandular tissue.

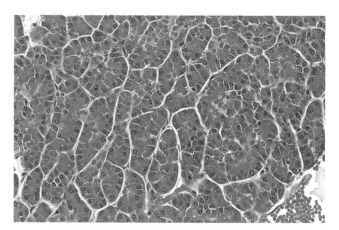

Figure 30.11   Other acini have tubular configurations and exhibit interanastomosing loops when studied by serial sectioning.

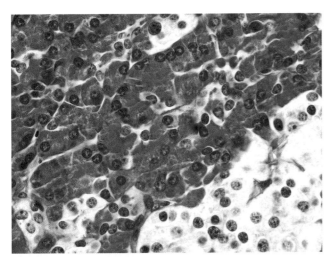

Figure 30.12 Zymogen granules are positive with periodic acid-Schiff's stain with diastase pretreatment. Islet cells (*lower right*) are negative.

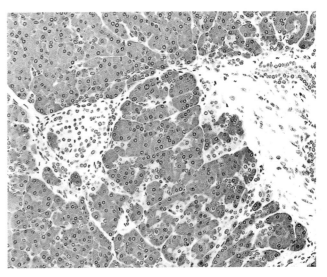

Figure 30.13 Immunohistochemical staining for trypsin results in intense labeling of acinar cells but not ductal and islet cells. Faint luminal labeling of ductal cells may be seen due to deposition of luminal enzymatic secretions on the apical cell surfaces (*upper right*).

content in the acinar cells immediately adjacent to islets compared with those distant from islets, perhaps as a reflection of regional variations in islet hormone levels (76,77).

Zymogen granules stain positively with periodic acid-Schiff (PAS) stain and are resistant to diastase digestion (Figure 30.12). Acinar cells also can be demonstrated using stains for butyrate esterase, which is positive in the presence of enzymatically active lipase (38). Immunohistochemical labeling for pancreatic enzymes such as trypsin, chymotrypsin, lipase, amylase, and elastase is positive in acinar cells (Figure 30.13) and, with the exception of amylase, these are also sensitive markers for acinar differentiation in pancreatic neoplasms (38–40, 78). Each individual zymogen granule contains all of the various digestive enzymes, usually in a proenzyme form (79,80). Keratins detected by

the CAM 5.2 antibody (cytokeratins 8 and 18) are present in acinar cells; however, there is no labeling with the AE1 antibody nor is there with antibodies against cytokeratins 7, 19, and 20 (Figure 30.14). Mucins are not produced, and immunohistochemical labeling for glycoproteins such as DUPAN-2, CEA, and CA19.9 is negative. Finally, endocrine specific antibodies such as chromogranin and synaptophysin are negative as well.

Ultrastructural examination shows features characteristic of active exocrine secretion. The RER is arranged in parallel stacks and fills the basal cytoplasm (Figure 30.15). Scattered mitochondria and free polyribosomes are present between RER cisternae (81). The Golgi apparatus is situated in the

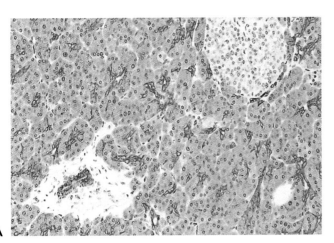
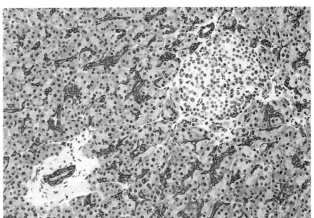

A   **B**

Figure 30.14 Immunohistochemical labeling for keratins. **A.** The CAM 5.2 antibody shows diffuse labeling of acinar cells and ductal cells, the latter being more intensely positive. **B.** The AE1/AE3 antibodies label only ductal cells. Islet cells show only focal faint labeling with any of these antibodies.

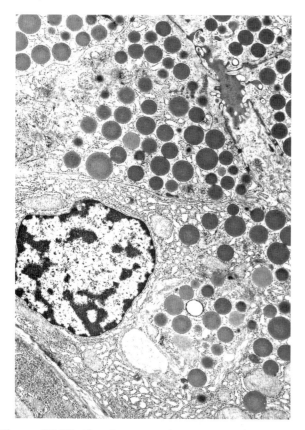

Figure 30.15 The ultrastructural appearance of acinar cells. These polarized cells have abundant parallel stacks of rough endoplasmic reticulum with interspersed mitochondria in the basal cytoplasm. Homogeneous electron-dense zymogen granules are concentrated in the apical cytoplasm underlying the lumina. The luminal spaces are lined by short microvilli. Adjacent acinar cells are joined to one another and to the centroacinar cells (*) by apical junctional complexes. The centroacinar cells have lucent cytoplasm devoid of secretory granules.

central region of the cytoplasm near the nucleus. Immature electron-dense zymogen granules emanate from the *trans* side of the Golgi apparatus. Larger round, homogeneous mature zymogen granules are present within the apical cytoplasm. They measure 250 to 1000 nm and have limiting membranes closely apposed to the dense secretory content. Upon stimulation, the membranes of the secretory granules fuse with the apical plasma membrane, expelling the contents into the lumen; the excess cell membranes are then recycled to the Golgi apparatus (82,83). Accumulated secretions are often present within the lumina, sometimes with crystal formation. The luminal membranes have sparse, short microvilli containing inner microfilaments that are continuous with the terminal web of filaments beneath the apical membrane (81). Adjacent acinar cells are joined by apical junctional complexes composed of zonula occludens- and zonula adherens-type junctions, whereas desmosomes (macula adherens junctions) join cells along the basal aspects of their lateral membranes (14,81). Each acinus is surrounded by a continuous basement membrane.

Ducts

The ductal system of the pancreas serves to transport the acinar cell secretions to the duodenum. The ductal epithelial cells secrete water, chloride, and bicarbonate to buffer the acidity of the pancreatic juices and stabilize the proenzymes until activation within the duodenum. The ductal system is subdivided into five portions: centroacinar cells, intercalated ducts, intralobular ducts, interlobular ducts (large and small), and main ducts (84). The ductal system begins with the centroacinar cells, which are small, relatively inconspicuous, flat to cuboidal cells with pale or lightly eosinophilic cytoplasm and central oval nuclei (Figure 30.16). Centroacinar cells are located in the middle of the acini, where they partially border

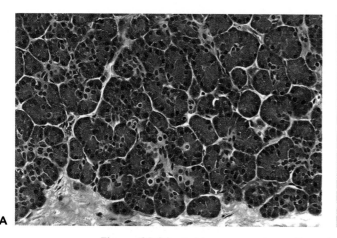
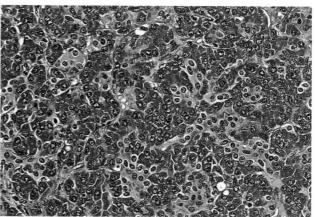

A   B

Figure 30.16 **A.** Most centroacinar cells are inconspicuous small cells with minimal cytoplasm and oval nuclei situated in the center of the acini. **B.** In other regions the centroacinar cells may be more prominent, with more abundant lightly eosinophilic cytoplasm. Centroacinar cells constitute the beginning of the ductal system and convey the secretions of acinar cells to the intercalated ducts.

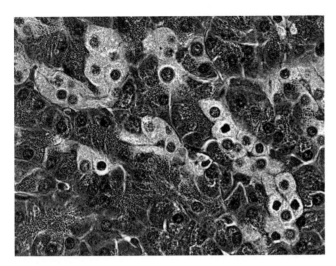

Figure 30.17 Some centroacinar cells are enlarged and have oncocytic cytoplasm, a variation of uncertain significance.

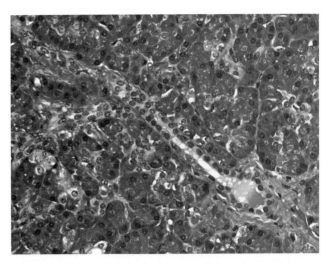

Figure 30.18 The ductal system within the lobules consists of innumerable intercalated ducts that fuse to form intralobular ducts. The cytologic appearance of the intercalated and intralobular ductal cells resembles that of the centroacinar cells, and the transition from one to the next is imperceptible. Only minimal collagenized stroma surrounds the intralobular ducts (*lower right*).

the acinar lumina along with the acinar cells, to which they are joined by tight junctions. Ultrastructurally, the centroacinar cells have cytoplasm largely devoid of organelles, with only scattered mitochondria; no zymogen, neurosecretory, or mucigen granules are present. Relative to the acinar cells, the cytoplasm is less dense and rough endoplasmic reticulum is minimal. The cell surfaces contain scattered short microvilli similar to those on the adjacent acinar cells. Adjacent cells are joined by abundant junctional complexes, and there are often complex interdigitations between them. Some centroacinar cells have more abundant granular oncocytic cytoplasm (Figure 30.17) that reflects numerous mitochondria (84,85); the significance of this variation is unknown.

The lumen surrounded by acinar and centroacinar cells drains into the intercalated ducts, which are the smallest ducts outside the acini (Figure 30.18). The cells lining the intercalated ducts resemble the centroacinar cells. They are cuboidal and have central oval nuclei with indistinct nucleoli. Mucins are not detected with Alcian blue or mucicarmine stains in centroacinar or intercalated duct cells. The intercalated ducts fuse to form the intralobular ducts, and the transition is imperceptible. The cells lining the intralobular ducts are essentially identical to those of the intercalated ducts, although the nuclei are round rather than oval (Figure 30.18). Neither intercalated nor intralobular ducts have a significant collagenous matrix surrounding them. The ductal cells rest directly on the basement membrane and lack both myoepithelial and basal cells; thus, in contrast to several other organs, the presence or absence of these cells cannot be used to help distinguish benign ducts from invasive pancreatic ductal adenocarcinoma.

Once the ducts leave the lobules, they become enveloped by a variably thick rim of collagen and are termed interlobular ducts (Figure 30.19). The interlobular ductal cells have slightly more cytoplasm than those of the intralobular ducts

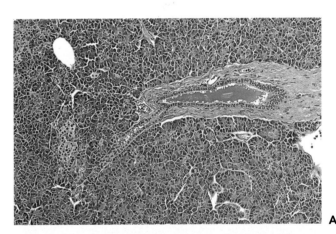

A

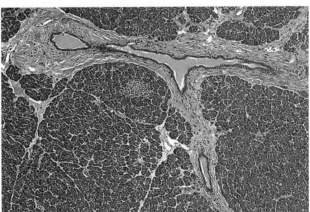

B

Figure 30.19 **A.** Intralobular ducts come together to form interlobular ducts. **B.** The interlobular ducts are surrounded by a variably thick rim of dense fibrous tissue and carry the pancreatic secretions to the major ducts, receiving tributaries of small interlobular ducts as they pass through the connective tissue septa of the gland.

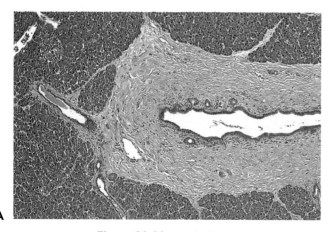 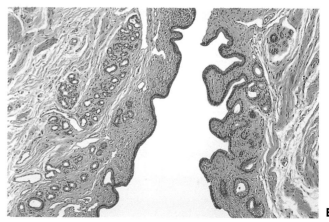

Figure 30.20   **A.** The largest interlobular ducts are surrounded by a thick rim of collagen. **B.** Small lobular aggregates of ductules are present within the wall of the larger ducts.

and assume a low columnar shape in the larger ducts. As in the smaller ducts, cytoplasmic mucin is not detectable by routine histology in intralobular or interlobular ductal cells; mucinous cytoplasm visible by routine histology is considered a pathological change (see below). However, some cytoplasmic mucin may be found using special stains. As the interlobular ducts approach the main pancreatic ducts (of Wirsung or Santorini), they develop an increasingly thick collagenous wall within which lobular aggregates of small ductules may be seen, resembling the ductules of Beale that surround the major bile ducts (Figure 30.20).

The main pancreatic ducts receive numerous tributaries of interlobular ducts (Figure 30.21). The lining epithelium remains flat, without papillary projections, except in the very distal duct within the ampulla, where simple papillae are found (Figure 30.22). The cells are low columnar with basal round nuclei. In these large ducts, there may be apical cytoplasmic clearing, reflecting mucin, but tall columnar cells with obvious abundant mucin are not normally found,

and special stains or electron microscopy are often needed to identify the mucin (84). The mucins of the intralobular and smaller interlobular ductal cells are predominantly sulphomucins and stain positively with Alcian blue at pH 1.0 (Figure 30.23) (55,86). In the cells of the larger ducts, there are fewer sulfomucins and more neutral mucins and sialomucins (86). There is relatively frequent cell exfoliation in the main duct, perhaps reflecting a high turnover rate due to injury; degenerating cells may be observed within the epithelium by electron microscopy (81). The thick connective tissue wall contains numerous periductal ductules, as well as fascicles of smooth muscle (1).

Other than the appearance of increasing numbers of mucigen granules and increased exocrine secretory apparatus (RER, mitochondria, and Golgi) in the larger ducts, the ultrastructural appearance of the ductal cells resembles that of the centroacinar cells (Figures 30.24–30.25). In ductal cells from the level of the small interlobular ducts, single long kinocilia project from the cell surfaces (81,84); cross

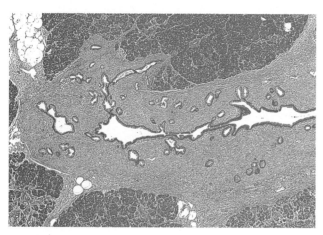

Figure 30.21   Numerous interlobular ducts join the main pancreatic duct along its course.

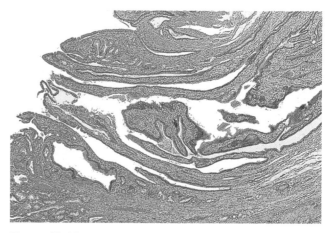

Figure 30.22   As the main pancreatic duct enters the ampulla of Vater, the ductal epithelium forms broad, simple papillae known as the valves of Santorini.

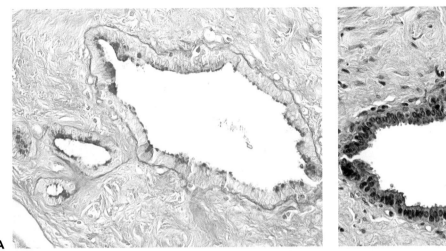
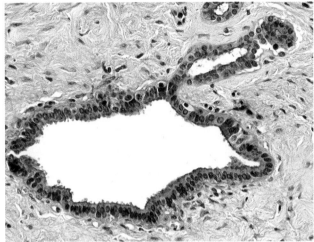

Figure 30.23 **A.** The cells of the intralobular and smaller interlobular ducts contain mucin in the apical cytoplasm that stains positively with Alcian blue/PAS. **B.** Staining with mucicarmine shows a similar distribution of mucin.

sections of these cilia may be observed within the lumina of the ducts (Figure 30.24). The cilia are connected to basal bodies in the paranuclear cytoplasm and may function in mixing and propulsion of the pancreatic secretions (81).

Ductal cells contain cytokeratins 7, 8, 18, and 19; hence, they are immunohistochemically reactive with the AE1, AE3, and CAM 5.2 antibodies, in addition to anti-

bodies against the specific individual cytokeratins (Figure 30.14). They do not express cytokeratin 20. Enzyme and endocrine markers are also negative. Carbonic anhydrase is detectable in ductal cells, reflecting their role in fluid and ion transport (87); most is detected in intercalated and intralobular ducts (88), although ducts of larger caliber may weakly express this enzyme (Figure 30.26).

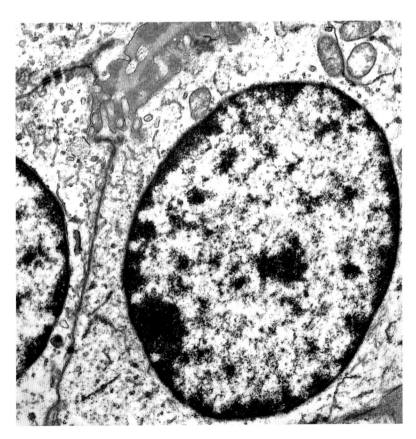

Figure 30.24 Ultrastructural appearance of intralobular ductal cells. The cytoplasm resembles that of centroacinar cells, with an electron-lucent appearance and scattered mitochondria and rough endoplasmic reticulum. In the smaller ducts, mucigen granules are largely absent. The luminal surface exhibits short microvilli. In addition, scattered cilia are present, the cross section of which may be seen within the lumen (*top*).

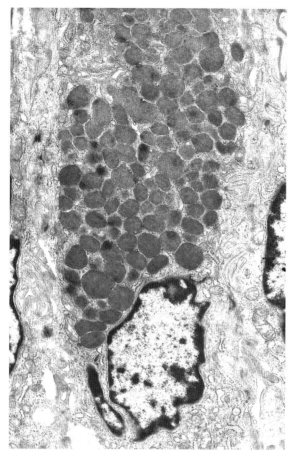

Figure 30.25 In the larger ducts, more abundant mucigen granules accumulate within the apical cytoplasm. These granules vary in size and have irregular contours and heterogeneous, variably electron-dense secretory contents. There are complex interdigitations of the lateral membranes between adjacent cells.

Other markers of ductal cells include antibodies against CA19-9, DUPAN-2, cystic fibrosis transmembrane conductance regulator (CFTR), and N-terminal gastrin-releasing peptide (N-GRP) (89–93). Normal ducts do not label with antibodies to carcinoembryonic antigen when monoclonal antisera are used (94) and also fail to label for B72.3 and CA125. Members of the MUC family of glycoproteins are variably expressed; MUC1 is present in smaller intralobular and intercalated ducts, MUC6 is expressed in centroacinar cells and intercalated ducts; MUC2 and MUC5AC are not normally expressed (95,96).

Islets of Langerhans

The endocrine component of the pancreas constitutes only 1 to 2% of the volume of the gland in adults (1,77) but about 10% in the newborn (55,97). The vast majority of endocrine cells are found in the over one million islets of Langerhans, first described by Paul Langerhans in 1869. Although islets are distributed throughout the pancreas, they are somewhat

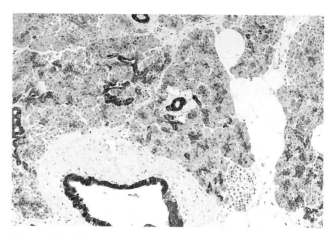

Figure 30.26 Immunohistochemical staining for carbonic anhydrase. In this preparation, there is staining of ductal cells of all sizes, including centroacinar, intercalated duct, and intralobular and interlobular ductal cells.

more numerous in the tail (98). Apparently random variations in islet concentration may occur from one lobule to the next, resulting in the appearance of plentiful islets in one area and sparse islets in an adjacent region (Figure 30.27).

The apparent volume of islets observed in histologic sections also varies with the age of the individual and the presence and extent of exocrine atrophy, as commonly occurs in chronic pancreatitis. In the fetus and neonate, the relative volume of endocrine cells far outmeasures that of the adult, especially in the portions derived from the dorsal lobe (Figure 30.28) (99).

Two types of islets are found. Most (90%) are the compact islets: sharply circumscribed nests usually measuring 75 to 225 μm, although islets as small as 50 μm or as large as 280 μm also may be found (100). Compact islets are found predominantly in the body and tail of the gland, with fewer in the head. The second type of islet, the diffuse islet, is essentially restricted to the posteroinferior head of the gland derived from the embryonic ventral lobe (101,102). These islets are much less numerous than the compact islets and may measure up to 450 μm.

Despite the circumscribed appearance of the compact islets, they are actually composed of interdigitating trabeculae that appear as small lobules in cross section (100). The cells of the compact islets have uniform round nuclei with coarsely clumped chromatin and inconspicuous nucleoli (Figure 30.29). The cytoplasm is pale and amphophilic. Occasional islet cells have nuclei two to four times the size of their neighbors, although no irregularities of shape or chromatin pattern are present. These nuclei have a 4n or 8n DNA content and have been shown to occur exclusively in β cells (103); they do not have any pathologic significance. Mitotic figures are only rarely encountered in normal islets (104). The islets contain numerous small vessels, although these capillary-sized vessels are almost inapparent by light microscopy. Essentially all of the islet cells contact the vasculature. In

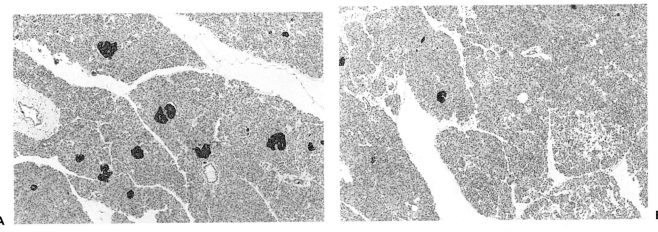

Figure 30.27 As highlighted by immunohistochemical labeling for chromogranin, the concentration of islets varies considerably from one lobule (**A**) to the next (**B**).

contrast to those supplying the acinar tissue, the capillaries of the islets have a fenestrated endothelium (1). A thin layer of connective tissue separates the compact islets from the surrounding acinar tissue, but they are not truly encapsulated.

Diffuse islets have a trabecular appearance, with winding cords of cells intermingled among acini (Figure 30.30A). Because they are less commonly encountered and have a pseudoinfiltrative appearance, they may be mistakenly regarded as neoplastic, an occurrence even more likely in the setting of chronic pancreatitis. In addition to the architectural differences already mentioned, the diffuse islets contain columnar cells within the trabecula. The cytoplasm is basophilic, the nuclei are somewhat hyperchromatic, and there may be more prominent nucleoli than in the compact islets (Figure 30.30B).

Each endocrine cell produces only one specific peptide hormone. The four major peptides produced by islet cells are insulin, glucagon, somatostatin, and pancreatic

polypeptide (105). Although some pancreatic endocrine neoplasms produce ectopic peptides such as gastrin or vasoactive intestinal polypeptide, these are not found in normal islet cells. Classical histochemical staining was used to distinguish the different cell types. Aldehyde-fuchsin stains insulin-secreting β cells, the Grimelius silver stain labels glucagon-secreting α cells, and the Hellerstrom-Hellman silver stain identifies somatostatin-secreting δ cells. Immunohistochemical labeling with antibodies against insulin, glucagon, somatostatin, and pancreatic polypeptide provides a more specific method to distinguish the cell types. There is a fairly consistent distribution of the cell types within the compact islets. The β cells are more centrally located, whereas the α cells populate the periphery of the islets (Figures 30.31–30.32). Beta cells constitue 60 to 70% and α cells make up 15 to 20% of the compact islets,

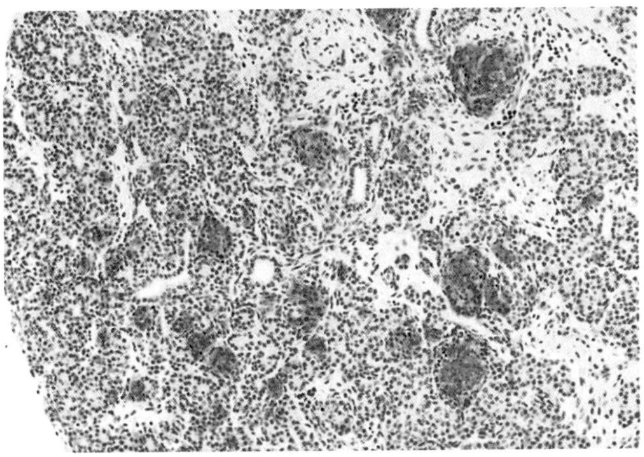

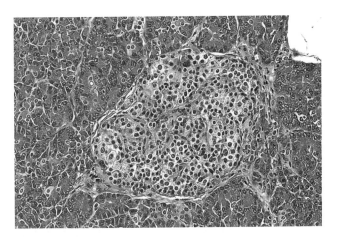

Figure 30.29 Compact islets consist of round to oval, generally circumscribed collections of endocrine cells. Small capillaries separate the islet into lobules. The nuclei have a stippled chromatin pattern, and there is moderate amphophilic cytoplasm. Some islet cells contain enlarged nuclei several times the size of those in the neighboring cells.

Figure 30.28 A fetal pancreas stained immunohistochemically for chromogranin. Note the abundance of endocrine cells relative to acinar cells at this stage of development.

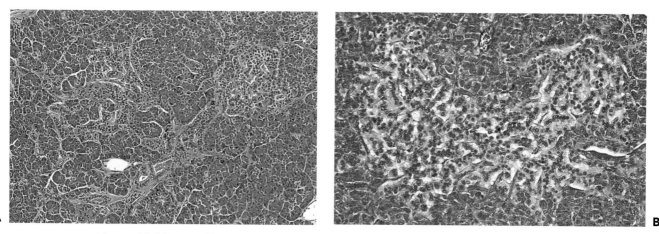

Figure 30.30 **A.** Diffuse islets are composed of trabeculae of endocrine cells interspersed between adjacent acini. **B.** The borders of the diffuse islets are ill defined. The cells have somewhat basophilic cytoplasm.

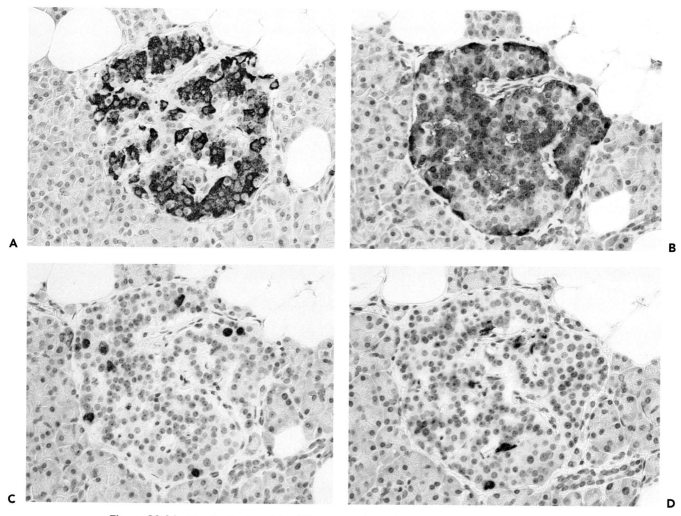

Figure 30.31 The distribution of the different peptide-producing cells within the islets of Langerhans. Beta cells (labeled for insulin) are the most numerous (**A**) and are situated in the central regions of the islet. Alpha cells (labeled for glucagon) are generally arranged around the periphery (**B**). Delta cells (labeled for somatostatin) (**C**) and PP cells (labeled for pancreatic polypeptide) (**D**) are much less numerous and do not display an obvious pattern of arrangement.

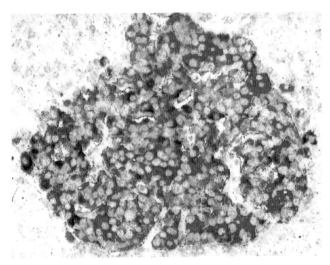

Figure 30.32 Triple immunohistochemical labeling of a compact islet for insulin (red-brown reaction product), glucagon (violet reaction product), and somatostatin (green reaction product) shows the characteristic distribution of the different cell types.

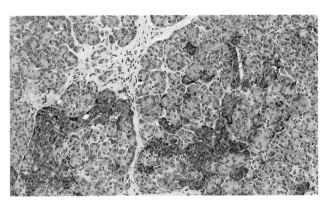

Figure 30.33 Immunohistochemistry for pancreatic polypeptide shows positive staining in most of the cells in the diffuse islets.

whereas the δ cells are much less numerous (100,106). Alpha cells are generally found in close contact with δ cells (42), and PP cells are rare in the compact islets, being concentrated in the diffuse islets where they constitute the majority (70%) of the cells (Figure 30.33) (107,108). The remaining cells of the diffuse islets are largely β cells (20%), with minor amounts of α and δ cells (5% of each). The difference in proportion of cell types between the compact and diffuse islets reflects their different embryologic origins (101,102). The relative proportion of the different peptide-producing cells also varies with age; for instance, the ratio of β to δ cells in the compact islets is manyfold higher in adults than in infants, in whom δ cells constitute one-third of the islet cell population (97,109). All of the islet cells also

express general endocrine markers such as neuron-specific enolase, CD56 (neural cell adhesion molecule), synaptophysin, and chromogranin (Figure 30.34). The last marker is expressed more intensely in α cells than in β cells, and the pattern of labeling also reflects the characteristic distribution of the cell types in the compact islets.

Keratins generally are not detected in islet cells by immunohistochemistry, although there may be some faint labeling with CAM 5.2. Enzymes also are not detectable. Progesterone and CD99 receptors are expressed in normal islets as well as in some pancreatic endocrine neoplasms (110–112). The homeodomain protein Pdx1, a transcription factor important in pancreatic development, is also expressed in adult islet cells.

Ultrastructural examination of the islets shows polygonal cells joined by tight and gap junctions, suggesting that there may be electronic or metabolic coupling between adjacent cells (42,100). Scattered desmosomes are also present. The cytoplasm contains all of the organelles necessary for protein synthesis, including RER, mitochondria, and

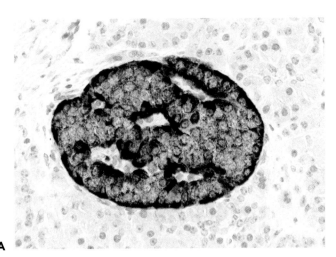

A

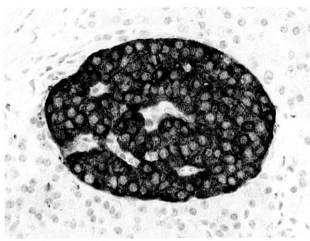

B

Figure 30.34 Alpha cells stain more intensely for chromogranin than do β cells (**A**), whereas all of the islet cells stain uniformly for synaptophysin (**B**).

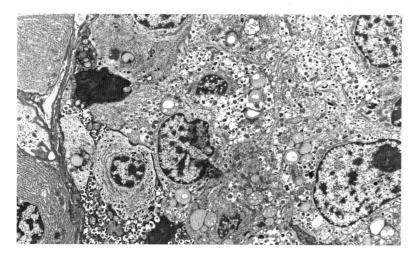

Figure 30.35 Ultrastructural appearance of islets of Langerhans. The islets are circumscribed and separated from the adjacent acinar cells (*left*). The peptide granules are randomly distributed within the cytoplasm. Lipid inclusions (ceroid bodies) are found within the β cells.

Golgi apparatus; however, the abundant parallel arrays of RER characteristic of acinar cells are absent (Figure 30.35). The granules are also more randomly distributed within the cytoplasm, with some concentration in the basal cytoplasm adjacent to the capillaries into which they are secreted. The granule sizes and morphologies are relatively specific for each cell type (105,113). Alpha cell granules measure 200

to 300 nm and contain an eccentrically located, dense core within a less dense outer region that is separated from the limiting membrane by a thin halo (Figure 30.36A). Beta cells contain 225- to 375-nm granules with either a finely granular or a crystalline core surrounded by a wide halo underlying the limiting membrane (Figure 30.36B). Cytoplasmic lipid inclusions (or ceroid bodies) are often found in β

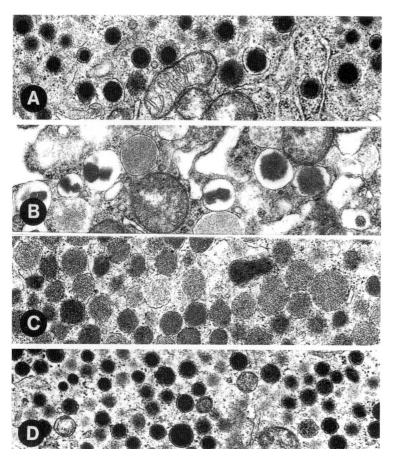

Figure 30.36 Ultrastructural appearance of islet cell granules. **A.** Alpha cell granules are round and contain an eccentric electron-dense core within a less dense peripheral region. There is a thin halo beneath the limiting membrane. **B.** Beta cell granules are polymorphous and contain crystalline cores with a wide halo beneath the limiting membrane. **C.** Delta cell granules are round with a moderately dense core surrounded by a very thin halo. **D.** The granules of PP cells are smaller and have homogenous hyperdense cores. Reprinted with permission from: Terada T, Ohta T, Sasaki M, Nakanuma Y, Kim YS. Expression of MUC apomucins in normal pancreas and pancreatic tumours. *J Pathol* 1996;180:160–165.

cells (Figure 30.35) (42). Delta cell granules are slightly smaller (170 to 220 nm) than α cell granules and have a uniformly dense core (Figure 30.36C). Delta cells have cytoplasmic processes extending toward the α and β cells, presumably allowing local paracrine release of somatostatin in addition to systemic release into the bloodstream (100). The PP cells of the ventrally derived portion of the pancreas have 180- to 220-nm granules of variable shape and density, whereas the PP cell granules of the remainder of the pancreas are smaller (120 to 150 nm) and more homogeneous (Figure 30.36D) (55). The cells are separated from the fenestrated endothelial cells of the capillaries only by the basement membranes of both cells and minimal interstitial material (42).

Extrainsular Endocrine Cells

In addition to the endocrine cells of the islets of Langerhans, there are small numbers of individual endocrine cells within the ducts and scattered among the acini (Figure 30.37). These extrainsular endocrine cells are especially abundant during infancy, but they constitute less than 10% of the total pancreatic endocrine cell population in the adult (55). The ductal endocrine cells are most commonly detected in the main and larger interlobular ducts and are rare in the smaller ducts (84,114). Some of them border the lumina and are joined to neighboring ductal cells by tight junctions (115), whereas others are situated between the ductal cells and the basement membrane. They may secrete peptides directly into the pancreatic ducts, accounting for the detection of endocrine peptides in pancreatic juice (115). Specific peptides may be found, especially insulin, somatostatin, and pancreatic polypeptide (114,116). Some of the extrainsular endocrine cells in the larger ducts also

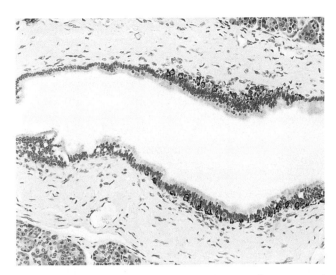

Figure 30.38 The number of ductal endocrine cells is increased in areas showing proliferation (the earliest stage of pancreatic intraepithelial neoplasia, PanIN-1) of the ductal epithelium (*right*).

produce serotonin (116); these cells may be the origin of the extremely rare true carcinoid tumors of the pancreas (117,118). The number of ductal endocrine cells appears to increase in the presence of proliferation of the ductal epithelium (Figure 30.38) (114).

Connective Tissues

In the normal adult pancreas, there is little connective tissue between the lobules and almost none within them. In the neonatal pancreas, mesenchymal tissue comprises nearly 30% of the volume of the gland; it gradually decreases during infancy (97). The acini are surrounded by basement membranes, but very little other collagen is present (Figure 30.39).

Small portal vessels exist that deliver hormonal secretions from the islets directly to the exocrine elements of the gland (76,77,119,120). A complex capillary network surrounds the acini, and accompanying nerve fibers may be found. The acini and ducts are innervated by bundles of unmyelinated nerves that travel through the interlobular connective tissues. In most cases the nerve endings are separated from the acinar or ductal cells by the basement membrane, although in some cases direct contact with the basal cell membrane of acinar cells may be seen (84). Islets are innervated by both sympathetic and parasympathetic fibers; in addition, there are peptidergic fibers from the autonomic ganglia. Some of the periacinar nerves produce neuropeptide Y, whereas vasoactive intestinal polypeptide–containing nerves are found within islets and adjacent to ducts (121). Other peptides found in pancreatic nerves include substance P, cholecystokinin, and calcitonin gene–related peptide (121). Small autonomic

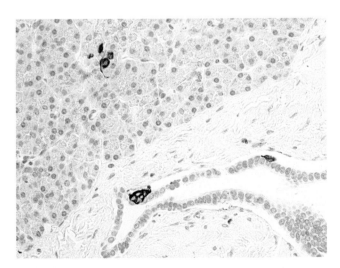

Figure 30.37 Extrainsular endocrine cells within the ducts and between the acini are only detectable with immunohistochemical labeling for chromogranin.

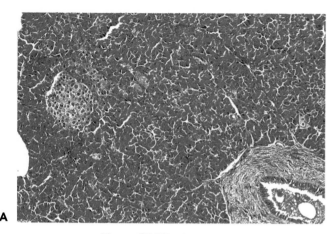
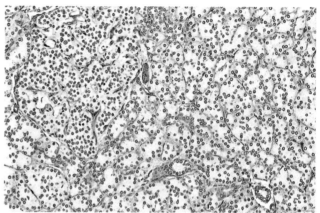

Figure 30.39 Connective tissues are minimal within the pancreas. **A.** Collagen is largely restricted to the tissues surrounding the interlobular ducts, with only thin bands extending into the lobules (trichrome). **B.** Immunohistochemical staining for type IV collagen shows that an extensive network of basement membranes surrounds each acinus and duct and accompanies the capillaries within the islets (*upper left*).

ganglia are located between clusters of acini (Figure 30.40). Paraganglia also may be found occasionally in the peripancreatic tissues. The muscular arteries run in the interlobular connective tissue, away from the centrally located pancreatic ducts. This separation of the ducts and muscular arteries is maintained in chronic pancreatitis, and presence of a gland close to a muscular artery suggests that the gland is malignant (122).

In almost every individual, there are some adipocytes within the pancreas. The proportion of the gland composed of fat varies from 3 to 20% (6). The amount of adipose tissue in the pancreas varies with the nutritional state and the age of the individual, older or overweight individuals having more intrapancreatic fat (123). The portions of the gland derived from the dorsal lobe may have more intraparenchymal fat than those from the ventral lobe (124,125).

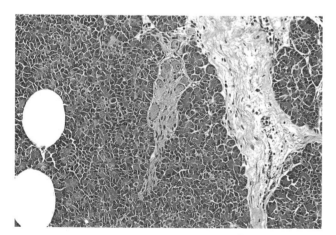

Figure 30.40 Small autonomic ganglia are located within lobules of acinar tissue.

Recently a population of vitamin A–storing fibroblast-like stromal cell has been described (126). These pancreatic "stellate cells" are biologically and morphologically similar to hepatic stellate (or Ito) cells, and activation of these cells appears to play a major role in the production of extracellular matrix proteins during the development of fibrosis in chronic pancreatitis (126). Another recently described stromal cell type is the interstitial cell of Cajal. Pancreatic interstitial cells of Cajal have the same morphological and immunophenotypic properties as do those in the tubular gastrointestinal tract, including immunohistochemical labeling for CD117 (127).

Cytological Features

Normal pancreatic epithelial cells are commonly encountered in cytological preparations such as fine needle aspiration specimens. In aspirates of normal pancreas, acinar cells predominate over other elements. However, most fine needle aspirations are performed to diagnose solid or cystic neoplasms, and any nonneoplastic epithelium in these specimens usually originates from areas of chronic pancreatitis within or adjacent to the neoplasm, where acinar elements are atrophic and ducts remain. Thus, nondiagnostic aspirates of pancreatic adenocarcinoma often contain relatively few acini and moderate amounts of ductal epithelium. Atypia in this ductal epithelium can present a diagnostic pitfall.

Cytologically, acinar cells appear predominantly as cohesive, small grape-like clusters with scattered single cells and occasional stripped nuclei (Figure 30.41) (128,129). The round, regular nuclei are usually central to eccentric and have uniform chromatin and variably prominent or even conspicuous nucleoli. The polygonal cells have abundant granular cytoplasm that stains blue-green with the standard

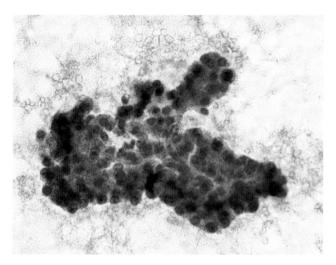

Figure 30.41 Cytology of normal acinar cells. There are grape-like clusters of cohesive cells with basal round nuclei having prominent nucleoli. The eosinophilic zymogen granules are apparent in the apical cytoplasm.

Papanicolaou stain and purple with the Romanowsky's stain. The individual granules may be visible depending on the specific stain. The Romanowsky's stain also reveals scattered small cytoplasmic vacuoles. The architectural arrangement of the cells is key to differentiating benign acinar cells from an acinar neoplasm, the latter generally forming large sheets and clusters as opposed to the small, uniform grape-like clusters of benign acini.

Normal ductal epithelium appears cytologically as large, flat cohesive sheets of epithelium containing round, uniform, evenly spaced nuclei that impart a honeycombed appearance (Figure 30.42) (128,129). The cytoplasm of these cells can best be seen when the epithelium is present in

strips, yielding a "picket fence" arrangement, or in sheets with a sharp luminal edge. Ductal cells have round to oval nuclei with even chromatin and generally small, inconspicuous nucleoli. The dense, nongranular and nonvacuolated cytoplasm stains aqua-blue with the Papanicolaou stain and more indigo-blue to purple with the Romanowsky's stain. Features consistent with a nonneoplastic process on cytology include cohesion and nuclei with uniform size, shape, spacing, and chromatin pattern. Abundant mucinous cytoplasm may be seen in ductal cells with low-grade pancreatic intraepithelial neoplasia (see below), but mucinous ductal epithelium also raises the possibility of a mucinous cystic neoplasm, an intraductal papillary mucinous neoplasm, or even an infiltrating adenocarcinoma.

Islet cells are rarely appreciable in aspirate smears. Islet cells are uniform and polygonal with round nuclei, coarsely clumped chromatin, inconspicuous nucleoli, and pale amphophilic cytoplasm.

MINOR ALTERATIONS

A number of minor alterations may affect various components of the pancreas due to physiologic changes, response to injury, or aging. Some of these changes are so subtle that they may be overlooked, but others may be confused for a neoplastic process. Recognition of these potential diagnostic pitfalls is essential for the accurate interpretation of biopsies and is complicated by the fact that many of these alterations may accompany pancreatic neoplasms.

Acinar Cells

Acinar cell nodules are common incidental findings that consist of circumscribed clusters of acini showing cytoplasmic or nuclear differences from the surrounding acini (130,131). Alternative terms include atypical acinar cell nodule, focal acinar transformation, eosinophilic degeneration, and focal acinar cell dysplasia (13,55,132,133). The last term suggests the lesion may be preneoplastic, but there is no proof of neoplastic alterations in acinar cell nodules in humans, where they are found in nearly half of nontumorous pancreata (134). The lesions are more prevalent in adults, suggesting that they are acquired (132). Although sometimes larger, acinar cell nodules are often similar in size to compact islets, with which they may be confused.

Two types of acinar cell nodules exist (131). The more common is the eosinophilic type, which appears as an abnormally pale, eosinophilic cluster of acini (Figure 30.43A). At high power, the cells are larger than the adjacent normal acinar cells, and the deep basophilia of the basal cytoplasm is lacking. The cytoplasm also may be vacuolated. The nuclei appear normal or hyperchromatic. This change is due to

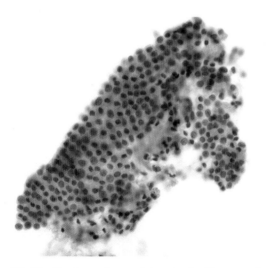

Figure 30.42 Cytology of normal ductal cells. There are sheets of evenly arranged cells with the characteristic honeycombed appearance. The nuclei are round and uniform.

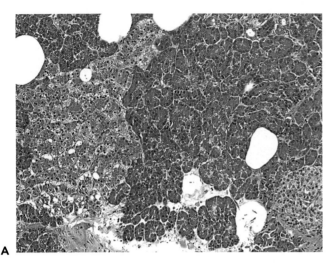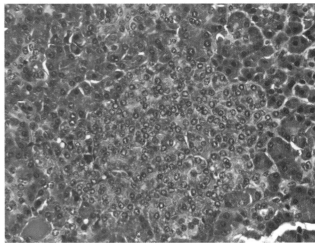

A   B

Figure 30.43 Atypical acinar cell nodules. **A.** The eosinophilic type is more common and consists of a collection of acini showing loss of basophilia in the basal cytoplasm and hyperchromasia of the nuclei. The eosinophilic granules within the apical cytoplasm are maintained. An islet of Langerhans, with which these lesions may be confused, is present at lower right. **B.** The basophilic type of atypical acinar cell nodule exhibits an increased nucleus to cytoplasm ratio with loss of eosinophilic granularity of the apical cytoplasm. Some degree of nuclear atypia is also present.

dilatation of the RER (135) and may be a result of localized hypoxia or other degenerative phenomena. The other less common type of acinar cell nodule, the basophilic type, exhibits a loss of the eosinophilic zymogen granules from the apical cytoplasm, as well as an increased nucleus-to-cytoplasm ratio (Figure 30.43B). Nuclear enlargement, mild atypia, and prominent nucleoli also may be seen. The reason for such localized depletion of zymogen granules is unclear.

Acinar ectasia refers to the dilatation of acinar lumina that may occur during active secretion (1) or due to ductal obstruction (133). Acinar ectasia is also a relatively common finding at autopsy, where it is associated with premortem uremia, septicemia, and dehydration (13,136,137). Acinar ectasia often involves an entire lobular unit. The ectatic acini resemble small ductules, with flattened lining cells, but some of the cells are still recognizable as acinar cells that have lost most of their zymogen granules (Figure 30.44). Centroacinar cells also line the dilated lumina and may proliferate (137). The dilated lumina often contain retained eosinophilic secretions.

Metaplastic changes less commonly involve the acini than the ducts; they include replacement by mucinous cells or squamous cells (138). Proliferating centroacinar cells may appear to replace the acinar cells, especially in the presence of early atrophy (133). The possibility that acinar cells may transform into centroacinar or ductular cells ("acinar to ductal metaplasia") has been suggested, especially in animal models of pancreatic neoplasia (139), but the occurrence of acinar to ductal metaplasia in humans is speculative (140).

Ductal Cells

Many metaplastic changes may affect the pancreatic ducts, including squamous, oncocytic, goblet cell (intestinal), and acinar metaplasia. However, the most common alteration in ductal cells, especially those of the medium-sized and large pancreatic ducts, is the replacement of the cuboidal, nonmucinous epithelium with tall columnar cells containing abundant luminal mucin that is easily appreciable on routinely stained slides (Figure 30.45A), resembling gastric foveolar or pyloric gland cells (141–143). For many years, this alteration was regarded as mucinous

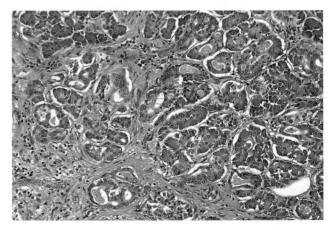

Figure 30.44 In acinar ectasia, the acinar lumina are dilated and filled with eosinophilic secretions. The lining cells have a flattened appearance, often resembling small ductules cells more than acinar cells.

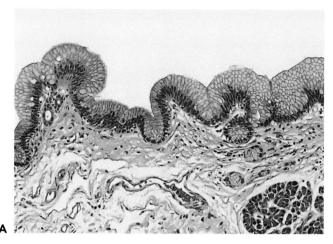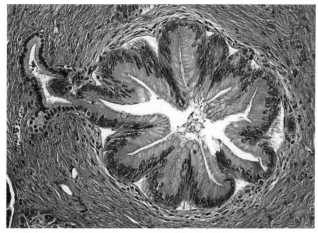

Figure 30.45 Pancreatic intraepithelial neoplasia (PanIN)-1. **A.** In PanIN-1A, the normal cuboidal to low columnar ductal epithelial cells are replaced by tall columnar cells containing abundant apical mucin. The nuclei remain basally located and show minimal pseudostratification. **B.** PanIN-1B has similar cytological features but demonstrates papilla formation. Note the transition to normal ductal epithelium (*left*).

metaplasia (or mucous cell hypertrophy, or pyloric gland metaplasia). The change is present in up to half of nontumorous pancreata (13,16,133,142,144,145) and is usually more prevalent in the head of the gland (144). The ductal epithelium may remain flat, or there may be formation of micropapillae or true papillae with fibrovascular cores (Figure 30.45B). The lesion may involve a single ductal profile or may extend into clusters of ductules adjacent to larger ducts. The latter circumstance results in the appearance of collections of small back-to-back tubules of mucinous cells and has been termed adenomatous hyperplasia (141); it is

particularly associated with areas of chronic pancreatitis (Figure 30.46). With the increasing knowledge of the molecular genetic events that occur in pancreatic ductal adenocarcinomas, it has become increasingly apparent over the past decade that these mucinous changes in the ductal epithelium share some of the genetic abnormalities of invasive carcinomas (such as activating mutations in codon 12 of the *KRAS* oncogene and telomere shortening (146–151)) and that they form the beginning of a spectrum of preinvasive neoplasia that also includes ductal lesions with increased degrees of cytoarchitectural atypia

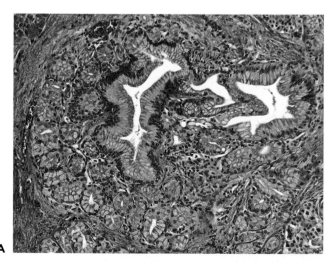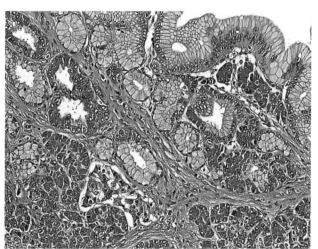

Figure 30.46 **A.** PanIN-1 may involve aggregates of small ductules around larger ducts, resulting in clusters of mucinous glands, a finding previously referred to as adenomatous hyperplasia (Cubilla AL, Fitzgerald PJ. Morphological lesions associated with human primary invasive nonendocrine pancreas cancer. *Cancer Res* 1976;36 (pt 2):2690–2698.). **B.** Because the smallest components of the ductal system are involved, cells with PanIN-1 may abut adjacent acinar cells.

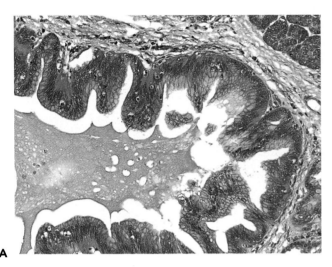
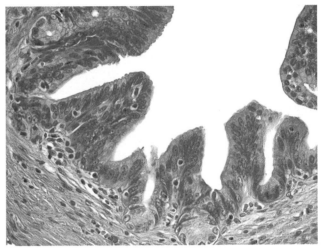

Figure 30.47 **A.** PanIN-2 is characterized by pseudostratified nuclei showing focal loss polarity. **B.** At higher power, the nuclei are enlarged, moderately atypical, and overlapping.

(141,142,145,152–154). Thus, the lesions previously designated as mucinous metaplasia are now regarded to be the earliest stage of pancreatic intraepithelial neoplasia (or PanIN) and are termed PanIN-1 (155,156). Since not all mucinous ductal lesions have detectable oncogene mutations, it is possible that a histologically indistinguishable subset is not truly neoplastic; thus, an alternative designation is PanIN/L-1, the L referring to "lesion". The PanIN-1 lesions with flat epithelium are referred to as PanIN-1A; those with micropapillae or true papillae are referred to as PanIN-1B.

Ductal proliferative lesions with greater degrees of cytoarchitectural atypia are considered higher grades of PanIN. Most PanIN-2 lesions (previously designated as atypical hyperplasia or moderate dysplasia) are micropapillary, but some may be flat; PanIN-2 shows nuclear abnor-

malities, including early loss of polarity with full-thickness pseudostratification as well as nuclear crowding, enlargement, and hyperchromasia (Figure 30.47). Mitoses are found rarely and, when present, are basal and morphologically normal. The PanIN-3 lesions (previously designated carcinoma in situ or severe dysplasia) demonstrate more significant architectural and cytological atypia (Figure 30.48). These lesions are usually papillary or micropapillary, although rarely they may be flat. Cribriforming, budding off of clusters of cells into the lumen, and luminal necrosis may occur. Also, the nuclei show complete loss of polarity and are enlarged, hyperchromatic, and irregular. The nucleus-to-cytoplasm ratio is increased. Nucleoli can be prominent, and mitoses are usually identifiable, including atypical forms (155,156). Higher grade PanINs contain more of the mutations of invasive carcinomas, including

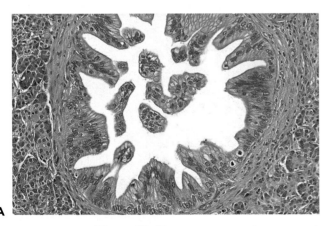
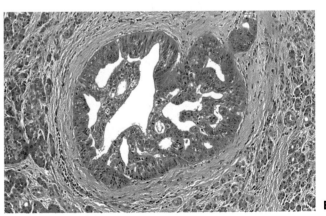

Figure 30.48 **A.** In PanIN-3, there is complete loss of polarity, with budding of disorganized cellular clusters into the ductal lumen. The nuclei are markedly irregular and vary in morphology between adjacent cells. Increased mitoses are present. **B.** In another focus, architectural abnormalities include cribriforming, and there is extreme nuclear atypia.

inactivating mutations in *p16/CDKN2A* (present at the PanIN2 stage), *SMAD4*, *TP53*, and *BRCA2* (all present in PanIN-3). Also, hypermethylation of the *ppENK*, *TSLC1*, and *p16* genes has been demonstrated in PanINs, the prevelance increasing from PanIN-1 through PanIN-3 (146–151). The proliferation rate, as measured by immunohistochemical staining for Ki-67, increases with increasing grades of PanIN (157).

Multiple grades of PanIN tend to coexist within the same pancreas, with gradual transitions from one to the next. All grades of PanINs are associated with invasive ductal adenocarcinomas (92,141,142), and PanIN-3 is usually only found in pancreata also harboring an invasive ductal adenocarcinoma (141,142), although it can occur in a pancreas without invasive carcinoma. Along with the genetic data, these observations support the concept that PanINs progress to carcinoma, but the frequency and time course of progression is unknown. The cells in foci of PanIN produce largely neutral mucins and sialomucins; sulfomucins are less abundant than in normal ductal cells (55). The histochemical and immunohistochemical profile of the mucins in these cells resembles that of the superficial gastric mucosa in some cases or of the pyloric glands in others (93,143). Because there is little morphologic difference between these two mucin-producing cells types, pyloric gland differentiation may not be distinguishable from gastric foveolar differentiation by routine microscopy. The morphological progression from PanIN-1 to PanIN-3 is also accompanied by increasingly abnormal expression of tumor-associated glycoproteins such as CEA, B72.3, and CA125 (92).

Up to one-third of pancreata exhibit squamous metaplasia (16,133,154). Although squamous metaplasia may occur in the larger interlobular and main ducts, it is most common in the intralobular and intercalated ducts, and metaplastic cells may extend into the center of the acini (Figure 30.49). It is exceptional for squamous metaplasia

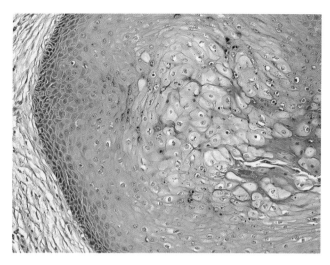

Figure 30.50 Squamous metaplasia of the ducts with keratinization, an uncommon finding.

to exhibit keratinization or a granular cell layer, which occurs most commonly in the setting of advanced chronic pancreatitis (Figure 30.50). For this reason, the terms *multilayered metaplasia* and *transitional metaplasia* have been suggested for this lesion (133). Histologically, the stratified squamous epithelium appears immature, with only minimal flattening of the superficial layers. There may be retention of a luminal mucinous cell layer. In the smaller ducts and ductules, the metaplastic epithelium may fill the lumen, virtually obliterating it. In most instances, squamous metaplasia is associated with chronic pancreatitis; there is no known preneoplastic significance.

Oncocytic changes are common in centroacinar cells, and oncocytic metaplasia may affect intercalated and intralobular ducts as well (85,158,159). The oncocytic cells have abundant granular eosinophilic cytoplasm (reflecting the accumulation of mitochondria), and the nuclei may be

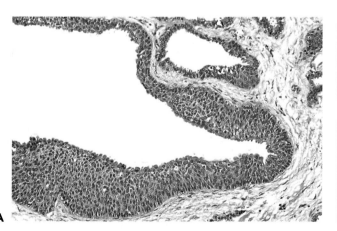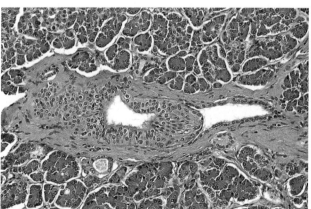

Figure 30.49 Squamous metaplasia of the ducts. **A.** There are multiple layers of immature-appearing squamous cells without keratinization. The process may involve larger ducts. **B.** In this example, there is partial involvement of a small interlobular duct.

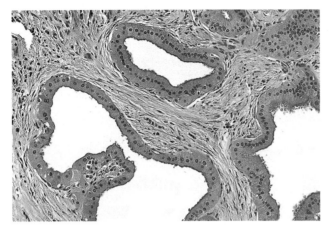

Figure 30.51 Oncocytic changes involving small ducts. In this example, there is associated fibrosing pancreatitis.

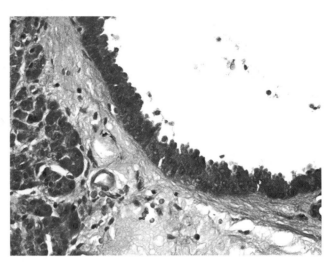

Figure 30.53 This small interlobular duct shows partial acinar metaplasia, with slightly enlarged acinar cells replacing the normal cuboidal ductal epithelium.

enlarged and contain prominent nucleoli (Figure 30.51). Involvement of clusters of small ductules may occur. Like mucinous and squamous metaplasia, oncocytic metaplasia may be associated with chronic inflammatory processes, or it may occur in the absence of other specific abnormalities (16,160). It has been suggested that oncocytic changes in the ducts may be a preneoplastic alteration (161), but molecular genetic abnormalities have yet to be identified in this lesion.

Goblet cells may be found within the ductal epithelium, especially in the main ducts near the ampulla of Vater (1,86). In addition, isolated goblet cells may appear in smaller ducts, presumably as a metaplastic change (Figure 30.52) (133,138). In contrast to PanIN-1, the mucin-containing goblet cells occur singly and are more flask-shaped. Presumably they reflect an intestinal metaplastic phenotype rather than the gastric phenotype of PanIN. Replacement of the ductal epithelium with mucinous cells having all of the histologic and immunohistochemical features of intestinal epithelium has been described (161) but

appears to be rare. True intestinal-type epithelium, with pseudostratified cells having elongate nuclei and expressing MUC2 and CDX2 by immunohistochemistry, is commonly found in intraductal papillary mucinous neoplasms (162,163), which may extend into smaller ducts, but this phenomenon is neoplastic and therefore not regarded as intestinal metaplasia of the ducts.

Sometimes small ducts may demonstrate partial or complete replacement by acinar cells. When this process is very localized, it has been referred to as acinar metaplasia. However, larger neoplasms composed of cystic spaces lined by benign acinar cells, designated as acinar cell cystadenomas, have also been described (164), and the distinction of microscopic examples of this neoplasm (which represent a significant proportion of the reported cases) from acinar metaplasia is somewhat arbitrary. In acinar metaplasia the acinar cells occur singly or in clusters within the ducts, and they exhibit the same appearance as their normally situated counterparts (Figure 30.53). Immunohistochemical labeling for trypsin or chymotrypsin facilitates identification of acinar metaplasia, although the granular apical cytoplasmic staining of true acinar cells must be distinguished from the labeling of deposited intraluminal enzyme secretions on the surface of ductal cells (Figure 30.13).

Another frequent alteration of the ducts is ectasia. Ectatic ducts are generally (but not invariably) found in association with chronic pancreatitis in older patients (13,16,165), often due to ductal obstruction. The ectatic ducts range up to several millimeters in size and occasionally are recognizable grossly. Dilatation of the main pancreatic duct to more than 4 mm is found in 16% of patients at autopsy (13). Because ectatic ducts are often tortuous and the dilatation may be localized, they may appear as single or multiple small cysts (retention cysts) in cross section (Figure 30.54A). Careful study of serial sections shows the

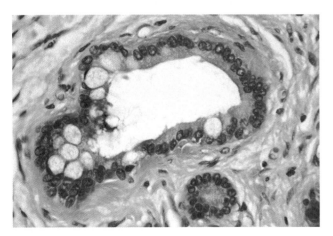

Figure 30.52 Goblet cell metaplasia involving a small duct. Flask-shaped goblet cells are distinct from the mucinous columnar cells of low grade PanIN.

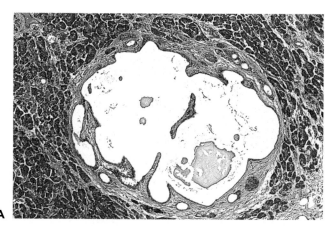 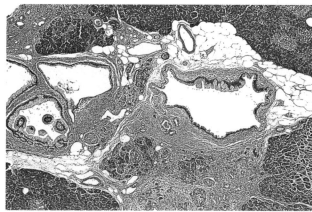

A B

Figure 30.54 Duct ectasia. The dilated ducts may be lined by a flattened cuboidal epithelium resembling normal ductal epithelium (**A**), or there may be involvement by PanIN (**B**). In the latter circumstance, the lesion merges morphologically with intraductal papillary-mucinous neoplasm.

continuity with the ductal system. Retention cysts are usually grossly evident and may reach several centimeters in diameter. The lining epithelium may harbor PanIN, usually PanIN-1 but sometimes higher grade lesions as well (Figure 30.54B). Retention cysts with PanIN may be difficult to distinguish from intraductal papillary mucinous neoplasms (IPMNs) (166–170), and attempts have been made to reach a consensus on diagnostic criteria (156). In general, multicystic lesions with micropapillae or true papillae are regarded as IPMNs, whereas solitary cysts with flat epithelium represent retention cysts with PanIN.

Islet Cells

Islet hyperplasia is defined as an absolute increase in the size or number of islets relative to the normal islet volume at a given age. Individual compact islets larger than 250 μm in diameter are regarded to be hyperplastic (171). However, making an assessment that there is an increase in the total volume of islet tissue in the pancreas is difficult. There are a number of conditions, most associated with pancreatic atrophy, that can result in the appearance of increased numbers of islets when in fact the islet volume is not increased but rather the volume of exocrine elements has decreased (see below). Plus, the density of islets varies in different regions of the pancreas. Thus, some objective assessment of islet volume must be made for a diagnosis of islet hyperplasia, rather than just a casual observation of "numerous" islets. Conditions associated with islet hyperplasia in infancy include Beckwith-Wiedemann syndrome, maternal diabetes, erythroblastosis fetalis, and hyperinsulinemic hypoglycemia (55); cases have also been described in adults with hyperinsulinism (172). Islet hyperplasia may occur either by proliferation of islet cells or by neoformation of islet cells from uncommitted progenitors (42). The distribution of the different peptide cell types is usually main-

tained, although there may be a relative increase in the number of β cells, some of which may show hypertrophy.

Nesidioblastosis is a descriptor of the morphologic findings accompanying functional disorders of β cells associated with hyperinsulinemic hypoglycemia in the absence of an insulinoma (173–176). This condition generally occurs in neonates and infants, where it is known as persistent neonatal hyperinsulinemic hypoglycemia (PNHH); a similar condition occurs rarely in adults. Morphologic abnormalities include hypertrophic β cells within the islets; close association of islet cells with small pancreatic ducts (ductuloinsular complexes), particularly in neonates; and abnormal aggregation of islets. Both focal and diffuse types are described (173). In focal nesidioblastosis, there is a localized nodular lesion that may resemble an insulinoma, but more often there is simply an aggregate of ill-formed islet-like clusters associated with small ductules (Figure 30.55).

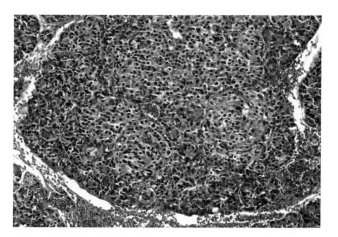

Figure 30.55 The pancreas from an infant with persistent neonatal hyperinsulinemic hypoglycemia shows the focal form of nesidioblastosis. There is localized aggregation of islets separated by thin bands of acini.

Some of the nuclei within the lesion are enlarged. The islets in the remaining pancreas are normal. The diffuse form of nesidioblastosis shows islet abnormalities throughout the gland without discrete localized aggregation of islets. The principal finding is the presence of enlarged, hyperchromatic β-cell nuclei. The size of nuclei in β cells varies somewhat in normal neonates; but, in nesidioblastosis, there is a 40% increase in nuclear volume compared with age-matched controls. By immunohistochemistry, the islets in both focal and diffuse types of nesidioblastosis retain their normal complements of peptide cell types. Genetically, PNHH is associated with a number of different mutations in genes such as *ABCC8* and *KCNJ11* that encode the ATP-sensitive potassium channel (K_{ATP}) in the cell membrane of β cells, demonstrating that this disorder clearly has a functional basis and does not simply reflect an increase in β-cell mass (177–180).

The apparent increase in number of islets that occurs secondary to exocrine atrophy has been termed islet aggregation and is not a result of hyperplasia. With the progressive atrophy that occurs in chronic pancreatitis, eventually most of the acini and many of the ducts disappear, leaving only residual islets embedded in fibrous or adipose tissue (Figure 30.56) (140). This phenomenon may be widespread in patients with significant chronic pancreatitis, or it may only involve one lobule of the gland. In addition to the clustering of islets, some degree of islet cell proliferation may occur (181); however, islet aggregation should be distinguished from true islet cell hyperplasia. The clustering of islets in regions of severe atrophy may resemble a solid tumorlike process with a nesting pattern, reminiscent of a pancreatic endocrine neoplasm (Figure 30.57). Individual islets may be found in the peripancreatic adipose tissue. The appearance of infil-

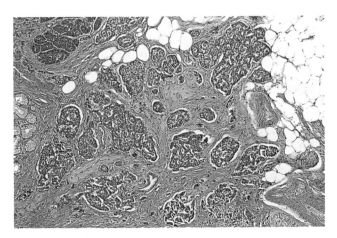

Figure 30.57 When advanced atrophy of exocrine elements occurs, aggregation of the remaining endocrine elements may simulate a neoplasm. The nests of cells may be poorly circumscribed and separated by bands of fibrous tissue, with extension into peripancreatic adipose tissue.

trative growth is even more marked when the process involves the regions of the head of the pancreas containing the diffuse islets; these islets lack the insular arrangement of the compact islets from the tail, appearing as small clusters, trabeculae, and individual cells when the exocrine elements undergo atrophy (Figure 30.58). In contrast to most pancreatic endocrine neoplasms, the border of foci of islet aggregation is ill defined. The surrounding pancreas often exhibits areas of pancreatitis that are less advanced, with incomplete acinar atrophy. In problematic cases, immunohistochemical labeling for the specific peptides may be helpful. In islet aggregation, the normal peptide cell types are present, in roughly normal numbers and distribution, although the relative proportions of α and PP cells may be increased (106,181). Although more than one peptide may be expressed in endocrine neo-

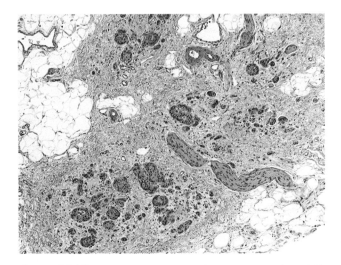

Figure 30.56 Islet aggregation involving compact islets. With extreme atrophy, there is complete loss of exocrine elements, leaving the clustered islets embedded in fibrous stroma.

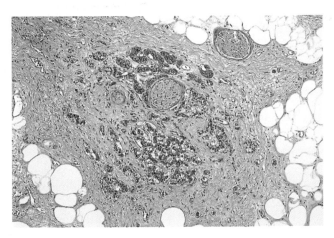

Figure 30.58 Exocrine atrophy in areas containing diffuse-type islets results in a pseudoinfiltrative pattern of individual cells and trabeculae.

plasms, it is exceptional for all of the normal peptides to be found in normal numbers, and there may be expression of peptides not found in normal islets (vasoactive intestinal polypeptide or gastrin). Bear in mind that the diffuse islets have a different normal peptide cell constitution (abundance of PP cells) from that of the compact islets (Figure 30.59). Another pseudoneoplastic property of islet cells in chronic pancreatitis is perineural invasion (Figure 30.60). Small clusters of islet cells may surround nerves, simulating the perineural invasion that is so common in pancreatic ductal adenocarcinoma. Fortunately, benign glands only exceptionally rarely exhibit perineural invasion. Immunohistochemical labeling for chromogranin may be used to distinguish benign perineural invasion by islet cells from adenocarcinoma.

The appearance of dilated blood-filled spaces within the islets (Figure 30.61) has been referred to as peliosis insulis. Although reported in a pancreas from a patient with

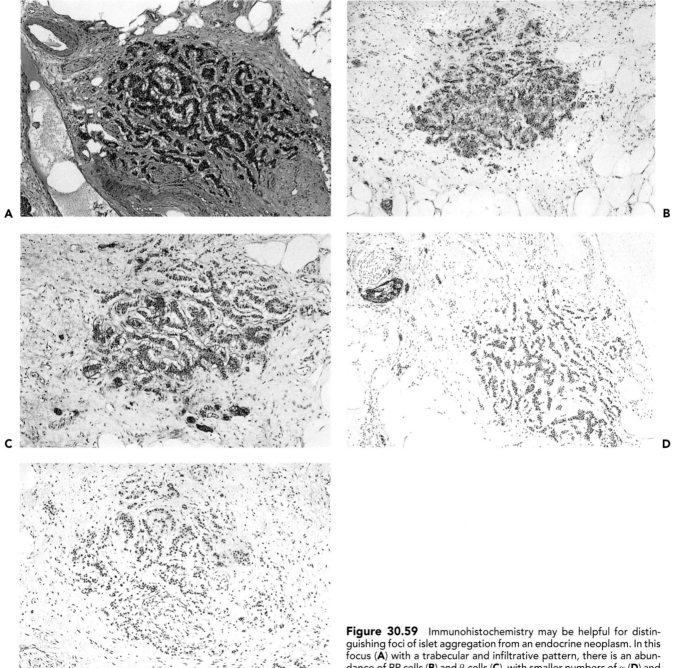

Figure 30.59 Immunohistochemistry may be helpful for distinguishing foci of islet aggregation from an endocrine neoplasm. In this focus (**A**) with a trabecular and infiltrative pattern, there is an abundance of PP cells (**B**) and β cells (**C**), with smaller numbers of α (**D**) and δ (**E**) cells, a composition typical of nonneoplastic diffuse type islets.

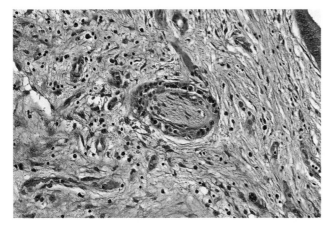

Figure 30.60 Perineural invasion by islet cells in chronic pancreatitis may simulate carcinoma.

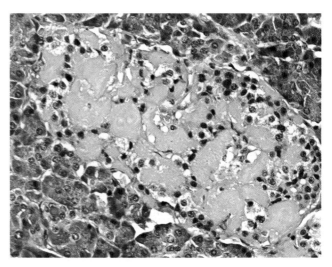

Figure 30.62 Amyloid-like hyalinization of the perivascular tissue may be seen in the islets, especially in older patients with type II diabetes. The surrounding acinar tissue is not fibrotic.

multiple endocrine neoplasia-I (MEN-I) and harboring multiple pancreatic endocrine neoplasms (182), peliosis insulis usually occurs in otherwise normal pancreata. It is of unclear etiology and significance. The blood-filled spaces are not observed to be lined by endothelium ultrastructurally.

Perivascular deposition of amyloid or amyloid-like material may be seen in islets of older individuals (Figure 30.62), especially in association with non–insulin-dependent (type II) diabetes mellitus (183). Insular amyloid is biochemically different from systemic amyloid, and there is no association between insular amyloidosis and systemic amyloidosis. In insular amyloidosis, the hyalinized stroma is limited to the islets. In patients with generalized fibrosis of the pancreatic parenchyma due to chronic pancreatitis or other causes, the islets also may be involved (insular fibrosis); however, the hyalinized stroma in these cases has no ultrastructural features of amyloid (183).

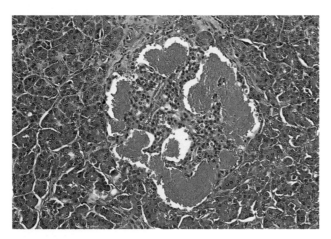

Figure 30.61 The appearance of dilated, blood-filled spaces within the islets has been called peliosis insulis. It is probably of no clinical significance.

Chronic Pancreatitis, Atrophy, and Fibrosis

Several different types of chronic pancreatitis exist, with etiologies including chronic alcoholism, ductal obstruction, autoimmune disorders, malnutrition, and genetic predisposition (184–190). Although the distribution of the disease within the pancreas varies with the different types, the histologic features of most types (except for autoimmune pancreatitis) are similar, especially at the end stages when fibrosis and atrophy are prominent (16). In fact, microscopic foci of fibrosis and atrophy (histologic chronic pancreatitis) are common incidental findings in pancreatic resection specimens or at autopsy, and the pathologic findings often reported as "focal chronic pancreatitis" are only loosely related to the clinical disease of chronic pancreatitis.

When chronic pancreatitis is localized, it may mimic pancreatic carcinoma clinically, radiographically, and grossly, and the resultant histological patterns also frequently simulate neoplasia. Early in the process, the fibrosis is largely around the periphery of the lobules, there is minimal acinar atrophy, and chronic inflammatory cells are evident (Figure 30.63A). The glands may be enlarged. However, as chronic pancreatitis progresses, the fibrosis involves the entire lobule, with marked distortion of the architecture. There is progressive exocrine atrophy, with eventual complete loss of acinar elements. The ducts become ectatic and irregularly shaped (Figure 30.63B). Ultimately, even the ducts are lost, leaving only the islets. In experimental pancreatitis induced by duct ligation, acinar atrophy occurs by necrosis and apoptosis (191,192), resulting in closely packed lobules of ductular structures. Small ductules and islets remaining after acinar atrophy become encircled and distorted by the fibrous tissue

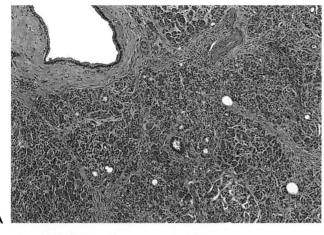

A

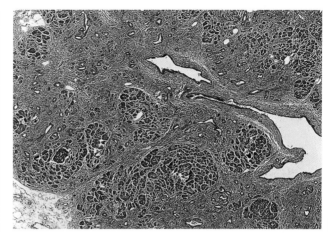

B

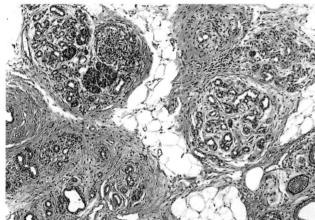

C

Figure 30.63 Progressive changes in chronic pancreatitis. **A.** In the early stages, the fibrosis is largely limited to the periductal and septal areas of the gland. The lobules show prominence of ductules. There are scattered aggregates of chronic inflammatory cells. **B.** As the pancreatitis progresses, the amount of fibrosis is increased, entrapping small lobules of residual acinar tissue. The ducts are ectatic. **C.** In the terminal stages, most of the acinar tissue is atrophic, leaving lobular aggregates of small ductules and islets within a fibrotic and fatty stroma.

(Figure 30.63C), often acquiring a pseudoinfiltrative appearance. Ductuloinsular complexes may be found (Figure 30.64). As the gland is replaced by fibrous tissue, it decreases in size and acquires a woody consistency. Inflammatory cells are sparse at this stage and may be aggregated

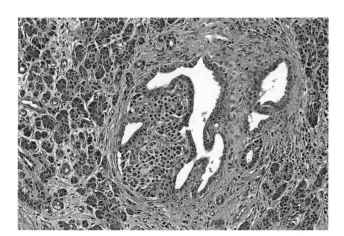

Figure 30.64 A ductuloinsular complex in an adult with mild chronic pancreatitis. Small ductules are surrounded by nests of endocrine cells, a finding that does not necessarily reflect true islet cell hyperplasia.

around small nerves (133). Duct ectasia, calcification, and intraductal calculi may occur (193), especially in pancreatitis of alcoholic etiology. The ducts may show PanIN, although the presence of intraepithelial neoplasia is not necessarily related to the chronic pancreatitis (142); and, other than the congenital type, chronic pancreatitis per se is only associated with a small increased risk for pancreatic cancer (194). It is possible that the chronic pancreatitis commonly accompanying ductal adenocarcinoma is secondary to ductal obstruction by the tumor rather than representing a preexisting condition.

The distinction of chronic pancreatitis from infiltrating ductal adenocarcinoma on the basis of biopsies can be very challenging. The distorted ducts and ductules in areas of fibrosis closely resemble the pattern of ductal adenocarcinoma, and the fibrotic stroma may simulate the desmoplastic stroma often accompanying carcinoma. Features that support the interpretation of chronic pancreatitis include a retention of the lobular arrangement of the small collections of ductules, normal location of the glands, and uniformity of nuclear morphology from one cell to the next (Figures 30.65A–C). Features that conversely favor the diagnosis of carcinoma include haphazardly arranged individual angulated glands infiltrating the

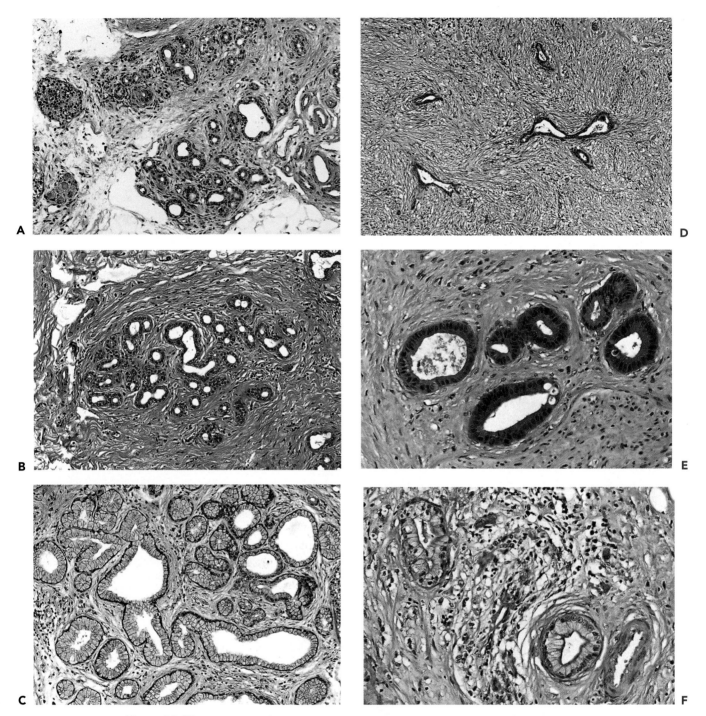

Figure 30.65 Comparison of ductules in atrophic chronic pancreatitis with well-differentiated ductal adenocarcinoma. **A.** In chronic pancreatitis, there is preservation of the lobular arrangement of small ductules, with larger branching ductules surrounded by collections of smaller tubular glands. Some residual islets of Langerhans are also present. **B.** At higher power, the cells are generally uniform, with round nuclei having a similar cytologic appearance from cell to cell. **C.** In areas showing mucinous metaplasia, there may not be as obvious a lobular arrangement. However, the glands retain a benign cytologic appearance and have uniformly basally oriented nuclei. **D.** In infiltrating adenocarcinoma, the lobular arrangement of the glands is lost. There is a haphazard configuration of angulated glands within a desmoplastic stroma. **E.** In some instances, there may not be significant stromal desmoplasia, and the glands may retain rounded contours. However, there is variability in cytologic appearance from one cell to the next, with occasional macronucleoli, loss of polarity, and mitotic figures. **F.** Some individual glands of infiltrating carcinoma may be almost impossible to distinguish from benign ductules. This remarkably well-differentiated gland (*lower right*) contrasts with an adjacent gland showing marked loss of nuclear polarity. The abnormal location of the gland adjacent to a muscular artery is another clue that it is malignant.

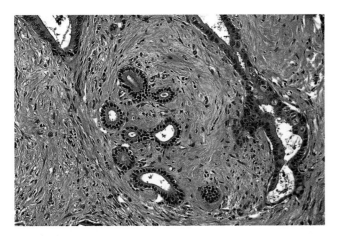

Figure 30.66 It is helpful to identify two populations of cells in specimens harboring an infiltrating adenocarcinoma. In this example, a lobular collection of benign ductules contrasts with irregularly shaped glands of adenocarcinoma.

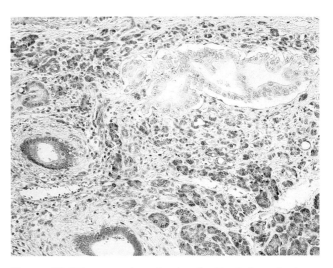

Figure 30.67 Immunohistochemisty for Dpc4 shows both nuclear and cytoplasmic labeling in normal acini and ducts, whereas the invasive carcinoma has complete absence of labeling.

stroma, glands in abnormal locations [adjacent to muscular arteries (122), in the perineurium, within vessels, or immediately apposed to adipocytes], significant cytological abnormalities (variation in shape and size of nuclei from one cell to the next, macronucleoli, loss of nuclear polarity), and individual cells or small cell clusters in the stroma (Figures 30.65D–F, 30.66). It is helpful when two cytologically distinct populations of cells are found in the biopsy, since some of nuclear features of well-differentiated carcinomas are very subtle unless compared with a second population of clearly benign glands. Unfortunately, biopsy samples of the pancreas are frequently small, and it is uncommon for all of the characteristic features to be present. Even if carcinoma is present, it may only be represented by two or three glands. Furthermore, needle biopsy samples are sometimes subjected to frozen section examination, which may introduce artifacts complicating the interpretation. Even for the experienced observer, there may be cases having rare atypical glands that cannot be confidently diagnosed as benign or malignant. Performance of serial sections sometimes reveals additional diagnostic features. Immunohistochemistry also can be useful to document some of the abnormalities characteristic of carcinoma. Most benign glands do not express CEA, B72.3, CA125, or p53 at immunohistochemically detectable levels (92), and they will all show normal intact labeling for the Dpc4 protein. By contrast, most pancreatic cancers express CEA, 75% label for B72.3, 50 to 75% for p53, 45% for CA125, and 55% show complete loss of Dpc4 expression (Figure 30.67) (195). Expression of mesothelin also supports a diagnosis of carcinoma (196).

Atrophy of pancreatic parenchyma due to long-standing ductal obstruction is often associated with infiltration by adipose tissue. Only rare islets may be found between lobules of fat in extreme cases (Figure 30.68). A primary form of fatty infiltration is Shwachman syndrome, an extremely rare autosomal recessive syndrome affecting the pancreas, bone marrow, and skeleton (197). An enlarged gland may result, but the amount of parenchymal tissue is reduced and exocrine insufficiency is present (16). The term *lipomatosis* has been applied to pancreata containing more than 25% adipose tissue (Figure 30.69). The distribution of the adipose tissue is generally not uniform. Lipomatosis is usually associated with parenchymal atrophy and is more common in older individuals (13). Other associations include adult-onset diabetes and generalized atherosclerosis, conditions that are also more prevalent in the elderly. Pancreatic lipomatosis is not associated with generalized obesity (13).

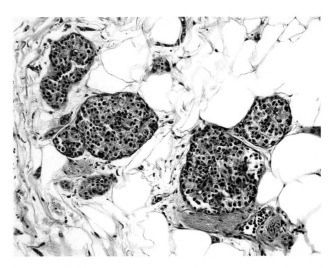

Figure 30.68 With extreme atrophy, the residual islets of Langerhans may be completely surrounded by adipose tissue.

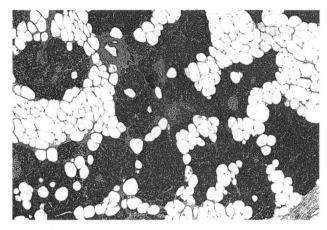

Figure 30.69 In pancreatic lipomatosis, adipose tissue comprises more than 25% of the volume of the gland. As in this case, the remaining parenchyma may not necessarily show changes of atrophic chronic pancreatitis.

REFERENCES

1. Fawcett DW. *Bloom and Fawcett: A Textbook of Histology.* 12th ed. New York: Chapman & Hall; 1994.
2. Moore KL. *Clinically Oriented Anatomy.* Baltimore: Williams & Wilkins; 1980.
3. Lack EE. *Pathology of the Pancreas, Gallbladder, Extrahepatic Biliary Tract, and Ampullary Region.* New York: Oxford University Press; 2003.
4. Skandalakis LJ, Rowe JS Jr, Gray SW, Skandalakis JE. Surgical embryology and anatomy of the pancreas. *Surg Clin North Am* 1993;73:661–697.
5. Pansky B. Anatomy of the pancreas. Emphasis on blood supply and lymphatic drainage. *Int J Pancreatol* 1990;7:101–108.
6. Bockman DE. Anatomy of the pancreas. In: Go VL, Brooks FP, DiMagno EP, Gardner JD, Lebenthal E, Scheele GA, eds. *The Exocrine Pancreas: Biology, Pathobiology and Diseases.* New York: Raven Press; 1986:1–7.
7. Ibukuro K. Vascular anatomy of the pancreas and clinical applications. *Int J Gastrointest Cancer* 2001;30:87–104.
8. Navas V, O'Morchoe PJ, O'Morchoe CC. Lymphatic system of the rat pancreas. *Lymphology* 1995;28:4–20.
9. Cubilla AL, Fortner J, Fitzgerald PJ. Lymph node involvement in carcinoma of the head of the pancreas area. *Cancer* 1978;41:880–887.
10. Deki H, Sato T. An anatomic study of the peripancreatic lymphatics. *Surg Radiol Anat* 1988;10:121–135.
11. Evans BP, Ochsner A. The gross anatomy of the lymphatics of the human pancreas. *Surgery* 1954;36:177–191.
12. Nagakawa T, Kobayashi H, Ueno K, et al. The pattern of lymph node involvement in carcinoma of the head of the pancreas. A histologic study of the surgical findings in patients undergoing extensive nodal dissections. *Int J Pancreatol* 1993;13:15–22.
13. Stamm BH. Incidence and diagnostic significance of minor pathologic changes in the adult pancreas at autopsy: a systematic study of 112 autopsies in patients without known pancreatic disease. *Hum Pathol* 1984;15:677–683.
14. Heitz PU, Beglinger C, Gyr K. Anatomy and physiology of the exocrine pancreas. In: Kloeppel G, Heitz PU, eds. *Pancreatic Pathology.* New York: Churchill-Livingstone; 1984:3–21.
15. Birnstingl M. A study of pancreaticography. *Br J Surg* 1959;47:128–139.
16. Cubilla AL, Fitzgerald PJ. Tumors of the exocrine pancreas. In: Hartmann WH, Sobin LH, eds. *Atlas of Tumor Pathology.* 2nd series, fascicle 19. Washington, DC: Armed Forces Institute of Pathology; 1984.
17. Kozu T, Suda K, Toki F. Pancreatic development and anatomical variation. *Gastrointest Endosc Clin N Am* 1995;5:1–30.
18. Baggenstoss AH. Major duodenal papilla. Variations of pathologic interest and lesions of mucosa. *Arch Pathol* 1938;26:853–868.
19. DiMagno EP, Shorter RG, Taylor WF, Go VL. Relationships between pancreaticobiliary ductal anatomy and pancreatic ductal and parenchymal histology. *Cancer* 1982;49:361–368.
20. Flati G, Flati D, Porowska B, Ventura T, Catarci M, Carboni M. Surgical anatomy of the papilla of Vater and biliopancreatic ducts. *Am Surg* 1994;60:712–718.
21. Frierson HF Jr. The gross anatomy and histology of the gallbladder, extrahepatic bile ducts, Vaterian system, and minor papilla. *Am J Surg Pathol* 1989;13:146–162.
22. Corliss CE. *Patten's Human Embryology: Elements of Clinical Development.* New York: McGraw-Hill; 1976.
23. Lebenthal E, Lev R, Lee PC. Prenatal and postnatal development of the human exocrine pancreas. In: Go VL, Brooks FP, DiMagno EP, Garder, Lebenthal E, Scheele GA, eds. *The Exocrine Pancreas: Biology, Pathobiology, and Diseases.* New York: Raven Press; 1986:33–43.
24. Edlund H. Pancreas: how to get there from the gut? *Curr Opin Cell Biol* 1999;11:663–668.
25. Ahlgren U, Jonsson J, Edlund H. The morphogenesis of the pancreatic mesenchyme is uncoupled from that of the pancreatic epithelium in IPF1/PDX1-deficient mice. *Development* 1996;122:1409–1416.
26. Song SY, Gannon M, Washington MK, et al. Expansion of Pdx1-expressing pancreatic epithelium and islet neogenesis in transgenic mice overexpressing transforming growth factor alpha. *Gastroenterology* 1999;117:1416–1426.
27. Gradwohl G, Dierich A, LeMeur M, Guillemot F. Neurogenin3 is required for the development of the four endocrine cell lineages of the pancreas. *Proc Natl Acad Sci U S A* 2000;97:1607–1611.
28. Murtaugh LC, Melton DA. Genes, signals, and lineages in pancreas development. *Annu Rev Cell Dev Biol* 2003;19:71–89.
29. Naya FJ, Huang HP, Qiu Y, et al. Diabetes, defective pancreatic morphogenesis, and abnormal enteroendocrine differentiation in BETA2/neuroD-deficient mice. *Genes Dev* 1997;11:2323–2334.
30. Schwitzgebel VM, Scheel DW, Conners JR, et al. Expression of neurogenin3 reveals an islet cell precursor population in the pancreas. *Development* 2000;127:3533–3542.
31. Krapp A, Knofler M, Ledermann B, et al. The bHLH protein PTF1-p48 is essential for the formation of the exocrine and the correct spatial organization of the endocrine pancreas. *Genes Dev* 1998;12:3752–3763.
32. Murtaugh LC, Stanger BZ, Kwan KM, Melton DA. Notch signaling controls multiple steps of pancreatic differentiation. *Proc Natl Acad Sci U S A* 2003;100:14920–14925.
33. Hebrok M. Hedgehog signaling in pancreas development. *Mech Dev* 2003;120:45–57.
34. Conklin JL. Cytogenesis of the human fetal pancreas. *Am J Anat* 1962;111:181–193.
35. Chong JM, Fukayama M, Shiozawa Y, et al. Fibrillary inclusions in neoplastic and fetal acinar cells of the pancreas. *Virchows Arch* 1996;428:261–266.
36. Laitio M, Lev R, Orlic D. The developing human fetal pancreas: an ultrastructural and histochemical study with special reference to exocrine cells. *J Anat* 1974;117(pt 3):619–634.
37. Hassan MO, Gogate PA. Malignant mixed exocrine-endocrine tumor of the pancreas with unusual intracytoplasmic inclusions. *Ultrastruct Pathol* 1993;17:483–493.
38. Klimstra DS, Heffess CS, Oertel JE, Rosai J. Acinar cell carcinoma of the pancreas. A clinicopathologic study of 28 cases. *Am J Surg Pathol* 1992;16:815–837.
39. Klimstra DS, Rosai J, Heffess CS. Mixed acinar-endocrine carcinomas of the pancreas. *Am J Surg Pathol* 1994;18:765–778.
40. Klimstra DS, Wenig BM, Adair CF, Heffess CS. Pancreatoblastoma. A clinicopathologic study and review of the literature. *Am J Surg Pathol* 1995;19:1371–1389.
41. Tucker JA, Shelburne JD, Benning TL, Yacoub L, Federman M. Filamentous inclusions in acinar cell carcinoma of the pancreas. *Ultrastruct Pathol* 1994;18:279–286.
42. Kloppel G, Lenzen S. Anatomy and physiology of the endocrine pancreas. In: Kloppel G, Heitz PU, eds. *Pancreatic Pathology.* New York: Churchill-Livingstone; 1984:133–153.

43. Robb P. The development of the islets of Langerhans in the human foetus. *Q J Exp Physiol Cogn Med Sci* 1961;46:335–343.

44. Clark A, Grant AM. Quantitative morphology of endocrine cells in human fetal pancreas. *Diabetologia* 1983;25:31–35.

45. Grasso S, Palumbo G, Fallucca F, Lanzafame S, Indelicato B, Sanfilippo S. The development and function of the endocrine pancreas of fetuses and infants born to normal and diabetic mothers. *Acta Endocrinol Suppl (Copenh)* 1986;277:130–135.

46. Albores-Saavedra J, Gould EW, Angeles-Angeles A, Henson DE. Cystic tumors of the pancreas. *Pathol Annu* 1990;25(pt 2):19–50.

47. Compagno J, Oertel JE. Mucinous cystic neoplasms of the pancreas with overt and latent malignancy (cystadenocarcinoma and cystadenoma). A clinicopathologic study of 41 cases. *Am J Clin Pathol* 1978;69:573–580.

48. Stoffers DA, Zinkin NT, Stanojevic V, Clarke WL, Habener JF. Pancreatic agenesis attributable to a single nucleotide deletion in the human IPF1 gene coding sequence. *Nat Genet* 1997;15:106–110.

49. Kiernan PD, ReMine SG, Kiernan PC, ReMine WH. Annular pancreas: May Clinic experience from 1957 to 1976 with review of the literature. *Arch Surg* 1980;115:46–50.

50. Lloyd-Jones W, Mountain JC, Warren KW. Annular pancreas in the adult. *Ann Surg* 1972;176:163–170.

51. Newman BM, Lebenthal E. Congenital abnormalities of the exocrine pancreas. In: Go VL, Brooks FP, DiMagno EP, Gardner JD, Lebenthal E, Scheele GA, eds. *The Exocrine Pancreas: Biology, Pathobiology, and Diseases.* New York: Raven Press; 1986:773–782.

52. England RE, Newcomer MK, Leung JW, et al. Case report: annular pancreas divisum—a report of two cases and review of the literature. *Br J Radiol* 1995;68:324–328.

53. Ravitch MM, Woods AC Jr. Annular pancreas. *Ann Surg* 1950;132:1116–1127.

54. Dowsett JF, Rode J, Russell RC. Annular pancreas: a clinical, endoscopic, and immunohistochemical study. *Gut* 1989;30:130–135.

55. Solcia E, Capella C, Kloppel G. Tumors of the pancreas. In: Rosai J, Sobin LH, eds. *Atlas of Tumor Pathology.* 3rd series, fascicle 20. Washington, DC: Armed Forces Institute of Pathology; 1996.

56. Dawson W, Langman J. An anatomical-radiological study on the pancreatic duct pattern in man. *Anat Rec* 1961;139:59–68.

57. Cotton PB. Pancreas divisum. *Pancreas* 1988;3:245–247.

58. Stern CD. A historical perspective on the discovery of the accessory duct of the pancreas, the ampulla "of Vater" and pancreas divisum. *Gut* 1986;27:203–212.

59. Leese T, Chiche L, Bismuth H. Pancreatitis caused by congenital anomalies of the pancreatic ducts. *Surgery* 1989;105(pt 1):125–130.

60. Kimura K, Ohto M, Saisho H, et al. Association of gallbladder carcinoma and anomalous pancreaticobiliary ductal union. *Gastroenterology* 1985;89:1258–1265.

61. Kinoshita H, Nagata E, Hirohashi K, Sakai K, Kobayashi Y. Carcinoma of the gallbladder with an anomalous connection between the choledochus and the pancreatic duct. Report of 10 cases and review of the literature in Japan. *Cancer* 1984;54:762–769.

62. Krishnamurty VS, Rajendran S, Korsten MA. Bifid pancreas. An unusual anomaly associated with acute pancreatitis. *Int J Pancreatol* 1994;16:179–181.

63. Pang LC. Pancreatic heterotopia: a reappraisal and clinicopathologic analysis of 32 cases. *South Med J* 1988;81:1264–1275.

64. Barbosa J, Dockerty MB, Waugh JM. Pancreatic heterotropia: surgical cases. *Proc Mayo Clin* 1946;21:246–255.

65. Lai EC, Tompkins RK. Heterotopic pancreas. Review of a 26 year experience. *Am J Surg* 1986;151:697–700.

66. Dolan RV, ReMine WH, Dockerty MB. The fate of heterotopic pancreatic tissue. A study of 212 cases. *Arch Surg* 1974;109:762–765.

67. Laughlin EH, Keown ME, Jackson JE. Heterotopic pancreas obstructing the ampulla of Vater. *Arch Surg* 1983;118:979–980.

68. Tsunoda T, Eto T, Yamada M, et al. Heterotopic pancreas: a rare cause of bile duct dilatation—report of a case and review of the literature. *Jpn J Surg* 1990;20:217–220.

69. Seifert G. Congenital anomalies. In: Kloppel G, Heitz PU, eds. *Pancreatic Pathology.* New York: Churchill-Livingstone; 1984:22–26.

70. Goldfarb WB, Bennett D, Monafo W. Carcinoma in heterotopic gastric pancreas. *Ann Surg* 1963;158:56–58.

71. Persson GE, Boiesen PT. Cancer of aberrant pancreas in jejunum. Case report. *Acta Chir Scand* 1988;154:599–601.

72. Tanimura A, Yamamoto H, Shibata H, Sano E. Carcinoma in heterotopic gastric pancreas. *Acta Pathol Jpn* 1979;29:251–257.

73. Landry ML, Sarma DP. Accessory spleen in the head of the pancreas. *Hum Pathol* 1989;20:497.

74. Albores-Saavedra J. The pseudometastasis. *Patologia (Mex)* 1994;32:63–71.

75. Akao S, Bockman DE, Lechene de la Porte P, Sarles H. Three-dimensional pattern of ductuloacinar associations in normal and pathological human pancreas. *Gastroenterology* 1986;90:661–668.

76. Henderson JR, Daniel PM, Fraser PA. The pancreas as a single organ: the influence of the endocrine upon the exocrine part of the gland. *Gut* 1981;22:158–167.

77. Williams JA, Goldfine ID. The insulin-acinar relationship. In: Go VL, Brooks FP, DiMagno EP, Gardner JD, Lebenthal E, Scheele GA, eds. *The Exocrine Pancreas: Biology, Pathobiology, and Diseases.* New York: Raven Press; 1986:347–360.

78. Hoorens A, Lemoine NR, McLellan E, et al. Pancreatic acinar cell carcinoma. An analysis of cell lineage markers, p53 expression, and Ki-ras mutation. *Am J Pathol* 1993;143:685–698.

79. Bendayan M, Roth J, Perrelet A, Orci L. Quantitative immunocytochemical localization of pancreatic secretory proteins in subcellular compartments of the rat acinar cell. *J Histochem Cytochem* 1980;28:149–160.

80. Kraehenbuhl JP, Racine L, Jamieson JD. Immunocytochemical localization of secretory proteins in bovine pancreatic exocrine cells. *J Cell Biol* 1977;72:406–423.

81. Kern HF. Fine structure of the human exocrine pancreas. In: Go VL, Brooks FP, DiMagno EP, Gardner JD, Lebenthal E, Scheele GA, eds. *The Exocrine Pancreas: Biology, Pathobiology, and Diseases.* New York: Raven Press; 1986:9–19.

82. Palade G. Intracellular aspects of the process of protein synthesis. *Science* 1975;189:347–358.

83. Romagnoli P. Increases in apical plasma membrane surface paralleling enzyme secretion from exocrine pancreatic acinar cells. *Pancreas* 1988;3:189–192.

84. Kodama T. A light and electron microscopic study on the pancreatic ductal system. *Acta Pathol Jpn* 1983;33:297–321.

85. Greider MH. Oxyphil cells of the human pancreas. *Anat Rec* 1967;157:251.

86. Roberts PF, Burns J. A histochemical study of mucins in normal and neoplastic human pancreatic tissue. *J Pathol* 1972;107:87–94.

87. Schulz I. Electrolyte and fluid secretion in the exocrine pancreas. In: Johnson LR, ed. *Physiology of the Gastrointestinal Tract.* Vol 2. New York: Raven Press; 1981:795–819.

88. Spicer SS, Sens MA, Tashian RE. Immunocytochemical demonstration of carbonic anhydrase in human epithelial cells. *J Histochem Cytochem* 1982;30:864–873.

89. Atkinson BF, Ernst CS, Herlyn M, Steplewski Z, Sears HF, Koprowski H. Gastrointestinal cancer-associated antigen in immunoperoxidase assay. *Cancer Res* 1982;42:4820–4823.

90. Borowitz MJ, Tuck FL, Sindelar WF, Fernsten PD, Metzgar RS. Monoclonal antibodies against human pancreatic adenocarcinoma: distribution of DU-PAN-2 antigen on glandular epithelia and adenocarcinomas. *J Natl Cancer Inst* 1984;72:999–1005.

91. Haglund C, Lindgren J, Roberts PJ, Nordling S. Gastrointestinal cancer-associated antigen CA 19-9 in histological specimens of pancreatic tumours and pancreatitis. *Br J Cancer* 1986;53:189–195.

92. Klimstra DS, Hameed MR, Marrero AM, Conlon KC, Brennan MF. Ductal proliferative lesions associated with infiltrating ductal adenocarcinoma of the pancreas. *Int J Pancreatol* 1994;16:224–225.

93. Sessa F, Bonato M, Frigerio B, et al. Ductal cancers of the pancreas frequently express markers of gastrointestinal epithelial cells. *Gastroenterology* 1990;98:1655–1665.

94. Kim JH, Ho SB, Montgomery CK, Kim YS. Cell lineage markers in human pancreatic cancer. *Cancer* 1990;66:2134–2143.

95. Balague C, Gambus G, Carrato C, et al. Altered expression of MUC2, MUC4, and MUC5 mucin genes in pancreas tissues and cancer cell lines. *Gastroenterology* 1994;106:1054–1061.

96. Terada T, Ohta T, Sasaki M, Nakanuma Y, Kim YS. Expression of MUC apomucins in normal pancreas and pancreatic tumours. *J Pathol* 1996;180:160–165.

97. Rahier J, Wallon J, Henquin JC. Cell populations in the endocrine pancreas of human neonates and infants. *Diabetologia* 1981;20:540–546.

98. Wittingen J, Frey CF. Islet concentration in the head, body, tail and uncinate process of the pancreas. *Ann Surg* 1974;179:412–414.

99. Stefan Y, Grasso S, Perrelet A, Orci L. A quantitative immunofluorescent study of the endocrine cell populations in the developing human pancreas. *Diabetes* 1983;32:293–301.

100. Grube D, Bohn R. The microanatomy of human islets of Langerhans, with special reference to somatostatin (D-) cells. *Arch Histol Jpn* 1983;46:327–353.

101. Malaisse-Lagae F, Stefan Y, Cox J, Perrelet A, Orci L. Identification of a lobe in the adult human pancreas rich in pancreatic polypeptide. *Diabetologia* 1979;17:361–365.

102. Stefan Y, Grasso S, Perrelet A, Orci L. The pancreatic polypeptide-rich lobe of the human pancreas: definitive identification of its derivation from the ventral pancreatic primordium. *Diabetologia* 1982;23:141–142.

103. Ehrie MG, Swartz FJ. Diploid, tetraploid and octaploid beta cells in the islets of Langerhans of the normal human pancreas. *Diabetes* 1974;23:583–588.

104. Lecompte PM, Merriam JC Jr. Mitotic figures and enlarged nuclei in the Islands of Langerhans in man. *Diabetes* 1962;11:35–39.

105. Pelletier G. Identification of four cell types in the human endocrine pancreas by immunoelectron microscopy. *Diabetes* 1977;26:749–756.

106. Bommer G, Friedl U, Heitz PU, Kloppel G. Pancreatic PP cell distribution and hyperplasia. Immunocytochemical morphology in the normal human pancreas, in chronic pancreatitis and pancreatic carcinoma. *Virchows Arch A Pathol Anat Histol* 1980;387:319–331.

107. Orci L, Baetens D, Ravazzola M, Stefan Y, Malaisse-Lagae F. Pancreatic polypeptide and glucagon: non-random distribution in pancreatic islets. *Life Sci* 1976;19:1811–1815.

108. Orci L, Malaisse-Lagae F, Baetens D, Perrelet A. Pancreatic-polypeptide-rich regions in human pancreas. *Lancet* 1978;2:1200–1201.

109. Orci L, Stefan Y, Malaisse-Lagae F, Perrelet A. Instability of pancreatic endocrine cell populations throughout life. *Lancet* 1979;1:615–616.

110. Fellinger EJ, Garin-Chesa P, Triche TJ, Huvos AG, Rettig WJ. Immunohistochemical analysis of Ewing's sarcoma cell surface antigen p30/32MIC2. *Am J Pathol* 1991;139:317–325.

111. Hochwald SN, Zee S, Conlon KC, et al. Prognostic factors in pancreatic endocrine neoplasms: an analysis of 136 cases with a proposal for low-grade and intermediate-grade groups. *J Clin Oncol* 2002;20:2633–2642.

112. Weidner N, Tjoe J. Immunohistochemical profile of monoclonal antibody O13: antibody that recognizes glycoprotein p30/32MIC2 and is useful in diagnosing Ewing's sarcoma and peripheral neuroepithelioma. *Am J Surg Pathol* 1994;18:486–494.

113. Kloppel G. Endokrines pankreas und diabetes mellitus. In: Doerr W, Seifert G, eds. *Spezielle Pathologische Anatomie*. Vol 14. Berlin: Springer; 1981:523–728.

114. Chen J, Baithun SI, Pollock DJ, Berry CL. Argyrophilic and hormone immunoreactive cells in normal and hyperplastic pancreatic ducts and exocrine pancreatic carcinoma. *Virchows Arch A Pathol Anat Histopathol* 1988;413:399–405.

115. Bendayan M. Presence of endocrine cells in pancreatic ducts. *Pancreas* 1987;2:393–397.

116. Oertel JE, Heffess CS, Oertel YC. Pancreas. In: Sternberg SS, ed. *Histology for Pathologists*. New York: Raven Press; 1992:657–668.

117. Patchefsky AS, Solit R, Phillips LD, et al. Hydroxyindole-producing tumors of the pancreas. Carcinoid-islet cell tumor and oat cell carcinoma. *Ann Intern Med* 1972;77:53–61.

118. Wilson RW, Gal AA, Cohen C, DeRose PB, Millikan WJ. Serotonin immunoreactivity in pancreatic endocrine neoplasms (carcinoid tumors). *Mod Pathol* 1991;4:727–732.

119. Chey WY. Hormonal control of pancreatic exocrine secretion. In: Go VL, Brooks FP, DiMagno EP, Gardner JD, Lebenthal E, Scheele GA, eds. *The Exocrine Pancreas: Biology, Pathobiology, and Diseases.* New York: Raven Press; 1986:301–313.

120. Henderson JR, Daniel PM. A comparative study of the portal vessels connecting the endocrine and exocrine pancreas, with a discussion of some functional implications. *Q J Exp Physiol Cogn Med Sci* 1979;64:267–275.

121. Adeghate E, Donath T. Distribution of neuropeptide Y and vasoactive intestinal polypeptide immunoreactive nerves in normal and transplanted pancreatic tissue. *Peptides* 1990;11:1087–1092.

122. Sharma S, Green KB. The pancreatic duct and its arteriovenous relationship: an underutilized aid in the diagnosis and distinction of pancreatic adenocarcinoma from pancreatic intraepithelial neoplasia. A study of 126 pancreatectomy specimens. *Am J Surg Pathol* 2004;28:613–620.

123. Olsen TS. Lipomatosis of the pancreas in autopsy material and its relation to age and overweight. *Acta Pathol Microbiol Scand A* 1978;86A:367–373.

124. Orci L, Stefan Y, Malaisse-Lagae F, Perrelet A, Patel Y. Pancreatic fat. *N Engl J Med* 1979;301:1292.

125. Suda K, Mizuguchi K, Hoshino A. Differences of the ventral and dorsal anlagen of pancreas after fusion. *Acta Pathol Jpn* 1981;31:583–589.

126. Jaster R. Molecular regulation of pancreatic stellate cell function. *Mol Cancer* 2004;3:26.

127. Popescu LM, Hinescu ME, Ionescu N, Ciontea SM, Cretoiu D, Ardelean C. Interstitial cells of Cajal in pancreas. *J Cell Mol Med* 2005;9:169–190.

128. Centeno BA, Pitman MB. Neoplasms of the exocrine and endocrine pancreas. In: Centeno BA, Pitman MB, eds. *Fine Needle Aspiration Biopsy of the Pancreas*. Boston: Butterworth-Heinemann; 1999:109–160.

129. Hruban RH, Pitman MB, Klimstra DS. Tumors of the pancreas. In: Silverberg SG, Sobin LH, eds. *Atlas of Tumor Pathology*. 4th series. Washington, DC: Armed Forces Institute of Pathology; 2006.

130. Shinozuka H, Lee RE, Dunn JL, Longnecker DS. Multiple atypical acinar cell nodules of the pancreas. *Hum Pathol* 1980;11:389–391.

131. Tanaka T, Mori H, Williams GM. Atypical and neoplastic acinar cell lesions of the pancreas in an autopsy study of Japanese patients. *Cancer* 1988;61:2278–2285.

132. Longnecker DS, Hashida Y, Shinozuka H. Relationship of age to prevalence of focal acinar cell dysplasia in the human pancreas. *J Natl Cancer Inst* 1980;65:63–66.

133. Oertel JE. The pancreas. Nonneoplastic alterations. *Am J Surg Pathol* 1989;13(suppl 1):50–65.

134. Longnecker DS, Shinozuka H, Dekker A. Focal acinar cell dysplasia in human pancreas. *Cancer* 1980;45:534–540.

135. Kodama T, Mori W. Atypical acinar cell nodules of the human pancreas. *Acta Pathol Jpn* 1983;33:701–714.

136. Baggenstoss AH. The pancreas in uremia: a histopathologic study. *Am J Pathol* 1948;24:1003–1017.

137. Walters MN. Studies on the exocrine pancreas. I. nonspecific pancreatic ductular ectasia. *Am J Pathol* 1964;44:973–981.

138. Walters MN. Goblet-cell metaplasia in ductules and acini of the exocrine pancreas. *J Pathol Bacteriol* 1965;89:569–572.

139. Schmid RM. Acinar-to-ductal metaplasia in pancreatic cancer development. *J Clin Invest* 2002;109:1403–1404.

140. Bockman DE, Boydston WR, Anderson MC. Origin of tubular complexes in human chronic pancreatitis. *Am J Surg* 1982;144:243–249.

141. Cubilla AL, Fitzgerald PJ. Morphological lesions associated with human primary invasive nonendocrine pancreas cancer. *Cancer Res* 1976;36(pt 2):2690–2698.

142. Kloppel G, Bommer G, Ruckert K, Seifert G. Intraductal proliferation in the pancreas and its relationship to human and experimental carcinogenesis. *Virchows Arch A Pathol Anat Histol* 1980;387:221–233.

143. Roberts PF. Pyloric gland metaplasia of the human pancreas. A comparative histochemical study. *Arch Pathol* 1974;97:92–95.

144. Allen-Mersh TG. Pancreatic ductal mucinous hyperplasia: distribution within the pancreas, and effect of variation in ampullary and pancreatic duct anatomy. *Gut* 1988;29:1392–1396.

145. Mukada T, Yamada S. Dysplasia and carcinoma in situ of the exocrine pancreas. *Tohoku J Exp Med* 1982;137:115–124.

146. Brat DJ, Lillemoe KD, Yeo CJ, Warfield PB, Hruban RH. Progression of pancreatic intraductal neoplasias to infiltrating adenocarcinoma of the pancreas. *Am J Surg Pathol* 1998;22:163–169.

147. Goggins M, Hruban RH, Kern SE. BRCA2 is inactivated late in the development of pancreatic intraepithelial neoplasia: evidence and implications. *Am J Pathol* 2000;156:1767–1771.

148. Maitra A, Adsay NV, Argani P, et al. Multicomponent analysis of the pancreatic adenocarcinoma progression model using a pancreatic intraepithelial neoplasia tissue microarray. *Mod Pathol* 2003;16:902–912.

149. Moskaluk CA, Hruban RH, Kern SE. p16 and K-ras gene mutations in the intraductal precursors of human pancreatic adenocarcinoma. *Cancer Res* 1997;57:2140–2143.

150. van Heek NT, Meeker AK, Kern SE, et al. Telomere shortening is nearly universal in pancreatic intraepithelial neoplasia. *Am J Pathol* 2002;161:1541–1547.

151. Wilentz RE, Iacobuzio-Donahue CA, Argani P, et al. Loss of expression of Dpc4 in pancreatic intraepithelial neoplasia: evidence that DPC4 inactivation occurs late in neoplastic progression. *Cancer Res* 2000;60:2002–2006.

152. Klimstra DS, Longnecker DS. K-ras mutations in pancreatic ductal proliferative lesions. *Am J Pathol* 1994;145:1547–1550.

153. Kozuka S, Sassa R, Taki T, et al. Relation of pancreatic duct hyperplasia to carcinoma. *Cancer* 1979;43:1418–1428.

154. Pour PM, Sayed S, Sayed G. Hyperplastic, preneoplastic and neoplastic lesions found in 83 human pancreases. *Am J Clin Pathol* 1982;77:137–152.

155. Hruban RH, Adsay NV, Albores-Saavedra J, et al. Pancreatic intraepithelial neoplasia: a new nomenclature and classification system for pancreatic duct lesions. *Am J Surg Pathol* 2001;25:579–586.

156. Hruban RH, Takaori K, Klimstra DS, et al. An illustrated consensus on the classification of pancreatic intraepithelial neoplasia and intraductal papillary mucinous neoplasms. *Am J Surg Pathol* 2004;28:977–987.

157. Klein WM, Hruban RH, Klein-Szanto AJ, Wilentz RE. Direct correlation between proliferative activity and dysplasia in pancreatic intraepithelial neoplasia (PanIN): additional evidence for a recently proposed model of progression. *Mod Pathol* 2002;15:441–447.

158. Tasso F, Picard D. Sur les oncocytes du pancreas humain. *C R Soc Biol (Paris)* 1969;163:1855–1858.

159. Tasso F, Sarles H. Canalicular cells and oncocytes in the human pancreas. Comparative study on the normal condition and in chronic pancreatitis [article in French]. *Ann Anat Pathol (Paris)* 1973;18:277–300.

160. Frexinos J, Ribet A. Oncocytes in human chronic pancreatitis. *Digestion* 1972;7:294–301.

161. Albores-Saavedra J, Wu J, Crook T, Amirkhan RH, Jones L, Hruban RH. Intestinal and oncocytic variants of pancreatic intraepithelial neoplasia. A morphological and immunohistochemical study. *Ann Diagn Pathol* 2005;9:69–76.

162. Adsay NV, Merati K, Andea A, et al. The dichotomy in the preinvasive neoplasia to invasive carcinoma sequence in the pancreas: differential expression of MUC1 and MUC2 supports the existence of two separate pathways of carcinogenesis. *Mod Pathol* 2002;15:1087–1095.

163. Adsay NV, Merati K, Basturk O, et al. Pathologically and biologically distinct types of epithelium in intraductal papillary mucinous neoplasms: delineation of an "intestinal" pathway of carcinogenesis in the pancreas. *Am J Surg Pathol* 2004;28:839–848.

164. Zamboni G, Terris B, Scarpa A, et al. Acinar cell cystadenoma of the pancreas: a new entity? *Am J Surg Pathol* 2002;26:698–704.

165. Komatsu K. Pancreatographical and histopathologic study of dilatations of the pancreas ductules with special references to cystic dilatation. *Juntendoo Med J* 1974;19:250–269.

166. Agostini S, Choux R, Payan MJ, Sastre B, Sahel J, Clement JP. Mucinous pancreatic duct ectasia in the body of the pancreas. *Radiology* 1989;170:815–816.

167. Nagai E, Ueki T, Chijiiwa K, Tanaka M, Tsuneyoshi M. Intraductal papillary mucinous neoplasms of the pancreas associated with so-called "mucinous ductal ectasia." Histochemical and immunohistochemical analysis of 29 cases. *Am J Surg Pathol* 1995;19:576–589.

168. Nishihara K, Fukuda T, Tsuneyoshi M, Kominami T, Maeda S, Saku M. Intraductal papillary neoplasm of the pancreas. *Cancer* 1993;72:689–696.

169. Sessa F, Solcia E, Capella C, et al. Intraductal papillary-mucinous tumours represent a distinct group of pancreatic neoplasms: an investigation of tumour cell differentiation and K-ras, p53 and c-erbB-2 abnormalities in 26 patients. *Virchows Arch* 1994;425:357–367.

170. Tian FZ, Myles J, Howard JM. Mucinous pancreatic ductal ectasia of latent malignancy: an emerging clinicopathologic entity. *Surgery* 1992;111:109–113.

171. Solicia E, Capella C, Kloppel G. Tumors of the endocrine pancreas. In: Rosai J, Sobin LH, eds. *Atlas of Tumor Pathology*, 3rd series, farciche 20. Washington, DC: Armed Forces Institute of Pathology; 1997:145–196.

172. Weidenheim KM, Hinchey WW, Campbell WG Jr. Hyperinsulinemic hypoglycemia in adults with islet-cell hyperplasia and degranulation of exocrine cells of the pancreas. *Am J Clin Pathol* 1983;79:14–24.

173. Goossens A, Gepts W, Saudubray JM, et al. Diffuse and focal nesidioblastosis. A clinicopathological study of 24 patients with persistent neonatal hyperinsulinemic hypoglycemia. *Am J Surg Pathol* 1989;13:766–775.

174. Stanley CA, Thornton PS, Ganguly A, et al. Preoperative evaluation of infants with focal or diffuse congenital hyperinsulinism by intravenous acute insulin response tests and selective pancreatic arterial calcium stimulation. *J Clin Endocrinol Metab* 2004;89:288–296.

175. Suchi M, MacMullen C, Thornton PS, et al. Histopathology of congenital hyperinsulinism: retrospective study with genotype correlations. *Pediatr Dev Pathol* 2003;6:322–333.

176. Thomas PM, Cote GJ, Wohllk N, et al. Mutations in the sulfonylurea receptor gene in familial persistent hyperinsulinemic hypoglycemia of infancy. *Science* 1995;268:426–429.

177. Clayton PT, Eaton S, Aynsley-Green A, et al. Hyperinsulinism in short-chain L-3-hydroxyacyl-CoA dehydrogenase deficiency reveals the importance of beta-oxidation in insulin secretion. *J Clin Invest* 2001;108:457–465.

178. Glaser B, Kesavan P, Heyman M, et al. Familial hyperinsulinism caused by an activating glucokinase mutation. *N Engl J Med* 1998;338:226–230.

179. Reinecke-Luthge A, Koschoreck F, Kloppel G. The molecular basis of persistent hyperinsulinemic hypoglycemia of infancy and its pathologic substrates. *Virchows Arch* 2000;436:1–5.

180. Stanley CA, Lieu YK, Hsu BY, et al. Hyperinsulinism and hyperammonemia in infants with regulatory mutations of the glutamate dehydrogenase gene. *N Engl J Med* 1998;338:1352–1357.

181. Bartow SA, Mukai K, Rosai J. Pseudoneoplastic proliferation of endocrine cells in pancreatic fibrosis. *Cancer* 1981;47:2627–2633.

182. Kovacs K, Horvath E, Asa SL, Murray D, Singer W, Reddy SS. Microscopic peliosis of pancreatic islets in a woman with MEN-1 syndrome. *Arch Pathol Lab Med* 1986;110:607–610.

183. Kloppel G. Islet histopathology in diabetes mellitus. In: Kloppel G, Heitz PU, eds. *Pancreatic Pathology*. New York: Churchill-Livingstone; 1984:154–192.

184. Castellani C, Bonizzato A, Rolfini R, Frulloni L, Cavallini GC, Mastella G. Increased prevalence of mutations of the cystic fibrosis gene in idiopathic chronic and recurrent pancreatitis. *Am J Gastroenterol* 1999;94:1993–1995.

185. Gorry MC, Gabbaizedeh D, Furey W, et al. Mutations in the cationic trypsinogen gene are associated with recurrent acute and chronic pancreatitis. *Gastroenterology* 1997;113:1063–1068.

186. Ito T, Nakano I, Koyanagi S, et al. Autoimmune pancreatitis as a new clinical entity. Three cases of autoimmune pancreatitis with effective steroid therapy. *Dig Dis Sci* 1997;42:1458–1468.

187. Kloppel G, Maillet B. Pathology of acute and chronic pancreatitis. *Pancreas* 1993;8:659–670.

188. Lilja P, Evander A, Ihse I. Hereditary pancreatitis—a report on two kindreds. *Acta Chir Scand* 1978;144:35–37.

189. Whitcomb DC, Gorry MC, Preston RA, et al. Hereditary pancreatitis is caused by a mutation in the cationic trypsinogen gene. *Nat Genet* 1996;14:141–145.

190. Yoshida K, Toki F, Takeuchi T, Watanabe S, Shiratori K, Hayashi N. Chronic pancreatitis caused by an autoimmune abnormality. Proposal of the concept of autoimmune pancreatitis. *Dig Dis Sci* 1995;40:1561–1568.

191. Abe K, Watanabe S. Apoptosis of mouse pancreatic acinar cells after duct ligation. *Arch Histol Cytol* 1995;58:221–229.

192. Walker NI. Ultrastructure of the rat pancreas after experimental duct ligation. I. The role of apoptosis and intraepithelial macrophages in acinar cell deletion. *Am J Pathol* 1987;126:439–451.

193. Gyr K, Heitz PU, Beglinger C. Pancreatitis. In: Kloppel G, Heitz PU, eds. *Pancreatic Pathology*. New York: Churchill-Livingstone; 1984:44–72.

194. Lowenfels AB, Maisonneuve P, Cavallini G, et al. Pancreatitis and the risk of pancreatic cancer. International Pancreatitis Study Group. *N Engl J Med* 1993;328:1433–1437.

195. Tascilar M, Offerhaus GJ, Altink R, et al. Immunohistochemical labeling for the Dpc4 gene product is a specific marker for adenocarcinoma in biopsy specimens of the pancreas and bile duct. *Am J Clin Pathol* 2001;116:831–837.

196. Argani P, Iacobuzio-Donahue C, Ryu B, et al. Mesothelin is overexpressed in the vast majority of ductal adenocarcinomas of the pancreas: identification of a new pancreatic cancer marker by serial analysis of gene expression (SAGE). *Clin Cancer Res* 2001;7:3862–3868.

197. Seifert G. Lipomatous atrophy and other forms. In: Kloppel G, Heitz PU, eds. *Pancreatic Pathology*. New York: Churchill-Livingstone; 1984:27–31.

HEMATOPOIETIC SYSTEM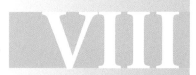

LYMPH NODES

31

Paul van der Valk   Chris J.L.M. Meijer

INTRODUCTION

The lymph nodes are an integral part of the immune system, a complex system whose job is to adequately deal with foreign substances (1). "Dealing with" here is taken in the broadest sense: it can mean either ignoring an antigen entirely (i.e., tolerance) or mounting a destructive reaction to the antigen, clearing it from the system. In certain areas of the body, an effective elimination is, of course, vitally important. This is certainly true for lymph nodes in areas where antigens serve no purpose and are therefore best eliminated. In contrast, in areas such as the gastrointestinal tract, reactivity against food antigens is not always advantageous, and tolerance is often the better response. As lymph nodes deal with antigens, their histology reflects the

(re)activity of the immune system; the nature of the antigen determines whether a reaction will be mounted against it but also determines what effector cells will be employed. This will be reflected in the morphology of the lymph nodes, as will be discussed later.

As the entire body is continually confronted with antigens, lymph nodes are required throughout the body and are concentrated in areas draining organs with environmental contact. The skin has numerous draining lymph nodes, partly grouped in areas where lymphatics converge, such as the axillary, cervical, and inguinal regions. The gastrointestinal tract and the airways have small collections of lymphoid cells in their mucosal surfaces (the so-called mucosa-associated lymphoid tissue, or MALT), as well as draining lymph nodes in the mesenteric or the mediastinal and hilar regions (2–5). Drainage from extra-abdominal areas is through the para-iliac and para-aortic nodes. All these systems converge on a single lymphatic channel, the thoracic duct, which returns the lymphatic fluid to the bloodstream. The only organ where no lymphatics are found is the brain, which drains its extracellular fluid via the cerebrospinal fluid or the extra-parenchymatous Virchow-Robin space.

Under antigenic pressure, lymph nodes can become apparent in areas where they are usually not found. Whether this appearance is actually an enlargement of very small lymph nodes already present or de novo formation of a lymph node is uncertain.

EMBRYOLOGY/DEVELOPMENTAL CHANGES

Relatively little is known about the embryonic development of lymph nodes. They seem to arise from the lymphatic sacs, which in turn develop from the venous system. From the sacs, a lymphatic plexus forms; and, as early as the first trimester, small collections of lymphoblasts can be found in association with this plexus (6). In the second trimester, differentiation into cortex and medulla begins to take place, gradually forming the familiar compartmentalized structure of the lymph node parenchyma. This process is probably also under the influence of nonlymphoid cells (such as macrophages and interdigitating dendritic cells) and mesenchymally derived cells (such as follicular dendritic cells and, perhaps, fibroblastic reticulum cells). After the compartmentalization of the lymph node is completed, no other changes take place except those that follow antigenic challenge.

GROSS FEATURES

Reactive lymph nodes are mostly small structures, round or reniform in shape. When clinically detectable, they are usually enlarged due to some degree of stimulation. Normally, they do not exceed a diameter of 1 cm, although during immune reactions they can become considerably larger. A diameter of more than 3 cm, however, is unusual (though not unheard of) in benign lymph nodes and should raise the suspicion of malignancy. The cut surface of a lymph node is a pink-brown in color and homogenous. A white ("fish meat") aspect or distinct nodularity is suspicious for maligancy (lymphoma). In lymph node dissection specimens, the lymph nodes often consist of small rims of parenchyma enclosing fatty tissue. They can be difficult for pathologists to spot grossly; but, in those cases, their resistance to the palpating finger gives them away.

ANATOMY

Blood Supply

Arterioles enter the lymph node through the hilus, branch, and then rapidly form a plexus of capillaries in the parenchyma. Subtle differences exist at the level of the basement membrane between the capillaries in the follicles and those in the paracortex. Laminin-5 is found exclusively in the basement membranes of the follicular compartment (7). It is also very likely that, at the level of the endothelial cells, differences in expression of surface markers (such as chemokine receptors) also exist, though these have not yet been formally demonstrated. Such differences likely play a role in the positioning of lymphocytes in the differing nodal compartments.

Venous drainage channels accompany the arterioles. The postcapillary venules in the lymph nodes are special, as they are the main route for the entrance of lymphocytes homing to the lymph nodes. They will be discussed in more detail later.

Lymphatics

The lymph node is positioned in the lymphatic system. The afferent lymphatics enter the lymph node through the capsule, draining into the subcapsular sinus. This sinus is lined by endothelial cells, but the system of branching sinuses arising from it no longer has an endothelial lining. Further discussion of the different cell types in the sinuses follows below.

LIGHT MICROSCOPY: THE DIFFERENT COMPARTMENTS, HISTOLOGY, AND FUNCTION

Examination of a sectioned lymph node at low power reveals more or less clearly defined areas or compartments (Figure 31.1A); most obvious are the follicles, generally rounded structures with pale centers and a dark rim. The centers often show a mottled appearance. The follicles are mainly present in the cortical area (i.e., the outer area of the lymph node just below the capsule). Occasionally follicles are found in the deeper regions. Between the follicles and extending to the deeper parenchyma is an ill-defined area, the paracortex or paracortical area, recognizable by its rather pronounced vessels, the epithelioid or high endothelial venules, the specialized postcapillary venules mentioned earlier. On occasion, this area shows a mottling not unlike that of the follicles (Figure 31.1B). In the medullary region of the lymph node, if present in the specimen, low power shows dark areas separated by lighter staining ones, often in a somewhat reticular pattern. The dark areas are the

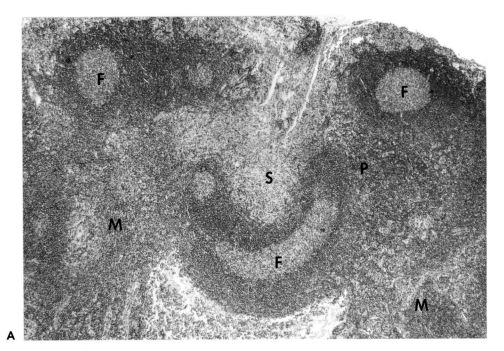

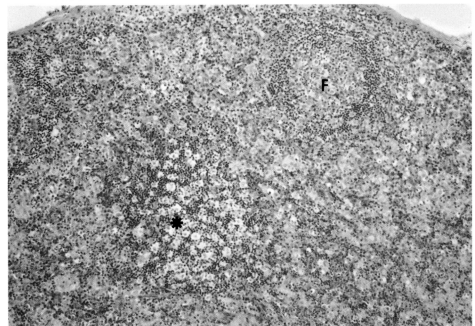

Figure 31.1   A. Low-power view of lymph node (periodic acid-Schiff stained, paraffin-embedded section). This "smiling" picture illustrates the four different compartments of the lymph node. In the upper corners and in the middle of the bottom (the "eyes and mouth") the follicles (*F*) are seen. The paracortical area (*P*) here is fairly small; usually there is more paracortex present. The less sharply defined sections where light and dark areas are juxtaposed represent the medullary cords (*M*, dark) and sinuses (*S*, light). **B.** Low-power view of another lymph node (H&E; paraffin-embedded section). In the upper right there is a follicle (*F*) recognizable. The rest of the picture shows paracortical area, with considerable influx of macrophages and interdigitating dendritic cells. In the center the typical mottling of the paracortex is seen (*).

medullary cords, where plasma cells and, with appropriate stains, mast cells are found. The lighter areas between these sheets of dark-staining small lymphocytes are the sinuses, filled with histiocytes whose ample pale cytoplasm imparts the lighter coloration to this region. The sinuses run through the entire parenchyma but are especially visible in the medullary zone and directly beneath the capsule.

These different areas can be easily recognized on low-power microscopy (Figure 31.1A), but it must be stressed that their representation varies greatly in different specimens and not rarely, for instance, the medullary cords are not found.

As humans are in constant contact with antigens, a lymph node is virtually always stimulated to some degree, and the increase in one area caused by this stimulation will often be at the cost of the volume of the other compartments (Figure 31.2). Such stimulation will not only increase the size of one compartment (and decrease the size of the others), but it will also cause a shift in the cellular composition. This usually means an increase in the proliferative fraction of each compartment, the blast cells (8). This adaptability to the constantly changing antigenic challenges explains the variety in "normal" lymph node histology: almost all lymph nodes that come under the

microscope are stimulated to some degree. Each of the four different compartments, follicle, medullary cords, paracortical area, and sinuses, is discussed separately.

The Follicle

Distinction must be made between primary and secondary follicles. Primary follicles are aggregates of small, dark-staining lymphoid cells. In these primary follicles, a germinal center can develop, turning them into secondary follicles. Thus, the mantle zone around the follicle center has the same characteristics as the original primary follicle. The outer portion of the mantle zone is somewhat less densely packed than the inner layer. This outer rim is sometimes called the marginal zone (9), largely based on a very loose resemblance to the splenic marginal zone and on the fact that marginal zone lymphomas tend to localize perifollicularly. However, if the marginal zone exists in the lymph node, it is difficult to distinguish except when it is expanded in benign or lymphomatous proliferations (10).

In the follicle center, an immunologic reaction takes place that is called, after its location, the follicle center cell reaction. It requires the cooperation of follicular dendritic cells (FDCs), lymphoid cells, and tingible body macrophages (Figure 31.3A–B). The function of the reaction is the generation of B cells that have been affinity-selected against an antigen (i.e., that produce an antibody with the best possible fit to the antigen) and that can function either as a direct precursor for antibody-producing plasma cells or as (long-term) memory cells.

Follicular Dendritic Cells

Follicular dendritic cells (FDCs; previously called dendritic reticulum cells) trap antigens on their surface and present them to B cells (11,12). Because these cells can retain antigen on their surfaces, it was postulated they provide a long-lasting reaction to that antigen, which may be important for immune memory (13); however, this is controversial, and other functions have been proposed (14). Follicular dendritic cells are difficult to recognize in light microscopic sections; they were first described by electron microscopy and later by enzyme and immunohistochemistry (Figure 31.3C) (12,15–17). They have a large but inconspicuous nucleus with very fine, almost vesicular chromatin and a small nucleolus. Not infrequently, they are or appear binucleated, with the nuclei pressed together. The cytoplasm is largely invisible with the light microscope; but, in ultrathin sections and with immunohistochemistry, they appear to have many long and slender cytoplasmic protrusions. These are linked to the protrusions of other FDCs via (hemi)desmosomes, thus forming a round network with a fingerprint-like configuration. In this way, they are responsible for the shape of the follicle. Their origin is still a matter of debate; a deriva-

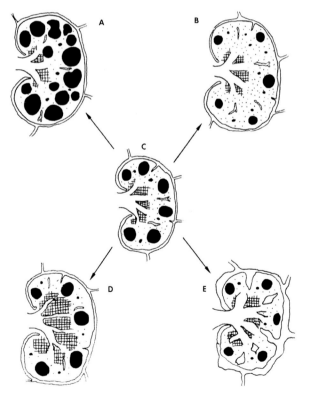

Figure 31.2 Schematic representation of the lymph node with enlargement of the four different compartments, respectively the follicular (**A**), the paracortical (**B**), the medullary (**D**) and the sinusoidal (**E**) compartments. **C** represents an unstimulated lymph node.

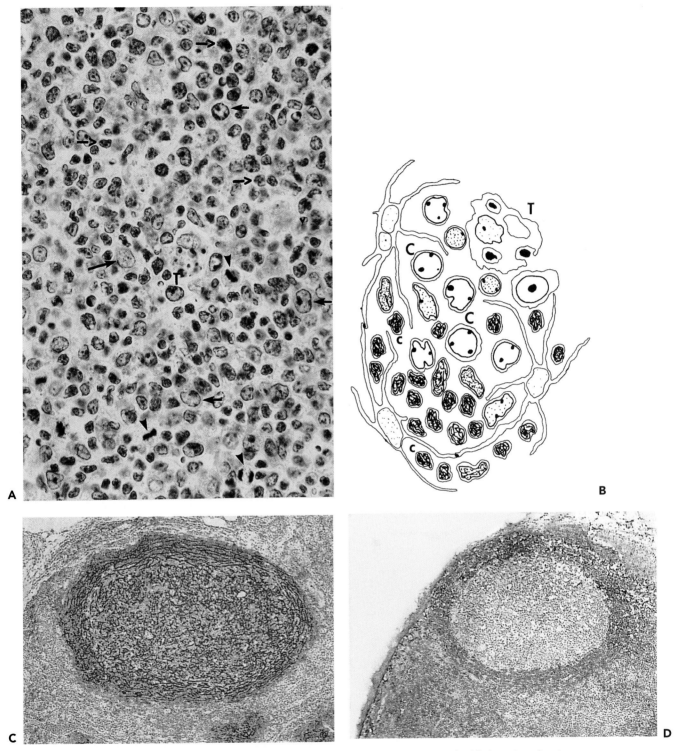

Figure 31.3 The follicular compartment. **A**. Giemsa-stained, plastic-embedded section, showing the pleomorphism of the follicle center. All typical elements are present: mitotic figures (*arrowheads*); a tingible body macrophage (*T*) with phagocytized debris, staining intensely black; blastic cells (*short arrows*); small follicle center cells (*open arrows*), and a follicular dendritic cell (FDC) (*long arrow*). **B.** Diagrammatic representation of a follicle, stressing the FDC morphology. Other elements are tingible body macrophage (*T*) and blastic (*C*) and small (*c*) lymphoid cells. **C.** Frozen section stained with a CD35 antibody against the C3b-receptor on FDCs. Note the somewhat fingerprint-like pattern of the FDC lattice. **D.** Frozen section stained for IgD. The mantle cells are positive; the cells in the center are not.

tion from the mononuclear phagocyte system was proposed (18), as was an origin from the perivascular mesenchyme (19), possibly via a circulating mesenchymal stem cell (20).

Lymphoid Cells

The lymphoid cells of the primary follicle and the mantle zone have small, slightly irregular nuclei, with condensed, dark-staining chromatin. They have scanty cytoplasm and, consequently, are packed closely together. The outer rim of the mantle zone, the marginal zone equivalent of the lymph node, houses cells that are slightly bigger and less densely packed, but they have the same dark nuclei (9). All of these cells are B cells, staining with antibodies to CD20, 22, and 24. They also express IgM on their surface, and the mantle zone cells proper also express IgD simultaneously (Figure 31.3D) (17,21–23). In the germinal center, distinctive B cells can be found:

1. Blast cells with large vesicular nuclei and several small but distinct nucleoli, often located at the nuclear membrane. When they are round, they have a small rim of basophilic cytoplasm, especially well-appreciated in cytologic preparations. These are the proliferative cells of the follicle; where they predominate, mitotic figures are easily found. Also, because of their basophilic cytoplasm, areas where they are in the majority appear dark (the dark zone of the follicle).
2. After the blast phase of proliferation, the cells gradually become smaller and get more irregular nuclei. As they get smaller, they lose their nucleoli and the chromatin condenses. This leads to cells that are almost indistinguishable from the mantle cells; small, irregular cells with dark-staining nuclei and virtually invisible cytoplasm. These cells are less densely packed, and the areas where they predominate (the light zones) appear a little lighter than the dark zones. Naturally, cells in transition between large round to small irregular are frequent, giving rise to a particularly polymorphic cellular picture, with a mixture of cells that are large, medium-sized, or small, round or irregular and with vesicular or condensed chromatin.
3. A smaller portion of the cells are medium-sized to large, with a finely dispersed chromatin and inconspicuous nucleoli and scanty but intensely basophilic cytoplasm (lymphoblasts).
4. Other lymphoid cells include occasional plasma cells and "immunoblasts" (i.e., very large blastic cells with big vesicular nuclei and single centrally placed nucleoli) and small, dark-staining lymphocytes (a little smaller than the small follicle center cells themselves), probably representing T lymphocytes. The number of these various cells varies considerably. On occasion, plasma cells can be quite numerous; also, T lymphocytes can outnumber the B lymphocytes in the follicle.

As follicle center cells are B cells, too, they react with the same markers as mentioned for the mantle and marginal zone cells (with the exception of IgD). In addition, they are mostly positive for the markers CD10 and Bcl-6, considered markers of follicle center cells (23).

Tingible-Body Macrophages

Tingible-body macrophages (TBMs) are large cells with abundant, pale cytoplasm. The cytoplasm contains phagocytized debris and apoptotic bodies from surrounding lymphocytes that have died in the selection process that takes place in the follicle (see Function section, below). Tingible-body macrophages have large nuclei, with finely dispersed chromatin. Because their nuclear size is fairly constant, they can be used as an internal "yardstick" to compare to the nuclear size of the surrounding lymphocytes, especially in lymphomas (nuclei as big or bigger than a TBM nucleus means a large-cell lymphoma). The cytoplasm of TBMs is often very clear, and therefore their presence causes clear/white spots in the tissue, a mottling colorfully described as the "starry sky" pattern. It should be noted that this highly characteristic feature, often used to distinguish between benign and malignant, is in fact a fixation artifact. In some fixatives, such as sublimate-formaldehyde or B5, this starry sky pattern is not seen!

Variations of the Follicular Pattern

From the above information, a characteristic pattern for the morphology of the follicle emerges: a more or less round or oval area, with a dark outer edge (the mantle zone) and a lighter center, that shows mottling and, upon closer inspection, a very polymorphic cytologic picture and many mitotic figures. Sometimes zonation is seen, with the dark zone directed inwards, the light zone directed more to the capsule of the node. As it is very dependent on how the follicle is cut in the section, this zonation is often not seen (15,24).

Variations occur in the shape of the follicles and in their composition. An important cause for variation is time: the pattern described above takes time to evolve. In the beginning, the follicle consists largely of blasts, with smaller follicle center cells appearing as the follicle center cell reaction runs its course (24).

In reactive conditions, follicles can become very large and coalesce; HIV lymphadenopathy is a good example of this phenomenon (25,26,27) (Figure 31.4). Their composition can also vary somewhat. Changes that occur with malignancy are discussed later. With involution, the follicle can become hyalinized and atrophic, or it can be overrun by T lymphocytes, a phenomenon known as progressive transformation of the germinal center (15,28). This can

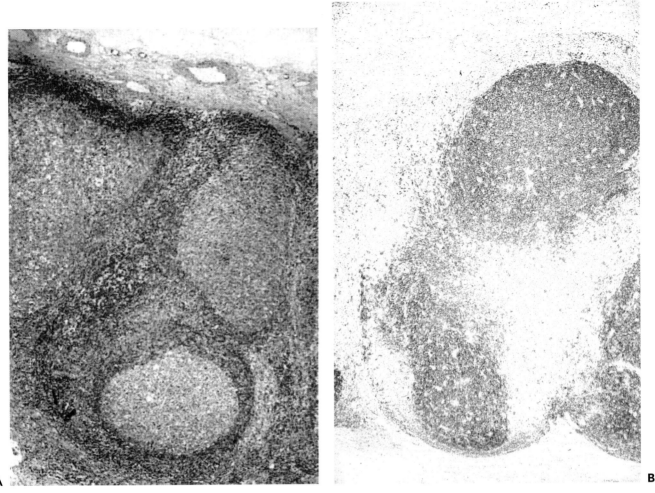

Figure 31.4 HIV-induced follicular hyperplasia. **A.** Very large and irregularly shaped follicles dominate the picture (H&E; paraffin-embedded section). **B.** Two follicles are seen, with ragged borders showing beginning follicular disintegration (CD20 stain).

make the follicle difficult to recognize. It is only by their remnant round shape (and by special stains for FDCs) that they may be recognized as follicles. Fortunately, this somewhat alarming-appearing feature usually involves only a few follicles at the same time, so the presence of nearby normal follicles is reassuring.

The Medullary Cords

The medullary cords are found in the hilar region of the lymph node, between the sinuses. The cellular composition of this compartment is described next (Figure 31.5).

Lymphoid Cells

Small lymphocytes make up the majority of cells in the medullary cords. They have small, more or less round nuclei

and a scant-to-moderate amount of cytoplasm. In some cells, the chromatin is clumped and peripherally distributed in the nucleus, similar to the plasma cell nucleus, though the typical "clock face" chromatin of a mature plasma cell is not seen. Cells with this kind of chromatin tend to have more cytoplasm and sometimes even a perinuclear hof, clearly indicative of plasmacytoid differentiation. These are called lymphoplasmacytoid or lymphoplasmacytic cells. Immunologically, the cells can be identified with CD20 and, even better with CD79a, general B cell markers. Staining for immunoglobulins can sometimes show cytoplasmic IgM and light chains. Many of the cells with less cytoplasm and irregular nuclei are T lymphocytes (CD2-, 3-, 5-, and 7-positive), necessary to modulate or drive the process of antibody formation that takes place in the medullary cords. The blast cells of this process, the immunoblasts, are striking, though infrequent. They have large vesicular nuclei with a large, centrally located nucleolus and abundant basophilic

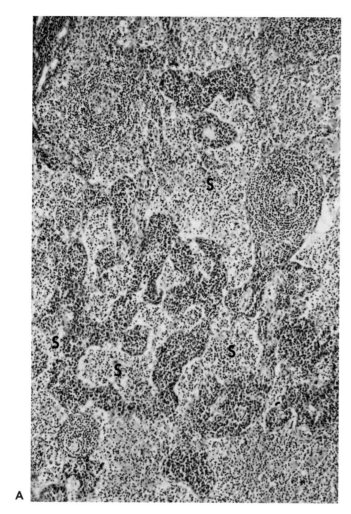

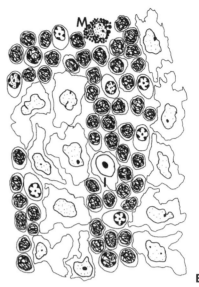

Figure 31.5 Medullary cords. **A.** The sheets and ribbons of dark-staining cells are the medullary cords, containing small lymphocytes and plasma cells; they are separated by the lighter staining areas, the sinuses (*S*) (H&E; paraffin-embedded section). **B.** Schematic representation, also depicting an immunoblast (*I*) and a mast cell (*M*).

cytoplasm. Plasma cells are also present but in varying number. They are distinctive cells, with their small round nuclei having a "clock face" chromatin pattern due to small clumps of dark chromatin at the nuclear membrane, like the numbers on a dial. The nucleus is eccentrically located in the cytoplasm, with a perinuclear hof or small zone of cytoplasmic clearing. The outer rim of the cytoplasm is deeply basophilic. Under some conditions, plasma cells accumulate immunoglobulins in their cytoplasm, forming so-called Russell bodies, globular structures that stain positive with PAS and that can indent the nucleus if they reach sufficient size. Plasma cells are CD20-negative but retain their CD79a expression and are, of course, positive for cytoplasmic immunoglobulins. Plasma cells will also (paradoxically) label for epithelial membrane antigen (EMA).

Macrophages

Macrophages are fairly scarce in the medullary cords. They have medium-sized to large irregular nuclei and abundant cytoplasm. They are not as avidly phagocytic as the TBMs from the follicle center, perhaps because they are differen-

tiated more toward antigen-handling and presentation then for phagocytosis.

Other Cell Types

T lymphocytes were already mentioned. The mast cell is the other cell type that can be found—especially in the medullary cords, where they can be easily demonstrated with a metachromatic dye such as a Giemsa stain. Their characteristic purple granulation permits easy recognition. The granules generally obscure the nucleus.

The Paracortex

The paracortex, or paracortical area, was the last compartment to be described and named (29), probably because its boundaries are indistinct and the area best appreciated in less commonly used fixatives, such as Zenker's or sublimate-formaldehyde. Nevertheless, it has some typical structural elements that allow easy recognition—the epithelioid venules and the interdigitating dendritic cell (IDC) (Figure 31.6).

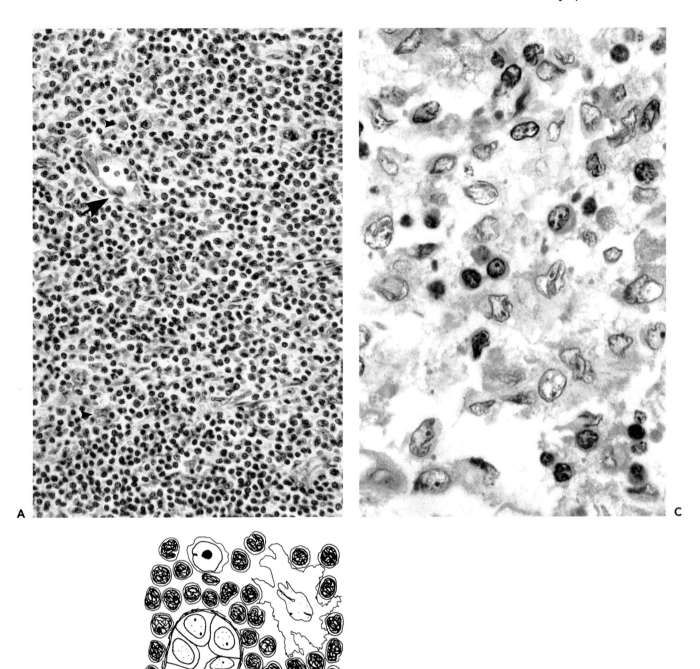

A

B

C

Figure 31.6   The paracortex. **A.** An epithelioid venule is seen (*arrow*); small lymphocytes dominate the picture, with an occasional blast present; interdigitating dendritic cells (IDCs), with their markedly irregular, grooved, and pale nuclei are scattered throughout the area (*arrowheads*) (H&E; paraffin-embedded section). **B.** Schematic representation. Note the typical IDC. **C.** This section demonstrates an increase in IDCs, characteristically displaying their irregular pale nuclei and abundant cytoplasm (lymph node with dermatopathic lymphadenopathy)(Giemsa; plastic-embedded section).

Epithelioid (Postcapillary or High Endothelial) Venules

These highly distinct vessels are found only in the paracortex; they are lined with plump cuboidal or even cylindrical endothelial cells with fairly large oval nuclei, with vesicular chromatin and indistinct nucleoli. Sometimes the lumina of these vessels appear to be obliterated by the endothelium. These vessels have long since been recognized as the port of entrance for bloodborne lymphocytes to the lymph node parenchyma (30,31). Therefore, they play a crucial role in recirculation, distribution, and homing of lymphocytes in different lymphoid organs, a process mediated by specific homing receptors on the lymphocyte surface, that react with organ-specific ligands (or vascular addressins) on the endothelial cell surface (32–35) (Figure 31.7). In this process chemokines also play an important role (36,37).

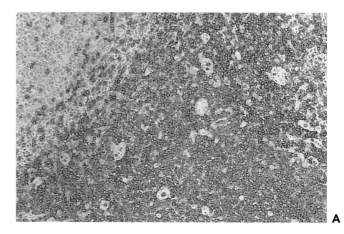

A

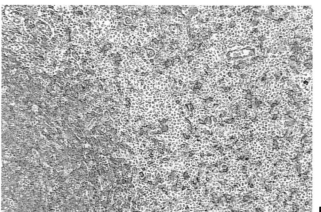

B

Figure 31.8 Immunohistochemistry of paracortex. **A.** The vast majority of the cells in the paracortex stain positive for CD3 (frozen section). In the upper left corner, a segment of a follicle (B-cell area) is seen. **B.** Here, the IDCs stain positive for HLA-DR (frozen section); they are larger and show more cytoplasm than the group of follicular (B) cells on the left.

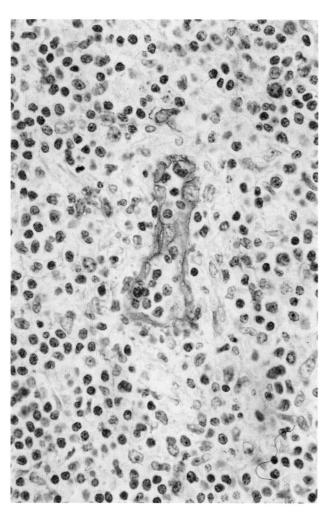

Figure 31.7 Paracortical area with a highlighted epithelioid venule. Lymphocytes are seen adhering to the endothelium and passing through the vessel wall (HECA 452 stain).

Interdigitating Dendritic Cells

Interdigitating dendritic cells (IDCs) are large cells with large and bizarre nuclei having deep clefts and folds. The chromatin pattern is delicate, almost transparent, and nucleoli are inconspicuous. The cytoplasm is abundant, pale, and with ill-defined borders (Figure 31.6C). Electron microscopy shows protrusions, broad and veil-like, in contrast to the thin processes of the FDC. Contact points are lacking. Furthermore, IDCs have a typical organelle of undetermined function: the tubulovesicular system (15). When present in large numbers IDCs cause a mottling of the paracortex.

The IDC is a bone marrow-derived cell, intimately related to the Langerhans cell of the skin, which it closely resembles, both morphologically and functionally (38–41). Both are antigen-presenting cells to T lymphocytes, important to initiate and/or maintain immune responses. Immunologically, these cells are best demonstrated in stains for S-100 protein or by HLA-DR, among the class II–negative T lymphocytes (Figure 31.8).

Lymphoid Cells

The cytology of the paracortex is somewhat variable; but, in the majority of cases, small T lymphocytes predominate. They have small, irregular nuclei with coarse chromatin and little cytoplasm. They are demonstrated with stains for CD2, 3 (Figure 31.8), 5, and 7 and are either CD4- or CD8-positive, with CD4-positive cells outnumbering the CD8-positive ones. Blast cells are present in varying numbers; they are large cells with vesicular nuclei of a varying shape.

Other Cell Types

The fibroblastic reticulum cell (FRC) is often found at the edge of the paracortex (15). It is a somewhat functionally enigmatic cell that forms reticulin fibers involved in the transport of cytokines and/or antigens through the parenchyma. This so-called FRC conduit system is an effective means of spreading important activating molecules throughout the entire lymph node (42).

The Sinuses

The sinuses are the structures carrying the lymphatic fluid from the afferent lymphatics through the lymph node to the efferent lymph vessels. The afferent lymph vessels drain into the subcapsular sinus, a structure at least partly lined by endothelium. As the sinuses traverse through the lymph node, they lose their endothelial lining and acquire a "lining" of macrophages (43). The macrophages in the sinuses are similar to macrophages elsewhere. They are large cells with large, irregular, and vesicular nuclei, a low nuclear-to-cytoplasmic ratio, and signs of phagocytotic activity.

Apart from the macrophages, which look the same here as elsewhere in the lymph node, small lymphocytes are also found in the sinuses (Figures 31.5A, 31.9A). In addition, occasional neutrophils or eosinophils can be found here as well.

Mention must be made of two other cell types. The first is the so-called sinus-lining cell, an ill-defined cell type that is primarily recognized with immunohistochemical stains for keratins. It is found in the area of the subcapsular sinus and has a coarsely dendritic morphology (44). Its nature is unclear; but, in evaluating lymph node sections for metastatic tumor, it is important to be aware of these cells and not confuse them with tumor cells. The second is the so-called immature sinus histiocyte, a misnomer as these are B lymphocytes (Figure 31.9B and C). These cells are primarily seen in certain reactive conditions in which they can partially fill the sinuses. They have small, more lymphoid appearing nuclei but have ample cytoplasm. Also called monocytoid B cells (another unfortunate name!), they are indeed B-lymphocytes, probably marginal zone cells (45,46).

FUNCTION

Each of the above-described compartments has a specific function, housing its own immunological reaction. Together these reactions make up the individual's immunologic integrity.

1. In the follicle, the follicle center cell reaction takes place. In this reaction the naïve B lymphocytes are exposed to antigen (on the FDC surface), and they adapt their antigen receptor (the immunoglobulin) to make a perfect fit to the presented antigen by a process called somatic hypermutation. This involves rearranging their immunoglobulin receptor genes through a partially trial-and-error process. Thus, some of the changes are actually for the worse and decrease the fit. Such cells are ruthlessly eliminated through apoptosis (hence the many apoptotic cells in this compartment). Eventually though, a perfect fit is achieved, and the cell is rescued from elimination by expressing the anti-apoptotic Bcl-2 molecule. Normal follicles, where selection takes place, are therefore negative for Bcl-2. Typically, several clones are developing in a single follicle, making it an oligoclonal proliferation (47).

   Through this complicated molecular biologic process of antibody selection, the follicle center cell reaction results in B cells that express high avidity antibodies on their surface. These cells can recirculate through the body as memory cells, spreading immune competence through the entire body and waiting for another encounter with the antigen; others go to the medullary cords or to the bone marrow to enter the plasma cell reaction and develop into plasma cells that produce antibodies for secretion.

2. In the medullary cords, the plasma cell reaction takes place. As mentioned above, it leads to the formation of plasma cells and the secretion of antibodies. The antibody production in the lymph node does not substantially contribute to the level of circulating antibodies, but it may be locally important, for instance for fixing antibodies on FDCs.

3. In the paracortex, we find the specific cellular response that generates antigen-specific effector T lymphocytes of the various subsets: helper cells, suppressor cells, regulatory cells, memory cells, and maybe more (32). The cellular processes here are still poorly understood. It is likely that T-cell memory, cytokine production, and a number of other reactions take place in the paracortex, but little is known about this. Its role in the delayed-type contact hypersensitivity is well-recognized (29).

4. The sinuses, with their abundant macrophages, are a filtering system, clearing foreign substances from the lymph. Given their ability to handle antigens, a function in antigen-presenting might be plausible, but little is known about this.

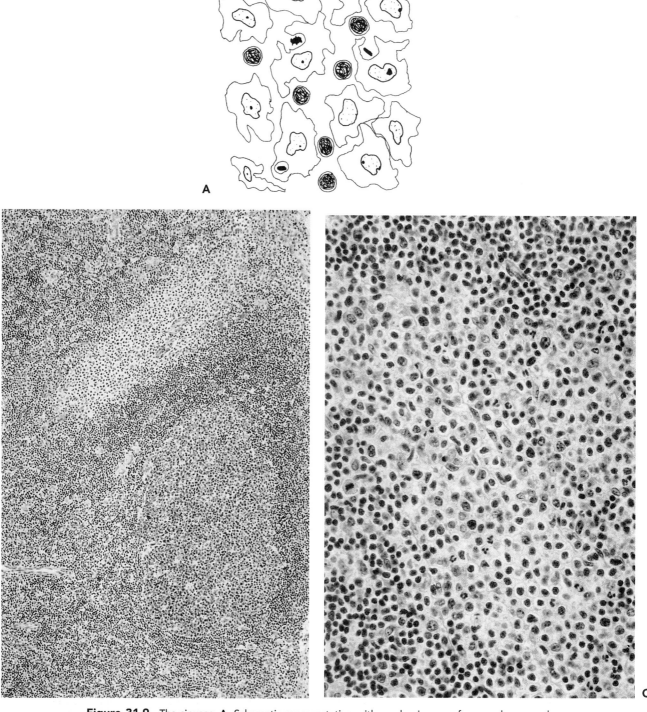

Figure 31.9 The sinuses. **A.** Schematic representation with predominance of macrophages and some lymphocytes. **B.** Low-power view of immature sinus histiocytosis, recognizable as the pale area to the upper left of the central follicle. **C.** Detail of B, showing the cells to be somewhat larger than the dark, small lymphocytes and having fairly abundant cytoplasm.

CHANGES IN COMPARTMENTS: BENIGN VERSUS MALIGNANT

The differential diagnosis of benign and malignant lesions is important in the discussion of normal lymph node histology for two reasons: (a) it is naturally of the utmost importance for the surgical pathologist to decide between benign and malignant, and (b) it is often difficult to distinguish between these two. The first goes without saying; the second can be clarified somewhat.

Though a link between normal tissue and the tumors arising from them has been self-evident for epithelial neoplasms, the same insight for lymphomas and lymph node structure was slow to arrive. However, this has been firmly established through careful morphologic and immunologic studies. We now regard the (non-Hodgkin's) lymphomas as malignant counterparts of the normal immunologic reactions to antigens that take place in the different compartments of the lymphoid tissues (15,48–50). Lymphoma cells have similar morphologic, immunologic, and functional characteristics when compared with normal cells. This explains why a malignant process can resemble a reactive condition so closely. Table 31.1 relates some of the benign variations in normal histology to their malignant counterparts. As this chapter deals with normal histology and many excellent texts have been written on lymphomas, we will discuss this matter only briefly.

Follicular Changes

The most important issue here is the distinction between follicular hyperplasia and follicular lymphoma. The term *follicular hyperplasia* covers a large number of conditions, most of which are difficult to differentiate from each other on morphologic grounds. Thus, it occurs in: (a) lymph nodes in the vicinity of a (bacterial) inflammation [e.g., tonsillitis but also in syphilis (51)]; (b) in autoimmune diseases, such as rheumatoid arthritis and systemic lupus erythematosus (52,53); (c) viral infections, such as HIV (25,26); and (d) in a number of idiopathic conditions,

such as Castleman's disease, multicentric angiofollicular hyperplasia, reactive lymph node hyperplasia with giant follicles (54–57). (It is by no means clear that these are all separate entities.) Sometimes special stains can help in elucidating causation (spirochetal stains, p24 for HIV). In essence, the follicles are all more or less the same, so they are taken together here.

The most important morphologic criteria arguing for a benign lesion, mentioned in the literature (15,53, 58–62) are:

1. Cellular pleiomorphism of the follicle center
2. Presence of TBMs
3. High number of mitotic figures
4. Well-defined mantle zone
5. Differences in size and shape of the follicles
6. Low number of follicles per surface area and predominant cortical localization
7. Well-developed and intact FDC networks in the follicle center
8. Zonation of the follicles, with clear dark and light zone

Despite this impressive list of criteria it may not be possible in all cases, even by an experienced pathologist, to distinguish reliably between benign and malignant on morphologic features alone. Therefore, there are some additional roles from immunohistochemistry and molecular biology (63). Features of malignancy by these techniques include: (a) demonstration of light chain restriction by immunohistochemistry (expression of either κ- or λ- light chain by follicular lesions is considered proof of malignancy); (b) expression of Bcl-2 by follicle center cells; (c) demonstration of clonality by detection of rearrangement of immunoglobulin genes, either by Southern blotting or by polymerase chain reaction (PCR) analysis; and (d) demonstration of a t(14;18) translocation (perhaps not 100% proof but a very strong argument).

Even with these additional techniques, it is not possible to diagnose all cases with certainty. It is good to realize that the majority of the lymph nodes encountered by pathologists are quickly scanned and interpreted, and rarely cause diagnostic problems. However, a high index of suspicion is

TABLE 31.1

BENIGN COMPARTMENTAL ENLARGEMENT AND THEIR MALIGNANT COUNTERPARTS

Compartment	Benign	Malignant
Follicle	Follicular hyperplasia	Follicular lymphomas
Paracortex	Paracortical hyperplasia	T-NHL
	Dermatopathic lymphadenopathy	Mycosis fungoides
Medullary cords	Medullary hyperplasia	Lymphoplasmacytic lymphoma
	Reactive plasmocytosis	Plasmacytoma
Sinuses	Sinus histiocytosis	Malignant histiocytosis

probably a good general attitude, simply because of the occasional treacherous similarities between benign and malignant follicular processes.

Changes in the Medullary Cords

Two distinctions can be important when examining changes in medullary cords. The first is reactive plasmacytosis (Figure 31.10) versus plasmacytoma. Preserved lymph node architecture and the presence of plasma cell precursors strongly favor the diagnosis of a reactive condition (15). In rare doubtful cases, immunohistochemistry can clinch the diagnosis by demonstrating light chain restriction. Second, expansion of the medullary cords, a rare event in itself, can be mimicked by a lymphoplasmacytic lymphoma. In rare instances, this lymphoma does not efface the architecture but expands the medullary cords. If the expansion is sufficient to arouse suspicion, marker studies can settle this easily, again by showing light chain restriction. It is good to realize that demonstrating clonality in paraffin sections may be difficult due to diffusion artifacts. The intercellular fluid is rich in immunoglobulins, and these can diffuse into the cells of a specimen if fixation is delayed. Subsequent fixation will trap the polyclonal

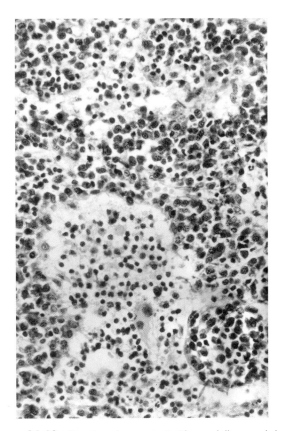

Figure 31.10 Reactive plasmacytosis. The medullary cords here consist almost entirely of plasma cells; sinuses are patent, a sign of preserved lymph node structure (H&E; paraffin-embedded section).

immunoglobulins inside the cells, potentially obscuring monoclonality. In practice, when a lesion is clearly monoclonal, this will be demonstrable; however, caution must be taken in interpreting immunoglobulin stains.

Changes in the Paracortex

Paracortical hyperplasia can take three forms, each with their own differential diagnostic considerations.

1. *Expansion of the paracortex by predominantly small lymphocytes, usually with an increase in epithelioid venules.* Distinctive features, suggestive of malignancy are cellular monotony and destruction of lymph node architecture by the proliferation. Immunohistochemical features that may be supportive are: (a) demonstration of an aberrant phenotype (e.g., strong predominance of CD4 or CD8), loss of markers that are normally present (such as CD7 or CD5), or expression of markers normally not expressed by lymph node T cells (such as CD1); and (b) demonstration of clonality by molecular biology [i.e., Southern blotting or PCR analysis of the T cell receptor chains (64,65)].

2. *Expansion with an increase of blasts.* This can be seen in viral infections or following vaccinations, as well as in some drug reactions (the antiepileptic drugs featured prominently here) (53,60,66,67). The changes can be histologically very alarming for malignancy. In some conditions, even necrosis can occur, such as in Kikuchi's histiocytic necrotizing lymphadenitis (68). On occasion, the changes can exhibit a nodular pattern (69). In such cases, a preserved architecture should raise the possibility of a benign condition, regardless of the histologic picture. Simple analysis with immunohistochemistry will reveal blasts of B-cell origin next to blasts of T-cell origin; also mitotic cells labelled by both B-cell and T-cell markers argue strongly for a benign proliferation and against a peripheral T-cell lymphoma. A differential diagnosis with Hodgkin's disease is also sometimes a consideration; Reed-Sternberg cells can be found in reactive conditions. Therefore, this differential can be very problematic. It should be kept in mind, however, that cases of Hodgkin's disease with intact lymph node architecture are rare. In short, this pattern can be extremely difficult to interpret; a combination of clinical history, morphology, immunophenotyping, and molecular biology (demonstration of clonality) must bring about a final diagnosis.

3. *Dermatopathic lymphadenopathy.* In this pattern, seen in lymph nodes draining skin areas with itching skin disorders, the paracortex is expanded by a marked increase in IDCs and Langerhans cells (70,71). It is mentioned here, because the skin lymphomas, mycosis fungoides, and the Sézary syndrome, when they involve the lymph nodes, will do so in the background of a dermatopathic lymphadenopathy. This problem will

thus arise only in the setting of a patient known to suffer from one of these skin lymphomas. That does not make the problem easier in itself. The only way to arrive at the diagnosis is to make a careful search for the diagnostic large cerebriform mononuclear cells, which can be difficult to find (72,73). Their demonstration is clinically very relevant (74). Immunohistochemistry and molecular biology unfortunately are not helpful here (75).

Sinusoidal Changes

Sinusoidal changes are very common in lymph node specimens. Lymph nodes draining tumors or inflammatory areas often show sinus histiocytosis. Typical conditions showing a sinusoidal pattern include sinus histiocytosis with massive lymphadenopathy (76,77) and Langerhans cell histiocytosis (60,78). The former condition is a peculiar clinicopathological entity in which the histiocytes seem to engulf large numbers of lymphocytes in their cytoplasm without destroying them, a phenomenon dubbed emperipolesis. This is a highly characteristic finding. The latter can also cause a (mostly but not always benign) sinus histiocytosis. The typical features of Langerhans cells, with their deeply grooved nuclei and the admixture with eosinophils, are important clues. Immunohistochemistry with CD1 (and S-100) will prove the true nature of the cells. Malignant conditions in the sinuses are almost always easily recognized on histology as frankly malignant. Metastatic carcinoma or melanoma, large-cell anaplastic lymphoma (79), and malignant histiocytosis (80) all can be difficult to distinguish from one another, but doubts about their malignancy are rare.

As mentioned above, the sinuses can be filled with immature sinus histiocytes or monocytoid B cells. A malignant equivalent is nodal marginal zone B-cell lymphoma (81). A predominant sinusoidal localization of such a lymphoma is rare but can occur. Demonstration of clonality is helpful and necessary in such cases.

Finally a particular sinusoidal pattern involving vessels can be seen on occasion, often as a reaction of the lymph node to ischemia or irradiation. This pattern is called vascular transformation of the sinuses and can show some histological variation, from a delicate vascular pattern to a more spindle-cell proliferation resembling Kaposi's sarcoma (82).

Combined Patterns

Follicular, medullary, paracortical, and sinusoidal patterns often occur simultaneously, and any combination is possible. As combined patterns are extremely rare in lymphomas, any combination argues for a benign condition. For example, *Toxoplasma* and Epstein-Barr virus infections often cause combined patterns. If suspicions of a malig-

nancy arise, the same criteria as mentioned for the single patterns apply.

In addition a number of other patterns may occur, such as granulomatous patterns. As this chapter cannot aspire to completeness and this is not a treatise on benign conditions of the lymph node, they will not be discussed further.

ARTIFACTS

A number of extrinsic and intrinsic factors can influence lymph node histology. Though they are not patterns, they can cause considerable difficulties in evaluating histology and are therefore mentioned here.

Technical Artifacts

Lymph node tissue is vulnerable and easily damaged in processing. Undue pressure on a specimen during dissection can cause considerable crushing artifact, to the point of obliterating morphology completely. *Specimens with extensive crushing artifacts should best not be evaluated.* Differences are already subtle, and no chance should be taken with poor material.

Another disturbing artifact is fixation related. It occurs especially in large specimens or if processing is too quick. If the fixation time in formalin is too short, only the outer edge of the specimen is fixed. The central part will not be reached by the formalin and will be fixed in the alcohol of the dehydrating series. This causes a marked difference in the histologic appearance of outer and inner segments. The inner segment shows loss of cohesion, and cells appear more shrunken and hyperchromatic (Figure 31.11). Great care should be taken in evaluating such specimens.

Intrinsic Artifacts

Though the lymph node architecture described above is found in all nodes throughout the body, in some areas typical changes can be found, mostly the result of repeated inflammation or reactions. These changes are most often seen in inguinal nodes and take the form of deposits of fibrotic material that can distort the normal architecture. This should be kept in mind when evaluating such specimens. Similarly, in retroperitoneal lymph nodes, hyalinization can be found.

HANDLING OF LYMPH NODE SPECIMENS

In an area where morphologic differences are (very) subtle, additional techniques can be decisive in making a diagnosis. In the past, this meant having snap-frozen material

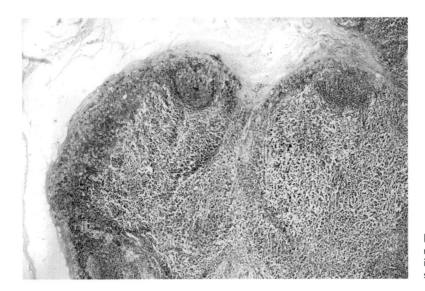

Figure 31.11 Fixation artifact. Edge of the specimen is properly fixed; the center, fixed in alcohol during the dehydration procedure, shows loss of tissue structure.

available to do marker studies and/or Southern blotting. However, at the moment, all commonly used markers in characterizing lymphoid tissues and their tumors are applicable on formalin-fixed, paraffin-embedded material. In addition, though Southern blotting is still the most sensitive and reliable technique, PCR analysis with multiple primers is a good alternative for molecular biologic evaluation of gene rearrangements and translocation. Nevertheless, it is still good policy to ask clinicians to send in lymph node specimens fresh and to snap-freeze a part of the specimen. It is no longer necessary to use a special fixative for immunohistochemistry (Bouin's fixative, sublimate-formaldehyde, B5, Sensofix, zinc-containing fixatives, among others); most of these are toxic and damage DNA to such a degree that molecular biologic analysis becomes impossible. It can be helpful to make touch imprints, by *carefully* pressing the cut surface of a specimen against a slide. The cytological picture can be helpful, especially in cases where the histology is not so good.

Electron microscopy is not particularly helpful in diagnosing lymphoid lesions, whether benign or malignant. For very rare lesions, tumors of dendritic cells for instance, this may be of assistance, and it is a small effort to slice off a very small and thin fragment for fixation in glutaraldehyde. However, and this is a general principle, *if a specimen is small, any manipulation is a risk of damaging the cells in the lesion severely and should be kept to a minimum or even avoided altogether.*

If circumstances so dictate, consider sending a piece of tissue to the microbiology department for culture.

For research purposes—and if the size of the specimen allows it—a cell suspension can be made. Routine use of cell suspensions to perform marker analysis is not to be encouraged. One loses the morphologic control of the lesion and its cells, which is extremely important.

SPECIAL TECHNIQUES AND PROCEDURES

Immunohistochemistry can hardly be described as a very special technique, given its omnipresence in pathologic diagnostics. It is, however, not always used properly. Therefore, we will stress the basic rules for this important additional technique.

1. <u>Always</u> *use positive and negative controls.* Given the problems with endogenous peroxidase, alkaline phosphatase, or biotin activity/presence and the very real possibility of technical mistakes, they are absolutely essential.
2. *Use panels of antibodies.* Because no single antibody is absolutely specific for one molecule and cross-reactions can be very confusing, it is sound policy to use a well-constructed panel in which individual staining results will confirm each other. Panels for classification of lymphoid lesions have been reported (83,84); they are primarily in use for classification of lymphoma but are also useful for benign lymphoid lesions and distinguishing between benign and malignant.
3. *Use the morphology.* Immunohistochemistry is an additional technique; one should always be extremely cautious if morphology and immunohistochemistry are at odds. Also, morphology can direct the interpretation of the immunohistochemistry, for instance by looking at the immunophenotype of those cells that are considered the tumor cells. In lymphoid lesions, there are always a lot of admixed cells that are also of lymphoid origin. The best example is that of a paracortical expansion where the blasts prove to be of B-cell origin with the immunohistochemistry, a strong argument for a benign process.

4. *Use your common sense.* This goes without saying. It is curious, however, how often this essential piece of advice is ignored!

By and large, similar advice goes for the use of molecular biology in the evaluation of lymphoid lesions. Controls, common sense, and the use of several primer pairs or techniques to confirm test results are equally as important here as they are for immunohistochemistry. The demonstration of clonality must be considered a (strong) argument for malignancy; however, not all clonal lesions are malignant and certainly will not behave in a malignant fashion, the obvious example being monoclonal gammopathy of undetermined significance (85). Again, the data must be interpreted in their entire context.

Even lineage determination (e.g., by demonstration of immunoglobulins or T-cell receptor rearrangements) is not absolute. The terms *lineage infidelity* and *lineage promiscuity* already suggest that there are exceptions to the rule that only B cells rearrange immunoglobulin genes and only T cells rearrange T-cell receptor genes (86–90). Obviously, additional techniques are invaluable in the analysis of lymphoid lesions, but only if they are properly used!

REFERENCES

1. Hall JG. The functional anatomy of lymph nodes. In: Stansfeld AG, ed. *Lymph Node Biopsy Interpretation.* Edingburgh: Churchill Livingstone; 1985:1–25.
2. Parrott DMV. The gut as a lymphoid organ. *Clin Gastroenterol* 1976;5:211–228.
3. McDermott MR, Bienenstock J. Evidence for a common mucosal immunologic system. I. Migration of B immunoblasts into intestinal, respiratory, and genital tissues. *J Immunol* 1979;122:1892–1898.
4. Sminia T, Plesch BE. An immunohistochemical study of cells with surface and cytoplasmic immunoglobulins in situ in Peyer's patches and lamina propria of rat small intestine. *Virchows Arch B Cell Pathol Incl Mol Pathol* 1982;40:181–189.
5. Azzali G. Structure, lymphatic vascularization and lymphocyte migration in mucosa-associated lymphoid tissue. *Immunol Rev* 2003;195:178–189.
6. O'Rahilly R, Müller F. *Human Embryology and Teratology.* New York: Wiley-Liss; 1992.
7. Jaspars LH, van der Linden HC, Scheffer GL, Scheper RJ, Meijer CJLM. Monoclonal antibody 4C7 recognizes an endothelial basement membrame component that is selectively expressed in capillaries of lymphoid follicles. *J Pathol* 1993;170:121–128.
8. Taylor CR. Classification of lymphomas: "new thinking" on old thoughts. *Arch Pathol Lab Med* 1978;102:549–554.
9. van den Oord JJ, de Wolf-Peters C, Desmet VJ. The marginal zone in the human reactive lymph node. *Am J Clin Pathol* 1986;86:475–479.
10. Nathwani BN, Hernandez AM, Drachenberg MR. Diagnostic significance of morphologic patterns of lymphoid proliferations in lymph nodes. In: Knowles DM, ed. *Neoplastic Hematopathology.* 2nd ed. Philadelphia: Lippincott Williams & Wilkins; 2001:507–536.
11. Nossal GJ, Abbot A, Mitchell J, Lummus Z. Antigens in immunity. XV. Ultrastructural features of antigen capture in primary and secondary lymphoid follicles. *J Exp Med* 1968;127:277–290.
12. Park CS, Choi YS. How do follicular dendritic cells interact intimately with B cells in the germinal centre? *Immunology* 2005;114:2–10.
13. Donaldson SL, Kosco MH, Szakal AK, Tew JG. Localization of antibody-forming cells in draining lymphoid organs during long-term maintenance of the antibody response. *J Leukoc Biol* 1986;40:147–157.
14. Haberman AM, Shlomchik MJ. Reassessing the function of immune-complex retention by follicular dendritic cells. *Nat Rev Immunol* 2003;3:757–764.
15. Parl I. The cytologic, hystologic, and functional bases for a modern classification of lymphomas. In: Lubarsch O, Henke F. Handbuch der speziellen pathologischen Anatomie und Histologie I/3/B. Berlin: Springer-Verlag; 1978:1–72.
16. Naiem M, Gerdes J, Abdulaziz Z, Stein H, Mason DY. Production of a monoclonal antibody reactive with human dendritic reticulum cells and its use in the immunohistological analysis of lymphoid tissue. *J Clin Pathol* 1983;36:167–175.
17. van der Valk P, van der Loo EM, Jansen J, Daha MR, Meijer CJLM. Analysis of lymphoid and dendritic cells in human lymph node, tonsil and spleen. A study using monoclonal and heterologous antibodies. *Virchows Arch B Cell Pathol Incl Mol Pathol* 1984;45:169–185.
18. Gerdes J, Stein H, Mason DY, Ziegler A. Human dendritic reticulum cells of lymphoid follicles: their antigenic profile and their identification as multinucleated giant cells. *Virchows Arch B Cell Pathol Incl Mol Pathol* 1983;42:161–172.
19. Beranek JT, Masseyeff R. Hyperplastic capillaries and their possible involvement in the pathogenesis of fibrosis. *Histopathology* 1986;10:543–551.
20. van Nierop K, de Groot C. Human follicular dendritic cells: function, origin and development. *Semin Immunol* 2002;14:251–257.
21. Stein H, Bonk A, Tolksdorf G, Lennert K, Rodt H, Gerdes J. Immunohistologic analysis of the organization of normal lymphoid tissue and non-Hodgkin's lymphomas. *J Histochem Cytochem* 1980;28:746–760.
22. Hsu SM, Jaffe ES. Phenotypic expression of B-lymphocytes. I. Identification with monoclonal antibodies in normal lymphoid tissue. *Am J Pathol* 1984;114:387–395.
23. Knowles DM. Immunophenotypic markers useful in the diagnosis and classification of hematopoietic neoplasms. In: Knowles DM, ed. *Neoplastic Hematopathology.* 2nd ed. Philadelphia: Lippincott Williams & Wilkins; 2001:93–226.
24. van den Oord JJ. The immune response in the human lymph node. A morphological, enzyme, and immunohistochemical study (Thesis). Leuven, Belgium: University of Leuven; 1985.
25. Ewing EP, Chandler GW, Spira TJ, Bynes RK, Chan WC. Primary lymph node pathology in AIDS and AIDS-related lymphadenopathy. *Arch Pathol Lab Med* 1985;109:977–981.
26. Stanley MW, Frizzera G. Diagnostic specificity of histologic features in lymph node biopsy specimens from patients at risk for the acquired immunodeficiency syndrome. *Hum Pathol* 1986;17:1231–1239.
27. Chadburn A, Metroka C, Mouradian J. Progressive lymph node histology and its prognostic value in patients with acquired immunodeficiency syndrome and AIDS-related complex. *Hum Pathol* 1989;20:579–587.
28. Chang CC, Osipov V, Wheaton S, Tripp S, Perkins SL. Follicular hyperplasia, follicular lysis, and progressive transformation of germinal centers. A sequential spectrum of morphologic evolution in lymphoid hyperplasia. *Am J Clin Pathol* 2003;120:322–326.
29. Oort J, Turk JL. A histological and autoradiographic study of lymph nodes during the development of contact sensitivity in the guinea pig. *Br J Exp Pathol* 1965;46:147–154.
30. Gowans JL, Knight J. The route of recirculation of lymphocytes in the rat. *Proc R Soc Lond Ser B Biol Sci* 1964;159:257–282.
31. Chin YH, Carey GD, Woodruff JJ. Lymphocyte recognition of lymph node high endothelium. IV. Cell surface structures mediating entry into lymph nodes. *J Immunol* 1982;129:1911–1915.
32. Stevens SK, Weismann IL, Butcher EC. Differences in the migration of B and T lymphocytes: organ-selective localization in vivo and the

role of lymphocyte-endothelial cell recognition. *J Immunol* 1982;128:844–851.

33. Butcher ES, Scollay RG, Weissman IL. Organ specificity of lymphocyte migration: mediation by highly selective lymphocyte interaction with organ-specific determinants on high endothelial venules. *Eur J Immunol* 1980;10:556–561.

34. Pals ST, Kraal G, Horst E, de Groot A, Scheper RJ, Meijer CJLM. Human lymphocyte-high endothelial venule interaction: organ-selective binding of T and B lymphocyte populations to high endothelium. *J Immunol* 1986;137:760–763.

35. Wiedle G, Dunon D, Imhof BA. Current concepts in lymphocyte homing and recirculation. *Crit Rev Clin Lab Sci* 2001;38:1–31.

36. Lopez-Giral S, Quintana NE, Cabrerizo M, et al. Chemokine receptors that mediate B cell homing to secondary lymphoid tissues are highly expressed in B cell chronic lymphocytic leukemia and non-Hodgkin lymphomas with widespread nodular dissemination. *J Leukoc Biol* 2004;76:462–471.

37. Schaerli P, Moser B. Chemokines: control of primary and memory T-cell traffic. *Immunol Res* 2005;31:57–74.

38. Kamperdijk EW, Raaymakers EM, de Leeuw JH, Hoefsmit EC. Lymph node macrophages and reticulum cells in the immune response. I. The primary response to paratyphoid vaccine. *Cell Tissue Res* 1978;192:1–23.

39. Groscurth P. Non-lymphatic cells in the lymph node cortex of the mouse. I. Morphology and distribution of the interdigitating cells and the dendritic reticular cells in the mesenteric lymph node of adult ICR mouse [article in German]. *Pathol Res Pract* 1980;169:212–234.

40. Thorbecke GJ, Silberberg-Sinakin I, Flotte TJ. Langerhans cells as macrophages in skin and lymphoid organs. *J Invest Dermatol* 1980;75:32–43.

41. Hoefsmit EC, Duijvestijn AM, Kamperdijk EW. Relation between Langerhans cells, veiled cells, and interdigitating cells. *Immunobiology* 1982;161:255–265.

42. Anderson AO, Shaw S. T cell adhesion to endothelium: the FRC conduit system and other anatomic and molecular features which facilitate the adhesion cascade in lymph node. *Semin Immunol* 1993;5:271–282.

43. Forkert PG, Thliveris JA, Bertalanffy FD. Structure of sinuses in the human lymph node. *Cell Tissue Res* 1977;183:115–130.

44. Wacker HH, Frahm SO, Heidebrecht HJ, Parwaresch R. Sinus lining cells of the lymph nodes recognized as a dendritic cell type by the monoclonal antibody Ki-M9. *Am J Pathol* 1997;151:423–434.

45. Cardoso De Almeida P, Harris NL, Bhan AK. Characterization of immature sinus histiocytes (monocytoid cells) in reactive lymph nodes by use of monoclonal antibodies. *Hum Pathol* 1984;15:330–335.

46. Sheibani K, Fritz RM, Winberg CD, Burke JS, Rappaport H. "Monocytoid" cells in reactive follicular hyperplasia with and without multifocal histiocytic reactions: an immunohistochemical study of 21 cases including suspected cases of toxoplasmic lymphadenitis. *Am J Clin Pathol* 1984;81:453–458.

47. MacLennan IC. Germinal centers. *Annu Rev Immunol* 1994;12:117–139.

48. Lennert K. Follicular lymphoma. A tumor of the germinal centers. In: Akazaki K, Rappaport H, Bernard CW, Bennett JM, Ishikawa E, eds. *Malignant Diseases of the Hematopoietic System. Gann Monograph on Cancer Research.* Vol 15. Tokyo: University of Tokyo Press; 1973:217–231.

49. Lukes RJ, Collins RD. A functional approach to the classification of malignant lymphomas. *Recent Results Cancer Res* 1974;46:18–30.

50. Mann RB, Jaffe ES, Bernard CW. Malignant lymphomas—a conceptual understanding of morphologic diversity. A review. *Am J Pathol* 1979;94:105–191.

51. Evans N. Lymphadenitis of secondary syphilis: its resemblance to giant follicular lymphadenopathy. *Arch Pathol* 1944;37:175–179.

52. Nosanchuk JS, Schnitzer B. Follicular hyperplasia in lymph nodes from patients with rheumatoid arthritis. A clinicopathologic study. *Cancer* 1969;24:243–254.

53. Ioachim HL, Ratech H. *Ioachim's Lymph Node Pathology.* 3rd ed. Philadelphia: Lippincott Williams & Wilkins; 2002.

54. Keller AR, Holchholzer L, Castleman B. Hyaline-vascular and plasma-cell types of giant lymph node hyperplasia of the mediastinum and other locations. *Cancer* 1972;29:670–683.

55. Osborne BM, Butler JJ, Variakojis D, Kott M. Reactive lymph node hyperplasia with giant follicles. *Am J Clin Pathol* 1982;78:493–499.

56. Weisenburger DD, Nathwani BN, Winberg CD, Rappaport H. Multicentric angiofollicular lymph node hyperplasia: a clinicopathologic study of 16 cases. *Hum Pathol* 1985;16:162–172.

57. Martino G, Cariati S, Tintisona O, et al. Atypical lymphoproliferative disorders: Castleman's disease. Case report and review of the literature. *Tumori* 2004;90:352–355.

58. Schnitzer B. Reactive lymphoid hyperplasias. In: Jaffe ES, ed. *Surgical Pathology of the Lymph Nodes and Related Organs.* Philadelphia: WB Saunders; 1995:98–132.

59. Rappaport H. Tumors of the hematopoietic system. In: *Atlas of Tumor Pathology.* 3rd series, fascicle 8. Washington, DC: Armed Forces Institute of Pathology; 1966.

60. Dorfman RF, Warnke R. Lymphadenopathy simulating the malignant lymphomas. *Hum Pathol* 1974;5:519–550.

61. Nathwani BN, Winberg CD, Diamond LW, Bearman RM, Kim H. Morphologic criteria for the differentiation of follicular lymphoma from florid reactive follicular hyperplasia. A study of 80 cases. *Cancer* 1981;48:1794–1806.

62. Mann RB. Follicular lymphoma. In: Jaffe ES, ed. *Surgical Pathology of the Lymph Nodes and Related Organs.* Philadelphia: WB Saunders; 1985:252–282.

63. Harris NL, Ferry JA. Follicular lymphoma and related disorders (germinal center lymphomas). In: Knowles DM, ed. *Neoplastic Haematology.* 2nd ed. Baltimore: Lippincott Williams & Wilkins; 2001:823–853.

64. Picker LJ, Weiss LM, Medeiros LJ. Immunophenotypic criteria for the diagnosis of non-Hodgkin's lymphoma. *Am J Pathol* 1987;128:181–201.

65. Catovsky D, Ralfkiaer E, Muller-Hermelink HK. T-cell prolymphocytic leukaemia. In: Jaffe ES, Harris NL, Stein H, Vardiman JW, eds. *World Health Organization Classification of Tumours: Pathology and Genetics of Tumours of Haematopoietic and Lymphoid Tissues.* Lyon, France: IARC Press; 2001:195–196.

66. Saltstein SL, Ackerman LV. Lymphadenopathy induced by anticonvulsant drugs and mimicking clinically and pathologically malignant lymphomas. *Cancer* 1959;12:164–182.

67. Hartsock RJ. Postvaccinial lymphadenitis. Hyperplasia of lymphoid tissue that simulates malignant lymphomas. *Cancer* 1968;21:632–649.

68. Kuo TT. Kikuchi's disease (histiocytic necrotizing lymphadenitis). A clinicopathologic study of 79 cases with an analysis of histologic subtypes, immunohistology, and DNA ploidy. *Am J Surg Pathol* 1995;19:798–809.

69. van den Oord JJ, de Wolf-Peeters C, Desmet VJ, Takahashi K, Ohtsuki Y, Akagi T. Nodular alteration of the paracortical area. An in situ immunohistochemical analysis of primary, secondary, and tertiary T-nodules. *Am J Pathol* 1985;120:55–66.

70. van der Oord JJ, de Wolf-Peeters C, de Vos R, Desmet VJ. The paracortical area in dermatopathic lymphadenitis and other reactive conditions of the lymph node. *Virchows Arch B Cell Pathol Incl Mol Pathol* 1984;45:289–299.

71. Burke JS, Sheibani K, Rappaport H. Dermatopathic lymphadenopathy. An immunophenotypic comparison of cases associated and unassociated with mycosis fungoides. *Am J Pathol* 1986;123:256–263.

72. Scheffer E, Meijer CJLM, von Vloten WA. Dermatopathic lymphadenopathy and lymph node involvement in mycosis fungoides. *Cancer* 1980;45:137–148.

73. Colby TV, Burke JS, Hoppe RT. Lymph node biopsy in mycosis fungoides. *Cancer* 1981;47:351–359.

74. van Doorn R, van Haselen CW, van Voorst Vader P, et al. Mycosis fungoides: disease evolution and prognosis of 309 Dutch patients. *Arch Dermatol* 2000;136:504–510.

75. Willemze R, Scheffer E, Meijer CJLM. Immunohistochemical studies using monoclonal antibodies on lymph nodes from patients with mycosis fungoides and Sézary's syndrome. *Am J Pathol* 1986;120:46–54.

76. Rosai J, Dorfman RF. Sinus histiocytosis with massive lymphadenopathy. A newly recognized benign clinicopathological entity. *Arch Pathol* 1969;87:63–70.

77. Rosai J, Dorfman RF. Sinus histiocytosis with massive lymphadenopathy: pseudolymphomatous benign disorder. Analysis of 34 cases. *Cancer* 1972;30:1174–1188.

78. Callihan TR. Langerhans'cell histiocytosis (Histiocytosis X). In: Jaffe ES, ed. *Surgical Pathology of the Lymph Nodes and Related Organs.* Philadelphia: WB Saunders; 1995:534–559.

79. Delsol G, Ralfkiaer E, Stein H, Wright D, Jaffe ES. Anaplastic large cell lymphomas. In: Jaffe ES, Harris NL, Stein H, Vardiman JW, eds. *World Health Organization Classification of Tumours: Pathology and Genetics of Tumours of Haemotopoietic and Lymphoid Tissues.* Lyon, France: IARC Press; 2001:230–235.

80. Pileri SA, Grogan TM, Harris NL, et al. Tumours of histiocytes and accessory dendritic cells: an immunohistochemical approach to classification from the International Lymphoma Study Group based on 61 cases. *Histopathology* 2002;41:1–29.

81. Sheibani K, Sohn CC, Burke JS, Winberg CD, Wu AM, Rappaport H. Monocytoid B-cell lymphoma. A novel B-cell neoplasm. *Am J Pathol* 1986;124:310–318.

82. Chan JK, Warnke RA, Dorfman RF. Vascular transformation of sinuses in lymph nodes. A study of its morphological spectrum and distinction from Kaposi's sarcoma. *Am J Surg Pathol* 1991;15:732–743.

83. Oudejans JJ, van der Valk P. Immunohistochemical classification of T cell and NK cell neoplasms. *J Clin Pathol* 2002;55:892.

84. Oudejans JJ, van der Valk P. Immunohistochemical classification of B cell neoplasms. *J Clin Pathol* 2003;56:193.

85. Grogan TM, Van Camp B, Kyle RA, Muller-Hermelink HK, Harris NL. Plasma cell neoplasms. In: Jaffe ES, Harris NL, Stein H, Vardiman JW, eds. *World Health Organization Classification of Tumours: Pathology and Genetics of Tumours of Haemotopoietic and Lymphoid Tissues.* Lyon, France: IARC Press; 2001:142–156.

86. Ha K, Minden M, Hozumi N, Gelfland EW. Immunoglobulin gene rearrangement in acute myelogenous leukemia. *Cancer Res* 1984;44:4658–4660.

87. Rovigatti U, Mirro J, Kitchingman G, et al. Heavy chain immunoglobulin gene rearrangement in acute non-lymphocytic leukemia. *Blood* 1984;63:1023–1027.

88. Waldmann TA, Davis MM, Bongiovanni KF, Korsmeyer SJ. Rearrangements of genes for the antigen receptor on T cells as markers of lineage and clonality in human lymphoid neoplasms. *N Engl J Med* 1985;313:776–783.

89. Asou N, Matsuoka M, Hattori T, et al. T cell gamma gene rearrangements in hematologic neoplasms. *Blood* 1987;69:968–970.

90. Zuniga M, D'Eustachio P, Ruddle NH. Immunoglobulin heavy chain gene rearrangement and transcription in murine T cell hybrids and T lymphomas. *Proc Natl Acad Sci U S A* 1982;79:3015–3019.

Spleen

32

J. Han J. M. van Krieken   Attilio Orazi

INTRODUCTION

Historically, the human spleen has attracted attention from poets as a producer of melancholy. Galen (131–201 AD) called the human spleen an enigmatic organ, a notion that has persisted for a long time. In the seventeenth century, Malpighi described, macroscopically, the splenic lymphoid follicles as white pulp against a background of red pulp. In 1857, Billroth published one of the first histologic studies of the human spleen in which he divided the red pulp into cord tissue and venous sinuses (1). Still, until the second half of the twentieth century, the spleen was considered a rather useless reservoir for blood cells and was hardly studied. In the 1970s, by using electron microscopy, Weiss was able to elucidate the fine structure of the organ, which gave insights into the red pulp function (2,3). During the same period, Nieuwenhuis, Ford, and Keuning performed immunologic function studies on rat spleen (4–6), and Veerman published a detailed description of the white pulp of

the rat spleen (7). A complete summary of the organization and functions of the spleen is provided by Weiss in 1988, in the sixth and last edition of his *Textbook of Histology* (Cell and Tissue Biology) (8).

Nevertheless, many pathologists still lack a clear understanding of the normal histology and functions of the human spleen. This is due to several reasons. The organ is extremely vulnerable to autolysis, which often makes histologic findings in postmortem specimens difficult to interpret and of limited teaching value. Surgically removed spleens are suitable, if processed without delay. However, since the number of splenectomies performed in most institutions is relatively scarce, it is not surprising that pathologists may feel uncomfortable when interpretating splenic pathology as a result of a lack of familiarity with splenic histologic features.

Another source of confusion with respect to the structure and function of the human spleen is in the terminology and definitions applied to this organ, which are still largely based on studies of animal spleens. The human and animal spleens do not have an identical architecture; for example, in the human spleen, the periarteriolar lymphocyte sheath and the marginal sinus as described in rodent spleens are not present. Furthermore, certain definitions (e.g., of the marginal zone) vary widely from author to author (9,10).

The next problem is the large variations that occur in the "normal" spleen. The spleen is a compartimentalized organ (Table 32.1). Stimulation of one of the many functions of the spleen can lead to morphologic changes in the compartment that is mainly responsible for that function. The normal spleen therefore can show wide variation. As one of us has shown in a previously published study, it is essential to define a normal control population if one undertakes histologic studies in the spleen in specific disorders (11). For example, a morphometric analysis showed that spleens removed incidentally during abdominal surgery (i.e., for highly selective vagotomy or early gastric cancer) differed from traumatically ruptured spleens; we therefore excluded the latter from our "normal" group. All these problems sometimes make it difficult to differentiate physiologic from pathologic changes.

Part of this chapter is based on a previous study, performed by one of the authors, of methylmethacrylate sections of more than 400 surgically removed human spleens and our immunohistochemical experience using frozen (12,13) and/or paraffin-embedded tissue.

PRENATAL AND DEVELOPMENTAL CHANGES

During embryogenesis, the spleen can be recognized from about the fifth week of gestation, and blood vessels appear in it by the ninth week. Red and white pulp cannot be distinguished until the ninth month. The functional role of the spleen during prenatal development varies widely from that of the adult spleen, and this is reflected in the microscopic anatomy of the organ. Hematopoiesis was considered to take place in the fetal spleen (and liver) and to contribute largely to blood cell formation in the fetus until the sixth month of gestation, but it has been shown that, in fact, the spleen functions at most as a site of maturation for hematopoietic precursors derived from the peripheral blood (14,15). In adults, one may see foci of hematopoietic cells (extramedullary hematopoiesis) in the spleen in many reactive conditions (e.g., sepsis), as well as in disorders of the bone marrow associated with myelofibrosis. Extramedulary hematopoiesis as seen in the spleen is also referred to as myeloid metaplasia.

TABLE 32.1

SUMMARY OF SPLENIC HISTOLOGY, FUNCTION, AND RELATIONSHIP TO LYMPH NODE COMPARTMENTS

Spleen Compartment	Description	Function/Composition	Equivalent in Lymph Node
White pulp			
T-cell area	Irregular area of small lymphocytes containing lymph vessels bordering arteries	Predominant CD4 lymphocytes	Paracortex
B-cell follicle	Round area of small lymphocytes surrounded by medium-sized lymphocytes (a germinal center may be present)	Production of Ig-producing cells and probably memory cells	Follicle
Perifollicular zone	Area between white and red pulp containing many erythrocytes and lacking a normal sinusoidal structure	Place of retarded blood flow with interaction of blood cells, cells, antigens, and antibodies	Medulla (?)
Red Pulp			
Sinuses/cord tissue with sheathed capillaries	Tissue containing a meshwork of sinuses (with interrupted basement membrane) and capillaries, partly sheathed	Removal of particles from blood cells. Possible place of interaction of new antigens with reticulum cells	Sinus: partly high endothelial venule Sheathed capillary: medullary sinus
Nonfiltering area	Area of red pulp tissue lacking capillaries and containing lymphocytes	Probably place of onset of immune reaction	Medulla or compartment of primary follicles
Perivascular rim	Small area along the vessel tree containing lymphocytes and plasma cells	Probably connected to lymphatics	Medulla (?)

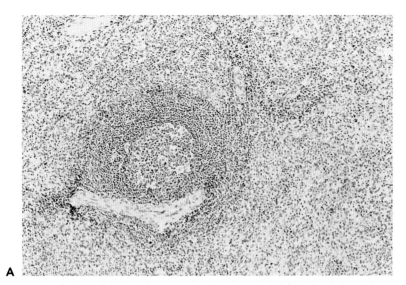

A

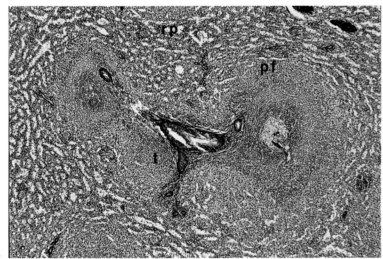

B

Figure 32.1 Spleen removed in idiopathic thrombocytopenic purpura. **A.** Formalin-fixed paraffin embedding (H&E, original magnification ×40). **B.** Methylmethacrylate embedding (methenamine-silver/H&E, original magnification ×40). Overview of red and white pulp showing central arteriole with T-cell area, a primary follicle, and a secondary follicle containing a germinal center. Note the absence of the marginal zone around the T-cell area and the presence of the erythrocyte-rich (pink) perifollicular zone surrounding both the T- and B-cell compartment of the white pulp. Note the lack of detail on the structure of the red pulp and the difficult discernable perifollicular zone in standard H&E section. (*rp*, red pulp; *pf*, perifollicular zone)

The immune system develops during fetal growth, and this development continues after birth (16). This functional maturation is reflected by the morphology: until birth the splenic white pulp does not contain follicles and marginal zones. There are immature B cells in clusters and T cells scattered throughout the organ. Their numbers increase with the developmental age of the fetus; and, from the end of the second semester onward, B- and T-cell areas can be recognized (17,18). Phagocytosis can be demonstrated at the twelfth week of gestation (14,15).

Developmental changes of the spleen are very familiar. The presence of accessory spleens (so-called splenculi, small extra pieces of spleen tissue with the complete and normal histology of the red and white pulp) can be found in at least 25% of autopsies. In disorders being treated with splenectomy, these splenculi may lead to recurrence of the disease.

Rare but well known is the polysplenia associated with immotile cilia syndrome (19). In this syndrome, left-right orientation of thoracal and abdominal organs may be abnormal, and the spleen at the right side is often divided into many small pieces, generally having normal function. This is not to be confused with acquired splenosis, in which many small fragments of spleen are present after trauma. Congenital asplenia, which is exceedingly rare, is associated with abnormalities of the cardiovascular system.

APOPTOSIS

In the development of the spleen, apoptosis does not seem to play an important role, but the lymphoid compartment, as in other lymphoid tissues, shows extensive apoptosis, especially in the germinal centers of the B-cell follicles. This is illustrated in Figure 32.1, where the "starry sky" phenomenon can be observed. The starry sky cells are macrophages that phagocytose remnants of lymphocytes that are dying through apoptosis, generally because they have an unsuccessful gene rearrangement of the antigen receptor or because of the fact that the produced immunoglobulin recognizes autoantigen. This physiologic process is important in the protection against autoimmune diseases. The Bcl-2 protein that protects against certain forms of apoptosis (see Chapter 1), which is expressed in most B and T cells, is lacking in germinal center B cells, rendering them susceptible for apoptosis. In follicular lymphoma the t(14;18) translocation leads to aberrant expression of Bcl-2 in the tumor cells. This is sometimes helpful in the recognition of follicular lymphoma in the spleen for the following reasons. Because the spleens of patients over about 20 years of age only rarely contain active germinal centers, the distinction between a primary follicle and follicular lymphoma can be difficult. Furthermore, the involvement of the spleen by follicular lymphoma is often nodular but does not lead to the disturbance of the architecture that is so noticeable in the lymph nodes involved by follicular lymphoma. Because spleens are often received after fixation, immunoglobulin light chain restriction is not possible by immunohistochemistry, immunofluorescence, or flow cytometry.

Apoptosis also plays an important role in mantaining a normal number and function of T cells. In cases of autoimmune lymphoproliferative syndrome (a pediatric disorder due to a genetic defect of FAS or FAS ligand that is associated with splenomegaly and autoimmunity), a decreased rate of apoptosis in T lymphocytes is responsible for the marked degree of lymphoid hyperplasia seen in the T-cell rich areas of the spleen.

GROSS FEATURES/ORGAN WEIGHT

The human spleen is a bean-shaped organ surrounded by a smooth capsule covered by the peritoneum. In contrast to several species, the capsule does not contain smooth muscle fibers and therefore does not have the capability of undergoing contraction in response to acute blood loss. The spleen in animals such as dogs and cats has an important red blood cell reservoir function. By undergoing rapid contraction, the spleen can squeeze out its red blood cell reservoir and, by doing so, produce a rapid increase in the amount of circulating blood. The surface may be covered with fibrotic or even calcified plaques, the cause of which is unknown. It is not uncommon to find several grooves at the outer surface that have no clinical significance. The weight of the spleen is highly variable (20). In adults, the spleen generally weighs 150 to 250 g; but, in the elderly, the spleen is often substantially smaller, even when there is no apparent hypofunction.

On the cut surface, the red and white pulp can be discerned, the latter consisting of small (less than or equal to 2-mm) nodules. It is important to realize that involvement of the spleen in malignant lymphoma often is observed foremost in the white pulp (21), which becomes enlarged but often not to a great extent. Therefore, the spleen should be cut up into small sections (less than or equal to 5 mm).

ANATOMY

Blood Supply

Blood reaches the spleen via the splenic artery, a large branch of the celiac artery, and enters the spleen through four to six branches; their number and location is, however, highly variable. Venous outflow occurs via four to six venous branches. These combine, within the lienorenal ligament to form the splenic vein, which drains into the portal vein (22). This is why portal hypertension can produce "congestive" splenomegaly. The blood flow within the spleen is highly specialized and relates to the different functions of the spleen.

Nerves

The spleen is innervated by nonmyelinated fibers from the major splanchnic nerves and the celiac plexus (23). These nerve fibers run along the splenic artery. Innervation in human spleens is less extensive than in cat and dog spleens, and this might be related to the important reservoir function of the spleen in these animals, as previously mentioned.

Lymphatics

No afferent lymphatic vessels are present in the spleen. Its lymph drainage occurs via hilar lymph nodes and lymph nodes in the gastrosplenic ligament. The lymph then flows through lymphatics along the splenic artery to the celiac lymph nodes along the celiac artery. The lymphatics in the spleen are described below.

LIGHT MICROSCOPY

Vascular Tree

After entering at the hilus, the splenic artery branches like a tree (24). Within the splenic parenchyma, these arterial branches, called trabecular arteries, are accompanied by veins and lymph vessels and surrounded by collagenous fibers. These vessels containing fibrous structures are usually referred to as trabeculae or septa, a term which is inappropriate to describe what in essence are perivascular collagen cuffs. Real, albeit short, true septa are also present in the spleen. These are connected to the capsule, lack inside vessels, and only extend for a short length into the splenic tissue. Foci of condensed reticular fibers devoid of vessels are found throughout the red pulp. The condensed reticulum appears to be in direct continuity with the reticular meshwork of the surrounding red pulp; they may represent areas of collapse or involution of the red pulp tissue.

Trabecular arteries branch to form central arteries and arterioles that are no longer accompanied by veins and are surrounded not by a collagenous cuff but rather by lymphatic tissue predominantly composed of T lymphocytes. This lymphatic compartment, which is usually referred to as periarterial or periarteriolar lymphoid sheath (PALS) is present around the vessels and becomes smaller toward the capillary ending. The arterioles are usually described as branching into penicillary arterioles, which run in parallel. In humans, however, this phenomenon seems to be restricted to involuted specimens in which the disappearance of tissue between arterioles has left them lying close to each other.

Branching of arterioles and capillaries often occurs at right angles, as can frequently be seen in sections. Reconstructions based on serial sections have shown that the terminal end of the capillary forms a peculiar and specifically splenic structure (25,26) (Figures 32.2–32.3). These structures are known by several names, determined partly by the species in which they have been studied, for example, sheathed capillaries, Hülsekapillaren, ellipsoids, or peri-

arteriolar macrophage sheaths. In humans, they are present in the red pulp and the perifollicular zone and are generally referred to as sheathed capillaries. The sheathed capillary is surrounded by a "sheath" of mononuclear phagocytes and rare reticulum cells. Because autolysis is so rapid, visualization of the sheathed capillaries in particular is dependent on adequate tissue processing. The endothelial lining of the capillary ends abruptly in a string of concentrically arranged macrophages. Blood cells coming from an arteriole have to pass through the sheathed capillary on their way to the lumen of the sinus, which they reach by slowly percolating through the cord macrophages and red pulp stroma (open circulation), and then via the slits in the basement membrane of the sinus (3,27). Although no direct anatomic connection between the arteriolar ends and the sinuses has been demonstrated, a proportion of the arteriolar branches may end in close opposition to walls of the sinuses, allowing a more rapid circulation (close circulation) of at least a portion of the blood flow. The red pulp sinuses are considered as the first part of the splenic venous tree.

The localization of the sheathed capillaries at the end of the arterial tree seem perfect for their functioning as a filtering unit.

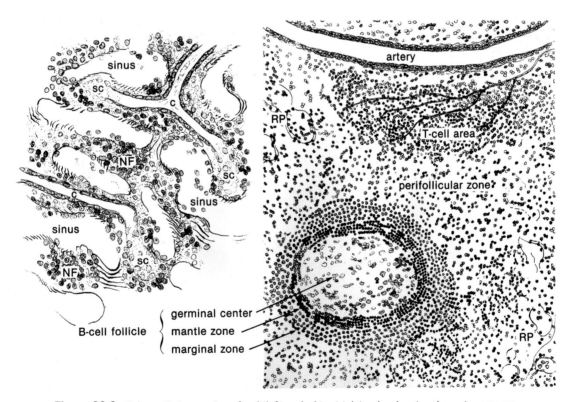

Figure 32.2 Schematic impression of red (*left*) and white (*right*) pulp, showing the main compartments and structures of the human spleen. The capillaries (*c*) end as sheathed capillaries (*sc*) without direct communication with the sinuses. The nonfiltering areas (*NF*) are bordered by sinuses and are devoid of (sheathed) capillaries. The perifollicular zone surrounds the white pulp (follicle and T-cell area) and lacks fully developed sinuses. Note the zoning in the B-cell but not in the T-cell compartment. The T-cell area contains a lymphatic plexus. (*Left*, original magnification ×250; *right*, original magnification ×100.)

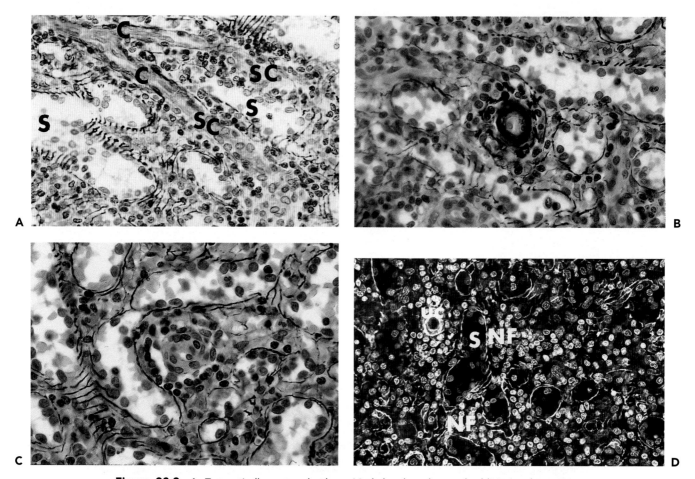

Figure 32.3 **A.** Traumatically ruptured spleen. Methylmethacrylate embedding (methenamine-silver/H&E, original magnification ×400). Capillary transitioning into sheathed capillary. Note the proximity to, but lack of connection with, the sinuses. (*C*, capillary (unsheathed); *SC*, sheathed capillary; *S*, sinus) **B.** Same specimen as in A (original magnification ×1000). Detail of unsheathed capillary. **C.** Same specimen as in A (original magnification ×1000). Detail of sheathed capillary. **D.** Same specimen as in A (original magnification ×250). Detail of the red pulp showing sinuses in cord tissue. Note the nonfiltering areas devoid of capillaries and completely surrounded by sinuses. (*Uc*, unsheathed capillary; *S*, sinus; *NF*, nonfiltering area)

Within the sinusoidal meshwork, there are large sinuses that open directly into veins running along the arteries in the collagenous cuff.

Small efferent lymph vessels can be found in the T-lymphocyte compartment of the white pulp in about two-thirds of the spleens. They are not seen in the surrounding perifollicular zone. A reconstruction from serial sections showed that these lymph vessels form a network around arterioles and eventually follow the arterial tree to the hilar region (9,28).

Red Pulp

Seventy-five percent of the volume of the spleen is made up of red pulp (26). The two-dimensional picture given by conventional histology sections suggests that the red pulp is largely composed of cordal macrophages, interconnected by their cytoplasmic processes to form a reticular meshwork that provides structural support to the venous sinuses. Serial sections have shown, however, that the red pulp contains also a loose reticular framework, is rich in capillaries, and contains the terminal ends of the penicillary arterioles (Figure 32.3D). The sinuses account for about 30% of the red pulp (26). The sinus endothelial cells are surrounded by almost circular strands of discontinuous basement membrane that is predominantly composed of collagen IV and laminin, known as the ring fibers (Figure 32.4). The ring fibers are both interconnected among themselves and anchored to the dendritic processes of the cordal macrophages and splenic (fibroblastic) reticulum cells. Stromal fibers and reticulum cells running throughout the red pulp cords also contribute to provide structural support to this splenic area (the reticular meshwork of the red pulp).

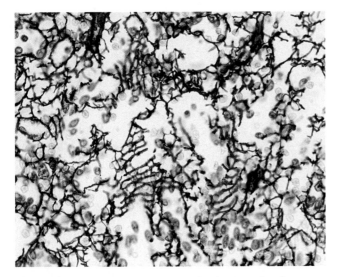

Figure 32.4 Normal spleen with red pulp stained with an antibody against collagen IV showing the ring fibers surrounding the sinuses (original magnification ×250).

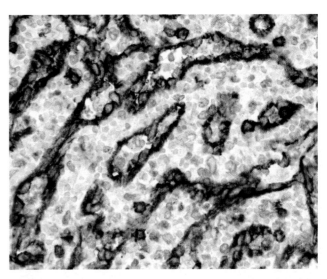

Figure 32.5 Normal spleen, red pulp stained with anti-CD8 showing the positive sinus endothelial cells (original magnification ×400).

A subpopulation of reticulum cells that express nerve growth factor receptor is found predominantly in periarteriolar location (29). These cells, most likely representing adventitial reticulum cells similar to those present in the adventitia of blood vessels, also have been observed within the stroma of bone marrow and lymph nodes (30). Myoid reticulum cells (smooth muscle actin–positive, or SMA-positive) are found scattered throughout the red pulp. These cells are, however, much more concentrated within the marginal zone of the lymphoid follicles and in the PALS (31–33). Whether the SMA-positive red pulp cells correspond to fibroblastic reticulum cells that have undergone myofibroblastic differentiation, or are a truly separate population, is unclear at this time. The red pulp sinuses themselves form a complex network of their own with many interconnections and bulblike extensions with blind ends, the latter of which project into the cord tissue [see Figure 4 of van Krieken et al. (26)].

The sinuses are lined by elongated, flat endothelial cells with typical bean-shaped nuclei having a longitudinal cleft; these cells are also known as littoral cells. Immunoperoxidase studies have shown positivity for endothelial markers and, unique among other endothelial cells, to CD8 (Figure 32.5) and often CD68 and CD21. Parts of the endothelial lining react also with a monoclonal antibody that also immunostains high endothelial venules in the lymph node (van Krieken JHJM, unpublished observation).

The preponderant function of red pulp is blood filtration. However, in serial sections, one might notice that a fair amount of the red pulp tissue does not include capillary endings, including sheathed capillaries, and that these areas are surrounded only by sinuses. Small aggregates of lymphocytes (both B and T) and mononuclear phagocytes

are present (Figure 32.3), which means that these nonfiltering areas of the red pulp should be regarded as a previously unrecognized splenic lymphoid compartment in addition to the white pulp. Morphometrically, the size of this lymphoid, nonfiltering red pulp compartment seems to be comparable to that of the white pulp (26). Newly formed white pulp follicles might originate from the small lymphoid aggregates of these nonfiltering areas.

Blood cells can only reach these areas by passing through large stretches of red pulp tissue or, which seems more likely, via influx from the sinus by passing through the sinus endothelium. A retrograde return of lymphocytes from the venous sinus lumen back into the splenic tissue is known for the rat spleen, where lymphocytes migrate through the walls of what is called the marginal sinus into the white pulp. This type of sinus is histologically not discernable in the white pulp of the human spleen. In humans, the role played in the rat by the marginal sinus in the exchange of lymphocytes between the sinusoidal circulation and the splenic lymphoid compartment might be played by the previously described blind-ended bulblike extensions of the red pulp sinuses, representing a splenic endothelial component with high endothelial venulelike characteristics. This hypothesis is supported by the observation that, in humans, splenic follicles are surrounded by a perifollicular zone, a distinct splenic compartment containing erythrocyte-filled vascular spaces. The perifollicular zone sinuses differ from the typical red pulp sinuses in their enhanced expression of CD34. Recent evidence has suggested that this zone may represent the entry compartment for recirculating lymphocytes into the white pulp since it is capable of supporting influx and local proliferation of lymphoreticular cells, particularly CD4-positive T lymphocytes

(33). It has been recently suggested that the entry of these cells may be dependent on the presence in the perifollicular area of specialized reticulum cells with an endothelial-like phenotype secreting lymphokines and guiding the T cells into the PALS (33).

White Pulp

The white pulp consists of B- and T-cell lymphoid compartments (11) (Figure 32.1). The B-cell compartment mainly consists of the splenic lymphoid follicles. These are composed of a germinal center (only found in secondary follicles) directly surrounded by a ring of small lymphocytes, called the mantle zone or corona, which in turn is surrounded by the marginal zone that contains medium-sized lymphocytes (Figure 32.6). The germinal centers have similar features to those found in other lymphoid organs. They are formed by a scaffold of follicular dendritic cells that express CD21, CD23, CD35, and the low-affinity nerve growth factor receptor. The B cells of the germinal centers express CD20, CD19, CD10, and CD79a but not CD5. They have a high proliferation activity with Ki-67 and do not express Bcl-2. The T lymphocytes present within germinal centers are predominantly CD4-positive; tingible-body macrophages are CD68-positive. Mantle zones consist predominantly of CD5-positive small lymphocytes that are IgM-, IgD-, Ki-B3–, and DBA.44-positive and alkaline phosphatase–negative (Figure 32.7). The marginal zone lymphocytes are, in contrast, positive with alkaline phosphatase and are IgD-, Ki-B3–, and DBA.44-negative (34). The marginal zone also contains a population of macrophages that are functionally distinct from the cord histiocytes of the red pulp, which, at

least in animal models, seem to be important in maintaining the anatomic structure of the marginal zone by attracting newly differentiated marginal zone B lymphocytes into it. These cells move into the marginal zone area from the germinal center, where they derive from a common follicular/marginal zone precursor B cell (35).

The reticulin framework of the marginal zone is characterized by the presence of numerous SMA-positive reticulum cells arranged in a concentric meshwork pattern. The marginal zone SMA-positive cells continue into the T-cell zones, where reticulum cells, exhibiting the same immunophenotype, form the reticular framework of the PALS. Cells with SMA positivity are also seen, although less frequently, in the perifollicular zone and throughout the red pulp. These cells become more prominent in the presence of red pulp congestion, such as seen in cases of fibrocongestive splenomegaly (Figure 32.8) (29,36). Contractile capability may be important for a scaffoldlike reticular structure capable of being reversibly stretched around lymphoid follicles as they expand and contract within the PALS.

In the rat spleen, the mantle and marginal zones are separated by a marginal sinus that can easily be seen by light microscopic examination. It plays an essential role in the splenic immune function as the site of entry of lymphocytes and antigens (37). This dividing sinus is not discernible in humans, at least by light microscopy. Recently, by using electron microscopy, a marginal sinuslike structure was described (38), although, surprisingly, it seems to be absent in active follicles (39). However, neither the exact location nor functional properties of this structure are known.

The light microscopic differences with rodent spleens has led to confusion in the definition of follicular structures

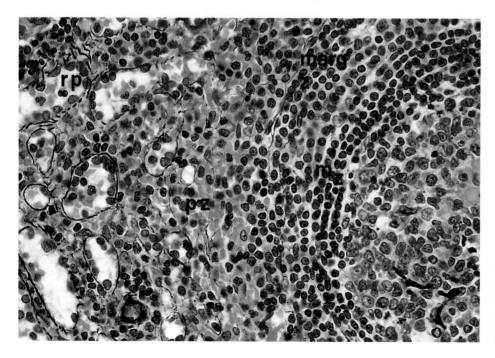

Figure 32.6 Same specimen as in Figure 32.3. A secondary follicle (germinal center to the right) borders the red pulp. (*mz*, mantle zone; *margz*, marginal zone; *pz*, perifollicular zone; *rp*, red pulp; original magnification ×100)

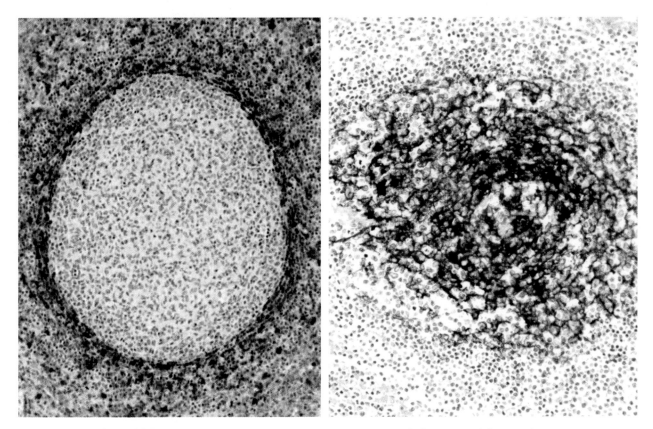

Figure 32.7 Normal spleen showing the positive mantle zone cells for DBA.44 (*left*, original magnification ×40) and the dendritic cells stained for CD21 (*right*, original magnification ×40).

of the human spleen. The term *marginal zone* has been used with different meanings (11,40–42). Some investigators use the term to refer to the ring of medium-sized lymphocytes that surrounds the outer border of the mantle zone; few others have included the mantle zone, still others only the

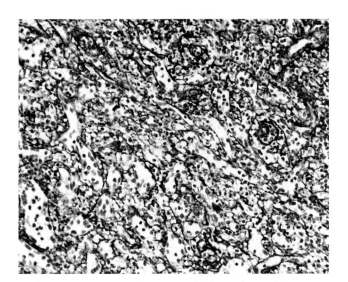

Figure 32.8 Spleen in fibrocongestive splenomegaly showing increased expression for smooth muscle actin (original magnification ×100).

bordering area between the red and white pulp, and sometimes even the zone surrounding the T-cell areas (PALS). We prefer to reserve the term *marginal zone* for the unique splenic structure that encases from the outside the IgD- and IgM-positive small lymphocytes of the mantle zone (in the secondary follicle) or of the primary follicle. We refer to the bordering area between the red and white pulp as the perifollicular zone. The same definitions are used in the extensive Japanese literature on the histology of the human spleen. However, the Japanese investigators call our marginal zone the inner marginal zone and refer to the perifollicular zone as the outer marginal zone. Because of the totally different architecture and cell population of these two structures, we find it preferable to use different names.

The T-cell areas lie around arterioles but are not as regularly arranged as in the PALS seen in the rodent spleen (Figure 32.9). The arterioles are not constantly covered by these cylindrical lymphoid cuffs; they can be seen "naked" traversing follicles and even germinal centers.

In humans, the PALS are rather irregular aggregates of small polymorphic T lymphocytes, most of which express CD4 reactivity (T-helper/inducer lymphocytes). The T-cell areas are also surrounded by a perifollicular-like zone. The follicles sometimes border T-cell areas, with which they share a common perifollicular zone.

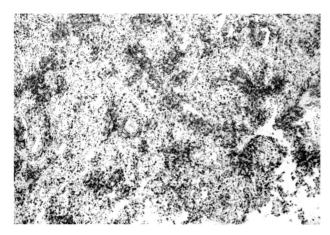

Figure 32.9 Normal spleen stained with anti-CD3 antibody (original magnification ×40) showing the somewhat loosely organized T-cell compartment.

Perifollicular Zone

The perifollicular zone (PFZ) is a specialized compartment of the red pulp that is associated with its own reticular stroma; PFZ is found both at the outside of the white pulp marginal zone (in the follicles) and at the periphery of the T-cell areas (PALS). In the PFZ, the reticular fibers are more widely spaced than in the rest of the red pulp (Figures 32.2 and 32.6). In silver-stained plastic sections, the PFZ can be identified by the paucity of basal membrane strands and by the presence of a vascular pattern that is different from the one seen in the rest of the red pulp. At the outer border of this area, red pulp sinuses are more widely spaced than elsewhere, and a rich network of capillaries, including sheathed capillaries, is present. The PFZ contains a considerable numbers of erythrocytes and leukocytes.

The PFZ zone at the outside of the white pulp stands out in silver-stained sections but may be poorly visible in routine hematoxylin- and eosin (H&E)-stained sections. However, since the PFZ contains a large number of erythrocytes, it can be recognized by its deeply congested appearance around the densely packed lymphocytes of the T- and B-cell areas (Figure 32.1A). The erythrocytes are seen more regularly in PFZ than in the red pulp sinuses; the red pulp sinuses outside the PFZ often appear to be less filled with these cells than the cord tissue.

The PFZ, which makes up about 8% of the spleen, contains a mixture of blood cells comparable with that of the peripheral blood. It has been suggested that this area is responsible for the passage of the about 10% of the splenic blood, which is known to have a retarded flow (11).

FLOW CYTOMETRY

The spleen has been only rarely investigated by flow cytometry. Recently, we have looked at the immunophenotypic characteristics of the human spleen lymphocytes and have established reference values for those cells in normal and reactive spleens (43). Altough the results obtained showed B- and T-antigen patterns of expression comparable to those seen in other lymphoid organs, a few differences were noted (Table 32.2). In contrast to the thymus and bone marrow, the spleen contains only very rare Tdt-positive lymphoid precursors. Within the Bcell subsets, the spleen shows a frequency of CD19-positive/CD20-negative B cells that is higher than in the peripheral blood or lymph node. This corresponds to the presence, in the spleen, of a sizable proportion of early plasma cells (CD138-negative) as well as more mature plasma cells. Other findings included a significant population of CD20/CD5–positive B cells, accounting for approximately 10% of the B lymphocytes; the presence of CD4/CD8 ratio of 1.2:1 (lower than in the blood but similar to the one seen in lymph node) and a mean number of γ/δ-positive T cells (of all CD3-positive cells) of 6% in normal and 10% in reactive spleens. While in the peripheral blood, NK/T cells account for less than 6% of the CD3-positive circulating lymphocytes, our study showed a relatively high frequency of these cells in the spleen. Similar results have been observed in the liver by others and support the concept that spleen and liver lymphocytes have specific, although yet unknown, immunoregulatory functions (43).

ULTRASTRUCTURE

Electron microscopy (especially scanning electron microscopy), including the use of microcasts from the vasculature, has elucidated largely the functional microanatomy of the spleen. These studies have shown the routes that blood cells take through the spleen and have also clearly illustrated the pitting function of the spleen (removal of inclusions in erythrocytes) exerted by the sinusoids. In spleen examined in a diagnostic-oriented setting, however, there is hardly if ever the necessity of using ultrastructural studies.

FUNCTION

The human spleen has several important functions. However, splenectomy in general does not lead to impaired health, except for an increased risk of overwhelming postsplenectomy infections caused by encapsulated bacteria (e.g., pneumococci). The reason for this is that many functions of the spleen, at least in adults, can be taken over by other organs.

In humans, the spleen is involved in the primary immune response to bloodborne antigens and polysaccharide antigens; it also acts as a regulator of immune reactions elsewhere in the body. It contains a specific environment that facilitates the binding of antibodies and antigens; cells or microorganisms covered by antibodies are trapped and destroyed in the spleen, as are erythrocytes that have decreased flexibility and lowered osmotic resistance

TABLE 32.2
EXPRESSION OF SURFACE AND INTRACELLULAR MARKERS BY HUMAN SPLEEN LYMPHOCYTES

Cell Marker	Normal (cadaveric) Spleen		Reactive (nonmalignant) Spleen		
	N	Mean ± s.d. (%)	N	Mean ± s.d.(%)	P-value[a]
CD2	14	38±10	12	50±14	0.015
CD3		31±9		43±14	0.009
CD4		17±8		23±7	NS
CD5		32±8		42±13	0.028
CD7		37±11		44±12	NS
CD8		14±5		19±7	0.028
CD4/CD8 ratio		1.2±3		1.2±0.2	NS
CD10		1±1		1±1	NS
CD11c		28±10		25±10	NS
CD13		1±1		1±1	NS
CD16/56+CD3−		15±7		12±5	NS
CD16/56+CD3+		5±2		5±4	NS
CD19		55±11		45±14	0.04
CD20		49±9		42±12	NS
CD20+CD5+		8±6		11±7	NS
CD23		34±13		35±12	NS
CD30		1±1		1±1	NS
CD34		2±2		2±1	NS
CD38		79±13		83±12	NS
CD103		2±1		2±1	NS
cy CD79a		52±12		44±10	NS
HLA-DR		71±11		71±12	NS
IgM		42±14		40±17	NS
IgG		5±5		3±2	NS
IgA		9±7		6±2	NS
IgD		36±12		35±12	NS
FMC7		38±13		30±10	NS
Kappa (κ)		28±5		25±8	NS
Lambda (λ)		21±5		17±6	NS
Kappa/Lambda (κ/λ)		1.3±0.2		1.4±0.2	NS
cy Kappa (cy κ)		31±6		29±8	NS
cy Lambda (cy λ)		22±5		16±6	NS
cy TdT		<1		<1	NS
TCR alpha/beta (TCR α/β)		29±9		37±12	NS
TCR gamma/delta (TCR γ/δ)		2±2		5±1	NS

[a] NS, not significant ($P>0.05$).

(1,44–50). Each of these functions takes place in a specific splenic compartment, which is capable of undergoing rapid changes in its size and composition, even under physiologic conditions. Therefore, the main splenic functions to be considered include blood filtering, immunologic function, hematopoiesis, and reservoir.

Filter Function

The location and specialized anatomy of the spleen is especially suitable for its function as a filter of the blood. Normal blood cells are capable of traversing the barrier of macrophages of the sheathed capillary, the red pulp cord macrophages, and the sinus endothelium (collectively, the filtering unit of the spleen) at a speed comparable to that of the blood in the capillary bed of other organs. However, in cases in which the flexibility of the red blood cell is diminished (e.g., by aging, intoxication, or congenital defects), the macrophages of the splenic filtering unit can eliminate the abnormal cell by ingesting it. The filtering function includes a process known as pitting, a term which is used to describe the removal of inclusions, such as nuclear remnants known as Howell-Jolly (H-J) bodies, from erythrocytes without destroying the cell. The presence of H-J bodies in circulating erythrocytes in the peripheral blood indicates the presence of splenic hypofunction (e.g., splenectomized patients).

In addition to red blood cells, the macrophages of the spleen can readily take up bacteria, antigens, and immune complexes. The spleen is capable of filtering out reticulocytes, platelets, hematopoietic stem cells, lymphocytes, and dendritic cells from the blood and provides the proper microambient conditions for their further differentiation. Also, it sequesters monocytes from the blood and facilitates their transformation into splenic macrophages (8).

Immunologic Function

The spleen plays a more important role in the development of the immune system, but even in adults the spleen is still involved in B- and T-lymphocyte production and differentiation. The spleen receives B and T cells from the recirculating lymphocyte pool and sorts them into dedicated compartments such as the follicles and the PALS, where they can interact with antigens and antigen-presenting cells and become capable of mounting effective immune responses.

The marginal zone is a component of the B-cell follicle and is a remarkably larger compartment in the spleen than elsewhere (e.g., tonsils). Although the exact physiologic function(s) of the marginal zone is still unclear (42), its main immunologic role relates to the thymus-independent rapid response to bloodborne microorganisms; since these are rapidly trapped in the spleen and brought directly into contact with numerous immunocompetent cells, the spleen is well situated for this task.

Hematopoiesis

In rodents, the spleen has a large hematopoietic function, but this is not the case in humans. As described above, the hematopoietic function is only present in the fetal spleen; in the adult spleen, hematopoiesis does not occur (15). Hematopoietic cells encountered in the adult spleen originate from circulating, marrow-derived, progenitors/early precursors that become entrapped in the spleen and are capable of undergoing further differentiation. When this "physiologic" phenomenon reaches pathologic relevance by causing splenomegaly, it is termed splenic myeloid metaplasia or extramedullary hematopoiesis. Although splenic myeloid metaplasia can be seen in many different conditions, the most striking examples of this condition can be observed in patients with chronic idiopathic myelofibrosis (15).

Reservoir Function

The human spleen contains about 300 mL of blood. This is a relatively small amount, in contrast to that seen in a dog or cat. In these animals, the spleen functions as an important blood reservoir; and in situations where more blood is needed, its rapid contraction can increase substantially the amount of circulating blood cells. It is highly doubtful that this function occurs at all in humans, whose splenic capsule lacks a significant component of smooth muscle fibers. The spleen, however, does function as a reservoir for factor VIII of the clotting system, platelets, granulocytes, and iron.

AGING DIFFERENCES

In infancy and childhood, the immune system is not yet fully developed, and this is also reflected in the histology of the spleen. The marginal zone is observed as a separate compartment only after four months of age; moreover, the marginal zone B cells in the spleen of infants have a different phenotype (lack CD21; IgD- and IgM-positive) compared with adult marginal zone B cells (51). An important age difference, in our experience, is the regular occurrence of germinal centers in the white pulp of normal spleens in patients younger than 20 years; older patients have been shown to have only rare secondary follicles (9). The often mentioned age-dependent atrophic change has only been documented in patients in their eighth decade of life (11).

Hyalinization of vessels in the spleen is seen frequently, even in very young children and, therefore, does not represent a pathologic finding (52).

DIFFERENTIAL DIAGNOSIS

In the spleen, compartmentalized lymphoid tissue (white pulp) is interwoven by the filtering red pulp. Each splenic compartment reacts to external stimuli with physiologic changes in its composition and histology. As in the lymph node, the line between pathologic and impressive but essential physiologic reactions is vague. The amount of white pulp, for instance, varied from 5 to 22% of the total splenic tissue in a normal control group (11).

As previously mentioned, normal blood cells can pass undamaged through the barrier of macrophages of the sheathed capillary and the red pulp cord tissue as well as the sinus endothelium (i.e., the filtering unit of the spleen) at a speed comparable with that of the blood flow in the capillary bed of other organs. However, when the flexibility of the blood cells is diminished (e.g., by aging, intoxication, or congenital defects), the red pulp macrophages can ingest the abnormal cells. In this process, the sheathed capillaries seem to lose their macrophages, which spread out into the surrounding red pulp or enter the sinuses to be transported to the liver. In cases characterized by chronic stimulation of the filtering function, it can be demonstrated that the amount and length of the capillaries increase in parallel with the hypertrophy of the red pulp, whereas the sheathed capillaries are less readily seen in the sections (26). In idiopathic thrombocytopenic purpura (ITP), remnants of phagocytosed thrombocytes can be seen as periodic acid-Schiff (PAS)-positive fragments in cord macrophages. If blood cells are covered by immunoglobulins or immuno-complexes, parts of the cell membrane can be removed by the sinus endothelium by "pitting and culling," giving rise to a spherocyte. This happens in a fashion similar to the removal of nuclear remnants, as previously described (15).

In septicemia, the filtering compartment may show morphologic findings (activation and hyperplasia of macrophages) indistinguishable from those seen in cases of acute or chronic hemolysis; these changes are most likely induced by the presence of circulating immunocomplexes, fragmented cells, or antibody-coated cells. In these conditions, postmortem autolysis of the activated macrophages can lead to early disintegration of the red pulp cells and stroma. The septic spleen at autopsy thus probably represents an artifact that can be the result of, but is not specific for, sepsis; it, especially, should not be diagnosed as splenitis. True splenitis, in which the spleen contains an inflammatory response to a local noxious agent such as in typhoid fever or tropical diseases, is rare in the Western hemisphere. Lymphoplasmacytoid cells and plasma cells normally rim arteries and arterioles and extend along red pulp capillaries. This perivascular cellular rim also may contain some macrophages or small epithelioid granulomas, the significance of which is unclear. The perivascular presence of plasma is a normal finding and by no means justifies a diagnosis of splenitis, nor does the diffuse influx of granulocytes throughout the red pulp in specimens resected during prolonged surgery.

The effects of chronic venous congestion are not clear. In our preliminary studies in patients dying with chronic cardiac disease, the so-called effect of chronic cardiac congestion on the lymphoid and filtering compartments appears more likely to be the effect of concomitant infections or is therapy mediated. In chronic venous congestion due to portal hypertension, the sinuses are normal in size but contain fewer buds and appear rigid. The amount of cord tissue and the number of capillaries are both decreased; in the cord tissue, an increase of reticular fibers (fibrocongestive splenomegaly) and increased expression of smooth muscle actin in reticulum cells is seen (26,36). Infarcts in the splenic tissue are microscopically more irregularly defined and poorly demarcated than could be expected macroscopically due to the intricate distribution of the splenic vessels. In three-dimensional reconstructions, capillaries from different arterioles are seen to cross each other with overlapping territories.

Primary tumors of the spleen are rare. Metastatic carcinoma seems especially to occur in neuroendocrine tumors, including small cell carcinoma of the lung, with a conspicuous tendency for intrasinusoidal spread. Malignant lymphomas exhibit a homing pattern to specific splenic compartments dependent on the type of lymphoma, similar to that observed in other lymphoid organs (21). In non-lymphomatous hematopoietic malignancies involving the spleen, their distribution pattern is similar to that observed in the bone marrow: extramedullary erythropoiesis and megakaryopoiesis are found primarily along and within the sinuses of the red pulp, whereas myelomonopoiesis is found in proximity of the capillaries within the cord tissue. Blastic infiltration seen in cases of acute leukemia can be found anywhere in the spleen.

SPECIMEN HANDLING

The spleen is quite vulnerable and, due to the large numbers of macrophages and granulocytes, may undergo rapid autolysis. Proper and rapid fixation is therefore important, and this goal is not reached when the entire organ is put into formalin. For proper handling, the specimen has to be received fresh, and handling has to be rapid. The organ is weighed and the surface examined. After that, the organ is cut into small slices of 0.5 cm. Then the cut surface is inspected carefully for nodules larger than normal white pulp. Ideally pieces should be frozen for flow cytometry, cryostat section immunohistochemistry, or other techniques. When no abnormalities are seen, at least three or four blocks are taken out randomly and processed for microscopic examination.

HISTOLOGIC TECHNIQUE

Routine paraffin embedding leads to shrinkage and loss of cellular detail. Because routine H&E staining often does not yield sufficient information, the use of appropriate histology techniques, such as plastic embedding (53), methenamine-silver/H&E stain (54), or at least, PAS and Gomori's reticulin stains, is necessary for an adequate morphologic analysis of the splenic microarchitecture (Figure 32.10).

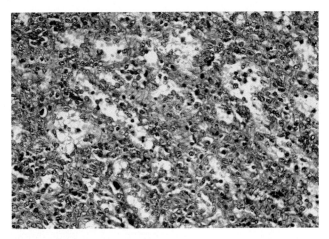

Figure 32.10 Same specimen as in Figure 32.1. Detail of red pulp showing with some difficulty the structure of the sinuses (PAS stain, paraffin-embedded, original magnification ×200).

SPECIAL PROCEDURES

The spleen is only rarely removed for diagnostic purposes. Staging laparotomy is no longer part of the required diagnostic workup of a patient with Hodgkin's disease. Therefore, splenic pathology may be seen as an unsuspected incidental finding in a patient splenectomized for other reasons (e.g., chronic idiopathic thrombocytopenia, trauma). Not uncommonly, splenic lymphoma may be discovered as an incidental finding. A high degree of suspiciousness of the grossing pathologist is necessary in these case since, for optimal lymphoma diagnosis, it is often necessary to apply techniques that require fresh/frozen tissue, such as flow cytometry, frozen tissue immunohistochemistry, molecular analysis, and/or cytogenetics (Figure 32.8).

In view of the frequent lack of fresh specimens, clonality assessment in a spleen is usually done by immunohistochemistry applied to paraffin-embedded tissue, looking for a restricted pattern of immunoglobulin light chain expression in B cells. This is one of the most important "special techniques" used in routine diagnostic laboratories. In addition, clonality can also be established by using a polymerase chain reaction–based technique for detecting immunoglobulin gene rearrangement, which can also be succesfully applied to paraffin-embedded tissue (55).

Immunohistochemistry can also be necessary to characterize other hematopoietic and nonhematopoietic tumors, the latter primary or metastatic, which can occur (although infrequently) in the spleen. In storage disorders such as Gaucher's disease, electron microscopy can be of additional value, although biochemical analysis is considered by most experts as the most practical and specific approach.

CONCLUSION

The human spleen has always been a somewhat enigmatic organ. Studies of its histology must be based on carefully selected, surgically excised "normal" spleens. The organ should be processed immediately and appropriately for optimal results.

Previous studies by one of us of a large series of spleens with adequate histologic techniques and with reconstruction based on serial sections has shown that the spleen is a highly compartmentalized organ (Table 32.1). Each compartment has its own structure and cell populations and often a separate function. The old division into red and white pulp is probably oversimplified and should be expanded.

Human and animal spleens are different in many important structural aspects; data extrapolation from animal studies to humans is therefore problematic and often unwarranted.

REFERENCES

1. Crosby WH. The spleen. In: Wintrobe MM, ed. *Blood, Pure and Eloquent.* New York: McGraw-Hill; 1980:96–138.
2. Chen L, Weiss L. Electron microscopy of the red pulp of human spleen. *Am J Anat* 1972;134:425–458.
3. Weiss L. The spleen. In: Greep RO, Weiss L, eds. *Histology.* 3rd ed. New York: McGraw-Hill; 1973:545–573.
4. Nieuwenhuis P, Keuning FJ. Germinal centres and the origin of the B-cell system. II. Germinal centres in the rabbit spleen and popliteal lymph nodes. *Immunology* 1974;26:509–519.
5. Nieuwenhuis P, Ford WL. Comparative migration of B- and T-lymphocytes in the rat spleen and lymph nodes. *Cell Immunol* 1976;23:254–267.
6. Ford WL. Lymphocyte migration and immune responses. *Prog Allergy* 1975;19:1–59.
7. Veerman AJ, van Ewijk W. White pulp compartments in the spleen of rats and mice. A light and electron microscopic study of lymphoid and non-lymphoid celltypes in T- and B-areas. *Cell Tissue Res* 1975;156:417–441.
8. Weiss L. The spleen. In: Weiss L, ed. *Cell and Tissue Biology: A Textbook of Histology.* 6th ed. Baltimore: Urban & Schwarzenberg; 1988:517–538.
9. van Krieken JH, te Velde J, Kleiverda K, Leenheers-Binnendijk L, van de Velde CJ. The human spleen: a histological study in splenectomy specimens embedded in methylmethacrylate. *Histopathology* 1985;9:571–585.
10. Scothorne RJ. The spleen: structure and function. *Histopathology* 1985;9:663–669.
11. van Krieken JH, te Velde J, Hermans J, Cornelisse CJ, Welvaart K, Ferrari M. The amount of white pulp in the spleen: a morphometrical study done in methacrylate-embedded splenectomy specimens. *Histopathology* 1983;7:767–782.
12. van Krieken JHJM. *The architecture of the human spleen.* Academic thesis. Pijnacker, The Netherlands: Dutch Efficiency Bureau; 1985.
13. van Krieken JH, te Velde J. Immunohistology of the human spleen: an inventory of the localization of lymphocyte subpopulations. *Histopathology* 1986;10:285–294.
14. Wolf BC, Luevano E, Neiman RS. Evidence to suggest that the human fetal spleen is not a hematopoietic organ. *Am J Clin Pathol* 1983;80:140–144.
15. Neiman RS, Orazi A. *Disorders of the Spleen.* 2nd ed. Philadelphia: WB Saunders; 1999.
16. Timens W, Rozeboom T, Poppema S. Fetal and neonatal development of human spleen: an immunohistological study. *Immunology* 1987;60:603–609.
17. Jones JF. Development of the spleen. *Lymphology* 1983;16:83–89.
18. Namikawa R, Mizuno T, Matsuoka H, et al. Ontogenic development of T and B cells and non-lymphoid cells in the white pulp of human spleen. *Immunology* 1986;57:61–69.
19. Moller JH, Nakib A, Anderson RC, Edwards JE. Congenital cardiac disease associated with polysplenia. A developmental complex of bilateral "left-sidedness." *Circulation* 1967;36:789–799.
20. Myers J, Segal RJ. Weight of the spleen. I. Range of normal in a nonhospital population. *Arch Pathol* 1974;98:33–35.
21. van Krieken JH, Feller AC, te Velde J. The distribution of non-Hodgkin's lymphoma in the lymphoid compartments of the human spleen. *Am J Surg Pathol* 1989;13:757–765.
22. Seufert RM. *Chirurgie der Milz.* Stuttgart, Germany: Enke-Verlag; 1983.
23. Tischendorf F. *Blutgefäss und Lympfgefässapparat Innersekretorische Drusen. Die Milz.* Berlin: Springer-Verlag; 1969.
24. Snook T. A comparative study of the vascular arrangements in mammalian spleens. *Am J Anat* 1950;87:31–77.
25. Buyssens N, Paulus G, Bourgeois N. Ellipsoids in the human spleen. *Virchows Arch A Pathol Anat Histopathol* 1984;403:27–40.
26. van Krieken JH, te Velde J, Hermans J, Welvaart K. The splenic red pulp: a histomorphometrical study in splenectomy specimens embedded in methylmethacrylate. *Histopathology* 1985;9:401–416.
27. Heusermann U, Stutte HJ. Comparative histochemical and electron microscopic studies of the sinus and venous walls of the

human spleen with special reference to the sinus–venous connections. *Cell Tissue Res* 1975;163:519–533.

28. Fukuda T. Deep lymphatics of the spleen. *Tohoku J Exp Med* 1963;79:281–292.

29. Orazi A, O'Malley DP, Thomas JL, Czader M. Stromal changes in reactive and malignant disorders of the spleen. *Mod Pathol* 2004;17:264A.

30. Cattoretti G, Schiro R, Orazi A, Soligo D, Colombo MP. Bone marrow stroma in humans: anti-nerve growth factor receptor antibodies selectively stain reticular cells in vivo and in vitro. *Blood* 1993;81:1726–38.

31. Pinkus GS, Warhol MJ, O'Connor EM, Etheridge CL, Fujiwara K. Immunohistochemical localization of smooth muscle myosin in human spleen, lymph node, and other lymphoid tissues. Unique staining patterns in splenic white pulp and sinuses, lymphoid follicles, and certain vasculature, with ultrastructural correlations. *Am J Pathol* 1986;123:440–453.

32. Toccanier-Pelte MF, Skalli O, Kapanci Y, Gabbiani G. Characterization of stromal cells with myoid features in lymph nodes and spleen in normal and pathologic conditions. *Am J Pathol* 1987;129:109–118.

33. Steiniger B, Barth P, Hellinger A. The perifollicular and marginal zones of the human splenic white pulp: do fibroblasts guide lymphocyte immigration? *Am J Pathol* 2001;159:501–512.

34. van Krieken JH, von Schilling C, Kluin PM, Lennert K. Splenic marginal zone lymphocytes and related cells in the lymph node: a morphologic and immunohistochemical study. *Hum Pathol* 1989;20:320–325.

35. Pillai S, Cariappa A, Moran ST. Marginal Zone B lymphocytes. *Annu Rev Immunol* 2005;23:161–196.

36. Kraus MD. Splenic histology and histopathology: an update. *Semin Diagn Pathol* 2003;20:84–93.

37. Sasou S, Satodate R, Katsura S. The marginal sinus in the perifollicular region of the rat spleen. *Cell Tissue Res* 1976;172:195–203.

38. Schmidt EE, MacDonald IC, Groom AC. Microcirculatory pathways in normal human spleen, demonstrated by scanning electron microscopy of corrosion casts. *Am J Anat* 1988;181:253–266.

39. Schmidt EE, MacDonald IC, Groom AC. Changes in splenic microcirculatory pathways in chronic idiopathic thrombocytopenic purpura. *Blood* 1991;78:1485–1489.

40. Takasaki S. Light microscopic, scanning and transmission electron microscopic, and enzyme histochemical observations on the boundary zone between the red pulp and its surroundings in human spleens. *Tokyo Yikekai Med J* 1979;94:553–568.

41. Yamamoto K, Arimasa N, Yamamoto T, Tokuyama K, Kobayashi T, Itoshima T. Scanning electron microscopy of the perimarginal cavernous sinus plexus of the human spleen. *Scan Electron Microsc* 1979;3:763–768.

42. Kraal G. Cells in the marginal zone of the spleen. *Int Rec Cytol* 1992;132:31–74.

43. Colovai AI, Giatzikis C, Ho EK, et al. Flow cytometric analysis of normal and reactive spleen. *Mod Pathol* 2004;17:918–927.

44. Koyama S, Aoki S, Deguchi D. Electron microscopic observations of the splenic red pulp with special reference to the pitting function. *Mie Med J* 1964;14:143–188.

45. Sampson D, Grotelueschen C, Kauffman HM Jr. The human splenic suppressor cell. *Transplantation* 1975;20:362–367.

46. Videbaok A, Christensen BE, Jonsson V. *The Spleen in Health and Disease.* Chicago: Year Book Medical; 1983.

47. Wyler DJ. The spleen in malaria. In: Evered D, Whelan J, eds. *Malaria and the Red Cell.* London: Pitman; 1983.

48. Van Krieken JH, Breedveld FC, te Velde J. The spleen in Felty's syndrome: a histological, morphometrical, and immunohistochemical study. *Eur J Haematol* 1988;40:58–64.

49. Claassen E. Histological organization of the spleen: implications for immune functions of the spleen (38th forum in immunology). *Res Immunol* 1991;142:315–372.

50. van Rooijen N, Claassen E, Kraal G, Dijkstra C. Cytological basis of immune functions of the spleen. Immunocytochemical characterization of lymphoid and non-lymphoid cells involved in the "in situ" immune response. *Prog Histochem Cytochem* 1989; 19:1–71.

51. Timens W, Boes A, Rozeboom-Uiterwijk T, Poppema S. Immaturity of the human splenic marginal zone in infancy. Possible contribution to the deficient infant immune response. *J Immunol* 1989;143:3200–3206.

52. Lindley RP. Splenic arteriolar hyalin in children. *J Pathol* 1986; 148:321–325.

53. te Velde J, Burkhardt R, Kleiverda K, Leenheers-Binnendijk L, Sommerfeld W. Methyl-methacrylate as an embedding medium in histopathology. *Histopathology* 1977;1:319–330.

54. Jones DB. Nephrotic glomerulonephritis. *Am J Pathol* 1957;33: 313–329.

55. van Dongen JJ, Langerak AW, Bruggemann M, et al. Design and standardization of PCR primers and protocols for detection of clonal immunoglobulin and T-cell receptor gene recombinations in suspect lymphoproliferations: report of the BIOMED-2 Concerted Action BMH4-CT98-3936. *Leukemia* 2003;17:2257–2317.

Bone Marrow

S. N. Wickramasinghe

INTRODUCTION

The bone marrow is a large and complex organ that is distributed throughout the cavities of the skeleton. The total mass of the bone marrow of an adult has been estimated to be 1600 to 3700 g, exceeding that of the liver. About half this mass consists of hematopoietically inactive fatty marrow (which appears yellow) and the remainder of hematopoietically active marrow (which appears red). Although essentially hematopoietically inactive, even fatty marrow contains a few scattered microscopic foci of hematopoietic cells. The functions of hematopoietic marrow include: (a) the formation and release of various types of blood cells (hematopoiesis),

mast cells, osteoclasts and some endothelial progenitor cells; (b) the phagocytosis and degradation of circulating particulate material such as microorganisms and abnormal or senescent red cells and leukocytes; and (c) antibody production. Recent studies indicate that, in addition to hematopoietic stem cells, the marrow contains mesenchymal stem cells that can differentiate under appropriate conditions into adipocytes, hepatocytes, osteoblasts and osteocytes, chondrocytes, skeletal and cardiac muscle cells, kidney cells and neural cell lineages, but the interpretation of some of the data is still being debated (1). The nonhematopoietic marrow serves as a large store of reserve lipids. The various functions of hematopoietic marrow are based on a high degree of structural organization. However, this organization is labile, altering rapidly in response to many stimuli.

TECHNIQUES FOR STUDYING THE MARROW

The microscopic structure of the human bone marrow can be studied during life by performing a trephine biopsy of the posterior superior iliac spine or anterior iliac crest. This provides a core of bone and associated marrow. The biopsy specimen is commonly fixed in 10% neutral buffered formalin for 6 to 18 hr (depending on its width) but may be fixed in Zenker's solution for a minimum of 4 hr or in B5 (formalin and mercury chloride) for 4 hr. The fixed specimen is decalcified in 10% formic acid and 1% formalin or in one of a number of other decalcifying reagents. It is then processed in the usual manner and embedded in paraffin (2–4). Decalcification and paraffin embedding result in some shrinkage of marrow tissue, loss of the activity of cellular enzymes, and, sometimes, blurring of nuclear staining. In addition, certain decalcification procedures cause leaching of the iron stores (i.e., of the hemosiderin present within macrophages). However, the reactivity of some antigens with antibody is retained.

Histologic studies also can be performed on aspirated marrow. Two methods are in use. The first is to allow the marrow to clot before fixation and subsequent processing to paraffin. The clot sections obtained usually show only a few marrow fragments within a large mass of clotted blood. The second approach is to concentrate the marrow fragments by filtration or some other procedure before processing. This approach yields better preparations than do clot sections.

Sections of paraffin-embedded marrow fragments or decalcified bone cores are cut to a thickness of 3 to 5 μm and are routinely stained with hematoxylin and eosin (H&E), with the Giemsa's stain, by a silver impregnation technique for reticulin, and by Perls' acid ferrocyanide method for hemosiderin (Prussian blue reaction). They may also be stained by the periodic acid-Schiff (PAS) reaction for glycogen or glycoprotein. A Leder's stain for chloroacetate esterase may be performed on sections of marrow fragments but works poorly on decalcified specimens (2). A limited range of antibodies can be used for immunohistochemical studies on formalin- or B5-fixed, paraffin-embedded sections of trephine biopsy specimens, using an immunoalkaline phosphatase or immunoperoxidase method. The most useful antibodies and the cell types they recognize are given in Table 33.1 (5–11).

TABLE 33.1

SOME MONOCLONAL AND POLYCLONAL ANTIBODIES THAT CAN BE USED IN IMMUNOHISTOCHEMICAL STUDIES ON SECTIONS OF DECALCIFIED, PARAFFIN-EMBEDDED TREPHINE BIOPSIES OF THE MARROW

Antibody	Antigen	Cellular Specificity in Normal Tissue
Anti-CD34, QBEND10	CD34	Hematopoietic stem and progenitor cells, endothelial cells
Leu-M1	CD15	Neutrophil granulocyte series[a], monocytes
Antilysozyme	Lysozyme	Neutrophil granulocyte series[a], monoblasts, monocytes, macrophages
NP57	Neutrophil elastase	Neutrophil promyelocytes and myelocytes (strong), neutrophil metamyelocytes and granulocytes (weak), monocytes
Antimyeloperoxidase	Myeloperoxidase	Neutrophil granulocyte series[a]
Antilactoferrin	Lactoferrin	Neutrophil myelocytes to granulocytes
PG-M1, KP–1	CD68	Monocytes, macrophages
Antiglycophorin A or C	Glycophorin A or C	Erythroid series
Antihemoglobin A	Hemoglobin A	Erythroid series
Antifactor-VIII–related antigen	von Willebrand factor	Megakaryocytes, endothelial cells
Y2/51	CD61, GP IIIa	Megakaryocytes, platelets
PD7/26, 2B11, antileucocyte common antigen	CD45	T and B lymphocytes, macrophages, granulocytes (weak)
UCHL 1	CD45 RO	T lymphocytes
Anti-CD3	CD3	T lymphocytes
L26	CD20	B lymphocytes, activated B lymphocytes
Anti-CD79a (JCB117)	CD79a	B lymphocytes
Anti-Ig light chain (κ or λ)	Light chain	Plasma cells, immunoblasts, B lymphocytes (weak)
Anti-Ig heavy chain	Heavy chain	Plasma cells, immunoblasts, B lymphocytes (weak)
Leu–7	CD57	Natural killer cells, some cytotoxic T lymphocytes
AA1	Mast cell tryptase	Mast cells
Ki–67, MIB–1	Ki-67 nuclear protein	Proliferating cells

[a] Other than normal myeloblasts

The cores obtained by trephine biopsy also may be fixed in a mixture containing formaldehyde, methanol, and glucose phosphate buffer and embedded in methyl methacrylate without decalcification (4,12–15). Semithin sections (1–3 μm thick) of the undecalcified methyl methacrylate–embedded material then may be cut using a special heavy-duty microtome. Such sections show cellular features in much greater detail than do paraffin-embedded sections but have no antigenic or enzymic reactivity. On the other hand, if the core is appropriately fixed and embedded in glycol methacrylate (a water-miscible plastic) or a mixture of methyl and glycol methacrylate, a number of antigen epitopes and enzyme activities are preserved (16–18).

Methyl methacrylate–embedded semithin sections may be stained (after removing the methacrylate) with H&E or gallamine blue–Giemsa for cellular detail, Gomori's stain for reticulin fibers, PAS stain, Berlin blue stain for iron, and Ladewig's and Goldner's stains for osteoid, calcified bone, and connective tissue (14,15,19–21). Trephine biopsy cores that are embedded in a mixture of methyl methacrylate and glycol methacrylate may be used for the demonstration of chloroacetate esterase, acid phosphatase, peroxidase, nonspecific esterase, and alkaline phosphatase, as well as for the immunohistochemical detection of some antigens (16,17).

For immunohistochemical studies with the widest range of antibodies, frozen sections of trephine biopsy cores must be used (22,23). However, such sections show less cytologic detail than paraffin-embedded sections and tend to become distorted, making interpretation difficult. The distortion when cutting frozen sections can be reduced using a special supporting medium such as Histocon (Polysciences; Warrington, Pennsylvania), which does not impair antigenic reactivity.

The trephine biopsy core can be used to prepare several imprints by gently touching it with glass slides before fixation for histology. The imprints so obtained are used for detailed investigations into the morphology and other characteristics of individual marrow cells. However, such studies are best performed on smears of aspirated marrow. In adults, marrow is aspirated from the posterior superior iliac spine or the iliac crest. In children, marrow is usually aspirated from the posterior superior iliac spine and, in the case of patients less than 1 year of age, also from the upper end of the medial surface of the tibia just below and medial to the tibial tuberosity. The imprints from the trephine biopsy core and marrow smears are usually stained by a Romanowsky method such as the May-Grünwald-Giemsa (MGG) stain and also by Perls' acid ferrocyanide method. The smears also may be briefly fixed under conditions that preserve enzyme activity and antigenic sites and used to perform cytochemical and immunocytochemical studies. The details of these techniques and their value in hematologic diagnosis have been discussed by Hayhoe and Quaglino (24). Antibodies useful in immunocytochemical studies of appropriately fixed smears include those listed in Table 33.1, as well as several others such as those against CD2 (a pan-T marker), CD19 (a pan-B marker), and CD41 or CD42b (megakaryocyte lineage markers).

A thorough study of the marrow requires examination of both marrow smears and tissue sections. Marrow smears are the best preparations for the study of cellular detail but provide little information on intercellular relationships and the organization of the marrow. Histologic sections provide this information and are therefore superior to marrow smears for the detection of tumor infiltration, granulomas, amyloidosis, and necrosis of the marrow. They are essential for studying the distribution and quantity of extracellular reticulin and collagen fibers and may show vascular lesions (e.g., in thrombotic thrombocytopenic purpura and polyarteritis nodosa).

When electron microscopic studies are to be performed, an aliquot of a marrow aspirate is mixed with heparinized Hanks' solution. A few marrow fragments are then removed without delay and placed in a solution of 2.5 to 4% glutaraldehyde in 0.1 M phosphate buffer (pH 7.3). Alternatively, 1-mm pieces of the trephine biopsy core are fixed in glutaraldehyde for 1 hr, after which the marrow is gently teased out of the bone using a dissecting microscope.

In this chapter, unless otherwise stated, the descriptions of cells in marrow smears apply to smears stained by a Romanowsky method. The electron microscopic data relate to ultrathin sections stained with uranyl acetate and lead citrate. Such sections were prepared from marrow fragments that were fixed in glutaraldehyde and postfixed in osmium tetroxide.

GENERAL FEATURES OF HEMATOPOIESIS

Blood cells are produced in the embryo and fetus and throughout postnatal life. In the developing fetus and growing child, the total number of hematopoietic cells and blood cells increases progressively with time. By contrast, the hematopoietic systems of healthy adults are examples of steady-state cell renewal systems. In such systems, a relatively constant rate of loss of mature blood cells from the circulation is balanced by the production of new blood cells at the same rate. The number of hematopoietic cells and blood cells therefore remains constant.

New blood cells are eventually derived from a small number of hematopoietic stem cells (25), which are estimated to constitute 1 in 10^4 nucleated marrow cells. These cells have two properties: (a) the ability to mature into all types of blood cell and (b) an extensive capacity to generate new stem cells and thus to maintain their own number (self-renewal). In humans, the existence of pluripotent hematopoietic stem cells with both the above properties has been demonstrated by the success of bone marrow transplantation. The marrow also contains primitive cells that form "cobblestone" foci of myelopoiesis under stromal cells in long-term marrow cultures (limited to 8–20 weeks); these do not have the capacity for extensive self-renewal or for long-term lymphopoiesis and are therefore considered to be more differentiated than stem cells. The pluripotent stem cells (25–27) give rise to lymphoid stem cells and multipotent myeloid stem cells. They may also give rise to endothelial cells (28). The lymphoid stem cells mature into all types of lymphocytes. The myeloid stem cells mature into neutrophil, eosinophil, and basophil granulocytes, monocytes, erythrocytes, platelets, mast cells, and osteoclasts. The immediate progeny of the lymphoid and myeloid stem cells are usually termed hematopoietic progenitor cells. The myeloid progenitor cells are committed to one, two, or a few hematopoietic differentiation pathways (i.e., are unipotent, bipotent, or oligopotent) and have only a limited capacity for self-renewal. The most immature of the myeloid progenitor cells are oligopotent. Such cells undergo a progressive restriction of their differentiation potential such that the most mature progenitor cells are committed to only a single line of differentiation. Hematopoietic progenitor cells have been identified and characterized by their ability to form colonies containing cells of one or more hematopoietic lineages in vitro and are therefore called colony-forming units (CFUs) or colony-forming cells (CFC). These generate colonies containing a mixture of granulocytes, erythroblasts, macrophages, and megakaryocytes and are, therefore, termed CFU-GEMM. There is some indirect evidence for the presence of tripotent hematopoietic cells (CFU-E mega baso) that give rise to erythroblasts, megakaryocytes, and basophil granulocytes. Bipotent hematopoietic progenitor cells that give rise to colonies containing granulocytes and macrophages are termed CFU-GM. There are also bipotent progenitor cells generating colonies containing a mixture of erythroblasts and megakaryocytes (CFU-E mega). The unipotent progenitor cells that give rise to neutrophil granulocytes, eosinophil granulocytes, basophil granulocytes, macrophages, erythroblasts, and megakaryocytes are described as CFU-G, CFU-eo, CFU-baso, CFU-M, CFU-E, and CFU-mega, respectively. These develop into the most immature of the morphologically recognizable blood cell precursors in the marrow. Thus, CFU-G develop into myeloblasts, CFU-eo into eosinophil promyelocytes, CFU-baso into basophil promyelocytes, CFU-M into monoblasts, CFU-E into pronormoblasts, and CFU-mega into megakaryoblasts. The stem cells and progenitor cells are found in both the blood and the marrow but cannot be identified on morphologic criteria. The characteristics of the various types of morphologically recognizable hematopoietic cell found in the marrow are described later in this chapter. The relationships between the different categories of cell involved in hematopoiesis are illustrated in Figure 33.1.

Small numbers of bone marrow-derived hematopoietic stem cells and early hematopoietic progenitor cells circulate in the blood and these can "home" to the marrow.

Two processes are involved in the formation of all types of blood cells. These are the progressive acquisition of the biochemical, functional, and morphologic characteristics of the particular cell type (i.e., differentiation) and cell proliferation. The latter results in the production of a large number of mature cells from a single cell committed to one or more differentiation pathways. Differentiation occurs at all stages of hematopoiesis, and cell proliferation occurs in the hematopoietic stem cells, progenitor cells and, except in the megakaryocytic lineage, in the more immature morphologically recognizable precursor cells. The nearly mature blood cells seem to enter the circulation mainly by passing through the endothelial cells of the marrow sinusoids.

REGULATION OF HEMATOPOIESIS

Hematopoietic stem cells and early progenitor cells show low-level expression of transcription factors and genes specific to several hematopoietic lineages (multilineage priming). Commitment to a single lineage involves enhancement of transcription factors controlling the gene expression programs specific to that lineage and permanent silencing by those transcription factors of gene programs required for differentiation down other lineages.

The mechanisms underlying the commitment of a stem cell to differentiate are not yet fully understood (29,30). According to one model, the probability of a stem cell undergoing self-renewal or differentiation is a stochastic process. Environmental signals (soluble factors, cell-cell and cell–extracellular matrix interactions) mediated by specific receptor-ligand interactions operate only by influencing stem cell and progenitor cell apoptosis (and, thus, survival) and proliferation. Another model proposes that all decisions taken by stem cells and progenitor cells are determined by environmental signals. Bone marrow stromal cells (e.g., macrophages, nonphagocytic reticular or fibroblastoid cells, adipocytes, endothelial cells) play a major role in generating such signals; they provide niches for the attachment of stem cells and their progeny, are a source of the extracellular matrix involved in such attachment, and secrete various membrane-bound and soluble stimulatory hematopoietic growth factors and inhibitory cytokines (29,31,32).

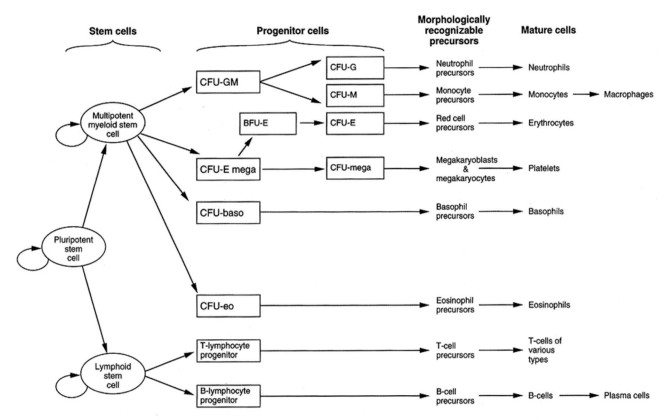

Figure 33.1 Model of hematopoiesis showing the relationships between the various types of stem cell, progenitor cell, and morphologically recognizable precursor cell. (*BFU*, E, erythroid burst-forming units; *CFU*, colony-forming units; *E*, erythroblasts; *GM*, granulocytes and macrophages; *eo*, eosinophil granulocytes; *baso*, basophil granulocytes; *mega*, megakaryocytes; *G*, neutrophil granulocytes; *M*, macrophages)

Stem cells and early hematopoietic progenitor cells interact via specific cell surface receptors with multilineage hematopoietic growth factors. The latter include stem cell factor (Steel factor, kit ligand), interleukin-1 (IL-1) and IL-6 for the pluripotent stem cells, and stem cell factor, thrombopoietin, IL-3 (multi-CSF) and granulocyte-macrophage–colony stimulating factor (GM-CSF) for the multipotent myeloid stem cells. The regulation of later progenitor cells and the morphologically recognizable hematopoietic cells is dependent both on multilineage growth factors and lineage-specific growth factors such as G-CSF, M-CSF, IL-5 (influencing CFU-eo), thrombopoietin and IL11 (influencing CFU-mega), and erythropoietin (mainly influencing late BFU-E and CFU-E). The growth factors influencing lymphocyte progenitor cells and precursors include IL-2, IL-4, IL-5, IL-6, IL-7, and IL-11 for the B lineage and IL-2, IL-3, IL-4, IL-7, and IL-10 for the T lineage.

Hematopoietic growth factors are glycoproteins and influence the survival, proliferation, and differentiation of their target cells via second messengers. In their absence, the target cells undergo programmed cell death (apoptosis). Some growth factors such as G-CSF and GM-CSF not only regulate hematopoiesis but also enhance the function of the mature cells. Most hematopoietic growth factors are produced by bone marrow stromal cells and T lymphocytes, either constitutively (e.g., M-CSF production by fibroblastoid cells and endothelial cells) or after their activation by various signals. Thus, fibroblastoid cells and endothelial cells that have been activated by macrophage-derived IL-1 or tumor necrosis factor (TNF) and endotoxin-stimulated macrophages produce M-CSF, GM-CSF, G-CSF, IL-6, and stem cell factor. Antigen- or IL-1– activated T cells produce IL-3, IL-5, and GM-CSF.

The main organ of erythropoietin production in postnatal life is the kidney, and the probable site of synthesis appears to be peritubular cells. About 10% of the erythropoietin is produced in the liver, which is the main organ of synthesis in the fetus. There is an oxygen sensor in the peritubular cells of the kidney, and the production of erythropoietin is inversely proportional to the degree of oxygenation of renal tissue. A limited amount of data suggest that there also may be paracrine or autocrine erythropoietin production in the bone marrow. The erythropoietin receptor is upregulated at the late BFU-E and CFU-E stages, and signalling through this receptor is required to prevent apoptosis.

In addition to the stimulatory cytokines mentioned above, inhibitors (negative regulators) of hematopoiesis are produced by macrophages, fibroblastoid cells, and endothelial cells. These include transforming growth factor-$\beta 1$ (TGF-$\beta 1$), which inhibits multilineage progenitor cells, early erythroid progenitors, and megakaryocytes; TNF-α, which inhibits the proliferation of granulocyte precursors; interferon-α, which inhibits megakaryocyte progenitors; and macrophage inflammatory protein-1α (MIP-1α), which inhibits the proliferation of stem cells.

HEMATOPOIESIS IN THE EMBRYO AND FETUS: DEVELOPMENT OF THE BONE MARROW

Studies in experimental animals have shown that hematopoietic stem cells responsible for embryonic (primitive) hematopoiesis develop in the yolk sac. Those responsible for fetal and postnatal (definitive) hematopoiesis are considered to arise in the aorto-gonad-mesonephros region by some investigators and the yolk sac by others (33–35). The stem cells migrate through the blood stream to colonize the fetal liver and other fetal tissues.

In the human embryo, erythropoietic cells first appear within the blood islands of the yolk sac about 19 days after fertilization (36,37). A few megakaryocytes are found in these blood islands during the sixth and seventh weeks of gestation. Yolk sac erythropoiesis is megaloblastic and results in the production of nucleated red cells (Figure 33.2) that contain three embryonic hemoglobins (25), namely, hemoglobins Gower I ($\zeta_2\varepsilon_2$), Gower II ($\alpha_2\varepsilon_2$), and Portland I ($\zeta_2\gamma_2$), and, in later embryos, hemoglobin F ($\alpha_2\gamma_2$).

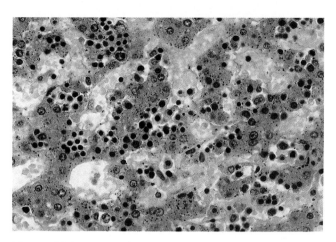

Figure 33.3   Fetal liver tissue obtained postmortem showing erythropoietic activity. The erythroblasts are found extravascularly, both within the hepatic cords and between the cords and the sinusoidal endothelial cells. The brown material within hepatocytes is formalin pigment, a common postmortem fixation artifact. (H&E.)

Hematopoietic foci develop in the hepatic cords during the sixth week of gestation, and the liver becomes the major site of erythropoiesis in the middle trimester of pregnancy (38,39). During this period, about half the nucleated cells of the liver consist of erythropoietic cells (Figure 33.3). A few granulocytopoietic cells and megakaryocytes also are found in this organ. Fetal hepatic erythropoiesis is normoblastic and gives rise to nonnucleated red cells containing hemoglobin F. These red cells are considerably larger than the red cells of adults. The number of erythropoietic cells in the liver decreases progressively after the seventh month of gestation; a few cells persist until the end of the first postnatal week.

Marrow cavities are formed as a result of the erosion of bone or calcified cartilage by blood vessels and cells from the periosteum (37). The first marrow cavity to develop is that of the clavicle (at about 2 months gestational age). After the formation of the marrow cavities, the vascular connective tissue present within them becomes colonized by circulating hematopoietic stem cells. The latter generate erythropoietic cells during the third and fourth months of gestation, the order of appearance of erythropoietic cells being the same as the order of formation of the marrow cavities. After the sixth month, the bone marrow becomes the major site of hematopoiesis (40). Erythropoiesis in fetal bone marrow is normoblastic and results in the production of nonnucleated red cells, which contain hemoglobins F and A ($\alpha_2\beta_2$) and which are larger than adult red cells. The fetal bone marrow is the predominant site of intrauterine granulocytopoiesis and megakaryocytopoiesis. In this tissue, the myeloid/erythroid ratio (i.e., the ratio of the number of neutrophil precursors plus neutrophil granulocytes to the number of

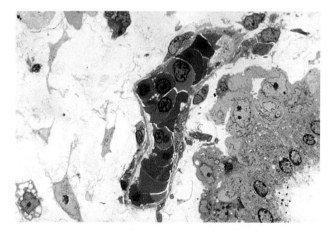

Figure 33.2   Semithin section of a plastic-embedded chorionic villus biopsy sample obtained at 7 weeks of gestation, showing a blood vessel containing nucleated embryonic red cells (toluidine blue).

erythroblasts) remains constant at about 1:4 after 6.5 months of gestation (40).

POSTNATAL CHANGES IN THE DISTRIBUTION OF RED MARROW AND IN THE TYPE OF HEMOGLOBIN

At birth, all the marrow cavities contain red, hematopoietic marrow. Furthermore, the red marrow contains only a few fat cells. After the first four years of life, an increasing number of fat cells appears between the hematopoietic cells, particularly in certain regions of the marrow, and these regions eventually become yellow and virtually devoid of hematopoietic cells (41,42). Zones of yellow, fatty marrow are found just below the middle of the shafts of the long bones between the ages of 10 and 14 years and, subsequently, extend in both directions, distal spread being more rapid than proximal spread. By the age of about 25 years, hematopoietic marrow is confined to the proximal quarters of the shafts of the femora and humeri, the skull bones, ribs, sternum, scapulae, clavicles, vertebrae, pelvis, and the upper half of the sacrum. Although the distribution of hematopoietic marrow remains essentially unaltered throughout adult life, its fat cell content increases slightly with increasing age and more substantially after the age of 70 years, in association with a gradual expansion of the volume of the marrow cavities.

The percentages of hemoglobins F and A in the blood of full-term neonates are, respectively, 50 to 85% and 15 to 50%. The proportion of hemoglobin F decreases postnatally at different rates in different individuals, but adult levels of less than 1% are reached in nearly all children by the age of 2.5 years.

Because young children have red marrow containing few fat cells in virtually all their marrow cavities, a rapid increase in hematopoietic tissue in this age group is presumably accommodated mainly by a reduction in the proportion of marrow space occupied by sinusoids. If the increase in the rate of hematopoiesis is substantial and prolonged (e.g., in congenital hemolytic anemias), there is an increase in the total volume of the marrow cavities and the reestablishment of extramedullary hematopoiesis in organs such as the liver, spleen, and lymph nodes (43). The expansion of the marrow cavities leads to skeletal abnormalities, such as frontal and parietal bossing, dental deformities, and malocclusion of the teeth. It also causes thinning of the cortex, which may lead to fractures after minor trauma. In adults, increased hematopoiesis is initially associated with the replacement of fat cells in red marrow by hematopoietic cells and also with the spread of red marrow into marrow cavities normally containing yellow marrow (43). If the increase in hematopoiesis is marked, extramedullary hematopoiesis may develop.

STRUCTURAL ORGANIZATION OF HEMATOPOIETIC MARROW

The marrow cavities of most bones contain trabeculae of cancellous bone. The inner surface of the cortex and the outer surfaces of the trabeculae are lined by the endosteum, which consists of a single layer of cells supported on a delicate layer of reticular connective tissue. In most areas of the endosteum, the cells consist of very flat bone-lining cells (endosteal lining cells), but in some areas they consist of osteoblasts or osteoclasts. The marrow, which is located between the trabeculae, is supplied with an extensive microvasculature and some myelinated and nonmyelinated nerve fibers. It does not have a lymphatic drainage (44). The space between the small blood vessels contains a few reticulin fibers and a variety of cell types. The latter include fat cells, precursors of red cells, granulocytes, monocytes and platelets, lymphocytes, plasma cells, macrophages (phagocytic reticular cells), nonphagocytic reticular cells, and mast cells (4,45).

Blood Supply

One or more nutrient canals penetrate the shafts of the long bones obliquely. Each canal contains a nutrient artery and one or two nutrient veins. After entering the marrow, the nutrient artery divides into ascending and descending branches, which coil around the central longitudinal vein, the main venous channel of the marrow. The ascending and descending arteries give off numerous arterioles and capillaries that travel radially toward the endosteum and often open into a plexus of sinusoids (25). The sinusoids drain through a system of collecting venules and larger venous channels into the central longitudinal vein, which in turn drains mainly into the nutrient veins. In the diaphyses of long bones containing yellow fatty marrow, the nutrient artery gives off relatively few branches until it reaches the lower edge of the red marrow, where it breaks up into numerous vessels that penetrate the hematopoietic tissue. Many blood vessels of various sizes supply the marrow within flat and cuboidal bones, entering the marrow cavity via one or more large nutrient canals, as well as through numerous smaller canals.

There are interconnections between the blood supply of the bone marrow and bone through an endosteal network of blood vessels. This network communicates both with the periosteal vessels via fine veins passing through the bone and with branches of the nutrient artery. Furthermore, studies in experimental animals have shown that many capillaries derived from the nutrient artery enter Haversian canals but swing back into the marrow and open into sinusoids or venules (46,47). There has been much speculation as to whether blood reaching the marrow from the bone contains one or more

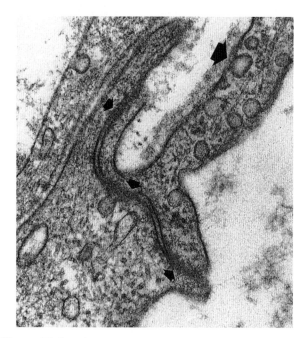

Figure 33.4   Electron micrograph of part of the wall of a sinusoid from normal bone marrow. There are three tight junctions (*small arrows*) at the area of contact between two adjacent endothelial cells. Several pinocytotic vesicles (*large arrow*) are present both at the luminal and abluminal surface of one of the endothelial cells, and a single pinocytotic vesicle is present at the outer surface of the adventitial cell.

hematopoietic factors derived from the bone or endosteal cells.

The sinusoids of human bone marrow have thin walls consisting of an inner complete layer of flattened endothelial cells with little or no underlying basement membrane and an outer incomplete layer of adventitial cells (48). The endothelial cells are characterized by the presence of numerous small pinocytotic vesicles along both their luminal and abluminal surfaces (Figure 33.4). The nucleus is flattened and contains moderate quantities of nuclear membrane–associated condensed chromatin. The cytoplasm also contains ribosomes, rough endoplasmic reticulum (RER), mitochondria, some microfilaments, a few lysosomes, and occasional fat droplets. Adjacent endothelial cells overlap and may interdigitate extensively. These areas of contact are characterized by (a) a strictly parallel alignment of the membranes of the interacting cells with a narrow gap between the opposing membranes and (b) short stretches in which the membranes fuse together, forming tight junctions (not true desmosomes). There is an increased electron density of the cytoplasm immediately adjacent to and on both sides of the tight junctions (Figure 33.4). Some endothelial cells show alkaline phosphatase activity. Endothelial cells contain no stainable iron except when the iron stores are increased. They produce extracellular matrix, stem cell factor, IL6, GM-CSF, IL-1α, IL-11, and G-CSF and are thus intimately involved with the regulation

of hematopoiesis. Endothelial cells of the sinusoids allow the bidirectional migration of progenitor cells and hematopoietic stem cells through them by a mechanism involving specific binding molecules.

Adventitial cells project long peripheral cytoplasmic processes, which may be closely associated with some extracellular reticulin fibers. Some of these processes lie along the sinusoidal surface, and others protrude outward between hematopoietic cells. Thus, adventitial cells are a type of reticular cell (i.e., form part of the cytoplasmic network or reticulum of the marrow stroma). The cytoplasm of adventitial cells contains ribosomes, RER, some pinocytotic vesicles, a few electron-dense lysosomes, occasional fat globules, and numerous microfilaments that are often arranged in bands. The latter are usually situated within the peripheral cytoplasmic processes. The cytoplasm of some adventitial cells appears very electron lucent. Adventitial cells stain strongly for alkaline phosphatase.

Nerve Supply

In the case of a long bone, the nerve supply enters the bone marrow mainly via the nutrient canal but also through a number of epiphyseal and metaphyseal foramina. Bundles of nerve fibers travel together with the nutrient artery and its branches and supply the smooth muscle in such vessels or, occasionally, terminate between hematopoietic cells (49).

Extracellular Matrix (Connective Tissue)

Normal marrow contains a scanty incomplete network of fine branching reticulin fibers between the parenchymal cells (Figure 33.5). A higher concentration of thicker fibers is found in and around the walls of the larger arteries and

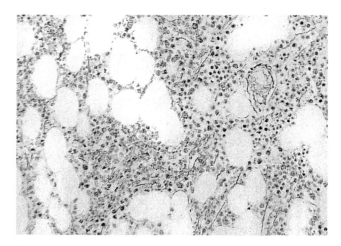

Figure 33.5   Section of a decalcified, paraffin-embedded trephine biopsy core from a hematologically normal adult, showing a scant network of fine reticulin fibers. The upper right-hand quadrant of the photomicrograph shows a circular arrangement of fibers associated with a blood vessel. (Silver impregnation of reticulin.)

near the endosteum; such fibers are continuous with the fibers in the parenchyma. Other extracellular matrix components produced by stromal cells include fibronectin, vascular cell adhesion molecule (VCAM)-1, vitronectin, thrombospondin, and proteoglycans such as heparan sulphate and chondroitin sulphate.

Stromal Cells

The stromal cells comprise (a) osteoblasts, bone marrow fat cells (adipocytes), and nonphagocytic reticular cells (including myofibroblasts), all of which are derived from mesenchymal stem cells within the marrow; (b) osteoclasts, macrophages, and mast cells that are derived from the myeloid hematopoietic stem cell; and (c) endothelial cells (discussed above) that are derived either from the hematopoietic stem cell or a more primitive marrow cell that also gives rise to hematopoietic stem cells (28). Some stromal cells are intimately involved in the regulation of hematopoiesis.

Osteoblasts and Osteoclasts

Osteoblasts are present in the endosteum in areas of deposition of osseous matrix (osteoid). In histologic sections, osteoblasts are cuboidal or pyramidal and have eccentric nuclei. Their cytoplasm is markedly basophilic and contains a large round pale zone. Osteoblasts are frequently found in a continuous layer, usually one or two cells thick, and appear like an area of epithelium. They become surrounded by the osteoid they produce and thus eventually become osteocytes. Osteoclasts are large multinucleate cells involved in bone resorption and are often found in shallow excavations on the surface of the bone, termed Howship's lacunae. Osteoblasts arise from progenitor cells closely associated with the endosteal lining cells. Although it is usually considered that osteoblast progenitor cells are not derived from hematopoietic stem cells, recent studies in mice indicate that osteoblasts and hematopoietic cells arise from a common primitive marrow cell (50). Osteoblasts produce cytokines such as IL6, G-CSF, and GM-CSF that influence hemopoiesis (51). Osteoclasts originate from the myeloid hematopoietic stem cells. The relationship between the osteoclast progenitor cell and other hematopoietic progenitor cells (e.g., CFU-GEMM, CFU-GM, CFU-M) is not yet clear (52).

Romanowsky-stained normal marrow smears may contain groups of osteoblasts or individual osteoclasts. In such preparations, osteoblasts have an oval or elongated shape and are 20 to 50 μm in diameter. They have abundant basophilic cytoplasm, often with somewhat indistinct margins, and a single small eccentric nucleus with only small quantities of condensed chromatin and with one to three nucleoli. The cytoplasm contains a rounded

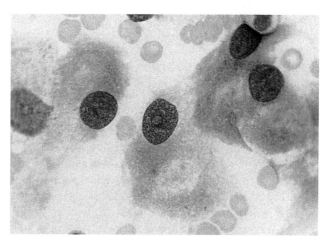

Figure 33.6 Group of osteoblasts from a May-Grünwald-Giemsa (MGG)–stained smear of normal bone marrow.

pale area corresponding to the Golgi apparatus, which often is situated some distance from the nucleus (Figure 33.6). Osteoblasts stain positively for alkaline phosphatase activity. They superficially resemble plasma cells, but the latter are smaller, contain heavily stained clumped chromatin, and have a Golgi zone situated immediately adjacent to the nucleus. Osteoclasts appear as giant multinucleate cells with abundant pale blue cytoplasm containing many azurophilic (purple-red) granules (Figure 33.7). The individual nuclei are rounded in outline, uniform in size, contain a single prominent nucleolus, and do not overlap. Osteoclasts are strongly acid phosphatase positive. They must be distinguished from the other polyploid giant cells in the marrow, the megakaryocytes. These are usually not multinucleate but contain a single large lobulated nucleus.

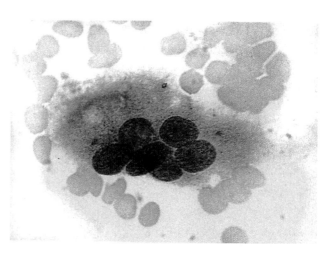

Figure 33.7 A multinucleate osteoclast from an MGG-stained smear of normal bone marrow.

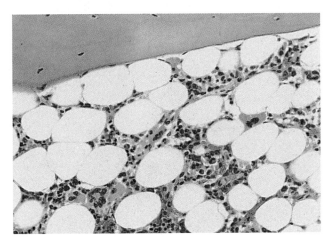

Figure 33.8   Section of a decalcified, paraffin-embedded trephine biopsy core from a hematologically normal adult. About 70% of the area of marrow tissue in this photomicrograph is occupied by fat cells. There may be a substantial variation in cellularity in different parts of the same section. (H&E.)

Fat Cells

The number of fat cells in hematopoietic bone marrow varies markedly with age (53,54). In normal adults, 30 to 70% of the area of a histologic section of hematopoietic marrow consists of fat cells (Figures 33.8–33.9). Fat cells are the largest cells in the marrow, and sections of such cells have average diameters of about 85 μm. Ultrastructural studies show that these cells have a single large fat globule at their center and a narrow rim of cytoplasm at their periphery. This cytoplasmic rim contains a flattened nucleus, several small lipid droplets, ribosomes, strands of endoplasmic reticulum, and several mitochondria. The fat cells of the bone marrow only have small quantities of reticulin and collagen fibers around them. They are in intimate

contact with vascular channels, macrophages, and all types of hematopoietic cells. Marrow fat cells seem to be formed by the accumulation of lipid within adventitial cells, other nonphagocytic reticular cells, and, possibly, sinus endothelial cells. Whenever there is an increase or decrease in the number of hematopoietic cells in bone marrow, there is a corresponding decrease or increase, respectively, of the number of fat cells so that the intersinusoidal space within marrow cavities is always fully occupied by cells. The mechanisms underlying this inverse relationship between the mass of fat cells and hematopoietic cells in the marrow are uncertain. In severe anorexia nervosa or cachexia secondary to chronic disorders, such as tuberculosis or carcinoma, there is a marked reduction in fat cells, often together with a reduction in hematopoietic tissue. In these conditions, the space normally occupied by cells is filled with a gelatinous extracellular substance composed of acid mucopolysaccharide (55).

Macrophages (Phagocytic Reticular Cells)

The bone marrow contains many macrophages. The frequency of this cell type is best appreciated in sections of trephine biopsies stained for an antigen found in macrophages such as CD68 (Figure 33.10) or in electron micrographs of ultrathin sections of marrow fragments rather than in smears of aspirated bone marrow. In H&E-stained sections of trephine biopsies, macrophages appear as moderately large cells with abundant cytoplasm. In Romanowsky-stained marrow smears, they appear as irregularly shaped cells 20 to 30 μm in diameter and have a round or oval nucleus with pale, lacelike chromatin and one or more large nucleoli. The cytoplasm is voluminous, stains pale blue, and contains azurophilic granules, vacuoles, and variously sized inclusions consisting of

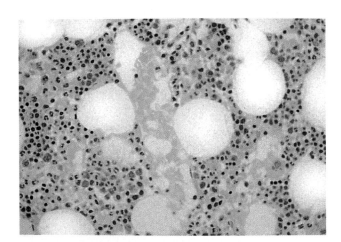

Figure 33.9   Semithin section of an undecalcified, plastic-embedded trephine biopsy core from a hematologically normal adult. A wide sinusoid containing red cells is seen passing vertically between some fat cells. (H&E.)

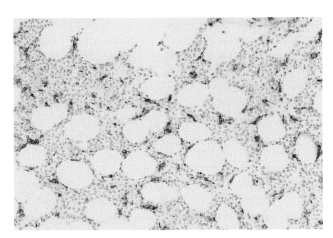

Figure 33.10   Immunohistochemical demonstration of macrophages in a section of a paraffin-embedded trephine biopsy core from a hematologically normal subject. The section was reacted with the monoclonal antibody PG-M1 (against CD68) and the reaction visualized using an immunoperoxidase technique.

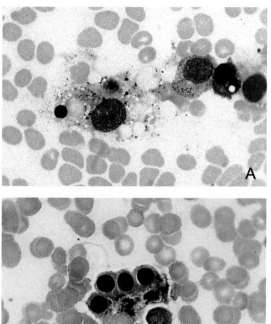

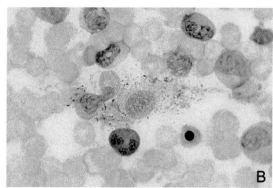

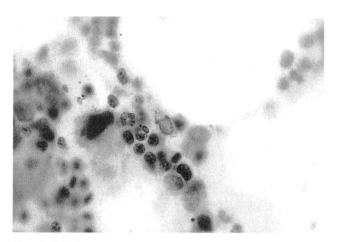

Figure 33.11 Macrophages from normal bone marrow smears. **A.** Macrophage containing a black extruded erythroblast nucleus and several intracytoplasmic inclusions of various shapes, sizes, and staining characteristics. The large pale rounded inclusions may represent degraded red cells (MGG). **B.** Macrophage containing several PAS-positive cytoplasmic granules, together with a PAS-negative late erythroblast and several PAS-positive neutrophil myelocytes and granulocytes. **C:** Macrophage showing strong α-naphthyl acetate esterase activity, surrounded by six unreactive erythroblasts. The diazonium salt of fast blue BB was used as the capture agent.

phagocytosed material (Figure 33.11A). Macrophages are derived from monocytes and, therefore, eventually from the hematopoietic stem cells.

In unstained smears and sections of normal marrow and in Giemsa- or H&E-stained sections, macrophages may show refractile yellow-brown hemosiderin-containing intracytoplasmic inclusions, which vary between 0.5 and 4 μm in diameter. These appear as blue or blue-black granules when stained by Perls' acid ferrocyanide method. This stain also may color the entire cytoplasm a diffuse pale blue (Figure 33.12). The amount of iron-positive granules within the marrow fragments on a marrow smear (Figure 33.13) or the amount in a histologic section of a trephine biopsy sample may be assessed semiquantitatively and is a useful guide to the total iron stores in the body (56). Stainable iron is absent or virtually absent in iron deficiency (with or without anemia) and increased in conditions such as hereditary hemochromatosis or transfusion-induced iron overload. Macrophages contain PAS-positive material and are strongly positive for α-naphthyl acetate esterase

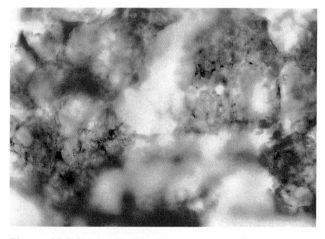

Figure 33.12 Section of a paraffin-embedded normal marrow fragment (*clot section*). The macrophage in the center shows blue hemosiderin-containing intracytoplasmic granules and a diffuse bluish coloration of the cytoplasm (Perls' acid ferrocyanide reaction).

Figure 33.13 Marrow fragment from a normal marrow smear stained by Perls' acid ferrocyanide reaction. The dark blue granular material represents hemosiderin within macrophages.

(Figure 33.11B–C) and acid phosphatase. They do not stain for α-naphthol AS-D chloroacetate esterase activity (57), and most do not stain with Sudan black. Some macrophages appear to stain positively for alkaline phosphatase activity.

Ultrastructural studies of marrow fragments show that macrophages form long cytoplasmic processes at their periphery and that such processes extend for considerable distances between various types of hematopoietic cells (Figure 33.14). Some cytoplasmic processes protrude through the endothelial cell layer into the sinusoidal lumen (Figure 33.15) and appear to be involved in recognizing and phagocytosing circulating microorganisms and senescent or damaged erythrocytes and granulocytes. The nucleus often has an irregular outline and contains small to moderate quantities of nuclear membrane–associated condensed chromatin. The cytoplasm has many strands of RER, scattered ferritin molecules, a well-developed Golgi apparatus, several mitochondria, a number of small or medium-sized homogeneous electron-dense primary lysosomes of variable shape, and a number of large inclusions. Some of the latter have a complex ultrastructure with both electron-dense and electron-lucent areas and myelin figures and may contain numerous ferritin and hemosiderin molecules; these appear to represent secondary lysosomes with residual material from phagocytosed cells (Figure 33.16). Other large inclusions can be recognized readily as granulocytes (Figure 33.17), extruded erythroblast nuclei, and erythrocytes at various stages of degradation. A few reticulin fibers may be found in contact with parts of the cell surface.

Macrophages are present within erythroblastic islands (Figure 33.11C), plasma cell islands, and lymphoid nodules

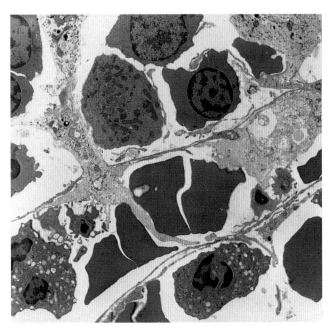

Figure 33.15 Electron micrograph of a sinusoid from a normal bone marrow. A process of macrophage cytoplasm is seen protruding through the lining endothelial cell into the sinusoidal lumen. Serial sectioning of this sinusoid showed that the mass of macrophage cytoplasm occupying the right-hand side of the sinusoidal lumen connected transendothelially with a second extrasinusoidal cytoplasmic process. Both processes arose from the same macrophage.

but also may occur elsewhere in the marrow parenchyma. Some are found immediately adjacent to the endothelial cells of sinusoids, forming part of the adventitial cell layer. Bone marrow macrophages not only function as phagocytic cells but also generate various hematopoietic growth factors

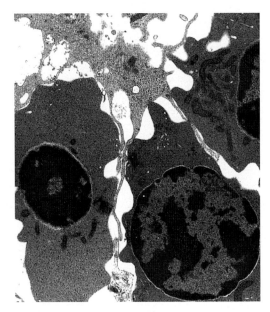

Figure 33.14 Electron micrograph of three erythroblasts from a normal marrow showing fine processes of macrophage cytoplasm extending between the cells.

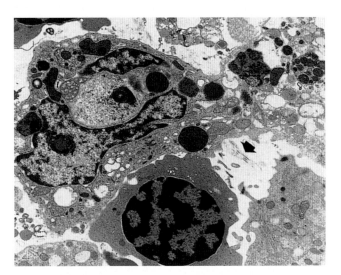

Figure 33.16 Electron micrograph of a macrophage lying next to an early polychromatic erythroblast in a normal bone marrow. The nucleus of the macrophage is irregular in outline, and its cytoplasm contains several inclusions and vacuoles. Some of the inclusions are ultrastructurally complex and probably represent secondary lysosomes. There are some reticulin fibers (*arrow*) near the macrophage.

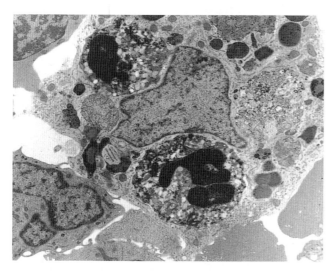

Figure 33.17 Electron micrograph of a macrophage from normal bone marrow. The cytoplasm contains two phagocytosed neutrophils and a large number of other inclusions of varying size, shape, and appearance.

(e.g., c-kit ligand or stem cell factor, M-CSF, IL-1, and G-CSF) and are thus involved in short-range regulation of lymphopoiesis and myelopoiesis. They presumably also are involved in antigen processing.

Nonphagocytic Reticular Cells

In Romanowsky-stained marrow smears, nonphagocytic reticular cells have an irregular or spindle shape and resemble macrophages except that they lack large intracyto-plasmic inclusions. Light microscope cytochemical and histochemical data indicate that these cells are PAS- negative, strongly positive for alkaline phosphatase, negative for acid phosphatase, negative or only weakly positive for α-naphthyl acetate esterase, and negative for stainable iron. Thus, there seems to be some overlap between the cytochemical characteristics of nonphagocytic reticular cells and macrophages (57,58). In the case of mice and rats, however, light and electron microscopic cytochemical data have clearly established the existence of two distinct types of reticular cells in the marrow stroma: (a) fibroblast-like nonphagocytic reticular cells that have cell membrane–associated alkaline phosphatase and no acid phosphatase and (b) macrophage-like phagocytic reticular cells that are positive for acid phosphatase but not for alkaline phosphatase (59).

Electron microscopic studies of nonphagocytic reticular cells in human bone marrow (48,60,61) have shown that, like macrophages, these cells extend branching cytoplasmic processes between hematopoietic cells and are in contact with extracellular reticulin fibers (Figure 33.18). However, unlike macrophages, they do not have secondary lysosomes or have only an occasional secondary lysosome. They may contain variable numbers of filaments or a few small fat globules in their cytoplasm. The intracytoplasmic filaments sometime occur in bundles, and the cells are then ultra-structurally indistinguishable from adventitial cells. It is possible that the nonphagocytic reticular cells comprise a number of different cell types including fibroblasts or my-ofibroblasts, adventitial cells, and cells whose functions have not yet been defined. Myeloid cell and B-lymphoid progenitors are located adjacent to myofibroblasts.

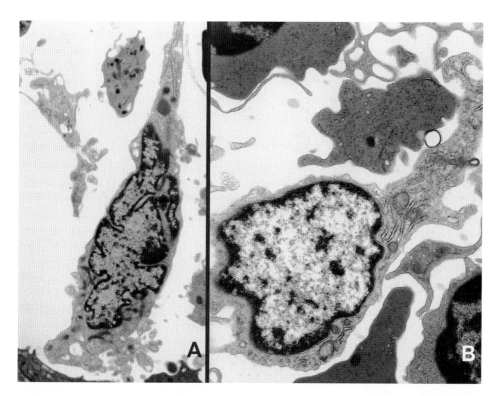

Figure 33.18 Electron micrographs of two nonphagocytic reticular cells from normal bone marrow. The nuclear outline of one of these cells (**A**) shows several deep clefts and that of the other (**B**) is less irregular.

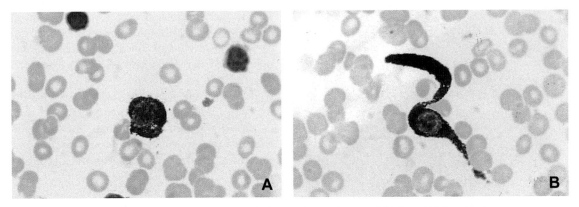

Figure 33.19 Two mast cells, one rounded (**A**) and one elongated (**B**) from MGG-stained smears of bone marrow.

At least some of the nonphagocytic reticular cells arise from a mesenchymal stem cell capable of giving rise to colonies of fibroblast-like or myofibroblast-like cells in vitro. As mentioned earlier, nonphagocytic reticular cells appear to play an important role in the microenvironmental regulation of hematopoiesis, both by binding to primitive hematopoietic cells (62) and by producing certain hematopoietic growth factors both constitutively and in response to stimulation by monokines (63). In mice and presumably also in humans, they synthesize collagen (types I and III) and fibronectin.

Mast Cells

Mast cells tend to be found in association with the periphery of lymphoid follicles and the adventitia of small arteries and adjacent to the endosteal cells of bone trabeculae and the endothelial cells of sinusoids.

It is now known that the hematopoietic stem cells generate morphologically unrecognizable progenitors of mast cells within the bone marrow (64) and that the most mature of these cells enter the blood (65,66). The circulating cells, which still lack mast cell granules, migrate into the tissues, where they proliferate and mature into mast cells. Mast cells and basophils appear not to share a common early progenitor cell (67).

Unlike the granules of basophils, which are very water soluble, those of mast cells are much less so. Nevertheless, mast cells are not easily recognized in sections of marrow stained with H&E. By contrast, they are readily identified in sections stained with the Giemsa stain. In such sections, mast cells have round, oval, or spindle-shaped outlines and many dark purple cytoplasmic granules. The nucleus is often oval and may be situated eccentrically. Immunochemical staining can be performed using the antibody AA1, which reacts with mast cell tryptase (10) and does not cross-react with basophils. In Romanowsky-stained marrow smears, mast cells vary between 5 and 25 μm in their long axis and tend to have an ovoid or elongated shape

(Figure 33.19A–B). The cytoplasm is packed with coarse purple-black to red-purple granules; but, unlike in basophil granulocytes, the granules seldom overlie the nucleus. The nucleus is small, round or oval, and either centrally or eccentrically located. It contains less condensed chromatin than that of a basophil granulocyte. The granules of mast cells are rich in heparin and stain metachromatically with toluidine blue. Mast cells are also peroxidase negative, PAS positive, acid phosphatase positive, and α-naphthol AS-D chloroacetate esterase positive. Unlike basophil granulocytes, mast cells are capable of mitosis.

In the electron microscope, the granules of mast cells vary considerably in appearance. They may be homogeneously electron dense, have areas of increased electron density at their centers, or contain parallel arrangements, whorls, or scrolls of a crystalline or fibrillar structure (Figures 33.20A–B). The nucleus contains moderate quantities of condensed chromatin. In addition to the numerous granules, the cytoplasm contains some mitochondria, a few short strands of endoplasmic reticulum, occasional lipid droplets, and some fibrils.

Hematopoietic Cells

Lymphocytes and Plasma Cells

Histologic sections of normal marrow show nodules of small lymphocytes that are 0.08 to 1.2 mm in diameter and contain occasional reticular cells (68) (Figure 33.21A), as well as much smaller lymphoid aggregates; these nodules and aggregates are usually found in the intertrabecular and perivascular areas and are rarely found immediately adjacent to trabeculae. Paratrabecular nodules and aggregates are characteristic of infiltration by malignant lymphoid cells. In normal marrow, the prevalence of lymphoid nodules increases with age. About 20% of such nodules are irregular in outline, poorly circumscribed, and often contain several fat cells and a few eosinophils between the lymphocytes; they do not contain germinal centers, and their

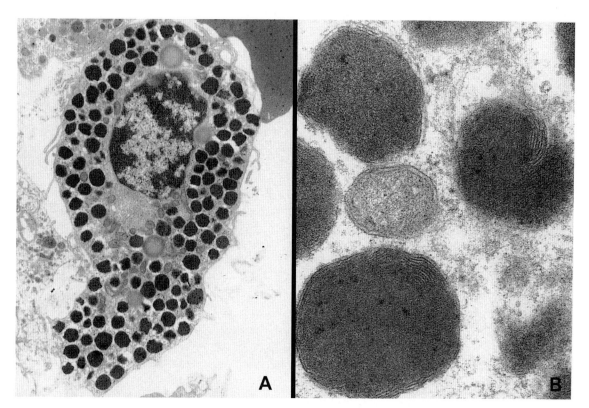

Figure 33.20 Electron micrographs of mast cells from normal bone marrow. **A.** The cytoplasm is packed with characteristic granules and contains four lipid droplets. **B.** Granules from a mast cell at high magnification showing parallel lamellae.

reticulin content is normal for marrow or only slightly increased. The remaining 80% are rounded or oval, well circumscribed, and compact, and they have a follicular structure with blood vessels at their center and some plasma cells and mast cells toward their periphery. Well-developed germinal centers are seen in about 5% of the sections.

Lymphocytes extend between surrounding fat cells, and the entire nodule may be surrounded by eosinophils. The reticulin content of such a lymphoid nodule is clearly increased (Figure 33.21B). Immunohistochemical studies indicate that the lymphocytes within such nodules are of both T and B phenotypes (mainly T).

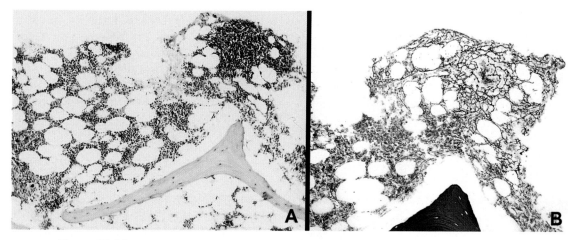

Figure 33.21 Lymphoid nodule in a paraffin-embedded trephine biopsy core from a woman without any evidence of a lymphoproliferative disorder. **A.** Section stained with hematoxylin and eosin showing a nodule (*top right*) incorporating fat cells at its periphery. **B.** Parallel section stained by a silver impregnation technique, showing increased reticulin in the nodule (photographed at higher magnification than A).

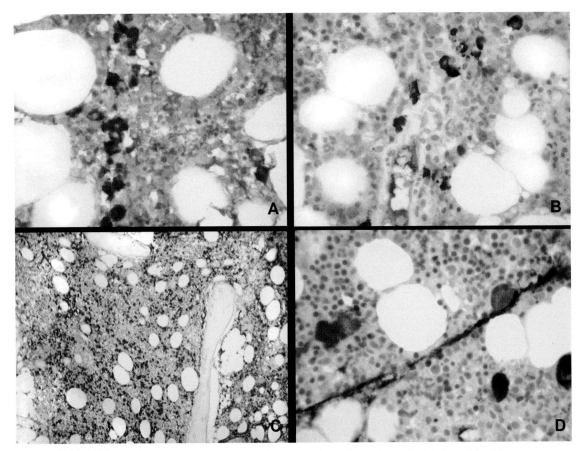

Figure 33.22 Immunohistochemical studies on sections of paraffin-embedded trephine biopsy cores. The reactions were visualized using an immunoalkaline phosphatase method. **A.** Section reacted with anti-Ig κ light chains, showing plasma cells aligned along a blood vessel. **B.** Section reacted with anti-Ig λ light chains showing a cluster of plasma cells. There are fewer positive plasma cells with anti-λ chain than anti-κ chain antibody. **C.** Section reacted with antimyeloperoxidase antibody showing positively-stained promyelocytes and more mature cells of the neutrophil granulocyte series. Note the presence of stained cells along the endosteal surface of the bone trabeculum. **D.** Section reacted with antibody against factor VIII–related antigen showing positively stained megakaryocytes and linearly arranged endothelial cells. One of the megakaryocytes is closely apposed to the blood vessel. (Courtesy of Dr. Alex Rice, Department of Histopathology, St. Mary's Hospital, London).

T and B lymphocytes (with more T than B cells) and plasma cells also are found unassociated with lymphoid nodules. Lymphocytes are found scattered between hematopoietic cells, and plasma cells are often present in small groups, surrounding a central macrophage or sheathing some small blood vessels. There are more κ than λ light chain–positive plasma cells (Figure 33.22A–B).

Precursors of Red Cells, Granulocytes, Monocytes, and Platelets

The early granulocytopoietic cells (myeloblasts and promyelocytes) mainly are found near the endosteum of bone trabeculae and the adventitial aspects of arterioles (Figure 33.22C). Maturing granulocyte precursors radiate outward from these sites, and the neutrophil granulocytes often are found in the center of intertrabecular areas, adjacent to sinusoids. A few promyelocytes and myeloctyes are present singly or in small clusters at sites away from bone

trabeculae and blood vessels. Erythroblasts and megakaryocytes are also found away from the endosteum. The erythroblasts occur in one or two layers surrounding one or two central macrophages; the late erythroblasts and marrow reticulocytes usually are situated next to sinusoids. The megakaryocytes usually lie near sinusoids (Figure 33.22D) and protrude cytoplasmic processes into their lumina; these processes discharge platelets directly into the microcirculation.

HEMATOPOIETIC CELLS: CHARACTERISTICS IN MARROW SMEARS AND ULTRASTRUCTURE

Neutrophil Precursors

The earliest morphologically recognizable neutrophil precursor is termed the myeloblast. The successive cytologic

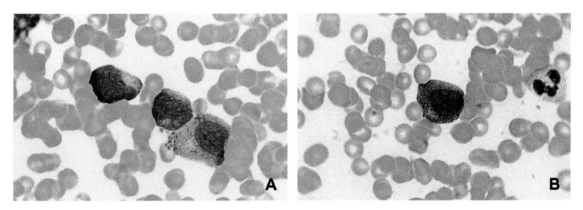

Figure 33.23 Neutrophil precursors from an MGG-stained normal marrow smear. **A.** A myeloblast, an early promyelocyte, and a late promyelocyte/early myelocyte. **B.** A promyelocyte and a neutrophil granulocyte.

classes through which myeloblasts mature into circulating neutrophil granulocytes are termed neutrophil promyelocytes, neutrophil myelocytes, neutrophil metamyelocytes, juvenile neutrophils, and marrow neutrophil granulocytes (Figures 33.23–33.24). Cell division occurs in myeloblasts, promyelocytes, and myelocytes but not in more mature cells.

A myeloblast is 10 to 20 μm in diameter. It has a large rounded nucleus with finely dispersed chromatin and two to five nucleoli. The nucleus-to-cytoplasm ratio is moderately high, and the cytoplasm is basophilic and nongranular. It is likely that only some myeloblasts mature into neutrophil promyelocytes and that others mature into eosinophil or basophil promyelocytes.

Neutrophil promyelocytes are larger than myeloblasts and have basophilic cytoplasm containing a few to several purple-red (azurophilic) granules. The nuclear chromatin pattern is slightly coarser than in myeloblasts, and there may be prominent nucleoli. The neutrophil myelocytes are characterized by the presence in their cytoplasm of

many fine light pink (neutrophilic) granules in addition to some azurophilic granules; the neutrophilic granules also are termed *specific granules*. The nucleus is often eccentric and is round, oval, or slightly indented. The nuclear chromatin is coarsely granular, and the nucleoli are indistinct. The cytoplasm occupies a larger fraction of the cell volume than in promyelocytes; it initially appears pale blue but subsequently becomes predominantly pink. The progressive reduction of cytoplasmic basophilia during the maturation of a myeloblast to a mature myelocyte results largely from a reduction of blue-staining cytoplasmic RNA. The neutrophil metamyelocyte has a C-shaped nucleus and an acidophilic cytoplasm containing numerous fine neutrophilic granules. Few or no azurophilic granules are seen. Juvenile neutrophils (also called band or stab forms) have U-shaped or long, relatively narrow, bandlike nuclei that are often twisted into various configurations. The nuclei contain large clumps of condensed chromatin and may show one or more partial constrictions along their length. These constrictions become progressively more complete and eventually develop into the fine strands of chromatin that are typical of the segmented nuclei of marrow and blood neutrophil granulocytes. Most neutrophil granulocytes have two to five nuclear segments that are joined together by such strands. Some of the neutrophil granulocytes of females have a drumsticklike nuclear appendage (representing an inactivated X chromosome) attached to one of the nuclear segments.

Cytochemistry

When stained by the PAS reaction, myeloblast cytoplasm shows a diffuse, pale red-purple tinge, sometimes with fine granules of the same color. Myeloblasts either do not stain with Sudan black or show a few small sudanophilic granules near the nucleus. They are also peroxidase-negative and, usually, α-naphthol AS-D chloroacetate esterase–negative. The cytoplasm of neutrophil promyelocytes and

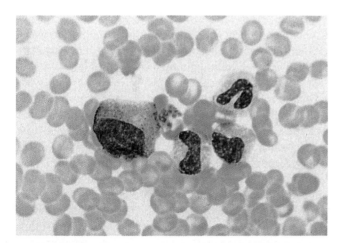

Figure 33.24 Two neutrophil myelocytes (one large and one small), a neutrophil metamyelocyte, and a juvenile neutrophil (stab form) from a normal marrow smear.

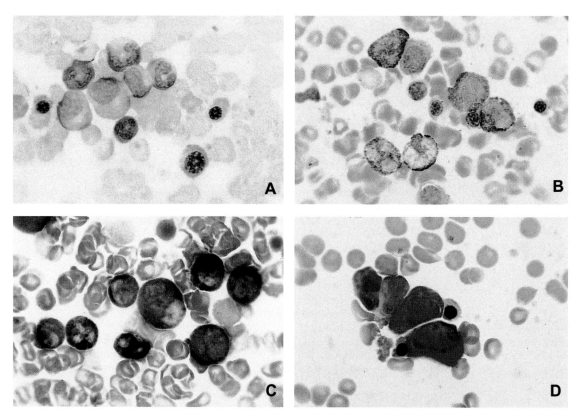

Figure 33.25 Cytochemical reactions of neutrophil precursors and neutrophil granulocytes. **A.** Faint PAS positivity in neutrophil myelocytes and stronger positivity in neutrophil granulocytes. The three erythroblasts are PAS negative. **B.** Sudan black positivity in two neutrophil myelocytes, one eosinophil myelocyte, a neutrophil metamyelocyte, and a neutrophil granulocyte. The lymphocytes and erythroblasts are sudanophobic. **C.** Strong peroxidase positivity in neutrophil myelocytes and granulocytes; p-phenylene diamine and catechol were used as the substrate. **D.** Alpha-naphthol AS-D chloroacetate esterase positivity in three neutrophil myelocytes and a neutrophil granulocyte. The two erythroblasts have not stained. The diazonium salt of fast violet-red LB was used as the capture agent.

more mature cells of the neutrophil series stain positively with the PAS reagent, with Sudan black, and with reactions for peroxidase and α-naphthol AS-D chloroacetate esterase activity. A granular staining pattern is produced with all these cytochemical reactions (Figure 33.25). The intensity of staining increases in cell classes of increasing maturity with the PAS reaction and, to a lesser extent, with Sudan black. Promyelocytes and neutrophil myelocytes, but not neutrophil granulocytes, stain for α-naphthyl acetate esterase activity and, more weakly, for α-naphthyl butyrate esterase activity. Acid phosphatase activity is present in cells at and after the promyelocyte stage; this activity is strongest in the immature cells and weak in neutrophil granulocytes. A few neutrophil metamyelocytes stain weakly for alkaline phosphatase activity, and segmented neutrophil granulocytes stain with a variable intensity (weak to strong) (24, 69–71). Immunocytochemical studies indicate that both lysozyme (muramidase) and elastase are present in promyelocytes and all of the more mature cells of the neutrophil series and that lactoferrin is present in neutrophil myelocytes, metamyelocytes, and granulocytes.

Ultrastructure

Myeloblasts show no special ultrastructural features (72–75). The nucleus has one or more well-developed nucleoli and shows only slight peripheral chromatin condensation. The cytoplasm contains many ribosomes but only a few strands of endoplasmic reticulum and a poorly developed Golgi apparatus. By contrast, the cytoplasm of a promyelocyte is much more complex, being rich in ribosomes, RER, and mitochondria. It also contains a highly developed Golgi apparatus. During the maturation of a promyelocyte to a neutrophil granulocyte, there is a progressive increase in the degree of condensation of nuclear chromatin; a progressive reduction in the quantity of ribosomes, RER, and mitochondria; a diminution of the Golgi apparatus after the myelocyte stage; and the accumulation of large quantities of glycogen at the metamyelocyte and

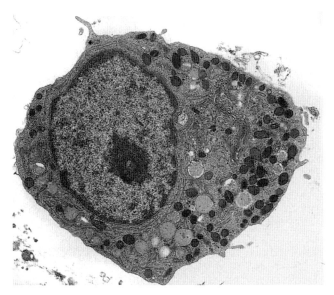

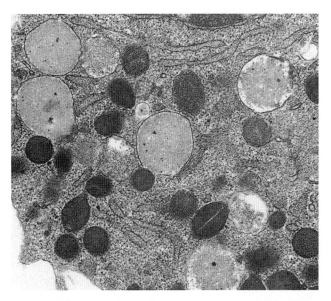

Figure 33.26 Electron micrograph of an immature neutrophil myelocyte from normal bone marrow. The nucleus contains a prominent nucleolus and a small quantity of nuclear membrane–associated condensed chromatin. The cytoplasm contains several strands of endoplasmic reticulum, a prominent paranuclear Golgi apparatus, and two ultrastructurally distinct types of granules.

Figure 33.27 Part of the cytoplasm of the cell in Figure 33.26 at higher magnification. Two types of granules can be clearly recognized. These are (a) rounded or elliptical, very electron-dense primary granules (formed at the promyelocyte stage) and (b) larger, rounded, less electron-dense secondary granules (formed at the myelocyte stage).

granulocyte stages. The cytoplasm of a promyelocyte characteristically contains a variable number of immature and mature primary granules. Mature primary granules are elliptical, measure 0.5 to 1.0 μm in their long axis, are electron dense, and contain peroxidase, lysozyme, elastase, α1 antitrypsin, and sulphated mucosubstances. Some have a core with a linear periodic substructure. Ultrastructurally different granules, the secondary granules, are found in addition to primary granules at the neutrophil myelocyte stage (Figures 33.26–33.27). Secondary granules are larger and less electron dense than primary granules, have rounded outlines, tend to undergo a variable degree of extraction, and are only peroxidase positive if a high concentration of diaminobenzidine is used at alkaline pH. They contain lysozyme and vitamin B$_{12}$ binding protein. Another variety of granule, known as tertiary granules, is present at and after the metamyelocyte stage. These granules are small (0.2–0.5 μm in their long axis), pleomorphic (including rounded, elongated, or dumbbell-shaped forms), and peroxidase negative. Their electron density is usually between that of primary and secondary granules (Figure 33.28). Other electron microscopic cytochemical studies have shown that acid phosphatase is present in primary granules but not in secondary or tertiary granules. The above data on the distribution of peroxidase and acid phosphatase suggest that secondary and tertiary granules do not arise from the modification of primary granules but are synthesized de novo at the myelocyte and metamyelocyte stages, respectively (72). Immunoelectron microscopy has demonstrated that lactoferrin is only found in some of the

granules at and after the neutrophil myelocyte stage. The alkaline phosphatase activity in neutrophil granulocytes is present within small membrane-bound intracytoplasmic vesicles called phosphosomes.

The primary granules observed with the electron microscope correspond to the azurophilic granules seen in Romanowsky-stained smears, and the secondary and tertiary

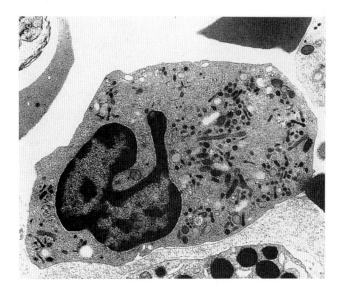

Figure 33.28 Electron micrograph of a neutrophil granulocyte from a normal bone marrow. In addition to some primary and secondary granules, the cytoplasm contains several small pleomorphic tertiary granules.

granules correspond to the neutrophilic or specific granules. Although primary granules are present in all granule-containing cells of the neutrophil series, they lose their azurophilic property and are therefore not detectable by light microscopy at and after the metamyelocyte stage.

Eosinophil and Basophil Precursors

The eosinophil and basophil granulocytes develop through stages that are essentially similar to those through which the neutrophil granulocytes develop. The earliest morphologically recognizable precursors are cells in which a few eosinophil or basophil granules have formed, that is, the eosinophil promyelocytes and basophil promyelocytes. Eosinophil promyelocytes have rounded nuclei with dispersed chromatin and nucleoli and contain two types of granules: large red-orange (eosinophilic) granules and large bluish granules. Eosinophil myelocytes (Figure 33.29), metamyelocytes, and granulocytes have only large eosinophilic granules. Basophil myelocytes, metamyelocytes, and granulocytes are characterized by the presence of large, round, deeply basophilic granules that often overlie the nucleus (Figure 33.30); the more mature granules stain metachromatically with toluidine blue. The majority of circulating eosinophil and basophil granulocytes have two nuclear segments.

Cytochemistry

The granules of eosinophil and basophil granulocytes and their precursors do not stain by the PAS reaction (24,76). However, PAS-positive deposits are found between the specific granules in both cell lineages. The periphery of the eosinophil granules of all cells of the eosinophil series stains strongly with Sudan black, and the core stains weakly or not at all. Basophil granules are strongly sudanophilic in

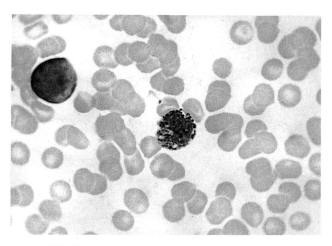

Figure 33.30 Basophil granulocyte from an MGG-stained normal marrow smear.

basophil promyelocytes and myelocytes, but the degree of sudanophilia decreases with increasing maturity; in mature basophils, the granules either do not stain or stain metachromatically (reddish). Peroxidase and acid phosphatase but not lysozymes are demonstrable in the eosinophil granules in all eosinophil precursors and eosinophils. Human eosinophil peroxidase is biochemically and immunochemically distinct from myeloperoxidase, the type of peroxidase present in the neutrophil series. In the basophil series, the granules are strongly positive for peroxidase in basophil promyelocytes and myelocytes, weakly positive in basophil metamyelocytes, and almost negative in basophil granulocytes. Basophil granules stain positively for acid phosphatase. Basophil and eosinophil granulocytes are essentially negative for α-naphthol AS-D chloroacetate esterase and α-naphthyl butyrate esterase.

Eosinophil granules contain eosinophil cationic proteins and an arginine- and zinc-rich major basic protein that are involved in the killing of metazoan parasites. The major basic protein also stimulates basophils and mast cells to release histamine. Other constituents of eosinophil granules include histaminase and arylsulfatase, which are involved in the modulation of immediate-type hypersensitivity reactions. Basophil granules contain chondroitin sulfate and heparin sulfate, which account for their property of staining metachromatically (red-violet) with toluidine blue. They also contain histamine, one of the substances released when immunoglobulin E (IgE)-coated basophils react with specific antigen.

Ultrastructure

On the basis of their electron microscopic features, two types of eosinophil granules, termed primary and secondary granules, are recognized (75,77). Primary granules are large, rounded, homogeneous, and electron dense, and

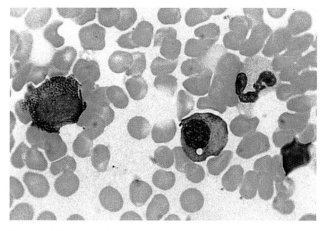

Figure 33.29 Cells from an MGG-stained normal bone marrow smear. The cell types shown are, from left to right, an eosinophil myelocyte, a plasma cell, a neutrophil granulocyte, and a lymphocyte.

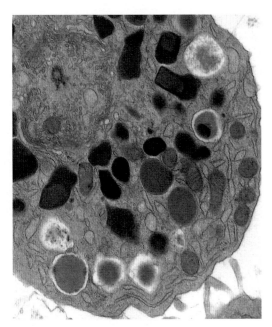

Figure 33.31 Electron micrograph of part of the cytoplasm of an early eosinophil myelocyte. A centriole surrounded by well-developed Golgi saccules, several strands of rough endoplasmic reticulum, and a number of large granules are seen. Some of the granules are homogeneously electron dense (primary granules), but others have a central crystalloid (secondary granules).

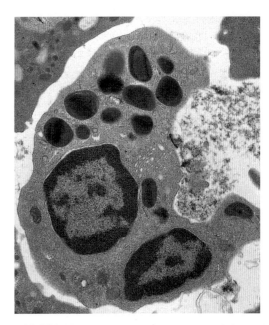

Figure 33.32 Electron micrograph of an eosinophil granulocyte from normal bone marrow. The majority of the cytoplasmic granules are crystalloid-containing secondary granules. Note that the uppermost granule is unusual in that its crystalloid stains more lightly than the surrounding granule matrix.

secondary granules contain a central electron-dense crystalloid inclusion consisting largely of polymerized major basic protein. It is generally held that the primary granules mature into secondary granules. Early eosinophil promyelocytes contain only primary granules, but more mature promyelocytes contain many primary and a few secondary granules. Eosinophil myelocytes contain some primary and several secondary granules (Figure 33.31). By contrast, the majority of the granules in eosinophil metamyelocytes and granulocytes are secondary granules (Figure 33.32). The primary granules of eosinophil promyelocytes are larger and more rounded than the primary granules of neutrophil promyelocytes and promonocytes.

Cells of the basophil series contain characteristic basophil granules, which are prone to undergo varying degrees of extraction during processing for electron microscopy (Figure 33.33). Basophil granules are made up of numerous, closely packed, fine rounded particles (Figure 33.34); the particles are about 20 nm in diameter in mature basophils and slightly smaller in basophil promyelocytes and myelocytes.

Monocyte Precursors

The morphologically recognizable cells belonging to the monocyte series are the monoblasts, promonocytes, marrow monocytes, and blood monocytes. The blood monocytes are not end cells but develop further in the tissues to become macrophages. Certain data suggest that macrophages and

osteoclasts have a common progenitor. All these cells are considered to constitute the mononuclear phagocyte system. In this system, cell division occurs mainly in the monoblasts and promonocytes.

Monoblasts are similar in appearance to myeloblasts except that their nuclei may be slightly indented or lobulated.

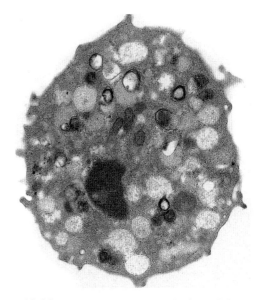

Figure 33.33 Electron micrograph of a basophil granulocyte from a normal bone marrow. The granules have been markedly extracted during processing, but the characteristic closely packed rounded particles can still be recognized in several of the granules.

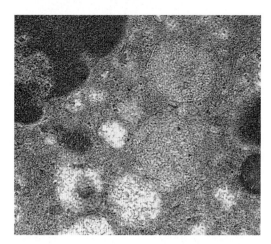

Figure 33.34   Electron micrograph illustrating the particulate ultrastructure of basophil granules at high magnification.

They have small quantities of agranular deeply basophilic cytoplasm and can only be reliably distinguished from other types of blast cells by cytochemical and other special techniques (Figure 33.35). Promonocytes are larger, have a lower nucleus-to-cytoplasm ratio, and contain less basophilic cytoplasm than monoblasts; their cytoplasm contains a few azurophilic granules. Promonocytes usually have a large, rounded, cleft or lobulated nucleus with the chromatin appearing as a fine network. Nucleoli may or may not be visible.

Marrow monocytes and blood monocytes have a lower nucleus-to-cytoplasm ratio (<1), a less basophilic cytoplasm, and a larger number of azurophilic granules than promonocytes. The cytoplasm is pale gray-blue, has a ground glass appearance, and may contain vacuoles. The

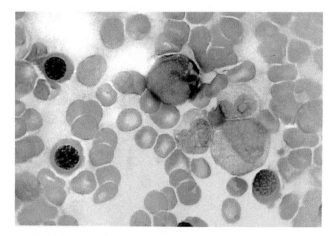

Figure 33.35   A cell with strong α-naphthyl acetate esterase activity from a normal marrow smear (the diazonium salt of fast blue BB was used as the capture agent). This cell has a slightly convoluted nucleus and relatively little cytoplasm and is most probably a monoblast or early promonocyte.

nucleus is eccentrically placed and may be oval, kidney-shaped, horseshoe-shaped, or lobulated; the chromatin has a skeinlike or lacy appearance.

Cytochemistry

Some normal monocytes show several fine or moderately coarse PAS-positive granules and sudanophilic granules and a few peroxidase-positive granules scattered in their cytoplasm (24,71,78). Monocytes do not stain for alkaline phosphatase but stain strongly for acid phosphatase. They contain lysozyme.

Monocytes are α-naphthol AS-D chloroacetate esterase negative but are α-naphthyl acetate esterase (nonspecific esterase) positive. Alpha-naphthyl acetate esterase activity is present not only in monocytes and macrophages, but also in other myeloid cells, including neutrophil promyelocytes and myelocytes, megakaryocytes, and immature red cell precursors. Alpha-naphthyl butyrate esterase activity is stronger than α-naphthyl acetate esterase activity in monocytes and macrophages and is much weaker in the other types of myeloid cells mentioned above. Both the α-naphthyl acetate and the α-naphthyl butyrate esterase activities of monocytes are inhibited by fluoride; in granulocytes and their precursors, these enzyme activities are fluoride insensitive.

Ultrastructure

The earliest monocyte precursor that can be identified on ultrastructural criteria (72,75) is the promonocyte. The nucleus of this cell has only small quantities of nuclear membrane–associated condensed chromatin and has one or more nucleoli. The cytoplasm contains many ribosomes, a moderate number of mitochondria, several strands of RER, bundles of fibrils, a prominent Golgi apparatus, and a few characteristic cytoplasmic granules. The strands of endoplasmic reticulum are shorter and less abundant than in neutrophil promyelocytes. Two types of cytoplasmic granules are seen in promonocytes: (a) immature granules, which have a central zone of flocculent electron-dense material and a clear peripheral zone, and (b) mature granules, which are smaller than the immature granules, vary considerably in size and shape, and are homogeneously electron dense (Figures 33.36–33.37). The maturation of promonocytes first into marrow monocytes and then into blood monocytes is associated with some increase in the quantity of condensed chromatin in the nucleus, a progressive reduction in the number of ribosomes, RER, and fibrils in the cytoplasm, and an increase in the number of cytoplasmic granules. Most or all of the granules of marrow monocytes and all the granules of blood monocytes are of the mature type. Ultrastructural cytochemical studies have shown that some large round granules have acid phosphatase activity and that such granules are more frequent in promonocytes than

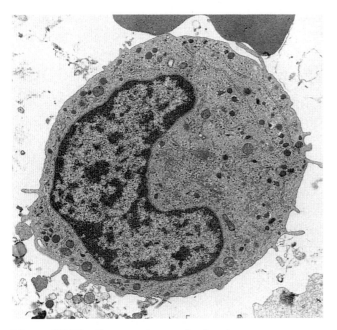

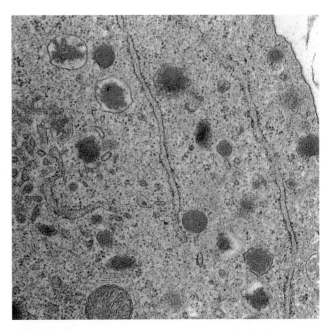

Figure 33.36 Electron micrograph of an immature monocyte from normal bone marrow. The cytoplasm contains many small mature granules and a few immature granules (see Figure 33.37). Several short cytoplasmic processes can be seen at the periphery of the cell.

Figure 33.37 A higher-power view of part of the cytoplasm of the cell in Figure 33.36 showing a few immature-looking granules with an electron-dense central zone and an electron-lucent peripheral zone. There are also some small, uniformly electron-dense mature granules.

monocytes. All the promonocyte granules and some of the monocyte granules are peroxidase positive.

Red Cell Precursors

In this chapter, the term *erythroblast* is used to describe any nucleated red cell precursor, normal or pathologic, and the term *normoblast* to describe all cells that have the morphologic characteristics of the erythroblasts found in normal bone marrow. The terms used to describe various classes of normal red cell precursor are, in order of increasing maturity, pronormoblast, basophilic normoblast, early polychromatic normoblast, late polychromatic normoblast, marrow reticulocyte, and blood reticulocyte (Figure 33.38). Cell division occurs only in the first three of these cytologic classes. Marrow samples containing normoblasts are said to show normoblastic erythropoiesis.

Pronormoblasts are large cells with a diameter of 12 to 20 μm. They have rounded nuclei and moderate quantities of agranular cytoplasm that stains intensely basophilic except for a pale area (corresponding to the Golgi apparatus) adjacent to the nucleus. The nuclear chromatin has a finely stippled or fine reticular appearance, and there are one or more prominent nucleoli. The basophilic normoblasts resemble pronormoblasts except that their nuclear chromatin is slightly more condensed and consequently has a coarsely granular appearance. The early polychromatic normoblasts are smaller than basophilic normoblasts and have a smaller

nucleus and a lower nucleus-to-cytoplasm ratio. The cytoplasm is polychromatic and agranular, and the nucleus contains several medium-sized clumps of condensed chromatin, particularly adjacent to the nuclear membrane. The polychromasia results from the presence of moderate quantities of cytoplasmic RNA (which stains blue), as well as of hemoglobin (which stains red). Late polychromatic normoblasts are even smaller and show a further reduction in the ratio of the area of the nucleus to the area of the cytoplasm. The cytoplasm is predominantly orthochromatic but still has a grayish tinge (i.e., is faintly polychromatic). The nucleus is small and eccentric and contains large clumps of condensed chromatin. The nuclear diameter is less than about 6.5 μm. When mature, late polychromatic normoblasts extrude their nuclei and become marrow reticulocytes; the extruded nuclei are rapidly phagocytosed and degraded by adjacent macrophages. The marrow reticulocyte is irregular in outline and has faintly polychromatic cytoplasm. It is motile and soon enters the marrow sinusoids. When marrow and blood reticulocytes are stained supravitally with brilliant cresyl blue, the ribosomal RNA responsible for their polychromasia precipitates into a basophilic reticulum (hence the term *reticulocyte*). Reticulocytes circulate in the blood for one to two days before becoming mature red cells. The average volume of blood reticulocytes is 20% larger than that of red cells. The latter are circular, biconcave, and acidophilic (i.e., stain red) and, in dried fixed smears, have an average diameter of 7.2 μm (range: 6.7–7.7 μm).

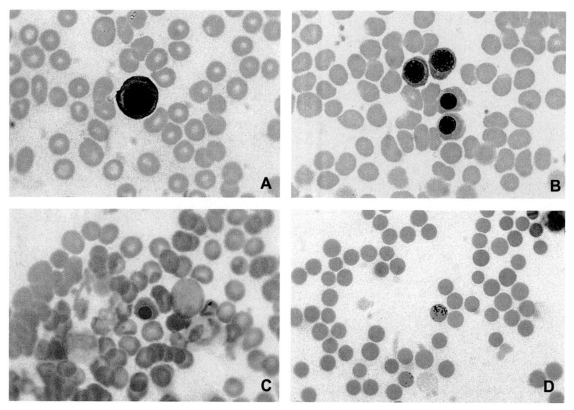

Figure 33.38 Red cell precursors from a normal bone marrow smear (**A–C**) and a reticulocyte from normal peripheral blood (**D**). A. Pronormoblast. B. Two early polychromatic normoblasts and two late polychromatic normoblasts. C. A sideroblast showing a fine, barely visible blue siderotic granule. (A and B, MGG stain; C, Perls' acid ferrocyanide reaction; D, supravital staining with brilliant cresyl blue.)

Cytochemistry

Normal erythroblasts are PAS negative. They also fail to stain with Sudan black and are peroxidase negative. Most nucleated red cells are α-naphthol AS-D chloroacetate esterase negative, but occasional cells show a few positive granules. A few α-naphthol butyrate esterase–positive granules are seen in some nucleated red cells of all degrees of maturity; the positive granules are sometimes seen at the nuclear margin. Coarse acid phosphatase–positive paranuclear granules are frequently present in all types of erythroblasts.

In normal bone marrow smears stained by Perls' acid ferrocyanide method, 20 to 90% of the polychromatic erythroblasts contain one to five small blue-black granules that are usually just visible at high magnification (Figure 33.38C). These iron-containing (siderotic) granules are randomly distributed within the cytoplasm and correspond to the siderosomes seen under the electron microscope. Erythroblasts containing siderotic granules are termed *sideroblasts*. In iron deficiency anemia and, to a lesser extent, in the anemia of chronic disorders, the percentage of sideroblasts is decreased. In conditions associated with an increased percentage saturation of transferrin (e.g., hemolytic anemias), the average number of siderotic granules per cell and the average size of such granules are increased.

Ultrastructure

All nucleated red cell precursors are characterized by the presence of small surface invaginations that develop into intracytoplasmic vesicles (rhopheocytotic vesicles) (75) (Figure 33.39). The nucleus of the pronormoblast has a small quantity of nuclear membrane–associated condensed chromatin (Figure 33.40). The cytoplasm is of low-electron density and contains numerous ribosomes, a moderately well-developed Golgi apparatus, several mitochondria, some strands of endoplasmic reticulum, and small numbers of scattered ferritin molecules. It also contains a few pleomorphic electron-dense acid phosphatase–positive lysosomal granules, which are usually arranged in a group near the Golgi saccules. During the maturation of a pronormoblast into a late polychromatic normoblast (Figure 33.41), the following changes are seen: (a) a steady increase in the quantity of condensed chromatin, (b) a gradual increase in the electron density of the cytoplasmic matrix due to the synthesis of increasing quantities of hemoglobin, (c) a progressive reduction in the number of ribosomes in the cytoplasm, (d) a reduction in the number and size of the mitochondria, and (e) an increasing tendency for some of the intracytoplasmic ferritin molecules to aggregate and form siderosomes (Figures 33.42–33.43). Small autophagic

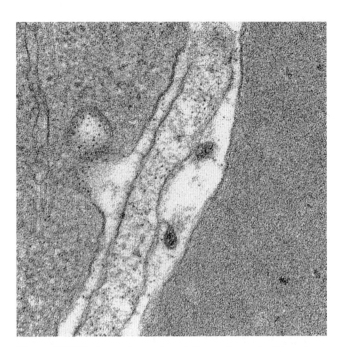

Figure 33.39 Part of an early polychromatic erythroblast showing a rhopheocytotic surface invagination with a few adherent ferritin molecules. A rhopheocytotic vesicle containing several ferritin molecules is closely apposed to the surface invagination. A narrow process of ferritin-containing macrophage cytoplasm is present between the erythroblast displaying rhopheocytosis and the adjacent cell.

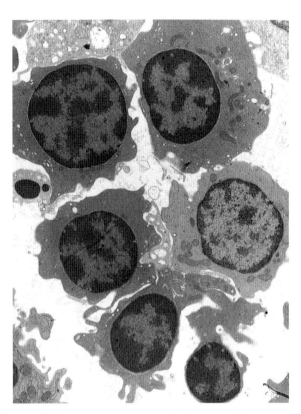

Figure 33.41 Electron micrograph of a group of six erythroblasts at various stages of maturation. Note that maturation is associated with an increase in the electron density of the cytoplasm. The lowermost cell is a late erythroblast about to extrude its nucleus.

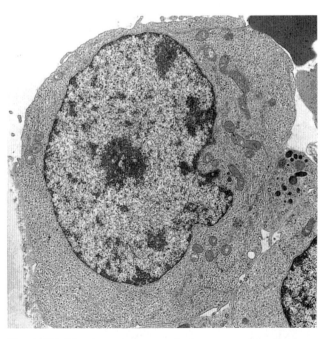

Figure 33.40 Electron micrograph of a pronormoblast from normal bone marrow. The nucleus contains very small quantities of condensed chromatin and has a prominent nucleolus. The cytoplasm is relatively electron lucent and rich in polyribosomes.

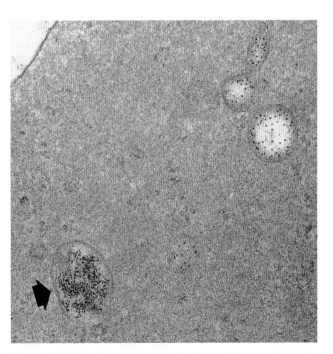

Figure 33.42 Electron micrograph of part of the cytoplasm of a polychromatic erythroblast from normal bone marrow. The cytoplasm shows a membrane-bound accumulation of ferritin and hemosiderin (siderosome) (*arrow*) and a few ferritin-containing rhopheocytotic vesicles.

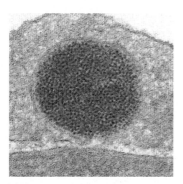

Figure 33.43 Part of a polychromatic erythroblast from a normal marrow showing a membrane-bound siderosome that is much more densely packed with ferritin and hemosiderin molecules than the siderosome in Figure 33.42.

vacuoles are found in 22% and slight to substantial degrees of myelinization of the nuclear membrane in 12% of erythroblast profiles (79). Other data shown by electron microscopic studies of the erythron are that (a) part of the cell's cytoplasmic membrane and a narrow rim of hemoglobin-containing cytoplasm completely surrounds the extruded erythroblast nucleus (Figure 33.44); (b) the marrow reticulocytes enter the sinusoids by passing through, rather than between, endothelial cells (Figure 33.45); and (c) whereas reticulocytes contain ribosomes and mitochondria, mature red cells do not.

Dyserythropoiesis and Ineffective Erythropoiesis

Most of the erythroblasts in normal bone marrow are uninucleate and do not display any unusual morphologic

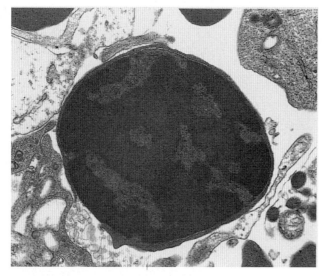

Figure 33.44 Electron micrograph of an extruded erythroblast nucleus. Note that the nucleus is surrounded by a rim of hemoglobin-containing cytoplasm and lies in close contact with processes of macrophage cytoplasm.

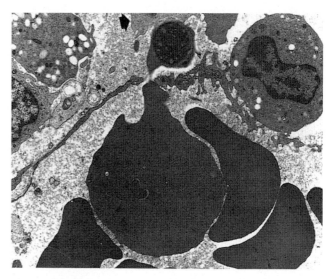

Figure 33.45 Electron micrograph illustrating an uncommon mechanism of formation of a reticulocyte. Whereas nuclear expulsion often occurs extravascularly and the resulting reticulocytes then enter a sinusoid, the cytoplasm of the late erythroblast shown has passed through the endothelial cell of the sinusoid before nuclear expulsion. The nucleus of this erythroblast has not passed through the narrow passage in the endothelial cell and presumably will be severed from the rest of the cell and phagocytosed by the macrophage (*arrow*) lying in contact with it. Thus, in this erythroblast, nuclear expulsion appears to occur during entry of the future reticulocyte into the sinusoid.

features. However, when 400 to 1,000 consecutive erythroblasts (excluding mitoses) were studied in bone marrow smears from each of 10 healthy volunteers with stainable iron in the bone marrow, 0 to 0.57% (mean: 0.31%) were found to be binucleate, 0.7 to 4.8% (mean: 2.4%) showed intererythroblastic cytoplasmic bridges, 0 to 0.9% (mean: 0.24%) showed cytoplasmic stippling, and 0 to 0.7% (mean: 0.39%) showed cytoplasmic vacuolation. In addition, 0 to 0.55% (mean: 0.22%) had markedly irregular nuclear outlines or karyorrhectic nuclei, and 0 to 0.39% (mean: 0.18%) contained Howell-Jolly bodies (micronuclei), a marker of chromosome breaks (80) (Figure 33.46). In another study of 15 healthy males in which 5,000 erythroid cells (including mitoses) were assessed per subject, 0.14% ± 0.04 (SD) were found to be binucleate or multinucleate cells or to be pluripolar mitoses (81). A number of other unusual morphologic features are seen in some erythroblast profiles when the marrow is examined with the electron microscope. These include short stretches (250–910 nm) of duplication of the nuclear membrane in 2% of the profiles, short (260–520 nm) intranuclear clefts in 1.7%, and iron-laden mitochondria in less than 0.2% (79). The above-mentioned light and electron microscopic features are sometimes described as dyserythropoietic changes, with the implication that they are morphologic manifestations of a minor disturbance of

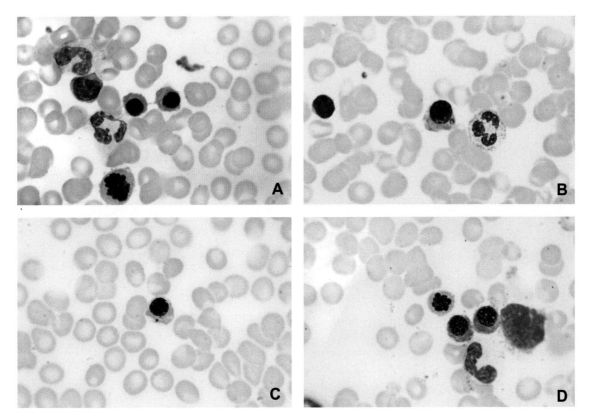

Figure 33.46 Morphologic evidence of dyserythropoiesis in bone marrow smears from healthy volunteers. **A.** Intererythroblastic cytoplasmic bridge. **B.** Large Howell-Jolly body in an early polychromatic erythroblast. **C.** Two smaller Howell-Jolly bodies in a late polychromatic erythroblast. **D.** Karyorrhexis in a late polychromatic erythroblast.

proliferation or maturation in the affected cells. In many congenital or acquired disorders characterized by grossly disordered erythropoiesis, the proportion of erythroblasts showing these dyserythropoietic changes is increased, and some erythroblasts show various dyserythropoietic changes not seen in normal marrow (43). The latter include nonspecific abnormalities, such as large autophagic vacuoles and extensive intranuclear clefts, as well as abnormalities that are specific for certain diseases or groups of diseases.

The phrase *ineffective erythropoiesis* is used to describe the loss of potential erythrocytes due to the phagocytosis and destruction of developing erythroblasts within the bone marrow. The extent of ineffective erythropoiesis in normal bone marrow is small (25). In a number of conditions such as homozygous β-thalassemia and the megaloblastic anemias, there is a gross increase in the ineffectiveness of erythropoiesis; some of the abnormal erythroblasts undergo apoptosis prior to phagocytosis. In such conditions, erythroblasts at various stages of degradation may be recognized within marrow macrophages, both by light and electron microscopy. Apoptosis at the late BFU-E and CFU-E stages is thought to be a major factor controlling the rate of erythropoiesis.

Megakaryocytes

The majority of the cells of the megakaryocyte series are larger than other hematopoietic cells and have polyploid DNA contents. The earliest morphologically recognizable cells in this series are called megakaryoblasts. These are 20 to 30 μm in diameter and have a single large, oval, kidney-shaped, or lobed nucleus that is surrounded by a narrow rim of intensely basophilic agranular cytoplasm. The nucleus contains several nucleoli. Megakaryoblasts (group I megakaryocytes) mature into promegakaryocytes (group II megakaryocytes), which in turn develop into granular megakaryocytes (group III megakaryocytes). Promegakaryocytes are larger than megakaryoblasts and have a larger volume of cytoplasm relative to that of the nucleus. They possess a single large multilobed nucleus with the overlapping lobes arranged in a C-shaped formation. The cytoplasm is less basophilic than that of megakaryoblasts and contains a few azurophilic granules that are usually grouped within the concavity formed by the overlapping nuclear lobes. The granular megakaryocytes (Figure 33.47) are up to 100 μm in diameter and have abundant pale-staining cytoplasm containing many azurophilic granules. The nucleus has multiple lobes, and these become

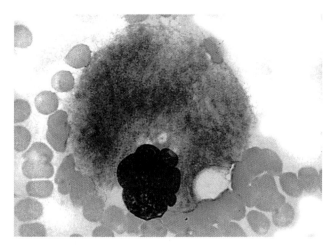

Figure 33.47 Granular megakaryocyte from an MGG-stained normal bone marrow smear.

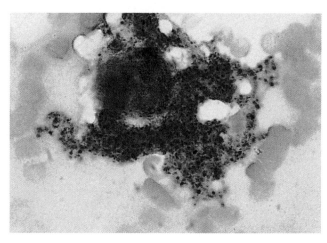

Figure 33.48 Megakaryocyte from a normal bone marrow smear showing large quantities of PAS-positive material.

fairly tightly packed together before the shedding of platelets. The nuclear chromatin has a coarse-grained appearance. Platelets are formed by the fragmentation of cytoplasmic processes of the mature granular megakaryocytes. When platelet formation is completed, a bare nucleus remains.

Mature platelets are usually 2 to 3 μm in diameter and are irregular in outline. The cytoplasm stains pale blue and has a number of azurophilic granules at its center. Newly formed platelets are slightly larger than mature ones.

About 40% of megakaryoblasts, 20% of promegakaryocytes, and 2% of granular megakaryocytes synthesize DNA (82). However, cell division is probably uncommon in megakaryoblasts and is not seen in the other two cell types. The occurrence of cycles of DNA replication without cytokinesis results in the characteristic polyploidy of these cells. The total DNA contents of megakaryoblasts range between 4c and 32c and of promegakaryocytes and granular megakaryocytes between 8c and 64c (1c = the haploid DNA content). There is a positive correlation between the nuclear area and DNA content of megakaryocytes.

Cytochemistry

When stained by the PAS reaction, megakaryocytes show a diffuse and finely granular positivity over both the nucleus and the perinuclear and intermediate zones of the cytoplasm (24,69–71). These positive areas also contain varying numbers of densely positive blocks (Figure 33.48). A narrow peripheral zone of the cytoplasm is often PAS negative, and this may be surrounded by clumps of positive granules within attached platelets. Within platelets, PAS-positive material appears as scattered, lightly staining fine granules at the periphery and as clumps of darkly staining coarse granules at the center. Megakaryocytes and platelets are usually unstained by Sudan black, but occasional megakary-

ocytes may show a diffuse positivity with fine positive granules scattered both in the cytoplasm and over the nucleus. Megakaryocytes and platelets display strong acid phosphatase activity.

Peroxidase activity cannot be demonstrated in megakaryocytes by light microscopy but can be demonstrated in a characteristic distribution using the electron microscope.

Megakaryocytes show no α-naphthol AS-D chloroacetate esterase activity. However, they have substantial α-naphthyl acetate esterase activity (Figure 33.49) and weaker α-naphthyl butyrate esterase activity; the latter generates many coarse or fine positive granules in the cytoplasm and over the nucleus.

Ultrastructure

The nucleus of a megakaryoblast has two or more lobes, very little condensed chromatin, and prominent nucleoli (75,83,84). The cytoplasm contains large numbers of ribosomes, scattered RER, several mitochondria, and a few

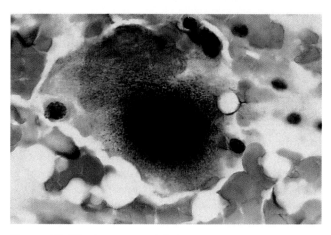

Figure 33.49 Strong α-naphthyl acetate esterase activity in a normal megakaryocyte.

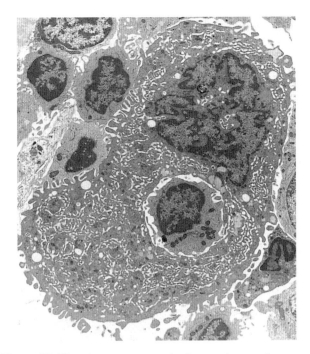

Figure 33.50 Electron micrograph of a granular megakaryocyte from normal bone marrow. The cytoplasm contains a lymphocyte that appears to be traveling through the megakaryocyte (emperipolesis).

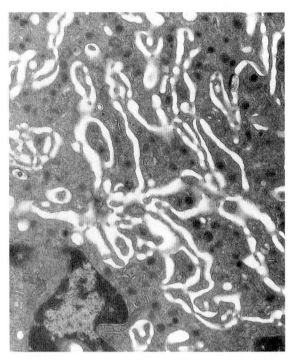

Figure 33.51 Electron micrograph of a part of the intermediate zone of the cytoplasm of a granular megakaryocyte, showing the extensive demarcation membrane system, demarcating granule-containing future platelet areas.

membrane-lined vesicles representing the beginning of the demarcation membrane system (DMS). The cytoplasm also contains a well-developed Golgi apparatus within a deep nuclear indentation. A few immature α granules and a few lysosomal vesicles containing acid phosphatase and arylsulfatase are present near the Golgi apparatus. The maturation of megakaryoblasts into promegakaryocytes and granular megakaryocytes (Figure 33.50) is accompanied by a progressive increase in the quantity of nuclear membrane–associated condensed chromatin, an increase in the number of a granules, a progressive development of the DMS, and a reduction in the number of ribosomes, RER, and mitochondria. Megakaryocyte maturation also is accompanied by the formation of increasing quantities of glycogen in the cytoplasm; the glycogen particles often are found in large clumps. The DMS is an extensive system of membrane-lined cytoplasmic sacs, which arises as invaginations of the surface membrane; it demarcates areas of cytoplasm that eventually become platelets (Figure 33.51).

Three zones can be recognized in the extensive cytoplasm of a granular megakaryocyte (Figure 33.50): (a) a narrow perinuclear zone containing the Golgi apparatus and some of the ribosomes, RER, and mitochondria, (b) a wide intermediate zone containing many ovoid, electron-dense a granules, numerous sacs of the DMS, lysosomal vesicles, ribosomes, RER, and mitochondria, and (c) a narrow outer zone that is devoid of organelles. Mature granular megakaryocytes protrude cytoplasmic processes

that lie near to or within marrow sinusoids. Platelets are formed by the fragmentation of these processes, the platelet membranes being made up of membranes of the DMS.

Ultrastructural cytochemical studies of the oxidation of 3,3′-diaminobenzidine have demonstrated a platelet peroxidase (PPO) in the endoplasmic reticulum and perinuclear space but not in the Golgi apparatus of megakaryoblasts and megakaryocytes and in the dense bodies and dense tubular system of platelets (85). A few small rounded cells present in normal marrow also have PPO activity in the endoplasmic reticulum and perinuclear space and have been identified as promegakaryoblasts (86). Platelet peroxidase appears to be distinct from myeloperoxidase.

Some normal megakaryocytes display the phenomenon of emperipolesis (87,88). This term is used to describe the movement of one cell type within the cytoplasm of another. The cytoplasm of an affected megakaryocyte may contain one or more cells of a number of types, including neutrophil and eosinophil granulocytes and their precursors, lymphocytes, erythroblasts, and red cells (Figure 33.50). The physiologic relevance of megakaryocyte emperipolesis is uncertain; one suggestion has been that certain marrow cells may enter the circulation via the processes of megakaryocyte cytoplasm that protrude into marrow sinusoids.

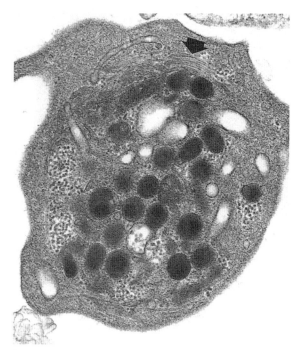

Figure 33.52 Electron micrograph of a platelet from normal blood. The platelet has been sectioned near, rather than at, the equatorial plane and, consequently, shows only part of the circumferential band of microtubules (*arrow*). The section also shows the electron-lucent vesicles of the surface-connected canalicular system, several platelet granules, a few mitochondria, and numerous clumps of glycogen molecules.

Nonactivated platelets are biconvex and have a smooth surface. Their shape is maintained by an equatorial bundle of microtubules situated below the cell membrane, as well as by microfilaments found between various organelles. Other structures found in the cytoplasm include various types of granules, mitochondria, a surface-connected canalicular system, the dense tubular system, and many glycogen particles, which may occur singly or in clumps (Figure 33.52).

Four types of cytoplasmic granule are recognized, namely, the α granules, λ granules (lysosomal granules), δ granules, and peroxisomes (75,89,90). The α and λ granules are moderately electron dense and can be distinguished from each other only by ultrastructural cytochemistry; for example, λ granules have acid phosphatase activity and α granules do not. Substances present in α granules include β-thromboglobulin, platelet factor 4, platelet-derived growth factor, fibrinogen, fibronectin, von Willebrand factor, and thrombospondin. In addition to acid phosphatase, the λ granules contain β-glucuronidase and arylsulfatase. The δ granules (dense granules) are smaller and much more electron dense than α granules and often have a peripheral electron-lucent zone, which gives them a bull's-eye appearance. They contain serotonin, calcium, and the storage pool of ADP and ATP. The peroxisomes are smaller than the α and λ granules; they are moderately electron dense and contain catalase.

The surface-connected canalicular system is an extensive system of electron-lucent intracytoplasmic canaliculi and saccules that open to the exterior at multiple sites on the cell membrane. This canalicular system provides a large surface through which various substances, including granule contents, could be discharged extracellularly. The channels of the dense tubular system are shorter and narrower than those of the surface-connected canalicular system and contain material with an electron density similar to that of the cytoplasm. The dense tubular system contains platelet peroxidase and seems to be derived from the endoplasmic reticulum of megakaryocytes. It is an important site of synthesis of thromboxane A_2, which is involved in the release of granule contents. It is also rich in calcium and may regulate various calcium-dependent reversible reactions such as the activation of actomyosin and the polymerization of tubulin.

Lymphocytes and Plasma Cells

All lymphocytes are eventually derived from the lymphoid stem cells present in the marrow, which are in turn derived from the pluripotent hematopoietic stem cells. The lymphoid stem cells generate both B-cell progenitors and T-cell progenitors. The former mature through a number of antigen-independent intermediate stages into B cells; this maturation occurs within the microenvironment of the marrow. The newly formed B cells travel via the blood into the B-cell zones of peripheral lymphoid tissue. Either the lymphoid stem cells or early T-cell progenitors migrate from the marrow through the blood into the thymus. Here, these cells undergo antigen-independent maturation into T cells, and those T cells that recognize self are deleted. The mature T cells then travel through the blood into the T-cell zones of the peripheral lymphoid organs. The mature B and T lymphocytes that enter the peripheral lymphoid tissue are triggered into division when they react with specific antigen in the presence of appropriate accessory cells. Their progeny develop into effector cells or memory cells. In the case of B cells, the effector cell is an antibody-secreting plasma cell. Antigen-dependent proliferation of B cells occurs in normal marrow and results in the presence of plasma cells in this tissue.

Immunohistochemical studies show that the ratio of T cells to B cells in normal adult marrow is around 3:1. The light and electron microscopic appearances of bone marrow lymphocytes are indistinguishable from those of other lymphocytes in the body. Some T and B lymphocytes have fine or coarse PAS-positive granules arranged in one to four (usually one or two) rings around the nucleus, and occasional cells have large clumps of PAS-positive material. Lymphocytes are peroxidase negative and α-naphthol AS-D chloroacetate esterase negative, and over 99% of cells are alkaline phosphatase negative. Some lymphocytes show a positive paranuclear dot when stained for α-naphthyl butyrate esterase; this staining is unaffected by fluoride. A substantial proportion of normal lymphocytes show either a paranuclear dot or diffuse granular positivity when stained for acid phosphatase. A paranuclear dot is found in both T cells and B cells but more frequently in T cells.

Plasma Cells

Plasma cells seen in smears of normal bone marrow vary considerably in size and appearance. Most are 14 to 20 μm in diameter and have deep blue cytoplasm. The cytoplasm has a pale paranuclear area corresponding to the Golgi apparatus and may contain one or more vacuoles (Figure 33.53A–B). The nucleus is small relative to the volume of cytoplasm, contains moderate quantities of condensed chromatin, and is eccentrically located. Although most plasma cells are uninucleate, a few are binucleate or multinucleate. Some normal plasma cells have other features. For example, occasional cells may contain one or a few large rounded acidophilic, PAS-positive cytoplasmic inclusions (Russell bodies) or several smaller slightly basophilic rounded inclusions (Mott cells, grape cells, or morular cells). Some plasma cells have many pleomorphic cytoplasmic inclusions and, consequently, appear reticulated (Figure 33.53C). Others have eosinophilic cytoplasm, usually at the periphery, but sometimes in the entire cell (flaming cell); when the

eosinophilia is confined to the periphery, it contrasts markedly with the intense basophilia of the rest of the cytoplasm. Occasional plasma cells have azurophilic rods that resemble Auer rods present in acute myeloid leukemia but that are PAS, Sudan black, and peroxidase negative. Plasma cells show strong acid phosphatase activity, particularly around the nucleus and over the Golgi zone. They do not stain for α-naphthol AS-D chloroacetate esterase.

The electron microscope shows that the eccentric rounded nucleus of a plasma cell contains a variable quantity of condensed chromatin (Figures 33.54–33.55A) and a well-developed nucleolus (Figure 33.55A). The presence of moderately large clumps of nuclear membrane–associated condensed chromatin gives the nuclei of mature plasma cells a cartwheel or clock face appearance in histologic sections (but not in marrow smears). The cytoplasm contains numerous long flattened sacs of RER that are arranged either parallel to each other (Figure 33.56), concentrically, or spirally; the sacs are distended to varying extents with a granular, moderately electron-dense material, consisting mostly of immunoglobulin. The cytoplasm also contains mitochondria, a large Golgi apparatus situated immediately adjacent to the nuclear membrane (Figure 33.54), and a few small or medium-sized membrane-bound electron-dense granules. The latter are often found near the Golgi complex, contain acid phosphatase, and appear to be primary lysosomes. Occasional cells contain larger cytoplasmic inclusions that vary markedly in size, electron density, and shape

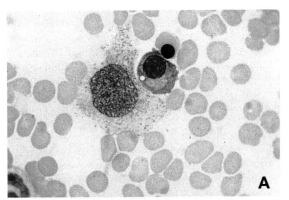

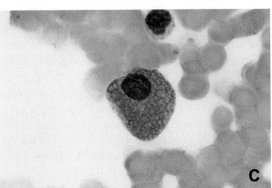

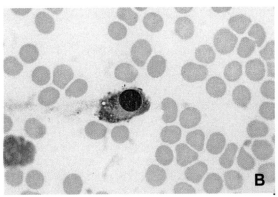

Figure 33.53 Various appearances of plasma cells in a smear of normal bone marrow. A prominent pale paranuclear zone and cytoplasmic vacuoles are seen in (**A**) and (**B**). The cytoplasm in (**C**) has a reticular appearance. The other cells in (A) are a nonphagocytic reticular cell and a late polychromatic erythroblast.

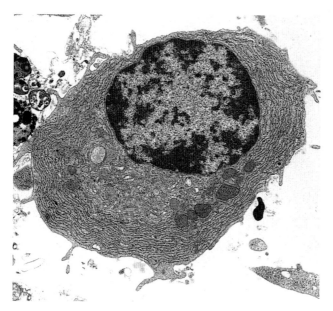

Figure 33.54 Electron micrograph of a plasma cell from a normal bone marrow showing numerous parallel sacs of rough endoplasmic reticulum and a very prominent Golgi apparatus immediately adjacent to the nucleus. The nucleus has moderate quantities of condensed chromatin.

and are often lined by RER. Many of these inclusions are rounded, elliptical, or irregular in outline, but a few are rhomboidal or needlelike and have a crystalline structure (Figure 33.55B–D). Thus, the various types of cytoplasmic inclusion seen under the light microscope appear to be formed by the accumulation of unusually large quantities of immunoglobulin within regions of the RER.

HEMATOPOIETIC CELLS: CHARACTERISTICS IN HISTOLOGIC SECTIONS

In H&E-stained sections of formalin-fixed paraffin-embedded trephine biopsies, insufficient cytoplasmic basophilia and nuclear detail is seen to enable reliable distinction between myeloblasts, neutrophil promyelocytes, neutrophil myelocytes, and early erythroblasts. However, neutrophil metamyelocytes and band cells can be recognized by their C- or U-shaped nuclei and neutrophil granulocytes by the presence of two or more darkly staining nuclear lobes or segments lying together (Figure 33.57). In histologic sections, the fine chromatin strands that join the nuclear lobes of granulocytes usually are not seen. The cytoplasm of neutrophil myelocytes and metamyelocytes stains pale pink and that of neutrophil granulocytes a very pale pink. The granules contained within cells of the neutrophil series stain poorly and are usually difficult to see. Neutrophil promyelocytes and myelocytes can be reliably distinguished from imma-

ture cells belonging to other cell lineages by immunohistochemical staining of neutrophil series–specific antigens such as neutrophil elastase (Table 33.1). In sections of paraffin-embedded marrow fragments, the neutrophil promyelocytes/myelocytes, metamyelocytes, and granulocytes are stained by Leder's stain for chloroacetate esterase (Figure 33.58A). These cells are also stained, both in sections of marrow fragments and trephine biopsy cores, by the PAS reaction (Figure 33.58B). Eosinophil myelocytes, metamyelocytes, and myelocytes can be readily recognized by their red-orange cytoplasm, resulting from the presence of large eosinophilic granules (Figure 33.57). Because basophil granules are water soluble, their contents become extracted during routine fixation for histologic studies. Consequently, basophil granulocytes cannot be seen in histologic sections processed in the usual way.

Erythroblasts of varying degrees of maturity are found in distinctive clumps. Pronormoblasts and basophilic normoblasts are large cells with rounded nuclei containing nucleoli. They only show slight cytoplasmic basophilia when stained by H&E and thus resemble early granulocyte precursors; their identification is therefore based largely on their association with groups of more mature erythroblasts. The late erythroblasts contain rounded heavily stained nuclei showing little structural detail and have moderate quantities of poorly staining cytoplasm, usually with a distinct cytoplasmic membrane. They may show clear halos around the nucleus as a consequence of the shrinkage of the cytoplasm (Figure 33.59). Lymphocytes do not show this artifact. Erythroblasts can be reliably identified by immunohistochemical staining of glycophorins A and C and of hemoglobin A (Table 33.1, Figure 33.60).

The Giemsa stain is superior to H&E for identifying myeloblasts and promyelocytes as well as pronormoblasts and basophilic normoblasts, staining their cytoplasm blue. However, it is still not possible to reliably distinguish myeloblasts from promyelocytes. In Giemsa-stained sections, pronormoblasts have more basophilic cytoplasm than do other blasts and promyelocytes (Figure 33.61).

Lymphocytes may be difficult to distinguish from late erythroblasts in histologic sections of paraffin-embedded trephine biopsy cores except when present in lymphoid nodules. They have a narrow rim of slightly basophilic (Giemsa) or poorly staining (H&E) cytoplasm, indistinct cytoplasmic margins, and a clumped nuclear chromatin pattern. The nuclei of lymphocytes are less perfectly rounded and more variable in size and shape and show more structural detail than those of late erythroblasts. In H&E-stained sections, plasma cells can be identified by the presence of slightly or moderately basophilic cytoplasm, an eccentric nucleus with a cartwheel or clock face chromatin pattern, and a pale paranuclear zone corresponding to the Golgi apparatus. In Giemsa-stained sections, the cytoplasm of many plasma cells stains a deep blue and, consequently, the pale Golgi zone is especially prominent.

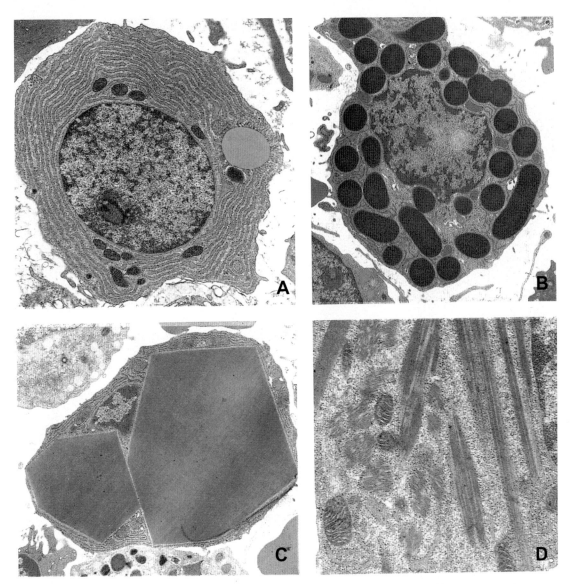

Figure 33.55 Different ultrastructural appearances of plasma cells from normal bone marrow. **A.** Cell with a prominent nucleolus, small quantities of condensed chromatin, several perinuclear mitochondria, some electron-dense material within all the sacs of rough endoplasmic reticulum (RER), and a single large, round, relatively electron-lucent intracytoplasmic inclusion lined by RER. **B.** Cell with multiple rounded or elliptical electron-dense intracytoplasmic inclusions lined by RER. **C.** Cell with two polygonal inclusions lined by RER. **D.** Cell with needlelike crystalline inclusions. The inclusions in (A–C) probably result from the accumulation of large quantities of altered immunoglobulin within sacs of RER.

Megakaryocytes are readily recognized by their large size, light or dark pink cytoplasm, and lobulated nucleus in sections stained either with hematoxylin and eosin or Giemsa (Figure 33.62). In sections of normal bone marrow they are present in clusters of two to five cells and are usually not found in a paratrabecular position. Small numbers of bare megakaryocyte nuclei, with convolutions and a considerable quantity of condensed chromatin, also are seen.

B and T lymphocytes, plasma cells (Figure 33.22A–B), and megakaryoctyes (Figure 33.22D) can be identified immunohistochemically, and megakaryoblasts can be reliably identified only in this way (Table 33.1). Using the monoclonal antibody Y2/51 which is directed against Gp IIIa, the mean value for the total number of megakaryocytes and megakaryoblasts in 15 normal subjects was $24/mm^2$ (range: 14–38) and for megakaryoblasts alone it was $2.8/mm^2$ (range: 1.2–4.9) (91).

As has already been mentioned, much more cytologic detail and especially nuclear detail can be seen in semithin sections of undecalcified plastic-embedded trephine cores (Figure 33.63) than in convention sections of decalcified paraffin-embedded cores (Figure 33.62A).

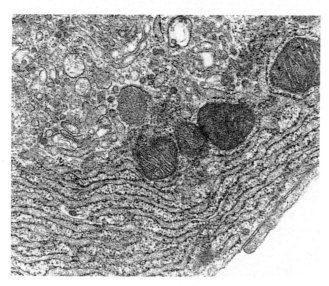

Figure 33.56 Electron micrograph showing part of the Golgi apparatus and some of the sacs of RER from the plasma cell in Figure 33.54, at higher magnification. Four mitochondria are also present.

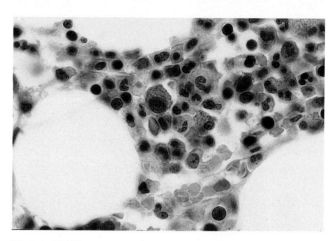

Figure 33.57 Neutrophil promyelocytes/myelocytes, metamyelocytes, stab cells, and granulocytes in a section of a paraffin-embedded trephine biopsy core from a hematologically normal subject. The two cells with large orange granules belong to the eosinophil granulocyte series. (H&E.)

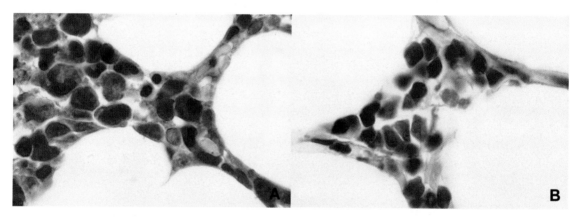

Figure 33.58 Histochemistry of neutrophil series. **A.** Section of a paraffin-embedded marrow fragment from a hematologically normal subject showing cytoplasmic chloroacetate esterase activity in neutrophil promyelocytes/myelocytes and metamyelocytes but not in two erythroblasts (Leder's stain). **B.** Section of a paraffin-embedded trephine biopsy core showing PAS positivity in neutrophil granulocytes and their precursors.

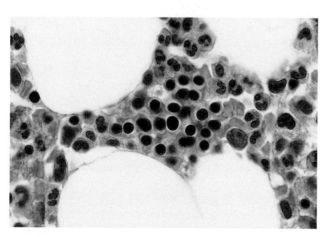

Figure 33.59 Section of a paraffin-embedded trephine biopsy core from a hematologically normal adult showing a group of early and late polychromatic erythroblasts with halos around their nuclei. (H&E.)

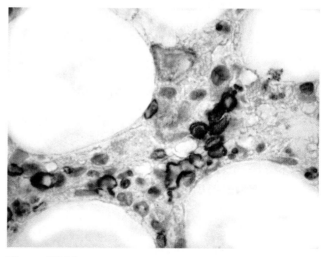

Figure 33.60 Immunohistochemical demonstration of erythroblasts in a section of a paraffin-embedded trephine biopsy core. The section was reacted with antiglycophorin A antibody and the reaction visualized using an immunoalkaline phosphatase method. Courtesy of Dr. Alex Rice.)

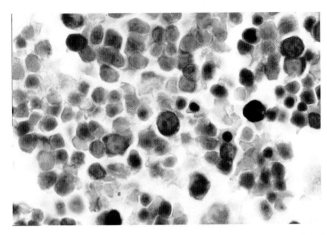

Figure 33.61 Giemsa-stained section of a paraffin-embedded marrow fragment from a patient with erythroid hyperplasia due to a congenital dyserythropoietic state. The cell in the center with deep blue cytoplasm and prominent nucleoli is a proerythroblast. The photomicrograph also shows a few other proerythroblasts, several basophilic erythroblasts, and some early and late polychromatic erythroblasts.

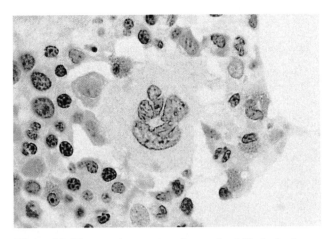

Figure 33.63 Semithin section of an undecalcified, plastic-embedded trephine biopsy core showing a megakaryocyte and adjacent marrow cells. When compared with Figure 33.62A, this semithin section shows considerably more cellular detail, especially nuclear detail. The cytoplasmic granules of cells of the eosinophil series are clearly seen; these are stained red-orange. (H&E.)

CELLULARITY OF THE MARROW

The term *marrow cellularity* usually is defined as the proportion of the area of a histologic section excluding bone occupied by hematopoietic cells (by cells other than fat cells). Cellularity is usually assessed by point counting using an eyepiece with a graticule (histomorphometry) or, more accurately, by computerized image analysis (92). The shrinkage of tissue subjected to decalcification and paraffin embedding results in the cellularity of paraffin-embedded sections being about 5% lower than in plastic-embedded sections (93).

In healthy subjects, cellularity varies with age (53,54). In neonates, there are very few fat cells in the marrow, and the cellularity approaches 100%. Cellularity decreases steadily in the first three decades and stabilizes at 30 to 70% between the ages of 30 and 70 years. During the eighth decade of life, cellularity decreases further and may be less than 20%; this reduction is largely caused by a reduction in bone volume and a consequent increase in the volume of the marrow cavities.

In assessing cellularity, it should be noted that cellularity varies markedly from one intertrabecular space to the next in a single biopsy specimen so that a reliable estimate requires the examination of at least five such spaces (i.e., a biopsy core of greater than 2 cm). Furthermore, the immediate subcortical marrow of the ilium is frequently less cellular than deeper marrow. A study of postmortem biopsy samples from 100 normal subjects who died suddenly without evidence of bone or marrow disease showed only slight differences in the cellularity at different hematopoietic sites. The percentage cellularity ($\pm$ SD) in biopsies from the anterior iliac crest, posterior iliac crest, lumbar vertebrae, and sternum were, 60 $\pm$ 6, 62 $\pm$ 7, 64 $\pm$ 7, and 61 $\pm$ 8, respectively (94).

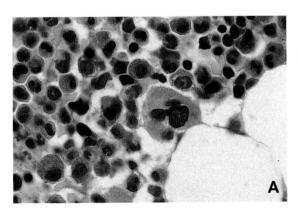
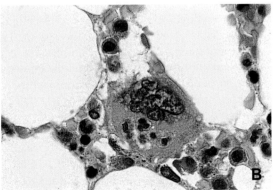

Figure 33.62 Two megakaryocytes from a section of a paraffin-embedded sample of clotted normal marrow (*clot section*). The cells in (**A**) showing a slight orange tinge are eosinophils and their precursors. The megakaryocyte in (**B**) displays emperipolesis. (H&E.)

	TABLE 33.2		

DIFFERENTIAL COUNTS[a] ON MARROW SMEARS FROM 28 HEALTHY ADULTS AGED BETWEEN 20 AND 29 YEARS

	Percentages		
Cell Type	**Mean**	**95% Confidence Limits**	**Observed Range**
Myeloblasts	1.21	0.75–1.67	0.75–1.80
Promyelocytes	2.49	0.99–3.99	1.00–3.75
Myelocytes			
Neutrophil	17.36	11.54–23.18	12.25–22.65
Eosinophil	1.37	0–2.85	0.25–3.45
Basophil	0.08	0–0.21	0.00–0.25
Metamyelocytes			
Neutrophil	16.92	11.40–22.44	11.45–23.60
Eosinophil	0.63	0.07–1.19	0.25–1.30
Juvenile neutrophil granulocytes (stab forms)	8.70	3.58–13.82	4.85–13.95
Granulocytes			
Neutrophil	13.42	4.32–22.52	8.70–8.95
Eosinophil	0.93	0.21–1.65	0.45–1.55
Basophil	0.20	0–0.48	0.05–0.50
Monocytes	1.04	0.36–1.72	0.65–2.10
Plasma cells	0.46	0–0.96	0.10–0.95[b]
Lymphocytes	14.60	6.66–22.54	9.35–25.05
Basophilic erythropoietic cells	0.92	0.40–1.44	0.50–1.60
Early polychromatic normoblasts	6.76	2.56–10.96	3.30–12.20
Late polychromatic normoblasts	11.58	6.16–17.0	7.85–19.55
Reticular cells	0.24	0–0.54	0.05–0.65

[a]Two thousand cells were studied in each individual.
[b]The observed range in 63 cases, aged 20–93 years, was 0.10–2.00%.
From: Jacobson KM. Untersuchungen über das knochenmarkspunktat bei normalen individuen verschiedener altersklassen. *Acta Med Scand* 1941;106:417–446.

MARROW DIFFERENTIAL COUNT

During the first day of life, the erythroblasts account for 18.5 to 65% (mean: 40%) of the nucleated cells in a marrow smear. Over the next 8 to 10 days, this figure decreases progressively to 0 to 20.5% (mean: 8%). After a period of erythroblastopenia lasting about three weeks, the percentage of erythroblasts increases again, reaching values of 6.5 to 31.5% (mean: 16%) at the age of 3 months (95). These changes are caused by an increase in arterial oxygen saturation soon after birth and the consequent suppression of erythropoietin production. Erythropoietin production increases again 6 to 13 weeks later when the hemoglobin concentration in the blood decreases to about 11 g/dL. The proportion of granulocytes and their precursors ranges between 20 and 73% (mean: 46%) of the nucleated marrow cells on the first day of life (95), increases during the next three weeks, and then decreases again to reach a stable value of about 55% after the second month. The average value for the proportion of lymphocytes in the marrow increases from 12% during the first two days of life, to 33% at seven to ten days, and 47% at one month. The lymphocyte percentage then remains stable until the end of the first year, after which it decreases slowly to 19% at 4 to 4.5 years, which is only slightly higher than the adult value of 15% (95-98). Plasma cells are infrequent in the neonate, accounting for up to 0.4% (mean: 0.016%) of nucleated marrow cells (99). They gradually increase in number to reach a mean value of 0.386% at the age of 12 to 15 years (5000 cell differential count). When 300 to 500 consecutive marrow cells are assessed in each case, the prevalence of plasma cells in healthy adults is 0.4 to 4.0%.

The differential count on 2000 consecutive nucleated cells in bone marrow smears from normal adults is given in Table 33.2 (100). The mean and range for the myeloid/erythroid ratio in healthy adults are 3.1 and 2.0:8.3, respectively (101).

REFERENCES

1. Preston SL, Alison MR, Forbes SJ, Direkze NC, Poulsom R, Wright NA. The new stem cell biology: something for everyone. *Mol Pathol* 2003;56:86–96.

2. Rywlin AM. *Histopathology of the Bone Marrow*. Boston: Little, Brown & Co.; 1976.

3. Krause JR, ed. *Bone Marrow Biopsy*. Edinburgh: Churchill Livingstone;1981.

4. Bartl R, Frisch B. Normal bone marrow: histology, histochemistry and immunohistochemistry. In: Wickramasinghe SN, McCullough J, eds. *Blood and Bone Marrow Pathology*. Edinburgh: Churchill Livingstone; 2003:53–69.

5. Andrade RE, Wick MR, Frizzera G, Gajl-Peczalska KJ. Immunophenotyping of hematopoietic malignancies in paraffin sections. *Hum Pathol* 1988;19:394–402.

6. Pulford KA, Erber WN, Crick JA, et al. Use of monoclonal antibody against human neutrophil elastase in normal and leukaemic myeloid cells. *J Clin Pathol* 1988;41:853–860.

7. Gatter KC, Cordell JL, Turley H, et al. The immunohistological detection of platelets, megakaryocytes and thrombi in routinely processed specimens. *Histopathology* 1988;13:257–267.

8. Kubic VL, Brunning RD. Immunohistochemical evaluation of neoplasms in bone marrow biopsies using monoclonal antibodies reactive in paraffin-embedded tissue. *Mod Pathol* 1989;2: 618–629.

9. van der Valk P, Mullink H, Huijgens PC, Tadema TM, Vos W, Meijer CJ. Immunohistochemistry in bone marrow diagnosis. Value of a panel of monoclonal antibodies on routinely processed bone marrow biopsies. *Am J Surg Pathol* 1989;13:97–106.

10. Walls AF, Jones DB, Williams JH, Church MK, Holgate ST. Immunohistochemical identification of mast cells in formaldehyde-fixed tissue using monoclonal antibodies specific for tryptase. *J Pathol* 1990;162:119–126.

11. Horny HP, Wehrmann M, Steinke B, Kaiserling E. Assessment of the value of immunohistochemistry in the subtyping of acute leukemia on routinely processed bone marrow biopsy specimens with particular reference to macrophage-associated antibodies. *Hum Pathol* 1994;25:810–814.

12. te Velde J, Burkhardt R, Kleiverda K, Leenheers-Binnendijk L, Sommerfeld W. Methyl-methacrylate as an embedding medium in histopathology. *Histopathology* 1977;1:319–330.

13. Burkhardt R. Bone marrow histology. In: Catovsky D, ed. *The Leukemic Cell (Methods in Hematology)*. Edinburgh: Churchill Livingstone; 1981:49–86.

14. Frisch B, Lewis SM, Burkhardt R, Bartl R. *Biopsy Pathology of Bone and Bone Marrow*. London: Chapman & Hall; 1985.

15. Frisch B, Bartl R. Atlas of bone marrow pathology. In: Gresham GA, ed. *Current Histopathology*. Vol 15. Dordrecht, The Netherlands: Kluwer Academic; 1990.

16. Beckstead JH, Halverson PS, Ries CA, Bainton DF. Enzyme histochemistry and immunohistochemistry on biopsy specimens of pathologic human bone marrow. *Blood* 1981;57:1088–1098.

17. Beckstead JH. The bone marrow biopsy: a diagnostic strategy. *Arch Pathol Lab Med* 1986;110:175–179.

18. Archimbaud E, Islam A, Preisler HD. Immunoperoxidase detection of myeloid antigens in glycolmethacrylate-embedded human bone marrow. *J Histochem Cytochem* 1987;35:595–599.

19. Burkhardt R. Präparative Voraussetzungen zur klinischen Histologie des menschlichen Knochenmarks. I. Mitteilung. *Blut* 1966;13:337–357.

20. Burkhardt R. Präparative Voraussetzungen zur klinischen Histologie von Knochenmark und Knochen. II. Ein neues Verfahren zur histologischen Präparation von Biopsien aus Knochenmark und Knochen. *Blut* 1966;14:30–46.

21. Burkhardt R. *Bone Marrow and Bone Tissue. Color Atlas of Clinical Histopathology*. Berlin: Springer-Verlag; 1971.

22. Wood GS, Warnke RA. The immunologic phenotyping of bone marrow biopsies and aspirates: frozen section techniques. *Blood* 1982;59:913–922.

23. Falini B, Martelli MF, Tarallo F, et al. Immunohistological analysis of human bone marrow trephine biopsies using monoclonal antibodies. *Br J Haematol* 1984;56:365–386.

24. Hayhoe FGJ, Quaglino D. *Haematological Cytochemistry*. 2nd ed. Edinburgh: Churchill Livingstone; 1988.

25. Wickramasinghe SN. *Human Bone Marrow*. Oxford: Blackwell Scientific; 1975.

26. Gordon MY. Human haemopoietic stem cell assays. *Blood Rev* 1993;7:190–197.

27. Ogawa M. Hematopoiesis. *J Allergy Clin Immunol* 1994;94: 645–650.

28. Baron MH. Hemangioblasts in adults? *Blood* 2004;103:1

29. Verfaillie C. Regulation of hematopoiesis. In: Wickramasinghe SN, McCullough J, eds. *Blood and Bone Marrow Pathology*. Edinburgh: Churchill Livingstone; 2003:71–85.

30. Krause DS. Regulation of hematopoietic stem cell fate. *Oncogene* 2002;21:3262–3269.

31. Lord BI, Dexter TM, ed. Growth factors in haemopoiesis. *Baillieres Clin Haematol* 1992;5.

32. Brenner M, ed. Cytokines and growth factors. *Baillieres Clin Haematol* 1994;7.

33. Moore MA, Metcalf D. Ontogeny of the haemopoietic system: yolk sac origin of in vivo and in vitro colony forming cells in the developing mouse embryo. *Br J Haematol* 1970;18:279–296.

34. Dzierzak E, Medvinsky A, de Bruijn M. Qualitative and quantitative aspects of haematopoietic cell development in the mammalian embryo. *Immunol Today* 1998;19:228–236.

35. Palis J, Robertson S, Kennedy M, Wall C, Keller G. Development of erythroid and myeloid progenitors in the yolk sac and embryo proper of the mouse. *Development* 1999;126:5073–5084.

36. Bloom W, Bartelmez GW. Hematopoiesis in young human embryos. *Am J Anat* 1940;67:21–53.

37. Kelemen E, Calvo W, Fliedner TM. *Atlas of Human Hemopoietic Development*. Berlin: Springer-Verlag; 1979.

38. Gilmour JR. Normal haemopoiesis in intrauterine and neonatal life. *J Pathol Bacteriol* 1941;52:25–55.

39. Emura I, Sekiya M, Ohnishi Y. Two types of immature erythrocytic series in the human fetal liver. *Arch Histol Jpn* 1983;46: 631–643.

40. Kalpaktsoglou PK, Emery JL. Human bone marrow during the last three months of intrauterine life. A histological study. *Acta Haematol* 1965;34:228–238.

41. Piney A. The anatomy of the bone marrow with special reference to the distribution of the red marrow. *Br Med J* 1922;2:792–795.

42. Custer RP, Ahlfeldt FE. Studies on the structure and function of bone marrow. II. Variations in cellularity in various bones with advancing years of life and their relative response to stimuli. *J Lab Clin Med* 1932;17:960–962.

43. Wickramasinghe SN, McCullough J, eds. *Blood and Bone Marrow Pathology*. Edinburgh: Churchill Livingstone; 2003.

44. Munka V, Gregor A. Lymphatics and bone marrow. *Folia Morphol (Praha)* 1965;13:404–412.

45. Bain BJ, Clark DM, Lampert IA, Wilkins BS. *Bone Marrow Pathology*. 3rd ed. Oxford: Blackwell Science; 2001.

46. Branemark PI. Bone marrow microvascular structure and function. *Adv Microbiol* 1968;1:1–65.

47. De Bruyn PPH, Breen PC, Thomas TB. The microcirculation of the bone marrow. *Anat Rec* 1970;168:55–68.

48. Wickramasinghe SN. Observations on the ultrastructure of sinusoids and reticular cells in human bone marrow. *Clin Lab Haematol* 1991;13:263–278.

49. Miller MR, Kasahara M. Observations on the innervation of human long bones. *Anat Rec* 1963;145:13–17.

50. Dominici M, Pritchard C, Garlits JE, Hofmann TJ, Persons DA, Horwitz EM. Hematopoietic cells and osteoblasts are derived from a common marrow progenitor after bone marrow transplantation. *Proc Natl Acad Sci U S A* 2004;101:11761–11766.

51. Benayahu D, Horowitz M, Zipori D, Wientroub S. Hemopoietic functions of marrow-derived osteogenic cells. *Calcif Tissue Int* 1992;51:195–201.

52. Chambers TJ. Regulation of osteoclast development and function. In: Rifkin BR, Gay CV, eds. *Biology and Physiology of the Osteoclast*. Boca Raton, FL: CRC Press; 1992:105–128.

53. Sturgeon P. Volumetric and microscopic pattern of bone marrow in normal infants and children. III. Histologic pattern. *Pediatrics* 1951;7:774–781.

54. Hartsock RJ, Smith EB, Petty CS. Normal variations with aging of the amount of hematopoietic tissue in bone marrow from the anterior iliac crest. A study made from 177 cases of sudden death examined by necropsy. *Am J Clin Pathol* 1965;43:326–331.

55. Tavassoli M, Eastlund DT, Yam LT, Neiman RS, Finkel H. Gelatinous transformation of bone marrow in prolonged self-induced starvation. *Scand J Haematol* 1976;16:311–319.

56. Gale E, Torrance J, Bothwell T. The quantitative estimation of total iron stores in human bone marrow. *J Clin Invest* 1963;42:1076–1082.

57. Trubowitz S, Masek B. A histochemical study of the reticuloendothelial system of human marrow—its possible transport role. *Blood* 1968;32:610–628.

58. Burgio VL, Magrini U, Ciardelli L, Pezzoni G. An enzyme-histochemical approach to the study of the human bone-marrow stroma. *Acta Haematol* 1984;71:73–80.

59. Westen H, Bainton DF. Association of alkaline-phosphatase-positive reticulum cells in bone marrow with granulocytic precursors. *J Exp Med* 1979;150:919–937.

60. Tanaka Y. An electron microscopic study of non-phagocytic reticulum cells in human bone marrow. I. Cells with intracytoplasmic fibrils. *Nippon Ketsueki Gakkai Zasshi* 1969;32:275–286.

61. Biermann A, Graf von Keyserlingk D. Ultrastructure of reticulum cells in the bone marrow. *Acta Anat (Basel)* 1978;100:34–43.

62. Tsai S, Patel V, Beaumont E, Lodish HF, Nathan DG, Sieff CA. Differential binding of erythroid and myeloid progenitors to fibroblasts and fibronectin. *Blood* 1987;69:1587–1594.

63. Broudy VC, Zuckerman KS, Jetmalani S, Fitchen JH, Bagby GC Jr. Monocytes stimulate fibroblastoid bone marrow stromal cells to produce multilineage hematopoietic growth factors. *Blood* 1986;68:530–534.

64. Kirshenbaum AS, Kessler SW, Goff JP, Metcalfe DD. Demonstration of the origin of human mast cells from CD34+ bone marrow progenitor cells. *J Immunol* 1991;146:1410–1415.

65. Zucker-Franklin D, Grusky G, Hirayama N, Schnipper E. The presence of mast cell precursors in rat peripheral blood. *Blood* 1981;58:544–551.

66. Denburg JA, Richardson M, Telizyn S, Bienenstock J. Basophil/mast cell precursors in human peripheral blood. *Blood* 1983;61:775–780.

67. Kempuraj D, Saito H, Kaneko A, et al. Characterization of mast cell-committed progenitors present in human umbilical cord blood. *Blood* 1999;93:3338–3346.

68. Rywlin AM, Ortega RS, Dominguez CJ. Lymphoid nodules of bone marrow: normal and abnormal. *Blood* 1974;43:389–400.

69. Rheingold JJ, Wislocki GB. Histochemical methods applied to hematology. *Blood* 1948;3:641–655.

70. Gibb RP, Stowell RE. Glycogen in human blood cells. *Blood* 1949;4:569–579.

71. Rozenszajn L, Leibovich M, Shoham D, Epstein J. The esterase activity in megaloblasts, leukaemic and normal haemopoietic cells. *Br J Haematol* 1968;14:605–610.

72. Scott RE, Horn RG. Ultrastructural aspects of neutrophil granulocyte development in humans. *Lab Invest* 1970;23:202–215.

73. Bainton DF, Ullyot JL, Farquhar MG. The development of neutrophilic polymorphonuclear leukocytes in human bone marrow. *J Exp Med* 1971;134:907–934.

74. Cawley JC, Hayhoe FGJ. *Ultrastructure of Haemic Cells. A Cytological Atlas of Normal and Leukaemic Blood and Bone Marrow.* London: WB Saunders; 1973.

75. Bessis M. *Living Blood Cells and Their Ultrastructure.* Berlin: Springer-Verlag; 1973.

76. Parwaresch MR. *The Human Blood Basophil.* Berlin: Springer-Verlag; 1976.

77. Scott RE, Horn RG. Fine structural features of eosinophile granulocyte development in human bone marrow. *J Ultrastruct Res* 1970;33:16–28.

78. Leder LD. The origin of blood monocytes and macrophages. A review. *Blut* 1967;16:86–98.

79. Wickramasinghe SN, Hughes M. Globin chain precipitation, deranged iron metabolism and dyserythropoiesis in some thalassaemia syndromes. *Haematologia (Budap)* 1984;17:35–55.

80. Wickramasinghe SN, Lee MJ, Furukawa T, Eguchi M, Reid CD. Composition of the intra-erythroblastic precipitates in thalassaemia and congenital dyserythropoietic anaemia (CDA): identification of a new type of CDA with intra-erythroblastic precipitates not reacting with monoclonal antibodies to α- and β-globin chains. *Br J Haematol* 1996;93:576–585.

81. Němec J, Polák H. Erythropoietic polyploidy. I. The morphology of polyploid erythroid elements and their incidence in healthy subjects. *Folia Haematol Int Mag Klin Morphol Blutforsch* 1965;84:24–40.

82. Queisser U, Queisser W, Spiertz B. Polyploidization of megakaryocytes in normal humans, in patients with idiopathic thrombocytopenia and with pernicious anaemia. *Br J Haematol* 1971;20:489–501.

83. Jean G, Lambertenghi-Deliliers G, Ranzi T, Poirier-Basseti M. The human bone marrow megakaryocyte. An ultrastructural study. *Haematologia (Budap)* 1971;5:253–264.

84. Breton-Gorius J, Reyes F. Ultrastructure of human bone marrow cell maturation. *Int Rev Cytol* 1976;46:251–321.

85. Breton-Gorius J. The value of cytochemical peroxidase reactions at the ultrastructural level in haematology. *Histochem J* 1980;12:127–137.

86. Breton-Gorius J, Gourdin MF, Reyes F. Ultrastructure of the leukemic cell. In: Catovsky D, ed. *The Leukemic Cell (Methods in Hematology).* Edinburgh: Churchill Livingstone; 1981:85–128.

87. Larsen TE. Emperipolesis of granular leukocytes within megakaryocytes in human hemopoietic bone marrow. *Am J Clin Pathol* 1970;53:485–489.

88. Rozman C, Vives-Corrons JL. On the alleged diagnostic significance of megakaryocytic "phagocytosis" (emperipolesis). *Br J Haematol* 1981;48:510.

89. White JG. Current concepts of platelet structure. *Am J Clin Pathol* 1979;71:363–378.

90. Berndt MC, Castaldi PA, Gordon S, Halley H, McPherson VJ. Morphological and biochemical confirmation of gray platelet syndrome in two siblings. *Aust N Z J Med* 1983;13:387–390.

91. Thiele J, Wagner S, Weuste R, et al. An immunomorphometric study of megakaryocyte precursor cells in bone marrow tissue from patients with chronic myeloid leukemia (CML). *Eur J Haematol* 1990;44:63–70.

92. Al-Adhadh AN, Cavill I. Assessment of cellularity in bone marrow fragments. *J Clin Pathol* 1983;36:176–179.

93. Kerndrup G, Pallensen G, Melsen F, Mosekilde L. Histomorphometrical determination of bone marrow cellularity in iliac crest biopsies. *Scand J Haematol* 1980;24:110–114.

94. Bartl R, Frisch B. *Biopsy of Bone in Internal Medicine: An Atlas and Sourcebook (Current Histopathology).* Vol 21. Dordrecht, The Netherlands: Kluwer Academic; 1993.

95. Gairdner D, Marks J, Roscoe JD. Blood formation in infancy. Part I. The normal bone marrow. *Arch Dis Child* 1952;27:128–133.

96. Glaser K, Limarzi LR, Poncher HG. Cellular composition of the bone marrow in normal infants and children. *Pediatrics* 1950;6:789–824.

97. Diwany M. Sternal marrow puncture in children. *Arch Dis Child* 1940;15:159–170.

98. Rosse C, Kraemer MJ, Dillon TL, McFarland R, Smith NJ. Bone marrow cell populations of normal infants: the predominance of lymphocytes. *J Lab Clin Med* 1977;89:1225–1240.

99. Steiner ML, Pearson HA. Bone marrow plasmacyte values in childhood. *J Pediatr* 1966;68:562–568.

100. Jacobsen KM. Untersuchungen über das knochenmarkspunktat bei normalen individuen verschiedener altersklassen. *Acta Med Scand* 1941;106:417–446.

101. Young RH, Osgood EE. Sternal marrow aspirated during life. Cytology in health and in disease. *Arch Intern Med* 1935;55:186–203.

GENITOURINARY TRACT

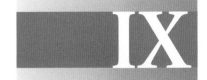

Kidney

34

William L. Clapp   *Byron P. Croker*

INTRODUCTION

The kidney has an intricate structure that underlies its diverse roles of excreting waste products, regulating body fluid and solute balance, regulating blood pressure, and secreting hormones. A familiarity with the basic structure of the kidney facilitates the evaluation and comprehension of diseases and functional disorders that can affect the kidney. The structure of the normal human kidney is considered in this chapter. Although the focus is on the human kidney, analogous renal structures in other mammalian species are discussed or illustrated when pertinent.

PEDIATRIC KIDNEY

Renal enthusiasts, especially developmental biologists and pathologists, have long been fascinated with how a kidney develops from primitive mesoderm into such a wondrously complex organ. A basic understanding of nephrogenesis provides a framework to enhance our knowledge of congenital kidney disease. The human kidney is structurally immature at the time of birth, and important morphologic changes occur during infancy and childhood. Pathologists not familiar with the histologic peculiarities of the pediatric kidney may mistake normal findings for abnormalities or fail to observe significant abnormalities of renal maturation. The following section covers the pediatric kidney,

focusing first on kidney development prior to birth, and second, on the kidney after birth.

Kidney Development

During development, cells proliferate, migrate, differentiate, die, and interact with other cells to form tissues and organs. These different aspects of cell behavior are controlled by genes in a temporal and spatial manner. The kidney has long been considered an excellent model system for the study of organogenesis. However, when one considers the elaborate architecture and heterogenous cellular elements of the organ, it is not surprising that understanding the mechanisms of kidney development remains a considerable challenge. Detailed reviews of kidney development are available for more information (1–12).

Embryonic Kidneys

Organogenesis begins during the third week of human embryogenesis with the initial formation of the central nervous and cardiovascular systems. The urogenital system represents the last organ system to develop. Kidney development goes through three successive stages: pronephros, mesonephros and metanephros. All three systems develop from the intermediate mesoderm, located between the dorsal somites and lateral plate mesoderm and extending from the cervical to the caudal regions of the embryo. The

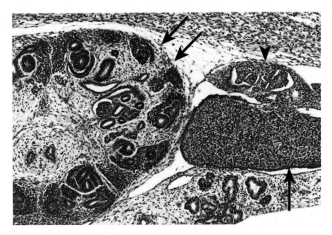

Figure 34.1 Mesonephros amd metanephros. The mesonephros (*arrowhead*) contributes somatic cell lineages to the gonadal ridge (*single arrow*), which will develop into the gonad. Early nephron formation is present in the metanephros (*double arrows*), whose development is dependent on the presence of the mesonephros. Reprinted with permission from: Murphy WM, Grignon DJ, Perlman EJ. Tumors of the kidney, bladder, and related urinary structures. In: *Atlas of Tumor Pathology*. 4th series, fascicle 1. Washington, DC: Armed Forces Institute of Pathology; 2004.

pronephros and mesonephros are transient structures in mammals. However, all three systems are essential for the formation of each subsequent organ and are dependent on the presence of the preceeding structure. The mesonephros forms before the pronephros regresses, and the metanephros develops before the mesonephros disappears (Figure 34.1). This developmental scheme may be likened to a wave of nephrogenesis moving in a cervical to caudal direction through the intermediate mesoderm. Some genes that regulate metanephric kidney development are also believed to be involved in forming the earlier embryonic kidneys.

Pronephros

The pronephros develops in the cervical region at the end of the third week of human gestation. However, most of our knowledge of the pronephros has come from the study of lower vertebrates (13,14). The pronephros consists of a glomus (glomerulus-like structure), tubules, and a duct. The glomus, not physically connected to the tubules, projects into the coelomic cavity and filters blood.

Ciliated tubules, called nephrostomes, open into the coelom and collect the filtrate. The nephrostomes connect to proximal tubules, which empty into a distal tubule that joins the pronephric duct. In humans, the pronephros is a rudimentary organ and does not function. As the pronephric duct extends caudally, the glomus and tubules regress. However, the pronephric duct persists and becomes the mesonephric duct.

Mesonephros

The human mesonephros develops in the middle of the fourth week of gestation as a thoracic organ. Considerable

variation in structure and function of the mesonephros exists, even among mammalian species (15). The human mesonephros contains 20 to 40 nephrons, consisting of glomeruli directly connected to tubules, with proximal and distal segments, some of which directly connect to the mesonephric duct (wolffian duct). The distal mesonephric duct fuses with the cloaca, a precursor of the urinary bladder. In some mammals, two sets of mesonephric tubules exist. The caudal tubules, representing the majority of the mesonephric nephrons, never fuse with the mesonephric duct, whereas the more cephalad tubules are connected to the duct. Moreover, mice deficient for the Wilms' tumor suppressor gene, *WT1*, lack the caudal set of mesonephric tubules but develop the cephalad ones (16). Thus, *WT1* appears to regulate only caudal mesonephric development, which may have some molecular events similar to metanephric development since both require *WT1* for formation. The excretory function of the human mesonephros is believed to be limited. As observed with the pronephros, the mesonephros undergoes apoptosis and degenerates (17).

In the male, some mesonephric tubules form the efferent ducts of the epididymis, whereas the mesonephric duct gives rise to the duct of the epididymis, the seminal vesicle, and the ejaculatory duct. In females, the mesonephros undergoes dissolution, with the epoöphoron, paroöphoron, and Gartner's duct remaining as vestigial structures. Evidence has emerged indicating the mesonephros contributes cell lineages for other organ systems. A region including the dorsal aorta, gonad, and mesonephros (AGM) is the first site in which adult-type hematopoietic stem cells are generated (18,19).

Metanephros

Overview

The metanephros, the definitive and permanent kidney, develops from an inductive interaction between the ureteric bud and the mesenchyme of the caudal intermediate mesoderm, called the metanephric mesenchyme, or blastema. During the fifth week of gestation, the first step in metanephric development occurs. Factors expressed by the metanephric mesenchyme induce the ureteric bud, a branch of the caudal mesonephric duct, to grow dorsally until it encounters the mesenchyme. The ureteric bud undergoes iterative branching to form the renal pelvis, calyces, and collecting ducts. Induced by the ureteric bud, the metanephric mesenchyme differentiates into the glomeruli, proximal and distal tubules, and Henle's loops. Thus, cells of the metanephric kidney originate from two different lineages to form the collecting ducts and nephrons. The reciprocal inductive interaction between the ureteric bud and the metanephric mesenchyme is the central process of metanephrogenesis. For detailed information, the reader is directed to the classic light microscopic (1–3), microdissection (4–6), and experimental (7,8) studies.

Formation of the Renal Pelvis and Calyces

The complex three-dimensional branching pattern of the ureteric bud and its derivatives creates an elaborate renal architecture. The ureteric bud and its branches consist of a tubule portion, which elongates, and an actively growing ampullary tip. Various types of branching have been observed, including bifid and trifid branching from the ampullary tip and different modes of lateral branching (Oliver's "closed and open divided" models) from the tubule portion of the ureteric bud. The complexity of branching morphogenesis varies according to the period of nephrogenesis and also among mammalian species (4–6,20–22).

The first three to five generations of ureteric bud branches form the renal pelvis, with more divisions occurring in the poles than in the midpolar region (Figure 34.2). Urine production is accompanied by progressive dilatation and coalescence of the earlier branches to form the early pelvic-calyceal system by 11 to 12 weeks. Subsequent generations of branches form the calyces. Extensive tissue remodeling of the calyceal system occurs. By 11 to 14 weeks, the calyces become compressed between the expanding renal pelvis and the aggregation of nephrons induced by collecting ducts in the developing papillae. The minor calyces convert from a bulbous configuration to their definitive cuplike shape, and the papillae become conical (Figure 34.3). The fate of the very first nephrons formed, presumably induced by and attached to the first generations of the ureteric bud that form the pelvis and calyces, remains a question. They are believed to either degenerate or attach to a later generation branch that elongates eventually to reach the juxtamedullary cortex.

Formation of the Collecting System

At eight weeks, the first nephrons can be observed attached to ureteric bud branches. The organogenetic processes of collecting duct branching/elongation and nephron differentiation occur simultaneously. Collecting duct morphogenesis has been divided into four periods (5). In the first period, from the fifth to the fourteenth week of gestation,

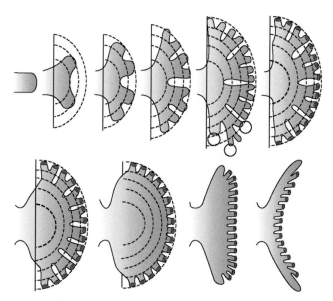

Figure 34.3 Diagram illustrating later branches of ureteric bud forming a minor calyx and papilla. *Circles* indicate generation branches that may expand to form part of the calyx or, if not expanding, form papillary ducts. The expanding pelvis and the peripheral zone of differentiating nephrons compress the original saccular cavity, producing the cuplike shape of the calyx and the conical configuration of the papilla. Modified with permission from: Potter EL. *Normal and Abnormal Development of the Kidney.* Chicago: Year Book; 1972.

branching occurs from the ampullary tips, and individual nephrons remain attached to their ampullae. In an iterative bifurcation model of branching, one of the two new ampullae retains the old nephron whereas the other induces the formation of a new one. The second period, weeks 14 through 22, is characterized by the formation of arcades. Ampullae rarely branch, but single elongating tips repeatedly induce new nephrons while carrying attached older nephrons. As new nephrons are formed, the connecting tubule of the older nephron merges its point of attachment away from the ampulla to the connecting tubule of the newer nephron. Repetition of this process results in three to seven nephrons forming around a single ampulla, joined to one another in an arcade by their connecting tubules. Arcades are associated with juxtamedullary nephrons in the inner cortex of the fully developed kidney.

In the third period, weeks 20 through 36, the ampullae advance beyond the attachment point of the arcade, toward the outer surface. The ampullae do not branch but induce five to seven nephrons, each of which will have a direct connection to the developing collecting tubule. This type of nephron attachment predominates in the outer cortex of the mature kidney (Figure 34.4). Since nephrons retain contact with their ampullae of origin, either through arcades or directly, the longitudinal growth of the collecting tubules positions the attached glomeruli in the cortex. In the fourth period, beginning at 32 to 36 weeks, the ampullae disappear, and no new nephrons form. Normally, nephrogenesis does not occur beyond 36 weeks of gestation. The last

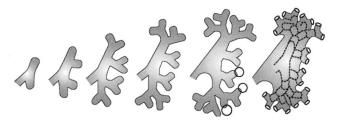

Figure 34.2 Diagram depicting early branches of ureteric bud that dilate and coalesce to form the renal pelvis. Examples of third, fourth, and fifth generation branches are *circled*. Modified with permission from: Potter EL. *Normal and Abnormal Development of the Kidney.* Chicago: Year Book; 1972.

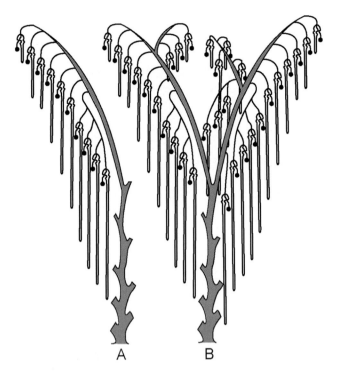

Figure 34.4 Diagram demonstrating the pattern of nephrons and collecting tubules at birth. **A.** The most common arrangement is for each collecting tubule to have a single arcade composed of three to five nephrons and five to seven nephrons individually attached. **B.** Depending on the division of the ampullary tips, other variations are possible. Modified with permission from: Potter EL. *Normal and Abnormal Development of the Kidney.* Chicago: Year Book; 1972.

nephrons formed are in the outer cortex with their glomeruli near the renal capsule.

Nephron Formation

Over 100 years ago, investigations by Herring and Huber provided a fairly accurate morphologic view of human nephron development (Figure 34.5) (1,2). They were also prescient in regard to some mechanisms of nephrogenesis; for example, the development of glomerular capillaries. From eight weeks of gestation, the nephrons and collecting duct system develop together. The stages in individual nephron development do not vary and occur continuously throughout the periods of collecting duct formation. The formation of nephrons can be divided into two phases: the induction stage and the morphogenetic stage (7,8,23). In the induction stage, the mesenchyme condenses around the ampullary tips in response to inducing signals from the ureteric bud. Two types of mesenchymal condensates form in this induction stage prior to epithelial differentiation of the mesenchyme (24). The first condensate, called the *cap*, closely surrounds each ampullary tip. A short time later, another condensate, termed the *pretubular aggregate*, forms at the lateral edges of the ampullary tip, below the cap. At the stage of ureteric bud

division, forming a T-shaped structure, two pretubular aggregates may be observed, one on each side of the T bud. The caps and pretubular aggregates can be distinguished by histology. The cap is believed to regulate ureteric bud branching, whereas the pretubular aggregate is destined to form the nephron.

The morphogenetic stage of nephron formation involves several complex phases (Figure 34.5). First, the cells of the pretubular aggregate undergo a mesenchyme-to-epithelium transition, characterized by expression of epithelial markers and synthesis of basement membrane matrix glycoproteins. The cells develop intercellular junctions and become polarized and surrounded by a basal lamina, forming a structure termed the *vesicle*. A central cavity may be observed in the vesicle. Soon after formation, the vesicle fuses to the ureteric duct epithelium, and a continuous basal lamina surrounds both the vesicle and the duct. Opposite the area of fusion between the vesicle and the ureteric duct, a vascular cleft develops representing the site where the glomerular capillaries will emerge. The vesicle becomes a comma-shaped tubular structure. Another crevice forms near the fusion between the comma structure and the ureteric duct. After elongation and folding, an S-shaped figure (representing an early nephron) forms (Figure 34.6). At this stage, the S-shaped body is already compartmentalized into distinct cell types that are arranged into three areas. The vascular cleft lies below the upper and middle limbs of the S-shaped body and above the lower limb. The upper limb (connected to the ureteric duct) and the middle limb (also known as *Stoerk's complex*) generate the proximal and distal convoluted tubules and the loops of Henle. The lower limb, most distant from the ureteric bud, differentiates into the parietal and visceral epithelium of the glomerulus.

Active nephron formation occurs across the developing renal cortex in a band, known as the *nephrogenic zone* (termed the *neogenic zone* in early studies) (Figures 34.7–34.9). After nephron formation ceases, generally by 36 weeks of gestation, the nephrogenic zone disappears (Figure 34.10). The growth of the collecting ducts and the incremental formation of nephrons result in a centrifugal developmental pattern extending through the renal cortex. The earliest nephrons to form are found in the juxtamedullary zone of cortex, whereas the last nephrons to develop are in the outer cortex. This principle is fundamental to understanding postnatal structural changes in the kidney and is sometimes useful in the timing of developmental disturbances in the cortex. For example, a disturbance during the early months of development may result in an abnormality of the entire cortical thickness, whereas one that occurs in the last half of gestation may involve only the outermost layers of cortical nephrons. In summary, the coincident processes of ureteral-derived epithelial branching and nephron formation largely establish the basic architectural organization of the kidney.

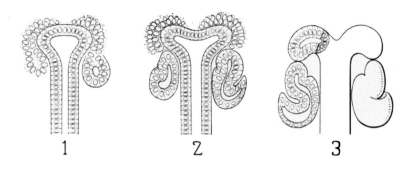

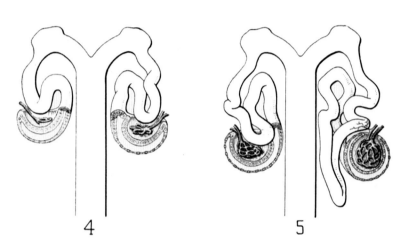

Figure 34.5 Huber's schematic drawings of nephron development. **1.** Condensation stage with the cap and the pretubular aggregate. A renal vesicle (*right*) is present. **2.** Comma-shaped body. **3.** S-shaped body. 4. Early glomerular capillary development, Bowman's capsule formation and tubule elongation. 5. Glomerular and tubule maturation (*right*). Reprinted from: Huber GC. On the development and shape of uriniferous tubules of certain of the higher mammals. *Am J Anat* 1905;4(suppl):1–98.

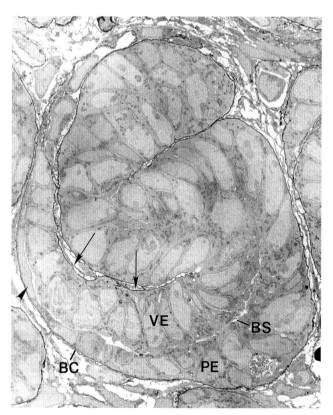

Figure 34.6 Electron micrograph of S-shaped figure from newborn mouse kidney. The basement membranes are rendered black by labeling with anti-laminin IgG conjugated to horseradish peroxidase. The vascular cleft (*arrows*), visceral epithelial cells (*VE*), Bowman's space (*BS*), parietal epithelial cells (*PE*), and Bowman's capsule (*BC*) can be seen. The visceral epithelial cells will differentiate into podocytes. Some parietal epithelial cells are becoming squamous (*arrowhead*) and will line Bowman's capsule. The epithelial cells above the vascular cleft will give rise to the proximal tubules, loops of Henle, and distal convoluted tubules. (Magnification ×5000.) Modified with permission from: Clapp WL, Abrahamson DR. Development and gross anatomy of the kidney. In: Tisher CC, Brenner BM, eds. *Renal Pathology*. 2nd ed. Philadelphia: JB Lippincott; 1994:3–59.

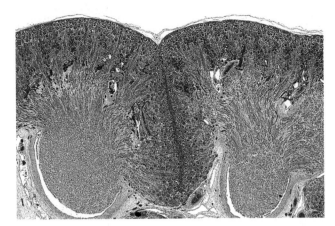

Figure 34.7 Developing kidney at 21 weeks of gestation showing two medullary pyramids with surrounding cortex. The nephrogenic zone represents a thin layer outlining the peripheral aspects of the lobes, both at the surface and in the midplane of the septa (column) of Bertin, between the two renal lobes.

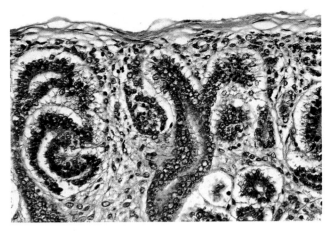

Figure 34.9 Higher magnification of same field as in Figure 34.7. In the center, pretubular aggregates (early renal vesicles) are present on either side of the ureteric duct. An early S-shaped body is present (*left*).

Glomerulogenesis

To appreciate how some glomerular diseases arise or how the glomerulus responds to injury, an understanding of glomerular development is indispensable. Glomerular development proceeds through a sequence of structures described as vesicle, comma-shaped, S-shaped, capillary loop, and maturing glomerulus stages (9,25,26). The vesicle and comma-shaped stages were discussed previously. At the S-shaped stage, the lower limb beneath the vascular cleft separates into two layers (lips) divided by a narrow developing Bowman's space (Figure 34.6). Lining the upper, internal lip are the visceral epithelial cells, which will differentiate into podocytes. On the opposite side of Bowman's space, the cells of the lower, outer lip will become the parietal epithelial cells lining Bowman's capsule.

During the S-shaped stage, microvessels can often be identified within the vascular cleft of the S-figure. Because this vascular cleft is the site where the glomerular capillaries emerge, the origin of the microvessels has generated considerable study. A long-standing question has been whether the glomerular endothelial cells have an *angiogenic* or a *vasculogenic* origin. Earlier evidence favored the process of angiogenesis, whereby endothelial cells sprout from external vessels that grow into the kidney. More recent studies

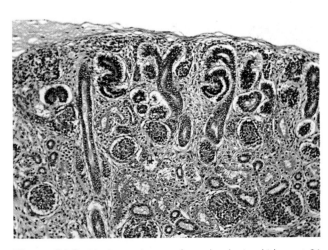

Figure 34.8 Nephrogenic zone from developing kidney at 26 weeks of gestation illustrating several stages of nephron formation.

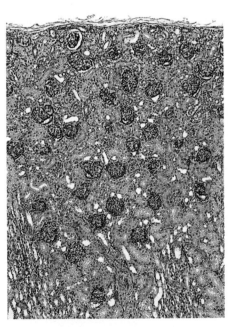

Figure 34.10 Newborn kidney (40 weeks of gestation). Note the absence of a nephrogenic zone. Some glomeruli are near the renal capsule.

provide compelling evidence for a vasculogenic mechanism, whereby endothelial cells of the early glomerular capillaries originate from intrinsic angioblasts, likely derived from the metanephric mesenchyme (27,28). Release of growth factors, such as vascular endothelial growth factor (VEGF), from the immature podocytes may attract the angioblasts, expressing VEGF receptors (as Flk1) into the vascular clefts. Other signaling systems such as the angiopoietin (ligand)-Tie (receptor) axis also play a role in endothelial cell and vascular development (29). At this stage, the endothelial cells contain few fenestrae. The early podocytes are cuboidal or columnar, whereas the parietal epithelial cells are already flattening. Situated between the endothelial and podocyte layers are two basement membranes. The basement membrane beneath the podocytes is usually thicker and more continuous than the one underneath the endothelial cells.

During the capillary loop stage, the capillaries start to fill out into an expanding Bowman's space. The endothelial cells flatten and develop numerous fenestrae. The podocytes develop a complex cellular architecture as they become terminally differentiated and cease to undergo mitosis. They flatten and form cytoplasmic primary processes, which in turn, extend foot processes that interdigitate with those from adjacent podocytes and adhere to the developing glomerular basement membrane (GBM). Intercellular junctional complexes are present at the apical membranes between podocytes. With foot process development, these junctions migrate down the lateral surfaces of the emerging foot processes and disappear, when they are either replaced by or converted into the slit diaphragms (26). Slit diaphragms, specialized intercellular junctions, bridge the space between adjacent foot processes. The slit diaphragm is connected to the podocyte cytoskeleton as part of a multifunctional protein complex that includes nephrin, CD2-associated protein (CD2AP), and podocin (30,31). Nephrin is the protein encoded by the *NPHS1* gene that is mutated in congenital nephrotic syndrome of the Finnish type, which is associated with loss of the slit diaphragm, abnormal foot processes, and massive proteinuria (32). Thus, the slit diaphragm is critical for maintaining podocyte architecture and the glomerular filtration barrier. The dual GBM, synthesized by both the endothelium and podocytes, is still present, but areas of fusion between the two membranes are found. Beginning during the capillary loop stage, a complex series of transitions in the GBM protein composition occurs. There is developmental switching of both type IV collagen and laminin isoforms in the GBM, events which are essential for forming normal glomerular capillaries (26,33).

Glomeruli in the maturing stage resemble adult glomeruli by histology but are smaller in diameter. The podocytes of the maturing glomeruli may have a cuboidal appearance. A single fused GBM predominates, and areas of dual unfused basement membranes are rarely seen. At this time, the synthesis of components for the GBM is largely by the podocytes. In areas where foot process interdigitation is continuing, irregular outpocketings of basement membrane are found beneath the podocytes. These outpocketings, or loops, reflect newly synthesized GBM that will be deposited into the existing GBM.

The development of the mesangium occurs relatively later in glomerulogenesis. Although the mesangial cells likely derive from the metanephric mesenchyme, their origin is not entirely clear. The mesangial cell precursors are distinct from the VEGF receptor expressing angioblasts that differentiate into the glomerular endothelial cells. However, the emergence of mesangial cells in the glomerulus is dependent on platelet-derived growth factor-B (PDGF-B), produced by podocytes and endothelial cells, and its receptor, PDGF receptor-B (PDGF-RB), expressed on mesangial cells (34).

Development of the Juxtaglomerular Apparatus

In the human mesonephros, a complete juxtaglomerular apparatus has not been observed, although renin-expressing cells have been noted (35). Renin expression in the metanephric kidney has been detected as early as eight weeks of gestation, and renin mRNA levels are significantly higher in the developing kidney than in the adult organ (35,36). In the developing kidney, renin-expressing cells are found in intrarenal arteries, including the arcuate and interlobular arteries. As development progresses, the distribution of renin-expressing cells shifts from the larger vessels to the juxtaglomerular apparatus—primarily to the terminal afferent arteriole—in the mature kidney (37,8). However, within the afferent arterioles themselves, heterogeneous patterns of renin expression exist (39). The juxtaglomerular (JG) cell, as a cellular component of the mature juxtaglomerular apparatus, is located in the wall of the terminal afferent arteriole close to the glomerulus. Studies of the embryonic origin and lineage of JG cells have demonstrated that JG cells originate from renin-expressing precursor cells of the metanephric blastema rather than an extrarenal source (40). Furthermore, studies have provided in vivo genetic evidence that renin precursor cells, in addition to differentiating into JG cells, can also differentiate into non–renin-expressing cells, such as vascular smooth muscle cells and glomerular mesangial cells (41).

Development of the Interstitium

Compared to other parenchymal components, there is far less known about the interstitium (stroma) in kidney development. In addition to providing a structural framework around the other components, an emerging view is that the developing interstitium plays an essential role in nephron and collecting duct differentiation (42–44). A traditional view is that cells of the metanephric mesenchyme not induced by the ureteric bud will become interstitial (stroma) cells. However, it is now believed that stroma cells arise from different cell lineages within the metanephric mesenchyme and also separate from the mesenchyme. A loose stroma containing spindle-shaped cells surrounds the early ureteric bud branches and early nephrons and is known as the primary interstitium (or clear-cell type stroma). As nephrogenesis proceeds, a cortical interstitium and a medullary interstitium, each with distinct cellular phenotypes, forms. Although the interstitial cells resemble fibroblasts, dendritic cells, macrophages, or lymphocytes according to morphologic and immunophenotypical findings, their origins and functions are mysterious (45–47). There is accumulated evidence to indicate that signals emanating from cells in the interstitium as well as the renal capsule are essential for normal nephron and collecting duct development (42–44). These important stromal cell–expressed molecules include Foxd1, RARα, RARβ2, FGF-7, BMP4, Pod1 and Pbx1 (Table 34.1).

Structural fibers extending between the ureteric bud ampulla and the renal capsule may represent a morphologic correlate that in part mediates the signals between the developing collecting duct and the capsule (48).

Apoptosis

In addition to prominent cell proliferation in the nephrogenic zone of the cortex, cell proliferation also contributes to the differentiation of the medullary tubules (49,50). Considering the widespread nature of apoptosis during embryologic development, it is not surprising that it occurs in kidney organogenesis. However, unlike the well-known function of apoptosis in the formation of nonwebbed digits, the biologic role of apoptosis in kidney development is not as apparent. During normal nephrogenesis, apoptosis has been observed within uninduced metanephric mesenchyme (51,52), comma-shaped bodies (53), developing tubules (52,54,55), stromal cells surrounding the tubules (51), and immature glomeruli (56). As shown by several

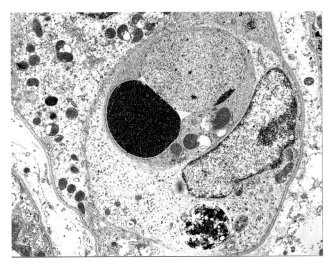

Figure 34.12 Electron micrograph of a postnatal medullary collecting duct illustrating a phagocytosed apoptotic body composed of a nucleus with condensed chromatin and organelle remnants (magnification ×1200; courtesy of Dr. Jin Kim).

genetic defects in signaling between the mesenchyme and ureteric bud (Table 34.1), the metanephric mesenchyme is programmed to undergo massive apoptosis if it fails to be induced by the ureteric bud. At later stages of kidney development, apoptosis plays a role in remodeling the cell composition of medullary collecting ducts (54) and in the differentiation of the loops of Henle (55). Intercalated cells, involved in urine acidification, are removed from the developing medullary collecting duct by apoptosis or simple extrusion from the epithelium (Figures 34.11–34.12) (54). Also, in developing glomeruli, endothelial cells are removed by apoptosis during capillary lumen formation (55), and apoptosis can be observed in the parietal epithelium during glomerular development (Figure 34.13).

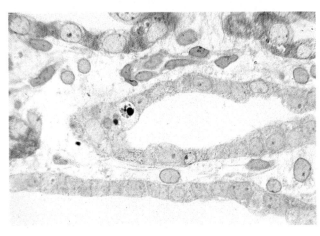

Figure 34.11 Developing medullary collecting duct in a postnatal kidney. After etching with sodium methoxide, toluidine blue is removed from normal nuclei but remains in the nuclear fragments of apoptotic bodies (magnification ×300; courtesy of Dr. Jin Kim).

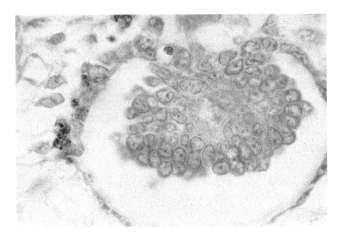

Figure 34.13 Micrograph from cortical nephrogenic zone of a fetal kidney demonstrating labeling for apoptosis in parietal epithelium of a developing glomerulus. Cells with fragmented DNA are identified by a Tdt-mediated dUTP-biotin nick end-labeling (TUNEL) immunoperoxidase method. (Courtesy of Dr. Jin Kim.)

There are disparate findings considering the quantitative scale of apoptosis during nephrogenesis (52,57). However, a role for apoptosis during nephrogenesis is further evidenced by the fact that mice deficient for *Bcl-2*, the major antiapoptotic regulator, have fulminant apoptosis of the metanephric mesenchyme, develop multiple cysts, and die of renal failure (58). Considering the above findings and the complex morphogenetic processes occurring during nephrogenesis, it seems likely that apoptosis plays a role in sculpting the kidney.

Molecular Regulation of Kidney Development

To make a kidney requires an orchestration of numerous complex cellular and molecular events. Several experimental approaches and model systems have enhanced our understanding of kidney development. A variety of in vitro studies have been valuable, including organic culture of metanephric rudiments, pioneered by Grobstein (7), and cell cultures of individual nephrogenic lineages. Gene targeting studies such as gene ablation in mice ("knockout" mice) have provided powerful in vivo evidence for the role of certain genes in nephrogenesis. A detailed review of the molecular aspects of nephrogenesis is beyond the scope of this chapter, but several reviews are available (9–12,59–61). Table 34.1 outlines some of the genes involved in mammalian kidney development, their encoded protein functions, their normal expression in the developing kidney, and the mutant kidney phenotypes that result from their ablation in mice. In addition, the known human syndromes caused by naturally occurring mutations in these genes are noted. The genes are listed under the cellular process (specification of nephrogenic mesenchyme, cell survival, cell proliferation, ureteric bud branching, mesenchymal-to-epithelial transition, glomerulogenesis and nephron differentiation) in which they are believed to have an important function (60). Where some of the genes are temporally positioned (upstream or downstream to one another) in the functional cascade of kidney organogenesis remains to be determined.

Compelling evidence exists to indicate that some genes, for example *WT1*, *Pax 2*, and *Pod1*, play multiple roles during nephrogenesis. Note that these particular genes are placed under more than one nephrogenic cellular process in Table 34.1. The listing of the genes in Table 34.1 is based predominantly on in vivo genetic evidence. The generation of knockout mice using homologous recombination in embryonic stem cells has been very informative. However, embryonic lethality and pleiotropic phenotypes may occur, preventing an analysis of the significance of the targeted gene in nephrogenesis. Creating "conditional" knockout mice by disrupting genes only in specific renal cell types using site-specific DNA recombinase systems (e.g., Cre-lox P system) will provide important insights into kidney development (62). Moreover, some of the mutant kidney phenotypes will serve as valuable models for human disease.

In the near future, a list similar to Table 34.1 will be significantly lengthened. There will be a greater appreciation for the multiple roles that some genes have during nephrogenesis. However, our understanding of the cellular and molecular events that underlie the dynamics of kidney formation will be enhanced. In addition to a morphogenetic role during kidney organogenesis, some genes have an important physiologic function in the adult kidney. Also, the tabulated genes and their encoded proteins will no doubt be useful as lineage- or cell-specific markers to study renal diseases, including tumors.

Gross Anatomy

Kidney Position and Blood Supply

Upon formation, the metanephric kidneys are situated close to each other in the pelvis at the level of the upper sacrum. Between the sixth and ninth weeks of gestation, the kidneys are found further apart and at higher levels in the abdomen until they reach their final upper lumbar position (178). This "ascent" of the kidneys is believed to result largely from differential growth of the caudal part of the embryo away from the kidneys (179,180). However, others have argued that the cephalad movement of the kidneys is active and not caused by differential growth of the vertebral column (181). With this migration, the renal hilum, where the main vessels enter and exit, rotates from a ventral orientation to face anteriomedially. Initially, the kidneys receive their blood supply from branches of the common iliac arteries. With their ascension, the kidneys are supplied by arteries originating from progressively higher levels of the distal aorta (178). The question of whether some of these vessels anastomose in a periaortic plexus is not well studied (182). As the ascending kidneys receive new branches from the aorta, the older, caudal branches undergo involution. Persistence of these inferior vessels may result in accessory renal arteries. The most cephalad branches arising from the abdominal aorta become the permanent main renal arteries.

Kidney Weight and Configuration

The various reference values reported for fetal and neonatal kidney weights correspond relatively closely, despite potential variability due to factors such as the social and economic status and the level of health care in a given population (183–188). Separate values from nonmacerated and macerated cases are available (188), as well as values using prefixation (187,188) and postfixation weighing (183,186) of the kidneys. Data for the combined weight (right and left) of the kidneys during the second

TABLE 34.1
GENES INVOLVED IN KIDNEY DEVELOPMENT

Developmental Process Gene (Human syndrome)	Function	Expression in Normal Developing Kidney	Mutant Kidney Phenotype (Mouse)	Reference
Specification of the Nephrogenic Mesenchyme				
Lim 1	Transcription factor	Intermediate mesoderm, nephric duct, mesonephros, ureteric bud, collecting ducts, pretubular aggregates, S-shaped bodies, podocytes	Absent pro-, meso-, and metanephros (Lim 1 required at multiple steps of kidney development)	(63–65)
Eya1 (Mutations in branchiooto-renal [BOR] syndrome)	Transcription coactivator (interacts with Six1)	Intermediate mesoderm, uninduced and induced metanephric mesenchyme	Intact pro- and mesonephros, but absent metanephric blastema, renal agenesis	(66–68)
Six1 (Mutations in branchiooto-renal [BOR] syndrome)	Transcription factor (interacts with Eya1)	Uninduced and induced metanephric mesenchyme and collecting tubules	Ureteric bud forms but does not fully invade metanephric mesenchyme, which undergoes apoptosis, renal agenesis	(69–70)
Sall 1 (Mutations in Townes-Brocks syndrome)	Transcription factor	Mesonephros, induced metanephric mesenchyme	Ureteric bud forms but does not fully invade metanephric mesenchyme, which undergoes apoptosis, renal hypoplasia, or agenesis	(71)
Hoxa11, Hoxd11	Transcription factors	Intermediate mesoderm, metanephric mesenchyme	Impaired ureteric bud branching, renal hypoplasia in Hoxa11/Hoxd11 double mutants	(72,73)
Pax 2	Transcription factor	Intermediate mesoderm, nephric duct, mesonephros, ureteric bud, induced metanephric mesenchyme	Intact nephric duct but mesonephric tubules and ureteric bud fail to form, renal agenesis	(74–76)
WT1	Transcription factor	Intermediate mesoderm, mesonephros, uninduced and induced metanephric mesenchyme, comma- and S-shaped bodies, podocytes	Absent caudal mesonephros, ureteric bud fails to form, metanephric mesenchyme undergoes apoptosis, renal agenesis	(77,78)
Foxc1/2	Transcription factor	Intermediate mesoderm, mesonephros, uninduced and induced metanephric mesenchyme	Double ureters with one a hydroureter, duplex kidneys (Foxc1/Foxc2 compound heterozygous mutants similar to Foxc1 homozygous mutants)	(79,80)
Slit2	Secreted protein	Mesonephric duct, anterior intermediate mesoderm, ureteric bud tips	Supernumerary ureteric buds, hydroureter, fused multiple kidneys	(81)
Robo2	Transmembrane (receptor for Slit2)	Intermediate mesoderm, induced metanephric mesenchyme	Supernumerary ureteric buds, hydroureter, fused multiple kidneys	(81)
Cell Survival				
BMP7	Growth factor	Mesonephric duct, ureteric bud, induced metanephric mesenchyme, distal tubules, comma-and S-shaped bodies, podocytes	Increased apoptosis in metanephric mesenchyme, decreased ureter bud branching, hydroureter, severe renal hypoplasia	(82–84)
FGF-8	Growth factor	Pretubular aggregates, vesicles, tubule progenitors in S body	Increased apoptosis in S body precursors, truncated nephrons, severe renal hypoplasia	(85,86)

(continued)

TABLE 34.1
(CONTINUED)

Developmental Process Gene (Human syndrome)	Function	Expression in Normal Developing Kidney	Mutant Kidney Phenotype (Mouse)	Reference
Bcl-2	Antiapoptotic factor	Ureteric bud, induced metanephric mesenchyme, parietal epithelium of Bowman's capsule, tubules and collecting ducts	Increased apoptosis especially in metanephric mesenchyme, cysts in tubules and collecting ducts, severe renal hypoplasia.	(87,88)
AP-2β	Transcription factor	Distal tubules and collecting ducts	Increased apoptosis and cyst formation in distal tubules and collecting ducts	(89,90)
Pax-2 (Heterozygous mutations in renal-coloboma syndrome)	Transcription factor	Intermediate mesoderm, nephric duct, mesonephros, ureteric bud, induced metanephric mesenchyme	Heterozygous *Pax-2* mutations result in increased apoptosis in collecting ducts, reduced ureteric branching, hypoplastic kidneys	(91–93)
Cell Proliferation				
FGF-7	Growth factor	Interstitial fibroblasts or stroma surrounding ureteric bud and developing collecting ducts	Decreased growth of ureteric bud and collecting ducts, decreased number of nephrons, renal hypoplasia	(94)
N-Myc	Transcription factor	Induced metanephric mesenchyme	Decreased cell proliferation, decreased ureteric bud tips and nephrons, renal hypoplasia	(95)
Glypican-3 (Mutations in Simpson-Golabi-Behmel syndrome)	Heparan sulfate proteoglycan	All metanephric mesenchyme and ureteric bud derivatives	Increased cell proliferation in cortical collecting ducts, increased apoptosis in medullary collecting ducts, renal medullary cystic dysplasia	(96,97)
Branching of the Ureteric Bud				
GDNF	Growth factor	Intermediate mesoderm, mesonephros, induced metanephric mesenchyme, pretubular aggregates	Ureteric bud fails to form or has abnormal branching, renal hypoplasia or agenesis	(98–100)
c-ret	GF receptor (TK) (receptor for GDNF)	Mesonephric duct, ureteric bud and tips of ureteric bud	Similar to GDNF-deficient mice	(101,102)
GFRα1	GF coreceptor (forms signaling complex with GDNF and c-ret)	Induced metanephric mesenchyme, pretubular aggregates, mesonephric duct, ureteric bud and tips of ureteric bud	Similar to GDNF-deficient mice	(103)
GDF11	Growth factor	Mesonephric duct, uninduced and induced metanephric mesenchyme, ureteric bud and branches	No ureteric bud formation, metanephric mesenchyme undergoes apoptosis, renal hypoplasia or agenesis	(104)
Sprouty1	Receptor (TK) antagonist	Mesonephric duct, ureteric bud and tips of ureteric bud	Supernumerary ureteric buds, multiple ureters, multiplex kidneys	(105)
Emx2	Transcription factor	Intermediate mesoderm, mesonephric duct, mesonephros, ureteric bud, comma- and S-shaped bodies	Ureteric bud invades metanephric mesenchyme but fails to dilate or branch, no induction of mesenchyme, renal agenesis	(106)

(continued)

TABLE 34.1
(CONTINUED)

Developmental Process Gene (Human syndrome)	Function	Expression in Normal Developing Kidney	Mutant Kidney Phenotype (Mouse)	Reference
RARα, RARβ2	Transcription factors	RARα—ureteric bud, metanephric mesenchyme, stroma RARβ2—stroma only	Decreased ureteric bud branching (defective stroma signaling) in RARα/β2 double mutants, renal hypoplasia	(107,108)
BMP4	Bone morphogenetic protein	Stromal mesenchymal cells around ureteric bud branches	Reduced and ectopic ureteral branching, ectopic ureterovesical junction, hydroureter, double collecting ducts, hypo/dysplastic kidneys (heterozygous BMP4 null mice)	(109)
Pod1	Transcription factor	Induced metanephric mesenchyme, stromal cells and podocytes	Decreased ureteric branching, arrest in tubular and glomerular differentiation, renal hypoplasia	(110)
Heparan sulfate 2-sulfotransferase	Enzyme (synthesis of heparan sulfate, a component of HS proteoglycan)	Mesonephric duct, transient in ureteric bud, metanephric mesenchyme	Ureteric bud outgrowth but no branching, no condensation of metanephric mesenchyme, renal agenesis	(111)
Integrin α8	Transmembrane adhesion receptor	Intermediate mesoderm, induced metanephric mesenchyme, pretubular aggregates	Limited ureteric bud invasion of metanephric mesenchyme, decreased ureteric branching, renal hypoplasia or agenesis	(112)
Integrin α3β1	Transmembrane adhesion receptor	Ureteric bud, collecting ducts, podocytes	Decreased branching of medullary collecting ducts, microcystic proximal tubules, defective glomerulogenesis	(113)
Pbxl	Transcription factor	Induced metanephric mesenchyme and stromal cells	Decreased and irregular ureteric bud branching, large mesenchymal condensates, renal hypoplasia or unilateral agenesis	(114)
Grem1	Bone morphogenetic protein (BMP) antagonist	Intermediate mesoderm, mesonephric duct, metanephric mesenchyme	Ureteric bud forms but fails to invade metanephric mesenchyme, which undergoes apoptosis, renal agenesis	(115)
Wnt11	Secreted glycoprotein	Ureteric bud tips	Loss of ureteric tips, reduced ureteric branching, renal hypoplasia	(116)
Formin (Mutations in mice cause the limb deformity syndrome)	Protein that regulates cytoskeleton function	Mesonephric duct, mesonephros, ureteric bud, metanephric mesenchyme	Decreased ureteric bud outgrowth, renal hypoplasia, unilateral or bilateral renal agenesis	(117)
Angiotensinogen (Agt)	Renin substrate	Ureteric bud, stroma, S-shaped bodies, glomeruli, proximal tubules	Hypoplastic papillae, hydronephrosis, thickened blood vessels, reduced blood pressure	(118,119)
Renin	Enzyme (cleaves Agt to form angiotensin I)	Developing arcuate and interlobular arteries and afferent arterioles, restricted to juxtaglomerular apparatus with maturity	Hypoplasic papillae, hydronephrosis, thickened blood vessels, reduced blood pressure	(120,121)

(continued)

TABLE 34.1
(CONTINUED)

Developmental Process Gene (Human syndrome)	Function	Expression in Normal Developing Kidney	Mutant Kidney Phenotype (Mouse)	Reference
Angiotensin converting enzyme (ACE)	Enzyme (converts angiotensin I to angiotensin II)	Glomeruli, proximal tubules and collecting ducts, small arteries	Hypoplastic papillae, hydronephrosis, thickened blood vessels, reduced blood pressure	(122)
Angiotensin II receptor, type 1 (AT₁)	Angiotensin II receptor	Ureteric bud, stroma, S-shaped bodies, proximal tubules, collecting ducts	Hypoplastic papillae, hydronephrosis, thickened blood vessels, reduced blood pressure	(123,124)
Angiotensin II receptor, type 2 (AT₂)	Angiotensin II receptor	Stroma adjacent to ureteric bud stalk	3% have abnormalities, duplicated collecting system, and hydronephrotic upper pole	(125,126)
Mesenchymal-to-Epithelial Transition				
Wnt4	Secreted glycoprotein	Pretubular aggregates, comma-shaped body, distal S-shaped body	Ureteric bud branching occurs, no mesenchymal-epithelial transition, renal agenesis	(127)
Wnt9b	Secreted glycoprotein	Mesonephric duct, ureteric bud and collecting ducts but not branching tips	No mesenchymal-epithelial transition, renal agenesis	(128)
Foxd1(BF2)	Transcription factor	Interstitial stroma cells	Decreased ureteric bud branching, large mesenchymal condensates, abnormal renal capsule, small fused pelvic kidneys	(129,130)
Pod1	Transcription factor	Induced metanephric mesenchyme, stromal cells and podocytes	Increased size of induced mesenchymal condensates, arrest in tubular and glomerular differentiation, renal hypoplasia	(131)
Fras1 (Mutations in Fraser syndrome)	Extracellular matrix (ECM) protein	Basal side of ureteric ducts	Ureteric bud invades metanephric mesenchyme but decreased induction, apoptosis of mesenchyme, renal hypoplasia or agenesis	(132,133)
Grip1	Cytoplasmic protein (interacts with Fras1)	Basal side of ureteric ducts	Similar abnormal phenotype as in Fras1-deficient mice	(134)
Cadherin-6 (K-cadherin)	Transmembrane adhesion protein	Renal vesicle, proximal end of comma- and S-shaped bodies, developing proximal tubules and Henle's loops	Delayed fusion of some comma-shaped bodies to ureteric bud leading to loss of nephrons	(135)
Glomerulogenesis				
WT1 (Mutations in WAGR, Denys-Drash, and Frasier syndromes)	Transcription factor	Intermediate mesoderm, mesonephros, uninduced and induced metanephric mesenchyme, S-shaped body, podocytes	Disturbed podocyte differentiation, glomerulosclerosis	(136–138)
PDGF-B	Growth factor	Glomerular endothelial cells and podocytes	Dilated glomerular capillaries with no mesangial cells	(139)
PDGFR-β	Growth factor receptor (receptor for PDGF-B)	Glomerular mesangial cells	Dilated glomerular capillaries with no mesangial cells	(140)
Notch2	Transmembrane receptor	Developing collecting ducts, comma- and S-shaped bodies, podocytes	Abnormal glomeruli arrested at capillary loop stage, with disorganized podocytes and no mesangial cells	(141)

(continued)

851

TABLE 34.1
(CONTINUED)

Developmental Process Gene (Human syndrome)	Function	Expression in Normal Developing Kidney	Mutant Kidney Phenotype (Mouse)	Reference
VEGF-A	Growth factor	S-shaped bodies, podocytes, collecting ducts	Small glomeruli, lack capillary loops, few endothelial cells	(142)
Laminin α5	Basement membrane protein	Basement membranes of ureteric bud, developing tubules and glomerular basement membrane (GBM)	Abnormal glomeruli with displaced endothelial and mesangial cells, and clustered podocytes	(143)
Laminin β2	Basement membrane protein	Glomerular basement membranes beginning at capillary loop stage	Absence of podocyte foot processes, proteinuria	(144)
Laminin α3β1	Transmembrane adhesion receptor	Ureteric bud, collecting ducts, podocytes	Glomerular capillary loops dilated and fewer in number, loss of podocyte foot processes, dual GBMs (failure of fusion)	(113)
Collagen IVα3 (Mutations in Alport syndrome)	Basement membrane protein	Forms heterodimer with α4 (IV) and α5 (IV) chains in GBM from capillary stage onward	Thinning and "basket-weave" thickening of GBMs	(145–147)
Nephrin (Mutations in Congenital nephrotic syndrome of Finnish type)	Transmembrane protein	Podocyte filtration slit diaphragm	Foot process effacement, absent filtration slit diaphragms, proteinuria	(148)
CD2AP	Adapter protein (interacts with nephrin)	Podocyte filtration slit diaphragm domain	Irregular foot processes, absent filtration slit diaphragms, proteinuria	(149)
Podocin (Mutations in autosomal recessive steroid resistant nephrotic syndrome)	Membrane protein (interacts with nephrin)	Podocyte filtration slit diaphragm domain	Irregular foot processes, absent filtration slit diaphragms, proteinuria	(150)
α-Actinin (Mutations in autosomal dominant focal segmental glomerulosclerosis [FSGS])	Cross-links actin filaments	Podocyte filtration slit diaphragm domain	Foot process effacement, GBM duplication, proteinuria, and FSGS	(151,152)
TRPC6 (Mutations in autosomal dominant FSGS)	Cation-channel	Podocyte filtration slit diaphragm domain	Foot process effacement and FSGS (humans)	(153,154)
Neph1	Transmembrane protein (interacts with nephrin)	Podocyte filtration slit diaphragm	Foot process effacement, proteinuria	(155)
FAT1	Protocadherin	Podocyte filtration slit diaphragm	Foot process effacement	(156)
Lmx1b (Mutations in nail patella syndrome)	Transcription factor	Podocytes	Abnormal foot processes, absent filtration slit diaphragms	(157,158)
Podocalyxin	CD34-related transmembrane protein	Podocyte apical membrane domain	Abnormal podocytes, foot process effacement, absent filtration slit diaphragms, anuria	(159)

(continued)

TABLE 34.1
(CONTINUED)

Developmental Process Gene (Human syndrome)	Function	Expression in Normal Developing Kidney	Mutant Kidney Phenotype (Mouse)	Reference
GLEPP1 (Ptpro)	Receptor tyrosine phosphatase	Podocyte apical membrane domain	Shortened and widened podocyte foot processes, reduced glomerular filtration rate	(160)
Kreisler (Krml1/MafB)	Transcription factor	Podocytes, initially at capillary loop stage	Abnormal podocyte differentiation with no foot processes	(161)
Tubular Differentiation				
PKD1 (polycystin-1) (Mutations in autosomal dominant polycystic kidney disease [ADPKD])	Transmembrane protein (adhesion receptor, in cilia, interacts with polycystin-2)	Developing nephron segments and collecting ducts	Renal cysts arising from developing nephron segments and collecting ducts	(162–165)
PKD2 (polycystin-2) (Mutations in autosomal dominant polycystic kidney disease [ADPKD])	Transmembrane protein (calcium channel, in cilia, interacts with polycystin-1)	Developing nephron segments and collecting ducts	Renal cysts arising from developing nephron segments and collecting ducts	(166,167)
Frem2 (Mutations in Fraser syndrome)	Extracellular matrix (ECM) protein	Mesonephros, ureteric bud especially at tips, tubule derivatives	Cysts of collecting ducts and thick ascending limbs	(168)
Cox-2 (Cyclooxygenase-2)	Enzyme (prostaglandin synthesis)	Developing collecting ducts, S-shaped bodies, macula densa, cortical thick ascending limb, medullary interstitial cells	Progressive postnatal outer cortical dysplasia, tubular cysts, and glomerular hypoplasia	(169,170)
EGFR	Growth factor receptor (TK)	Mesonephric duct, ureteric bud, collecting ducts	Dilatation of collecting ducts, uremia	(171,172)
Brn1	Transcription factor	Renal vesicle, comma- and S-shaped bodies, developing Henle's loop (HL), distal convoluted tubule (DCT), macula densa (MD)	Disrupted differentiation of HLs, MD, and DCT	(173)
Psen1/Psen2	Presinilins-(transmembrane protein with γ-secretase activity)	Developing early nephron structures	Renal vesicles and pretubular aggregates form, but no comma- or S-shaped bodies; proximal tubules and glomeruli fail to form (Psen1/Psen2 double null mutant mice with human PSEN1 transgene)	(174,175)
Tensin	Adhesion protein (phosphoprotein, binds actin)	Proximal and distal tubules (adult kidney)	Hydronephrosis, cystic dilatation of proximal tubules	(176)
R-cadherin	Transmembrane adhesion protein	Induced metanephric mesenchyme, renal vesicle, comma- and S-shaped bodies	Dilatation and cytoplasmic vacuolization of proximal tubules	(177)

(FSGS, focal segmental glomerulosclerosis; GBM, glomerular basement membrane)

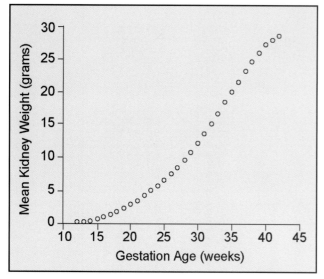

Figure 34.14 Mean combined (right and left) weight of kidneys from second and third trimester fetuses and neonates. Modified with permission from: Hansen K, Sung CJ, Huang C, Pinar H, Singer DB, Oyer CE. Reference values for second trimester fetal and neonatal organ weights and measurements. *Pediatr Dev Pathol* 2003;6:160–167.

and third trimesters are shown in Figure 34.14. Different reference values published for combined kidney weights during infancy and childhood also favorably compare (183,189). The data of Emery and Mithal (183) are illustrated (Figure 34.15).

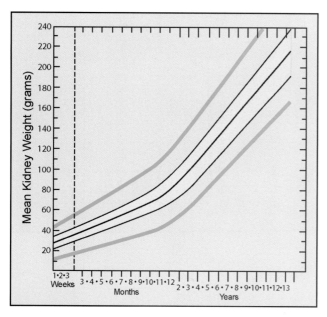

Figure 34.15 Mean combined (right and left) weight of kidneys at various postnatal ages. The middle black line represents the means. The 50th percentile (yellow band) and 95th percentile (blue lines) ranges are shown. Modified with permission from: Emery JL, Mithal A. The weights of kidneys in late intra-uterine life and childhood. *J Clin Pathol* 1960;13:490–493.

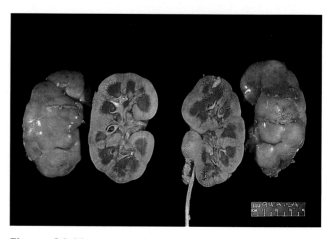

Figure 34.16 Gross appearance of newborn kidneys. The rounded configuration with a relatively deeper sinus, characteristic of the infantile kidney, is seen on the sectioned surface. Fetal lobations are prominent on the external surface.

The newborn kidney has a shorter, more rounded configuration than that of the adult. The upper and lower poles project further medially, so the renal sinus is relatively deeper in the infant (Figures 34.16–34.17) (190). The renal sinus of infants contains much less fat and connective tissue than in the adult, and the cortical septa (columns) of Bertin approach much closer to the pelvic-calyceal system. Figure 34.17 illustrates the process of "unrolling" of the renal poles during childhood, as the kidney assumes the more elongated configuration observed in adults. This change in configuration produces a shallower renal sinus with partial exteriorization of the pelvis. As the pelvic-calyceal system assumes a more exterior position, it also becomes displaced further from the parenchyma lining the sinus. The additional space created between the pelvic-calyceal system and the cortical columns of Bertin is normally filled with fat, which increases in quantity as the kidney approaches maturity.

Fetal Lobations

A renal lobe consists of a medullary pyramid and its surrounding cortical parenchyma (Figures 34.7, 34.16). The centrilobar cortex covers the base of a pyramid, whereas the septal cortex surrounds the sides of a pyramid. Thus, a septum (column) of Bertin represents the confluence of two layers of septal cortex from two adjacent lobes. Although a lobe does not represent a functional renal unit, it may be viewed as an anatomic organizational unit (191). Lobation begins in the human kidney at six to seven weeks and proceeds to maximun development with an average of 14 lobes at 28 weeks of gestation (192,193). At this stage, generally 14 papillae and calyces are present, corresponding with the same number of lobes. Deep clefts on the surface separate the lobes. After the twenty-eighth week, a process of variable lobar fusion decreases the number of surface fissures, papillae, and calyces. The degree of calyceal fusion is greater than papillae fusion. In full-term infant kidneys, the mean

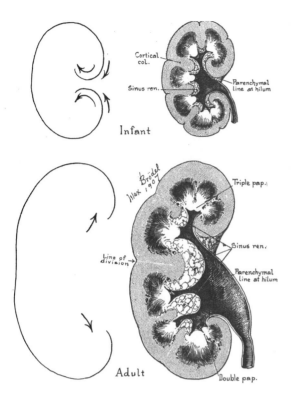

Infant

Adult

Figure 34.17 Max Brödel's classic illustration of the process of unrolling of the kidney in postnatal life (from Kelley HA, Burnam CF. *Diseases of the Kidneys, Ureters, and Bladder.* Vol.1. New York: Appleton; 1925). The rounded configuration of the infantile organ becomes elongated as the upper and lower poles diverge and pelvic-calyceal structures are partially everted from their original position within the renal sinus. The space thus created within the renal sinus is filled by fat, which is far more abundant in the adult kidney than in the infant kidney.

number reported for calyces is 9 and for papillae, it is 11 (193). Considerably more lobar fusion, creating compound papillae, occurs in the polar regions than in the midpolar region, where simple papillae are more likely to be retained.

The surface of the neonatal kidney is divided into polygons by prominent fissures that correspond roughly, although not precisely, to the lobar outlines (Figure 34.16). These fetal lobations usually decrease in prominence with advancing age, persisting longer on the ventral surface than the dorsal surface of the organ. Although there is considerable individual variation in the chronology of their disappearance, they are usually inconspicuous by 4 to 5 years of age (194). The only valid generalization is that fetal lobations usually diminish in number and prominence in the first few years of life, but they remain apparent, especially on the ventral surfaces, in a significant proportion of adult kidneys. In one study, one or more interlobar fissures were detected in up to 50% of adult kidneys (193). In older children and adults, it is important to distinguish persistent fetal lobations from cortical scars. Fetal lobation is a more accurate term than fetal lobulation because a lobule is an architectural feature of the cortex, primarily observed on the histologic level.

Histology

Cortical Architecture

The developing renal cortex has unique temporal and spatial features of organization. Each generation of nephrons, most easily observed histologically by the glomeruli, forms a "layer" over the preceeding generation. The earliest formed nephrons are situated in the inner cortex (juxtamedullary) near the future medulla, whereas the nephrogenic zone in the outer cortex (superficial) contains the last nephrons formed. Between the thirty-second and thirty-sixth weeks of gestation, nephron formation ceases and the nephrogenic zone disappears. Although the nephrogenic zone persists in kidneys of children born prematurely (195,196), evidence suggests that postnatal nephrogenesis is suboptimal and does not occur after 40 days (197).

The histologic features of the developing renal cortex have been used as an index of fetal maturation (196). The ratio of the width of the nephrogenic zone to the width of the remaining cortex decreases in a linear fashion as the birth weight increases (185,198). This approach has been used to detect infants with reduced intrauterine growth in whom this ratio is less than expected for the birth weight. Using glomeruli as representative of nephrons, studies have employed counting the number of layers (or rows) of glomeruli from inner to outer cortex as a method to evaluate nephrogenesis (199–201). Each successive layer is assumed to represent a new glomerular "generation." These estimates are performed on well-oriented sections that are orthogonal to the cortex and display a well-defined corticomedullary junction.

The studies are in fair agreement between gestations of 24 to 36 weeks, in which the average number of rows (nephron generations) of glomeruli are as follows: 5 to 7 (24 weeks), 8 to 9 (28 weeks), 9 to 10 (32 weeks), and 10 to 14 (36 weeks). After the full complement of nephrons is attained by the normal fetus, subsequent renal growth reflects hypertrophy and maturation of the nephrons. As tubules elongate and increase in diameter, they become interposed between glomeruli. The glomeruli in the outer cortex of newborns are crowded together (Figure 34.10), whereas the older, more mature glomeruli deeper in the cortex are more widely separated. This process of tubular growth not only separates glomeruli from one another, but it also tends to separate them from the cortical surface near where they originally developed. In a normal term newborn, one observes many glomeruli very close to the renal capsule (Figure 34.10). By about 2 months of age, the process of nephron growth has begun to separate the outermost glomeruli, and a narrow zone largely devoid of glomeruli develops beneath the renal capsule (Figure 34.18). This latter zone has been termed the *cortex corticis* (202). The cortex corticis becomes progressively wider during childhood (Figure 34.19). Although it is normal to find an occasional glomerulus adjacent to the

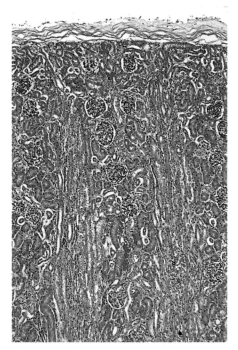

Figure 34.18   Renal cortex at 2 months of age. Glomeruli in the outer cortex are becoming more widely spaced due to tubular elongation. Superficial glomeruli are beginning to separate from the renal capsule, the first indication of the cortex corticis.

capsular surface in normal infants and children, the presence of numerous very superficial glomeruli suggests defective renal growth during late fetal or early postnatal life. Abnormally crowded glomeruli also can be an important clue to defects in nephron growth and differentiation, which may involve only the outer cortex or the entire cortical mantle. Thus, the cortical architecture may be viewed as a record of the developmental history of the kidney.

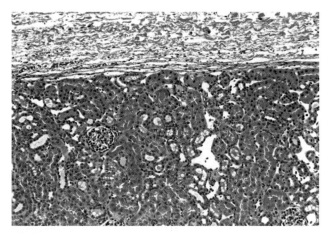

Figure 34.19   Micrograph of well-developed renal cortex corticis. The zone without glomeruli beneath the distinct renal capsule is evident. Reprinted with permission from: Murphy WM, Grignon DJ, Perlman EJ. Tumors of the kidney, bladder, and related urinary structures. In: *Atlas of Tumor Pathology*. 4th series, fascicle 1. Washington, DC: Armed Forces Institute of Pathology; 2004.

The cortex is subdivided into distinctly demarcated *lobules* by radially oriented groups of tubules termed *medullary rays* that extend from the base of the pyramids upward into the cortex (Figure 34.20). A lobule is defined as the cortical domain surrounding a medullary ray. Despite their name, the medullary rays (of Ferrein) actually are part of the cortex and contain the straight segments of the proximal tubule, the thick ascending limbs, and the collecting ducts. Medullary rays usually extend to near the cortical surface in infants but not in older children. The presence of complete medullary rays is a good indicator that the plane of a given section is perpendicular and reflective of the true thickness of the cortex. Medullary ray nodules are complex tangled tubular configurations commonly seen in the medullary rays of infants during the early months of life, being most prominent between 1 and 6 months of age (Figure 34.21) (203). These structures apparently represent a normal transitory developmental phenomenon of variable prominence, which is pathologic only when extreme.

Nephron Number

The number of nephrons in a kidney is determined in utero. The final number is dependent on gestational age and a favorable intrauterine environment. Unbiased, precise stereological methods have been used to count glomeruli, which serve as a surrogate for nephron number. One study of human intrauterine renal growth revealed the glomerular number increased from 15,000 at 15 weeks of gestation to 740,000 by 40 weeks (204). The greatest rate of nephron induction has been observed between 15 to 17 weeks of

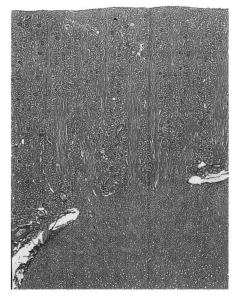

Figure 34.20   Kidney at 21 months of age. This perpendicularly oriented section illustrates the full length of several medullary rays that extend from the corticomedullary junction to a level near the cortex corticis. Each medullary ray marks the center of a cortical lobule.

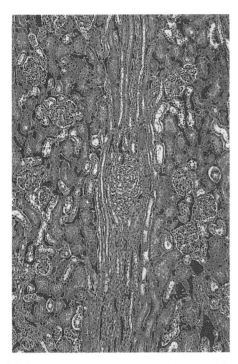

Figure 34.21 Medullary ray nodule. In the center of the micrograph, a tangled cluster of collecting ducts forms a nodule near the midportion of a medullary ray. This structure is usually transitory, being uncommon in the first month of life and extremely rare after 1 year of age.

gestation; however, approximately 60% of the total nephrons are believed to form during the third trimester (204). Nephron number, inferred from glomerular number estimates in children and adults without renal disease, is strongly correlated with birth weight (205). Intrauterine growth retardation has been shown to impair nephron formation, as measured in fetuses and in infants dying within a year of birth (206,207).

It is apparent that a kidney having a quantitative abnormality, such as low nephron number, may not demonstrate an obvious defect of nephron spatial topography on histologic examination. However, studies have demonstrated an inverse correlation between the number of glomeruli and mean glomerular volume, suggesting glomeruli increase in size to compensate for an innate low nephron number (205,207). Large glomeruli may be susceptible to scarring. Glomerulomegaly has been used as an adverse factor to assess the risk of disease progression in childhood nephrotic syndrome (208). Thus, increased glomerular size (volume or area) may be useful as an indicator for nephron deficiency in individuals susceptible to renal disease.

Until a few years ago, each human kidney was believed to contain one million nephrons. It is now appreciated that there is a remarkably wide variation in total nephrons per kidney among "normal" adults, ranging from as low as 227,000 to over 2,000,000 (209–211). Nephron endowment is programmed in the perinatal period, capping the nephron number in an individual's lifetime. Some time ago, Brenner et al. (212) postulated that an inborn deficit of nephrons predisposes to acquired renal disease, including hypertension, in adults. A study showing that hypertensive individuals had fewer nephrons but a larger glomerular volume than age-matched normotensive controls supports this hypothesis (213). The endowment of nephrons from nephrogenesis and the developmental origins of renal disease are fertile areas for investigation.

Glomerular Maturation and Growth

Newly formed glomeruli are structurally distinctive, and their evolution toward a mature form is a gradual process. Because the period of glomerular development spans a six- to seven-month period of fetal life, a spectrum of maturational stages is normally present in infant kidneys. As mentioned before, this spectrum is organized in a temporal-spatial manner in the cortex. Familiarity with normal glomerular maturation can facilitate an assessment of the renal developmental status in infants. Dramatic changes in glomerular structure and size occur through the early months and years of life. For convenience of study, several stages of glomerular development have been defined in studies (214–217). Figure 34.22 shows representative glomeruli from the midcortical region of infants and children from birth to 9 years of age to illustrate the maturational changes. Figure 34.22A shows the characteristic appearance of recently formed glomeruli from a term newborn infant. In addition to their small size, the most obvious distinctions from mature glomeruli are the simple character of the tufts with relatively few capillary loops and the layer of cuboidal cells surfacing the visceral layer of the tuft. This cuboidal layer, representing developing podocytes, is often continuous and covers most of the circumference of the tufts. Ultrastructurally, these primitive podocytes are closely approximated to one another and often lack foot processes (Figure 34.23A). The glomerular basement membrane (GBM) is thin and two lamina densa structures, representing basal laminae produced by endothelial cells and podocytes prior to their fusion into a single lamina, may be focally observed. The thickness of the GBM increases progressively with age (Figure 34.23). The approximate values for GBM thickness during childhood range as follows: 100 to 130 nm in fetal kidneys; 170 nm ($\pm$ 30) at birth; 208 nm ($\pm$ 24) at 1 year; 245 nm ($\pm$ 49) at 2 years; 268 nm ($\pm$ 43) at 6 years; and 300 nm ($\pm$ 42) by 10 years (216,218,219). The growth rate is greatest prior to 2 years of age. In contrast to adults, the GBM thickness in children appears less sex dependent (206). The data of Volger and colleagues, illustrating the increase in GBM (Figure 34.24A) and lamina densa widths (Figure 34.24B) with age are shown. Further GBM growth in adolescence, which is less documented, must occur to reach the adult GBM thickness in men (373 nm $\pm$ 42) and women (326 nm $\pm$ 45) (220).

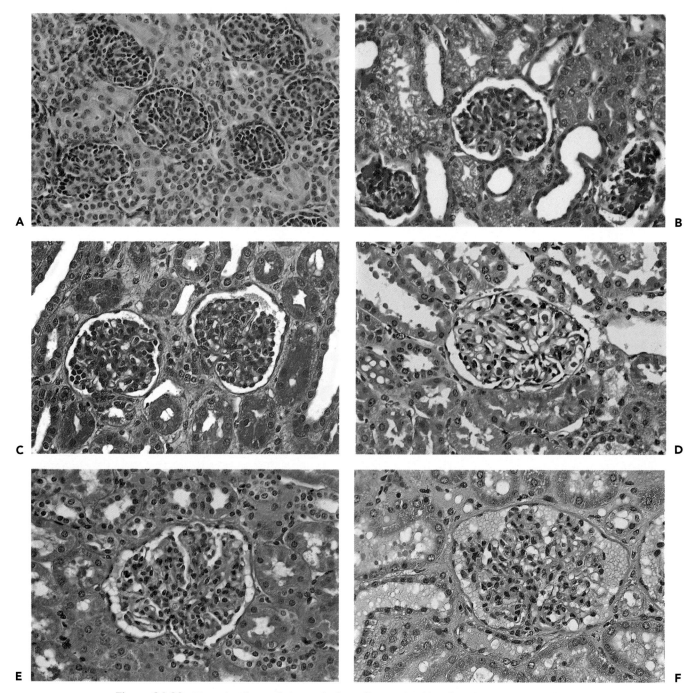

Figure 34.22   Normal midcortical glomeruli of six infants and children from birth to 9 years of age. All the micrographs were taken at the same magnification. **A.** Newborn. **B.** 6 months. **C.** 11 months. **D.** 21 months. **E.** 5 years. **F.** 9 years.

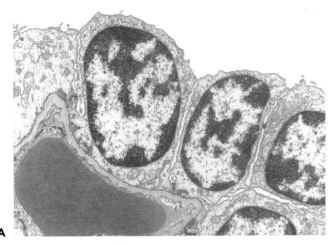
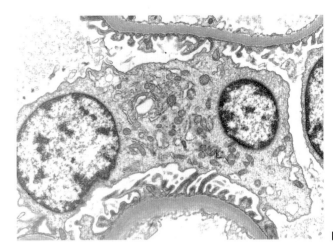

A

B

Figure 34.23 **A.** Electron micrograph of a normal glomerulus from an infant 2 months of age. Note the continuous layer of primitive podocytes lacking foot processes and the thin glomerular basement membrane. **B.** Mature glomerulus from a patient 16 years of age, photographed at the same magnification as in A. There is prominent foot process development, and the glomerular basement membrane is distinctly thicker than in the infant. (Courtesy of Dr. Gary W. Mierau.)

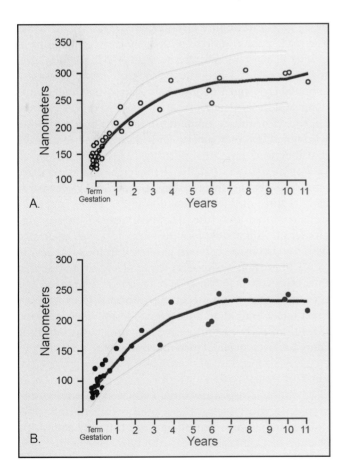

Figure 34.24 Thickness of glomerular basement membrane (GBM) in children. **A.** Total thickness of GBM. **B.** Thickness of lamina densa (LD) portion of GBM. The thickness of both the total GBM and the LD increases rapidly in early childhood and slows in growth after 3 years of age. The mean GBM and LD thicknesses (red lines) and the 95th percentile ranges (yellow lines) are shown. Modified with permission from: Volger C, McAdams J, Homan SM. Glomerular basement membrane and lamina densa in infants and children: an ultrastructural evaluation. *Pediatr Pathol* 1987;7:527–534.

The continuous cuboidal layer of cells is transient as the maturing podocytes flatten over the surfaces of the developing capillaries. A few small clusters of cuboidal podocytes remain in infant glomeruli (Figure 34.22 B–C). After a glomerulus has been in existence for more than 12 months, remnants of the cuboidal layer are usually not seen in normally developed glomeruli. In 1940, Gruenwald and Popper suggested that some podocytes may be sloughed into Bowman's space as part of the maturation process (214). In fact, several studies have demonstrated that podocytes are shed from the glomerulus and excreted in the urine in various glomerular diseases, as well as in healthy individuals (221,222). Moreover, most of the urinary podocytes are viable as evidenced by their ability to grow in culture under in vitro conditions. Whether podocyturia occurs in the normal neonate and infant remains to be established. The above podocyte alterations are coincident with the emergence of more conspicuous capillary loops (Figure 34.22 C–D). Eventually, the capillary loops are arranged into lobules (Figure 34.22 E–F). However, an occasional glomerulus with the small size and immature appearance of a neonatal glomerulus may be observed in older infants, especially in the outer one-third of the cortex (Figure 34.25).

Glomerular growth during childhood has been evaluated in several investigations (223–227). In these studies, the source of renal tissue (postmortem or biopsy specimen), the observational technique (histology or microdissection), and the morphometric method varied. However, it is well established that glomerular size increases from birth into adolescence. Spouster and Emery (225) reported that the midcortical and juxtamedullary mean glomerular area in fetuses actually decreased between 12 and 20 weeks gestation. After this initial decrease, the

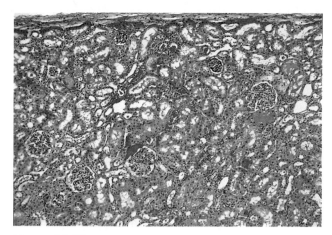

Figure 34.25 Persistent immature glomeruli at 12 months of age. Two miniature glomeruli with cuboidal cells at the periphery of the tuft are present near the renal capsule. Small numbers of defective glomeruli can be found in infant kidneys, but they are destined to undergo sclerosis and involution.

glomeruli remained at the same size until birth, after which they steadily grew. Moore et al. (226) observed that the mean glomerular diameter in normal children increased from 112 to 167 μm between birth and 15 years of age, averaging 3.6 μm per year during this period. Akaoka et al. (227) found that the mean glomerular tuft area in children with minimal change nephrotic syndrome and recurrent hematuria, increased from 6,600 μm² to 11,000 μm² between 2 and 15 years of age. In the latter study, the glomerular capillary lumina area did not correlate with the glomerular tuft area, whereas the number of capillaries per glomerulus showed a positive correlation with the glomerular tuft area. Although some of the glomeruli were not normal in this study, the findings support the concept that glomerular growth occurs by an increase in the number or length of capillaries rather than by hemodynamic capillary dilatation.

Juxtamedullary glomeruli are larger than superficial glomeruli at birth and during infancy. However, some uncertainty exists regarding these regional differences in glomerular size in later childhood and young adults. Some authors have observed no size difference between juxtamedullary and superficial glomeruli by the fourteenth to thirty-sixth postnatal month (223,225), whereas others have found a size difference persists until at least 15 years of age (224,226). Methodological differences in the studies or the wide variation in glomerular size existing among individuals (228) may account for these disparate findings.

Investigations using stereological methods have provided estimates for the number of cells in glomeruli. Steffes et al. (229) observed that the total number of cells per glomerulus increased along with the mean glomerular volume in comparing normal individuals younger than 20 years of age to those greater than 20 years. The number of endothelial cells and mesangial cells increased with age, whereas the number of podocytes remained unchanged with age. These results are consistent with the large amount of animal data indicating that mature podocytes are largely terminally differentiated and do not replicate. This concept is also supported by the expression pattern of cell cycle regulatory proteins during glomerulogenesis (230–232). The proliferation marker Ki-67 is expressed in podocyte precursors in comma- and S-shaped bodies, but its expression is markedly reduced in podocytes of the glomerular capillary loop stage. The cyclin-dependent kinase (CDK) inhibitors p27 and p57 are absent in the comma- and S-shaped bodies but expressed in maturing podocytes of the capillary loop stage, as well as in mature podocytes in adult kidneys. These findings suggest the CDK inhibitors are involved with arresting the cell cycle of podocytes at the capillary loop stage and maintaining the fully mature podocytes in a quiescent differentiated state.

Early Juxtamedullary Glomeruli

The maturational process in the very early generations of glomeruli may be accelerated because, even in very young fetuses, these juxtamedullary glomeruli rarely possess a cuboidal layer and are considerably larger than their immediate superficial neighbors. Attention was drawn to these large juxtamedullary glomeruli in humans by Kampmeier, who noted that they subsequently disappeared, suggesting that they were transient structures (233). Tsuda observed in human fetuses that the diameter of juxtamedullary glomeruli were nearly twice that of superficial glomeruli as early as three months of gestation (199). Emery and Macdonald noted that the disappearance of these large glomeruli, in the early months after birth, was associated with the presence of scarred glomeruli in the same region (234). These findings support Kampmeier's suggestion that they represent a transient population of nephrons. It is presumed that these precociously formed glomeruli are functionally important during fetal life and likely undergo involution early in the postnatal period. Relatively little study has been made of these interesting structures.

Glomerulosclerosis in Infants

Glomerulosclerosis in infantile kidneys is commonly observed. In most cases, it is a presumably normal phenomenon that must be distinguished from the pathologic changes of glomerular disease. In 1909, Herxheimer concluded that sclerotic glomeruli usually represented defective development of glomeruli in otherwise normal kidneys and were not manifestations of a disease process (235). Other investigators have suggested this context of glomerulosclerosis might result from a vascular origin, excretion of toxic substances, or renal infection (236,237).

Emery and Macdonald conducted thorough studies of glomerulosclerosis in children's kidneys that were considered morphologically within normal limits (234). Their series of 475 cases included kidneys from fetuses at 24 weeks of gestation to children 15 years of age. The percentage of sclerotic glomeruli in each kidney was most often in the range of 1 to 2% (65% of cases), although higher percentages from 3 to 10% affected glomeruli (30% of cases) were observed. The proportion of infants having sclerotic glomeruli was age dependent. Scarred glomeruli occurred in 25 to 40% of kidneys from late fetuses and newborns. They were detected in 70% of kidneys by 2 months of age, remaining near this level throughout the first year. Afterwards, their incidence steadily declined and was about 10% of children at 6 years of age.

Emery and Macdonald found that sclerotic glomeruli localized to two areas; the deep inner cortex (juxtamedullary zone near the arcuate vessels) and the superficial outer cortex (near the capsule). Sclerotic glomeruli in the juxtamedullary zone were more common in the first six months of life than in older children. Affected glomeruli in the outer cortex were most prominent in the first two years after birth. The presence of scarred glomeruli in the juxtamedullary zone coincided with the disappearance of the large glomeruli seen in this region during the months after birth, as discussed previously. Thus, it appears the sclerosing glomeruli in the juxtamedullary zone represent the involution of the large glomeruli that localize to this zone during nephrogenesis. The glomerular scarring in the outer cortex near the capsule likely reflects a different etiologic process that, if linked to nephrogenesis, is probably occurring relatively late. In a study of 800 infant kidneys, Thomas reported a similar distribution pattern of sclerotic glomeruli in the cortex (238). The general consensus is that these lesions are defects of development but without functional or clinical significance. Their major significance for pathologists is that they not be interpreted as evidence of glomerular disease, unless their number is considerably above the usual range (greater than 20%) mentioned above.

A typical example of infantile glomerulosclerosis is illustrated in Figure 34.26. The scarred glomeruli may occur singly or in small groups. They are usually smaller than normal, immature in appearance, and variably hyalinized. The afferent arteriole is often thickened, and periglomerular fibrosis may be present as well as some chronic inflammatory cells in the interstitium. In later stages, only a small globule of hyalin material in a small focus of sclerosis without capillary lumens may be seen. The tubules associated with the sclerotic glomeruli often contain proteinaceous material and apparently disappear along with the glomeruli.

Ectopic Glomeruli

In the kidneys from fetuses and infants, glomeruli are often found outside the confines of the renal parenchyma, either in the renal sinus (Figure 34.27) or in the connective tissue around interlobar vessels. These *ectopic* glomeruli occur in

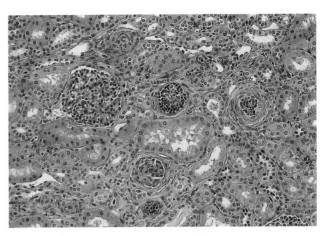

Figure 34.26 Infantile glomerulosclerosis at 9 months of age. One small, developmentally immature glomerulus is seen near the center, and two adjacent glomeruli are undergoing involutional sclerosis.

several mammalian species as well as in young humans (239). They appear to degenerate during postnatal life and are not found in adult human kidneys. It has been suggested that some vessels supplying the pelvic mucosa and medulla may be derived from degenerated ectopic glomeruli (239,240). The ectopic glomeruli may represent the early large juxtamedullary glomeruli, described by Kampmeier, that have persisted at least until infancy rather than degenerate.

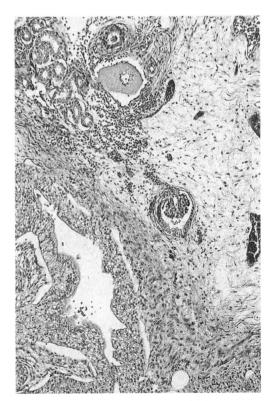

Figure 34.27 Ectopic glomerulus in the renal sinus.

Tubular Maturation and Growth

There is less known about the maturation and growth of tubules between birth and adulthood compared to glomeruli. Although all tubular segments increase in size during postnatal maturation, the proximal convoluted tubules undergo very prominent elongation and increased tortuosity (5). The results of microdissection studies reported from two laboratories were fairly similar (223,241). The mean lengths of proximal tubules observed were: about 2 mm at birth, 3.5 mm at 3 months, 6.5 mm at 1 year of age, 7.7 mm at 2 years, and 12.0 mm at 12 years. The mean proximal tubular length of 20 mm in adult kidney indicates that proximal tubule elongation continues through adolescence and young adulthood. Proximal tubules at birth are less uniform in size than glomeruli. Proximal tubules in the outer cortex of the newborn kidney were observed to be the shortest, those in the midcortex intermediate in length, and those from the juxtamedullary cortex the longest, consistent with a centrifugal pattern of development (223). These regional differences in proximal tubules decreased significantly after 1 month of age and disappeared by 14 months. Whether tubular function, such as solute and volume reabsorption, of the maturing proximal tubules from different cortical regions also follows a centrifugal pattern of maturation remains uncertain (242). It is interesting that in the adult kidney, the proximal tubules from the outer cortex have been observed to be longer than those from the mid- and juxtamedullary cortex (223). The ratio of glomerular surface area to proximal tubular volume was proposed as a theoretical anatomic correlate of functional glomerulotubular balance, that is, the balance between the capacity of the glomerulus to filter and the tubule to reabsorb the filtrate (223). Values for this ratio (28 in the term newborn kidney, 13 in the 3-month kidney, 6 in the 6-month kidney, and 3 in the adult kidney) suggested morphologic dominance of glomeruli over tubules early in life until the tubules, in effect, "grew up to their glomeruli" (223). However, it is difficult to correlate these morphologic ratios with experimental functional data indicating proportionate increases in glomerular filtration rate (GFR) and proximal tubule reabsorption after birth, consistent with maintenance of glomerulotubular balance during postnatal maturation (243).

During postnatal maturation, the loops of Henle undergo striking elongation (5). The newborn kidney lacks a well-formed inner medulla and contains loops of Henle that are relatively short (2,4,5). At birth, the loops of Henle are shortest in the younger nephrons, whereas longer loops belong to the older nephrons. As the kidney increases in size after birth, the loops of Henle elongate, the medullary interstitium increases, and the medulla becomes separated into outer and inner zones. From birth until full maturation, loops of Henle may increase in length as much as three-fold. In the mature kidney, the location of the tips of the loops of Henle relates to the age of their associated nephrons. The loops of the last-formed nephrons (outer cortex) reach the junction between the outer and inner medulla and are known as short loops of Henle. In contrast, the loops of the earliest formed nephrons (juxtamedullary cortex) extend deep into the inner medulla near the tip of the papilla and are referred to as long loops of Henle. Prior to birth, thin portions of loops of Henle are only observed in the long loops of Henle. These thin portions are present in the *descending* limbs of the long loops of Henle and continue to lengthen after birth. *Descending* thin limbs are not seen in short loops of Henle until after birth. Only long loops of Henle develop *ascending* thin limbs, which are derived from the thick ascending limbs, likely by an ascending process of apoptotic remodeling (55,244).

ADULT KIDNEY

Gross Anatomy

The kidneys lie within the retroperitoneum and extend from the twelfth thoracic (T12) to the third lumbar (L3) vertebrae, with the right kidney usually slightly more caudad. They are situated within the perirenal space, which contains abundant fat and is traversed by fine fibrous septae (245–247). Visualization of the renal fascia with radiologic procedures has been reported in normal individuals (248,249). Each kidney weighs 125 to 170 grams in men and 115 to 155 grams in women (250). If differences in body build are considered, kidney weight correlates best with body surface area, whereas age, sex, and race have less influence (251). Each kidney is 11 to 12 cm in length, 5 to 7.5 cm in width, and 2.5 to 3 cm in thickness. The left kidney tends to be slightly larger and may demonstrate irregularities of the lateral contour from compression by the spleen in up to 10% of normal individuals (252). A glistening tough fibroelastic capsule surrounds the kidney.

In the hilar region, the main renal artery branches to form anterior and posterior divisions (Figure 34.28), which in turn divide into segmental arteries that supply the apical, upper, middle, lower, and posterior segmental regions of the parenchyma (253,254). No collateral circulation has been demonstrated between the segmental arteries. Some of the so-called accessory arteries actually represent normal segmental arteries with an early origin from the main-stem renal artery or aorta (254). Therefore, ligation of such a segmental artery in the belief that it is an accessory vessel results in necrosis of the corresponding parenchymal segment. The intrarenal veins do not follow a segmental distribution, and there are numerous anastomoses of the veins throughout the kidney. There are variable drainage patterns of the large extra-renal veins that join to form the main renal vein (255). A relatively common occurrence is a posterior primary venous tributary, whose retropelvic

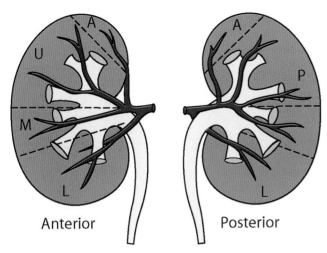

The human kidney is a multipapillary type of mammalian kidney (256), with the medulla divided into 8 to 18 striated conical masses called pyramids (Figure 34.29). The striated appearance reflects the parallel linear orientation of the loops of Henle and collecting ducts. The base of each pyramid is located at the corticomedullary junction, whereas the apex extends toward the renal pelvis, forming a papilla. The tip of each papilla is perforated by 20 to 70 small openings (6) that represent the distal ends of the collecting ducts (of Bellini). The cortex is about 1 cm in thickness, encircles the base of each pyramid, and extends downward between pyramids to form the septa (columns) of Bertin. Despite well-described radiologic features (257, 258), an enlarged septum of Bertin on occasion has been clinically mistaken for a renal tumor. Longitudinal striations extending from the base of the pyramids out into the cortex are termed the medullary rays (of Ferrein). Regardless of their name, they are actually part of the cortex and are formed by the straight segments of the proximal tubules (PSTs), the thick ascending limbs (TALs), and the collecting ducts. The medullary rays may be visualized during excretory urography in conditions with tubular fluid stasis (259).

A single pyramid with its surrounding cortical parenchyma constitutes a renal lobe (191,260) (Figure 34.30). The human kidney has an average of 14 lobes (102). During development, variable lobar fusion leads to coalescence of some papillae and remodeling of the corresponding calyces, gradually reducing the number of papillae and calyces. The mean number of calyces and papillae

Figure 34.28 Diagram of the vascular supply of the human kidney. The anterior division of the renal artery divides into three segmental branches that supply the upper (*U*) and middle (*M*) segments of the anterior surface and most of the lower (*L*) segment. The small apical (*A*) segment is usually supplied by a branch from the anterior division. The posterior division of the renal artery supplies the posterior (*P*) segment, which represents more than half of the posterior surface of the kidney. Modified with permission from: Graves FT. The anatomy of the intrarenal arteries and its application to segmental resection of the kidney. *Br J Surg* 1954;42:132–139.

position should be remembered during renal surgical intervention. An outer pale region (the cortex) and an inner darker region (the medulla) can be distinguished on the cut surface of a bisected kidney. The presence of glomeruli and convoluted tubules results in the cortex having a more granular appearance.

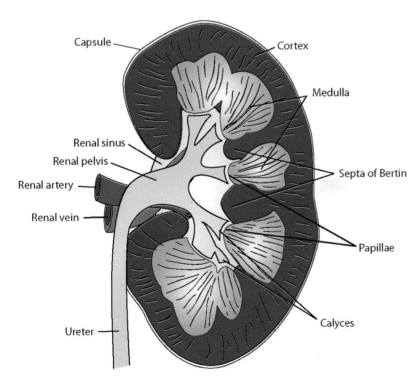

Figure 34.29 Diagram of a bisected kidney illustrating major anatomic structures.

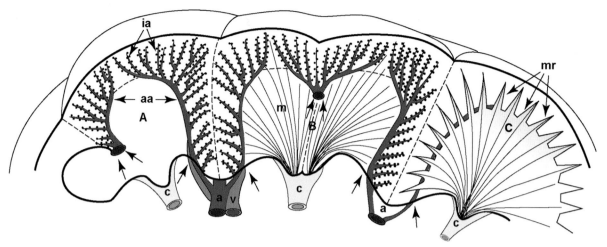

Figure 34.30 Diagram of three renal lobes. **A.** Arcuate (*aa*) and interlobular (*ia*) arteries. **B.** Cortex and medulla (*m*) are illustrated in a double lobe with fused double papillae. **C.** Lobe showing medullary rays (*mr*). A septum of Bertin represents the approximation of two layers of septal cortex from two adjacent lobes. (*Small double arrows* in A and B, subsidiary septal arteries; *single arrows*, location where arcuate vessels enter the renal parenchyma; *a*, interlobar arteries; *v*, interlobar vein; *c*, calyces). Modified with permission from: Hodson CJ. The renal parenchyma and its blood supply. *Curr Probl Diagn Radiol* 1978; 7:1–32.

reported is 9 and 11, respectively (193). There is a greater degree of lobar fusion in the polar regions than in the mid-polar region of the kidney. A degree of persistent fetal lobation may be observed in some adult kidneys.

There are two main types of renal papillae (261). Simple papillae drain only one lobe and have convex tips containing small, often slitlike orifices. Compound papillae drain two or more adjacent fused lobes and have flattened, ridged, or concave tips with round, often gaping orifices. The distribution of papillae types within the kidney is related to the embryologic pattern of fusion involving the lobes, papillae, and calyces (Figure 34.31). It is believed that the more open orifices of compound papillae are less capable of preventing intrarenal reflux (262), which may be associated with an increase in intrapelvic pressure. This concept is supported by the observation that pyelonephritic scars associated with intrarenal reflux are present more commonly in the renal poles, where the compound papillae predominantly occur.

The renal pelvis is the saclike expansion of the upper ureter. Two or three outpouchings or major calyces (infundibula) extend from the pelvis and divide into the minor calyces, into which the papillae protrude. In addition, elaborate leaflike extensions, termed fornices, extend from the minor calyces into the medulla, and secondary pouches increase the pelvic surface area (263).

The renal sinus is located on the medial or concave aspect of each kidney (Figure 34.32) (264,265). It contains the renal pelvis, the major renal arteries and veins, the lymphatics, and neural structures that supply the kidney. The renal hilus is the entry into the sinus. Fat fills the renal sinus

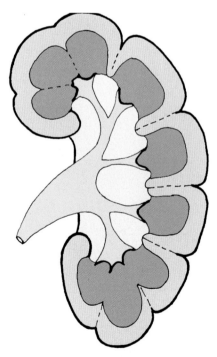

Figure 34.31 Schematic representation of the lobar architecture. In the polar regions, there is a greater degree of lobe fusion, resulting in the formation of compound papillae and calyces and the loss of septal cortex. The individual lobes tend to be retained in the midpolar region, and the septal cortex extends between renal pyramids, as septa of Bertin, to the renal sinus. Modified with permission from: Hodson CJ. The renal parenchyma and its blood supply. *Curr Probl Diagn Radiol* 1978; 7:1–32.

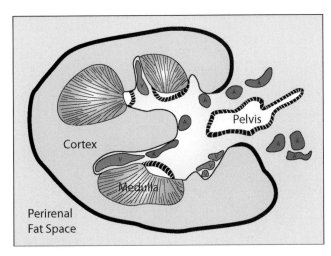

Figure 34.32 Diagram of kidney cross section, showing the renal sinus which is filled with fat (yellow). The renal sinus contains the pelvic-calyceal system and the major renal vessels. The renal capsule (thick black line) surrounds the convex surface of the kidney but disappears from the cortical surface as the latter enters the renal sinus. The cortical surfaces, including the septa of Bertin, facing the renal sinus lack a capsule. The capsule surrounding the pelvic-calyceal system is indicated by a cross-hatched thick black line. The capsule covering the calyces, appears to extend over the medullary pyramids on cross section, and it envelopes the renal pelvis as well. Modified with permission from: Murphy WM, Grignon DJ, Perlman EJ. Tumors of the kidney, bladder, and related urinary structures. In: *Atlas of Tumor Pathology*. 4th series, fascicle 1. Washington, DC: Armed Forces Institute of Pathology; 2004.

and is contiguous with the perirenal fat. Within the renal sinus, the renal capsule does not enclose the cortical parenchymal surface. Beckwith called attention to the importance of the renal sinus as a pathway for tumor dissemination in Wilms' tumor (266), and this has also been shown in renal cell carcinomas (267,268). A detailed description of the gross anatomy of the kidney is provided elsewhere (9).

Nephron

The structural and functional unit of the kidney is the nephron, which consists of the renal corpuscle (glomerulus and Bowman's capsule), proximal tubule, thin limbs, and distal tubule, all of which originate from the metanephric blastema. The total number of nephrons in a human kidney varies markedly among normal individuals (209–211). Although a tenfold variation in nephron number has been reported, the usual range is about 600,000 to 1,200,000 nephrons per kidney. Nephrons can be classified according to the position of their glomeruli in the cortex or the length of their loop of Henle (Figure 34.33). In the former scheme, superficial, midcortical, and juxtamedullary nephrons are distinguished. Superficial nephrons have glomeruli located in the outer cortex, and their efferent arterioles usually ascend to the cortical surface. The glomeruli of juxtamedullary nephrons are located immediately above

the corticomedullary junction in the inner cortex, and their efferent arterioles form the descending vasa recta. The glomeruli of midcortical nephrons are situated in the midcortex above the juxtamedullary region but below the superficial nephrons.

In the more commonly used classification, there are two main populations of nephrons: those with a short loop of Henle and those with a long loop. The length of the loop of

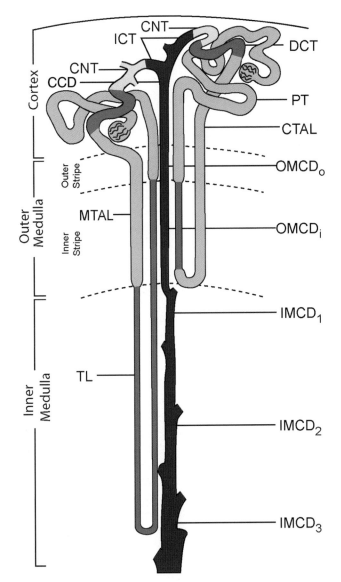

Figure 34.33 Diagram illustrating the segments of the nephron and the zones of the kidney. (*PT*, proximal tubule; *TL*, thin limb of Henle's loop; *MTAL*, medullary thick ascending limb; *CTAL*, cortical thick ascending limb; *DCT*, distal convoluted tubule; *CNT*, connecting tubule; *ICT*, initial collecting tubule; *CCD*, cortical collecting duct; *OMCD_o*, collecting duct in outer stripe of outer medulla; *OMCD_i*, collecting duct in inner stripe of outer medulla; *IMCD_1*, outer third of inner medullary collecting duct; *IMCD_2*, middle third of inner medullary collecting duct; *IMCD_3*, inner third of inner medullary collecting duct. Modified with permission from: Madsen KM, Tisher CC. Structural-functional relationships along the distal nephron. *Am J Physiol* 1986;250(pt 2):F1–F15.

Henle is generally related to the location of its parent glomerulus in the cortex. The short loops form their bend at various levels within the inner stripe of the outer medulla, whereas the long loops of Henle enter and turn back within the inner medulla. Although there are numerous gradations between these two main types of nephrons, there are seven times more short than long loop nephrons in human kidneys (269). A correlation between the urinary concentrating ability and the relative length of the medulla has been established in several mammalian kidneys (270).

The connecting tubule, a transitional segment, joins the nephron to the collecting duct system, which originates from the ureteric bud. Although not correct in a strict anatomic sense, for practical considerations, the term *nephron* is commonly used to include the connecting segment and entire collecting duct. The collecting duct system can be divided into the cortical, outer medullary, and inner medullary collecting ducts (271,272). Structural and functional heterogeneity exist along the nephron (273). Internephron heterogeneity refers to the differences between analogous segments in superficial and juxtamedullary nephrons. Intranephron or axial heterogeneity may be defined as the differences between early and successive later portions of an individual nephron segment.

Architecture

The renal cortex can be divided into lobules. A renal lobule consists of a centrally positioned medullary ray and its surrounding cortical parenchyma, containing all nephrons draining into the collecting ducts of the medullary ray. In contrast to lobules of other organs, renal lobules are not distinctly separated by fine connective tissue septa; therefore, they are difficult to distinguish histologically. Furthermore, because it has been difficult to establish any structural-functional significance, the concept of the renal lobule is not commonly used.

The nephron segments and blood vessels in the cortex and medulla have a specific geometric arrangement (274). This intricate architecture allows integration (axial) of complex transport functions along the length of a specific nephron segment, as well as integration (regional) between different nephron segments in a specific region or zone (275).

Two architectural regions of the renal cortex can be distinguished: the cortical labyrinth and the medullary rays (Figure 34.34). The cortical labyrinth represents a continuous parenchymal zone that surrounds the regularly distributed medullary rays. Glomeruli, proximal and distal convoluted tubules, interlobular vessels (also termed cortical radial vessels), and a rich capillary network are situated in the cortical labyrinth. The large majority of convoluted tubular profiles are proximal tubules. Connecting tubules of juxtamedullary nephrons fuse and form so-called arcades, which are adjacent to the interlobular vessels within the cortical labyrinth. Individual nephrons with their interlob-

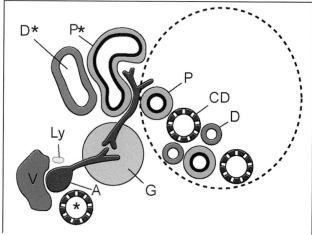

Figure 34.34 Diagram of architectural regions of the renal cortex. A medullary ray is encircled by the *dotted line*, and the cortical labyrinth is outside the *dotted line*. The proximal straight (*P*) and distal straight ascending limb (*D*) tubules and the collecting ducts (*CD*) are located in the medullary ray. The adjacent cortical labyrinth contains the interlobular vessels: arteries (*A*), veins (*V*), and lymphatics (*Ly*); arcades (*) of connecting tubules; glomeruli (*G*); and the proximal (*P**) and distal (*D**) convoluted tubules. Modified with permission from: Kriz W, Kaissling B. Structural organization of the mammalian kidney. In: Seldin DW, Giebisch D, eds. *The Kidney: Physiology and Pathophysiology*. 3rd ed. Philadelphia: Lippincott Williams & Wilkins; 2000:587–654.

ular vessels, glomeruli, and attached tubular segments, are difficult to distinguish in this complex topography by histology. The medullary rays (Figures 34.35–34.36) contain the proximal and distal straight tubules and collecting ducts, all of which enter into the medulla. The distal straight tubules are the thick ascending limbs. Within an individual medullary ray, the straight tubules of superficial nephrons are situated centrally, the straight tubules of midcortical nephrons are localized peripherally, and the collecting ducts occupy a position between the two groups. The straight tubules of juxtamedullary nephrons decend directly into the medulla without ever entering the medullary rays.

The localization of specific segments of the nephrons at various levels in the medulla account for the division of the medulla into an outer and inner zone, with the former subdivided into an inner and outer stripe (Figure 34.33). The relative tissue volumes for the cortex and the outer and inner medulla are 70, 27, and 3% respectively (272).

The outer stripe of the outer medulla is relatively thin. It contains the terminal portions of the proximal straight tubules, the thick ascending limbs, and the collecting ducts. The outer stripe is also distinguished by the absence of thin limbs of Henle. Glomeruli are not present in the medulla. In contrast to the outer stripe, the inner stripe of the outer medulla is thicker. It contains thin descending limbs, thick ascending limbs, and collecting ducts. It is further characterized by the absence of the proximal straight tubules. Aggregations of descending and ascending vasa recta, known as vascular bundles, develop in the

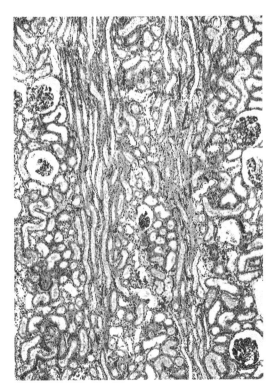

Figure 34.35 Longitudinal section of cortex demonstrating two linear aggregates of tubules representing medullary rays (original magnification ×50).

outer stripe but are located predominantly in the inner stripe. Compared with the kidneys of some mammals with very high urine concentrating ability, the human kidney has a simple medulla (274). In contrast to the complex medulla, the vascular bundles of the simple medulla do not fuse to form larger vascular structures, and they do not incorporate the descending thin limbs of short loops (Figure 34.37). The inner medulla contains the thin descending and thin ascending limbs of long loops, as well

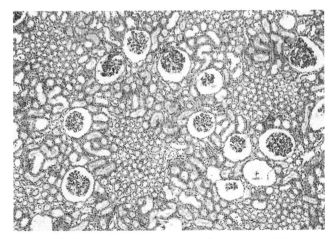

Figure 34.36 Cross section of cortex illustrating medullary rays that are regularly distributed within the cortical labyrinth (original magnification ×50).

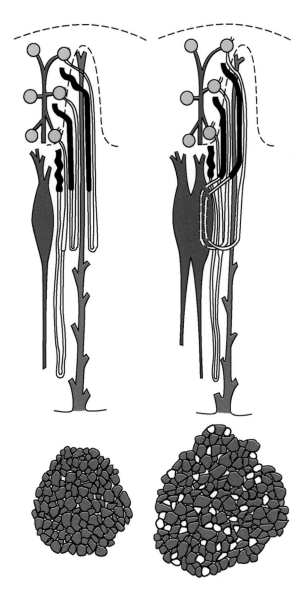

Figure 34.37 Schematic diagram demonstrating the simple and complex types of medulla. **Upper left:** In the simple medulla, the loops of Henle remain separate from the vascular bundle (purple). The vascular bundle itself (**lower left** cross section) contains only descending (red) and ascending (blue) vasa recta. **Upper right:** In the complex medulla, the descending thin limbs (DTLs) of short loops of Henle descend within the vascular bundles (purple), which tend to fuse. Therefore, the complex bundles (**lower right** cross section) contain the DTLs of short loops (white) in addition to descending (red) and ascending (blue) vasa recta. Modified with permission from: Jamison RL, Kriz W. *Urinary Concentrating Mechanism: Structure and Function.* New York: Oxford University Press;1982.

as the collecting ducts. Thick ascending limbs are absent in the inner medulla.

Parenchyma

An accurate morphologic evaluation of the kidney requires a detailed systematic examination of the glomeruli, tubules, interstitium, and blood vessels of the renal parenchyma. A standard nomenclature for structures of the kidney exists (276). A detailed approach to the histopathologic evaluation of the kidney has been described (277), and technical guidelines for handling the renal biopsy are available (278,279). The following discussion emphasizes normal morphologic aspects and structural-functional relationships in the kidney. The reader is directed to detailed discussions for more information (274,280).

Glomerulus

Overview

In 1666, Malpighi first described the glomeruli and demonstrated their continuity with the renal vasculature (281,282). About 175 years later, Bowman elucidated in detail the capillary architecture of the glomerulus and the continuity between its surrounding capsule and the proximal tubule (283,284). The renal corpuscle consists of a tuft of interconnected capillaries and an enclosing capsule named after Bowman. The term *glomerulus* is commonly used to refer to the glomerular capillary tuft and Bowman's capsule, although the term *renal corpuscle* is more accurate in a strict anatomic sense. The glomerulus does not simply represent a ball of capillaries. Providing structural support for the capillary tuft is a central region termed the mesangium, which contains cells and their surrounding matrix material. The capillaries are lined by a

thin layer of endothelial cells, contain a basement membrane, and are covered by epithelial cells (also called podocytes) that form the visceral layer of Bowman's capsule. The parietal epithelium is continuous with the visceral epithelium at the vascular pole where the afferent arteriole enters the glomerulus and the efferent arteriole exits. The glomerulus somewhat resembles a blind-pouched extension (Bowman's capsule) of the proximal tubule invaginated by a tuft of capillaries (Figure 34.38) (285). The cavity situated between the two epithelial layers of Bowman's capsule is called Bowman's space, or the urinary space. At the urinary pole, this space and the parietal layer of Bowman's capsule continue into the lumen and epithelium of the proximal tubule. The glomerular tuft originates from the afferent arteriole, which enters the glomerulus at the vascular pole and divides into several lobules. Anastomoses are believed to exist between individual capillaries within a lobule, as well as between lobules (274,286,287).

The efferent arteriole is formed by rejoined capillaries and leaves the glomerulus at the vascular pole. In contrast to the afferent arteriole, the efferent arteriole has a more continuous intraglomerular segment. The glomerulus is responsible for the ultrafiltration of plasma. The glomerular filtration barrier consists of the fenestrated endothelium, the peripheral glomerular basement membrane (GBM), and the slit diaphragms between the podocyte foot processes.

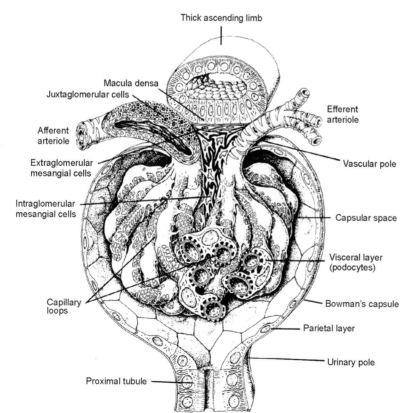

Figure 34.38 Schematic three-dimensional representation of the glomerulus. Modified with permission from: Geneser F. *Textbook of Histology*. Philadelphia: Lea & Febiger; 1986.

The glomerulus has a round configuration and an average diameter of about 200 μm (274,280). Although the diameter of juxtamedullary glomeruli has been reported up to 20 to 50% greater than that of superficial glomeruli (274), other researchers have found no significant size difference between these glomerular populations in the normal adult kidney (288). It has been reported that the glomeruli in solitary functioning kidneys are significantly larger than those in control patients with two kidneys (289). Although the glomerulus has a lobular architecture, the lobulation is often inconspicuous in light microscopic sections. An accentuated degree of lobulation may be more prominent in autopsy kidneys than in biopsy specimens (277). An apparent increase in the number of glomerular cells can be observed with an increased section thickness, therefore an accurate assessment of glomerular cellularity requires histologic sections 2 to 4 μm thick (Figure 34.39). Generally, the presence of more than three cells in a mesangial area away from the vascular pole constitutes hypercellularity. The delicate character of the glomerular capillary walls can be observed on thin histologic and frozen sections (Figure 34.40) (290).

Global glomerulosclerosis may occur as part of aging, without renal disease. The mean percentage of global glomerulosclerosis in normal kidneys was reported as follows: less than 1% between 1 and 20 years of age; 2% between 20 and 40 years; 7% between 40 and 60 years; and 11% between 60 and 80 years (291–293). There are no differences between the sexes in the development of glomerulosclerosis in aging humans (294). The 90th percentile for global glomerulosclerosis may be generally estimated for any age by subtracting 10 from half the patient's age (293).

Endothelial Cells

A thin fenestrated endothelium lines the glomerular capillaries. By light microscopy, the endothelial cells have light eosinophilic cytoplasm and slightly oval nuclei. Their nuclei are present within the capillary lumina. The

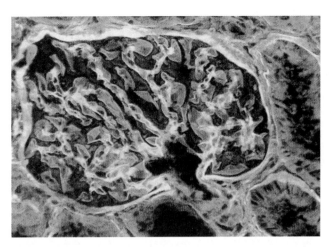

Figure 34.40 Fluorescent micrograph of an H&E-stained frozen section. Note the delicate character of the glomerular capillaries. (Courtesy of Dr. Stephen M. Bonsib.)

endothelial cells are extremely attenuated around the capillary lumen, and the thicker portions of the cells containing the nuclei lie adjacent to the mesangium away from the urinary space. The cytoplasm contains microtubules, microfilaments, and intermediate filaments (295). The attenuated portion of endothelial cytoplasm is perforated by fenestrae 70 to 100 nm in diameter (286). It has been argued that endothelial fenestrae do not simply arise from fusion of plasma membrane invaginations, called caveolae (296). It has been widely stated that glomerular endothelial fenestrae lack diaphragms, but thin bridging diaphragms have been observed when certain methods of fixation are used (297). The endothelial cell surface carries a negative charge because of the presence of polyanionic glycoproteins, including podocalyxin, a major sialoprotein of glomerular endothelial cells and podocytes (298,299). Results from recent studies have suggested that glomerular endothelial cells have a glycocalyx surface layer about 60 nm thick, and this surface coat fills the fenestrae forming "sieve plugs" (300,301). There is emerging evidence that the glomerular endothelial glycocalyx may be an important component of the glomerular filtration barrier (302,303). Vascular endothelial growth factor (VEGF), produced by podocytes, is an important regulator of glomerular endothelial cell function; VEGF induces fenestrae and increases permeability of endothelial cells, both in vivo and in vitro (304,305).

Current evidence indicates that maintenance of glomerular endothelial differentiation appears dependent on podocyte-derived VEGF (306). Glomerular endothelial cells synthesize nitric oxide (NO) and endothelin-1, a vasoconstrictor (307). There is strong expression of CD34 in glomerular endothelial cells (Figure 34.41).

Mesangial Cells

The mesangium, composed of mesangial cells and their surrounding matrix, is observed as a periodic acid-Schiff

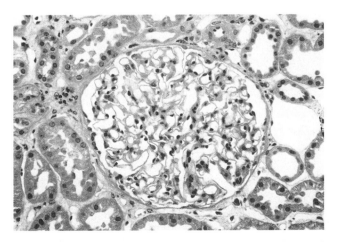

Figure 34.39 Glomerulus exhibiting round configuration and normal cellularity (original magnification ×250).

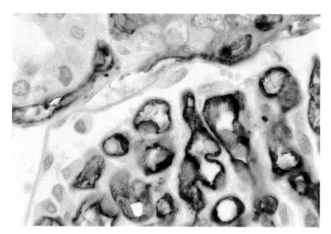

Figure 34.41 Glomerular endothelium showing immunoreactivity for CD34. Some peritubular capillaries show staining along the upper border. (CD34 immunoperoxidase, original magnification ×300.)

(PAS)- and methenamine silver-positive structural support for the glomerular capillary loops (Figure 34.42). By light microscopy, the mesangial cells usually can be distinguished by their mesangial location and dark-staining nuclei. Ultrastructurally, they are irregular in shape and have elongated cytoplasmic processes that may extend between the endothelium and the glomerular basement membrane. The mesangial cell processes have microfilaments that contain actin, myosin, and α-actinin (308,309). With smooth muscle contractile properties, the mesangial cell has been proposed to be a specialized pericyte that likely modulates glomerular filtration (310). Whereas the endothelium forms a continuous layer around the inner circumference of the glomerular capillary, the basement membrane and the visceral epithelial cell layer do not completely encircle the capillary but enclose the mesangial matrix and cells between the capillaries (Figure 34.43). The mesangial matrix is similar but not identical to the GBM and contains

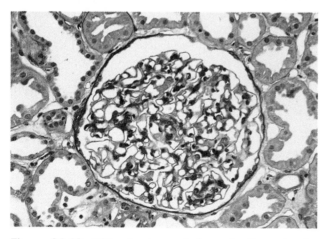

Figure 34.42 PAS-stained normal glomerulus illustrating the PAS-positive mesangium within the central regions of the glomerular capillaries (original magnification ×250).

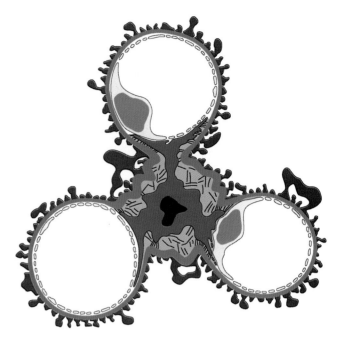

Figure 34.43 Schematic diagram illustrating the relationship between the mesangium and the glomerular capillaries. The visceral epithelial cell (podocyte) cytoplasm (red) and endothelial cell cytoplasm (yellow) are depicted. Note that the glomerular basement membrane (green) encloses the mesangium and its attached capillaries. The central mesangial cell is represented by dark brown cytoplasm and a black nucleus, and the mesangial matrix is represented by the tan fibrillar texture. The cytoplasmic processes of mesangial cells are connected to the glomerular basement membrane directly or indirectly by microfibrils in the mesangial matrix. Modified with permission from: Kriz W, Elger M, Lemley K, Sakai T. Structure of the glomerular mesangium: a biomechanical interpretation. *Kidney Int Suppl* 1990;30:S2–S9.

several types of collagen, as well as fibronectin and small proteoglycans. The matrix is especially rich in microfibrils, unbranched, noncollagenous structures that contain fibrillins and microfibril-associated glycoproteins (MAGPs) (311,312). The presence of microfibril-mediated attachments between mesangial cell processes and the GBM suggests that the mesangial cell and the GBM represent a biomechanical functional unit (313–315). It has been proposed that the contractile apparatus of the mesangium appears to maintain the structure of the capillary walls by counteracting the distention caused by the intracapillary hydraulic pressure (316). The mesangial cell also has phagocytic capability and plays a role in the clearance of macromolecules and debris from the mesangium (317). Mesangial cells can respond to, as well as generate, a variety of molecules, including interleukin-1, platelet-derived growth factor, and arachidonic acid metabolites, which may play a central role in the response to glomerular injury (318). It is recognized that a small subpopulation of cells in the mesangium are bone marrow-derived macrophages and play a role in immune responsiveness (Figure 34.44) (319–321). Occasional leukocytes are observed in the

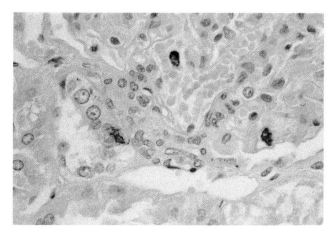

Figure 34.44 KP-1 immunohistochemical stain illustrating that a small percentage of cells in the mesangium label as tissue monocytes. (KP-1 immunoperoxidase, original magnification ×210.)

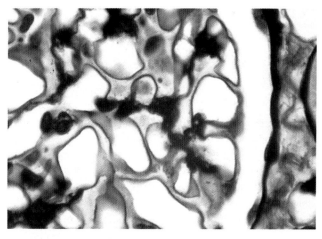

Figure 34.46 Higher magnification micrograph demonstrating thin regular glomerular basement membranes of peripheral capillary loops. (Silver methenamine stain, original magnification ×1250.)

normal glomerulus and label with leukocyte common antigen (CD45 and CD45RB) staining (322–324).

Interestingly, it has been demonstrated that mesangial cells residing in the extraglomerular mesangial region of the juxtaglomerular apparatus (JGA) may migrate and repopulate the intraglomerular mesangium upon glomerular injury (325).

Glomerular Basement Membrane

The glomerular basement membrane (GBM) can be demonstrated on light microscopy by PAS and methenamine silver stains (Figure 34.45). The silver preparation is more specific. Examination of a normal peripheral capillary loop away from the vascular pole and the mesangium shows a delicate basement membrane (Figure 34.46). Hematoxylin and eosin (H&E) and PAS preparations may stain capillary luminal contents and the cytoplasm of the endothelial and podocyte cell layers, resulting in an apparent thickening of the GBM. The basement membrane is situated between the endothelium and the podocytes in the glomerular capillary wall. On ultrastructural examination, the GBM consists of a central dense layer (the lamina densa) and two surrounding thinner electron-lucent layers (the lamina rara interna and the lamina rara externa). In comparison with laboratory animals, the electron-lucent layers appear less prominent in the human glomerulus (Figure 34.47). This may be due in part to different fixation conditions.

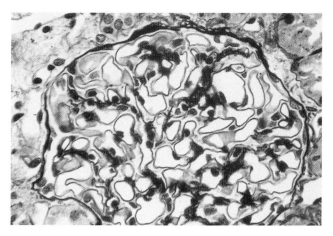

Figure 34.45 Silver methenamine-stained normal glomerulus illustrating the silver-positive glomerular basement membrane and positive basement membrane of Bowman's capsule (original magnification ×500).

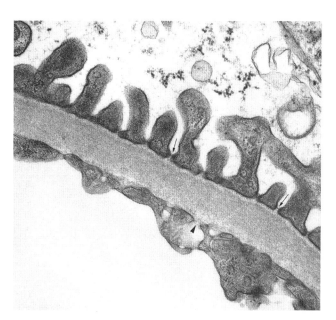

Figure 34.47 Transmission electron micrograph of a glomerulus. Bowman's space is above and the capillary lumen is below the glomerular capillary wall. A fenestra or pore (*arrowhead*) in the endothelium is evident. Note the regular alignment of the foot processes of the podocytes. Filtration slit diaphragms (*arrows*) are present between individual foot processes. The glomerular basement membrane consists primarily of the lamina densa. The electron-lucent lamina rara interna and lamina rara externa are not prominent (original magnification ×48,000).

The adult GBM ranges between 310 and 380 nm in mean thickness (326–328). It is significantly thicker in men (mean 373 nm) than in women (mean 326 nm) and increases in width until the fourth decade of life (220). Quantitative data on the normal adult glomerular capillary structure include the following values: mean glomerular volume of 1.38×10^6 μm^3, average capillary diameter of 6.75 μm, and capillary filtration surface/glomerulus of 200×10^3 μm^2 (329).

The major components of the GBM include type IV collagen, laminin, nidogen (also called entactin), and proteoglycans, including perlecan and agrin (26). Collagen IV is the major constituent of the GBM. Six chains, $\alpha 1(IV)$ through $\alpha 6(IV)$, make up the collagen IV protein family (330,331). Three chains of collagen IV self-associate to form triple-helical molecules called protomers. Despite many possible combinations, the six chains of collagen IV form only three types of protomers, which are designated as $\alpha 1.\alpha 1.\alpha 2(IV)$, $\alpha 3.\alpha 4.\alpha 5(IV)$, and $\alpha 5.\alpha 5.\alpha 6(IV)$. The triple helical protomers unite at the noncollagenous domain (NC1) at the carboxy terminus to form hexamers, which in turn, assemble to form a polymerized network that serves as a scaffold for integration of other GBM components (330,331). Three canonical sets of hexamers form three distinct networks in basement membranes: the $\alpha 1.\alpha 1.\alpha 2(IV)$–$\alpha 1.\alpha 1.\alpha 2(IV)$, the $\alpha 3.\alpha 4.\alpha 5(IV)$–$\alpha 3.\alpha 4.\alpha 5(IV)$, and the $\alpha 1.\alpha 1.\alpha 2(IV)$–$\alpha 5.\alpha 5.\alpha 6(IV)$ networks (332). The $\alpha 3.\alpha 4.\alpha 5(IV)$–$\alpha 3.\alpha 4.\alpha 5(IV)$ network predominates in the adult GBM, and mutations of the genes encoding the $\alpha 3$, $\alpha 4$, and $\alpha 5(IV)$ chains cause Alport syndrome (333). In Goodpasture syndrome, autoantibodies are targeted to the $\alpha 3(IV)$ chain (333).

Laminins are heterotrimers composed of three chains; α, β and γ. Laminin-11, containing the $\alpha 5$, $\beta 2$, and $\gamma 1$ chains, is the major laminin isoform in the adult GBM (33). Nidogen/entactin binds to laminin and is present in the GBM (334). Proteoglycans consist of glycosaminoglycan (GAG) chains bound to a core protein (335). They are primarily responsible for the negative charge of the GBM (336,337). Of three heparan sulfate proteoglycans, agrin (338) and collagen type XVIII (339) are more abundant in the GBM than is perlecan (340). Bamacan, a chondroitin sulfate proteoglycan, is present in the immature GBM but disappears from the adult GBM, remaining in the mesangial matrix (341).

Podocytes

The podocytes (visceral epithelial cells) are the largest cells in the glomerulus. By light microscopy, they are positioned on the outside of the glomerular capillary wall, often bulge into the urinary space, and have prominent nuclei and abundant light eosinophilic cytoplasm. Scanning electron microscopy shows that the podocytes have long cytoplasmic ramifications, the primary processes that surround the glomerular capillaries and divide into individual foot

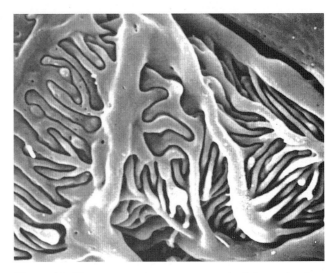

Figure 34.48 Scanning electron micrograph of glomerulus illustrating the primary processes of podocytes wrapping around the capillary loops. Note the interdigitation of the foot processes (original magnification ×13,000; courtesy of Dr. Jill W. Verlander).

processes (Figure 34.48) (342). The foot processes cover the capillary wall, contact the lamina rara externa of the GBM, and interdigitate with foot processes from different podocytes. It is generally believed that the cell body and primary processes of the podocyte are not directly attached to the GBM and are suspended within Bowman's space. There is morphologic evidence for an even more complex cytoarchitecture of the podocyte. Neal et al. (343) demonstrated foot processes (termed anchoring processes) directly between the podocyte cell body and the GBM. Moreover, their study characterized three distinct compartments of Bowman's space. The subpodocyte space (SPS), first described by Gautier et al. in 1950 (344), exists as a restricted area under the podocyte cell body and is associated with a reported 60% of the glomerular filtration surface (343). The interpodocyte space (IPS) was characterized as a narrow anastomosing region interconnecting the subpodocyte space with the main peripheral Bowman's space (343). The physiologic role of these podocyte partitions of Bowman's space remains to be clarified. By transmission electron microscopy, the cells have abundant rough endoplasmic reticulum, a well-developed Golgi apparatus, and prominent lyosomes. There are numerous intermediate filaments, microtubules, and microfilaments in the cytoplasm (295). The intermediate filaments (vimentin, desmin) and microtubules predominate in the cell body and primary processes, whereas the foot processes contain a dense microfilament contractile apparatus (345–347). The latter, containing actin, myosin, α-actinin, talin, and vinculin, connects to the intermediate filaments and microtubules of primary processes (348).

This ultrastructural arrangement of contractile proteins may allow the podocytes to play an active role in modifying the glomerular filtration surface area. Although the GBM is synthesized by both endothelial cells and podocytes, the latter play a greater role in the adult (349).

The adjacent foot processes near the GBM are separated by a 30- to 40-nm space termed the filtration pore (or slit), which is bridged by a thin extracellular structure called the filtration slit diaphragm. On ultrastructural examination, the slit diaphragm has always attracted the attention of pathologists. Over 30 years ago, based on electron microscopy, Karnovsky and co-workers proposed an isoporous zipperlike structural model for the slit diaphragm (350–352). In this model, a central filament, corresponding to the central dot of the diaphragm on cross section, is connected to the adjacent foot processes by spaced crossbridges, between which are rectangular pores. Recent three-dimensional reconstruction of the slit diaphragm by electron tomography has provided results that generally agree with the Karnovsky model (353). The electron tomographic study showed that the slit diaphragm consists of a network of winding strands, about 30 to 35 nm long, which merge centrally into a longitudinal density. The strands, which create a slit diaphragm thickness between 5 and 10 nm, surround pores that are the same size or smaller than albumin molecules. The pores appear more irregular than previously supposed.

The slit diaphragm appears unique but shares similarities with tight and adherens junctions (354,355). It separates the different membrane surfaces of the podocyte. Podocytes, similar to other epithelial cells, are polarized with distinct membrane domains (356) (Figure 34.49). The basal membrane domain and the apical membrane domain are located below and above the slit diaphragm, respectively. The slit diaphragm area (including the bridging diaphragm, adjacent podocyte foot process membrane, and cytoplasm) may also be considered a surface domain, a very specialized one.

A major advance in our understanding of the podocyte was the identification of the protein nephrin, encoded by *NPHS1*, the gene mutated in congenital nephrotic syndrome of the Finnish type (30,32). Nephrin, a transmembrane adhesion protein of the immunoglobulin superfamily, localizes to strands of the slit diaphragm (353,357). Lack of nephrin in humans or animals leads to the loss of the slit diaphragm, foot process effacement, and massive proteinuria (32,148). An increasing number of other proteins localize to the slit diaphragm domain, where they interact with nephrin and other partners, forming a multifunctional complex (Figure 34.50) (348,356,358–360). Some proteins are present in the actual slit diaphragm itself. For example, there is evidence nephrin and Neph1, a protein similar to nephrin, each form homodimers and form heterodimeric interactions with each other in the slit diaphragm (361–364).

Another member in the Neph protein family, Neph2, localizes to the slit diaphragm, homodimerizes, and forms heterodimers with nephrin but not with Neph1 (365). Other proteins are present in the podocyte cytoplasm or plasma membrane adjacent to the slit diaphragm. For example, members of the membrane-associated guanylate kinase (MAGUK) family of scaffolding proteins (including MAGI-1, MAGI-2, CASK, and ZO-1) localize adjacent to the slit diaphragm (358–360). These scaffolding proteins connect junctional membrane proteins to the actin cytoskeleton and signaling cascades. In addition, multiple adherens junction–associated proteins (AJAP) (including α-actinin, IQGAP1, αII spectrin, and βII spectrin) are also components of this expanding nephrin-associated multiprotein complex (358–360).

Mutations or deficiencies of genes encoding some of the proteins that comprise the slit diaphragm domain complex, including nephrin (32,148), Neph1 (155), Fat1 (156), podocin (150), CD2AP (149), α-actinin (151,152), and TRPC6 (153,154), cause glomerular diseases in humans and animals as characterized by absent slit diaphragms, foot process effacement, and proteinuria (Table 34.1). In addition to functioning as a critical barrier to

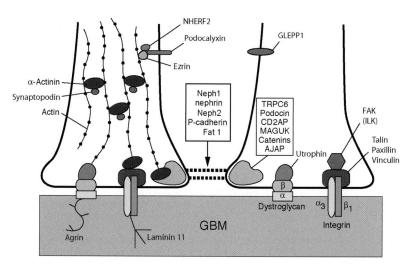

Figure 34.49 Schematic drawing of the membrane domains of the podocyte: the filtration slit diaphragm, basal membrane, and apical membrane domains. Molecular interactions within these domains of the podocyte foot processes are represented. See the text for further explanations. Modified from: Pavenstadt H, Kriz W, Kretzler M. Cell biology of the glomerular podocyte. *Physiol Rev* 2003;83:253–307; Kerjaschki D. Caught flat-footed: podocyte damage and the molecular bases of focal glomerulosclerosis. *J Clin Invest* 2001;108:1583– 1587.

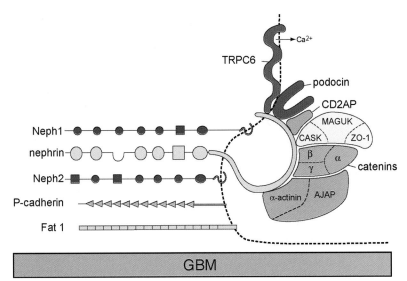

Figure 34.50 Schematic drawing of a working model of the podocyte filtration slit diaphragm domain. The *left* side portrays the molecular composition of the slit diaphragm itself, which spans between adjacent foot processes. The *right* side illustrates the molecular interactions of the nephrin-associated multiprotein complex within the podocyte foot process membrane and cytoplasm. See the text for further explanations. Modified from: Pavenstadt H, Kriz W, Kretzler M. Cell biology of the glomerular podocyte. *Physiol Rev* 2003;83:253–307; Kerjaschki D. Caught flat-footed: podocyte damage and the molecular bases of focal glomerulosclerosis. *J Clin Invest* 2001;108:1583–1587; Huber TB, Benzing T. The slit diaphragm: a signaling platform to regulate podocyte function. *Curr Opin Nephrol Hypertens* 2005;14:211–216; Lehtonen S, Ryan JJ, Kudlicka K, Iino N, Zhou H, Farquhar MG. Cell junction-associated proteins IQGAP1, MAGI-2, CASK, spectrins, and alpha-actinin are components of the nephrin multiprotein complex. *Proc Natl Acad Sci U S A* 2005;102: 9814–9819.

filtration, the slit diaphragm appears to regulate actin cytoskeletal dynamics in the foot processes (366). For example, α-actinin, an important protein in the slit diaphragm domain, interacts with synaptopodin (another actin-associated protein) to facilitate the formation of long unbranched parallel actin filaments in differentiated podocytes (367). The slit diaphragm also functions as a signaling center (368). For example, nephrin and CD2AP interact to stimulate antiapoptotic signaling in podocytes by activating the serine/threonine kinase AKT (369).

The basal membrane domain, the "sole" of the podocyte foot process, is embedded in the underlying GBM (Figure 34.49). Two types of surface receptors in the basal membrane, integrins and dystroglycan, anchor the foot processes by binding to their ligands in the GBM (370,371). The α3β1 integrin binds to collage type IV, laminin, and nidogen/entactin, whereas dystroglycan binds to laminin, agrin, and perlecan (348). Both integrins and dystroglycan are coupled by adapter molecules to the actin cytoskeleton. The integrins bind the talin, paxillin, vinculin complex (346), and dystroglycan binds utrophin (371). The induction of cellular responses from integrin-ligand interactions, known as "outside-in" signaling, is believed to be mediated by FAK (focal adhesion kinase) and ILK (integrin-linked kinase) (348,372). Similar to the filtration slit domain, an intact basal membrane domain is required to maintain foot process integrity.

The apical membrane domain, above the slit diaphragm, has a prominent glycocalyx surface of negatively charged glycoproteins (Figure 34.49) (373). These include podocalyxin (374) and GLEPP1 (375). Podocalyxin interacts with a complex composed of ezrin and NHERF2 (Na$^+$/H$^+$ exchanger-regulatory factor 2), which in turn, associates with the actin cytoskeleton (376,377). Genetic evidence exists indicating podocalyxin is important for foot process stability (159). The development of the glomerulus

as a vascular structure distinct from the remainder of the nephron is reflected in the intrarenal distribution of intermediate filaments. Vimentin is present in glomerular endothelial and mesangial cells and podocytes (Figures 34.51–34.52) (347,378–381).

Human podocytes often do not stain for desmin, however rat podocytes may show desmin expression, especially in response to injury (381,382). The glomerular tuft does not stain for keratins.

The Wilms' tumor suppressor gene, *WT1*, plays an indispensable role in the regulation of cell growth and differentiation during early nephrogenesis. Embryonic mice homozygous for a targeted mutation of *WT1* fail to develop kidneys (77). Striking evidence also exists for the importance of *WT1* in glomerular podocyte differentiation. During kidney development, *WT1* expression is detected in the metanephric mesenchyme and becomes stronger in the

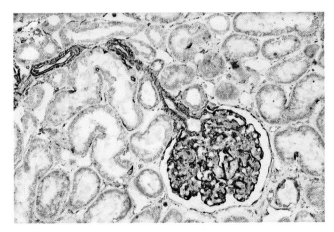

Figure 34.51 Vascular structures including the glomerulus are heavily labeled with antibody to vimentin. Tubular and interstitial components show weaker and sparse labeling. (Vimentin immunoperoxidase, original magnification ×62.)

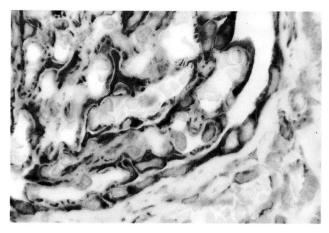

Figure 34.52 Prominent expression of vimentin is seen in glomerular endothelium, podocytes, and parietal epithelium. (Vimentin immunoperoxidase, original magnification ×300.)

renal vesicle, but highest levels occur during glomerulus formation within the podocyte cell layer (383,384). Expression of the *WT1* protein, a transcription factor, in the nuclei of podocytes does not disappear with glomerular maturation but persists in the adult kidney (Figure 34.53). Greater than 95% of patients with the Denys-Drash syndrome (nephrotic syndrome and genital anomalies and/or Wilms' tumor), characterized by shrunken glomeruli with hypertrophied podocytes, have point mutations affecting the zinc finger DNA-binding domain of *WT1* (385). These findings provide a functional link between a molecular defect of *WT1* and podocyte pathology and suggest that *WT1* has a role in maintenance of podocyte structure and function in the mature kidney.

Glomerular Filtration Barrier

The glomerular capillary wall functions as a filter that is selective for the size and charge of molecules. To pass through the capillary wall, a molecule must journey along an extra-

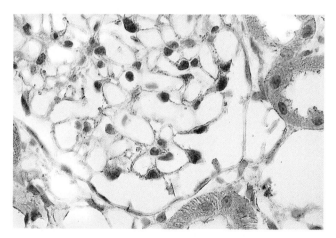

Figure 34.53 Light micrograph demonstrating expression of the WT1 protein in podocyte nuclei of an adult glomerulus. (WT1 immunoperoxidase, original magnification ×210.)

cellular pathway through the fenestrated endothelium, the GBM, and the filtration slit diaphragm. Historically, the GBM has been considered the main barrier to filtration. More recently, the role of the podocyte slit diaphragm has emerged. The permeability of the glomerular capillary wall to water and small molecules is very high, whereas its permeability to molecules the size of albumin and larger is very low. Studies employing mathematical modeling have suggested that the GBM and filtration slits contribute equally to the total resistance to water filtration (386). A model incorporating ultrastructural data has shown that the slit diaphragm is the most restrictive part of the barrier to the filtration of macromolecules (387).

Mutations or deficiencies of genes encoding proteins of the filtration slit diaphragm domain, including nephrin and several of its interacting protein partners, result in massive proteinuria, providing genetic evidence for the crucial role of the slit diaphragm in glomerular permselectivity (348,358). Although the protein networks within the GBM contribute to the size selectivity of the filtration barrier, the slit diaphragm appears to be the most important size-selective filter.

The GBM has been favored as the principal structure responsible for the charge-selective permeability of the glomerular capillary wall (388). This charge selectivity in the GBM has been associated with the presence of polyanionic molecules, such as heparan sulfate proteoglycans. Therefore, it was somewhat surprising that mice deficient for the heparan sulfate side chains of Perlecan were found to have no morphologic GBM defects and exhibited no proteinuria (389).

However, since agrin appears to be the major heparan sulfate proteoglycan in the GBM (338), it will be important to evaluate its contribution to the charge barrier in the GBM. The distribution of negatively charged molecules in the cellular layers of the glomerular capillary wall are also likely important. Experimental removal of polyanionic sialic acids from the plasma membrane of podocytes leads to proteinuria (390). Although relatively neglected, there is emerging evidence that negative charges within the glomerular endothelial glycocalyx may play a role in charge selectivity (302,303).

The "integrated view" of the glomerular filtration barrier is that the endothelium, the GBM, and the podoctyes and their slit diaphragms do not act independently but are linked to one another in a functional unit. Each of these components is important for normal glomerular filtration. Detailed reviews of the the filtration barrier are available (391–393).

Parietal Epithelial Cells

The parietal layer of Bowman's capsule consists of relatively flat squamous epithelial cells. They have prominent proliferative potential (394). Keratins, cadherens, and the transcription factor Pax-2 are expressed in parietal epithelial

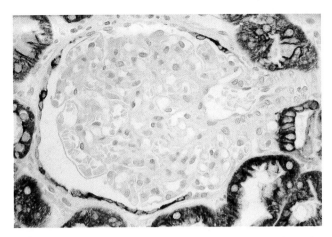

Figure 34.54 Keratin expression is not observed in the glomerular tuft, but immunoreactivity is seen in the parietal epithelial cells. The vascular pole is on the *right*. The macula densa (*far right center*) and other tubule segments are immunoreactive for keratin. (CAM 5.2 immunoperoxidase, original magnification ×120.)

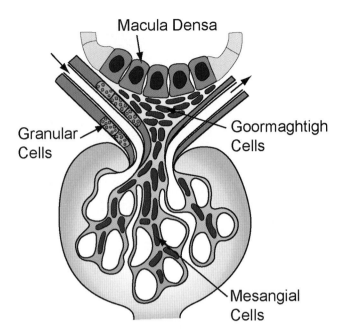

Figure 34.55 The basic components of the juxtaglomerular apparatus. Modified with permission from: Kriz W, Kaissling B. Structural organization of the mammalian kidney. In: Seldin DW, Giebisch D, eds. *The Kidney: Physiology and Pathophysiology*. 3rd ed. Philadelphia: Lippincott Williams & Wilkins; 2000:587–654.

cells (Figure 34.54) (347,379–381,395). Cytokeratin 8 has been reported to be a marker for activated parietal epithelial cells (394). The cells are 0.1 to 0.3 μm in height but may increase to 2 to 3.5 μm at the nucleus (284). The epithelium rests on the basement membrane of Bowman's capsule, which has been reported to range from 1,200 to 1,500 nm in thickness and may have a lamellated appearance (284). In contrast to the GBM, the basement membrane of Bowman's capsule expresses the α6 chain of type IV collagen, which is part of the α1.α1.α2(IV)–α5.α5. α6(IV) network (396), and bamacan, a chondroitin sulfate proteoglycan (397).

Peripolar Cells

A peripolar cell, situated between the visceral and parietal epithelial cell layers at the origin of the glomerular tuft in Bowman's space, has been most commonly observed in sheep but also identified in humans (398–401). However, these cells have been detected only in approximately 1% of human glomeruli by light microscopy (399). Ultrastructurally, the peripolar cell contains multiple membrane-bound electron-dense secretory type granules. It has been proposed that this cell represents a component of the juxtaglomerular apparatus (398). The exact function of the peripolar cells is unknown, but they may have a secretory function and discharge their contents into Bowman's space.

Juxtaglomerular Apparatus

The juxtaglomerular apparatus (JGA), discovered by Golgi (402), is situated at the vascular pole of the glomerulus and includes the afferent and efferent arterioles, extraglomerular mesangial region, and macula densa (MD)

(Figure 34.55). The JGA is the major structural unit of the renin-angiotensin system. Although the general outline of this anatomical unit usually can be observed in light microscopic sections (Figure 34.56), histochemical or immunocytochemical methods are usually required to demonstrate the distinctive juxtaglomerular granular cells. These cells tend to occur in clusters and are most

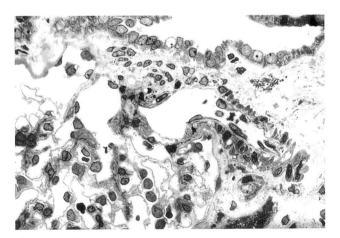

Figure 34.56 Light micrograph depicting the juxtaglomerular apparatus. From the top to the bottom of the micrograph are the macula densa, extraglomerular mesangium, afferent arteriole, and glomerulus (original magnification ×750; courtesy of Dr. Luciano Barajas). Reprinted with permission from: Barajas L, Salido EC, Smolens P, Hart D, Stein JH. Pathology of the juxtaglomerular apparatus including Bartter's syndrome. In: Tisher CC, Brenner BM, eds. *Renal Pathology with Clinical and Functional Correlations*. 2nd ed. Philadelphia: JB Lippincott; 1994:948–978.

abundant in the wall of the afferent arteriole, but they are also found in the wall of the efferent arteriole and the extraglomerular mesangial region (403–405). Ultrastructural analysis shows the presence of myofilaments, attachment bodies, a well-developed endoplasmic reticulum and Golgi apparatus, and numerous membrane-bound granules (Figure 34.57). The granules are variable in shape and size. It is believed that the smaller, often rhomboid-shaped granules with a crystalline substructure (called protogranules) observed in the Golgi region represent mature granules. Renin and angiotensin II have been immunolocalized to the granules of these cells (406,407). Renin release occurs by exocytosis. It is believed to be modulated by adrenergic nerve activity (408,409). The extraglomerular mesangium, also called the lacis or the cells of Goormaghtigh, is located between the afferent and efferent arterioles and has extensive contact with the basal surface of the MD. This extraglomerular region is continuous with the intraglomerular mesangium, and the Goormaghtigh's cells are similar in ultrastructure to the mesangial cells. There are numerous gap junctions between the extraglomerular mesangial cells and the cells of the intraglomerular mesangium and glomerular arterioles (410,411). These morphologic features and the central position within the JGA suggest that the extraglomerular mesangium may represent the structural-functional link between the MD and the glomerular arterioles and mesangium. The MD represents a plaque of specialized tubular cells within the cortical thick ascending limb of Henle adjacent to the hilus of the glomerulus. The cells are low columnar and may protrude into the tubular lumen (Figure 34.58). By electron microscopy, they have apical nuclei, cellular organelles largely lateral to and beneath the nuclei, and basal cellular processes that inter-

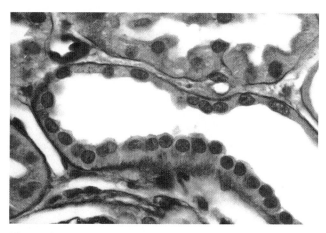

Figure 34.58 Macula densa characterized as a morphologically distinct plaque of low columnar cells with apically situated nuclei (PAS stain, original magnification ×750).

digitate with the extraglomerular mesangial cells. The lateral intercellular spaces between the MD cells vary in width but usually are more dilated compared with the lateral intercellular spaces of other nephron segments (412). In contrast with contiguous portions of the thick ascending limb, there is evidence that the MD lacks epidermal growth factor and Tamm-Horsfall protein but may be water permeable (Figure 34.59) (413–415).

The anatomic arrangement of the juxtaglomerular apparatus is suited for functional regulation of the adjacent structures. The MD plays a role in tubuloglomerular feedback, a mechanism whereby luminal concentrations of

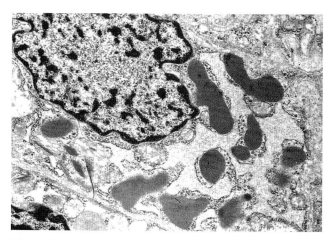

Figure 34.57 Electron micrograph of a juxtaglomerular granular cell. Note the prominent cytoplasmic membrane-bound granules (original magnification ×19,000; courtesy of Dr. Luciano Barajas). Reprinted with permission from: Barajas L, Bloodworth JMB Jr, Hartroft PM. Endocrine pathology of the kidney. In: Bloodworth JMB Jr, ed. *Endocrine Pathology: General and Surgical.* 2nd ed. Baltimore: Williams & Wilkins; 1982:723–766.

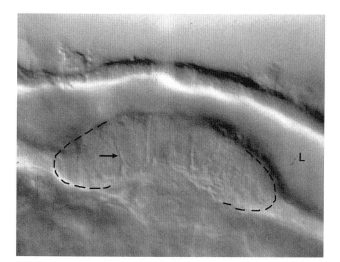

Figure 34.59 Differential interference contrast image of an isolated thick ascending limb segment perfused in vitro. The tubular lumen (L) and macula densa (dashed lines enclose the ends of the macula densa plaque) are observed. In response to a reduction in tubular luminal osmolality, there is dilatation of the lateral intercellular spaces (arrow) in the macula densa, suggesting increased water flow (original magnification ×1250) Modified with permission from: Kirk KL, Bell PD, Barfuss DW, Ribadeneira M. Direct visualization of the isolated and perfused macula densa. *Am J Physiol* 1985;248(pt 2):F890–F894.

sodium and/or chloride are sensed by the MD, leading to the transfer of a signal to the glomerular arterioles to regulate the glomerular filtration rate (GFR) (416). For example, increased luminal salt concentration at the MD results in a decreased GFR. The neuronal isoform of nitric oxide synthase (nNOS) and the cyclooxygenase enzyme COX-2 immunolocalize to the MD (417–419). There is evidence that both nitric oxide (NO)- and COX-2–generated prostaglandins play a role in the signaling between the MD and the renin-secreting cells in the afferent arteriole (420,421).

Proximal Tubule

The proximal tubule is divided into an initial convoluted portion (PCT), the pars convoluta, and a straight portion (PST), the pars recta. The convoluted portion forms several coils around its parent glomerulus in the cortex and continues into the straight portion, which is located in the medullary ray.

The human proximal tubule is approximately 14 mm in length (422). In histologic sections of the cortex, sectioned profiles of proximal convoluted tubules represent the major parenchymal component. The appearance of the cortex and especially the proximal tubules varies, according to the method of fixation. A decrease in blood pressure results in decreased filtration and renal volume (423,424). After immersion fixation of excised pieces of renal tissue, the cortex has a more homogeneous compact appearance, and there is collapse of the proximal tubular lumens (Figure 34.60) (425). Free nuclei and vesicular membranous material may be observed in the proximal tubular lumens. Fixation of an experimental functioning kidney in situ by rapid freezing, dripping of fixative on the renal surface, or vascular perfusion results in more conspicuous intertubular interstitial spaces and widely open lumens of the proximal tubules. The cells of the proximal tubule are cuboidal to low colum-

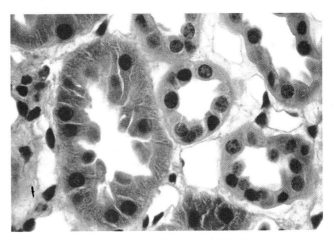

Figure 34.61 Cross section of a proximal tubule (*left* of *center*). The proximal tubular cells are taller and more eosinophilic than the cells of the distal nephron segments (*right*). (Original magnification ×750.)

nar with eosinophilic, often granular cytoplasm and round nuclei situated in the center or near the base of the cells (Figure 34.61). The lateral cell borders are indistinct because of extensive interdigitations of lateral cellular processes from adjacent cells (Figure 34.62). In the basal part of the cells there are vertical striations that represent numerous elongated mitochondria. Cytoplasmic apical vacuoles and granules correspond to a well-developed endocytic-lysosomal apparatus. There is a prominent PAS-positive luminal brush border composed of the numerous densely packed long microvilli (Figure 34.63). The brush border, apical cytoplasmic vacuoles, and basal striations are less prominent in the pars recta. Lectins have been used as selective probes to delineate renal tubular segments (426–428).

Although a certain degree of nonspecificity has been reported, the lectin *Lotus tetragonolobus* has been used as a marker of proximal tubular epithelium (Figure 34.64).

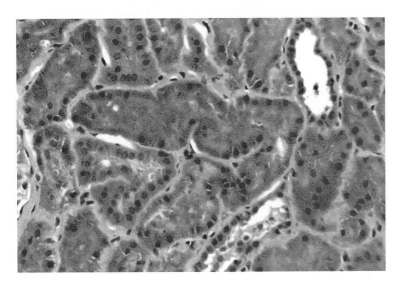

Figure 34.60 Immersion-fixed renal biopsy specimen demonstrating diffuse collapse of the proximal tubular lumens. Note the patent lumens of the distal nephron segments. (Original magnification ×250.)

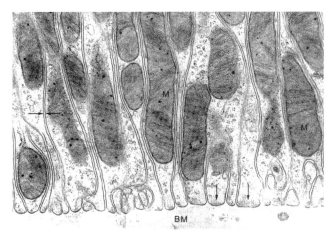

Figure 34.62 Electron micrograph illustrating extensive interdigitation of cellular processes in the basal region of proximal tubular cells. The mitochondria (*M*) are elongated. The width of the extracellular space (*opposing arrows*) is constant, and there are bundles of cytoplasmic filaments (*single arrows*) adjacent to the basement membrane (*BM*) (original magnification ×40,000). Reprinted with permission from: Maunsbach AB, Christensen EI. Functional ultrastructure of the proximal tubule. In: Windhager EE, ed. *Handbook of Physiology. Renal Physiology.* New York: Oxford University Press; 1992:41–107.

Keratins 8 and 18 are expressed in both the convoluted and straight portions of the proximal tubule, whereas keratin 19 is focally expressed in the straight portion (379,380,429). The specific expression of the cell adhesion protein cadherin-6 in the proximal tubule has been reported (430).

In most mammals, distinct segments of the tubule portion of the nephron can be distinguished by structural and functional differences. The structural differences have been characterized mainly on the ultrastructural level (431). However, these tubule segments often can be detected on light microscopy because of their known distribution within specific zones of the kidney (Figure 34.33). In

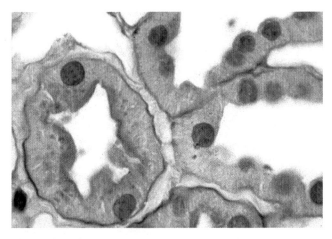

Figure 34.63 PAS-stained cross section of proximal tubule to the left of the center of the micrograph. Note the prominent PAS-positive brush border (original magnification ×1250).

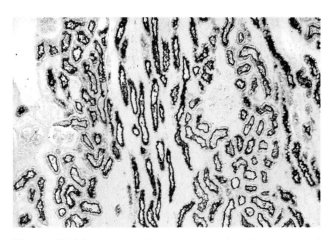

Figure 34.64 Staining of the brush border of the proximal tubules with lectin *Lotus tetragonolobus*. The distal nephron segments and glomeruli are negative. (Courtesy of Dr. Randolf A. Hennigar.)

general, the degree of tubule segmentation has not been characterized in detail in the human kidney. In several mammals, the proximal tubule can be divided into three morphologically distinct segments (Figure 34.65) (431). The S_1 segment originates at the glomerulus and constitutes one-half to two-thirds of the pars convoluta. The S_2 segment represents the remainder of the pars convoluta and the initial part of the pars recta. The S_3 corresponds to the remainder of the pars recta and is located in the inner cortex and outer stripe of the outer medulla. Although a pars convoluta and a pars recta have been described in the human kidney (432), the segmentation of the proximal tubule into three divisions has not been closely examined.

The cells in the S_1 segment have a tall brush border, a well-developed endocytic lysosomal apparatus, numerous elongated mitochondria, and extensive basolateral invaginations and interdigitations.

The cells in the S_2 segment are similar to those in the S_1 segment; however, the brush border is shorter, and the endocytic organelles, mitochondria, and basolateral invaginations and interdigitations are less prominent (Figure 34.66). The cells in the S_3 segment are more cuboidal and have relatively fewer endocytic organelles, small mitochondria, and inconspicuous membrane invaginations and interdigitations. The length of the brush border in the S_3 segment varies among species.

The proximal tubule is responsible for the reabsorption of about 60% of the glomerular ultrafiltrate. The reabsorption of chloride, bicarbonate, glucose, amino acids, and fluid is coupled to the active transport of sodium (433). An excellent correlation exists along the length of the proximal tubule between the elaborately developed basolateral membrane expressed as surface area (Figure 34.67), the high sodium potassium (Na^+/K^+)-ATPase activities that are localized to the basolateral membrane, and the capacity

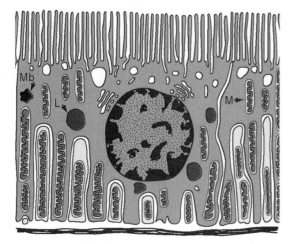

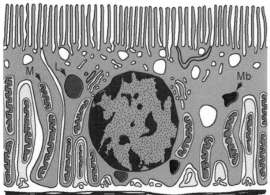

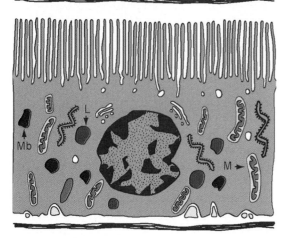

Figure 34.65 Schematic diagram of the three segments of the proximal tubule: **upper**, S$_1$; **middle**, S$_2$; **lower**, S$_3$. The prominent basolateral processes are lined with mitochondria. The interdigitating cellular processes that come from adjacent cells are shaded lighter. (*Mb*, microbody; *M*, mitochondrion; *L*, lysosome) Modified with permission from: Maunsbach AB, Christensen EI. Functional ultrastructure of the proximal tubule. In: Windhager EE, ed. *Handbook of Physiology. Renal Physiology.* New York: Oxford University Press; 1992:41–107.

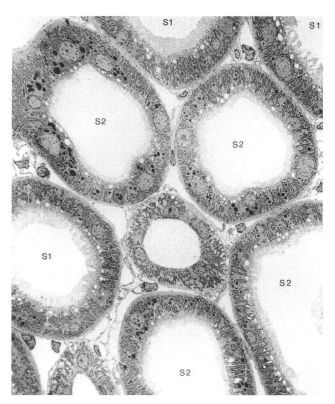

Figure 34.66 Electron micrograph of rat renal cortex. The cells in the S$_1$ segment are taller and have a more prominent brush border than the cells in the S$_2$ segment (original magnification ×1870). Reprinted with permission from: Maunsbach AB, Christensen EI. Functional ultrastructure of the proximal tubule. In: Windhager EE, ed. *Handbook of Physiology. Renal Physiology.* New York: Oxford University Press; 1992:41–107.

to transport sodium and ions (434,435). The α1β1 heterodimer is the main Na$^+$/K$^+$-ATPase isozyme of the kidney, but the α2- and α3-isoforms have been detected (436,437). This sodium pump–mediated active transport of Na$^+$ out of the cell across the basolateral membrane establishes a lumen-to-cell concentration gradient for Na$^+$.

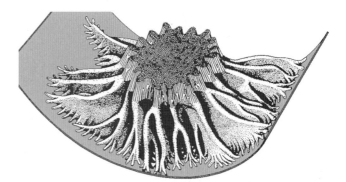

Figure 34.67 Three-dimensional schematic drawing of the proximal convoluted tubule illustrating the complex basal and lateral cellular processes that interdigitate with those from adjacent cells. Modified with permission from: Welling LW, Welling DJ. Shape of epithelial cells and intercellular channels in the rabbit proximal nephron. *Kidney Int* 1976;9:385–394.

The transport of Na$^+$ from the lumen into the proximal tubule cell, down its concentration gradient, is mediated by the Na$^+$/H$^+$ exchanger, NHE3, expressed in the brush border (438,439). The numerous mitochondria located in close proximity to the plasma membrane provide a source for the cellular energy required for active transport. In general, the intrinsic rates at which fluid and solutes are transported decrease along the proximal tubule from S$_1$ to S$_3$. The discovery of the aquaporins, a family of water channel proteins, has enhanced our understanding of the kidney's role as the primary organ that regulates water balance (440,441). Aquaporin-1 (AQP1), abundant in both the apical and basolateral membranes of the proximal tubule, is believed to mediate osmotic water permeability in this segment (442,443).

The well-developed endocytic-lysosomal apparatus in the proximal tubule (Figure 34.68) plays an important role in reabsorption and degradation of albumin and low-molecular weight proteins filtered by the glomerulus (444). Proteins are absorbed by endocytosis and transferred through the endosomal compartment to the lysosomes, where they are degraded. This is a selective process dependent upon the size and charge of the protein molecule (445–447). The capacity for protein degradation decreases from the S$_1$ to the S$_3$ segment (448). Upon exposure to an acidic environment in the endosomes (449), the internalized ligand-receptor complexes are segregated, and the receptors are recycled back to the luminal membrane via small vacuolar structures, termed apical dense tubules (450). Megalin and cubilin are multiligand endocytic receptors expressed throughout the endocytic apparatus of the proximal tubule (451). The receptors function independently but also interact as a dual complex to facilitate the uptake of albumin (452), as well as numerous ligands, including low-molecular weight proteins, vitamin-binding proteins, hormones, lipoproteins, and drugs (453).

The normal adult kidney has a relatively low rate of cell turnover with little proliferation (454–456). However, renal cell proliferation is accelerated during hypertrophy and following injury. Histologic assessment of cell proliferation can be made by determining a mitotic index or immunostaining with an antibody that detects proteins present during the cell cycle (457). During recovery after tubular injury, such as ischemia or toxin exposure, cell proliferation in tubular cells, especially in the proximal tubule, increases markedly (Figure 34.69) (458,459). Apoptosis has been documented in the adult kidney during the repair response to various forms of tubular injury, including ischemia, toxic insults, and hydronephrosis (Figure 34.70) (460–463).

Thin Limbs of Henle's Loop

The transition of the thin limbs of Henle's loop with other nephron segments marks the borders between certain zones of the kidney (Figure 34.33). Between the outer and inner stripes of the outer medulla, there is an abrupt transition from the proximal tubule to the descending thin limb (DTL) of Henle's loop. Short-looped nephrons have only a short DTL located in the inner stripe of the outer medulla. Near the hairpin turn of the short loop, the DTL continues into the thick ascending limb. Long-looped

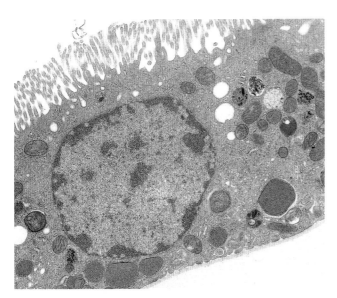

Figure 34.68 Electron micrograph illustrating an isolated perfused S$_2$ segment of the rabbit proximal tubule. Note the endocytic compartment consisting of coated pits and vesicles, apical tubules, small endocytic vesicles, and larger endocytic vacuoles. The lysosomes are heterogeneous and contain electron-dense material. The mitochondria are numerous (original magnification ×15, 000). Reprinted with permission from: Clapp WL, Park CH, Madsen KM, Tisher CC. Axial heterogeneity in the handling of albumin by the rabbit proximal tubule. *Lab Invest* 1988;58:549–558.

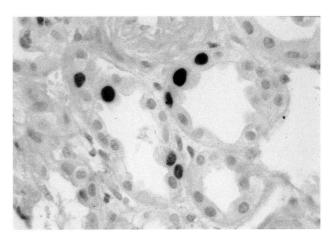

Figure 34.69 Biopsy of kidney allograft with cyclosporin A toxicity. Normally there is sparse labeling for Ki-67, a nuclear protein expressed by proliferating cells. In this example, there is a prominent increase in labeling of the tubular nuclei. (Ki-67 immunoperoxidase, original magnification ×210.)

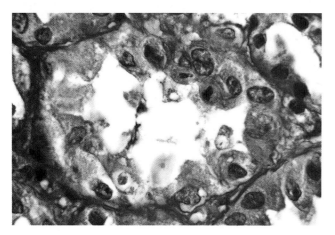

Figure 34.70 Micrograph from same case as in Figure 34.69. Several apoptotic nuclei are present (1 to 2 o'clock positions) in the tubular epithelium. (PAS stain, original magnification ×300).

nephrons have both a long DTL and a long ascending thin limb (ATL). The long DTL traverses the inner stripe of the outer medulla and enters the inner medulla, whereas the long ATL resides entirely within the inner medulla. At the border between the outer and inner medulla, the long ATL continues into the thick ascending limb. By light microscopy, the thin limb is lined with a flat, simple epithelium about 1 to 2 μm thick (Figure 34.71). The lenticularly shaped nucleus bulges slightly into the lumen. Four types of epithelium have been described in the thin limb in several mammals (Figure 34.72) (272,464). It is not known if four types exist in humans, but at least two different types of epithelium have been demonstrated (465). Type I is present in the DTL of short-looped nephrons. It is an extremely thin, simple epithelium with few cellular interdigitations and cell organelles. Type II epithelium lines the initial part of the DTL of long-looped nephrons located in the outer medulla. This epithelium exhibits species variation and is

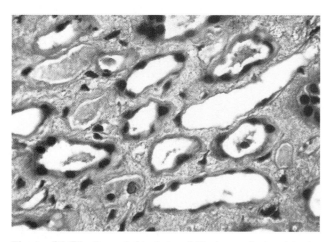

Figure 34.71 Several thin limbs of Henle are depicted in the center of the light micrograph. The lining epithelium is extremely attenuated, and the nuclei protrude into the lumens (original magnification ×500).

Type I

Type II

Type III

Type IV

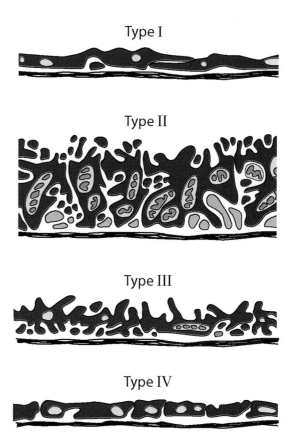

Figure 34.72 Schematic drawing of the four types of epithelium in the thin limbs of Henle's loop. (The interdigitating cellular processes that come from adjacent cells are shaded lighter.) Modified with permission from: Madsen KM, Tisher CC. Anatomy of the kidney. In: Brenner BM, ed. *Brenner and Rector's The Kidney.* 7th ed. Philadelphia: WB Saunders; 2004:3–72.

characterized by taller cells, short microvilli, and more prominent cell organelles than in the other epithelial types. In the rat and mouse, type II epithelium is complex and characterized by extensive lateral interdigitations; whereas in the rabbit and human kidney, the interdigitations are less prominent (272). Type III epithelium, found in the DTL of long-looped nephrons in the inner medulla, is composed of simple cells with few organelles and without lateral interdigitations. Type IV epithelium forms the bends of the long loops and lines the entire ATL in the inner medulla. It is characterized by low, flattened cells with few organelles and no microvilli but abundant lateral interdigitations. Thin limb epithelium has been reported to be immunoreactive for keratins 7, 8, 18, and 19 (379,380).

The thin limb of Henle's loop plays an important role in the countercurrent multiplication component of urinary concentration. Physiologic studies have demonstrated that the DTL is permeable to water but has low permeability to sodium chloride, whereas the thin ascending limb is largely impermeable to water but has a high permeability to sodium chloride (272,466). These physiologic investigations are supported by immunohistochemical studies. The aquaporin water channel protein, AQP1, is prominently expressed in the DTL but not in the ATL (442,467). The kidney-specific chloride channel C1C-K1 is expressed exclusively in the ATL (468,469). Mice and humans lacking AQP1 (470,471) and mice deficient for C1C-K1 (472) have impaired urine concentrating ability. In the passive model proposed by Kokko and Rector (473) and Stephenson (474), a hypertonic medullary interstitium concentrates sodium chloride in the DTL by extraction of water. The fluid that then enters the ATL has a higher sodium chloride concentration, resulting in passive salt absorption and dilution of the fluid of the ATL. Thus, the thin limb contributes to the maintenance of a hypertonic medullary interstitium and delivers a dilute fluid to more distal segments. The morphologic features of a simple epithelium with few organelles in the ATL are consistent with the lack of demonstrable active transport in this segment.

Distal Tubule

The distal tubule consists of three distinct segments: the thick ascending limb of Henle's loop (TAL), the macula densa (MD), and the distal convoluted tubule (DCT) (Figure 34.33). The MD, as previously discussed (in the section entitled Juxtaglomerular Apparatus), is a specialized plaque of cells within the TAL. In short-looped nephrons, the transition from the descending thin limb to the TAL occurs before the hairpin turn. In long-looped nephrons, the transition from the thin ascending limb to the TAL marks the border between the inner medulla and the inner stripe of the outer medulla. The TAL can be divided into a medullary (MTAL) and a cortical segment (CTAL). The cells are eosinophilic and cuboidal, and the round nucleus tends to be located in the apical region and causes a bulge of the cell into the lumen (Figure 34.73). Similar to the proximal

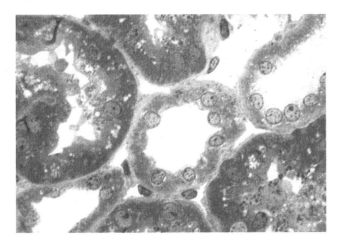

Figure 34.73 Light micrograph demonstrating a cross section of a thick ascending limb in the center. There is no brush border, and the cells are lower than the adjacent proximal tubular cells. (Toluidine blue-stained, 1-μm Epon section, original magnification ×750.)

tubule cells, the cells of the TAL have indistinct lateral cell borders because of elaborate basolateral membrane invaginations and interdigitations. They also have cytoplasmic basal striations because of elongated mitochondria. These morphologic features are characteristic for epithelial cells involved in active transport. However, in contrast to the proximal tubule, the cells are lower and less eosinophilic, and there is no brush border in the TAL. As the TAL ascends into the cortex, there is a gradual decrease in cell height, basolateral membrane area, and size of the mitochondria (475). Scanning electron microscopy has shown two luminal surface configurations of cells in the TAL (476). Cells with a relatively smooth surface are most commonly found in the medullary segment, whereas cells with a rough surface due to luminal microprojections and apical lateral membrane invaginations predominate in the cortical segment. The functional significance of these structural findings remains unexplained. The TAL continues into the distal convoluted tubule just beyond the MD. The cells of the TAL synthesize Tamm-Horsfall protein and secrete it into the tubular lumen (414). This segment expresses keratins 8 and 18 (378,380,429), and also kidney-specific (Ksp) cadherin (477).

An important function of the TAL is the active reabsorption of sodium chloride. There is a correlation between structure and function in the ascending limb. The basolateral membrane surface area, the Na^+/K^+-ATPase activity, and the reabsorptive capacity for sodium chloride are all greater in the medullary segment than in the cortical segment of the TAL (433,475,478). The reabsorption of sodium chloride in both the medullary and cortical segments of the TAL is mediated by a bumetanide-sensitive $Na^+/K^+/2Cl^-$ cotransporter (BSC-1), which localizes to the TAL apical plasma membrane (479). This reabsorption of salt coupled with the water impermeability of the TAL results in a hypertonic interstitium and delivery of a hypotonic fluid to more distal tubular segments.

The DCT begins just beyond the MD in the cortex and represents the terminal part of the distal tubule. The cells of the DCT are similar to those of the TAL and contain numerous mitochondria. However, the DCT cells are taller, characteristically have nuclei closer to the lumen, and lack lateral interdigitations in the apical region between adjacent cells (Figure 34.74). In comparison with the proximal tubule, the cells of the DCT are lower and less eosinophilic, have a less prominent apical endocytic apparatus, and lack a brush border. More nuclei are observed in a cross section than in the proximal tubule, and the lumen is normally open. The epithelium of the DCT shows immunoreactivity for keratins 8, 18, and 19 (379,429) and for Ksp-cadherin (477). In the DCT, reabsorption of sodium chloride is mediated by the Na^+/Cl^- cotransporter, TSC, which localizes to the apical plasma membrane and apical cytoplasmic vesicles (480,481). The cotransporter TSC, the target of thiazide diuretics, is distinct from the cotransporter BSC-1,

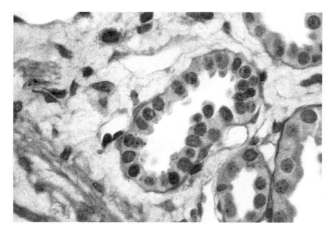

Figure 34.74 Light micrograph showing a distal convoluted tubule. Note the absence of a brush border and the nuclei situated close to the lumen. (PAS stain, original magnification ×750.)

present in the thick ascending limb. Biochemical studies have demonstrated that the DCT has a higher level of Na$^+$/K$^+$-ATPase activity than any other tubular segment (116). Morphologic and physiologic studies have provided evidence that the DCT, similar to the TAL, is relatively impermeable to water but responsible for the reabsorption of sodium chloride (482–484).

Connecting Segment

The connecting segment (or tubule) is a transitional segment that joins the DCT with the collecting duct system. In superficial nephrons, the connecting segment (CS) continues directly into an initial collecting tubule (Figure 34.75). In contrast, the connecting segments of juxtamedullary nephrons and of many midcortical nephrons join to form an arcade that ascends in the cortex before draining into an initial collecting tubule. In humans, most nephrons empty individually into initial collecting tubules (272).

Fourteen percent of the nephrons are connected to arcades, and each arcade consists of about three nephron attachments (6). Each cortical collecting tubule receives an average of 11 nephrons (6). In most species, including humans, the CS contains different cell types as a result of an intermixing of cells from the adjacent DCT and cortical collecting duct (485). The connecting tubule cell is the most characteristic cell type of this transitional segment. They display ultrastructural features intermediate between the DCT cells and the principal cells of the cortical collecting duct and contain deep true infoldings of the basal cell membrane (486). The connecting tubule cell appears to be the only cell type in the kidney (of those thus far identified) that shows immunoreactivity for the proteolytic enzyme kallikrein (487,488). The physiologic relevance of this finding remains uncertain. Various types of intercalated cells, similar to those in the cortical collecting duct, are also present in the

CS and are likely involved in tubular acid-base regulation. The CS is an important site of potassium secretion regulated by mineralocorticoids (484). An ATP-sensitive K$^+$ channel, ROMK, localizing to the apical membrane of connecting tubule cells, likely mediates the potassium secretion (489,490). The expression of a Na$^+$/Ca^{2+} exchanger and a Ca^{2+}-ATPase in the basolateral membrane of the connecting tubule cells suggests the CS has a significant role in calcium reabsorption (491,492).

Collecting Duct

The collecting duct begins in the cortex and descends to the tip of the papilla, also called the area cribrosa, where the inner medullary segments terminate as the ducts of Bellini. These terminal collecting duct segments were apparently described by Eustachio nearly 100 years before the observation of Bellini (493). During its course, there is an increase in diameter from the cortical portion to the terminal segments at the area cribrosa. The collecting duct can be divided into the cortical (CCD), outer medullary (OMCD), and inner medullary collecting ducts (IMCD). Significant cellular heterogeneity exists along the collecting duct (271). Although there is a degree of nonspecificity, the lectins *Dolichos biflorus* and *Arachis hypogaea* have been used as markers for collecting duct epithelium (Figure 34.76) (427). The distal tubules and collecting ducts show variable but generally more intense staining for keratins than do the proximal tubules (Figures 34.77–34.78). Keratins 8, 18, and 19 are prominently expressed throughout the cortical and medullary collecting ducts (379,380,429). There is less

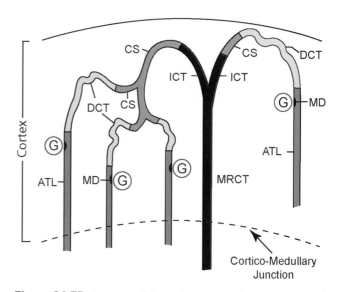

Figure 34.75 Diagram of the various anatomic arrangements of the distal tubule connecting to the cortical collecting duct in superficial, midcortical and juxtamedullary nephrons. (*G,* glomerulus; *ATL,* ascending thick limb (of Henle); *MD,* macula densa; *DCT,* distal convoluted tubule; *CS,* connecting segment; *ICT,* initial collecting tubule; *MRCT,* medullary ray collecting tubule)

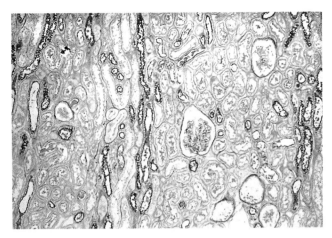

Figure 34.76 Staining of the collecting ducts and thick ascending limbs with lectin *Arachis hypogaea*. The proximal tubules and glomeruli are negative. (Courtesy of Dr. Randolf A. Hennigar.)

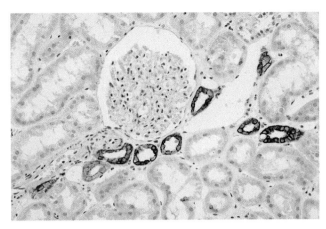

Figure 34.78 Detection of keratin expression varies depending on the specificity and dilution of the antibody. In this micrograph, there is prominent immunoreactivity of the distal tubules and collecting ducts. (35βH11 immunoperoxidase, original magnification ×62.)

staining for keratin 7. Scattered keratin 7- and 19-negative cells have been observed to be intercalated cells (379). Keratins 5/6, 17, and 20, as well as vimentin, are restricted primarily to medullary collecting ducts (429). There is less immunoreactivity for Ksp-cadherin in collecting ducts compared to the thick ascending limbs and distal convoluted tubules (477).

Cortical Collecting Duct

The cortical collecting duct can be subdivided further into the initial collecting tubule and the medullary ray portion. By light microscopy, the epithelium of the cortical collecting duct consists of cuboidal cells with distinct lateral cell borders and central round nuclei (Figure 34.79). The lumen is prominently open, and there is no brush border. The cortical collecting duct is composed of principal cells

and intercalated cells. Principal cells are mainly responsible for salt and water transport, and the intercalated cells are involved in acid-base regulation. It is difficult to distinguish principal cells from intercalated cells on H&E paraffin sections. The principal cells on light microscopy have an extremely light or clear cytoplasm. By electron microscopy, the principal cells have relatively few cell organelles and no interdigitations of lateral cellular processes from adjacent cells, which accounts for the distinct cell borders observed on light microscopy (Figure 34.80). However, there are prominent infoldings of the basal plasma membrane, which gives the basal region an accentuated clear appearance on light microscopy (494). The principal cell has a fairly smooth luminal surface with short microvilli and a single cilium by scanning electron microscopy (Figure 34.88).

Principal cells are involved in sodium reabsorption and potassium secretion. Sodium reabsorption is mediated by

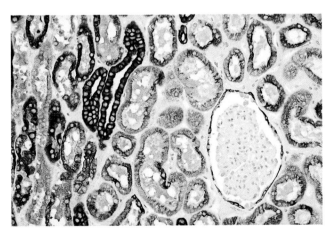

Figure 34.77 Distal tubules, collecting ducts, proximal tubules, and parietal epithelium lining Bowman's capsule showing expression of keratins. The distal tubules and collecting ducts label more intensely than do the proximal tubules. (CAM 5.2 immunoperoxidase, original magnification ×62.)

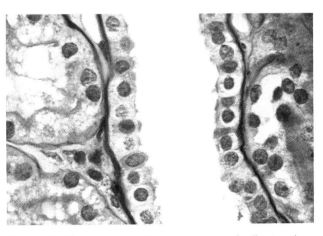

Figure 34.79 Micrograph illustrating a cortical collecting duct. Note the distinct lateral cell orders (original magnification ×500).

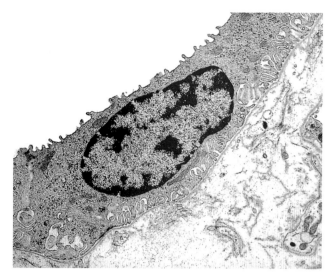

Figure 34.80 Electron micrograph of principal cell from the collecting duct. Note the relatively prominent infoldings of the basal plasma membrane (original magnification ×12,500).

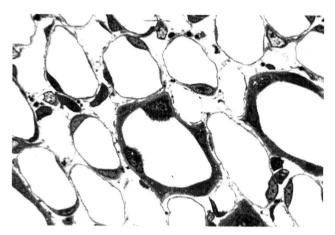

Figure 34.81 Light micrograph of the outer medulla showing intercalated cells in the collecting ducts. The intercalated cells exhibit a bulging apical surface covered with microprojections and dark-staining cytoplasm. (One-micron toluidine blue-stained Epon section, original magnification ×160.)

an amiloride-sensitive sodium channel, ENaC, located in the apical membrane of principal cells throughout the entire collecting duct (495,496). Experimental conditions of dietary potassium loading or mineralocorticoid stimulation have shown increases in potassium secretion and Na^+/K^+-ATPase activity in the cortical collecting duct, along with an increase in the surface area of the basolateral membrane of the principal cells (497–501). These findings indicate that the principal cells are involved in potassium secretion in the cortical collecting duct. The entire collecting duct becomes permeable to water in the presence of the antidiuretic hormone vasopressin. After vasopressin binds to its receptor on the basolateral membrane of principal cells (502), small apical cytoplasmic tubulovesicles (called aggrephores) containing the aquaporin water channel AQP2 are shuttled to the apical membrane, which markedly increases water permeability (503,504). The presence of the aquaporin water channels AQP3 and AQP4 in the basolateral membranes of principal cells facilitate the final exit of water into the interstitium (505,506).

The intercalated or "dark" cells are interspersed in the lining epithelia of the collecting duct. Although intercalated cells usually represent the minority cell type in epithelia where they are found, they constitute 30 to 40% of the cells in the cortical collecting duct in some mammals (271,280). They are also present in the connecting segment, the outer medullary collecting duct, and the initial portion of the inner medullary collecting duct. Intercalated cells may be identified on 1-μm thick toluidine blue-stained Epon sections by their densely staining cytoplasm and their often convex luminal surface covered with numerous microprojections (Figure 34.81). The darkly staining cytoplasm is due in part to the presence of relatively more organelles, especially mitochondria. Two distinct popula-

tions of intercalated cells, types A and B, have been described in the cortical collecting duct of mammals (507,508). On ultrastructural examination, the type A intercalated cells have prominent microprojections of the apical membrane and extensive tubulovesicular structures in the apical cytoplasm (Figure 34.82). In comparison with the type A cells, the type B intercalated cells have a denser cytoplasm, more mitochondria, a smaller apical membrane area, a small number of microprojections on the apical surface, more spherical vesicular structures throughout the cytoplasm (but fewer vesicles beneath the apical membrane), and a larger basolateral membrane surface area (Figure 34.83). By scanning electron microscopy, the type A cells have a large convex luminal surface covered with numerous complex microprojections called microplicae (Figure 34.84), whereas the type B cells display a small angular luminal surface with relatively small microvilli (Figure 34.85) (508). The type B intercalated cells may be inconspicuous on scanning electron microscopy. More recently, a third type of intercalated cell has been characterized in the cortical

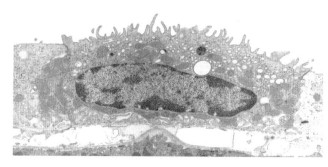

Figure 34.82 Electron micrograph of a type A intercalated cell in the cortical collecting duct. Note the prominent tubulovesicular membrane compartment in the apical cytoplasm and the numerous microprojections on the luminal surface. (Original magnification ×11, 800; courtesy of Dr. Jill W. Verlander.)

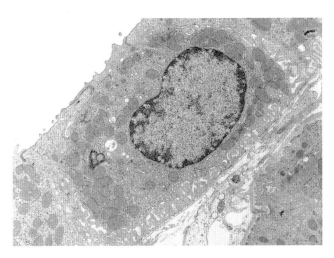

Figure 34.83 Electron micrograph of a type B intercalated cell in the cortical collecting duct. There are numerous vesicles throughout the cytoplasm, and the basolateral membrane is prominent. Note the paucity of microprojections on the luminal surface. Compared to the type A intercalated cell, there are fewer vesicles beneath the apical membrane. (Original magnification ×11,800; courtesy of Dr. Jill W. Verlander.)

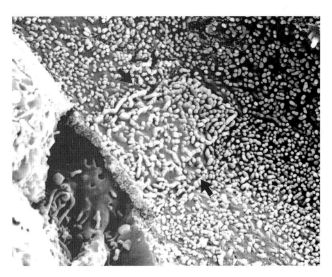

Figure 34.85 Scanning electron micrograph of the luminal surface of a cortical collecting duct. A type B intercalated cell (*arrows*) displays a small angular luminal surface covered with short microprojections, mainly microvilli. (Original magnification ×15,000; courtesy of Dr. Jill W. Verlander.)

collecting duct of some mammals (509,510). They account for 40 to 50% of intercalated cells in the mouse connecting segment and initial collecting duct. The non-A–non-B intercalated cells are larger than type A and type B intercalated cells, have abundant mitochondria, and have prominent apical microprojections similar to those of type A cells. Compared to the type A and B intercalated cells, the non-A–non-B intercalated cells have been studied in fewer species, mainly the rat and mouse. There are significant differences in the prevalence and distribution of the different types of intercalated cells throughout the connecting

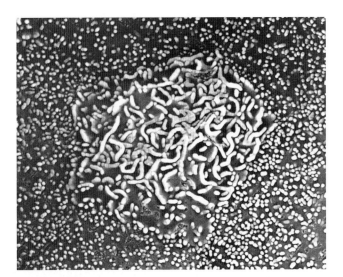

Figure 34.84 Scanning electron micrograph of the luminal surface of a type A intercalated cell in the cortical collecting duct. The type A cell is well demarcated and has a large luminal surface covered primarily with microplicae but also microvilli. (Original magnification ×15,000; courtesy of Dr. Jill W. Verlander.).

segment and cortical collecting duct among mammalian species (280).

Intercalated cells are typified by their high levels of carbonic anhydrase, the enzyme that catalyzes the interconversion of carbon dioxide (CO_2) to bicarbonate (HCO_3^-), suggesting they are involved in urine acidification (511). Physiologic studies have demonstrated that the cortical collecting duct reabsorbs bicarbonate in acid-loaded animals (512) and secretes bicarbonate in alkali-loaded animals (513). In a study of experimental acute respiratory acidosis, there was a striking increase in the apical membrane surface area of the type A intercalated cells, whereas no morphologic changes were observed in the type B cells (508).

Studies have immunolocalized the vacuolar-type proton pump H^+-ATPase in the apical membrane (514–516) and the Cl^-/HCO_3^- exchanger, AE1 (Band 3), in the basolateral membrane (507,516–518) of type A intercalated cells. These findings indicate that type A cells are responsible for H^+ secretion in the cortical collecting duct. The immunolocalization of the H^+-ATPase to the basolateral membrane of type B intercalated cells (515,516) and the physiologic evidence for an apical Cl^-/HCO_3^- exchange in these cells (519) indicate that type B cells are involved in bicarbonate secretion. Evidence has accumulated to indicate that the apical Cl^-/HCO_3^- exchange in the type B cell is mediated by the protein pendrin, which immunolocalizes to the apical membrane and apical cytoplasmic vesicles of the B cell (520–522). Furthermore, the renal cortical expression of pendrin is increased in alkali-loaded animals and decreased in acid-loaded animals (523). Type B intercalated cells are most numerous in the cortical collecting duct. Pendrin is not in the same protein family as AE1 (524). Mutations of the gene encoding pendrin result in

Pendred's syndrome, a disorder mainly associated with a thyroid goiter and deafness (525). The non-A–non-B intercalated cells express pendrin in the apical membrane and cytoplasmic vesicles like type B intercalated cells but also express the H^+-ATPase in the apical membrane-like type A intercalated cells (522,526). It is unclear whether the non-A–non-B cells function as H^+- or HCO_3^--secreting cells or possibly switch between these two functions. Thus, the types of intercalated cells may be defined by their cellular distribution of the H^+-ATPase and the presence or absence of the anion exchangers, AE1 and pendrin (527). Alternatively, it has been proposed that intercalated cells exhibit a high degree of plasticity and may reverse their apical-basolateral polarity in response to changes in the acid-base status (528). For example, it has been reported that type B intercalated cells can convert to type A cells in response to metabolic acidosis (529).

Outer Medullary Collecting Duct

The collecting duct traverses the outer medulla without receiving tributaries. The outer medullary collecting duct is lined by principal cells and intercalated cells (Figure 34.86). The principal cells in this segment are similar to those in the cortical collecting duct but are taller and have fewer organelles and basal membrane infoldings. The intercalated cells constitute 18 to 40% of the cells in the outer medullary collecting duct in some species and gradually decrease along this segment (530,531). The intercalated cells in the outer

medullary collecting duct resemble the type A intercalated cells in the cortical collecting duct but are taller and have a less dense cytoplasm.

The outer medullary collecting duct plays a major role in urine acidification. An increase in the surface area of the apical plasma membrane of the intercalated cells in this segment has been demonstrated after hydrogen ion stimulation (532,533). The apical and basolateral membranes of these cells label with antibodies against the H^+-ATPase and the chloride/bicarbonate exchanger, respectively (514,518). These findings suggest that the intercalated cells in the outer medullary collecting duct are responsible for hydrogen ion secretion. In addition, this segment may be an important site of potassium reabsorption. The functional presence of H^+/K^+-ATPase activity in the outer medullary collecting duct (534,535) and the immunohistochemical (536) and in situ hybridization (537,538) localization of H^+/K^+-ATPase in the intercalated cells of this segment indicate that these cells are involved in potassium reabsorption in exchange for hydrogen ion secretion.

Inner Medullary Collecting Duct

The inner medullary collecting duct (IMCD) represents the terminal portion of the collecting duct. Although the IMCD is often called the papillary collecting duct, only the inner two-thirds of the IMCD are located in the papilla.

Descending through the inner medulla, the collecting ducts join in successive fusions, which result in an arborescent architectural arrangement. There is a significant increase in diameter and height of the epithelium as the ducts descend (539). The height of the cells increases gradually from cuboidal to columnar (Figure 34.87). However, in the terminal portion of the human inner medulla there is often an abrupt transition between collecting ducts lined with cuboidal cells and the ducts of Bellini, which are composed of tall columnar cells.

Structural and functional heterogeneity exist along the IMCD (539). It can be subdivided arbitrarily into three por-

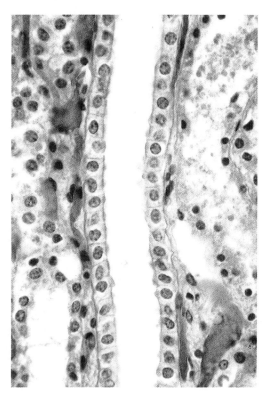

Figure 34.86 Light micrograph illustrating longitudinal section of an outer medullary collecting duct (original magnification ×250).

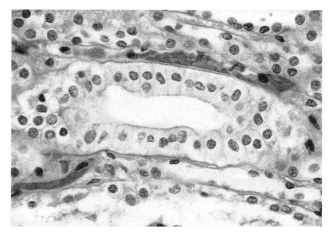

Figure 34.87 Micrograph illustrating columnar cells of the collecting duct in the inner medulla (original magnification ×500).

tions: the outer third (IMCD$_1$), middle third (IMCD$_2$), and inner third (IMCD$_3$). However, there is physiologic evidence for the division of the IMCD into two functionally distinct segments, which are termed the initial IMCD and the terminal IMCD (540,541).

The initial IMCD is the outer segment and mainly corresponds to the IMCD$_1$, whereas the terminal IMCD includes most of the IMCD$_2$ and the IMCD$_3$. The initial IMCD consists mainly of principal cells that are similar in structure to the principal cells in the OMCD. In the rat, intercalated cells similar to the type A intercalated cells in the OMCD comprise approximately 10% of the cells in the initial IMCD (Figure 34.88) (542). Intercalated cells are rare to absent in the initial IMCD of the human (485) and rabbit (530). The terminal IMCD is composed of mainly one cell type, the IMCD cell. Compared with principal cells, the IMCD cells are taller and have lighter staining cytoplasm containing numerous ribosomes, small lysosomes in the basal cytoplasm, and fewer infoldings of the basal plasma membrane (Figure 34.89) (543). By scanning electron microscopy, the IMCD cells display more numerous small microvilli and lack the central cilium characteristic of principal cells (Figure 34.90).

The inner medullary collecting duct has an important role in urinary concentration. The reabsorption of urea and

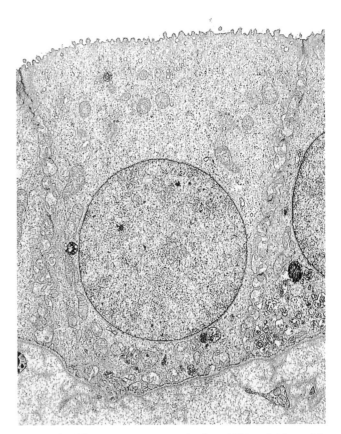

Figure 34.89 Electron micrograph of an IMCD cell. The cell is tall, has extensive lateral membranes, and exhibits small stubby microvilli. Infoldings of the basal plasma membrane are not prominent. (Original magnification ×12,500.) Reprinted with permission from: Clapp WL, Madsen KM, Verlander JW, Tisher CC. Morphologic heterogeneity along the rat inner medullary collecting duct. *Lab Invest* 1989;60:219–230.

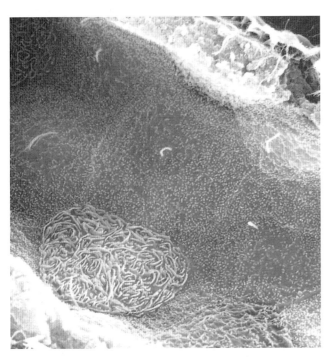

Figure 34.88 Scanning electron micrograph of the inner medullary collecting duct. The intercalated cell is round and exhibits a convex luminal surface covered with microplicae without cilia. The adjacent principal cells are characterized by short microvilli and a single central cilium on their luminal surface. (Original magnification ×12,000.) Reprinted with permission from: Clapp WL, Madsen KM, Verlander JW, Tisher CC. Morphologic heterogeneity along the rat inner medullary collecting duct. *Lab Invest* 1989;60:219–230.

water in this segment causes the formation of a concentrated urine. Physiologic studies demonstrated that urea and water permeabilities are low in the initial IMCD and relatively high in the terminal IMCD (540,541). Water permeability is increased by vasopressin in both subsegments and is mediated by the aquaporin water channel AQP2 present in the apical membrane of the IMCD cells (503). Vasopressin increases urea permeability only in the terminal IMCD. The urea transporters UT-A1 and UT-A3 immunolocalize to the terminal IMCD and mediate urea transport in this segment (544–546). There is evidence that the IMCD is also involved in urine acidification. Acid secretion mediated by an H$^+$/K$^+$-ATPase has been demonstrated in isolated perfused segments from this region, although no immunoreactivity for this transport protein has been demonstrated in the IMCD (547).

Interstitium

The renal interstitium consists of an extracellular matrix containing sulfated and nonsulfated glucosaminoglycans and interstitial cells (548). In humans, estimates of the relative

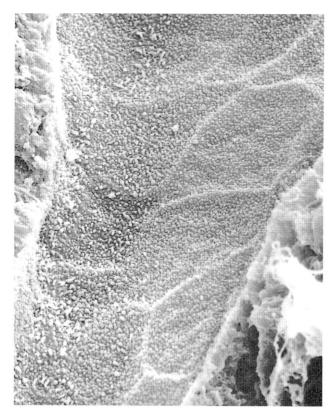

Figure 34.90 Scanning electron micrograph of the terminal IMCD. The entire luminal surface of the IMCD cells is covered with abundant short microvilli. There is an absence of cilia. (Original magnification ×12,500). Reprinted with permission from: Clapp WL, Madsen KM, Verlander JW, Tisher CC. Morphologic heterogeneity along the rat inner medullary collecting duct. *Lab Invest* 1989;60:219–230.

cortical interstitial volume range from 5 to 20%, with a mean of 12% (549–551). A significant increase with age has been reported (551). The peritubular interstitial tissue in the normal cortex is inconspicuous on light microscopy, and the tubules and capillaries often have a back-to-back architectural appearance (Figure 34.91). Types I and III collagen and fibronectin are present (552). The periarterial connective tissue constitutes a loose sheath around the intrarenal arteries and contains the lymphatic vessels (553). The periarterial connective tissue should not be overinterpreted as representing focal interstitial fibrosis in the cortex. Two types of cortical interstitial cells have been described: a fibroblast-like cell and a lymphocyte-like cell (548). The fibroblast-like cells show immunoreactivity for ecto-5-nucleotidase (5-NT) (554). These 5-NT-postive interstitial fibroblasts are the erythropoietin-producing cells in the kidney (555,556).

The relative volume of the renal interstitium increases from the cortex to the tip of the papilla. The interstitial volume has been reported from 10 to 20% in the outer medulla to approximately 30 to 40% at the papillary tip in some species (557). This appreciable amount of interstitium in the medulla should not be mistaken for interstitial

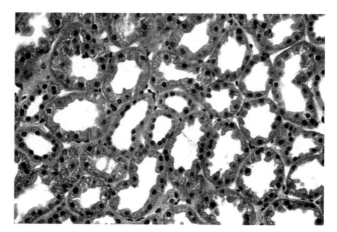

Figure 34.91 Biopsy specimen of the cortex of a kidney donated for transplantation. Note the compact arrangement of the tubules and the limited amount of interstitial tissue. (Original magnification ×250.)

fibrosis by the pathologist. The medullary interstitium has a gelatinous appearance on light microscopy (Figure 34.92). The interstitial cells in the medulla include lymphocyte-like cells virtually identical to the ones in the cortex, pericytes situated near the descending vasa recta, and prominent lipid-containing cells mainly localized to the inner medulla (548). The latter, the renomedullary interstitial cells, are often arranged in rows between the loop of Henle and the vasa recta, have irregular, long cytoplasmic processes, and contain lipid inclusions. These cells can be observed on 1-μm thick toluidine blue-stained sections of the inner medulla. The lipid droplets contain mainly triglycerides that are rich in unsaturated fatty acids, including arachidonic acid, phospholipids, and cholesterol (548). In addition to the synthesis of the extracellular matrix of the interstitium, the renomedullary interstitial cells are believed to contribute to the endocrine-like antihypertensive function of the renal medulla (558,559).

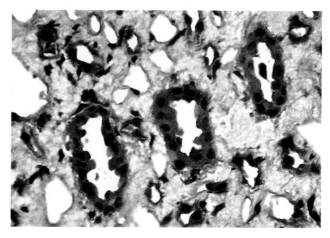

Figure 34.92 Renal biopsy specimen illustrating the inner medulla. Note the prominent amount of interstitium surrounding the tubules. (Original magnification ×500.)

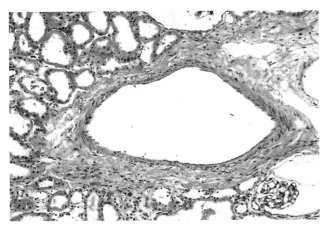

Figure 34.93 Micrograph of the corticomedullary junction illustrating an arcuate artery (original magnification ×125).

Vasculature

A detailed description of the renal vasculature is available (560). The segmental arteries, originating from the anterior and posterior divisions of the main renal artery, divide to form the interlobar arteries, which course toward the cortex along the septa of Berlin between adjacent renal pyramids. At the corticomedullary junction, the interlobar arteries give rise to the arcuate arteries, which follow a gently curved course along the base of the pyramids parallel to the kidney surface (Figure 34.93). The interlobular arteries branch sharply from the arcuate arteries and ascend in the cortex in a radial fashion toward the renal surface. Because the renal lobules cannot be clearly distinguished, it has been recommended that the interlobular arteries be called cortical radial arteries (276,560).

Most afferent arterioles originate from the interlobular arteries, and each supplies a single glomerulus. The angle of origin of the afferent arterioles becomes less recurrent and more open as the interlobular arteries extend to the outer

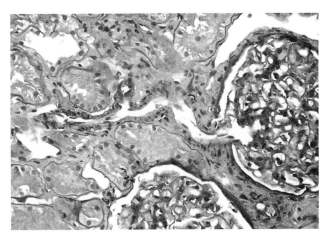

Figure 34.95 Micrograph depicting the transverse course of an afferent arteriole supplying a glomerulus. (PAS stain, original magnification ×250.)

cortex (Figure 34.94) (561). The length of the afferent arterioles is variable; average values of 170 to 280 μm have been reported (Figure 34.95) (562,563). Some rare branches of the intrarenal arteries that do not terminate in glomeruli, the so-called aglomerular vessels, may result from degeneration of the connected glomeruli (561). Aglomerular arterioles near the corticomedullary junction have been observed to enter the medulla, and shunt arterioles between afferent and efferent arterioles have been reported (564–566).

The wall structure of the intrarenal arteries and the proximal portion of the afferent arterioles resembles that of blood vessels of the same size elsewhere in the body. The endothelium stains for factor VIII–related antigen (Figure 34.96) (567,568) and CD34 (Figure 34.97) (569,570), whereas the muscularis stains for smooth muscle actin (Figure 34.98) (571) and vimentin.

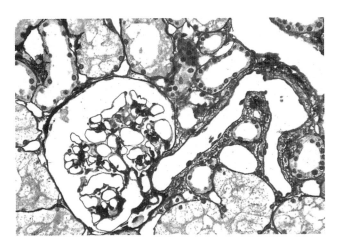

Figure 34.94 Juxtamedullary glomerulus with a connected hilar arteriole. Note the recurrent angle of the arteriole. (Silver methenamine stain, original magnification ×250.)

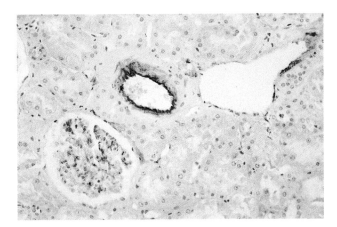

Figure 34.96 Factor VIII is produced by endothelium. The micrograph shows factor VIII immunoperoxidase staining of a medium-sized artery (*center*), vein (*right*), and glomerulus (*left*) (original magnification ×62).

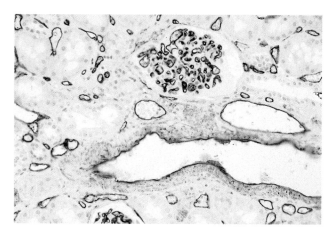

Figure 34.97   CD34 immunoperoxidase staining demonstrates a greater variety of vascular structures that label more intensely than with factor VIII. In the micrograph, arteries, veins, glomeruli, and peritubular capillaries are immunoreactive (original magnification ×62).

The efferent arterioles from the glomeruli branch to form a complex postglomerular microcirculation (Figure 34.99). Although gradations exist, three basic types of efferent arterioles may be distinguished (572,573). The superficial or outer cortical efferent arterioles are fairly long and divide into extensive capillary networks that supply the convoluted tubules of the cortical labyrinth. These capillaries are readily identified by CD34 and smooth muscle actin staining (Figures 34.98, 34.100–34.101). The midcortical efferent arterioles are variable in length and supply the cortical labyrinth and the straight tubules of the medullary rays. With the exception of the outer cortex, there is dissociation between the tubule segments and the efferent arterioles of their parent glomeruli. In the midcortex and inner cortex, tubule segments are supplied by capillaries of efferent arterioles from other glomeruli

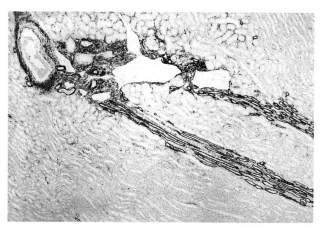

Figure 34.98   Smooth muscle actin immunoperoxidase stain illustrating a labeled large artery (*upper left*) and arterioles at the corticomedullary junction and two positive-stained columns of vasa recta (*midright*) penetrating the medulla. Two venous profiles (*upper center*) have minimal muscularis. (Original magnification ×11.)

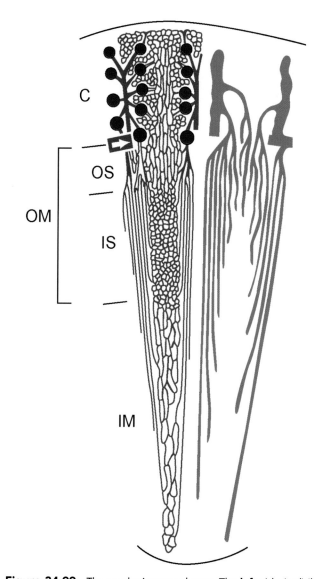

Figure 34.99   The renal microvasculature. The **left** side (red) illustrates the arterial vessels, glomeruli, and capillaries. An interlobular artery originates from an arcuate artery (*white arrow*) and gives rise to the afferent arterioles, which supply the glomeruli (dark brown). The efferent arterioles of the superficial and midcortical glomeruli supply the capillary plexuses of the cortical labyrinth and the medullary rays. The efferent arterioles of the juxtamedullary glomeruli descend into the medulla and form the descending vasa recta, which supply the adjacent capillary plexuses. Note the prominence of the capillary plexus in the inner stripe of the outer medulla. The **right** side (blue), which may be superimposed on the left side, displays the venous system. The ascending vasa recta drain the medulla and empty into the arcuate and interlobular veins, which drain the cortex. The vasa recta from the inner medulla ascend within the vascular bundles, whereas most vasa recta from the inner stripe ascend between the bundles. (*C*, cortex; *OM*, outer medulla; *OS*, outer stripe; *IS*, inner stripe; *IM*, inner medulla) Modified with permission from: Kriz W, Kaissling B. Structural organization of the mammalian kidney. In: Seldin DW, Giebisch D, eds. *The Kidney: Physiology and Pathophysiology*. 3rd ed. Philadelphia: Lippincott Williams & Wilkins; 2000:587–654.

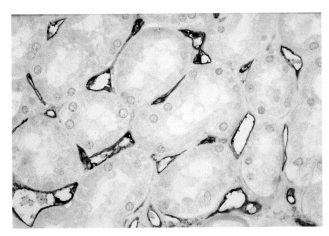

Figure 34.100 The extensive cortical peritubular capillary network is shown by endothelial labeling with CD34 antibody. (CD34 immunoperoxidase, original magnification ×120.)

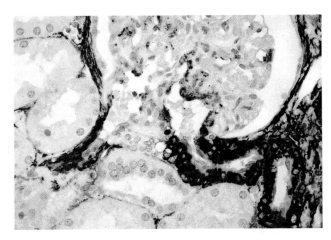

Figure 34.102 Smooth muscle actin immunoperoxidase of a superficial glomerulus delineating the more prominent smooth muscle investment of the afferent arteriole (*right*) compared with the efferent arteriole (*left*) (original magnification ×120).

(574,575). The efferent arterioles from juxtamedullary nephrons descend and supply the entire medulla. In contrast to the efferent arterioles of superficial and midcortical glomeruli (Figure 34.102), those from juxtamedullary glomeruli are larger in diameter, display more layers of smooth muscle cells, and have more endothelial cells on cross sections (274,560).

In the outer stripe of the outer medulla, the efferent arterioles of juxtamedullary nephrons divide to form the descending vasa recta that descend in the vascular bundles but at intervals leave the bundles to form capillary plexuses. The ascending (or venous) vasa recta drain the renal medulla. The ascending vasa recta from the inner medulla join the vascular bundles, whereas most from the inner stripe of the outer medulla ascend between the bundles (560). This architectural arrangement creates a functional separation of the blood flow to the outer and inner medulla. The close proximity of the arterial descending and

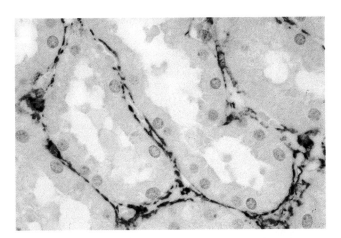

Figure 34.101 Smooth muscle actin expression complements and parallels the CD34 expression in documenting the cortical peritubular capillaries. (Smooth muscle actin immunoperoxidase, original magnification ×120.)

venous ascending vasa recta within the vascular bundles permits effective countercurrent exchange (274,560). The ascending vasa recta at the corticomedullary junction empty into the arcuate and interlobular veins (Figure 34.98), which do form extensive anastomoses, in contrast to the arcuate arteries.

The interlobular veins, which accompany the interlobular arteries, drain the cortex and empty into the arcuate veins. In sections the intrarenal veins have less musculature than comparably sized veins in other organs (Figure 34.98). The arcuate veins empty into the interlobar veins, which converge to form a single renal vein that exits at the hilus of the kidney.

Lymphatics

The lymphatic vessels of the kidney are embedded in the loose periarterial connective tissue in the cortex (Figure 34.103) (576–578). They are not prominent on routine histologic sections. The lymphatics originate as small vessels around the interlobular arteries and empty into arcuate and interlobar lymphatics, which finally drain into larger lymph vessels at the renal hilus. The interlobar and hilar lymphatics possess valves. Lymphatics are not believed to exist in the renal medulla (560,578). There is a less prominent subcapsular network of lymphatic vessels that appears to communicate with the major intrarenal lymphatics within the cortex (578). It has been proposed that the periarterial spaces and the lymphatics may function as a unit to allow exchange with the venous system and serve as a route for the intrarenal distribution of hormones and inflammatory cells (579). Several markers of lymphatic endothelium are now available including: VEGFR-3 (receptor for VEGF-C, VEGF-D, lymphatic angiogenic factor), LYVE-1 (a CD44 homologous hyaluronate receptor), Prox-1 (lymphatic

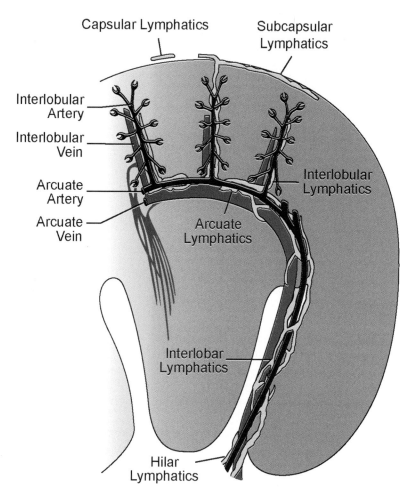

Capsular Lymphatics

Subcapsular Lymphatics

Interlobular Artery

Interlobular Vein

Arcuate Artery

Arcuate Vein

Interlobular Lymphatics

Arcuate Lymphatics

Interlobar Lymphatics

Hilar Lymphatics

Figure 34.103 The lymphatic vessels of the kidney. The arteries (red), veins (blue), and lymphatics (yellow) are illustrated. The lymphatics are primarily distributed in the cortex, although a subcapsular network is also present. Note the absence of the lymphatics in the medulla. Modified with permission from: Madsen KM, Tisher CC. Anatomy of the kidney. In: Brenner BM, ed. *Brenner and Rector's The Kidney.* 7th ed. Philadelphia: WB Saunders; 2004:3–72.

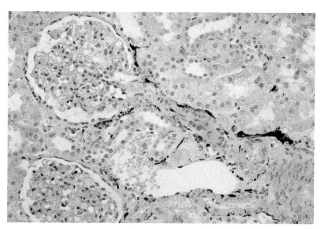

Figure 34.104 S-100 immunoperoxidase stain demonstrating nerves extending along the afferent arteriole to the vascular pole of the glomerulus (original magnification ×62).

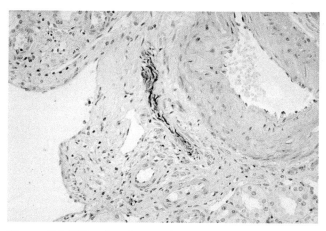

Figure 34.105 Phosphoneurofilament (pNF) immunoperoxidase stain showing a nerve between an artery (*right*) and a vein (*left*) (original magnification ×62).

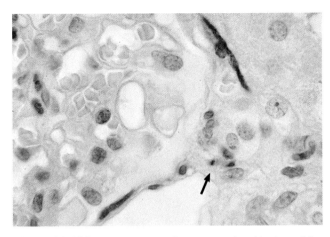

Figure 34.106 Two axons are demonstrated in this view of the vascular pole of a glomerulus (*center*). One axon has a longitudinal profile (*upper right*), and the other is observed in cross-section as a dot (*arrow*). (pNF immunoperoxidase, original magnification ×300.)

vessel transcription factor), and podoplanin (a membrane mucoprotein) (580).

Nerves

The kidney is innervated by adrenergic fibers mainly derived from the celiac plexus (581). The nerve fibers generally accompany the arteries and arterioles in the cortex and outer medulla (582). Staining for myelin by S-100 (Figure 34.104) or for peripheral axons with antibodies against phosphoneurofilament (pNF) (Figure 34.105) demonstrates the nerve fibers (583–586). There is prominent innervation of the juxtaglomerular apparatus (Figure 34.106) (587). The efferent arterioles and the descending vasa recta are accompanied by nerve fibers as long as they contain a surrounding smooth muscle layer (588). Although the direct relationship of nerve terminals to tubules is somewhat controversial, autoradiographic studies have provided evidence for monoaminergic innervation of cortical tubules (589,590).

ACKNOWLEDGMENTS

We are most grateful to Dr. Bruce Beckwith, whose figures and text from the previous edition of this book were in considerable measure retained. Dr. Beckwith has not only advanced our understanding of pediatric tumors, especially Wilms' tumor, but also provided insights into normal and abnormal kidney development. We also thank Roger Hoover of the University of Florida Biomedical Media Services and Ron Irby of the North Florida–South Georgia Veterans Health System for their expert and dedicated assistance with the figures.

REFERENCES

1. Herring PT. The development of the Malpighian bodies of the kidney, and its relation to pathological changes which occur in them. *J Pathol Bacteriol* 1900;6:459–496.
2. Huber GC. On the development and shape of uriniferous tubules of certain of the higher mammals. *Am J Anat* 1905;4(suppl):1–98.
3. Felix W. The development of the urogenital organs. In: Kiebel F, Mall FP, eds. *Manual of Human Embryology.* Vol. 2. Philadelphia: JB Lippincott; 1912:752–979.
4. Peter K. *Untersuchungen über Bau und Entwicklung der Niere.* 2nd ed. Jena, Germany: Verlag Gustav Fischer; 1927.
5. Potter EL. *Normal and Abnormal Development of the Kidney.* Chicago: Year Book; 1972.
6. Oliver J. *Nephrons and Kidneys: A Quantitative Study of Developmental and Evolutionary Mammalian Renal Architectonics.* New York: Harper & Row; 1968.
7. Grobstein C. Inductive interaction in the development of the mouse metanephros. *J Exp Zool* 1955;130:319–340.
8. Saxen L. *Organogenesis of the Kidney.* Cambridge: Cambridge University Press; 1987.
9. Clapp WL, Abrahamson DR. Development and gross anatomy of the kidney. In: Tisher CC, Brenner BM, eds. *Renal Pathology.* 2nd ed. Philadelphia: JB Lippincott; 1994:3–59.
10. Risdon RA, Woolf AS. Development of the kidney. In: Jennette JC, Olson JL, Schwartz MM, Silva FG, eds. *Heptinstall's Pathology of the Kidney.* 5th ed. Philadelphia: Lippincott-Raven; 1998:67–84.
11. Vize PD, Woolf AS, Bard JB. *The Kidney: From Normal Development to Congenital Disease.* San Diego: Academic Press; 2003.
12. Bush KT, Stuart RO, Nigam SK. Developmental biology of the kidney. In: Brenner BM, ed. *Renner & Rector's the Kidney.* 7th ed. Philadelphia: WB Saunders; 2004:73–103.
13. Jones EA. *Xenopus:* a prince among models for pronephric kidney development. *J Am Soc Nephrol* 2005;16:313–321.
14. Drummond IA. Kidney development and disease in the zebrafish. *J Am Soc Nephrol* 2005;16:299–304.
15. Sainio K. Development of the mesonephric kidney. In: Vize PD, Woolf AS, Bard JB, eds. *The Kidney. From Normal Development to Congenital Disease.* San Diego: Academic Press; 2003:75–86.
16. Sainio K, Hellstedt P, Kreidberg JA, Saxen L, Sariola H. Differential regulation of two sets of mesonephric tubules by WT-1. *Development* 1997;124:1293–1299.
17. Pole RJ, Qi BQ, Beasley SW. Patterns of apoptosis during degeneration of the pronephros and mesonephros. *J Urol* 2002;167:269–271.
18. Medvinsky A, Dzierzak E. Definitive hematopoiesis is autonomously initiated by the AGM region. *Cell* 1996;86:897–906.
19. Kumaravelu P, Hook L, Morrison AM, et al. Quantitative developmental anatomy of definitive haematopoietic stem cells/long-term repopulating units (HSC/RUs): role of the aorta-gonad-mesonephros (AGM) region and the yolk sac in colonisation of the mouse embryonic liver. *Development* 2002;129:4891–4899.
20. Davies J. Development of the ureteric bud. In: Vize PD, Woolf AS, Bard JB, eds. *The Kidney: From Normal Development to Congenital Disease.* San Diego: Academic Press; 2003:165–179.
21. al-Awqati Q, Goldberg MR. Architectural patterns in branching morphogenesis in the kidney. *Kidney Int* 1998;54:1832–1842.
22. Watanabe T, Costantini F. Real-time analysis of ureteric bud branching morphogenesis in vitro. *Dev Biol* 2004;271:98–108.
23. Bard J. The metanephros. In: Vize PD, Woolf AS, Bard JB, eds. *The Kidney: From Normal Development to Congenital Disease.* San Diego: Academic Press; 2003:139–148.
24. Sariola H, Sainio K, Bard J. Fates of the metanephric mesenchyme. In: Vize PD, Woolf AS, Bard JB, eds. *The Kidney: From Normal Development to Congenital Disease.* San Diego: Academic Press; 2003:181–193.
25. Abrahamson DR. Glomerulogenesis in the developing kidney. *Semin Nephrol* 1991;11:375–389.
26. Abrahamson DR, Wang R. Development of the glomerular capillary and its basement membrane. In: Vize PD, Woolf AS, Bard JBL, eds. *The Kidney: From Normal Development to Congenital Disease.* San Diego: Academic Press; 2003:221–249.

27. Robert B, St John PL, Hyink DP, Abrahamson DR. Evidence that embryonic kidney cells expressing flk-1 are intrinsic, vasculogenic angioblasts. *Am J Physiol* 1996;271(pt 2):F744–F753.

28. Robert B, St John PL, Abrahamson DR. Direct visualization of renal vascular morphogenesis in Flk1 heterozygous mutant mice. *Am J Physiol* 1998;275(pt 2):F164–F172.

29. Woolf AS, Yuan HT. The development of kidney blood vessels. In: Vize PD, Woolf AS, Bard JB, eds. *The Kidney: From Normal Development to Congenital Disease.* San Diego: Academic Press; 2003: 251–266.

30. Tryggvason K. Unraveling the mechanisms of glomerular ultrafiltration: nephrin, a key component of the slit diaphragm. *J Am Soc Nephrol* 1999;10:2440–2445.

31. Ly J, Alexander M, Quaggin SE. A podocentric view of nephrology. *Curr Opin Nephrol Hypertens* 2004;13:299–305.

32. Kestila M, Lenkkeri U, Mannikko M, et al. Positionally cloned gene for a novel glomerular protein—nephrin—is mutated in congenital nephrotic syndrome. *Mol Cell* 1998;1:575–582.

33. Miner JH. Building the glomerulus: a matricentric view. *J Am Soc Nephrol* 2005;16:857–861.

34. Betsholtz C, Lindblom P, Bjarnegard M, Enge M, Gerhardt H, Lindahl P. Role of platelet-derived growth factor in mesangium development and vasculopathies: lessons learned from platelet-derived growth factor and platelet-derived growth factor receptor mutations in mice. *Curr Opin Nephrol Hypertens* 2004;13:45–52.

35. Celio MR, Groscurth P, Inagami T. Ontogeny of renin immunoreactive cells in the human kidney. *Anat Embryol (Berl)* 1985;173:149–155.

36. Gomez RA, Lynch KR, Chevalier RL et al. Renin and angiotensinogen gene expression in maturing rat kidney. *Am J Physiol* 1988;254(pt 2):F582–F587.

37. Minuth M, Hackenthal E, Poulsen K, Rix, Taugner R. Renin immunocytochemistry of the differentiating juxtaglomerular apparatus. *Anat Embryol (Berl)* 1981;162:173–181.

38. Gomez RA, Lynch KR, Sturgill BC, et al. Distribution of renin mRNA and its protein in the developing kidney. *Am J Physiol* 1989;257(pt 2):F850–F858.

39. Reddi V, Zaglul A, Pentz ES, Gomez RA. Renin-expressing cells are associated with branching of the developing kidney vasculature. *J Am Soc Nephrol* 1998;9:63–71.

40. Sequeira Lopez ML, Pentz ES, Robert B, Abrahamson DR, Gomez RA. Embryonic origin and lineage of juxtaglomerular cells. *Am J Physiol Renal Physiol* 2001;281:F345–F356.

41. Sequeira Lopez ML, Pentz ES, Nomasa T, Smithies O, Gomez RA. Renin cells are precursors for multiple cell types that switch to the renin phenotype when homeostasis is threatened. *Dev Cell* 2004;6:719–728.

42. Alcorn D, Maric C, McCausland J. Development of the renal interstitium. *Pediatr Nephrol* 1999;13:347–354.

43. Levinson R, Mendelsohn C. Stromal progenitors are important for patterning epithelial and mesenchymal cell types in the embryonic kidney. *Semin Cell Dev Biol* 2003;14:225–231.

44. Cullen-McEwen LA, Caruana G, Bertram JF. The where, what and why of the developing renal stroma. *Nephron Exp Nephrol* 2005;99:e1–e8.

45. Sundelin B, Bohman SO. Postnatal development of the interstitial tissue of the rat kidney. *Anat Embryol (Berl)* 1990;182: 307–317.

46. Maric C, Ryan GB, Alcorn D. Embryonic and postnatal development of the rat renal interstitium. *Anat Embryol (Berl)* 1997;195: 503–514.

47. Marxer-Meier A, Hegyi I, Loffing J, Kaissling B. Postnatal maturation of renal cortical peritubular fibroblasts in the rat. *Anat Embryol (Berl)* 1998;197:143–153.

48. Schumacher K, Strehl R, De Vries U, Groene HJ, Minuth WW. SBA-positive fibers between the CD ampulla, mesenchyme, and renal capsule. *J Am Soc Nephrol* 2002;13:2446–2453.

49. Nadasdy T, Lajoie G, Laszik Z, Blick KE, Molnar-Nadasdy G, Silva FG. Cell proliferation in the developing human kidney. *Pediatr Dev Pathol* 1998;1:49–55.

50. Cha JH, Kim YH, Jung JY, Han KH, Madson KM, Kim J. Cell proliferation in the loop of Henle in the developing rat kidney. *J Am Soc Nephrol* 2001;12:1410–1421.

51. Koseki C, Herzlinger D, al-Awqati Q. Apoptosis in metanephric development. *J Cell Biol* 1992;119:1327–1333.

52. Coles HS, Burne JF, Raff MC. Large-scale normal cell death in the developing rat kidney and its reduction by epidermal growth factor. *Development* 1993;118:777–784.

53. Winyard PJ, Nauta J, Lirenman DS, et al. Deregulation of cell survival in cyctic and dysplastic renal development. *Kidney Int* 1996;49:135–146.

54. Kim J, Cha JH, Tisher CC, Madsen KM. Role of apoptotic and nonapoptotic cell death in removal of intercalated cells from developing rat kidney. *Am J Physiol* 1996;270(pt 2):F575–F592.

55. Kim J, Lee GS, Tisher CC, Madsen KM. Role of apoptosis in development of the ascending thin limb of the loop of Henle in rat kidney. *Am J Physiol* 1996;271(pt 2):F831–F845.

56. Fierlbeck W, Liu A, Coyle R, Ballermann BJ. Endothelial cell apoptosis during glomerular capillary lumen formation in vivo. *J Am Soc Nephrol* 2003;14:1349–1354.

57. Foley GD, Bard JB. Apoptosis in the cortex of the developing mouse kidney. *J Anat* 2002;210:477–484.

58. Veis DJ, Sorenson CM, Shutter JR, Korsmeyer SJ. Bcl-2-deficient mice demonstrate fulminant lymphoid apoptosis, polycystic kidneys, and hypopigmented hair. *Cell* 1993;75:229–240.

59. Cho EA, Dressler GR. The formation and development of nephrons. In: Vize PD, Woolf AS, Bard JB, eds. *The Kidney: From Normal Development to Congenital Disease.* San Diego: Academic Press; 2003:195–210.

60. Carroll TJ, McMahon AP. Overview: the molecular basis of kidney development. In: Vize PD, Woolf AS, Bard JB, eds. *The Kidney: From Normal Development to Congenital Disease.* San Diego: Academic Press; 2003:343–376.

61. Yu J, McMahon AP, Valerius MT. Recent genetic studies of mouse kidney development. *Curr Opin Genet Dev* 2004;14:550–557.

62. Gawlik A, Quaggin SE. Conditional gene targeting in the kidney. *Curr Mol Med* 2005;5:527–536.

63. Karavanov AA, Karavanova I, Perantoni A, Dawid IB. Expression pattern of the rat Lim-1 homeobox gene suggests a dual role during kidney development. *Int J Dev Biol* 1998;42:61–66.

64. Tsang TE, Shawlot W, Kinder SJ, et al. Lim1 activity is required for intermediate mesoderm differentiation in the mouse embryo. *Dev Biol* 2000;223:77–90.

65. Kobayashi A, Kwan KM, Carroll TJ, McMahon AP, Mendelsohn CL, Behringer RR. Distinct and sequential tissue-specific activities of the LIM-class homeobox gene Lim1 for tubular morphogenesis during kidney development. *Development* 2005;132: 2809–2823.

66. Xu PX, Adams, J, Peters H, Brown MC, Heaney S, Maas R. Eya1-deficient mice lack ears and kidneys and show abnormal apoptosis of organ primordia. *Nat Genet* 1999;23:113–117.

67. Sajithlal G, Zou D, Silvius D, Xu PX. Eya 1 acts as a critical regulator for specifying the metanephric mesenchyme. *Dev Biol* 2005;284:323–336.

68. Li X, Oghi KA, Zhang J, et al. Eya protein phosphatase activity regulates Six1-Dach-Eya transcriptional effects in mammalian organogenesis. *Nature* 2003;426:247–254.

69. Xu PX, Zheng W, Huang L, Maire P, Laclef C, Silvius D. Six1 is required for the early organogenesis of mammalian kidney. *Development* 2003;130:3085–3094.

70. Ruf RG, Xu PX, Silvius D, et al. SIX1 mutations cause branchio-oto-renal syndrome by disruption of EYA1-SIX1-DNA complexes. *Proc Natl Acad Sci U S A* 2004;101:8080–8095.

71. Nishinakamura R, Matsumoto Y, Nakao K, et al. Murine homolog of SALL1 is essential for ureteric bud invasion in kidney development. *Development* 2001;128:3105–3115.

72. Patterson LT, Pembaur M, Potter SS. Hoxa11 and Hoxd11 regulate branching morphogenesis of the ureteric bud in the developing kidney. *Development* 2001;128:2153–2161.

73. Wellik DM, Hawkes PJ, Capecchi MR. Hox11 paralogous genes are essential for metanephric kidney induction. *Genes Dev* 2002;16:1423–1432.

74. Dressler GR, Deutsch U, Chowdhury C, Nornes HO, Gruss P. Pax2, a new murine paired-box-containing gene and its expression in the developing excretory system. *Development* 1990; 109:787–795.

75. Torres M, Gomez-Pardo E, Dressler GR, Gruss P. Pax-2 controls multiple steps of urogenital development. *Development* 1995; 121:4057–4065.

76. Brophy PD, Ostrom L, Lang KM, Dressler GR. Regulation of ureteric bud outgrowth by Pax2-dependent activation of the glial derived neurotrophic factor gene. *Development* 2001;128:4747–4756.

77. Kreidberg JA, Sariola H, Loring J, et al. WT-1 is required for early kidney development. *Cell* 1993;74:679–691.

78. Donovan MJ, Natoli TA, Sainio K, et al. Initial differentiation of the metanephric mesenchyme is independent of WT1 and the ureteric bud. *Dev Genet* 1999;24:252–262.

79. Kume T, Deng K, Hogan BL. Murine forkhead/winged helix genes Foxc1 (Mf1) and Foxc2 (Mfh1) are required for the early organogenesis of the kidney and urinary tract. *Development* 2000;127: 1387–1395.

80. Kume T, Deng K, Hogan BL. Minimal phenotype of mice homozygous for a null mutation in the forkhead/winged helix gene, Mf2. *Mol Cell Biol* 2000;20:1419–1425.

81. Grieshammer U, Ma L, Plump AS, Wang F, Tessier-Lavigne M, Martin GR. SLIT2-mediated ROBO2 signaling restricts kidney induction to a single site. *Dev Cell* 2004;6:709–717.

82. Dudley AT, Lyons KM, Robertson EJ. A requirement for bone morphogenetic protein-7 during development of the mammalian kidney and eye. *Genes Dev* 1995;9:2795–2807.

83. Luo G, Hofmann C, Bronckers AL, Sohocki M, Bradley A, Karsenty G. BMP-7 is an inducer of nephrogenesis, and is also required for eye development and skeletal patterning. *Genes Dev* 1995;9:2808–2820.

84. Godin RE, Takaesu NT, Robertson EJ, Dudley AT. Regulation of BMP7 expression during kidney development. *Development* 1998;125:3473–3482.

85. Grieshammer U, Cebrian C, Ilagan R, Meyers E, Herzlinger D, Martin GR. FGF8 is required for cell survival at distinct stages of nephrogenesis and for the regulation of gene expression in nascent nephrons. *Development* 2005;132:3847–3857.

86. Perantoni AO, Timofeeva O, Naillat F, et al. Inactivation of FGF8 in early mesoderm reveals an essential role in kidney development. *Development* 2005;132:3859–3871.

87. Sorenson CM, Rogers SA, Korsmeyer SJ, Hammerman MR. Fulminant metanephric apoptosis and abnormal kidney development in bcl-2-deficient mice. *Am J Physiol* 1995;268(pt 2):F73–F81.

88. Sorenson CM, Padanilam B, Hammerman MR. Abnormal postpartum renal development and cytogenesis in the bcl-2 (-/-) mouse. *Am J Physiol* 1996;271:F184–F193.

89. Moser M, Pscherer A, Roth C, et al. Enhanced apoptotic cell death of renal epithelial cells in mice lacking transcription factor AP-2 beta. *Genes Dev* 1997;11:1938–1948.

90. Moser M, Dahmen S, Kluge R, et al. Terminal renal failure in mice lacking transcription factor AP-2 beta. *Lab Invest* 2003;83: 571–578.

91. Favor J, Sandulache R, Neuhauser-Klaus A, et al. The mouse Pax2[1Neu] mutation is identical to a human PAX2 mutation in a family with renal-coloboma syndrome and results in developmental defects of the brain, ear, eye, and kidney. *Proc Natl Acad Sci U S A* 1996;93:13870–13875.

92. Porteous S, Torban E, Cho N-P, et al. Primary renal hypoplasia in humans and mice with PAX2 mutations: evidence of increased apoptosis in fetal kidneys of Pax2[1Neu] +/− mutant mice. *Hum Mol Genet* 2000;9:1–11.

93. Torban E, Eccles MR, Favor J, Goodyer PRl. PAX2 suppresses apoptosis in renal collecting duct cells. *Am J Pathol* 2000;157: 833–842.

94. Qiao J, Uzzo R, Obara-Ishihara T, Degenstein L, Fuchs E, Herzlinger D. FGF-7 modulates ureteric bud growth and nephron number in the developing kidney. *Development* 1999;126:547–554.

95. Bates CM, Kharzai S, Erwin T, Rossant J, Parada LF. Role of N-myc in the developing mouse kidney. *Dev Biol* 2000;222:317–325.

96. Cano-Gauci DF, Song HH, Yang H, et al. Glypican-3-deficient mice exhibit developmental overgrowth and some of the abnormalities typical of Simpson-Golabi-Behmel syndrome. *J Cell Biol* 1999;146:255–264.

97. Grisaru S, Cano-Gauci D, Tee J, Filmus J, Rosenblum ND. Glypican-3 modulates BMP- and FGF-mediated effects during renal branching morphogenesis. *Dev Biol* 2001;231:31–46.

98. Sanchez MP, Silos-Santiago L, Frisen J, He B, Lira SA, Barbacid M. Renal agenesis and the absence of enteric neurons in mice lacking GDNF. *Nature* 1996;382:70–73.

99. Pichel JG, Shen L, Sheng HZ, et al. Defects in enteric innervation and kidney development in mice lacking GDNF. *Nature* 1996;382:73–76.

100. Moore MW, Klein RD, Farinas I, et al. Renal and neuronal abnormalities in mice lacking GDNF. *Nature* 1996;382:76–79.

101. Schuchardt A, D'Agati V, Larsson-Blomberg L, Costantini F, Pachnis V. Defects in the kidney and enteric nervous system of mice lacking the tyrosine kinase receptor Ret. *Nature* 1994;367:380–383.

102. Schuchardt A, D'Agati V, Pachnis V, Costantini F. Renal agenesis and hypodysplasia in ret-k-mutant mice result from defects in ureteric bud development. *Development* 1996;122:1919–1929.

103. Enomoto H, Araki T, Jackman A, et al. GFR alpha1-deficient mice have deficits in the enteric nervous system and kidneys. *Neuron* 1998;21:317–324.

104. Esquela AF, Lee SJ. Regulation of metanephric kidney development by growth/differentiation factor 11. *Dev Biol* 2003;257:356–370.

105. Basson MA, Akbulut S, Watson-Johnson J, et al. Sprouty1 is a critical regulator of GDNF/RET-mediated kidney induction. *Dev Cell* 2005;8:229–239.

106. Miyamoto N, Yoshida M, Kuratani S, Matsuo I, Aizawa S. Defects of urogenital development in mice lacking Emx2. *Development* 1997;124:1653–1664.

107. Mendelsohn C, Batourina E, Fung S, Gilbert T, Dodd J. Stromal cells mediate retinoid-dependent functions essential for renal development. *Development* 1999;126:1139–1148.

108. Batourina E, Gim S, Bello N, et al. Vitamin A controls epithelial/mesenchymal interactions through Ret expression. *Nat Genet* 2001;27:74–78.

109. Miyazaki Y, Oshima K, Fogo A, Hogan BL, Ichikawa I. Bone morphogenetic protein 4 regulates the budding site and elongation of the mouse ureter. *J Clin Invest* 2000;105:863–873.

110. Quaggin SE, Schwartz L, Cui S, et al. The basic-helix-loop-helix protein Pod1 is critically important for kidney and lung organogenesis. *Development* 1999;126:5771–5783.

111. Bullock SL, Fletcher JM, Beddington RS, Wilson VA. Renal agenesis in mice homozygous for a gene trap mutation in the gene encoding heparan sulfate 2-sulfotransferase. *Genes Dev* 1998;12: 1894–1906.

112. Muller U, Wang D, Denda S, Meseses JJ, Pederson RA, Reichardt LF. Integrin alpha-8/beta-1 is critically important for epithelial-mesenchymal interactions during kidney morphogenesis. *Cell* 1997;88:603–613.

113. Kreidberg JA, Donovan MJ, Goldstein SL, et al. Alpha 3 beta 1 integrin has a crucial role in kidney and lung organogenesis. *Development* 1996;122:3537–3547.

114. Schnabel CA, Godin RE, Cleary ML. Pbx1 regulates nephrogenesis and ureteric branching in the developing kidney. *Dev Biol* 2003;254:262–276.

115. Michos O, Panman L, Vintersten K, Beier K, Zeller R, Zuniga A. Gremlin-mediated BMP antagonism induces the epithelial-mesenchymal feedback signaling controlling metanephric kidney and limb organogenesis. *Development* 2004;131:3401–3410.

116. Majumdar A, Vainio S, Kispert A, McMahaon J, McMahon AP. Wnt11 and Ret/Gdnf pathways cooperate in regulating ureteric branching during metanephric kidney development. *Development* 2003;130:3175–3185.

117. Maas R, Elfering S, Glaser T, Jepeal L. Deficient outgrowth of the ureteric bud underlies the renal agenesis phenotype in mice manifesting the limb deformity (ld) mutation. *Dev Dyn* 1994;199: 214–228.

118. Niimura F, Labosky PA, Kakuchi J, et al. Gene targeting in mice reveals a requirement for angiotensin in the development and maintenance of kidney morphology and growth factor regulation. *J Clin Invest* 1995;96:2947–2954.

119. Nagata M, Tanimoto K, Fukamizu A, et al. Nephrogenesis and renovascular development in angiotensinogen-deficient mice. *Lab Invest* 1996;75:745–753.

120. Yanai K, Saito T, Kakinuma Y, et al. Renin-dependent cardio-vascular functions and renin-independent blood-brain barrier functions revealed by renin-deficient mice. *J Biol Chem* 2000; 275:5–8.

121. Takahashi N, Lopez ML, Cowhig JE Jr, et al. Ren1c homozygous null mice are hypotensive and polyuric, but heterozygotes are indistinguishable from wild-type. *J Am Soc Nephrol* 2005;16: 125–132.

122. Esther CR Jr, Howard TE, Marino EM, Goddard JM, Capecchi MR, Bernstein KE. Mice lacking angiotensin-converting enzyme have low blood pressure, renal pathology, and reduced male fertility. *Lab Invest* 1996;7:953–965.

123. Tsuchida S, Matsusaka T, Chen X, et al. Murine double nullizygotes of the angiotensin type 1A and 1B receptor genes duplicate severe abnormal phenotypes of angiotensinogen nullizygotes. *J Clin Invest* 1998;101:755–760.

124. Oliverio MI, Kim HS, Ito M, et al. Reduced growth, abnormal kidney structure, and type 2 (AT_2) angiotensin receptor-mediated blood pressure regulation in mice lacking both AT_{1A} and AT_{1B} receptors for angiotensin II. *Proc Natl Acad Sci U S A* 1998;95: 15496–15501.

125. Nishimura H, Yerkes E, Hohenfellner K, et al. Role of the angiotensin type 2 receptor gene and congenital anomalies of the kidney and urinary tract, CAKUT, of mice and men. *Mol Cell* 1999;3:1–10.

126. Oshima K, Miyazaki Y, Brock JW III, Adams MC, Ichikawa I, Pop JC IV. Angiotensin type II receptor expression and ureteral budding. *J Urol* 2001;166:1848–1852.

127. Stark K, Vainio S, Vassileva G, McMahon AP. Epithelial transformation of metanephric mesenchyme in the developing kidney regulated by Wnt-4. *Nature* 1994;372:679–683.

128. Carroll TJ, Park JS, Hayashi S, Majumdar A, McMahon AP. Wnt9b plays a central role in the regulation of mesenchymal to epithelial transitions underlying organogenesis of the mammalian urogenital system. *Dev Cell* 2005;9:283–292.

129. Hatini V, Huh SO, Herzlinger D, Soares VC, Lai E. Essential role of stromal mesenchyme in kidney morphogenesis revealed by targeted disruption of Winged Helix transcription factor BF-2. *Genes Dev* 1996;10:1467–1478.

130. Levinson RS, Batourina E, Choi C, Vorontchikhina M, Kitajewski J, Mendelsohn CL. Foxd1-dependent signals control cellularity in the renal capsule, a structure required for normal renal development. *Development* 2005;132:529–539.

131. Cui S, Schwartz, Quaggin SE. Pod1 is required in stromal cells for glomerulogenesis. *Dev Dyn* 2003;226:512–522.

132. McGregor L, Makela V, Darling SM, et al. Fraser syndrome and mouse blebbed phenotype caused by mutations in FRAS1/Fras1 encoding a putative extracellular matrix protein. *Nat Genet* 2003;34:203–208.

133. Vrontou S, Petrou P, Meyer BI, et al. Fras1 deficiency results in cryptophthalmos, renal agenesis and blebbed phenotype in mice. *Nat Genet* 2003;34:209–214.

134. Takamiya K, Kostourou V, Adams S, et al. A direct functional link between the multi-PDZ domain protein GRIP1 and the Fraser syndrome protein Fras1. *Nat Genet* 2004;36:172–177.

135. Mah SP, Saueressig H, Goulding M, Kintner C, Dressler GR. Kidney development in cadherin-6 mutants: delayed mesenchyme-to-epithelial conversion and loss of nephrons. *Dev Biol* 2000; 223:38–53.

136. Patek CE, Fleming S, Miles CG, et al. Murine Denys-Drash syndrome: evidence of podocyte de-differentiation and systemic mediation of glomerulosclerosis. *Hum Mol Genet* 2003;12:2379–2394.

137. Gao F, Maiti S, Sun G, et al. The Wt1^{+R394W} mouse displays glomerulosclerosis and early-onset renal failure characteristic of human Denys-Drash syndrome. *Mol Cell Biol* 2004;24:9899–9910.

138. Hammes A, Guo JK, Lutsch G, et al. Two splice variants of the Wilms' tumor 1 gene have distinct functions during sex determination and nephron formation. *Cell* 2001;106:319–329.

139. Leveen P, Pekny M, Gebre-Medhin S, Swolin B, Larsson E, Betsholtz C. Mice deficient for PDGF B show renal, cardiovascular, and hematological abnormalities. *Genes Dev* 1994;8: 1875–1887.

140. Soriano P. Abnormal kidney development and hematological disorders in PDGF beta-receptor mutant mice. *Genes Dev* 1994;8:1888–1896.

141. McCright B, Gao X, Shen L, et al. Defects in development of the kidney, heart and eye vasculature in mice homozygous for a hypomorphic Notch2 mutation. *Development* 2001;128:491–502.

142. Eremina V, Sood M, Haigh J, et al. Glomerular-specific alterations of VEGF-A expression lead to distinct congenital and acquired renal diseases. *J Clin Invest* 2003;111:707–716.

143. Miner JH, Li C. Defective glomerulogenesis in the absence of laminin alpha5 demonstrates a developmental role for the kidney glomerular basement membrane. *Dev Biol* 2000;217:278–289.

144. Noakes PG, Miner JH, Gautam M, Cunningham JM, Sanes JR, Merlie JP. The renal glomerulus of mice lacking s-laminin/laminin beta 2: nephrosis despite molecular compensation by laminin beta 1. *Nat Genet* 1995;10:400–406.

145. Cosgrove D, Meehan DT, Grunkemeyer JA, et al. Collagen COL4A3 knockout: a mouse model for autosomal Alport syndrome. *Genes Dev* 1996;10:2981–2992.

146. Miner JH, Sanes JR. Molecular and functional defects in kidneys of mice lacking collagen alpha 3(IV): implications for Alport syndrome. *J Cell Biol* 1996;135:1403–1413.

147. Lu W, Phillips CL, Killen PD. Insertional mutation of the collagen genes Col4a3 and Col4a4 in a mouse model of Alport syndrome. *Genomics* 1999;61:113–124.

148. Putaala H, Soininen R, Kilpelainen P, Wartiovaara J, Tryggvason K. The murine nephrin gene is specifically expressed in kidney, brain and pancreas: inactivation of the gene leads to massive proteinuria and neonatal death. *Hum Mol Genet* 2001; 10:1–8.

149. Shih NY, Li J, Karpitskii V, et al. Congenital nephrotic syndrome in mice lacking CD2-associated protein. *Science* 1999;286:312–315.

150. Roselli S, Heidet L, Sich M, et al. Early glomerular filtration defect and severe renal disease in podocin-deficient mice. *Mol Cell Biol* 2004;24:550–560.

151. Kaplan JM, Kim SH, North KN, et al. Mutations in ACTN4, encoding alpha-actinin-4, cause familial focal segmental glomerulosclerosis. *Nat Genet* 2000;24:251–256.

152. Kos CH, Le TC, Sinha S, et al. Mice deficient in alpha-actinin-4 have severe glomerular disease. *J Clin Invest* 2003;111:1683–1690.

153. Winn MP, Conlon PJ, Lynn KL, et al. A mutation in the TRPC6 cation channel causes familial focal segmental glomerulosclerosis. *Science* 2005;308:1801–1804.

154. Reiser J, Polu KR, Moller CC, et al. TRPC6 is a glomerular slit diaphragm-associated channel required for normal renal function. *Nat Genet* 2005;37:739–744.

155. Donoviel DB, Freed DD, Vogel H, et al. Proteinuria and perinatal lethality in mice lacking NEPH1, a novel protein with homology to NEPHRIN. *Mol Cell Biol* 2001;21:4829–4836.

156. Ciana L, Patel A, Allen ND, et al. Mice lacking the giant protocadherin mFAT1 exhibit renal slit junction abnormalites and a partially penetrant cyclopia and anophthalmia phenotype. *Mol Cell Biol* 2003;23:3575–3582.

157. Chen H, Lun Y, Ovchinnikov D, et al. Limb and kidney defects in Lmxb1 mutant mice suggest an involvement of LMX1B in human nail patella syndrome. *Nat Genet* 1998;19:51–55.

158. Miner JH, Morello R, Andrews KL, et al. Transcriptional induction of slit diaphragm genes by Lmx1b is required in podocyte differentiation. *J Clin Invest* 2002;109:1065–1072.

159. Doyonnas R, Kershaw DB, Duhme C, et al. Anuria, omphalocele, and perinatal lethality in mice lacking the CD34-related protein podocalyxin. *J Exp Med* 2001;194:13–27.

160. Wharram BL, Goyal M, Gillespie PJ, et al. Altered podocyte structure in GLEPP1(Ptpro)-deficient mice associated with hypertension and low glomerular filtration rate. *J Clin Invest* 2000;106: 1281–1290.

161. Sadl VS, Jin F, Yu J, et al. The mouse Kreisler (Krml1/MafB) segmentation gene is required for differentiation of glomerular visceral epithelial cells. *Dev Biol* 2002;249:16–29.

162. Lu W, Peissel B, Babakhanlou H, et al. Perinatal lethality with kidney and pancreas defects in mice with a targeted Pkd1 mutation. *Nat Genet* 1997;17:179–181.

163. Lu W, Fan X, Basora N, et al. Late onset of renal and hepatic cysts in Pkd1-targeted heterozygotes. *Nat Genet* 1999;21: 160–161.

164. Boulter C, Mulroy S, Webb S, Fleming S, Brindle K, Sanford R. Cardiovascular, skeletal, and renal defects in mice with a targeted disruption of the Pkd1 gene. *Proc Natl Acad Sci U S A* 2001;98: 12174–12179.

165. Chauvet V, Qian F, Boute N, et al. Expression of PKD1 and PKD2 transcripts and proteins in human embryo and during normal kidney development. *Am J Pathol* 2002; 160:973–983.

166. Wu G, Markowitz GS, Li L, et al. Cardiac defects and renal failure in mice with targeted mutations in Pkd2. *Nat Genet* 2000;24: 75–78.

167. Wu G, D'Agati V, Cai Y, et al. Somatic inactivation of Pkd2 results in polycystic kidney disease. *Cell* 1998;93:177–188.

168. Jadeja S, Smyth I, Pitera JE, et al. Identification of a new gene mutated in Fraser syndrome and mouse myelencephalic blebs. *Nat Genet* 2005;37:520–525.

169. Morham SG, Langenbach R, Loftin CD, et al. Prostaglandin synthase 2 gene disruption causes severe renal pathology in the mouse. *Cell* 1995;83:473–482.

170. Norwood VF, Morham SG, Smithies O. Postnatal development and progression of renal dysplasia in cyclooxygenase-2 null mice. *Kidney Int* 2000;58:2291–2300.

171. Threadgill DW, Dlugosz AA, Hansen LA, et al. Targeted disruption of mouse EGF receptor: effect of genetic background on mutant phenotypes. *Science* 1995;269:230–234.

172. Bernardini N, Bianchi F, Lupetti M, Dolfi A. Immunohistochemical localization of the epidermal growth factor, transforming growth factor alpha, and their receptor in the human mesonephros and metanephros. *Dev Dyn* 1996;206:231–238.

173. Nakai S, Sugitani Y, Sato H, et al. Crucial roles of Brn1 in distal tubule formation and function in mouse kidney. *Development* 2003;130:4751–4759.

174. Wang P, Pereira FA, Beasley D, Zheng H. Presenilins are required for the formation of comma- and S-shaped bodies during nephrogenesis. *Development* 2003;130:5019–5029.

175. Cheng HT, Miner JH, Lin M, Tansey MG, Roth K, Kopan R. Gamma-secretase activity is dispensable for mesenchyme-to-epithelium transition but required for podocyte and proximal tubule formation in developing mouse kidney. *Development* 2003;130:5031–5042.

176. Lo SH, Yu QC, Degenstein L, Chen LB, Fuchs E. Progressive kidney degeneration in mice lacking tensin. *J Cell Biol* 1997;136: 1349–1361.

177. Dahl U, Sjodin A, Larue L, et al. Genetic dissection of cadherin function during nephrogenesis. *Mol Cell Biol* 2002;22:1474–1487.

178. Moore KL, Persaud TVN. *The Developing Human: Clinically Oriented Embryology.* 7th ed. Philadelphia: WB Saunders; 2003.

179. Gruenwald P. The normal changes in the position of the embryonic kidney. *Anat Rec* 1943;85:163–176.

180. Friedland GW, de Vries P. Renal ectopia and fusion. Embryologic basis. *Urology* 1975;5:698–706.

181. Muller F, O'Rahilly R. Somitic-vertebral correlation and vertebral levels in the human embryo. *Am J Anat* 1986;177:3–19.

182. Bremer JL. The origin of the renal artery in mammals and its anomalies. *Am J Anat* 1915;18:179–200.

183. Emery JL, Mithal A. The weights of kidneys in late intra-uterine life and childhood. *J Clin Pathol* 1960;13:490–493.

184. Gruenwald P, Minh HN. Evaluation of body and organ weights in perinatal pathology. I. Normal standards derived from autopsies. *Am J Clin Pathol* 1960;34:247–253.

185. Singer DB, Sung CJ, Wigglesworth JS. Fetal growth and maturation: with standards for body and organ development. In: Wigglesworth JS, Singer DB, eds. *Textbook of Fetal and Perinatal Pathology.* 2nd ed. Oxford: Blackwell; 1998:8–40.

186. Guihard-Costa AM, Menez F, Delezoide AL. Organ weights in human fetuses after formalin fixation: standards by gestational age and body weight. *Pediatr Dev Pathol* 2002;5:559–578.

187. Hansen K, Sung CJ, Huang C, Pinar H, Singer DB, Oyer CE. Reference values for second trimester fetal and neonatal organ weights and measurements. *Pediatr Dev Pathol* 2003;6: 160–167.

188. Maroun LL, Graem N. Autopsy standards of body parameters and fresh organ weights in nonmacerated and macerated human fetuses. *Pediatr Dev Pathol* 2005;8:204–217.

189. Coppoletta JM, Wolbach SB. Body length and organ weights of infants and children. *Am J Pathol* 1933;9:55–70.

190. Kelley HA, Burnam CF. *Diseases of the Kidneys, Ureters, and Bladder.* Vol.1. New York: Appleton; 1925.

191. Hodson J. The lobar structure of the kidney. *Br J Urol* 1972;44: 246–261.

192. Löfgren F. *Das topographische System der Malpighischen Pyramiden der Menschenniere.* Uppsala, Sweden: Lund Hakan Ohlssons Boktryckeri; 1949.

193. Sykes D. The morphology of renal lobulations and calices, and their relationship to partial nephrectomy. *Br J Surg* 1964;51:294–304.

194. Crelin ES. *Functional Anatomy of the Newborn.* New Haven, CT: Yale University Press; 1976.

195. Campos ES. Pathological changes in the kidney in congenital syphilis. *Johns Hopkins Hosp Bull* 1923;34:253–263.

196. Potter EL, Thierstein ST. Glomerular development in the kidney as an index of fetal maturity. *J Pediatr* 1943;22:695–706.

197. Rodriguez MM, Gomez AH, Abitbol CL, Chandar JJ, Duara S, Zilleruelo G. Histomorphometric analysis of postnatal glomerulogenesis in extremely preterm infants. *Pediatr Dev Pathol* 2004; 7:17–25.

198. Singer DB, Klish W. Morphometric studies of the renal glomerulogenic zone. *Am J Pathol* 1970;59:32a.

199. Tsuda S. Histologic investigation of the foetal kidney. *Jap J Obstet Gynecol* 1934;17:337–341.

200. Dorovini-Zis K, Dolman CL. Gestational development of brain. *Arch Pathol Lab Med* 1977;101:192–195.

201. Hinchliffe SA, Sargent PH, Chan YF, et al. "Medullary ray glomerular counting" as a method of assessment of human nephrogenesis. *Pathol Res Pract* 1992;188:775–782.

202. Peter K. Harnorgane, Organe Uropoietica. In: Peter K, Wetzel G, Heiderich F, eds. *Handbuch der Anatomie des Kindes.* Vol. 2. Munich: JF Bergmann; 1938:1–41.

203. Benjamin DR, Beckwith JB. Medullary ray nodules in infancy and childhood. *Arch Pathol* 1973;96:33–35.

204. Hinchliffe SA, Sargent PH, Howard CV, Chan YF, van Velzen D. Human intrauterine renal growth expressed in absolute number of glomeruli assessed by the disector method and Cavalieri principle. *Lab Invest* 1991;64:777–784.

205. Hughson M, Farris AB III, Douglas-Denton R, Hoy WE, Bertram JF. Glomerular number and size in autopsy kidneys: the relationship to birth weight. *Kidney Int* 2003;63:2113–2122.

206. Hinchliffe SA, Lynch MR, Sargent PH, Howard CV, van Velzen D. The effect of intrauterine growth retardation on the development of renal nephrons. *Br J Obstet Gynaecol* 1992;99:296–301.

207. Manalich R, Reyes L, Herrera M, Melendi C, Fundora I. Relationship between weight at birth and the number and size of renal glomeruli in humans: a histomorphometric study. *Kidney Int* 2000;58:770–773.

208. Fogo A, Hawkins EP, Berry PL, et al. Glomerular hypertrophy in minimal change disease predicts subsequent progression to focal glomerular sclerosis. *Kidney Int* 1990;38:115–123.

209. Nyengaard JR, Bendtsen TF. Glomerular number and size in relation to age, kidney weight, and body surface in normal man. *Anat Rec* 1992;232:194–201.

210. Merlet-Benichou C, Gilbert T, Vilar J, Moreau E, Freund N, Lelievre-Pegorier M. Nephron number: variability is the rule. Causes and consequences. *Lab Invest* 1999;79:515–527.

211. Hoy WE, Hughson MD, Bertram JF, Douglas-Denton R, Amann K. Nephron number, hypertension, renal disease, and renal failure. *J Am Soc Nephrol* 2005;16:2557–2564.

212. Brenner BM, Garcia DL, Anderson S. Glomeruli and blood pressure. Less of one, more of the other? *Am J Hypertens* 1988;1(pt 1): 335–347.

213. Keller G, Zimmer G, Mall G, Ritz E, Amann K. Nephron number in patients with primary hypertension. *N Eng J Med* 2003;348: 101–108.

214. Gruenwald P, Popper H. The histogenesis and physiology of the renal glomerulus in early postnatal life: histological examination. *J Urol* 1940;43:452–459.

215. MacDonald MS, Emery JL. The late intrauterine and postnatal development of human renal glomeruli. *J Anat* 1959;93:331–340.

216. Vernier RL, Birch-Andersen A. Studies of the human fetal kidney. I. Development of the glomerulus. *J Pediatr* 1962;60:754–768.

217. Thony HC, Luethy CM, Zimmermann A, et al. Histological features of glomerular immaturity in infants and small children with normal or altered tubular function. *Eur J Pediatr* 1995; 154(suppl 4):S65–S68.

218. Volger C, McAdams J, Homan SM. Glomerular basement membrane and lamina densa in infants and children: an ultrastructural evaluation. *Pediatr Pathol* 1987;7:527–534.

219. Ramage IJ, Howatson AG, McColl JH, Maxwell H, Murphy AV, Beattie TJ. Glomerular basement membrane thickness in children: a stereologic assessment. *Kidney Int* 2002;62:895–900.

220. Steffes MW, Barbosa J, Basgen JM, Sutherland DE, Najarian JS, Mauer SM. Quantitative glomerular morphology of the normal human kidney. *Lab Invest* 1983;49:82–86.

221. Vogelmann SU, Nelson WJ, Myers BD, Lemley KV. Urinary excretion of viable podocytes in health and renal disease. *Am J Physiol Renal Physiol* 2003;285:F40–F48.

222. Petermann AT, Krofft R, Blonski M, et al. Podocytes that detach in experimental membranous nephropathy are viable. *Kidney Int* 2003;64:1222–1231.

223. Fetterman GH, Shuplock NA, Philipp FJ, Gregg HS. The growth and maturation of human glomeruli and proximal convolutions from term to adulthood: studies by microdissection. *Pediatrics* 1965;35:601–619.

224. Zolnai B, Palkovits M. Glomerulometrics III. Data referring to the growth of the glomeruli in man. *Acta Biol Sci Hung* 1965; 15:409–423.

225. Souster LP, Emery JL. The sizes of renal glomeruli in fetuses and infants. *J Anat* 1980;130(pt 3):595–602.

226. Moore L, Williams R, Staples A. Glomerular dimensions in children under 16 years of age. *J Pathol* 1993;171:145–150.

227. Akaoka K, White RH, Raafat F. Human glomerular growth during childhood: a morphometric study. *J Pathol* 1994;173: 261–268.

228. Samuel T, Hoy WE, Douglas-Denton R, Hughson MD, Bertram JF. Determinants of glomerular volume in different cortical zones of the human kidney. *J Am Soc Nephrol* 2005;16:3102–3109.

229. Steffes MW, Schmidt D, McCrery R, Basgen JM; International Diabetic Nephropathy Study Group. Glomerular cell number in normal subjects and in type 1 diabetic patients. *Kidney Int* 2001;59:2104–2113.

230. Combs HL, Shankland SJ, Setzer SV, Hudkins KL, Alpers CE. Expression of the cyclin kinase inhibitor, p27^{kip1}, in developing and mature human kidney. *Kidney Int* 1998;53:892–896.

231. Nagata M, Nakayama K, Terada Y, Hoshi S, Watanabe T. Cell cycle regulation and differentiation in the human podocyte lineage. *Am J Pathol* 1998;153:1511–1520.

232. Hiromura K, Haseley LA, Zhang P, et al. Podocyte expression of the CDK-inhibitor p57 during development and disease. *Kidney Int* 2001;60:2235–2246.

233. Kampmeier OF. The metanephros or so-called permanent kidney in part provisional and vestigial. *Anat Rec* 1926;33:115–120.

234. Emery JL, Macdonald MS. Involuting and scarred glomeruli in the kidneys of infants. *Am J Pathol* 1960;36:713–723.

235. Herxheimer G. Uber hyaline Glomeruli der Neugeborenen und Sauglinge. *Frankfurt Ztschr Path* 1909;2:138–152.

236. Schwarz L. Weitere Beitrage zur Kenntnis der anatomischen Nierenveranderungen der Neugeborenen und Sauglinge. *Virchows Arch Path Anat* 1928;267:654–689.

237. Friedman HH, Grayzel DM, Lederer M. Kidney lesions in stillborn and newborn infants. "Congenital glomerulosclerosis." *Am J Pathol* 1942;18:699–713.

238. Thomas MA. Congenital glomerulosclerosis. *Pathology* 1969;1: 105–112.

239. Moffat DB, Fourman J. Ectopic glomeruli in the human and animal kidney. *Anat Rec* 1964;149:1–7.

240. MacCallum DB. The bearing of degenerating glomeruli on the problem of the vascular supply of the mammalian kidney. *Am J Anat* 1939;65:69–103.

241. Darmady EM, Prince J, Stranack F, Offer J. The proximal convoluted tubule in the renal handling of water. *Lancet* 1964;2: 1254–1257.

242. Evan AP, Larsson L. Morphologic development of the nephron. In: Edelmann CM Jr, Bernstein J, Meadow SR, Spitzer A, Travis LB, eds. *Pediatric Kidney Disease.* 2nd ed. Boston: Little Brown & Co; 1992:19–48.

243. Satlin LM, Woda CB, Schwartz GJ. The development of function in the metanephric kidney. In: Vize PD, Woolf AS, Bard JB, eds. *The Kidney: From Normal Development to Congenital Disease.* San Diego: Academic Press; 2003:267–325.

244. Neiss WF. Histogenesis of the loop of Henle in the rat kidney. *Anat Embryol (Berl)* 1982;164:315–330.

245. Raptopoulos V, Kleinman PK, Mark S Jr, Synder M, Silverman PM. Renal fascial pathway: posterior extension of pancreatic effusions within the anterior pararenal space. *Radiology* 1986;158: 367–374.

246. Tobin CE. The renal fascia and its relation to the transversalis fascia. *Anat Rec* 1944;89:295–311.

247. Kunin M. Bridging septa of the perinephric space: anatomic, pathologic, and diagnostic considerations. *Radiology* 1986;158: 361–365.

248. Kochkodan EJ, Hagger AM. Visualization of the renal fascia: a normal finding in urography. *AJR Am J Roentgenol* 1983;140: 1243–1244.

249. Parienty RA, Pradel J, Picard JD, Ducellier R, Lubrano JM, Smolarski N. Visibility and thickening of the renal fascia on computed tomograms. *Radiology* 1981;139:119–124.

250. Wald H. The weight of normal adult human kidneys and its variability. *Arch Pathol Lab Med* 1937;23:493–500.

251. Kasiske BL, Umen AJ. The influence of age, sex, race, and body habitus on kidney weight in humans. *Arch Pathol Lab Med* 1986; 110:55–60.

252. Frimann-Dahl J. Normal variations of the left kidney. An anatomical and radiologic study. *Acta Radiol* 1961;55:207–216.

253. Graves FT. The anatomy of the intrarenal arteries and its application to segmental resection of the kidney. *Br J Surg* 1954;42:132–139.

254. Graves FT, Graves D. *Anatomical Studies for Renal and Intrarenal Surgery.* Bristol, England: John Wright; 1986.

255. Satyapal KS. Classification of the drainage patterns of the renal veins. *J Anat* 1995;186(pt 2):329–333.

256. Sperber I. Studies on the mammalian kidney. *Zool Bidrag Uppsala* 1944;22:249–432.

257. Hodson CJ, Mariani S. Large cloisons. *AJR Am J Roentgenol* 1982;139:327–332.

258. Lafortune M, Constantin A, Breton G, Vallee C. Sonography of the hypertrophied column of Bertin. *AJR Am J Roentgenol* 1986;146:53–56.

259. Bigongiari LR, Patel SK, Appelman H, Thombury JR. Medullary rays. Visualization during excretory urography. *Am J Roentgenol Ther Nucl Med* 1975;125:795–803.

260. Hodson CJ. The renal parenchyma and its blood supply. *Curr Probl Diagn Radiol* 1978;7:1–32.

261. Ransley PG, Risdon RA. Renal papillary morphology in infants and young children. *Urol Res* 1975;3:111–113.

262. Ransley PG. Intrarenal reflux: anatomical, dynamic and radiologic studies—part I. *Urol Res* 1977;5:61–69.

263. Schmidt-Nielsen B. The renal pelvis. *Kidney Int* 1987;31:621–628.

264. Murphy WM, Grignon DJ, Perlman EJ. Tumors of the kidney, bladder, and related urinary structures. In: *Atlas of Tumor Pathology.* 4th series, fascicle 1. Washington, DC: Armed Forces Institute of Pathology; 2004.

265. Amis ES Jr, Cronan JJ. The renal sinus: an imaging review and proposed nomenclature for sinus cysts. *J Urol* 1988;139:1151–1159.

266. Beckwith JB. National Wilms Tumor Study: an update for pathologists. *Pediatr Dev Pathol* 1998;1:79–84.

267. Bonsib SM, Gibson D, Mhoon M, Greene GF. Renal sinus involvement in renal cell carcinomas. *Am J Surg Pathol* 2000;24: 451–458.

268. Bonsib SM. The renal sinus is the principal invasive pathway: a prospective study of 100 renal cell carcinomas. *Am J Surg Pathol* 2004;28:1594–1600.

269. Oliver J. *Architecture of the Kidney in Chronic Bright's Disease.* New York: Hoeber; 1939.

270. Schmidt-Nielsen B, O'Dell R. Structure and concentrating mechanism in the mammalian kidney. *Am J Physiol* 1961;200:1119–1124.

271. Madsen KM, Tisher CC. Structural-functional relationships along the distal nephron. *Am J Physiol* 1986;250(pt 2):F1–F15.

272. Jamison RL, Kriz W. *Urinary Concentrating Mechanism: Structure and Function.* New York: Oxford University Press;1982.

273. Sands JM, Kokko JP, Jacobson HR. Intrarenal heterogeneity: vascular and tubular. In: Seldin DW, Giebisch D, eds. *The Kidney: Physiology and Pathophysiology.* 2nd ed. New York: Raven Press; 1992:1087–1155.

274. Kriz W, Kaissling B. Structural organization of the mammalian kidney. In: Seldin DW, Giebisch D, eds. *The Kidney: Physiology and Pathophysiology.* 3rd ed. Philadelphia: Lippincott Williams & Wilkins; 2000:587–654.

275. Knepper M, Burg M. Organization of nephron function. *Am J Physiol* 1983;244:F579–F589.

276. Kriz W, Bankir L. A standard nomenclature for structures of the kidney. The Renal Commission of the International Union of Physiological Sciences (IUPS). *Kidney Int* 1988;33:1–7.

277. Croker BP, Tisher CC. Indications for and interpretation of the renal biopsy: evaluation by light, electron and immunofluorescence microscopy. In: Schrier RW, ed. *Diseases of the Kidney.* 8th ed. Philadelphia: Lippincott Williams & Wilkins; 2006.

278. Pirani CL, Croker BP. Handling and processing of renal biopsy and nephrectomy specimens. In: Tisher CC, Brenner BM, eds. *Renal Pathology. With Clinical and Functional Correlations.* 2nd ed. Philadelphia: JB Lippincott; 1994:1683–1694.

279. Walker PD, Cavallo T, Bonsib SM; Ad Hoc Committee on Renal Biopsy Guidelines of the Renal Pathology Society. Practice guidelines for the renal biopsy. *Mod Pathol* 2004;17:1555–1563.

280. Madsen KM, Tisher CC. Anatomy of the kidney. In: Brenner BM, ed. *Brenner and Rector's The Kidney.* 7th ed. Philadelphia: WB Saunders; 2004:3–72.

281. Malpighi M. *De Viscerum Structura Exercitatio Anatomica.* Bonn, Germany: De Liene; 1666.

282. Hayman JM Jr. Malpighi's "Concerning the structure of the kidneys." *Ann Med Hist* 1925;7:242–263.

283. Bowman W. On the structure and use of the Malpighian bodies of the kidney, with observations on the circulation through that gland. *Philos Trans R Soc Lond* 1842;132:57–80.

284. Fine LG. William Bowman's description of the glomerulus. *Am J Nephrol* 1985;5:437–440.

285. Geneser F. *Textbook of Histology.* Philadelphia: Lea & Febiger; 1986.

286. Jorgensen F. *The Ultrastructure of the Normal Human Glomerulus.* Copenhagen: Munksgaard; 1966.

287. Tisher CC, Brenner BM. Structure and function of the glomerulus. In: Tisher CC, Brenner BM, eds. *Renal Pathology. With Clinical and Functional Correlations.* 2nd ed. Philadelphia: JB Lippincott; 1994:143–161.

288. Newbold KM, Sandison A, Howie AJ. Comparison of size of juxtamedullary and outer cortical glomeruli in normal adult kidney. *Virchows Arch A Pathol Anat Histopathol* 1992;420:127–129.

289. Newbold KM, Howie AJ, Koram A, ADu D, Michael J. Assessment of glomerular size in renal biopsies including minimal change nephropathy and single kidneys. *J Pathol* 1990;160:255–258.

290. Bonsib SM, Reznicek MJ. Renal biopsy frozen section: a fluorescent study of hematoxylin and eosin-stained sections. *Mod Pathol* 1990;3:204–210.

291. Kaplan C, Pasternak B, Shah H, Gallo G. Age-related incidence of sclerotic glomeruli in human kidneys. *Am J Pathol* 1975;80:227–234.

292. Kappel B, Olsen S. Cortical interstitial tissue and sclerosed glomeruli in the normal human kidney, related to age and sex. A quantitative study. *Virchows Arch A Pathol Anat Histol* 1980;387:271–277.

293. Smith SM, Hoy WE, Cobb L. Low incidence of glomerulosclerosis in normal kidneys. *Arch Pathol Lab Med* 1989;113:1253–1255.

294. Neugarten J, Gallo G, Silbiger S, Kasiske B. Glomerulosclerosis in aging humans is not influenced by gender. *Am J Kidney Dis* 1999;34:884–888.

295. Vasmant D, Maurice M, Feldmann G. Cytoskeleton ultrastructure of podocytes and glomerular endothelial cells in man and in the rat. *Anat Rec* 1984;210:17–24.

296. Sorensson J, Fierlbeck W, Heider T, et al. Glomerular endothelial fenestrae in vivo are not formed from caveolae. *J Am Soc Nephrol* 2002;13:2639–2647.

297. Rostgaard J, Qvortrup K. Electron microscopic demonstrations of filamentous sieve plugs in capillary fenestrae. *Microvasc Res* 1997;53:1–13.

298. Horvat R, Hovoka A, Dekan G, Poczewski H, Kerjaschki D. Endothelial cell membranes contain podocalyxin—the major sialoprotein of visceral glomerular epithelial cells. *J Cell Biol* 1986;102:484–491.

299. Kerjaschki D, Sharkey DJ, Farquhar MG. Identification and characterization of podocalyxin—the major sialoprotein of the renal glomerular epithelial cell. *J Cell Biol* 1984;98:1591–1596.

300. Rostgaard J, Qvortrup K. Sieve plugs in fenestrae of glomerular capillaries—site of the filtration barrier? *Cells Tissue Organs* 2002;170:132–138.

301. Hjalmarsson C, Johansson BR, Haraldsson B. Electron microscopic evaluation of the endothelial surface layer of glomerular capillaries. *Microvas Res* 2004;67:9–17.

302. Ciarimboli G, Hjalmarsson C, Bokenkamp A, Schurek HJ, Haraldsson B. Dynamic alterations of glomerular charge density in fixed rat kidneys suggest involvement of endothelial cell coat. *Am J Physiol Renal Physiol* 2003;285:F722–F730.

303. Jeansson M, Haraldsson B. Morphological and functional evidence for an important role of the endothelial cell glycocalyx in the glomerular barrier. *Am J Physiol Renal Physiol* 2006;290:F111–F116.

304. Roberts WG, Palade GE. Increased microvascular permeability and endothelial fenestration induced by vascular endothelial growth factor. *J Cell Sci* 1995;108(pt 6):2369–2379.

305. Esser S, Wolburg K, Wolburg H, Breier G, Kurzchalia T, Risau W. Vascular endothelial growth factor induces endothelial fenestrations in vitro. *J Cell Biol* 1998;140:947–959.

306. Ballermann BJ. Glomerular endothelial cell differentiation. *Kidney Int* 2005;67:1668–1671.

307. Ballermann BJ, Marsden PA. Endothelium-derived vasoactive mediators and renal glomerular function. *Clin Invest Med* 1991; 14:508–517.

308. Becker CG. Demonstration of actomyosin in mesangial cells of the renal glomerulus. *Am J Pathol* 1972;66:97–110.

309. Drenckhahn D, Schnittler H, Nobiling R, Kriz W. Ultrastructural organization of contractile proteins in rat glomerular mesangial cells. *Am J Pathol* 1990;137:1343–1351.

310. Schlondorff D. The glomerular mesangial cell: an expanding role for a specialized pericyte. *FASEB J* 1987;1:272–281.

311. Sterzel RB, Hartner A, Schlotzer-Schrehardt U, et al. Elastic fiber proteins in the glomerular mesangium in vivo and in cell culture. *Kidney Int* 2000;58:1588–1602.

312. Schaefer L, Mihalik D, Babelova A, et al. Regulation of fibrillin-1 by biglycan and decorin is important for tissue preservation in the kidney during pressure-induced injury. *Am J Pathol* 2004;165: 383–396.

313. Mundel P, Elger M, Sakai T, Kriz W. Microfibrils are a major component of the mesangial matrix in the glomerulus of the rat kidney. *Cell Tissue Res* 1988;254:183–187.

314. Sakai T, Kriz W. The structural relationship between mesangial cells and basement membrane of the renal glomerulus. *Anat Embryol (Berl)* 1987;176:373–386.

315. Kriz W, Elger M, Lemley K, Sakai T. Structure of the glomerular mesangium: a biomechanical interpretation. *Kidney Int Suppl* 1990;30:S2–S9.

316. Kriz W, Elger M, Mundel P, Lemley KV. Structure-stabilizing forces in the glomerular tuft. *J Am Soc Nephol* 1995;5:1731–1739.

317. Michael AF, Keane WF, Raij L, Vernier RL, Mauer SM. The glomerular mesangium. *Kidney Int* 1980;17:141–154.

318. Sterzel RB, Lovett DH. Interactions of inflammatory and glomerular cells in the response to glomerular injury. In: Wilson

CB, Brenner BM, Stein JH, eds. *Immunopathology of Renal Disease.* New York: Churchill Livingstone; 1988:137–173.

319. Schreiner GF, Kiely JM, Cotran RS, Unanue FR. Characterization of resident glomerular cells in the rat expressing Ia determinants and manifesting genetically restricted interactions with lymphocytes. *J Clin Invest* 1981;68:920–931.

320. Falini B, Flenghi L, Pileri S, et al. PG-M1: a new monoclonal antibody directed against a fixative-resistant epitope on the macrophage-restricted form of the CD68 molecule. *Am J Pathol* 1993;142:1359–1372.

321. Imasawa T, Utsunomiya Y, Kawamura T, et al. The potential of bone marrow-derived cells to differentiate to glomerular mesangial cells. *J Am Soc Nephrol* 2001;12:1401–1409.

322. Hall PA, d'Ardenne AJ, Stansfeld AG. Paraffin section immunohistochemistry. I. Non-Hodgkin's lymphoma. *Histopathology* 1988;13:149–160.

323. Streuli M, Morimoto C, Schrieber M, Schlossman SF, Saito H. Characterization of CD45 and CD45R monoclonal antibodies using transfected mouse cell lines that express individual human leukocyte common antigens. *J Immunol* 1988;141:3910–3914.

324. Pulido R, Cebrian M, Acevedo A, de Landazuri MO, Sanchez-Madrid F. Comparative biochemical and tissue distribution study of four distinct CD45 antigen specificities. *J Immunol* 1988;140:3851–3857.

325. Hugo C, Shankland SJ, Bowen-Pope DF, Couser WG, Johnson RJ. Extraglomerular origin of the mesangial cell after injury. A new role of the juxtaglomerular apparatus. *J Clin Invest* 1997;100:786–794.

326. Jorgensen F, Weis Bentzon M. The ultrastructure of the normal human glomerulus; thickness of glomerular basement membranes. *Lab Invest* 1968;18:42–48.

327. Osawa G, Kimmelstiel P, Seiling V. Thickness of glomerular basement membranes. *Am J Clin Pathol* 1966;45:7–20.

328. Osterby R. Morphometric studies of the peripheral glomerular basement membrane in early juvenile diabetes. I. Development of initial basement membrane thickening. *Diabetologia* 1972;8:84–92.

329. Ellis EN, Mauer SM, Sutherland DE, Steffes MW. Glomerular capillary morphology in normal humans. *Lab Invest* 1989;60:231–236.

330. Hudson BG, Reeders ST, Tryggvason K. Type IV collagen: structure, gene organization, and role in human diseases. Molecular basis of Goodpasture and Alport syndromes and diffuse leiomyomatosis. *J Biol Chem* 1993;268:26033–26036.

331. Abrahamson DR, Vanden Heuvel GB, Clapp WL. Nephritogenetic antigens in the glomerular basement membrane. In: Neilson EG, Couser WG, eds. *Immunologic Renal Diseases.* Philadelphia: Lippincott-Raven; 1997:217–234.

332. Hudson BG. The molecular basis of Goodpasture and Alport syndromes: beacons for the discovery of the collagen IV family. *J Am Soc Nephrol* 2004;15:2514–2527.

333. Hudson BG, Tryggvason K, Sundaramoorthy M, Neilson EG. Alport's syndrome, Goodpasture's syndrome, and type IV collagen. *N Eng J Med* 2003;348:2543–2556.

334. Katz A, Fish AJ, Kleppel MM, Hagen SG, Michael AF, Butkowski RJ. Renal entactin (nidogen): isolation, characterization and tissue distribution. *Kidney Int* 1991;40:643–652.

335. Iozzo RV. Basement membrane proteoglycans: from cellar to ceiling. *Nat Rev Mol Cell Biol* 2005;6:646–656.

336. Farquhar MG. The glomerular basement membrane. A selective macromolecular filter. In: Hay ED, ed. *Cell Biology of Extracellular Matrix.* 2nd ed. New York: Plenum; 1991:365–418.

337. Mahan JD, Sisson-Ross SS, Vernier RL. Anionic sites in the human kidney: ex vivo perfusion studies. *Mod Pathol* 1989;2:117–124.

338. Groffen AJ, Ruegg MA, Dijkman H, et al. Agrin is a major heparan sulfate proteoglycan in the human glomerular basement membrane. *J Histochem Cytochem* 1998;46:19–27.

339. Halfter W, Dong S, Schurer B, Cole GJ. Collagen XVIII is a basement membrane heparan sulfate proteoglycan. *J Biol Chem* 1998;273:25404–25412.

340. Groffen AJ, Hop FW, Tryggvason K, et al. Evidence for the existence of multiple heparan sulfate proteoglycans in the human

glomerular basement membrane and mesangial matrix. *Eur J Biochem* 1997;247:175–182.

341. McCarthy KJ, Bynum K, St John PL, Abrahamson DR, Couchman JR. Basement membrane proteoglycans in glomerular morphogenesis: chondroitin sulfate proteoglycan is temporally and spatially restricted during development. *J Histochem Cytochem* 1993;41:401–414.

342. Arakawa M. A scanning electron microscope of the human glomerulus. *Am J Pathol* 1971;64:457–466.

343. Neal CR, Crook H, Bell E, Harper SJ, Bates DO. Three-dimensional reconstruction of glomeruli by electron microscopy reveals a distinct restrictive urinary subpodocyte space. *J Am Soc Nephrol* 2005;16:1223–1235.

344. Gautier A, Bernhard W, Oberling C. [The existence of a pericapillary lacunar apparatus in the malpighian glomeruli revealed by electronic microscopy]. *CR Seances Soc Biol Fil* 1950;144:1605–1607.

345. Andrews PM, Bates SB. Filamentous actin bundles in the kidney. *Anat Rec* 1984;210:1–9.

346. Drenckhahn D, Franke R. Ultrastructural organization of contractile and cytoskeletal proteins in glomerular podocytes of chicken, rat, and man. *Lab Invest* 1988;59:673–682.

347. Holthofer H, Miettinen A, Lehto V, Lehtonen E, Virtanen I. Expression of vimentin and cytokeratin types of intermediate filament proteins in developing and adult human kidneys. *Lab Invest* 1984;50:552–529.

348. Pavenstadt H, Kriz W, Kretzler M. Cell biology of the glomerular podocyte. *Physiol Rev* 2003;83:253–307.

349. Abrahamson D. Structure and development of the glomerular capillary wall and basement membrane. *Am J Physiol* 1987;253(pt 2):F783–F794.

350. Rodewald R, Karnovsky MJ. Porous substructure of the glomerular slit diaphragm in the rat and mouse. *J Cell Biol* 1974;60:423–433.

351. Karnovsky MJ, Ryan GB. Substructure of the glomerular slit diaphragm in freeze-fractured normal rat kidney. *J Cell Biol* 1975;65:233–236.

352. Schneeberger EE, Levey RH, McCluskey RT, Karnovsky MJ. The isoporous substructure of the human glomerular slit diaphragm. *Kidney Int* 1975;8:48–52.

353. Wartiovaara J, Ofverstedt L-G, Khoshnoodi J, et al. Nephrin strands contribute to a porous slit diaphragm scaffold as revealed by electron tomography. *J Clin Invest* 2004; 114:1475–1483.

354. Schnabel E, Anderson JM, Farquhar MG. The tight junction protein ZO-1 is concentrated along slit diaphragms of the glomerular epithelium. *J Cell Biol* 1990;111:1255–1263.

355. Reiser J, Kriz W, Kretzler M, Mundel P. The glomerular slit diaphragm is a modified adherens junction. *J Am Soc Nephrol* 2000;11:1–8.

356. Kerjaschki D. Caught flat-footed: podocyte damage and the molecular bases of focal glomerulosclerosis. *J Clin Invest* 2001;108:1583–1587.

357. Ruotsalainen V, Ljungberg P, Wartiovaara J, et al. Nephrin is specifically located at the slit diaphragm of glomerular podocytes. *Proc Natl Acad Sci U S A* 1999;96:7962–7967.

358. Huber TB, Benzing T. The slit diaphragm: a signaling platform to regulate podocyte function. *Curr Opin Nephrol Hypertens* 2005;14:211–216.

359. Lehtonen S, Ryan JJ, Kudlicka K, Iino N, Zhou H, Farquhar MG. Cell junction-associated proteins IQGAP1, MAGI-2, CASK, spectrins, and alpha-actinin are components of the nephrin multiprotein complex. *Proc Natl Acad Sci U S A* 2005;102:9814–9819.

360. Hirabayashi S, Mori H, Kansaku A, et al. MAGI-1 is a component of the glomerular slit diaphragm that is tightly associated with nephrin. *Lab Invest* 2005;85:1528–1543.

361. Gerke P, Huber TB, Sellin L, Benzing T, Walz G. Homodimerization and heterodimerization of the glomerular podocyte proteins nephrin and NEPH1. *J Am Soc Nephrol* 2003;14:918–926.

362. Khoshnoodi J, Sigmundsson K, Ofverstedt L-G, et al. Nephrin promotes cell-cell adhesion through homophilic interactions. *Am J Pathol* 2003;163:2337–2346.

363. Barletta GM, Kovari IA, Verma RK, Kerjaschki D, Holzman LB. Nephrin and Neph1 co-localize at the podocyte foot process

intercellular junction and form cis hetero-oligomers. *J Biol Chem* 2003;278:19266–19271.

364. Liu G, Kaw B, Kurfis J, Rahmanuddin S, Kanwar YS, Chugh SS. Neph1 and nephrin interaction in the slit diaphragm is an important determinant of glomerular permeability. *J Clin Invest* 2003;112:209–221.

365. Gerke P, Sellin L, Kretz O, et al. NEPH2 is located at the glomerular slit diaphragm, interacts with nephrin and is cleaved from podocytes by metalloproteinases. *J Am Soc Nephrol* 2005;16: 1693–1702.

366. Oh J, Reiser J, Mundel P. Dynamic (re)organization of the podocyte actin cytoskeleton in the nephrotic syndrome. *Pediatr Nephrol* 2004;19:130–137.

367. Asanuma K, Kim K, Oh J, et al. Synaptopodin regulates the actin-bundling activity of alpha-actinin in an isoform-specific manner. *J Clin Invest* 2005;115:1188–1198.

368. Benzing T. Signaling at the slit diaphragm. *J Am Soc Nephrol* 2004;15:1382–1391.

369. Huber TB, Hartleben B, Kim J, et al. Nephrin and CD2AP associate with phosphoinositide-3-OH kinase and stimulate AKT-dependent signaling. *Mol Cell Biol* 2003;23:4917–4928.

370. Kerjaschki D, Ojha PP, Susani M, et al. A beta1-integrin receptor for fibronectin in human kidney glomeruli. *Am J Pathol* 1989; 134:481–489.

371. Regele HM, Fillipovic E, Langer B, et al. Glomerular expression of dystroglycans is reduced in minimal change nephrosis but not in focal segmental glomerulosclerosis. *J Am Soc Nephrol* 2000;11: 403–412.

372. Hannigan GE, Leung-Hagesteijn C, Fitz-Gibbon L, et al. Regulation of cell adhesion and anchorage-dependent growth by a new beta1-integrin-linked protein kinase. *Nature* 1996; 379:91–96.

373. Barisoni L, Mundel P. Podocyte biology and the emerging understanding of podocyte diseases. *Am J Nephrol* 2003;23:353–360.

374. Sawada H, Stukenbrok H, Kerjaschki D, Farquhar MG. Epithelial polyanion (podocalyxin) is found on the sides but not the soles of the foot processes of the glomerular epithelium. *Am J Pathol* 1986;125:309–318.

375. Wiggins RC, Wiggins JE, Goyal M, Wharram BL, Thomas PE. Molecular cloning of cDNAs encoding human GLEPP1, a membrane protein tyrosine phosphatase: characterization of the GLEPP1 protein distribution in human kidney and assignment of the GLEPP1 gene to human chromosome 12p 12-p13. *Genomics* 1995;27:174–181.

376. Takeda T, McQuistan T, Orlando RA, Farquhar MG. Loss of glomerular foot processes is associated with uncoupling of podocalyxin from the actin cytoskeleton. *J Clin Invest* 2001;108: 289–301.

377. Orlando RA, Takeda T, Zak B, et al. The glomerular epithelial cell anti-adhesin podocalyxin associates with the actin cytoskeleton through interactions with ezrin. *J Am Soc Nephrol* 2001;12:1589–1598.

378. Stamenkovic I, Skalli O, Gabbiani G. Distribution of intermediate filament proteins in normal and diseased human glomeruli. *Am J Pathol* 1986;125:465–475.

379. Moll R, Hage C, Thoenes W. Expression of intermediate filament proteins in fetal and adult human kidney. Modulations of intermediate filament patterns during development and in damaged tissue. *Lab Invest* 1991;65:74–86.

380. Oosterwijk E, van Muijen GNP, Oosterwijk-Wakka JC, Warnaar SO. Expression of intermediate-sized filaments in developing and adult human kidney and in renal cell carcinoma. *J Histochem Cytochem* 1990;38:385–392.

381. Yaoita E, Franke WW, Yamamoto T, Kawasaki K, Kihara I. Identification of renal podocytes in multiple species: higher vertebrates are vimentin positive/lower vertebrates are desmin positive. *Histochem Cell Biol* 1999;111:107–115.

382. Floege J, Alpers CE, Sage EH, et al. Markers of complement-dependent and complement-independent glomerular visceral epithelial injury in vivo. Expression of antiadhesive proteins and cytoskeletal changes. *Lab Invest* 1992;67:486–497.

383. Pritchard-Jones K, Fleming S, Davidson D, et al. The candidate Wilms' tumor gene is involved in genitourinary development. *Nature* 1990;346:194–197.

384. Mundlos S, Pelletier J, Darveau A, Bachmann M, Winterpacht A, Zabel B. Nuclear localization of the protein encoded by the Wilms' tumor gene WT1 in embryonic and adult tissues. *Development* 1993;119:1329–1341.

385. Pelletier J, Bruening W, Kashtan CE. Germline mutations in the Wilms' tumor suppressor gene are associated with abnormal urogenital development in Denys-Drash syndrome. *Cell* 1991;67: 437–447.

386. Drummond MC, Deen WM. Structural determinants of glomerular hydraulic permeability. *Am J Physiol* 1994;266(pt 2):F1–F12.

387. Edwards A, Daniels BS, Deen WM. Ultrastructural model for size selectivity in glomerular filtration. *Am J Physiol* 1999;276(pt 2): F892–F902.

388. Kanwar YS, Liu ZZ, Kashihara N, Wallner EI. Current status of the structural and functional basis of glomerular filtration and proteinuria. *Semin Nephrol* 1991;11:390–413.

389. Rossi M, Morita H, Sormunen R, et al. Heparan sulfate chains of perlecan are indispensable in the lens capsule but not in the kidney. *EMBO J* 2003;22:236–245.

390. Gelberg H, Healy L, Whiteley H, Miller LA, Vimr E. In vivo enzymatic removal of alpha 2—6-linked sialic acid from the glomerular filtration barrier results in podocyte charge alteration and glomerular injury. *Lab Invest* 1996;74:907–920.

391. Deen WM, Lazzara MJ, Myers BD. Structural determinants of glomerular permeability. *Am J Physiol Renal Physiol* 2001;281: F579–F596.

392. Haraldsson B, Sorensson J. Why do we not all have proteinuria? An update of our current understanding of the glomerular barrier. *News Physiol Sci* 2004;19:7–10.

393. Tryggvason K, Wartiovaara J. How does the kidney filter plasma? *Physiology (Bethesda)* 2005;20:96–101.

394. Dijkman H, Smeets B, van der Laak J, Steenbergen E, Wetzels J. The parietal epithelial cell is crucially involved in human idiopathic focal segmental glomerulosclerosis. *Kidney Int* 2005;68: 1562–1572.

395. Ohtaka A, Ootaka T, Sato H, Ito S. Phenotypic change of glomerular podocytes in primary focal segmental glomerulosclerosis: developmental paradigm? *Nephrol Dial Transplant* 2002; 17(suppl 9):11–15.

396. Peissel B, Geng L, Kalluri R, et al. Comparative distribution of the alpha 1(IV), alpha 5(IV), and alpha 6(IV) collagen chains in normal human adult and fetal tissues and in kidneys from X-linked Alport syndrome patients. *J Clin Invest* 1995;96:1948–1957.

397. Couchman JR, Kapoor R, Sthanam M, Wu RR. Perlecan and basement membrane-chondroitin sulfate proteoglycan (bamacan) are two basement membrane chondroitin/dermatan sulfate proteoglycans in the Engelbreth-Holm-Swarm tumor matrix. *J Biol Chem* 1996;271:9595–9602.

398. Ryan GB, Coghlan JP, Scoggins BA. The granulated peripolar epithelial cell: a potential secretory component of the renal juxtaglomerular complex. *Nature* 1979;277:655–656.

399. Gall JA, Alcorn D, Butkus A, Coghlan JP, Ryan GB. Distribution of glomerular peripolar cells in different mammalian species. *Cell Tissue Res* 1986;244:203–208.

400. Gardiner DS, Lindop GB. The granular peripolar cell of the human glomerulus: a new component of the juxtaglomerular apparatus? *Histopathology* 1985;9:675–685.

401. Ryan GB, Alcorn D, Coghlan JP, Hill PA, Jacobs R. Ultrastructural morphology of granule release from juxtaglomerular myoepithelioid and peripolar cells. *Kidney Int Suppl* 1982;12:S3–S8.

402. Golgi C. Annotazioni intorno all'istologia dei reni dell'uomo e di altri mammiferi e sull'istogenesi: dei canalicoli oriniferi. *Atti R Accad Naz Lincei Rendiconti* 1889;5:337–342.

403. Barajas L. Anatomy of the juxtaglomerular apparatus. *Am J Physiol* 1979;237:F333–F343.

404. Barajas L, Bloodworth JMB Jr, Hartroft PM. Endocrine pathology of the kidney. In: Bloodworth JMB Jr, ed. *Endocrine Pathology: General and Surgical.* 2nd ed. Baltimore: Williams & Wilkins; 1982:723–766.

405. Barajas L, Salido EC, Smolens P, Hart D, Stein JH. Pathology of the juxtaglomerular apparatus including Bartter's syndrome. In: Tisher CC, Brenner BM, eds. *Renal Pathology with Clinical and Functional Correlations.* 2nd ed. Philadelphia: JB Lippincott; 1994:948–978.

406. Cantin M, Gutkowska J, Lacasse J, et al. Ultrastructural immunocytochemical localization of renin and angiotensin II in the juxtaglomerular cells of the ischemic kidney in experimental renal hypertension. *Am J Pathol* 1984;115:212–224.

407. Taugner R, Mannek E, Nobiling R, et al. Coexistence of renin and angiotensin II in epithelioid cell secretory granules of rat kidney. *Histochemistry* 1984;81:39–45.

408. Barajas L, Wang P. Localization of tritiated norepinephrine in the renal arteriolar nerves. *Anat Rec* 1979;195:525–534.

409. Kopp UC, DiBona GF. Neural regulation of renin secretion. *Semin Nephrol* 1993;13:543–551.

410. Pricam C, Humbert F, Perrelet A, Orci L. Gap junctions in mesangial and lacis cells. *J Cell Biol* 1974;63:349–354.

411. Taugner R, Schiller A, Kaissling B, KRiz W. Gap junctional coupling between the JGA and the glomerular tuft. *Cell Tissue Res* 1978;186:279–285.

412. Kaissling B, Kriz W. Variability of intercellular spaces between macula densa cells: a transmission electron microscopic study in rabbits and rats. *Kidney Int Suppl* 1982;12:S9–S17.

413. Salido EC, Barajas L, Lechago J, Laborde NP, Fisher DA. Immunocytochemical localization of epidermal growth factor in mouse kidney. *J Histochem Cytochem* 1986;34:1155–1160.

414. Sikri KL, Foster CL, MacHugh N, Marshall RD. Localization of Tamm-Horsfall glycoprotein in the human kidney using immunofluorescence and immunoelectron microscopical techniques. *J Anat* 1981;132(pt 4):597–605.

415. Kirk KL, Bell PD, Barfuss DW, Ribadeneira M. Direct visualization of the isolated and perfused macula densa. *Am J Physiol* 1985;248(pt 2):F890–F894.

416. Schnermann J. Homer W. Smith Award lecture. The juxtaglomerular apparatus: from anatomical peculiarity to physiological relevance. *J Am Soc Nephrol* 2003;14:1681–1694.

417. Wilcox CS, Welch WJ, Murad F, et al. Nitric oxide synthase in macula densa regulates glomerular capillary pressure. *Proc Natl Acad Sci U S A* 1992;89:11993–11997.

418. Mundel P, Bachmann S, Bader M, et al. Expression of nitric oxide synthase in kidney macula densa cells. *Kidney Int* 1992;42:1017–1019.

419. Harris RC, McKanna JA, Akai Y, Jacobson HR, Dubois RN, Breyer MD. Cyclooxygenase-2 is associated with the macula densa of rat kidney and increases with salt restriction. *J Clin Invest* 1994;94:2504–2510.

420. Welch WJ, Wilcox CS, Thomson SC. Nitric oxide and tubuloglomerular feedback. *Semin Nephrol* 1999;19:251–262.

421. Harris RC, Breyer MD. Physiological regulation of cyclooxygenase-2 in the kidney. *Am J Physiol Renal Physiol* 2001;281:F1–F11.

422. Rouiller C. General anatomy and histology of the kidney. In: Rouiller C, Muller AF, eds. *The Kidney: Morphology, Biochemistry, Physiology*. New York: Academic Press; 1969:61–156.

423. Swann HG. The functional distention of the kidney: a review. *Tex Rep Biol Med* 1960;18:566–595.

424. Hodson CJ. Physiological changes in size of the human kidney. *Clin Radiol* 1961;12:91–94.

425. Parker MV, Swann HG, Sinclair JG. The functional morphology of the kidney. *Tex Rep Biol Med* 1962;20:425–445.

426. Faraggiana T, Malchiodi F, Prado A, Churg J. Lectin-peroxidase conjugate reactivity in normal human kidney. *J Histochem Cytochem* 1982;30:451–458.

427. Hennigar RA, Schulte BA, Spicer SS. Heterogeneous distribution of glycoconjugates in human kidney tubules. *Anat Rec* 1985;211:376–390.

428. Silva FG, Nadasdy T, Laszik Z. Immunohistochemical and lectin dissection of the human nephron in health and disease. *Arch Pathol Lab Med* 1993;117:1233–1239.

429. Skinnider BF, Folpe AL, Hennigar RA, et al. Distribution of cytokeratins and vimentin in adult renal neoplasms and normal renal tissue: potential utility of a cytokeratin antibody panel in the differential diagnosis of renal tumors. *Am J Surg Pathol* 2005;29:747–754.

430. Paul R, Ewing CM, Robinson JC, et al. Cadherin-6, a cell adhesion molecule specifically expressed in the proximal renal tubule and renal cell carcinoma. *Cancer Res* 1997;57:2741–2748.

431. Maunsbach AB, Christensen EI. Functional ultrastructure of the proximal tubule. In: Windhager EE, ed. *Handbook of Physiology. Renal Physiology*. New York: Oxford University Press; 1992:41–107.

432. Tisher CC, Bulger RE, Trump BF. Human renal ultrastructure. I. Proximal tubule of healthy individuals. *Lab Invest* 1966;15:1357–1394.

433. Moe OW, Baum M, Berry CA, et al. Renal transport of glucose, amino acids, sodium, chloride and water. In: Brenner BM, ed. *Brenner & Rector's The Kidney*. 7th ed. Philadelphia: WB Saunders; 2004:413–452.

434. Welling LW, Welling DJ. Shape of epithelial cells and intercellular channels in the rabbit proximal nephron. *Kidney Int* 1976;9:385–394.

435. Welling LW, Welling DJ. Relationship between structure and function in renal proximal tubule. *J Electron Microsc Tech* 1988;9:171–185.

436. Ahn KY, Madsen KM, Tisher CC, Kone BC. Differential expression and cellular distribution of mRNAs encoding alpha- and beta-isoforms of Na^+-K^+-ATPase in rat kidney. *Am J Physiol* 1993;265(pt 2):F792–F801.

437. Clapp WL, Bowman P, Shaw GS, Patel P, Kone BC. Segmental localization of mRNAs encoding Na^+-K^+-ATPase alpha- and beta-subunit isoforms in rat kidney using RT-PCR. *Kidney Int* 1994;46:627–638.

438. Biemesderfer D, Pizzonia J, Abu-Alfa A, et al. NHE3: a Na^+/H^+ exchanger isoform of renal brush border. *Am J Physiol* 1993;265(pt 2):F736–F742.

439. Amemiya M, Loffing J, Lotscher M, Kaissling B, Alpern RJ, Moe OW. Expression of NHE-3 in the apical membrane of rat renal proximal tubule and thick ascending limb. *Kidney Int* 1995;48:1206–1215.

440. Agre P, King LS, Yasui M, et al. Aquaporin water channels—from atomic structure to clinical medicine. *J Physiol* 2002;542(pt 1):3–16.

441. King LS, Kozono D, Agre P. From structure to disease: the evolving tale of aquaporin biology. *Nat Rev Mol Cell Biol* 2004;5:687–698.

442. Nielsen S, Smith BL, Christensen EI, Knepper MA, Agre P. CHIP28 water channels are localized in constitutively water-permeable segments of the nephron. *J Cell Biol* 1993;120:371–383.

443. Maunsbach AB, Marples D, Chin E, et al. Aquaporin-1 water channel expression in human kidney. *J Am Soc Nephrol* 1997;8:1–14.

444. Maack T. Renal filtration, transport, and metabolism of proteins. In: Seldin D, Giebisch G, eds. *The Kidney: Physiology and Pathophysiology*. 3rd ed. Philadelphia: Lippincott Williams & Wilkins; 2000:2235–2267.

445. Christensen EI, Rennke HG, Carone FA. Renal tubular uptake of protein: effect of molecular charge. *Am J Physiol* 1983;244:F436–F441.

446. Park CH, Maack T. Albumin absorption and catabolism by isolated perfused proximal convoluted tubules of the rabbit. *J Clin Invest* 1984;73:767–777.

447. Park CH. Time course and vectorial nature of albumin metabolism in isolated perfused rabbit PCT. *Am J Physiol* 1988;255(pt 2):F520–F528.

448. Clapp WL, Park CH, Madsen KM, Tisher CC. Axial heterogeneity in the handling of albumin by the rabbit proximal tubule. *Lab Invest* 1988;58:549–558.

449. Larsson L, Clapp WL III, Park CH, Cannon JK, Tisher CC. Ultrastructural localization of acidic compartments in cells of isolated rabbit PCT. *Am J Physiol* 1987;253(pt 2):F95–F103.

450. Christensen EI. Rapid membrane recycling in renal proximal tubule cells. *Eur J Cell Biol* 1982;29:43–49.

451. Christensen EI, Birn H. Megalin and cubilin: synergistic endocytic receptors in renal proximal tubule. *Am J Physiol Renal Physiol* 2001;280:F562–F573.

452. Birn H, Fyfe JC, Jacobsen C, et al. Cubilin is an albumin binding protein important for renal tubular albumin reabsorption. *J Clin Invest* 2000;105:1353–1361.

453. Christensen EI, Birn H. Megalin and cubilin: multifunctional endocytic receptors. *Nat Rev Mol Cell Biol* 2002;3:256–266.

454. Olsen S, Solez K. Acute tubular necrosis and toxic renal injury. In: Tisher CC, Brenner BM, eds. *Renal Pathology with Clinical and Functional Correlations*. 2nd ed. Philadelphia: JB Lippincott; 1994:769–809.

455. Nadasdy NT, Laszik Z, Blick KE, Johnson LD, Silva FG. Proliferative activity of intrinsic cell populations in the normal human kidney. *J Am Soc Nephrol* 1994;4:2032–2039.

456. Droz D, Zachar D, Charbit L, Gogusev J, Chretein Y, Iris L. Expression of the human nephron differentiation molecules in renal cell carcinomas. *Am J Pathol* 1990;137:895–905.

457. Gerdes J, Becker MHG, Key G, Cattoretti G. Immunohistochemical detection of tumor growth fraction (Ki-67 antigen) in formalin-fixed and routinely processed tissues. *J Pathol* 1992; 168:85–86.

458. Witzgall R, Brown D, Schwarz C, Bonventre JV. Localization of proliferating cell nuclear antigen, vimentin, c-Fos, and clusterin in the postischemic kidney. Evidence for a heterogenous genetic response among nephron segments, and a large pool of mitotically active and dedifferentiated cells. *J Clin Invest* 1994;93: 2175–2188.

459. Kliem V, Johnson RJ, Alpers CE, et al. Mechanisms involved in the pathogenesis of tubulointerstitial fibrosis in 5/6-nephrectomized rats. *Kidney Int* 1996;49:666–678.

460. Gobe GC, Axelsen RA. Genesis of renal tubular atrophy in experimental hydronephrosis in the rat. Role of apoptosis. *Lab Invest* 1987;56:273–281.

461. Gobe GC, Axelsen RA, Searle JW. Cellular events in experimental unilateral ischemic renal atrophy and in regeneration after contralateral nephrectomy. *Lab Invest* 1990; 63:770–779.

462. Schumer M, Colombel MC, Sawczuk IS, et al. Morphologic, biochemical, and molecular evidence of apoptosis during the reperfusion phase after brief periods of renal ischemia. *Am J Pathol* 1992;140:831–838.

463. Shimizu A, Yamanaka N. Apoptosis and cell desquamation in repair process of ischemic tubular necrosis. *Virchows Arch B Cell Pathol Incl Mol Pathol* 1993;64:171–180.

464. Dieterich HJ, Barrett JM, Kriz W, Bulhoff JP. The ultrastructure of the thin loop limbs of the mouse kidney. *Anat Embryol (Berl)* 1975;147:1–18.

465. Bulger RE, Tisher CC, Myers CH, Trump BF. Human renal ultrastructure. II. The thin limb of Henle's loop and the interstitium in healthy individuals. *Lab Invest* 1967;16:124–141.

466. Knepper MA, Gamba G. Urine concentration and dilution. In: Brenner BM, ed. *Brenner & Rector's The Kidney*. 7th ed. Philadelphia: WB Saunders; 2004:599–636.

467. Nielsen S, Pallone T, Snith BL, Christensen EI, Agre P, Maunsbach AB. Aquaporin-1 water channels in short and long loop descending thin limbs and in descending vasa recta in rat kidney. *Am J Physiol* 1995;268(pt 2):F1023–F1037.

468. Uchida S, Sasaki S, Nitta K, et al. Localization and functional characterization of rat kidney-specific chloride channel, C1C-K1. *J Clin Invest* 1995;95:104–113.

469. Takeuchi Y, Uchida S, Marumo F, Sasaki S. Cloning, tissue distribution, and intrarenal localization of C1C chloride channels in human kidney. *Kidney Int* 1995;48:1497–1503.

470. Ma T, Yang B, Gillespie A, Carlson EJ, Epstein CJ, Verkman AS. Severely impaired urinary concentrating ability in transgenic mice lacking aquaporin-1 water channels. *J Biol Chem* 1998;273: 4296–4299.

471. King LS, Choi M, Fernandez PC, Cartron JP, Agre P. Defective urinary-concentrating ability due to a complete deficiency of aquaporin-1. *N Eng J Med* 2001;345:175–179.

472. Matsumura Y, Uchida S, Kondo Y, et al. Overt nephrogenic diabetes insipidus in mice lacking the CLC-K1 chloride channel. *Nat Genet* 1999;21:95–98.

473. Kokko JP, Rector FC Jr. Countercurrent multiplication system without active transport in inner medulla. *Kidney Int* 1972;2: 214–223.

474. Stephenson JL. Concentration of urine in a central core model of the renal counterflow system. *Kidney Int* 1972;2:85–94.

475. Kone BC, Madsen KM, Tisher CC. Ultrastructure of the thick ascending limb of Henle in the rat kidney. *Am J Anat* 1984;171: 217–226.

476. Allen F, Tisher CC. Morphology of the ascending thick limb of Henle. *Kidney Int* 1976;9:8–22.

477. Shen SS, Krishna B, Chirala R, Amato RJ, Truong LD. Kidney-specific cadherin, a specific marker for the distal portion of the nephron and related renal neoplasms. *Mod Pathol* 2005;18: 933–940.

478. Garg LC, Knepper MA, Burg MB. Mineralocorticoid effects on Na-K-ATPase in individual nephron segments. *Am J Physiol* 1981;240:F536–F544.

479. Nielsen S, Maunsbach AB, Ecelbarger CA, Knepper MA. Ultrastructural localization of Na-K-2Cl cotransporter in thick ascending limb and macula densa of rat kidney. *Am J Physiol* 1998;275(pt 2):F885–F893.

480. Bachmann S, Velazquez H, Obermuller N, Reilly RF, Moser D, Ellison DH. Expression of the thiazide-sensitive Na-Cl cotransporter by rabbit distal convoluted tubule cells. *J Clin Invest* 1995;96:2510–2514.

481. Plotkin MD, Kaplan MR, Verlander JW, et al. Localization of the thiazide-sensitive Na-Cl cotransporter, rTSC1, in the rat kidney. *Kidney Int* 1996;50:174–183.

482. Woodhall PB, Tisher CC. Response of the distal tubule and cortical collecting duct to vasopressin in the rat. *J Clin Invest* 1973;52:3095–3108.

483. Gross JB, Imai M, Kokko JP. A functional comparison of the cortical collecting tubule and the distal convoluted tubule. *J Clin Invest* 1975;55:1284–1294.

484. Kaissling B. Structural aspects of adaptive changes in renal electrolyte excretion. *Am J Physiol* 1982;243:F211–F226.

485. Myers CE, Bulger RE, Tisher CC, Trump BF. Human ultrastructure. IV. Collecting duct of healthy individuals. *Lab Invest* 1966; 15:1921–1950.

486. Kaissling B, Kriz W. Structural analysis of the rabbit kidney. *Adv Anat Embryol Cell Biol* 1979;56:1–123.

487. Vio CP, Figueroa CD. Subcellular localization of renal kallikrein by ultrastructural immunocytochemistry. *Kidney Int* 1985;28: 36–42.

488. Barajas L, Powers K, Carretero O, Scicli AG, Inagami T. Immunocytochemical localization of renin and kallikrein in the rat renal cortex. *Kidney Int* 1986;29:965–970.

489. Mennitt PA, Wade JB, Ecelbarger CA, Palmer LG, Frindt G. Localization of ROMK channels in the rat kidney. *J Am Soc Nephrol* 1997;8:1823–1830.

490. Xu JZ, Hall AF, Peterson LN, Bienkowski MJ, Eessalu TE, Hebert SC. Localization of the ROMK protein on apical membranes of rat kidney nephron segments. *Am J Physiol* 1997;273(pt 2): F739–F748.

491. Reilly RF, Shugrue CA, Lattanzi D, Biemesderfer D. Immunolocalization of the Na^+/Ca^{2+} exchanger in rabbit kidney. *Am J Physiol Renal Physiol* 1993;265:F327–F332.

492. Borke JL, Caride A, Verma AK, Penniston JT, Kumar R. Plasma membrane calcium pump and 28-kDa calcium binding protein in cells of rat kidney distal tubules. *Am J Physiol* 1989;257(pt 2): F842–F849.

493. Fine LG. Eustachio's discovery of the renal tubule. *Am J Nephrol* 1986;6:47–50.

494. Welling LW, Evan AP, Welling DJ. Shape of cells and extracellular channels in rabbit cortical collecting ducts. *Kidney Int* 1981;20: 211–222.

495. Duc C, Farman N, Canessa CM, Bonvalet JP, Rossier BC. Cell-specific expression of epithelial sodium channel alpha, beta, and gamma subunits in aldosterone-responsive epithelia from the rat: localization by in situ hybridization and immunocytochemistry. *J Cell Biol* 1994;127(pt 2):1907–1921.

496. Hager H, Kwon TH, Vinnikova AK, et al. Immunocytochemical and immunoelectron microscopic localization of alpha-, beta-, and gamma-ENaC in rat kidney. *Am J Physiol Renal Physiol* 2001;280:F1093–F1096.

497. Stanton BA, Biemesderfer D, Wade JB, Giebisch G. Structural and functional study of the rat nephron: effects of potassium adaptation and depletion. *Kidney Int* 1981;19:36–48.

498. Petty KJ, Kokko JP, Marver D. Secondary effect of aldosterone on Na-KATPase activity in the rabbit cortical collecting tubule. *J Clin Invest* 1981;68:1514–1521.

499. Mujais SK, Chekal MA, Jones WJ, Hayslett JP, Katz AI. Regulation of renal Na-K-ATPase in the rat: Role of the natural mineralo- and glucocorticoid hormones. *J Clin Invest* 1984;73:13–19.

500. Kaissling B, Le Hir M. Distal tubular segments of the rabbit kidney after adaptation to altered Na- and K-intake. I. Structural changes. *Cell Tissue Res* 1982;224:469–492.

501. Wade JB, O'Neil RG, Pryor JL, Boulpaep EL. Modulation of cell membrane area in renal collecting tubules by corticosteroid hormones. *J Cell Biol* 1979;81:439–445.

502. Kirk KL, Buku A, Eggena P. Cell specificity of vasopressin binding in renal collecting duct: computer-enhanced imaging of a fluorescent hormone analog. *Proc Natl Acad Sci U S A* 1987;84:6000–6004.

503. Nielsen S, DiGiovanni SR, Christensen EI, Knepper MA, Harris HW. Cellular and subcellular immunolocalization of vasopressin-regulated water channel in rat kidney. *Proc Natl Acad Sci U S A* 1993;90:11663–11667.

504. Nielsen S, Chou CL, Marples D, Christensen EI, Kishore BK, Knepper MA. Vasopressin increases water permeability of kidney collecting duct by inducing translocation of aquaporin-CD water channels to plasma membrane. *Proc Natl Acad Sci U S A* 1995;92:1013–1017.

505. Ecelbarger CA, Terris J, Frindt G, et al. Aquaporin-3 water channel localization and regulation in rat kidney. *Am J Physiol* 1995;269(pt 2):F663–F672.

506. Hasegawa H, Ma T, Skach W, Matthay MA, Verkman AS. Molecular cloning of a mercurial-insensitive water channel expressed in selected water-transporting tissues. *J Biol Chem* 1994;269:5497–5500.

507. Schuster VL, Bonsib SM, Jennings ML. Two types of collecting duct mitochondria-rich (intercalated) cells: lectin and band 3 cytochemistry. *Am J Physiol* 1986;251(pt 1):C347–C355.

508. Verlander JW, Madsen KM, Tisher CC. Effect of acute respiratory acidosis on two populations of intercalated cells in the rat cortical collecting duct. *Am J Physiol* 1987;253(pt 2):F1142–F1156.

509. Teng-umnuay P, Verlander JW, Yuan W, Tisher CC, Madsen KM. Identification of distinct subpopulations of intercalated cells in the mouse collecting duct. *J Am Soc Nephrol* 1996;7:260–274.

510. Kim J, Kim YH, Cha JH, Tisher CC, Madsen KM. Intercalated cell subtypes in connecting tubule and cortical collecting duct of rat and mouse. *J Am Soc Nephrol* 1999;10:1–12.

511. Lonnerholm G. Histochemical demonstration of carbonic anhydrase activity in the human kidney. *Acta Physiol Scand* 1973;88:455–468.

512. McKinney TD, Burg MB. Bicarbonate absorption by rabbit cortical collecting tubules in vitro. *Am J Physiol* 1978;234:F141–F145.

513. McKinney TD, Burg MB. Bicarbonate secretion by rabbit cortical collecting tubules in vitro. *J Clin Invest* 1978;61:1421–1427.

514. Brown D, Gluck S, Hartwig J. Structure of the novel membrane-coating material in proton-secreting epithelial cells and identification as an H^+ATPase. *J Cell Biol* 1987;105:1637–1648.

515. Brown D, Hirsh S, Gluck S. An H^+-ATPase in opposite plasma membrane domains in kidney epithelial cell subpopulations. *Nature* 1988;331:622–624.

516. Alper SL, Natale J, Gluck S, Lodfish HF, Brown D. Subtypes of intercalated cells in rat kidney collecting duct defined by antibodies against erythroid band 3 and renal vacuolar H^+-ATPase. *Proc Natl Acad Sci U S A* 1989;86:5429–5433.

517. Drenckhahn D, Schluter K, Allen DP, Bennett V. Colocalization of band 3 with ankyrin and spectrin at the basal membrane of intercalated cells in the rat kidney. *Science* 1985;230:1287–1289.

518. Verlander JW, Madsen KM, Low PS, Allen DP, Tisher CC. Immunocytochemical localization of band 3 protein in the rat collecting duct. *Am J Physiol* 1988;255(pt 2):F115–F125.

519. Weiner ID, Hamm LL. Regulation of intracellular pH in the rabbit cortical collecting tubule. *J Clin Invest* 1990;85:274–281.

520. Royaux IE, Wall SM, Karniski LP, et al. Pendrin, encoded by the Pendred syndrome gene, resides in the apical region of renal intercalated cells and mediates bicarbonate secretion. *Proc Natl Acad Sci U S A* 2001;98:4221–4226.

521. Soleimani M, Greeley T, Petrovic S, et al. Pendrin: an apical $Cl^-/OH^-/HCO_3^-$ exchanger in the kidney cortex. *Am J Physiol Renal Physiol* 2001;280:F356–F364.

522. Kim YH, Kwon TH, Frische S, et al. Immunocytochemical localization of pendrin in intercalated cell subtypes in rat and mouse kidney. *Am J Physiol Renal Physiol* 2002;283:F744–F754.

523. Frische S, Kwon TH, Frokiaer J, Madsen KM, Nielsen S. Regulated expression of pendrin in rat kidney in response to chronic NH_4Cl or $NaHCO_3$ loading. *Am J Physiol Renal Physiol* 2003;284:F584–F593.

524. Romero MF. Molecular pathophysiology of SLC4 bicarbonate transporters. *Curr Opin Nephrol Hypertens* 2005;14:495–501.

525. Everett LA, Glaser B, Beck JC, et al. Pendred syndrome is caused by mutations in a putative sulphate transporter gene (PDS). *Nat Genet* 1997;17:411–422.

526. Wall SM, Hassell KA, Royaux IE, et al. Localization of pendrin in mouse kidney. *Am J Physiol Renal Physiol* 2003;284:F229–F241.

527. Wall SM. Recent advances in our understanding of intercalated cells. *Curr Opin Nephrol Hypertens* 2005;14:480–484.

528. Schwartz GJ, Barasch J, Al-Awqati Q. Plasticity of functional epithelial polarity. *Nature* 1985;318:368–371.

529. Schwartz GJ, Tsuruoka S, Vijayakumar S, Petrovic S, Mian A, Al-Awqati Q. Acid incubation reverses the polarity of intercalated cell transporters, an effect mediated by hensin. *J Clin Invest* 2002;109:89–99.

530. LeFurgey A, Tisher CC. Morphology of rabbit collecting duct. *Am J Anat* 1979;115:111–124.

531. Hansen GP, Tisher CC, Robinson RR. Response of the collecting duct to disturbances of acid-base and potassium balance. *Kidney Int* 1980;17:326–337.

532. Madsen KM, Tisher CC. Cellular response to acute respiratory acidosis in rat medullary collecting duct. *Am J Physiol* 1983;245:F670–F679.

533. Madsen KM, Tisher CC. Response of intercalated cells of rat outer medullary collecting duct to chronic metabolic acidosis. *Lab Invest* 1984;51:268–276.

534. Garg LC, Narang N. Ouabain-insensitive K- adenosine triphosphatase in distal nephron segments of the rabbit. *J Clin Invest* 1988;81:1204–1208.

535. Wingo CS. Active proton secretion and potassium absorption in the rabbit outer medullary collecting duct. Functional evidence for proton-potassium-activated adenosine triphosphatase. *J Clin Invest* 1989;84:361–365.

536. Wingo CS, Madsen KM, Smolka A, Tisher CC. H-K-ATPase immunoreactivity in cortical and outer medullary collecting duct. *Kidney Int* 1990;38:985–990.

537. Ahn KY, Kone BC. Expression and cellular localization of mRNA encoding the "gastric" isoform of H^+-K^+-ATPase α-subunit in rat kidney. *Am J Physiol* 1995;268(pt 2):F99–F109.

538. Campbell-Thompson ML, Verlander JW, Curran KA, et al. In situ hybridization of H-K-ATPase B-subunit mRNA in rat and rabbit kidney. *Am J Physiol* 1995;269(pt 2):F345–F354.

539. Madsen KM, Clapp WL, Verlander JW. Structure and function of the inner medullary collecting duct. *Kidney Int* 1988;34:441–454.

540. Sands JM, Knepper MA. Urea permeability of mammalian inner medullary collecting duct system and papillary surface epithelium. *J Clin Invest* 1987;79:138–147.

541. Sands JM, Nonoguchi H, Knepper MA. Vasopressin effects on urea and H_2O transport in inner medullary collecting duct subsegments. *Am J Physiol* 1987;253(pt 2):F823–F832.

542. Clapp WL, Madsen KM, Verlander JM, Tisher CC. Intercalated cells of the rat inner medullary collecting duct. *Kidney Int* 1987;31:1080–1087.

543. Clapp WL, Madsen KM, Verlander JW, Tisher CC. Morphologic heterogeneity along the rat inner medullary collecting duct. *Lab Invest* 1989;60:219–230.

544. Nielsen S, Terris J, Smith CP, Hediger MA, Ecelbarger CA, Knepper MA. Cellular and subcellular localization of the vasopressin-regulated urea transporter in rat kidney. *Proc Natl Acad Sci U S A* 1996;93:5495–5500.

545. Shayakul C, Knepper MA, Smith CP, DiGiovanni SR, Hediger MA. Segmental localization of urea transporter mRNAs in rat kidney. *Am J Physiol* 1997;272(pt 2):F654–F660.

546. Terris JM, Knepper MA, Wade JB. UT-A3: localization and characterization of an additional urea transporter isoform in the IMCD. *Am J Physiol Renal Physiol* 2001;280:F325–F332.

547. Wall SM, Truong AV, DuBose TD Jr. H$^+$-K$^+$-ATPase mediates net acid secretion in rat terminal inner medullary collecting duct. *Am J Physiol* 1996;271(pt 2):F1037–F1044.

548. Bohman SO. The ultrastructure of the renal medulla and the interstitial cells. In: Cotran RS, ed. *Tubulo-Interstitial Nephropathies*. New York: Churchill Livingstone; 1983:1–34.

549. Hestbech J, Hansen HE, Amdisen A, Olsen S. Chronic renal lesions following long-term treatment with lithium. *Kidney Int* 1977;12:205–213.

550. Bohle A, Grund KE, Mackensen S, Tolon M. Correlations between renal interstitium and level of serum creatinine. Morphometric investigations of biopsies in perimembranous glomerulonephritis. *Virchows Arch A Pathol Anat Histol* 1977;373:15–22.

551. Kappel B, Olsen S. Cortical interstitial tissue and sclerosed glomeruli in the normal human kidney, related to age and sex. A quantitative study. *Virchows Arch A Pathol Anat Histol* 1980;387: 271–277.

552. Mounier F, Foidart JM, Gubler MC. Distribution of extracellular matrix glycoproteins during normal development of human kidney. An immunohistochemical study. *Lab Invest* 1986;54:394–401.

553. Lemley KV, Kriz W. Anatomy of the renal interstitium. *Kidney Int* 1991;39:370–381.

554. Kaissling B, Hegyi I, Loffing J, Le Hir M. Morphology of interstitial cells in the healthy kidney. *Anat Embryol (Berl)* 1996;193: 303–318.

555. Bachmann S, Le Hir M, Eckardt KU. Colocalization of erythropoietin mRNA and ecto-5-nucleotidase immunoreactivity in peritubular cells of the rat renal cortex indicates that fibroblasts produce erythropoietin. *J Histochem Cytochem* 1993;41:335–341.

556. Maxwell PH, Osmond MK, Pugh CW, et al. Identification of the renal erythropoietin-producing cells using transgenic mice. *Kidney Int* 1993;44:1149–1162.

557. Pfaller W. Structure function correlation in rat kidney. Quantitative correlation of structure and function in normal and injured rat kidney. *Adv Anat Embryol Cell Biol* 1982;70:1–106.

558. Muirhead EE. Antihypertensive functions of the kidney. Arthur C. Corcoran memorial lecture. *Hypertension* 1980;2:444–464.

559. Muirhead EE. Discovery of the renomedullary system of blood pressure control and its hormones. *Hypertension* 1990;15:114–116.

560. Lemley KV, Kriz W. Structure and function of the renal vasculature. In: Tisher CC, Brenner BM, eds. *Renal Pathology with Clinical and Functional Correlations.*. 2nd ed. Philadelphia: JB Lippincott; 1994:981–1026.

561. Fourman J, Moffat DB. *The Blood Vessels of the Kidney*. Oxford, England:Blackwell Scientific; 1971.

562. More RH, Duff GL. The renal arterial vasculature in man. *Am J Pathol* 1951;27:95–117.

563. Edwards JG. Efferent arterioles of glomeruli in the juxtamedullary zone of the human kidney. *Anat Rec* 1956;125:521–529.

564. Casellas D, Mimran A. Shunting in renal microvasculature of the rat. A scanning electron microscopic study of corrosion casts. *Anat Rec* 1981;201:237–248.

565. Ljungqvist A. Ultrastructural demonstration of a connection between afferent and efferent juxtamedullary glomerular arterioles. *Kidney Int* 1975;8:239–244.

566. Ljungqvist A. Fetal and postnatal development of the intrarenal arterial pattern in man. A microangiographic and histologic study. *Acta Paediatr* 1963;52:443–464.

567. Mukai K, Rosai J, Burgdorf WH. Localization of factor VIII-related antigen in vascular endothelial cells using an immunoperoxidase method. *Am J Surg Pathol* 1980;4:273–276.

568. Sanfilippo F, Pizzo SV, Croker BP. Immunohistochemical studies of cell differentiation in a juxtaglomerular tumor. *Arch Pathol Lab Med* 1982;106:604–607.

569. Fina L, Molgaard HV, Robertson D, et al. Expression of the CD34 gene in vascular endothelial cells. *Blood* 1990;75:2417–2426.

570. Civin CL, Trischmann TM, Fackler MJ, et al. Summary of CD34 cluster workshop section. In: Knapp W, ed. *Leucocyte Typing IV*. London: Academic Press; 1989:818–825.

571. Gabbiani G, Schmid E, Winter S, et al. Vascular smooth muscle cells differ from other smooth muscle cells: predominance of vimentin filaments and a specific alpha-type actin. *Proc Natl Acad Sci U S A* 1981;78:298–302.

572. Rollhäuser H, Kriz W, Heinke W. Das Gefäss–System der Rattenniere. *Z Zellforsch Mikrosk Anat* 1964;64:381–403.

573. Kriz W, Barrett JM, Peter S. The renal vasculature: anatomical-functional aspects. In: Thurau K, ed. *Kidney and Urinary Tract Physiology II*. Baltimore: University Park Press; 1976:1–21.

574. Beeuwkes R III, Bonventre JV. Tubular organization and vascular-tubular relations in the dog kidney. *Am J Physiol* 1975;229: 695–713.

575. Beeuwkes R. Vascular-tubular relationship in the human kidney. In: Leaf A, Giebisch G, Bolis L, Gorini S, eds. *Renal Pathophysiology: Recent Advances*. New York: Raven Press; 1980: 155–163.

576. Pierce EC. Renal lymphatics. *Anat Rec* 1944;90:315–335.

577. Bell RD, Keyl MJ, Shrader FR, Jones EW, Henry LP. Renal lymphatics: the internal distribution. *Nephron* 1968;5:454–463.

578. Kriz W, Dieterich HJ. Das lymphagefass system der niere bei einigen saugetieren: licht-und elektronenmikroskopische untersuchungen. *Z Anat Entwickl Gesch* 1970;131:111–147.

579. Kriz W. A periarterial pathway for intrarenal distribution of renin. *Kidney Int Suppl* 1987;20:S51–S56.

580. Colvin RB. Emphatically lymphatic. *J Am Soc Nephrol* 2004;15: 827–829.

581. Mitchell GA. The nerve supply of the kidneys. *Acta Anat (Basel)* 1950;10:1–37.

582. Gosling JA. Observations on the distribution of intrarenal nervous tissue. *Anat Rec* 1969;163:81–88.

583. Stefansson K, Wollmann RL, Jerkovic M. S-100 protein in soft-tissue tumors derived from Schwann cells and melanocytes. *Am J Pathol* 1982;106:261–268.

584. Nakajima T, Watanabe S, Sato Y, Kameya T, Hirota T, Shimosato Y. An immunoperoxidase study of S-100 protein distribution in normal and neoplastic tissues. *Am J Surg Pathol* 1982;6:715–727.

585. Trojanowski JQ, Lee VM, Schlaepfer WW. An immunohistochemical study of human central and peripheral nervous system tumors, using monoclonal antibodies against neurofilaments and glial filaments. *Hum Pathol* 1984;15:248–257.

586. Lee VM, Carden MJ, Schlaepfer WW. Structural similarities and differences between neurofilament proteins from five different species as revealed using monoclonal antibodies. *J Neurosci* 1986;6:2179–2186.

587. Barajas L. Innervation of the renal cortex. *Fed Proc* 1978;37: 1192–1201.

588. Fourman J. The adrenergic innervation of the efferent arterioles and the vasa recta in the mammalian kidney. *Experientia* 1970;26:293–294.

589. Barajas L, Powers K, Wang P. Innervation of the renal cortical tubules: a quantitative study. *Am J Physiol* 1984;247(pt 2): F50–F60.

590. Barajas L, Powers K. Innervation of the thick ascending limb of Henle. *Am J Physiol* 1988;255(pt 2):F340–F348.

Urinary Bladder, Ureter, and Renal Pelvis

35

Victor E. Reuter

INTRODUCTION

The urinary bladder is an epithelial-lined muscular viscus that has the ability to distend and accommodate up to 400 to 500 mL of urine without a change in intraluminal pressure. In addition, it is able to initiate and sustain a contraction until the organ is empty. Interestingly, micturition may be initiated or inhibited voluntarily despite the involuntary nature of the organ. The ureters are epithelial lined muscular tubes designed to transport urine from the kidneys to the urinary bladder with the aid of peristalsis. The renal pelvis represents the expanded proximal end of the ureter and serves to collect the urine excreted from the kidney and to transport it to the ureter proper.

EMBRYOLOGY

The cloaca is divided by the urorectal septum into a dorsal rectum and a ventral urogenital sinus [1,2]. It is this urogenital sinus that will give rise to the majority of the urinary bladder; it is aided by the caudal migration of the cloacal membrane, which will close the infraumbilical portion of the abdominal wall. The caudal portions of the mesonephric ducts become dilated and eventually fuse with the urogenital sinus in the midline dorsally, contributing to the formation of the bladder trigone. While these ducts contribute initially to the formation of the mucosa of the trigone, this is subsequently entirely replaced by endodermal epithelium of the urogenital sinus. The gradual absorption of the mesonephric ducts bring about the separate opening of the ureters into the urinary bladder in the area of the trigone. During embryologic development, the allantois regresses to completely form a thick, epithelial-lined tube, the urachus, which extends from the umbilicus to the apex (dome) of the bladder [1]. Before or shortly after birth, the urachus involutes further becoming simply a fibrous cord. Pathologists commonly refer to this fibrous cord, which extends from the dome of the bladder to the umbilicus, as the urachal remnant, but it should be called the median umbilical ligament since "urachal remnant" refers to remnants of the epithelial lining of the urachus that occasionally persist

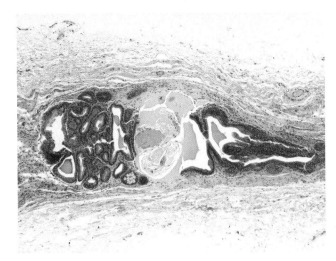

Figure 35.1 Urachal remnants within the median umbilical ligament.

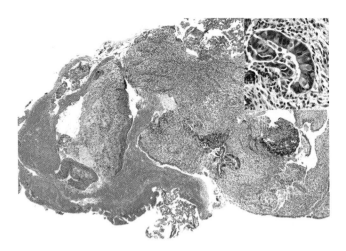

Figure 35.2 Endometriosis involving the ureteral wall. This female patient presented with hematuria and was thought to have a primary ureteral neoplasm. Insert shows an endometriotic gland at higher magnification.

within the median umbilical ligament (Figure 35.1). The epithelial lining of the urachus is urothelium, similar to that of the urinary bladder and ureter, but it frequently undergoes metaplastic change that is mostly of a glandular nature.

The epithelium of the urinary bladder is endodermally derived from the cranial portion of the urogenital sinus in continuity with the allantois. The lamina propria, the muscularis propria, and the adventitia develop from the adjacent splanchnic mesenchyme. These facts are important in understanding the histogenesis and nomenclature of lesions arising from the epithelial surface, as well as the bladder wall. For example, glandular features within benign (cystitis glandularis, nephrogenic adenoma) and malignant (adenocarcinoma) urothelium is not due to mesodermal or müllerian rests within the trigone but come about through a process of metaplasia and are a reflection of histologic plasticity (multipotentiality) of the urothelium. Since the mesonephric ducts involute totally during embryologic development, it is wrong to refer to tumors with mixed epithelial and sarcomatoid features arising in the bladder epithelium as mesodermal mixed tumors. They are, in fact, "endodermal mixed" tumors and are usually called sarcomatoid carcinomas (3). Very rarely, müllerian rests may be identified in the wall of the bladder and ureters or in the surrounding soft tissues in the form of endometriosis, endocervicosis, or endosalpingiosis (so-called müllerianosis) (4–7) (Figure 35.2).

The ureters develop by branching and elongation of the ureteric bud (metanephric diverticulum), which begins as a dorsal bud from the mesonephric duct (1,2). The stalk of the ureteric bud becomes the ureter, while the cranial end forms the renal pelvis, calyces, and collecting tubules. The epithelium of the ureter and renal pelvis, although histologically identical to that of the bladder, is of mesodermal derivation.

ANATOMIC CONSIDERATIONS

Bladder

In the adult, the empty urinary bladder lies within the anteroinferior portion of the pelvis minor, inferior to the peritoneum. In infants and children, it is located in part within the abdomen, even when empty (8). It begins to enter the pelvis major at about 6 years of age and will not be found entirely within the pelvis minor until after puberty. Nevertheless, in adults, as the bladder fills it will distend and ascend into the abdomen, at which time it may reach the level of the umbilicus.

The bladder lies relatively free within the fibrofatty tissues of the pelvis except in the area of the bladder neck, where it is firmly secured by the pubovesical ligaments in the female and the puboprostatic ligaments in the male (8,9). The relative freedom of the rest of the bladder permits expansion superiorly as the viscus fills with urine.

The empty bladder in an adult has the shape of a four-sided inverted pyramid and is enveloped by the vesical fascia (8). The superior surface faces superiorly and is covered by the pelvic parietal peritoneum (Figures 35.3–35.4). The posterior surface, also known as the base of the bladder, faces posteriorly and inferiorly. It is separated from the rectum by the uterine cervix and the proximal portions of the vagina in females and by the seminal vesicles and the ampulla of the vasa deferentia in males. These posterior anatomic relationships are very important clinically. Since the majority of vesicle neoplasms arise in the posterior wall adjacent to the ureteral orifices, invasive tumor may extend into adjacent soft tissue and organs (Figure 35.5A). The intimate relationship to the previously mentioned organs explains why hysterectomy and partial vaginectomy are commonly performed at the time of radial cystectomy in

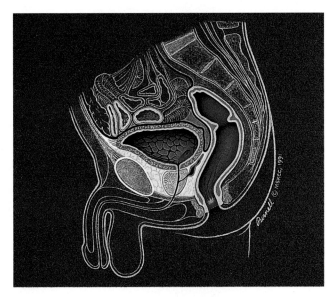

Figure 35.3 Anatomical relationships of the urinary bladder in males.

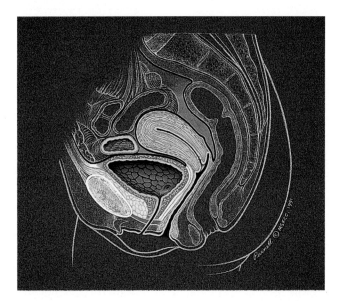

Figure 35.4 Anatomical relationships of the urinary bladder in females.

women. Similarly, we know that perivesical and seminal vesicle involvement is a bad prognostic sign in bladder carcinoma in males (10–12), a reflection of high pathologic stage. It is important to note that seminal vesicles may contain carcinoma without invasion, and this occurs in cases of in situ urothelial carcinoma involving prostatic and ejaculatory ducts and extending into the seminal vesicle epithelium. The latter is a rare occurrence, but these patients do not appear to have a similarly bad prognosis unless prostatic stromal invasion is present. The two inferolateral surfaces of the bladder face laterally, inferiorly, and anteriorly and are in contact with the fascia of the levator ani muscles. The most anterosuperior point of the bladder is known as the apex, and it is located at the point of contact

of the superior surfaces and the two inferolateral surfaces. The apex (dome) marks the point of insertion of the median umbilical ligament and consequently is the area where urachal carcinomas are located (Figures 35.3–35.4).

The trigone is a complex anatomic structure located at the base of the bladder and extending to the posterior bladder neck. In the proximal and lateral aspects of the trigone, the ureters enter into the bladder (ureteral orifices) obliquely. The muscle underlying the mucosa in this region is a combination of smooth muscle of the longitudinal layer of the intramural ureter and detrusor muscle (13–17). The intramural ureter is surrounded by a fibromuscular sheath (Waldeyer's sheath) that is fused into the ureteral muscle. This fibromuscular tissue fans out in the area of the

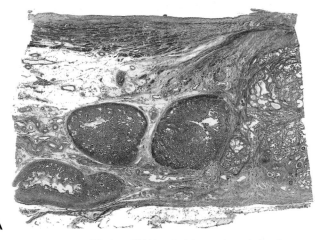

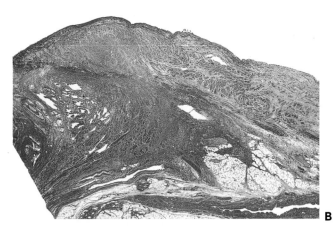

A   B

Figure 35.5 Bladder neck and distal trigone. **A.** The seminal vesicles are separated from the muscularis propria of the trigone by a scant amount of soft tissue. **B.** The muscularis propria merges with the prostate in the bladder neck area. The central (circular) fibers will predominate in this area and form the internal sphincter. The outer longitudinal layer contributes somewhat to the formation of the prostate musculature.

trigone and mixes with the detrusor muscle, thus fixing the intramural ureter to the bladder. As the bladder distends, the surrounding musculature exerts pressure on the obliquely oriented intramural ureter, producing closure of the ureteral lumen and thus avoiding reflux of urine.

The most distal portion of the bladder is called the bladder neck, and it is marked by the area where the posterior and the inferolateral walls converge and open into the urethra. In the male, the bladder neck merges with the prostate gland, and one may occasionally observe several prostatic ducts present in this area. It is important to recognize the existence of these ducts since their involvement by carcinoma should not be mistaken with invasive carcinoma. The bladder neck is formed with contributions from the trigonal musculature (inner longitudinal ureteral muscle and Waldeyer's sheath), the detrusor musculature, and the urethral musculature (13–18). The internal sphincter is located in this general area, with major contributions from the middle circular layer of the detrusor muscle (Figure 35.5B).

The bladder bed (structures on which the bladder neck rests) is formed posteriorly by the rectum in males and vagina in females (Figures 35.3 and 35.4). Anteriorly and laterally it is formed by the internal obturator and levator ani muscles, as well as the pubic bones. These structures may be involved in advanced tumors occupying the anterior, lateral, or bladder neck regions and render the patient inoperable.

The main arterial blood supply of the bladder comes from the inferior vesical arteries that branch from the internal iliacs (19,20). The umbilical arteries and its branches (the superior vesical arteries) also supply the bladder, as do the obturator and inferior gluteal arteries and, in females, the uterine and vaginal arteries. The veins of the urinary bladder drain into the internal iliac veins and form the vesical venous plexus. In the male, this plexus envelops the bladder base, prostate, and seminal vesicles and connects with the prostatic venous plexus. In females, it covers the bladder neck and urethra and communicates with the vaginal plexus. Lymphatic drainage is through the external and internal lymph nodes although drainage of portions of the bladder neck region may be through the sacral or common iliac nodes.

The urinary bladder is supplied by both sympathetic and parasympathetic nerves, which form the vesical nerve plexus (19,20). The former are derived from T_{11} through L_2 nerves and play no role in micturition. On the other hand, the parasympathetic nerves come from S_2 through S_4 and travel to the bladder via the pelvic nerve and inferior hypogastric plexus. These nerves are important to micturition since they contract the fibers of the muscularis propria, which in turn produces traction upon the bladder neck and opens the internal sphincter of the bladder. In fact, it is believed that micturition is initiated by voluntary relaxation of the perineal muscles and the striated muscle of the external sphincter located along the urethra. This action decreases urethral resistance and triggers contraction of the smooth muscle of the trigone and remaining bladder, closing the ureteral orifices and increasing the hydrostatic pressure within the viscus (9,21). These facts account for the difficulty in starting micturition while whistling. The bladder also contains sensory nerves that travel along the pelvic and hypogastric nerves and account for the sensation of pain as the bladder becomes too distended.

Ureters

The ureters measure approximately 30.0 cm in length, equally divided between the abdomen (retroperitoneum) and pelvis (22–27). The abdominal ureter takes a vertical course downward and medially on the anterior surface of the psoas muscle, covered by adventitia that is in fact an extension of Gerota's fascia. The pelvic ureter can be subdivided into a longer parietal and a shorter intravesical portion. The parietal portion is intimately related to the peritoneum. It descends posterolaterally; and, as it approaches the bladder base, it becomes medially directed to reach the urinary bladder. The ureters enter the base of the bladder obliquely and empty into the bladder at the ureteral orifices. The distal parietal portion and the intravesical segments are enveloped in a fibromuscular sheath (Waldeyer's sheath), which aids in fixing the ureter to the bladder (see description of the trigone).

The ureteral blood supply is quite diverse (19,22). Depending on the anatomic level, it receives blood from branches of the renal, abdominal aortic, gonadal, hypogastric, vesical, and uterine arteries, which form a richly intercommunicating plexus of vessels surrounding the tube. Venous drainage is variable but tends to follow a pattern similar to the arterial distribution. Lymphatic drainage is also quite complex. The upper portions drain into the lateral aortic lymph nodes, the middle portion drains into the common iliac lymph nodes, and the inferior portion drains into either the common, external, or internal iliac lymph nodes.

Renal Pelvis

As previously mentioned, the renal pelvis has its origin in the cranial portion of the ureteric bud, together with the calyces and collecting ducts. The renal pelvis lies primarily within the renal hilum, a space formed medially when one draws a vertical plane through the medial aspects of the upper and lower poles of the kidney (Figure 35.6). Within the hilum is the renal sinus, a space within the medial and antral portion of the kidney occupied by the renal pelvis, renal vessels and nerves, renal calyces, and fat. The fibrous capsule that lines the kidney passes over the lips of the hilum and lines the renal sinus, becoming continuous with the renal calyces. Within the renal sinus, the renal pelvis divides into two and rarely three major calyces, which in turn divide into 7 to 14 minor calyces. Urine from the distal collecting ducts within the renal

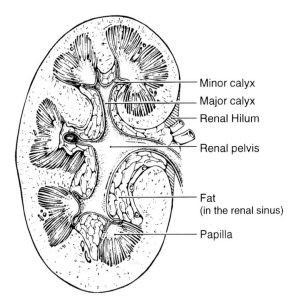

Figure 35.6 Anatomical relationships of the renal pelvis. Notice that the pelvis is mostly within the renal hilum (medial shaded area) and the renal sinus.

Minor calyx
Major calyx
Renal Hilum
Renal pelvis
Fat
(in the renal sinus)
Papilla

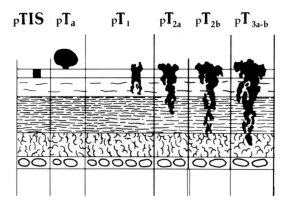

Figure 35.8 Pathologic staging of bladder cancer. This classification follows the recommendations of the American Joint Committee on Cancer (AJCC). In addition, prostatic stromal invasion is considered stage pT_4.

medulla (ducts of Bellini) flows into the minor calyces at the tips of the renal papillae (area cribrosa) (Figures 35.6 and 35.7). The blood supply of the renal pelvis comes from branches of the renal arteries, and the venous drainage follows a similar distribution. Its lymphatic drainage is into the renal hilar lymph nodes.

Microscopic Anatomy

The urinary bladder, ureter, and renal pelvis for the most part have a similar anatomic composition, the innermost layer being an epithelial lining and, extending outward, a lamina propria, smooth muscle (muscularis propria), and adventitia. The superior surface of the bladder comes in contact with parietal peritoneum and hence has a serosa. The anatomic landmarks are used clinically and pathologically to stage patients with urothelial cancer in order to choose therapy

and estimate survival (Figure 35.8). For this reason, it is important to accurately identify them microscopically.

Urothelium

The urinary bladder, ureters, and renal pelvis are lined by so-called transitional epithelium. This name was coined because its histologic appearance was transitional between nonkeratinizing squamous and pseudostratified columnar. Many histologists and pathologists have suggested urothelium as a more appropriate term.

The thickness of the urothelium will vary according to the degree of distension and anatomical location. It may be only two or three cell layers thick along the minor calyces. In the contracted bladder, it is usually six to seven cells thick and in the ureter three to five cells thick. One can identify three regions: the superficial cells that are in contact with the urinary space, the intermediate cells, and the basal cells that lie on a basement membrane (28,29) (Figure 35.9). In the distended bladder, the urothelium

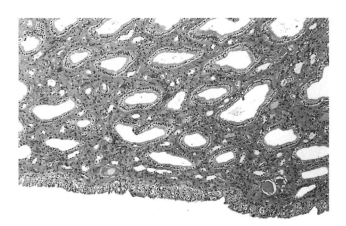

Figure 35.7 Renal papilla. Distal collecting ducts open into the urothelium covering the papillae.

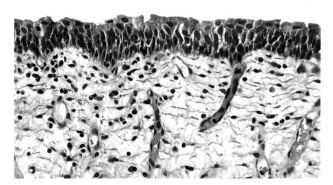

Figure 35.9 Normal urothelium. The mucosa may be up to seven cells thick in the bladder, but thickness will vary as a consequence of distension and other factors. The superficial (umbrella) cells have ample eosinophilic cytoplasm.

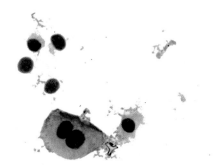

Figure 35.10 Urine cytology preparation stained with monoclonal antibody CD-15. A large, binucleated umbrella cell expresses the antigen identified by this antibody, while other normal urothelial cells do not.

may be only two to three cells thick and flattened with their long axis horizontal to the basement membrane. In practice, the thickness of the urothelium is dependent not only in the degree of distension but also on the plane on which the tissue is cut. If the cut is tangential to the basement membrane, it is possible to generate an artificially thick mucosa. For these and other reasons, we feel that urothelial thickness is of marginal or no utility in the assessment of urothelial neoplasms.

Superficial cells are in contact with the urinary space. They are large, elliptical cells that lie umbrella-like over the smaller intermediate cells (28–31). They may be binucleated and have abundant eosinophilic cytoplasm (Figure 35.10). In the distended bladder, they become flattened and barely discernible. While the presence of these cells is taken as a sign of normalcy of the urothelium, one must be aware that they may become detached due to superficial erosion during instrumentation or tissue processing in the prosecting area. Conversely, it is possible to see umbrella cells overlying frank carcinoma. In summary, the presence or absence of superficial cells cannot be used as a determining factor of malignancy.

Ultrastructural studies have shown the superficial urothelial cells to be quite unique. The luminal surface is lined by a cytoplasmic membrane that is three layers thick, having two electron-dense layers and a central lucent layer (Figure 35.11A). The two dense layers are said to be unequal thickness; for this reason, the membrane is known as the asymmetric unit membrane (AUM) (30–34). In reality, while the trilaminar arrangement of the cytoplasmic membrane can be readily observed, it is difficult to see the asymmetry of the dense layers. The membrane contains frequent invaginations, giving it a scalloped

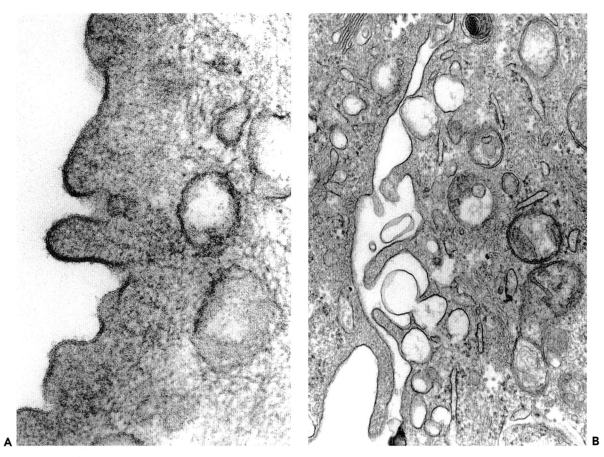

Figure 35.11 Ultrastructure of the urothelium. **A.** Detail of the luminal surface of a urothelial cell from a 1-year-old infant. The trilaminar cell membrane does not appear to be asymmetric (×136,000). **B.** Vesicles communicating with the apical/lateral surface of a urothelial cell (×54,000).

appearance. The superficial (luminal) cytoplasm contains vesicles that are also lined by AUM (Figure 35.11B). During the process of distention, these invaginations and vesicles are incorporated into the surface membrane, thus increasing the surface area and maintaining the structural integrity of the urothelium.

The intermediate cell layer may be up to five cells thick in the contracted bladder, where they are oriented with the long axis perpendicular to the basement membrane. The nuclei are oval and have finely stippled chromatin with absent or minute nucleoli. There is ample cytoplasm, which may be vacuolated. The cytoplasmic membranes are distinct, and these cells are attached to each other by desmosomes. In the distended state, this layer may be inconspicuous or only one cell thick and flattened. The basal layer is composed of cuboidal cells that are evident only in the contracted bladder and which lie on a thin but continuous basement membrane composed of a lamina lucida, lamina densa, and anchoring fibrils (35). All normal urothelial cells may contain glycogen, but only the superficial cells are occasional mucicarminophilic.

Urothelial Variants and Benign Urothelial Proliferations

While the above microscopic and ultrastructural features describe normal urothelium, we know there are many benign morphologic variants. Koss studied 100 grossly normal bladders obtained postmortem (36). Of these, 93% had Brunn's nests, cystitis cystica, or squamous metaplasia.

The most common urothelial variant is the formation of Brunn's nests, which represent invaginations of the surface urothelium into the underlying lamina propria (Figure 35.12). In some cases these solid nests of benign-appearing urothelium may lose continuity with the surface. They become cystic due to accumulation of cellular debris or mucin, and the term *cystitis cystica* has been coined to describe this phenomenon. The lining epithelium of these small cysts is composed of one or several layers of flattened transitional or cuboidal epithelium. In some cases, the epithelial lining undergoes glandular metaplasia, giving rise to what is called cystitis glandularis (Figure 35.12). The cells become cuboidal or columnar and mucin secreting; some are transformed into goblet cells. These processes also occur in the renal pelvis and ureter, where they are called pyelitis or ureteritis cystica (or glandularis), respectively (Figure 35.13).

Brunn's nests, cystitis cystica, and cystitis glandularis represent a continuum of proliferative or reactive changes seen along the entire urothelial tract, and it is common to see all three in the same tissue sample (Figure 35.12). Most investigators believe that they occur as a result of local inflammatory insult (36–38). Nevertheless, these proliferative changes are seen in the urothelium of patients with no evidence of local inflammation, so that it is possible that they also represent either normal histologic variants or

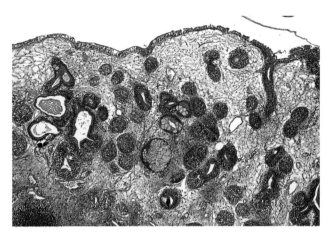

Figure 35.12 Bladder urothelium exhibiting proliferative changes, including Brunn's nests and cystitis glandularis.

the residual effects of old inflammatory processes (39,40). The high incidence of these proliferative changes in normal bladder suggests that they are not likely to be premalignant changes and that there is no cause-and-effect relationship between their presence and the appearance of bladder cancer. It is true that one or all of these changes are commonly present in biopsy specimens containing bladder cancer; but, the coexistence may be coincidental, or the cancer itself may be producing the local inflammatory insult that causes them. The fact that exceptional cases may occur in which carcinoma clearly arises within the epithelium of these reactive lesions does not alter this argument (41,42).

Metaplasia refers to a change in morphology of one cell type into another that is considered aberrant for that location. Urothelium frequently undergoes either squamous or glandular metaplasia, presumably as a response to chronic inflammatory stimuli such as urinary tract infection, calculi, diverticula, or frequent catheterization (37,40).

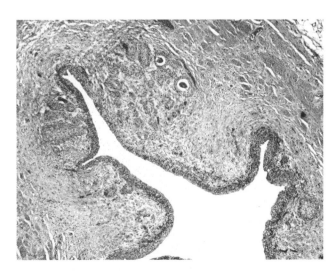

Figure 35.13 Brunn's nests involving a ureter. Notice that the nests are more numerous and irregularly oriented compared to what is commonly seen in the bladder.

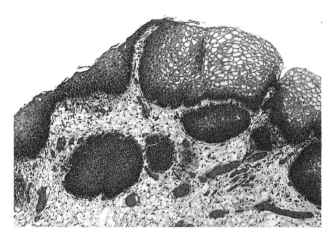

Figure 35.14 Squamous epithelium in the trigone of a woman. In this setting squamous epithelium is so common that it is considered to be a normal urothelial variant.

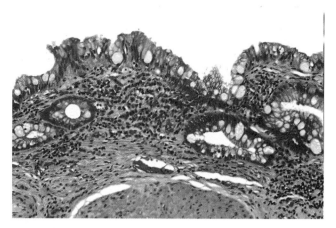

Figure 35.15 Intestinal metaplasia. The individual cells are morphologically identical to intestinal-type epithelium, even at the electron microscopic level.

Squamous epithelium in the area of the trigone is a common finding in women. It is characterized by abundant intracytoplasmic glycogen and lack of keratinization, making it histologically similar to vaginal or cervical squamous epithelium (Figure 35.14). In this particular setting, most of us believe that squamous epithelium should be regarded as a variant of urothelium rather than metaplasia. Squamous metaplasia may occur at other sites and at times may undergo keratinization and even exhibit parakeratosis and a granular layer. Squamous metaplasia is not preneoplastic per se, but patients with keratinizing squamous metaplasia must be monitored closely since some may progress to squamous carcinoma (43).

The most common site of glandular metaplasia of the urothelium is the bladder, in the form of cystitis glandularis. Nevertheless, it may also occur within surface urothelium elsewhere in the urinary tract, usually as a response to chronic inflammation or irritation and also in cases of bladder exstrophy (44,45). The epithelium is composed of tall columnar cells with mucin-secreting goblet cells (Figure 35.15), strikingly similar to colonic or small intestinal epithelium in which one might identify even Paneth's cells. In this setting, we should use the term intestinal metaplasia. As with squamous metaplasia, glandular metaplasia is not of itself a precancerous lesion but may eventually undergo neoplastic transformation in exceptional cases (45). Patients should be monitored accordingly.

So-called nephrogenic adenoma is a distinct metaplastic lesion characterized by aggregates of cuboidal or hobnail cells with clear or eosinophilic cytoplasm and small discrete nuclei without prominent nucleoli (46). These cells line thin papillary fronds on the surface or form tubular structures within the lamina propria of the bladder (Figure 35.16). The tubules are often surrounded by a thickened and hyalinized basement membrane. Variable numbers of acute and chronic inflammatory cells are commonplace within the bladder wall.

Nephrogenic adenoma is thought to be secondary to an inflammatory insult or local injury (46–50). It was originally described in the trigone and given its name because it was thought to arise from mesonephric rests. We now know that nephrogenic adenoma may occur anywhere in the urothelial tract, although it is most common in the bladder. It is important in that it may present as an exophytic mass mimicking carcinoma grossly and suggesting adenocarcinoma microscopically. The benign histologic appearance of the cells arranged in characteristic tubules surrounded by a prominent basement membrane should provide the correct diagnosis. A very interesting publication described nephrogenic adenomas of the bladder in patients who underwent renal transplantation (51). The authors demonstrated the adenomatous lesions and the donor kidneys were clonal, suggesting that they developed through a process of shedding of donor renal tubule cells followed by implantation and proliferation within

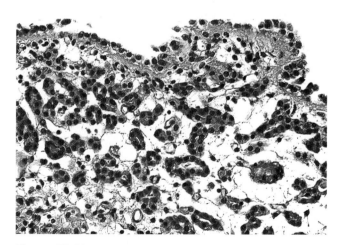

Figure 35.16 Nephrogenic adenoma. This proliferative urothelial lesion is characterized by aggregates of cuboidal cells with scant eosinophilic cytoplasm forming small tubules within the lamina propria. It may exhibit an exophytic, papillary growth.

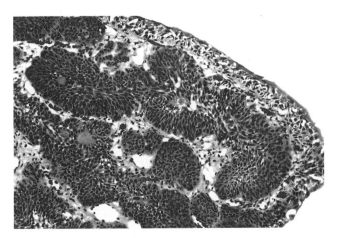

Figure 35.17 Inverted papilloma. This proliferative urothelial lesion is characterized by invaginated cords and nests of transitional epithelium within the lamina propria.

the bladder. While this is interesting, it is certainly not the usual mechanism by which they develop.

Inverted papillomas are relatively rare lesions that may occur anywhere along the urothelial tract and may be confused clinically and pathologically with transitional-cell carcinoma (52,53). In order of decreasing frequency, they occur in the bladder, renal pelvis, ureter, and urethra (54–60). Patients usually present with hematuria. Cystoscopically, the lesions are polypoid and either sessile or pedunculated. The mucosal surface is smooth or nodular and without villous or papillary fronds. Microscopically, the surface epithelium is compressed but otherwise unremarkable. It is undermined by invaginated cords and nests of transitional epithelium that occupy the lamina propria (Figure 35.17). The accumulation of these endophytic growths gives the lesion its characteristic polypoid gross appearance. The urothelial cells forming the cords are benign, exhibiting normal maturation and few mitoses. They are similar to the cells of bladder papillomas, differing only in that the epithelial cords are endophytic and consequently more closely packed. Frequently the cells are oval or spindle-shaped. Epithelial nests may become centrally cystic, dilated, and even lined by cuboidal epithelium.

These cords of transitional epithelium in the lamina propria represent invagination, not invasion. As such, there are no fibrous reactive changes within the stroma. Although mitotic figures can be seen, they are rare, regular, and located at or near the basal layer of the epithelium. Inverted papillomas are discrete lesions and do not exhibit an infiltrative border (54,55). One must be careful not to confuse a nested type of urothelial carcinoma infiltrating the lamina propria with an inverted papilloma.

The etiology of inverted papilloma is unclear. Most investigators feel that, similar to other proliferative lesions such as Brunn's nests and cystitis cystica, they are a reactive, proliferative process secondary to a noxious insult. They are not premalignant, although in exceptional cases they have

been associated with carcinoma (56–58). Given the rarity of this association, we consider it incidental.

Lamina Propria

The lamina propria lies between the mucosal basement membrane and the muscularis propria. It is composed of dense connective tissue containing a rich vascular network, lymphatic channels, sensory nerve endings, and a few elastic fibers (20,28,32). In the deeper aspects of the lamina propria, of the urinary bladder and ureter, the connective tissue is loose, allowing the formation of thick mucosal folds when the viscus is contracted (Figures 35.18–35.19). Its thickness varies with the degree of distention and is generally thinner in the areas of the trigone and bladder neck. In fact, in patients with urinary outflow obstruction (i.e., prostatic hyperplasia), the bladder neck may contain muscularis propria directly beneath the mucosa, with the lamina propria being virtually indiscernible (Figure 35.5B). Lamina propria is also absent beneath the urothelium lining the renal papillae in the renal pelvis and is quite thin along the minor calyces (Figure 35.20).

In the midportion of the lamina propria of the bladder lie intermediate-sized arteries and veins. Wisps of smooth muscle are commonly found in the lamina propria and usually are associated with these vessels (61,62) (Figures 35.21A and 35.21B). These fascicles of smooth muscle are not connected to the muscularis propria; they appear as isolated bundles but may form a discontinuous thin layer of muscle. The anatomic relationship of these fibers to the overlying urothelium can be severely disrupted by inflammation or prior therapeutic intervention when they may be seen juxtaposed to the basement membrane (Figure 35.21C). Uncommonly, these muscle fibers may present as a continuous layer of muscle within the lamina propria, thus forming a true muscularis mucosae (62). In evaluating surgical and

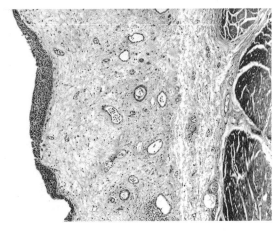

Figure 35.18 Lamina propria. It is composed of connective tissue, vascular structures, sensory nerves, and elastic fibers. Notice that the superficial connective tissue is denser than the deep portion.

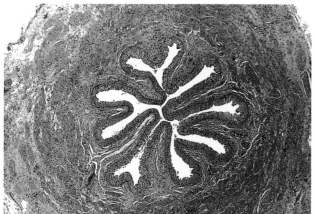

Figure 35.19 Cross section of mid-ureter. The elastic fibers and loose connective tissue within the lamina propria impart a festooned appearance to the urothelium. Notice that the different layers of the muscularis propria are indiscernible.

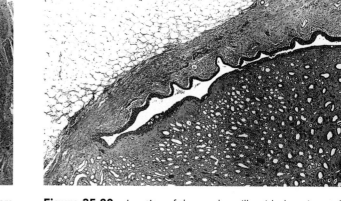

Figure 35.20 Junction of the renal papilla with the minor calyx. Notice the absence of the lamina propria along the papilla and a very thin lamina propria and muscularis propria along the minor calyx.

biopsy material, every effort should be made to distinguish these superficial muscle fascicles from muscularis propria since a failure to do so will lead to errors in tumor staging and treatment. A pathologist should not sign out a biopsy as "transitional cell carcinoma invading muscle" because he/she is not giving useful information as to the depth of

invasion. In fact, many urologists are unaware of the existence of a superficial muscle layer (muscularis mucosae) so that the above diagnosis will lead the urologist to treat the patient as a deeply invasive tumor (stage pT_2 or greater) when in fact the patient has superficially invasive disease (stage pT_1). Occasionally one may encounter fat within the

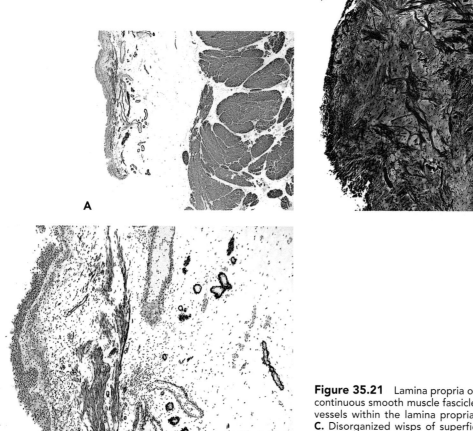

Figure 35.21 Lamina propria of the urinary bladder. **A. and B.** Discontinuous smooth muscle fascicles are adjacent to intermediate size vessels within the lamina propria (anti–actin monoclonal antibody). **C.** Disorganized wisps of superficial smooth muscle lie directly beneath the urothelium at the site of a prior biopsy. (Transurethral resection biopsy [TURB] specimen.)

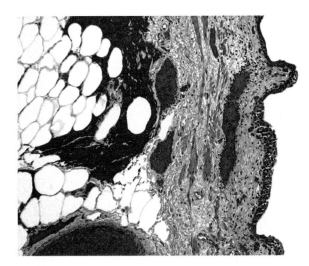

Figure 35.22 Mature adipose tissue within the lamina propria of the urinary bladder.

lamina propria and muscularis (63) (Figure 35.22). At this time, it is unclear whether this is due to the patient's body habitus, but its presence should not be misinterpreted by pathologists as evidence of perivesical fat.

Pathologists are surprised to learn that, in terms of prognosis and treatment, urologists and urologic oncologists lump noninvasive (T_a) and superficially invasive (T_1) into a single category. It is my opinion that this is due greatly to the fact that we, as pathologists, do not agree as to what constitutes lamina propria invasion. There are many cases of pT_1 disease that are unequivocal, but there are an equal number in which invasion is, at best, questionable. Pathologists' interpretation in the latter group is inconsistent and not reproducible. While this confusion is partly due to the lack of orientation of transurethral biopsy specimens and to disruption of the normal histologic architecture by tumor or prior therapy, it is clear that better parameters are needed to make this distinction.

Muscularis Propria

The muscularis propria is said to be composed of three smooth muscle coats, inner and outer longitudinal layers, and a central circular layer. In fact, these layers can only be identified consistently in the area of the bladder neck. In other areas, the longitudinal and circular layers mix freely and have no definite orientation. In the ureter, the muscularis propria is thicker distally, and the proximal portion contains only two layers (64). In the renal pelvis, the muscularis propria becomes thinner along the major and minor calyces, and no orientation of the muscle fibers is evident. No muscular fibers are evident between the urothelium and the renal medulla at the level of the renal papillae (Figures 35.7, 35.20). Within the renal sinus, the muscularis propria is surrounded by variable amounts of fat (Figures 35.6, 35.23). This fact is rarely mentioned by pathologists at the

time of evaluating urothelial tumors arising in the renal pelvis. Many cases are signed out as "invading renal hilar fat" or "invading perirenal fat," when in fact the invasion is solely into the fat within the renal sinus. The significance of this finding remains to be determined (65).

In the contracted bladder, the muscle fibers are arranged in relatively coarse bundles that are separated from each other by moderate to abundant connective tissue containing blood vessels, lymphatics, and nerves. Mature adipose tissue may also be present. Very infrequently, one may see nests of paraganglia, usually associated with neural or vascular structures (Figure 35.24A). The cells are arranged in discrete nests or cords and have clear or granular cytoplasm with round or vesicular nuclei. They should not be confused with invasive carcinoma. Immunohistochemical stains for cytokeratins are negative but for chromogranin are positive (Figure 35.24B).

Similar to other layers, the thickness of the muscularis propria will vary from patient to patient, with age, and with the degree of distention (Figures 35.25A–B). In fact, Jequier and Rousseau (66) performed sonographic measurements of the bladder wall thickness in 410 urologically normal children and 10 adults. They found that the bladder wall thickness varied mostly with the state of bladder filling and only minimally with age and gender. The bladder wall had a mean thickness of 2.76 mm when empty and 1.55 mm when distended.

For staging purposes, the muscularis propria has been divided into two segments, superficial and deep (T_{2a} and T_{2b}, respectively) (Figure 35.8). No anatomical landmarks can be used to make this distinction so it must be done by direct visualization on the light microscope. Prior transurethral resection will alter the anatomy of the site and mask normal landmarks, making proper staging difficult—if not impossible.

Bladder diverticula are relatively common, yet their etiology remains controversial. Most investigators agree that they occur secondary to increased intravesical pressure as a

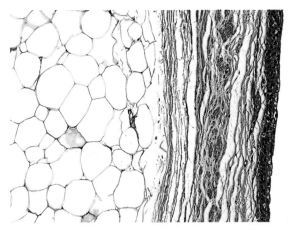

Figure 35.23 Urothelial wall along the minor calices. Thin layers of lamina propria and muscularis propria are surrounded by fat within the renal sinus.

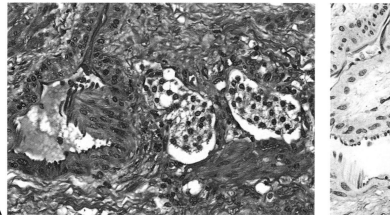
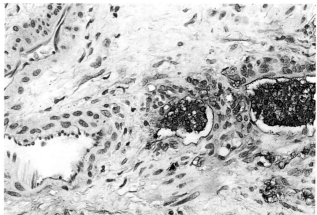

Figure 35.24 Nests of paraganglia within the bladder wall. **A.** The cells are small, have vesicular nuclei and clear cytoplasm, and are seen adjacent to neural or vascular structures. They should not be confused with invasive carcinoma. **B.** Immunostain for chromogranin A can clarify the issue.

result of obstruction distal to the diverticulum (67–69). The obstruction brings about compensatory muscle hypertrophy and eventual mucosal herniation in areas of weakness. Others feel that at least some diverticula are a consequence of congenital defects in the bladder musculature, citing as evidence cases of diverticula in young patients without evidence of obstruction (69,70). The most common sites of diverticula are (a) adjacent to the ureteral orifices, (b) the bladder dome (probably related to an urachal remnant), and (c) the region of the internal urethral orifice. Grossly, one sees distortion of the external surface of the bladder. The diverticula may be widely patent but are usually narrow in symptomatic patients. The mucosa adjoining the diverticulum is usually hyperemic or ulcerated.

There may be epithelial hyperplasia and hypertrophy of the muscularis propria. Very commonly, there is inflammation involving the lamina propria and muscularis. The wall of the diverticulum itself consists of urothelium and underlying connective tissue, similar to the bladder mucosa with lamina propria (Figure 35.26). Few, if any, muscle fascicles of the muscularis propia will be identified in the majority of cases of acquired diverticula, although muscularis mucosae may be present. The true "congenital" diverticulum contains a thinned outer muscle layer. Infrequently, the epithelium lining the sac will undergo squamous or glandular metaplasia due to local irritation associated with urine stasis, infection, or stone. In these cases, it is not unusual for the diverticular wall to become extensively fibrotic.

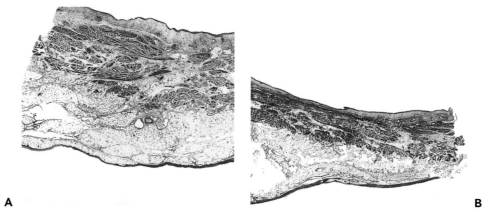

Figure 35.25 Full thickness section of the bladder. **A.** Notice the irregular thickness of the lamina propria. The three layers of muscle comprising the muscularis propria cannot be clearly defined. In contradistinction to the muscularis propria of the gut, there are ample amounts of soft tissue between muscle bundles in the bladder. **B.** Cross section of distended bladder. The overall thickness of the viscus is diminished as compared to the contracted bladder. Both the lamina propria and muscularis propria become more compact.

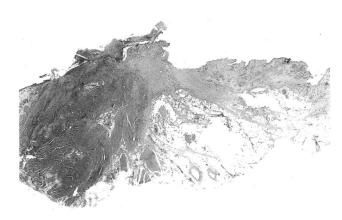

Figure 35.26 Bladder diverticulum. To the left is inflamed but anatomically normal bladder wall, while in the center and to the right one sees total absence of the muscularis propria. Perivesical soft tissue comes in contact with the inflamed, fibrotic, and thickened lamina propria.

Major complications of bladder diverticula include infection, lithiasis, and carcinoma. It is believed that 2 to 7% of patients with bladder diverticula will develop an associated neoplasm, presumed secondary to the chronic inflammatory stimuli mentioned above (71,72). Ureteral diverticula are rare and are asymptomatic if uncomplicated (73). They are not seen in the renal pelvis.

REFERENCES

1. Moore K. The urinary system. In: Moore K, ed. *The Developing Human: Clinically Oriented Embryology.* Philadelphia: WB Saunders; 1982.
2. Kissane JM. Development and structure of the urogenital system. In: Murphy WM, ed. *Urological Pathology.* Philadelphia: WB Saunders; 1989;1–33.
3. Eble JN, Sauter G, Epstein JI, Sesterhenn IA, eds. *World Health Organization Classification of Tumors: Pathology and Genetics of Tumors of the Urinary System and Male Genital Organs.* Lyon, France: IARC Press; 2004.
4. Clement PB, Young RH. Endocervicosis of the urinary bladder. A report of six cases of a benign mullerian lesion that may mimic adenocarcinoma. *Am J Surg Pathol* 1992;16:533–542.
5. Young RH, Clement PB. Mullerianosis of the urinary bladder. *Mod Pathol* 1996;9:731–737.
6. Comiter CV. Endometriosis of the urinary tract. *Urol Clin North Am* 2002;29:625–635.
7. Chapron C, Boucher E, Fauconnier A, Vieira M, Dubuisson JB, Vacher-Lavenu MC. Anatomopathological lesions of bladder endometriosis are heterogeneous. *Fertil Steril* 2002;78:740–742.
8. Moore KL. The pelvis and perineum. In: Moore KL, ed. *Clinically Oriented Anatomy.* 2nd ed. Baltimore: Williams & Wilkins; 1985.
9. Tanagho E. Anatomy of the lower urinary tract. In: Campbell MF and Walsh PC, eds. *Campbell's Urology.* 6th ed. Philadelphia: WB Saunders; 1992.
10. Mahadevia PS, Koss LG, Tar IJ. Prostatic involvement in bladder cancer. Prostate mapping in 20 cystoprostatectomy specimens. *Cancer* 1986;58:2096–2102.
11. Utz DC, Farrow GM, Rife CC, Segura JW, Zincke H. Carcinoma in situ of the bladder. *Cancer* 1980;45(suppl 7):1842–1848.
12. Ro JY, Ayala AG, el-Naggar A, Wishnow KI. Seminal vesicle involvement by in situ and invasive transitional cell carcinoma of the bladder. *Am J Surg Pathol* 1987;11:951–958.
13. Tanagho EA, Smith DR, Meyers FH. The trigone: anatomical and physiological considerations. II. In relation to the bladder neck. *J Urol* 1968;100:633–639.
14. Tanagho EA, Meyers FH, Smith DR. The trigone: anatomical and physiological considerations. I. In relation to the ureterovesical junction. *J Urol* 1968;100:623–632.
15. Shehata R. A comparative study of the urinary bladder and the intramural portion of the ureter. *Acta Anat (Basel)* 1977;98:380–395.
16. Politano VA. Ureterovesical junction. *J Urol* 1972;107:239–242.
17. Elbadawi A. Anatomy and function of the ureteral sheath. *J Urol* 1972;107:224–229.
18. Tanagho EA, Smith DR. The anatomy and function of the bladder neck. *Br J Urol* 1966;38:54–71.
19. Moore KL, Dalley AF. *Clinically Oriented Anatomy.* 5th ed. Baltimore: Lippincott Williams & Wilkins; 2005.
20. Weiss L. *Cell and Tissue Biology: A Textbook of Histology.* 6th ed. Baltimore: Urban & Schwarzenberg; 1988.
21. Fletcher TF, Bradley WE. Neuroanatomy of the bladder-urethra. *J Urol* 1978;119:153–160.
22. Olson CA. Anatomy of the upper urinary tract. In: Campbell MF and Walsh PC, eds. *Campbell's Urology.* 5th ed. Philadelphia: WB Saunders; 1986.
23. Hanna MK, Jeffs RD, Sturgess JM, Barkin M. Ureteral structure and ultrastructure. Part I. The normal human ureter. *J Urol* 1976;116:718–724.
24. Kaye KW, Goldberg ME. Applied anatomy of the kidney and ureter. *Urol Clin North Am* 1982;9:3–13.
25. Motola JA, Shahon RS, Smith AD. Anatomy of the ureter. *Urol Clin North Am* 1988;15:295–299.
26. Notley RG. Ureteral morphology: anatomic and clinical considerations. *Urology* 1978;12:8–14.
27. Crelin ES. Normal and abnormal development of ureter. *Urology* 1978;12:2–7.
28. Koss LG. Tumors of the urinary bladder. In: *Atlas of Tumor Pathology.* 2nd series, fascicle 11. Washington, DC: Armed Forces Institute of Pathology; 1975.
29. Fawcett DW. *Bloom and Fawcett: A Textbook of Histology.* 11th ed. Philadelphia: WB Saunders; 1986.
30. Hicks RM. The function of the golgi complex in transitional epithelium. Synthesis of the thick cell membrane. *J Cell Biol* 1966;30:623–643.
31. Battifora H, Eisenstein R, McDonald JH. The human urinary bladder mucosa. An electron microscopic study. *Invest Urol* 1964;12:354–361.
32. Fawcett DW, Raviola E, eds. *Bloom and Fawcett: A Textbook of Histology.* 12th ed. New York: Chapman & Hall; 1994.
33. Koss LG. The asymmetric unit membranes of the epithelium of the urinary bladder of the rat. An electron microscopic study of a mechanism of epithelial maturation and function. *Lab Invest* 1969;21:154–168.
34. Newman J, Antonakopoulos GN. The fine structure of the human fetal urinary bladder. Development and maturation. A light, transmission and scanning electron microscopic study. *J Anat* 1989;166:135–150.
35. Alroy J, Gould VE. Epithelial-stromal interface in normal and neoplastic human bladder epithelium. *Ultrastruct Pathol* 1980;1:201–210.
36. Koss LG. Mapping of the urinary bladder: its impact on the concepts of bladder cancer. *Hum Pathol* 1979;10:533–548.
37. Mostofi FK. Potentialities of bladder epithelium. *J Urol* 1954;71:705–714.
38. Morse HD. The etiology and pathology of pyelitis cystica, ureteritis cystica and cystitis cystica. *Am J Pathol* 1928;4:33–50.
39. Goldstein AM, Fauer RB, Chinn M, Kaempf MJ. New concepts on formation of Brunn's nests and cysts in urinary tract mucosa. *Urology* 1978;11:513–517.
40. Wiener DP, Koss LG, Sablay B, Freed SZ. The prevalence and significance of Brunn's nests, cystitis cystica and squamous metaplasia in normal bladders. *J Urol* 1979;122:317–321.
41. Edwards PD, Hurm RA, Jaeschke WH. Conversion of cystitis glandularis to adenocarcinoma. *J Urol* 1972;108:568–570.

42. Lin JI, Yong HS, Tseng CH, Marsidi PS, Choy C, Pilloff B. Diffuse cystitis glandularis. Associated with adenocarcinomatous change. *Urology* 1980;15:411–415.

43. Tannenbaum M. Inflammatory proliferative lesion of urinary bladder: squamous metaplasia. *Urology* 1976;7:428–429.

44. Engel RM, Wilkinson HA. Bladder exstrophy. *J Urol* 1970;104: 699–704.

45. Nielsen K, Nielsen KK. Adenocarcinoma in exstrophy of the bladder—the last case in Scandinavia? A case report and review of literature. *J Urol* 1983;130:1180–1182.

46. Bhagavan BS, Tiamson EM, Wenk RE, Berger BW, Hamamoto G, Eggleston JC. Nephrogenic adenoma of the urinary bladder and urethra. *Hum Pathol* 1981;12:907–916.

47. Navarre RJ Jr, Loening SA, Platz C, Narayana A, Culp DA. Nephrogenic adenoma: a report of 9 cases and review of the literature. *J Urol* 1982;127:775–779.

48. Molland EA, Trott PA, Paris AM, Blandy JP. Nephrogenic adenoma: a form of adenomatous metaplasia of the bladder. A clinical and electron microscopical study. *Br J Urol* 1976;48:453–462.

49. Ford TF, Watson GM, Cameron KM. Adenomatous metaplasia (nephrogenic adenoma) of urothelium. An analysis of 70 cases. *Br J Urol* 1985;57:427–433.

50. Satodate R, Koike H, Sasou S, Ohori T, Nagane Y. Nephrogenic adenoma of the ureter. *J Urol* 1984;131:332–334.

51. Mazal PR, Schaufler R, Altenhuber-Muller R, et al. Derivation of nephrogenic adenomas from renal tubular cells in kidney-transplant recipients. *N Engl J Med* 2002;347:653–659.

52. DeMeester LJ, Farrow GM, Utz DC. Inverted papillomas of the urinary bladder. *Cancer* 1975;36:505–513.

53. Henderson DW, Allen PW, Bourne AJ. Inverted urinary papilloma: report of five cases and review of the literature. *Virchows Arch A Pathol Anat Histol* 1975;366:177–186.

54. Caro DJ, Tessler A. Inverted papilloma of the bladder: a distinct urological lesion. *Cancer* 1978;42:708–713.

55. Anderstrom C, Johansson S, Pettersson S. Inverted papilloma of the urinary tract. *J Urol* 1982;127:1132–1134.

56. Lazarevic B, Garret R. Inverted papilloma and papillary transitional cell carcinoma of urinary bladder: report of four cases of inverted papilloma, one showing papillary malignant transformation and review of the literature. *Cancer* 1978;42: 1904–1911.

57. Whitesel JA. Inverted papilloma of the urinary tract: malignant potential. *J Urol* 1982;127:539–540.

58. Stein BS, Rosen S, Kendall AR. The association of inverted papilloma and transitional cell carcinoma of the urothelium. *J Urol* 1984;131:751–752.

59. Assor D. Inverted papilloma of the renal pelvis. *J Urol* 1976;116:654.

60. Lausten GS, Anagnostaki L, Thomsen OF. Inverted papilloma of the upper urinary tract. *Eur Urol* 1984;10:67–70.

61. Dixon JS, Gosling JA. Histology and fine structure of the muscularis mucosae of the human urinary bladder. *J Anat* 1983;136 (pt 2):265–271.

62. Ro JY, Ayala AG, el-Naggar A. Muscularis mucosa of urinary bladder. Importance for staging and treatment. *Am J Surg Pathol* 1987;11:668–673.

63. Philip AT, Amin MB, Tamboli P, Lee TJ, Hill CE, Ro JY. Intravesical adipose tissue: a quantitative study of its presence and location with implications for therapy and prognosis. *Am J Surg Pathol* 2000;24:1286–1290.

64. Notley RG. The musculature of the human ureter. *Br J Urol* 1970;42:724–727.

65. Olgac S, Mazumdar M, Dalbagni G, Reuter VE. Urothelial carcinoma of the renal pelvis: a clinicopathologic study of 130 cases. *Am J Surg Pathol* 2004;28:1545–1552.

66. Jequier S, Rousseau O. Sonographic measurements of the normal bladder wall in children. *AJR Am J Roentgenol* 1987; 149:563–566.

67. Miller A. The aetiology and treatment of diverticulum of the bladder. *Br J Urol* 1958;30:43–56.

68. Kertsschmer HL. Diverticula of the urinary bladder: a clinical study of 236 cases. *Surg Gynecol Obstet* 1940;71: 491–503.

69. Fox M, Power RF, Bruce AW. Diverticulum of the bladder: presentation and evaluation of treatment of 115 cases. *Br J Urol* 1962;34:286–298.

70. Barrett DM, Malek RS, Kelalis PP. Observations on vesical diverticulum in childhood. *J Urol* 1976;116:234–236.

71. Abeshouse BS. Primary carcinoma in a diverticulum of the bladder: a report of four cases and a review of the literature. *J Urol* 1943;49:534–547.

72. Faysal MH, Freiha FS. Primary neoplasm in vesical diverticula. A report of 12 cases. *Br J Urol* 1981;53:141–143.

73. Cochran ST, Waisman J, Barbaric ZL. Radiographic and microscopic findings in multiple ureteral diverticula. *Radiology* 1980;137:631–636.

Prostate

36

John E. McNeal

EMBRYOLOGY AND DEVELOPMENT OF THE PROSTATE

The prostate appears in early embryonic development as a condensation of mesenchyme along the course of the pelvic urethra. By 9 weeks of embryonic life, a number of features that are characteristic of adult contour and location are evident (Figure 36.1). The mesenchymal condensation is most dense along the posterior (rectal) aspect of the urethra and distal (apical) to its midpoint. This is the only region where highly condensed mesenchyme is in immediate contact with urethral lining epithelium, and only here is the urethra lined by a tall columnar epithelium (1). Between its midpoint and the bladder neck, the proximal urethral segment shows a sharp anterior angulation. However, the strip of highly condensed mesenchyme continues directly proximally to a dome-shaped base, leaving a gap between condensed prostatic mesenchyme and proximal urethra.

The ejaculatory ducts penetrate the mesenchyme toward the future verumontanum, which is located at the urethral midpoint. This is wolffian duct tissue, but its stroma is indistinguishable from the remaining prostatic mesenchyme, which is mainly derived from the urogenital sinus (2). However, that portion of the mesenchyme that surrounds the ejaculatory ducts and expands proximally to occupy nearly the entire prostate base is distinguishable in the adult as the central zone, which is probably also derived from the wolffian duct, as are the seminal vesicles (1). In this concept, the prostate is of dual embryonic derivation.

At about 10 weeks, epithelial buds begin to branch, mainly posteriorly and laterally from the posterior and lateral walls of the distal urethral segment into the condensed mesenchyme. Recent computer reconstructions of serially sectioned specimens have shown that the branching pattern that is established initially is identical to that described for the adult later in this chapter (3).

This developmental program is activated by androgen secreted by the fetal testes. However, the eventual size of the neonatal prostate—less than 1 cm in diameter—is predetermined by the stroma as a programmed number of stromal cell divisions, after which the stroma ceases to have further inductive influence on the branching duct system.

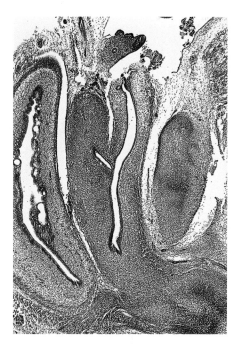

Figure 36.1 Embryonic prostate, age 9 weeks, in the sagittal plane of the pelvis. Urethra (narrow central lumen) is angulated to the right at the midpoint, where the ejaculatory duct approaches from above left. A vertical strip of highly condensed prostate mesenchyme contacts the posterior urethral wall only distal to the ejaculatory ducts. The prostate is flanked by the rectum (*left*) and pubis (*right*). Duct buds have not yet formed.

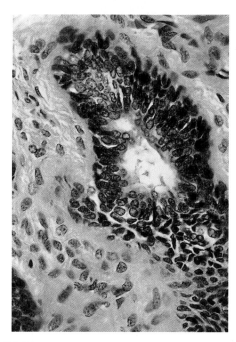

Figure 36.2 Prepubertal prostatic duct lined by epithelium with multiple layers of nuclei and showing no cytoplasmic differentiation.

GENERAL RELATIONSHIPS: THE GLANDULAR PROSTATE

Postnatally the prostate grows at a slow rate, reaching less than 2 cm in diameter by the time of puberty. During this period, the ducts and acini are lined by epithelium, which undergoes little change from the neonatal period. Gland spaces are lined by cells that are crowded with multilayered dark nuclei (Figure 36.2). There is a superficial resemblance to adult postinflammatory atrophy, but the histologic features are quite different.

The pubertal growth acceleration and maturation of the prostate gland appears not to be complete until at least 20 years of age. The average prostate by this time measures about 4.5 cm in width, 3.5 to 4.0 cm in length, and 3 cm in thickness. In most men over 50 years of age, there is focal resumption of growth as benign nodular hyperplasia (BPH). This process increases the thickness of the gland prominently and affects its length the least; in massive BPH, however, the prostate becomes nearly spherical, with a diameter of 6 cm or more. Dissections show that BPH represents enlargement of only a single tiny region of the gland. In fact, the normal mass of the glandular portion of the prostate after subtraction of the BPH-prone region remains at nearly constant mean volume until 70 years of age or more. However, the range about the mean increases in men more than 50 years of age, suggesting that the normal non-BPH glandular prostate may continue enlarging into old age rather than undergoing atrophy.

The human prostate gland is a composite organ, made up of several glandular and nonglandular components. These different tissues are tightly fused together within a common capsule so that gross dissections are difficult and unreliable. Anatomic features are best demonstrated by examination of cut sections in carefully selected planes (4,5). The nonglandular tissue of the prostate is concentrated anteromedially and is responsible for much of the anterior convexity of the organ. The contour of the glandular prostate approximates a disk with lateral wings that fold anteriorly to partially encircle the nonglandular tissue. There are four distinct glandular regions, each of which arises from a different segment of the prostatic urethra.

The urethra is a primary reference point for describing anatomic relationships. These relationships are best visualized in a sagittal plane of section (Figure 36.3). The prostatic urethra is divided into proximal and distal segments of approximately equal length by an abrupt anterior angulation of its posterior wall at the midpoint between the prostate apex and bladder neck (1,6). The angle of deviation is roughly 35 degrees, but it is quite variable and is greater in men with nodular hyperplasia. The base of the verumontanum protrudes from the posterior urethral wall at the point of angulation. The verumontanum bulges into the urethral lumen along its posterior wall for about half the length of the distal segment and tapers distally to form the crista urethralis.

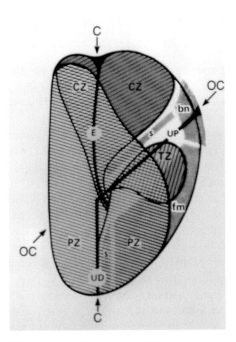

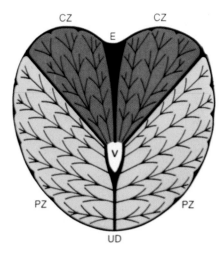

Figure 36.4 Coronal section diagram of prostate showing location of central zone (*CZ*) and peripheral zone (*PZ*) in relation to the distal urethral segment (*UD*), verumontanum (*V*), and ejaculatory ducts (*E*). The branching pattern of prostatic ducts is indicated; subsidiary ducts provide uniform density of acini along entire main duct course.

Figure 36.3 Sagittal diagram of distal prostatic urethral segment (*UD*), proximal urethral segment (*UP*), and ejaculatory ducts (*E*) showing their relationships to a sagittal section of the anteromedial nonglandular tissues [bladder neck (*bn*), anterior fibromuscular stroma (*fm*), preprostatic sphincter (*s*), distal striated sphincter (*s*)]. These structures are shown in relation to a three-dimensional representation of the glandular prostate [central zone (*CZ*), peripheral zone (*PZ*), transition zone (*TZ*)]. Coronal plane (*C*) of Figure 36.4 and oblique coronal plane (*OC*) of Figure 36.5 are indicated by arrows.

The distal urethral segment receives the ejaculatory ducts and the ducts of about 95% of the glandular prostate; it is, therefore, the only segment that is primarily involved in ejaculatory function. The ejaculatory ducts extend proximally from the verumontanum to the base of the prostate, following a course that is nearly a direct extension of the long axis of the distal urethral segment, although usually offset a few millimeters posteriorly.

A coronal plane of section along the course of the ejaculatory ducts and distal urethral segment provides the best demonstration of the anatomic relationships between the two major regions of the glandular prostate (7) (Figure 36.4). The peripheral zone comprises about 65% of the mass of the normal glandular prostate. Its ducts exit from the posterolateral recesses of the urethral wall along a double row extending from the base of the verumontanum to the prostate apex. The ducts extend mainly laterally in the coronal plane, with major branches that curve anteriorly and minor branches that curve posteriorly (Figure 36.4). The central zone comprises about 30% of the glandular prostate mass. Its ducts arise in a small focus on the convexity of the verumontanum and immediately surrounding the ejaculatory duct orifices. The ducts branch directly toward the base of the prostate along the course of the ejaculatory ducts, fanning out mainly in the coronal

plane to form a conical structure that is flattened in the anteroposterior dimension. The base of the cone comprises almost the entire base of the prostate. The most lateral central zone ducts run parallel to the most proximal peripheral zone ducts, separated only by a narrow band of stroma.

The proximal segment of the prostatic urethra is best visualized in an oblique coronal-plane section running along its long axis from the base of the verumontanum to the bladder neck (Figure 36.5). Normally, the proximal urethral segment is related to only about 5% of the prostatic glandular tissue, and almost all of this is represented by the transition zone (8). This zone consists of two independent small lobes whose ducts leave the posterolateral recesses

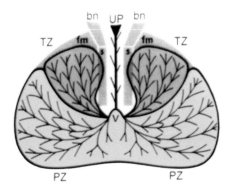

Figure 36.5 Oblique coronal section diagram of prostate showing location of peripheral zone (*PZ*) and transition zone (*TZ*) in relation to proximal urethral segment (*UP*), verumontanum (*V*), preprostatic sphincter (*s*), bladder neck (*bn*), anterior fibromuscular stroma (*fm*), and periurethral region with periurethral glands. Branching pattern of prostatic ducts is indicated: the medial transition zone ducts penetrate into the sphincter.

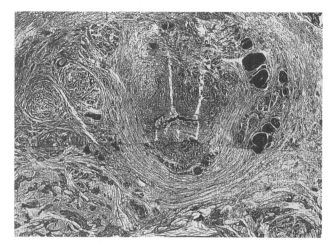

Figure 36.6 Preprostatic sphincter in section transverse to long axis of proximal urethral segment. The sphincter is most compact dorsal to the urethra (*below*) and separates periurethral tissue (*dark central area*) from central zone glands (*bottom, right,* and *left*). Laterally, transition zone glands are embedded in the sphincter. They show cystic change (*right*) and nodule formation (*left*).

of the urethral wall at a single point, just proximal to the point of urethral angulation and at the lower border of the preprostatic sphincter. The sphincter is a sleeve of smooth muscle fibers surrounding the proximal urethral segment (6,8) (Figure 36.6). The main ducts of the transition zone extend laterally around the distal border of the sphincter and curve sharply anteriorly, arborizing toward the bladder neck immediately external to the preprostatic sphincter. Main duct branches fan out laterally and ventrally toward the apex but not dorsally above the plane of the urethra. The most medial ducts and acini of the transition zone curve medially to penetrate into the sphincter (Figure 36.6).

The periurethral gland region is only a fraction of the size of the transition zone. It consists of tiny ducts and abortive acinar systems scattered along the length of the proximal urethral segment and arborizing exclusively inside the confines of the preprostatic sphincter. These glands lie within the longitudinal periurethral smooth muscle stroma.

The peripheral zone is the most susceptible region to inflammation (7) and is the site of origin of most carcinomas (9). Some cancers arise in the transition zone, and most tumors found incidentally at transurethral resection (TUR) represent this site of origin (10,11).

The transition zone and periurethral region are the exclusive sites of origin of BPH (8). Most cases consist almost entirely of transition zone enlargement, so-called lateral lobe hyperplasia. Benign nodular hyperplasia in the periurethral region seldom attains significant mass, except as the occasional midline dorsal nodule at the bladder neck that protrudes into the bladder lumen. The above anatomic descriptions have gained acceptance over the past 10 years, replacing a number of previous anatomic models that suffered from less accurate descriptions of morphologic detail (12,13).

GENERAL RELATIONSHIPS: NONGLANDULAR TISSUE

The nonglandular tissues of the prostate are the preprostatic sphincter, striated sphincter, anterior fibromuscular stroma, and prostatic capsule. The nerves and vascular supply are also included in this section.

The preprostatic sphincter consists of precisely parallel, compact ring fibers forming a cylinder whose proximal end abuts against the detrusor muscle surrounding the urethra at the bladder neck. The coarsely interwoven, somewhat randomly arranged smooth muscle bundles of the detrusor contrast sharply with the uniform arrangement of the sphincter fibers, but there is no boundary between the two structures.

The preprostatic sphincter is thought to function during ejaculation to prevent retrograde flow of seminal fluid from the distal urethral segment. It also may have resting tone that maintains closure of the proximal urethral segment (6). Dorsal to the urethra, the sphincter is compact, but laterally its fibers spread apart and mingle with the small ducts and acini of the medial transition zone (Figure 36.6) (8). Anterior and ventral to the urethra, its fibers do not form identifiable complete rings but blend with the tissue of the anterior fibromuscular stroma. The anterior fibromuscular stroma is an apron of tissue that extends downward from the bladder neck over the antero-medial surface of the prostate, narrowing to join the urethra at the prostate apex (8) (Figures 36.3, 36.7). Its

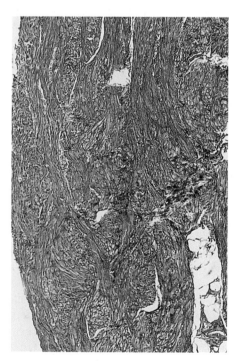

Figure 36.7 Texture of anterior fibromuscular stroma in an area with little fibrous component. Muscle bundles are coarse and interwoven (trichrome stain).

lateral margins blend with the prostate capsule along the line where the capsule covers the most anteriorly projecting border of the peripheral zone (Figure 36.5). Its deep surface is in contact with the preprostatic sphincter and transition zone proximally and with the striated sphincter distally. It is composed of large compact bundles of smooth muscle cells that are similar to those of the bladder neck and blend with them at its proximal extent. The smooth muscle fibers are more random in orientation than those of the bladder neck, but they tend to be aligned more or less vertically. They are often separated by bands of dense fibrous tissue.

The anterior fibromuscular stroma is distinguished from the capsule of the prostate by its thickness, its coarse interwoven muscle bundles, and its rough external surface. Microscopically its external aspect shows interdigitation of the muscle bundles along its surface with the adipose tissue of the space of Retzius.

Between the verumontanum and the prostate apex, there is a striated sphincter of small, uniform, compactly arranged striated muscle fibers. It is best developed near the apex and is continuous with the external sphincter below the prostate apex (6,14). The sphincter is incomplete posterolaterally, where its semicircular fibers anchor into the anterior glandular tissue of the peripheral zone rather than encircling the posterior aspect of the urethra. Its degree of development and precise anatomic relationships are variable between prostates. Near the apex in some prostates, individual striated fibers may penetrate deeply into the glandular tissue of the peripheral zone. Consequently, most of the length of the prostatic urethra is provided with sphincteric muscle. The distal striated sphincter is incomplete posteriorly, and the proximal smooth muscle sphincter is probably incomplete anteriorly.

The prostatic capsule envelopes most of the external surface of the prostate, and the terminal acini of the central zone and peripheral zone abut on the capsule. The terminal acini of the transition zone abut on the anterior fibromuscular stroma, and the periurethral glands never reach the prostate surface (8,11). At the prostate apex, there is a defect in the capsule anteriorly and anterolaterally. Here the most distal fibers of the anterior fibromuscular stroma and the striated sphincter together often mingle with the prostatic glandular tissue anterolateral to the urethra, and the relative extent of these three tissue components may vary considerably between prostates. Hence, if carcinoma at the prostate apex invades anteriorly, it may occasionally be difficult to determine whether it has invaded beyond the boundary of the gland. However, around most of the circumference of the apex, the capsule is complete up to the border of the periurethral stroma, where the urethra penetrates the prostate surface. Even with extensive BPH, a thin compressed rim of peripheral zone tissue enclosed by capsule usually still forms the apical prostate boundary except anterior and anterolateral to the urethra.

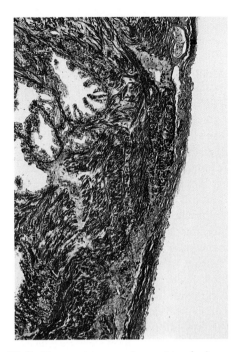

Figure 36.8 The prostate capsule consists of a layer of mainly transverse smooth muscle bundles (red), which is of variable thickness and blends with periacinar smooth muscle bundles at the capsule's poorly defined inner aspect (*left*). Collagen fibers (blue) are always present and usually concentrated in a thin compact membrane at the external capsular border (*right*) (trichrome stain).

The capsule of the prostate ideally consists of an inner layer of smooth muscle fibers, mainly oriented transversely, and an outer collagenous membrane. However, the relative and absolute amounts of fibrous and muscle tissue and their arrangement vary considerably from area to area (Figure 36.8) (15,16). At the inner capsular border, transverse smooth muscle blends with periacinar smooth muscle, and clear separation between them cannot be identified either microscopically or by gross dissection. The distance from terminal acinus to prostate surface is variable even between different regions within a single prostate, and the proportion and arrangement of collagenous tissue is inconstant except for the most superficial layer, which appears to form a thin continuous collagenous membrane over the prostate surface. Consequently, except for its external surface, the prostate capsule cannot be regarded as a well-defined anatomic structure with constant features. In contrast to the kidney, there is no inner membrane surface that can be stripped in evaluating capsule penetration by prostatic carcinoma; there are no reliable landmarks for determining the depth of capsule invasion. However, it has been proposed that only complete penetration with perforation through the capsule surface may be related to prognosis in prostatic carcinoma (16,17). Hence, penetration of cancer into the capsule without perforation is not of clinical importance.

Over the medial half of the posterior (rectal) surface of the prostate, the thickness of the capsule is increased by its fusion to Denonvilliers' fascia (Figures 36.9–36.10). This is a thin, compact collagenous membrane whose smooth posterior surface rests directly against the muscle of the rectal wall (18). The capsule is typically fused to the inner aspect of the fascia, obliterating any trace of its original surface except for occasional remnants of an interposed adipose layer that embryonically covered the anterior aspect of the fascia. In the adult, there remain only scattered microscopic islands of fat, usually forming a layer that is only one adipose cell thick.

Smooth muscle fibers are found to a variable extent in Denonvilliers' fascia, but they usually course vertically, in contrast to the predominant transverse muscle fibers of the adherent capsule. In some prostates, the smooth muscle of Denonvilliers' fascia is gathered into a thick, flattened vertical band at the midline, where it easily may be mistaken in a radical prostatectomy specimen for muscle of the rectal wall. This is an important distinction because carcinoma invading such a longitudinal muscle bundle may still be confined within the prostate and should not be considered

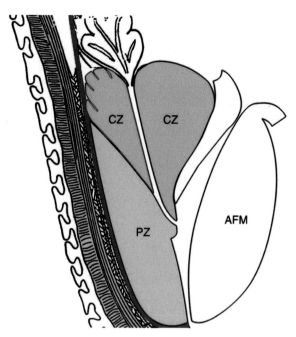

Figure 36.10   Relationships of Denonvilliers' fascia (narrow red band) to sagittal plane of prostate (yellow and orange; *right*) and to rectal smooth muscle (brown; *left*). (*CZ*, central zone; *PZ*, peripheral zone; *AFM*, anterior fibromuscular fascia)

to have invaded the rectum. Wherever the capsule and fascia are fused, it is the surface of the fascia rather than the capsule surface that presents a barrier to the spread of carcinoma.

Superiorly, Denonvilliers' fascia extends above the prostate to cover the posterior surface of the seminal vesicles, but it is only loosely adherent to them (Figure 36.9–36.10). Laterally, the fascia leaves the posterior capsule where the prostate surface begins to deviate anteriorly, and it continues in a coronal plane to anchor against the pelvic sidewalls. So the prostate and seminal vesicles are suspended along the anterior aspect of this fascial membrane as the uterus is suspended from the broad ligament in the female. This can be demonstrated in the radical prostatectomy specimen after surgery for carcinoma. If the specimen is picked up at the right and left superior margins, its posterior aspect is a smooth-surfaced triangular membrane whose apex coincides with the prostate apex and whose base is a transverse line above the seminal vesicles. Any surgical defect in the fascia potentially compromises the complete resection of the tumor because tears in the fascia tend to extend through the adherent capsule and into the gland.

Where Denonvilliers' fascia separates from the prostate capsule posterolaterally, the space between them is filled with adipose tissue in a thick layer between the anterior aspect of the fascia and the posterolateral capsular surface of the prostate. The autonomic nerves, from the pelvic plexus

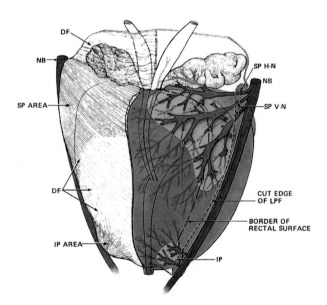

Figure 36.9   Distribution of nerve branches to the prostate, right posterolateral view. Nerves within the neurovascular bundle (*NB*) (red) branch to supply the prostate (brown) in a large superior pedicle (*SP*) at the prostate base and a small inferior pedicle (*IP*) at the prostate apex. Nerve branches (orange) leave the lateral pelvic fascia (not shown) to travel in Denonvilliers' fascia (*DF*), which has been cut away from the right half of the prostate. Nerve branches from the superior pedicle fan out over a large pedicle area. A small horizontal subdivision (*H-N*) crosses the base to midline; a large vertical subdivision (*V-N*) fans out extensively over the prostate surface as far distally as midprostate. Branches continue their course within the prostate after penetration into the capsule within a large nerve penetration area (green). A small inferior pedicle has a limited ramification and nerve penetration area (green). (*LPF*, lateral pelvic fascia)

to the seminal vesicles, prostate, and corpora cavernosa of the penis, travel in this fatty layer. The nerves, along with the blood vessels to the prostate, originate from the paired neurovascular bundles that course vertically along the pelvic sidewalls just anterior to the junction of Denonvilliers' fascia with the pelvis (Figure 36.9) (19). Most of the nerve branches to the prostate leave the neurovascular bundle at a single level just above the prostate base and course medially as the superior pedicle. These nerve branches fan out to penetrate the superior pedicle insertion area of the capsule, which is centered at the lateral aspect of the prostate base posteriorly (19,20). The insertion area does not usually extend far onto the rectal surface but extends toward the prostate apex as far as the midprostate. Some nerve trunks travel medially across the prostate base, sending branches into the central zone, but the majority of nerve branches fan out distally and penetrate the capsule at an oblique angle.

Most examples of capsule penetration by cancer represent tumor extension through the capsule along perineural spaces (20). Because of the oblique retrograde nerve pathway toward the prostate base, perforation though the full capsule thickness most commonly occurs near or even above the superior border of the cancer within the gland. Because of the boundaries of the superior pedicle insertion area plus the additional thickness of Denonvilliers' fascia overlying the capsule posteromedially, penetration of cancer directly through the rectal surface of the prostate is uncommon.

Before supplying the corpora cavernosa, nerve branches leave the neurovascular bundle at the prostate apex in the very small inferior pedicle and penetrate the capsule directly in a small apical insertion area located laterally and posterolaterally (20). Here the distance from neurovascular bundle to prostate capsule is narrowed to only a few millimeters. The prostate apex is the most common location for positive surgical margins at radical prostatectomy. This may result from capsule penetration along inferior pedicle nerves by cancers that are located near the apex, but it most commonly results from inadvertent surgical incision into the prostate. In this area, the surgeon is most concerned to stay close to the prostate capsule in order to spare the nerves involved in erectile function (21,22).

Arterial branches follow the nerve branches from the neurovascular bundle; they spread over the prostate surface and penetrate the capsule to extend directly inward toward the distal urethral segment between the radiating duct systems of the central and peripheral zones (23,24). A major arterial branch enters the prostate at each side of the bladder neck and runs toward the verumontanum parallel to the course of the proximal urethral segment. It supplies the periurethral region and medial transition zone. Transurethral resection regularly obliterates this arterial branch and all the tissue supplied by it (23).

ARCHITECTURAL PATTERNS OF THE GLANDULAR PROSTATE

The biologic role of the prostate calls for the slow accumulation and occasional rapid expulsion of small volumes of fluid. These requirements are optimally met by a muscular organ having a large storage capacity and low secretory capacity. In such an organ, the different morphology of ducts and acini found in organs of high secretory capacity, such as the pancreas, would appear to be of limited value. Accordingly, the prostatic ducts are morphologically identical to the acini except for their geometry, and both appear to function as distensible secretory reservoirs. Within each prostate zone, the entire duct–acinar system, except for the main ducts near the urethra, is lined by columnar secretory cells of identical appearance between ducts and acini. Immunohistochemical staining for prostate-specific antigen (PSA) and prostatic acid phosphatase (PAP) shows uniform granular staining of all ductal and acinar cells (Figure 36.11). In view of these considerations, there is probably no functional duct–acinar distinction in the prostate, and it is unlikely that there is any morphologic or biologic distinction between carcinomas of ductal versus acinar origin.

Except for the main transition zone ducts, which terminate at the anterior fibromuscular stroma, the main ducts of the prostate originate at the urethra and terminate near the capsule (4,7,8) (Figures 36.4–36.5). Because ducts and acini within each zone have comparable caliber, spacing,

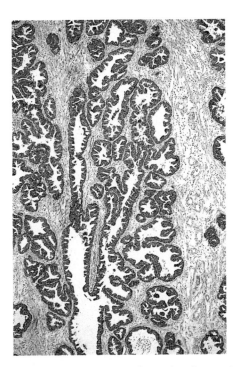

Figure 36.11 Ducts and acini of peripheral zone, immunostained with anti-PSA and showing uniform distribution of protein throughout the cytoplasm of all ducts and acini.

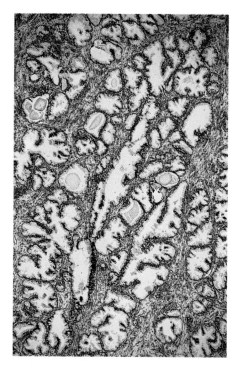

Figure 36.12 Subsidiary duct and branches in peripheral zone, terminating in small rounded acini with undulating borders. Ducts and acini have similar calibers and histologic appearances.

and histologic appearance, ducts, ductules, and acini cannot reliably be distinguished microscopically except in sections cut along the ductal long axis. Hence, abnormalities of architectural pattern are identified in routine sections mainly by deviations from normal size and spacing of glandular units.

The main excretory duct orifices of the peripheral zone arise from the urethral wall about every 2 mm along a double lateral line extending the full 1.5 cm length of the distal urethral segment. A cluster of three or four subsidiary ducts arise about every 2 mm along the course of each main excretory duct from urethra to capsule. They branch at angles of about 15 degrees and extend only a short distance, re-branching and giving rise to groups of acini (Figure 36.12). Hence, acini tend to be distributed with nearly uniform density along the course of the main duct between urethra and capsule, except that no acini are found immediately adjacent to the urethra. Conversely, beneath the capsule all glands are acinar. The architecture in the transition zone is similar to the peripheral zone. However, there is more extensive arborization because the main ducts arise from the urethra in a small focus.

The duct origins of the transition zone and periurethral glands from the proximal urethral segment represent a proximal continuation of the double lateral line of the peripheral zone duct origins along the distal urethral segment. However, periurethral ducts also originate anteriorly and posteriorly. This accounts for the presentation of peri-

urethral gland BPH as a dorsal midline bladder neck mass, whereas the lateral locations of transition zone BPH masses reflect the constant location of their main ducts (8).

In the peripheral zone and transition zone, ducts and acini are usually 0.15 to 0.3 mm in diameter and have simple rounded contours that are not perfectly circular because of prominent undulations of the epithelial border (5,7). The undulations mainly reflect the presence of corrugations of the wall, which presumably allow expansion of the lumina as secretory reservoirs. An important criterion for the diagnosis of many highly differentiated prostatic carcinomas is their tendency toward precisely round or oval glandular contours (25,26), reflecting a loss of reservoir function.

Central zone ducts and acini are distinctively larger than those of the peripheral zone and transition zone and may be up to 0.6 mm in diameter or larger (Figure 36.13). Unlike the peripheral zone, both ducts and acini of the central zone become progressively larger toward the capsule at the prostate base, where they often exceed 1 mm in diameter. There is also a gradient of increasing density of acini toward the base. Both of these gradients reflect the great expansion of central zone cross-sectional area from a small focus on the verumontanum to almost the entire prostate base. Near the urethra, the central zone ducts have few branches and lack distinctive histologic features. Hence, they may not be recognizable in transverse planes of section near the base of the verumontanum. Acini are clustered into lobules around a central subsidiary duct,

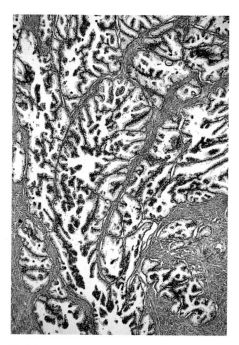

Figure 36.13 Subsidiary ducts and acini in the central zone form a compact lobule with flattened gland borders and prominent intraluminal ridges.

which is distinguishable from the acini in cross section only by its central location. Ducts and acini are polygonal in contour. Many of the corrugations in their walls are exaggerated into distinctive intraluminal ridges with stromal cores, which partially subdivide acini.

Glandular subdivisions within a given duct branch in the central zone are separated by narrow bands of distinctively compact smooth muscle fibers, whereas broader bands separate different branches. The normal overall ratio of epithelium to stroma here (lumens excluded) is roughly 2:1. The epithelial to stromal ratio of the peripheral zone and transition zone is close to 1:1. In the peripheral zone, the more abundant stroma is loosely woven, with randomly arranged muscle bundles separated by indistinct spaces containing loose, finely fibrillar collagenous tissue. Between the glandular spaces in a given duct branch, stroma is as abundant as between different branches.

There is an abrupt contrast in stromal morphology that delineates the boundary between central zone and peripheral zone and a similar contrast between peripheral zone and transition zone (11) (Figures 36.14–36.16). The transition zone stroma is composed of compact interlacing smooth muscle bundles (Figures 36.14, 36.16). This stromal density contrasts sharply with the adjacent loose peripheral zone stroma, but it blends with the stromas of the preprostatic sphincter and anterior fibromuscular stroma. Stromal distinctions are less evident in older prostates and may be obliterated by disease (27,28).

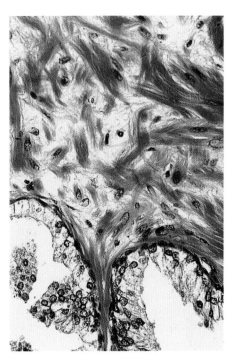

Figure 36.15 Peripheral zone acini set in loosely woven fibromuscular stroma. Secretory cells are more regular than in central zone, with smaller basal nuclei and pale cytoplasm. Basal cells are visible.

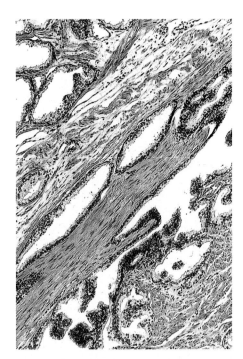

Figure 36.14 Border between the peripheral zone (*above*) and transition zone shows contrast in stromal texture and a band of smooth muscle at the zone boundary. Glandular histology is similar between zones.

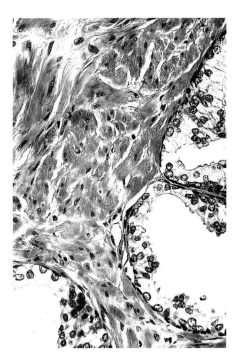

Figure 36.16 Transition zone acini set in a compact stroma composed of interlacing, coarse, smooth muscle bundles. Acinar histology is identical to that in the peripheral zone. Basal cells are visible.

CYTOLOGIC FEATURES OF THE GLANDULAR PROSTATE

As with other glandular organs, the secretory cells throughout the prostate are separated from the basement membrane and stroma by a layer of basal cells. These cells are markedly elongated and flattened parallel to the basement membrane and have slender, filiform dark nuclei and usually little or no discernible cytoplasm (29) (Figures 36.15–36.16). They are typically quite inconspicuous; and, in routine preparations, the basal cell envelope may appear incomplete or even absent around individual ducts or acini. However, immunohistochemical staining for basal cell–specific keratin or for p63 antibody shows the envelope to be complete, even where no basal cells are identified with routine stains (30). These stains are consistently negative in the cells of invasive malignant glands (31) because basal cells are absent.

Basal cells are not myoepithelial cells analogous to those of the breast because, by electron microscopy, they do not contain muscle filaments (29). Logically, myoepithelial cells would appear to be functionally superfluous in a muscular organ (29). Basal cells have been found to be the proliferative compartment of the prostate epithelium, normally dividing and maturing into secretory cells (32–34). Using immunostaining for proliferating cell nuclear antigen as a marker for cycling cells, roughly 1% of basal cells and 0.1% of secretory cells were labeled in each zone, and there was no difference between ducts and acini. Eighty-three percent of all labeled cells were basal cells, even though they comprised only 30% of the total epithelial cell population (34).

In all zones of the prostate, the epithelium contains a small population of isolated, randomly scattered endocrine–paracrine cells (35) that are rich in serotonin-containing granules and contain neuron-specific enolase. Subpopulations of these cells also contain a variety of peptide hormones, such as somatostatin, calcitonin, and bombesin. They rest on the basal cell layer between secretory cells but do not typically appear to extend to the lumen or may send a narrow apical extension to the lumen. They often have laterally spreading dendritic processes. They are not reliably identifiable microscopically except with immunohistochemical and other special stains. Their specific role in prostate biology is unknown, but they presumably have paracrine function, perhaps in response to neural stimulation. Like similar cells in the lung and other organs, they occasionally give rise to small cell carcinomas, which do not contain PSA or PAP (36). Not infrequently, however, small cell carcinoma arises as a variant morphologic pattern within adenocarcinomas that elsewhere contain PSA and PAP; peptide hormones are found only in the small cell component (36). Hence, the status of these cells as an independent lineage is doubtful in the prostate.

The secretory cells of the prostate contribute a wide variety of products to the seminal plasma. PSA and PAP are produced by the secretory cells of the ducts and acini of all zones. Pepsinogen II (37) and tissue plasminogen activator (38) are normally produced only in the ducts and acini of the central zone. Lactoferrin is also exclusively a secretory product of the central zone, except in areas of inflammation where both the cells and secretions anywhere in the prostate may produce this substance (39). Lectin staining for cell membrane carbohydrates also shows significant differences between the two zones (40). It has been suggested that the central zone may be specialized for the production of enzymes whose substrates are secreted by the peripheral zone (38), but probable substrates have not been identified. In fact, no secretory product has so far been identified that is produced exclusively by the peripheral zone or transition zone.

The cytoplasm of the normal secretory cell in all zones is similar in appearance and is dominated by the universal abundance of uniform small clear secretory vacuoles. Vacuoles in peripheral zone and transition zone cytoplasm are packed at nearly maximum density (41), whereas, in the central zone, a more abundant dense cytoplasm is associated with a somewhat wider vacuole spacing and lower vacuole density. Because the secretory vacuoles appear empty by routine microscopy, peripheral zone and transition zone cells are pale to clear, and central zone cells are typically somewhat darker.

However, the appearance of normal cell cytoplasm on tissue sections is strongly influenced by staining technique and by the type of fixative used. In the peripheral zone and transition zone, light hematoxylin and eosin (H&E) staining after formalin fixation shows that normal cells are "clear cells" in which a faint network of pale-staining cytoplasmic partitions between vacuoles can be visualized with careful scrutiny under high magnification (Figure 36.17). Only an occasional cell shows complete outlines that define numerous intact vacuoles, but immunostaining with PSA or PAP on the same tissue sharply outlines all the cytoplasmic vacuolar partitions and shows no evidence of protein within the vacuoles. Denser H&E staining not only darkens the partitions but also enhances diffuse staining throughout the cytoplasm, which obscures both the clear cell appearance and the visualization of the vacuoles.

The contents of the apparently empty vacuoles consist partly of lipid, as judged by interpretation of fat stains on fresh frozen sections, but there is also a nonlipid component. With H&E staining after fixation in glutaraldehyde or the commercial fixative Ultrim (American Histology Reagent Co., Stockton, CA), the clear vacuoles are replaced by brightly staining red granules. The nature of the stained product is probably related to spermine, a low-molecular weight alkaline substance. Using these alternate fixatives, immunostaining for protein such as PSA or PAP is still negative within vacuole lumens.

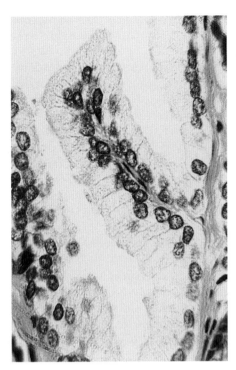

Figure 36.17 Peripheral zone epithelium showing clear cells in which cytoplasm is barely discernible as composed of a sheet of small empty vacuoles with delicate pale partitions.

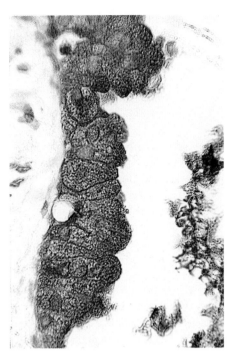

Figure 36.18 Peripheral zone epithelium immunostained with anti-PSA. Protein is concentrated in a reticulated pattern that spares vacuole lumens and accentuates portions of vacuole partitions.

Vacuoles are usually reduced or absent in the cytoplasm in dysplasia (prostatic intraepithelial neoplasia) (41) (Figure 36.3) and in most invasive carcinomas of Gleason's grade 3 or higher. In Gleason's grades 1 and 2 cancer, as well as some areas in grade 3 cancer, cytoplasmic vacuoles are retained, and these tumors have been referred to as clear cell carcinomas.

The secretory lining of peripheral zone glands conveys an orderly appearance, with a single layer of columnar cells having basally oriented nuclei. In most glands, however, the epithelial row shows considerable random variation between neighboring cells in the ratio of cell height to width and in apparent cell volume. Nuclear location also varies from the basal cell aspect to the mid-portion of the cell. The luminal cell border is consequently often uneven, and its roughness is accentuated by frequent cells whose luminal aspect is irregular and frayed. Prostate-specific antigen stain shows a reticular pattern diffusely throughout the cytoplasm (Figure 36.18).

These deviations from uniformity and the resulting slightly untidy pattern of the normal epithelial strip appear intimately related to secretory function. Cytokeratin immunostaining of secretory cells shows that the cytoskeleton does not extend as far as the luminal aspect of each cell (Figure 36.19); it usually terminates somewhat above the midportion of the cell level in a sharp transverse line whose level from cell to cell defines a more uniform thickness of

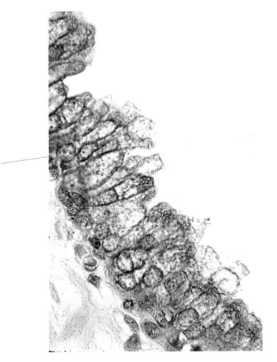

Figure 36.19 Peripheral zone epithelium immunostained with antibody to secretory cell cytokeratin. Normal epithelial cells appear quite variable in size and shape, and some nuclei are displaced from cell base. Cytokeratin is accentuated toward luminal border, but at lower right and upper middle, clusters of cells have attached apocrine compartments lumenward, which have no cytokeratin staining and accentuate the irregularity of luminal epithelial border.

the epithelial row than the full thickness that is stained by H&E. All of the cell contents toward the lumen from this transverse line appear to represent an isolated apocrine secretion compartment having diminished or absent cytoskeleton. As much as one-third of the total height of some cells may belong to this apocrine compartment. Lumenward from the terminal line of the keratin cytoskeleton, neighboring cells may lose their lateral adhesion and are sometimes separated by a narrow cleft. The indistinct luminal aspect of some cells appears to represent disintegration of this apical portion of the cell in situ. Release of contents of apocrine secretion into the lumen by fragmentation while still attached to the cell is the characteristic mode of peripheral zone and transition zone secretions; release of intact apocrine sacs from the underlying cell is rarely seen.

The morphologic appearance of normal peripheral zone epithelium is closely mimicked by only that minority of clear cell well-differentiated carcinomas that retain abundant cytoplasmic clear vacuoles, often Gleason's grades 1 and 2 (25,26). However, these malignant cells usually differ from normal peripheral zone in having a sharply defined luminal plasma membrane that lies at the same height between epithelial cells and traces an even transverse line around the gland perimeter (Figure 36.20). Thus, the frag-

menting apocrine compartment is usually absent; and, correspondingly, the cytoskeleton as visualized by keratin immunostaining the entire cytoplasm. Also, these malignant clear cells are of more nearly equal dimensions and contours than their benign counterparts, and nuclei are more strictly localized at the cell base. In dysplasia and in most grade 3 carcinomas, secretory vacuoles are much reduced or absent; cell cytoplasm is correspondingly dark (41).

Central zone epithelium, by contrast, shows an accentuation of the mild disorder of cell arrangement of the peripheral zone/transition zone (Figure 36.21). Here the epithelium is variably thickened by prominent cell crowding. Nuclei, which are usually larger than in the peripheral zone, are often displaced further from the cell base than in the peripheral zone and may give the illusion of stratification in more crowded areas. Cell height is often quite variable, and because the luminal cell border usually is intact rather than disintegrating, irregular protrusion of cell apices into the lumen is prominent. Apocrine secretion in the central zone may be identical to that in the peripheral zone, but often it is characterized by intact spherical sacs in the gland lumen, containing no vacuoles, and staining more densely than the parent cell. They tend to remain intact after secretion as dense luminal spheres (Figure 36.21).

The dark cytoplasm, thickened variable epithelium, and complex architecture in the central zone may be misinterpreted as atypical hyperplasia or dysplasia on needle

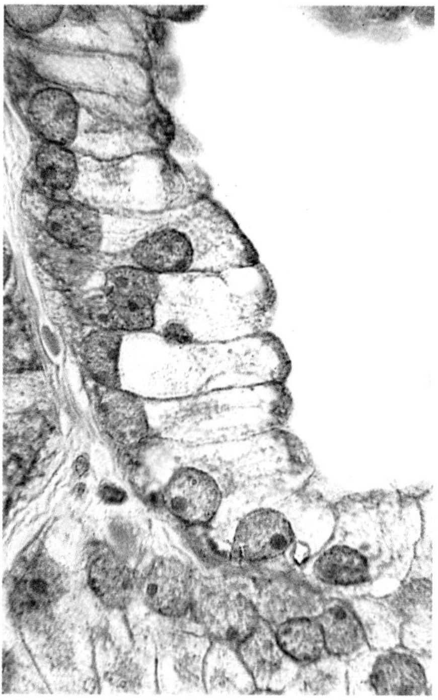

Figure 36.20 Clear cell carcinoma immunostained with antibody to secretory cell cytokeratin shows stronger cytokeratin accentuation at a luminal epithelial border, which is more even than in Figure 36.19, and lacks the apocrine secretory compartment. Cells are larger and more uniform than in Figure 36.19, with more basally located nuclei.

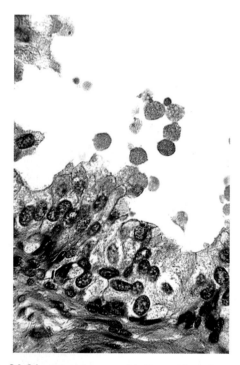

Figure 36.21 Central zone epithelium with dark cytoplasmic staining in an area of active apocrine secretion. Clear vacuoles are absent from apocrine secretion. Nuclei appear crowded and disordered, lying at different levels.

biopsies. However, the distinctive histologic features plus the absence of nuclear size variability, hyperchromasia, and loss of polarity rule against dysplasia. The central zone is not often sampled by needle biopsies because its maximum extent is mainly restricted close to the prostate base.

Unique specialized secretory structures called lacunae are also common in the central zone (39). These are tiny round lumens that appear to lie entirely within the epithelial cell layer, isolated from the main duct–acinar lumen system (Figures 36.22–36.23). A complete layer of flattened epithelial cells is seen to surround each lacuna, but these lacunar cells have no apparent contact with stroma. They only abut onto surrounding secretory cells. Lacunae are a specialized apparatus for lactoferrin production and storage, as demonstrated by immunohistochemical staining.

The central zone appears to represent a separate glandular organ within the prostate capsule. Aside from its unique morphologic features, its ducts arise from the urethra separately from the double lateral line of the remainder of the prostate. In addition, its ducts are in close anatomic proximity to the ejaculatory ducts and seminal vesicles. It has been suggested that the central zone may arise embryonically as an intrusion of wolffian duct stroma around the ejaculatory ducts into an organ that is otherwise of urogenital sinus origin (7). Pepsinogen II (37) and lactoferrin (39) are secreted by both the central zone and seminal vesicles but are not found under normal conditions in the peripheral or transition zones.

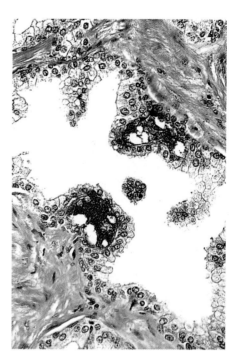

Figure 36.23 Central zone gland immunostained with anti-lactoferrin. Lacunae on both sides of the lumen are densely stained, but cell cytoplasm is negative.

DEVIATIONS FROM NORMAL HISTOLOGY

Beyond the age of 30 years, many prostates begin to show a variety of focal deviations from normal morphology (4,7,27,28). Their prevalence, extent, and severity progressively increase with age so that most prostates by the seventh decade of life are quite heterogeneous in histologic composition. Although these deviant histologic patterns seldom have clinical significance, their distinction from adenocarcinoma or BPH is sometimes difficult.

Early morphologic studies concluded that focal atrophy in the prostate was a manifestation of aging and was seen as early as 40 years of age. In fact, focal atrophy in the prostate is often the consequence of previous inflammation rather than aging (4,7). The number and extent of atrophic foci tend to be greater in older men, but their histologic appearance is identical to that of isolated foci found as early as 30 years of age. The histologic features are identical to those produced by chronic bacterial prostatitis, but no etiologic agent has been identified in the vast majority of cases, most of which appear to be asymptomatic.

Postinflammatory atrophy is an extremely common lesion and is mainly a disease of the peripheral zone, where its distribution is sharply segmental along the ramifications of a duct branch (4,7). It is characterized by a marked shrinkage of ducts and acini with periglandular fibrosis and variable distortion of architecture (Figures 36.24–36.25).

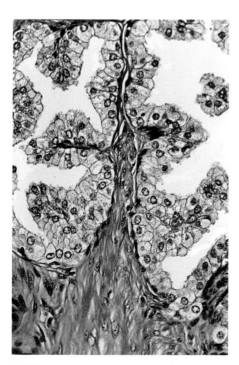

Figure 36.22 Central zone with dense muscle bundles, dark basal cells, and opaque cytoplasm.

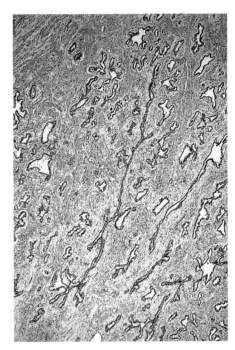

Figure 36.24   Focus of postinflammatory atrophy in peripheral zone. Duct–acinar architecture is apparent but distorted by marked gland shrinkage, with reduced luminal area and periglandular fibrosis.

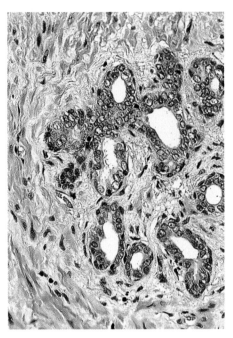

Figure 36.25   Tiny distorted glands of postinflammatory atrophy. Irregular contours and large nuclei mimic carcinoma; however, cytoplasm is scant, and there are periglandular collagenous rings.

Glandular units may be drawn together into clusters or spread out into a pattern suggesting invasive carcinoma. In addition to the presence of tiny distorted glands, the resemblance to cancer is further increased by the fact that nuclei may remain relatively large with occasional small nucleoli.

In contrast to carcinoma, cell cytoplasm is usually much reduced in volume, and evidence of the original duct–acinar architecture often can be detected. Furthermore, there is usually residual inflammation, with scattered round cells in the adjacent stroma. Finally, there is sometimes an admixture of glands showing the earlier active phase of the process, with prominent periductal and periacinar chronic inflammatory infiltrate and less prominent gland shrinkage.

Cystic atrophy is another common focal lesion that is typically found in the peripheral zone and is segmental in distribution. The markedly enlarged acini with flattened epithelium and the segmental distribution suggest an obstructive cause (Figure 36.26). However, obstruction is not typically demonstrable, and the stroma between glands is usually attenuated rather than compressed by luminal expansion. This suggests that stromal atrophy may be the main pathogenetic event.

The histologic hallmark of BPH is the expansile nodule, produced by the budding and branching of newly formed duct–acinar structures (Figure 36.27), by the focal proliferation of stroma, or by a combination of both elements (4,5,8,42). It mainly affects the transition zone, with occasional contribution from the periurethral region.

Individual BPH nodules rarely become larger than 1.6 cm in greatest diameter; and, in any prostate, median nodule diameter is almost always less than 8 mm. An exception is produced in massive BPH by secondary nodule enlargement due to cystic dilatation of component glands.

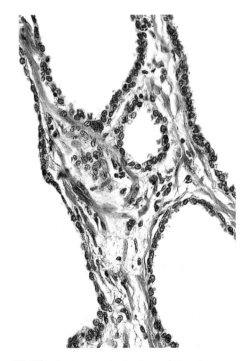

Figure 36.26   Cystic atrophy in the peripheral zone.

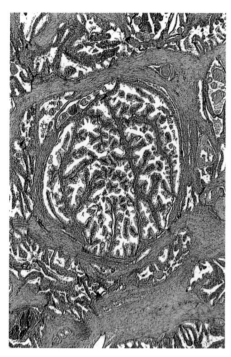

Figure 36.27 Very small, gland-rich benign nodular hyperplasia nodule arising from dense stroma.

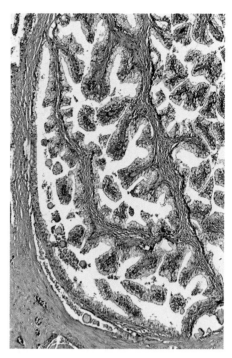

Figure 36.28 Small BPH nodule with increase of epithelial to stromal ratio to roughly 2:1 and surrounded by normal transition zone with epithelial to stromal ratio far below 1.

Grossly BPH is usually recognized as a globular mass replacing each transition zone and composed of numerous individual nodules embedded within a diffusely hyperplastic transition zone tissue (Figure 36.28). Only the nodular component is recognizable histologically as a deviation from normal pattern; internodular tissue, even when increased in amount, is not distinguishable microscopically from normal transition zone.

The enlargement of transition zone BPH produces a characteristic progressive deformity of overall prostate contour (Figure 36.29). The tissue lateral and posterior to the prostatic urethra (central zone and peripheral zone) is relatively unyielding, and expansion is directed anteriorly and toward the apex at the selective expense of stretching and thinning of the anterior fibromuscular stroma. This produces a predominant increase in the thickness (anteroposterior dimension) of the gland. The anterolateral wings of the peripheral zone where they taper to join the anterior fibromuscular stroma (Figure 36.5) are compressed and thinned concomitant with increase of overall prostate width, but posterior and lateral peripheral zones are not significantly thinned except in massive BPH.

The central zone is the least compressed region, but it is pulled forward over the BPH mass, accompanied by characteristic lengthening of the proximal urethral segment. As the urethra lengthens, its angulation at the midpoint increases, sometimes approaching 90 degrees (Figure 36.29). Increased angulation produces a more globular anteroapical compartment, which accommodates a larger BPH mass. The

mucosa of the lateral urethral walls is compressed between the two opposed transition zone masses, and its surface area is stretched to a larger expanse as the transition zone masses expand (Figure 36.30).

Basal cell hyperplasia is most often seen as a secondary change in BPH nodules or inflammatory foci (33). The basal cells of ducts and acini become rounded with oval nuclei, and they form a multilayered lining that stains for

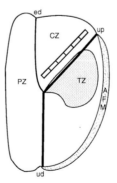
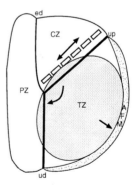

Figure 36.29 Sagittal diagrams of prostate showing main features of deformity produced by transition zone BPH. Transition zone (*TZ*) is bounded by the distal urethral segment (*ud*), proximal urethral segment (*up*), and anterior fibromuscular stroma (*FM*) (see Figure 36.3). Only the last leg of this triangular compartment yields easily to the pressure of transition zone expansion. Increased angulation and lengthening of urethra produce a more spherical compartment with increased capacity. *Arrows* indicate main features of deformity. (*CZ*, central zone; *PZ*, peripheral zone; *ed*, ejaculatory duct)

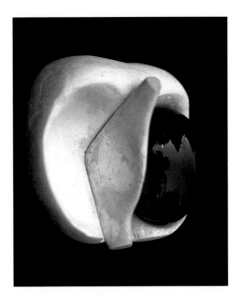

Figure 36.30   Model of prostate with severe BPH seen in three-quarter frontal view. The transition zone mass on far side (blue) shows growth mainly anteriorly and toward the apex. BPH mass has been removed on the near side, showing concavity in the peripheral zone caused mainly by stretching and thinning of the anterolateral margin. The urethra shows prominent increased angulation, with anterior stretching of lateral walls between BPH masses.

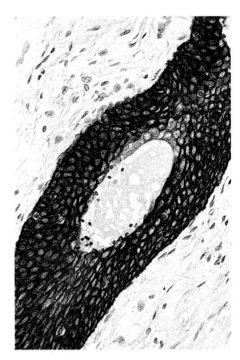

Figure 36.31   Prostatic duct with basal cell hyperplasia immunostained with antibody to basal cell–specific cytokeratin. Basal cells create multiple layers, but a single luminal layer is secretory and remains unstained.

basal cell–specific cytokeratin (Figure 36.31). There is typically a single luminal row of columnar secretory cells that stain positive for PSA.

In BPH, basal cell hyperplasia is common at the margin of nodule infarcts, where presumably it represents a reaction to ischemia. Consistent with this proposal is the finding of smooth muscle atrophy and replacement by fibroblastic stroma in these areas. Much more commonly, basal cell hyperplasia is found in BPH nodules without frank infarction, but the almost invariable presence of fibroblastic stroma and smooth muscle atrophy suggest that ischemia may be etiologic here also. Gland shrinkage also usually accompanies these foci and may suggest a superficial resemblance to carcinoma.

Dysplasia is a type of morphologic change seen in any prostate zone and characterized by focal enlargement of individual cells in an area with rounded dark nuclei showing changes characteristic of adenocarcinoma and occasionally showing features intermediate between cancer, dysplasia ducts, and acini (Figures 36.32–36.33).

EVALUATION OF RADICAL PROSTATECTOMY SPECIMENS

Normal morphologic features can be difficult to evaluate in the age group in which radical prostatectomy is usually performed. Landmarks are often obscured or distorted by retrogressive changes with aging or inflammation, whereas some prostates retain the normal appearance of the third

decade of life, and some show increased glandular epithelial activity with or without atypia. Not infrequently, the morphologic appearance of any zone seems unrelated to the changes in other zones. Difficulties of interpretation are compounded when all sections are cut in the same plane

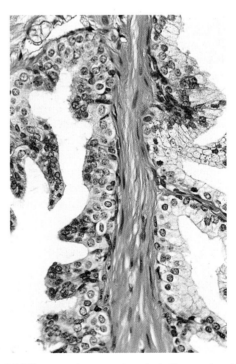

Figure 36.32   Central zone with right half normal and left half showing mild dysplasia.

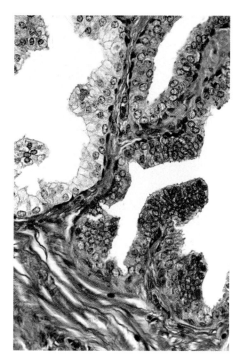

Figure 36.33 Central zone with left half showing mild dysplasia and right half showing severe dysplasia.

rather than different planes designed for optimum visualization of each zone.

Transverse planes of section, perpendicular to the rectal surface are the most common type of routine prostate sectioning, partly because they are the easiest to cut. They are also nearly parallel to the plane of many ultrasound and magnetic resonance images. They show much the same relationships as the oblique coronal planes except that the urethra is never seen along its long axis. It is important to review the expected appearance of transverse planes at different levels because of the considerable differences encountered.

Transverse sections distal to the base of the verumontanum demonstrate the transition zone at most levels of section toward the apex in most men over 50 years of age, even when there are few nodules to signify BPH (8,42). Diffuse transition zone enlargement accompanying nodule development is nearly universal with age, and expansion is mainly anterior and toward the apex. The boundary between the transition zone and peripheral zone is often visualized more clearly by ultrasound imaging than by histologic study. Microscopically the difference in texture of the stroma between the two zones is the most important evidence for the location of the boundary between them, but it may not be apparent at all points.

The boundary of the transition zone with the peripheral zone seldom extends closer than 1.0 cm to the posterior (rectal) prostate surface. If there has been a previous TUR, the resection cavity usually extends mainly anteriorly from the posterior urethral wall. Significantly, the TUR often spares the lateral portion of the transition zone, sometimes with residual nodules, and the transition zone boundary remains intact.

Proximal to the base of the verumontanum, only one or two sections still show a transition zone unless there is a large mass of BPH tissue. The ejaculatory ducts now appear on these proximal sections, with the utricle between them. The dorsal, compact transverse portion of the preprostatic sphincter may be seen just anterior to the ejaculatory ducts. The sphincter and urethral lumen progress more anteriorly at each level of section cephalad until they reach the anterior tissue border at the bladder neck.

The bladder neck lies a variable number of sections below (apical to) the highest transverse section cut at the prostate base (Figure 36.34). The central zone may not be apparent histologically until the bladder neck level of section or higher. It usually appears suddenly between two transverse levels of section separated by only 3 mm. This is because the central zone is an inverted flared cone whose apical region near the verumontanum consists predominantly of main duct branches that cannot be readily distinguished from those of other zones. At the transverse level where it is first recognizable, the anterior portion of the central zone may lie directly above the area occupied by the transition zone in the section just one level below, and the transition zone is usually no longer visible. The central zone has a more distinctive histologic appearance in sections toward the base because of the rather abrupt increase in size and number of branches. The most basal section is usually almost entirely composed of central zone and consists mostly of acini that are distinctively large, polygonal, and closely packed (14).

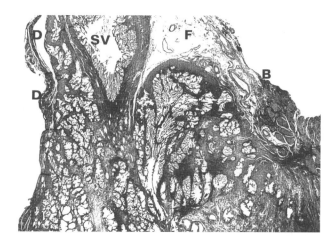

Figure 36.34 Parasagittal section of prostate base located almost at midline. Bladder neck smooth muscle above the level of bladder neck lumen is seen as a small dark patch (*B*) at far right. A layer of fat (*F*) covers the dome-shaped surface of the anterior central zone (*top center*). All glandular tissue within is central zone. One main duct (*center*) is seen in profile as it flares out toward the base, generating elaborate acinar structures. Behind the seminal vesicle (*SV*), the posterior central zone extends more celaphad as a narrow plate. Denonvilliers' fascia (*D*) is not adherent behind the seminal vesicles but blends with the capsule below.

As the seminal vesicles leave the prostate base, they extend laterally along its basal surface (Figure 36.9). Often there is no capsule between the two organs, at least for the medial centimeter or more of the seminal vesicle. The degree of fusion between the two muscular walls is variable between prostates, but there is frequently no boundary whatever between the two organs medially, and only one millimeter of common muscular wall may separate the most basal central zone gland lumen from the seminal vesicle lumen.

The origin of the ejaculatory ducts at the junction of seminal vesicles and vas deferens is surrounded by central zone glandular tissue and usually situated so that about two-thirds of the central zone mass is anterior to the ejaculatory ducts. However, it is quite common for the ejaculatory ducts to be situated more posteriorly; occasionally they enter the prostate on the rectal surface and entirely posterior to the central zone.

The most basal transverse section of prostate usually has some bladder neck muscular wall at its anterior extent (Figure 36.34). Behind this muscle is a strip of fat that lies between the seminal vesicles and the bladder and rests on top of the most anterior aspect of the central zone. That portion of the central zone anterior to the ejaculatory ducts usually terminates at a lower level than the posterior portion, and the latter extends further cephalad as a thin plate between seminal vesicles and Denonvilliers' fascia (Figure 36.35). The strip of fat contains the large nerve trunks extending medially from the autonomic ganglia of the superior pedicle, which is situated lateral to the central zone at this level. When cancer penetrates the capsule at the prostate base, it is often seen within the fatty strip between bladder neck and central zone. Less often, it is associated with the nerves and ganglia of the superior pedicle lateral to the gland. Occasionally cancer extends above the prostate base posteri-

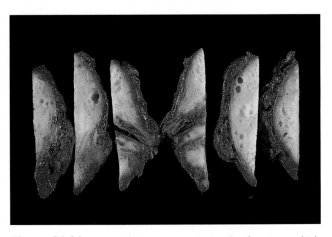

Figure 36.36 Apex of prostate seen grossly after 6-mm thick apical block has been subsectioned parasagittally at 3-mm intervals. Orientation of sections and localization of lesions are easily demonstrated, and cuts through the capsule are nearly perpendicular to the apical surface.

orly within the layers of Denonvillier's fascia. In large cancers, these three routes of extension—anteriorly, laterally, and posteriorly—often fuse with cancer in the seminal vesicle to produce a confluent mass of tumor above the prostate base.

At the apex of the prostate, sections should be taken as serial parasagittal subsections of a 6-mm thick block (Figure 36.36). This procedural modification sacrifices the transverse sectioning of the last level, which would lie 3 mm above the apex. However, it creates the advantage of showing the apical prostate tissue in planes that are more nearly perpendicular to the apical capsule surfaces, so that penetration of cancer can be more easily evaluated. In this area, where positive surgical margins are relatively common and capsule layers may be indistinct, such an advantage is important. Anterior to the urethra and for a narrow span anterolaterally, there is no capsule but only the distal end of the anterior fibromuscular stroma. Here there is a variable admixture of glands, striated muscle, and smooth muscle, and evaluation of capsule penetration is difficult. This is an area where adequate surgical resection is particularly difficult, and a positive margin may occasionally be created by transection of a small anterior cancer that was incidental, whereas the clinically detected cancer was elsewhere and has been successfully removed.

CONSIDERATIONS IN TRANSURETHRAL RESECTION AND NEEDLE BIOPSY SPECIMENS

Tissue distortion by heat coagulation near the edges of TUR chips can create important diagnostic problems that occasionally may be insurmountable. Basal cell hyperplasia,

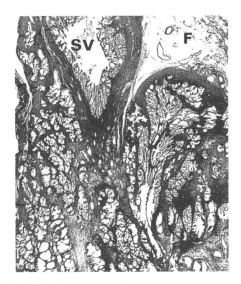

Figure 36.35 High power of central zone showing vertical course of ducts. (*SV*, seminal vesicle; *F*, fat)

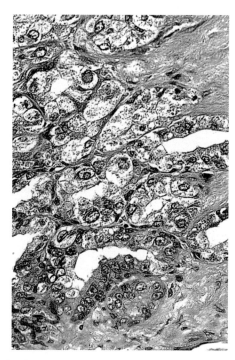

Figure 36.37 Benign tubular invaginations from the wall of the intraprostatic seminal vesicle showing architectural and cytologic features that suggest carcinoma. Note the characteristic yellow-brown cytoplasmic granules.

adenomatous hyperplasia, inflammatory atrophy, and fragments of BPH nodules with small glands may be indistinguishable from carcinoma. Loss of nuclear detail occurs to a greater depth into the chip than obvious cell distortion. Hence, small foci of cancer may be more difficult to diagnose because of the artifactual absence of nucleoli. Gleason has indicated that the identification of occasional nucleoli larger than 1 μm in diameter is an important criterion for distinguishing well-differentiated cancer from adenosis (26).

The same problems are seen in needle biopsies, where the artifact is presumably due to compression rather than heat. The presence of artifact is usually limited to loss of nuclear detail and is more subtle because areas of severe tissue distortion are not often represented.

The regions of the prostate sampled by TUR and by needle biopsy tend to be quite different. Most needle biopsies represent peripheral zone tissue. Unless a special effort is made, the needle seldom reaches the central zone or the more anterior portions of the transition zone.

In the majority of cases, TUR specimens consist of transition zone tissue, urethral and periurethral tissues, bladder neck fragments, and anterior fibromuscular stroma (42). The preprostatic sphincter is always present but usually not identifiable. Occasionally, fragments of the proximal end of the striated sphincter are present. Our study of radical prostatectomy specimens post-TUR has shown that the resection usually does not extend beyond the transition zone boundary into the central or peripheral zones,

and usually not all the transition zone tissue has been removed (42).

Occasionally, peripheral zone or central zone tissue may be sampled at TUR. Central zone fragments show distinctive architectural and cytologic features described above. They are not infrequently accompanied by fragments of ejaculatory duct, intraprostatic vas deferens, and/or seminal vesicle. The tiny tubular outgrowths from the walls of these structures may be misinterpreted as adenocarcinoma when seen in tangential sections that do not reveal the main lumen (Figure 36.37). This impression may be further encouraged by the frequent presence of enlarged dark nuclei of bizarre contour. The presence of golden brown cytoplasmic granules, which may be few and inconspicuous, helps to establish the true diagnosis. Uniform negative staining for PSA and PAP are confirmatory.

ACKNOWLEDGMENT

Dr. McNeal, the author of this chapter, passed away in November 2005. Dr. Ronald Cohen, who worked closely with Dr. McNeal for 10 years and is most familiar with Dr. McNeal's work, was asked to proofread and answer questions associated with this chapter. Dr. Cohen is Associate Professor on the Faculty of Medicine at University of Western Australia as well as Director of Pathology at Uropath both in Perth, Western Australia.

REFERENCES

1. McNeal JE. Developmental and comparative anatomy of the prostate. In: Grayhack J, Wilson J, Scherbenske M, eds. *Benign Prostatic Hyperplasia.* DHEW publication no. (NIH) 76–1113. Washington, DC: Department of Health, Education and Welfare; 1975:1–10.
2. Cunha GR, Donjacour AA. Mesenchymal–epithelial interactions in the growth development of the prostate. In: Lepor H, Ratliff TL, eds. *Urologic Oncology.* Boston: Kluwer Academic; 1989:159–175.
3. Timms BG, Mohs TV, Didio LJ. Ductal budding and branching patterns in the developing prostate. *J Urol* 1994;151:1427–1432.
4. McNeal JE, Stamey TA, Hodge KK. The prostate gland: morphology, pathology, ultrasound anatomy. *Monogr Urol* 1988;9:36–54.
5. McNeal JE. Anatomy of the prostate and morphogenesis of BPH. *Prog Clin Biol Res* 1984;145:27–53.
6. McNeal JE. The prostate and prostatic urethra: a morphologic synthesis. *J Urol* 1972;107:1008–1016.
7. McNeal JE. Regional morphology and pathology of the prostate. *Am J Clin Pathol* 1968;49:347–357.
8. McNeal JE. Origin and evolution of benign prostatic enlargement. *Invest Urol* 1978;15:340–345.
9. McNeal JE. Origin and development of carcinoma in the prostate. *Cancer* 1969;23:24–34.
10. McNeal JE, Price HM, Redwine EA, Freiha FS, Stamey TA. Stage A versus Stage B adenocarcinoma of the prostate: morphologic comparison and biological significance. *J Urol* 1988;139:61–65.
11. McNeal JE, Redwine EA, Freiha FS, Stamey TA. Zonal distribution of prostatic adenocarcinoma: correlation with histologic patterns and direction of spread. *Am J Surg Pathol* 1988;12:897–906.
12. Villers A, Steg A, Boccon–Gibod L. Anatomy of the prostate: review of different models. *Eur Urol* 1991;20:261–268.
13. Blacklock NJ. Anatomical factors in prostatitis. *Br J Urol* 1947; 46:47–54.

14. Myers RP, Goellner JR, Cahill DR. Prostate shape, external striated urethral sphincter and radical prostatectomy: the apical dissection. *J Urol* 1987;138:543–550.

15. Ayala AG, Ro JY, Babaian R, Troncoso P, Grignon DJ. The prostatic capsule: does it exist? Its importance in the staging and treatment of prostatic carcinoma. *Am J Surg Pathol* 1989;13:21–27.

16. McNeal JE, Villers AA, Redwine EA, Freiha FS, Stamey TA. Capsular penetration in prostate cancer: significance for natural history and treatment. *Am J Surg Pathol* 1990;14:240–247.

17. McNeal JE, Bostwick DG, Kindrachuk RA, Redwine EA, Freiha FS, Stamey TA. Patterns of progression in prostate cancer. *Lancet* 1986;1:60–63.

18. Villers A, McNeal JE, Freiha FS, Boccon-Gibod L, Stamey TA. Invasion of Denonvilliers' fascia in radical prostatectomy specimens. *J Urol* 1993;149:793–798.

19. Lepor H, Gregerman M, Crosby R, Mostofi FK, Walsh PC. Precise localization of the autonomic nerves from the pelvic plexus to the corpora cavernosa: a detailed anatomical study of the adult male pelvis. *J Urol* 1985;133:207–212.

20. Villers A, McNeal JE, Redwine EA, Freiha FS, Stamey TA. The role of perineural space invasion in the local spread of prostatic adenocarcinoma. *J Urol* 1989;142:763–768.

21. Catalona WJ, Dresner SM. Nerve-sparing radical prostatectomy: extraprostatic tumor extension and preservation of erectile function. *J Urol* 1985;134:1149–1151.

22. Eggleston JC, Walsh PC. Radical prostatectomy with preservation of sexual function: pathological findings in the first 100 cases. *J Urol* 1985;134:1146–1148.

23. Flocks RH. The arterial distribution within the prostate gland: its role in transurethral prostatic resection. *J Urol* 1937;37:524–525.

24. Clegg EV. The vascular arrangements within the human prostate gland. *Br J Urol* 1956;28:428–435.

25. Gleason DF. Histologic grading and clinical staging of prostatic carcinoma. In: Tannenbaum M, ed. *Urologic Pathology: The Prostate.* Philadelphia: Lea & Febiger; 1977:171–197.

26. Gleason DF. Atypical hyperplasia, benign hyperplasia and well differentiated adenocarcinoma of the prostate. *Am J Surg Pathol* 1985;9(suppl):53–67.

27. McNeal JE. Age-related changes in the prostatic epithelium associated with carcinoma. In: Griffiths K, Pierrepoint CG, eds. *Some Aspects of the Aetiology and Biochemistry of Prostatic Cancer.* Cardiff, Wales: Tenovus; 1970:23–32.

28. McNeal JE. Aging and the prostate. In: Brocklehurst JC, ed. *Urology in the Elderly.* Edinburgh: Churchill Livingstone; 1984:193–202.

29. Mao P, Angrist A. The fine structure of the basal cell of human prostate. *Lab Invest* 1966;15:1768–1782.

30. Brawer MK, Peehl DM, Stamey TA, Bostwick DG. Keratin immunoreactivity in the benign and neoplastic human prostate. *Cancer Res* 1985;45:3663–3667.

31. Bostwick DG, Brawer MK. Prostatic intra-epithelial neoplasia and early invasion in prostate cancer. *Cancer* 1987;59:788–794.

32. Dermer GB. Basal cell proliferation in benign prostatic hyperplasia. *Cancer* 1978;41:1857–1862.

33. Cleary KR, Choi HY, Ayala AG. Basal cell hyperplasia of the prostate. *Am J Clin Pathol* 1983;80:850–854.

34. McNeal JE, Haillot O, Yemoto C. Cell proliferation in dysplasia of the prostate: analysis by PCNA immunostaining. *Prostate* 1995;27:258–268.

35. di Sant'Agnese PA. Neuroendocrine differentiation in prostatic carcinoma. *Cancer* 1995;75:1850–1859.

36. Ro JY, Tetu B, Ayala AG, Ordonez NG. Small cell carcinoma of the prostate. II. Immunohistochemical and electron microscopic studies of 18 cases. *Cancer* 1987;59:977–982.

37. Reese JH, McNeal JE, Redwine EA, Samloff IM, Stamey TA. Differential distribution of pepsinogen II between the zones of the human prostate and the seminal vesicle. *J Urol* 1986;136:1148–1152.

38. Reese JH, McNeal JE, Redwine EA, Stamey TA, Freiha FS. Tissue type plasminogen activator as a marker for functional zones, within the human prostate gland. *Prostate* 1988;12:47–53.

39. Reese JH, McNeal JE, Goldenberg L, Redwine EA, Sellers RG. Distribution of lactoferrin in the normal and inflamed human prostate: an immunohistochemical study. *Prostate* 1992;20:73–85.

40. McNeal JE, Leav I, Alroy J, Skutelsky E. Differential lectin staining of central and peripheral zones of the prostate and alterations in dysplasia. *Am J Clin Pathol* 1988;89:41–48.

41. deVries CR, McNeal JE, Bensch K. The prostatic epithelial cell in dysplasia: an ultrastructural perspective. *Prostate* 1992;21:209–221.

42. Price H, McNeal JE, Stamey TA. Evolving patterns of tissue composition in benign prostatic hyperplasia as a function of specimen size. *Hum Pathol* 1990;21:578–585.

Testis and Excretory Duct System

Thomas D. Trainer

INTRODUCTION

The adult testes are paired organs that lie within the scrotum suspended by the spermatic cord (Figure 37.1). The average weight of each is 15 to 19 g, the right usually being 10% heavier than the left (1). The scrotal covering layers are skin, dartos muscle and Colles' fascia, an external spermatic fascia, and the parietal layer of the tunica vaginalis (Figure 37.2). The dartos muscle, of the nonstriated type, is closely attached to the overlying skin but glides freely over the underlying loose fascial layer.

SUPPORTING STRUCTURES

The supporting structures of the testis consist of a tough capsule (the tunica) and a number of fibrous septa that extend from the inner surface of the tunica into the parenchyma and divide the testis into approximately 250 lobules, or compartments. The posterior portion of the testis not covered by the capsule is called the mediastinum, which contains blood vessels, nerves, lymphatics, and the extratesticular portion of the rete testis. The capsule has three distinctive layers: the outer serosa, or tunica vaginalis; the thick, collagenous tunica albuginea; and the inner tunica vasculosa. The tunica vaginalis consists of a flattened layer of mesothelial cells overlying a well-developed basement membrane. It forms a sac with two components; a visceral portion covering the testis and head of the epididymis and a parietal portion, formed as the lining reflects posteriorly and superiorly at the mediastinum and epididymis and then covers the internal spermatic fascia. Infrequently, transitional or squamous metaplasia of the surface epithelium may be present (2). The tunica albuginea is composed of a layer of collagen fibers, within which are embedded fibroblasts, myocytes, mast cells, nerve

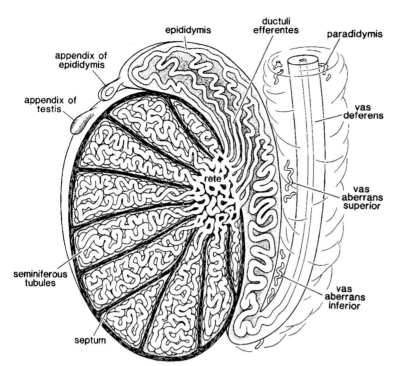

Figure 37.1 Diagrammatic view of testis, epididymis, and portion of ductus (vas) deferens.

fibers, and nerve endings resembling Meissner's corpuscles. The myocytes, found primarily in the posterior aspect of the testis, undergo regular contractions and cause a transient increase in intratesticular pressure. The tunica vasculosa, a loose connective tissue layer containing blood vessels and lymphatics, sends septa into the testicular parenchyma to form the individual lobules. Blood vessels passing through the tunica do so in an oblique plane, which may or may not have some significance with respect to blood flow within the testis. It is well known that the pulse pressure in the testicular parenchyma is extraordinarily low. The tunica varies greatly in thickness with age, averaging 300 µg at birth, 400 to 450 µg in young adults, and 900 to 950 µg in men over 65 years of age (3).

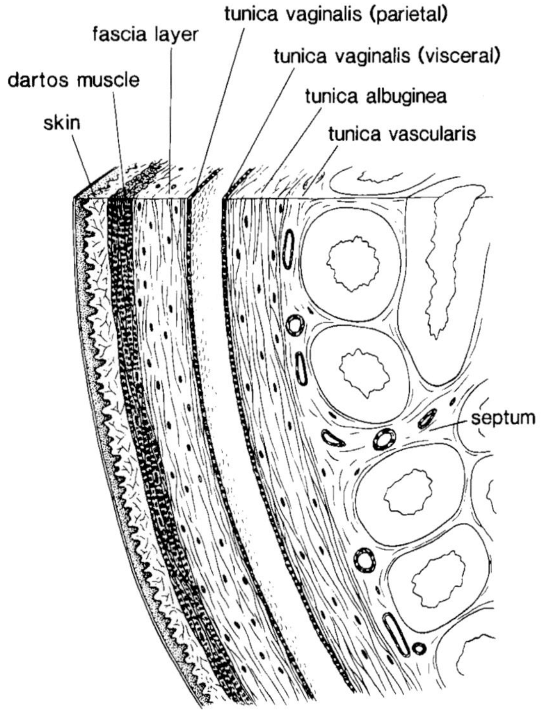

SEMINIFEROUS TUBULES

Each lobule of the testis contains one to four seminiferous tubules (Figure 37.1). The individual tubule is a highly convoluted, closed loop structure, with numerous communications between the arms of the loop but without any blind endings or branches. Each arm of the loop empties into the septal portion of the rete testis, although infrequently seminiferous tubules may empty directly into the mediastinal rete. The total length of seminiferous tubules in each testis has been estimated between 299 and 981 m, with an average around 540 m (4). The average tubule diameter in young adults is 180 µm (± 30). The usual open testicular biopsy may encompass tubules from up to five lobules along with portions of the intervening septa. It is important not to interpret the latter as foci of interstitial fibrosis. The seminiferous tubules are composed of germ cells in varying stages of differentiation and Sertoli cells. Each tubule has a distinctive basement membrane and a thin lamina propria (Figure 37.3).

Figure 37.2 Scrotal covering layers and capsule of testis.

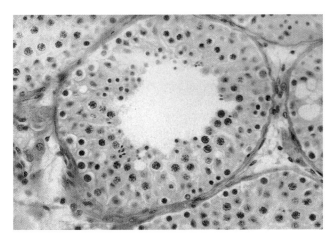

Figure 37.3 A cross-sectional view of seminiferous tubule and interstitium. Germ cell maturation is variable around the tubule, a normal finding.

SERTOLI CELLS

Sertoli cells play important and very different roles in the fetal and adult testes, and these divergent roles are reflected in their proliferative activity, cell protein markers, and the nature of cellular intermediate filaments at these periods of the cell's life span. Adult Sertoli cells are nondividing cells. Their number is important since they have the capacity to nurture only a fixed number of germ cells. Genetic, hormonal, and environmental factors appear to play significant roles in determining the final number of Sertoli cells in the adult testis (5). These tall, irregular, columnar cells, with their bases attached to the underlying basal lamina, have an abundant but relatively inconspicuous cytoplasm and an ill-defined cytoplasmic membrane on light microscopic examination. The cells send intricate cytoplasmic extensions around the germ cell elements and continuously alter their contours to accommodate the changing size and shape of the germ cells that they cradle. Adult Sertoli cell nuclei have round to slightly irregularly shapes, with a highly folded nuclear membrane, a homogeneous chromatin distribution, and a prominent, round nucleolus (Figure 37.4). These features are in sharp contast to those of the prepubertal and fetal Sertoli cells, which have an oval or elongated nucleus, a smoothly contoured nuclear membrane, and an inconspicuous nucleolus (Figure 37.15). The Sertoli cell nuclei represent about 10% of the nuclei in a normal adult tubule cross section. They are located toward the basal side of the tubule and lie just central to the nuclei of the spermatogonia and preleptotene spermatocytes. The cytoplasm may contain lipid vacuoles and/or granular eosinophilic material. Much of the phagocytosed material represents remnants of the residual bodies of the spermatid or degenerated earlier germ cell forms. Adult Sertoli cells contain vimentin as intermediate filaments, whereas embryonic and prepubertal Sertoli cells also contain cytoker-

atins 8 and 18 (6). The transient appearance of cytokeratins is of interest in view of the report of a malignant Sertoli cell tumor containing both cytokeratins and vimentin (7). Low-molecular weight cytokeratins also may be identified in some of the Sertoli cells of atrophic tubules of the adult testis (8), in Sertoli cells of tubules containing in situ germ cell neoplasia (9), and in Sertoli cells of the contralateral testis of patients with germ cell neoplasms. These Sertoli cells have an immature morphological appearance and appear to be part of the testicular dysgenesis syndrome described recently (10). Adult Sertoli cells, unlike fetal or prepubertal Sertoli cells, express androgen receptors within their nuclei but, at the same time, have lost their expression of cytoplasmic anti-müllerian hormone (5,11). A wide variety of other molecules are produced by the Sertoli cells, including inhibin/activin, insulin-like growth factor, platelet-derived growth factor, transforming growth factor, interleukins 1 and 6, and neurofilament proteins (12,13). Still unclear is whether or not the fetal Sertoli cell produces a substance or employs some other mechanism that serves to eventually bring the fetal germ cell into mitotic arrest. Those germ cells that fail to reach the fetal testis or the female germ cells in the ovary do not appear to be exposed to this undefined Sertoli cell product and consequently become arrested in the early phase of the first meiotic division (14,15). Present in the cytoplasm are the crystalloids of Charcot-Böttcher (16). These bundles of filamentous structures, located primarily in the basal portion of mature Sertoli cells, are best seen by ultrastructural examination but occasionally are large enough to be seen by light microscopic studies (Figure 37.5). Ultrastructurally, they appear to merge with vimentin-labeled intermediate filaments, both of which are increased in the cryptorchid testes and the Sertoli cell–only syndrome (9).

At puberty, a tight junction complex forms between adjacent Sertoli cells, dividing the seminiferous tubule into

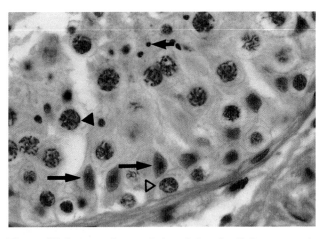

Figure 37.4 Seminiferous tubule with Sertoli cells (**long arrows**), spermatogonia (Δ), primary spermatocytes (▲), and spermatids (**short arrow**).

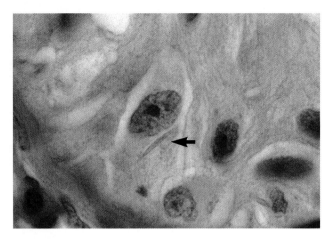

Figure 37.5 Sertoli cell with intracytoplasmic Charcot-Böttcher crystalloids (**arrow**) from a patient with germ cell aplasia. Note the prominent nucleolus and slightly wrinkled nuclear membrane.

basal and adluminal compartments; the former contains spermatogonia and preleptotene spermatocytes, and the latter holds the remaining primary spermatocytes, secondary spermatocytes, and spermatids. A transient, intermediate compartment is formed by adjacent Sertoli cells as germ cells move from the basal compartment to the adluminal compartment. A tight junction complex forms behind the germ cells to seal off the intercellular space, thereby ensuring the integrity of the Sertoli cell barrier (17). This junction forms the major blood-testis barrier, preventing access of bloodborne constituents to the germ cells in the adluminal compartment except through the Sertoli cell cytoplasm. Still unclear is the mechanism that serves to promote the movement of germ cells from the basal compartment to the adluminal compartment.

Other cell connections between adjacent Sertoli cells include gap junctions, desmosomes (rarely), and ectoplasm specialization sites (18). Intercellular junctionlike structures are present between Sertoli cells and germ cells, presumably serving as the conduit by which the Sertoli cell plays a role in the regulation of spermatogenesis.

GERM CELLS

Germ cells are derived from tissues in the posterior wall of the yolk sac and migrate in early embryonic life to the gonadal ridge (19). Deviations in this migration route account for the appearance in abnormal locations of tumors derived from these cells (Figure 37.6). The germ cell elements comprise the bulk of the cells seen in the adult seminiferous tubule (Figures 37.3–37.4). Maturation in humans covers a period of 70 ± 4 days (20), with no evidence that this time requirement is altered by age or pathologic states. The undifferentiated spermatogonia lie in the basal compartment and undergo proliferation and

renewal. Some of them become committed to the process of spermatogensis and give rise to primary spermatocytes, heralding the first meiotic division of spermatogenesis. The earliest of the primary spermatocytes, the preleptotene forms, are also located in the basal compartment. The preleptotene spermatocytes are then moved by an unknown signal into the adluminal compartment, where they sequentially become leptotene, zygotene, pachytene, and diplotene primary spermatocytes, this phase of the cycle involving a period of 24 days (21). After this relatively long period of gametogenesis, the first meiotic division occurs with the formation of secondary spermatocytes. These cells have an extremely short half-life and soon undergo the second meiotic division to form haploid spermatids, which are then converted into spermatozoa through a series of complex steps of metamorphosis (Figure 37.7).

Until spermatozoa are formed, all progeny of a spermatogonium committed to going through the meiotic process are connected together by a narrow cytoplasmic bridge that permits sharing of cytoplasmic organelles and allow for simultaneous maturation of interconnected cells. Of interest is the lack of these intercellular connections in seminomas and intratubular germ cell neoplasm but their occasional presence in spermatocytic seminomas (22). A failure of cell separation, a form of dysmaturation, is reflected in the tubular lumen and seminal fluid by the presence of multinucleated spermatids or multiheaded spermatozoa. In the late spermatid phase, excess cytoplasm is discarded by the spermatid and is phagocytosed by the enveloping Sertoli cells. The sloughing of germ cells into the seminiferous tubule lumen and the presence of immature and abnormal forms observed in patients with varicocele and other pathologic states suggest a failure of Sertoli cell regulation of this maturation process. One must take care to separate this pathologic sloughing process from the arti-

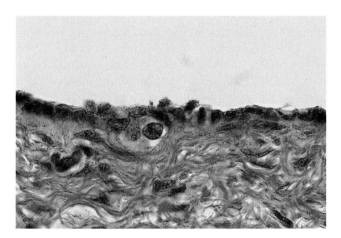

Figure 37.6 Germ cells located immediately beneath the mesothelial lining cells of the process vaginalis of a 16-week fetus.

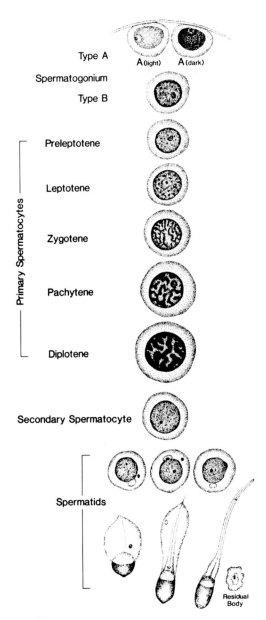

Type A
Spermatogonium
A (light)   A (dark)
Type B

Preleptotene

Leptotene

Zygotene

Pachytene

Diplotene

Primary Spermatocytes

Secondary Spermatocyte

Spermatids

Residual
Body

Figure 37.7 Steps in spermatogenesis.

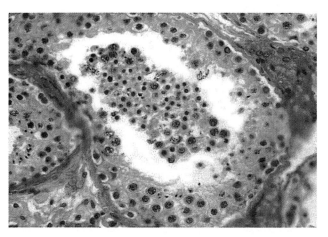

Figure 37.8 Seminiferous tubule with artifactual sloughing of germ cell elements into tubule lumen.

factual sloughing that frequently occurs in open biopsy specimens (Figure 37.8).

Maturation of germ cells proceeds in an ordered, nonrandom fashion along the length of the seminiferous tubule. Groups of evolving germ cells of one level of development tend to be found in association with developing germ cells of another level of development at any point along the tubule. Clermont (23) described 14 cell association patterns in the rat testis and 6 such cell associations in humans. In the rat, a given cross section of seminiferous tubule shows only one cell association around the circumference of the tubule, whereas in humans up to three cell associations may be seen in a tubule cross section. Initially this arrangement of cell clusters was considered to form an

overlapping helical pattern along the length of the tubule (24). That view has been recently challenged (25). Of practical importance is the need to recognize that not all stages of differentiation of germ cells may be seen in any one cross-sectional view of a seminiferous tubule. Mature spermatozoa and late spermatids may be seen in one portion of a tubule cross section, and the opposite wall may show maturation only to the early spermatid level (Figure 37.3). It has been recognized for many years that not all spermatogonia or spermatocytes progress to become spermatozoa and that apoptotic or degenerative changes in these precursor cells can be seen regularly in the seminiferous tubules (26). This normal physiologic process should not be mistaken for maturation arrest. The germ cell elements can be recognized with relative ease, and one should be able to distinguish spermatogonia, primary spermatocytes, secondary spermatocytes, and spermatids.

Spermatogonia are located in the basal compartment of the seminiferous tubule, the basal portion of most of the cells being in contact with the tubule basement membrane. They have been subdivided into three types, mainly on the basis of the nuclear chromatin pattern, as type A dark, type A light, and type B. Type A dark cells have a central nuclear cleared area, referred to as the nuclear vacuole, and contain glycogen in their cytoplasm. The type B cells tend to have a more coarsely clumped chromatin pattern than either of the type A cells. It should be pointed out that the nuclear chromatin pattern differences among these spermatogonia is usually evident only with fixatives such as Zencker-formal and that fixatives such as Bouin's produce coarse clumping in the nuclei of all of the spermatogonial subtypes, making subtyping difficult (23). The spermatogonia nuclei are oval to round and contain one or two easily identifiable nucleoli (Figure 37.9). Within the cytoplasm in a perinuclear location are the crystalloids of Lubarsch. These structures, measuring up to 3.0 μm in length, may be found in adults and infants as early as the fifth postnatal week.

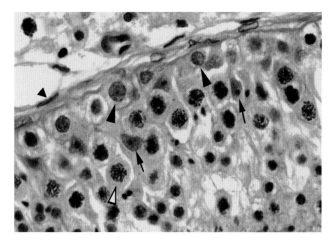

Figure 37.9 Portion of seminiferous tubule showing spermatogonia (**solid arrowhead**), primary spermatocytes (**open arrowhead**), Sertoli cells (**arrow**), and fibromyocyte of tunica propria (**solid triangle**). The smaller cells in the lower right are mainly secondary spermatocytes and early spermatids.

They are composed of a mixture of parallel arrays of fibrils 80 to 150 Å thick and ribosome-like granules (27).

The classification of primary spermatocytes is based on the alteration of the nuclear chromatin pattern (23). These cells are distinctive because of the doubling of the amount of DNA in their nuclei as a result of the duplication of each chromosome into chromatid pairs in preparation for the first meiotic division. The leptotene primary spermatocytes are characterized by a change in the chromatin pattern into a filamentous structure with a fine-beaded arrangement. Zygotene spermatocytes have an even coarser granularity of the chromosome filaments, and there is a tendency for the chromatin material to gather eccentrically within the nucleus. Pachytene and diplotene spermatocytes are the most easily recognized of the primary spermatocytes because of their large size and their prominent nucleus, containing thick, short chromatin filaments (Figure 37.9).

Secondary spermatocytes, having an extremely short half-life, make up only a small minority of the cells seen in a cross section of the tubule. Their nuclei, substantially smaller than in the primary spermatocytes, have a finely granular chromatin pattern and a haploid number of chromosomes but a diploid amount of DNA because of the presence of the chromatid pairs. These cells, located near the tubule lumen, differ only slightly in appearance from the very early spermatids with which they are closely associated. (Figures 37.4, 37.9).

The spermatids have a heavily stained granular pattern to the nucleus and, if the plane of section is appropriate, a slight depression on the surface of the cell, representing the beginning of the acrosome. The late spermatid form is characterized by a change in the nucleus, first to an oval shape with highly condensed chromatin material, then to an elongated form, and eventually assuming the configuration of the nucleus of a mature spermatozoon. One of the last steps in the maturation process is the separation of the interconnected progeny.

Elaborate methods have been developed for quantitatively assessing the germ cell elements and the relationship of spermatogenesis to seminal fluid sperm density (28–32). The method of Johnson (29) applies a score of 1 to 10 for each tubule cross section examined. The criteria are as follows: 10, complete spermatogenesis and perfect tubules; 9, many spermatozoa present but disorganized spermatogenesis; 8, only a few spermatozoa present; 7, no spermatozoa but many spermatids present; 6, only a few spermatids present; 5, no spermatozoa or spermatids present but many spermatocytes present; 4, only a few spermatocytes present; 3, only spermatogonia present; 2, no germ cells present; 1, neither germ cells nor Sertoli cells present. The mean score count should be at least 8.90 with an average of 9.38, and 60% or more of the tubules should score at 10.

Two relatively simple methods are helpful to the surgical pathologist. The first method (32) involves establishing a germ cell to Sertoli cell ratio by counting at least 30 tubule cross sections. This ratio is relatively constant at approximately 13:1 in young healthy men. An average of 10 to 12 Sertoli cells per tubule cross section is considered normal, and approximately half the germ cell elements within the tubule should be in the spermatid stage. An assumption is made that the Sertoli cell population is stable throughout adult life. A reasonably good assessment of the presence or absence of hypospermatogenesis or maturation arrest can be made with this technique. A second method involves counting spermatids per tubule cross section (33). Only the mature spermatids, that is those with oval nuclei and dark, densely stained chromatin, are counted. Excellent correlations have been made with seminal fluid sperm counts. A spermatid/tubule cross section count of 45 corresponds to a seminal fluid sperm count of 85×10^6/mL. Spermatid/tubule counts of 40, 20, and 6 to 10 correspond to sperm counts of 45, 10, and 3×10^6/mL, respectively. A minimum of 20 tubules must be counted.

INTERSTITIUM

The interstitium of the testis accounts for 25 to 30% of the testicular mass. It can be divided loosely into intertubular and peritubular regions. Within the former are Leydig cells, blood vessels, lymphatics, nerves, macrophages, and mast cells. The macrophages are often found in close association with Leydig cells (34), where the two cells form complex cell-cell interdigitations. There is increasing evidence for an important paracrine role for macrophages in Leydig cell function (35). Surrounding each seminiferous tubule in a sheathlike fashion is the lamina propria or tunica propria, which consists of an inner basal lamina, surrounded by a zone of multilayered spindle-shaped cells, intermingled with collagen and elastic fibers (Figure 37.9). The outermost two layers of cells stain for vimentin and actin but not for desmin. The inner layers of three to five cells stain intensely for desmin as well as actin and vimentin, findings that are characteristic of myofibroblasts (36). These same cells also contain androgen receptors in their nuclei (11). Elastic fibers first appear at puberty in the outermost layer of the lamina propria (37). There is a striking absence of elastic fibers in the lamina propria of sclerotic tubules in patients with Klinefelter's syndrome, in contrast to their abundance in the lamina propria of patients with postpubertal tubular sclerosis of multiple other causes (38).

A common finding in patients with oligozoospermia or azoospermia due to primary testicular failure is the accumulation of eosinophilic, acellular material in the lamina propria. This material is an admixture of increased collagen fibers, elastic fibrils, and basement membrane–like material (39). The peritubular tissue of patients with hypogonadotropic hypogonadism is underdeveloped, having only one or two layers of myoid cells mixed with a few collagen fibers. In contrast, there is a large accumulation of collagen in the lamina propria of some of the seminiferous tubules of adult patients with cryptorchidism.

LEYDIG CELLS

Adult Leydig cells, the source of testicular androgens, only rarely undergo mitotic division (40). They are found singly and in clusters within the interstitium of the testis; some lie immediately adjacent to capillaries, whereas others lie close to the peritubular myofibrocytes (Figure 37.10). They also may be seen in the tunica albuginea, epididymis, spermatic cord, and mediastinum of the testis. They are often located in intimate association with

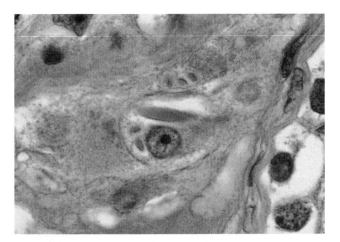

Figure 37.10   Leydig cells in interstitium of testis. An eosinophilic crystalloid of Reinke and abundant lipofuscin are prominent features in the cytoplasm of the Leydig cell in the center of this field.

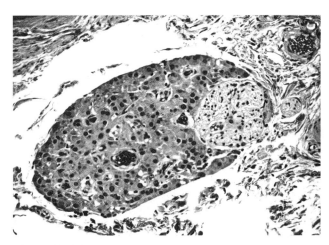

Figure 37.11   Leydig cells in intimate association with a nerve in the hilus of the testis.

large nerve fibers, sometimes as a large cluster adjacent to the nerve (Figure 37.11) and, at other times, scattered randomly throughout the nerve fiber (41). They may be found at these sites in the fetus as well as the adult. The single nucleus of the cell is round and vesicular, with one to two eccentrically located nucleoli. Occasional binucleated cells are present. The cytoplasm is usually abundant and stains intensely with acid dyes. Lipid droplets and lipofuscin pigment are found in the cytoplasm, first appearing at the time of puberty and increasing in prominence in the aging testis. The characteristic intracytoplasmic Reinke crystalloids are present only in the postpubertal state (Figure 37.10). Their presence is highly variable in the normal testis, and they are frequently absent in Leydig cell tumors. The nature of the material is still unknown, although it is presumed to represent a protein product of the cell (42). The crystalloids stain negatively for actin, vimentin, and desmin.

Quantitation of Leydig cells has been a difficult parameter to assess. Several indices have been used: mean Leydig cell number or Leydig cell cluster number per seminiferous tubule; mean number of Leydig cells per Leydig cell cluster; Leydig cell to Sertoli cell ratio; and ratio of Leydig cell area to seminiferous tubule area (43). Heller et al. (44), using the Leydig cell to Sertoli cell ratio, found a value of 0.39 and a range of 0.19 to 0.72. In that same study, they also determined the average number of Sertoli cells per tubular cross section to be 10.03 ± 0.6. They made an assumption that the Sertoli cell population was stable in their calculation of the Leydig cell population. As a rule, normal adults should have four to five Leydig cells for each tubular cross section.

Vimentin represents the predominant intermediate filament, but actin filaments and neurofilament triplet proteins have also been identified in both Leydig and Sertoli cells (13). Androgen receptors are found within the nuclei but at a much lower intensity than found in Sertoli cells

(11). Calretinin, a protein found primarily in the cytoplasm and to a lesser extent in the nucleus, has been shown to be a reliable marker for normal and neoplastic Leydig cells. Theca interna cells of the ovary stain equally well, but Sertoli cells, granulosa cells, and theca externa cells stain little or not at all (45). Relaxin-like factor, also known as the Leydig cell insulin-like factor, stains strongly in the cytoplasm of Leydig cells, as well as theca interna cells and hilar cells in the ovary (46,47). Leydig cells stain positively for S-100, glial fibrillary acidic protein (48), synaptophysin, chromogranin A-B, and neuron-specific enolase but not for vimentin or desmin. A subpopulation of cells will stain intensely for nestin, an intermediate filament seen mainly in nerve and muscle progenitor cells (49). The presence of these substances undoubtedly indicates an important paracrine function that Leydig cells share with Sertoli cells, peritubular cells, macrophages, and nerves.

VASCULAR SUPPLY

The blood supply to the testis is derived primarily from the internal spermatic (testicular) artery with a smaller contribution from the branches of the vasal portion of the internal (superior) vesicle artery. The testicular artery, arising from the aorta immediately distal to the renal artery, is highly coiled and extremely long relative to its diameter. It has a low pulse pressure as it enters the testis (50). The artery plays an important role in thermal regulation via countercurrent heat exchange with the veins of the pampiniform plexus. The combination of this vascular heat exchange and the heat lost via the thin scrotal covering layers serves to maintain the testicular temperature 2°C below body temperature. Arterial branches of the testicular artery arborize over the surface of the testis, penetrate the capsule, and pass in a centripetal fashion within the septa to the mediastinum, where they form a dense cluster. Only a few branches enter the lobules from these centripetal arteries. From the mediastinum, the small arterial segments then pass in a centrifugal fashion within the parenchyma, where they branch into arterioles and capillaries. The veins run either centrifugally or centripetally to the capsule or mediastinum, respectively, and eventually anastomose posteriorly to form the pampiniform plexus of the testicular vein. Biopsy specimens of the testis of patients with varicoceles often show a striking sclerosis of vascular walls (51). These changes appear to involve both arteries and veins. The significance of these vascular alterations with respect to seminiferous tubule function in patients with varicoceles is uncertain.

At puberty, there is extensive development of the intratesticular microvascular architecture, the most notable features being a marked coiling of the arteries and a great expansion of the peritubular capillary network. Unlike other capillaries of the systemic system, the testicular capillary walls have a prominent basement membrane and an incomplete outer layer of pericytes (52). Arteriovenous anastomoses occur in two locations: (a) beneath the tunica albuginea between branches of the centripetal artery and vein and (b) deep within the parenchyma between branches of the centrifugal artery and vein. The role of these anastomoses is unknown.

The capillary network appears to have a very structured arrangement with respect to the Leydig cells and the seminiferous tubules, ramifying around and within the Leydig cell-macrophage clusters and then penetrating the tunica propria of the seminiferous tubules. Not all areas of the tubule wall appear to be supplied with this elaborate network, and the reason for this is still unclear. The capillaries then reenter the loose interstitium as postcapillary venules, where they receive other capillaries coming from the Leydig cell clusters (53). The intralobular veins then enter the septa, where they move either to the mediastinum or to the tunica vasculosa.

There is a remarkable species-to-species variation in the distribution of lymphatic channels in the testis (54). In humans, ill-defined lymphatic spaces are found in the interstitium adjacent to Leydig cell clusters, but a peritubular lymphatic network is lacking. The lymphatic channels drain into the septa and thence to either the capsule or the mediastinum, where they join on the posterior aspect of the testis. They then anastomose with lymphatic channels from the epididymis, enter the spermatic cord, and drain into the periaortic lymph nodes.

FETAL AND PREPUBERTAL TESTIS

The fetal testis becomes recognizable at seven to eight weeks of gestation, at which time primitive testicular cords become evident. By the ninth week, the primordial germ cells, having migrated from their extraembryonal origin at the base of the allantois, have found their way into the cords, and are now referred to as gonocytes. These mitotically active cells, with a round nucleus and a prominent nucleolus, are scattered throughout the tubuli but usually are found in the center, surrounded by immature Sertoli cells (Figures 37.12–37.13). During the latter half of fetal life and the first six months after birth, the gonocytes undergo a maturation process in which they enter mitotic arrest. They become larger, acquire more cytoplasm, develop a prominent nucleus with a coarse chromatin pattern, and migrate to the periphery of the tubule to reach the basal lamina. At this time, these cells are variously referred to as prespermatogonia, prospermatogonia, M (multiplying) spermatogonia, T (transitional) spermatogonia, or simply spermatogonia (Figure 37.14). At birth, the germ cells average 4 per tubule cross section, two-thirds of them being gonocytes. At 45 days there are about

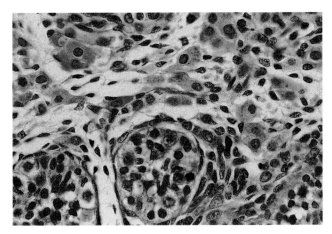

Figure 37.12 Fetal testis of 20 weeks' gestation, with numerous Leydig cells throughout the interstitium.

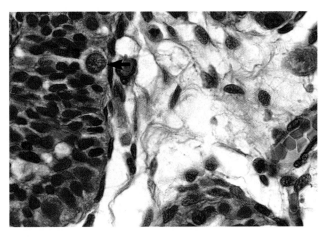

Figure 37.14 Testis of an 11-month-old child. A spermatogonium is present adjacent to the basement membrane (**arrow**). The interstitium contains undifferentiated spindle cells.

equal numbers of gonocytes and spermatogonia, with an average of 4 to 5 per tubule cross section (55). By the sixth postnatal month, virtually all of the germ cells are spermatogonia. This transition from the fetal stem cell pool to the adult stem cell pool is an important first step in the germ cell maturation process and appears to be defective in patients with cryptorchidism (56). From the age of one to four years, the number of germ cells average 1 to 2 per tubule cross section, and this number should double between the ages of 5 and 8 years (55). Although for the most part kept in mitotic arrest until just prior to puberty, occasional germ cells may be found in infancy, childhood, and even in the fetus that have entered the meiotic phase to form spermatocytes or even spermatids. In early puberty, repeated waves of incomplete spermatogenesis take place, with an orderly processs of complete maturation not appearing until the end of puberty (57). Several studies have demonstrated a marked diminution in the number of germ cells in the prepubertal cryp-

torchid testis (Figure 37.15) and a less predictable decrease of germ cells in the truly ectopic testis (27,58).

Gonocytes and, less commonly, spermatogonia express a number of markers that are employed in evaluating germ cell neoplasms in adults, including the cytoplasmic placenta-like alkaline phosphatase (PLAP), the cell membrane proto-oncogene receptor c-kit, and the nuclear transcriptional regulator Oct3/4 (also known as Oct3 and Pou5F1). These markers first appear early in the first few weeks of gestation and gradually disappear at birth or soon thereafter. They are not seen in Leydig, Sertoli, or interstitial cells nor are they found in normal adult germ cells. Beginning at about the twentieth week of gestation, PLAP is the first to decrease, followed by Oct3/4, and then by c-kit. These declines correspond to the maturation process of the gonocytes into spermatogonia. Since the rate of disappearance is different for these markers, it is possible to observe germ cells staining positive for all three of these markers

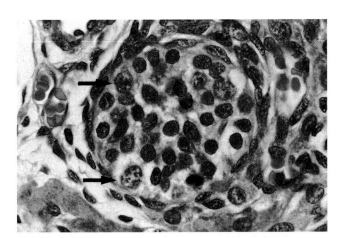

Figure 37.13 Same testis as shown in Figure 37.12. Note the mitotic figure, probably of a Sertoli cell. Larger cells (**arrows**) are undifferentiated germ cells. The remaining cells are immature Sertoli cells.

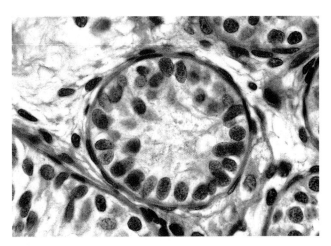

Figure 37.15 Thirteen-year-old prepubertal boy with bilateral cryptorchidism. Mature Leydig cells are absent in the interstitium. The tubules lack a lumen. The Sertoli cells are immature, and germ cells are absent.

simultaneously, positive staining only for c-kit and Oct-4 and not PLAP, or positive staining only for c-kit. Corresponding to their mitotic activity and eventual entry into mitotic arrest, gonocytes and spermatogonia both reveal strong nuclear staining with Ki-67 throughout gestation but with only a few cells reacting after birth (59).

At 20 weeks of fetal life, the testis is characterized by abundant, well-developed Leydig cells filling the interstitium (Figure 37.12). The seminiferous tubules are solidly filled with Sertoli cells and germ cells, measure 45 to 50 μm in diameter, and lack a well-defined lumen (60). The postnatal tubules slowly increase in size to reach a prepubertal diameter of 64 μm (range: 43–70μm), at which time lumens begin to appear (61).

Fetal Sertoli cells outnumber germ cells in a ratio of 7:1 (61) and undergo active mitotic division during this period. Unlike its adult counterpart, the immature Sertoli cell has an oval to round nucleus and an inconspicuous nucleolus (Figure 37.13). Vimentin and cytokeratins 8 and 18 are expressed in the cytoplasm, as noted above. Nuclear androgen receptors are not identified.

Early studies had suggested that the Sertoli cell is mitotically inactive after birth, but stereologic studies indicate their number increases from 260 million late in fetal life, to 1,500 million between 3 months and 10 years, and to 3,700 million in the adult testis (62). They account for 95% of the tubule mass, with the germ cells comprising the other 5%. The testis shows a sixfold increase in size in the first year after birth, primarily as a result of Sertoli cell proliferation and the marked lengthening of the seminiferous tubules rather than a significant increase in tubule diameter (57). To a lesser degree, Sertoli cells continue to proliferate until puberty. Sertoli cells per cross section average 30 in the fetal testis after 20 weeks, increase to 42 at the fourth postnatal month, decrease to 26 at age 13 years, and to 12 to 15 in the adult testis (27,60). At puberty there is a fivefold increase in Sertoli cell volume, at which time Charcot-Böttcher crystalloids first appear. The cryptorchid testis commonly contains microscopic collections, or "congeries," of very immature Sertoli cells, having either a round or fusiform-shaped nucleus and an inconspicuous nucleolus (Figure 37.16) (63).

The early prepubertal lamina propria is relatively undeveloped and is separated from the tubules by a thin basement membrane that lacks the knoblike thickening and splitting of the adult testis. The collagen fiber layer is relatively thin, and only one or two spindle-shaped cells are seen in the outer portion of the lamina propria.

Leydig cells are first recognizable by the eighth week of fetal life and become prominent in the fetal testis at 14 to 18 weeks of gestation (Figure 37.12), after which there is a progressive decline in number, with few mature-appearing Leydig cells being evident at birth. A second wave of Leydig cells appears at two to three months of neonatal life, corresponding to the activation of the hypothalamus/pituitary/gonad

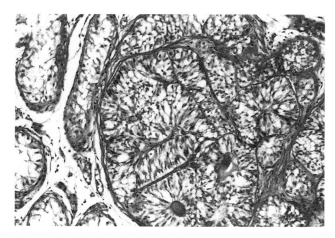

Figure 37.16 Sertoli cell collections, or congeries. The tubules are composed of immature Sertoli cells and lack both germ cells and lumens.

axis (64). This population is a mix of cells, some with the characteristics of mature Leydig cells, smaller cells with a round nucleus and fairly prominent nuleolus but without the prominent eosinophilic cytoplasm of typical adult Leydig cells, and spindle cells. After this second phase of Leydig cell activity ends at about the fourth neonatal month, only spindle cells (Figure 37.14) are recognized until just before puberty, when the precursor Leydig cells progressively differentiate and eventually take on the appearance of adult Leydig cells. Still unclear is whether adult Leydig cells are derived from dedifferentiated fetal Leydig cells or from the primitive fibroblast cell population (64,65).

AGING TESTIS

There is a general consensus that a decline in testicular function occurs with advancing age. These physiologic changes are matched by involutional changes in the testicular parenchyma, including hypospermatogenesis, peritubular fibrosis, and hyalinization of the seminiferous tubules. A few sclerotic tubules are found occasionally in the normal adult testis (66), but larger, focal, or diffuse areas of sclerosis are distinctly pathologic. Although the total number of peritubular cells is maintained in elderly men, there is a sharp decline in the proportion of cells that stain positively for desmin and actin (36).

Thickening of the testicular arterial walls with hyalinization, sometimes seen in otherwise normal testes, is found in over 90% of testes in which there are large zones of tubular fibrosis. The capillary bed in the aged testis becomes sparse and poorly organized (67). These vascular changes probably play a causal role in the peritubular sclerosis and tubular hyalinization.

Substantial controversy exists regarding the Leydig cell population in the aging testis (68–71). According to

Neaves et al. (72), Leydig cell numbers and size both progressively decline with advancing age, the total Leydig cell population decreasing by 50% during the first 30 years of adult life. The production of testosterone by Leydig cells is relatively maintained despite a loss of total Leydig cell mass, probably because of the large reserve of these cells in the adult testis. When the Leydig cell mass decreases to a certain threshold point, daily sperm production is depressed. The aged Leydig cell contains large amounts of lipofuscin pigment and numerous vacuoles within the cytoplasm.

Abnormal sperm maturation, sloughing of germ cells into the tubule lumen, degeneration of germ cell elements, and Sertoli cell lipid accumulation and cytoplasmic vacuolization are frequent findings in the aged testis. Earlier studies indicated that the Sertoli cell population is stable throughout the postpubertal years (73,74). However, Johnson et al. (75) found that men 20 to 48 years of age had significantly more Sertoli cells per tubule cross section than did men 50 to 85 years of age, and there was a relatively constant relationship between Sertoli cells and germ cells in both age groups. Furthermore, these investigators suggested that the decline in spermatozoa production in the elderly may be due to a decrease in Sertoli cell function and mass. Sertoli cells of those tubules demonstrating hypospermatogenesis have increased amounts of vimentin microfilaments and the reappearance of cytokeratins 8 and 18, suggesting that the reversion to the intermediate filament pattern of the fetal/prepubertal testis is related to the alteration of the normal spermatogenic process (6).

RETE TESTES

The rete testis, a network of channels at the hilus of the testis, receives the luminal contents of the seminiferous tubules (Figure 37.1). It is divided into three components: the septal portion containing the tubuli rete, the mediastinal rete, and the extratesticular portion also known as the bullae retis (76,77). The tubuli rete are short tubules, 0.5 to 1.0 mm in length, that connect the two ends of the seminiferous tubule loop to the mediastinum testis. The terminal end of the seminiferous tubule usually consist only of Sertoli cells, forming an epithelial pluglike structure as it protrudes into the rete lumen (Figure 37.17). There are approximately 1,500 entrances of seminiferous tubules into the rete. A few tubules may enter the mediastinal rete directly without intervening tubuli rete. The mediastinal rete is a cavernous network of interconnecting channels that exits from the testis to form several dilated, vesicular channels or antechamber-like structures called the bullae retis. These structures, measuring up to 3.0 mm in width, anastomose together to form the ductuli efferentia.

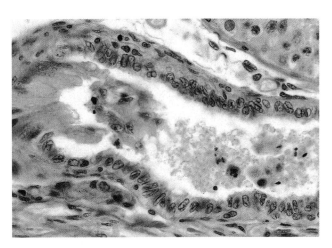

Figure 37.17 Junction of septal rete testis and terminal end of seminiferous tubule. Note the Sertoli cells "pouting" into the lumen of the rete. Rete epithelium is a low columnar type.

The rete epithelium is a simple squamous or low columnar type (Figure 37.17), the luminal surface of which is studded with microvilli. Each cell contains a single, central flagellum that is inconspicuous on light microscopic examination. The epithelium sits on a relatively thick basal lamina, beneath which are a few fibroblasts and myoid cells intermixed with collagen and elastic fibers. Traversing the mediastinum and the extratesticular rete are epithelium-covered columns or strands called chordae retis. These columns, often appearing as islands on a cross section of the rete testis (Figure 37.18), vary greatly in length (15–100 μm) and thickness (5–40 μm) and serve to connect opposing walls of the chambers. The cytoplasm of the rete epithelium contains keratin and vimentin intermediate filaments, the former being located primarily in the apical portion of the cell and the latter being found in the basal region. The keratins, primarily of low-molecular weight types, can be first identified at the tenth week of fetal life and precede

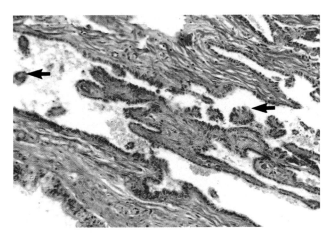

Figure 37.18 Rete testis, mediastinal portion, with irregular cavernous channels and cross sections of intratubular chordae (**arrows**).

the appearance of vimentin by two to three weeks (78). One would expect coexpression of these two intermediate filaments in the rare carcinoma of the rete or in hyperplasia of the rete. However, a report of nine cases of hyperplasia of the rete testis showed strong cytokeratin and epithelial membrane antigen staining but a negative reaction for vimentin (79). Sometimes found with hyperplastic or otherwise normal rete are hyalin refractile, eosinophilic globules, which are periodic acid-Schiff (PAS) positive, sometimes α1-antitrypsin positive, but α-fetoprotein negative (80). These should not be confused with the globules produced by yolk sac tumors of the testis. The rete epithelium, as well that of efferent ductules and the caput (head) of the epididymis, also contains receptors for estrogen, progesterone, and androgen (81), the presence of estrogen receptors perhaps accounting for the hyperplasia of the rete and efferent ductules seen in patients undergoing sex-reversal procedures (82).

The rete serves multiple functions: (a) as a mixing chamber for the contents of the seminiferous tubules, (b) as a pressure gradient between the seminiferous tubules and the epididymis, (c) as a possible source of as yet unknown components of the seminal fluid, and (d) as a reabsorptive site of proteins from the luminal contents (83).

DUCTULI EFFERENTIA

The ductuli efferentia consist of five to six tubules that arise from the extratesticular rete testis (Figure 37.1) (84). They are involved primarily in resorption of fluid and do not appear to store spermatozoa for any length of time. These tubules aggregate to form a significant portion of the caput of the epididymis proper (Figure 37.19). Unlike the body of the epididymis, the lumens have an undulating border. The cells of the efferent ductules are composed of ciliated and nonciliated columnar cells, basal cells, and

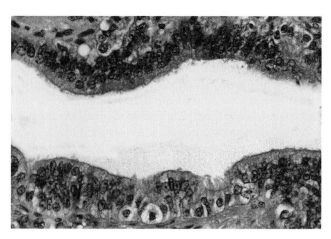

Figure 37.20 Epithelium of efferent ductulus. The columnar epithelial cells are mixed with basal cells and occasional intraepithelial lymphocytes, giving the epithelium a pseudostratified appearance.

scattered intraepithelial lymphocytes, giving the epithelium a pseudostratified appearance (Figure 37.20). Occasional cells with a Paneth cell–like appearance are seen (Figure 37.21). These numerous and brightly eosinophilic globules are PAS positive and diastase resistant and chromogranin A negative; they most likely represent prominent lysosomes. They are less frequently seen in the rest of the epididymis and are most often encountered in patients with epididymal obstruction (85). Coexpression of low-molecular weight cytokeratins and vimentin, as well as epithelial membrane antigen, is evident within the epithelial cytoplasm (78).

The epithelium sits on a thick basement membrane, surrounding which is a coat of smooth muscle cells and fibroblasts, as well as a few scattered macrophages. Intraluminal macrophages, actively phagocytizing spermatozoa, are occasionally present, particularly when duct obstruction exists.

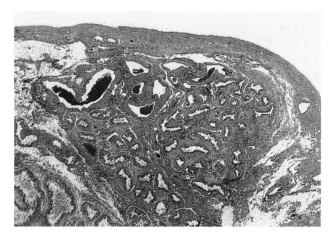

Figure 37.19 Caput (head) of epididymis, showing cross sections of distal portions of ductuli efferentia (**upper right**) and epididymis (**lower left**).

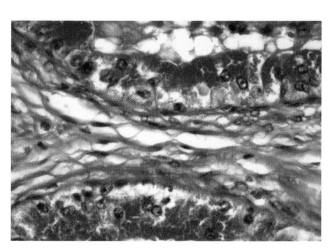

Figure 37.21 Epithelium of ductulus with prominent Paneth cell–like intracytoplasmic vacuoles.

EPIDIDYMIS

The epididymis, a highly coiled, tubular structure, can be divided anatomically into caput, corpus, and cauda portions (Figure 37.1). The epididymis plays an important role in (a) sperm transport, (b) sperm maturation, including the acquisition of motility, (c) sperm concentration, and (d) sperm storage. The average sperm transit time through the epididymis in humans is 12 days (86). The transport mechanism is by way of muscle contractions of the thick, muscular coat that surrounds the epididymal tubules. There is extensive reabsorption of intraluminal fluid, particularly in the caput portion of the epididymis. Most of the sperm are stored in the caudal segment until ejaculation occurs, and it is in this location in humans that sperm maturation takes place (87). Many spermatozoa apparently undergo senescence and degeneration in the cauda via an unknown mechanism.

The epithelium of the epididymis consists of tall columnar or principal cells, basal cells, clear cells, tall slender or apical cells rich in mitochondria (apical mitochondria-rich cells), and scattered intraepithelial lymphocytes and macrophages (88). The principal cells, comprising over 95% of the columnar cells, have straight stereocilia (Figure 37.22), which are tall and nearly obliterate the lumen in the caput but become progressively shorter as the cauda is reached. The principal cells stain strongly for vimentin, epithelial membrane antigen (EMA), and acid phosphatase. Both basal and principal cells stain positively for low-molecular weight cytokeratins, with more intense staining in the corpus and cauda sections than the caput region (89). In cryptorchid testes the intensity of staining of low-molecular weight keratins, particularly cytokeratin 18, is markedly diminished (90). Intense CD10 paraluminal staining of the columnar cells

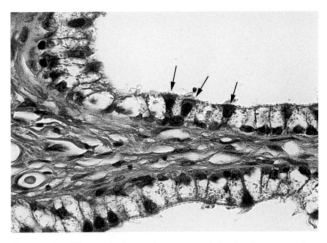

Figure 37.23 Epithelium of caput epididymis, demonstrating clear cells and apical mitochondrial-rich cells (**arrows**).

is evident both in the epididymis and vas deferens, a finding that has been utilized to ascertain the possible origin of glandular structures found adjacent to the epididymis or vas deferens (91). The intensity of the vimentin staining progressively declines in the cauda section (89). The mitochondria-rich apical cells, located primarily in the caput, show intense staining for cytokeratins and acid phosphatase and less intense reactivity for EMA and vimentin. Their configuration varies from slender cells extending from the basement membrane to the lumen to those that appear to be located only in the apex of the duct (Figure 37.23). Small foci of epithelium may rarely have the appearance of prostatic epithelium, including positive immunostaining for prostate-specific antigen. Whether this process represents metaplasia or ectopia is unclear (92). Epididymal cells may contain lipofuscin pigment, which tends to be more prominent in the caput segment and is particularly evident when there is obstruction of the epididymis (93). The lumens are generally round and regular. In up to 50% of individuals, a cribriform pattern is seen, which may represent either a normal variation or a hyperplastic process (85,94). Importantly, this changes should not be mistaken for intraepididymal spread from a testicular germ cell tumor or a primary epididymal carcinoma. The absence of either prominent nucleoli or mitoses should be helpful features supporting a benign process.

Intranuclear, eosinophilic, PAS–positive, and diastase-resistant inclusions (Figure 37.24), measuring 1 to 14 μm, are found in the columnar cells of the adult epididymis as well as throughout the vas and seminal vesicles. Electron microscopic examination shows the electron-dense globules to be enclosed by a single membrane and to lack any features suggesting viral structures (95). They are most common in the distal epididymis and adjacent vas and least common in the ampulla of the vas and seminal vesicles.

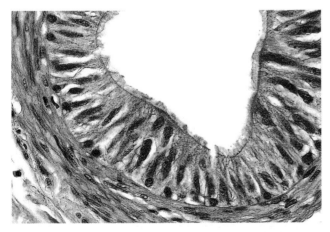

Figure 37.22 Epithelium of epididymis. Compare the tall columnar cells of the epididymis with the pseudostratified cells of the efferent ductulus. A few intraepithelial lymphocytes are present. The stereocilia are somewhat short, indicating the caudal segment. A layer of muscle cells forms the wall.

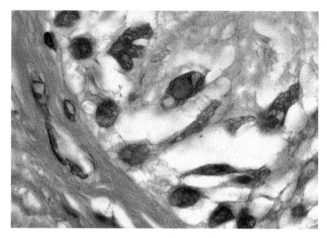

Figure 37.24 Intranuclear inclusions present in the epithelium of the epididymis. Similar inclusions are found in the epithelium of the ductus (vas) deferens.

The epididymis is supported by a thick basement membrane, surrounding which is a well-defined muscular coat. The latter plays an important role in sperm movement through the epididymis. Mast cells are found throughout the connective tissue of the epididymis in a pattern similar to that seen in the tunica and interstitium of the testis (96), being numerous in infancy, decreasing in childhood, and then increasing at the time of puberty. A progressive decline in numbers occurs in adulthood.

DUCTUS (VAS) DEFERENS

The ductus (vas) deferens, a tubular structure arising from the caudal portion of the epididymis, measures 30 to 40 cm in length. The distal 4 to 7 cm portion is enlarged to form the ampulla. The latter joins the excretory duct of the seminal vesicle to form the ejaculatory duct (Figure 37.25). The adult vas is lined by a pseudostratified, columnar epithelium, composed of columnar cells and basal cells by light microscopic examination. Ultrastructural studies show four different cell types: principal cells, pencil or peg cells, mitochondria-enriched cells, and basal cells. The luminal surface of the columnar cell is lined by tall stereocilia throughout most of the vas (97). These stereocilia are substantially shorter and sparser in the ampullary region. Prominent intranuclear inclusions, as described above in the epididymis, may be seen (95). In addition, occasional lipid-positive vacuoles are present within the cytoplasm. The epithelium of the vas is thrown into folds, which are relatively simple in the proximal vas (Figure 37.26) but become much more complicated in the ampullary segment (Figure 37.27). The ampulla has highly complex infoldings and many outpocketings or diverticula that reach into the muscle coat. Beneath the epithelium of the vas is a loose, connective tissue stroma that, after puberty, contains a well-defined, circumferentially oriented layer of elastic fibers (98). These fibers, lacking in infants and children, become frayed and fragmented in the aged vas. The muscle coat is an extraordinary thick structure with inner and outer longitudi-

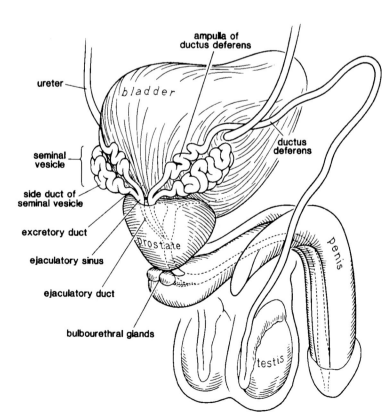

Figure 37.25 Diagram of excretory duct system from the vas to the ejaculatory ducts.

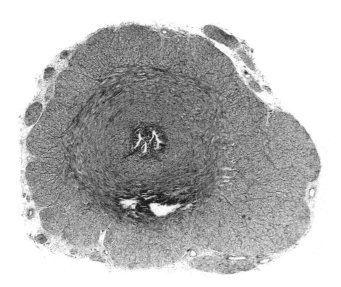

Figure 37.26 Proximal ductus (vas) deferens. This cross section shows a thick muscle coat, tiny lumen, and slightly folded mucosa.

nal coats and a middle oblique or circular zone. The entire muscle mass progressively decreases as one approaches the ampulla, although the inner longitudinal layer becomes somewhat thicker as one progresses distally (97). The epithelium in the ampulla contains significant amounts of lipofuscin pigment and rather closely resembles the epithelium seen in the seminal vesicles. Active phagocytosis of degenerated spermatozoa has been demonstrated in the ampullary region of a number of mammalian species (99).

SEMINAL VESICLES

The seminal vesicles are paired, highly coiled, tubular structures, lying posterolateral to the base of the bladder and in a parallel path with the ampulla of the vas deferens (Figure 37.25). Each vesicle measures 3.5 to 7.5 cm in length and

1.2 to 2.4 cm in thickness in the adult. The main duct, which is duplicated in approximately 10% of individuals, measures 10 to 15 cm in length when unraveled. Six to eight first-order side ducts extend off the main duct, and several secondary side ducts are derived from these. The upper part of the main duct is bent backward in a hooklike fashion. A short excretory duct combines with the ampulla of the vas to form the ejaculatory duct (Figure 37.25). The wall of the seminal vesicle has a thin external longitudinal and a thicker internal circular muscle layer. The mucosal folds, relatively simple and shallow in infancy and childhood, become highly complex and alveolus-like in the reproductive years (Figure 37.28) and are blunted in the aged vesicle. The lumen may contain a few sloughed epithelial cells and debris. Commonly seen within the lumens are eosinophilic secretions, often with crystalloid structures. The latter usually have a platelike arrangement but sometimes appear as smaller crystalloids similar to those seen in the lumens of well-differentiated prostate carcinomas. Their significance is unknown, but one should be aware of their presence in biopsies where the seminal vesicle is inadvertently sampled (100). Spermatozoa, refluxed from the ejaculatory duct, occasionally may be present, although they are not normally stored within the seminal vesicles.

The vesicle epithelium is composed of columnar and basal cells. The former have short microvilli projecting from the surface. The cytoplasm characteristically contains a large amount of lipofuscin pigment, a feature important in recognizing these cells obtained by needle biopsy or aspiration cytology studies of the prostate. Similar lipofuscin pigment is found in the ampulla of the ductus deferens and in the epithelium of the ejaculatory ducts. The pigment has been divided into two different types, based on its appearance. Type 1 consists of coarse, highly refractile, golden brown granules of uniform diameter (1–2 μg). Type 2 granules are much more variable in size (0.25–4 μg), faintly or nonrefractile and yellow-brown, grey-brown, blue, or pink.

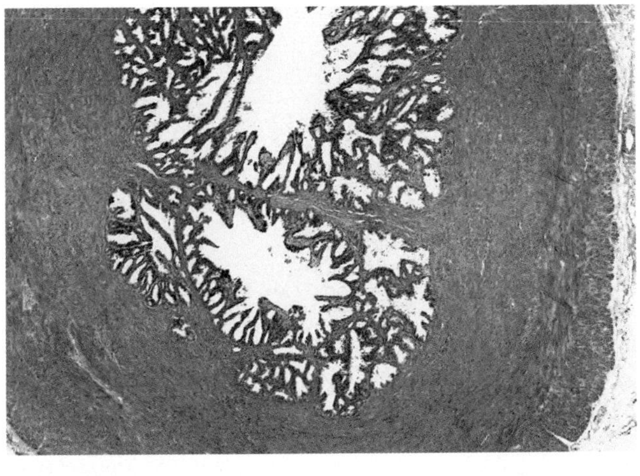

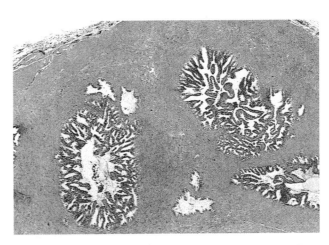

Figure 37.27 Ampullary region of ductus (vas) deferens. Note the complex folding and outpouching of the mucosa into the muscular coat.

Figure 37.28 Seminal vesicle: alveolus-like arrangement of mucosal folds and cross sections of side ducts.

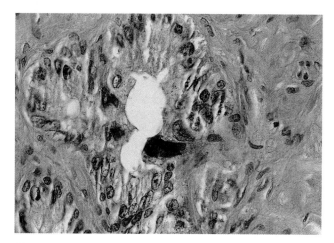

Figure 37.29 Seminal vesicle epithelium. Tall columnar cells line the lumen. A single hyperchromatic "monster" cell is present. These cells should not be mistaken for malignant cells.

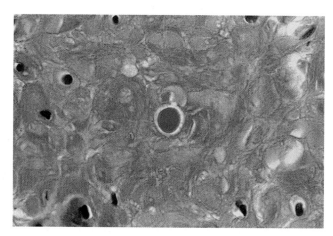

Figure 37.30 Muscle coat of seminal vesicle showing a hyalin globule, which probably represents a degenerated smooth muscle cell.

Both types 1 and 2 granules are found in the seminal vesicle, vas, and ejaculatory ducts, whereas only the type 2 granules are found in prostatic epithelium (101).

An unusual feature of the seminal vesicular epithelium is the presence of peculiar, monstrous epithelial cells (Figure 37.29). Similar cells may be seen in the ampulla of the vas and, less commonly, more proximally in the vas or epididymis. These cells have enlarged, hyperchromatic, and often irregularly shaped nuclei and are found in approximately three-quarters of adult seminal vesicles. They are not seen in infants or children. Their genesis is unknown but may be related to endocrine influences, similar to the Arias-Stella cells seen in gestational endometrium. Because these cells may be encountered in both needle biopsy and aspiration biopsy specimens, the surgical pathologist must be alert to avoid identifying them as malignant cells (102).

Also encountered in the muscle portion of the seminal vesicle are hyalin, pink globules (Figure 37.30), thought to represent degenerating smooth muscle cells. They also may be seen occasionally in the muscular coat of the vas and within the prostatic parenchyma (103).

EJACULATORY DUCTS

The ejaculatory ducts are short (1.5 cm) paired ducts, arising from the confluence of the excretory duct of the seminal vesicle and the ampulla of the vas, that quickly converge and enter the prostate (Figure 37.31). They run through the central zone of the prostatic parenchyma and enter the posterior aspect of the distal prostatic urethra at the verumontanum (104). The outer portions of the ejaculatory ducts have a thin muscle coat that progressively becomes more attenuated as the ducts pass through the prostate. The epithelium of the ejaculatory ducts resembles that of the seminal vesicle and ampulla of the vas (Figure 37.32). On occasion, a needle biopsy of the prostate will sample a portion of one of these ducts, making it imperative that the surgical pathologist be aware of the characteristics of these cells. The presence and character of the lipofuscin pigment in the cytoplasm should give a clue to the cell origin. Immunoperoxidase stains for prostate-specific antigen demonstrate a sharp contrast between the positively stained prostatic parenchyma and the negatively stained cells of the intraprostatic ejaculatory ducts (Figure 37.33).

TESTICULAR APPENDAGES

The testicular and paratesticular appendages are remnants of either the mesonephric duct or the paramesonephric (müllerian) duct (77). The four testicular appendages are

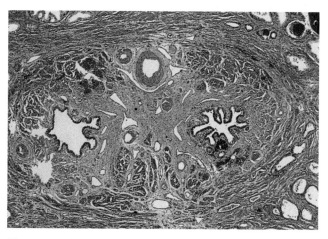

Figure 37.31 Paired ejaculatory ducts within the prostatic parenchyma. This section is adjacent to the verumontanum of the prostatic urethra.

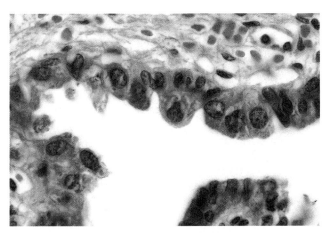

Figure 37.32 Epithelium of prostatic portion of ejaculatory duct. This epithelium may be encountered in a needle biopsy or aspiration biopsy of the prostate and should not be misinterpreted as malignant.

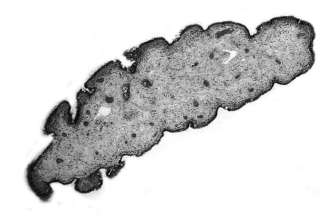

Figure 37.34 Appendix testis. This specimen was an incidental finding in a surgically removed testis. It was pedunculated and measures 0.9 cm in greatest length.

the appendix testis (hydatid of Morgagni), appendix epididymis, vas aberrans (organ of Haller), and paradidymis (organ of Giraldes) (Figure 37.1).

The appendix testis, a remnant of the cranial portion of the müllerian duct, is attached to the tunica vaginalis on the anterosuperior aspect of the testis just below the caput of the epididymis. Occasionally, it is attached to both the testis and the epididymis. It is most often sessile and either oval or fan-shaped (approximately 90%) and, less commonly, pedunculated (approximately 10%) and measures 0.5 to 2.5 cm in greatest dimension (Figure 37.34) (105,106). It is occasionally represented by only a slight roughening or a calcified thickening of the tunica vaginalis. Approximately 80% of individuals have an appendix testis, with bilaterality in one-third of them. The appendix is covered by a cuboidal or columnar epithelium, which may be ciliated

(Figure 37.35). The structure has a highly vascular fibrous core, containing variable numbers of smooth muscle cells. Tubular invaginations and small glandlike structures may also be found in the stroma. Rarely, a macroscopic cyst may be present. Because of its pedunculated structure, the appendix testis can become twisted, causing hemorrhagic infarction and producing severe testicular pain (107). This event occurs most often in prepubertal or pubertal boys and may be related to the presence of androgen and estrogen receptors known to be present in the appendix epithelium (and the appendix epididymis) and the possible growth of the appendix as a result of stimulation by androgens and estrogens at this period of time (108).

The appendix epididymis (Figure 37.36), a remnant of the most cranial portion of the mesonephric duct, is present in approximately 25% of testes (106). It is almost invariably cystic, the vesicle lumen being filled with amorphous protein secretions. The epithelium lining the cyst is

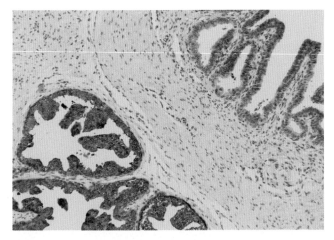

Figure 37.33 Intraprostatic ejaculatory duct (**right**) and adjacent prostatic tissue (**left**). Prostate-specific antigen immunoperoxidase from the central zone of the prostate is used to demonstrate strongly positive cytoplasmic staining of the prostatic secretory cells and negative staining of ejaculatory duct epithelium.

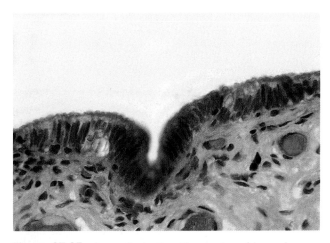

Figure 37.35 Appendix testis with covering of low columnar, nonciliated epithelium.

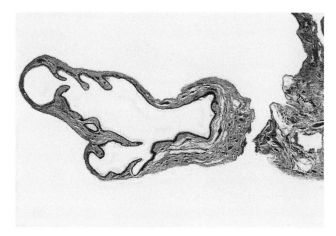

Figure 37.36 Appendix epididymis. A pedunculated cystic structure is attached to the caput of the epididymis.

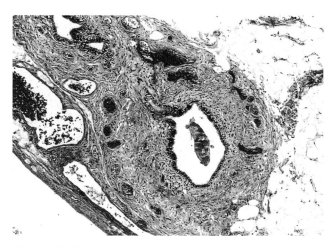

Figure 37.38 Vas aberrans inferior. A tubular structure is found near the caudal portion of the epididymis.

columnar and often ciliated (Figure 37.37). The external surface is covered by a flattened layer of serosal cells. Because it may be pedunculated, it is also subject to torsion and infarction.

The other appendicular structures are derived from remnants of either the mesonephric tubules or the paramesonephric ducts and are variably encountered in the fat, usually as microscopic incidental findings. These are the vas aberrans inferior, the vas aberrans superior, and the paradidymis. They all have somewhat similar histologic features, with a low columnar epithelium lining a small cystic space and a thin muscular coat. Some investigators collectively refer to these structures as the paradidymis (109). The vas aberrans inferior is a tubular structure (Figure 37.38) located near the junction of the vas and the caudal portion of the epididymis and which may or may not communicate with either structure.

The vas aberrans superior is a small collection of tubules located near the caput or body of the epididymis. It may communicate with the epididymis or the rete testis. Remnants of the vas aberrans may be the origin of cord cysts, seen sporadically in isolated individuals, in patients whose mothers had been treated with diethylstilbestrol (110), or in patients with von Hippel-Lindau syndrome (111).

The paradidymis is represented by one or more tubules embedded in the spermatic cord, adjacent to the ductus (vas) deferens, and near the caput of the epididymis. These tubules may be encountered in a section of the wall of an inguinal hernia sac and should not be mistaken for a portion of the ductus deferens (112). The relatively thick muscle coat of the true vas should allow for the correct interpetation. Rarely, macroscopic cysts may form in the spermatic cord (113).

Although not part of the paradidymis, infrequently one may find adrenal cortical rests in the fat of the spermatic

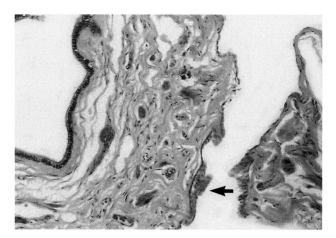

Figure 37.37 Appendix epididymis. Low columnar epithelium lines the cystic space. The outer covering of simple squamous epithelium has become stratified at the point of attachment to the caput of the epididymis (**arrow**).

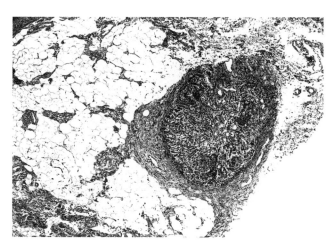

Figure 37.39 Adrenal cortical rest in fat adjacent to the epididymis.

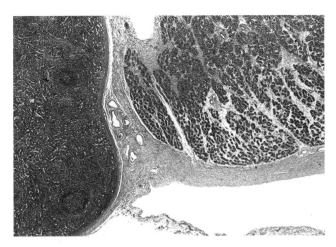

Figure 37.40 Splenogonadal fusion of a cryptorchid testis in a 3-year-old child. Spleen is on the left and gonad on the right.

cord, adjacent to the vas, the epididymis or the rete testis (Figure 37.39). Very rarely, adrenal medullary tissue may also be present. Even less commonly seen is splenogonadal fusion, in which the splenic and gonadal anlages fuse in early embryonal life. This process is almost always on the left side and most commonly is found as an incidental finding in a cryptorchid testis (Figure 37.40). Occasionally it presents as a mass in the scrotum or inguinal canal.

GUBERNACULUM

The gubernaculum has been the center of attention with respect to the descent of the testis since it was first described by John Hunter in 1762, and its specific role is still being debated. In the fetus, this cylindrical, gelatinous structure is attached cranially to the testis and epididymis (Figure 37.41) and caudally to the anterior abdominal wall at the

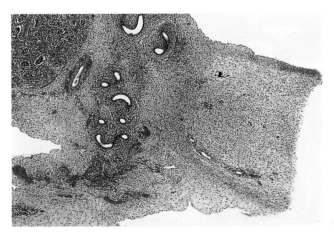

Figure 37.41 Gubernaculum and cranial attachment to epididymis and testis in a 26-week-old fetus.

site of the inguinal canal. Just before the descent of the testis through the inguinal canal, the gubernaculum increases in net weight disproportionately to the testis, supporting the theory that this structure plays a crucial role in this phase of the passage of the testis into the scrotum.

Histologically, the fetal gubernaculum is composed of a loose undifferentiated mesenchymal tissue similar to Wharton's jelly. Large amounts of glycosaminoglycans fill the extracellular space and separate the individual spindle cells. At the periphery of the gubernaculum, where it attaches to the inguinal wall, a few striated muscle cells can be identified. These fibers are derived from the developing cremaster muscle. The cranial portion of the early fetal gubernaculum is completely devoid of striated muscle. After the testis descends into the scrotum, the gubernaculum undergoes degenerative changes, loses much of the intercellular matrix, and becomes infiltrated by blood vessels, collagen fibers, and striated muscle.

REFERENCES

1. Handelsman DJ, Staraj S. Testicular size: the effects of aging, malnutrition, and illness. *J Androl* 1985;6:144–151.
2. Brennan MB, Scrigley JR. Brenner tumors of the testis and paratestis. *J Urol Pathol* 1999;10:219–228.
3. Sosnik H. Studies of the participation of the tunica albuginea and rete testis (TA and RT) in the quantitative structure of human testis. *Gegenbaurs Morphol Jahrb* 1985;131:347–356.
4. Lennox B, Ahmad RN, Mack WS. A method for determining the relative total length of the tubules in the testis. *J Pathol* 1970;102:229–238.
5. Sharpe R, McKinnell C, Kivlin C, Fisher JS. Proliferation and functional maturation of Sertoli cells, and their relevance to disorders of testis function in adulthood. *Reproduction* 2003;125: 769–784.
6. de Miguel M, Bethencourt F, Arenas M, Fraile B, Paniagua R. Intermediate filaments in the Sertoli cells of the ageing human testis. *Virchows Arch* 1997;431:131–138.
7. Nielsen K, Jacobsen GK. Malignant Sertoli cell tumour of the testis: an immunohistochemical study and a review of the literature. *APMIS* 1988;96:755–760.
8. Stosiek P, Kasper M, Karsten U. Expression of cytokeratins 8 and 18 in human Sertoli cells of immature and atrophic seminiferous tubules. *Differentiation* 1990;43:66–70.
9. Rogatsch H, Jezek D, Hittmair A, Mikuz G, Feichtinger H. Expression of vimentin, cytokeratin, and desmin in Sertoli cells of human fetal, cryptorchid, and tumour-adjacent testicular tissue. *Virchows Arch* 1996;427:497–502.
10. Hoei-Hansen C, Holm M, Rajpert-De Meyts E, Skakkebaek NE. Histological evidence of testicular dygenesis in contralateral biopsies from 218 patients with testicular germ cell cancer. *J Pathol* 2003;200:370–374.
11. Suaraz-Quian CA, Martinez-Garcia F, Nistal M, Regadera J. Androgen receptor distribution in adult human testis. *J Clin Endocrinol Metab* 1999;84:350–358.
12. Emerich D, Hemendinger R, Halberstadt C. The testicular-derived Sertoli cell: cellular immunoscience to enable transplantation. *Cell Transplant* 2003;12:335–349.
13. Davidoff M, Middendorff R, Pusch W, Muller D, Wichers S, Holstein AF. Sertoli and Leydig cells of the human testis express neurofilament triplet proteins. *Histochem Cell Biol* 1999;111: 173–187.
14. McLaren A. Studies on mouse germ cells inside and outside the gonad. *J Exp Zool* 1983;228:167–171.

15. Rey R. Regulation of spermatogenesis. *Endocr Dev* 2003;5:38–55.
16. Schulze C. Sertoli cells and Leydig cells in man. *Adv Anat Embryol Cell Biol* 1984;88:1–104.
17. Dym M. The fine structure of the monkey (Macaca) Sertoli cell and its role in maintaining the blood–testis barrier. *Anat Rec* 1973;175:639–656.
18. Russell LD, Peterson RN. Sertoli cell junctions: morphological and functional correlates. *Int Rev Cytol* 1985;94:177–211.
19. Witschi E. Migration of the germ cells of human embryos from the yolk sac to the primitive gonadal fold. *Contrib Embryol* 1948;32:67–80.
20. Heller CG, Clermont Y. Kinetics of the germinal epithelium in man. *Recent Prog Horm Res* 1964;20:545–575.
21. Kerr JB, de Kretser DM. The cytology of the human testis. In: Burger MD, de Kretser D, eds. *The Testis*. New York: Raven Press; 1981:141–169.
22. Gondos B. Ultrastructure of developing and malignant germ cells. *Eur Urol* 1993;23:68–75.
23. Clermont Y. Kinetics of spermatogenesis in mammals: seminiferous epithelium cycle and spermatogonial renewal. *Physiol Rev* 1972;52:198–236.
24. Schulze W, Riemer M, Rehder U, Hohne K. Computer-aided three-dimensional reconstructions of the arrangement of primary spermatocytes in human seminiferous tubules. *Cell Tissue Res* 1986;244:1–8.
25. Johnson L, McKenzie KS, Snell JR. Partial wave in human seminiferous tubules appears to be a random occurrence. *Tissue Cell* 1996;28:127–136.
26. Bartke A. Apoptosis of male germ cells, a generalized or a cell type-specific phenomenon? *Endocrinology* 1995;136:3–4
27. Hadziselimovic F. Ultrastructure of normal and cryptorchid testis development. *Adv Anat Embryol Cell Biol* 1977;53:3–71.
28. Johnson L, Petty CS, Neaves WB. The relationship of biopsy evaluations and testicular measurements to over-all daily sperm production in human testes. *Fertil Steril* 1980;34:36–40.
29. Johnsen SG. Testicular biopsy score count—a method for registration of spermatogenesis in human testis: normal values and results in 335 hypogonadal males. *Hormones* 1970;1:2–25.
30. Weissbach L, Ibach B. Quantitative parameters for light microscopic assessment of the tubuli seminiferi. *Fertil Steril* 1976;27:836–847.
31. Zuckerman Z, Rodriguez-Rigau LJ, Weiss D, Chowdhury AK, Smith KD, Steinberger E. Quantitative analysis of the seminiferous epithelium in human testicular biopsies, and the relation of spermatogenesis to sperm density. *Fertil Steril* 1978;30:448–455.
32. Skakkebaek NE, Heller CG. Quantification of human seminiferous epithelium. I. Histological studies in 21 fertile men with normal chromosome. *J Reprod Fertil* 1973;32:379–389.
33. Silber SJ, Rodriguez-Rigau LJ. Quantitative analysis of testicular biopsy: determination of partial obstruction and prediction of sperm count after surgery for obstruction. *Fertil Steril* 1981;36:480–485.
34. Miller SC, Bowman BM, Rowland HG. Structure, cytochemistry, endocytic activity, and immunoglobulin (Fc) receptors of rat testicular interstitial-tissue macrophages. *Am J Anat* 1983;168:1–13.
35. Hutson JC. Testicular macrophages. *Int Rev Cytol* 1994;149:99–143.
36. Arenas MI, Bethencourt FR, De Miguel MP, Fraile B, Romo E, Paniagua R. Immunocytochemical and quantitative study of actin, desmin and vimentin in the peritubular cells of the testes from elderly men. *J Reprod and Fertil* 1997;110:183–193.
37. De Menezes AP. Elastic tissue in the limiting membrane of the human seminiferous tubule. *Am J Anat* 1977;150:349–373.
38. Nistal M, Paniagua R. Non-neoplastic diseases of the testis. In: Bostwick DG, Elbe JN, eds. *Urologic Surgical Pathology*. St Louis: Mosby; 1997:457–465.
39. de Kretser DM, Kerr JB, Paulsen CA. The peritubular tissue in the normal and pathological human testis: an ultrastructural study. *Biol Reprod* 1975;12:317–324.
40. Amat P, Paniagua R, Nistal M, Martin A. Mitosis in adult human Leydig cells. *Cell Tissue Res* 1986;243:219–221.
41. Nistal M, Paniagua R. Histogenesis of human extraparenchymal Leydig cells. *Acta Anat (Basel)* 1979;105:188–197.
42. Nagano T, Otsuki I. Reinvestigation of the fine structure of Reinke's crystal in the human testicular interstitial cell. *J Cell Biol* 1971;51:148–161.
43. Weiss DB, Rodriguez-Rigau L, Smith KD, Chowdhury A, Steinberger E. Quantitation of Leydig cells in testicular biopsies of oligospermic men with varicocele. *Fertil Steril* 1978;30:305–312.
44. Heller CG, Lalli MF, Pearson JE, Leach DR. A method for the quantification of Leydig cells in man. *J Reprod Fertil* 1971;25:177–184.
45. Cao Q, Jones J, Li M. Expression of calretinin in human ovary, testis, and ovarian sex cord-stromal tumors. *Int J Gynecol Pathol* 2001;20:346–352.
46. Ivell R. Biology of the relaxin-like factor (RLF). *Rev Reprod* 1997;2:133–138.
47. Bamberger A, Ivell R, Balvers M, et al. Relaxin-like factor (RLF): a new specific marker for Leydig cells in the ovary. *Int J Gynecol Pathol* 1999;18:163–168.
48. Davidoff MS, Middendorff R, Kofuncu E, Muller D, Jezek D, Holstein AF. Leydig cells of the human testis possess astrocyte and oligodendrocyte marker molecules. *Acta Histochem* 2002;104:39–49.
49. Lobo M, Arenas M, Alonso J, et al. Nestin, a neuroectodermal stem cell marker molecule, is expressed in Leydig cells of the human testis and in some specific cell types from human testicular tumours. *Cell Tissue Res* 2004;316:369–376.
50. Kormano M, Suoranta H, Reijonen K. Blood supply to testis and excurrent ducts. In: Raspe G, ed. *Advances in the Biosciences*. Vol 10. Oxford, England: Pergamon Press; 1972:72–83.
51. Andres T, Trainer T, Lapenas D. Small vessel alterations in the testes of infertile men with varicocele. *Am J Clin Pathol* 1981;76:378–384.
52. Fawcett DW, Leak LV, Heidger PM Jr. Electron microscopic observations on the structural components of the blood–testis barrier. *J Reprod Fertil Suppl* 1979;10:105–122.
53. Ergun S, Stingl S, Holstein A. Microvasculature of the human testis in correlation to Leydig cells and seminiferous tubules. *Andrologia* 1994;26:255–262.
54. Fawcett DW, Neaves WB, Flores MN. Comparative observations on intertubular lymphatics and the organization of the interstitial tissue of the mammalian testis. *Biol Reprod* 1973;9:500–532.
55. Hadziselimovic F, Thommen J, Girard J, Herzog B. The significance of postnatal gonadotropin surge for testicular development in normal and cryptorchid testes. *J Urol* 1986;136(pt 2):274–276.
56. Huff, DS, Fenig DM, Canning DA, Carr MG, Zderic SA, Snyder HM III. Abnormal germ cell development in cryptorchidism. *Horm Res* 2001;55:11–17.
57. Chemes H. Infancy is not a quiescent period of testicular development. *Int J Androl* 2001;24:2–7.
58. Nistal M, Paniagua R, Queizan A. Histologic lesions in undescended ectopic obstructed testes. *Fertil Steril* 1985;43:455–462.
59. Honecker F, Stoop H, de Krijger R, Chris Lau YF, Bokemeyer C, Looijenga LH. Pathobiological implications of the expression of markers of testicular carcinoma in situ by fetal germ cells. *J Pathol* 2004;203:849–857.
60. Waters B, Trainer T. Development of the human fetal testis. *Pediatr Pathol Lab Med* 1996;16:9–23.
61. Muller J, Skakkebaek NE. Quantification of germ cells and seminiferous tubules by stereological examination of testicles from 50 boys who suffered sudden death. *Int J Androl* 1983;6:143–156.
62. Cortes D, Muller J, Skakkebaek NE. Proliferation of Sertoli cells during development of the human testis assessed by stereological methods. *Int J Androl* 1987;10:589–596.
63. Symington T, Cameron K. Endocrine and genetic lesions. In: Pugh CB, ed. *Pathology of the Testis*. Oxford, England: Blackwell Scientific; 1976:259–303.
64. Nistal M, Paniagua R, Regadera J, Santamaria L, Amat P. A quantitative morphological study of human Leydig cells from birth to adulthood. *Cell Tissue Res* 1986;246:229–236.
65. Prince F. Commentary. The triphasic nature of Leydig cell development in humans, and comments on nomenclature. *J Endocrinol* 2001;168:213–216.
66. Paniagua R, Nistal M, Amat P, Rodriguez M, Martin A. Seminiferous tubule involution in elderly men. *Biol Reprod* 1987;36:939–947.

67. Suoranta H. Changes in the small blood vessels of the adult human testis in relation to age and to some pathological conditions. *Virchows Arch A Pathol Anat* 1971;352:165–181.
68. Kothari LK, Gupta AS. Effect of ageing on the volume, structure and total Leydig cell content of the human testis. *Int J Fertil* 1974;19:140–146.
69. Sokal Z. Morphology of the human testes in various periods of life. *Folia Morphol* 1964;23:102–111.
70. Sargent JW, McDonald JR. A method for the quantitative estimate of Leydig cells in the human testis. *Proc Staff Meet Mayo Clin* 1948;23:249–254.
71. Kaler LW, Neaves WB. Attrition of the human Leydig cell population with advancing age. *Anat Rec* 1978;192:513–518.
72. Neaves WB, Johnson L, Petty C. Seminiferous tubules and daily sperm production in older adult men with varied numbers of Leydig cells. *Biol Reprod* 1987;36:301–308.
73. Rowley MJ, Heller CG. Quantitation of the cells of the seminiferous epithelium of the human testis employing the Sertoli cell as a constant. *Z Zellforsch Mikrosk Anat* 1971;115:461–472.
74. Steinberger A, Steinberger E. Replication pattern of Sertoli cells in maturing rat testis in vivo and in organ culture. *Biol Reprod* 1971;4:84–87.
75. Johnson L, Zane RS, Petty CS, Neaves WB. Quantification of the human Sertoli cell population: its distribution, relation to germ cell numbers, and age-related decline. *Biol Reprod* 1984;31:785–795.
76. Roosen-Runge EC, Holstein AF. The human rete testis. *Cell Tissue Res* 1978;189:409–433.
77. Srigley J. The paratesticular region: histoanatomic and general considerations. *Semin Diagn Pathol* 2000;17:258–269.
78. Dinges H, Zatloukal K, Schmid C, Mair S, Wirnsberger G. Co-expression of cytokeratin and vimentin filaments in rete testis and epididymis. An immunohistochemical study. *Virchows Arch A Pathol Anat Histopathol* 1991;418:119–127.
79. Hartwick RY, Ro JY, Srigley JR, Ondonez NG, Ayala AG. Adenomatous hyperplasia of the rete testis: a clinicopathologic study of nine cases. *Am J Surg Pathol* 1991;15:350–357.
80. Jones E, Murray S, Young R. Cysts and epithelial proliferations of the testicular collecting system (including rete testis). *Semin Diagn Pathol* 2000;17:270–293.
81. Hittmair A, Zelger B, Obrist P, Dirnhofer S. Ovarian Sertoli-Leydig cell tumor: a SRY gene-independent pathway of pseudomale gonadal differentiation. *Hum Pathol* 1997;28:1206–1210.
82. Sapino A, Pagani A, Godano A, Bussolati G. Effects of estrogens on the testis of transsexuals: a pathological and immunocytochemical study. *Virchows Arch A* 1987;411:409–414.
83. Hinton BT, Keefer DA. Evidence for protein absorption from the lumen of the seminiferous tubule and rete of the rat testis. *Cell Tissue Res* 1983;230:367–375.
84. Saitoh K, Terada T, Hatakeyama S. A morphological study of the efferent ducts of the human epididymis. *Int J Androl* 1990;160:369–376.
85. Shah V, Ro J, Amin M, Mullick S, Nazeer T, Ayala AG. Histologic variations in the epididymis: findings in 167 orchiectomy specimens. *Amer J Surg Path* 1998;22:990–996.
86. Rowley MJ, Teshima F, Heller CG. Duration of transit of spermatozoa through the human male ductular system. *Fertil Steril* 1970;21:390–396.
87. Hinrichsen MJ, Blaquier JA. Evidence supporting the existence of sperm maturation in the human epididymis. *J Reprod Fertil* 1980;60:291–294.
88. Regadera J, Cobo P, Paniagua R, Martinez-Garcia F, Palacios J, Nistal M. Immunohistochemical and semiquantitative study of the apical mitochondria-rich cells of the human prepubertal and adult epididymis. *J Anat* 1993;183(pt 3):507–514
89. Kasper M, Stosiek P. Immunohistochemical investigation of different cytokeratins and vimentin in the human epididymis from the fetal period up to adulthood. *Cell Tissue Res* 1989;257:661–664.
90. De Miguel M, Marino J, Gonzalez-Peramato P, Nistal M, Regadera J. Epididymal growth and differentiation are altered in human cryptorchidism. *J Androl* 2001;22:212–225.
91. Cerilli L, Sotelo-Avila C, Mills S. Glandular inclusions in inguinal hernia sacs: morphologic and immunohistochemical distinction from epididymis and vas deferens. *Am J Surg Pathol* 2003;27:469–476.
92. Lee LY, Tzeng J, Grosman M, Unger PD. Prostate gland-like epithelium in the epididymis: a case report and review of the literature. *Arch Pathol Lab Med* 2004;128:e60–e62.
93. Rajalakshmi M, Kumar B, Kapur M, Pal P. Ultrastructural changes in the efferent duct and epididymis of men with obstructive infertility. *Anat Rec* 1993;237:199–207.
94. Oliva E, Young R. Paratesticular tumor-like lesions. *Semin Diagn Pathol* 2000;17:340–358.
95. Madara JL, Haggitt RC, Federman M. Intranuclear inclusions of the human vas deferens. *Arch Pathol Lab Med* 1978;102:648–650.
96. Nistal M, Santamaria L, Paniagua R. Mast cells in the human testis and epididymis from birth to adulthood. *Acta Anat (Basel)* 1984;119:155–160.
97. Paniagua R, Regadera J, Nistal M, Abaurrea MA. Histological, histochemical and ultrastructural variations along the length of the human vas deferens before and after puberty. *Acta Anat (Basel)* 1981;111:190–203.
98. Paniagua R, Regadera J, Nistal M, Santamaria L. Elastic fibres of the human ductus deferens. *J Anat* 1983;137(pt 3):467–476.
99. Murakami M, Nishida T, Shiromoto M, Inokuchi T. Scanning and transmission electron microscopic study of the ampullary region of the dog vas deferens, with special reference to epithelial phagocytosis of spermatozoa and latex beads. *Anat Anz* 1986;162:289–296.
100. Shah R, Lee M, Giraldo A, Amin M. Histologic and histochemical characterization of seminal vesicle intraluminal secretions. *Arch Pathol Lab Med* 2001;125:141–145.
101. Shidham V, Lindholm P, Kajdacsy-Balla A, Basir Z, George V, Garcia FU. Prostate-specific antigen expression and lipochrome pigment granules in the differential diagnosis of prostatic adenocarcinoma versus seminal vesicle-ejaculatory duct epithelium. *Arch Pathol Lab Med* 1999;123:1093–1097.
102. Kuo T, Gomez LG. Monstrous epithelial cells in human epididymis and seminal vesicles: a pseudomalignant change. *Am J Surg Pathol* 1981;5:483–490.
103. Kovi J, Jackson MA, Akberzie ME. Unusual smooth muscle change in the prostate. *Arch Pathol Lab Med* 1979;103:204–205.
104. McNeal JE. Normal histology of the prostate. *Am J Surg Pathol* 1988;12:619–633.
105. Rolnick D, Kawanoue S, Szanto P, Bush IM. Anatomical incidence of testicular appendages. *J Urol* 1968;100:755–756.
106. Sahni D, Jit I, Joshi K, Jeev S. Incidence and structure of the appendices of the testis and epididymis. *J Anat* 1996;189(pt 2):341–348.
107. Skoglund RW, McRoberts JW, Ragde H. Torsion of testicular appendages: presentation of 43 new cases and a collective review. *J Urol* 1970;104:598–600.
108. Samnakay N, Cohen R, Orford J, King P, Davies R. Androgen and oestrogen receptor status of the human appendix testis. *Pediatr Surg Int* 2003;19:520–524.
109. Sadler TW. *Langman's Medical Embryology.* 7th ed. Baltimore: Williams & Wilkins; 1995:293.
110. Whitehead ED, Leiter E. Genital abnormalities and abnormal semen analysis in male patients exposed to diethylstilbestrol in utero. *J Urol* 1981;125:47–50.
111. Bernstein J, Gardner KD Jr. Renal cystic disease and renal dysplasia. In: Walsh PC, Gittes RF, Permutter AD, Stamey TA, eds. *Campbell's Urology.* 5th ed. Vol 2. Philadelphia: WB Saunders; 1986:1760–1803.
112. Popek E. Embryonal remnants in inguinal hernia sacs. *Hum Pathol* 1990;21:339–349.
113. Wollin M, Marshall F, Fink M, Malhotra R, Diamond D. Aberrant epididymal tissue: a significant clinical entity. *J Urol* 1987;138:1247–1250.

Penis and Distal Urethra

38

Elsa F. Velazquez   Christopher J. Cold

José E. Barreto   Antonio L. Cubilla

INTRODUCTION

Three cylindrical, firmly adherent, tubular erectile tissues (the corpora cavernosa and the corpus spongiosum) and the pendulous urethra are the basic constituents of the penis that can be subdivided into a distal portion that includes glans, coronal sulcus, and foreskin and a proximal portion, the corpus or shaft (1) (Figure 38.1). The vast majority of penile carcinomas arise from the distal portion of the organ (Figure 38.2).

DISTAL PENIS

Glans

ANATOMIC LEVELS OF THE GLANS (FIGURE 38.2)

Epithelium

Lamina Propria

Corpus Spongiosum

Tunica Albuginea*

Corpus Cavernosum*

* The distal portions of the corpora cavernosa encased by the tunica albuginea are part of the glans in 77% of the cases.

Anatomic Features

The conically shaped glans, covered by a pink smooth mucous membrane, is the most distal portion of the organ and shows in its central and ventral region, the meatus urethralis. The expanded anterior end of the corpus spongiosum, which has the shape of an obtuse cone similar to the cap of a mushroom, is the central and main tissue of the glans. It is molded over and attached to the blunt extremity of the corpora cavernosa and extends farther over their dorsal than their ventral surfaces (1). The base of this conus is an elevated rim or border, the corona, occupying 80% of the circumferential head of the glans; it is interrupted in the ventral portion of the glans by the mucosal fold of the

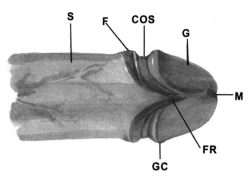

Figure 38.1 The penis can be subdivided in a distal portion that includes glans (*G*), coronal sulcus (*COS*), and foreskin (*F*) and a proximal portion, the corpus or shaft (*S*). (*M* urethral meatus; *GC*, glans corona; *FR*, frenulum)

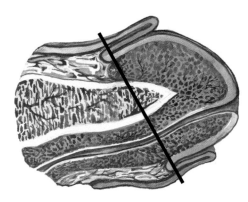

Figure 38.3 The distal portion of corpora cavernosa encased by the tunica albuginea is part of the glans in the majority of cases. The diagonal line passing through the coronal sulcus divides glans from shaft.

frenulum (Figure 38.1). The diameter of the corona is wider than the shaft and the remainder of the glans. Within the corpus spongiosum, there is the distal portion of the urethra that opens at the summit of the glans as a vertical, slit-like external orifice termed the urethral meatus (Figures 38.1–38.2). Normal anatomical structures frequently found in sexually active males and commonly located in the proximal glans are called pearly penile papules, hirsutoid papillomas, or papillomatosis corona penis or glandis (2–5). Grossly, they appear as 1- to 3-mm skin-colored, domed papules evenly distributed circumferentially around the corona and extending proximally on each side of the frenulum. They may be mistaken for warts and be the source of much anxiety for worried adolescents (2).

Considering the glans as the distal tissues to a line passing through the coronal sulcus, the distal portions of the

corpora cavernosa encased by the tunica albuginea extend out into the glans in approximately 77% of the cases (Figure 38.3) (6). However, since they are the main constituents of the shaft, they are discussed in detail in that section.

Microscopic and Immunohistochemical Features

Epithelium

Both circumcised and intact (uncircumcised) men have partially keratinized stratified squamous epithelium five to six layers thick (Figure 38.4). Some textbooks state that the circumcised glans is much thicker and more keratinized than in an intact man, but no well-controlled studies support this belief. The superficial cells usually contain no glycogen. The normal squamous epithelium is usually positive for the cytokeratins AE1/AE3, 34Be12 and CK7, and the epithelial membrane antigen (EMA). It is negative for the cytokeratins CAM 5.2 and CK20. Langer-

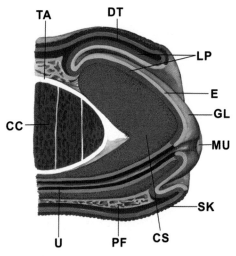

Figure 38.2 Diagram illustrating the distal portion of the penis, which includes glans (*GL*), coronal sulcus, and foreskin. (*E*, epithelium; *LP*, lamina propria; *CS*, corpus spongiosum; *TA*, tunica albuginea; *CC*, corpus cavernosum; *DT*, dartos; *SK*, skin; *U*, urethra; *MU*, meatus urethralis; *PF*, penile, or Buck's, fascia.

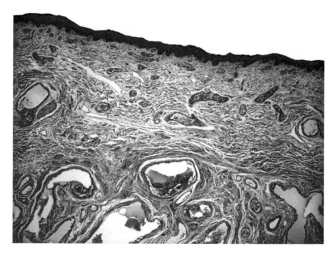

Figure 38.4 The three layers of the glans are noted: partially keratinized stratified squamous epithelium, lamina propria, and corpus spongiosum.

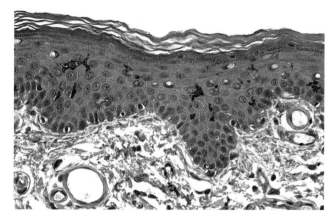

Figure 38.5 CD1a immunostain highlights the presence of scattered Langerhans cells in the glans epithelium.

hans cells are found scattered among keratinocytes, and they are increased in number in different inflammatory conditions. Langerhans cells express S-100 protein and CD1a (Figure 38.5). Very rare Merkel cells are also present, and they are very difficult to demonstrate by routine or immunohistochemical techniques. They are usually negative for chromogranin and positive for CK20 (7). The glans epithelium and the mucosal epithelium of the foreskin appear to not contain melanocytes (8,9). Rarely, mucus-producing cells can be noted in the perimeatal region of the glans epithelium (10). They may be the source of the adenosquamous carcinoma of the glans penis. Intraepithelial free nerves ending close to the surface of the epithelium are noted (11). No adnexal or glandular structures are present in the glans. Histologically, the pearly penile papules appear like fibrovascular papillary projections lined by squamous epithelium (Figure 38.6) (2). No koilocytosis is seen in these structures.

Lamina Propria

The lamina propia is the prolongation of the foreskin lamina propria and separates the corpus spongiosum from the glans epithelium. In the glans, the loose connective tissue of the penile fascia and the fibrous tunica albuginea are lacking so that the lamina propria adheres firmly to the underlying corpus spongiosum (Figure 38.4) (12). The connective tissue of the lamina propria is somewhat similar to that of the corpus spongiosum, although it is more compact and contains fewer peripheral nerve bundles and elastic fibers than the erectile structure. The transition between lamina propria and corpus spongiosum is sometimes difficult to determine at medium or high magnifications. However, at low power or even after a careful gross inspection or with a magnifying lens, this delimitation is evident and follows a line corresponding to the geographic limit of the extension of venous sinuses of the corpus spongiosum. The thickness of the lamina propria varies from 1 mm at the glans corona to 2.5 mm near the meatus. Scattered specialized genital corpuscles are identifed in the lamina propria underneath the squamous epithelium. These genital corpuscles are found mainly in the glans corona and frenulum and may be less numerous in the glans when compared to the foreskin. Additional quantitative studies are needed to confirm or deny this belief. A predominance of free nerve endings over the genital corpuscles has been described in the glans (8,13). A few dermal Merkel cells have been identified at the end of the free nerves.

Corpus Spongiosum

The corpus spongiosum is the principal tissue component of the glans penis and is composed of specialized venous sinuses (Figure 38.7). In the glans, the erectile tissue has the character of a dense, venous plexus (12). As compared to the corpora cavernosa, the interstitial fibrous connective tissue of the corpus spongiosum is more abundant and

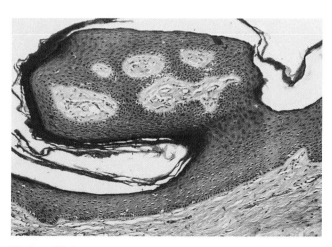

Figure 38.6 Pearly penile papule appears histologically as a papillary structure with a fibrovascular core lined by squamous epithelium with no evidence of koilocytosis.

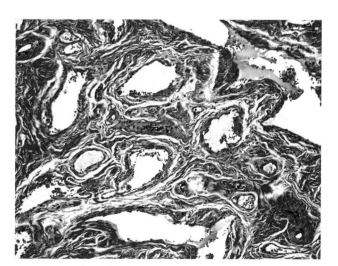

Figure 38.7 Glans. Higher power view of the corpus spongiosum showing specialized venous sinuses.

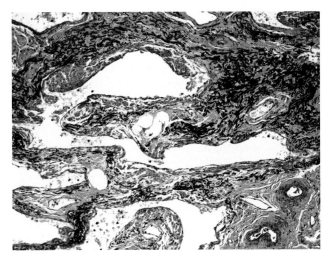

Figure 38.8 Corpus spongiosum. The interstitial fibrous connective tissue is more abundant and contains more elastic fibers than in the corpus cavernosum. Note the presence of nutritional veins and arteries in the interstitium of this erectile tissue. (Van Giesson's elastic stain.)

contains more elastic fibers and less smooth muscle bundles (14,15) (Figures 38.8–38.9). The stroma between the vascular spaces is a loose fibrous tissue containing some nerve endings and lymphatic vessels. In this erectile tissue, we also find nutritional veins and arteries (Figure 38.8).

Coronal Sulcus

ANATOMIC LEVELS OF THE CORONAL SULCUS

Epithelium
Lamina Propria
Buck's Fascia

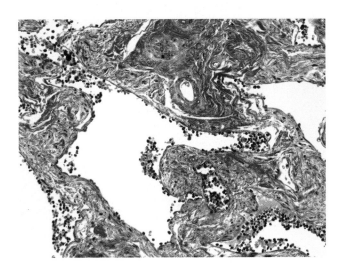

Figure 38.9 Corpus spongiosum. The interstitial fibrous connective tissue contains fewer smooth muscle fibers than does the corpus cavernosum (Masson's trichrome).

Anatomic Features

The coronal sulcus is a narrow and circumferential cul-de-sac located proximal to the glans corona (Figure 38.1–38.2). It is found in both lateral and dorsal aspects of the penis but not in the ventral region, which is occupied by the frenulum, a mucosal fold that fixes the foreskin to the inferior portion of the glans, just below the urethral meatus. The mucous membrane of the glans continues to cover this region as well as the inner surface of the foreskin.

Microscopic and Immunohistochemical Features

Three histologic layers are seen in the coronal sulcus: (a) the squamous epithelium, identical to the glans epithelium; (b) a thin lamina propria, or chorion, which is a prolongation of the foreskin and glans lamina propria; and (c) Buck's fascia and the point of insertion of some of smooth muscle fibers coming from the penile body dartos (Figure 38.10).

The coronal sulcus has been reported as the most frequent site of so-called Tyson's glands (1,14,16–20), described as modified sebaceous glands and reported as responsible for smegma production. Smegma represents epithelial debris and secretions collected in this space (21). There has been some question about the existence of the Tyson's glands (8,21,22). Several studies with numerous tissue sections failed to demonstrate these glands (21,23). We could not find Tyson's glands in a pathologic study of 67 totally sectioned penises removed for carcinoma of the penis. Apparently the original descriptions by Tyson (24) were based on primate studies that could not be confirmed in humans. After circumcision, occasionally some sebaceous glands can be found in the mucosa adjacent to the skin. They are probably skin sebaceous glands misplaced after surgery. Sebaceous glands associated with or without

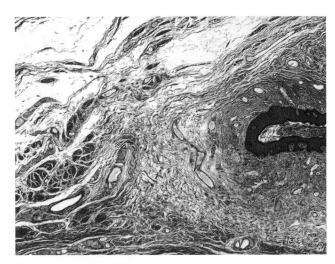

Figure 38.10 A section of the coronal sulcus. Histologic components of both glans and penile body are present. This specimen from an uncircumcised person (a portion of the foreskin is seen on top) shows the squamous epithelium (*right*), lamina propria below, then Buck's fascia and dartos smooth muscle bundles (*left*).

hair follicles are found in the penile shaft and cutaneous aspect of the foreskin. We have observed the presence of sebaceous glands that are nonrelated to hair follicles at the mucocutaneous junction of the foreskin and adjacent mucosa but not in the coronal sulcus. The presence of sebaceous gland hyperplasia or ectopic sebaceous glands (Fordyce's condition) is more frequent on the penile shaft and foreskin but may also occur in the glans (2).

Foreskin

ANATOMIC LEVELS OF THE FORESKIN

Epidermis
Dermis
Dartos
Lamina propria
Epithelium

Anatomic Features and Circumcision

The foreskin, or prepuce, is a unique genital structure of primates that has been present for over 65 million years, and it is present in all living primates and most mammals. The foreskin is the prolongation of the shaft's skin and normally covers most of the glans, reflecting beyond itself and transforming into a mucosal inner surface. This mucous membrane covers the coronal sulcus as well as the surface of the glans (Figures 38.1–38.2). Grossly, the adult foreskin shows a cutaneous surface that is dark and wrinkled and a mucosal surface that is pink to tan (Figure 38.11).

From very early years to the present, there have been discussions and controversies regarding the role of the foreskin and the importance of circumcision (25–28), a type of surgery known to mankind as early as 12,000 BCE and prac-

ticed for religious or tribal rites by, among others, Egyptians, Jews, Muslims, and Aztecs (29,30). Although circumcision has been practiced for thousands of years, circumcision of infants has only been practiced for approximately 4000 years, as described in Genesis 17. Circumcision on the eighth day represents a mark of the covenant between God and the Jewish people. Genesis 17 marks a significant change in the circumcision ritual since before this time circumcision was always performed on young boys and adolescents. Preputial functions are related to protection of the glans from external irritation or contamination, and it has been shown that the foreskin is normal erogenous tissue (8,31,32).

In addition, it has been demonstrated that the squamous mucosa of the glans, coronal sulcus, and foreskin are fused during the embryologic development of the penis (Figure 38.12), and they can be considered as one tissue compartment. The fused mucosa of the glans and inner lining of the foreskin separate gradually over the years (8). Most newborn males show an unretracted foreskin at the time of delivery (33). When boys reach the age of 5 to 6 years, the foreskin can be completely retracted in most cases beyond the level of the glans corona, but in some cases this can be done only at puberty. According to these observations, a tight preputial orifice due to an immature preputial plate does not represent an adhesion but a normal stage of penile development. Therefore, neonatal circumcision before the foreskin has naturally separated involves tearing the common prepuce/glans mucosa apart, with the possible complications of excoriation and injury to the glans and ablation of the frenular artery and meatal stenosis (8).

On the other hand, different studies have been published suggesting that circumcision may reduce the risk of penile carcinoma, urinary tract infection, common sexually transmitted diseases, and human immunodeficiency virus

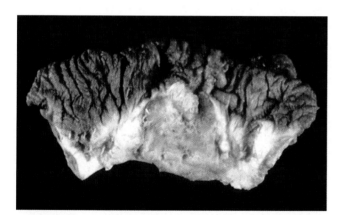

Figure 38.11 Gross appearance of an adult foreskin (prepuce). The cutaneous surface (*top*) is darker and more wrinkled. The mucosa (*bottom*) is pale beige and slightly irregular. A squamous cell carcinoma is present in the mucosal surface, the most common location of preputial carcinomas.

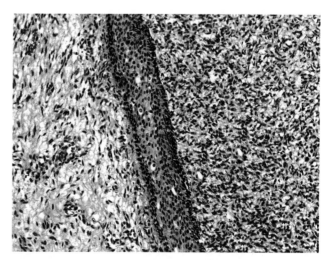

Figure 38.12 Fused squamous mucosa of the glans, coronal sulcus, and foreskin during the embryologic development of the penis. Note the common immature epithelial plate (*center*). The dense stromal cells of the glans will form the corpus spongiosum (*right*). The lamina propria of the glans is not yet formed. The foreskin is on the left.

infection (25,34,35). It has also been proposed that the mucosal inner surface of the foreskin from newborns shows a propensity to be colonized by fimbriated bacteria, with the subsequent occurrence of serious urinary tract infection (36). A recent study suggested that male circumcision is beneficial because it is associated with a reduced risk of penile HPV (human papillomavirus) infection and, in the case of men with a history of multiple sexual partners, a reduced risk of cervical cancer in their current female partner (37). However, it appears clear that the risk of sexually transmitted disease, including HPV infection, correlates with sexual behavior, and behavioral factors appear to be a far more important risk factor than circumcision status.

Review of existing literature supports that most children who are uncircumcised do well from a medical standpoint and, thus, the question of whether U.S. health care practitioners are subjecting neonates to an unnecessary surgical procedure remains (35). The clearest medical benefit of circumcision is the relative reduction in the risk for a urinary tract infection, especially in early infancy. Although this risk is real, the absolute numbers are small (risk ranges from 1 in 100 to 1 in 1000). Most of the other medical benefits of circumcision probably can be realized without circumcision as long as access to clean water and proper penile hygiene are achieved (35). Moreover, proper hygiene and access to clean water has been shown to reduce the rate of development of squamous cell carcinoma of the penis in the uncircumcised population (38), and the American Academy of Pediatrics stated that the benefits of male circumcision are not significant enough to merit its routine use. (35).

In adult populations, the variable length of the foreskin has motivated some studies, especially those related to the relation of length and amount of smegma in the balanopreputial sulcus (25,30,39). Phimosis is found in 4% of boys 6 to 17 years of age, but with a diminishing incidence in later years (from 8% in the 6- to 7-year-old group to 1% in the 16- to 17-year-old group) (39). In nonphimotic boys, where the preputial space can be inspected, smegma is present in 5% of the cases. Production of smegma appears to increase in quantity in the 16- to 17-year-old group (39). In a recent prospective study in a high-risk population, we found that long phimotic foreskins were significantly more frequent in patients with penile carcinoma as compared with the general population (25). Coexistence of a long foreskin and phimosis may explain the high incidence of penile cancer in some geographic regions, and circumcision in patients with long and phimotic foreskins living in high-risk areas may be indicated (25). However, additional studies are necessary to confirm whether the length of the foreskin is a significant risk factor, when all other known risk factors (multiple sex partners, foreskin tears, lack of indoor plumbing, tobacco use, etc.) are controlled. Also, studies in nonmestizo populations, in particular European countries that have low circumcision and low cancer rates, would be interesting.

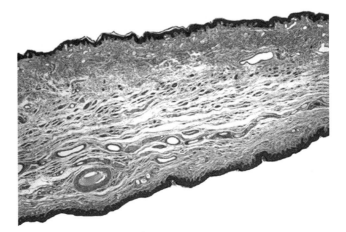

Figure 38.13 Full-thickness of the foreskin showing all five layers: keratinized stratified squamous epithelium (*top*), dermis, dartos, submucosa, and squamous epithelium of the mucosal portion (*bottom*).

Microscopic and Immunohistochemical Features

The male foreskin is formed by a midline collision of ectoderm, neuroectoderm, and mesenchyme, resulting in a pentalaminar structure (8). There are five layers in the histologic evaluation of the foreskin (Figure 38.13):

1. The epidermis consists of a keratinized stratified squamous cell epithelium that is similar to the epidermis seen in the cutaneous tegument. Melanocytes, Langerhans cells, and Merkel cells are also present. Compared to the mucosal epithelium, the epidermis is thinner with better developed rete ridges and usually a pigmented basal layer (Figure 38.14). Vellous hairs, sebaceous, and sweat glands may be seen connected to the epidermis.

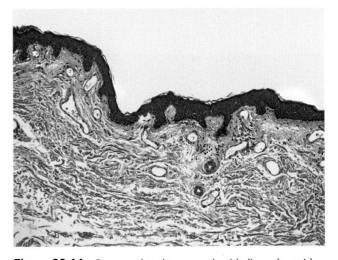

Figure 38.14 Compared to the mucosal epithelium, the epidermis is thinner with better developed rete ridges and usually a pigmented basal layer. The ductal portion of sweat glands connected to the epidermis can be appreciated in this photomicrograph.

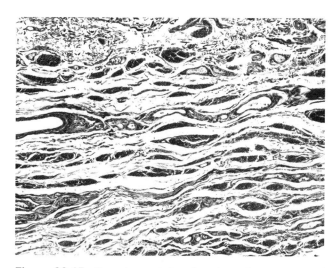

Figure 38.15 Smooth muscle bundles, the main component of the preputial dartos, are shown in red (Masson's trichrome).

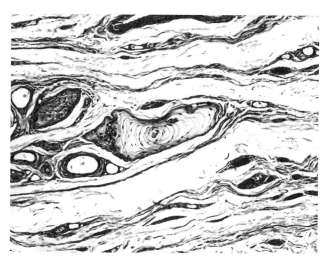

Figure 38.17 A Vater-Pacini corpuscle is present deep in the dartos layer of the foreskin.

2. The dermis of the foreskin consists of connective tissue with blood vessels and nerve bundles. Meissner corpuscles are present in the dermal papillae and a few Vater-Pacini corpuscles in deeper areas. Few vellous hair structures and sebaceous and sweat glands are noted, and they are not present beyond the dartos. The dermis appears to have more elastic fibers than does the lamina propria.

3. The dartos consists of smooth muscle fibers invested with elastic fibers, and it is the central axis of the foreskin (Figure 38.15). From the foreskin, the delicate penile dartos muscle surrounds the penile shaft and is continuous with the scrotal dartos muscle. Similar to the penile body dartos, the smooth muscle fibers vary in their disposition. At the level of the edge of the foreskin, the fibers are transversely arranged to form a sphincter to close this edge over the anterior end of the glans. There are numerous nerve endings in close association with the smooth muscle fibers (Figure 38.16). Nerve bundle density in the foreskin was noted to be highest in the ventral preputial tissue (mean: 17.9 bundles/nm) as opposed to lateral (8.6/nm) or dorsal (6.2/nm) tissues (40). A few Vater-Pacini corpuscles may be found scattered between these nerve bundles (Figure 38.17).

4. The lamina propria, or chorion, is composed of a vascular connective tissue looser than the glans lamina propria. Scattered genital corpuscles and free nerve endings are seen in the lamina propria immediately underneath the epithelium. The genital corpuscles are usually found in clusters of three to five (Figure 38.18). Some authors believe that the corpuscular receptors are more numerous at the mucocutaneous junction of the foreskin; this assertion needs further study (8,31). The mucosal lamina propria is devoid of lanugo hair follicles and sweat and sebaceous glands. We have observed

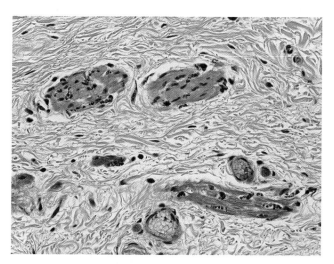

Figure 38.16 Neurofilament immunostain highlights numerous free nerve endings associated with smooth muscle bundles in the foreskin dartos.

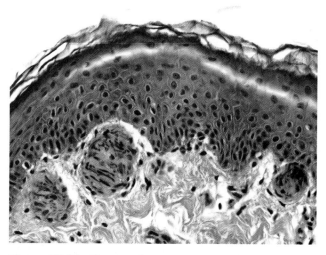

Figure 38.18 The genital corpuscles are usually found in clusters of three to five underneath the mucosal epithelium, in the lamina propria of the foreskin (neurofilament immunostain).

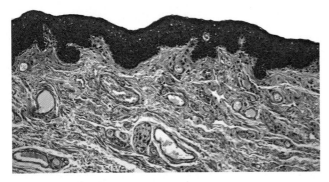

Figure 38.19 The squamous epithelium of the mucosal portion of the foreskin is usually thicker with more irregular and broad rete ridges than in the cutaneous portion. Adnexal structures are absent.

a few specimens with rare sebaceous glands unrelated to hair structures at the mucocutaneous junction and immediately adjacent foreskin mucosa, but it is not clear if these represent ectopic glands or variation of normal anatomy.

5. The squamous epithelium (Figure 38.19), which is identical to and a prolongation of the glans and coronal sulcus' epithelia except that the basal layer shows a progressive pigmentation toward the free edge of the foreskin where it reaches the skin epidermis. The immunohistochemical features of this epithelium are identical to the glans squamous epithelium. Langerhans and Merkel cells are present but not melanocytes. Intraepithelial nerves have been described (8,11).

PROXIMAL PENIS (OR SHAFT)

ANATOMICAL LEVELS OF THE PENILE SHAFT

Epidermis
Dermis
Dartos
Buck's fascia
Tunica Albuginea
Corpora cavernosa
Corpus spongiosum

Anatomic Features

The penile shaft, body, or corpus, of the penis is mainly composed of three cylindrical masses of erectile tissue, the two corpora cavernosa and a corpus spongiosum with central urethra (Figure 38.20A–B). The posterior portion of the corpora cavernosa are two divergent and gradually tapering structures, called the crura, that insert in the ischiopubic bone from where they converge to fuse at the level of the inferior portion of the pubic symphysis. The distal three-fourths of the two corpora cavernosa are intimately bound together and make up the greater part of the shaft of the penis. They retain a uniform diameter in the shaft and terminate anteriorly in a bluntly rounded extremity, being embedded in a cap formed by the corpus spongiosum of the glans (1). The erectile tissue of the corpora cavernosa is a vast, spongelike system of irregular vascular spaces fed by the afferent arteries and drained by the efferent veins. In the flaccid condition of the organ, the cavernous spaces contain little blood and appear as collapsed irregular clefts. In erection they become large cavities engorged with blood under pressure (14).

The corpora cavernosa are surrounded by a firm, thick, fibrous envelope, the tunica albuginea. In the flaccid state the tunica albuginea measures 2 to 3 mm in thickness and becomes thinner (about 0.5 mm) during erection. On longitudinal sections of the organ, the albuginea covering the corpora cavernosa terminates in a ">"-shaped pattern variably ending beyond or at the level of coronal sulcus or, less frequently, behind it (Figure 38.20A–B) (6). The tunica albuginea enveloping the corpora cavernosa is thicker and less elastic than that surrounding the corpus spongiosum (14,15). The superficial longitudinal fibers of the tunica albuginea form a single tube that encloses both corpora cavernosa while the deep fibers are arranged circularly around each corpus, forming the septum of the penis by their junction in the median plane (Figure 38.21) (1). The septum is thick and complete in the proximal shaft and discontinous distally. A shallow groove that marks their junction on the upper surfaces lodges the deep dorsal vein of the penis.

The corpus spongiosum and central urethra are located in the concave space on the undersurface of both corpora cavernosa (Figure 38.21). The middle portion of the corpus spongiosum located in the penile shaft is a uniform cylinder somewhat smaller than the corpus cavernosum. At its ends, it expands, the distal extremity forming the glans and the proximal forming the bulb. The urethra enters the corpus spongiosum 1 to 2 cm from the posterior extremity of the bulb by piercing the dorsal surface. The bulb is just superficial to the urogenital diaphragm, and its posterior portion projects backward towards the anus beyond the entrance of the urethra.

The three cylindrical structures forming the penile shaft are covered by a thin, delicate, and elastic skin. Beneath the dermis, there is a discontinuous smooth muscle layer called the dartos (Figure 38.21) embedded in a thin layer of connective tissue corresponding to the superficial fascia of the classical descriptions. Between the dartos and the albuginea, there is a highly elastic yellowish tubelike sheath encasing all three corpora cavernosa and spongiosum; this is designated as Buck's fascia (deep penile fascia of the classical descriptions) (Figures 38.20A–B, 38.21). A septum of fascia extends inward between the corpora cavernosa and the corpus spongiosum, providing separate tubular investments for these columns of erectile tissue and dividing the penis into its dorsal (corpora cavernosa) and ventral (corpus spongiosum)

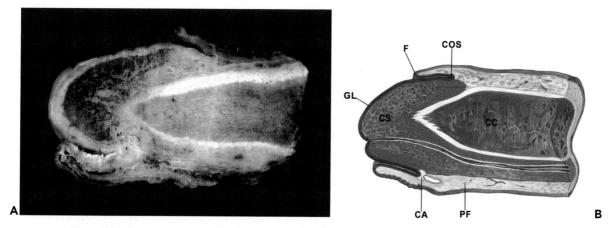

Figure 38.20 Gross picture (**A**) and diagram (**B**) of two longitudinal sections of a partial penectomy specimen with a small squamous cell carcinoma (CA) located in the coronal sulcus (COS). The albuginea (in white) surrounds the corpus cavernosum. The diagram from a parallel but more central section of the same specimen, illustrates the urethra running within the corpus spongiosum. (F, foreskin; GL, glans; PF, Buck's fascia; CS, corpus spongiosum; CC, corpus cavernosum).

portions as can be also seen via CT (computed tomography) or MRI (magnetic resonance imaging) (41). When using the terms *fascia* or *penile fascia* in this chapter, we are referring to the Buck's fascia since the superficial fascia is just part of the connective tissue surrounding the dartos.

Microscopic Features

Skin

The skin covering the penile shaft is rugged and elastic. It shows a thin epidermis composed of a few cell layers and

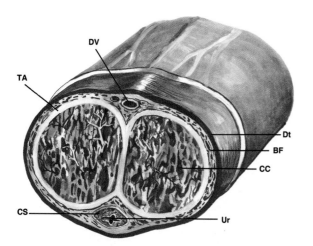

Figure 38.21 Cross section of the penis illustrating both corpora cavernosa (*CC*), each surrounded by the tunica albuginea (*TA*); they form the septum of the penis by their junction in the median plane. A shallow groove that marks their junction on the upper surfaces lodges the deep dorsal vein of the penis (*DV*). The dorsal arteries are located on both sides of the vein. Note the corpus spongiosum (*CS*) and central urethra (*Ur*) located in the concave space on the undersurface of both corpora cavernosa. (*BF*, Buck's fascia; *Dt*, dartos)

minimal keratinization. The epidermal papillae are thin and deep. The basal layer is hyperpigmented. Hair follicles are present in the dermis of the penile body and are more numerous in the proximal body. Hair follicles and other adnexa can extend out to the cutaneous foreskin in some individuals. They are scanty and contain no piloerector muscle. There are a few sebaceous glands not related to hair follicles. Occasionally there are also poorly developed sweat glands.

Dartos

The penile dartos is composed of a discontinuous layer of smooth muscle fibers, variably arranged in transverse and longitudinal branches. Some bundles end at the balanopreputial sulcus while others run farther to become the preputial dartos. The dartos is embedded in a loose fibrovascular connective tissue with numerous nerve bundles that correspond to the superficial penile fascia of the classical anatomic description, and it is the skin equivalent of the penile hypodermis but without adipose tissue (1). The penile dartos, similar to scrotal smooth muscle fibers, produces a retraction of genital structures when the exterior temperature falls.

Buck's Fascia

The Buck's fascia is a fibroelastic continuous membrane that encases the corpora cavernosa and the corpus spongiosum. It is composed of loose connective tissue with numerous blood vessels and peripheral nerve bundles running within and beneath it. Vater-Pacini corpuscles are often seen in the penile fascia. The yellow color is related to the numerous elastic fibers and adipose tissue present in the fascia (Figure 38.22). The skin and dartos slide over this fascia. The Buck's fascia is a well-developed sheath of close up fibrovascular tissue that is very important from the

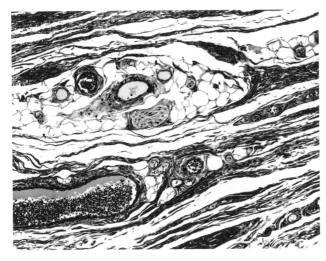

Figure 38.22 The Buck's fascia is composed of loose connective tissue with adipose cells and numerous blood vessels and peripheral nerve bundles.

surgical pathology point of view since it is a frequent pathway of tumor invasion in penile cancer progression (42). This is most likely due to the loose quality of this tissue and the presence of numerous lymphovascular and neural structures. Some investigators point to Buck's fascia as the site of origin of Peyronie's disease (43).

Tunica Albuginea

The tunica albuginea is a thick sheath of partially hyalinized collagen fibers covering both the corpora cavernosa and corpus spongiosum. It is a poorly vascular structure, with only a few branches of circumflex vessels traversing through it, as demonstrated by factor VIII and CD31 immunostains. It is mainly composed of collagen fibers arranged in an outer longitudinal and an inner circular layer (14,15). The outer layer, which appears to determine the variation in the thickness and strength of the tunica, is absent in the ventral portion of the corpus spongiosum, transforming this portion of tunica into a vulnerable area to perforation. This anatomic aspect probably explains why most prostheses tend to extrude in this area (44). The tunica albuginea forms an incomplete fibrous septum separating both corpora cavernosa. The collagen fibers are wavy in the flaccid state and become straight during erection. The fibers are arranged in such a way so as to permit some elasticity necessary for erection. Elastic fibers are rare in the tunica albuginea of the corpora cavernosa. The tunica albuginea surrounding the corpus spongiosum is thinner and contains more elastic fibers than the one around the corpora cavernosa. In some unusual cases of Fournier's gangrene (45), an infection of the lower urinary tract can spread to the corpus spongiosum. Eventually the tunica albuginea may be penetrated; and, with involvement of Buck's fascia, the infection can rapidly spread to

the dartos and directly extend to Colles' scrotal fascia and Scarpa's fascia of the anterior abdominal wall. The infection can spread to the buttocks, thigh, and ischiorectal space (46). The tunica albuginea is probably the real barrier to infiltration of squamous cell carcinoma, contrary to the old concept that the Buck's fascia was the barrier to the spread of the cancer (47).

Corpora Cavernosa

The corpora cavernosa are the main anatomic structures used during erection. The substance of the corpora cavernosa consists of a three-dimensional network of trabeculae. These are composed of connective tissue and smooth muscle and are covered by endothelium, creating a network of interanastomosing vascular spaces between them. These spaces tend to be larger in the more central parts of each corpus cavernosum and smaller at their periphery (14,15). It seems that the smooth muscle bundles are the main component of the trabeculae in the corpora cavernosa (Figure 38.23). There is a highly structured criss-crossing of interconnected fibers and spaces that are tensed as the cylinder expands during erection (48,49). This creates an internal strength and rigidity that is far greater than that possible in a hollow tube filled to equivalent pressure. This specialized network appears to be necessary for erection (49). In the flaccid state, the vascular spaces are 1-mm slits that increase several times in diameter with erection. The interconnection between the venous sinuses is so wide that if a contrast is injected at one point, both corpora cavernosa can be immediately and completely visualized. The precise nature of vascular connections between the corpora cavernosa and corpus spongiosum remains controversial. Cavernospongious arterial anastomoses were described by different authors; however, their physiological role in erection remains unknown (50). These arterial anastomoses could explain

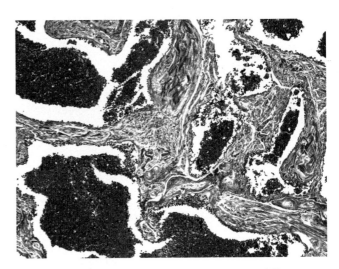

Figure 38.23 Corpus cavernosum. The interstitial fibrous connective tissue contains more smooth muscle fibers than in the corpus spongiosum (Masson's trichrome).

how drugs penetrate into the corpora cavernosa via the corpus spongiosum after transurethral diffusion (50,51). No arteriovenous shunts or venous connections were found between the corpora cavernosa and the corpus spongiosum (51).

A progressive increase of collagen fibers and decrease of smooth muscle and elastic fiber may be seen in the cavernous trabeculae over the course of time (52).

Corpus Spongiosum

In the corpus spongiosum of the shaft, there are widely interconnected, branching vascular spaces separated by trabeculae. These vascular spaces of variable caliber are lined by endothelial cells and are surrounded by a thin layer of smooth muscle fibers. These fibers coalesce in various extraluminal parts of the vessels to form the subendothelial cushions or polsters. Toward the urethra, the lacunae become continuous with a mucosal plexus of veins; at the periphery, they communicate with the venous network of the albuginea (12). Compared to the corpus spongiosum of the shaft, the substance of the glans corpus spongiosum is made up of convolutions of large veins rather than spaces separated by trabeculae (15).

The main differences between corpus spongiosum and corpora cavernosa from the penile shaft are that the blood spaces in the corpus spongiosum, unlike those of the corpora cavernosa, are the same size in peripheral and central areas and the trabeculae between them contain more elastic fibers, whereas smooth muscle bundles are relatively scarce when compared to the trabeculae of the corpora cavernosa (Figure 38.24) (14,15). However, there is variability and sometimes it can be difficult to distinguish corpus cavernosum from spongiosum by histology alone.

DISTAL URETHRA

ANATOMIC LEVELS OF THE URETHRA AND PERIURETHRAL TISSUES

Urethral Epithelium
Lamina Propria
Corpus Spongiosum
Tunica Albuginea
Buck's Fascia

Anatomic Features

The distal (anterior) urethra consists of the bulbous and penile (pendulous) segments. The 3- to 4-cm bulbous urethra is located between the inferior margin of the urogenital diaphragm and the penoscrotal junction and courses in the root of the penis within the bulb of the corpus spongiosum.

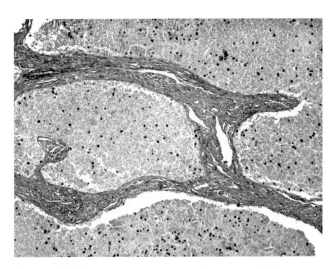

Figure 38.24 Corpus cavernosum. The interstitial fibrous connective tissue contains fewer elastic fibers than does the corpus spongiosum (van Giesson elastic stain).

The penile urethra measures approximately 15 cm in length and extends from the penoscrotal junction to the external meatus; it is closely associated to the corpus spongiosum that forms a protective cylindrical sheath around it (1,10,20). The distal 4 to 6 mm of the penile urethra corresponds to the fossa navicularis, a distal saccular expansion that is contiguous to the urethral meatus. The penile urethra has a more central position within the corpus spongiosum, in contrast to the more dorsally positioned bulbous urethra. The mucosa of the distal urethra has numerous recesses, called Morgagni's lacunae, which extend deeply into the mucin-secreting Littré's glands that are present in the lateral walls of the bulbous and penile urethra. A stellate-shaped lumen can be noted in cross section of the penile urethra owing to these folds of epithelium and lamina propria (Figures 38.25A–B). From the surgical pathology point of view the urethra with surrounding periurethral tissues is an important margin to be carefully evaluated in partial penectomy specimens with penile carcinoma since is the most frequent positive resection margin, as was shown in a recent review of penectomies with carcinoma (42). The anatomical levels at the urethral margin of resection are: epithelium, lamina propria, periurethral corpus spongiosum, tunica albuginea, and Buck's fascia (Figure 38.25B).

Microscopic and Immunohistochemical Features

Urethral Epithelium

There are two conflicting embryological explanations of the differentiation of the distal urethra: the ectodermal ingrowth theory (the distal urethra originates in the ectoderm, penetrating from glans to urethra) and the endodermal differentiation theory (distal urethra is formed by differentiation of endodermal tissues from urethra to

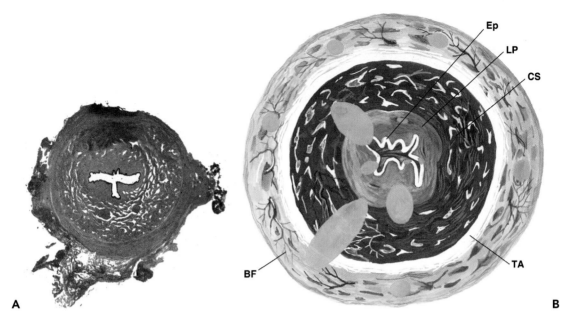

Figure 38.25 **A.** Cross section of the penile urethra and periurethral tissues. Note the stellate-shaped lumen at the center. **B.** Diagrammatic cross section of penile urethra and periurethral tissues. The anatomical levels at the urethral margin of resection are epithelium (*Ep*), lamina propria (*LP*), peri-urethral corpus spongiosum (*CS*), tunica albuginea (*TA*) and Buck's fascia (*BF*).

glans) (53,54). Independently of the embryogenesis, there are histological differences between the epithelium of the anterior urethra and the classical transitional urothelium of the posterior urethra and the urinary tract. The fossa navicularis is lined by nonkeratinizing squamous epithelium, and it is similar and continuous to the epithelium covering the glans penis. In the pendulous and bulbous urethra, the surface cell layer is columnar without the "umbrella" cells noted in bladder urothelium and prostatic urethra. In addition to the columnar cells, the epithelium of the anterior urethra is composed of 4 to 15 stratified layers of uniform small cells, usually categorized as stratified or pseudostratified columnar epithelium (Figure 38.26). The distinctive epithelium appears to be related to the squamous rather than to the transitional urothelium. This would explain the high frequency of squamous metaplasias, as well as the predominance of carcinomas of squamous type in the anterior urethra compared with a much higher frequency of transitional cell carcinomas in the prostatic urethra. The tumors in the membranous portion of the posterior urethra are more similar to those of the bulbous urethra. Adenocarcinomas preferentially arise in the bulbomembranous urethra; however, squamous cell carcinomas are significantly more frequent than adenocarcinomas in these portions (10). The frequent finding of intraepithelial precancerous lesions in the penile urethras of patients with penile squamous cell carcinoma is noteworthy because it indicates that the urethra participates either as a mechanical pathway of penile cancer progression in a continuous manner or as an independent site of primary tumor growth in discontinuous lesions (54).

Immunohistochemical studies show that the penile urethral epithelium expresses CK7, 34Be12, and p63 but is negative for CK20. The CK7 immunostain is positive in the upper layers of the epithelium, including the columnar cells (Figure 38.27), in contrast to the expression of p63 and 34Be12 that is mostly seen in basal and parabasal cells but not in the superficial layer of columnar cells (Figures 38.28–38.29). Occasional chromogranin-positive cells may be found close to the basal membrane by immunohistochemical stains.

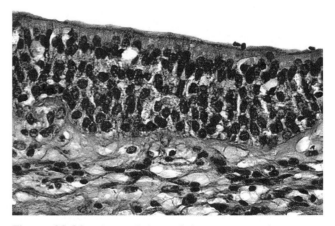

Figure 38.26 The epithelium of the anterior urethra is composed of columnar cells overlying 4 to 15 stratified layers of uniform small cells, usually categorized as stratified or pseudostratified columnar epithelium.

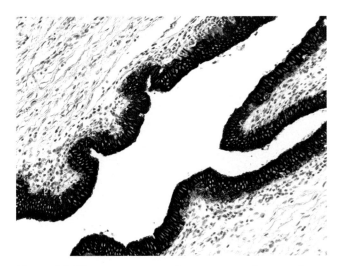

Figure 38.27 The expression of CK7 is seen in the upper layers of the urethral epithelium, including the columnar cells.

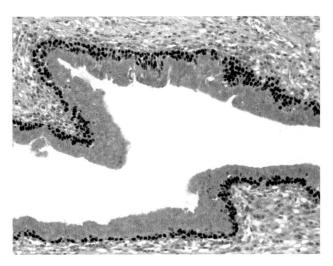

Figure 38.29 Urethral epithelium. In contrast to the superficial layers, basal and parabasal cells show p63 nuclear expression.

Urethral and Periurethral Glands

There are two different types of glands in the anterior urethra: the intra- or juxtaepithelial glands, with a dense eosinophilic cytoplasm and rounded basal nuclei, and the classical mucinous Littré's glands, with clear mucinous cytoplasm and basally compressed nuclei resembling pyloric glands of the gastrointestinal tract (Figure 38.30). There are histologic transitions from the intra- or juxtaepithelial glands with dense eosinophilic cytoplasm to more mucinous cells.

The recesses of the urethra (Morgagni's lacunae) are lined by paraurethral mucinous Littré's glands. Littré's glands are tubuloacinous mucous structures located along the full length of the corpus spongiosum, in close relation with erectile tissue (Figure 38.31). Littré's glands end in the urethra at the level of the intraepithelial lacunae. Some cysts have been described as originating in the parameatal Littré's glands

(55). Inflammation of Littré's glands can clinically simulate a tumor (56). Cohen et al. recognized the normal presence of prostatic epithelial cells in periurethral glands along the penile urethra. These "minor prostatic glands" may be entirely composed of prostatic cells or, more commonly, mixed prostatic and mucinous epithelium (57) (Figure 38.32). The same authors suggested that these glands may be partially responsible for the minimal but persistently elevated levels of serum PSA (prostate-specific antigen) in some cases of successful radical prostactectomy (57).

The bulbourethral or Cowper's, glands are two small structures deeply located at the level of the membranous (or bulbous) urethra where they terminate in two small ducts (58). They are mucous-acinous structures (Figure 38.33). The clear cells of these glands can be confused with prostatic carcinoma in a core needle biopsy specimen.

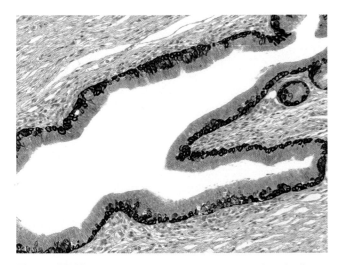

Figure 38.28 Urethral epithelium. Basal and parabasal cells express 34Be12. The superficial layers are negative.

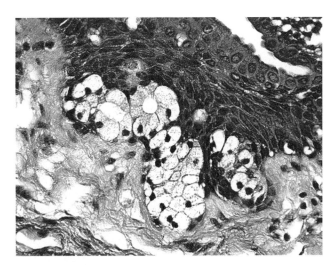

Figure 38.30 Penile urethra. A section illustrating intraepithelial mucinous glandular structures.

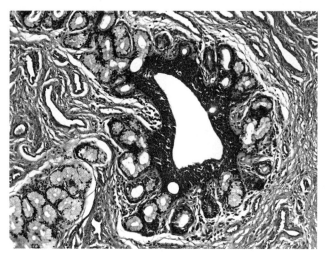

Figure 38.31 Penile urethra. Photomicrograph illustrating a cluster of tubular and acinar Littré's mucous glands.

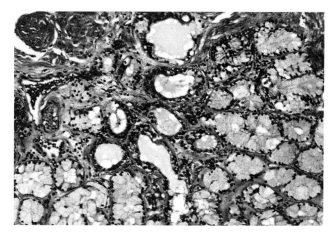

Figure 38.33 Bulbourethral (Cowper's) gland. Specimen was taken from autopsy and shows acinous-mucous structures, which are located deeply in the membranous urethra. (Courtesy Dr. Victor Reuter, Memorial Sloan-Kettering Cancer Center.)

Lamina Propria

The urethral lamina propria is a thin layer of loose fibrous and elastic tissue. Genital corpuscles are identified in the lamina propria of the most distal portion of the urethra, which is lined by squamous epithelium; however, they are not seen in other portions of the penile urethra. We have seen cases of lichen sclerosus affecting the glans and extending into the lamina propria of the anterior urethra (54).

The corpus spongiosum, tunica albuginea, and Buck's fascia were discussed in a previous section.

ARTERIES

The arteries of the penis are branches of the internal pudenda, which is a branch of the iliac. There are two systems: the dorsal and the cavernous arteries. The dorsal

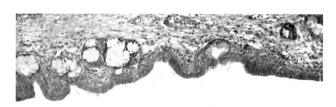

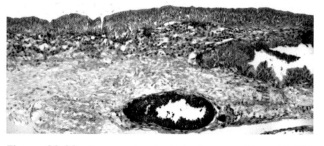

Figure 38.32 Some periurethral glands are positive with PSA (prostate-specific antigen) immunostain.

arteries are located from the base of the penis near and on both sides of the dorsal profunda vein within Buck's fascia and in the superior groove formed by the corpora cavernosa (Figure 38.21). Small-caliber branches, or circumflex arteries, irrigate the corpora cavernosa and the periurethral corpus spongiosum. They also perforate the albuginea to reach the corpora. The terminal branches irrigate the glans, and collateral branches provide the skin nutrients. Cavernous arteries penetrate the corpora cavernosa at the site where the corpora join, and they run longitudinally near the central septum, which divides the corpora. From the cavernous arteries originate the vasa vasorum, small arteries that irrigate the erectile tissues. The helicine branches also originate from the cavernous arteries, and they are responsible for filling the vascular spaces during the process of erection; their name derives from the fact that they are coiled and twisted along the trabeculae when the penis is flaccid (59,60). These arteries have thick muscular walls; and, in addition, many possess inner thickenings of longitudinal muscle fibers that bulge into their lumina. Many of the terminal branches of the helicine arteries open directly into the spaces of the erectile tissue.

VEINS

The superficial veins are irregularly distributed and easily noted under the skin. They end in the superficial dorsal vein; this vascular structure runs straight from the foreskin to the base of the penis. It drains the foreskin venous blood and the skin and is located in the space between the dermis and Buck's fascia. The deeper venous system, for which the axis is the deep dorsal vein, runs along the superficial dorsal vein but in a plane separated by the Buck's fascia (Figure 38.21). The circumflex veins originate in the periurethral corpus spongiosum and terminate in the deep dorsal vein system. Similarly, there are veins originating in the corpora cavernosa that, after forming a small plexus at the base of the penis, terminate in the internal pudendal vein. The cavernous venous system, unlike the venous drainage from the glans penis, delays venous drainage and in doing so assists in maintaining erections (61).

Penile erection is a vascular phenomenon that results from trabecular smooth muscle relaxation, arterial dilation, and venous restriction. In further support of the concept of restriction of outflow is the observation that the walls of the circumflex veins are unusually muscular. In addition, these veins exhibit unique specializations of their lumina caller *polsters*. These are local accumulations of fibroblasts and smooth muscle cells beneath the endothelium that form conspicuous longitudinal thickenings or ridges that can be followed throughout hundreds of serial sections. These are believed to have a role in constricting the lumen and retarding venous outflow during erection (14). There are, however, controversies regarding the real presence and significance of the polsters in the penile veins and arteries, and some authors have proposed that they represent degenerative changes (62).

The deep dorsal vein of the penis has a connection with the vertebral veins, hence it is possible for metastases to make their way to the vertebrae or even to the skull and brain without going through the heart and lungs. Pyogenic organisms may be transported by the same route (1).

LYMPHATICS

The lymphatics of the foreskin spring from a network that covers its internal and external surfaces; they arise from the lateral aspect and converge dorsally with the skin of the shaft lymphatics to form 4 to 10 vessels that run toward the pubis, where they diverge to drain into the right and left superficial inguinal lymph nodes. The lymphatics draining the glands form a rich network that, beginning in the lamina propia, course toward the frenulum, where they coalesce with two or three trunks from the distal urethra to form several collecting trunks following the coronal sulcus. A collar of lymphatics entirely surrounds the corona, forming two or three trunks that run along the dorsal surface of the penis deep to the fascia and accompanied by the deep dorsal vein. At the presymphyseal region they form a rich anastomosing plexus draining into superficial and deep inguinal lymph nodes (63). The male urethra has a dense plexus in the muscosa. The lymphatic capillaries are especially abundant around the fossa navicularis (1). The lymphatics of the urethra, corpus spongiosum, and corpora cavernosa run toward the ventral surface of the body of the penis, reaching the raphe and the dorsum, where they run with the dorsal vein and end in the superficial and deep inguinal lymph nodes.

NERVES

The nerves originate in the sacral and lumbar plexuses. Peripheral nerves run along the arteries. Dorsal nerves are located external to the arteries, giving circumflex branches to the corpora cavernosa (64,65). The terminal branches end in the glans and foreskin. The dorsal nerve of the penis, the principal somatosensory nerve innervating the penis, consists of two populations of axons, one to innervate the penile shaft and urethra and the other to innervate the glans. Urethral innervation by the dorsal nerve of the penis supports the view that urethral afferent impulses are a component of reflex ejaculatory activity. The pattern of glanular innervation by the dorsal nerve of the penis identifies the glans as a sensory end organ for sexual reflexes. The undulating character of the dorsal nerve of the penis is a mechanism by which the nerve can accommodate to significant changes in penile length with erection (64). The dorsal nerve of the penis supplies the glans in most men, but branches of the perineal nerve can supply the ventral penis, frenulum, and periurethral area in some men.

REFERENCES

1. Clemete CD, ed. *Gray's Anatomy of the Human Body*. 30th ed. Philadelphia: Lea & Febiger; 1985.
2. Bunker CB. *Male Genital Skin Disease*. Philadelphia: Elsevier Saunders; 2004.
3. Hyman AB, Brownstein MH. Tyson's "glands." Ectopic sebaceous glands and papillomatosis penis. *Arch Dermatol* 1969;99:31–36.
4. Tanenbaum MH, Becker SW. Papillae of the corona of the glans penis. *J Urol* 1965;93:391–395.
5. Winer JH, Winer LH. Hirsutoid papillomas of the coronal margin of glans penis. *J Urol* 1955;74:375–378.
6. Cubilla AL, Piris A, Pfannl R, Rodriguez I, Aguero F, Young RH. Anatomic levels: important landmarks in penectomy specimens: a detailed anatomic and histologic study based on examination of 44 cases. *Am J Surg Pathol* 2001;25:1091–1094.
7. Moll I, Kuhn C, Moll R. Cytokeratin 20 is a general marker of cutaneous Merkel cells while certain neuronal proteins are absent. *J Invest Dermatol* 1995;104:910–915.
8. Cold CJ, Taylor JR. The prepuce. *BJU Int* 1999;83(suppl1):34–44.
9. Tuncali D, Bingul F, Talim B, Surucu S, Sahin F, Aslan G. Histologic characteristics of the human prepuce pertaining to its clinical behavior as a dual graft. *Ann Plast Surg* 2005;54:191–195.
10. Young RH, Srigley JR, Amin MB, Ulbright TM, Cubilla AL. Tumors of the prostate gland, seminal vesicles, male urethra and penis. In: *Atlas of Tumor Pathology*. 3rd series, fascicle. Washington, DC: Armed Forces Institute of Pathology; 2000.
11. Montagna W, Kligman AM, Carlisle KS. *Atlas of Normal Human Skin*. New York Springer-Verlag; 1992.
12. Kelly DE, Wood RL, Enders AC. *Bailey's Textbook of Microscopic Anatomy*. 18th ed. Baltimore: Williams & Wilkins; 1984.
13. Halata Z, Munger BL. The neuroanatomical basis for the protopathic sensibility of the human glans penis. *Brain Res* 1986;371:205–230.
14. Fawcett DW. In: *Bloom and Fawcett: A Textbook of Histology*. 11th ed. Philadelphia: WB Saunders; 1986.
15. Ham AW, Cormack DH. *Histology*. 8th ed. Philadelphia: JB Lippincott Company; 1979.
16. Hyman AB, Brownstein MH. Tyson's "glands." Ectopic sebaceous glands and papillomatosis penis. *Arch Dermatol*. 1969;99:31–6.
17. Poirier P, Charpy A. Traité d'Anatomie humaine. Paris: Masson et Cie, 1901:183.

18. Saalfeld E. Ueber die Tyson'schen drüsen. *Arch Mikr Anat* 1899:212–218.

19. Tandler J, Dömeny P. Ueber Tyson'schen drüsen. *Wiener Klin Wochen* 1898;23:555–556.

20. Testut L, Latarjet A. *Tratado de Anatomía Humana*, Vol 4. 9th ed. Barcelona: Salvat; 1959.

21. Parkash S, Jeyakumar S, Subramanyan K, Chaudhuri S. Human subpreputial collection: its nature and formation. *J Urol* 1973;110:211–212.

22. Keith A, Shillitoe A. The preputial or odoriferous glands of man. *Lancet* 1904;1:146–148.

23. Sprunk H. Ueber die vermeintlichen Tyson'schen drauusen [dDissertation]. University of Königsberg. Germany; 1897.

24. Tyson E. The anatomy of a pygmy compared with that of a monkey, an ape and a man. London: University of London Press; 1699.

25. Velazquez EF, Bock A, Soskin A, Codas R, Arbo M, Cubilla AL. Preputial variability and preferential association of long phimotic foreskins with penile cancer: an anatomic comparative study of types of foreskin in a general population and cancer patients. *Am J Surg Pathol* 2003;27:994–998.

26. Weiss C. Motives for male circumcision among preliterate and literate people. *J Sex Res* 1966;2:69–88.

27. Winberg J, Bollgren I, Gothefors L, Herthelius M, Tullus K. The prepuce: a mistake of nature? *Lancet* 1989;1:598–599.

28. Wynder EL, Licklider SD. The question of circumcision. *Cancer* 1960;13:442–445.

29. Arellano-Arroyo A. La cirugía entre los aztecas [tThesis]. Facultad de Medicina, Universidad Nacional Autonoma de Mexico, Ciudad de Mexico, Mexico; 1962.

30. Riveros M. Cancer del pene. Artes Gráficas Zamphirópolos. *Asuncion* 1968.

31. Taylor JR, Lockwood AP, Taylor AJ. The prepuce: specialized mucosa of the penis and its loss to circumcision. *Br J Urol* 1996;77:291–295.

32. Winkelmann RK. The erogenous zones: their nerve supply and its significance. *Mayo Clin Proc* 1959;34:39–47.

33. Ben-Ari J, Merlob P, Mimouni F, Reisner SH. Characteristics of the male genitalia in the newborn: penis. *J Urol* 1985;134:521–522.

34. Dillner J, von Krogh G, Horenblas S, Meijer CJ. Etiology of squamous cell carcinoma of the penis. *Scand J Urol Nephrol Suppl* 2000;205:189–193.

35. Lerman SE, Liao JC. Neonatal circumcision. *Pediatr Clin North Am* 2001;48:1539–1557.

36. Fussell EN, Kaack MB, Cherry R, Roberts JA. Adherence of bacteria to human foreskins. *J Urol* 1988;140:997–1001.

37. Castellsague X, Bosch FX, Munoz N, et al. Male circumcision, penile human papillomavirus infection, and cervical cancer in female partners. *N Engl J Med* 2002;346:1105–1112.

38. Frisch M, Friis S, Kjaer SK, Melbye M. Falling incidence of penis cancer in an uncircumcised population (Denmark 1943–90). *BMJ* 1995;311:1471.

39. Oster J. Further fate of the foreskin: incidence of preputial adhesions, phimosis, and smegma among Danish schoolboys. *Arch Dis Child* 1968;43:200–203.

40. Modwing R, Valderrama E. Immunohistochemical analysis of nerve distributions pattern within preputial tissues. *J Urol* 1989;141(suppl 1):489A.

41. Hricak H, Marotti M, Gilbert TJ, et al. Normal penile anatomy and abnormal penile condition: evaluation with MR imaging. *Radiology* 1988;169:683–690.

42. Velazquez EF, Soskin A, Bock A, Codas R, Barreto JE, Cubilla AL. Positive resection margins in partial penectomies: sites of involvement and proposal of local routes of spread of penile squamous cell carcinoma. *Am J Surg Pathol* 2004;28:384–389.

43. Mostofi FK, Davis C Jr. Male reproductive system and prostate. In: Kissane JM, ed. *Anderson's Pathology.* 8th ed. Vol 1. St. Louis: CV Mosby; 1985.

44. Hsu GL, Brock G, Martínez-Pineiro L, von Heyden B, Lue TF, Tanagho EA. Anatomy and strength of the tunica albuginea: its relevance to penile prosthesis extrusion. *J Urol* 1994;151:1205–1208.

45. Fournier AJ. Gangrene foudroyante de la verge. *Semaine Med* 1883;3:345–348.

46. Spirnack JP, Resnick MI, Hampel N, Persky L. Fournier's gangrene: report of 20 patients. *J Urol* 1984;131:289–291.

47. Oota K. Cancer of the penis in Japan. *Rev Inst Nac Cancer (Mexico)* 1964;15:289–292.

48. Goldstein AMB, Meehan JP, Zakhary R, Buckley PA, Rogers FA. New observations on microarchitecture of corpora cavernosa in man and possible relationship to mechanism of erection. *Urology* 1982;20:259–266.

49. Zinner NR, Sterling AM, Coleman RV, Ritter RC. The role of internal structure in human penile rigidity. *J Urol* 1989;141:221A.

50. Droupy S, Giuliano F, Jardin A, Benoit G. Cavernospongious shunts: anatomical study of intrapenile vascular pathways. *Eur Urol* 1999;36:123–128.

51. Vardi Y, Saenz de Tejada I. Functional and radiologic evidence of vascular communication between the spongiosal and cavernosal compartments of the penis. *Urology* 1997;49:749–752.

52. Fontana D, Rolle L, Lacivita A, et al. Modificazioni anatomo-funzionali dei corpi cavernosi nell'anziano. *Arch Ital Urol Androl* 1993;65:483–486.

53. Kurzrock EA, Baskin LS, Cunha GR. Ontogeny of the male urethra: theory of endodermal differentiation. *Differentiation* 1999;64:115–122.

54. Velazquez EF, Soskin A, Bock A, Codas R, Cai G, Cubilla AL. Epithelial abnormalities and precancerous lesions of anterior urethra in patients with penile carcinoma. A report of 89 cases. *Mod Pathol* 2005;18:917–923.

55. Shiraki IW. Parameatal cysts of the glans penis: a report of 9 cases. *J Urol* 1975;114:544–548.

56. Krawitt LN, Schechterman L. Inflammation of the periurethral glands of Littre simulating tumor. *J Urol* 1977;118:685.

57. Cohen RJ, Garrett K, Golding JL, Thomas RB, McNeal JE. Epithelial differentiation of the lower urinary tract with recognition of the minor prostatic glands. *Hum Pathol* 2002;33:905–909.

58. Bourne CW, Kilcoyne RF, Kraenzler EJ. Prominent lateral mucosal folds in the bulbous urethra. *J Urol* 1981;126:326–330.

59. Breza J, Aboseif SR, Orvis BR, Lue TF, Tanagho EA. Detailed anatomy of penile neurovascular structures: surgical significance. *J Urol* 1989;141:437–443.

60. Krane RJ. Sexual function and dysfunction. In: Walsh PC, Gittes R, Perlmutter AD, Stamey TA, eds. *Campbell's Urology.* 5th ed. Vol 1. Philadelphia: WB Saunders; 1986:700–735.

61. Fitzpatrick T. The corpus cavernosum intercommunicating venous drainage system. *J Urol* 1975;113:494–496.

62. Benson GS, McConnell JA, Schmidt WA. Penile polsters: functional structures or atherosclerotic changes? *J Urol* 1981;125:800–803.

63. Cunéo B, Marcille M. Note sur les lymphatiques du gland. *Bull Soc Anat Paris* 1901;76:671–674.

64. Yang CC, Bradley WE. Peripheral distribution of the human dorsal nerve of the penis. *J Urol* 1998;159:1912–1916.

65. Lepor H, Gregerman M, Crosby R, Mostofi FK, Walsh PC. Precise localization of the autonomic nerves from the pelvic plexus to the corpora cavernosa: a detailed anatomical study of the adult male pelvis. *J Urol* 1985;133:207–212.

FEMALE GENITAL SYSTEM

Vulva

Edward J. Wilkinson   Nancy S. Hardt

CLINICAL PERSPECTIVE

Vulvar symptoms are a common cause of clinical visits to gynecologists and family practitioners. Complaints may include pruritus, burning, external dyspareunia, and a visible or palpable mass (1,2). The majority of sexually transmitted infections, as well as many granulomatous and dermatological diseases, may involve the vulva (2,3,4). Graft-versus-host disease (5) and contact dermatitis (6,7) may create symptoms requiring evaluation of the vulva and vagina. The vulva (pudendum femininum) is also a crucial area for detailed examination in cases of reported rape, sexual abuse, or female circumcision (8). Ambiguous genitalia and genital anomalies challenge the clinician and demand critical examination of the patient and the external genitalia. Clitoral enlargement in the newborn resulting from adrenal genital syndrome, maternal exposure to exogenous androgens, maldevelopment of the clitoris, benign tumors, and other conditions, such as the Lawrence-Seip syndrome (3,9,10), may result in ambiguous-appearing external genitalia. Clitoromegaly may occur in adulthood due to malignancy or endocrinopathy (11).

Surgical approaches to vulvar diseases are evolving as a result of better understanding of vulvar anatomy and sexual function. Clitoral specimens are submitted less frequently in cases of infant genital ambiguity now that follow-up studies have indicated that permanent loss of function and sensation may result (12,13,14,15,16). In radical surgery for carcinoma of the vulva, the clitoris may be surgically spared if clinical examination does not indicate tumor involvement of that structure (17). The techniques for sentinel node evaluation used in other cancers are now applied to carcinomas of the vulva, permitting removal of less normal tissue from lymph node drainage fields (18,19,20).

Cytologic evaluation of the vulva may complement biopsy in special cases such as extramammary Paget's disease (21) and distinguishing disorders that may clinically resemble Paget's disease (22).

SPECIAL TECHNIQUES IN CLINICAL EVALUATION

Direct examination of the vulva requires adequate illumination and is enhanced by the use of a ring light or magnifying glass (23). The use of higher magnification, using a colposcope, enhances the identification of small condyloma acuminatum, vestibular papillae, vulvar intraepithelial neoplasia and superficial lacerations, microulcerations, and contusions after sexual assault (24). In cases in which condyloma acuminatum or vulvar intraepithelial neoplasia is suspected, the use of 3% acetic acid (white vinegar) is of value. Gauze sponges soaked in acetic acid are applied for approximately five minutes, followed by prompt examination. The principle of this technique is that abnormal epithelium, especially condyloma acuminatum and vulvar intraepithelial neoplasia, becomes white immediately after exposure to acetic acid. This is related to poorly understood differences between normal epithelium and human papillomavirus–associated lesions. The color change to white after application of the dilute acetic acid is referred to as aceto-whitening, and the epithelium so changed is referred to as aceto-white epithelium. This procedure has gained wide acceptance in the evaluation of the cervical transformation zone during colposcopic examination to enhance identification of cervical intraepithelial neoplasia and carcinoma. However, its use on the vulva has two serious limitations. First, when ulcers or fissures are present on the vulva, the application of 3% acetic acid may be associated with pain and thus is unacceptable to the patient. Second, the vulvar vestibular epithelium is normally somewhat aceto-white. The inexperienced clinician may misinterpret this aceto-whitening as abnormal or as condyloma acuminatum. A biopsy is then performed of the vestibular epithelium and submitted as condyloma acuminatum. The vestibular epithelium in women of reproductive age is normally glycogenated (see section on Vulvar Vestibule) and can be misinterpreted by the unwary pathologist as koilocytosis suggestive of condyloma acuminatum, resulting in both improper diagnosis and improper therapy for the patient. Inflammation within the vestibule may be associated with epithelial spongiosis, which also may be confused with koilocytosis.

The use of 1% toluidine blue O also has been used to assist in the recognition of areas requiring biopsy when invasive carcinoma is suspected (23). A solution of 1% toluidine blue O is applied to the areas in question, which then are rinsed with 1% acetic acid. Areas with ulceration, parakeratosis, and carcinomas without a keratinized surface retain the blue stain. In principle, toluidine blue O is a DNA stain, and as such it is retained where cell nuclei are present (3,23). This test has limited usefulness in that false-positive staining patterns occur, usually due to benign superficial ulceration or fissures. The test may be falsely negative when the carcinoma or intraepithelial neoplasm has a keratinized surface. For these reasons, the test is no longer commonly used.

In addition to direct visualization techniques, imaging studies are increasingly applied in the vulvar assessment of female sexual response and have increased our understanding of the three-dimensional anatomy of that region. These include duplex Doppler ultrasound (25) and magnetic resonance imaging (26,27,28)

From the pathologist's perspective, the majority of vulvar specimens that are examined are either diagnostic biopsies, excisional biopsies, or partial superficial or deep, or total superficial or deep vulvectomy specimens submitted as treatment for vulvar intraepithelial neoplasia, Paget's disease, carcinoma, melanoma, and other diseases (3). An understanding of the normal histology of the vulva enhances interpretive skills and assists in arriving at an appropriate diagnosis.

ANATOMY

The female external genitalia can be defined as that portion of the female anatomy external to the hymen, extending anteriorly to include the mons pubis, posteriorly to the anus, and laterally to the inguinal–gluteal folds. Included are the mons pubis, clitoris, labia minora, labia majora, vulvar vestibule and vestibulovaginal bulbs, urethral meatus, hymen, Bartholin's and Skene's glands and ducts, and vaginal introitus (Figure 39.1). The anterior investment of the clitoris includes the prepuce, which represents the anterior fusion of the labia minora and overlays the clitoris anteriorly, and the frenulum, which passes posteriorly and ends in its attachment to the flattened posterior aspect of the clitoris. Posteriorly, the labia minora end in the fourchette, or frenulum of the labia. The labia majora lie lateral to the intralabial sulcus and medial to the inguinal-gluteal fold. Anteriorly, the hair-bearing lateral aspects of the labia majora blend with the mons pubis, and posteriorly, the labia majora end in the perineal body. The hair follicles of the labia majora are absent in its medial portion; however, the sebaceous gland elements are retained medial and posterior to the labia minora at the junction with the vulvar vestibule at Hart's line (29,30) (Figure

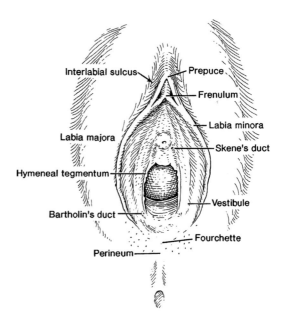

Figure 39.1 Topography of the vulva.

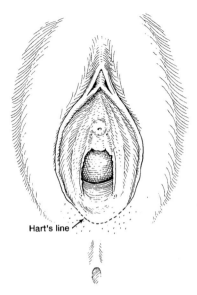

Hart's line

Figure 39.2   The vulvar vestibule and the position of Hart's line. Hart's line can be found on the medial aspect of the labia majora, extending in a curvilinear manner from the most inferior posterior portion of the labia minora to the vaginal fourchette.

39.2). These sebaceous gland elements open directly to the epithelial surface in this portion of the vulva and can be observed as small, slightly pale to yellow elevations of the epithelium, known as Fordyce's spots.

Normal vulvar epithelium varies in thickness from 0.27 ± 0.14 mm. When involved by vulvar intraepithelial neoplasia, the thickness of the epithelium with vulvar intraepithelial neoplasia (VIN) is reported from 0.52 ± 0.23 mm (31). The vulvar epithelium, especially that of the lateral labia minora, labia majora, and perineal body, contains melanocytes that are distributed among the basal cells of the epithelium in a ratio from 1:5 to 1:10 basal keratinocytes (32). Increased pigmentation of these areas during pregnancy relate to increased melanin production secondary to the effects of gestational hormones.

Langerhans cells are relatively abundant in the vulvar epithelium, where they are more prevalent than within the vagina or cervix. They are present predominantly in the suprabasal layers of vulvar epithelium, with a median number of 18.7 per 100 basal squamous cells (33). They are present in keratinized and nonkeratinized epithelium, as well as within skin appendages. These dendritic cells are bone marrow–derived and can express HLA-DR antigens and Fc and C3 receptors and are capable of activating T lymphocytes as an afferent component of the immune response of the vulvar epithelium (34). Langerhans cells are also thought to be associated with control of keratinocyte maturation (35). The topical T-lymphocyte inhibitor, pimecrolimus, has recently been used to effectively treat vulvar lichen sclerosus in a 10-year-old girl. Lichen sclerosus is a dermatosis that is considered to be T-lymphocyte mediated (36).

Merkel cells are neuroendocrine cells that are present in vulvar epithelium, as well as most other skin sites. These cells are involved in paracrine regulation of skin function (37). Merkel cell tumors of the vulva have been reported (38).

Lymphocytes are also commonly found in the dermis and submucosal areas of the vulva in small numbers and are located primarily in a perivascular area within the superficial tissues. Intraepithelial lymphocytes are infrequently seen in normal vulvar epithelium (33).

Vulvar Vestibule

The vulvar vestibule is defined as that portion of the vulva that extends from the exterior surface of the hymen to the frenulum of the clitoris anteriorly, the fourchette posteriorly, anterolaterally to the labia minora, and posterolaterally to Hart's line, on the medial aspects of the labia majora (Figures 39.1–39.2). The vestibular fossa (fossa navicularis) is that posterior portion of the vestibule, from the hymen to the fourchette, that is somewhat concave as compared with the remainder of the vestibule. Unlike the remainder of the vulvar epithelium, which is of ectodermal origin, the epithelium of the vulvar vestibule is of endodermal origin. One exception is the portion of the vulvar vestibular epithelium anterior to the urethra, which some think is of ectodermal origin (39). The vulvar vestibule is predominantly nonkeratinized stratified squamous epithelium, which peripherally blends with the thinly keratinized squamous epithelium of the labia minora, the medial labia majora at Hart's line, the prepuce, and the fourchette. Although the vestibular epithelium has an embryonic origin similar to that of the distal urethra of the male, the epithelium is not of a typical transitional type with associated surface umbrella cells. Rather, it is a stratified squamous epithelium that is rich in glycogen in women of reproductive age, similar to the mucosa of the vagina and ectocervix (Figure 39.3).

Both the vaginal opening and the urethral orifice are within the vestibule. Also within the vulvar vestibule are gland openings from both the major and minor vestibular glands, as well as the paired opening of the periurethral Skene's ducts. Skene's ducts are the homologues of the male prostate gland. The major vestibular gland, or Bartholin's gland (glandula vestibularis major), is of ectodermal origin and consists of bilateral tubuloalveolar glands located beneath the hymen, labia minora, and labia majora in the posteriolateral area of the vulva. Bartholin's gland corresponds to the male bulbourethral glands, or Cowper's glands. The epithelial cells of Bartholin's gland acini consist of mucus-secreting columnar cells (40,41) (Figure 39.4). The secretion of these acini empty into Bartholin's duct, which measures approximately 2.5 cm in length and enters the vestibule immediately exterior (distal) and adjacent to the hymen in a posteriolateral location. Bartholin's duct is lined by transitional epithelium

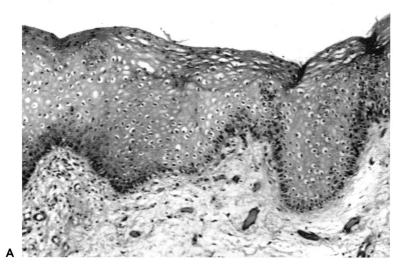

A

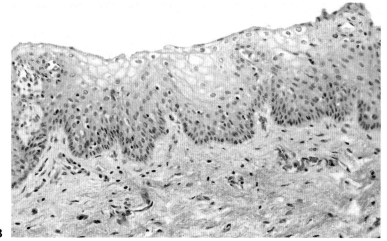

B

Figure 39.3 **A.** Vulvar vestibule with adjacent prominent vascular submucosa. Superficial thin-walled vessels are prominent and are found within the delicate fibrous stroma. A few lymphocytes are seen scattered in the superficial submucosa. **B.** Epithelium of the vulvar vestibule of a 27-year-old woman. Note that the epithelium is stratified squamous and that the superficial cells have cytoplasmic clearing, reflecting the glycogen-rich epithelium.

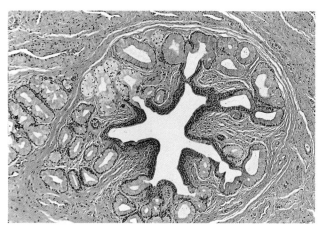

Figure 39.4 Bartholin's gland acini are lined with a columnar epithelium. The adjacent branching Bartholin's duct is present adjacent to the gland.

that is adjacent to columnar epithelium as it arises from the gland (Figure 39.5) to adjoin the nonkeratinized stratified squamous epithelium of the vulvar vestibule in the distal end of the duct (41) (Figure 39.6). Within the Bartholin duct epithelium, argentaffin cells also can be identified, predominantly concentrated within the transitional ductal epithelial cell area and absent in the secretory gland area (42). Cysts that arise in the area of Bartholin's gland are primarily a result of dilation of Bartholin's duct (3,43).

The periurethral, or Skene's, glands also enter the vulvar vestibule as paired gland openings found immediately adjacent to and posterolateral to the urethra. These glands, with their adjacent ducts, are generally not more than 1.5 cm in length. These periurethral glands are analogous to the male prostate gland and are lined with a pseudostratified mucus-secreting columnar epithelium. The ducts of Skene's glands are lined with transitional-type epithelium that joins with the stratified squamous epithelium of the vestibule at the gland orifices. A cyst of Skene's duct may result from obstruction of the duct.

The minor vestibular glands (glandulae vestibulares minores) consist of simple tubular glands that enter directly to

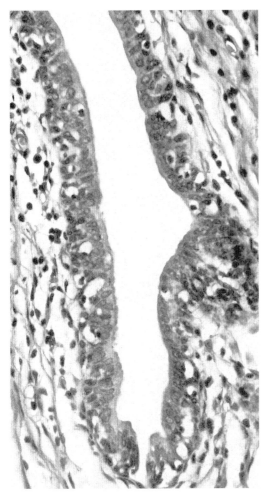

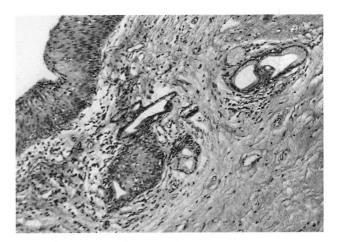

Figure 39.7   Minor vestibular glands of the vulvar vestibule. The vulvar vestibular glands are simple glands with a mucus-secreting columnar epithelial lining. Near their exit at the vestibular surface the glands have a stratified squamous epithelium. Vascular vestibular stroma surrounds the superficial gland elements.

the mucosal surface of the vestibule (Figure 39.7). They are analogous to the glands of Littré of the male urethra (39). Minor vestibular glands are small and shallow, with a maximum depth of 2.27 mm (44). These glands are lined with a mucus-secreting columnar epithelium that merges with the stratified squamous epithelium of the vestibule (44,45,46) identified minor vestibular glands within the vestibule in 47% of women studied in an autopsy-related series. We found minor vestibular glands in vulvar vestibulectomy specimens for vestibulitis in 66% of our cases (44). In the women with identifiable minor vestibular glands, Robboy et al. identified minor vestibular glands within the vestibule in 42% of women studied in an autopsy-related series (46). When present, the number ranged from 1 to over 100, with the majority having 2 to 10 identifiable minor vestibular glands. Although these glands were found to be distributed throughout the vestibule, they were found in greater numbers in the posterior vestibule,

Figure 39.5   Bartholin's duct near the gland. Bartholin's duct has a transitional-like epithelial lining, with columnar cells near the surface, similar to the columnar cells lining the gland acini.

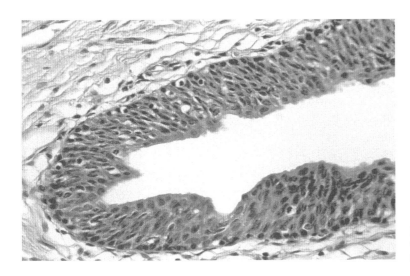

Figure 39.6   Bartholin's duct near its exit to the vulvar vestibule. At this location the duct is lined by stratified squamous epithelium, without surface columnar cells.

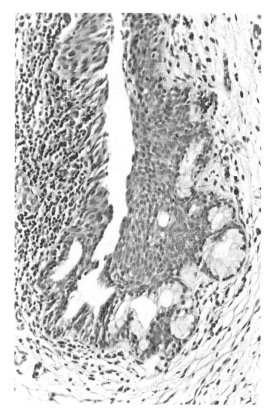

Figure 39.8 Vestibular gland with squamous metaplasia near the vestibular surface. Moderate chronic inflammation, consisting predominantly of lymphocytes, is seen adjacent to the gland and is consistent with vulvar vestibulitis.

just anterior to the fourchette. Minor vestibular glands have been described as having ducts composed of transitional epithelium; however, this epithelium is essentially the same epithelium and borders that of the adjacent vulvar vestibule, which is stratified squamous epithelium without surface umbrella cells. Minor vestibular glands may undergo squamous metaplasia, similar to that seen within the endocervix, where the mucus-secreting epithelial cells lining the glandular epithelium are replaced by stratified squamous epithelium (Figure 39.8). This metaplastic epithelium may completely replace the glandular epithelium, resulting in the formation of a vestibular cleft (44) (Figure 39.9). Obstruction of a minor vestibular gland associated with this metaplastic process may result in accumulation of mucous secretion within the simple tubular gland, leading to the formation of a vulvar mucous cyst (44,45,46). Vestibular adenomas have been described arising from these minor vestibular glands (47,48). Severe external dyspareunia, including vulvodynia, may be associated with inflammation of the vulvar vestibule, a poorly understood condition referred to as vulvar vestibulitis (1,44,49).

Urethral Orifice (Meatus Urinarius)

The urethra has a transitional epithelial lining that merges with the stratified squamous epithelium at the urethral

orifice. The periurethral glands of Huffman enter into the urethra throughout most of its length (50). Obstruction or inflammation of these periurethral glands may result in a urethral diverticulum or periurethral abscess. Partial prolapse of the urethra results in a polypoid mass, often referred to as a urethral caruncle. The mucosa may become ulcerated, and the underlying stroma may become inflamed with vascular dilation and engorgement; however, it otherwise retains the normal histology of the urethra.

Hymen

The hymen marks the distalmost extent of the vagina and the most proximal boundary of the vulvar vestibule. The hymen may be imperforate, round, annular, septate, cribriform, or porous (2). On the vaginal surface, the hymen has a nonkeratinized stratified squamous epithelium, which is glycogenated upon estrogen exposure, as seen in women of reproductive age, newborn female infants, and postmenopausal women receiving estrogen therapy. On the vulvar surface the vestibular epithelium appears similar to the vaginal epithelium in women of reproductive age (Figures 39.3, 39.10). The hymenal ring contains some Merkel tactile disks for touch and moderate numbers of free nerve endings, which are pain receptors; the hymenal ring lacks other receptors that are present in the labia majora (51,52).

In rare cases of imperforate hymen, the hymen lacks its normal opening. This leads to accumulation of menstrual exodus in the vagina, resulting in vaginal distension (1) with menstrual products, a condition referred to as hematocolpos. Coitus, or the routine use of intravaginal tampons, results in tears in the hymen, which result in small soft hymenal tags referred to as carunculae hymenales, or carunculae myrtiformes (34,53). On the external hymen and on the

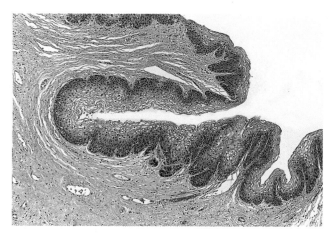

Figure 39.9 Vulvar vestibular cleft. The vulvar vestibular cleft has a stratified squamous epithelial lining, similar to the vulvar vestibule. These clefts appear to arise as a result of squamous metaplasia of vestibular glands.

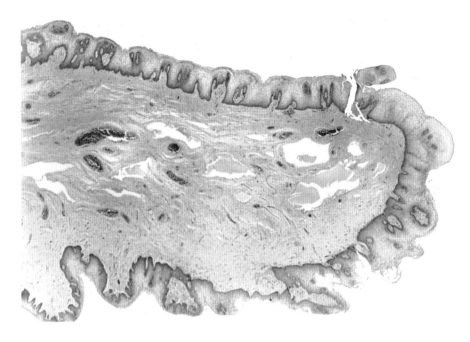

Figure 39.10 Cross section of the hymen of a 26-year-old woman. The epithelium of the vaginal (*upper*) and vestibular (*lower*) surfaces of the hymen is a stratified squamous epithelium, which is nonkeratinized and glycogen rich. The fibrovascular component of the hymen supports the epithelium.

vulvar vestibule, small papillae may be identified, which are referred to as vestibular papillae. Multiple papillae are seen in the condition known as vestibular papillomatosis (54). Such papillae within the vestibule are generally considered a variant of normal anatomy and are infrequently associated with human papillomavirus. Solitary or isolated asymptomatic papillae on the hymen usually represent a normal anatomic variant (55) (Figure 39.11).

Clitoris

The clitoris is the descendant of the embryonic phallus, homologous to the corpus cavernosum of the male penis. It is immediately anterior to the frenulum, at the junction of the labia minora, and it is enfolded by the prepuce. The clitoris measures approximately 2 cm in its long axis and consists of two crura and a glans clitoridis. The crura are composed

of erectile tissue similar to that in the corpora cavernosa of the male (3,4). They consist of cavernous veins surrounded by longitudinal smooth muscle, as well as small centrally placed muscular arteries, enveloped by the tunica albuginea. The tunica albuginea is composed of wavy collagen fibers and straight elastic fibers. Peripheral to the tunica albuginea is the loose connective tissue that supports the nerves and receptors of this area. The glans clitoridis is covered with squamous mucosa without glands, rete, or papillae (40,52,56). The cavernous tissue of the corpus spongiosum of the male does not have its counterpart in the clitoris; it is found instead in the vascular erectile tissue of the labia minora (Figure 39.12). The clitoris contains nerve endings in lesser amount than seen in the labia majora, although Pacinian corpuscles are abundant. Peritrichous nerve endings for touch reception are absent. The other receptors are present, although their distribution is highly variable (52). Other touch receptors, namely, Meissner's corpuscles and Merkel tactile disks, are present in reduced numbers in the clitoris, as compared with the labia majora or mons pubis. Pacinian corpuscles, for pressure reception, are present in large numbers (52). The free nerve endings for pain reception are found throughout the vulva and in relatively high concentrations in the clitoris, labia majora, and mons pubis (52). Ruffini's and Dogiel-Krause corpuscles, which may be associated with temperature or sexual sensation, are found throughout the vulva but not in the hymenal ring (52).

Labia Minora

The bilateral labia minora derive from the embryonic medial folds (genital folds) and lie lateral to the vulvar vestibule and medial to the labia majora, bounded by the

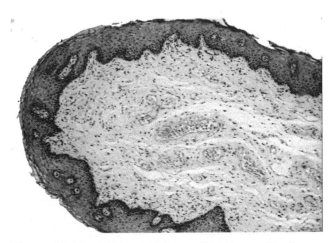

Figure 39.11 Vulvar vestibular papillae. The papillae have a stratified squamous epithelial surface and fibrovascular stalks.

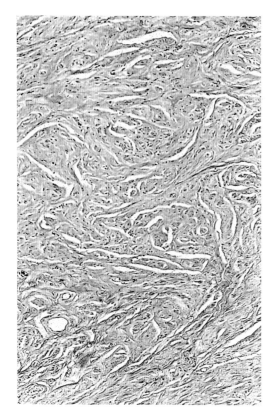

Figure 39.12 Erectile tissue of the labia minora.

intralabial sulcus. The epithelium of the labia minora is of ectodermal origin. The labia minora have their male embryologic counterpart in the penile corpus spongiosum (34). The minora measure approximately 5 cm in length and 0.5 cm in thickness; however, their length can vary considerably. The epithelium of the labia minora is of the stratified squamous type; it is not keratinized on its vestibular surface but has a thin keratin layer lateral from Hart's line.

Most of the epithelium of the labia minora does not contain skin appendages; however, in some individuals, the lateral labia minora may contain sweat and/or sebaceous glands (56). The epithelium of the labia minora may be somewhat pigmented, especially in lateral and posterior areas (Figure 39.13). Beneath the epithelium is highly vascular, loose connective tissue that is rich in elastic fibers. Posterior and deep to the labia minora are the vestibular bulbs (bulbi vestibuli), which are composed of erectile tissue and are invested by the bulbocavernous muscles. The labia minora contain erectile tissue and thus are highly vascular, yet they lack adipose tissue. The vessels and erectile tissue are supported by a rich elastic fiber component. The nerve endings within the labia majora are similar to those found within the clitoris, yet Meissner's corpuscles and Merkel tactile disks occur in larger numbers than usually identified within the clitoris (52).

Congenital enlargement of the labia minora may occur and may be asymmetrical. Enlargement also may be secondary to irritation, chronic edema or minor trauma. Surgical reduction of the labia minora or local excision for therapeutic reasons does not appear to impede normal sexual function or response; however, excision of the labia minora for female circumcision is associated with introital stenosis, vulvar keratinous cysts, and sexual and urinary dysfunction (8,57).

Labia Majora

The labia majora arise from the embryonic lateral folds (genital folds, labial folds), which arise lateral to the cloacal plate and do not fuse (39). The epithelium is ectodermally derived from the urogenital sinus. The endodermally derived epithelium of the vestibule joins with the ectodermally derived epithelium of the medial labial majora. This junction is apparently at Hart's line, where the epithelium of the medial (inner) labia majora joins the nonkeratinized squamous epithelium of the vestibule (29,30). In the male, the labial (scrotal) folds fuse to form the scrotum. This fusion usually occurs by 74 days of gestation (crown-rump length approximately 71 mm) (39). In the female, the labia

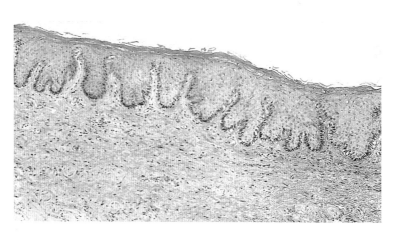

Figure 39.13 Lateral labia minora biopsy from a 27-year-old white woman. Within this area, the labia minora contain no skin appendages. The epithelium is pigmented, and melanocytes and pigmented basal epithelial cells are seen in the basal layer. The stratified squamous epithelium has a thinly keratinized surface. Beneath the epithelium, there is an elastic fiber–rich stroma without fat or skin appendages. Moderate numbers of small vessels can be seen. Deeper tissue is demonstrated in Figure 39.12.

majora merge with the mons pubis anteriorly and with the perineal body posteriorly. The labia majora lie immediately lateral and parallel to the labia minora, separated by the intralabial sulcus. In the medial posterior positions, the labia majora are bounded by the vulvar vestibule. Laterally, they merge with the inguinal-gluteal folds, which separate the labia from the medial aspect of the thighs. Although minor asymmetry of the labia majora is considered to be normal, marked asymmetry may be early evidence of neurofibromatosis (58). Chronic inflammation, varicosities, edema, Bartholin's cysts, and benign or malignant tumors also may be associated with asymmetry of the labia majora.

Aging changes related to the labia majora include an increase in size of the labia with puberty, primarily related to increased fat within the labia. In addition, there are dramatic changes in hair growth during puberty (see Mons Pubis discussion, below) (59). After menopause, there is a progressive loss of hair follicles and consequent loss of labial hair (60) as well as shrinkage of the labia majora. This is primarily related to loss of fat within the labia (34).

In addition to age-related changes, changes occur in the labia majora that are related to parity. During gestation, the influence of gestational hormones, especially progesterone, results in vascular dilation and stasis within the labia (52). These gestational changes may result in the development of vulvar venous varicosities (61).

Similar to other hair follicles, each follicle of the vulva has a hair root surrounded by the dermal root sheath, which invests the root sheath of the hair follicle. The inner root sheath is composed of an external clear epithelial cell layer (Henle's layer) and an inner granular epithelial cell layer (Huxley's layer). The hair matrix matures to the formed hair of the hair shaft, where the hair has an outer cuticle with a cortex and medulla. The hair papilla is found at the base of the hair root, protruding into and partially surrounded by the matrix of the hair. The papilla is supported by the dermal root sheath (40,56,62,63). Hair follicles are a portion of the pilosebaceous unit, which includes sebaceous glands.

In the labia majora, sebaceous glands can be found with and without associated hair follicles. The sebaceous glands are alveolar and arranged in a lobular manner, vested by collagen fibers. The cells of the sebaceous glands secrete in a holocrine manner, with the more mature cells accumulating sebaceous secretion (sebum) within their cytoplasm. The secretion is released as the cells undergo necrosis. The secretion may be released adjacent to the hair shaft in the pilosebaceous unit or directly to the surface when no hair shaft is present. There are two types of sweat gland: apocrine and merocrine (40,56,62,63). Apocrine glands are tubular and have a columnar secretory epithelium characterized by a prominent eosinophilic granular cytoplasm. These glands secrete by release of cytoplasmic secretion and are associated with scent production. The scent associated with these sudoriferous glands is related to bacterial growth supported by the secretory products (56,62). Beneath the epithelial layer, myoepithelial cells are identified. These myoepithelial cells are arranged about the periphery of the gland, and their contraction promotes expression of the secretory contents from the gland lumen. The ducts of the apocrine glands are similar to those of the merocrine glands but may secrete into the upper hair follicle rather than to the skin surface when present in hair-bearing skin.

The merocrine glands are eccrine glands that produce clear watery sweat. The secretory cells have a pale, slightly granular cytoplasm and an outer layer of myoepithelial cells. The glands are simple and coiled and are found deep to the reticular dermis. The sweat duct is lined by cuboidal epithelium two-cells thick, and the double epithelial cell layer is lost as it joins with the stratified epithelial surface. Unlike sebaceous and apocrine glands, merocrine glands are not significantly stimulated by the sex hormones. [For further discussion on the histology of the skin elements, the reader is referred to Chapter 1 in this volume and to texts on histology (40,56,62,63).]

The epithelium of the posterolateral aspects of the labia majora, peripheral to Hart's line, is thinly keratinized and pigmented (Figure 39.14). At the posterior fourchette, the

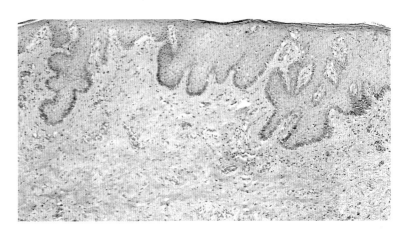

Figure 39.14 Posterior medial labia majora of a 27-year-old white woman peripheral to Hart's line. This pigmented portion of the labia majora has a stratified squamous epithelium with a thin keratinized surface. The epithelium has deeper rete ridges than seen in the minora. The dermis is elastic fiber rich and moderately vascular. Sebaceous gland–bearing skin was immediately adjacent to this area and has a moderately vascular dermis.

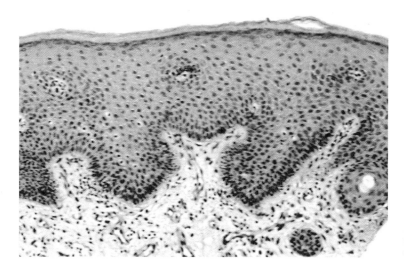

Figure 39.15 Posterior vulvar forchette. The epithelium has a thinly keratinized surface, moderately deep rete, and some melanin pigmentation within the basal cells.

retia are relatively deeper than in the posterior lateral area (Figure 39.15). Pigmented cells are seen at the basal layer in this area (Figure 39.16). A granular layer may be present immediately beneath the keratinized surface (stratum corneum). The granular layer arises from the underlying prickle cell (spinous cell) layer of the stratified squamous epithelium, with the stratum malpighii overlying the basal layer. The basal layer (stratum germinativum) is present immediately adjacent to the basement membrane (35,64). The medial hairless surfaces of the labia majora contain an abundance of sebaceous glands, which end at Hart's line. These glands are not associated with hair-bearing pilosebaceous units and open directly onto the epithelial surface, with a short nonkeratinized epithelium-lined duct joining with the keratinized epithelial surface (Figure 39.17). Sebaceous glands within the labia majora may have a depth of up to 2.03 mm (65). Keratinous (epithelial) cysts may be associated with these sebaceous gland elements (3,57). Sebaceous glands are not found medial to Hart's line (Figure 39.2). At the midportion of the labia majora, hair follicles are associated with the sebaceous gland elements. Hair follicles within the labia majora may be as deep as 2.38 mm (65) (Figures 39.18–39.19). Apocrine and eccrine sweat glands are found associated with the hair-bearing areas of the vulva but are generally absent in the vestibule and medial non–hair-bearing areas of the medial labia majora (Figure 39.20). Deeper within the dermis of the labia majora, a delicate muscle layer (tunica dartos labialis) is present. Beneath this layer is a fascial layer that has a prominent elastic fiber component (52). The fascial layer is associated with a prominent adipose layer in women of reproductive age.

Within the deep anterior labia majora, immediately adjacent to the inguinal canal, the round ligament joins with the deep longitudinal smooth muscle layer (cremaster muscle) of the labia majora (52). The round ligament

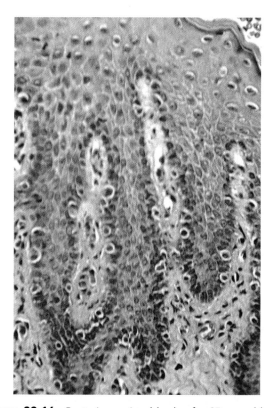

Figure 39.16 Posterior perineal body of a 27-year-old white woman. The skin at the perineal body is pigmented, and melanocytes and pigmented keratinocytes are present within the basal layer. The epithelium is stratified squamous epithelium, which has a thin keratin layer. The perinuclear halos present within the epithelial cells are normally seen and should not be confused with koilocytosis. Small clear cells are seen in the epithelial stromal junction within many of the retia.

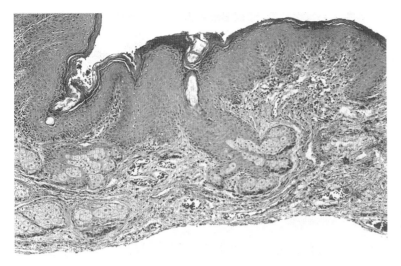

Figure 39.17 Labia majora, medial portion, with sebaceous gland elements exiting directly to the skin surface. The epithelium of the medial labia majora has a thin keratin and granular layer. The sebaceous glands may be seen clinically as Fordyce's spots.

may include entrapped peritoneum (processus vaginalis), which can become cystically dilated and result in a cyst of the canal of Nuck (3). These peritoneum-lined cysts are typically encountered in the anterior portion of the labia majora, adjacent to or within the inguinal canal.

The epithelium of the labia majora is rich in nerve endings and contains touch receptors, including Meissner's corpuscles, Merkel tactile disks, and peritrichous nerve endings (52). Pacinian corpuscles for pressure sensation are present within the fatty layer of the labia majora, as well as within the labia minora, clitoris, and mons pubis. Free nerve endings for pain reception are also present within the epithelium, as well as within muscle cells and blood vessels (51,52). Ruffini's corpuscles are seen throughout the subcutaneous tissue of the labia majora, labia minora, clitoris, and mons pubis. They are absent in the hymen. Their exact

function in the vulva is uncertain; however, they may be temperature receptors and/or receptors for sexual stimuli (52). Dogiel-Krause receptors have a distribution similar to that of Ruffini's corpuscles; however, they are present in a relatively smaller concentration in the mons pubis and labia majora (52).

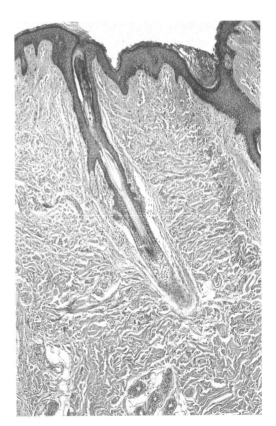

Figure 39.19 Labia majora, lateral, with hair follicle and sweat gland elements. The sweat gland duct is seen adjacent to the portion of the hair follicle.

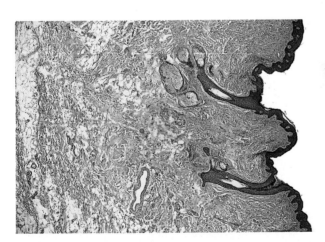

Figure 39.18 Labia majora, midportion, with underlying dermis and deep fatty tissue. The thickness of the dermis can be seen in this section of the labia majora. A few deep hair follicles can be seen within the elastic fiber–rich dermis. The dermal junction with the deep fatty tissue is irregular.

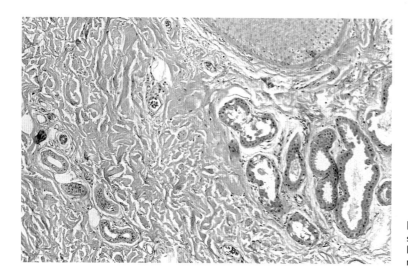

Figure 39.20 Labia majora with apocrine glands and sweat ducts adjacent to a hair follicle. Moderate vascularity of the collagen-rich dermis of the labia majora surrounds these sweat gland elements.

Medial to the labia majora, within the sulcus between the labia majora and minora (sulcus interlabialis), anogenital mammary-like glands are present that may give rise to cysts within the intralabial sulcus; they also may involve the medial aspect of the labia majora. These glands, and the cyst described, are lined with a cuboidal to columnar epithelium with an underlying myoepithelium. The myoepithelial cells are immunoreactive for smooth muscle actin and S-100 antigen, as well as low-molecular weight keratin. The superficial luminal epithelial cells are of an apocrine type, with visible "snouts" (Figure 39.21). These cells are immunoreactive for low-molecular weight keratin and human milk fat globule antigen. Individual cells are also immunoreactive for carcinoembryonic antigen and S-100 antigen. Estrogen and progesterone receptors have been detected in these cells. Mucus-containing or ciliated cells are not present, distinguishing the cysts of anogenital mammary-like glands from vestibular mucous cysts, Müllerian-related cysts or ciliated cysts, or Bartholin's gland. The lack of a stratified squamous epithelium or transitional epithelium distinguishes them from Bartholin's duct cysts, keratinous cysts, or vestibular glandular cysts that have undergone squamous metaplasia (66). There is evidence that these glands are the origin of fibroadenoma, hidradenoma papilliferum, milk cysts, and apparent ectopic breast tissue that have been described in the vulva (rather than being from true ectopic breast tissue) (67).

Mons Pubis (Mons Veneris)

The mons pubis has its origin in the embryonic genital medial cranial swellings (39). The subcutaneous tissue of mons pubis becomes more prominent with the onset of puberty, when there is a progressive increase in fat tissue beneath the mons. There is also a dramatic increase in hair growth of the mons pubis and labia majora.

Aging changes related to the mons pubis include hair growth changes that have been summarized and staged by Tanner in the following sequence (59). Stage 1 is characterized by no visible pubic hair growth. In stage 2, a small amount of pubic-type hair is seen on the midportion of the mons pubis, and some similar hair may be seen on the labia majora. In stage 3, the mons pubis hair growth is more prominent, both in the amount of hair and the coarseness of the hair. In stage 4, the hair growth over the mons pubis is similar to the adult, with the exception that the upper lateral corners of hair growth are lacking. Stage 5 characterizes the adult pubic hair pattern (59). The adult hair growth distribution is reached between the ages of 12 and 17 years (34). There can be substantial variability in the amount and character of the pubic hair (escutcheon) related to racial and genetic factors; however, pubic-type hair growth generally does not extend above a horizontal line drawn between, and 2 cm above, the uppermost limits of the genitofemoral folds (60,68). Hair follicle depth within the vulva is greatest in the mons pubis, where hair follicle depth has been measured up to 2.72 mm (65). The mons pubis is richly endowed with nerve receptor types that were previously described for the labia majora (52).

Lymphatic Drainage

The vulvar tissues drain to lymph nodes in the femoral and inguinal lymph node chains. The anterior labia minora and clitoris drain through channels anterior and superior to these structures to join lymphatics from the prepuce and labia majora. These channels course laterally to inguinal and femoral nodes (69). In some cases, lymphatic channels from a lateral site may drain to the contralateral node group, which has clinical relevance in planning therapy for malignancies of the vulva. The most common site of metastasis from vulvar malignancies are the superficial inguinal nodes. In general 8 to 10 nodes are found in this area, with superior oblique (above the ligament of Poupart) and inferior ventral (between the ligament of Poupart and the saphenous vein and fascia lata) divisions. Midline structures, such as the

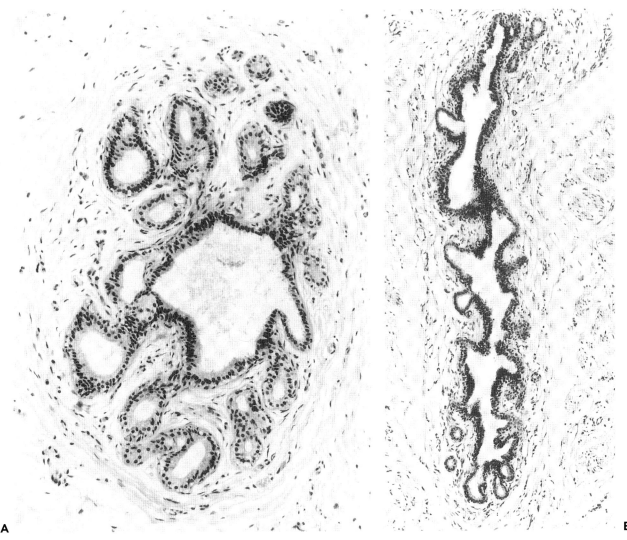

Figure 39.21 Mammary-like anogenital gland with main duct (**A** and **B**) and small acini (**A**). The epithelial lining is composed of a two-layered epithelium with underlying myoepithelial cell layer and a low columnar epithelial luminal epithelium. Reprinted with permission from: van der Putte SC. Mammary-like glands of the vulva and their disorders. *Int J Gynecol Pathol* 1994;13:150–160.

clitoris and the midline perineum, drain bilaterally. A second path of lymphatic drainage from the clitoris involves urethral lymphatics and lymphatics draining the dorsal vein of the clitoris. These channels lead inferior to the symphysis pubis through the anogenital diaphragm to join the lymphatic plexus of the anterior bladder surface. Ultimately, these channels terminate in the interiliac and obturator nodes or course superiorly to the femoral and internal iliac nodes. Deep pelvic nodes are not generally involved unless the superficial inguinal nodes are involved.

Sentinel lymph node mapping in the assessment of vulvar carcinoma and melanoma, employing intraoperative lymphoscintigraphy (technetium-99m–labelled nanocolloid) with or without blue dye (patent blue V) is gaining in application to assess inguinal lymph node status. Microscopic assessment of the lymph nodes picking up the colloid/dye is performed to plan appropriate lymph node resection related to the vulvar surgery. When nodes are found to be negative by this technique, the patient may be spared radical inguinal-femoral lymphadenectomy (18).

Obstruction of vulvar lymphatics, related surgical interruption, or inflammation (such as secondary to Crohn's disease) may result in lymphangiectasia of the vulva. This condition may present with leakage of clear fluid from the vulva, associated with multiple small, glistening, superficial clustered vesicles on the vulvar skin, resembling frog spawn. Some degree of epithelial and dermal edema is also typically present (70).

Arterial Supply

The major arterial supply of the vulva originates with the superficial and deep external pudendal arteries (branching from the femoral artery) and the internal pudendal arteries (branching from internal iliac arteries). The pudendal artery has anterior and posterior labial branches. Circulation to the clitoris is separate and emanates from the deep arteries of the clitoris. The anterior vaginal artery supplies the vestibule and Bartholin's gland areas (3).

Venous Supply

Major venous drainage of the vulva is primarily from the bilateral internal iliac veins, which drain into the external iliac venous system. The internal iliac veins drain both parietal and visceral venous systems. The parietal tributaries of the internal iliac vein include the internal obturator, internal pudendal veins, superior and inferior glutal veins, sciatic vein, and ascending lumbar veins. The visceral branches drain pelvic organs, including the uterine, ovarian, and vaginal venous systems. In a study of this drainage in 79 specimens, a single internal iliac vein was present on the side studied in 73% of the cases; in 29% of the cases, two separate iliac veins drained into the external iliac vein; and, in one case, the internal iliac vein drained directly to the inferior vena cava (71). Vulvar varices are identified in approximately 2% of women seeking care in a vein clinic; such varices correlate with insufficiency of the internal iliac venous system and also involve the tributaries of the internal iliac vein as well as the saphenous vein (71).

Nerve Supply

The major nerves of the vulva are from the anterior and posterior labial nerves. The anterior nerve is a branch of the ilioinguinal nerve, and the posterior labial branch is from the pudendal nerve. The clitoral nerve supply is from the dorsal nerve of the clitoris and the cavernous nerves of the clitoris. Branches of the cavernous nerves, arising from the vaginal nerve plexus, join the clitoral dorsal nerve at the hilum of the clitoral bodies. The dorsal nerve of the clitoral bundle branches from the pudendal nerve. The two clitoral bodies, beneath the pubic arch, separate to form the two clitoral crura. Immunohistochemical studies have demonstrated that the dorsal nerves form two bundles that are extensively distributed along the lateral aspects of the clitoral bodies at the eleven and one o'clock positions but are sparse at the twelve o'clock position. These join distally to form a single clitoral body. The densest nerve groups that enter the glans clitoris are found on the dorsal aspect of the clitoris, with a concentration of nerves under the epithelium of the glans clitoris (72). The vestibule shares the clitoral nerve supply (3,52).

REFERENCES

1. Haefner HK, Collins ME, Davis GD, et al. The vulvodynia guideline. *J Lower Genital Tract Disease* 2005;9:40–51.

2. Kaufman RH, Friedrich EG, Gardner HL. *Benign Diseases of the Vulva and Vagina*. 3rd ed. Chicago: Year Book Medical; 1989.

3. Wilkinson EJ, Xie DL. Benign diseases of the vulva. In: Kurman RJ, ed. *Blaustein's Pathology of the Female Genital Tract*. 5th ed. New York: Springer-Verlag; 2002:37–98.

4. Ridley CM. General dermatological conditions and dermatoses of the vulva. In: Ridley CM. *The Vulva*. New York, Churchill Livingstone; 1998:138–211.

5. Spiryda LB, Laufer MR, Soiffer RJ, Antin JA. Graft-versus-host disease of the vulva and/or vagina: diagnosis and treatment. *Biol Blood Marrow Transplant* 2003;9:760–765.

6. Farage MA, Bjerke DL, Mahony C, Blackburn KL, Gerberick GF. Quantitative risk assessment for the induction of allergic contact dermatitis: uncertainty factors for mucosal exposures. *Contact Dermatitis* 2003;49:140–147.

7. Nardelli A, Degreef H, Goossens A. Contact allergic reactions of the vulva: a 14-year review. *Dermatitis* 2004;15:131–136.

8. Thabet SM, Thabet AS. Defective sexuality and female circumcision: the cause and the possible management. *J Obstet Gynaecol Res* 2003;29:12–19.

9. Janaki VR, Premalatha S, Rao N, Thambiah AS. Lawrence-Seip syndrome. *Br J Dermatol* 1980;103:693–696.

10. Seely JR, Seely BL, Bley R Jr, Altmiller CJ. Localized chromosomal mosaicism as a cause of dysmorphic development. *Am J Hum Genet* 1984;36:899–903.

11. Hanna SJ, Kaiser L, Muneer A, Nottingham JF, Kunkler RB. Squamous cell carcinoma of the bladder presenting as vulvitis and cliteromegaly. *Gynecol Oncol* 2004;95:722–723.

12. Creighton SM, Minto CL, Steele SJ. Objective cosmetic and anatomical outcomes at adolescence of feminising surgery for ambiguous genitalia done in childhood. *Lancet* 2001;358: 124–125.

13. Baskin LS. Anatomical studies of the female genitalia: surgical reconstructive implications. *J Pediatr Endocrinol Metab* 2004;17: 581–587.

14. Lee PA, Witchel SF. Genital surgery among females with congenital adrenal hyperplasia: changes over the past five decades. *J Pediatr Endocrinol Metab* 2002;15:1473–1477.

15. Crouch NS, Minto CL, Laio LM, Woodhouse CR, Creighton SM. Genital sensation after feminizing genitoplasty for congenital adrenal hyperplasia: a pilot study. *BJU Int* 2004;93:135–138.

16. Minto CL, Liao LM, Woodhouse CR, Ransley PG, Creighton SM. The effect of clitoral surgery on sexual outcome in individuals who have intersex conditions with ambiguous genitalia: a cross-sectional study. *Lancet* 2003;361:1252–1257.

17. Chan JK, Sugiyama V, Tajalli TR, et al. Conservative clitoral preservation surgery in the treatment of vulvar squamous cell carcinoma. *Gynecol Oncol* 2004;95:152–156.

18. Hakam A, Nasir A, Raghuwanshi R, et al. Value of multilevel sectioning for improved detection of micrometastases in sentined lymph nodes in invasive squamous cell carcinoma of the vulva. *Anticancer Res* 2004;24:1281–1286.

19. Moore RG, Granai CO, Gajewski W, Gordinier M, Steinhoff MM. Pathologic evaluation of inguinal sentinel lymph nodes in vulvar cancer patients: a comparison of immunohistochemical staining versus ultrastaging with hematoxylin and eosin staining. *Gynecol Oncol* 2003;91:378–382.

20. Moore RG, DePasquale SE, Steinhoff MM, et al. Sentinel node identification and the ability to detect metastatic tumor to inguinal lymph nodes in squamous cell cancer of the vulva. *Gynecol Oncol* 2003;89:475–479.

21. Yu BK, Lai CR, Yen MS, Tou NF, Chao KC, Yuan CC. Extramammary Paget's disease found by abnormal vulvar brush sampling. *Eur J Gynaecol Oncol* 2002;23:35–36.

22. Brown HM, Wilkinson EJ. Cytology of secondary vulvar Paget's disease of urothelial origin: a case report. *Acta Cytol* 2005;49: 71–74.

23. Wilkinson EJ, Stone IK. *Atlas of Vulvar Disease*. Baltimore: Williams & Wilkins; 1995.

24. Mancino P, Parlavecchio E, Melluso J, Monti M, Russo P. Introducing colposcopy and vulvovaginoscopy as routine examinations for victims of sexual assault. *Clin Exp Obstet Gynecol* 2003;30: 40–42.

25. Bechara A, Bertolino MV, Casabe A, et al. Duplex Doppler ultrasound assessment of clitoral hemodynamics after topical administration of alprostadil in women with arousal and orgasmic disorders. *J Sex Marital Ther* 2003;29(suppl 1):1–10.

26. Suh DD, Yang CC, Cao Y, Garland PA, Maravilla KR. Magnetic resonance imaging anatomy of the female genitalia in premenopausal and postmenopausal women. *J Urol* 2003;170:138–144.

27. Deliganis AV, Maravilla KR, Heiman JR, et al. Female genitalia: dynamic MR imaging with use of MS-325 initial experiences evaluating female sexual response. *Radiology* 2002;225:791–799.

28. Maravilla KR, Cao Y, Heiman JR, et al. Noncontrast dynamic magnetic resonance imaging for quantitative assessment of female sexual arousal. *J Urol* 2005;173:162–166.

29. Hart DB. *Selected Papers in Gynaecology and Obstetrics.* Edinburgh, Scotland: W&AK Johnston; 1893.

30. Dickinson RL. *Human Sex Anatomy.* 2nd ed. Baltimore: Williams & Wilkins; 1949.

31. Benedet JL, Wilson PS, Matisic J. Epidermal thickness and skin appendage involvement in vulvar intraepithelial neoplasia. *J Reprod Med* 1991;366:608–612.

32. Hu F. Melanocyte cytology in normal skin. In: Ackerman AB, ed. *Masson Monographs in Dermatology-1.* New York: Masson; 1981.

33. Edwards JN, Morris HB. Langerhans' cells and lymphocyte subsets in the female genital tract. *Br J Obstet Gynaecol* 1985;92:974–982.

34. McLean JM. Anatomy and physiology of the vulva. In: Ridley CM, ed. *The Vulva.* New York: Churchill Livingstone; 1988:39–65.

35. MacKie RM. *Milne's Dermatopathology.* 2nd ed. London: Hodder Arnold; 1984.

36. Goldstein AT, Marinoff SC, Christopher K. Pimecrolimus for the treatment of vulvar lichen sclerosus: a report of 4 cases. *J Reprod Med* 2004;49:778–780.

37. Gould VE, Moll R, Moll I, Lee I, Franke WW. Biology of disease. Neuroendocrine (Merkel) cells of the skin: hyperplasias, dysplasias, and neoplasms. *Lab Invest* 1985;52:334–352.

38. Bottles K, Lacey CG, Goldberg J, Lanner-Cusin K, Hom J, Miller TR. Merkel cell carcinoma of the vulva. *Obstet Gynecol* 1984;63:S61–S65.

39. Robboy SJ, Bently RC, Russell P. Embryology of the female genital tract and disorders of abnormal sexual development. In: Kurman RJ, ed. *Blaustein's Pathology of the Female Genital Tract.* 5th ed. New York: Springer-Verlag; 2002:3–26.

40. Bloom W, Fawcett DW. *A Textbook of Histology.* 10th ed. Philadelphia: WB Saunders; 1975:904–905.

41. Rorat E, Ferenczy A, Richart RM. Human bartholin gland, duct, and duct cyst. Histochemical and ultrastructural study. *Arch Pathol* 1975;99:367–374.

42. Fetissof F, Berger G, Dubois MP, et al. Endocrine cells in the female genital tract. *Histopathology* 1985;9:133–145.

43. Word B. Office treatment of cyst and abscess of Bartholin's gland duct. *South Med J* 1968;61:514–518.

44. Pyka RE, Wilkinson EJ, Friedrich EG Jr, Croker BP. The histology of vulvar vestibulitis syndrome. *Int J Gynecol Oncol* 1988;7:249–257.

45. Friedrich EG Jr, Wilkinson EJ. Mucous cysts of the vulvar vestibule. *Obstet Gynecol* 1973;42:407–414.

46. Robboy SJ, Ross JS, Prat J, Keh PC, Welch WR. Urogenital sinus origin of mucinous and ciliated cysts of the vulva. *Obstet Gynecol* 1978;51:347–351.

47. Fowler WC Jr, Lawrence H, Edelman DA. Paravestibular tumor of the female genital tract. *Am J Obstet Gynecol* 1981;139:109–111.

48. Axe S, Parmley T, Woodruff JD, Hlopak B. Adenomas in minor vestibular glands. *Obstet Gynecol* 1986;68:16–18.

49. Friedrich EG Jr. Vulvar vestibulitis syndrome. *J Reprod Med* 1987;32:110–114.

50. Huffman JW. The detailed anatomy of the paraurethral ducts in the adult human female. *Am J Obstet Gynecol* 1948;55:86–101.

51. Krantz KE. Innervation of the human vulva and vagina: a microscopic study. *Obstet Gynecol* 1958;12:382–396.

52. Krantz KE. The anatomy and physiology of the vulva and vagina and the anatomy of the urethra and bladder. In: Philipp EE, Barnes J, Newton M, eds. *Scientific Foundations of Obstetrics and Gynaecology.* Chicago: Year Book; 1977:65–78.

53. Novak ER, Woodruff JD. Novak's *Gynecologic and Obstetric Pathology.* 7th ed. Philadelphia: WB Saunders; 1974.

54. Growdon WA, Fu YS, Lebherz TB, Rapkin A, Mason GD, Parks G. Pruritic vulvar squamous papillomatosis: evidence for human papillomavirus etiology. *Obstet Gynecol* 1985;66:564–568.

55. Bergeron C, Ferenczy A, Richart RM, Guralnick M. Micropapillomatosis labialis appears unrelated to human papillomavirus. *Obstet Gynecol* 1990;76:281–286.

56. Amenta PS. *Elias-Pauly's Histology and Human Microanatomy.* 5th ed. New York: John Wiley & Sons; 1987:502–503.

57. Junaid TA, Thomas SM. Cysts of the vulva and vagina: a comparative study. *Int J Gynaecol Obstet* 1981;19:239–243.

58. Friedrich EG Jr, Wilkinson EJ. Vulvar surgery for neurofibromatosis. *Obstet Gynecol* 1985;65:135–138.

59. Tanner JM. *Growth at Adolescence.* 2nd ed. Oxford: Blackwell; 1962.

60. Barman JM, Astore J, Pecoraro V. The normal trichogram of people over 50 years. In: Montagna W, Dobson RL, eds. *Advances in Biology of Skin. Vol. IX. Hair Growth.* Oxford, England: Pergamon Press; 1969.

61. Gallagher PG. Varicose veins of the vulva. *Br J Sex Med* 1986;13:12–14.

62. Geneser F. *Textbook of Histology.* Philadelphia: Munksgaard/Lea & Febiger; 1986:616–617.

63. Leeson CR, Leeson TS, Paparo AA. *Textbook of Histology.* 5th ed. Philadelphia: WB Saunders; 1985:485–486.

64. Zelickson AS. *Electron Microscopy of Skin and Mucous Membranes.* Springfield, IL: Charles C Thomas; 1963.

65. Shatz P, Bergeron C, Wilkinson EJ, Arseneau J, Ferenczy A. Vulvar intraepithelial neoplasia and skin appendage involvement. *Obstet Gynecol* 1989;74:769–774.

66. van der Putte SC, van Gorp LH. Cysts of mammary-like glands in the vulva. *Int J Gynecol Pathol* 1995;14:184–188.

67. van der Putte SC. Mammary-like glands of the vulva and their disorders. *Int J Gynecol Pathol* 1994;13:150–160.

68. Lunde O. A study of body hair density and distribution in normal women. *Am J Phys Anthropol* 1984;64:179–184.

69. Parry-Jones E. Lymphatics of the vulva. *J Obstet Gynaecol Br Commonw* 1963;70:751–765.

70. Handfield-Jones SE, Prendiville WJ, Norman S. Vulval lymphangiectasia. *Genitourin Med* 1989;65:335–337.

71. LaPage PA, Villavicencio JL, Gomez ER, Sheridan MN, Rich NM. The valvular anatomy of the iliac venous system and its clinical implications. *J Vasc Surg* 1991;14:678–683.

72. Yucel S, De Souza A Jr, Baskin LS. Neuroanatomy of the human female lower urogenital tract. *J Urol* 2004;172:191–195.

Vagina

Stanley J. Robboy   Rex C. Bentley

INTRODUCTION

Tissue from the vagina is infrequently examined via biopsy. Excluding the vaginal cuff removed for cervical disease, most biopsies and surgical operations are for infection, small intramural growths, intrauterine exposure to diethylstilbestrol (DES), or, in older women, squamous cell cancer and its precursors. This chapter addresses the gross, microscopic, and ultrastructural anatomy of the normal vagina. The embryologic discussion focuses on developmental perturbations, which provide insights into normal and microscopic anatomy.

EMBRYOLOGIC CHANGES

The paired müllerian (paramesonephric) ducts appear about the thirty-seventh day postconception as funnel-shaped openings of celomic epithelium (1,2). These develop into paired, undifferentiated tubes that later grow caudally, using the already formed wolffian (mesonephric) ducts as a guidewire to reach the level of the future hymen (Figure 40.1). The absence of this occurrence, the incidence of which is about 1 in 5,000 newborn girls, results in the Mayer-Rokitansky-Kuster-Hauser syndrome (absence of the vagina and cervix with usually only the remnants of the uterine horns) or complete absence of the müllerian derivatives [vagina, uterus, and fallopian tubes] (3).

At about day 54, the paired müllerian ducts fuse, becoming a straight uterovaginal canal (primordia of uterine corpus, cervix, and vagina), the lining of which is an immature columnar (Müllerian) epithelium (Figure 40.2) (4). The above changes occur in both female and male embryos. If the fetus is a male, the indifferent gonads become anatomically distinct testes at around day 44. The testis is important for two products it makes. One, müllerian-inhibiting substance (MIS), affects the future of the müllerian ducts. The other, testosterone, affects the future of the wolffian ducts. Shortly after the testes become distinct, Sertoli cells initiate MIS production, a protein in the large transforming growth factor-β family, in amounts effective to cause the müllerian ducts to regress through a process of programmed cell death (5,6). If the embryo is female, testes do not develop. Because there is then no MIS, the müllerian ducts are not inhibited from developing and thus grow without impedance to become the uterine tubes, uterus, and vagina.

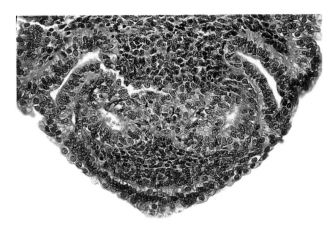

Figure 40.1 Region of urogenital sinus disclosing the tips of two central müllerian ducts that have grown down the (outer) paired wolffian ducts (circa day 54). The cytologic features of the cells comprising both types of duct are indistinguishable on light microscopy at early stages of development. Reprinted with permission from: Robboy SJ, Ellington KS. *Pathology of the Female Genital Tract in Kodachrome Slides.* 2nd ed. Durham, NC: Gyn-Path Associates; 1996.

In contradistinction to MIS, which acts as an inhibitor, testosterone stimulates and is required to promote wolffian duct growth. In the male, the critical period for testosterone stimulation begins early in the tenth week (circa day 71) and causes the embryonic wolffian ducts to differentiate into epididymis, seminal vesicle, and ductus (vas) deferens. If there are no testes (as in the female) and testosterone stimulation has not occurred by the close of the critical window (circa day 84), the wolffian ducts wither and become vestigial remnants, which in the adult are found deep in the vaginal wall.

Until near the end of week 10 (to about day 66) the uterovaginal canal, with its solid tip already in contact with the urogenital sinus, continues to elongate caudally, still remaining as a simple tube lined by columnar epithelium (Figure 40.2). Beginning in the eleventh week, the epithelium stratifies, becoming several layers thick. Under one theory, the squamous cells are believed to derive from the urogenital sinus, invading the common tube from below and growing up the muscular scaffold to completely replace the müllerian epithelium to the level of the external cervical os (7). The transition from müllerian to squamous epithelium occurs at about the time when nuclear estrogen receptors appear in the vaginal stroma (8,9).

Stratification of the squamous epithelium lining the uterovaginal canal heralds formation of the so-called vaginal plate (circa the eleventh week). The proliferation progressively occludes the canal beginning caudally and extending cranially. Studies with latex-injected specimens indicate that even the lateral wings of the vaginal plate may become occluded, but a central lumen persists, especially in the upper vagina.

During the thirteenth week (91 days), cervical glands develop; they exhibit a wavy architectural appearance but cytologically are minimally differentiated. By the fourteenth week, the caudal vagina increases markedly in size (Figure 40.3). During the fifteenth week, the solid epithelial anlage of the anterior and posterior vaginal fornices appear. Starting with the sixteenth week, the squamous epithelium lining the vagina and the exocervix begins to mature, thus resembling the lining of the adult vagina. The epithelium thickens and glycogenates, features most likely related to increased maternal and hence fetal estrogen levels. As the cells mature, they lose cellular adhesiveness and desquamate, heralding the canalization of the vaginal plate and thus the onset of the final gross adult structure of the vagina. By the eighteenth to twentieth week, the development of the vagina is complete.

Why columnar epithelium with an embryonic appearance should initially line the müllerian system and later be replaced by squamous epithelium remains of teleologic interest. The answer to the mechanism may lie in the vaginal wall stroma. Prior work in the mouse has shown that differentiation of the lower genital tract epithelium is dependent on the stroma on which it grows (10). For example, uterine epithelium, when grown intermingled with neonatal vaginal stroma, develops histotypic features of vagina. In contrast, vaginal epithelium, if grown with

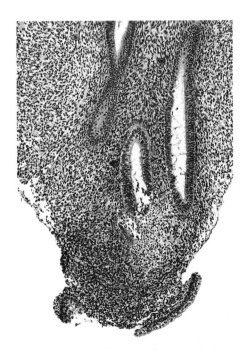

Figure 40.2 Single müllerian tube flanked by two wolffian ducts (circa day 67). The cytologic features of the cells comprising both types of duct are indistinguishable on light microscopy at early stages of development. Reprinted with permission from: Robboy SJ, Ellington KS. *Pathology of the Female Genital Tract in Kodachrome Slides.* 2nd ed. Durham, NC: Gyn-Path Associates; 1996.

neonatal uterine stroma, develops a uterine phenotype. The final epithelium has cytosolic proteins characteristic of the induced rather than original epithelial source.

Additional evidence that the vaginal stroma plays a key role in epithelial differences comes from embryologic appearance of estrogen receptors. Among various body organs tested, the receptors are detected only in the genital tract. They appear in the mesenchyme at the tenth week, just before the müllerian epithelium is normally replaced by squamous epithelium of sinus origin (8). Epithelial labeling appears later (sixteenth week), at the time when the sinus (squamous) epithelium begins to mature and accumulate large quantities of glycogen. Interestingly, the stroma probably plays a key role in the action of MIS as well; the receptor for MIS is located in the stroma surrounding the müllerian duct rather than in the müllerian epithelium (11).

The developmental morphology of the vaginal mucosa and the inductive properties of the stroma supporting the vaginal mucosa are complex. For example, a hitherto unrecognized band of subepithelial stroma was described in 1973 that extended from the endocervix to the vulva (Figure 40.4) (12). It is 0.5 to 5 mm thick in mature females and most prominent in the endocervix. It is from this zone that fibroepithelial polyps seem to arise, an entity of no apparent physiologic function but which clinically should not be confused with malignant tumor (13,14).

Should the squamous epithelium described above fail during the critical weeks of embryonic life to replace the

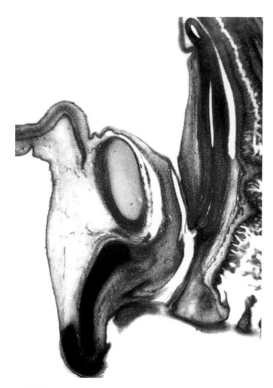

Figure 40.3 Sagittal section of pelvis at 16 weeks, showing vagina, bladder, urethra, and urogenital sinus. The lower genital tract is a straight longitudinal tube; and, at this stage, the vagina and cervix cannot be distinguished. Reprinted with permission from: Robboy SJ, Ellington KS. *Pathology of the Female Genital Tract in Kodachrome Slides.* 2nd ed. Durham, NC: Gyn-Path Associates; 1996.

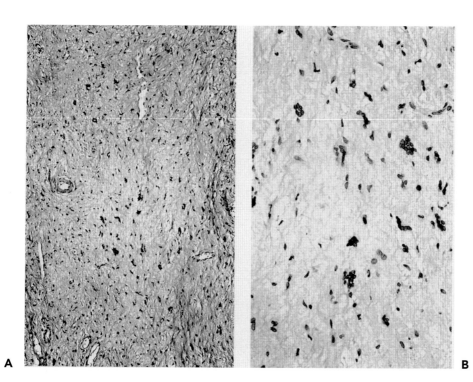

Figure 40.4 Bandlike area composed of loose connective tissue and multinucleated cells running the length of the vagina. **A.** Low-power view. **B.** High-power view. Reprinted with permission from: Fu YS. *Pathology of the Uterine Cervix, Vagina and Vulva.* 2nd ed. Philadelphia: WB Saunders; 2002.

A

B

original columnar cells lining the vagina, the columnar cells remain in an arrested state of development until sometime around puberty, when they may further differentiate into the adult-type epithelium usually seen in biopsy material. It is conjectured that the tuboendometrial type of epithelium is the basic form of epithelium supported by the vaginal mesenchyme. In fact, it may be that this type of epithelium is the basic type of müllerian epithelium supported throughout the female genital tract, manifesting as serous cells in the uterine tube, endometrioid cells in the uterine corpus, and tuboendometrial cells in the vagina—cells that are quite similar. In the cervix, a tuboendometrial layer of epithelium also lies deep to and as a cuff about the luminal layer of mucinous epithelium (15); the tuboendometrial layer, which is continuous with the lining of the corpus, is readily observed in hysterectomy specimens but is located too deep to be detected on biopsy. In fetuses where the vaginal lining has become squamous (older than 10 weeks), the inner stromal zone is obvious in the uterine tube, endometrium, and endocervix and tapers, appearing to end at the squamocolumnar junction of the cervix and vagina. Part of this layer may correspond to the most superficial stromal layer in the adult vagina described above. The original tuboendometrial layer is the origin of glandular remnants in the vagina of adults (adenosis).

GROSS FEATURES

The vagina (from the Latin for sheath) extends from the vestibule of the vulva to the uterus, lying posterior (dorsal) to the urinary bladder and anterior (ventral) to the rectum. It's axis averages 30 degrees with the vertical, arching slightly posteriocranially, and more than 90 degrees with the uterus (Figure 40.5). The anterior wall averages 8 cm in length and the posterior wall 11 cm, with the cervix filling the 3 cm difference. In early life, the vagina is constricted distally, dilated in the middle, and narrowed proximally. It surrounds the exocervix and forms vaultlike fornices between its cervical attachment and the lateral wall. In the adult, the anterior and posterior walls are slack and remain in contact with each other, whereas the lateral walls remain fairly rigid and separated. This is thought to give an H-shaped appearance to the vaginal canal on cross section (16), although with three-dimensional imaging with magnetic resonance imaging (MRI), a "W" shape is now also recognized (1). During intercourse, the position of the uterus and bladder change relative to the vagina (17).

Posteriorly, the upper one-fourth of the vagina is related to the rectouterine space (i.e., the cul-de-sac or pouch of Douglas), which is covered with peritoneum. The middle half of the vagina is closely apposed to the rectum, separated only by fibrofatty adventitia and the rectovaginal septum. The lower one-fourth of the vagina is separated from the anal canal by anal and rectal sphincters, as well as the interposing perineal body, which contains the origin of the bulbocavernous and superficial transverse perineal muscles.

The urinary bladder and urethra lie anterior to the vagina. The urethra courses approximately one-third of its length on the vagina and then enters into the vaginal wall to become an inseparable part of it, usually terminating with its external meatus at the introitus. Typically, the meatus is outwardly directed, but not uncommonly it is directed into the outermost vagina. The ureters course along both sides of the upper one-third of the vagina until entering the bladder wall.

The vagina opens into the vestibule formed from the urogenital sinus. The vestibule lies beneath the urethra and between the inner margins of the labia minora. The vagina, urethra, and ducts of Bartholin's glands open into the vestibule. The size and shape of the vaginal orifice are related to the state of the hymen. When the inner edges of

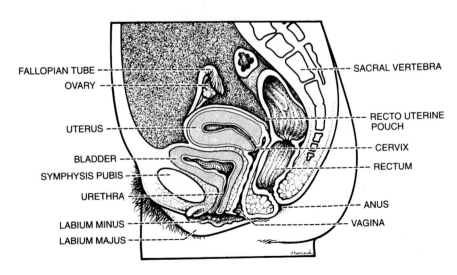

FALLOPIAN TUBE
OVARY
UTERUS
BLADDER
SYMPHYSIS PUBIS
URETHRA
LABIUM MINUS
LABIUM MAJUS

SACRAL VERTEBRA
RECTO UTERINE POUCH
CERVIX
RECTUM
ANUS
VAGINA

Figure 40.5 Structural relationships of the vagina. Its axis forms an angle of more than 90 degrees with the uterus. Reprinted with permission from: Zaino R, Robboy SJ, Kurman RJ. Diseases of the vagina. In: Kurman RJ, ed. *Blaustein's Pathology of the Female Genital Tract*. New York: Springer-Verlag; 2002:151–206.

the hymen are apposed, the vaginal opening resembles a cleft. When stretched, the hymen may persist in the form of a ringlike structure about the readily recognized vaginal orifice. (See Chapter 39 for the anatomy of the hymenal region.)

ANATOMY

Ligaments

The vaginal supports are intimately related to the uterus, urethra, bladder, and rectum (18). The lateral supports are called cardinal ligaments, the posterior supports sacrouterine ligaments. They originate where the isthmus of the uterine cervix and the uterine corpus meet and course outward, fanlike to the lateral and posterior pelvic walls. The isthmic fibers turn upward onto the uterus and downward onto the vagina. These ligaments, the connective tissues surrounding the vessels on the lateral vaginal walls, and the close proximity of the rectum, bladder, and urethra all contribute to support the vagina within the pelvis.

Blood Supply

The blood supply to the vagina is complex, with extensive anastomoses maintaining an adequate blood supply to all areas of the vagina in the event that injury restricts any single route of supply. The internal iliac (hypogastric) artery is the principal source of blood cranially as branches of the uterine arteries and caudally as branches of the middle hemorrhoidal arteries and pudendal arteries. Beginning cranially, the uterine artery gives off a descending branch, the cervicovaginal artery. Several branches supply the cervix. Lower branches supply the vagina. The vaginal arteries, which lie lateral to the vagina, send branches to both the anterior and posterior surfaces. The lower vagina receives its supply from ascending branches of the middle hemorrhoidal arteries and pudendal arteries, which also divide to send rami to the anterior and posterior vaginal walls. In toto, the extensive rami form a plexus around the vagina from which arise the median arteries, the azygos vaginal arteries on the anterior and posterior walls. A rich venous plexus also surrounds the vagina and communicates with the vesicle, pudendal, and hemorrhoidal venous plexuses, which empty into the internal iliac veins.

Nerves

The autonomic system of the pelvis originates in the superior hypogastric plexus. The middle hypogastric plexus, which passes into the pelvis, divides at the level of the S1 (sacral) vertebra into branches that pass to both sides of

the pelvis and initiate the inferior hypogastric plexus. The inferior hypogastric plexus, a divided continuation of the middle hypogastric plexus, the superior hypogastric plexus, and the presacral nerve, descends into the pelvis in a position posterior to the common iliac artery and anterior to the sacral plexus; it curves laterally and finally enters the sacrouterine ligament. The medial segment of the primary division of the sacral nerves (S2–S5), as it sends fibers into the pelvic plexus located within the sacrouterine folds, appears to contain both sympathetic (inferior hypogastric plexus) and parasympathetic (nervi erigentes) components. An extension of this plexus, located in the base of the broad ligament and supplied by the middle vesical artery, contains many ganglia. Most nerves enter the uterus near the isthmus. A lesser number descend along the lateral vagina, a pattern similar to the arteries that supply the vagina.

Lymphatic Drainage

The vaginal lymphatic system, despite the simplified view given here, is highly variable (Figure 40.6) (19). The lymphatics begin as a delicate plexus of small channels involving the entire mucosa and lamina propria and then drain into a deep muscular network. They terminate in a perivaginal plexus from which arise collecting trunks, which themselves coalesce into several larger channels.

The lymph drainage follows patterns that reflect functionally diverse geographic regions. The lymphatics of the upper anterior wall join those of the cervix, where they follow the cervical vessels to the uterine artery and accompany it to terminate in the medial chain of the external iliac

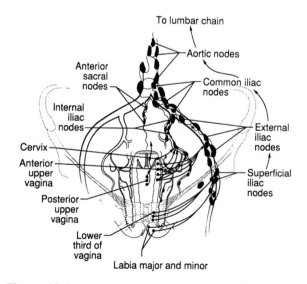

Figure 40.6 Lymphatic drainage of the vagina. Reprinted with permission from: Moore TR, Reiter RC, Rebar RW, Baker VV, eds. *Gynecology and Obstetrics: A Longitudinal Approach.* New York: Churchill Livingstone; 1993.

nodes. The lymph from the posterior vagina drains into deep pelvic, rectal, and aortic nodes. The lymphatics of the lower vagina, which also include the hymenal region, follow two distinct courses. One passes to the interiliac nodes in company with the upper vaginal discharge. The other traverses the paravesical space, carrying lymph to the deepest portions of the pelvis and draining into the inferior gluteal nodes near the origin of the vaginal or internal pudendal artery. The channels that anastomose with those of the vulva drain to the superficial iliac nodes. In summary, as a practical matter, one can generalize that tumors in the upper vagina will spread like cervical carcinoma to involve obturator and both internal and external iliac nodes. In contrast, tumors in the lower vagina will tend to involve superficial iliac (inguinal) and deep pelvic nodes, similar to vulvar cancer.

LIGHT MICROSCOPY

Epithelium

The vaginal wall consists of three principal layers: mucosa (epithelial and submucosal stroma), muscle, and adventitia. The epithelium is about 0.4 mm thick and, on gross examination, exhibits a characteristic pattern of folds or rugae separated by furrows of variable depth. There are two longitudinal (anterior and posterior) and multiple transverse furrows. The rugal pattern of the vaginal mucosa, which contributes to the organ's elasticity, produces an undulating appearance on microscopic examination in contrast to the flat surface of the cervix. The rugae, which are more prominent in nulliparous than multiparous women, reinforce the gripping effect of the levator ani and vaginal constrictor muscles during intercourse. Nonkeratinized glycogenated squamous epithelium lines the luminal surface in a manner similar to cervical epithelium. The normal vaginal mucosa lacks glands. Its surface is lubricated both by fluids that pass directly through the mucosa and by cervical mucus.

The mature, stratified squamous epithelium can be subdivided into several layers, typical of squamous epithelia elsewhere in the body (Figure 40.7). From the base to the surface, they are the deep, intermediate, and superficial zones. The deep zone contains the basal cell layer and, above this, the parabasal layer. Both are the active proliferative compartments or germinal beds, as shown by the Ki-67 antigen, which is demonstrable during late G1, G2, and M phases of the cell cycle (Figure 40.8). The basal cell layer consists of a single layer of columnar-like cells, approximately 10 μm thick, the long axis of which is vertically arranged. The cells have a basophilic cytoplasm and relatively large oval nuclei. Mitoses may be present. Occasional melanocytes also are found.

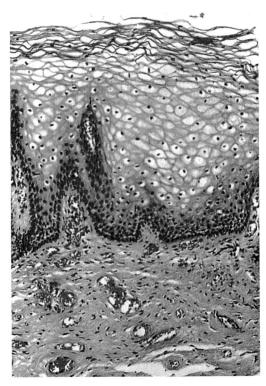

Figure 40.7 Mucosa of the adult vagina. Mature cells with glycogenic cytoplasm and pyknotic nuclei occupy most of the epithelial thickness. There is a single layer of dark basal cells and three to four layers of intermediate cells. Reprinted with permission from: Robboy SJ, Ellington KS. *Pathology of the Female Genital Tract in Kodachrome Slides.* 2nd ed. Durham, NC: Gyn-Path Associates; 1996.

The parabasal layer is poorly demarcated from the overlying cell layers. It consists usually of about two layers of small polygonal cells, having a total 14 μm thickness, often with intercellular bridges. The cells have basophilic cytoplasm, a relatively large, centrally placed, round nucleus, and occasional mitoses.

The intermediate cell layer is of variable thickness. The cells have prominent intercellular bridges, a naviculate configuration, and a long cell axis paralleling the surface. The cytoplasm is basophilic, although some glycogen may be present. The nuclei are round, oval, or irregular, with finely granular chromatin. This layer of cells has about 10 rows of cells of about 100 μm thickness.

The superficial layer is also of variable thickness. The cells are polygonal when viewed from above and flattened when viewed in cross section. The cytoplasm is acidophilic, and the nuclei are centrally located, small, round, and pyknotic. Keratohyalin granules are sometimes seen in the cytoplasm. This layer also contains about 10 rows of squamous cells.

Relatively little is known about the normal components of the epithelium itself. The submucosa contains a variety of mononuclear cells demonstrable by immunocytochemical

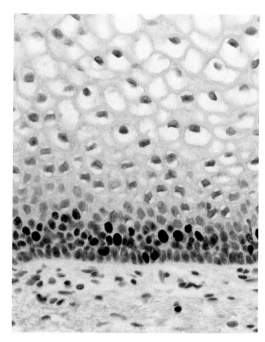

Figure 40.8 Ki-67 antigen, demonstrable during late G1, G2, and M phases of the cell cycle, in the basal and parabasal layers of the normal vaginal mucosa. Reprinted with permission from: Robboy SJ, Ellington KS. *Pathology of the Female Genital Tract in Kodachrome Slides.* 2nd ed. Durham, NC: Gyn-Path Associates; 1996.

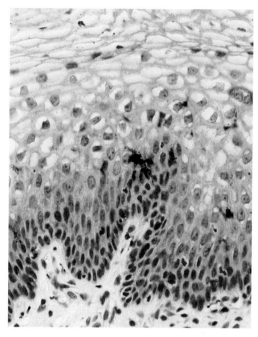

Figure 40.9 The dendritic processes of Langerhans cells. Reprinted with permission from: Robboy SJ, Ellington KS. *Pathology of the Female Genital Tract in Kodachrome Slides.* 2nd ed. Durham, NC: Gyn-Path Associates; 1996.

methods. The dendritic processes of Langerhans cells (about 4 per high power field) are distributed throughout the mucosa (20). We have found them largely in the deeper layers, but they can extend into the superficial fields (Figure 40.9). Both T8 and, to a lesser degree, T4 lymphocytes are also frequently found, whereas macrophages and B lymphocytes are relatively uncommon.

Epithelial Response to Hormones

Vaginal epithelial cells proliferate and mature in response to stimulation by ovarian or exogenous estrogenic hormones. Hence, it would seem that the total number of squamous cell layers would vary greatly during the normal menstrual cycle and as a woman passes through the various stages of the life cycle, that is, birth, childhood, reproduction, and the postmenopausal years. Earlier work indicated the high occurred at ovulation (average 45 layers). It built slowly during the proliferative phase and averaged 22 on day 10. After ovulation, the number receded to 33 on day 19 and to 23 on day 24 (21,22). More recent workers found there was a statistically significant decrease from 27.8 on days 1 to 5 and 28.1 on days 7 to 12 to 26.0 on days 19 to 24, but clinically this appears to be of little import (20).

Without hormonal stimulation, the cells atrophy (Figure 40.10). At the peak of estrogenic activity (i.e., just before ovulation), the superficial cells with abundant intracytoplasmic glycogen predominate, both on histologic

section and in smears (Figure 40.11). Lactobacilli metabolize the glycogen normally present in the vagina to lactic acid, which maintains an acid vaginal pH (about pH 4.4 during the late proliferative and secretory phases) (23).

Progesterone inhibits maturation of the vaginal epithelium. Consequently, intermediate cells predominate when the circulating levels of progesterone are high; for example, during the postovulatory phase of the menstrual cycle or during pregnancy. Estrogenic activity is low or absent before puberty and after the menopause; the vaginal

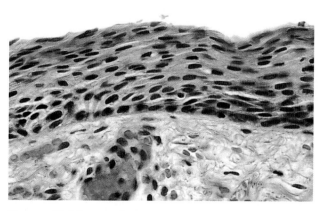

Figure 40.10 Atrophic vagina. Reprinted with permission from: Robboy SJ, Ellington KS. *Pathology of the Female Genital Tract in Kodachrome Slides.* 2nd ed. Durham, NC: Gyn-Path Associates; 1996.

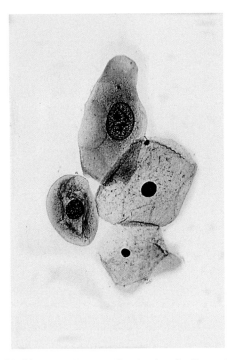

Figure 40.11 Vaginal smear, showing basal cell, two intermediate cells, and a superficial cell (Papanicolaou stain). Reprinted with permission from: Robboy SJ, Ellington KS. *Pathology of the Female Genital Tract in Kodachrome Slides.* 2nd ed. Durham, NC: Gyn-Path Associates; 1996.

epithelium fails to mature and hence remains thin. Parabasal and intermediate cells predominate in the vaginal smear. In the newborn child, the vaginal epithelium is frequently mature because of the influence of placental estrogens (Figure 40.12). Quantitative studies measuring the rate of change in the maturation index in the infant's vagina from birth to the atrophic state indicate that

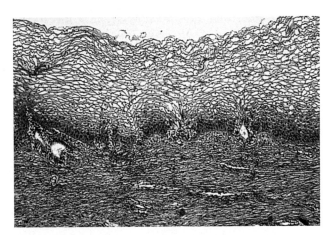

Figure 40.12 Vaginal mucosa of a near-term fetus. Mature cells predominate and cannot be distinguished from that of the adult (compare with Figure 40.7). In addition, two adenotic glands of the embryonic type are present. Reprinted with permission from: Robboy SJ, Ellington KS. *Pathology of the Female Genital Tract in Kodachrome Slides.* 2nd ed. Durham, NC: Gyn-Path Associates; 1996.

vaginal cells replace themselves in less than two weeks; that is, the time required for basal cells to work their way up and become desquamated superficial cells. Studies of the exocervix indicate that turnover there is also rapid (24).

The submucosa, or lamina propria, lies beneath the squamous epithelium. It contains elastic fibers and a rich venous and lymphatic network. Sometimes the superficial lamina propria discloses a bandlike zone of loose connective tissue that contains atypical polygonal to stellate stromal cells with scant cytoplasm (Figure 40.4). Many cells are multinucleated or have multilobulated hyperchromatic nuclei. Few are mononucleate. Mitoses are not observed. These atypical stromal cells are thought to give rise to fibroepithelial polyps, which have been observed within the cervix, vagina, and vulva. They have been shown to be fibroblastic in origin.

Vaginal Wall and Adventitia

The vaginal musculature is continuous with that of the uterus. The outer layers in muscle of both the uterus and vagina run longitudinally to pass out onto the lateral pelvic wall to form the superior and inferior surfaces, respectively, of the cardinal ligaments. The longitudinal muscle fibers continue to course the length of the vagina to the region of the hymenal ring, where they gradually disappear in the connective tissue. On the anterior vaginal wall, the longitudinal muscle fibers are displaced by the urethra more than diminished in number. The inner muscle layer of the vagina forms a spiral-like course, appearing in microscopic sections as somewhat circular in direction.

The adventitia is a thin coat of dense connective tissue adjoining the muscularis. The connective tissue of the adventitia merges with the stroma, connecting the vagina to the adjacent structures. This layer contains the many veins, lymphatics, nerve bundles, and small groups of nerve cells.

ULTRASTRUCTURE

On ultrastructural examination, the component layers are not sharply demarcated from each other. Rather, they may be somewhat difficult to distinguish because each layer has ill-defined limits and displays gradual changes in structure (25). In general the ultrastructural changes observed by transmission electron microscopy resemble those of the exocervix and mucosal squamous cells and are not further covered herein.

On scanning electron microscopic examination, the superficial cells appear large (50 μm in greatest dimension) and polygonal. The intercellular edges are narrow and dense and protrude slightly. The pattern of fine webbing and anastomotic intercellular bridges typifies nonkeratinized

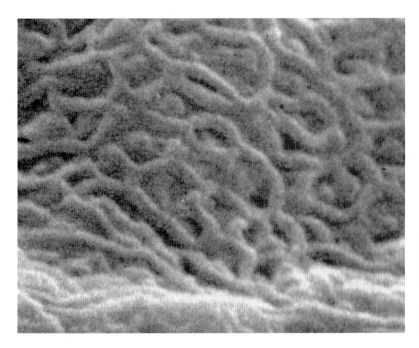

Figure 40.13 Intricate network of microridges on surface plasma membrane of most superficial squamous cells living in the normal vaginal lumen. Scanning electron microscopy (original magnification ×10,000). Reprinted with permission from: Ferenczy A, Richart RM. *Female Reproductive System: Dynamics of Scan and Transmission Electron Microscopy.* New York: John Wiley; 1974.

squamous epithelium, such as that observed in buccal mucosa. The key structure on the cell surface is the microridge, or in reality myriad microridges, which are interanastomotic longitudinal elevations of the plasma membrane 0.2 nm long and 0.1 nm high (Figure 40.13). Arranged in dense convolutions, they tie one cell to another, operating in a zipper-fastener principle. They are thought to provide surface adhesion. Desmosomes are prominent in these areas.

Microridge formation depends on the topographic configuration of disulfide-rich keratin or keratin precursors, which are absent in immature precursor cells, such as intermediate cells and young metaplastic squamous cells. From midcycle and early in the luteal phase, intercellular grooves widen. Porelike widening (porosites) of the intercellular crevices takes place where several cells interconnect. This porosity is thought to enhance continuity of the intercellular space system of the vaginal epithelium and the vaginal surface, thus permitting free passage of vaginal lubricating fluid.

Information about changes at the biochemical and immunological levels is relatively little, but clearly the cells at various levels show dramatic differences. Part may reflect degrees of cellular maturity. Part may reflect subcellular specialization. Like other epithelia, both squamous and glandular alike, the pattern of cytokeratin expression reflects the state and nature of differentiation of the epithelial cells. The vaginal mucosa reflects that of other nonkeratinized squamous epithelium. Cytokeratin 14 (CK14) is demonstrable in the basal layer and CK13 in the parabasal layer, the latter supporting a subpopulation of cells that express CK10 (26). In ways uncertain, the differentiating cells show changes that have other effects. One is its influence on bacterial binding, such that cellular receptors that

develop in the differentiated cells enhance adhesion of pathogenic bacteria. As one example, differentiated vaginal mucosal cells express receptors to *Escherichia coli* type 1 pili, which are surface-adhesive organelles (26). Such colonization where fecal *E. coli* are present in the vaginal introitus may be a key initial event leading to acute urinary infection. Another example is the presence of a surfactant protein (SP-A), which the human vaginal epithelial cells secrete. This factor, an important host defense, acts to facilitate micoorganism phagocytosis (27,28).

DIFFERENTIAL DIAGNOSIS AND SPECIAL ANATOMY

Wolffian Ducts

The wolffian duct, known otherwise as the mesonephric duct or Gartner's duct, is vestigial in the adult female (Figure 40.14). It begins to irreversibly wither if not stimulated to develop by testosterone before the thirteenth week postconception. This paired duct is most commonly situated in the lateral vaginal walls, although we have encountered it in all areas. Where encountered by chance in a radical vaginectomy specimen, the ducts are virtually always invisible grossly. Mitoses are absent. Usually it is a small duct or clusters of small glands about a duct. The lumen is filled frequently with a deeply eosinophilic, hyalinized secretion. The single layer of cells lining the duct is primarily composed of the cell nucleus. The cytoplasm is scant, relatively translucent, and lacks cilia. The nuclei frequently overlap. The chromatin is strikingly bland. On a

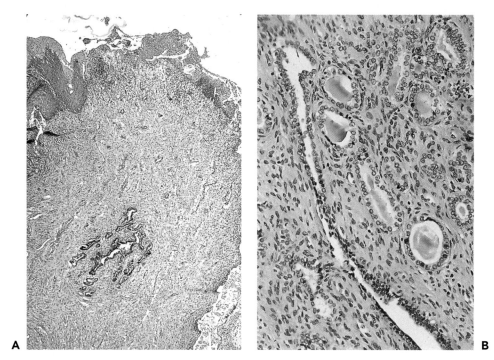

Figure 40.14 **A.** Vestigial wolffian duct remnants, deep in wall. **B.** Detail of central duct and arborized ductal terminals with eosinophilic secretions. Reprinted with permission from: Robboy SJ, Ellington KS. *Pathology of the Female Genital Tract in Kodachrome Slides.* 2nd ed. Durham, NC: Gyn-Path Associates; 1996.

clinical basis, individual ducts occasionally become cystic and macroscopically visible. In the cervix, these ducts rarely appear diffusely throughout the wall and appear as mesonephric hyperplasia or even adenoma (29). We also have seen rare cases where the neoplasm present appeared to be a true wolffian duct carcinoma.

Remnants of Müllerian Duct Epithelium (Adenosis)

The DES story began in 1938 when this nonsteroidal estrogen was synthesized and then gained popularity for the treatment of high-risk pregnancy. By 1971, up to two million women had taken the drug, at which time it was linked to the extremely rare development of clear cell adenocarcinoma of the vagina in young female offspring. Subsequently, about one-third of the exposed young women were found to have adenosis (presence of glandular tissue in the vagina). Both retrospective and prospective studies have shown that adenosis can be found in nonexposed women also, albeit rarely. In both exposed and nonexposed women, the adenosis is related to embryonic müllerian tissue that has remained entrapped and not been replaced by squamous epithelium during fetal life.

Adenosis appears in three forms. One type, the embryonic form, is exceedingly rare. The other two are the adult and common forms. In adenosis found during fetal life and in stillborns, but only rarely in adults, the glands are embryonic in character (Figures 40.12, 40.15) (30). They are small, usually at the epithelial–stromal interface, and are characterized by individual cells with small basal nuclei and copious bland cytoplasm that does not stain with either periodic acid-Schiff or mucicarmine.

It is believed that adenosis takes on its adult forms in women some time during puberty (31,32). Mucinous columnar cells, which by light and electron microscopy resemble those of the normal endocervical mucosa, comprise the glandular epithelium most frequently encountered as adenosis (62% of biopsy specimens with vaginal adenosis). This epithelium, because it frequently lines the surface of the vagina, is the type most commonly observed by colposcopy. Commonly, the mucinous columnar cells also line glands embedded in the lamina propria. This form of epithelium gives rise to the progestin-stimulated lesion, microglandular hyperplasia of the vagina (33).

Dark cells and light cells, often ciliated and resembling the lining cells of the uterine tube and endometrium, are found in 21% of specimens in the upper vagina with adenosis. This form of adenosis has been called tuboendometrial, although serous might be equally appropriate. The cells are usually found in glands in the lamina propria and not on the vaginal surface. Although adenosis

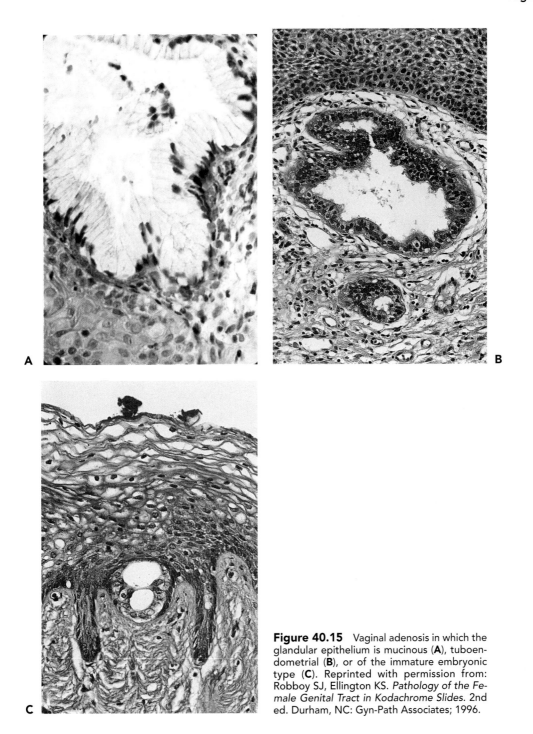

Figure 40.15 Vaginal adenosis in which the glandular epithelium is mucinous (**A**), tuboendometrial (**B**), or of the immature embryonic type (**C**). Reprinted with permission from: Robboy SJ, Ellington KS. *Pathology of the Female Genital Tract in Kodachrome Slides.* 2nd ed. Durham, NC: Gyn-Path Associates; 1996.

in the lower vagina is rare in absolute number, the percentage of biopsy specimens with adenosis that exhibits tuboendometrial rather than mucinous cells increases markedly in frequency in comparison with the more cranial aspects of the vagina. The tuboendometrial cell, which is benign, is the cell that we believe is related to clear cell adenocarcinoma, possibly through atypical adenosis, a transitional form (15,34). Mucinous glands and mucinous pools or droplets are encountered

frequently in the same biopsy specimen; mucinous and tuboendometrial cells are found together only occasionally in biopsy material. The tuboendometrial form of adenosis is the instrumental type of glandular cell induced by all regions of the müllerian duct, be it uterine tube, uterus, or vagina, whereas the mucinous cell is generally specific to the endocervix or, after DES exposure, to the deformed region of the cervix, which becomes ill-defined and includes what appears to be the upper vagina.

REFERENCES

1. Barnhart KT, Pretorius ES, Malamud D. Lesson learned and dispelled myths: three-dimensional imaging of the human vagina. *Fertil Steril* 2004;81:1383–1384.

2. Robboy SJ, Bentley RC, Russell P, Anderson MC. Embryology and Disorders of Sexual Development. In: Robboy SJ, Anderson MC, Russell P, eds. *Pathology of the Female Reproductive Tract*. London: Churchill Livingstone; 2002:819–860.

3. Aittomaki K, Eroila H, Kajanoja P. A population-based study of the incidence of mullerian aplasia in Finland. *Fertil Steril* 2001;76:624–625.

4. Lawrence WD, Whitaker D, Sugimura H, Cunha GR, Dickersin GR, Robboy SJ. An ultrastructural study of the developing urogenital tract in early human fetuses. *Am J Obstet Gynecol* 1992;167:185–193.

5. MacLaughlin DT, Donahoe PK. Mechanisms of disease: Sex determination and differentiation. *N Eng J Med* 2004;350:367–378.

6. Taguchi O, Cunha GR, Lawrence WD, Robboy SJ. Timing and irreversibility of Mullerian duct inhibition in the embryonic reproductive tract of the human male. *Dev Biol* 1984;106:394–398.

7. Ulfelder H, Robboy SJ. The embryologic development of the human vagina. *Am J Obstet Gynecol* 1976;126:769–776.

8. Taguchi O, Cunha GR, Robboy SJ. Expression of nuclear estrogen-binding sites within developing human fetal vagina and urogenital sinus. *Am J Anat* 1986;177:473–480.

9. Terruhn V. A study of impression moulds of the genital tract of female fetuses. *Arch Gynecol* 1980;229:207–217.

10. Kurita T, Cooke PS, Cunha GR. Epithelial-stromal tissue interaction in paramesonephric (Mullerian) epithelial differentiation. *Dev Biol* 2001;240:194–211.

11. Tsuji M, Shima H, Yonemura CY, Brody J, Donahoe PK, Cunha GR. Effect of human recombinant mullerian inhibiting substance on isolated epithelial and mesenchymal cells during mullerian duct regression in the rat. *Endocrinology* 1992;131:1481–1488.

12. Elliott GB, Elliott JD. Superficial stromal reactions of lower genital tract. *Arch Pathol* 1973;95:100–101.

13. Abdul-Karim FW, Cohen RE. Atypical stromal cells of lower female genital tract. *Histopathology* 1990;17:249–253.

14. Robboy SJ, Anderson MC, Russell P. Vagina. In: Robboy SJ, Anderson MC, Russell P, eds. *Pathology of the Female Reproductive Tract*. London: Churchill Livingstone; 2002:75–104.

15. Robboy SJ, Welch WR, Young RH, Truslow GY, Herbst AL, Scully RE. Topographic relation of cervical ectropion and vaginal adenosis to clear cell adenocarcinoma. *Obstet Gynecol* 1982;60:546–551.

16. Nichols DH, Randall CL. Pelvic anatomy of the living. In: Nichols DH, Randall CL, eds. *Vaginal Surgery*. 4th ed. Baltimore: Williams & Wilkins; 1996:1–42.

17. Faix A, Lapray JF, Courtieu C, Maubon A, Lanfrey K. Magnetic resonance imaging of sexual intercourse: initial experience. *J Sex Marital Ther* 2001;27:475–482.

18. Mostwin JL. Current concepts of female pelvic anatomy and physiology. *Urol Clin North Am* 1991;18:175–195.

19. Moore TR, Reiter RC, Rebar RW, Baker VV, eds. *Gynecology and Obstetrics: A Longitudinal Approach*. London: Churchill Livingstone; 1993.

20. Patton DL, Thwin SS, Meier A, Hooton TM, Stapleton AE, Eschenbach DA. Epithelial cell layer thickness and immune cell populations in the normal human vagina at different stages of the menstrual cycle. *Am J Obstet Gynecol* 2000;183:967–973.

21. Burgos MH, Roig de Vargas-Linares CE. Ultrastructure of the vaginal mucosa. In: Hafez ESE, Evans TN, eds. *The Human Vagina*. New York: North-Holland; 1978:63–93.

22. Steger RW, Hafez ESE. Age associated changes in vagina. In: Hafez ESE, Evans TN, eds. *The Human Vagina*. New York: North-Holland; 1978:95–108.

23. Eschenbach DA, Thwin SS, Patton DL, et al. Influence of the normal menstrual cycle on vaginal tissue, discharge, and microflora. *Clin Infect Dis* 2000;30:901–907.

24. Linhartova A. The height and structure of the cervical squamous epithelium in foetuses, newborns, and girls. *Cervix Low Female Genital Tract* 1989;7:37–48.

25. Ferenczy A, Richart RM. *Female Reproductive System: Dynamics of Scan and Transmission Electron Microscopy*. New York: John Wiley; 1974.

26. Klumpp DJ, Forrestal SG, Karr JE, Mudge CS, Anderson BE, Schaeffer AJ. Epithelial differentiation promotes the adherence of type 1-piliated Escherichia coli to human vaginal cells. *J Infect Dis* 2002;186:1631–1638.

27. MacNeill C, Umstead TM, Phelps DS, et al. Surfactant protein A, an innate immune factor, is expressed in the vaginal mucosa and is present in vaginal lavage fluid. *Immunology* 2004;111:91–99.

28. Wira CR, Fahey JV. The innate immune system: gatekeeper to the female reproductive tract. *Immunology* 2004;111:13–15.

29. Ferry JA, Scully RE. Mesonephric remnants, hyperplasia, and neoplasia in the uterine cervix: a study of 49 cases. *Am J Surg Pathol* 1990;14:1100–1111.

30. Robboy SJ, Hill EC, Sandberg EC, Czernobilsky B. Vaginal adenosis in women born prior to the diethylstilbestrol era. *Hum Pathol* 1986;17:488–492.

31. Robboy SJ. A hypothetic mechanism of diethylstilbestrol(DES)-induced anomalies in exposed progeny. *Hum Pathol* 1983;14:831–833.

32. Robboy SJ, Kaufman RH, Prat J, et al. Pathologic findings in young women enrolled in the National Cooperative Diethylstilbestrol Adenosis (DESAD) project. *Obstet Gynecol* 1979;53:309–317.

33. Robboy SJ, Welch WR. Microglandular hyperplasia in vaginal adenosis associated with oral contraceptives and prenatal diethylstilbestrol exposure. *Obstet Gynecol* 1977;49:430–434.

34. Robboy SJ, Young RH, Welch WR, et al. Atypical vaginal adenosis and cervical ectropion. Association with clear cell adenocarcinoma in diethylstilbestrol-exposed offspring. *Cancer* 1984;54:869–875.

Uterus and Fallopian Tubes

Michael R. Hendrickson   Kristen A. Atkins   Richard L. Kempson

INTRODUCTION

The fallopian tubes and uterus in many ways constitute a natural anatomic and functional unit. They both derive embryologically from the müllerian duct. Taken together, they provide the locations for the fusion of the descending egg and the ascending spermatozoon, the implantation of the resulting blastocyst, the incubation of the developing gestation, and they ultimately provide the mechanism for the delivery of the conceptus at term. They have a common anatomic organization and share common responses to a changing steroidal milieu. Looking beyond normal structure and function to pathology, the fallopian tube and the uterus, together with the ovarian surface epithelium, comprise what has been termed the extended müllerian system (1, 2), which gives rise to a common set of neoplasms and nonneoplastic metaplastic epithelial changes.

This chapter emphasizes those aspects of normal histology and immunohistochemistry relevant to the diagnostic pathologist and focuses on those features of the normal uterus and fallopian tubes that, because of their striking appearance or unfamiliarity, raise the issue of pathologic alterations.

Accounts of conventional light microscopic appearance of the fallopian tube and uterus have not changed substantially over the past several decades. This is in sharp contrast to the impressive gains in our knowledge of the biochemical and physiologic details of the normal function of these organs. Parallel advances have been made in microsurgery and radiologic imaging techniques. Increasing use of in vitro fertilization and embryo transfer technology has exploited these advances, and that in turn has prompted a return to many ancient questions: Why do women menstruate? What exactly does the endometrium do? Does it have an endocrine function? What are the functions of the many endometrial secretion products? Which of these endometrial contributions are essential to initiating and successfully sustaining a gestation? There has been an explosion of knowledge concerning the hormonal control of the reproductive system, fueled in large part by efforts to induce ovulation with pharmacologic agents. This has led in recent decades to a much more extensive knowledge of the neuroendocrine regulation of the menstrual cycle, the detailed anatomy and endocrinology of ovarian folliculogenesis, ovulation and corpus luteum function, the mechanism of action and genetics of steroid receptors, and the mechanisms responsible for normal menstrual bleeding. Paradoxically, most of this information is currently not of direct relevance to diagnostic pathologists. The practical orientation of this work notwithstanding, to ignore this knowledge would impart a distinctly dated character to this chapter. Therefore, we include a rough outline of some of this information and direct the interested reader to sources with a more detailed treatment of these issues.

This chapter first discusses the embryology and gross anatomy of the uterus and the fallopian tubes and then turns to the normal histology of the cervix, endometrium, myometrium, fallopian tube, and broad ligament.

EMBRYOLOGY

The uterus and fallopian tubes have a complex developmental history (3–11). For poorly understood reasons, precursors of both male and female internal genitalia are laid down early in each embryo in a manner analogous to the initial development of the bipotential gonad. This is known as the indifferent stage of genital development. Upon completion of this indifferent stage, definitive female differentiation is accompanied by regression of the male anlage, whereas male differentiation is accompanied by regression of the female anlage. Topographically, both of these systems are intimately related to the developing urinary tract, and, not surprisingly, anomalous development of the internal genitalia is often accompanied by anomalies of the urinary tract. Fetal sexual differentiation is completed during the first half of gestation; the last half is marked primarily by growth of the newly established genitalia. Relevant milestones have been summarized by Ramsey (12) (Figure 41.1).

The Indifferent Stage

By the 6th week of fetal life the urogenital sinus and the mesonephric (wolffian) ducts are well established. At this time the paired müllerian (paramesonephric) ducts begin their development. These structures are formed by an invagination of the celomic epithelium adjacent to that investing each developing ovary. The müllerian ducts are intimately related to the mesonephric ducts, and their normal formation appears in fact to be dependent on the presence of the mesonephros.

As the müllerian ducts grow caudally, they approach the midline where the distal portions fuse. Shortly after this fusion, the apposed medial duct walls disappear, bringing the two lumina into continuity to form a single cavity. Further downward growth of the fused müllerian structures (now termed the uterovaginal primordium) brings them into contact with the urogenital sinus. At this stage both the mesonephric ducts and the müllerian ducts are present in the fetus.

Female Differentiation

The differentiation of the indifferent internal genitalia into male or female structures depends on whether the fetus possesses ovaries or testes. In the male fetus, the Leydig cells and the Sertoli cells in the developing testes secrete testosterone and a nonsteroidal müllerian inhibiting substance respectively; the latter, antimüllerian hormone (ATM) is a member of the transforming growth factor-β family of glycoprotein differentiation factors (13). The net effect of this secretory activity is to ensure the persistence, differentiation, and growth of the mesonephric ducts to form the male genital system and the regression of the müllerian system. In the absence of a secreting testis (e.g., in a normal female fetus with ovaries or in a fetus with nonfunctioning gonads) the müllerian structures persist, whereas the mesonephric ducts regress. The nonfused portions of the müllerian ducts form the fallopian tubes; the fused segments develop into the uterus and probably the upper third of the vagina. Incomplete fusion of the caudal portion of the müllerian ducts results in a spectrum of uterovaginal abnormalities (14).

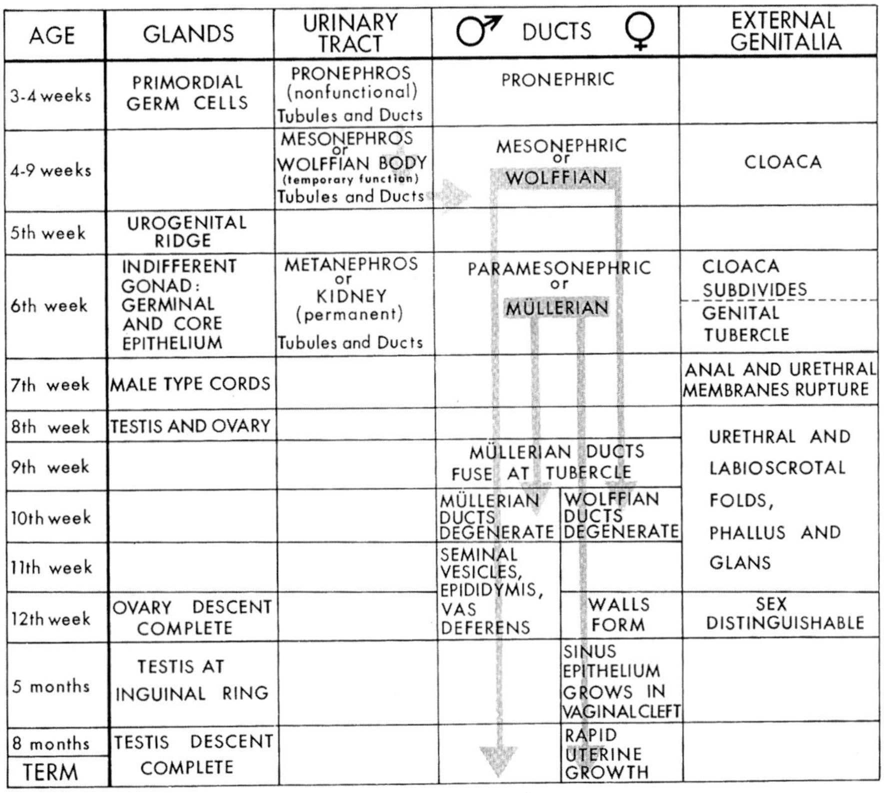

AGE	GLANDS	URINARY TRACT	♂ DUCTS	♀	EXTERNAL GENITALIA
3–4 weeks	PRIMORDIAL GERM CELLS	PRONEPHROS (nonfunctional) Tubules and Ducts	PRONEPHRIC		
4–9 weeks		MESONEPHROS or WOLFFIAN BODY (temporary function) Tubules and Ducts	MESONEPHRIC or WOLFFIAN		CLOACA
5th week	UROGENITAL RIDGE				
6th week	INDIFFERENT GONAD: GERMINAL AND CORE EPITHELIUM	METANEPHROS or KIDNEY (permanent) Tubules and Ducts	PARAMESONEPHRIC or MÜLLERIAN		CLOACA SUBDIVIDES / GENITAL TUBERCLE
7th week	MALE TYPE CORDS				ANAL AND URETHRAL MEMBRANES RUPTURE
8th week	TESTIS AND OVARY				URETHRAL AND
9th week			MÜLLERIAN DUCTS FUSE AT TUBERCLE		LABIOSCROTAL
10th week			MÜLLERIAN DUCTS DEGENERATE	WOLFFIAN DUCTS DEGENERATE	FOLDS,
11th week			SEMINAL VESICLES, EPIDIDYMIS, VAS DEFERENS		PHALLUS AND GLANS
12th week	OVARY DESCENT COMPLETE			WALLS FORM	SEX DISTINGUISHABLE
5 months	TESTIS AT INGUINAL RING			SINUS EPITHELIUM GROWS IN VAGINAL CLEFT	
8 months / TERM	TESTIS DESCENT COMPLETE			RAPID UTERINE GROWTH	

Figure 41.1 Chart showing interrelations and time sequence of events in the development of genitourinary system. Reprinted with permission from: Ramsey E. Embryology and developmental defects of the female reproductive tract. In: Danforth DN, Scott JR, eds. *Obstetrics and Gynecology.* 5th ed. Philadelphia: JB Lippincott; 1986:106–119.

By the 21st week, the uterus and vagina are well formed. In contrast to the adult cervix, the cervix of the prenatal uterus is disproportionately large and makes up two thirds of the length of the organ. The second half of gestation is marked by uterine growth; from the 28th week to birth, a period of approximately 10 weeks, the fetal uterus doubles in size. However, the earlier cervicocorpus disproportion is maintained into childhood.

The events described above are driven, at least in part, by the expression of secreted ligands of the wingless (WNT) gene family and transcriptional regulators of the homeobox (HOX) gene family (13,15).

GROSS ANATOMY

Premenarchal Uterus and Fallopian Tubes

Neonatal Period

At birth the uterus averages about 4 cm in length, and its bulk and shape are dominated by its disproportionately large cervix (the cervicofundal ratio is approximately 3–5:1) (Figure. 41.2). The impact of the maternal hormonal environment is reflected in the markedly thickened rugal vaginal mucosa typically present at birth and, to a certain extent, in the histologic appearance of the endometrium, which is most often proliferative or weakly secretory. Maternal estrogen also results in cervical squamous cell maturation with glycogen storage. These mucosal changes regress shortly after birth (16–18).

Infancy

Uterine growth continues into the second year of life, at which time it reaches a plateau that persists until the premenarchal growth spurt at about 9 years of age. Until approximately age 13, the cervix continues to account for greater than half of the uterine length.

Adult Uterus and Fallopian Tubes

General Relations and Attachments

The uterus is located anterior to the rectum and posterior to the bladder (Figure. 41.3). It is covered anteriorly and posteriorly by a reflection of pelvic peritoneum that continues laterally to form the anterior and posterior leaves of the broad

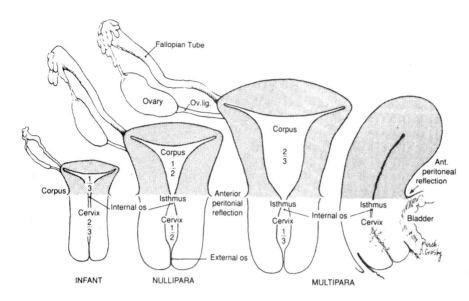

Figure 41.2 Drawings illustrating comparative sizes of prepubertal, mature nonparous, and parous uteri. The relative proportions of uterine corpus and cervix are seen to change with age and parity. Frontal and sagittal sections are presented. (After Ranice W. Crosby.) Reprinted with permission from: Ramsey E. Development of the human uterus and relevance to the adult condition. In: Chard T, Grudzinskas JG, eds. *The Uterus.* New York: Cambridge University Press; 1994: 41–53.

ligament. The posterior peritoneal reflection forms the uterine wall of the pouch of Douglas and covers a longer segment of the uterine isthmus than does the anterior peritoneal reflection. The tentlike broad ligaments house the major uterine vessels and the efferent lymphatic trunks; they also contain the fallopian tubes at their apices. Each ovary is attached to the ipsilateral uterine cornu by the utero-ovarian ligament, which is situated posterolateral and inferior to the uterine attachment of the fallopian tubes. The round ligaments arise anterolateral and inferior to the attachment of the fallopian tubes and pass anteriorly to insert into the canal of Nuck. These anatomic relations are of obvious im-

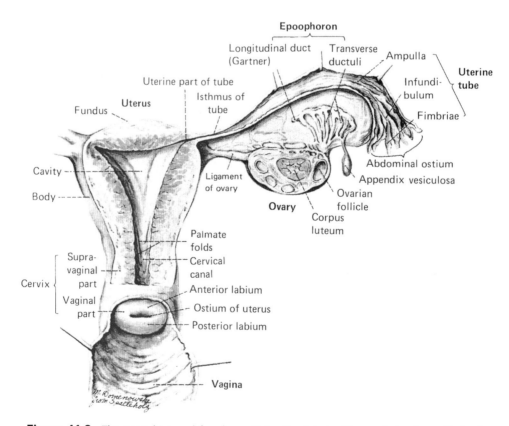

Figure 41.3 The normal internal female genitalia. Reprinted with permission from: Crafts R, Krieger H. Gross anatomy of the female reproductive tract, pituitary, and hypothalamus. In: Danforth D, Scott J, eds. *Obstetrics and Gynecology.* Philadelphia: JB Lippincott; 1986:64.

portance to the surgeon but also of value to the pathologist because they often enable proper orientation of the hysterectomy specimen. The anterior surface of the uterus is distinguished by its longer "bare" region (i.e., lacking peritoneum) and the anteriorly directed stump of the round ligament. The posterior surface is more extensively covered by peritoneum, and the utero-ovarian ligament is attached to the posterior cornual aspect of the uterus. The uterus is anchored to its surroundings by a number of connective tissue bands; notable among them are the cardinal, uterosacral, and pubocervical ligaments (11,18–20).

Gross Anatomic Features of the Uterus

The adult nulliparous uterus is a hollow, pear-shaped muscular organ weighing 40 to 80 g and measuring approximately 7 to 8 cm along its long axis, 5.0 cm at its broadest extent (cornu to cornu), and 2.5 cm in anteroposterior dimension. These measurements vary considerably as a function of age, phase of the menstrual cycle, and parity. In general, high parity and youth are positively correlated with increasing uterine size (21). The adult uterus consists of an expanded body, the corpus, and a smaller cervix. That portion of the corpus cephalad to a line connecting the origin of the two fallopian tubes is called the fundus. The cornua are the two lateral regions of the fundus associated with the intramural portion of the fallopian tubes. The remainder of the corpus tapers from the fundus into the isthmus or the lower uterine segment, which shares histologic features with both of the uterine segments that it bridges: the uterine corpus and the endocervix. The existence of an anatomically and functionally significant lower uterine segment has been disputed by some authorities (22). The uterine cavity has the approximate configuration of the uterus, but its internal dimensions are much smaller, reflecting the substantial thickness of the uterine wall. The cavity is triangular, and the apices of this potential space are continuous with the lumina of the fallopian tubes at the two cornua and with the endocervical canal at the internal os. The length of the cavity is approximately 6.0 cm. Again, these measurements vary considerably with the age and parity of the individual (23). The cervix is roughly cylindrical and normally measures approximately 3 to 4 cm in length (24). It is pierced through its center by the endocervical canal. Traditionally, the endocervical canal has been described as having an external os that opens onto the exocervix and an internal os that separates the endocervical canal from the endometrial cavity. Although the former is a reasonable anatomic landmark, the latter is not because grossly, the transition from endometrial cavity to endocervix is gradual, without abrupt anatomic demarcation between endocervix and endometrium. This is histologically mirrored by the gradual transition of the mucosa in this region from endocervical type to endometrial type. The mucosal surface of the endocervical canal is deeply clefted to form the plicae

palmatae. The lateral connective tissue attachments of the uterus are referred to as the parametria; they contain vessels, nerves, lymphatics, and lymph nodes.

The normal myometrium consists of two strata: an outer longitudinal muscle layer covering the fundus and an inner circular submucosal muscle layer extending to surround the internal os and the tubal ostia. There is an interposed thick middle layer, richly populated by vessels and composed of randomly interdigitating fibers (25). The magnetic resonance imaging (MRI) correlate of these layers is the outer zone and the submucosal low intensity halo "junctional zone" (26,27). Functionally, the junctional zone appears to be more involved with menstruation while the outer zone assumes a prominent role in gestation and parturition.

Parenthetically, Toth has described two lateral subserosally situated longitudinal bands of distinctive muscle fibers, the fasciculus cervicoangularis (28,29). On occasion, epithelium that is immunohistochemically and histologically similar to cervical mesonephric remnants is present within this bundle, suggesting that these structures represent the vestiges of the wolffian (mesonephric) duct which is more commonly encountered in the cervical stroma ("mesonephric rests") and lateral vagina (Gardner's duct and derivative cysts).

Substantial deviations from the nulliparous adult uterus naturally occur throughout adult life. The uterus undergoes small-amplitude changes in size during the menstrual cycle, attaining its greatest volume during the secretory phase (27). During pregnancy, of course, the uterus enlarges much more dramatically to accommodate the growing conceptus. This growth is due largely to myocyte hypertrophy and hyperplasia, an increase in uterine vasculature, and in extracellular matrix; the net weight increases 10-fold during pregnancy. After delivery, uterine size rapidly decreases, and over the ensuing weeks a striking resorption of connective tissue occurs that is associated with a decrease in the size of individual myocytes (30). However, the uterus generally does not return completely to its nulliparous size and weight. Prior pregnancy (parity) can be deduced from several gross features. The multiparous nongravid uterus tends to weigh more in consequence of its thicker and more prominently layered muscular walls; this increase in weight is proportional to the patient's parity (21). The vasculature of the multiparous uterus tends to be more prominent. The most suggestive changes of previous pregnancy, however, are seen in the cervix. The nulliparous circular small external os is transformed after pregnancy into a slit that forms prominent anterior and posterior lips. In addition, healed cervical lacerations may be pronounced, and enough endocervical tissue may reside on the exocervix to give it a red granular appearance near the os. With the waning of ovarian hormone synthesis during the menopausal years, the uterus involutes and atrophies. This is reflected by a decrease in its weight and its dimensions. On occasion the endocervical canal is almost completely obliterated. Exogenous estrogens administered during this period sometimes maintain uterine weight artificially despite the loss of ovarian hormonal support.

Gross Anatomic Features of the Fallopian Tubes

The fallopian tubes are hollow, epithelium-lined muscular structures 11 to 12 cm in length that run through the apex of the broad ligament to span the uterine cornu medially and the ovary laterally. Each tube is divided into four anatomic segments. The intramural segment begins at the funnel-like uppermost recess of the uterine cornu and ends where the tube emerges from the uterine wall. The course of this 8-mm, pinpoint lumened segment varies from straight to highly convoluted (31). Beyond the uterine wall the proximal tube continues for 2 to 3 cm as the isthmus, a thick-walled, narrow-calibered segment that merges into a comparatively thin-walled expanded area, the ampulla. The distal tube ends in the trumpet-shaped infundibulum whose mouth opens into the peritoneal cavity and is fringed by approximately 25 fimbria. One of these, the ovarian fimbrium, attaches to the ovary. At the time of ovulation the infundibulum forms a cap over the ovarian surface to create the ovarian bursa. The tubal mucosa and the underlying endosalpingeal stroma are thrown up into longitudinal, branching folds (the plicae) whose branches increase in complexity from the isthmus to the infundibulum. The plicae terminate in the fimbria. At the time of ovulation the fimbria sweep over the surface of the ovary to facilitate egg capture (13,32–35).

Uterine and Tubal Vasculature

The major arterial supply of the uterus derives from the right and left uterine arteries, which arise from the corresponding hypogastric (internal iliac) arteries. The uterine artery divides into ascending and descending branches laterally at the level of the uterine isthmus. The ascending uterine artery anastomoses freely with the ovarian artery (a branch of the aorta) in the mesosalpinx, whereas the descending branch anastomoses with the vaginal arterial supply. Both the ascending and descending uterine arteries give rise to a complex network of circumferentially arranged subserosal arteries: the arcuate arteries. These, in turn, give rise to a series of radial arteries that penetrate the myometrium. Each of these radial vessels branches, in the inner third of the myometrium, into straight arteries (supplying the basalis) and spiral arteries that become the spiral arteries of the endometrium (36–38).

A striking characteristic of the adult intramyometrial uterine arteries is their marked tortuosity. This, no doubt, has to do with the variation in uterine size during reproductive life.

In the postmenopausal years, striking degenerative changes may be seen in the uterine arteries, including intimal proliferation, fibrosis, and medial calcification. The severity of these changes is typically out of proportion to degenerative changes in nonuterine arteries. The venous drainage of the uterus parallels its arterial supply.

Uterine and Tubal Lymphatics

Lymphatics are present in both the cervix and the corpus. In the endometrium these vessels are intimately associated with the glands of the functionalis. The myometrium and cervical stroma contain a complex labyrinth of lymphatics that course toward the subserosal plexus. The channels forming the latter ramify over the entire surface of the uterus, and the confluence of these channels forms the major efferent lymphatic trunks of the uterus. The chief interest in lymphatic drainage for the pathologist is as a guide to the dissemination of carcinoma. The major lymph node groups draining cervical and endometrial carcinoma are indicated in Figures 41.4 and 41.5.

In both the mucosal and muscular layers, lymphatic anastomoses exist between the cervical and corpus systems, and on occasion cervical carcinomas may take advantage of this route to spread to the corpus. Whether the converse is true is unclear. Moreover, whether or not corpus carcinoma, once having invaded the cervix, then behaves like cervical carcinoma in terms of its lymphatic metastatic distribution is also unclear, even though this is a common clinical

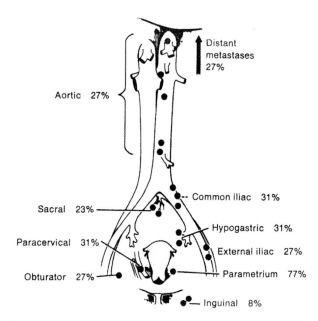

Figure 41.4 Percentage of involvement of draining lymph nodes in untreated patients with cervical cancer. Reprinted with permission from: Henriksen E. The lymphatic spread of carcinoma of the cervix and of the body of the uterus: a study of 420 necropsies. *Am J Obstet Gynecol* 1949;58:924–942.

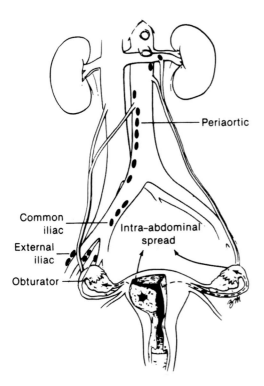

Figure 41.5 Paths of spread available to carcinoma of the endometrium. Not only may carcinoma cells metastasize to the pelvic and periaortic lymph nodes, but they also may spread through the fallopian tube to the peritoneum or they may invade through the myometrium into the broad ligament and ovary. Reprinted with permission from: DiSaia P, Creasman W, eds. *Clinical Gynecologic Oncology.* 3rd ed. St. Louis: CV Mosby; 1989:84–93.

assumption. Indeed, involvement of "cervical draining nodes" by endometrial carcinoma does not necessarily imply cervical involvement. For further detail, the reader is referred to specialty works and textbooks of gynecologic oncology (39–41).

Tubal lymphatics accompany the ovarian vessels and drain into nodes near the right and left renal veins and the presacral and common iliac nodes. Lymphatic spread of tubal malignancy may reach extrapelvic sites early in its dissemination (42,43).

UTERINE CERVIX

The uterine cervix (or "neck") is the elongate fibromuscular portion of the uterus that measures 2.5 to 3.0 cm. A part of this structure protrudes into the upper part of the vagina (vaginal part, portio vaginalis), whereas the remainder lies above the vaginal vault (supravaginal portion, portio supravaginalis). The outer surface of the vaginal portion of the cervix is known variously as the ectocervix or exocervix. It is covered, at least in part, by stratified squamous epithelium that is continuous with, and histologically identical to, the mucosa of the vaginal fornices. That portion of the

cervix, in relation to the endocervical canal, is known as the anatomic endocervix. The endocervical canal, lined for the most part by mucin-secreting epithelium that blends at one end with the squamous epithelium of the exocervix and with the epithelium of the lower uterine segment at its other end, brings the vagina into communication with the endometrial cavity. The anatomic opening of the endocervical canal onto the exocervix is known as the external os. In parous women, this most often takes on a slitlike configuration that serves to divide the exocervix into anterior and posterior lips (18,44). This particular geometry is thought to be important in uterine function during gestation (45). The upper limit of the endocervical canal is known as the internal os. This is not a distinct orifice; rather, there is a gradual, funnel-shaped widening of the endocervical canal and a transition from endocervical epithelium into the endometrial epithelium of the lower uterine segment. The junction of the endocervical glandular mucosa with the squamous epithelium of the exocervix is known as the squamocolumnar junction. This junction does not always lie at the external os; in fact, the squamocolumnar junction typically is located on the exocervix, where it can easily be inspected with the culposcope. This is further discussed in the section devoted to the transformation zone.

The uterine cervix obviously plays an important role in the anatomic support of the internal genitalia and plays an active role in labor and delivery, but arguably its primary role is the production of cervical mucous. Cervical mucous acts as a functional gate that prevents vaginal microorganisms from gaining access to the upper genital tract and (except for a small midcycle window before ovulation) denies sperm access to the uterus and fallopian tubes. At midcycle the chemical composition of the cervical mucous changes and its viscosity decreases. This has the effect of allowing the passage of sperm into the upper genital tract. These changes are the basis of the Spinnbarkeit and fern tests. In addition, the cervical mucous plays an important role in removing seminal plasma constituents (preventing sperm phagocytosis) and in providing a suitable environment for sperm storage, capacitation, and migration (46,47).

The following discussion first focuses on the epithelium of the exocervix, the endocervix, and the transformation zone and then turns to the stroma of the cervix and the changes that occur in the cervix during pregnancy.

Epithelium of the Exocervix

The squamous epithelium covering the exocervix is normally noncornified, and it grows, matures, and accumulates glycogen in its upper layers in response to circulating estrogens, most notably, estradiol (Figure 41.6). Because low blood levels of estrogen are the rule during childhood and the postmenopausal years, the squamous cells of the cervix do not proliferate or mature, and glycogen is not stored in the upper layers of the epithelium during these

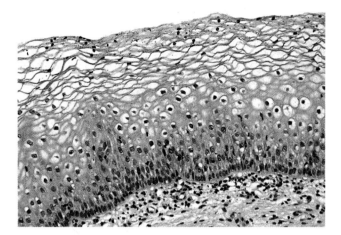

Figure 41.6 Mature squamous epithelium of the exocervix demonstrating a normal maturation sequence from basal cells to superficial cells. The cleared cytoplasm indicating glycogen storage should not be confused with koilocytosis.

periods unless estrogen is made available as a result of therapy or functioning ovarian tumors (18). In the immediate postnatal period, the squamous epithelium of the newborn cervix is fully mature due to maternal estrogen, but the epithelium quickly becomes atrophic and glycogen disappears as estrogen levels decrease.

The estrogenically stimulated cervical squamous epithelium of the sexually mature woman can be divided into three layers: the basal/parabasal cell layer, the midzone layer (or stratum spongiosum), and the superficial layer (Figure 41.6). The basal cell layer is composed of cells with scant cytoplasm and oval to cuboidal nuclei with dense chromatin. These cells are usually mitotically inactive and do not mark immunohistochemically with proliferation markers; for example, Ki-67 and proliferating cell nuclear antigen (PCNA) (48). The cells immediately above the basal layer comprise the lower portion of the midzone layer and are known as parabasal cells, a term often used in cytologic circles. The parabasal cells are somewhat larger than the basal cells due to their increased cytoplasm, and the nuclei have slightly less dense chromatin. In contrast to the basal layer, mitotic figures are usually present but are not abnormal or particularly numerous in the normal epithelium. This layer also displays proliferation markers (48). The midzone layer is composed of cells with even more abundant cytoplasm and somewhat smaller vesicular nuclei. These are known as intermediate cells. Glycogen accumulates in most intermediate cells, and this imparts a finely granular or clear appearance to the cytoplasm. The superficial cells contain small, rounded, regular pyknotic nuclei, and their cytoplasm is abundant and clear as a result of even greater glycogen accumulation. Keratinization occurs in both the superficial and intermediate cells and renders them flat and platelike when they are spread on a slide. The cytoplasmic clearing characteristic of normal intermediate and superficial cells is often perinuclear.

Because perinuclear clearing is also a feature of cells (koilocytes) infected by human papillomavirus (HPV), there is a potential for misinterpreting normal epithelial cells containing glycogen as abnormal. However, koilocytes not only feature perinuclear clearing of the cytoplasm, but their nuclei are larger, and these nuclei possess a more undulating nuclear membrane than do the nuclei found in intermediate and superficial cells (giving rise to the appearance of koilocytes sometimes described as "raisinoid" or "pruneoid"). Moreover, the nuclear chromatin of koilocytes has a ropy texture in contrast to the homogenous appearance of normal cells. The cervical squamous mucosa undergoes cyclic changes during the menstrual cycle similar to the estrogen–progesterone-induced changes in the vaginal mucosa, although the cells composing the latter are a more liable index of hormonal status. During the luteal phase and pregnancy, when progesterone levels are high, there is a predominance of intermediate cells.

The exocervical epithelium in postmenopausal women (not receiving a supplement of estrogen therapy) is composed mainly of basal and parabasal cells that feature scant cytoplasm and little or no cytoplasmic glycogen (Figure 41.7). The cells may have the same degree of nucleus-to-cytoplasm ratio shift toward the nucleus as do the cells composing cervical intraepithelial neoplasia (CIN). Consequently, atrophic epithelium is a part of the differential diagnosis of CIN, and care should be taken when a diagnosis of CIN is contemplated in a postmenopausal woman. However, the basal and parabasal cells in atrophic epithelia do not demonstrate the nuclear abnormalities and high mitotic index usually seen in the cells constituting the neoplastic epithelium in high grade CIN (high grade squamous intraepithelial lesion—SIL).

Endocrine cells have been identified in the squamous epithelium of the exocervix by immunohistochemical techniques; their function is unknown, but they are thought to give rise to the rare cervical carcinoid tumors (49–56). Langerhans cells also are present in the ectocervical epithelium, as well as in the transformation zone (57–59). They

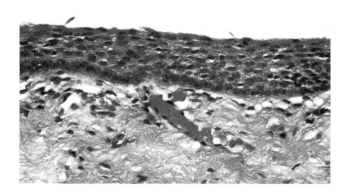

Figure 41.7 Postmenopausal atrophy of the cervical squamous epithelium. The immature cells can resemble the cells in high-grade squamous intraepithelial lesion—SIL (cervical intraepithelial neoplasia—CIN).

are involved in antigen presentation to T-lymphocytes. Melanin-containing cells have been reported in the cervical epithelium and provide a plausible cell of origin for the uncommon cervical melanoma and blue nevus (60).

Epithelium of the Endocervix

The anatomic endocervix extends from the external os to the internal os, but endocervical glandular epithelium is not exclusively limited to this anatomic area, particularly during the reproductive years. Rather, endocervical epithelium occupies significant regions of the anatomic exocervix during childhood and after the menarche. The shift of the endocervical epithelium out of the canal onto the exocervix is discussed in more detail below in the section devoted to the transformation zone.

The endocervix is lined by a single layer of mucin-secreting epithelium composed of cells with small, often basilar, nuclei above which is mucin-filled cytoplasm that imparts a "picket fence" appearance (Figure 41.8). Goblet cells are sometimes encountered (Figure 41.9). The nuclei are generally small, elongate, and have rather dense chromatin. They tend to overlap one another. When the endocervical epithelium has been damaged and is regenerating, the nuclei may become larger and more rounded, but mitotic figures are difficult to find in nonneoplastic endocervical cells (61). If one encounters endocervical epithelium containing easily found mitotic figures, consideration should be given to the possibility of a pathologic process such as well-differentiated carcinoma or carcinoma in situ, particularly if the nuclei are enlarged and nucleoli are prominent. Nucleoli are usually not prominent in resting endocervical cells, but they may become so during regeneration, pregnancy, and neoplastic transformation. Mitotic figures may be found in the constituent glandular cells of cervical endometriosis.

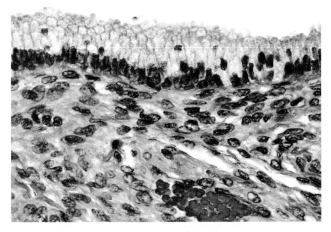

Figure 41.8 Normal endocervical mucosa with most nuclei in the characteristic basilar location. Enlargement of these nuclei and loss of apical mucin are features that should cause a closer inspection of the endocervical glands to ensure that neoplastic transformation is not present.

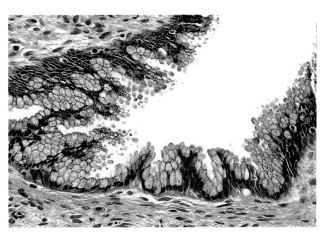

Figure 41.9 Goblet cells in the endocervix. Not infrequently, the nuclei of mucin-containing cells are displaced to the base of the cell and compressed by cytoplasmic mucin to produce a goblet cell. The presence of goblet cells and neuroendocrine cells in the normal endocervical mucosa tends to destabilize the conventional distinction in ovarian pathology between müllerian (i.e., cervical) mucinous and intestinal mucinous differentiation.

Other types of cells may be identified in the endocervical epithelium. Ciliated cells are almost always present and can be a useful marker of a benign process when the appearance of the endocervical glandular epithelium raises concerns about well-differentiated adenocarcinoma (62). When ciliated cells are numerous, the term "ciliary (or tubal) metaplasia" is often used (Figures 41.10A and 41.10B) (63–69). Ciliated cells themselves can develop enlarged dense nuclei and thus come to resemble neoplastic cells (Figure 41.10C). As a result, care should be taken to look for cilia before diagnosing in situ neoplastic transformation of the endocervix. Immunohistochemistry may be of aid in this distinction; Marques et al. found a combination of vimentin and carcinoembryonic antigen (CEA) helpful: adenocarcinoma in situ tended to be CEA positive and vimentin negative while the opposite was true for tubal metaplasia (70).

Subcolumnar reserve cells that have the potential to differentiate into ciliated and mucous secretory cells have been reported to populate the endocervix, even though there is evidence that the differentiated mucous cells are capable of division without the intercession of reserve cells (61,62). It is easy to confuse the lymphocytes that have populated the glandular epithelium with epithelial reserve cells (71).

Endocrine cells also are present within the endocervical epithelium. Their normal function is unclear, but it is generally held that they give rise to the endocrine neoplasms such as carcinoids and neuroendocrine carcinomas that occasionally are encountered in the cervix (49,54).

The endocervical epithelium not only lines the surface of the endocervical canal, it also dips, to a variable degree, into the underlying stroma to form elongate clefts

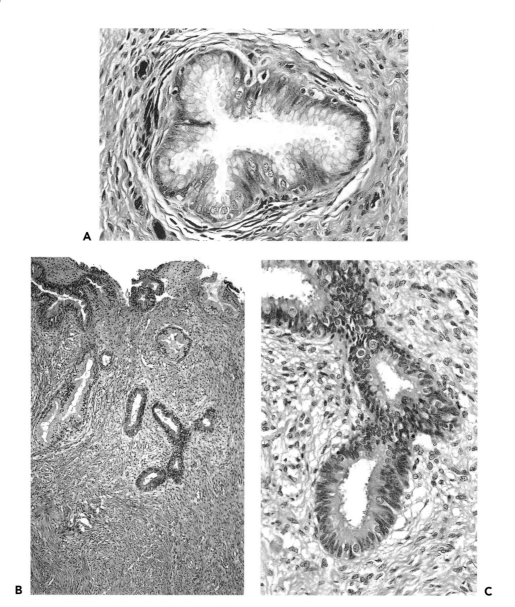

Figure 41.10 **A.** Ciliated cells in the endocervix. The normal cervical mucinous epithelium consists of an admixture of mucin-containing cells and a smaller population of ciliated cells. The population of ciliated cells undergoes cyclic variation with the menstrual cycle. **B.** Cervical tubal metaplasia. When ciliated cells are prominent they may simulate endocervical glandular dysplasia or carcinoma in situ. At low magnification the glands feature a prominence of nuclei, a feature shared with glandular dysplasia. **C.** Cervical tubal metaplasia. Higher magnification shows prominent cilia, the hallmark of ciliated cell metaplasia.

(Figure 41.11A). In histologic sections, these clefts typically are cut transversely, imparting the false impression that true endocervical glands are present within the stroma. However, true glands have different epithelia lining their ductal and secretory portions. In contrast, the endocervical mucosa has a more or less uniform appearance whether it lines the surface or the deep-lying "glands." Further evidence that these are not true glands was provided in an study conducted over 40 years ago by Fluhmann (72,73). He demonstrated, by means of serial sections and three-dimensional reconstructions, that what appeared to be

endocervical glands within the stroma are actually complex protrusions of the endocervical lining that form clefts into the underlying stroma. When the endocervical epithelium lining the stromal clefts proliferates, side channels grow out from the clefts, giving rise to a histologic pattern that even more closely suggests acini of glands (Figure 41.11B). Fluhmann labeled these side channels "tunnel clusters"; we also refer to them by a more euphonious designation: "Fluhmann's lumens." When secretion inspissates in tunnel clusters, either because of obstruction or because of the viscosity of the secretions, it appears as bright eosinophilic

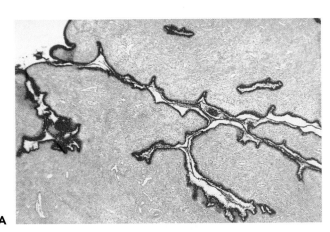
A

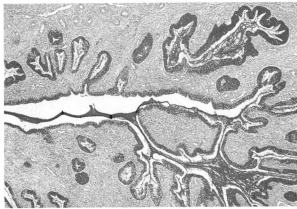
B

Figure 41.11 **A**. Tangential section of the endocervix stained with PAS to show how the gland clefts extend into the stroma and branch to form channels. **B**. When the endocervical mucosa undergoes hyperplasia and increases its surface area, as in pregnancy, the branches of the clefts proliferate and form even more collaterals ("tunnel clusters").

material, an eye-catching pattern resembling the thyroid (see Figure 41.16). Having now discharged our obligation to anatomic accuracy, we shall continue to use the terms endocervical "gland(s)" and "cleft(s)" interchangeably.

The depth to which benign endocervical glands can extend in the cervical stroma varies from cervix to cervix. They can be found as deep as 1 cm but usually are found at a depth of less than 5 mm (68,74,75). This anatomic variation becomes important when considering a diagnosis of "minimal deviation adenocarcinoma" (76,77). In this form of adenocarcinoma, the cytologic features differ only minimally from normal endocervical epithelium and the diagnosis depends to a large extent on the identification of abnormally shaped glands at an inappropriate depth within the cervical stroma. The trick here is to compare the depth of the glands in question with noncontroversially benign glands in the immediate neighborhood. Additionally useful in establishing a diagnosis of malignancy is a search for glands around nerves or vessels, an irregular "lobster claw" glandular configuration, and a granulation tissue stromal host response. We have not personally encountered a clinically malignant endocervical glandular proliferation that featured ciliated cells and, in our opinion, this finding argues strongly against a diagnosis of adenocarcinoma.

Endocervical cells show only minimal morphologic changes during the menstrual cycle, and even this amounts only to a shifting of the basally situated nuclei to a midcell position at the height of the proliferative phase. These minor cytologic changes are in contrast to the dramatic biochemical changes that occur within the endocervical cells during the menstrual cycle (46). Throughout the proliferative phase of the cycle, the endocervical cells secrete mucus of lower viscosity than at other times of the cycle. This is thought to aid penetration of the cervical canal by spermatozoa (46). When progesterone levels attain their zenith during the luteal phase, the endocervical glandular secre-

tion becomes thick and scant. It is at this stage that the secretion may become inspissated and more visible in histologic sections. During pregnancy the number of tunnel clusters increases, and when this phenomena is extreme the term "cervical glandular hyperplasia" is often used (78). Pregnancy also causes the secretions of the endocervical cells to thicken and form a mucous plug that blocks the endocervical canal (47,79).

Epithelium of the Transformation Zone

The endocervical mucosa shifts over the various divisions of the anatomic cervix throughout life (18,44,80). At birth, the endocervical mucosa resides on the exocervix in two thirds of infants but it quickly moves back into the anatomic endocervical canal where in most girls it remains until near the menarche. After the onset of puberty, the endocervical mucosa again moves out onto the exocervix, usually more prominently on the anterior portion than on the posterior part (Figure 41.12A). The mechanism whereby endocervical mucosa changes location is apparently a mechanical one caused by swelling of the stroma of the cervical tissue in response to hormonal stimulation. As the lips of the cervix swell, they roll anteriorly and posteriorly, pulling the endocervical mucosa out of the canal onto the exocervix. The exposed endocervical tissue is often referred to as ectropion. Because the exposed endocervical mucosa appears red and ulcerated to the naked eye, it also has been interpreted as an erosion. There is, in fact, no erosion of the mucosa, rather the process is one of physiologic ectopy. After menarchial ectropion occurs, the endocervical tissue is gradually replaced by squamous epithelium throughout the reproductive years. The area where the glandular tissue is being replaced by squamous epithelium is known as the transformation zone. The junction between the two types of epithelium is labeled the squamocolumnar junction

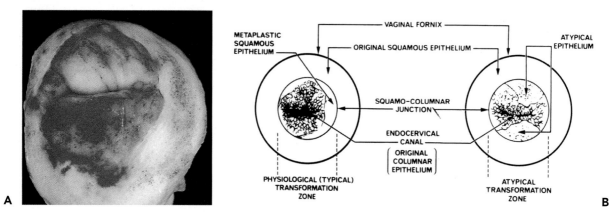

A

B

Figure 41.12 **A**. Multiparous cervix during the reproductive years. Note the slitlike configuration of the external os and the erythematous endocervical tissue out on the anatomic exocervix. This endocervical tissue undergoes conversion to squamous epithelium throughout the reproductive years. The squamocolumnar junction is visible as a sharp line between the white squamous epithelium and the erythematous glandular tissue. **B**. Diagram of the cervix demonstrating the transformation zone. On the left is a typical transformation zone in which metaplastic squamous epithelium is replacing endocervical columnar epithelium. "Squamocolumnar junction" refers to the original squamocolumnar junction. On the right is a nontypical transformation zone in which the metaplastic process is composed of dysplastic squamous cells and hence the process is cervical intraepithelial neoplasia. Reprinted with permission from: Fox H. *Haines and Taylor Obstetrical and Gynaecological Pathology*. 3rd ed. Philadelphia: WB Saunders; 1987.

(44,81). Two squamocolumnar junctions are usually recognized (Figure 41.12B). The original squamocolumnar junction is the point where the native (original) exocervical squamous epithelium joins the endocervical glandular epithelium and is out on the exocervix during the reproductive years (80). This junction is usually sharply defined and it is anatomically fixed. After squamous metaplasia has replaced endocervical tissue, the original squamocolumnar junction is the fusion point between the new squamous epithelium laid down in the transformation zone and the native squamous epithelium (Figure 41.13). The functional squamocolumnar junction is the point of active replacement of columnar endocervical epithelium by squamous cells. This junction is often irregular and patchy, and it changes its contours and its locations during reproductive life. The functional squamocolumnar junction is usually implied when the term "squamocolumnar junction" is used without a modifier and the area between the two squamocolumnar junctions is the transformation zone. During pregnancy, particularly the first pregnancy, even more endocervical tissue moves out onto the exocervix, enlarging the area of ectopic endocervical epithelium. This phenomenon also can occur during progestogen therapy.

Because endocervical glandular epithelium is present on the exocervix, the transformation zone can be visualized with the aid of a colposcope. This is fortunate because neoplastic change begins most commonly in the transformation zone, and neoplastic transformation is accompanied by structural alterations that can be recognized using the colposcope. The combination of papilloma virus detection, cytologic preparations, colposcopic examination, biopsy,

and local destruction of intraepithelial abnormalities in the transformation zone under colposcopic visualization is a powerful tool for the early detection and successful treatment of in situ neoplastic processes involving the cervix.

In the latter years of reproductive life the functional squamocolumnar junction reaches the area near the anatomic external os and, reversing its menarchal journey, begins to move up the anatomic endocervical canal. By the perimenopausal years, the squamocolumnar junction is usually concealed within the endocervical canal above the external os.

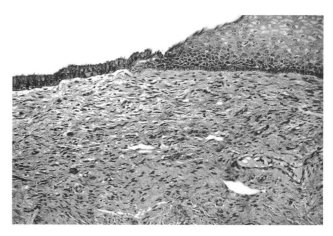

Figure 41.13 Squamocolumnar junction with a distinct transition from mature squamous epithelium on the right to endocervical glandular tissue on the left. Such a sharp change can be seen at the original squamocolumnar junction as well as the junction formed by squamous epithelium with endocervical tissue in the transformation zone when squamous epithelium is mature.

Two mechanisms are thought to be operative in transforming endocervical mucinous epithelium to squamous epithelium: squamous epithelialization and squamous metaplasia (3). The first involves the direct ingrowth of mature native squamous epithelium from the exocervix. This process is usually labeled "squamous epithelialization." During squamous epithelialization, mature squamous cells come to lie beneath the endocervical glandular cells. They push the endocervical cells off the basement membrane, and gradually the columnar cells degenerate and are sloughed. Squamous epithelialization initially spares the openings of the underlying endocervical glands, and at this stage the openings to the glands have the appearance of pores when examined with the colposcope. Eventually, the ingrowth of squamous epithelium involves the orifices of the glandular clefts and then it can extend for varying distances down into the cleft spaces (Figures 41.14 and 41.15). When this process involves the orifice, it may plug the opening and if the mucinous epithelium below continues to secrete, a mucin-filled cyst (Nabothian cyst) or tunnel clusters filled with eosinophilic secretion result (Figure 41.16). If squamous epithelialization involves the cleft and its ramifying tunnels, squamous epithelium will be surrounded by endocervical stroma. Consequently, histologic sections taken in an area of squamous epithelialization may show Nabothian cysts, mucification of tunnel clusters, and/or islands of benign squamous epithelium in the stroma beneath the surface epithelium.

When the endocervical clefts undergo squamous epithelialization, care must be taken not to confuse the deep-lying benign squamous cells with invasive carcinoma. Although the cells in squamous epithelialization may have enlarged nuclei and prominent nucleoli, they do not demonstrate the anaplasia, the pleomorphism, the chro-

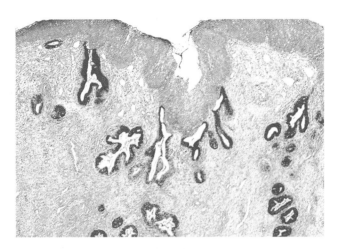

Figure 41.15 Conversion to squamous epithelium in the cervix may occur more rapidly on the surface than in the clefts, causing squamous epithelium to overlie endocervical gland clefts. When the newly laid down squamous epithelium blocks the orifices of the clefts, nabothian cysts or mucification of tunnel clusters, as seen in Figure 41.16, may result.

matin abnormalities, or the abnormal mitotic figures characteristic of invasive carcinoma. Moreover, the benign cells conform to the rounded configuration of the preexisting cleft and do not infiltrate the stroma irregularly. Typically there is no granulation tissue host response to squamous epithelialization, although chronic inflammation may be present. If squamous epithelialization involves tunnel clusters, small groups of squamous cells come to lie deep within the cervical stroma, imparting an architectural pattern that even more resembles infiltrating squamous cell carcinoma. Squamous epithelialization seems to be stimulated by chronic inflammation and local trauma, including cauterization or laser surgery.

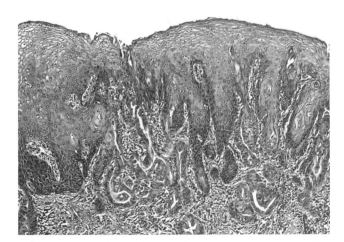

Figure 41.14 Squamous epithelialization of the endocervix. Note the mature squamous epithelium extending into endocervical gland clefts (PAS positive glandular structures surrounded by stroma). This process can mimic invasive carcinoma.

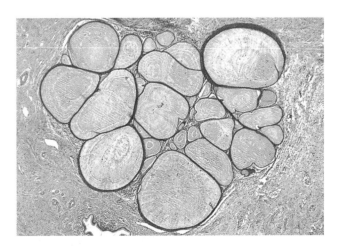

Figure 41.16 When the newly formed squamous epithelium in the transformation zone covers the endocervical gland cleft orifices and secretion continues, the tunnel clusters fill up with secretion that may become inspissated ("mucification").

The second mechanism thought to contribute to the conversion of endocervical mucinous epithelium to squamous epithelium entails first the proliferation of endocervical "reserve cells," and then the differentiation of these cells into squamous cells rather than mucin-producing cells (82). This process, known as squamous metaplasia or prosoplasia, can be distinguished from squamous epithelialization because, unlike the cells in squamous epithelialization, the reserve cells initially do not have squamous characteristics; rather, they appear as cuboidal cells with round nuclei growing beneath the mucinous epithelium (Figure 41.17). In fact, these cuboidal cells are identical in appearance to the basal or parabasal cells of the squamous epithelium. After the reserve cells proliferate and stratify, they differentiate into squamous cells that initially have only slightly increased amounts of cytoplasm (immature squamous metaplasia). Later the cells may fully mature to glycogen-containing squamous cells indistinguishable from the superficial cells of the exocervix (see Figure 41.13). Confusingly, "squamous metaplasia" is commonly used as a generic term for both metaplasia and squamous epithelialization.

Immature squamous metaplastic cells without fully developed squamous characteristics or glycogen accumulation can come to occupy most or all of the thickness of an epithelium (83,84) (Figure 41.18). Because fully mature squamous cells are not present toward the surface and because the cytoplasm of the immature cells is relatively scant and its nuclei often are elongate, immature squamous metaplasia can bear a close resemblance to high grade intraepithelial neoplasia (dysplasia–carcinoma in situ). However, the nuclei in immature squamous metaplasia are uniform, chromatin abnormalities are minimal at most, and nuclear contours are usually smooth. Although mitotic figures may be present, in

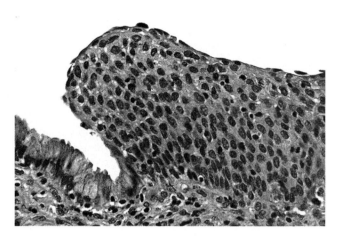

Figure 41.18 Immature squamous metaplasia on the right. The constituent cells do not demonstrate evidence of maturation and are similar to cells normally present in the basal layer of squamous epithelium. This type of metaplasia can be confused with high-grade squamous intraepithelial neoplasia.

immature squamous metaplasia abnormal forms are not found. The possibility of immature squamous metaplasia should be considered in each case where a diagnosis of intraepithelial neoplasia is contemplated.

Squamous metaplasia is usually patchy, giving rise to the characteristic irregularity of the functional squamocolumnar junction (Figures 41.19A, B). As squamous metaplasia proceeds, the islands of squamous cells form bridges to other centers of metaplasia, ultimately producing a solid area of squamous epithelium.

Whatever the mechanism—either squamous epithelialization or squamous metaplasia—squamous replacement of mucinous epithelium on the exocervix is a normal process that must be distinguished from in situ and invasive neoplasms. Features that are often found in neoplasia but not in metaplasia or epithelialization are moderate to marked pleomorphism, lack of maturation sequence (this may be present in immature squamous metaplasia), irregular nuclear outlines, and abnormal mitotic figures. Nucleoli are usually inconspicuous in cervical intraepithelial neoplasia but are often prominent in metaplasia, and epithelialization (a notable exception is immature squamous metaplasia), and reactive changes in response to cervicitis.

Cervical Stroma

In contrast to the wall of the uterine corpus, which is predominately muscular, the stroma of the exocervix is mainly fibrous tissue admixed with elastin through which run infrequent strands of smooth muscle (85–88). A large number of vessels course through the stroma. A rich capillary network interfaces with the epithelium at the stromal–epithelial junction. This interface is irregular and features

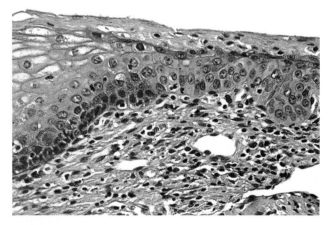

Figure 41.17 Functional squamocolumnar junction with metaplastic epithelium on the right. Note that in this example maturation has proceeded to the parabasal cell stage with abrupt keratinization rather than the normal maturation sequence to superficial cells as seen on the left.

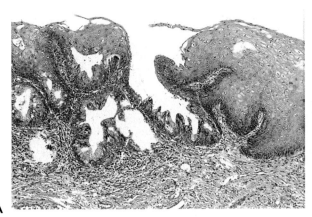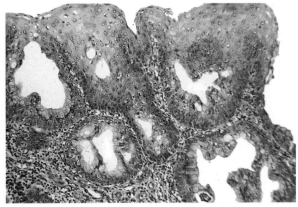

Figure 41.19 **A.** Islands of metaplastic squamous epithelium in the transformation zone at the functional squamocolumnar junction. These islands will eventually coalesce. **B.** Higher power photomicrograph of the area of squamous metaplasia demonstrated in A.

fingers of connective tissue containing vessels overlain by a squamous cell mucosa of variable thickness. Much of the endocervical stroma is also fibroelastic tissue, but at the upper end of the endocervix the superficial fibrous stroma blends imperceptibly into the endometrial stroma of the lower uterine segment. Consequently, the superficial stroma of the upper endocervix and the stroma of the lower uterine segment has a hybrid endometrial–cervical appearance. This can cause localization problems when it is important to determine whether a neoplastic process in a curettage specimen involves the endometrium or the endocervix, or both. We think the presence of unequivocal endometrial stroma, as determined by high cellularity (closely packed nuclei), should be present before interpreting tissue as originating from the endometrium on the basis of the stroma alone. Of course, if one type of normal glands is present, whether endocervical or endometrial, these glands can suggest the origin of the tissue, but both types of glands or even hybrid glands may be present in the transition area between the endocervix and the lower uterine segment. The endocervix contains a greater number of smooth muscle fibers in its deeper stroma than does the exocervix, and in the lower uterine segment these blend into the myometrium.

The cervix bridges the sterile environment of the uterine cavity and the microbiological jungle of the lower genital tract. It is not surprising that this important immunologic role (both humoral and cellular) would be marked by a conspicuous lymphoid presence (44). Thus, large numbers of T-lymphocytes normally populate the endocervical stroma (89). B-lineage lymphoid cells, manifest as either plasma cells or germinal centers, are also commonly encountered.

In addition, dendritic cells are numerous in the cervix; a subset of these are Langerhans cells (immature dendritic cells that express MHC class II antigens and the CD4 receptor on their surface) that are involved in internalizing antigen and presenting it to T-lymphocytes in the regional lymph nodes (58,90–92).

The relevance of these observations to the surgical pathologist is chiefly to discourage the overuse of "chronic cervicitis"; the presence of lymphoid tissue in the cervix is as normal as its presence in the small intestine.

In our opinion, a diagnosis of chronic cervicitis should be withheld unless the lymphoid infiltrate is very heavy and/or lymphoid nodules are numerous. Particularly important for the diagnosis of chronic cervicitis are large numbers of plasma cells. Scattered plasma cells are normal in the cervix. Acute cervicitis is not uncommon, but true inflammatory erosion or microabscesses are rare in the cervix.

Lymphocytes also may migrate into the endocervical epithelium, and in this location they may assume the appearance of "cleared cells." Such cells have been misconstrued as "reserve" cells in the past (71).

Remnants of the wolffian duct—commonly known as mesonephric rests—can be found in the endocervical stroma of the lateral portions of the cervix in about a third of women (93) (Figure 41.20A, B). Usually these are deep in the stroma, but occasionally they are found near the surface and they can even blend with the endocervical gland clefts. Mesonephric rests are tubular structures lined by a single row of cuboidal cells with a central, round, cytologically bland nucleus. Typically the tubules form lumens that contain hyalin-like, eosinophilic secretions. Architecturally, there is usually a central elongate duct surrounded by smaller tubules. The combination of deep stromal location, the hyalin-like secretions, and the cuboidal cells usually serves to make identification of mesonephric rests straightforward. Even though tunnel clusters may ramify from a central cleft and contain eosinophilic secretion, they are lined by endocervical mucin-producing cells. The importance of this vestigial structure lies in its mimicry of

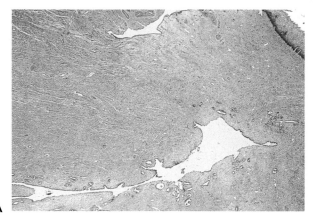
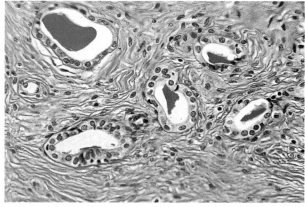

Figure 41.20 **A**. Mesonephric remnants in the cervix. A long cleftlike space deep in the stroma surrounded by tubules is the characteristic architectural finding. **B**. Ducts lined by bland cuboidal cells containing lumenal PAS-positive eosinophilic secretion are key features of mesonephric remnants. The blandness of the constituent cells and the organization around a central cleft are the most helpful features in distinguishing this from well-differentiated adenocarcinoma.

well-differentiated adenocarcinoma. Mitotic figures are usually absent in mesonephric rests and the chromatin of the cells is bland. Moreover, mesonephric rests do not exhibit the raggedly infiltrative growth of carcinoma even though they are located deep in the stroma. Rarely, atypical hyperplastic and neoplastic processes may involve mesonephric remnants (78,93,94). Mesonephric proliferations, benign and malignant, often express CD10 (95,96).

Multinucleated giant cells rarely are found in the normal superficial endocervical stroma. These cells have enlarged and sometimes bizarre-shaped nuclei with smudged chromatin similar to those seen in fibroepithelial stromal polyps (97). They should not be mistaken for a neoplasm (98–100).

Cervix During Pregnancy

During pregnancy the endocervical epithelium proliferates so that its mucus-secreting surface increases. This proliferation leads to both the formation of polypoid protrusions of endocervical epithelium into the endocervical canal and an increased number of tunnel clusters budding off preexisting clefts within the cervical stroma. The overall impression is one of an increase in the amount of endocervical tissue and, consequently, this normal process is often termed "endocervical glandular hyperplasia," or when numerous small glands are packed together, "microglandular hyperplasia." Identical changes can be produced by artificial progestogens. The endocervical mucus during pregnancy is thick and functions as a plug to seal off the endometrial cavity from the vagina (22,101). Arias-Stella reaction may be seen in the endocervical glandular cells (102). As in the endometrium, the large cells with prominent nucleoli characteristic of the Arias-Stella reaction can raise concern about clear cell carcinoma, but the absence of mitotic

figures and the gestational setting should quickly eliminate this possibility.

The stroma of the cervix undergoes a complex series of biochemical and biomechanical changes during pregnancy and parturition that taken together are known as cervical "ripening" (103). The initial change seems to be extensive destruction of collagen fibers by various collagenases accompanied by the accumulation of gel-like acid mucopolysaccharides. This process causes the cervix to soften, a process that reaches its zenith immediately before parturition. As a result, the cervix is easily effaced by the presenting part of the emerging infant. Thus, the usually cylindrical cervix is transformed into a thin saccular structure. The increased fluid in the cervical stroma during pregnancy causes the cervical lips to roll further out into the vagina, everting more of the endocervical mucosa beyond the external os. Squamous epithelialization and metaplasia rapidly ensue, and at the time of delivery there is often considerable immature squamous epithelium in the transformation zone. As noted previously, the cells in immature squamous metaplasia can closely resemble those found in intraepithelial neoplasia, so caution should be exercised when examining cervical specimens taken from pregnant women.

The cervical stromal cells, particularly those near the surface of the endocervical canal, may undergo decidual change during pregnancy (Figure 41.21A, B). Cervical decidual reaction is typically patchy, and at low power this focal replacement of the cervical stroma by aggregates of epithelioid cells can resemble invasive large cell nonkeratinizing carcinoma. Awareness of this physiologic process during pregnancy and close attention to the cytologic features of the suspect cells should avoid misdiagnosis (104).

Normal findings in the cervix that have relevance to histopathologic differential diagnosis are presented in Table 41.1.

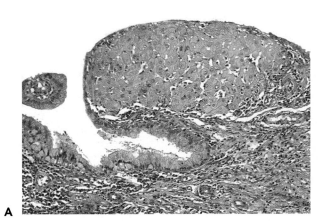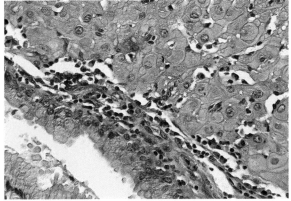

A   B

Figure 41.21 **A.** and **B.** Decidual reaction in the cervix. The sheetlike arrangement of the cells can mimic squamous cell carcinoma, but the nuclei are bland (see Figure 41.18).

ENDOMETRIUM

Tissue Sampling and Associated Problems

A variety of endometrial tissue sampling techniques are available to the clinician. These techniques differ with respect to their indications, their limitations, and their associated complications (105–113). Endometrial curettage (cervical dilation and endometrial curettage—D and C) entails the removal of most of the uterine mucosa by scraping with a sharp curette. Under ideal circumstances, the excision is complete or nearly complete. Endometrial biopsy (EMB) involves the removal of a more limited sample of tissue than does the complete curettage and is performed with a smaller curette. Single strips of endometrium are usually taken from both the anterior and the posterior fundal surfaces. Even though the sample is limited, the accuracy of diagnosis approximates that of the D and C. The chief advantage of this technique is that it does not require cervical dilation (and hence does not require anesthesia). EMB thus combines convenience and low cost, with little sacrifice in diagnostic accuracy. The major limitation of EMB lies in its inherent potential to miss focal lesions, such as polyps and localized carcinomas. Accordingly, when carcinoma is suspected clinically, a negative biopsy must be followed by a complete D and C, because only this technique ensures the absence of carcinoma. Hysteroscopy in combination with endometrial sampling is thought by some to increase the detection rate of uterine abnormalities (114); others disagree (115). If EMB is performed as part of an infertility workup (but see below), tissue should be obtained well into the presumed secretory phase; that is, 2 to 3 days before the time of the next menstrual period as estimated by clinical and laboratory findings. Although principle biopsy in the late luteal phase might destroy an early gestation, in practice this seems not to be the case (116).

Three artifacts of sectioning and tissue preparation should be mentioned at this point. A frequent finding in endometrial curettings is the "telescoped" gland, which is characterized by an "inside-out" gland within the lumen of a gland with a normal configuration. This artifact is seen when an intussuscepted or telescoped gland (produced by the traumatic removal of the tissue) is cross-sectioned, and it occurs most frequently in straight glands. Another artifact is the result of sectioning and involves the tangential cutting of a gland to produce a "pseudo-gland-within-gland" pattern. Confusion with adenocarcinoma can be avoided by attention to cytologic detail, comparison with surrounding glands, knowledge that the gland-within-gland pattern in carcinoma is usually extensive, and awareness of this topologic problem. A third artifact involves tangential sectioning of the endometrial surface to produce pseudocystic and pseudobudded glands. Poor fixation can sometimes result in the retraction of endometrial glands from their surrounding stromal envelope. Moreover, cytoplasmic vacuolization may be a result of autolysis and can simulate early secretory vacuolated epithelium.

Histology of the Normal Endometrium

The normal endometrium has a multiplicity of constantly changing normal patterns that depend on the nature and intensity of ovarian hormonal stimulation. The purpose of this section is to analyze the morphology of the normal nongravid endometrium in some detail from three points of view. First, we discuss regional variations, then the individual components of the endometrium; finally, using this background, we describe the temporal variations in the histology of the endometrium that occur throughout life.

TABLE 41.1

NORMAL FINDINGS IN THE CERVIX THAT HAVE RELEVANCE TO HISTOPATHOLOGIC DIFFERENTIAL DIAGNOSIS *(see text for additional differential diagnostic clues)*

Finding	Diagnostic Confusion	Suggestions for Resolution	References
Deeply situated normal endocervical gland clefts or Nabothian cysts	Minimal deviation adenocarcinoma (MDC)	Lobster claw configuration in MDC Ciliated cells in benign proliferations and almost always absent in malignant cervical glandular proliferations	68,74,75,262
Easily found mitotic figures in endocervical epithelium	Adenocarcinoma: invasive or in situ	Cytologic atypia in carcinoma Compare problematic epithelium with normal epithelium elsewhere	
In normal endocervical epithelium mitotic figures are rare. In squamous metaplasia and regenerating cervical epithelium mitotic figures may be numerous but abnormal forms are not present.			
Mesonephric remnants: mesonephric remnants, especially when florid, must be distinguished from invasive adenocarcinoma, especially minimal deviation adenocarcinoma.	Minimal deviation adenocarcinoma (MDC): mesonephric carcinoma	MDC often has an associated superficial component of ACIS The glands of mesonephric remnants are rounded and smooth contoured; those of carcinoma are usually jagged and infiltrative; the glands of Mesonephric remnants branch of a central, elongate, ductal structure, those of invasive adenocarcinoma are haphazard and lack a central originating duct.	93
Decidual reaction	Large cell nonkeratinizing squamous cell carcinoma	Mitotic figures, cytologic atypia in carcinoma	
Arias-Stella reaction	Clear cell carcinoma of the cervix/vagina	Arias-Stella reaction usually does not feature mitotic figures that are easily found in clear cell carcinoma. Maternal DES therapy was discontinued in the 1960s	102,223
Lower uterine segment vs. endocervical fragments: can make a difference when carcinoma (endocervical vs. endometrial) is found in curettings.		Differential curettage; imaging studies. Immunohistochemistry (stains for CEA and p16 often positive in endocervical carcinoma and negative in endometrial). Are not entirely reliable in the individual case but may be helpful.	
Squamous metaplasia and epithelialization involving cervical gland clefts	Invasive carcinoma	Assess nuclear features and evaluation for the presence or absence of infiltration	

(continued)

TABLE 41.1
(continued)

Finding	Diagnostic Confusion	Suggestions for Resolution	References
Endometriosis: benign endometrial glands and stroma	Adenocarcinoma: when stroma is inconspicuous Adenosarcoma: look for stromal mitotic figures	Think of the possibility of endometriosis Look for the missing component in additional levels Cytologic atypia is usually minimal in endometriosis but mitotic figures may be present	263–265
Microglandular adenosis and endocervical glandular hyperplasia	Adenocarcinoma	Prominent nucleoli and abnormal division figures are features of carcinoma. Easily found mitotic figures almost always are a carcinoma feature.	266,267
Immature squamous metaplasia	High-grade SIL: may mimic because nuclei of the cells are large and cytoplasm is relatively scant.	Look for nucleoli—often present in metaplasia, but often inconspicuous in CIN—and abnormal mitotic figures and abnormal chromatin patterns. Nucleoli may not be prominent *immature* squamous metaplasia	84
Glycogen storage in superficial squamous cells	Koilocytosis (HPV infection).	Koilocytic nuclei: (1) enlarged, (2) irregular nuclear membranes, (3) dense ropy chromatin.	
Tubal metaplasia: endocervical pithelium lined by prominent and numerous ciliated cells may suggest adenocarcinoma in situ or endometrioid carcinoma	Cervical adenocarcinoma in situ	Numerous mitoticfigures and abnormal mitotic figures are features for adeno CIS not tubal metaplasia. Look for ciliated cells; if numerous, the process is almost surely benign.	63–67,69
Multinucleated stromal giant cells: these may be a normal finding; probably myofibroblastic cells	Neoplasm, particularly sarcoma. Granulomatous inflammation	Look for abnormal mitotic figures, high cellularity, and granulomas.	

Reprinted with permission from: Young RH, Clement PB. Pseudoneoplastic glandular lesions of the uterine cervix. *Semin Diagn Pathol* 1991;8:234–249.

Regional Variations

The uterine lining can be divided into two regions on the basis of its morphology: the mucosa of the lower uterine segment and the mucosa of the corpus proper. The mucosa of the lower uterine segment (isthmus) is in general thinner than the fundal mucosa. The glands and stroma tend to be only sluggishly responsive to hormonal stimulation, and in consequence this portion of the endometrium most often lags behind the rest of the endometrium in its development. The morphologic transition from endocervical mucosa to lower uterine segment mucosa is gradual, and in fact the hybrid endocervical–endometrial appearance of both the glands and the stroma of the lower uterine segment serves to identify this zone in endometrial curettings (Figures 41.22).

The major portion of the uterine lining, the corpus mucosa proper, is normally fully responsive to hormonal stimulation. Two layers can be readily identified within the endometrium throughout this region: the lowermost is labeled the basalis and the overlying one the functionalis. The basalis is that zone of weakly proliferative glands and associated dense-spindled stroma immediately adjacent to the myometrium (Figure 41.23A, B). Characteristically, the junction of the basalis and myometrium is irregular, and smooth muscle and endometrial stroma interdigitate and blend together at this point (Figure 41.24). When florid, this irregularity may give the false impression that endometrial tissue is pathologically isolated within the myometrium. This deception is particularly important when evaluating the presence or absence of superficial myometrial invasion

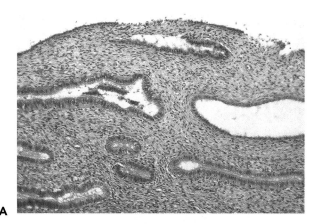
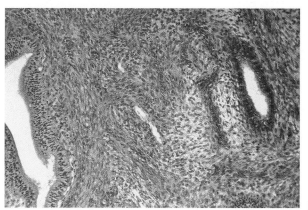

Figure 41.22 The lower uterine segment contains stroma and glands that are either hybrid between those seen in the endocervix and those in the fundus or a mixture of endometrial and endocervical glands and stroma. **A.** The stroma appears fibrous but more cellular than that typically found in the endocervix. **B.** An endometrial gland and an endocervical gland are found next to each other in this area of the lower uterine cervix.

in patients with endometrial adenocarcinoma. Of less importance is the confusion it creates in the diagnosis of adenomyosis. The basalis, despite its unimpressive, inactive, and undifferentiated appearance, plays a crucial role in the endometrial economy because it constitutes the "reserve cell layer" of the endometrium. After the bulk of the overlying functionalis is shed during menstruation, or after the functionalis is removed by curettage, the basalis and the residual deep functionalis are responsible for regenerating the endometrium. The remaining surface epithelium of the lower uterine segment also participates in this regeneration (117).

The appearance of the basalis is relatively constant throughout the menstrual cycle. Specifically, the glands usually appear weakly proliferative; that is, they possess pseudostratified elongate nuclei, rare mitotic figures, and dense, intensely basophilic chromatin. Most importantly, they lack secretory change (see Figure 41.23), and the stroma is spindled and nondecidualized. A notable exception to this generalization is the basalis during the latter half of pregnancy, which usually exhibits secretory glandular changes and stromal decidualization. The importance of recognizing the basalis of the endometrium lies in not mistaking it for the functionalis in a curettage specimen. This confusion would result in an erroneous impression that this weakly proliferative appearance represented the fully developed state of the functionalis.

It is the functionalis that exhibits the protean changes so characteristic of the normal endometrium. This layer has been traditionally divided into two strata—the compactum and the spongiosum—based on the morphologic

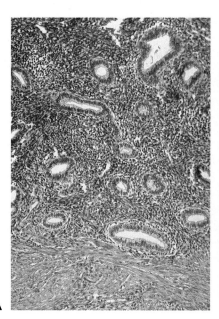
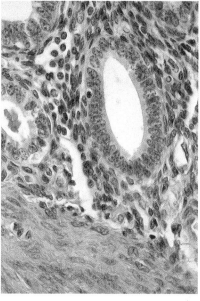

Figure 41.23 **A.** and **B.** The basalis of the endometrium is demonstrated. Throughout the menstrual cycle the basalis maintains a weakly proliferative appearance. As a result, dating of endometrium should be performed on fragments containing surface epithelium.

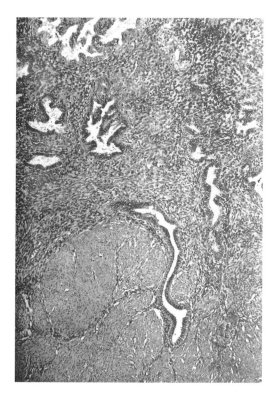

Figure 41.24 This is an example of an irregular endometrial—myometrial junction. This phenomenon is important to think about when determining whether or not adenocarcinoma is superficially invading the myometrium.

appearances of each during the late secretory phase of the menstrual cycle and during pregnancy. Unless otherwise specified, the term "endometrium" refers to the functionalis in the subsequent discussion.

Individual Components of the Endometrium

The normal endometrium consists of both epithelial (surface and glandular) and mesenchymal (stromal and vascular) elements, which during reproductive years first synchronously proliferate, then differentiate, and finally disintegrate at roughly monthly intervals.

Epithelial Elements

The endometrial glandular and surface epithelia are both composed of four morphologically distinct cells, two of which are functional variants of the same cell.

Proliferative and Basalis-Type Cells. The proliferative cells of the functionalis and the basalis-type cells are morphologically similar. These cells both have high nucleus-to-cytoplasm ratios and elongate sausage-shaped nuclei with dense chromatin and inconspicuous nucleoli. The cytoplasm is scant and generally basophilic to amphophilic (see Figure 41.33). Mitotic figures are common in the cells that compose the glands of the functionalis during the proliferative phase.

When proliferative cells are the predominant cell type composing the epithelium (as in the proliferative endometrium), the nuclei appear pseudostratified.

Secretory Cells. The characteristic cytoplasmic differentiation of the endometrial epithelial cell is nonmucinous secretion. Shortly after ovulation, secretory products accumulate in a subnuclear location in the proliferative cells; these products gradually shift to a supranuclear position and are ultimately discharged into the glandular lumens. This sequence of changes results in two easily recognizable secretory cell types: vacuolated and nonvacuolated secretory cells (see Figures 41.35B and 41.36C). Although vacuolated cells may have a nucleus similar to those seen in proliferative phase cells, the nonvacuolated secretory cells possess nuclei that are distinct from those seen in the undifferentiated proliferative phase cells. In contrast to the dense, intensely basophilic elongate nuclei of the proliferative cells, the nuclei of the nonvacuolated secretory cells are rounded and vesicular, they have uniformly dispersed chromatin, and occasionally nucleoli become prominent. The nonvacuolated secretory cells have uniform, moderately dense eosinophilic cytoplasm and often a frayed luminal border (see Figure 41.36C).

Another type of secretory cell is encountered, one that closely resembles the secretory cell of the uterine (fallopian) tube. This cell has an elongate nucleus with coarse chromatin, a moderate amount of densely eosinophilic cytoplasm, and a rounded luminal bleb similar to those found in apocrine glands. These cells are common in the surface epithelium and occasionally may line an entire endometrial gland. Some of these cells may in fact represent "exhausted" ciliated cells.

Ciliated Cells. The ciliated cells of the endometrium have received little emphasis in the past. However, they are consistently present in endometrial specimens and presumably represent one line of differentiation open to the basalis-type cell. These cells are more prominent near the uterine isthmus and during the proliferative phase (118,119).

Ciliated cells have distinctive round, smoothly contoured vesicular nuclei containing finely stippled chromatin (Figure 41.25). Although the nuclear features remain relatively unchanged throughout cell development, the configuration and location of ciliated cells vary as a function of the stage of ciliogenesis. The earliest identifiable ciliated cells are situated adjacent to the basal lamina of the gland and are roughly pyramidal in shape. They possess distinctively clear cytoplasm with central round nuclei. A rounded cytoplasmic zone containing eosinophilic fibrillary material can be identified with routine stains. This zone corresponds to the intracytoplasmic cilia seen with the electron microscope. When the growing ciliated cells reach the luminal surface, the cilia are exposed to the glandular lumen. Initially the

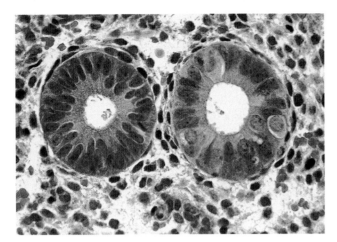

Figure 41.25 Proliferative phase glands with ciliated cells in the gland on the right. The round cell with clear cytoplasm at the 3-o'clock position has the characteristic appearance of ciliated cells before they have extruded their cilia into the glandular lumen. The other ciliated cells have a pyramidal shape.

luminal surface of the ciliated cell is concave, but as the cell continues its development, this surface becomes convex, and ultimately the cilia may pinch off as a merocrine secretion. During this stage the cell has a characteristic fusiform-to-pear shape. Ciliated cells can come to predominate the cellular population of glands, and when they do the term "ciliary metaplasia" has been used.

The Gland as a Whole. The normal endometrial gland is lined by the aforementioned cells arranged in a nonstratified cuboidal-to-columnar epithelium, which during the proliferative phase deceptively appears to be stratified (i.e., it is pseudostratified). During the early proliferative phase, the glands are straight and have narrow lumens (Figure 41.26). Beginning in the midproliferative period and lasting throughout the rest of the cycle, the glands exhibit increasing degrees of coiling, but not branching. This culminates in the serrated saw-toothed appearance of the glands in the late secretory and menstrual endometrium. The surface epithelium is composed predominantly of apocrine-like secretory cells and ciliated cells, and has a relatively constant appearance throughout the cycle.

Mesenchymal Elements

Cellular Elements

Endometrial Stroma

The endometrial stromal cell is the predominant cellular component of the stroma, and its appearance varies greatly with the stage of the menstrual cycle. During the early proliferative phase these cells have scant indistinct cytoplasm and dense oval-to-fusiform nuclei (Figure 41.27). As the menstrual cycle proceeds, the stromal cells become more elongate and acquire more cytoplasm. During the late proliferative phase and well into the secretory phase, electron microscopy shows increasing amounts of rough endoplasmic reticulum and both intra- and extracytoplasmic collagen. Toward the end of the secretory phase, the perivascular stromal cells become rounded, acquire more cytoplasm, and develop vesicular nuclei with occasionally prominent nucleoli. Cytoplasmic borders become more fully developed and gradually the entire endometrial stroma is transformed into sheets of cells, polygonal cells with sharp and distinct cytoplasmic borders, abundant cytoplasm, and centrally placed vesicular nuclei (Figure 41.28A, B).

This unique müllerian stromal transformation is called decidualization when fully developed (e.g., during pregnancy) and predecidualization when partially developed (e.g., during the late secretory phase of the menstrual cycle) (120). Ultrastructurally, the abundant cytoplasm of the decidual cell is populated by dilated rough endoplasmic

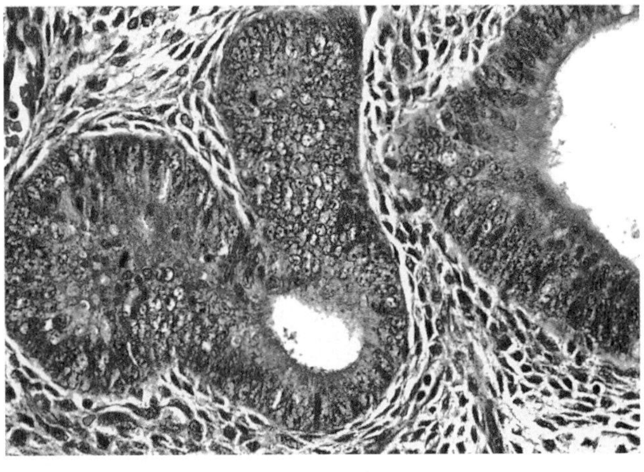

Figure 41.26 Proliferative phase glands and stroma. Note the elongate rather than rounded shape of the stromal cell nuclei. However, it is not uncommon for stromal cell nuclei to be elongate.

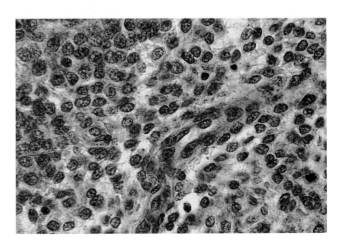

Figure 41.27 The proliferative phase endometrial stromal cells have scant, hard-to-discern cytoplasm and usually round nuclei (see Figure 41.26). Thin walled tubular blood vessels populate the endometrial stroma.

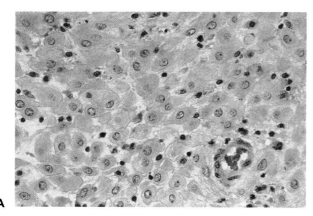 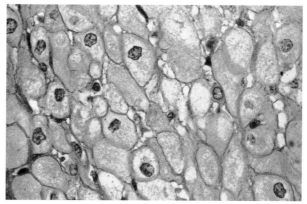

A   B

Figure 41.28 **A**. and **B**. These photomicrographs demonstrate decidual reaction during pregnancy. The cells have abundant cytoplasm and sharp cell margins.

reticulum, Golgi apparatus, and distinctly small mitochondria. Decidual cells form basal lamina and have complex intercellular interdigitations and tight junctions. The prominent intercellular borders are due to the accumulation of pericellular matrix (121).

Thus, the decidua is the specialized endometrium of pregnancy and plays an active role in implantation and in mediating the relationship between the fetoplacental unit and the mother. The decidua secretes a host of products (prolactin, relaxin, renin, insulin-like growth factors (IGFs) and insulin-like growth factor binding proteins (IGFBPs) involved in the paracrine and autocrine regulation of the feto-maternal interface (13,122). In short, the endometrium of pregnancy functions as an endocrine organ. In addition, decidual cells appear to be capable of phagocytosis and are thought to play a role dismantling the collagen scaffolding at the implantation site (106).

Hematolymphoid Cells

A second prominent cellular constituent, particularly in the late secretory phase and during pregnancy, is what historically has been referred to as the "stromal granulocyte" but is now known to be a uterine natural killer (uNK) cell (123). These are rounded cells with bilobed nuclei, and have pale cytoplasm that contains eosinophilic granules. Their immunoprofile differs from that of blood natural killer (NK) cells. Their number appears to be positively correlated with the degree of predicidualization or decidualization in the surrounding endometrium; indeed, the number of such cells was used by Noyes as a dating criterion. This close association has suggested to some workers that uNKs play a role in the control of trophoblast invasion and spiral artery remodelling in human pregnancy and suggest that uNK cells in the late secretory phase and in early decidua may be important in initiating and maintaining decidualization. Alternatively, the death of uNK cells might be an early event in the onset of endometrial breakdown at menstruation (124–126).

In addition to this unique uNK cell, the endometrium contains other leukocyte subsets whose precise composition is menstrual cycle-dependent. These subsets include neutrophils and eosinophils (both rare until the premenstrual phase); macrophages; mast cells, and T-lymphocyte populations (present throughout the cycle but increasing perimenstrually) (13,127,128). Lymphoid follicles are commonly seen in the basalis of normal endometria (Figure 41.29).

Plasma cells are routinely seen in postpartum endometrial samplings and as an associated feature in a variety of pathological settings (endometrial polyps, endometrial carcinoma, etc.) It has traditionally been held that, outside these settings, plasma cells are normally not present in the endometrium and when identified, suggest (usually subclinical) endometritis. Certainly this is plausible when large numbers are present, although recent studies have raised questions about the clinical relevance of scattered plasma cells (129,130). In fact, small numbers of

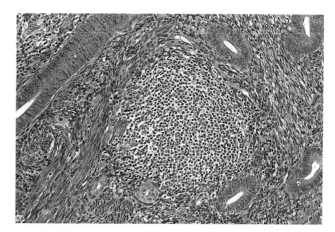

Figure 41.29 Lymphoid follicle. Scattered lymphoid follicles may be encountered in clinically normal women with otherwise unremarkable endometria. When present in large numbers and when associated with plasma cells, this finding is pathological.

B-lymphocytes and plasma cells can be detected in endometrial samples using flow cytometry (127).

Occasionally, cells with bean-shaped nuclei and abundant vacuolated lipid-containing cytoplasm are present in the stroma of endometria stimulated by estrogen. These are termed stromal foam cells and probably represent modifications of endometrial stromal cells (Figure 41.30). Similar appearing foam cells are seen as a component of an inflammatory infiltrate, particularly one produced by foreign material (e.g., keratin).

Reticulin Framework

The endometrial stromal cells elaborate a reticulin framework that becomes progressively denser as the endometrium develops during the menstrual cycle, so that by the late secretory phase each stromal cell is enmeshed in reticulin. This framework undergoes dissolution during menstruation. The stromal intercellular space is also rich in high-molecular-weight mucopolysaccharides during the midproliferative and late secretory phase.

Vascular Elements

The radial arteries of the endometrium derive from the myometrial arcuate system. As the radial arteries course toward the uterine cavity they give off basal branches and then continue as endometrial spiral arteries. The basal arteries are unresponsive to steroid hormones, whereas the spiral arteries respond to varying hormone levels both by proliferation and, during the luteal phase of the menstrual cycle, by intermittent contraction (131,132).

Angiogenesis, the formation of new vessels, is central to the menstrual cycle and to implantation and subsequent gestation. As concerns the menstrual cycle: there must be repair of the vessels ruptured during the menstrual phase, then rapid growth of vessels during the proliferative phase, further development of spiral arteries during the secretory phase and, to come full circle, the dismantling of the vasculature that leads into the menstrual phase (13). All these stages are closely monitored by activators and inhibitors (133–136).

During implantation and gestation, angiogenesis is again pivotal in negotiating the hookup of the feto-placental unit to the maternal circulation. This entails an extensive remodelling of the placental bed spiral arteries to form the utero-placental vessels (137,138).

Ultrastructural Features and Immunohistochemistry

Both transmission and scanning electron microscopic study of the endometrium has produced an immense body of literature (109,139,140). Despite its scientific interest and the high aesthetic quality of many of the electron micrographs, little of this literature is currently of diagnostic relevance to the surgical pathologist. Mention should be made of two distinctive ultrastructural features found in the early secretory glandular cell: the giant mitochondrion complex (141) and the nucleolar channel system (142). These two features seem to be the earliest postovulatory morphologic change in the endometrial glandular cell.

Normal endometrial and endocervical epithelium have some differences in their immunohistochemical profile. Endometrial glands are positive for low and high molecular weight cytokeratins, vimentin, and occasionally CEA while endocervical epithelium expresses CEA but is negative for vimentin and low-molecular-weight cytokeratin (96). The endometrial stroma and mesonephric remnants are typically strongly positive for CD10 while the endometrial and endocervical glands are not. Occasionally normal smooth muscle cells express CD10 and about 40% of leiomyomas contain CD10 positive cells usually focally. Both the endometrial stroma and smooth muscle express vimentin, muscle specific actin, smooth muscle actin, and Bcl-2. Smooth muscle cells typically express desmin and caldesmon, whereas endometrial stromal cells do not. The combination of desmin (or caldesmon) and CD10 can be helpful in distinguishing smooth muscle tumors from endometrial stromal sarcoma.

The endometrium produces many secreted proteins that serve local cell signaling functions important for the developing endometrium and embryo. There is a large and growing body of literature concerning these products of endometrium, a topic beyond the scope of this chapter. However, there have been a number of excellent recent reviews of this subject (13,107,143–146).

Temporal Variations

Unlike morphologically unchanging epithelia, such as vaginal or gastrointestinal mucosa, that have an essentially constant appearance throughout the cell's lifetime, the

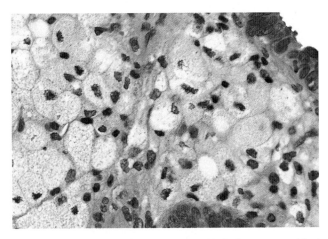

Figure 41.30 Stromal foam cells. Most likely these are modified endometrial stromal cells. In an inflammatory setting, stromal foam cells are probably macrophages.

endometrium undergoes dramatic temporal morphologic changes. The changes are cyclic and particularly striking during the reproductive years. These changes can be conveniently considered under six headings: newborn, premenarchal, perimenarchal, reproductive, perimenopausal, and postmenopausal years (107,147,148).

Newborn

The genitalia of the newborn girl respond to the high levels of circulating maternal and placental steroids by a transient burst of precocious development. The endometrium may be well developed and have either a proliferative or, less commonly, a secretory appearance. Within 2 weeks these changes have regressed, and the long hormonal quiescence of the premenarchal years begins. This quiescent period is characterized by a thin endometrium populated by inactive glands set within a spindled inactive stroma. Rarely, estrogen-secreting lesions of the ovary (follicular cysts, sex cord gonadal stromal tumors) may cause abnormal endometrial growth, with resulting abnormal bleeding as part of the syndrome of precocious pseudopuberty. The endometrium under these circumstances is proliferative or hyperplastic. That this phenomenon occurs suggests that the inactive appearance of the normal endometrium during this period results from an absence of hormonal stimulation rather than from transient end-organ unresponsiveness (10).

Menarche

The onset of uterine bleeding (menarche) is one of the many changes that signal the maturation of the reproductive system. In the United States, this usually occurs between 12 and 15 years of age. Characteristically, the perimenarchal period is marked by greater variability in the length of individual cycles than is seen in the reproductive years and by the occurrence of anovulatory cycles (148). Disordered proliferative endometria are commonly encountered in this setting (see section "Disordered Proliferative Endometrium").

Reproductive Years

The reproductive years are characterized by regularly occurring, roughly monthly, cycles, the end of which is signaled by menstrual bleeding (149,150). The dominant ovarian steroid secreted during the first half of the menstrual cycle is estradiol (E2), which induces endometrial proliferation. The second half of the cycle (beginning after ovulation) is hormonally dominated by both progesterone and estradiol, and this combination of hormones induces endometrial glandular secretion and stromal predecidualization. With the withdrawal of corpus luteum steroidal support, the endometrium is shed, setting the stage for the next cycle. These regularly recurring cycles may be interrupted by pregnancies, but after the termination of pregnancy, cycling is soon restored.

The biochemistry of the steroid molecules and their receptors that are responsible for the remarkable morphologic changes of the menstrual cycle have been the subject of intense study (151–153). Steroid molecules are hydrophobic and easily diffuse through cell membranes and freely enter all cells. The endometrium, vaginal mucosa, and other steroid-sensitive tissues are target organs by virtue of the presence of high-affinity, high-specificity, low-capacity saturable receptors for E2 and progesterone. These nucleus-based receptors are absent in nonresponsive cells. In addition to being highly responsive to circulating hormones, the endometrium also synthesizes substances such as glycoproteins that affect the hypothalamic-pituitary-ovary axis and the endometrium itself (see above). A detailed description of hormone regulation is beyond the scope of this chapter, but several excellent reviews on the topic have been published and can be found in the general references listed at the end of the chapter. In broad terms, the steroid molecule combines with the appropriate receptor, and the steroid–receptor complex becomes associated with a nonhistone nucleoprotein. The net effect of this linkage is to alter both qualitatively and quantitatively DNA-dependent RNA transcription. The consequence is an altered profile of protein biosynthesis. Furthermore, the unique response of a particular target cell type depends on what specific growth and differentiation program is initiated by the steroidal signal. The endometrium is a major target organ for this continual barrage of steroidal information. It responds by undergoing the dramatic morphologic alterations that constitute the normal menstrual cycle as well as producing proteins important for hypothalamic feedback, modulation of placental hormone secretion, regulation of macrophages, and regeneration after menses.

Morphology of the Normal Menstrual Cycle Endometrium

The first day of the menstrual cycle has conventionally been identified as the first day of menstrual flow. Menses usually lasts for less than 5 days and is followed by the endometrial proliferative phase, the length of which exhibits great variation (9–20 days), but on average it lasts for 10 days. After ovulation, the coordinated and highly predictable series of stromal and glandular changes characteristic of the secretory (luteal) phase takes place. The traditional view is that the length of this phase is constant (14 days), and it is this alleged constancy that provides the basis for endometrial dating. Due to the sensitivity and specificity of serum hormonal studies, it is now uncommon for the surgical pathologist to be called upon to date the endometrium for infertility purposes. However, given the prevalence of polycystic ovarian disease, dysfunctional uterine bleeding, and iatrogenic hormonal use and because some gynecologists want endometrial dating it remains important for the surgical pathologist to recognize when ovulation has occurred and the normal responses of the endometrium to various hormonal stimuli. The following discussion is a concise description of the normal menstrual cycle with more detailed information in the accompanying figures. (Figures 41.31 and 41.32, Table 41.2) (106,107,117,154–156).

Proliferative Endometrial Phase (Ovarian Follicular Phase)

The proliferative phase spans the time from the previous menstrual period to ovulation. The endometrium responds to rising estrogen levels by synchronous proliferation of glands, stroma, and vessels. During the first third of the proliferative phase (early proliferative), the rate of growth of all three of these elements is coordinated, and as a consequence both vessels and glands are noncoiled.

After a few days the growth of both glands and vessels outstrips that of the stroma; as a result, these tubular structures become coiled (mid- and late proliferative) (Figure 41.33).

The glands are lined by mitotically active pseudostratified columnar cells with high nuclear to cytoplasmic ratios and dense chromatin (Figure 41.34). Mitotic figures are almost always easy to find. These cells are present throughout the proliferative phase and even into early secretion. After about 10 to 11 days, irregular subnuclear vacuoles begin to appear. During the last 2 days mitotic activity decreases, glandular coiling becomes more prominent, and vacuoles are easily found.

The interval period is the 48 hours between ovulation and the presence of uniformly vacuolated cells indicative of postovulatory day 2. Mitotic figures are present during this period, and the cells retain their proliferative nuclear features.

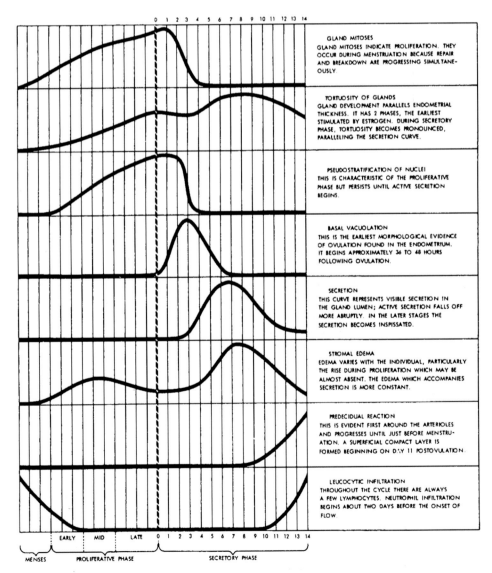

Figure 41.31 Approximate qualitative changes in eight morphologic criteria found to be most useful in dating human endometrium. Reprinted with permission from: Noyes R. Normal phases of the endometrium. In: Hertig A, Norris H, Abell M, eds. *The Uterus.* Baltimore: Williams & Wilkins; 1973:110–135.

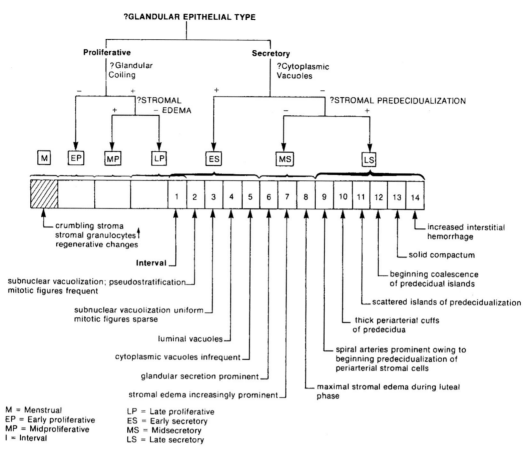

Figure 41.32 Decision tree for endometrial dating. Reprinted with permission from: Hendrickson M, Kempson R. *Surgical Pathology of the Uterine Corpus.* Philadelphia: WB Saunders; 1980.

Endometrial Secretory Phase (Ovarian Luteal Phase)

Ovulation is mediated by the luteinizing hormone (LH) surge, a synchronous burst of LH and follicle-stimulating hormone secretion that peaks on the 14th day of the ideal 28-day cycle. Ovulation occurs roughly 10 to 12 hours after this peak. The length of time from the last menstrual period to the day of ovulation for an individual woman is the length of her follicular phase. This surge of pituitary hormones initiates a complex series of events that results in the expulsion of the oocyte from the developed tertiary follicle and the transformation of the follicle into a corpus luteum. As a consequence of this transformation, the biosynthetic profile of the follicle changes, and both estradiol and large quantities of progesterone, are secreted. The biosynthetic lifetime of the corpus luteum defines the ovarian luteal phase that corresponds to endometrial secretory development. Both ovarian and endometrial luteal phases last 14 days on average, but this can be highly variable (see section "Relevance of Endometrial Dating to Diagnostic Surgical Pathologists").

The endometrium, which has proliferated and has been primed by estrogen, responds to the simultaneous stimulation of estrogen and progesterone by differentiating in a distinctive fashion. The morphologic changes can be divided into four periods: interval, early secretory, midsecretory, and late secretory (see Figure 41.32). The first 24 to 36 hours of the secretory phase are morphologically silent because the endometrium, for the most part, retains its late proliferative appearance, although scattered nonuniform subnuclear vacuoles may appear. This morphologically indeterminate endometrium is termed "interval." The first unequivocal light microscopic indication that ovulation has occurred is the presence of uniform subnuclear vacuoles involving more than 50% of the endometrial glands. Over the next few days these vacuoles shift from a subnuclear to a supranuclear location. By the fifth postovulatory day, most of the secretion has been discharged into the gland lumen. The morphologic hallmark then of the early secretory phase (postovulatory days 2 to 5) is the vacuolated gland (Figure 41.35A, B).

The midsecretory phase lasts from postovulatory days (PODs) 5 to 9 and is characterized by nonvacuolated, prominently coiled secretory glands set within a spindled edematous stroma. Luminal secretion is most prominent during this period, and the overall appearance is one of

TABLE 41.2
DECISION TREE FOR ENDOMETRIAL DATING

What type of gland is present?

A. Proliferative Gland (Early proliferative, midproliferative, late proliferative, interval)

    Is the gland straight or coiled?

      Straight: early proliferative

      Coiled: midproliferative, late proliferative, interval

    Is there stromal edema?

      Yes: midproliferative

      No: late proliferative, interval

    Are there scattered subnuclear vacuoles present, but with less than 50% of the glands
      exhibiting uniform subnuclear vacuolization?

      No: late proliferative

      Yes: interval—consistent with but not diagnostic of POD 1

B. Secretory Gland–Vacuolated (Early secretory)

    POD 2: Subnuclear vacuolization uniformly present, leading to exaggerated nuclear pseudo-
        stratification (greater than 50% of the glands exhibit uniform subnuclear
        vacuolization); mitotic figures frequent

    POD 3: Subnuclear vacuoles and nuclei uniformly aligned; scattered mitotic figures

    POD 4: Vacuoles assume luminal position; mitotic figures rare

    POD 5: Vacuoles infrequent; secretion in lumen of gland; cells have a nonvacuolated
        secretory appearance

C. Secretory Gland–Nonvacuolated (Midsecretory, late secretory, menstrual)

    Is there stromal predecidualization?

      No: midsecretory

    POD 6: Secretion prominent

    POD 7: Beginning stromal edema

    POD 8: Maximal stromal edema

      Yes: late secretory, menstrual

    Is there crumbling of the stroma?

      No: late secretory

    POD 9: Spiral arteries first prominent

    POD 10: Thick periarterial cuffs of predecidual

    POD 11: Islands of predecidual in superficial compactum

    POD 12: Beginning coalescence of islands of predecidual

    POD 13: Confluence of surface islands; stromal granulocytes prominent

    POD 14: Extravasation of red cells in stroma; prominence of stromal granulocytes

      Yes: menstrual

        crumbling stroma, hemorrhage

        intravascular fibrin thrombi

        stromal granulocytes prominent

        polymorphs present

        late menstrual: regenerative changes prominent

glandular crowding (157). The secretory cells usually have round somewhat vesicular nuclei. This serves to separate them from the nuclei found in early secretory phase cells (Figure 41.36A, B, C). The distinctive feature of the late secretory endometrium (PODs 10–14) is stromal predecidualization. This diagnostic stromal change is heralded by an increased prominence of the spiral arteries. By the 10th postovulatory day, cuffs of predecidual cells are present around these arteries, initially involving the part of the vessel adjacent to the surface of the endometrium (Figure 41.37A, B). Subsequently, islands of predecidual cells appear in the superficial compactum. By POD 13 these islands become confluent. The extent of predecidualization is roughly paralleled by the degree of stromal infiltration by stromal granulocytes, although some investigators have suggested that the intensity of this infiltration is more closely correlated with the time of onset of menses (158). The appearance of the glands during the late secretory phase is not significantly different from their appearance during the midsecretory phase. They are lined by nonvacuolated secretory cells with round vesicular nuclei, and during the later days of this period, the glands typically have the saw-toothed appearance sometimes referred to as secretory exhaustion. As the late secretory phase progresses, increasing numbers of secretory cells exhibit apoptosis and apoptotic bodies accumulate within stromal macrophages.

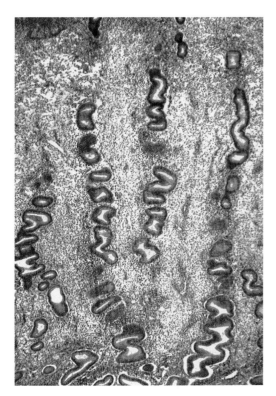

Figure 41.33 Midproliferative endometrium. Note the early coiling and synchronously developed glands.

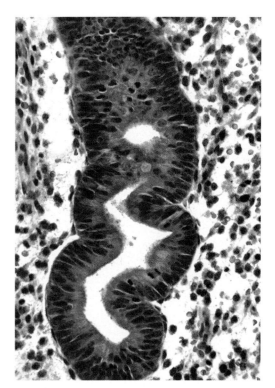

Figure 41.34 High-power view of a proliferative phase gland. The constituent cells are pseudostratified, and the characteristically elongate glandular nuclei have dense chromatin.

Menstruation

Menstrual Phase (cycle days 1–4). The abrupt withdrawal of both estrogen and progesterone accompanying the demise of the corpus luteum initiates menstrual bleeding. The molecular events initiating and guiding the controlled bleeding of menstruation are bewilderingly complex in contrast to the relatively straighforward light microscopic picture (159). The endometrium on the first day of menstrual bleeding (cycle day 1) is thin and compact. It is composed of the basalis and—relative to the fully developed secretory endometrium—a substantially shrunken, dense functionalis. The basalis maintains the relatively constant histologic appearance it has throughout the endometrial cycle. The shrinkage of the functionalis is largely due to "deflation" consequent on the withdrawal of interstitial fluid. The constituent glands and stroma of the functionalis fragment and crumble. Fibrin thrombi appears in vessels and within the

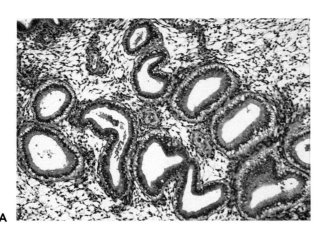

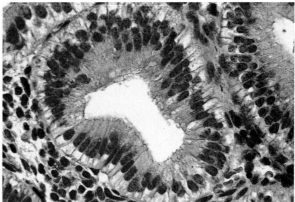

A B

Figure 41.35 **A**. and **B**. Early secretory endometrium with subnuclear vacuoles. The nuclei retain the dense chromatin of the proliferative phase. Uniformly present cytoplasmic vacuoles are the most useful marker of the first third of the secretory phase.

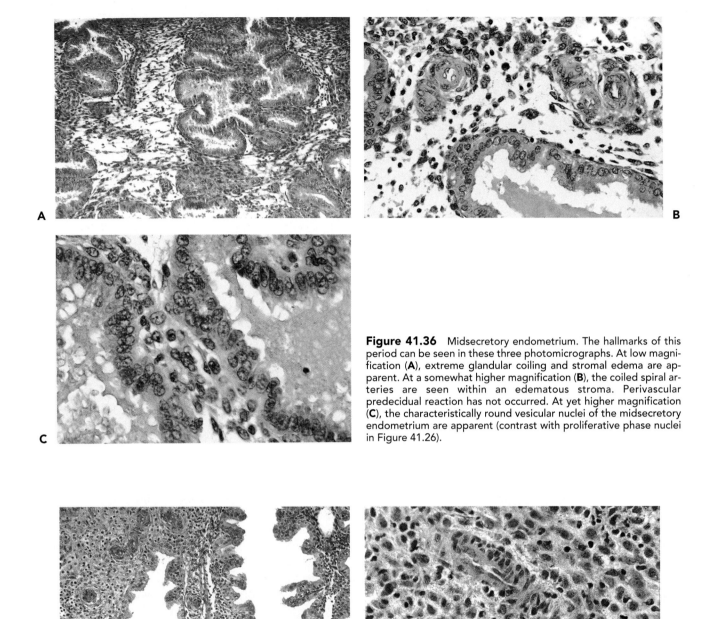

Figure 41.36 Midsecretory endometrium. The hallmarks of this period can be seen in these three photomicrographs. At low magnification (**A**), extreme glandular coiling and stromal edema are apparent. At a somewhat higher magnification (**B**), the coiled spiral arteries are seen within an edematous stroma. Perivascular predecidual reaction has not occurred. At yet higher magnification (**C**), the characteristically round vesicular nuclei of the midsecretory endometrium are apparent (contrast with proliferative phase nuclei in Figure 41.26).

Figure 41.37 Late secretory endometrium. At low magnification (**A**), the serrated appearance of the gland reflects their coiled state. The stroma cells have undergone predecidual reaction (**B**). Predecidual reaction begins around the spiral arteries, and this reaction serves to distinguish midsecretory endometria from late secretory endometria.

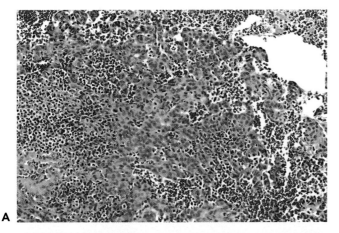

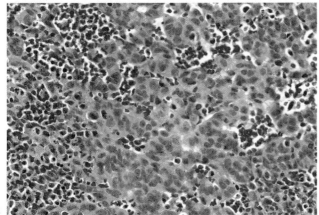

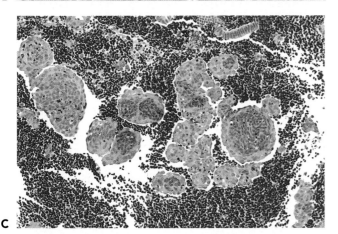

Figure 41.38 Stromal breakdown. Disintegrating endometrium may simulate endometrial malignancy. **A**. Sheets of disintegrating stromal cells may simulate an endometrial stromal neoplasm. **B**. Higher magnification shows individual cell necrosis and inflammation, findings that should raise the possibility of disintegrating nonneoplastic endometrium. **C**. Confirmation of this possibility is made by finding inflamed epithelium associated with degenerating stromal cells. In this case, characteristic epithelium-covered spherules are produced.

stroma. As the stroma disintegrates, the endometrial glands are randomly arranged and may artificially crowd together (Figure 41.38). The degenerative atypia of these glands, the necrotic background, and the close approximation of glands may suggest a diagnosis of malignancy. The general strategy of not making a diagnosis of malignancy when well-preserved glands and stroma are absent, should prevent such a mistake (Figure 41.39).

There is rapid onset of endometrial repair during this time. Numerous studies have demonstrated the outgrowth of epithelium from the stumps of the disrupted endometrial glands and ingrowth from the intact areas of the cornual and isthmic endometrium. This process begins during the 2nd or 3rd day and is completed by the 4th or 5th day. This early repair phase is thought by some to be estrogen independent as is the initial regrowth of the vasculature (160). In normal women, almost 50% of menstrual blood loss occurs on the first day (106,161,162).

Endometrial Morphology During the Luteal Phase of the Cycle of Conception

If implantation of a blastocyst occurs, it will be during the midsecretory phase (PODs 6–8), and this event is associated with a resurgence of glandular secretion and a persistence of stromal edema. After this time, biopsy findings will

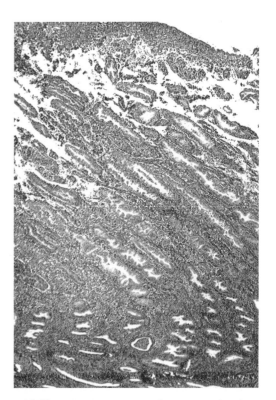

Figure 41.39 A low-power view of a menstrual endometrium showing the unresponsive basalis in the lower part of the photomicrograph and the functionalis disintegrating near the surface.

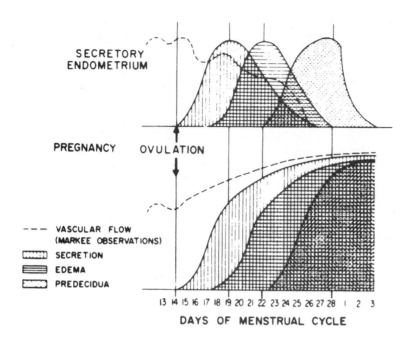

Figure 41.40 The transition from secretory to gestational endometrium is shown. The simultaneous occurrence of intense secretion, edema, and predecidual reaction and maintained vascular flow characterizes the early endometrial gestational responses. Reprinted with permission from: Arias-Stella J. Gestational endometrium. In: Hertig A, Norris H, Abell M, eds. *The Uterus.* Baltimore: Williams & Wilkins; 1973:185–212.

feature prominent glandular secretion (which in a non-gravid cycle would have subsided), stromal edema, and stromal predecidualization (Figure 41.40) (163, 164).

The developing predecidua is gradually converted to decidua after POD 14 of the luteal phase of conception. This transformation is complete by the end of the first month of gestation. The fully developed decidual reaction is distinctive. Almost all of the endometrial stroma is converted into pavementlike sheets of epithelioid cells with prominent cytoplasmic margins and central vesicular nuclei (see Figure 41.28). In the superficial portion of the functionalis, the glands are compressed and their lining becomes flattened and endothelium-like. This compact sheetlike zone, the zona compactum, overlies saw-toothed scalloped glands, the zona spongiosum, which continue to exhibit secretory features. Many of the glands in the spongiosum are lined by cells with enlarged nuclei that often have atypical nuclear features approaching those of the Arias-Stella reaction (Figure 41.41). Scattered 'stromal granulocytes' (uterine NK cells) are present. Decidual cells may exhibit substantial nuclear pleomorphism and cytologic atypia. This is particularly prominent in the region of the implantation site. In addition, this region is also infiltrated by intermediate trophoblastic cells, which normally have a bizarre cytologic appearance. These cells are positive for both keratin and hPL. The infiltration of decidua and the underlying myometrium by trophoblasts in the past has been termed "syncytial metritis," not a particularly felicitous label because the process has little to do with inflammation (Figure 41.42). Accordingly, the current term for this process is "implantation site reaction" and is diagnostic of intrauterine preg-

nancy (165). Both placental site reaction and decidual atypia may incorrectly suggest malignancy, but confusion with adenocarcinoma is avoided by noting the secretory setting of these findings as well as the clinical history.

Although a fully developed decidual reaction is a constant feature of intrauterine pregnancy, it is by no means a diagnostic finding. An identical decidual reaction may be seen in extrauterine (ectopic) pregnancy; also, it can be produced by progestational agents or can be associated with persistence of the corpus luteum unassociated with pregnancy (e.g., corpus luteum cyst). For this reason, intrauterine implantation should only be diagnosed in the presence

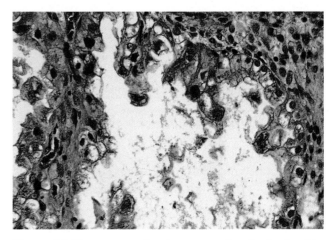

Figure 41.41 Gestational endometrium. This gland is lined by cells with enlarged dense nuclei characteristic of the Arias-Stella reaction.

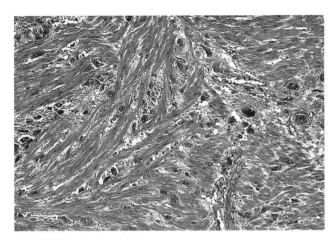

Figure 41.42 Myometrium beneath an implantation site containing infiltrating trophoblasts. This must not be misinterpreted as evidence of gestational trophoblastic disease.

of chorionic villi or the presence of intermediate trophoblasts associated with enlarged vessels replaced by hyalin, or with fragments of fibrinoid matrix (165).

Distressingly, on rare occasions, the finding of trophoblastic tissue in a curetting does not exclude an ectopic gestation and suggests that when clinical suspicion is high, the presence of either chorionic villi or an implantation site should not preclude further workup of a possible ectopic pregnancy (166).

Previous intrauterine pregnancy is strongly suggested in the postpartum endometrium by the presence of cuffs of hyalinized decidua around sclerotic ectatic spiral arteries. The decidual cells composing this cuff often have hyperchromatic smudged and degenerate nuclei, and the vessels are often thrombosed. These findings have been referred to as subinvolution of the placental site and can be responsible for postpartum hemorrhage (167). This presumably occurs because these severely altered vessels are incapable of contraction. With time, the foci of hyalinization shrink and the nuclei may disappear, leaving a small pink scar resembling an ovarian corpus atreticum. These distinctive foci have been referred to as pregnancy plaques, and they may persist in the basalis for many years. Similar lesions featuring intermediate trophoblasts have been termed placental site nodule and placental site plaque (167). Occasionally, a placental site nodule (PSN) or exaggerated placental site can be confused for a gestational trophoblastic tumor such as placental site trophoblastic tumor (PSTT) or epithelioid trophoblastic tumor (ETT). While conventional H&E morphology is still very useful in distinguishing placental site nodules and plaques, immunohistochemical profiles can also be helpful. Studies over the last decade have shown that there are a variety of intermediate trophoblasts involved in implantation and establishing vascular connections to the maternal blood flow. These trophoblasts seem to have distinct immunohistochemical properties, some of which are

shared with the cells of gestational trophoblastic tumors (GTTs). An exaggerated placental site is characterized by infiltration of individual cells with preservation of normal structures and mitoses essentially absent. Plancetal site trophoblastic tumors are characterized by mitotically active confluent masses of cells that disrupt normal architectures. All trophoblasts express pancytokeratins, so while this may be helpful in highlighting the trophoblasts it does little to predict the aggressive potential of the proliferation. Kurman et al. have established algorithms for evaluating placental site nodules and trophoblastic tumors, using a combination of human placental lactogen (hPL), p63 and Ki67. Briefly, the intermediate trophoblasts of an exaggerated placental site is hPL positive, p63 negative, and has a Ki67 activity of less than 1%. A PTT will have the same immunohistochemical profile except the Ki67 is much greater. The intermediate trophoblasts in a placental site nodule are hPL negative, p63 positive and have a Ki67 activity of less than 10%. Epitheloid trophoblastic tumor can sometimes be confused with a placental site nodule but has a Ki67 activity of greater than 10%. Occasionally, the diagnostic dilemma is between placental site nodule and squamous cell carcinoma; in this scenario, inhibin and cytokeratin 18 can be useful as PSNs are postitive for both of these antibodies while squamous cell carcinomas are negative (168–170).

Hyperprogestational states (particularly pregnancy) are sometimes associated with the distinctive glandular change to which Arias-Stella first drew attention in 1954 and that now bears his name (171,172). Most commonly this change is encountered in endometrial glands, but on occasion it may be present in foci of endometriosis or adenomyosis, in endocervical glands, in uterine (fallopian) tube epithelium, or in the glands within polyps. The Arias-Stella (AS) phenomenon characteristically involves a focus of tightly packed glands whose extreme coiling and collapse throw the lining epithelium into prominent papillary folds. This epithelium is composed of cells exhibiting marked nuclear pleomorphism and hyperchromatism. The nuclei typically have a smudged appearance. The cell cytoplasm may be strikingly hypervacuolated and cleared (clear cells) or densely eosinophilic (dark cells) (see Figure 41.41). One or the other cell type may predominate from area to area. Occasionally the eosinophilic cells may line the glands in a hobnail fashion. Mitotic figures only rarely are present. Elsewhere the endometrium usually exhibits the other changes one would anticipate with progestational stimulation, such as secretory glands and a stromal decidual reaction.

Less striking degrees of nuclear hyperchromasia, nuclear pleomorphism, and cytoplasmic vacuolization are, in our experience, constant features of the secretory glands of every pregnancy. The Arias-Stella reaction appears to represent the extreme end of the morphologic spectrum of the glandular epithelial changes seen in all pregnancies.

An endometrial Arias-Stella change may be present in a variety of clinical settings, including normal intrauterine pregnancy, extrauterine pregnancy, gestational trophoblastic disease, and persistent corpus luteum. In a retrospective review of patients coded as having Arias-Stella reaction, 16% had an extrauterine gestation. It also may be produced by the administration of ovulation-inducing drugs or progestational agents (171).

Because of the marked nuclear atypia of the epithelium lining the closely packed glands, the Arias-Stella phenomenon can be confused with adenocarcinoma, particularly with the architectural and cytologic features of clear cell carcinoma. This difficulty largely can be avoided by remembering that the Arias-Stella phenomenon occurs in a secretory setting; that is, more conventional secretory glands and decidualized or predecidualized stroma are usually found elsewhere in the specimen and the patient is premenopausal. Moreover, glandular mitotic figures tend not to be a prominent feature, although they may occasionally be encountered (173). Clear cell carcinoma (like any carcinoma) is fundamentally a proliferative process, and the constituent cells not only possess malignant features but also exhibit mitotic activity. Most importantly, clear cell carcinoma of the endometrium develops almost exclusively in postmenopausal women. Immunochemistry has been useful in separating the two; p53 and Ki-67 staining are absent in Arias-Stella (AS) and are present in clear cell carcinoma (174).

Occasionally in a gestational setting glandular nuclei may exhibit marked nuclear clearing reminiscent of herpetic infections (Figure 41.43) (175).

Endometrial Vasculature

The transition from the endometrium of early gestation to that of fully developed pregnancy is marked by the accelerated development of the endometrial vasculature, resulting in increased thickness of the spiral arteries, as reflected in their mean cross-sectional diameter (176,177).

Perimenopausal and Postmenopausal Years

With the waning of hormonal function in the fifth decade of life, a woman enters the perimenopause, during which time uterine bleeding characteristically again becomes erratic, and the length of time between bleeding episodes lengthens. Thus, both the perimenopause and the perimenarche may be marked by erratic ovarian function and consequent dysfunctional uterine bleeding (178).

The end of ovarian follicular development and ovulation results in cessation of the menstrual periods and the menopause. Thereafter, the uterus enters a second inactive period, and the endometrial glandular epithelium, as in the premenarchal years, is typically atrophic. However, the glandular architecture and thickness of the endometrium may vary considerably. Several different patterns may be seen in the peri- and postmenopausal endometrium, which are described in the following sections.

Atrophic Endometrium

Atrophic epithelium is nonstratified and composed of a single layer of flattened to cuboidal cells. Mitotic figures are not present, the nucleus-to-cytoplasm ratio is high, and there is usually no specific cytoplasmic differentiation, although cilia may be present occasionally. The defining and only constant feature of atrophic endometria is the atrophic epithelial lining of its constituent glands, which may have any configuration, including cystic dilatation and glandular crowding. The stroma is spindled and is neither predecidualized nor decidualized. The nuclei may be densely pyknotic (as in postmenopausal endometria or endometrial polyps) or plump (as in endometria associated with oral contraceptives). Stromal disintegration may be present (Figure 41.44) (179–181).

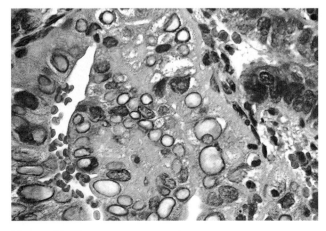

Figure 41.43 Nuclear clearing of the glandular cells in the endometrium may be seen in a gestational setting. This change should not be misconstrued as evidence of herpes virus infection.

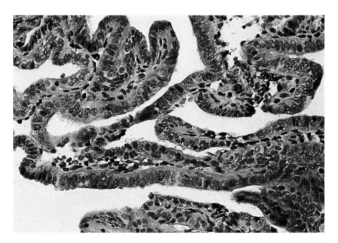

Figure 41.44 Endometrial atrophy as seen in an endometrial sampling. On occasion, atrophic surface epithelium may be removed in coiled masses and simulate hyperplasia because the glands are closely approximated. Reprinted with permission from: Hendrickson M, Kempson R. The uterine corpus. In: Sternberg S, ed. *Diagnostic Surgical Pathology*. New York: Raven; 1994:2091–2193.

Atrophic endometria can occur in a variety of clinical settings. It is the normal state during the premenarchal and later postmenopausal years. During the reproductive years, atrophic patterns may be seen in association with premature ovarian failure or, more commonly, in patients taking oral contraceptives.

Weakly Proliferative Endometrium

Weakly proliferative epithelium is nonstratified, although some degree of nuclear pseudostratification may be present, and its constituent cells are thin (pencil shape). This epithelium differs from the normal proliferative epithelium in the paucity of mitotic figures, the greater density of the nuclear chromatin, and, in the usual case, the overall lack of organization of the glands. The glands may be of any configuration, but the glands-to-stroma ratio is almost always near unity or there can be a slight stromal predominance. The stroma is spindled; stromal cell nuclei may be densely pyknotic or plump.

The morphologic variability of the weakly proliferative endometrium parallels that of the atrophic endometrium. The difference between them is solely based on the appearance of the epithelial cells: weakly proliferative rather than flattened or cuboidal. The clinical settings in which these two endometria occur overlap considerably. It is conceptually convenient to regard the weakly proliferative endometrium as lying on a continuum between normal and atrophic endometrium; the weakly proliferative patterns may then be conceived of as representing a transition between normal proliferation and atrophy. Weakly proliferative endometria are most often encountered in patients in the peri- or postmenopausal years; these endometria appear to be poorly supported by low levels of endogenous or exogenous estrogen. This pattern is normal in the hormonally hyporesponsive lower uterine segment of the normally cycling premenopausal women.

During the perimenopausal period some women are prone to chronic stromal breakdown due to the inconsistent hormonal milieu and anovulatory cycles. This can result in surface metaplasias such as eosinophilic or papillary metaplasia. The former is characterized by enlarged cells with abundant pink cytoplasm and conspicuous nccleoli. The latter often form small papillary aggregates which layer the surface epithelium but can be detached and free-floating in an endometrial sampling. When atypia is present in these cells, this benign process can be mistaken for serous papillary carcinoma or its precursor, endometrial intraepithelial neoplasia. In this setting Ki67 and p53 can be useful adjuvant tests as eosinophillic metaplasia has a low Ki67 index and is usually only weakly for p53 while EIC is often strongly positive for both. While this panel will not give a definitive answer, it can prove helpful in confirming the histologic impression (182).

Disordered Proliferative Endometrium

We regard "disordered proliferation" as the morphologic bridge spanning normaly proliferating endometrium and endometrial hyperplasia. It is the endometrial pattern encountered in women experiencing sporadic anovulatory cycles and thus is most commonly encountered in the perimenopausal and perimenarchal years. It is also commonly seen in women receiving estrogen therapy. Disordered proliferation differs from normal proliferation by virtue of a loss of synchrony of glandular development so that some glands are tubular, whereas others are cystically dilated or have complex shapes. Budding may be present so that there may be a shift in the glands-to-stroma ratio in favor of the glands, but this shift is never more than 2:1. When glandular predominance is so marked that there is a shift in the glands-to-stroma ratio of 3:1 in favor of the glands, a diagnosis of hyperplasia is warranted (Figure 41.45).

We think that disordered proliferation (in the sense above) represents the response of a normal endometrium to sporadic, unopposed estrogen stimulation. There is no evidence that this pattern is a marker for an increased risk for the subsequent development of endometrial carcinoma. Because the term "hyperplasia" connotes to many clinicians such an increased risk, we part company with those pathologists who include this pattern in the hyperplasia group.

Histologically, the variously shaped glands are lined by normal proliferative cells with elongate dense nuclei that are most often pseudostratified. Mitotic figures are usually present and may be numerous. Stromal cells are spindled with plump nuclei.

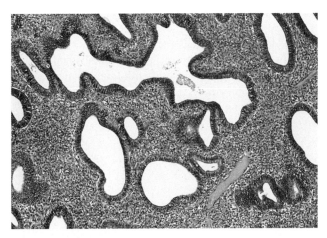

Figure 41.45 Disordered proliferation is the result of anovulatory cycles and is normal during the perimenopausal years. It is often found in the endometrium of women receiving estrogen therapy. Disordered proliferation is characterized by nonsynchronous growth of the glands including budding, but the glands-to-stroma ratio is unity or with a slight glandular predominance. This pattern of endometrial growth serves as a bridge between normal proliferation and hyperplasia.

Relevance of Endometrial Dating to Diagnostic Surgical Pathologists

The endometrial biopsy (EB) no longer plays the major role it used to play in the evaluation of the infertility patient for three reasons. First, historically, the EB's primary function was to serve as a bioassay for assessing a patient's endocrinological state; this role has been largely replaced by a variety of sophisticated and user-friendly direct methods of measuring circulating steroid and gonadotropin levels. Second, the EB's other function was to detect organic uterine disease. This role has been rendered irrelevant by the general availability of a large number of sophisticated imaging techniques. Finally, over recent years, many carefully controlled studies have established that, as a screening test for distinguishing fertile from infertile couples, the endometrial biopsy has poor test characteristics. That is, setting aside organic causes of infertility, the endometrial biopsy, functioning as a bioassay, is unreliable in separating fertile from infertile women. This is due largely to the substantial morphologic heterogeneity of the normally functioning endometrium (183–188).

The latest edition of a widely used infertility text asserts: "Taken together, the body of available evidence supports the conclusion that traditional endometrial histologic dating is not a valid diagnostic tool. Consequently, endometrial dating cannot be used to guide the clinical management of women with reproductive failure and should no longer be regarded as an important element of their evaluation" (189).

That said, the EB is still employed by some infertility specialists. In a recent survey of infertility physicians, 12% routinely ordered this test as part of the workup of the infertile couple, chiefly for its bioassay function (187,190).

Its deficiencies notwithstanding, the EB, when it is ordered for fertility evaluation, can provide much useful information. Its chief function is to determine whether ovulation has occurred and documenting anovulatory cycles points toward an ovarian factor in the patient's infertility. Again, organic reproductive tract disease may be detected on the endometrial biopsy; for example, endometrial poylps, leiomyomas, endometritis, hyperplasia, or carcinoma.

What modern studies *do* suggest is that the obsessive fine-tuning of the postovulatory morphologic date provides no useful clinical information. Historically, this fine-tuning of the postovulatory morphologic date was designed to detect luteal phase deficiency (LPD). Briefly, LPD can be thought of as a subtle form of ovulatory dysfunction manifested by a relatively short luteal phase. This results in low cumulative serum levels of progesterone in the luteal phase of the cycle and a consequent underdevelopment of secretory endometrium. LPD is a relatively uncommon syndrome, that (like congestive heart failure) has many etiologies. LPD is thought by many experts to be responsible for some cases of infertility and to be remediable by using a variety of techniques, chiefly ovulation induction (13, 189). Historically, LPD was defined in terms of a greater than 3-day disparity between the woman's *chronologic* date of ovulation and her endometrial *morphologic* date when this disparity occured more than sporadically. The diagnosis of this condition is now largely based on an assessment of the integrated luteal phase progesterone and not on a histological assessment of the endometrium (188,191,192).

What follows is a stripped down version of endometrial dating for those who are asked to provide a fine-tuned morphologic date (i.e., more than proliferative, early-, mid- or late-secretory); most endometrial biopsies do not require this.

The precise details of the morphologic patterns corresponding to standard cycle dates are presented in Table 41.2 and Figures 41.31 and 41.32.

Some general points are important to keep in mind when using these aids:

1) *Morphologic dates and chronological dates*

In evaluating the endometrium, it is important to carefully distinguish between the morphologic postovulatory date assigned to a morphologically normal endometrium and the chronologic postovulatory date (POD) (106,147, 193,194). The morphologic date is a summary characterization of the histologic development of the endometrium based on an assessment of glandular and stromal features. The morphologic findings may be summarized either in terms of postovulatory days, cycle days, or phases. For example, the morphologic pattern associated with a particular "standard" postovulatory day is assigned the number of that day; for example, POD 12 refers to the pattern seen on POD 12 of the "standard" cycle. Equivalently, this morphologic information can be conveyed using cycle day or phase (e.g., late secretory).

2) *Endometrial dating should be reported as a range of 2 days*

Research in the last two decades has shown the fallacy in using a standard 28 day cycle for all women. It is now known that both the follicular and leuteal phases vary among women (195). Adding to this biological heterogeneity is the poor interobserver reproducibility of the conventional Noyes' dating.

Noyes and Haman reported that two observers agreed on the same morphologic date 29% of the time, were within one day of each other in 63% of the cases, and were within 2 days of one another in 82% of cases (196). These results have been duplicated in more recent studies (154,197–199). As a consequence, the results of endometrial dating should be reported as a range of 2 days to reflect this variability.

3) *Determining whether the patient has ovulated*

Deciding whether a woman has ovulated by examining an endometrial biopsy (EMB) taken in what is presumed to be her late luteal phase is usually a trivial matter; the presence of a late secretory endometrium means ovulation. Deciding whether ovulation has occurred in the early luteal phase is more problematic. The characteristic light microscopic postovulatory secretory changes in the endometrium lag behind actual ovulation by at least 1 day. A biopsy on POD 2 usually reveals subnuclear vacuoles in the vast majority of glandular cells in the superficial functionalis but these may be spotty (interval pattern). Such vacuolization may be seen in late proliferative endometria as well as in other types of nonsecretory endometria and is, for this reason, not diagnostic of ovulation. Because of the ambiguous morphologic picture in the early postovulatory period, endometrial biopsies are usually obtained well into the presumed luteal phase of the cycle, preferably on PODs 11 to 13. We require uniform subnuclear vacuolization in 50% of the glands before diagnosing the earliest morphologic evidence of ovulation; this usually is present by POD 3.

4) *Some practical details*

Accurate endometrial dating requires attention to a number of details (193). Dating features should be sought only in fragments of endometrial functionalis, which are lined by surface epithelium; fragments of basalis and lower uterine segment should be ignored. The assigned date should be of the most developed area and should be based on features near the surface epithelium (the "egg's eye view" of Noyes) (193).

The preconditions for assigning a morphologic date to an endometrium are described as follows. Assigning a date to an EMB is obviously not possible in the absence of an adequate specimen, in a noncycling endometrium (e.g., nonsecretory pattern other than proliferative), in a patient being treated with medication that alters the morphology of the endometrium, or in an endometrium that is inflamed or that houses an intrauterine device. Thus, a precondition for applying the dating criteria is that one is dealing with a roughly normal endometrial pattern. Scanning power examination should establish the presence of pattern uniformity (apart from the expected variation due to sectioning randomly oriented fragments and normal out of phase curettage inhabitants such as fragments of the lower uterine segment, cervical epithelium, and stratum basalis), the absence of significant budding and branching of glands, and the absence of necrosis and inflammation. Examination at higher power should exclude the presence of significant epithelial nuclear atypia and the absence of significant numbers of stromal plasma cells.

A checklist for the contents of the pathology report of endometrial biopsies is provided in Table 41.3.

Endometrial–Myometrial Junction

The endometrial–myometrial junction is normally irregular, a phenomenon that must be kept in mind when assessing the presence or absence of myoinvasion by endometrial

---

TABLE 41.3

THE CONTENTS OF THE PATHOLOGY REPORT FOR AN INFERTILITY ENDOMETRIAL BIOPSY

Statement of the adequacy of the biopsy
  Suggest re-biopsy if:
    Sample is inadequate
    The endometrium is disintegrating and not clearly
      menstrual (i.e., postovulatory)
    The endometrium is disintegrating, postovulatory but
      otherwise undatable and the main
      concern is with the adequacy of the luteal phase
Statement about evidence of ovulation
Statement about pattern uniformity
An estimate of the endometrium's morphologic date (2-day
  interval)
Correlation with information about the chronological date
Statement about presence or absence of "organic disease"
  Inflammation
  Endometrial polyps
  Submucous leiomyomas

---

adenocarcinoma and in diagnosing superficial adenomyosis (see Figure 41.24).

Apoptosis and the Endometrium

The role of programmed cell death or apoptosis in the remodeling of the endometrium was mentioned earlier in this chapter. Apoptosis and its hormonal control in both human and animal endometrium is an area of active investigation by a number of groups (200–203).

Withdrawal of progesterone in the rabbit endometrium correlates with the development of apoptosis (204–207).

Bcl-2 is a protooncogene initially described in the (14, 18) translocation in follicular lymphoma. It has been shown to prolong cell survival by preventing apoptosis. Gompel et al. studied Bcl-2 expression immunohistochemically in the normal endometrium (208). They found that Bcl-2 predominated in glandular cells and reached a maximum at the end of the follicular phase but disappeared at the onset of secretory activity. Maia et al. found a precipitous drop in Bcl-2 after ovulation, further supporting an increase in Bcl-2 in response to estrogen and a decrease in response to progesterone (209). In addition, this group found an elevated p53 expression in the proliferative phase but a drop in the late luteal phase. These results strongly suggest hormone-dependent regulation of Bcl-2 expression and cell cycling.

The role of tumor necrosis factor alpha (TNF-α) in the induction of apoptosis was explored by Tabibzadeh et al. (210). They found that the TNF receptor as well as Fas protein were expressed in endometrial epithelium throughout the entire menstrual cycle and were most prominent in the basalis. They concluded that endometrial epithelium, by expressing receptors for TNF-α and Fas protein, can respond to ligands that regulate apoptosis.

Normal findings in the endometrium that have relevance to histopathologic differential diagnosis are shown in Table 41.4.

MYOMETRIUM

The bulk of the myometrium comprises smooth muscle cells, but an important contribution is made by extracellular components such as collagen and elastin. The smooth muscle within the corpus is more concentrated relative to collagen and elastin than the muscle in either the cervix or the lower uterine segment. This distribution of muscle is consistent with the passive role of the cervix during parturition; the uterine contents propelled by fundal contractions are thought to passively dilate a cervix previously softened by the action of collagenase. The uterine smooth muscle cells are spindled, with blunt-ended fusiform nuclei. Their cytoplasmic volume depends on whether the patient is pregnant (211–214). Scattered normal mitotic figures may be encountered, particularly during the secretory phase of the endometrial cycle (215). Characteristic ultrastructural features of smooth muscle include (a) numerous dense, 60- to 80-A myofilaments without cross striations, which almost fill the cytoplasm; (b) small round dense bodies along the trajectory of the filaments; (c) dense plaques arranged along the inner aspect of the plasma membrane; and (d) plasma membrane–related vesicles that may play a role in ionized calcium movement across the plasma membrane during contraction. In addition, there is the usual complement of cytoplasmic organelles, including smooth and rough endoplasmic reticulum, mitochondria, and a Golgi apparatus. Typically these organelles arrange themselves around the nucleus, which often has an irregular shape. These ultrastructural features reflect the dual function of the uterine myocyte: muscular contraction and collagen and elastin synthesis. The ultrastructural appearance varies with the levels of circulating steroidal hormones. In particular, estrogen appears to sharply increase myocyte protein synthesis. This correlates morphologically in an increased volume of rough endoplasmic reticulum and increased numbers of cytoplasmic contractile elements. The biochemistry and electrophysiology of the myometrium have been extensively reviewed (214,216,217). The histologic and ultrastructural appearance of smooth muscle cells differ substantially from those of the endometrial stromal cell. These differences are set out in Table 41.5. However, it should be noted that cells with a hybrid smooth muscle–stromal phenotype occur normally at the endometrial–myometrial junction and

that this phenotypic ambiguity is sometimes expressed by spindle cell neoplasms of the uterine corpus (218). Some uterine smooth muscle cells have been shown to express some classes of keratins (219–222). The immunohistochemical profile of myometrial cells is presented in Table 41.5.

Pregnancy-Related Changes

To accommodate the growing fetus and to prepare for its role in fetal expulsion, the uterus undergoes a 10-fold increase in size and weight during pregnancy both by hypertrophy and, to a much lesser extent, by hyperplasia. Normal mitotic figures are often increased and may be present in large numbers. Uterine growth during pregnancy appears to be largely promoted by estradiol, whereas progesterone probably functions to inhibit uterine contractions during gestation. The light microscopic appearance of the hypertrophied uterine smooth muscle cells of pregnancy is distinctive. They are enlarged and have abundant, rather glassy cytoplasm and vesicular elongate nuclei with occasionally prominent nucleoli. Changes occur in the ultrastructural appearance of the smooth muscle cells as well. In addition to an increase in size and the number of myofilaments, there is a striking increase in the number of gap junctions (223,224). These establish the contact between cells required for the coordinated uterine contractions that expel the term infant (225). These myometrial changes are closely coordinated with the dramatic structural changes of cervical "ripening" required for cervical effacement (see section "Uterine Cervix"). In the postpartum period, the uterus undergoes an extraordinary 85% reduction in weight within 3 weeks of delivery (25). This weight loss is primarily due to a reduction in individual cell volume rather than a reduction in cell number. In addition, a large amount of collagen is degraded over this brief period. Complete return of the uterus to the nulliparous weight does not occur if gestation has proceeded beyond the second trimester.

THE FALLOPIAN TUBE

Histology of the Fallopian Tube

The fallopian tube is lined by a nonstratified epithelium that is separated from the endosalpingeal stroma by a basement membrane. Each of the tubal segments is lined by a mixture of three basic cell types: ciliated cells, secretory cells, and intercalated (peg) cells (Figures 41.46A, B and 41.47). In recent years it has become apparent that the peg cell is, in reality, a stage in the cyclic variation during the menstrual cycle of the secretory cell (226). The relative number of these cells differs in each of the anatomic

TABLE 41.4

TABLE 41.4

NORMAL FINDINGS IN THE ENDOMETRIUM THAT HAVE RELEVANCE TO HISTOPATHOLOGIC DIFFERENTIAL DIAGNOSIS *(see text for additional differential diagnostic clues)*

Findings	Diagnostic Confusion	Suggestions for Resolution	References
"Glands within glands" can occur from trauma of D&C (telescoping) and tangential cutting	**Endometrial hyperplasia:** rolled up carpet effect may simulate the architectural complexity of hyperplasia or carcinoma	This artifact is usually only focal and often at the periphery or otherwise normal fragments of functionalis. Check that epithelium is identical to architecturally normal glands in the sample.	
Strips of normal surface epithelium Commonly seen with atrophic endometrium	**Endometrial/hyperplasia/carcinoma:** rolled up carpet effect may simulate the architectural complexity of hyperplasia or carcinoma	In contrast to hyperplasia and carcinoma, the rolled up atrophic endometrium is cytologically bland and mitotically inactive.	268
Lower uterine segment	**Dating problem:** the glands respond weakly at best to hormones and the stroma is often fibrous	Look for mucinous epithelial component. Unless the sample is inadequate for dating the endometrium, there will be other fragments around with an appearance more typical of functionalis.	
Normal basalis	**Dating problem:** the glands respond weakly at best to hormones and the stroma is inactive	When assigning a morphologic date to an endometrial fragment, use only glands in close approximation to surface epithelium	
Ciliated cells	**Adenocarcinoma:** intraepithelial ciliated cells have rounded pear-shaped contours and open, rounded nuclei with nucleoli	Look for cilia. Endometria containing ciliated cells have a polymorphous appearance; the cytologic features are uniform within each subpopulation of cells.	268
Foam cells	**Endometritis:** foam cells are commonly encountered in hypoestrogenic settings and are thought to be one differentiated form of endometrial stromal cells	Look for plasma cells to establish the diagnosis of chronic endometritis. Macrophages (xanthoma cells) with foamy cytoplasm may occur in the endometrium as a component of a chronic inflammatory process. Commonly seen as a reaction to a foreign body or to keratin (e.g., in setting of proliferations shedding keratin).	269
Arias-Stella reaction	**Adenocarcinoma:** particularly clear cell carcinoma	Clear cell carcinoma is most frequently encountered in postmenopausal women. Arias-Stella reaction usually does not feature mitotic figures, which are almost always easily found in clear cell carcinoma. A more difficult problem is distinguishing clear cell carcinoma from Arias-Stella reaction in a postmenopausal woman who is taking progestational medication.	171,173,174,223

(continued)

TABLE 41.4
(continued)

Findings	Diagnostic Confusion	Suggestions for Resolution	References
Implantation site	**Gestational trophoblastic disease:** early gestations may mimic choriocarcinoma. The often bizarre shapes of trophoblastic cells may raise the possibility of choriocarcinoma a molar gestation, or PSTT	Clinical history to establish time course of gestation Insistence on a bilaminar pattern of cytotrophoblast alternating with syncytiotrophoblast for choriocarcinoma, villi are not present in choriocarcinoma PSTT features.	
	Clinically relevant endometritis: a mixed plasmacytic–lymphocytic infiltrate is a normal finding at the implantation site	Clinically relevant gestational endomyometritis can occur but only rarely is diagnosed initially on endometrial samplings. The vast majority of cases of "chronic endometritis" seen in practice represent a clinically insignificant "physiologic" finding.	
Irregular endometrial–myometrial junction	**Adenomyosis:** glands and stroma surrounded by smooth muscle	Associated smooth muscle hypertrophy is a common feature of adenomyosis and not irregular junctions. Superficial myometrial location of suspected foci favors irregular junctions.	268
	Myoinvasive adenocarcinoma: the irregular junction, when expanded by hyperplasia or carcinoma, often simulates myoinvasive carcinoma Tangential sectioning often reinforces this impression	Absence of stromal host response that is usual in myoinvasive carcinoma. Presence of endometrial stroma or normal glands means irregular junction (or adenomyosis).	
Menstrual endometrium	**Adenocarcinoma:** "cytologic atypia" produced by degenerating, poorly preserved glandular elements	Obtain history; menstrual fragments have degenerating, not neoplastic, nuclei.	
	Endometrial stromal neoplasm: degenerating stroma may produce a pattern resembling endometrial stromal sarcoma with or without sex cord elements		
Lymphoid nodules	**Endometritis**	The presence of scattered lymphoid nodules does not correlate with significant clinical disease Large numbers of lymphoid nodules and germinal centers are usually associated with the conventional sine qua non of "chronic endometritis," the plasma cell.	
Stromal "granulocytes"	**Acute or chronic endometritis**	"Stromal granulocytes" are a normal feature of the late secretory endometrium and serve as one of the original Noyes dating criteria. In the fullness of time it has been established that these "granulocytes" are uterine NK cells (see text).	129,270–273

(continued)

TABLE 41.4
(continued)

Findings	Diagnostic Confusion	Suggestions for Resolution	References
		Clinically significant inflammation (of the type encountered in patients with established salpingitis) features the presence of easily found plasma cells and usually is accompanied by acute inflammation and necrosis of the surface epithelium.	
		Not infrequently, endometrial stromal cells or normal lymphoid constituents may have somewhat eccentric nuclei and amphophilic cytoplasm that mimics that of a plasma cell. This is usually a problem with one or two scattered cells in a fragment. Plasma cells have to be easily found before they amount to anything clinically.	
Nuclear ground glass appearance of nuclei of epithelial cells in gestational setting and with progestogen therapy	Herpes endometritis	Herpes endometritis is rare; obtain history. Immunohistochemistry may be helpful.	175

regions of the tube. In addition, many investigators believe that the numbers of the three types of cells within each of these anatomic regions undergo regular variations throughout the menstrual cycle (227–232). Ciliated cells are most prominent at the ovarian (distal) end of the tube—particularly in the fimbrial mucosa—and predominate during midcycle; their numbers diminish progressively to achieve a nadir at the time of menstruation (Figure 41.47). In a gestational cycle the number of cilia continue to decrease. Ciliary movement rather than muscular contractions is chiefly responsible for the movement of the egg toward the site of fertilization: the ampulloisthmic junction.

Secretory cells are most prominent toward the uterine end of the tube and undergo cyclic changes in cell height and appearance, reflecting their elaboration, accumulation, and discharge of oviduct secretions as the menstrual cycle proceeds. Most often they have ovoid, somewhat dense nuclei, and they may contain an apical vacuole (Figure 41.48A, B). The oviduct fluid secreted by these cells serves many important functions and has been the subject of a review (233).

Intercalated cells have been thought to represent either effete secretory cells or some type of reserve cells. They have a thin dense nucleus and little cytoplasm. Endocrine cells have been noted in the fallopian tube; their function is as mysterious here as it is in the uterus (234). The "basal cells" reported in the early literature have been shown to be lymphocytes, which may represent a tubal component of a mucosa-associated lymphoid system (235–239). Scattered lymphocytes and occasional lymphoid follicles should be considered to be within normal limits and constitute part of the mucosa-associated lymphoid system (240).

Ciliogenesis is promoted by estradiol and deciliation by progesterone. Prolonged exposure to progestogens (whether endogenously as in pregnancy or exogenously) or withdrawal of estrogen (as in the postmenopausal years) leads to epithelial atrophy. Postmenopausal estrogen administration leads to regrowth of cilia.

Mitotic figures are rarely seen in the fallopian tube epithelium, so no cyclic regeneration occurs as in the endometrium. Both the transmission and scanning electron microscopic appearance of the normal tubal mucosa have been extensively documented over the past two decades.

Of interest to the diagnostic pathologist are the abnormalities of ciliogenesis found in patients with Kartagener's syndrome (241,242).

TABLE 41.5

COMPARISON OF DIFFERENTIATED FEATURES FOR ENDOMETRIAL STROMAL CELLS AND SMOOTH MUSCLE CELLS

Technique	Endometrial Stromal Cells	Usual Smooth Muscle Cells	Epithelioid Smooth Muscle Cells	Endometrial Stroma with Epithelioid and/or Glandular Areas
Light microscopy Architectural features	Haphazardly arranged cells resembling normal proliferative phase endometrial stromal cells	Cells arranged in looping intersecting fascicles	Rounded or polygonal cells with moderate amount of cytoplasm	Biphasic pattern Stromal component (featuring cellular endometrial stroma or fibroblastic stroma) + Epithelioid component {• Trabecular epithelial pattern or • nests or • insular pattern or • Sertoli-like tubular pattern or • glands}
	Complex plexiform vascular pattern	Vascular component not complex	Foci of neoplasm often exhibit standard smooth muscle features	When the entire neoplasm has this biphasic appearance the term "uterine tumor resembling ovarian sex cord tumors" has been used When the change is focal within what is otherwise an endometrial stromal neoplasm (either stromal nodule or endometrial stromal sarcoma) the endometrial stromal diagnosis is supplemented with "with epithelioid or glandular areas"
	Hyalin sometimes abundant with a tendency to be glassy			
Cytological features Nucleus	Blunt, round-to-fusiform, uniform, bland	Elongate, cigar-shaped	Round, crumpled	Small, round and regular nuclei • Minimal nuclear pleomorphism • Only rare mitotic figures
Cytoplasm	Scanty on H&E and trichrome)	Moderate amount (on H&E and trichrome), typically fibrillar	Cytoplasm may be clear around the nucleus, clear at the periphery of the cell, or entirely clear	Scanty cytoplasm, or may have abundant eosinophilic or foamy (lipid-rich) cytoplasm
Immunohisto-chemistry	Normal endometrial stromal cells express CD10 and may express desmin; they are negative for cytokeratin and EMA.	Uterine smooth muscle cells express desmin and caldesmon. They also express CD10 (approximately 40%), CD34 (about a third), keratin (about 20%), and EMA (roughly half).	AE1 is positive in 40% of cases, desmin is positive in 80%, and CD34 in 10%.	Epithelioid areas are: • Muscle specific actin (HHF-35) positive • Vimentin positive • Cytokeratin positive
Immunohisto-chemistry References	274–279	219,222,276,277, 280–282	277,283	284–287

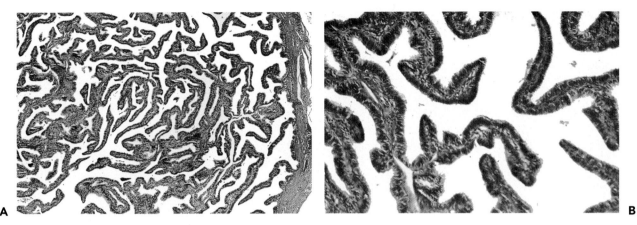

Figure 41.46   **A**. and **B**. Ampulla of the fallopian tube. Note the long slender plicae or folds resting on the muscularis.

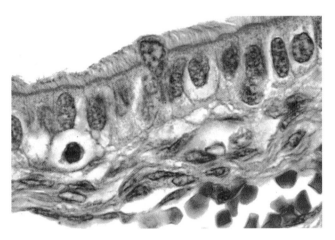

Figure 41.47   This high-power photomicrograph of tubal epithelium shows numerous ciliated cells with a compressed secretory cell nucleus above the level of the ciliated cells. The cell with clear cytoplasm is probably a lymphocyte.

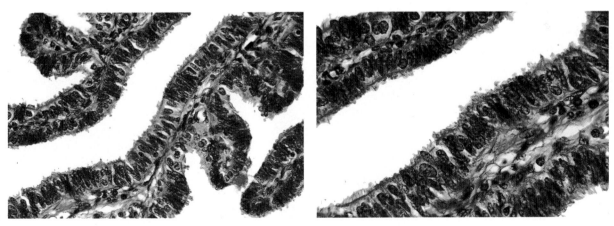

Figure 41.48   **A**. and **B**. In this area the tubal epithelial cells are crowded, a pattern that is common in the fallopian tube when ciliated cells are not numerous.

With the advent of genetic testing for BRCA-1 and BRCA-2 gene mutations, prophylactic salpingo-oophorectomies are being performed. Although there are no inherent morphological changes in the epithelium of a fallopian tube from a woman who harbors a BRCA-1 or BRCA-2 gene mutation, she is at an increased risk of having an in situ or invasive carcinoma. Therefore, in this setting the entire fallopian tube should be submitted for histological evaluation and scrutinized for occult malignancy (243, 244).

Myosalpinx

The myosalpinx is composed of an inner circular layer and an outer longitudinal layer. The isthmus near the uterotubal junction also possesses an inner longitudinal layer. The presence of the muscular layer can be particularly helpful to the pathologist when trying to distinguish a tubo-ovarian complex from an ovarian serous neoplasm.

Physiology

The details of the physiology of the tube are beyond the scope of this chapter; interested readers are referred to published reviews (229,245). Unresolved mysteries include how the sperm moves so rapidly from the vagina to the ampulla (in some cases within 5 minutes) and how the tube manages to orchestrate fertilization by ensuring that spermatozoa moving toward the ovary and an egg moving away from the ovary meet in the appropriate part of the fallopian tube.

Fallopian Tube in Pregnancy

The fallopian tube has already played its part when the fertilized ovum implants in the endometrium. It is now inactive throughout the gestational period. A muted version of endometrial decidual change often occurs in the endosalpingeal stroma during the latter part of pregnancy, while the epithelium of the fallopian tube undergoes atrophy (246) (Figure 41.49). The fallopian tube is the most common site of ectopic gestation. A review of physiologic factors in its development has been presented (247). Morphologic changes in the fallopian tube can be produced by birth control pills and of course tubal ligation (248–250).

Normal findings in the fallopian tubes that have relevance to histopathologic diagnosis can be found in Table 41.6.

Paraovarian and Paratubal Structures

The broad ligament and environs are populated by a variety of tubular and cystic structures with the propensity to form clinically or surgically noticeable cysts (38,251). These are indicated in Figure 41.50. Many are lined by müllerian-type epithelium. Walthard rests are universal

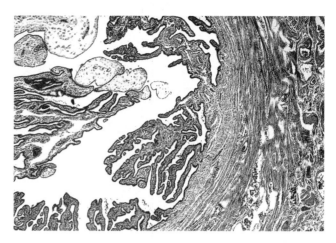

Figure 41.49 Fallopian tube containing decidual cells (upper left). The stromal cells of the plicae frequently undergo decidual change during pregnancy.

findings over the serosal surface of the fallopian tubes. They are lined by transitional-type epithelium. A more or less constant finding in sections that include the peritubal soft tissue are the tortuous remnants of the mesonephric ducts. These are lined by cuboidal epithelium and possess a fibromyovascular cuff.

SUPPLEMENTAL READINGS

A chronicle of the changing concepts of the uterus through the ages is provided by Ramsey (10), and a fascinating discussion of the role of preconceptions in filtering the "facts" of uterine anatomy is provided by Laqueur (252). There has been interesting speculation on the evolutionary purposes of menstruation (253,254).

Several textbooks of gynecological pathology provide coverage of normal uterine and fallopian tube anatomy and the differential diagnostic issues raised by departures from typical appearances.

Fox H, Wells M, eds. *Haines and Taylor Obstetrical and Gynaecological Pathology*. 5th ed. Edinburgh, Scotland: Churchill Livingstone; 2003.

Robboy S, Anderson M, Russell P. *Pathology of the Female Reproductive Tract*. New York: Churchill Livingstone; 2001.

Kurman RJ, ed. *Blaustein's Pathology of the Female Genital Tract*. 5th ed. New York: Springer-Verlag; 2002.

Several extensive treatises on reproductive endocrinology have been published or revised in recent years:

Strauss JF III, Barbieri RL. *Yen and Jaffe's Reproductive Endocrinology: Physiology, Pathophysiology, and Clinical Management*. 5th ed. Philadelphia: Elsevier Saunders; 2004.

Speroff L, Fritz MA, eds. *Clinical Gynecologic Endocrinology and Infertility*. 7th ed. Philadelphia: Lippincott Williams & Wilkins; 2004.

TABLE 41.6

NORMAL FINDINGS IN THE UTERINE (FALLOPIAN) TUBE AND UTERINE SEROSA THAT HAVE RELEVANCE TO HISTOPATHOLOGIC DIFFERENTIAL DIAGNOSIS (see text for additional differential diagnostic clues)

Finding	Diagnostic Confusion	Suggestions for Resolution	References when Relevant
Decidual reaction (usually encountered in postpartum tubal ligation specimens but may also be seen in the tubes of patients on progestational agents)	Do not misinterpret as carcinoma	Nuclei are bland in decidua	246,250
Endosalpingiosis	Distinguish from endometriosis and ovarian serous tumor of low malignant potential (borderline tumors)	Look for endometrial stroma to confirm diagnosis of endometriosis; look for complex papillae with micropapillae to confirm diagnosis of serous LMP.	
Crowded cells and dense nuclei	Carcinoma in situ	Carcinoma in situ features prominent nucleoli and abnormal mitotic figures. Nuclear atypia and glandular complexity can be significant in chronic salpingitis.	
Mucinous and eosinophilic metaplasia (may be associated with Peutz-Jeghers syndrome)	Carcinoma	Metaplasia lacks the architectural complexity, the nuclear atypia, and the mitotic activity of carcinoma.	288,289
Squamous metaplasia Walthard cell rests	Carcinoma	Metaplasia lacks the architectural complexity, the nuclear atypia, and the mitotic activity of carcinoma.	

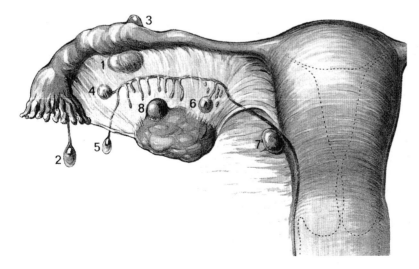

Figure 41.50 Topography of various cysts encountered in the female internal genitalia. 1, Paraovarian cyst of paramesonephric origin (type I); 2, hydatid cyst of Morgagni (paramesonephric origin); 3, subserosal müllerian cyst (paramesonephric origin); 4, paraovarian cyst of mesonephric origin (type II); 5, Kobelt's cyst (appendix vesiculosa); 6, cyst of the paroophoron; 7, duct cyst; 8, cyst of the rete ovarii. Reprinted with permission from: Janovski N, Paramanandhan T. *Ovarian Tumors, Tumors and Tumor-like Conditions of the Ovaries, Fallopian Tubes and Ligaments of the Uterus.* Philadelphia: WB Saunders; 1973:191–194.

Adashi EY, Rock JA, Rosenwaks Z, eds. *Reproductive Endocrinology, Surgery, and Technology.* Philadelphia: Lippincott-Raven; 1996.

Ferin M, Jewelewicz R, Warren M. *The Menstrual Cycle: Physiology, Reproductive Disorders, and Infertility.* New York: Oxford University Press; 1993.

Two monographs devoted exclusively to the biology of the uterus are listed as follows:

Chard T, Grudzinskas JG, eds. *The Uterus.* New York: Cambridge University Press; 1994.

Wynn RM, Jollie WP, eds. *Biology of the Uterus.* 2nd ed. New York: Plenum Medical Book Company; 1989.

More general treatments of the territory surveyed in this chapter with more emphasis on basic science issues and less emphasis on practical surgical pathology diagnostics are listed as follows:

Uterine Cervix

Wright TC, Ferenczy A. Anatomy and histology of the cervix. In: Kurman RJ, ed. *Blaustein's Pathology of the Female Genital Tract.* 5th ed. New York: Springer-Verlag; 2002: 207-224.

Singer A, Chow C. Anatomy of the cervix and physiological changes in cervical epithelium. In: Fox H, Wells M, eds. *Haines and Taylor Obstetrical and Gynaecological Pathology.* 5th ed. Vol 1. New York: Churchill Livingstone; 2003: 247-272.

Uterine Endometrium and Myometrium

Buckley CH. Normal endometrium and non-proliferative conditions of the endometrium. In: Fox H, Wells M, eds. *Haines and Taylor Obstetrical and Gynaecological Pathology.* 5th ed. New York: Churchill Livingstone; 2003: 391-441.

Giudice LC, Ferenczy A. The endometrial cycle: morphological and biochemical events. In: Adashi EY, Rock JA, Rosenwaks Z, eds. *Reproductive Endocrinology, Surgery, and Technology.* Vol 1. Philadelphia: Lippincott-Raven; 1996: 271-300.

Mutter GL, Ferenczy A. Anatomy and histology of the uterine corpus. In: Kurman RJ, ed. *Blaustein's Pathology of the Female Genital Tract.* 5th ed. New York: Springer-Verlag; 2002:383-420.

Warren M, Li T, Klentzeris D. Cell biology of the endometrium: histology, cell types and menstrual changes. In: Chard T, Grudzinskas J, eds. *The Uterus.* New York: Cambridge University Press; 1994:94-125.

Normal Gestational Findings

Shih I-M, Mazur MT, Kurman RJ. Gestational trophoblastic disease and related lesions. In: Kurman RJ, ed. *Blaustein's Pathology of the Female Genital Tract.* New York: Springer-Verlag; 2002:1193-1250.

Fallopian Tube

Brenner RM, Slayden OD. The fallopian tube cycle. In: Adashi EY, Rock JA, Rosenwaks Z, eds. *Reproductive Endocrinology, Surgery, and Technology.* Vol 1. Philadelphia: Lippincott-Raven; 1996:326-339.

Honoré L. Pathology of the fallopian tube and broad ligament. In: Fox H, Wells M, eds. *Haines and Taylor Obstetrical and Gynaecological Pathology.* 5th ed. New York: Churchill Livingstone; 2003:585-634.

Wheeler JE. Diseases of the fallopian tube. In: Kurman RJ, ed. *Blaustein's Pathology of the Female Genital Tract.* 5th ed. New York: Springer-Verlag; 2002:617-648.

REFERENCES

1. Lauchlan S. Metaplasias and neoplasias of Müllerian epithelium. *Histopathology* 1984;8:543–557.
2. Lauchlan SC. The secondary mullerian system revisited. *Int J Gynecol Pathol* 1994;13:73–79.
3. Moore K, Persaud TVN. *The Developing Human: Clinically Oriented Embryology.* 7th ed. Philadelphia: WB Saunders; 2003:207–221.
4. Acien P. Embryological observations on the female genital tract. *Hum Reprod* 1992;7:437–445.
5. O'Rahilly R. Prenatal human development. In: Wynn RM, Jolli WP, eds. *Biology of the Uterus.* 2nd ed. New York: Plenum Medical Book Company; 1989:35–56.
6. Jost A, Vigier B, Prepin J, Perchellet JP. Studies on sex differentiation in mammals. *Recent Prog Horm Res* 1973;29:1–41.
7. Gondos B. Development of the reproductive organs. *Ann Clin Lab Sci* 1985;15:363–373.
8. Szamborski J, Laskowska H. Some observations on the developmental histology of the human foetal uterus. *Biol Neonat* 1968;13:298–314.
9. Gray CA, Bartol FF, Tarleton BJ, et al. Developmental biology of uterine glands. *Biol Reprod* 2001;65:1311–1323.
10. Ramsey E. Development of the human uterus and relevance to the adult condition. In: Chard T, Grudzinskas JG, eds. *The Uterus.* New York: Cambridge University Press; 1994:41–53.
11. McLean JM. Embryology and anatomy of the female genital tract. In: Fox H, Wells M, eds. *Haines and Taylor Obstetrical and Gynaecological Pathology.* Edinburgh, Scotland: Churchill Livingstone; 2003:1–40.
12. Ramsey E. Embryology and developmental defects of the female reproductive tract. In: Danforth DN, Scott JR, eds. *Obstetrics and Gynecology.* 5th ed. Philadelphia: JB Lippincott; 1986:106–119.
13. Strauss JF III, Lessey BA. The structure, function, and evaluation of the female reproductive tract. In: Strauss JF III, Barbieri RL, eds. *Yen and Jaffe's Reproductive Endocrinology: Physiology, Pathophysiology, and Clinical Management.* 5th ed. Philadelphia: Elsevier Saunders; 2004:255–306.
14. Patton G, Kistner R. *Atlas of Infertility Surgery.* Boston: Little, Brown and Company; 1984.
15. Tulac S, Nayak NR, Kao LC, et al. Identification, characterization, and regulation of the canonical Wnt signaling pathway in human endometrium. *J Clin Endocrinol Metab* 2003;88: 3860–3866.
16. Haber HP, Mayer EI. Ultrasound evaluation of uterine and ovarian size from birth to puberty. *Pediatr Radiol* 1994;24:11–13.
17. Nussbaum A, Sanders R, Jones M. Neonatal uterine morphology as seen on real-time US. *Radiology* 1986;160:641–643.
18. Singer A, Chow C. Anatomy of the cervix and physiological changes in cervical epithelium. In: Fox H, Wells M, eds. *Haines and Taylor Obstetrical and Gynaecological Pathology.* Edinburgh, Scotland: Churchill Livingstone; 2003:247–272.
19. Eddy CA, Pauerstein CJ. Anatomy and physiology of the fallopian tube. *Clin Obstet Gynecol* 1980;23:1177–1193.

20. Williams PL, Warwick R, Dyson M, Bannister LH. *Gray's Anatomy of the Human Body.* 37th ed. New York: Churchill Livingstone; 1989.

21. Langlois PL. The size of the normal uterus. *J Reprod Med* 1970;4:220–228.

22. Calder AA. The cervix during pregnancy. In: Chard T, Grudzinskas JG, eds. *The Uterus.* New York: Cambridge University Press; 1994:288–307.

23. Kurz K, Tadesse E, Haspels A. In vivo measurements of uterine cavities in 795 women of fertile age. *Contraception* 1984;29:495–510.

24. Zemlyn S. The length of the uterine cervix and its significance. *J Clin Ultrasound* 1981;9:267–269.

25. Finn C, Porter D. *The Uterus.* Acton, MA: Publishing Sciences Group; 1975.

26. Togashi K, Nakai A, Sugimura K. Anatomy and physiology of the female pelvis: MR imaging revisited. *J Magn Reson Imaging* 2001;13:842–849.

27. Hoad CL, Raine-Fenning NJ, Fulford J, Campbell BK, Johnson IR, Gowland PA. Uterine tissue development in healthy women during the normal menstrual cycle and investigations with magnetic resonance imaging. *Am J Obstet Gynecol* 2005;192: 648–654.

28. Toth A. Studies on the muscular structure of the human uterus. II. Fasciculi cervicoangulares: vestigial or functional remnant of the mesonephric duct? *Obstet Gynecol* 1977;49:190–196.

29. Toth S, Toth A. Undescribed muscle bundle of the human uterus: fasciculus cervicoangularis. *Am J Obstet Gynecol* 1974;118: 979–984.

30. Huszar G, Naftolin F. The myometrium and uterine cervix in normal and preterm labor. *N Engl J Med* 1984;311:571–581.

31. Merchant RN, Prabhu SR, Chougale A. Uterotubal junction—morphology and clinical aspects. *Int J Fertil* 1983;28:199–205.

32. Vizza E, Correr S, Muglia U, Marchiolli F, Motta PM. The three-dimensional organization of the smooth musculature in the ampulla of the human fallopian tube: a new morpho-functional model. *Hum Reprod* 1995;10:2400–2405.

33. Croxatto HB. Physiology of gamete and embryo transport through the fallopian tube. *Reprod Biomed Online* 2002;4:160–169.

34. Talbot P, Geiske C, Knoll M. Oocyte pickup by the mammalian oviduct. *Mol Biol Cell* 1999;10:5–8.

35. Gordts S, Campo R, Rombauts L, Brosens I. Endoscopic visualization of the process of fimbrial ovum retrieval in the human. *Hum Reprod* 1998;13:1425–1428.

36. Greiss FC Jr, Rose JC. Vascular physiology of the nonpregnant uterus. In: Wynn R, Jollie W, eds. *Biology of the Uterus.* 2nd ed. New York: Plenum Medical Book Company; 1989:69–88.

37. Ramsey E. Vascular anatomy. In: Wynn R, Jollie W, eds. *Biology of the Uterus.* 2nd ed. New York: Plenum Medical Book Company; 1989:57–68.

38. Wydrzynski M. Anatomical principles of microsurgery of the tubal arteries. *Anat Clin* 1985;7:233–236.

39. DiSaia PJ, Creasman WT. *Clinical Gynecologic Oncology.* 5th ed. St. Louis: Mosby; 1997:viii, 657.

40. Major FJ, Blessing JA, Silverberg SG, et al. Prognostic factors in early-stage uterine sarcoma. A Gynecologic Oncology Group study. *Cancer* 1993;71(4 suppl):1702–1709.

41. Plentl A, Friedman E. *Lymphatic System of the Female Genitalia: The Morphologic Basis of Oncologic Diagnosis and Therapy.* Philadelphia: WB Saunders; 1971.

42. Klein M, Rosen A, Lahousen M, et al. Lymphogenous metastasis in the primary carcinoma of the fallopian tube. *Gynecol Oncol* 1994;55(pt 1):336–338.

43. Klein M, Rosen AC, Lahousen M, Graf AH, Rainer A. Lymphadenectomy in primary carcinoma of the fallopian tube. *Cancer Lett* 1999;147:63–66.

44. Wright TC, Ferenczy A. Anatomy and histology of the cervix. In: Kurman RJ, ed. *Blaustein's Pathology of the Female Genital Tract.* 5th ed. New York: Springer-Verlag, 2002:207–224.

45. Aspden RM. The importance of a slit-like lumen cross-section for the mechanical function of the cervix. *Br J Obstet Gynaecol* 1987; 94:915–916.

46. Gorodeski G. The cervical cycle. In: Adashi E, Rock J, Rosenwaks Z, eds. *Reproductive Endocrinology, Surgery, and Technology.* Philadelphia: Lippincott-Raven; 1996:301–324.

47. Gipson IK. Mucins of the human endocervix. *Front Biosci* 2001;6:D1245–D1255.

48. Konishi I, Fujii S, Nonogaki H, Nanbu Y, Iwai T, Mori T. Immunohistochemical analysis of estrogen receptors, progesterone receptors, Ki-67 antigen, and human papillomavirus DNA in normal and neoplastic epithelium of the uterine cervix. *Cancer* 1991;68:1340–1350.

49. Albores-Saavedra J, Gersell D, Gilks CB, et al. Terminology of endocrine tumors of the uterine cervix: results of a workshop sponsored by the College of American Pathologists and the National Cancer Institute. *Arch Pathol Lab Med* 1997;121: 34–39.

50. Fetisof F, Arbeille B, Boivin F, Sam-Giao M, Henrion C, Lansac J. Endocrine cells in ectocervical epithelium. An immunohistochemical and ultrastructural analysis. *Virchows Arch A Pathol Anat Histopathol* 1987;411:293–298.

51. Fetisof F, Berger G, Dubois MP, et al. Endocrine cells in the female genital tract. *Histopathology* 1985;9:133–145.

52. Fetisof F, Dubois MP, Heitz PU, Lansac J, Arbeille-Brassart B, Jobard P. Endocrine cells in the female genital tract. *Int J Gynecol Pathol* 1986;5:75–87.

53. Fetisof F, Heitzman A, Machet MC, Lansac J. Unusual endocervical lesions with endocrine cells. *Pathol Res Pract* 1993;189:928–939.

54. Fetisof F, Serres G, Arbeille B, de Muret A, Sam-Giao M, Lansac J. Argyrophilic cells and ectocervical epithelium. *Int J Gynecol Pathol* 1991;10:177–190.

55. Scully R, Aguirre P, DeLellis R. Argyrophilia, serotonin, and peptide hormones in the female genital tract and its tumors. *Int J Gynecol Pathol* 1984;3:51–70.

56. Chan JK, Tsui WM, Tung SY, Ching RC. Endocrine cell hyperplasia of the uterine cervix. A precursor of neuroendocrine carcinoma of the cervix? *Am J Clin Pathol* 1989;92:825–830.

57. Hussain LA, Kelly CG, Fellowes R, et al. Expression and gene transcript of Fc receptors for IgG, HLA class II antigens and Langerhans cells in human cervico-vaginal epithelium. *Clin Exp Immunol* 1992;90:530–538.

58. Miller CJ, McChesney M, Moore PF. Langerhans cells, macrophages and lymphocyte subsets in the cervix and vagina of rhesus macaques. *Lab Invest* 1992;67:628–634.

59. Morelli AE, di Paola G, Fainboim L. Density and distribution of Langerhans cells in the human uterine cervix. *Arch Gynecol Obstet* 1992;252:65–71.

60. Osamura RY, Watanabe K, Oh M. Melanin-containing cells in the uterine cervix: histochemical and electron-microscopic studies of two cases. *Am J Clin Pathol* 1980;74:239–242.

61. Hiersche HD, Nagl W. Regeneration of secretory epithelium in the human endocervix. *Arch Gynecol* 1980;229:83–90.

62. Gould PR, Barter RA, Papadimitriou JM. An ultrastructural, cytochemical, and autoradiographic study of the mucous membrane of the human cervical canal with reference to subcolumnar basal cells. *Am J Pathol* 1979;95:1–16.

63. Ismail SM. Cone biopsy causes cervical endometriosis and tubo-endometrioid metaplasia. *Histopathology* 1991;18:107–114.

64. Jonasson JG, Wang HH, Antonioli DA, Ducatman BS. Tubal metaplasia of the uterine cervix: a prevalence study in patients with gynecologic pathologic findings. *Int J Gynecol Pathol* 1992; 11:89–95.

65. Novotny DB, Maygarden SJ, Johnson DE, Frable WJ. Tubal metaplasia. A frequent potential pitfall in the cytologic diagnosis of endocervical glandular dysplasia on cervical smears. *Acta Cytol* 1992;36:1–10.

66. Pacey F, Ayer B, Greenberg M. The cytologic diagnosis of adenocarcinoma in situ of the cervix uteri and related lesions. III. Pitfalls in diagnosis. *Acta Cytol* 1988;32:325–330.

67. Suh KS, Silverberg SG. Tubal metaplasia of the uterine cervix. *Int J Gynecol Pathol* 1990;9:122–128.

68. Young RH, Clement PB. Pseudoneoplastic glandular lesions of the uterine cervix. *Semin Diagn Pathol* 1991;8:234–249.

69. Oliva E, Clement PB, Young RH. Tubal and tubo-endometrioid metaplasia of the uterine cervix. Unemphasized features that may cause problems in differential diagnosis: a report of 25 cases. *Am J Clin Pathol* 1995;103:618–623.

70. Marques T, Andrade LA, Vassallo J. Endocervical tubal metaplasia and adenocarcinoma in situ: role of immunohistochemistry for

71. Peters WM. Nature of "basal" and "reserve" cells in oviductal and cervical epithelium in man. *J Clin Pathol* 1986;39:306–312.

72. Fluhmann C. *The Cervix Uteri and Its Diseases.* Philadelphia: WB Saunders; 1961.

73. Fluhmann CF. The nature and development of the so-called glands of the cervix uteri. *Am J Obstet Gynecol* 1957;74: 753–768.

74. Clement PB, Young RH. Deep nabothian cysts of the uterine cervix. A possible source of confusion with minimal-deviation adenocarcinoma (adenoma malignum). *Int J Gynecol Pathol* 1989;8:340–348.

75. Teshima S, Shimosato Y, Kishi K, Kasamatsu T, Ohmi K, Uei Y. Early stage adenocarcinoma of the uterine cervix. Histopathologic analysis with consideration of histogenesis. *Cancer* 1985; 56:167–172.

76. Bertrand M, Lickrish GM, Colgan TJ. The anatomic distribution of cervical adenocarcinoma in situ: implications for treatment. *Am J Obstet Gynecol* 1987;157:21–25.

77. Gilks CB, Reid PE, Clement PB, Owen DA. Histochemical changes in cervical mucus-secreting epithelium during the normal menstrual cycle. *Fertil Steril* 1989;51:286–291.

78. Nucci MR. Symposium part III: tumor-like glandular lesions of the uterine cervix. *Int J Gynecol Pathol* 2002;21:347–359.

79. Lagow E, DeSouza MM, Carson DD. Mammalian reproductive tract mucins. *Hum Reprod Update* 1999;5:280–292.

80. McDonnell JM, Emens JM, Jordan JA. The congenital cervicovaginal transformation zone in sexually active young women. *Br J Obstet Gynaecol* 1984;91:580–584.

81. Burch DJ, Spowart KJ, Jesinger DK, Randall S, Smith SK. A dose-ranging study of the use of cyclical dydrogesterone with continuous 17 beta oestradiol. *Br J Obstet Gynaecol* 1995;102: 243–248.

82. Forsberg JG. Cervicovaginal epithelium: its origin and development. *Am J Obstet Gynecol* 1973;115:1025–1043.

83. Crum CP, Egawa K, Fu YS, et al. Atypical immature metaplasia (AIM). A subset of human papilloma virus infection of the cervix. *Cancer* 1983;51:2214–2219.

84. Duggan MA. Cytologic and histologic diagnosis and significance of controversial squamous lesions of the uterine cervix. *Mod Pathol* 2000;13:252–260.

85. Aspden RM. Collagen organisation in the cervix and its relation to mechanical function. *Coll Relat Res* 1988;8:103–112.

86. Kiwi R, Neuman MR, Merkatz IR, Selim MA, Lysikiewicz A. Determination of the elastic properties of the cervix. *Obstet Gynecol* 1988;71:568–574.

87. Leppert PC, Cerreta JM, Mandl I. Orientation of elastic fibers in the human cervix. *Am J Obstet Gynecol* 1986;155:219–224.

88. Leppert PC, Yu SY. Three-dimensional structures of uterine elastic fibers: scanning electron microscopic studies. *Connect Tissue Res* 1991;27:15–31.

89. Johansson EL, Rudin A, Wassen L, Holmgren J. Distribution of lymphocytes and adhesion molecules in human cervix and vagina. *Immunology* 1999;96:272–277.

90. Edwards JN, Morris HB. Langerhans' cells and lymphocyte subsets in the female genital tract. *Br J Obstet Gynecol* 1985;92:974–982.

91. Hughes RG, Norval M, Howie SE. Expression of major histocompatibility class II antigens by Langerhans' cells in cervical intraepithelial neoplasia. *J Clin Pathol* 1988;41:253–259.

92. Roncalli M, Sideri M, Gie P, Servida E. Immunophenotypic analysis of the transformation zone of human cervix. *Lab Invest* 1988;58:141–149.

93. Ferry JA, Scully RE. Mesonephric remnants, hyperplasia, and neoplasia in the uterine cervix. A study of 49 cases. *Am J Surg Pathol* 1990;14:1100–1111.

94. Seidman JD, Tavassoli FA. Mesonephric hyperplasia of the uterine cervix: a clinicopathologic study of 51 cases. *Int J Gynecol Pathol* 1995;14:293–299.

95. Oliva E. CD10 expression in the female genital tract: does it have useful diagnostic applications? *Adv Anat Pathol* 2004;11:310–315.

96. McCluggage WG, Oliva E, Herrington CS, McBride H, Young RH. CD10 and calretinin staining of endocervical glandular lesions, endocervical stroma and endometrioid adenocarcinomas of the uterine corpus: CD10 positivity is characteristic of, but not specific for, mesonephric lesions and is not specific for endometrial stroma. *Histopathology* 2003;43:144–150.

97. Nucci MR, Young RH, Fletcher CD. Cellular pseudosarcomatous fibroepithelial stromal polyps of the lower female genital tract: an underrecognized lesion often misdiagnosed as sarcoma. *Am J Surg Pathol* 2000;24:231–240.

98. Abdul-Karim FW, Cohen RE. Atypical stromal cells of lower female genital tract. *Histopathology* 1990;17:249–253.

99. Clement PB. Multinucleated stromal giant cells of the uterine cervix. *Arch Pathol Lab Med* 1985;109:200–202.

100. Metze K, Andrade LA. Atypical stromal giant cells of cervix uteri—evidence of Schwann cell origin. *Pathol Res Pract* 1991; 187:1031–1038.

101. Ledger WL, Anderson AB. The influence of steroid hormones on the uterine cervix during pregnancy. *J Steroid Biochem* 1987;27: 1029–1034.

102. Nucci MR, Young RH. Arias-Stella reaction of the endocervix: a report of 18 cases with emphasis on its varied histology and differential diagnosis. *Am J Surg Pathol* 2004;28:608–612.

103. Leppert PC. Anatomy and physiology of cervical ripening. *Clin Obstet Gynecol* 1995;38:267–279.

104. Pisharodi LR, Jovanoska S. Spectrum of cytologic changes in pregnancy. A review of 100 abnormal cervicovaginal smears, with emphasis on diagnostic pitfalls. *Acta Cytol* 1995;39:905–908.

105. Manganiello PD, Burrows LJ, Dain BJ, Gonzalez J. Vabra aspirator and pipelle endometrial suction curette. A comparison. *J Reprod Med* 1998;43:889–892.

106. Mutter GL, Ferenczy A. Anatomy and histology of the uterine corpus. In: Kurman RJ, ed. *Blaustein's Pathology of the Female Genital Tract.* 5th ed. New York: Springer-Verlag; 2002:383–420.

107. Giudice LC, Ferenczy A. The endometrial cycle: morphologic and biochemical. In: Adashi EY, Rock JA, Rosenwaks Z, eds. *Reproductive Endocrinology, Surgery, and Technology.* Philadelphia: Lippincott-Raven; 1996:271–300.

108. Buckley CH. Normal endometrium and non-proliferative conditions of the endometrium. In: Fox H, Wells M, eds. *Haines and Taylor Obstetrical and Gynaecological Pathology.* 5th ed. London: Churchill Livingstone; 2003:391–442.

109. Warren M, Li T, Klentzeris D. Cell biology of the endometrium: histology, cell types and menstrual changes. In: Chard T, Grudzinskas JG, eds. *The Uterus.* New York: Cambridge University Press; 1994:94–124.

110. Cooper JM, Erickson ML. Endometrial sampling techniques in the diagnosis of abnormal uterine bleeding. *Obstet Gynecol Clin North Am* 2000;27:235–244.

111. Chambers JT, Chambers SK. Endometrial sampling: When? Where? Why? With what? *Clin Obstet Gynecol* 1992;35: 28–39.

112. Mihm LM, Quick VA, Brumfield JA, Connors AF Jr, Finnerty JJ. The accuracy of endometrial biopsy and saline sonohysterography in the determination of the cause of abnormal uterine bleeding. *Am J Obstet Gynecol* 2002;186:858–860.

113. Revel A, Shushan A. Investigation of the infertile couple: hysteroscopy with endometrial biopsy is the gold standard investigation for abnormal uterine bleeding. *Hum Reprod* 2002;17: 1947–1949.

114. Tahir MM, Bigrigg MA, Browning JJ, Brookes ST, Smith PA. A randomised controlled trial comparing transvaginal ultrasound, outpatient hysteroscopy and endometrial biopsy with inpatient hysteroscopy and curettage. *Br J Obstet Gynaecol* 1999;106: 1259–1264.

115. Ben-Yehuda OM, Kim YB, Leuchter RS. Does hysteroscopy improve upon the sensitivity of dilatation and curettage in the diagnosis of endometrial hyperplasia or carcinoma? *Gynecol Oncol* 1998;68:4–7.

116. Hill GA, Herbert CM III, Parker RA, Wentz AC. Comparison of late luteal phase endometrial biopsies using the Novak curette or PIPELLE endometrial suction curette. *Obstet Gynecol* 1989;73(pt 1):443–445.

117. Ferenczy A, Bergeron C. Histology of the human endometrium: from birth to senescence. *Ann N Y Acad Sci* 1991;622:6–27.

118. Denholm R, More IA. Atypical cilia of the human endometrial epithelium. *J Anat* 1980;131(pt 2):309–315.

119. Comer MT, Andrew AC, Leese HJ, Trejdosiewicz LK, Southgate J. Application of a marker of ciliated epithelial cells to gynaecological pathology. *J Clin Pathol* 1999;52:355–357.

120. Kearns M, Lala P. Life history of decidual cells: a review. *Am J Reprod Immunol* 1983;3:78–82.

121. Iwahashi M, Muragaki Y, Ooshima A, Yamoto M, Nakano R. Alterations in distribution and composition of the extracellular matrix during decidualization of the human endometrium. *J Reprod Fertil* 1996;108:147–155.

122. Speroff L, Fritz MA. The uterus: embryology, histology, and endocrinology of the uterus and menstruation. Anatomical abnormalities and leiomyomas. In: Speroff L, Fritz MA, eds. *Clinical Gynecologic Endocrinology and Infertility.* 7th ed. Philadelphia: Lippincott Williams & Wilkins; 2004:113–144.

123. Whitelaw PF, Croy BA. Granulated lymphocytes of pregnancy. *Placenta* 1996;17:533–543.

124. Bulmer JN, Lash GE. Human uterine natural killer cells: a reappraisal. *Mol Immunol* 2005;42:511–521.

125. King A. Uterine leukocytes and decidualization. *Hum Reprod Update* 2000;6:28–36.

126. Kayisli UA, Guzeloglu-Kayisli O, Arici A. Endocrine-immune interactions in human endometrium. *Ann N Y Acad Sci* 2004;1034:50–63.

127. Givan AL, White HD, Stern JE, et al. Flow cytometric analysis of leukocytes in the human female reproductive tract: comparison of fallopian tube, uterus, cervix, and vagina. *Am J Reprod Immunol* 1997;38:350–359.

128. Tabibzadeh S. Proliferative activity of lymphoid cells in human endometrium throughout the menstrual cycle. *J Clin Endocrinol Metab* 1990;70:437–443.

129. Kiviat N, Wolner-Hanssen P, Eschenbach D, et al. Endometrial histopathology in patients with culture-proved upper genital tract infection and laparoscopically diagnosed acute salpingitis. *Am J Surg Pathol* 1990;14:167–175.

130. Achilles SL, Amortegui AJ, Wiesenfeld HC. Endometrial plasma cells: do they indicate subclinical pelvic inflammatory disease? *Sex Transm Dis* 2005;32:185–188.

131. Ramsey E. Vascular anatomy. In: Wynn RM, ed. *Biology of the Uterus.* New York: Plenum Press; 1977:59–76.

132. Ramsey E. Anatomy of the human uterus. In: Chard T, Grudzinskas JG, eds. *The Uterus.* New York: Cambridge University Press; 1994:18–40.

133. Gargett CE, Rogers PA. Human endometrial angiogenesis. *Reproduction* 2001;121:181–186.

134. Taylor RN, Lebovic DI, Hornung D, Mueller MD. Endocrine and paracrine regulation of endometrial angiogenesis. *Ann N Y Acad Sci* 2001;943:109–121.

135. Rees MC, Bicknell R. Angiogenesis in the endometrium. *Angiogenesis* 1998;2:29–35.

136. Albrecht ED, Pepe GJ. Steroid hormone regulation of angiogenesis in the primate endometrium. *Front Biosci* 2003;8:D416–D429.

137. Anin SA, Vince G, Quenby S. Trophoblast invasion. *Hum Fertil (Camb)* 2004;7:169–174.

138. Lyall F. Priming and remodelling of human placental bed spiral arteries during pregnancy—a review. *Placenta* 2005;26(suppl A):S31–S36.

139. Spornitz UM. The functional morphology of the human endometrium and decidua. *Adv Anat Embryol Cell Biol* 1992;124:1–99.

140. Cornillie FJ, Lauweryns JM, Brosens IA. Normal human endometrium. An ultrastructural survey. *Gynecol Obstet Invest* 1985;20:113–129.

141. Dockery P, Rogers AW. The effects of steroids on the fine structure of the endometrium. *Baillieres Clin Obstet Gynaecol* 1989;3:227–248.

142. Dockery P, Pritchard K, Warren MA, Li TC, Cooke ID. Changes in nuclear morphology in the human endometrial glandular epithelium in women with unexplained infertility. *Hum Reprod* 1996;11:2251–2256.

143. Paria BC, Reese J, Das SK, Dey SK. Deciphering the cross-talk of implantation: advances and challenges. *Science* 2002;296:2185–2188.

144. Tazuke SI, Giudice LC. Growth factors and cytokines in endometrium, embryonic development, and maternal: embryonic interactions. *Semin Reprod Endocrinol* 1996;14:231–245.

145. Mylonas I, Jeschke U, Wiest I, et al. Inhibin/activin subunits alpha, beta-A and beta-B are differentially expressed in normal human endometrium throughout the menstrual cycle. *Histochem Cell Biol* 2004;122:461–471.

146. Stavreus-Evers A, Koraen L, Scott JE, Zhang P, Westlund P. Distribution of cyclooxygenase-1, cyclooxygenase-2, and cytosolic phospholipase A2 in the luteal phase human endometrium and ovary. *Fertil Steril* 2005;83:156–162.

147. Speroff L, Fritz MA, eds. *Clinical Gynecologic Endocrinology and Infertility.* 7th ed. Philadelphia: Lippincott Williams & Wilkins; 2004.

148. Treloar A, Boynton R, Behn B, Brown BW. Variation of the human menstrual cycle through reproductive life. *Int J Fertil* 1967;12 (pt 2):77–126.

149. Hall J. Neuroendocrine control of the menstrual cycle. In: Strauss J, Barbieri R, eds. *Yen and Jaffe's Reproductive Endocrinology: Physiology, Pathophysiology, and Clinical Management.* Philadelphia: Elsevier Saunders; 2004:195–212.

150. Hodgen GD. Neuroendocrinology of the normal menstrual cycle. *J Reprod Med* 1989;34(1 suppl):68–75.

151. Koehler KF, Helguero LA, Haldosen LA, Warner M, Gustafsson JA. Reflections on the discovery and significance of estrogen receptor beta. *Endocr Rev* 2005;26:465–478.

152. Alberts B, Johnson A, Lewis J, Raff M, Roberts K, Walter P. Cell communication. In: Alberts B, Johnson A, Lewis J, Raff M, Roberts K, Walter P. *Molecular Biology of the Cell.* 4th ed. New York: Garland Science; 2002:831–906.

153. Rhen T, Cidlowski JA. Steroid hormone action. In: Strauss J, Barbieri R, eds. *Yen and Jaffe's Reproductive Endocrinology: Physiology, Pathophysiology, and Clinical Management.* 5th ed. Philadelphia: Elsevier Saunders; 2004:155–174.

154. Li T, Dockery P, Rogers A, Cooke I. How precise is histologic dating of endometrium using the standard dating criteria? *Fertil Steril* 1989;51:759–763.

155. Strauss JI, Gurpide E. The endometrium: regulation and dysfunction. In: Yen S, Jaffe R, eds. *Yen and Jaffe's Reproductive Endocrinology: Physiology, Pathophysiology and Clinical Management.* Philadelphia: WB Saunders; 1991:309–356.

156. Wynn RM. The human endometrium: cyclic and gestational changes. In: Wynn R, Jollie W, eds. *Biology of the Uterus.* 2nd ed. New York: Plenum Medical Book Company; 1989:289–332.

157. Milwidsky A, Palti Z, Gutman A. Glycogen metabolism of the human endometrium. *J Clin Endocrinol Metab* 1980;51:765–770.

158. Daly D, Tohan N, Doney T, Maslar I, Riddick D. The significance of lymphocytic-leukocytic infiltrates in interpreting late luteal phase endometrial biopsies. *Fertil Steril* 1982;37:786–791.

159. Critchley HO, Kelly RW, Brenner RM, Baird DT. The endocrinology of menstruation—a role for the immune system. *Clin Endocrinol (Oxf)* 2001;55:701–710.

160. Rogers PA, Lederman F, Taylor N. Endometrial microvascular growth in normal and dysfunctional states. *Hum Reprod Update* 1998;4:503–508.

161. Salamonsen LA. Tissue injury and repair in the female human reproductive tract. *Reproduction* 2003;125:301–311.

162. Ludwig H, Spornitz UM. Microarchitecture of the human endometrium by scanning electron microscopy: menstrual desquamation and remodeling. *Ann N Y Acad Sci* 1991;622:28–46.

163. Hertig A. Gestational hyperplasia of endometrium: a morphologic correlation of ova, endometrium, and corpora lutea during early pregnancy. *Lab Invest* 1964;13:1153–1191.

164. Parr M, Parr E. The implantation reaction. In: Wynn R, Jollie W, eds. *Biology of the Uterus.* 2nd ed. New York: Plenum Medical Book Company; 1989:233–278.

165. O'Connor D, Kurman R. Intermediate trophoblast in uterine curettings in the diagnosis of ectopic pregnancy. *Obstet Gynecol* 1988;72:665–670.

166. Gruber K, Gelven PL, Austin RM. Chorionic villi or trophoblastic tissue in uterine samples of four women with ectopic pregnancies. *Int J Gynecol Pathol* 1997;16:28–32.

167. Young RH, Kurman RJ, Scully RE. Placental site nodules and plaques. A clinicopathologic analysis of 20 cases. *Am J Surg Pathol* 1990;14:1001–1009.

168. Shih IM, Seidman JD, Kurman RJ. Placental site nodule and characterization of distinctive types of intermediate trophoblast. *Hum Pathol* 1999;30:687–694.

169. Shih IM, Kurman RJ. Ki-67 labeling index in the differential diagnosis of exaggerated placental site, placental site trophoblastic tumor, and choriocarcinoma: a double immunohistochemical staining technique using Ki-67 and Mel-CAM antibodies. *Hum Pathol* 1998;29:27–33.

170. Shih IM, Kurman RJ. p63 expression is useful in the distinction of epithelioid trophoblastic and placental site trophoblastic tumors by profiling trophoblastic subpopulations. *Am J Surg Pathol* 2004;28:1177–1183.

171. Arias-Stella J. The Arias-Stella reaction: facts and fancies four decades after. *Adv Anat Pathol* 2002;9:12–23.

172. Huettner PC, Gersell DJ. Arias-Stella reaction in nonpregnant women: a clinicopathologic study of nine cases. *Int J Gynecol Pathol* 1994;13:241–247.

173. Arias-Stella J Jr, Arias-Velasquez A, Arias-Stella J. Normal and abnormal mitoses in the atypical endometrial change associated with chorionic tissue effect [corrected]. *Am J Surg Pathol* 1994;18:694–701.

174. Vang R, Barner R, Wheeler DT, Strauss BL. Immunohistochemical staining for Ki-67 and p53 helps distinguish endometrial Arias-Stella reaction from high-grade carcinoma, including clear cell carcinoma. *Int J Gynecol Pathol* 2004;23:223–233.

175. Mazur M, Hendrickson M, Kempson R. Optically clear nuclei. An alteration of endometrial epithelium in the presence of trophoblast. *Am J Surg Pathol* 1983;7:415–423.

176. Lichtig C, Deutch M, Brandes J. Vascular changes of endometrium in early pregnancy. *Am J Clin Pathol* 1984;81:702–707.

177. Hustin J, Wells M. Pathology of the pregnant uterus. In: Fox H, Wells M, eds. *Haines and Taylor Obstetrical and Gynaecological Pathology*. 5th ed. Edinburgh, Scotland: Churchill Livingstone; 2003:1327–1357.

178. Taffe JR, Dennerstein L. Menstrual patterns leading to the final menstrual period. *Menopause* 2002;9:32–40.

179. Archer DF, McIntyre-Seltman K, Wilborn WW Jr, et al. Endometrial morphology in asymptomatic postmenopausal women. *Am J Obstet Gynecol* 1991;165:371–322.

180. Choo YC, Mak KC, Hsu C, Wong TS, Ma HK. Postmenopausal uterine bleeding of nonorganic cause. *Obstet Gynecol* 1985;66:225–228.

181. Moodley M, Roberts C. Clinical pathway for the evaluation of postmenopausal bleeding with an emphasis on endometrial cancer detection. *J Obstet Gynaecol* 2004;24:736–741.

182. Quddus MR, Sung CJ, Zheng W, Lauchlan SC. p53 immunoreactivity in endometrial metaplasia with dysfunctional uterine bleeding. *Histopathology* 1999;35:44–49.

183. Haney AF. Endometrial biopsy: a test whose time has come and gone. *Fertil Steril* 2004;82:1295–1296, 1301–1302.

184. Coutifaris C, Myers ER, Guzick DS, et al. Histological dating of timed endometrial biopsy tissue is not related to fertility status. *Fertil Steril* 2004;82:1264–1272.

185. Murray MJ, Meyer WR, Zaino RJ, et al. A critical analysis of the accuracy, reproducibility, and clinical utility of histologic endometrial dating in fertile women. *Fertil Steril* 2004;81:1333–1343.

186. Myers ER, Silva S, Barnhart K, et al. Interobserver and intraobserver variability in the histological dating of the endometrium in fertile and infertile women. *Fertil Steril* 2004;82:1278–1282.

187. Glatstein IZ, Harlow BL, Hornstein MD. Practice patterns among reproductive endocrinologists: further aspects of the infertility evaluation. *Fertil Steril* 1998;70:263–269.

188. Balasch J. Investigation of the infertile couple: investigation of the infertile couple in the era of assisted reproductive technology: a time for reappraisal. *Hum Reprod* 2000;15:2251–2257.

189. Speroff L, Fritz MA. Female infertility. In: *Clinical Gynecologic Endocrinology and Infertility*. 7th ed. Philadelphia: Lippincott Williams & Wilkins; 2004:1013–1069.

190. Glatstein IZ, Harlow BL, Hornstein MD. Practice patterns among reproductive endocrinologists: further aspects of the infertility evaluation. *Fertil Steril* 1998;70:263–269.

191. Balasch J, Fabregues F, Creus M, Vanrell J. The usefulness of endometrial biopsy for luteal phase evaluation in infertility. *Hum Reprod* 1992;7:973–977.

192. Peters AJ, Lloyd RP, Coulam CB. Prevalence of out-of-phase endometrial biopsy specimens. *Am J Obstet Gynecol* 1992;166(pt 1):1738–1746.

193. Noyes R. Normal phases of the endometrium. In: Hertig A, Norris H, Abell M, eds. *The Uterus*. Baltimore: Williams & Wilkins; 1973:110–135.

194. Noyes R, Hertig A, Rock J. Dating the endometrial biopsy. *Fertil Steril* 1950;1:3–25.

195. McNeely MJ, Soules MR. The diagnosis of luteal phase deficiency: a critical review [see comments]. *Fertil Steril* 1988;50:1–15.

196. Noyes R, Haman J. Accuracy of endometrial dating: correlation of endometrial dating with basal body temperature and menses. *Fertil Steril* 1953;4:504–517.

197. Li T, Rogers A, Lenton E, Dockery P, Cooke I. A comparison between two methods of chronological dating of human endometrial biopsies during the luteal phase, and their correlation with histologic dating. *Fertil Steril* 1987;48:928–932.

198. Gibson M, Badger GJ, Byrn F, Lee K, Korson R, Trainer T. Error in histologic dating of secretory endometrium: variance component analysis. *Fertil Steril* 1991;56:242–247.

199. Scott RT, Snyder RR, Strickland DM, et al. The effect of interobserver variation in dating endometrial histology on the diagnosis of luteal phase defects. *Fertil Steril* 1988;50:888–892.

200. Otsuki Y. Apoptosis in human endometrium: apoptotic detection methods and signaling. *Med Electron Microsc* 2001;34:166–173.

201. Kokawa K, Shikone T, Nakano R. Apoptosis in the human uterine endometrium during the menstrual cycle. *J Clin Endocrinol Metab* 1996;81:4144–4147.

202. Konno R, Igarashi T, Okamoto S, et al. Apoptosis of human endometrium mediated by perforin and granzyme B of NK cells and cytotoxic T lymphocytes. *Tohoku J Exp Med* 1999;187:149–155.

203. Sivridis E, Giatromanolaki A. New insights into the normal menstrual cycle-regulatory molecules. *Histol Histopathol* 2004;19:511–516.

204. Rotello RJ, Lieberman RC, Purchio AF, Gerschenson LE. Coordinated regulation of apoptosis and cell proliferation by transforming growth factor beta 1 in cultured uterine epithelial cells. *Proc Natl Acad Sci U S A* 1991;88:3412–3415.

205. Gerschenson LE, Rotello RJ. Apoptosis: a different type of cell death. *FASEB J* 1992;6:2450–2455.

206. Rotello RJ, Hocker MB, Gerschenson LE. Biochemical evidence for programmed cell death in rabbit uterine epithelium. *Am J Pathol* 1989;134:491–495.

207. Rotello RJ, Lieberman RC, Lepoff RB, Gerschenson LE. Characterization of uterine epithelium apoptotic cell death kinetics and regulation by progesterone and RU 486. *Am J Pathol* 1992;140:449–456.

208. Gompel A, Sabourin JC, Martin A, et al. Bcl-2 expression in normal endometrium during the menstrual cycle. *Am J Pathol* 1994;144:1195–1202.

209. Maia H Jr, Maltez A, Studart E, Athayde C, Coutinho EM. Ki-67, Bcl-2 and p53 expression in endometrial polyps and in the normal endometrium during the menstrual cycle. *BJOG* 2004;111:1242–1247.

210. Tabibzadeh S, Zupi E, Babaknia A, Liu R, Marconi D, Romanini C. Site and menstrual cycle-dependent expression of proteins of the tumour necrosis factor (TNF) receptor family, and BCL-2 oncoprotein and phase-specific production of TNF alpha in human endometrium. *Hum Reprod* 1995;10:277–286.

211. Cole W, Garfield R. Ultrastructure of the myometrium. In: Wynn R, Jollie W, eds. *Biology of the Uterus*. 2nd ed. New York: Plenum Medical Book Company; 1989:455–504.

212. Garfield R, Yallampalli C. Structure and function of uterine muscle. In: Chard T, Grudzinskas JG, eds. *The Uterus*. New York: Cambridge University Press; 1994:54–93.

213. Huszar G, Walsh M. Biochemistry of the myometrium and cervix. In: Wynn R, Jollie W, eds. *Biology of the Uterus*. 2nd ed. New York: Plenum Medical Book Company; 1989:355–402.

214. Kao C. Electrophysiological properties of uterine smooth muscle. In: Wynn R, Jollie W, eds. *Biology of the Uterus*. 2nd ed. New York: Plenum Medical Book Company; 1989:403–454.

215. Kawaguchi K, Fujii S, Konishi I, Nanbu Y, Nonogaki H, Mori T. Mitotic activity in uterine leiomyomas during the menstrual cycle. *Am J Obstet Gynecol* 1989;160:637–641.

216. Hamoir G. Biochemistry of the myometrium. In: Wynn R, ed. *Biology of the Uterus*. New York: Plenum Press; 1977:377–421.

217. Marshall J. The physiology of the myometrium. In: Hertig A, Norris H, Abell M, eds. *The Uterus*. Baltimore: Williams & Wilkins; 1973:89–109.

218. Oliva E, Clement PB, Young RH, Scully RE. Mixed endometrial stromal and smooth muscle tumors of the uterus: a clinicopathologic study of 15 cases. *Am J Surg Pathol* 1998;22: 997–1005.

219. Azumi N, Ben-Ezra J, Battifora H. Immunophenotypic diagnosis of leiomyosarcomas and rhabdomyosarcomas with monoclonal antibodies to muscle-specific actin and desmin in formalin-fixed tissue. *Mod Pathol* 1988;1:469–474.

220. Brown D, Theaker J, Banks P, Gatter K, Mason D. Cytokeratin expression in smooth muscle and smooth muscle tumours. *Histopathology* 1987;11:477–486.

221. Langloss J, Kurman R, Bratthauer G. *Expression of keratin by normal and neoplastic smooth muscle cells of the human uterus.* 1990.

222. Norton AJ, Thomas JA, Isaacson PG. Cytokeratin-specific monoclonal antibodies are reactive with tumours of smooth muscle derivation. An immunocytochemical and biochemical study using antibodies to intermediate filament cytoskeletal proteins. *Histopathology* 1987;11:487–499.

223. Clement PB, Young RH, Scully RE. Nontrophoblastic pathology of the female genital tract and peritoneum associated with pregnancy. *Semin Diagn Pathol* 1989;6:372–406.

224. Silverberg S, Kurman R. Tumors of the uterine corpus and gestational trophoblastic disease. 3rd series, fascicle 3. In: *Atlas of Tumor Pathology*. Washington, DC: Armed Forces Institute of Pathology; 1992:191–206.

225. Garfield RE, Hayashi RH. Appearance of gap junctions in the myometrium of women during labor. *Am J Obstet Gynecol* 1981; 140:254–260.

226. Brenner R, Slayden O. The fallopian tube cycle. In: Adashi E, Rock J, Rosenwaks Z, eds. *Reproductive Endocrinology: Surgery and Technology*. Vol 1. Philadelphia: Lippincott-Raven; 1996:325–339.

227. Bonilla-Musoles F, Ferrer-Barriendos J, Pellicer A. Cyclical changes in the epithelium of the fallopian tube. Studies with scanner electron microscopy (SEM). *Clin Exp Obstet Gynecol* 1983;10:79–86.

228. Donnez J, Casanas-Roux F, Caprasse J, Ferin J, Thomas K. Cyclic changes in ciliation, cell height, and mitotic activity in human tubal epithelium during reproductive life. *Fertil Steril* 1985;43: 554–559.

229. Jansen RP. Endocrine response in the fallopian tube. *Endocr Rev* 1984;5:525–551.

230. Lindenbaum ES, Peretz BA, Beach D. Menstrual-cycle-dependent and -independent features of the human fallopian tube fimbrial epithelium: an ultrastructural and cytochemical study. *Gynecol Obstet Invest* 1983;16:76–85.

231. Verhage HG, Bareither ML, Jaffe RC, Akbar M. Cyclic changes in ciliation, secretion and cell height of the oviductal epithelium in women. *Am J Anat* 1979;156:505–521.

232. Menezo Y, Guerin P. The mammalian oviduct: biochemistry and physiology. *Eur J Obstet Gynecol Reprod Biol* 1997;73:99–104.

233. Leese HJ. The formation and function of oviduct fluid. *J Reprod Fertil* 1988;82:843–856.

234. Sivridis E, Buckley C, Fox H. Argyrophil cells in normal, hyperplastic, and neoplastic endometrium. *J Clin Pathol* 1984;37: 378–381.

235. Constant O, Cooke J, Parsons CA. Reformatted computed tomography of the female pelvis: normal anatomy. *Br J Obstet Gynaecol* 1989;96:1047–1053.

236. de Castro A, Yebra C, Aznar F, et al. Measurement of the endometrial cavity length using Wing Sound I. *Adv Contracept* 1987;3:133–137.

237. Hricak H. MRI of the female pelvis: a review. *AJR Am J Roentgenol* 1986;146:1115–1122.

238. Morris H, Emms M, Visser T, Timme A. Lymphoid tissue of the normal fallopian tube—a form of mucosal-associated lymphoid tissue (MALT). *Int J Gynecol Pathol* 1986;5:11–22.

239. Boehme M, Donat H. Identification of lymphocyte subsets in the human fallopian tube. *Am J Reprod Immunol* 1992;28:81–84.

240. Kutteh WH, Blackwell RE, Gore H, Kutteh CC, Carr BR, Mestecky J. Secretory immune system of the female reproductive tract. II. Local immune system in normal and infected fallopian tube. *Fertil Steril* 1990;54:51–55.

241. Lurie M, Tur-Kaspa I, Weill S, Katz I, Rabinovici J, Goldenberg S. Ciliary ultrastructure of respiratory and fallopian tube epithelium in a sterile woman with Kartagener's syndrome. A quantitative estimation. *Chest* 1989;95:578–581.

242. Halbert SA, Patton DL, Zarutskie PW, Soules MR. Function and structure of cilia in the fallopian tube of an infertile woman with Kartagener's syndrome. *Hum Reprod* 1997;12:55–58.

243. Agoff SN, Mendelin JE, Grieco VS, Garcia RL. Unexpected gynecologic neoplasms in patients with proven or suspected BRCA-1 or -2 mutations: implications for gross examination, cytology, and clinical follow-up. *Am J Surg Pathol* 2002;26: 171–178.

244. Kauff ND, Satagopan JM, Robson ME, et al. Risk-reducing salpingo-oophorectomy in women with a BRCA1 or BRCA2 mutation. *N Engl J Med* 2002;346:1609–1615.

245. Lindblom B, Wilhelmsson L, Wikland M, Hamberger L, Wiqvist N. Prostaglandins and oviductal function. *Acta Obstet Gynecol Scand Suppl* 1983;113:43–46.

246. Green LK, Kott ML. Histopathologic findings in ectopic tubal pregnancy. *Int J Gynecol Pathol* 1989;8:255–262.

247. Pulkkinen MO, Talo A. Tubal physiologic consideration in ectopic pregnancy. *Clin Obstet Gynecol* 1987;30:164–172.

248. Donnez J, Casanas-Roux F, Ferin J. Macroscopic and microscopic studies of fallopian tube after laparoscopic sterilization. *Contraception* 1979;20:497–509.

249. Donnez J, Casanas-Roux F, Ferin J, Thomas K. Tubal polyps, epithelial inclusions, and endometriosis after tubal sterilization. *Fertil Steril* 1984;41:564–568.

250. Mills SE, Fechner RE. Stromal and epithelial changes in the fallopian tube following hormonal therapy. *Hum Pathol* 1980;11(5 suppl):583–585.

251. Blackwell PM, Fraser IS. Superficial lymphatics in the functional zone of normal human endometrium. *Microvasc Res* 1981;21: 142–152.

252. Laqueur T. *Making Sex: Body and Gender from the Greeks to Freud.* Cambridge, MA: Harvard University Press; 1990.

253. Profet M. Menstruation as a defense against pathogens transported by sperm. *Q Rev Biol* 1993;68:335–386.

254. Strassmann BI. The evolution of endometrial cycles and menstruation. *Q Rev Biol* 1996;71:181–220.

255. Crafts R, Krieger H. Gross anatomy of the female reproductive tract, pituitary, and hypothalamus. In: Danforth D, Scott J, eds. *Obstetrics and Gynecology*. Philadelphia: JB Lippincott; 1986:64.

256. Henriksen E. The lymphatic spread of carcinoma of the cervix and of the body of the uterus; a study of 420 necropsies. *Am J Obstet Gynecol* 1949;58:924–942.

257. DiSaia P, Creasman W, eds. *Clinical Gynecologic Oncology*. 3rd ed. St. Louis: CV Mosby; 1989:84–93.

258. Hendrickson M, Kempson R. *Surgical Pathology of the Uterine Corpus*. Philadelphia: WB Saunders; 1980.

259. Arias-Stella J. Gestational endometrium. In: Hertig A, Norris H, Abell M, eds. *The Uterus*. Baltimore: Williams & Wilkins; 1973:185–212.

260. Hendrickson M, Kempson R. The uterine corpus. In: Sternberg S, ed. *Diagnostic Surgical Pathology*. New York: Raven; 1994: 2091–2193.

261. Janovski N, Paramanandhan T. *Ovarian Tumors, Tumors and Tumor-like Conditions of the Ovaries, Fallopian Tubes and Ligaments of the Uterus*. Philadelphia: WB Saunders; 1973:191–194.

262. Anderson MC, Hartley RB. Cervical crypt involvement by intraepithelial neoplasia. *Obstet Gynecol* 1980;55:546–550.

263. Clement PB, Young RH, Scully RE. Stromal endometriosis of the uterine cervix. A variant of endometriosis that may simulate a sarcoma. *Am J Surg Pathol* 1990;14:449–455.

264. Clement PB. Pathology of endometriosis. *Pathol Annu* 1990; 25(pt 1):245–295.

265. Baker PM, Clement PB, Bell DA, Young RH. Superficial endometriosis of the uterine cervix: a report of 20 cases of a process that may be confused with endocervical glandular dysplasia or adenocarcinoma in situ. *Int J Gynecol Pathol* 1999;18:198–205.

266. Young RH, Scully RE. Atypical forms of microglandular hyperplasia of the cervix simulating carcinoma. A report of five cases and review of the literature. *Am J Surg Pathol* 1989;13:50–56.

267. Leslie KO, Silverberg SG. Microglandular hyperplasia of the cervix: unusual clinical and pathological presentations and their differential diagnosis. *Prog Surg Pathol* 1984;5:95–114.

268. Hendrickson MR, Longacre TA, Kempson RL. The uterine corpus. In: Mills SE, ed. *Diagnostic Surgical Pathology*. 4th ed. New York: Raven Press; 2004:2435–2542.

269. Russack V, Lammers R. Xanthogranulomatous endometritis. Report of six cases and a proposed mechanism of development. *Arch Pathol Lab Med* 1990;114:929–932.

270. Johannisson E, Parker R, Landgren B, Diczfalusy E. Morphometric analysis of the human endometrium in relation to peripheral hormone levels. *Fertil Steril* 1982;38:564–571.

271. Jones R, Mammel J, Shepard M, Fisher R. Recovery of chlamydia trachomatis from the endometrium of women at risk for chlamydial infection. *Am J Obstet Gynecol* 1986;155:35–39.

272. Poropatich C, Rojas M, Silverberg S. Polymorphonuclear leukocytes in the endometrium during the normal menstrual cycle. *Int J Gynecol Pathol* 1987;6:230–234.

273. Winkler B, Reumann W, Mitao M, Gallo L, Richart R, Crum C. Chlamydial endometritis. A histological and immunohistochemical analysis. *Am J Surg Pathol* 1984;8:771–778.

274. Farhood AI, Abrams J. Immunohistochemistry of endometrial stromal sarcoma (ESS). *Hum Pathol* 1991;22:224–230.

275. Binder SW, Nieberg RK, Cheng L, al-Jitawi S. Histologic and immunohistochemical analysis of nine endometrial stromal tumors: an unexpected high frequency of keratin protein positivity. *Int J Gynecol Pathol* 1991;10:191–197.

276. Dabbs DJ. *Diagnostic Immunohistochemistry*. New York: Churchill Livingstone; 2002.

277. Devaney K, Tavassoli FA. Immunohistochemistry as a diagnostic aid in the interpretation of unusual mesenchymal tumors of the uterus. *Mod Pathol* 1991;4:225–231.

278. Farhood AI, Abrams J. Immunohistochemistry of endometrial stromal sarcoma. *Hum Pathol* 1991;22:224–230.

279. Franquemont DW, Frierson HF Jr, Mills SE. An immunohistochemical study of normal endometrial stroma and endometrial stromal neoplasms. Evidence for smooth muscle differentiation. *Am J Surg Pathol* 1991;15:861–870.

280. Brown DC, Theaker JM, Banks PM, Gatter K, Mason D. Cytokeratin expression in smooth muscle and smooth muscle tumours. *Histopathology* 1987;11:477–486.

281. Gown AM, Boyd HC, Chang Y, Ferguson M, Reichler B, Tippens D. Smooth muscle cells can express cytokeratins of "simple" epithelium. Immunocytochemical and biochemical studies in vitro and in vivo. *Am J Pathol* 1988;132:223–232.

282. Ramaekers FC, Pruszczynski M, Smedts F. Cytokeratins in smooth muscle cells and smooth muscle tumours. *Histopathology* 1988;12:558–561.

283. Rizeq MN, van de Rijn M, Hendrickson MR, Rouse RV. A comparative immunohistochemical study of uterine smooth muscle neoplasms with emphasis on the epithelioid variant. *Hum Pathol* 1994;25:671–677.

284. Balaton AJ, Vuong PN, Vaury P, Baviera EE. Plexiform tumorlet of the uterus: immunohistological evidence for a smooth muscle origin. *Histopathology* 1986;10:749–754.

285. Sullinger J, Scully RE. Uterine tumors resembling ovarian sex-cord tumors. A clinicopathologic and immunohistochemical study [abstract]. *Mod Pathol* 1989;2:93A.

286. Lillemoe I, Perrone T, Norris H, Dehner L. Myogenous phenotype of epithelial-like areas in endometrial stromal sarcomas. *Arch Pathol Lab Med* 1991;115:215–219.

287. McCluggage WG, Shah V, Walsh MY, Toner PG. Uterine tumour resembling ovarian sex cord tumour: evidence for smooth muscle differentiation. *Histopathology* 1993;23:83–85.

288. Fetissof F, Berger G, Dubois MP, Philippe A, Lansac J, Jobard P. Female genital tract and Peutz-Jeghers syndrome: an immunohistochemical study. *Int J Gynecol Pathol* 1985;4:219–229.

289. Saffos RO, Rhatigan RM, Scully RE. Metaplastic papillary tumor of the fallopian tube—a distinctive lesion of pregnancy. *Am J Clin Pathol* 1980;74:232–236.

Ovary

Philip B. Clement

42

EMBRYOLOGY

Approximately 5 weeks after fertilization, a thickening of the coelomic epithelium (mesothelium) along the medial and ventral borders of the mesonephros leads to the formation of the genital ridge. The gonadal anlage forms as a result of continued proliferation of this epithelium and the subjacent mesenchyme (1). Simultaneously, primordial germ cells migrate to the gonad from the yolk sac endoderm, reaching the genital ridge during the fifth and sixth weeks of embryonic life (2). These cells (oogonia) undergo mitotic activity and become most numerous at midgestation; two-thirds of them will undergo atresia by term

(1,3). At 12 to 15 weeks' gestation, the oogonia begin meiosis and arrest in meiotic prophase, and are now referred to as primary oocytes (3–5).

At two months, the primitive gonad is recognizable as an ovary because, in contrast to the testis, it has remained basically unaltered. At 7 to 9 weeks' gestation, the outer zone of the ovary has enlarged to form the definitive cortex, which consists of confluent sheets of primitive germ cells admixed haphazardly with a smaller number of smaller pregranulosa cells (4,6). At 12 to 15 weeks, vascular connective tissue septa begin to radiate from the medullary mesenchyme into the inner portion of the cortex, and extend into the superficial part of the cortex by 20 weeks (5,6). The cortex thereby becomes divided into cellular groups composed of oocytes and pregranulosa cells (sex cords). Simultaneously, the pregranulosa cells begin to surround individual germ cells to form primordial follicles. Folliculogenesis begins in the inner part of the cortex at 14 to 20 weeks' gestation (2,3,5,7), and gradually extends to the outer cortex by the early neonatal period (8). The occasional follicles that mature into preantral and antral follicles in late gestation become surrounded by a condensation of mesenchymal cells that become the theca interna (4,7). The rete ovarii is present in the hilus as early as 12 weeks (5).

The origin of the gonadal sex cords (pregranulosa cells in the ovary and Sertoli cells in the testis) is controversial. Some investigators (2,4,8,9) believe that they are derived from the coelomic epithelium, while others (10) favor an origin from the "mesenchyme." Still others (11,12) believe that the gonadal blastema is too undifferentiated to classify as either epithelial or mesenchymal. More recent observations indicate that the sex cords are likely of mesonephric origin (13–16). Satoh (14) found that although rudimentary cord-like structures arise from coelomic epithelial cells, they disappear before contributing to the formation of the definitive sex cords, which are derived from cells that originate from the mesonephros.

GROSS ANATOMY

The ovaries are paired pelvic organs that lie on either side of the uterus close to the lateral pelvic wall, behind the broad ligament and anterior to the rectum. Each ovary is attached along its anterior (hilar) margin to the posterior aspect of the broad ligament by a double fold of peritoneum, the mesovarium; at its medial pole to the ipsilateral uterine cornu by the ovarian (or utero-ovarian) ligament; and from the superior aspect of its lateral pole to the lateral pelvic wall by the infundibulopelvic (or suspensory) ligament. The location of the ovary posterior to the broad ligament and a similar relationship of the ovarian ligament to the ipsilateral uterine (fallopian) tube aids in the determination of the laterality of a salpingo-oophorectomy specimen.

Prepubertal Ovaries

The ovary in the newborn is a tan, elongated, and flattened structure that lies above the true pelvis. It sometimes has a lobulated appearance with irregular edges (Figure 42.1A). It has approximate dimensions of 1.3 cm by 0.5 cm by 0.3 cm, and a weight of less than 0.3 gm (17–19). Throughout infancy and childhood, the ovary enlarges, increases in weight 30-fold, and changes in shape, so that by the time of puberty it has reached the size, weight, and shape of the adult ovary, and lies within the true pelvis (18,19). Inspection of the external and cut surfaces, particularly during the first few months of life and at puberty, may reveal

prominent cystic follicles (20) similar to those seen in polycystic ovary disease (Figure 42.1B).

Adult Ovaries

Adult ovaries are ovoid with dimensions of approximately 3.0 to 5 cm by 1.5 to 3.0 cm by .6 to 1.5 cm, and a weight of 5 to 8 gm. Their size and weight, however, vary considerably depending on their content of follicular derivatives. They have a pink-white exterior, which in early reproductive life is usually smooth (Figure 42.1C), but thereafter becomes increasingly convoluted. Three ill-defined zones are discernible on the cut surface: an outer cortex, an inner medulla, and the hilus. Follicular structures (cystic follicles, yellow corpora lutea, white corpora albicantia) are typically visible in the cortex and medulla.

Postmenopausal Ovaries

After the menopause, the ovaries typically shrink to approximately one half their size in the reproductive era (21). Their size varies considerably, however, with the number of ovarian stromal cells and unresorbed corpora albicantia (22). Most postmenopausal ovaries have a shrunken, gyriform, external appearance (Figure 42.1D), while some are more smooth and uniform. They have a firm consistency and a predominantly solid, pale cut surface, although occasional cysts measuring several millimeters in diameter (inclusion cysts) may be discernible within the cortex. Small white scars (corpora albicantia) are typically present within the medulla. Thick-walled blood vessels may be appreciable within the medulla and the hilus.

BLOOD SUPPLY

The ovarian artery, a branch of the aorta, courses along the infundibulopelvic ligament and the mesovarial border of the ovary where it anastomoses with the ovarian branch of the uterine artery. Approximately ten arterial branches from this arcade penetrate the ovarian hilus, becoming markedly coiled and branched as they course through the medulla (23). These helicine arteries possess longitudinal ridges of intimal smooth muscle along their length. At the corticomedullary junction, the medullary arteries and arterioles form a plexus from which smaller, straight cortical arterioles arise and penetrate the cortex in a radial fashion, perpendicular to the ovarian surface. The cortical arterioles branch and anastomose several times, forming sets of interconnected vascular arcades (23). These arcades give rise to capillaries that form dense networks within the theca layers of the ovarian follicles. The intraovarian veins accompany the arteries, becoming large and tortuous in the medulla and forming a hilar plexus that drains into the ovarian veins; the latter traverse the mesovarium and course

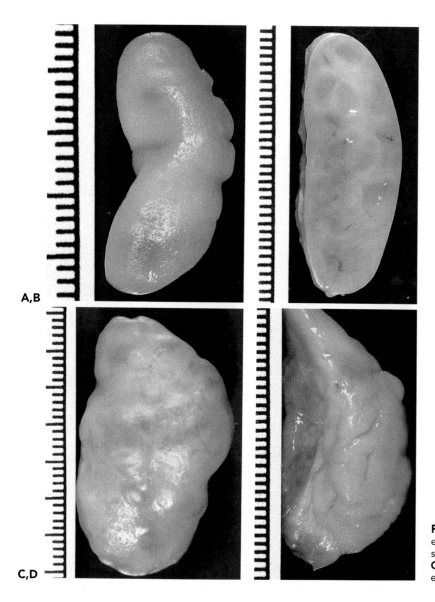

A,B

C,D

Figure 42.1 Gross appearance of ovary. **A.** Newborn, external aspect. **B.** Pubertal (age 15 years), sectioned surface. Note elongate shape and multiple cystic follicles. **C.** Adult (age 30), external aspect. **D.** Postmenopausal, external aspect. Note shrunken, gyriform appearance.

along the infundibulopelvic ligament (23). The ovarian veins also anastomose with tributaries of the uterine veins. The left and right ovarian veins drain into the left renal vein and the inferior vena cava respectively.

In postmenopausal women, the medullary blood vessels may appear particularly numerous and closely packed (Figure 42.2) and should not be mistaken for a hemangioma on microscopic examination. In addition, many of the same vessels may be calcified or have thickened walls and narrowed lumina due to medial deposition of a hyaline, amyloid-like material.

LYMPHATICS

The lymphatics of the ovary originate predominantly within the theca layers of the follicles. The granulosa layer of a maturing follicle is devoid of lymphatics in contrast to

its counterpart within the corpus luteum, which possesses a rich supply of lymphatics (24). The lymphatics pass through the ovarian stroma, independent of blood vessels, to drain into larger trunks that form a plexus at the hilus. Within the hilus, the lymphatics and blood vessels converge, with the former coiled around veins in a helicoid fashion. Four to eight efferent channels pass into the mesovarium where they converge to form the subovarian plexus, which, in turn, is joined by branches from the uterine (fallopian) tube and uterine fundus (24). Leaving the plexus, the drainage trunks diminish in number and size, passing along the free border of the infundibulopelvic ligament enmeshed with the ovarian veins. From there they accompany the ovarian vessels, juxtaposed to the psoas muscle, and drain into the upper para-aortic lymph nodes at the level of the lower pole of the kidney (24,25). The major lymphatic drainage of the ovary is therefore in a cephalad direction toward the para-aortic nodes. Accessory channels, however,

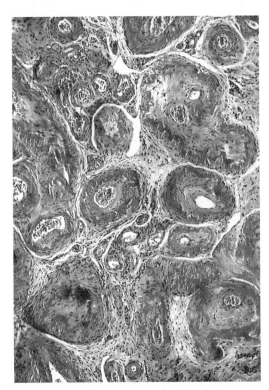

Figure 42.2 Numerous crowded thick-walled blood vessels within ovarian medulla of postmenopausal woman. Some of the vessels have an eosinophilic amyloid-like material within their walls.

may bypass the subovarian plexus, passing through the broad ligament to the internal iliac, external iliac, and interaortic lymph nodes, or in some females, via the round ligament to the iliac and inguinal lymph nodes (24,25). When the pelvic and para-aortic lymph nodes are extensively replaced by tumor, retrograde lymphatic flow may represent a rare mechanism of tumor spread to the ovaries.

NERVE SUPPLY

The nerve supply of the ovary arises from a sympathetic plexus that is enmeshed with the ovarian vessels in the infundibulopelvic ligament (26). Nerve fibers, which are predominantly nonmyelinated, accompany the ovarian artery, entering the ovary at the hilus. Delicate terminal fibers, many surrounding small arteries and arterioles, penetrate the medulla and cortex to terminate as plexuses surrounding the follicles (26,27). Adrenergic nerve fibers and terminals are in close contact with smooth muscle cells in the cortical stroma and theca externa. The physiological significance of ovarian sympathetic innervation is not clear, although it has been suggested that it may play a role in follicular maturation, follicular rupture, or both (26,28,29). In addition, catecholamines can stimulate progesterone production by the ovarian follicles and androgen production by the ovarian stroma in vitro (30).

SURFACE EPITHELIUM

Histology

The surface epithelium of the ovary consists of a single, focally pseudostratified layer of modified peritoneal cells. The cells vary from flat to cuboidal to columnar and several types may be seen in different areas of the same ovary (Figure 42.3). The surface cells are separated from the underlying stroma by a distinct basement membrane. This epithelium is extremely fragile and is almost always denuded in oophorectomy specimens because of undesirable rubbing of the surface by the surgeon and the pathologist, as well as lack of prompt fixation resulting in drying. Preserved epithelium is often confined to areas protected by surface adhesions or lining sulci.

Histochemical studies have demonstrated glycogen, as well as acid and neutral mucopolysaccharides, within surface epithelial cells (31,32). Seventeen-beta hydroxysteroid dehydrogenase activity, absent in extraovarian mesothelial cells, also has been demonstrated (31). The surface epithelial cells are immunoreactive for cytokeratin, Ber-EP4, Wilms' tumor gene (WT1), calretinin, desmoplakin, vimentin, transforming growth factor alpha, $\alpha v/\beta 3$ integrin (and its ligand vitronectin), α- and β-catenins, and receptors for estrogen, progesterone, follicle stimulating hormone, and epidermal growth factor (33–46).

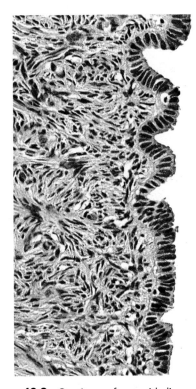

Figure 42.3 Ovarian surface epithelium composed of a single layer of columnar cells.

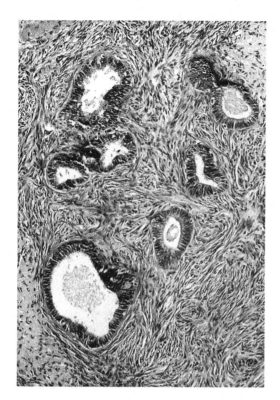

Figure 42.4 Epithelial inclusion glands within ovarian cortex.

Epithelial inclusion glands (EIGs) arise from cortical invaginations of the surface epithelium that have lost their connection with the surface. They often become cystic, resulting in epithelial inclusion cysts (EICs), which may be recognized on macroscopic examination; a diameter of 1 cm has been suggested as a dividing line between an EIC and the smallest cystadenoma. EIGs have been identified on microscopic examination of ovaries from all age groups, including fetuses, infants, and adolescents (47,48). Inclusion glands and cysts (EIGCs) become more numerous with age, and are common incidental findings in late reproductive and postmenopausal age groups. They are typically multiple, scattered singly or in small clusters throughout the superficial cortex (Figure 42.4); less commonly, extension into the deeper cortical or medullary stroma may occur. EIGCs are typically lined by a single layer of ciliated tubal-type columnar cells; psammoma bodies within their lumina or the adjacent stroma are occasionally present. Similar glands, with or without associated psammoma bodies, encountered on the ovarian surface, within periovarian adhesions, and on the extraovarian peritoneum and omentum, are designated "endosalpingiosis" (49). Less frequently, EIGCs may be lined by other müllerian epithelia (endometrioid, mucinous), or nonspecific columnar or flattened cells (50,51). EIGCs are probably the site of origin of most cystic surface epithelial tumors (52). One study (53) found that EIGCs were more common in ovaries contralateral to a unilateral ovarian carcinoma and that they

more often were lined by serous epithelium than in age-matched control patients without ovarian carcinoma. Dysplastic changes also have been described within EIGCs (52,54).

The histogenetic relationship between the ovarian surface epithelium, EIGCs, and tumors of epithelial type is reflected by the presence of markers associated with ovarian epithelial tumors within the normal surface epithelial cells and/or the cells lining EIGs. These have included WT1, E-cadherin, p53, CA 125, CA 19-9, CEA, hCG, MH99, placental lactogen, alpha-2 glycoprotein, beta-1 glycoprotein, placental alkaline phosphatase, human milk fat globule protein, and $\alpha v/\beta 3$ integrin/vitronectin (55–63). Hyperplasia and metaplasia of the surface epithelium, and of that within EIGs, are more common in women with polycystic ovarian disease and endometrial carcinoma (64), suggesting a possible hormonal basis in some cases.

Urothelial differentiation is also within the metaplastic potential of the ovarian surface epithelium and pelvic peritoneum. Such differentiation typically takes the form of Walthard nests of transitional cells, a common microscopic finding within the serosa or the immediately subjacent stroma of the uterine (fallopian) tube, mesosalpinx, and mesovarium, or less commonly, the ovarian hilus (Figure 42.5) (65–68). The larger nests frequently become cystic and may be lined by columnar mucinous cells. Brenner tumors are also characterized by urothelial differentiation;

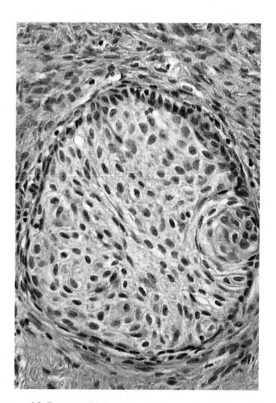

Figure 42.5 Walthard nest within ovarian hilus abutting medullary stroma.

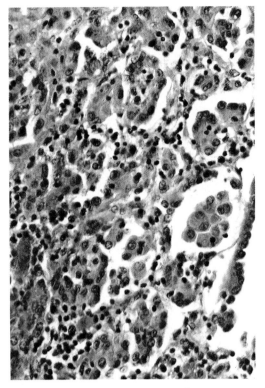

Figure 42.6 Hyperplastic mesothelial cells on ovarian surface. Note admixed inflammatory cells.

as many as one-half of those encountered by the pathologist are of microscopic size.

Hyperplastic mesothelial cells, usually a response to chronic pelvic inflammation, may involve the surface of the ovary and focally replace the ovarian surface epithelium. Florid examples exhibiting tubulopapillary (Figure 42.6) and pseudoinfiltrative patterns, as well as varying degrees of nuclear atypia, must be distinguished from a malignant mesothelioma or a primary ovarian or metastatic carcinoma.

Ultrastructure

The ultrastructural appearance of the ovarian surface epithelium is similar to that of the extraovarian peritoneum (69–71). The cell surfaces by scanning and transmission electron microscopy have dome-shaped apices covered by numerous, often branching, microvilli, occasional single cilia, and pinocytotic vesicles (Figure 42.7). The cytoplasm contains abundant polysomes, free ribosomes, abundant mitochondria, and bundles of intermediate filaments and tonofilaments. Lipid droplets are sometimes present in the basal cytoplasm. The nuclei have indented nuclear membranes and peripheral nucleoli. Straight or convoluted lateral plasma membranes are reinforced by luminal junctional complexes, scattered desmosomes, and desmosomal-tonofilament complexes. The membranes may be widely separated in areas creating dilated intercellular spaces (70). A well-developed basal lamina separates the surface epithelium from the underlying stroma.

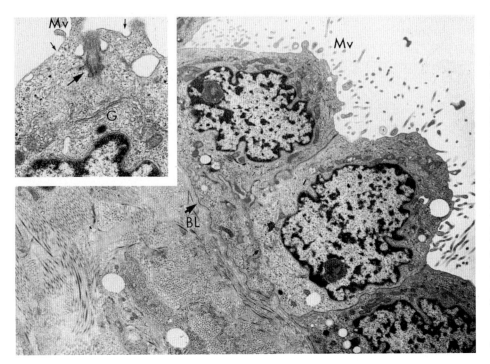

Figure 42.7 Electron micrograph of ovarian surface epithelium. The cells have numerous microvilli (Mv) and well-developed organelles in a perinuclear location. The nuclei have indented membranes and peripheral nucleoli. The lateral plasma membranes are reinforced by luminal junctional complexes and scattered desmosomes, but are occasionally widely separated producing dilated intercellular spaces. A well-defined basal lamina (BL) separates the cells from the underlying stroma (original magnification x6400). **Inset:** the surface microvilli are associated with micropinocytotic vesicles (short arrows) and occasional single cilia (long arrows). Note Golgi complex (G) (original magnification x22,000). Reprinted with permission from: Ferenczy A, Richart RM. *Female Reproductive System: Dynamics of Scan and Transmission Electron Microscopy.* New York: John Wiley & Sons; 1974.

STROMA

Histology

As the cortical and medullary stroma is continuous and similar in appearance, the boundary between these two zones is ill defined and arbitrary. The spindle-shaped stromal cells, which have scanty cytoplasm, are typically arranged in whorls or a storiform pattern (Figure 42.8). Fine cytoplasmic lipid droplets may be appreciable with special stains, especially in the late reproductive and postmenopausal age groups (72). Immunohistochemical stains reveal cytoplasmic vimentin, actin, and desmin (33,35,36,73,74). Stromal cells are separated by a dense reticulum network (Figure 42.8 inset) and a variable amount of collagen that is most abundant in the superficial cortex. Although the latter is frequently referred to as the tunica albuginea, it lacks the densely collagenous, almost acellular appearance and sharp delineation of the tunica albuginea of the testis.

A variety of other cells may be found within the ovarian stroma, most of which are probably derived from the cells of fibroblastic type. *Luteinized stromal cells*, which lie in the stroma at a distance from the follicles, are found singly or in small nests, most often in the medulla. They are polygonal cells with abundant eosinophilic to clear cytoplasm containing variable amounts of lipid, a central round nucleus, and a prominent nucleolus (Figure 42.9). These cells

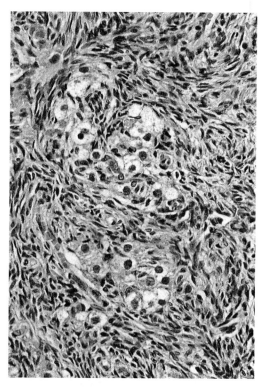

Figure 42.9 Luteinized stromal cells.

are typically immunoreactive for inhibin (75–79), calretinin (46,80), melan-A (81), CD10 (82), and occasionally, testosterone (83). The numbers of luteinized stromal cells increase during pregnancy and after the menopause; they are probably secondary to elevated levels of circulating gonadotropins during these periods (22,72). In one autopsy study, luteinized stromal cells were demonstrated after diligent searching in 13% of women under the age of 55 and in one-third of women over that age; the frequency of their detection increased with increasing degrees of stromal proliferation (22). More exhaustive sampling might indicate that luteinized stromal cells are a normal finding in the ovary, particularly in later life. In this age group, the presence of luteinized cells is not usually associated with clinical evidence of a hormonal disturbance. In some older women, but more often in younger patients, however, more striking degrees of stromal luteinization (stromal hyperthecosis) are frequently associated with androgenic and estrogenic manifestations. Occasionally in such cases, nodules of luteinized stromal cells may be appreciable on low-power microscopic examination (nodular hyperthecosis).

Enzymatically active stromal cells (EASC) are characterized by their oxidative and other enzymatic activity (72,84–86). The frequency of their detection and their numbers increase with age, occurring in over 80% of postmenopausal women, typically in the medulla (84,85). Some EASC correspond to luteinized stromal cells, but most cannot be distinguished from neighboring, nonreactive stromal cells in routine histologic preparations (84).

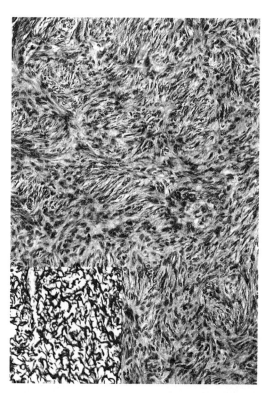

Figure 42.8 Ovarian stroma composed of whorls of plump spindle cells of fibroblastic type. **Inset:** note dense reticulum network (reticulin stain).

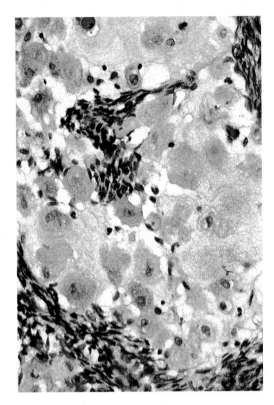

Figure 42.10 A nest of decidual cells within the ovarian stroma.

Decidual cells may occur singly, as small nodules, or as confluent sheets within the stroma of the superficial cortex or within periovarian adhesions (Figure 42.10). The appearance of the decidual cells is usually identical to eutopic decidua, but occasional examples may exhibit cytological atypia potentially mimicking metastatic carcinoma on histological examination (87–92). A network of capillaries and a sprinkling of lymphocytes are typically present within the decidual foci. A decidual reaction within the ovary is almost always a response of the ovarian stromal cells to elevated circulating or local levels of progesterone; progesterone receptors have been identified in the ovarian stromal cells (37). The process is seen most commonly in pregnancy, occurring as early as the ninth week of gestation, and by term is present in virtually all ovaries. Less commonly it may occur in association with trophoblastic disease, in patients treated with progestins, in the vicinity of a corpus luteum, or in association with hormonally active, hyperplastic or neoplastic ovarian lesions (22,87,89). Prior pelvic irradiation may be a predisposing factor by increasing the sensitivity of the stromal cells to hormonal stimulation (89). Foci of ovarian decidua have been occasionally described in both pre- and postmenopausal women with no obvious cause (22,89).

Foci of *smooth muscle* may be seen within the ovarian stroma (Figure 42.11), most commonly within perimenopausal or postmenopausal women (93). The smooth muscle is bilateral in about 25% of cases and usually is confined to a few microscopic fields. It is often associated with

other findings in the ovary, occurring with the hyperplastic ovarian stroma associated with stromal hyperthecosis or sclerocystic ovaries (94), and within the stroma surrounding nonneoplastic and neoplastic cysts, including endometriotic cysts. Rare endometriotic cysts may contain prominent amounts of smooth muscle ("endomyometriosis") (95). One study (93) found that almost 90% of women with ovarian smooth muscle metaplasia had uterine leiomyomas.

Nests of cells resembling *endometrial stromal cells* ("stromal endometriosis") occur within the ovarian stroma, usually in the absence of typical endometriosis (Figure 42.12) (96,97). Foci of mature *fat cells* may be encountered as an incidental histological finding within the subcapsular ovarian stroma (98,99); a possible association with obesity was noted in one study (99). Reinke-crystal-containing Leydig cells, presumably representing transformed stromal cells, may occur rarely, and are typically associated with stromal hyperthecosis or within the nonneoplastic stroma in or adjacent to an ovarian neoplasm (100–102). So-called *"neuroendocrine" or "APUD" type cells* have been demonstrated within the ovarian stroma in approximately 6% of normal women in one study (103). The cells occur in small groups in the corticomedullary stromal junction and are argyrophilic and argentaffinic. Their clinical significance and hormonal function, if any, is unknown, but it has been suggested that they may represent the cell of origin of rare primary ovarian carcinoid tumors not associated with teratomatous or mucinous elements.

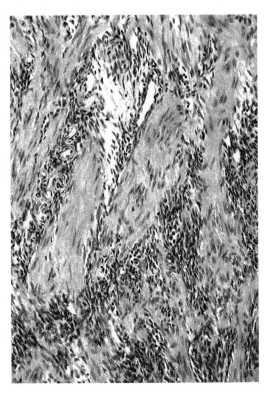

Figure 42.11 Smooth muscle cells within ovarian stroma.

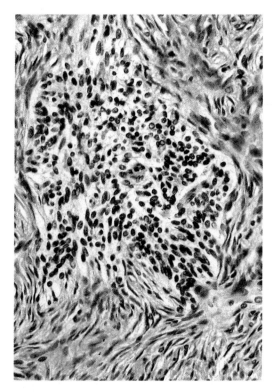

Figure 42.12   Focus of endometrial stromal cells ("stromal en-dometriosis") within ovarian cortex.

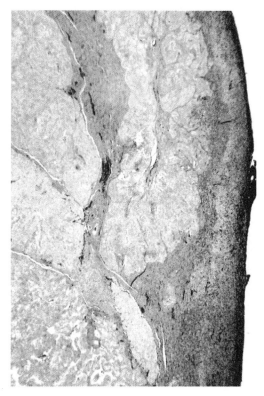

Figure 42.13   Atrophic postmenopausal ovary. The cortex is thin and multiple corpora albicantia are present within the medullla.

Aging Changes

Although there is typically a gradual increase in its volume from the fourth to the seventh decades (21,104), the ovarian stroma in postmenopausal women exhibits a wide spectrum of appearances (22,70,88). At one extreme, there is stromal atrophy manifested by a thin cortex and minimal amounts of medullary stroma (Figure 42.13). At the other extreme, there is marked stromal proliferation warranting the designation "stromal hyperplasia". Most postmenopausal subjects, however, exhibit varying degrees of nodular or diffuse proliferation of the cortical and medullary stromal cells that lie between these two extremes (Figure 42.14) (22,85), making the "normal" appearance difficult to define. Broad irregular areas of cortical fibrosis may be encountered in peri- and postmenopausal ovaries (22). When well-circumscribed, these foci resemble a small fibroma, but this designation is applied to lesions 1 cm or greater in diameter. A similar size limit could be used to distinguish between the foci of surface stromal papillarity commonly encountered in this age group (Figure 42.15) and serous surface papillomas. Cortical "granulomas" are common incidental microscopic findings in the late reproductive and postmenopausal age groups, having been demonstrated in up to 45% of women over the age of 40 (22,96,97,105–107). They consist of spherical circumscribed aggregates of epithelioid cells, lymphocytes, and

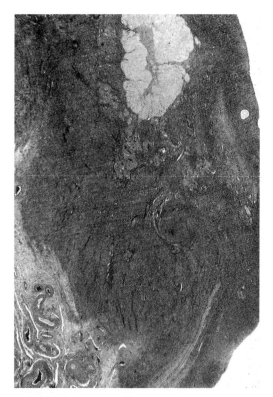

Figure 42.14   Postmenopausal ovary with a moderate degree of stromal proliferation.

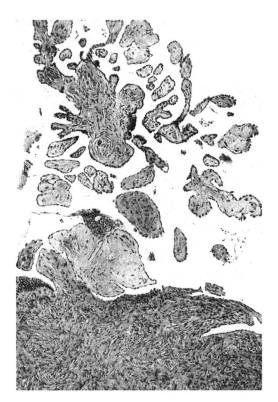

Figure 42.15 Papillary stromal projections from ovarian surface.

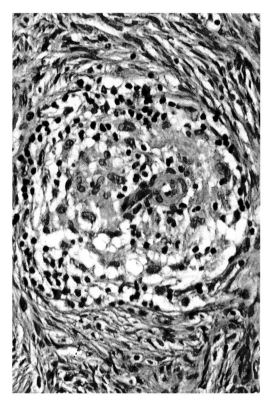

Figure 42.16 Cortical granuloma.

occasionally, multinucleated giant cells and anisotropic fat crystals (Figure 42.16). Cortical granulomas and the spherical, cloud-like, hyalin scars (Figure 42.17) present within the superficial cortical stroma of almost all post-menopausal ovaries are of uncertain histogenesis. It has been suggested that they may represent regressed foci of stromal endometriosis, ectopic decidua, or luteinized stromal cells.

Ultrastructure

Typical ovarian stromal cells have slender spindle-shaped nuclei and complex cytoplasmic processes (70,85). Their scant cytoplasm is rich in organelles required for collagen synthesis, including free ribosomes and mitochondria. Tropocollagen, concentrated at the periphery of the cytoplasm, is deposited in the extracellular space and eventually converted to collagen (Figure 42.18). Rows of micropinocytotic vesicles occur along the plasma membrane and desmosome-like attachments may be found between the cells (85). Luteinized stromal cells have abundant cytoplasm-containing lipid droplets and steroidogenic organelles, including smooth endoplasmic reticulum, mitochondria with tubular cristae, and Golgi (70,85,86,108). Some cells have ultrastructural features that are intermediate between those of fibroblasts and luteinized cells (70,85). Argyrophilic stromal cells have 300 to 750 nm, electron-dense, membrane-bound, cytoplasmic granules (103).

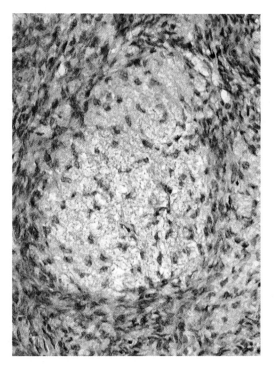

Figure 42.17 Hyalin scar.

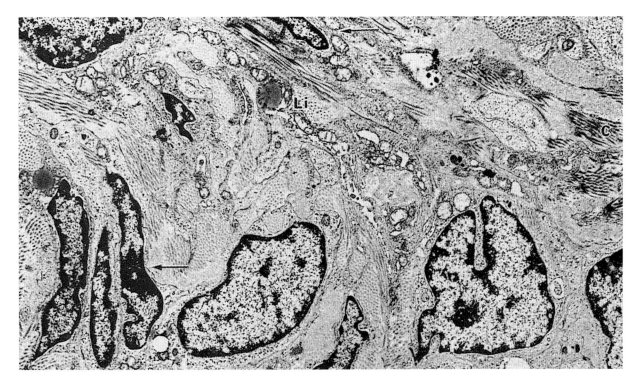

Figure 42.18 Electron micrograph of ovarian stromal cells. The cells are fibroblastic in type. C: collagen fibers; Mf: tropocollagen; R: free ribosomes; Li: lipid inclusions; upper arrow, perinuclear clustering of mitochondria (original magnification x3000).

Hormonal Aspects

Numerous studies have demonstrated the steroidogenic potential and the gonadotropin-responsiveness of the ovarian stroma in both pre- and postmenopausal women (109–121). In vitro incubation of ovarian stromal tissue indicates that its principal steroid product is androstenedione, in addition to smaller quantities of testosterone and dehydroepiandrosterone (122). In vitro production of androgens is enhanced by human chorionic gonadotropin (hCG), pituitary gonadotropins, and insulin, consistent with the presence of receptors for these hormones within the stromal cells (83,86,123). To what extent the ovarian stroma contributes to the androgen pool in normal premenopausal women is unknown, but it is likely that it is the source of small amounts of testosterone. With cessation of follicular activity at the time of the menopause, the ovarian stroma becomes, together with the adrenal glands, the major source of androgens. Testosterone and androstenedione are the major androgens secreted by the ovarian stroma in postmenopausal women (109–111,113,121), and in vitro and in vivo studies have shown that ovaries with stromal hyperplasia secrete more androstenedione, estrone, and estradiol than normal ovaries (114,116). Approximately 80% of the circulating androstenedione in postmenopausal women, however, is of adrenal origin (110). Despite a cessation of follicular synthesis of estradiol (E2) in postmenopausal subjects,

small amounts of this hormone are present in the circulation (probably derived from the adrenal glands) by peripheral conversion of estrone (110,124), and from the ovarian stroma itself (109,111,125). Estrone, however, becomes the major circulating estrogen after the menopause, derived predominantly from the peripheral aromatization of androstenedione that occurs in fat, muscle, liver, kidney, brain, and adrenals (110,125,126). Increased aromatization in postmenopausal women, likely due to high endogenous LH levels in these subjects, leads to a twofold increase in the daily production rate of estrone compared to that in premenopausal women; aromatization is also higher in obese subjects. In some postmenopausal women, sufficient estrogen is elaborated by this mechanism to prevent the clinical manifestations of estrogen withdrawal and to play a role in the genesis of endometrial carcinoma (104,110). An association between the degree of stromal proliferation and postmenopausal endometrial adenocarcinoma has been noted (104), and the ovarian stroma in postmenopausal women with endometrial adenocarcinoma produces more androgens in vitro than that of control subjects without endometrial cancer (127). The variations that exist in the ovarian steroid hormone output from one postmenopausal woman to another may correspond to similar variations in the morphologic appearance of the stroma in this age group, although no correlative functional and structural studies have been performed.

PRIMORDIAL FOLLICLES

Histology

The approximately 400,000 primordial follicles present at the time of birth fill the ovarian cortex (Figure 42.19). After this period, their numbers decrease progressively through the processes of atresia and folliculogenesis until their eventual disappearance that marks the end of the menopause. However, rare follicles may persist for several years after the cessation of menses, accounting for sporadic ovulation and occasional episodes of postmenopausal bleeding (128). In the reproductive era, primordial follicles are found scattered irregularly in clusters throughout a narrow band in the superficial cortex. They consist of a primary oocyte, measuring 40 to 70 μm in diameter, surrounded by a single layer of flattened, mitotically inactive, granulosa cells resting on a thin basal lamina (Figure 42.20). Rare primordial (and maturing) follicles may contain multiple oocytes, particularly in individuals who are less than 20 years of age (19,129–131). The oocyte is arrested at the dictyate stage of meiotic prophase at the time of birth, enters an interphase period until follicular maturation prior to ovulation, or undergoes degeneration during atresia (132). The large spherical nucleus of the oocyte has finely granular, uniformly dispersed chromatin and one or more dense, thread-like nucleoli (132); rare oocytes may have multiple nuclei (130,131).

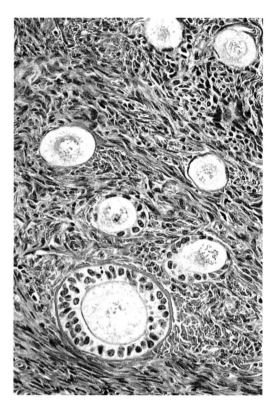

Figure 42.20 Primordial follicles (four at top of figure) and primary follicles (three at bottom of figure).

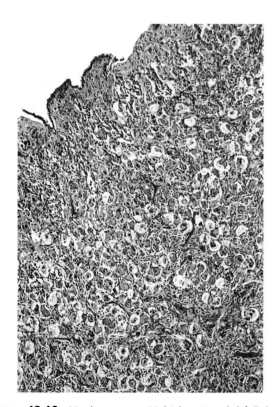

Figure 42.19 Newborn ovary. Multiple primordial follicles fill the ovarian cortex.

The cytoplasm of the oocyte contains a paranuclear, eosinophilic, crescent-shaped zone consisting of a complex of interrelated organelles, so-called Balbiani's vitelline body (BVB) (133,134). Within the vitelline body is a dark spot (the centrosome) surrounded by a halo, which in turn is flanked by darker, PAS-positive, granular zones rich in mitochondria (133,14). The cytoplasm of the oocyte lacks the abundant glycogen and the high alkaline phosphatase activity characteristic of the primordial germ cells and the oogonia of the embryonic gonad.

Ultrastructure

The granulosa cells of the primordial follicle have sparse organelles, occasional desmosomal attachments with each other, and microvillous projections that attach to the oocyte by tight apposition (70). Within the oocyte, the juxtanuclear centrosome of the BVB (Figure 42.21A) consists of dense granules, closely packed vesicles, and dense fibers that form a basket-like structure at the periphery of the centrosome (Figure 42.21B) (133,134). The centrosome is surrounded by a zone of smooth endoplasmic reticulum (ER) that represents the halo seen by light microscopy. More peripheral and constituting the rest of the BVB are a concentration of most of the oocyte's organelles, including multiple Golgi complexes, prominent compound aggre-

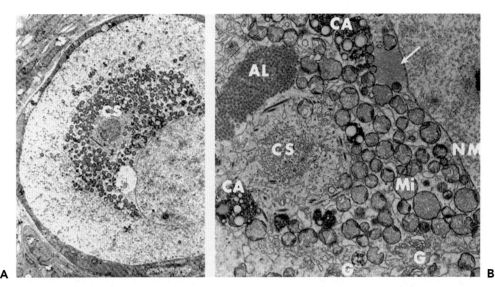

Figure 42.21 Electron micrograph of a primordial follicle. **A.** Balbiani's vitelline body consists of a juxtanuclear centrosome (CS) surrounded by a condensation of mitochondria, Golgi complexes, endoplasmic reticulum, and lysosomes (original magnification. x2400). **B.** Detailed view of Balbiani's vitelline body. A cluster of closely packed spiral fibrils (arrow) is attached to the nuclear envelope (NM). The centrosome (CS) is composed of dense granules, some arranged periodically on fine fibers, and small vesicles, with a peripheral zone of endoplasmic reticulum and dense fibers. Surrounding the centrosome are masses of mitochondria (Mi) and compound aggregates (CA). A stack of annulate lamellae (AL) is seen tangentially. Note the prominent endoplasmic reticulum in close association with multiple Golgi complexes at the periphery of the vitelline body. Reprinted with permission from: Hertig AT. The primary human oocyte: some observations on the fine structure of Balbiani's vitelline body and the origin of the annulate lamellae. *Am J Anat* 1968;122:107–137.

gates, numerous mitochondria intimately associated with sparsely granular ER, and annulate lamellae (Figure 42.21B) (133,134). The latter structures, which may be attached or immediately adjacent to the nucleus or free within the BVB, are constantly present in primary oocytes and other rapidly growing embryonal or neoplastic cells. They are arranged in stacks or concentric arrangements of up to 100 parallel, smooth, paired membranes that delineate greatly flattened cisternal spaces, 30 to 50 μm wide. At regularly spaced intervals, the paired membranes of each lamellar unit become fused with one another (132). When the lamellae are sectioned along a tangential plane, the sites of apposition of the membranes are seen as regularly spaced annuli 100 nm in diameter. At their periphery they are connected to the granular ER (133). The paired membranes of the annulate lamellae mimic the two leaflets of the nuclear membrane, and it is likely that they are formed from its outer leaflet (70,132,133). Their function is not known with certainty, but it has been suggested that they may have a role in nucleocytoplasmic exchange of substances related to metabolic activity or the transfer of genetic information (70,133).

In some oocytes, Golgi, ER, and mitochondria may also be found outside the vitelline body, closely applied to the entire circumference of the nucleus (133). Similarly, microtubules present throughout the oocyte cytoplasm are most prevalent around the circumference of the nuclear membrane. Bundles of spiral filaments occasionally abut the nuclear membrane (Figure 42.21B) or are seen in the more peripheral cytoplasm (134). A variety of different vacuoles may also be seen in the peripheral cytoplasm, some containing multiple small vesicles (133).

MATURING FOLLICLES

Histology and Ultrastructure

Folliculogenesis

Folliculogenesis refers to the continuous process occurring throughout reproductive life whereby cohorts of primordial follicles undergo maturation during each menstrual cycle. Follicular maturation begins during the luteal phase and continues throughout the follicular phase of the next cycle. Each month only one such follicle, the preovulatory (or dominant) follicle, achieves complete maturation, culminating in the release of the oocyte (ovulation). The other follicles that have begun the maturational process undergo atresia at earlier stages of their development. Folliculogenesis and atresia also occur prenatally, throughout childhood and during pregnancy, although maturing follicles rarely reach the preovulatory follicle stage during these periods (19,135–143).

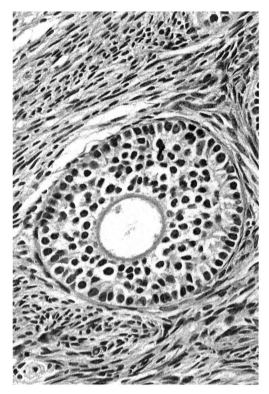

Figure 42.22 Preantral follicle. Several layers of granulosa cells surround the oocyte. A theca interna layer is not yet apparent.

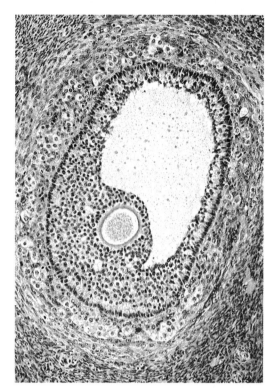

Figure 42.23 Mature follicle. Oocyte within cumulus oophorus projects into antrum. The theca layers are well developed.

The first morphological evidence of follicular maturation is the assumption of a cuboidal to columnar shape of the granulosa cells accompanied by enlargement of the oocyte (*primary follicle*) (Figure 42.20). Mitotic activity in the granulosa cells results in their stratification and three to five concentric layers around the oocyte (*secondary or preantral follicle*) (Figure 42.22). At this stage an

eosinophilic, PAS-positive, homogeneous, acellular layer, known as the zona pellucida, appears, encasing the oocyte. Its formation is usually attributed to the granulosa cells, but the oocyte may also play a role. At the end of its development, the zona pellucida is a 20 to 25 μm thick membrane rich in acid mucopolysaccharides and glycoprotein (Figures 42.22–42.25) (70). Preantral follicles measure from 50 to

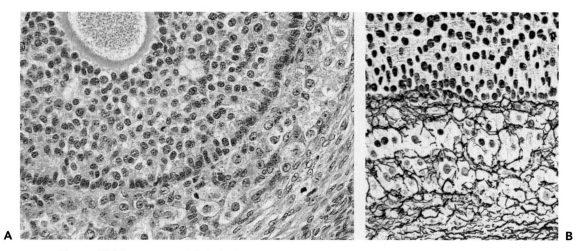

Figure 42.24 **A.** Mature follicle, high power view. The granulosa layer, which contains several Call-Exner bodies, abuts the zona pellucida of the oocyte. The granulosa layer is surrounded by a layer of luteinized theca interna cells. Note mitotic figures in granulosa and theca cells. **B.** There is a reticulum network in the theca interna layer, but an absence of reticulin in the granulosa layer.

400 μm in diameter, and as they increase in size, they migrate into the deeper cortex and medulla. Simultaneously, the surrounding ovarian stromal cells become specialized into several layers of theca interna cells and an outer, ill-defined layer of theca externa cells. Secretion of mucopolysaccharide-rich fluid by the granulosa cells results in their separation by fluid-filled clefts that eventually coalesce to form a single large cavity or antrum lined by several layers of granulosa cells (*tertiary, antral, or vesicular follicle*). The first evidence of antrum formation occurs in follicles that are 200 to 400 μm in diameter, after which the follicles progressively enlarge due to continued fluid secretion into the antrum. Concurrently, the oocyte enlarges to its definitive size and assumes an eccentric position at one pole of the follicle. At this site the granulosa cells proliferate to form the cumulus oophorus which, containing the oocyte in its center, protrudes into the antrum (*mature or Graafian follicle*) (Figure 42.23).

Ovulation

During each cycle, only a small number of mature follicles (<4 per ovary) reach a diameter of 4 to 5 mm by the mid-to late luteal phase; one of them will become the preovulatory follicle of the subsequent cycle (144,145). Late in follicular growth, the oocyte, its surrounding zona pellucida, and a single layer of radially-disposed, columnar granulosa cells (the corona radiata) detach from the cumulus oophorus and float in the antral fluid. The preovulatory follicle, shortly before ovulation, reaches a diameter of 15 to 25 mm (28,145) and partially protrudes from the ovarian surface at the eventual rupture point, or stigma. Here the overlying surface epithelial cells exhibit progressive flattening, degeneration, and desquamation. The stroma in this area becomes attenuated and almost avascular, with degeneration of the stromal cells, fragmentation of collagen fibers, and an accumulation of intercellular fluid (28). These surface epithelial and stromal changes that immediately precede ovulation may be secondary to local ischemia and the release of proteolytic enzymes and prostaglandins into the stroma. The preovulatory follicle then ruptures, possibly secondary to the contraction of the perifollicular smooth muscle cells, with liberation of the follicular fluid and oocyte (with its surrounding layers) into the peritoneal cavity. Following ovulation, the stigma is occluded by a mass of coagulated follicular fluid, fibrin, blood, granulosa and connective tissue cells; it is eventually converted to scar tissue.

Shortly before ovulation, the oocyte within the ovulatory follicle enters telophase of the first meiotic division. Chromosomal reduction occurs by migration of one-half the oocyte chromosomes into a portion of the oocyte cytoplasm that separates from the cell as the first polar body. The first meiotic division begun in fetal life is now complete, and the oocyte is now designated the secondary oocyte. Immediately after expulsion of the first polar body, the secondary oocyte enters the second meiotic division, arresting at metaphase until fertilization occurs.

Granulosa Layer

Granulosa cells are almost entirely formed from their embryonic precursors by the time of birth (19). Those within maturing and mature follicles are polyhedral cells 5 to 7 μm in diameter; the cells resting on the basement membrane are often columnar. The granulosa cells have pale, scanty cytoplasm, indistinct cell borders, and small, round to oval, hyperchromatic nuclei that typically lack nuclear grooves (Figure 42.24A) (146). Mitotic figures within granulosa cells are usually numerous in maturing follicles, decreasing in numbers prior to ovulation. Until the onset of luteinization several hours prior to ovulation, cytoplasmic lipid is absent (or sparse) as are steroidogenic histochemical patterns (147,148). The cytoplasm of granulosa cells of primary, secondary, and mature follicles is immunoreactive for cytokeratin, vimentin, inhibin, CD99, melan-A, müllerian inhibiting substance, WT1, and desmoplakin (33,35,36,75,77,78,81).

The granulosa cells typically surround small cavities, referred to as Call-Exner bodies (Figure 42.24A), which have a distinctive appearance, representing one of the most specific features of granulosa cells, both normal and neoplastic. Call-Exner bodies are delimited from the granulosa cells by a basal lamina, and typically contain a deeply eosinophilic, PAS-positive, filamentous material consisting of excess basal lamina (70). Unlike the theca layers, the granulosa layer of the maturing and Graafian follicles is avascular and devoid of a reticulum framework (Figure 42.24B).

Mitochondria with lamelliform cristae, granular ER, free ribosomes, and Golgi gradually increase in abundance within the granulosa cells of maturing follicles. These ultrastructural features suggest active protein synthesis. Histochemical and ultrastructural features (abundant smooth ER and mitochondria with tubular cristae) indicative of steroid biosynthesis are absent until shortly before ovulation (72,84,147–150). The granulosa cells of follicles of varying stages contain adhaerens junctions, gap junctions, and desmosomes between adjacent granulosa cells (35,70,132). The slender cytoplasmic extensions of the granulosa cells of the corona radiata that traverse the zona pellucida have gap junctions and puncta adhaerentia with the plasma membrane of the oocyte (Figure 42.25).

Theca Layers

In contrast to granulosa cells, theca cells differentiate continuously from the stromal cells at the periphery of developing follicles from fetal life until the end of the menopause. The thecal component of the antral follicle is

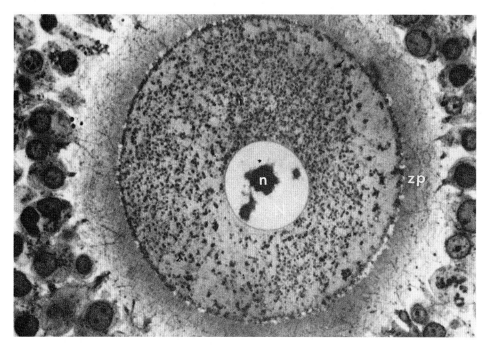

Figure 42.25 Maturing oocyte. Note the uniform distribution of the organelles and the row of dense granules in the cytoplasm immediately subjacent to the plasma membrane of the oocyte. A continuous zona pellucida (zp) surrounds the oocyte and separates it from the granulosa cells. Numerous cytoplasmic processes of the granulosa cells are visible within the zona pellucida. N, nucleolus. Thick section, OsO4 fixed, Epon-embedded, toluidine blue stain. Reprinted with permission from: Baca M, Zamboni L. The fine structure of the human follicular oocytes. *J Ultrastruct Res* 1967;19:354–381.

characterized by a well-developed theca interna and a less well-defined theca externa. The theca interna layer is three or four cells in thickness and lies external to the granulosa layer (Figure 42.24A) from which it is separated by a basement membrane. Unlike the granulosa cells of the developing and mature follicles, the theca interna cells typically have a luteinized or partially luteinized appearance (Figure 42.24A) and exhibit steroidogenic histochemical patterns (72,147–149). Luteinization of the theca interna of maturing follicles is particularly prominent during pregnancy. The round to polygonal cells are 12 to 20 micra in diameter and have abundant, eosinophilic to clear, vacuolated cytoplasm containing variable amounts of lipid; a central, round, vesicular nucleus typically contains a single, prominent nucleolus (Figure 42.24A). The cells differ from granulosa cells but resemble stromal cells in being immunoreactive for vimentin but not cytokeratin (36); theca cells are also immunoreactive for inhibin, calretinin, and melan-A (46,77,81). Mitotic figures are typically present with the theca cells of maturing follicles. The layer contains a rich vascular plexus consisting of dilated capillaries, as well as a dense reticulin network that surrounds each cell (Figure 42.24B). A tangential section through the theca interna may result in seemingly isolated nodules of luteinized theca cells that may occasionally be misinterpreted as foci of stromal luteinization.

The theca externa is an ill-defined layer of variable thickness that surrounds the theca interna and merges almost imperceptibly with the adjacent ovarian stroma. It is composed of circumferentially arranged collagen bundles, blood and lymphatic vessels, and plump spindle cells that lack steroidogenic histochemical features (151). The spindle cells of the theca externa are typically highly mitotic and may be

misinterpreted as fibrosarcoma, particularly when only the edge of the follicle is seen microscopically (Figure 42.26).

Ultrastructural examination of theca interna cells reveals the organelles associated with steroidogenesis, similar to those within granulosa-lutein cells. The theca externa cells,

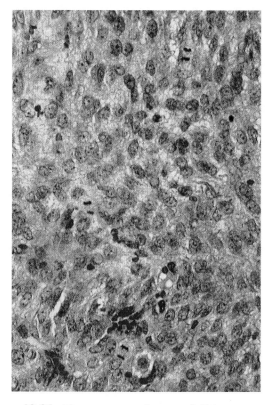

Figure 42.26 Theca externa of mature follicle composed of plump spindle cells. Note mitotic figures.

some of which exhibit smooth muscle differentiation, lack such organelles (152).

Hormonal Aspects

The initiation of folliculogenesis and early preantral follicular development is independent of gonadotropin influence, whereas the later stages of follicular maturation are under gonadotropin control. As a small antral follicle develops into a preovulatory follicle, the sequence of endocrine events within its antral fluid differs from most, if not all, other antral follicles in the same ovary (153,154). The early stages of this development are associated with an increase in FSH receptors and intrafollicular FSH within the preovulatory follicle (153–156). There is a concomitant increase in estradiol (E2) receptors within the granulosa cells and the E2 level within the follicular fluid. The latter reaches peak concentration (10,000 times the circulating level) during the mid- to late proliferative phase when plasma FSH falls to a basal level. At this stage the preovulatory follicle is self-sustaining, continuing to mature under the influence of intrafollicular FSH and E2 (118). During the late proliferative phase, plasma LH rises and LH-receptors within the granulosa cells of the preovulatory follicle (but not other follicles) become apparent (156). In contrast, LH-receptors are present within the theca cells of all follicles throughout the follicular phase. Eden et al. found concentrations of insulin-like growth factor (IGF1) to be significantly higher in the follicular fluid of preovulatory follicles than their matched cohorts, and suggested that IGF1 may have a role in the selection of the dominant follicle (157).

Whereas circulating E2 is likely derived from both the granulosa cells and the LH-stimulated theca cells, intrafollicular E2 is derived almost exclusively from the granulosa cells by both de novo synthesis and by FSH-dependent aromatization of theca-derived androstenedione (118,158). Aromatase activity is highest in the preovulatory follicle, thereby maintaining a high E2:androstenedione ratio (153,154,159). In contrast, follicles that will undergo atresia are FSH- and aromatase-deficient and have high androstenedione:E2 ratios within their intrafollicular fluid. High circulating estrogen levels initiate a preovulatory surge of plasma LH (160,161) that induces luteinization of the granulosa cells, an increase in intrafollicular progesterone (P) concentration, and a small preovulatory rise in circulating P (153,154,162). The rising plasma P level and the peaking estrogen level further augment the LH surge, as well as initiating a smaller increase in FSH, triggering ovulation. The latter has been estimated to occur 36 to 38 hours after the onset of the LH surge, 24 to 36 hours after the estradiol peak, and 10 to 12 hours after the LH peak (162).

The ovarian follicles also produce nonsteroidal hormones. Inhibin, a glycoprotein synthesized by the granulosa cells, is secreted into the follicular fluid and ovarian venous effluent in amounts that correlate with steroid levels (162–164). Inhibin, which is predominantly under the control of LH (165), reduces, by negative feedback, FSH secretion from the hypothalamic–pituitary unit. High concentrations of prorenin are present within the fluid of mature follicles (166), and their granulosa cells, as well as theca and stromal cells, are immunoreactive for renin and angiotensin II (167). The function, if any, of the renin–angiotensin system within the ovary is currently unknown.

CORPUS LUTEUM OF MENSTRUATION

Following ovulation on the fourteenth day of the typical 28-day menstrual cycle, and in the absence of fertilization, the collapsed ovulatory follicle becomes the corpus luteum of menstruation (CLM). When mature, the CLM is a 1.5 to 2.5 cm, round, yellow structure with festooned contours and a cystic center filled with a gray, focally hemorrhagic coagulum.

Histology

During the 14 days following ovulation, the CLM undergoes an orderly sequence of histological changes that allow an approximate estimation of its age. Corner has described these stages in detail, using endometrial histology and menstrual data to establish the age of the CLM (168,169). A subsequent study that correlated the histologic date of the CLM (using Corner's criteria) with the interval between the LH peak and the biopsy of the CLM, determined that the use of the histology of the CLM for retrospective timing of ovulation is subject to an error of variable magnitude due to unequal duration of each stage as well as considerable individual variation (170).

In contrast to the granulosa cells of the maturing and preovulatory follicles, the luteinized granulosa cells of the mature CLM (granulosa-lutein cells) are large, 30 to 35 micra, polygonal cells with abundant, pale, eosinophilic cytoplasm that may contain numerous small lipid droplets (Figures 42.27, 42.28) (151). The spherical nucleus contains one or two large nucleoli. The histochemical pattern of these cells varies with the age of the CLM, but is generally typical of steroid hormone-producing cells (72,148,149,171). The cytoplasm of luteinized granulosa cells contains vimentin, but in contrast to granulosa cells of maturing and mature follicles, little or no cytokeratin (35). The luteinized granulosa cells are also immunoreactive for inhibin and calretinin (46,77).

The theca interna forms an irregular and often interrupted layer several cells in thickness around the circumference of the CLM (Figure 42.27) and ensheathes the vascular septa that extend into its center (151). When these septa are cut in cross section, triangular-shaped nests of theca cells appear at intervals throughout the granulosa layer. In all but the earliest stages of the CLM, the theca lutein cells are approximately half the size of granulosa-lutein cells. They contain a round to oval nucleus with a

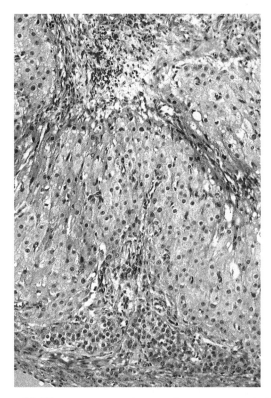

Figure 42.27 Mature corpus luteum of menstruation. The lining is composed of a thick layer of large granulosa-lutein cells and an outer, thinner layer of smaller theca-lutein cells. The cavity (top of figure) contains erythrocytes and fibrin.

single prominent nucleolus. Their less abundant, more darkly staining cytoplasm contains lipid droplets, which are usually larger than those in granulosa-lutein cells, and exhibits steroidogenic histochemical patterns (148), and immunoreactivity for inhibin, calretinin, and melan-A (46,77,81).

A third type of cell, the so-called "K" cell, occurs in small numbers within the theca interna of the mature follicle and appears in greater numbers within the granulosa layer of the early CLM (146). K cells persist until menstruation at which time they degenerate. They are characterized by a stellate shape, a deeply eosinophilic cytoplasm, and an irregular, hyperchromatic or pyknotic nucleus (Figure 42.28). The cytoplasm is uniformly sudanophilic due to the presence of phospholipid (146). K cells lack the histochemical patterns of steroidogenic cells and have been shown to be T-lymphocytes (172).

During the maturation of the CLM, capillaries originating from the theca interna layer penetrate the granulosa layer and reach the central cavity. Fibroblasts that accompany the vessels form an increasingly dense reticulum network within the granulosa layer as well as an inner fibrous layer that lines the central cavity (Figure 42.27) (32).

Involutional changes begin on the eighth or ninth day following ovulation (168). The granulosa-lutein cells decrease in size, develop pyknotic nuclei, and accumulate abundant cytoplasmic lipid (Figure 42.29). There is a

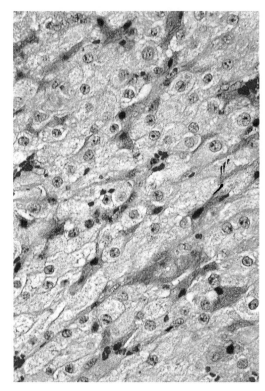

Figure 42.28 Mature corpus luteum of menstruation. K cells with darkly staining cytoplasm and pyknotic nuclei are interspersed between granulosa-lutein cells.

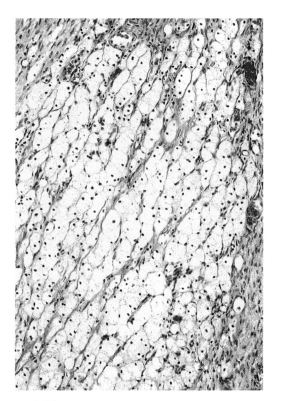

Figure 42.29 Degenerating corpus luteum of menstruation. Granulosa-lutein cells have pyknotic nuclei and abundant cytoplasmic lipid.

decrease in histochemical staining of enzymes associated with steroid biosynthesis and an increase in hydrolytic enzymes (149). Eventually the cells undergo dissolution and are phagocytosed (173). There is progressive fibrosis and shrinkage over a period of several months and eventual conversion to a corpus albicans.

Ultrastructure

At the ultrastructural level, luteinization is characterized by a gradually increasing content of steroidogenic organelles, specifically smooth ER and abundant mitochondria with tubular cristae (Figure 42.30) (151,173–176). The smooth ER exhibits a characteristic regional modification in the form of a folded-membrane complex consisting of highly-folded, radiating, tubular cisternae that communicate and interdigitate with adjacent cisternae (175). Well-developed, dispersed and perinuclear Golgi, free and bound ribosomes, lipid droplets, and lipofuscin pigment are also seen (Figure 42.30) (151,173–175). The cells are separated by a narrow space of variable width, but occasionally the outer leaflets of their plasma membranes become closely apposed and reinforced by desmosomal and pentilaminar tight junctional complexes (151,173,176). Nearly all the cells have a free surface that borders on a broad pericapillary space from which they are separated by an interrupted basal lamina (151). Many irregular microvillous cytoplasmic extensions project into these pericapillary, as well as the intercellular, spaces (Figure 42.30) (70,151,173,175). Occasional interdigitation of these microvilli between adjacent cells form intercellular channels (175). Underlying the microvilli is a narrow zone of cytoplasm filled with a network of filaments that also extend into the microvilli (151).

Theca-lutein cells are similar ultrastructurally to granulosa lutein cells except for the presence of localized per-inuclear Golgi and the absence of folded-membrane complexes, microvilli, and a network of fine filaments (151,175). The varying degrees of cell density appreciable on histological examination are also seen at the ultrastructural level and may represent a fixation artifact. The theca externa layer of the CLM does not differ significantly from that of the Graafian follicle.

The lutein cells of the degenerating CLM exhibit disorganization and fragmentation of the smooth ER, alterations of the mitochondria, and an increase in cytolysosomes (70). Lipid droplets are increased and irregular in size and show increased osmiophilia (173).

Hormonal Aspects

The formation and function of the CLM is under the control of LH, reflected by the high content of LH receptors within the granulosa-lutein cells (156,162). Receptors for FSH (140) and growth hormone (158) have also been identified in the corpus luteum, although their roles in luteal function are unknown. Although P is the major steroid formed in vivo and in vitro by the CLM, it also synthesizes (both in vitro and in vivo) estrone and E2, as well as androgens, mostly androstenedione (177).

After ovulation, LH, FSH, and E2 levels fall, but the LH concentration is sufficient to maintain the CLM, producing a mid-luteal peak in P and E2. If fertilization does not occur, the increased levels of P and estrogen through negative feedback result in a fall of LH and FSH to basal levels, a reduction in LH and FSH receptors within the CLM, and a marked decline in P and E2 synthesis after the 22nd day of the cycle (155,156,162,178,179). These changes are reflected by the morphological involution of the CLM and the onset of menses. Luteolysis appears to be estrogen related, possibly secondary to an estrogen-induced reduction in LH receptors or by enhancement of the luteolytic action

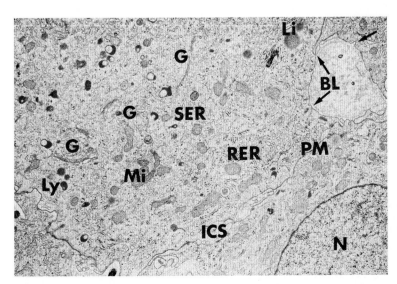

Figure 42.30 Electron micrograph of granulosa-lutein cell of a mature corpus luteum of menstruation. Note abundant smooth ER (SER), mitochondria (Mi), Golgi complex (G), rough ER (RER), lipid droplets (Li), and intercellular space (ICS). BL, basal lamina; N, nucleus of granulosa-lutein cell; Ly, lysosomes; PM, plasma membrane; arrows, micropinocytotic vesicle (original magnification x3600). Reprinted with permission from: Ferenczy A, Richart RM. *Female Reproductive System: Dynamics of Scan and Transmission Electron Microscopy*. New York: John Wiley & Sons; 1974.

of prostaglandins synthesized by the CLM (162,180). A nonsteroidal LH-receptor-binding-inhibitor, which increases in concentration during the luteal phase, may also play a role (162).

CORPUS LUTEUM OF PREGNANCY

Gross Appearance

On gross inspection, the corpus luteum of pregnancy (CLP) may be indistinguishable from the CLM, but is usually larger and bright yellow in contrast to the orange-yellow of the late CLM (181). The larger size, which may account for up to half the ovarian volume, is due primarily to the presence of a central cystic cavity that is filled with fluid or a coagulum composed of fibrin and blood (91,141,182). The cavity size, however, can be highly variable. If the central cyst results in a corpus luteum that is over 3 cm in diameter, the CLP (or less commonly a CLM) is designated a corpus luteum cyst; if less than this size, a cystic corpus luteum. When the cavity of a CLP is large, typically in the first trimester, the wall may lose its convolutions, becoming stretched and attenuated to the extent that it may consist focally of only the inner fibrous layer. Obliteration of the cavity usually begins by the fifth month and is typically completed by term (142). The CLP thus gradually decreases in size, and by the last trimester, it is not a conspicuous structure. During the puerperium, the CLP undergoes involution and conversion to a corpus albicans.

Histology

The CLP, in contrast to the CLM, does not mature in an orderly sequence that allows an estimation of its age; however, early and late stages are recognizable on histological examination.

Granulosa Layer

The first morphological evidence within the corpus luteum that conception has occurred is the absence of the regressive changes that normally appear in the CLM on the 8th or 9th days. Instead, the granulosa lutein cells enlarge, reaching their maximum size of 50 to 60 μm by 8 to 9 weeks' gestation. They assume a round or polyhedral shape with abundant eosinophilic cytoplasm, round to oval, vesicular nuclei, and one or two prominent nucleoli (142) (Figure 42.31A). The granulosa cells of the early CLP are characterized by cytoplasmic vacuoles that initially are tiny but eventually enlarge to occupy almost the entire cell, often with displacement and flattening of the nucleus (Figure 42.31A). The vacuoles tend to diminish in number and size as gestation progresses, and usually disappear after the 4th month. Fine, diffusely scattered, cytoplasmic lipid droplets are also commonly seen within the cells, particularly in early CLP. With increasing age of the corpus luteum, the droplets become fewer and larger (142).

Eosinophilic colloid or hyalin droplets within the granulosa cells of a CLP, which can be identified as early as 15 days after ovulation, are almost diagnostic of pregnancy; they may occur very rarely, however, within a CLM (142). These inclusions initially appear as small, round or irregu-

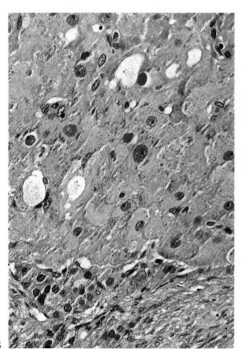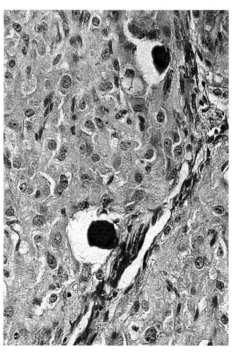

Figure 42.31 Corpus luteum of pregnancy. **A.** Note granulosa-lutein cells with large irregular vacuoles and densely eosinophilic hyalin body. Nests of theca cells are seen at bottom left. **B.** Focal calcification within a late corpus luteum of pregnancy.

A, B

lar, often multiple, droplets that enlarge, possibly by fusion of smaller droplets into one or several large bodies that may fill the entire cell (Figure 42.31A). They become more numerous as gestation progresses (182), although by term their numbers decrease as they undergo calcification, which continues into the puerperium (Figure 42.31B). It is likely that these calcified bodies eventually are resorbed, as they are not a feature of corpora albicantia.

K cells identical to those within CLM are typically found in the granulosa layer of the early CLP. They are most numerous in the second, third, and fourth months of gestation after which time they are rarely encountered (141,142,182).

Theca Layer

The theca interna is thickest in the early CLP at which time it resembles its counterpart in the CLM, surrounding the granulose-lutein layer and forming triangular-shaped, vascular septa that extend into the latter. In the CLP, the theca cells are polyhedral or round and approximately one fourth the size of the granulosa-lutein cells (Figure 42.31A). Their cytoplasm is more darkly staining and granular than in the latter, and is typically not vacuolated. Their nuclei are central, round, and more hyperchromatic than those of the granulosa cells; one or two prominent nucleoli are usually present. The characteristic colloid inclusions seen within the granulosa cells are absent or very rare within the theca cells. Occasional K cells may be seen in early pregnancy, but in smaller numbers than in the granulosa layer (146,182). After the 4th month, the theca interna and its trabeculae become much thinner as the theca cells become smaller and fewer in number, with darker, more irregular, oblong to spindle-shaped nuclei, so that they resemble fibroblasts (182). By term, the theca interna layer has almost completely disappeared.

Connective Tissue

As in the mature CLM, the central cystic cavity is typically lined by a layer of fibrous tissue, composed of variable numbers of fibroblasts, collagen and reticulin fibers, and blood vessels (126). Its thickness is highly variable, not only within the same CLP, but also from one CLP to another and from one phase of pregnancy to another (182). As noted, in some CLP with large cystic cavities, the granulosa layer is focally absent, and its wall is formed entirely by this fibrous layer. As gestation advances, the central cyst or coagulum is eventually obliterated by connective tissue that may exhibit focal hyalinization and calcification (141).

Reticulin staining reveals a pattern similar to that of the mature CLM; that is, a dense pattern within the theca interna and inner fibrous layer, and a sparser framework within the granulosa layer (142). In the early CLP, many, often large, vessels are present in the theca externa and

interna, from which emanate smaller vessels that penetrate the granulosa and inner fibrous layers. In the late CLP, the vessels develop sclerotic walls with luminal narrowing or obliteration (142,182). The amount of connective tissue around the vessels increases in proportion to the decreasing vascularization and regression of the theca interna layer.

Ultrastructure

The ultrastructural appearance of the CLP is similar to that of the CLM, and remains intact throughout pregnancy despite a reduction in its metabolic activity (183–185). The increased cell volume of the granulosa cells in the CLP is reflected by increased smooth ER that exhibits many folded-membrane complexes. There is also an increase in rough ER that is localized in stacks and characteristic concentric whorls not usually seen in the CLM (175,184). Electron-dense, 150 to 200 nm, membrane-bound granules are closely associated with the cisternae of the rough ER. Mitochondria, including large spherical mitochondria not seen in the CLM, are typically highly variable in their size, shape, and internal structure (175,184). The colloid or hyalin inclusions consist of homogeneous electron-opaque material that may surround occasional needle-shaped crystals (Figure 42.32). They typically have no relationship to any organelle, although occasional smaller hyalin bodies are surrounded by rough ER. The vacuoles seen by light microscopy are lined by attenuated microvilli and contain an electron-translucent material (183). Unlike the CLM, extensive bundles of microfilaments are typically encountered throughout the cytoplasm in most lutein cells, and become more prominent as pregnancy progresses (183,184). Collagen fibrils are encountered more frequently in the intercellular and perivascular spaces of the term CLP compared to the CLM.

Hormonal Aspects

Following fertilization, placental hCG stimulates P production by the granulosa-lutein cells. P concentration within the postovulatory corpus luteum increases six-fold, while the E2 level drops to 10% of that within the preovulatory follicle (153,154). HCG alone cannot maintain P secretion from the CLP for more than a few days, and the regulation of P secretion beyond that time is unknown. P production by the CLP begins to decline by the end of the second month of gestation with a concomitant increase of placental P production. However, in vivo and in vitro studies indicate that the CLP continues to produce P throughout the remainder of gestation, albeit in reduced amounts, consistent with the maintenance of its structural integrity until term (140,183,184,186,187). It is not known if P derived from the CLP has a biological role during this period or is redundant because of the massive P production by the placenta

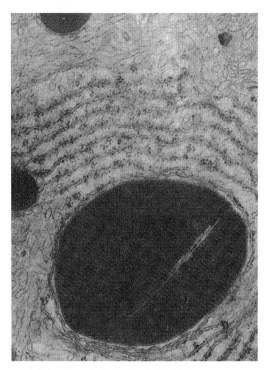

Figure 42.32 Hyalin bodies within a lutein cell from a corpus luteum of pregnancy consisting of homogeneous, electron-opaque material. Note needle-shaped cleft within the largest hyalin body. Some smaller hyalin bodies are surrounded by granular ER (original magnification x22,000). Reprinted with permission from: Adams EC, Hertig AT. Studies on the human corpus luteum. I. Observations on the ultrastructure of development and regression of the luteal cells during the menstrual cycle. *J Cell Biol* 1969;41:696–715.

ating corpus luteum and the young corpus albicans may contain macrophages laden with ceroid and hemosiderin pigment (192,193). The mature corpus albicans is a well-circumscribed structure with convoluted borders composed almost entirely of densely packed collagen fibers with occasional admixed fibroblasts (Figures 42.13, 42.33). Focal calcification and ossification may be occasionally encountered. Most corpora albicantia are eventually resorbed and replaced by ovarian stroma. Persistent corpora albicantia are typically found in the medulla of postmenopausal women (Figure 42.13) suggesting that this resorption process decelerates or terminates prior to the menopause.

ATRETIC FOLLICLES

Histology

Of the original 400,000 primordial follicles present at birth, approximately 400 mature to ovulation. The remaining 99.9% undergo atresia, a process that begins before birth and continues throughout reproductive life, but is most intense immediately after birth and during puberty and pregnancy (135–139,141,143). Factors that initiate atresia and determine which follicles will ultimately undergo atresia are unknown. The atretic process varies with the stage of follicular maturation that has been reached. Atresia of early follicles (primordial and preantral) begins with degenera-

(177,188). There is a rapid decline in function during the puerperium, reflecting falling hCG levels during this period.

Relaxin, a polypeptide hormone, is also produced during gestation and the puerperium by the CLP, probably under the control of hCG (188–191). The concentration of relaxin in ovarian vein plasma during pregnancy correlates with P levels. The placenta and uterus have also been suggested as additional, but less important, sources for this hormone. Its reported actions include cervical dilatation and softening, inhibition of uterine contractions, and relaxation of the pubic symphysis and other pelvic joints (188–191). Immunoreactivity for renin and angiotensin II, similar to that noted within the preovulatory follicle (see above), has been demonstrated within the CLP (167), consistent with the observation that prorenin, likely of ovarian origin, increases 10-fold in pregnant women soon after conception (166).

CORPUS ALBICANS

The regressing CLM is invaded by connective tissue that gradually converts it to a scar, the corpus albicans. The degener-

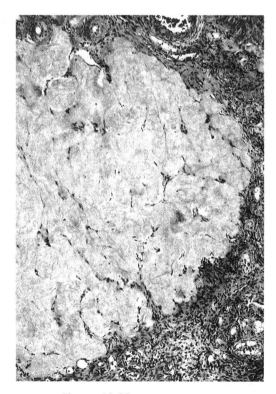

Figure 42.33 Corpus albicans.

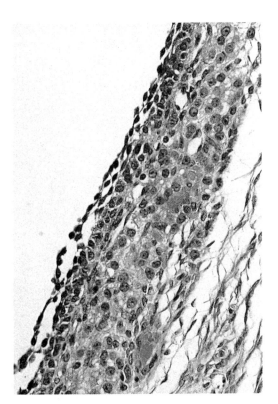

Figure 42.34 Lining of atretic cystic follicle composed of a thin inner layer of small, exfoliating granulosa cells and an outer, luteinized theca interna layer.

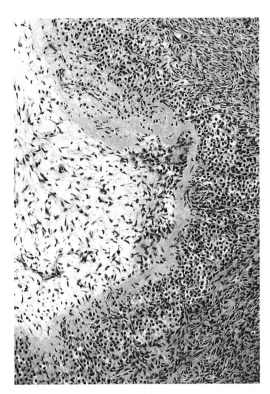

Figure 42.35 Atretic cystic follicle undergoing obliterative atresia. Loose connective tissue is replacing the central cavity. The wavy basement membrane ("glassy membrane") is thickened and hyalinized. A prominent layer of luteinized theca interna is evident.

tion of the oocyte manifested by nuclear changes (chromatin condensation, pyknosis, fragmentation) and cytoplasmic vacuolation. Degeneration of the granulosa cells soon follows and the follicle disappears without a trace. In contrast, atresia of follicles that have reached the antral stage of development is more complex and variable, but ultimately leads to obliterative atresia and the formation of a scar, the corpus fibrosum. The earliest evidence of this process is mitotic inactivity of the granulosa cells and a decrease in their numbers, manifested by thinning and focal exfoliation of the granulosa layer. Some follicles may persist for an indefinite period of time at this stage as atretic cystic follicles (Figure 42.34); those that exceed 3 cm are designated follicular cysts. Atretic cystic follicles and follicular cysts may persist for a number of years after the menopause (194,195). Atretic follicles are ultimately invaded by vascular connective tissue that eventually fills the central cavity (Figure 42.35). The oocyte may persist for an indefinite period of time but eventually degenerates. Concurrent with these changes, the basement membrane between the granulosa and theca interna layers becomes transformed into a thick, wavy, eosinophilic, hyalinized band, the so-called "glassy membrane" (Figures 42.35, 42.36). The theca interna layer typically persists, often with prominent luteinization (Figures 42.35, 42.36), until the late stages of

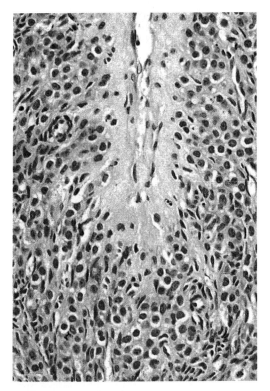

Figure 42.36 Edge of follicle in late stage of obliterative atresia. Hyalinized fibrous tissue occupies the central cavity and extends into the persistent luteinized theca interna layer.

atresia at which time cords and nests of theca cells become surrounded by proliferating connective tissue (Figure 42.36). Luteinization of both theca and granulosa layers is particularly striking in atretic follicles during infancy and childhood (196) and pregnancy (Figure 42.37) (142).

Microscopic proliferations of persistent granulosa cells within the centers of atretic follicles of pregnant, and less commonly nonpregnant women, may mimic small granulosa cell tumors (Figure 42.37), or rarely, Sertoli cell tumors (197). Similarly, structures resembling microscopic gonadoblastomas and sex cord tumors with annular tubules have been identified within atretic follicles in up to 35% of normal fetuses and infants (131,198,199). There is no evidence to suggest that any of these tumorlike proliferations represent early stages of neoplasia.

Continued shrinkage and hyalinization of an atretic follicle produces a serpiginous strand of hyalin tissue, the corpus fibrosum or atreticum (Figure 42.38). Like corpora albicantia, most corpora fibrosa are probably resorbed by the ovarian stroma.

Hormonal Aspects

In contrast to preovulatory follicles, the microenvironment of follicles undergoing atresia is predominantly androgenic, with high concentrations of intrafollicular

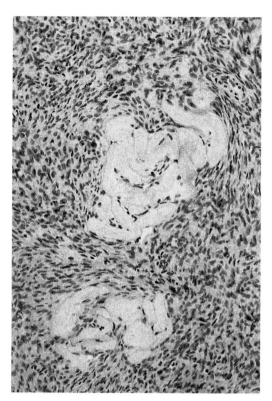

Figure 42.38   Two corpora fibrosa.

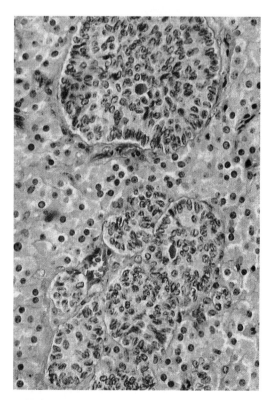

Figure 42.37   Atretic follicle in pregnancy. Within the center of the follicle is a proliferation of persistent granulosa cells surrounded by luteinized theca interna cells.

androstenedione and low concentrations of FSH and E2 (17,119,153,154,200). As noted, these follicles are deficient in granulosa cells, and the residual granulosa cells do not respond to FSH in vitro (145); both FSH- and LH-receptors are lower than in nonatretic follicles (156). Oocytes from atretic follicles are unable to complete the first meiotic division (145). It is likely that an androgenic intrafollicular milieu is the major factor that halts follicular growth and initiates atresia of that follicle.

HILUS CELLS

Histology

Ovarian hilus cells, morphologically identical to testicular Leydig cells (with the exception of a female chromatin pattern), are present during fetal life but not during childhood. They reappear at the time of puberty and are demonstrable in most postmenopausal women (201–203). Their number and location can be highly variable, and their numbers increase during pregnancy, with increasing age after the menopause, and with increasing degrees of ovarian stromal proliferation and stromal luteinization (22). Mild hilus cell hyperplasia is a relatively common incidental histological finding in postmenopausal women (85).

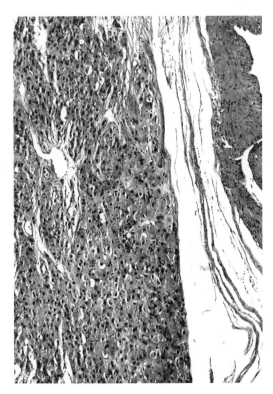

Figure 42.39 Nest of hilus cells adjacent to large vessel within the ovarian hilus.

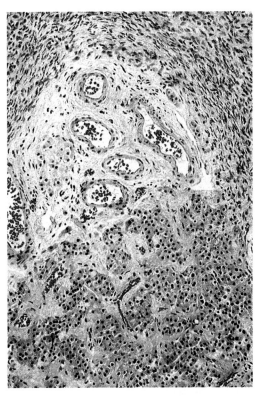

Figure 42.40 Nest of hilus cells with admixed small blood vessels abutting medullary stroma (top of figure).

Hilus cell aggregates of variable size and shape are typically found in the ovarian hilus and adjacent mesovarium (Figures 42.39, 42.40). They are more numerous in the lateral and medial poles of the hilus and near the junction of the ovarian ligament with the ovary, typically lying close to the junction of the hilus with the medullary stroma (Figure 42.40) (201). The aggregates are closely associated with large hilar veins and lymphatic sinusoids, and may form nodular protrusions into their lumina. Hilus cells characteristically ensheathe, or less commonly lie within, nonmedullated nerves (Figure 42.41), and occasionally surround the rete ovarii (201). Nests may also be present within the medullary stroma near the hilus, probably representing extensions of the hilus into the medulla. Also, as previously noted, cells of hilus-type may also occur rarely within the ovarian stroma at a distance from the hilus (stromal Leydig cells). Hilus cells also may be encountered rarely in the perisalpinx and fimbrial endosalpinx (204).

Hilus cells nests are unencapsulated, typically lying within loose connective tissue, or rarely ovarian-type stroma, within the hilus (101). The cells are 15 to 25 micra in diameter, round to oval, less commonly elongate, with abundant eosinophilic cytoplasm and a spherical vesicular nucleus with one or two prominent nucleoli (Figure 42.42). The nuclei, particularly in postmenopausal

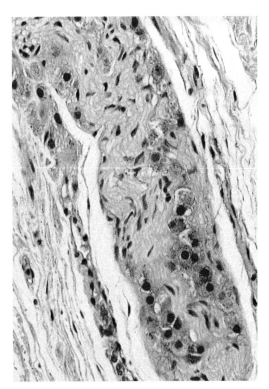

Figure 42.41 Perineural and intraneural hilus cells. Note fine brown lipochrome pigment within hilus cells.

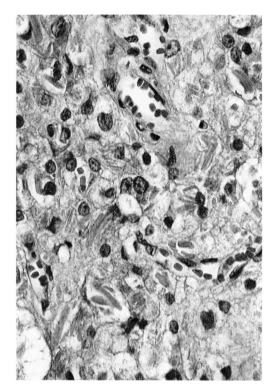

Figure 42.42 Hilus cells with Reinke crystals.

women, may have hyperchromatic, bizarre nuclei. Hilus cells are typically strongly immunoreactive for inhibin, calretinin, and melan-A (77,81).

Hilus cells contain specific crystals of Reinke, which are homogenous, eosinophilic, nonrefractile, rod-shaped structures, 10 to 35 μm in length, with blunt, but occasionally tapered, ends (Figure 42.42). The crystals typically lie in a parallel or stacked arrangement within a cell, and often are surrounded by a clear halo; occasionally they appear to extend through or overlie cell membranes. The crystals are unevenly distributed and are typically present in only a minority of cells; frequently they cannot be identified (205). Their visualization may be facilitated by the use of Masson's trichrome and iron hematoxylin methods that stain them magenta and black respectively. Additionally, the crystals fluoresce yellow when H&E stained sections are viewed by ultraviolet light (206). Also present within hilus cells, often in greater numbers than crystals, are spherical or ellipsoidal hyalin structures that have an otherwise identical appearance to crystals and probably represent their precursors. Elongated erythrocytes compressed within capillaries should not be confused with crystals and crystal-precursors. The cytoplasm of Leydig cells may also contain perinuclear eosinophilic granules, peripheral lipid vacuoles, and golden-brown lipochrome pigment (Figure

42.41). Delicate collagen fibrils surround each cell. Typically admixed with the hilus cells are fibroblasts and cells intermediate in appearance between the two cell types (207). The hilus cells and intermediate cells have intimate attachments to nerves, including true synaptic connections, suggesting that hilus cells may originate from hilar fibroblasts, possibly under the inductive influence of hilar nerves (201,207).

Hilus cells should be distinguished from adrenal cortical rests. The latter are extremely rare in the ovary (208), but are found in the mesovarium, and occasionally within the ovarian hilus, in approximately one-quarter of women (209). Their histologic appearance mimics that of the normal adrenal cortex, with most of the cells containing numerous lipid vacuoles.

Ultrastructure

Hilus cells have a steroidogenic ultrastructure consisting of prominent smooth endoplasmic reticulum and mitochondria with tubular cristae, as well as well developed Golgi, large lysosomes, and osmiophilic lipid inclusions (207). Reinke crystals have a true crystalline appearance composed of dense parallel hexagonal microtubules with a mean thickness of 12 nm separated by clear spaces 15 nm wide producing a "woven fabric" appearance (Figure 42.43) (207). The crystals are typically oriented in many directions in the same cell. They appear to be formed by progressive association of precrystalline units each of which is composed of bundles of four or five parallel filaments (Figure 42.43).

Typically found admixed with hilus cells are fibroblasts and cells intermediate in ultrastructural appearance between the two cell types. Hilus cells, and more commonly the intermediate cells, have intimate attachments to nerves in the form of simple membranous contacts, invaginations of axon terminals into hilus cells, or surface membrane thickenings resembling a true synapse (207).

Hormonal Aspects

The light and electron microscopic morphology and enzyme content of hilus cells are those of steroid hormone-producing cells, although to what extent hilus cells contribute to the steroid hormone pool in normal females is unknown (32,201). In vitro incubation studies indicate that the major steroid produced by ovarian hilus cells is androstenedione and that it is produced in amounts higher than that produced from ovarian stroma (210). Lesser amounts of E2 and P are also produced in vitro. Hilus cells are responsive in vivo to both exogenous and endogenous hCG stimulation, manifested by an increase in their numbers, cell size, and mitotic activity (202).

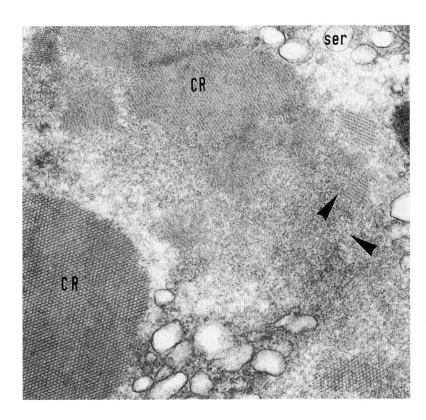

Figure 42.43 Reinke crystals with hexagonal internal pattern (CR) formed by association of precrystalline units (arrowheads); ser, smooth ER (original magnification x25,000). Reprinted with permission from: Laffargue P, Benkoel L, Laffargue F, Casanova P, Chamlian A. Ultrastructural and enzyme histochemical study of ovarian hilar cells in women and their relationships with sympathetic nerves. *Hum Pathol* 1978;9:649–659.

RETE OVARII

The rete ovarii, the ovarian analog of the rete testis, is present in the hilus of all ovaries. It consists of a network of irregular clefts, tubules, cysts, and intraluminal papillae, lined by an epithelium that varies from flat to cuboidal to columnar (Figure 42.44) (211,212). Solid cords of similar cells may also be seen. Characteristically, the rete is surrounded by a cuff of spindle-cell stroma similar to, but discontinuous from, the ovarian stroma (Figure 42.44).

The cytoplasm of the cells of the rete is immunoreactive for cytokeratin, EMA, vimentin, and desmoplakin (35,36,213). Ultrastructural examination has revealed two types of cells, one ciliated and the other nonciliated with apical microvilli (35). The cytoplasm contains many mitochondria, a moderate amount of rough ER, many free polyribosomes, and some glycogen. Numerous desmosomes with associated tonofilament bundles connect adjacent cells. The basal lamina is well defined.

The rete juxtaposes and may communicate with mesonephric tubules within the mesovarium (212). Rare hilar cysts originate from the rete, and small tumorlike proliferations of the rete have been referred to as "rete adenomas" (212,214). The transitional cell metaplasia that has been encountered in the rete epithelium may account for the occasional small hilar Brenner tumors that have been contiguous with and possibly derived from the rete (211).

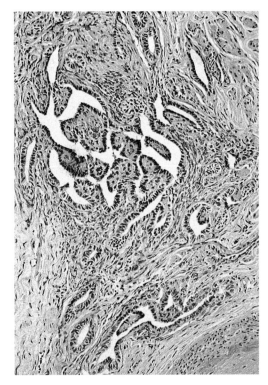

Figure 42.44 Rete ovarii.

REFERENCES

1. Baker TG, Sum W. Development of the ovary and oogenesis. *Clin Obstet Gynaecol* 1976;3:3–26.
2. Hoang-Ngoc M, Smadja A, Herve De Sigalony JP, Orcel L. Etude histologique de la gonade a differenciation ovarienne au cours de l'organogenese. *Arch Anat Cytol Pathol* 1989;37:201–207.
3. Gondos B, Bhiraleus P, Hobel CJ. Ultrastructural observations on germ cells in human fetal ovaries. *Am J Obstet Gynecol* 1971;110:644–652.
4. Gondos B. Cellular interrelationships in the human fetal ovary and testis. In: Federoff S, ed. *Prog Clin Biol Res. volume 59B. Eleventh International Congress of Anatomy: Advances in the Morphology of Cells and Tissues.* New York: Alan R. Liss Inc; 1981:373–381.
5. Konishi I, Fujii S, Okamura H, Parmley T, Mori T. Development of interstitial cells and ovigerous cords in the human fetal ovary: an ultrastructural study. *J Anat* 1986;148:121–135.
6. Gondos B. Surface epithelium of the developing ovary. Possible correlation with ovarian neoplasia. *Am J Pathol* 1975;81:303–321.
7. Rabinovici J, Jaffe RB. Development and regulation of growth and differentiated function in human and subhuman primate fetal gonads. *Endocr Rev* 1990;11:532–557.
8. Van Wagenen G, Simpson ME. *Embryology of the Ovary and Testis in Homo Sapiens and Macaca Mulatta.* New Haven: Yale University Press; 1965.
9. Fukuda O, Miyayama Y, Fujimoto T, et al. Electron microscopic study of the gonadal development in early human embryos. *Prog Clin Biol Res* 1989;296:23–29.
10. Pinkerton JH, McKay DG, Adams EC, Hertig AT. Development of the human ovary—a study using histochemical techniques. *Obstet Gynecol* 1961;18:152–181.
11. Gruenwald P. The development of the sex cords in the gonads of man and mammals. *Am J Anat* 1942;70:359–389.
12. Jirasek JE. Development of the genital system in human embryos and fetuses. In: Jirasek J. *Development of the Genital System and Male Pseudohermaphroditism.* Baltimore: Johns Hopkins Press; 1971:3–41.
13. Byskov AG. Differentiation of mammalian embryonic gonad. *Physiol Rev* 1986;66:71–117.
14. Satoh M. Histogenesis and organogenesis of the gonad in human embryos. *J Anat* 1991;177:85–107.
15. Wartenberg H. The influence of the mesonephric blastema on gonadal development and sexual differentiation. In: Byskov AG, Peters H, eds. *Development and Function of Reproductive Organs.* Amsterdam-Oxford-Princeton: Excerpta Medica; 1981:3–12.
16. Wartenberg H. Development of the early human ovary and role of the mesonephros in the differentiation of the cortex. *Anat Embryol (Berl)* 1982;165:253–280.
17. Nicosia SV. Morphological changes in the human ovary throughout life. In: Serra GB, ed. *The Ovary.* New York: Raven Press; 1983:57–81.
18. Pryse-Davies J. The development, structure and function of the female pelvic organs in childhood. *Clin Obstet Gynaecol* 1974;1:483–508.
19. Valdes-Dapena MA. The normal ovary of childhood. *Ann N Y Acad Sci* 1967;142:597–613.
20. Merrill JA. The morphology of the prepubertal ovary: relationship to the polycystic ovary syndrome. *South Med J* 1963;56:225–231.
21. Pavlik EJ, DePriest PD, Gallion HH, et al. Ovarian volume related to age. *Gynecol Oncol* 2000;77:410–412.
22. Boss JH, Scully RE, Wegner KH, Cohen RB. Structural variations in the adult ovary. Clinical significance. *Obstet Gynecol* 1965;25:747–764.
23. Reeves G. Specific stroma in the cortex and medulla of the ovary. Cell types and vascular supply in relation to follicular apparatus and ovulation. *Obstet Gynecol* 1971;37:832–844.
24. Plentl AA, Friedman EA. *Lymphatic System of the Female Genitalia.* Philadelphia: WB Saunders; 1971.
25. Eichner E, Bove ER. In vivo studies on the lymphatic drainage of the human ovary. *Obstet Gynecol* 1954;3:287–297.
26. Jacobowitz D, Wallach EE. Histochemical and chemical studies of the autonomic innervation of the ovary. *Endocrinology* 1967;81:1132–1139.
27. Owman C, Rosenbren E, Sjoberg N. Adrenergic innervation of the human female reproductive organs: a histochemical and chemical investigation. *Obstet Gynecol* 1967;30:763–773.
28. Balboni GC. Structural changes: ovulation and luteal phase. In: Serra GB, ed. *The Ovary.* New York: Raven Press; 1983:123–141.
29. Mohsin S. The sympathetic innervation of the mammalian ovary. A review of pharmacological and histochemical studies. *Clin Exp Pharmacol Physiol* 1979;6:335–354.
30. Dyer CA, Erickson GF. Norepinephrine amplifies human chorionic gonadotropin-stimulated androgen biosynthesis by ovarian theca-interstitial cells. *Endocrinology* 1985;116:1645–1652.
31. Blaustein A, Lee H. Surface cells of the ovary and pelvic peritoneum: a histochemical and ultrastructural comparison. *Gynecol Oncol* 1979;8:34–43.
32. McKay DG, Pinkerton JH, Hertig AT, Danzinger S. The adult human ovary: a histochemical study. *Obstet Gynecol* 1961;18:13–39.
33. Miettinen M, Lehto V, Virtanen I. Expression of intermediate filaments in normal ovaries and ovarian epithelial, sex cord-stromal, and germinal tumors. *Int J Gynecol Pathol* 1983;2:64–71.
34. Czernobilsky B, Moll R, Franke WW, Dallenbach-Hellweg G, Hohlweg-Majert P. Intermediate filaments of normal and neoplastic tissues of the female genital tract with emphasis on problems of differential tumor diagnosis. *Pathol Res Pract* 1984;179:31–37.
35. Czernobilsky B, Moll R, Levy R, Franke WW. Co-expression of cytokeratin and vimentin filaments in mesothelial, granulosa and rete ovarii cells of the human ovary. *Eur J Cell Biol* 1985;37:175–190.
36. Benjamin E, Law S, Bobrow LG. Intermediate filaments cytokeratin and vimentin in ovarian sex cord-stromal tumours with correlative studies in adult and fetal ovaries. *J Pathol* 1987;152:253–263.
37. Isola J, Kallioniemi OP, Korte JM, et al. Steroid receptors and Ki-67 reactivity in ovarian cancer and in normal ovary: correlation with DNA flow cytometry, biochemical receptor assay, and patient survival. *J Pathol* 1990;162:295–301.
38. Rodriguez GC, Berchuk A, Whitaker RS, Schlossman D, Clarke-Pearson DL, Bast RC Jr. Epidermal growth factor receptor expression in normal ovarian epithelium and ovarian cancer. II. Relationship between receptor expression and response to epidermal growth factor. *Am J Obstet Gynecol* 1991;164:745–750.
39. Jindal SK, Snoey DM, Lobb DK, Dorrington JH. Transforming growth factor alpha localization and role in surface epithelium of normal human ovaries and in ovarian carcinoma lines. *Gynecol Oncol* 1994;53:17–23.
40. Latza U, Niedobitek G, Schwarting R, Nekarda H, Stein H. Ber-EP4: new monoclonal antibody which distinguishes epithelia from mesothelial. *J Clin Pathol* 1990;43:213–219.
41. Shimizu M, Toki T, Takagi Y, Konishi I, Fujii S. Immunohistochemical detection of the Wilms' tumor gene (WT1) in epithelial ovarian tumors. *Int J Gynecol Pathol* 2000;19:158–163.
42. Carreiras F, Denoux Y, Staedel C, Sichel F, Gauduchon P. Expression and localization of αv integrins and their ligand vitronectin in normal ovarian epithelium and in ovarian carcinoma. *Gynecol Oncol* 1996;62:260–267.
43. Zheng W, Magid MS, Kramer EE, Chen YT. Follicle-stimulating hormone receptor is expressed in human ovarian surface epithelium and fallopian tube. *Am J Pathol* 1996;148:47–53.
44. Davies BR, Worsley SD, Ponder BA. Expression of E-cadherin, α-catenin and β-catenin in normal ovarian surface epithelium and epithelial ovarian cancers. *Histopathology* 1998;32:69–80.
45. Cruet S, Salamanca C, Mitchell GW, Auersperg N. $\alpha v \beta 3$ and vitronectin expression by normal ovarian surface epithelial cells: role in cell adhesion and cell proliferation. *Gynecol Oncol* 1999;75:254–260.
46. Cao QJ, Jones JG, Li M. Expression of calretinin in human ovary, testis, and ovarian sex cord-stromal tumors. *Int J Gynecol Pathol* 2001;20:346–352.
47. Blaustein A. Surface cells and inclusion cysts in fetal ovaries. *Gynecol Oncol* 1981;12(pt 1):222–233.

48. Blaustein A, Kantius M, Kaganowicz A, Pervez N, Wells J. Inclusions in ovaries of females aged day 1-30 years. *Int J Gynecol Pathol* 1982;1:145–153.

49. Zinsser KR, Wheeler JE. Endosalpingiosis in the omentum: a study of autopsy and surgical material. *Am J Surg Pathol* 1982;6: 109–117.

50. Mulligan RM. A survey of epithelial inclusions in the ovarian cortex of 470 patients. *J Surg Oncol* 1976;8:61–66.

51. Von Numers C. Observations on metaplastic changes in the germinal epithelium of the ovary and on the aetiology of ovarian endometriosis. *Acta Obstet Gynecol Scand* 1965;44:107–116.

52. Scully RE. Ovary. In: Henson DE, Albores-Saavedra J, eds. *The Pathology of Incipient Neoplasia. Major Problems in Pathology Series.* 2nd ed. Vol 28. Philadelphia: WB Saunders; 1993:279–300.

53. Mittal KR, Zeleniuch-Jacquotte A, Cooper JL, Demopoulos RI. Contralateral ovary in unilateral ovarian carcinoma: a search for preneoplastic lesions. *Int J Gynecol Pathol* 1993;12:59–63.

54. Hutson R, Ramsdale J, Wells M. p53 protein expression in putative precursor lesions of epithelial ovarian cancer. *Histopathology* 1995;27:367–371.

55. Blaustein A, Kaganowicz A, Wells J. Tumor markers in inclusion cysts of the ovary. *Cancer* 1982;49:722–726.

56. Charpin C, Bhan AK, Zurawski VR Jr, Scully RE. Carcinoembryonic antigen (CEA) and carbohydrate determinant 19-9 (CA 19-9) localization in 121 primary and metastatic ovarian tumors: an immunohistochemical study with the use of monoclonal antibodies. *Int J Gynecol Pathol* 1982;1:231–245.

57. Cordon-Cardo C, Mattes MJ, Melamed MR, Lewis JL Jr, Old LJ, Lloyd KO. Immunopathologic analysis of a panel of mouse monoclonal antibodies reacting with human ovarian carcinomas and other human tumors. *Int J Gynecol Pathol* 1985;4:121–130.

58. Kabawat SE, Bast RC Jr, Bhan AK, Welch WR, Knapp RC, Colvin RB. Tissue distribution of coelomic-epithelium-related antigen recognized by the monoclonal antibody OC125. *Int J Gynecol Pathol* 1983;2:275–285.

59. Nouwen EJ, Pollet DE, Schelstraete JB, et al. Human placental alkaline phosphatase in benign and malignant ovarian neoplasia. *Cancer Res* 1985;45:892–902.

60. Nouwen EJ, Hendrix PG, Dauwe S, Eerdekens MW, De Broe ME. Tumor markers in the human ovary and its neoplasms. A comparative immunohistochemical study. *Am J Pathol* 1987;126:230–242.

61. Mittal KR, Goswami S, Demopoulos RI. Immunohistochemical profile of ovarian inclusion cysts in patients with and without ovarian carcinoma. *Histochem J* 1995;27:119–122.

62. Maines-Bandiera SL, Auersperg N. Increased E-cadherin expression in ovarian surface epithelium: an early step in metaplasia and dysplasia? *Int J Gynecol Pathol* 1997;16:250–255.

63. Sundfeldt K, Piontkewitz Y, Ivarsson K, et al. E-cadherin expression in human epithelial ovarian cancer and normal ovary. *Int J Cancer* 1997;74:275–280.

64. Resta L, Scordari MD, Colucci GA, et al. Morphological changes of the ovarian surface epithelium in ovarian polycystic disease or endometrial carcinoma and a control group. *Eur J Gynaecol Oncol* 1989;10:39–41.

65. Bransilver BR. Ferenczy A, Richart RM. Brenner tumors and Walthard cell nests. *Arch Pathol* 1974;98:76–86.

66. Danforth DN. Cytologic relationship of Walthard cell rest to Brenner tumor of ovary and the pseudomucinous cystadenoma. *Am J Obstet Gynecol* 1942;43:984–996.

67. Roth LM. The Brenner tumor and the Walthard cell nest. An electron microscopic study. *Lab Invest* 1974;31:15–23.

68. Teoh TB. The structure and development of Walthard nests. *J Pathol Bacteriol* 1953;66:433–439.

69. Papadaki L, Beilby JO. The fine structure of the surface epithelium of the human ovary. *J Cell Sci* 1971;8:445–465.

70. Ferenczy A, Richart RM. *Female Reproductive System: Dynamics of Scan and Transmission Electron Microscopy.* New York: John Wiley & Sons; 1974.

71. Blaustein A. Peritoneal mesothelium and ovarian surface cells—shared characteristics. *Int J Gynecol Pathol* 1984;3:361–375.

72. Fienberg R, Cohen RB. A comparative histochemical study of the ovarian stromal lipid band, stromal theca cell, and normal ovarian follicular apparatus. *Am J Obstet Gynecol* 1965;92:958–969.

73. Czernobilsky B, Shezen E, Lifschitz-Mercer B, et al. Alpha smooth muscle actin (alpha-SM actin) in normal human ovaries, in ovarian stromal hyperplasia and in ovarian neoplasms. *Virchows Arch B Cell Pathol Incl Mol Pathol* 1989;57:55–61.

74. Lastarria D, Sachdev RK, Babury RA, Yu HM, Nuovo GJ. Immunohistochemical analysis for desmin in normal and neoplastic ovarian stromal tissue. *Arch Pathol Lab Med* 1990;114:502–505.

75. Matias-Guiu X, Pons C, Prat J. Mullerian inhibiting substance, alpha-inhibin, and CD99 expression in sex cord-stromal tumors and endometrioid ovarian carcinomas resembling sex cord-stromal tumors. *Hum Pathol* 1998;29:840–845.

76. Rishi M, Howard LN, Bratthauer GL, Tavassoli FA. Use of monoclonal antibody against human inhibin as a marker for sex cord-stromal tumors of the ovary. *Am J Surg Pathol* 1997;21: 583–589.

77. Pelkey TJ, Frierson HF Jr, Mills SE, Stoler MH. The diagnostic utility of inhibin staining in ovarian neoplasms. *Int J Gynecol Pathol* 1998;17:97–105.

78. Zheng W, Sung CJ, Hanna I, et al. α and β subunits of inhibin/activin as sex cord-stromal differentiation markers. *Int J Gynecol Pathol* 1997;16:263–271.

79. Hildebrandt RH, Rouse RV, Longacre TA. Value of inhibin in the identification of granulosa cell tumors of the ovary. *Hum Pathol* 1997;28:1387–1395.

80. McCluggage WG, Maxwell P. Immunohistochemical staining for calretinin is useful in the diagnosis of ovarian sex cord-stromal tumours. *Histopathology* 2001;38:403–408.

81. Jungbluth AA, Busam KJ, Gerald WL, et al. A103: An anti-melan-a monoclonal antibody for the detection of malignant melanoma in paraffin-embedded tissues. *Am J Surg Pathol* 1998; 22:595–602.

82. Oliva E, Vu Q, Young RH. CD10 expression in sex cord-stromal tumors (SCTs) and steroid cell tumors (StCTs) of the ovary. *Mod Pathol* 2002;15:204A.

83. Nagamani M, Hannigan EV, Dinh TV, Stuart CA. Hyperinsulinemia and stromal luteinization of the ovaries in postmenopausal women with endometrial cancer. *J Clin Endocrinol Metab* 1988; 67:144–148.

84. Scully RE, Cohen RB. Oxidative-enzyme activity in normal and pathologic human ovaries. *Obstet Gynecol* 1964;24:667–681.

85. Loubet R, Loubet A, Leboutet MJ. The ovarian stroma after the menopause: activity and ageing. In: de Brux J, Gautray JP, eds. *Clinical Pathology of the Ovary.* Boston: MTP Press Ltd; 1984:119–141.

86. Nakano R, Shima K, Yamoto M, Kobayashi M, Nishimori K, Hiraoka J. Binding sites for gonadotropins in human postmenopausal ovaries. *Obstet Gynecol* 1989;73:196–200.

87. Bassis ML. Pseudodeciduosis. *Am J Obstet Gynecol* 1956;72: 1029–1037.

88. Israel SL, Rubenstone A, Meranze DR. The ovary at term. I. Decidua-like reaction and surface cell proliferation. *Obstet Gynecol* 1954;3:399–407.

89. Ober WB, Grady HG, Schoenbucher AK. Ectopic ovarian decidua without pregnancy. *Am J Pathol* 1957;33:199–217.

90. Bersch W, Alexy E, Heuser HP, et al. Ectopic decidua formation in the ovary (so-called deciduoma). *Virch Archiv A* 1973;360: 173–177.

91. Starup J, Visfeldt J. Ovarian morphology in early and late human pregnancy. *Acta Obstet Gynecol Scand* 1974;53:211–218.

92. Herr JC, Heidger PM Jr, Scott JR, Anderson JW, Curet LB, Mossman HW. Decidual cells in the human ovary at term. I. Incidence, gross anatomy and ultrastructural features of merocrine secretion. *Am J Anat* 1978;152:7–27.

93. Doss BJ, Wanek SM, Jacques SM, Qureshi F, Ramirez NC, Lawrence WD. Ovarian smooth muscle metaplasia: an uncommon and possibly underrecognized entity. *Int J Gynecol Pathol* 1999;18:58–62.

94. Hughesdon PE. Morphology and morphogenesis of the Stein-Leventhal ovary and of so-called "hyperthecosis." *Obstet Gynecol Surv* 1982;37:59–77.

95. Scully RE. Smooth-muscle differentiation in genital tract disorders. *Arch Pathol Lab Med* 1981;105:505–507.

96. Hughesdon PE. The origin and development of benign stromatosis of the ovary. *J Obstet Gynaecol Br Commonw* 1972;79:348–359.

97. Hughesdon PE. The endometrial identity of benign stromatosis of the ovary and its relation to other forms of endometriosis. *J Pathol* 1976;119:201–209.

98. Hart WR, Abell MR. Adipose prosoplasia of ovary. *Am J Obstet Gynecol* 1970;106:929–931.

99. Honoré LH, O'Hara KE. Subcapsular adipocytic infiltration of the human ovary: a clinicopathological study of eight cases. *Eur J Obstet Gynaecol Reprod Biol* 1980;10:13–20.

100. Sternberg WH, Roth LM. Ovarian stromal tumors containing Leydig cells. I. Stromal-Leydig cell tumor and non-neoplastic transformation of ovarian stroma to Leydig cells. *Cancer* 1973;32:940–951.

101. Zhang J, Young RH, Arseneau J, Scully RE. Ovarian stromal tumors containing lutein or Leydig cells (luteinized thecomas and stromal Leydig cell tumors)—a clinicopathological analysis of fifty cases. *Int J Gynecol Pathol* 1982;1:270–285.

102. Rutgers JL, Scully RE. Functioning ovarian tumors with peripheral steroid cell proliferation: a report of twenty-four cases. *Int J Gynecol Pathol* 1986;5:319–337.

103. Hidvegi D, Cibils LA, Sorensen K, Hidvegi I. Ultrastructural and histochemical observations of neuroendocrine granules in nonneoplastic ovaries. *Am J Obstet Gynecol* 1982;143:590–594.

104. Snowden JA, Harkin PJ, Thornton JG, Wells M. Morphometric assessment of ovarian stromal proliferation—a clinicopathological study. *Histopathology* 1989;14:369–379.

105. Bigelow B. Comparison of ovarian and endometrial morphology spanning the menopause. *Obstet Gynecol* 1958;11:487–513.

106. Roddick JW Jr, Greene RR. Relation of ovarian stromal hyperplasia to endometrial carcinoma. *Am J Obstet Gynecol* 1957;73:843–852.

107. Woll E, Hertig AT, Smith GVS, Johnson LC. The ovary in endometrial carcinoma: with notes on the morphological history of the aging ovary. *Am J Obstet Gynecol* 1948;56:617–633.

108. Laffargue P, Adechy-Benkoel L, Valette C. Ultrastructure du stroma ovarien. *Ann d'Anat Pathol* 1968;13:381–402.

109. Aiman J, Forney JP, Parker CR Jr. Secretion of androgens and estrogens by normal and neoplastic ovaries in postmenopausal women. *Obstet Gynecol* 1986;68:1–5.

110. Chang RJ, Judd HL. The ovary after menopause. *Clin Obstet Gynaecol* 1981;24:181–191.

111. Dennefors BL, Janson PO, Knutson F, Hamberger L. Steroid production and responsiveness to gonadotropin in isolated stromal tissue of human postmenopausal ovaries. *Am J Obstet Gynecol* 1980;136:997–1002.

112. Greenblatt RB, Colle ML, Mahesh VB. Ovarian and adrenal steroid production in the postmenopausal woman. *Obstet Gynecol* 1976;47:383–387.

113. Judd HL, Judd GE, Lucas WE, Yen SS. Endocrine function of the postmenopausal ovary: concentration of androgens and estrogens in ovarian and peripheral vein blood. *J Clin Endocrinol Metab* 1974;39:1020–1024.

114. Judd HL, Lucas WE, Yen SSC. Effect of oophorectomy on circulating testosterone and androstenedione levels in patients with endometrial cancer. *Am J Obstet Gynecol* 1974;118:793–798.

115. Longcope C, Hunter R, Franz C. Steroid secretion by the postmenopausal ovary. *Am J Obstet Gynecol* 1980;138:564–568.

116. Lucisano A, Russo N, Acampora MG, et al. Ovarian and peripheral androgen and oestrogen levels in post-menopausal women: correlations with ovarian histology. *Maturitas* 1986;8:57–65.

117. Mattingly RF, Huang WY. Steroidogenesis of the menopausal and postmenopausal ovary. *Am J Obstet Gynecol* 1969;103:679–693.

118. McNatty KP, Makris A, DeGrazia C, Osathanondh R, Ryan KJ. The production of progesterone, androgens, and estrogens by granulosa cells, thecal tissue, and stromal tissue from human ovaries in vitro. *J Clin Endocrinol Metab* 1979;49:687–699.

119. McNatty KP, Smith DM, Makris A, et al. The intraovarian sites of androgen and estrogen formation in women with normal and hyperandrogenic ovaries as judged by in vitro experiments. *J Clin Endocrinol Metab* 1980;50:755–763.

120. Plotz EJ, Wiener M, Stein AA, Hahn BD. Enzymatic activities related to steroidogenesis in postmenopausal ovaries of patients with and without endometrial carcinoma. *Am J Obstet Gynecol* 1967;99:182–197.

121. Vermeulen A. The hormonal activity of the postmenopausal ovary. *J Clin Endocrinol Metab* 1976;42:247–253.

122. Rice BF, Savard K. Steroid hormone formation in the human ovary. IV. Ovarian stromal compartment; formation of radioactive steroids from acetate-1-14C and action of gonadotropins. *J Clin Endocrinol Metab* 1966;26:593–609.

123. Barbieri RL, Makris A, Randall RW, Daniels G, Kistner RW, Ryan KJ. Insulin stimulates androgen accumulation in incubations of ovarian stroma obtained from women with hyperandrogenism. *J Clin Endocrinol Metab* 1986;62:904–910.

124. Reed MJ, Beranek PA, Ghilchik MW, James VH. Conversion of estrone to estradiol and estradiol to estrone in postmenopausal women. *Obstet Gynecol* 1985;66:361–365.

125. Longcope C. Metabolic clearance and blood production rates of estrogens in postmenopausal women. *Am J Obstet Gynecol* 1971;111:778–781.

126. Grodin JM, Siiteri PK, MacDonald PC. Source of estrogen production in postmenopausal women. *J Clin Endocrinol Metab* 1973;36:207–214.

127. Nagamani M, Stuart CA, Doherty MG. Increased steroid production by the ovarian stromal tissue of postmenopausal women with endometrial cancer. *J Clin Endocrinol Metab* 1992;74:172–176.

128. Dawood MY, Strongin M, Kramer EE, Wieche R. Recent ovulation in a postmenopausal woman. *Int J Gynaecol Obstet* 1980;18:192–194.

129. Sherrer C, Gerson B, Woodruff JD. The incidence and significance of polynuclear follicles. *Am J Obstet Gynecol* 1977;128:6–12.

130. Gougeon A. Frequent occurrence of multiovular follicles and multinuclear oocytes in the adult human ovary. *Fertil Steril* 1981;35:417–422.

131. Manivel JC, Dehner LP, Burke B. Ovarian tumorlike structures, biovular follicles, and binucleated oocytes in children: their frequency and possible pathologic significance. *Pediatr Pathol* 1988;8:283–292.

132. Baca M, Zamboni L. The fine structure of the human follicular oocytes. *J Ultrastruct Res* 1967;19:354–381.

133. Hertig AT. The primary human oocyte: some observations on the fine structure of Balbiani's vitelline body and the origin of the annulate lamellae. *Am J Anat* 1968;122:107–137.

134. Hertig AT, Adams EC. Studies on the human oocyte and its follicle. I. Ultrastructural and histochemical observations on the primordial follicle stage. *J Cell Biol* 1967;34:647–675.

135. Curtis EM. Normal ovarian histology in infancy and childhood. *Obstet Gynecol* 1962;19:444–454.

136. Dekel N, David MP, Yedwab GA, Kraicer PF. Follicular development during late pregnancy. *Int J Fertil* 1977;22:24–29.

137. Govan ADT. Ovarian follicular activity in late pregnancy. *J Endocrinol* 1970;48:235–241.

138. Himelstein-Braw R, Byskov AG, Peters H, Faber M. Follicular atresia in the infant human ovary. *J Reprod Fertil* 1976;46:55–59.

139. Maqueo M, Goldzieher JW. Hormone-induced alterations of ovarian morphology. *Fertil Steril* 1966;17:676–683.

140. Mikhail G, Allen WM. Ovarian function in human pregnancy. *Am J Obstet Gynecol* 1967;99:308–312.

141. Nelson WW, Greene RR. The human ovary in pregnancy. *Int Abstr Surg* 1953;97:1–22.

142. Nelson WW, Greene RR. Some observations on the histology of the human ovary during pregnancy. *Am J Obstet Gynecol* 1958;76:66–90.

143. Peters H, Himelstein-Braw R, Faber M. The normal development of the ovary in childhood. *Acta Endocrinol (Copenh)* 1976;82:617–630.

144. McNatty KP, Hillier SG, van den Boogaard AM, Trimbos-Kemper TC, Reichert LE Jr, van Hall EV. Follicular development during the luteal phase of the human menstrual cycle. *J Clin Endocrinol Metab* 1983;56:1022–1031.

145. McNatty KP, Smith DM, Makris A, Osathanondh R, Ryan KJ. The microenvironment of the human antral follicle: interrelationships among the steroid levels in antral fluid, the population of granulosa cells, and the status of the oocyte in vivo and in vitro. *J Clin Endocrinol Metab* 1979;49:851–860.

146. White RF, Hertig AT, Rock J, Adams E. Histological and histochemical observations on the corpus luteum of human pregnancy with special reference to corpora lutea associated with early normal and abnormal ova. *Contrib Embryol* 1951;34:55–74.

147. Jones GE, Goldberg B, Woodruff JD. Histochemistry as a guide for interpretation of cell function. *Am J Obstet Gynecol* 1968;100:76–83.

148. Sasano H, Mori T, Sasano N, Nagura H, Mason JI. Immunolocalization of 3 beta-hydroxysteroid dehydrogenase in human ovary. *J Reprod Fertil* 1990;89:743–751.

149. Deane HW, Lobel BL, Romney SL. Enzymic histochemistry of normal human ovaries of the menstrual cycle, pregnancy, and the early puerperium. *Am J Obstet Gynecol* 1962;83:281–294.

150. Mestwerdt W, Muller O, Brandau H. Structural analysis of granulosa cells from human ovaries in correlation with function. In: Channing CP, Marsh JM, Sadler WA, eds. *Ovarian Follicular and Corpus Luteum Function: Advances in Experimental Medicine and Biology.* Vol 112. New York: Plenum Press; 1978.

151. Gillim SW, Christensen AK, McLennan CE. Fine structure of the human menstrual corpus luteum at its stage of maximum secretory activity. *Am J Anat* 1969;126:409–427.

152. Okamura H, Virutamasen P, Wright KH, Wallach EE. Ovarian smooth muscle in the human being, rabbit, and cat. Histochemical and electron microscopic study. *Am J Obstet Gynecol* 1972;112:183–191.

153. McNatty KP. Follicular determinants of corpus luteum function in the human ovary. In: Channing CP, Marsh JM, Sadler WA, eds. *Ovarian Follicular and Corpus Luteum Function: Advances in Experimental Medicine and Biology.* Vol 112. New York: Plenum Press; 1978:465–477.

154. McNatty KP. Cyclic changes in antral fluid hormone concentrations in humans. *Clin Endocrinol Metab* 1978;7:577–600.

155. Erickson GF. Normal ovarian function. *Clin Obstet Gynecol* 1978;21:31–52.

156. Shima K, Kitayama S, Nakano R. Gonadotropin binding sites in human ovarian follicles and corpora lutea during the menstrual cycle. *Obstet Gynecol* 1987;69:800–806.

157. Eden JA, Carter GD, Jones J, Alaghband-Zadeh J. Insulin-like growth factor 1 as an intra-ovarian hormone—an integrated hypothesis and review. *Aust N Z J Obstet Gynaecol* 1989;29:30–37.

158. McNatty KP, Makris A, De Grazia C, Osathanondh R, Ryan KJ. The production of progesterone, androgens and oestrogens by human granulosa cells in vitro and in vivo. *J Steroid Biochem* 1979;11:775–779.

159. Hillier SG. Intrafollicular paracrine function of ovarian androgen. *J Steroid Biochem* 1987;27:351–357.

160. Pauerstein CJ, Eddy CA, Croxatto HD, Hess R, Siler-Khodr TM, Croxatto HB. Temporal relationships of estrogen, progesterone, and luteinizing hormone levels to ovulation in women and infrahuman primates. *Am J Obstet Gynecol* 1978;130:876–886.

161. Yussman MA, Taymor ML. Serum levels of follicle stimulating hormone and luteinizing hormone and of plasma progesterone related to ovulation by corpus luteum biopsy. *J Clin Endocrinol Metab* 1970;30:396–399.

162. Futterweit W. *Polycystic Ovarian Disease: Clinical Perspectives in Obstetrics and Gynecology.* New York: Springer-Verlag; 1985.

163. Tanabe K, Gagliano P, Channing CP, et al. Levels of inhibin-F activity and steroids in human follicular fluid from normal women and women with polycystic ovarian disease. *J Clin Endocrinol Metab* 1983;57:24–31.

164. Tsonis CG, Messinis IE, Templeton AA, McNeilly AS, Baird DT. Gonadotropic stimulation of inhibin secretion by the human ovary during the follicular and early luteal phase of the cycle. *J Clin Endocrinol Metab* 1988;66:915–921.

165. McLachlan RI, Cohen NL, Vale WW, et al. The importance of luteinizing hormone in the control of inhibin and progesterone secretion by the human corpus luteum. *J Clin Endocrinol Metab* 1989;68:1078–1085.

166. Sealey JE, Glorioso N, Itskovitz J, Laragh JH. Prorenin as a reproductive hormone. New form of the renin system. *Am J Med* 1986;81:1041–1046.

167. Palumbo A, Jones C, Lightman A, Carcangiu ML, DeCherney AH, Naftolin F. Immunohistochemical localization of renin and angiotensin II in human ovaries. *Am J Obstet Gynecol* 1989;160:8–14.

168. Corner GW Jr. The histological dating of the human corpus luteum of menstruation. *Am J Anat* 1956;98:377–401.

169. Visfeldt J, Starup J. Dating of the human corpus luteum of menstruation using histological parameters. *Acta Pathol Microbiol Scand A* 1974;82:137–144.

170. Croxatto HD, Ortiz ME, Croxatto HB. Correlation between histologic dating of human corpus luteum and the luteinizing hormone peak—biopsy interval. *Am J Obstet Gynecol* 1980;136:667–670.

171. Wiley CA, Esterly JR. Observations on the human corpus luteum: histochemical changes during development and involution. *Am J Obstet Gynecol* 1976;125:514–519.

172. Hameed A, Fox WM, Kurman RJ, Hruban RH, Podack ER. Perforin expression in human cell-mediated luteolysis. *Int J Gynecol Pathol* 1995;14:151–157.

173. Adams EC, Hertig AT. Studies on the human corpus luteum. I. Observations on the ultrastructure of development and regression of the luteal cells during the menstrual cycle. *J Cell Biol* 1969;41:696–715.

174. Tamura M, Sasano H, Suzuki T, et al. Immunohistochemical localization of growth hormone receptor in cyclic human ovaries. *Hum Reprod* 1994;9:2259–2262.

175. Crisp TM, Dessouky DA, Denys FR. The fine structure of the human corpus luteum of early pregnancy and during the progestational phase of the menstrual cycle. *Am J Anat* 1970;127:37–69.

176. Green JA, Maqueo M. Ultrastructure of the human ovary. I. The luteal cell during the menstrual cycle. *Am J Obstet Gynecol* 1965;92:946–957.

177. LeMaire WJ, Conly PW, Moffett A, Spellacy WN, Cleveland WW, Savard K. Function of the human corpus luteum during the puerperium: its maintenance by exogenous human chorionic gonadotropin. *Am J Obstet Gynecol* 1971;110:612–618.

178. Centola GM. Structural changes: follicular development and hormonal requirements. In: Serra GB, ed. *The Ovary.* New York: Raven Press; 1983:95–111.

179. Rao CV. Receptors for gonadotropins in human ovaries. In: Muldoon T, Mahesh V, Perez-Ballester B, eds. *Recent Advances in Fertility Research Part A: Developments in Reproductive Endocrinology.* New York: Alan R. Liss; 1982:123–135.

180. Vijayakumar R, Walters WA. Ovarian stromal and luteal tissue prostaglandins, 17beta-estradiol and progesterone in relation to the phases of the menstrual cycle in woman. *Am J Obstet Gynecol* 1987;156:947–951.

181. Hertig AT. Gestational hyperplasia of endometrium. A morphologic correlation ova, endometrium, and corpora lutea during early pregnancy. *Lab Invest* 1964;13:1153–1191.

182. Visfeldt J, Starup J. Histology of the human corpus luteum of early and late pregnancy. *Acta Pathol Microbiol Scand A* 1975;83:669–677.

183. Adams EC, Hertig AT. Studies on the human corpus luteum. II. Observations on the ultrastructure of luteal cells during pregnancy. *J Cell Biol* 1969;41:716–735.

184. Green JA, Garcilazo JA, Maqueo M. Ultrastructure of the human ovary. II. The luteal cell at term. *Am J Obstet Gynecol* 1967;99:855–863.

185. Pedersen PH, Larsen JF. The ultrastructure of the human granulosa lutein cell of the first trimester of gestation. *Acta Endocrinol (Copenh)* 1968;58:481–496.

186. Le Maire WJ, Rice BF, Savard K. Steroid hormone formation in the human ovary: V. Synthesis of progesterone in vitro in corpora lutea during the reproductive cycle. *J Clin Endocrinol Metab* 1968;28:1249–1256.

187. Weiss G, Rifkin I. Progesterone and estrogen secretion by puerperal human ovaries. *Obstet Gynecol* 1975;46:557–559.

188. Weiss G, O'Byrne M, Hochman JA, Goldsmith LT, Rifkin I, Steinetz BG. Secretion of progesterone and relaxin by the human corpus luteum at midpregnancy and at term. *Obstet Gynecol* 1977;50:679–681.

189. Weiss G, O'Byrne EM, Steinetz BG. Relaxin: a product of human corpus luteum of pregnancy. *Science* 1976;194:948–949.

190. Schmidt CL, Black VH, Sarosi P, Weiss G. Progesterone and relaxin secretion in relation to the ultrastructure of human luteal cells in culture: effects of human chorionic gonadotropin. *Am J Obstet Gynecol* 1986;155:1209–1219.

191. Quagliarello J, Goldsmith L, Steinetz B, Lustig DS, Weiss G. Induction of relaxin secretion in nonpregnant women by human chorionic gonadotropin. *J Clin Endocrinol Metab* 1980;51:74–77.

192. Joel RV, Foraker AG. Fate of the corpus albicans: a morphologic approach. *Am J Obstet Gynecol* 1960;80:314–316.

193. Reagan JW. Ceroid pigment in the human ovary. *Am J Obstet Gynecol* 1950;59:433–436.

194. Centola GM. Structural changes: atresia. In: Serra GB, ed. *The Ovary.* New York: Raven Press; 1983:113–122.

195. Strickler RC, Kelly RW, Askin FB. Postmenopausal ovarian follicle cyst: an unusual cause of estrogen excess. *Int J Gynecol Pathol* 1984;3:318–322.

196. Kraus FT, Neubecker RD. Luteinization of the ovarian theca in infants and children. *Am J Clin Pathol* 1962;37:389–397.

197. Clement PB, Young RH, Scully RE. Ovarian granulosa cell proliferations of pregnancy: a report of nine cases. *Hum Pathol* 1988;19:657–662.

198. Kedzia H. Gonadoblastoma: structures and background of development. *Am J Obstet Gynecol* 1983;147:81–85.

199. Safneck JR, deSa DJ. Structures mimicking sex cord-stromal tumours and gonadoblastomas in the ovaries of normal infants and children. *Histopathology* 1986;10:909–920.

200. Bomsel-Helmreich O, Gougeon A, Thebault A, et al. Healthy and atretic human follicles in the preovulatory phase: differences in evolution of follicular morphology and steroid content of follicular fluid. *J Clin Endocrinol Metab* 1979;48:686–694.

201. Sternberg WH. The morphology, androgenic function, hyperplasia, and tumors of the human ovarian hilus cells. *Am J Pathol* 1949;25:493–521.

202. Sternberg WH, Segaloff A, Gaskill CJ. Influence of chorionic gonadotropin on human ovarian hilus cells, Leydig-like cells. *J Clin Endocrinol Metab* 1953;13:139–153.

203. Merrill JA. Ovarian hilus cells. *Am J Obstet Gynecol* 1959;78:1258–1271.

204. Honoré LH, O'Hara KE. Ovarian hilus cell heterotopia. *Obstet Gynecol* 1979;53:461–464.

205. Janko AB, Sandberg EC. Histochemical evidence for the protein nature of the Reinke crystalloid. *Obstet Gynecol* 1970;35:493–503.

206. Schmidt WA. Eosin-induced fluorescence of Reinke crystals. *Int J Gynecol Pathol* 1986;5:88–89.

207. Laffargue P, Benkoel L, Laffargue F, Casanova P, Chamlian A. Ultrastructural and enzyme histochemical study of ovarian hilar cells in women and their relationships with sympathetic nerves. *Hum Pathol* 1978;9:649–659.

208. Symonds DA, Driscoll SG. An adrenal cortical rest within the fetal ovary: report of a case. *Am J Clin Pathol* 1973;60:562–564.

209. Falls JL. Accessory adrenal cortex in the broad ligament: incidence and functional significance. *Cancer* 1955;8:143–150.

210. Dennefors BL, Janson PO, Hamberger L, Knutsson F. Hilus cells from human postmenopausal ovaries: gonadotrophin sensitivity, steroid and cyclic AMP production. *Acta Obstet Gynecol Scand* 1982;61:413–416.

211. Sauramo H. Development, occurrence, function and pathology of the rete ovarii. *Acta Obstet Gynecol Scand Suppl* 1954;33:29–46.

212. Rutgers JL, Scully RE. Cysts (cystadenomas) and tumors of the rete ovarii. *Int J Gynecol Pathol* 1988;7:330–342.

213. Woolnough E, Russo L, Khan MS, Heatley MK. An immunohistochemical study of the rete ovarii and epoophoron. *Pathology* 2000;32:77–83.

214. Gardner GH, Greene RR, Peckham B. Tumors of the broad ligament. *Am J Obstet Gynecol* 1957;73:536–555.

Placenta

43

Steven H. Lewis   Kurt Benirschke

INTRODUCTION

The placenta is problematic for the pathologist. Many normal histologic variations may be mistaken for pathology and conversely, important pathologic alterations may be difficult to discern. Unique in pathology, the placenta, as a specimen, provides data about two patients and has three different anatomic sources. It is fetal, yet mostly extraembryonic in its differentiation and has maternal attachments. The placenta may be pivotal in adjudicating the etiology of "bad babies" in litigation (1,2) but more importantly, an objective, thorough, well-documented analysis can provide data important for both maternal and neonatal care. Acknowledging the placenta's many histologic and pathologic varients, its complicated derivation and its role in legal cases, the pathologist should become accustomed to obtaining information from both pediatric and obstetrical providers. The relevance of varients and alterations viewed by the pathologist can thereby be better understood.

These complex considerations cannot be addressed without a thorough understanding of the placenta's normal structure, and it is to this end that this chapter is devoted. Pathologic entities are discussed to better demonstrate normal anatomy and histology. For more encyclopedic and complete discussions regarding placental pathology, the reader is directed elsewhere (1,2). It is easiest and most appropriate to describe (and for that matter, "report") the principal structural components of the placenta in a compartmentalized manner. These consist of the umbilical cord, the membranes (amnion and chorion), the villous parenchyma, and the maternal decidual tissue.

ROUTINE STORAGE, EXAMINATION, AND PROCESSING

After obstetric delivery, placentas may be stored at 4°C in a refrigerator before examination. The period of time for this storage generally should not exceed 1 week. Placentas should not be frozen before evaluation as freezing renders the gross examination difficult and histologic features are obscured. For refrigeration, suitable containers include cardboard buckets or styrofoam storage cups. It has been advocated by some to immediately fix the placenta in 10% buffered formalin for later examination (3). It should be noted that when this method of processing is used, placental weights increase by a factor of approximately 10% (4).

It should be underscored that although assessment of the placenta is considered in the pathologist's domain, it is the obstetrical provider who first visualizes the specimen. An educated clinician may aid the pathologist by submitting it. Otherwise it becomes "discarded." Most institutions do not perform histologic evaluation of all placentas from all deliveries and a discarded placenta can be of no use when problems are associated with pregnancy, labor and delivery, and the neonatal period. Labor and delivery suites should have a list of appropriate clinical and pathologic entities that require pathologic examination of the placenta (5). Because of the frequent turmoil in labor and delivery areas and because problems may often arise in neonates within the first few days of life, the week of storage of all placentas is highly important. It is common for academic institutions to perform histologic examination on approximately 10% to 20% of all delivered placentas.

The gross morphologic assessment of the placenta should be approached in a thorough, routine fashion. Our procedure for the gross assessment and sectioning of placentas is illustrated in Table 43.1.

The placenta is removed from its container and its shape is described. It is usually discoid, but additional lobes may be present. Next, it is convenient to note the location of insertion of the umbilical cord, describe its length and diameter, note irregularities in its contour and texture, describe its color, and note the number of vessels it contains. The cord is then amputated at its base, and representative sections are immersed in fixative.

Attention is next directed to the membranes (amnion and chorion), which are inspected for completeness. Usually, the placenta is delivered vaginally with the membranes surrounding the placental maternal surface ("Schultze"). The membranes are then manually reflected to their normal anatomic position and the smallest distance from the point of rupture to the placental disk (the narrowest width of membranes) is measured. When this measurement equals zero (after vaginal delivery), a low-lying or marginal placenta previa is implicated. The membranes are then assessed for their color, transparency, sheen, and surface irregularities, as well as for the presence of membranous vessels or accessory lobes. The membranes are then removed from the placental disk margin, keeping track of the point of rupture. This point is grasped with a toothed forceps and rolled in a concentric fashion to produce a "membrane roll." With the membranes rolled in such a fashion, the point of rupture can be identified histologically. The presence of inflammatory cells confined to this region suggests early mild chorioamnionitis. Representative sections are immersed in fixative.

The fetal surface of the placenta is next examined. Chorionic vascular thrombi, if present, and nodules or irregularities of the amnion are noted. The maternal surface of the placenta is inspected, and any blood clot that has settled in the storage container with the dependent portions of the organ is removed. Areas of blood clot that are adherent or discolored brown (indicating chronicity) and that are depressing the maternal surface are considered indicative of retroplacental hemorrhage (clinically designated as abruptio). Should this be noted, the dimensions or percentage of the maternal surface involvement are recorded. The organ is next weighed free of its cord and associated membranes. The average weight of the term placenta is approximately 400 to 600 g. Placental weight varies with neonatal weight and normal weights have been reviewed for all gestational ages (1). The average dimensions of the term placenta are approximately 18 × 16 × 2.3 cm.

The villous parenchyma is then inspected by sectioning the placenta at 1- to 2-cm intervals looking for irregularities in the parenchyma that indicate infarction, thrombi, or other pathologic entities. There are normally 16 to 20 cotyledonous units that do not have distinct functional correlates. An absent cotyledon may indicate a portion of retained placenta in utero. Representative sections of abnormal areas are blocked out, and areas of normal-appearing parenchyma (usually three) are placed into fixative along with the already sectioned membrane roll and umbilical cord.

The fixation of the materials for study is routine. We prefer to fix tissues in Bouin's solution for a period of 24 hours before trimming and submission for final processing. This process of fixation allows for excellent tissue penetration and ease of sectioning. In addition, it provides superior cytologic detail. The drawbacks to the Bouin's fixation are twofold. One is that if certain special studies are of interest (i.e., immunohistochemistry and in situ hybridization), Bouin's fixation may interfere with antigen–antibody reactions or nucleic acid hybridization. This problem may be eliminated by fixing tissues desired for such studies in Bouin's solution for only a limited period of time. For small uterine cervix biopsies, it has been shown that Bouin's fixation for less than 8 hours produces good results with in situ hybridization (6). The second problem with Bouin's fixation is that if in the final preparation lithium carbonate is omitted, increased extraneous pigment formation occurs.

Pathologists are accustomed to using 10% buffered formalin solution for the processing of most tissues, and this is not contraindicated in the processing of placentas. We find that when using formalin, the period of time required to create sufficient tissue hardness for proper sectioning delays processing and histologic resolution is somewhat inferior to that obtained with Bouin's fixation. It is our

TABLE 43.1
RECORDING FORMAT[a]

	Unit No:
	Name:
	Date of Birth: Sex:
	Location:
	Path. No:

	Date of Delivery:
	Date Received:
	Physician:
	Baby's Unit No:

Previous Specimens:

SPECIMEN: Placenta

CLINICAL INFORMATION: (Circle and fill in pertinent information)
NSVD   C-section   GA: _____ wk   DM class _____
Chorioamnionitis   Preeclampsia   Fetal distress
Newborn wt. _____ grams   5 min Apgar <7   Other: _____

GROSS DESCRIPTION:

Cord:	____ × ____ cm	Insertion:
	# pieces: _____	Vessel #: _____
Membranes:	complete/incomplete	Narrowest width: _____ cm
	clear/opaque	Meconium: old/recent/none
	vascular thrombi: present/none	Calcification: present/none
Parenchyma:	red/pale/friable	Abruptio: _____ %
	Infarct: _____ %	Weight: _____ grams
Dimensions:	____ × ____ × ____ cm	
Other:		

MICROSCOPIC DESCRIPTION: (___) slides evaluated.

DIAGNOSIS(ES):

Umbilical cord:

Membranes:

Villi:

Decidua:

Reviewed by:

Date Dictated:
Date Typed:
Print Date:

[a] This format is easily converted to a computerized final report that includes final microscopic diagnoses.

procedure to stain tissue sections with hematoxylin and eosin (H&E) or hematoxylin-phloxine and saffron (HPS). Other standard special stains may be used for the detection of specific infectious agents, secretory activity, or structural composition (silver stains, periodic acid-Schiff (PAS), Masson's trichrome, etc.). Furthermore, a host of immunohistochemical stains have been used to elucidate functions of specific placental cell types.

UMBILICAL CORD

Embryology

Specific embryologic considerations are germane to the understanding of the normal umbilical cord structure, including its frequent possession of embryologic remnants. The open region on the ventral surface of the developing embryo diminishes in size and then forms the early umbilicus. Through this structure extend both the yolk stalk and the body stalk, as well as the allantois. This cylindrical structure elongates, and its surface becomes covered by the expanding amnion. This is a single-layered epithelium on a layer of connective tissue. Therefore, the developing umbilical cord contains the yolk stalk, a pair of vitelline blood vessels, the allantois, and the allantoic blood vessels (two arteries and one vein) and is covered by amnionic epithelium. These anatomic relationships explain the presence of the omphalomesenteric duct (the connection between developing endoderm and the yolk sac) and the allantoic duct (which has its communication in early gestation with the urachus) within sections of proximal (fetal) umbilical cord.

Gross Morphology

The gross anatomic features of the umbilical cord that are of importance are the location of its insertion in the placental disk, its length, and the number of vessels. The presence of true knots (Figure 43.1) may be considered normal when there is no adverse outcome, yet this occurrence may lead to fetal demise when the knot is tight. The presence of vascular tortuosities (false knots) is common and rarely of clinical significance (Figure 43.2). The finding of meconium staining and the presence of surface plaques are definitely abnormal and are described below.

The normal umbilical cord is pearly white and somewhat translucent. The length of the umbilical cord has great significance, principally when it is excessively long or excessively short. Cord length has been shown to vary with gestational age, and measurements indicate that the cord elongates as gestation proceeds. At approximately 20 weeks' gestational age, the average cord length is 32 cm (7). The normal length of the umbilical cord at term has been

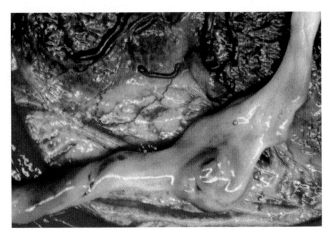

Figure 43.2 False knot. Note the unrelated abnormal membranous vessels connecting placental lobes.

determined to be, on average, between 55 and 65 cm (1,7–10) (Figure 43.3). The literature contains many articles that relate the significance of abnormal cord lengths with both in utero fetal activity and neonatal outcome. The reader is referred to an extensive review of the subject (1).

Histology

Histologic examination of the umbilical cord shows several distinct layers. On the surface is a well-defined single layer of amnionic epithelium. The epithelium is squamoid and, in the region of fetal cord insertion, often becomes multi-layered and closely resembles its epidermal contiguity. Electron microscopy studies performed on cord amnionic cells

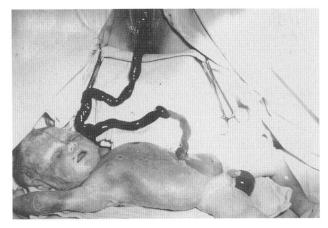

Figure 43.1 True knot, in this case, resulted in intrauterine fetal death. Reprinted with permission from: Benirschke K, Kaufmann P. *Pathology of the Human Placenta.* 3rd ed. New York: Springer-Verlag; 1995.

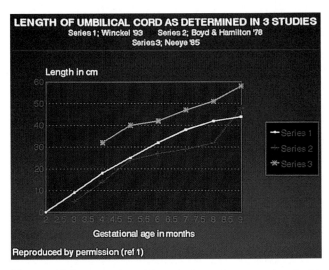

Figure 43.3 Normal cord length dimensions associated with changes in gestational age. Reprinted with permission from: Benirschke K, Kaufmann P. *Pathology of the Human Placenta.* 3rd ed. New York: Springer-Verlag; 1995.

have suggested that the epithelium is responsible for fluid equilibrium activities (11). True squamous metaplasia of the umbilical cord is considered a normal variant, and ultrastructural studies of this epithelium have shown morphologic similarities between this epithelium and the fetal epidermis (12).

Deep to the amnionic epithelium that comprises the surface of the cord is the substance of Wharton's jelly. This material largely is composed of mucopolysaccharides (hyaluronic acid and chondroitin sulfate). Ultrastructural examination of this material shows the presence of delicate interlacing microfibrils and sparse collagen. Mast cells are prominent. Their frequency is increased in the near periphery of the cord vasculature (13). In this same region, and in the cord in general, macrophages are rarely identified.

Embedded within the substance of Wharton's jelly are the umbilical vessels. There have been considerable interest and discussion focused on the identification of vasa vasorum and vascular neuronal innervation. Although the vasculature of the umbilical cord is of a considerable caliber, there are no vasa vasorum or lymphatic channels present in this structure. Studies investigating vascular innervation have concluded that no nerves are present within the umbilical cord. This has been borne out by electron microscopic studies (14). Occasionally, however, autonomic nerves are identified using acetylcholinesterase thiocholine techniques in the proximal (fetal) end of the cord (15). Such findings are compatible with the persistence of peripheral vagal neuronal elements associated with the ductus venosus, which are entrapped in the proximal portion of the umbilical cord. Certainly any neuronal vestiges found within the umbilical cord are best considered as remnants, and to date there has been no demonstration of their functional significance (16).

Since the yolk sac connects to the primitive midgut through the body stalk in early development, vestiges of this epithelium-lined duct are common in the umbilical cord. The persistence of the omphalomesenteric duct is characterized by a tubular structure present within Wharton's jelly and lined by a single layer of low cuboidal to columnar, mucin-secreting epithelium (Figure 43.4A–D). Remnants of the duct may form cystic structures that contain a variety of endodermally-derived epithelia, including pancreatic, intestinal (small and large), and gastric components. Such findings are rarely of any clinical significance, although secretory products of gastric origin resulted in umbilical vascular ulceration, hemorrhage, and fetal death in a case report described by Blanc and Allan (17).

The allantois differentiates as a protuberance from the yolk sac into the body stalk and is essential for the development of the umbilical vessels. This structure is incorporated into the anterior aspect of the hindgut, where it communicates with the urachus. Remnants of the allantoic duct are often found in sections of proximal umbilical cords. Its intimate relationship with the formation of

umbilical vessels explains its presence between the two umbilical arteries, when it is identified. These remnants rarely have clinical significance. The lining of this tract is often devoid of a lumen and consists of aggregates of epithelial cells with a variety of epithelia represented (transitional, bladder, and yolk sac–derived endodermally classified cells) (Figure 43.5).

The vasculature of the umbilical cord is composed of two arteries and a single vein. The arteries possess no internal elastic lamina and have a double-layered muscular wall. Each of these muscular layers is composed of a network of interlacing smooth muscle bundles. The vein does have an inner elastic lamina. As noted, no vasa vasorum are present. Remnants of the vitelline vasculature in the proximal portion of the cord sometimes may be observed in sections taken from this region. The umbilical vein, which generally has a larger diameter, possesses a thinner muscular coat consisting of a single layer of circular smooth muscle (Figure 43.6A, B).

Of further interest, distinguishing umbilical vasculature from other systemic vessels, is that no true vascular adventitia is found. Near the placental insertion, it is common to identify anastomotic channels between the two umbilical arteries (18,19) (Figure 43.7).

Transverse serial sections confirm that two umbilical arteries spiral in parallel around the umbilical vein. Often, multiple twists in the cord occur. The proposed origin of this spiraling has been extensively discussed; however, its true functional significance and origin remain to be definitively elucidated (1).

Pathologic Alterations

Distinguishing normal anatomy from pathologic entities is the essence of proper understanding of the normal anatomy and histology of the umbilical cord. Most pathology of the cord may be seen in the gross sense. Histology is confirmatory. A tight knot with notching indicating stricture associated with proximal vascular dilatation may result in fetal death. Interestingly, although true knots occur frequently and are associated with long cords, adverse outcomes are rare events; therefore, in most instances a true knot can be considered a normal variant. The absence of an umbilical artery is a well-established observation and easy to identify grossly or in histologic sections (Figure 43.8). This phenomenon has been found in approximately 1% of neonates. The association of this finding with congenital anomalies is well known, and these malformations often take the form of urinary tract malformations.

Persistence of a second (right) umbilical vein is an unusual phenomenon. The pathologist is cautioned in this regard. It is not unusual to find histologic sections identifying more than three vessels in an umbilical cord. This finding is related to commonly identified tortuosities. These tortuosities have been termed "false knots" (Figure 43.2) and have

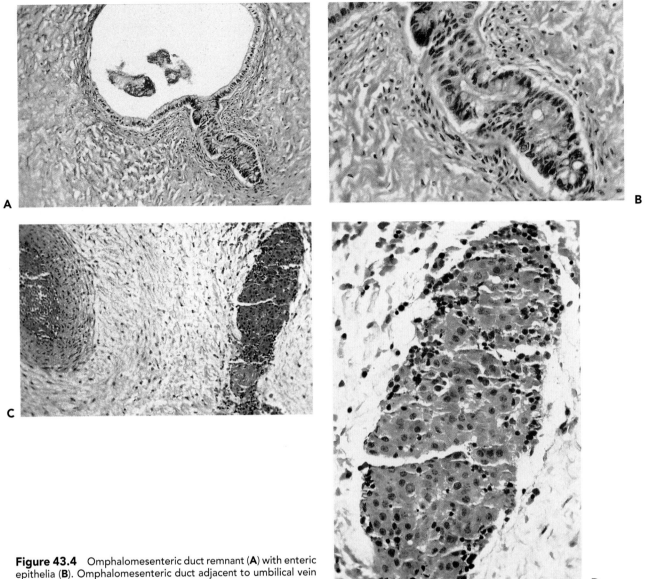

Figure 43.4 Omphalomesenteric duct remnant (**A**) with enteric epithelia (**B**). Omphalomesenteric duct adjacent to umbilical vein (**C**) with unusual finding of hepatic tissue (**D**).

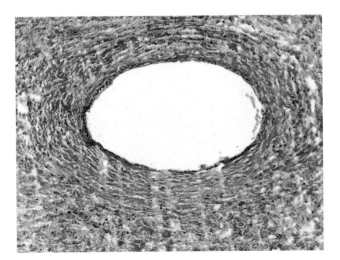

Figure 43.5 Allantoic duct remnant hematoxylin and eosin (H&E stain).

little clinical significance. An exception is that these vessels rarely may be prone to thrombosis.

The presence of thrombotic material in the vasculature of the umbilical cord is truly pathologic. The process may be related to the genesis of a single umbilical artery when it occurs in early gestation. Abnormal umbilical insertions may cause thrombosis.

Velamentous cord insertions are abnormal and are characterized by the presence of the umbilical vasculature implanting in the placental membranes as opposed to the usual implantation over the placental disk (Figure 43.9). These vessels course independently within the chorion and are unguarded by the protective substance of the umbilical cord (Wharton's jelly). Thrombosis thus results from pressure on those vessels by fetal parts, and these vessels are subject to injury at the time of spontaneous or, more commonly, artificial membrane rupture.

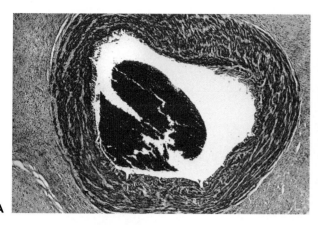

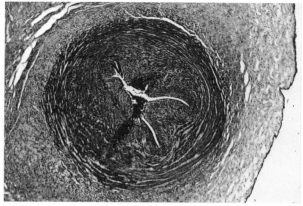

Figure 43.6 Umbilical vein (**A**) and artery (**B**) [hematoxylin-phloxine and saffron (HPS) stain].

Other abnormalities and pathologic findings of the umbilical cord (certainly to be distinguished from normal morphology and histology) that are of clinical importance are umbilical cord vascular rupture, complete absence of Wharton's jelly (Figure 43.10), and neoplasms of the umbilical cord [hemangioma (Figure 43.11) and teratoma, both unusual findings].

Most significant when considering normal histologic changes in the umbilical cord is the presence of hemorrhagic material in the perivascular region, which would suggest umbilical cord vascular rupture. Although true cord hematomas do occur on occasion (Figure 43.12), the presence of hemorrhage in this region is common and generally attributed to the mode of delivery of the placenta, with traction or clamping of the umbilical cord producing this artifactual finding (Figure 43.13).

Umbilical torsion and stricture are associated with excessive fetal movement and focal absence of Wharton jelly,

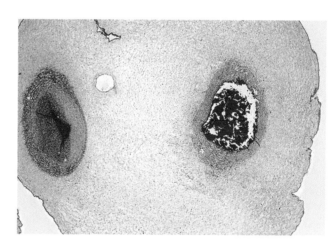

Figure 43.8 Single umbilical artery (HSP stain).

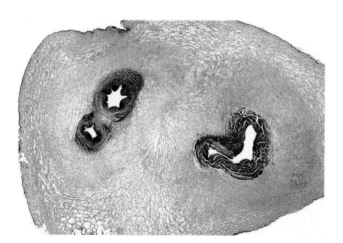

Figure 43.7 Normal proximal anastomosis of umbilical arteries rendering the appearance of a single umbilical artery.

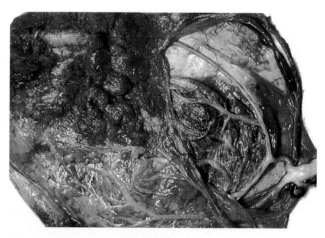

Figure 43.9 Velamentous insertion of umbilical cord. Umbilical vessels insert in membranes adjacent to the chorionic plate. In this case, the fetus exsanguinated after amniotomy and rupture of membranous vessels.

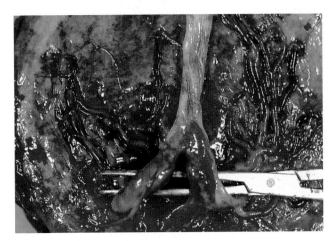

Figure 43.10 Furcate insertion of umbilical cord. Umbilical cord vessels insert into placental substance individually (UA, *left*; UA and UV, *right*) not surrounded by Wharton's jelly.

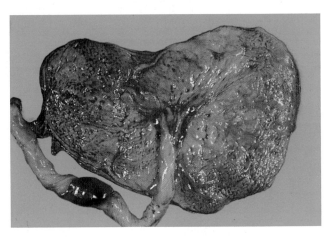

Figure 43.12 Hematoma of umbilical cord. This placenta was delivered by cesarean section and there was no traction or clamping of this segment of cord.

respectively. Both are associated with adverse outcomes (1). In the former, the normal twist or coiling of the cord becomes excessive. There is an association with long cords. The latter is less well understood but may at times be a function of torsion (Figure 43.14). Additionally, excessive coiling has been associated with increased fetal activity, cocaine use, abnormal fetal heart rate tracings and preterm deliveries (20). Nascent dimensions of cord width are therefore germane. There is little literature that actually defines the dimensions of normal cords, although published data correlate abnormalities associated with fat and thin cords (7,8) (Figure 43.15).

Another definitively pathologic entity that must be distinguished from normal histology is the presence of leukocytes within the cord substance. Such findings are indicative

of funisitis and are the result of inflammatory response to infectious antigens and recruitment through inflammatory pathways (Figure 43.16). When the process is prominent (severe) and with calcifications, the term *necrotizing funisitis* is applicable. Such severe pathology is indicative of chronic inflammation and may be seen in syphilis as well as other infections (1) (Figure 43.17). The identification of fungal elements about the umbilical cord are often difficult to discern from an overgrowth storage phenomenon. In this regard, the difficulty lies in the usual absence of associated inflammatory infiltrate. The cord, when involved, has white surface plaques. Fungal elements (i.e., *Candida albicans*) may be identified merely with hematoxylin and eosin stains, although special stains for fungi can be helpful when such pathology is suspect (1).

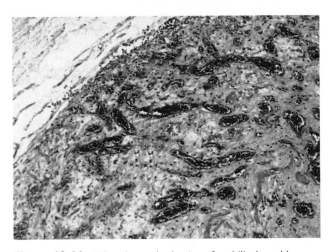

Figure 43.11 Dilated vascular lumina of umbilical cord hemangioma (HPS stain).

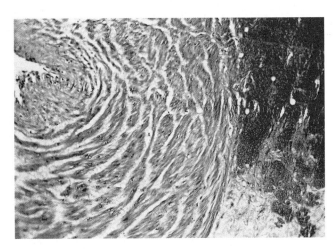

Figure 43.13 Perivascular hemorrhage located adjacent to umbilical artery found in the region of a cord clamp (HPS stain).

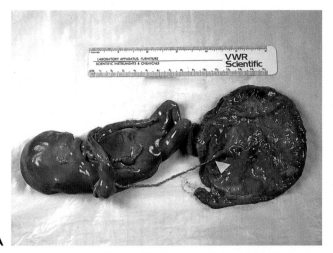
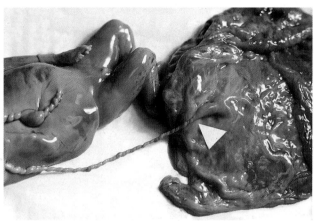

Figure 43.14 Excessive spiraling (**A**) leading to torsion (**B**) and stricture resulting in fetal death.

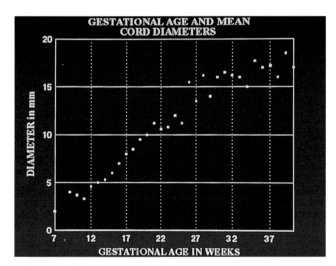

Figure 43.15 Mean cord width (as determined by ultrasound 2 cm from umbilical insertion) versus advancing gestational age (n = 100, p < 0.05). Reprinted with permission from: Lewis SH, Starr C. Cord width. *In Utero* (Unpublished).

Last, a finding in the cord that is notably pathologic is meconium-induced medial destruction (Figure 43.18A, B), which results from direct meconium toxicity and necrobiosis of vascular media (21). Associated vascular spasm and medial degeneration may adversely affect hemodynamics in the cord and chorionic vasculature.

RAMIFICATION OF CHORIONIC VASCULATURE

At this point it is convenient to discuss the ramification of the umbilical vessels in the chorionic plate. The umbilical cord inserts in a central or eccentric fashion. Although abnormal insertion at the margin (Battledore) and in the membranes (velamentous) comprises a small portion of cord insertions, both should be considered pathologic

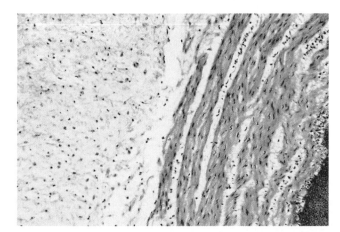

Figure 43.16 Acute funisitis. Polymorphonuclear leukocytes are present within the umbilical vein muscularis and adjacent Wharton's jelly.

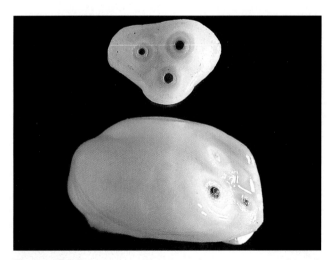

Figure 43.17 Necrotizing funisitis with intense perivascular malformations associated with calcification (peripheral white circular bands) may be seen in the gross.

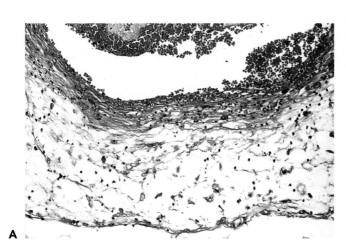

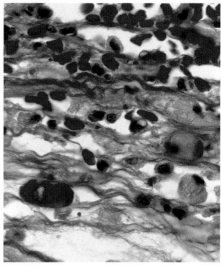

A B

Figure 43.18 Globular degenerated necrobiotic medial cells so effected by meconium. The process is focal and contrasts with adjacent normal myocytes. Luna Ishak stain (**A**). Intensified magnification for delineation (**B**). Reprinted with permission from: Rana J, Ebert GA, Kappy KA. Adverse perinatal outcome with an abnormal umbilical coiling index. *Obstet Gynecol* 1995;85:573–578.

and not normal variants insofar as they have been attributed to adverse outcomes when extensively analyzed (22).

The pattern of vascular ramification within the chorion is described as either magistral (characterized by large-diameter vessels, radially diminishing in caliber to the periphery of the placenta) or disperse (characterized by multiple small vessels emanating directly from the cord

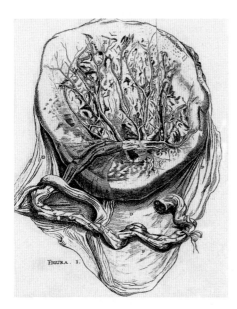

Figure 43.19 As early as the 1600s, Nicholas Hoboken recognized that chorionic arteries (H) overlie veins, and this was beautifully depicted in his painstaking drawings. These are the earliest accurate drawings of the human placenta known to exist.

insertion site). It is of interest that in the chorionic vasculature, no distinction can be made between branches of the umbilical vein and umbilical arteries using histologic criteria (in counterdistinction to the aforementioned description of differentiation between vein and artery in the umbilical cord). The only means of identifying which vessels are branches of arteries and which are veins is by noting their gross anatomic distribution. Arteries always cross over veins when observed from the fetal surface (Figure 43.19). The notation of such vascular relationships is of extreme significance when considering vascular anastomoses, as may be seen in some twin pregnancies (23).

The primary branches of the umbilical vasculature that course through the chorionic plate periodically dive beneath this stratum to establish the circulation of primary vascular ramifications ending in the terminal villi.

PATHOLOGIC ALTERATIONS OF THE CHORIONIC VASCULATURE

Abnormalities in the chorionic vasculature are similar to those found in the umbilical cord, the most significant being thrombosis of a chorionic vessel. During the gross examination of placentas so affected, the presence of thrombotic material may readily be identified by noting dilated vessels containing firm thrombotic substance. On the other hand, vascular thrombi may be more subtle and their appearance characterized only by the presence of faintly highlighted linear white streaks that parallel the peripheral

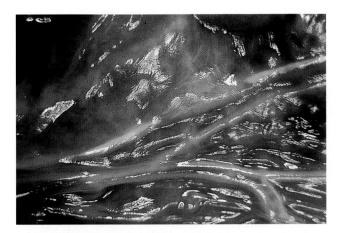

Figure 43.20 Chorionic vascular thrombosis characterized by a linear streak paralleling the vascular course (in this case a chorionic vein). Reprinted with permission from: Benirschke K, Kaufmann P. *Pathology of the Human Placenta*. 3rd ed. New York: Springer-Verlag; 1995.

margin of vessels involved (Figure 43.20). These findings can be confirmed histologically.

The presence of polymorphonuclear leukocytes migrating from the chorionic vasculature and from the umbilical vasculature is pathognomonic of chorionitis and umbilical cord funisitis, respectively. Findings of chorionitis are histologically similar to those aforementioned in acute funisitis (Figure 43.16).

MEMBRANES

Embryology

The placental membranes consist of the amnion and chorion. The amnion, which constitutes the innermost aspect of the embryonic cavity, develops from the margin of the embryonic disk. As the embryonic disk begins to take the form of a tube, the amnionic periphery also folds inward and its attachment to the ventral body is defined. The amnionic cavity subsequently develops by the process of cavitation. Elongation of the body stalk coincides with embryonic prolapse into the amnionic compartment. As development proceeds, the resultant cavity expands, and by 12 weeks from the last menstrual period the amniotic cavity completely occupies the chorionic sac. At this point, fusion occurs with the chorionic wall. This event is commonly identified by clinicians via routine ultrasonographic analysis of advancing gestations. At this gestational age, the potential space between the chorion and amnion is visibly obliterated. The amnionic cavity remains filled with amnionic fluid, which by the end of gestation amounts to approximately 1 L.

The chorion forms the base for the peripherally radiating villi and serves to encapsulate the embryo and developing amnion. As the early implantation embryo develops, the em-

bryonic tissues (the trophoblast and its mesodermal investments) continue to expand in a spherical fashion. The inner aspect of the condensation of mesoderm, which forms the inner capsular structure deep to the peripheral trophoblast, is also termed the chorion. In the region that becomes the placental disk proper, chorionic villi continue to develop beneath these structures, and the placenta proper or the chorion frondosum is defined. The region of the chorion that covers the expanded amnionic cavity forms what has been termed the chorionic laeve. This constitutes the reflected membranes and is discerned from the membranous covering of the chorionic plate. Chorionic villi in the region of the laeve (which delimits the sac containing amnionic fluid) atrophy by pressure, although remnants of villous tissue may be found in association with this structure. In the region of the chorion frondosum, the fetal blood vessels invest the chorionic plate. Such vessels only occur in the chorion; the amnion is an avascular structure.

Amnion and Chorion

Gross Morphology

The fetal membranes have a particular and characteristic appearance in normal deliveries. The sac, when viewed from the fetal surface, is clear and often has a bluish hue, and the amnion is devoid of vasculature. Remnants of atrophied vasculature may be seen in the overlying chorion and appear as filamentous streaks. The chorionic plate also has a characteristic blue sheen and, as described previously, the distribution of chorionic vessels has a characteristic appearance. The membranes of the chorionic plate are distinguished from the laeve as described above. It is not infrequent to find a peripheral nodule on the surface of the disk membranes. This normal nodule is the remnant of the fetal yolk sac (Figure 43.21).

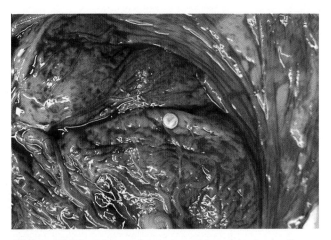

Figure 43.21 White nodule is the residua of the fetal yolk sac.

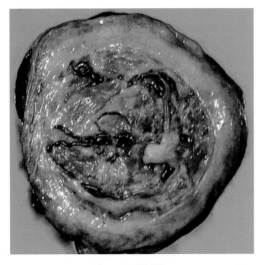
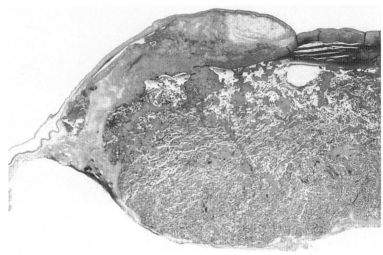

A

B

Figure 43.22 **A.** Circumvallate placenta. **B.** Note loose association of amnion peripheral to marginal subamnionic fibrin deposition. Reprinted with permission from: Benirschke K, Kaufmann P. *Pathology of the Human Placenta.* 3rd ed. New York: Springer-Verlag; 1995.

Gross Morphologic Alterations

Although chorionic vessels are normal in the chorion of the chorionic plate overlying the disk, the persistence of functional vasculature in the chorion laeve is aberrant and equates to membranous vessels. These vessels may connect lobes of placenta or relate to the membranous insertion of the umbilical cord (velamentous insertion as described above).

On occasion, the chorionic plate may possess a ring of fibrin that forms a concentric ridge between the insertion of the cord and the margin of the placental disk. This fibrin ring, which lies deep to the amnion, is indicative of an extrachorial placentation. Such a placentation is characterized by two forms: the circumvallate placentation and the circumarginate placentation. In the former, the membranes are reflected upon themselves at the ridge of the fibrin deposition. They then cover the remaining margin of the placental disk in a loose fashion (Figure 43.22A, B). In the circumarginate placenta, the ring of fibrin is present over the chorion, and the overlying amnion is not reflected upon itself at this fibrinous ring (Figure 43.23). The amnion thus extends to the margin of the placental disk, and its departure to form the amnionic sac occurs at this margin. It is currently felt that this fibrinous ring represents placental migration in conjunction with an enlarging uterus during the second trimester (so-called trophotropism) (1).

The common occurrence of squamous metaplasia on the amnionic surface can be identified grossly by its characteristic appearance. It is a normal finding unless its presence is extensive. Immersion of the placental membranes in water generally defines this area by its failure to become moist as opposed to the normal surrounding amnion. Thus, these areas are more clearly defined. In pathologic conditions, meta-

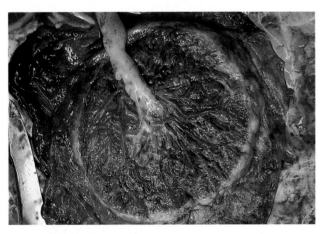

Figure 43.23 Circumarginate placenta. Note the close association of amnion to the disk peripheral to the fibrin ring.

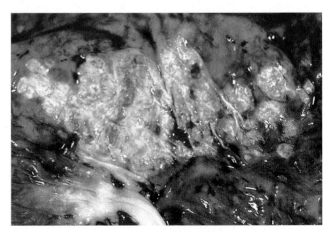

Figure 43.24 Extensive squamous metaplasia on the amnionic surface from a fetus with an encephalocele. It is believed that irritation from the encephalocele in this region produced the extensive metaplasia.

plasia in these regions may be pronounced, and large plaques and nodules may form (Figure 43.24). These nodules are distinguished from the truly pathologic condition of amnion nodosum by their failure to be easily denuded from the surface of the amnion by slight mechanical pressure.

The presence of amnion nodosum is characterized in the gross sense by the presence of multiple small papules on the amnionic surface (Figure 43.25). The clinical history is suggestive, and oligohydramnios characterizes these gestations. The small papules are easily removed from the amnionic surface by excoriation, and their substances are confirmed histologically by the presence of debris and degenerated squames. The origin of these cells is fetal epidermal, and their presence on the amnionic surface is related to apposition of this membrane and fetal skin in conditions where there is diminished amnionic fluid.

Amnionic bands are rare. The condition is responsible for in utero fetal part amputation and trauma and is a phenomenon that occurs in approximately one in 10,000 births. The occurrence is important because it demonstrates potential difficulties from abnormal amnionic membrane development. The precise mechanism is not known in most cases, but rupture of the amnion (most probably in the first trimester) allows the fetus to enter the chorionic sac. The remnants of amnion form the substance of the resulting amnionic bands. At term these placentas have highly opaque chorionic surfaces that reflect hyperplasia of this uncovered layer. The remaining amnionic epithelium is densely adherent to the umbilical cord from which it cannot be stripped. Only small amounts of amnion are present, which distinguishes this condition from artifactual disruption of the amnion from the chorionic plate during the delivery process (1,24,25). Occasionally, an abnormal "web" will be present at the base of the cord insertion, and this may limit normal cord movement (5) (Figure 43.26).

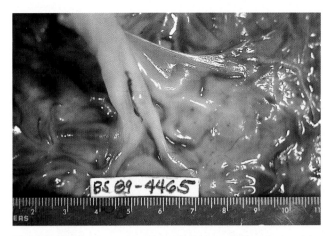

Figure 43.26 Amniotic web partially immobilizes the cord by limiting its movement at the cord base.

Amnion Histology

The amnion, the innermost layer of the amnionic cavity, is lined by a single layer of epithelial cells that resides on a basement membrane. The basement membrane is attached to an underlying thin layer of connective tissue (26) (Figure 43.27). The amnion, although adjacent to the chorion, is not truly fused to it and may be separated with minimum effort. This juxtaposition of the two membranous layers occurs at 12 weeks' gestational age (27) (Figure 43.28). Before this time, as the amnion develops, it is separated from the chorion by the so-called magma reticulare, which is a viscous and thixotropic gelatinous fluid. Stellate mesenchymal cells may be found within this subtance. These cells also have epithelial characteristics and have been stained immunohistochemically and found to be cytokeratin and vimentin positive (28).

The epithelial cell layer of the amnion is composed of one distinct cytologic type (29). The epithelium is a single layer, squamoid to cuboidal, and devoid of secretory activity. Ultrastructural studies show extensive microvillous projections (30). Multiple vesicular structures have been identified at the base of these epithelia. It has been postulated that these vesicles represent pinocytotic activity (11). This observation is important because, as stated earlier, the amnion possesses no vasculature. This also pertains to its mesenchymal component. Therefore, the cytologic components of this layer gain their nutrition from adjacent amnionic fluid, which in turn is rich in nutrients from transudation (from fetal vasculature) and fetal excretory products. In early gestation, this nutrition is derived from the magma reticulare. Channels that also have been considered responsible for fluid transmission (31) are felt to be the residua of epithelial cell loss. A postulate relating to cell loss may invoke a newly revitalized theoretical discussion (initiated by Virchow) that describes "apoptosis" as a form of programmed cell death. Such epithelial loss or "cell death by suicide" also has been noted in placental

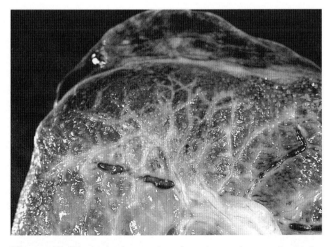

Figure 43.25 Multiple papules of amnion nodosum stipple the amnionic surface of this placenta from a gestation characterized by oligohydramnios.

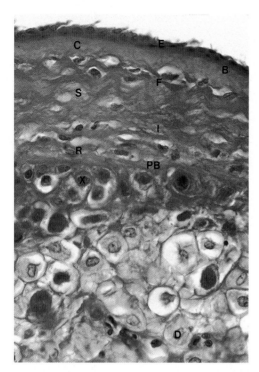

Figure 43.27 Flattened to cuboidal amnionic epithelial cells (E) adhere to their basement membrane (B). Beneath this is the compact layer of the amnion (C), which is acellular and may form a barrier to PMNs. The compact layer is rarely affected by edema and is probably the strongest amnionic layer. A fibroblastic layer (F) lies beneath the compact layer, and macrophages may be found. A spongy layer (S), relatively devoid of fibroblasts, separates the amnion from the chorion, although the two may merge imperceptibly. Often, an artifactual separation may be present near the plane of true fusion. The amnion usually measures from 0.2 to 0.5 mm in thickness (1). The most superficial layer of chorion is usually an incomplete cellular zone (I) that overlies a thick reticular layer (R). This layer is composed of fibroblasts and macrophages. Beneath the reticular layer is a pseudo–basement membrane (PB) overlying trophoblastic X cells (X) and then maternal decidua (D) (HPS stain).

components, including the wall of the yolk sac and in the endothelium of umbilical veins. Further investigation in these areas may enhance understanding of developmental biology and with refinement may be used for addressing future methodologies for the treatment of neoplasia (32,33).

Amnionic epithelial cells are attached to one another by desmosomes in freeze-fracture experiments (34). Furthermore, the amnionic epithelium attaches to the underlying basement membrane by hemidesmosomes (35).

Amnionic epithelial cells divide by mitosis (36). On occasion, multinucleated cells are identified. Morphometry studies have demonstrated that polyploid cells exist in this layer (37). Other karyotypic anomalies occur, and amniocentesis for chromosomal defects may yield false-positive results when these amnionic cells contaminate preparations (38).

Although the epithelium of the amnion does not actively secrete, lipid droplets have been noted within these cells, an observation that correlates with increasing gestational age (36,39,40). Glycogen also has been found within amnionic cells.

Squamous metaplasia is a common occurrence in the amnionic epithelium, especially near the insertion of the umbilical cord (Figure 43.29). This epithelium may become keratinized, and keratohyalin granules can be identified. Although this appears to result from irritation of the amnionic epithelial surface, these changes can be found in more than half of all term placentas (1).

Beneath the basement membrane of the amnionic epithelium, an additional component of the amnion is identified. This layer principally is divided into a compact and a fibroblastic region. The connective tissue within this region may harbor macrophages, which have been identified within the first trimester of pregnancy (41).

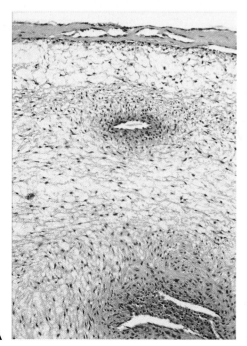

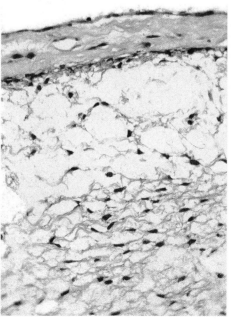

Figure 43.28 The separation between amnion and chorion is more apparent in early gestations as seen in this section from the chorionic plate of a 10- to 12-week placenta. The amnion is readily distinguished from the underlying chorion, which contains the easily identifiable chorionic vessels. Mesynchymal components are prominent (H&E stain).

A

B

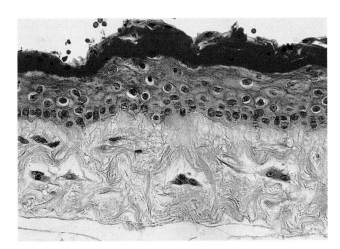

Figure 43.29 Squamous metaplasia of the amnion with hyperkeratosis (HPS stain).

Amnion Histopathology

Histologic abnormalities of the amnion are heralded by an abnormal gross appearance. For example, membranes that are stained green may reflect deposition of meconium. Amnionic membranes that are white may be indicative of polymorphonuclear leukocyte infiltration and acute chorioamnionitis (26) (Figure 43.30A, B).

Abnormalities of amnionic epithelial cells, although suggested by gross examination, can be confirmed by histologic assessment. Abnormalities that reflect degenerative changes are characterized by the presence of vacuolated cytoplasm and elongation to columnar forms. A rather rare and unusual finding associated with gastroschisis carries a pathognomonic histologic aberrancy of the amnion whereby amnionic epithelial cells contain innumerable vacuoles (1) (Figure 43.31).

Amnionic epithelial degeneration (Figure 43.32) is characteristic when meconium is present. Such findings may be confirmed when macrophages, present within the amnionic layer, contain meconium (a coarse brown pigment), which does not stain for iron (Figure 43.33). On the other hand, hemosiderin deposition may be found within the amnionic layer in macrophages, and this can be confirmed by the use of iron stains (i.e., Prussian blue).

Although there are no true tumors of the amnion, occasional cysts representing edema may be identified. Although they may be striking in their gross appearance, it must be recognized that no clinical significance can be identified. Occasional cysts of ectodermal and mesodermal tissue have been identified deep to the amnionic layer, but such findings are not considered true neoplasms. Teratomas have been described (42). These lesions probably represent degenerative acardiac twins (1), but the lack of directed differentiation from pluripotential stem cells could account for the former.

The papules of amnion nodosum are clearly pathologic and reflect, in most cases, decreased amnionic fluid. In such

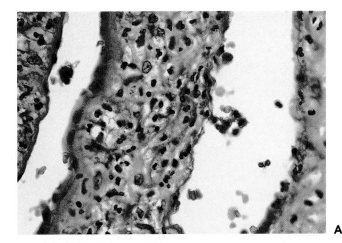

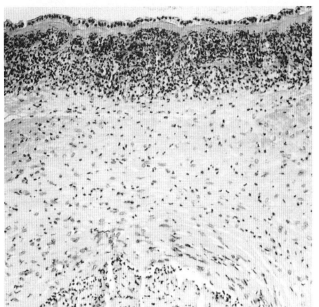

Figure 43.30 Acute chorioamnionitis in membrane roll (**A**) (HPS stain) and in chorionic plate (**B**) (H&E stain).

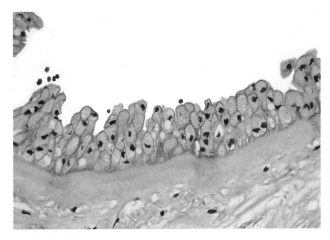

Figure 43.31 Unusual vacuolated elongated amnionic epithelial cells pathognomonic of gastroschisis. The pathophysiology is uncertain (H&E).

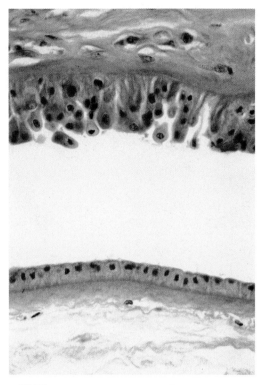

Figure 43.32 A twisted membrane roll with amnionic epithelial degeneration (*above*) and normal amnionic epithelium (*below*) (HPS stain).

Chorion Histology

The chorion is composed of a connective tissue membrane that carries the fetal vasculature. Its inner aspect is bounded by the outer layer of the amnion, and the outer aspect is directly associated with the trophoblastic villi that sprout from its surface. There are two distinct aspects of the chorion: the chorion frondosum and the chorion laeve. The chorion of the reflected membranes (chorion laeve) is composed of an inner cellular layer, a "reticular" layer, a "pseudo-basement membrane," and an outer trophoblastic layer (44) (Figure 43.27). The precise origin of the mesenchymal component of the chorion is not clear, but it is believed that this connective tissue is derived from the primitive streak and not the trophoblast (45,46) (Figure 43.28). Electron microscopy studies have shown the connective tissue cells adjacent to the amnion to be rich in endoplasmic reticulum (47,48). Macrophages and degenerative endothelial cells also have been described as part of the cytologic makeup of this layer (48). Acid mucopolysaccharides are prominent within the connective tissue matrix of the chorion (49). Although present in other regions of the placenta, type VI collagen is a prominent constituent of the chorionic layer (50). The chorion frondosum is similarly constituted but contains functional chorionic vessels and is bordered deeply by functional villi.

instances, vernix (desquamated epithelia from the fetus) forms minute nodules on the amnionic surface in this characteristic fashion (Figure 43.34). The lesions are composed of acellular debris and remnants of cells (43). The material within these papules is PAS and alcian blue positive.

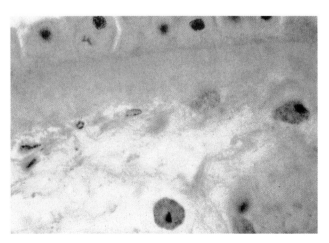

Figure 43.33 Amnionic epithelial degeneration overlies pigment-laden macrophages containing meconium (HPS stain).

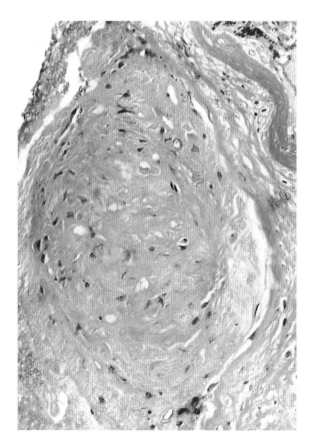

Figure 43.34 Amnion nodosum (H&E stain).

Chorion Histopathology

Pathology of the chorionic vasculature (described above in the context of its umbilical cord continuity) includes chorionitis and thromboses. The fetal chorionic vessels allow permeation of polymorphonuclear cells (PMNs) in response to intraamnionic bacterial antigens. Maternal PMNs also may be seen in the chorion laeve. In both cases, the amnion is later affected (Figure 43.30).

Chorionic cysts, which do not truly arise from the chorion proper, are derived from trophoblastic cytologic components (X cells). Multiple cysts may be present, bulging the fetal surface of the disk. These may appear terribly abnormal but in fact carry no significance in the form of true pathology (Figure 43.35). These cysts, which are commonly found in the chorionic plate and within placental septa, are discussed further below.

MULTIPLE GESTATION

The normal relationship of the placental membranes are germane to the understanding of twin or multiple-gestation placentations. These relationships are described briefly, but for a more complete discussion of twinning and associated pathological conditions, readers are referred to an extensive and detailed review of the topic (1).

The majority of twin placentas (incidences show a dependence on geographic location and ethnic background) are dizygotic. The dizygotic twin placenta has a variety of presentations: separate placentas or fused placentas. In the latter, the intervening membrane should be studied to distinguish dichorionic from monochorionic twin placentas. The intervening membrane of about 70% of monozygotic twin placentas is devoid of a chorion, and the term

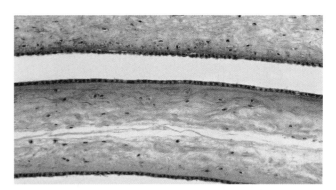

Figure 43.36 Intervening membrane from diamnionic monochorionic twin placenta. Note the absence of an intervening chorionic layer (HPS stain).

"diamnionic–monochorionic" (DiMo) is applicable (Figure 43.36). All DiMo placentas are monozygotic. In these gestations (DiMo), the shared chorion invests only the chorionic plate and is not present in the intervening membrane. In DiMo placentas, shared vascular districts between placentas are possible, and vein-to-vein and artery-to-artery anastomoses are the most common. Artery-to-vein anastomoses are relatively infrequent and are the etiology of the twin–twin transfusion syndrome (Figure 43.37A–D).

The diamnionic–dichorionic (DiDi) placenta is distinguished morphologically by examining the intervening membrane and noting the presence of two fused chorions beneath the two amnionic layers (Figure 43.38A, B). Most of these placentas are dizygotic; however, approximately 30% of DiDi twin placentas result from monozygotic twin implantations and are the result of splitting within 3 days of fertilization. Vascular anastomoses are reportable.

The complete absence of an intervening membrane (monoamnionic–monochorionic) in a twin gestation is also diagnostic of monozygotic twins. There, splitting of the embryo occurs later in gestation (at approximately 7 days of age), and although twin–twin transfusions can occur, these are less common than in DiMo placentations. The significant pathologic problems from these placentations result from cord entanglements, and fetal death is common. Even later separations result in fused twin fetuses (Siamese twins).

VILLI

Embryology

After formation of the blastocyst, the trophectoderm gives rise to extraembryonic trophoblastic villi. The organization of the inner cell mass gives rise to the embryo proper. The trophoblastic derivatives of the early implantation embryo

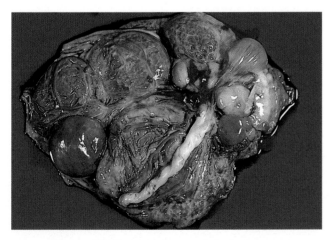

Figure 43.35 Multiple normal chorionic cysts.

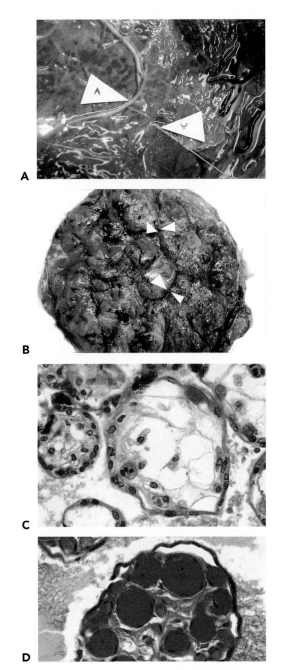

Figure 43.37 **A.** Twin–twin anastomosis characterized by artery-to-vein transfusion. **B.** Note pale anemic and edematous parenchyma of donor (left) and dark congested parenchyma of recipient (right). The arrowheads mark the vascular equator along the maternal surface. **C.** Villi from the anemic twin are edematous with abundant macrophages, and vascular spaces contain nucleated hematologic precursors denoting high-output failure and increased red cell production, respectively. **D.** Villi from plethoric twin are markedly congested (HPS stain). Characteristic "classic" twin–twin transfusion outcomes may not always occur. Although one twin may be smaller, hemoglobin may be increased in a paradoxical fashion suggesting shifts in flow before analysis. Reprinted with permission from: Benirschke K, Kaufmann P. *Pathology of the Human Placenta.* 3rd ed. New York: Springer-Verlag; 1995.

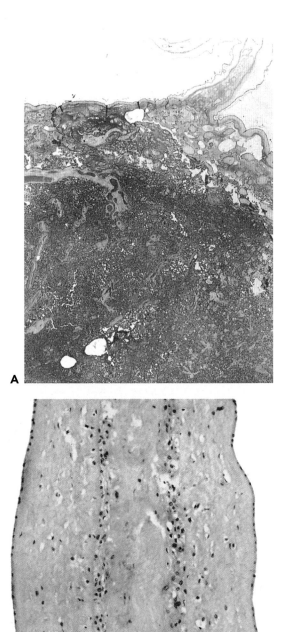

Figure 43.38 **A.** Diamnionic–dichorionic intervening membrane, site of fusion at chorionic plate ("T zone") (H&E stain). **B.** Note the more cellular intervening chorion separating the two layers of amnion (A) (HPS stain).

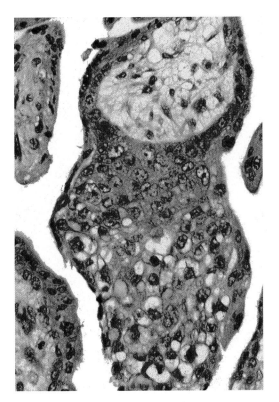

Figure 43.39 Polar trophoblastic proliferation comprising trophoblastic cell column. Many vacuolated X cells are identified (H&E stain).

the villus thins so that a syncytiovascular membrane forms the villous interface with the maternal intervillous blood. Deep to the trophoblast lies a basement membrane (also present in earlier villi), which in turn surrounds the villous mesenchyme. Deep to the villous mesenchyme, fetal blood courses within capillaries lined by endothelial cells supported on a basement membrane. These are the constituents of the "syncytial vascular membrane" separating fetal from maternal blood across which transport of essential nutrients and waste products must occur.

The course of development also has an impact on the mesenchyme. Early in development, when villi have a pronounced double trophoblastic cell layer, the mesenchyme is prominent. The cytologic constituents of this region alter with development. Before 6 weeks from the last menstrual period, capillary lumina are not readily identified (Figure 43.41). After this point, the development of vascularization within villous tissue becomes more pronounced. The vasculature is derived from branches of the stem vessels that connect with the vasculature of the chorionic plate. By about 8 weeks' gestational age (from the last menstrual period), only nucleated hematologic precursors are evident

are best characterized by discussing their structures and cell types. The trophoblastic villus forms the functional unit of the placenta. In the first trimester, trophoblastic villi are composed of an outer syncytiotrophoblastic layer and an inner cytotrophoblastic layer encompassing villous mesenchyme in which the fetal vasculature differentiates. Although the majority of the villus is surrounded by the characteristic two-cell layers, a polarity to the villi can be identified and their basal implantation regions are composed of additional trophoblastic constituents, which make up the trophoblastic cell columns (Figure 43.39). Cytotrophoblast gives rise to syncytiotrophoblast. The origin of X cells (which contribute to the trophoblastic cell columns and "percolate" into the maternal decidua along with syncytiotrophoblast) is less clearly understood.

As gestation progresses, the characteristic elements of the trophoblastic villus, as described from the early implantation, differentiate and develop to form a more functionally efficient unit. This occurs with gradual diminution in the size of peripheral branching villi. The tertiary villi, which stem from secondary villi, which in turn are derived from major stem villi, have a characteristic appearance (Figure 43.40A, B). The previously noted two-cell layer is less apparent, and the cytotrophoblast becomes much more difficult to identify. The overlying syncytiotrophoblast of

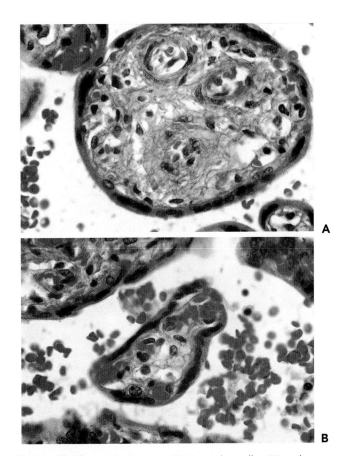

Figure 43.40 Third trimester villi. Secondary villus (**A**) and tertiary villus (**B**). Note that capillary lumina are more peripherally located in the tertiary villus. Furthermore, there is less prominent villous mesenchymal substance (HPS stain).

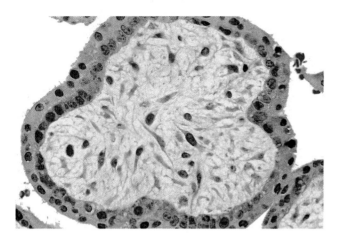

Figure 43.41   Villus from gestation of less than 6 weeks. No capillary lumina are present and no embryonic erythropoiesis is identified (H&E stain).

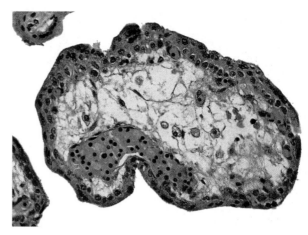

Figure 43.42   Trophoblastic villus at 8 weeks' gestation. Note only nucleated hematologic precursors present within villous capillary spaces (H&E stain).

within these villous capillary spaces (Figure 43.42). Many of these primitive blood cell precursors have their origin within the yolk sac. As gestational age progresses, there is a decrease in the number of nucleated hematologic precursors, such that between 10 and 12 weeks' gestational age (from the last menstrual period) only approximately 10% of these blood cells are nucleated. The near absence of nucleated hematologic precursors after 12 weeks is readily apparent in histologic sections (Figure 43.43). Surrounding the early villous vasculature, the villous mesenchyme is also prominent early in gestation. The mesenchymal structural units (primitive fibroblastic cells) form about 50% of the cells in this region. The remainder of cells are composed of members of the macrophage family. These cells bear antigens that characterize them as such (CD4, LeuM3, and a variety of other macrophage markers can be identified) (51).

The villous macrophages or so-called Hofbauer cells lose their prominence as gestation proceeds. The maturing tertiary villus, although it possesses this cell type, has fewer of them at term. The function of Hofbauer cells, although not completely understood, is important in water regulation activities, the transport of various nutrients and waste, and villous homeostasis. This cell type also may be important to immune regulatory functions as an intermediate in the processing of infectious agents that are blood borne.

Chorionic villi may be useful in prenatal diagnosis. Karyotype analysis may be assessed at 10 to 12 weeks' gestational age through chorionic villus sampling (CVS). It should be noted that although early diagnosis is often preferable (to later amniocentesis), several concerns exist. There have been controversies regarding limb reduction abnormalities, but the vast majority of evidence does not confirm this adverse event, especially in "experienced hands." Of genuine concern, CVS is not useful in the diagnosis of neural tube defects (amniotic fluid for α-fetoprotein deter-

mination is required) and fragile X syndrome, which also requires amniotic fluid due to alterations in methylation patterns found in trophoblast as compared with fetal squames (52).

Gross Morphology

The villous parenchyma is discoid and occupies the space beneath the chorionic plate. The substance of the parenchyma is red and "beefy." On sectioning, it appears homogeneous in contour and texture. Irregularities within the substance denote abnormalities within the villous parenchyma. Many abnormalities so identified are common, and in most instances, due to their frequent occurrence, they should be considered as normal varients (unless they are unduly prominent). Such entities include infarcts and perivillous fibrin deposition.

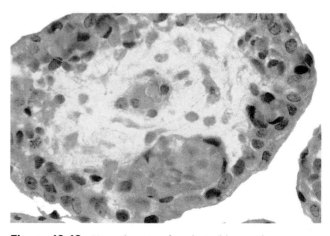

Figure 43.43   Near absence of nucleated hematologic precursors within villous capillaries after 12 weeks' gestation (H&E stain).

In addition to the perivillous fibrin deposition, other fibrinous depositions are common and are generally considered normal within the placenta. The so-called Langhans' stria, located below the chorionic plate, is probably related to alterations of materal intervillous blood flow. By virtue of its distance from the decidual vasculature, it tends to be more static.

Nitabuch's fibrin is present between the floor of the placenta and the maternal decidua. This layer was once believed to prevent allograft rejection, but now the precise nature and functional significance of this fibrin deposition are not clear.

On occasion, the placental parenchyma have spherical defects (usually 1 to 2 cm in greatest dimension), which represent so-called jet lesions. These cleared areas within the villous parenchyma represent pressure heads from maternal decidual vascular flow. It is not uncommon to histologically identify a small zone of acute infarction peripheral to these lesions.

Calcification is a common phenomenon in the mature placenta. Calcification has been used to diagnose placental maturity by ultrasonographic evaluation during pregnancy. Third-trimester gestations have an increase in the amount of calcium present in the placenta, and when calcifications are prominent, placentas are considered grade 3. A mature placenta detected by ultrasound does not necessarily denote fetal maturity. The appearance of calcium deposition in the gross sense is that of fine, pinhead-sized deposits of yellow–white, gritty material. Calcification of the placenta is a normal physiologic response to development and aging (53,54).

Gross Morphologic Alterations

Many placentas normally have some degree of infarction. When infarction roughly exceeds 10 to 15% of the placental surface, or when it is more central than peripheral, this should be considered pathologic. Infarcts are characterized grossly as either acute or "old." Acute infarcts are pale, poorly demarcated regions that are slightly granular on palpation. "Old" infarcts are white, often triangular, and they too are granular (Figure 43.44).

Infarcts evaluated grossly are distinguished from perivillous fibrin deposition. Upon palpation, infarcts are granular and firm. Perivillous fibrin, on the other hand, tends to be nodular and smooth. Further distinctions are made histologically, and these are described in detail below.

Intervillous thrombi also may be identified during the gross examination of the placenta. These triangular or diamond-shaped lesions within the placenta may consist of soft gelatinous red to white (depending on age of lesion) aggregates of collected blood. The lamellations of fibrin within this thrombotic material may be observed grossly. It is this aspect, as well as the gelatinous soft makeup of this material, that distinguishes these lesions

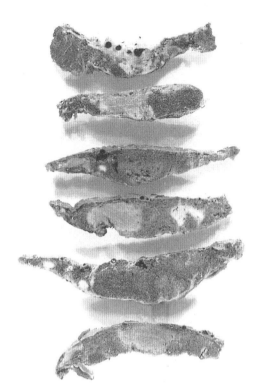

Figure 43.44 Multiple old infarcts from a hypertensive pregnancy.

from infarcts and perivillous fibrin deposition upon gross examination.

Histology

The histologic variations in placental architecture are largely dependent on the developmental state at which observations are made. The histology of the individual cell types involved directly in villous implantation is now described.

X cells, also termed intermediate trophoblasts, are major constituents of the cell columns that form the deepest structural components of the implantation site. These cytologic components of trophoblastic origin are unique with respect to other trophoblastic derivatives (syncytiotrophoblasts and cytotrophoblasts). X cells are secretorily distinct and produce human placental lactogen and major basic protein, and are electron microscopically distinct insofar as they contain large numbers of mitochondria with tubular cristae (55–57). Similar cell types are identified along with the chorion laeve (Figure 43.45A, B), and these cells have been characterized histologically as being eosinophilic or vacuolated; it was suggested that they represent two distinct subpopulations in this region (58). In the implantation site, these cells are morphologically distinguished from decidual elements in that their cytoplasm is generally darker and they

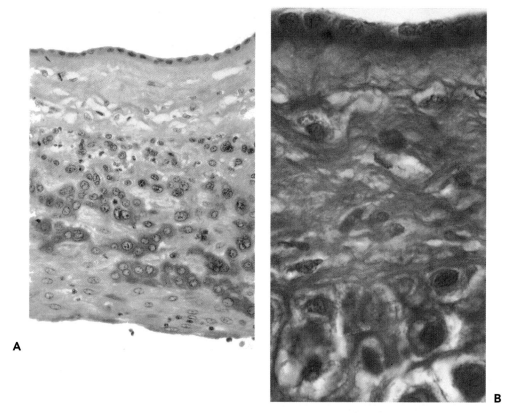

Figure 43.45 Prominent nonvacuolated X cells within the decidua of the chorionic laeve. Note their darker cytoplasm and occasional multinucleation (**A**) and vacuolated X cells deep in the chorion (**B**) (HPS stain).

are occasionally multinucleated. Furthermore, these cells tend to be more vacuolated then their neighboring decidual cells. Difficulty in distinguishing these cell types has resulted in some problems with the diagnosis of intrauterine pregnancy when these are the only trophoblastic cells present in currettage specimens. In the absence of villi, most pathologists confirm their diagnosis of intrauterine pregnancy (and hence generally exclude the possibility of a tubal pregnancy) based on the presence of multinucleated trophoblastic derivatives, which are more readily distinguished from the surrounding decidua. Should difficulty arise with morphologic assessment of the true nature of the uninuclear cells in question, immunohistochemical localization of human placental lactogen within X cells is helpful (59). This cell type is of important immunologic interest because it may be responsible for the synthesis of fibronectin (1). An excess of immature intermediate trophoblasts has been associated with preeclampsia and eclampsia (60).

An interesting normal finding within the placenta is the so-called chorionic cyst. These cysts occur in placental septae and are composed largely of decidua and X cells. The cysts are entirely lined by X cells. As noted above, such cysts also may be seen in the chorionic plate (Figure 43.35). On sectioning, gelatinous fluid may be present, and the major constituent of this fluid is one of the substances produced by X cells: major basic protein. The function of these cysts

is not known. They should not be considered pathologic when present (1).

The syncytiotrophoblast, the outer cell layer, possesses a brush border. Microvilli that constitute this border are felt to be involved in pinocytotic activity. Vacuoles within the cytoplasm of these cells are indicative of the absorptive and secretory activities of the syncytiotrophoblast. Syncytiotrophoblasts are composed of pyknotic (often multiple) nuclei that are hyperchromatic. In addition to the multiple vesicles present within this cell type, ultrastructural examinations show a cytoplasm that is rich in endoplasmic reticulum, mitochondria, lipid droplets, and Golgi bodies (61).

The cytotrophoblastic nuclei are more round and open. Tritiated thymidine incorporation experiments have shown that uptake and incorporation are confined to the cytotrophoblastic layer and not the syncytiotrophoblastic layer (62). On occasion, cytotrophoblasts may possess mitotic figures (Figure 43.46). Ultrastructurally, the cytotrophoblast has fewer organelles than does the syncytiotrophoblast. Most prominent are large mitochondria, which may be numerous.

Human placental lactogen may be localized within X cells and syncytiotrophoblasts. Human chorionic gonadotropin can be identified within syncytiotrophoblast cells, but not within cytotrophoblast cells (55,63).

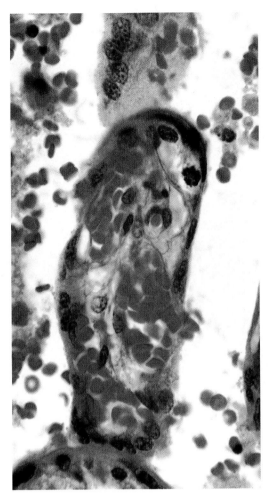

Figure 43.46 Sparse cytotrophoblast with rare mitotic figure in terminal villus from a third trimester placenta (HPS stain).

Histopathology

Various pathologic entities, which may be identified within the villous parenchyma at the histologic level, serve to better illustrate the normal histology of the placenta.

Infarcts, which are common in the placental substance, have a characteristic gross appearance. Acute infarcts are characterized histologically by the presence of faint staining villi, which are aggregated, compressed, or agglutinated to one another and have interspersed polymorphonuclear leukocytes within the intervillous space (Figure 43.47). (As described below, it is crucial to distinguish this inflammation from that which occurs in an intravellous fashion). Earlier forms of infarction may be characterized by the presence of villous agglutination and congestion, with lysis of intervillous maternal blood (Figure 43.48). In very advanced ("old") infarcts, complete absence of villous architecture is noted and a fuzzy outline of remaining villous constituents can be identified (Figure 43.49). No viable staining cells are identified, and an acute inflammatory infiltrate may persist. The placenta rarely undergoes "organization" or fibrosis. When acute infarcts resolve and

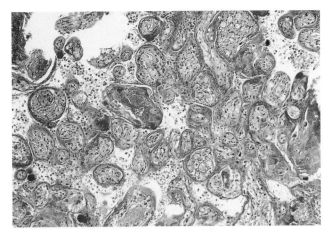

Figure 43.47 Acute infarct (HPS stain).

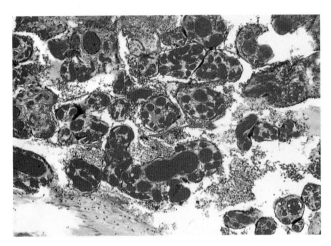

Figure 43.48 Villous vascular congestion may indicate early infarction or need to be more closely examined to exclude chorangiosis (HPS stain).

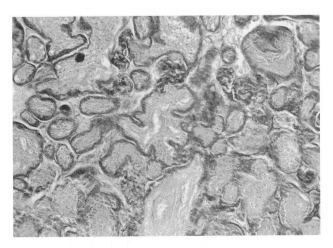

Figure 43.49 "Old" infarct (HPS stain).

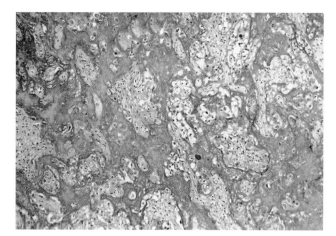

Figure 43.50 Increased perivillous fibrin. Note trophoblastic nuclear remnants encased in fibrin (HPS stain).

become "old," fibroblasts are generally lacking. It is for this reason that organization is not a term applied to the placenta. Classic organization as might apply to other organ systems undergoing ischemic change does not occur. The variance probably relates to the two distinct vascular supplies (maternal and fetal). Disturbance in maternal flow results in placental infarction.

Infarcts are distinguished from perivillous fibrin deposition histologically in that regions of the latter contain cytotrophoblastic nuclear remnants that are often prominent

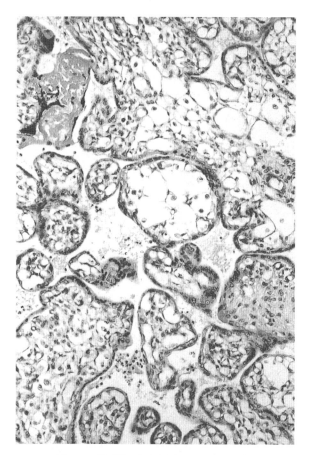

Figure 43.52 Focal edema (H&E stain).

(Figure 43.50). Intervillous thrombi are identified histologically by the presence of lamellated thrombotic material displacing neighboring villi (Figure 43.51).

Other abnormalities of the villous parenchyma include villous edema, where edema fluid displaces intravillous cytologic architecture; it is considered pathologic, especially in premature gestations (Figure 43.52) and has been reported as a cause of fetal ischemia. Its etiology is not clear (22). Tenney-Parker change is characteristic of placentas from preeclamptic gestations. This change is characterized by increased syncytial knotting on villi (Figure 43.53). These syncytial knots are best considered failed adaptive responses to low oxygen tension within the intervillous space. As noted above, increased intermediate trophoblasts also may be seen (60). Infarcts are not uncommon (1), and in preeclamptic/eclamptic gestations, decidual vasculopathy is also encountered and is discussed below.

Unusual appearances of villous vasculature take three unrelated forms. First, villous vasculature may be congested (Figure 43.48), and this may have no pathologic significance or may be indicative of early infarction. Second, increased numbers of villous capillaries, so-called chorangiosis, has been considered to be indicative of chronic hypoxic changes. The definition is precise, and in histologic terms three crite-

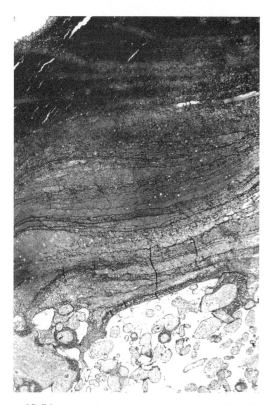

Figure 43.51 Intervillous thrombus. Note lamellated lines of Zahn (HPS stain).

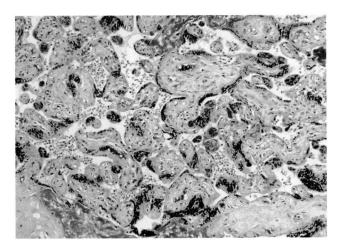

Figure 43.53 Increased syncytial knots in a hypertensive pregnancy (HPS stain).

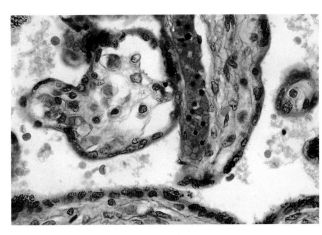

Figure 43.55 Fetal nucleated red blood cells are abnormal at term. There is associated focal villous edema (H&E stain).

ria (10 vessels/10 villi/10 fields at 10×) need to be met (64). Third, abnormal proliferations of villous vessels that form histologically hemangiomatous nodules, are termed chorioangiomas when present in the placenta (Figure 43.54A, B). These lesions have pathologic significance when prominent and may result in high-output cardiac failure in the fetus or microangiopathic hemolytic phenomena.

Dysmaturity of villi is also considered pathologic. Villi that show the characteristic two-cell layer of the first-trimester implantation, when present in third-trimester placentas, are indicative of abnormal developmental events. This change has been noted to occur in mothers who are diabetic.

Nucleated red blood cells are common in very early gestations, but as gestation proceeds, and especially in the third trimester, nucleated red blood cells should not be present. When present, fetal anemia with increased erythroid production should be suspected. Additionally, recent investigations have addressed the presence of nucleated red blood cells (in advanced-gestation placentas), correlating such findings with erythropoietin secretion by the fetus and concomitant fetal hypoxia (1) (Figure 43.55).

In patients with sickle cell disease, it is not unusual to find sickling of maternal erythrocytes within the intervillous spaces. This is promoted by diminished oxygen tension in the setting of abnormal maternal hemoglobin S. It is wise to correlate histopathologic findings with clinical status in that it has been reported that hypoxia during and after placental separation causes sickling (65) (Figure 43.56).

Inflammatory changes within villi are probably one of the most interesting aspects of placental pathology. These inflammatory changes herald the presence of infectious disease agents in many cases. The presence of syphilis and cytomegalovirus (CMV) should be considered when

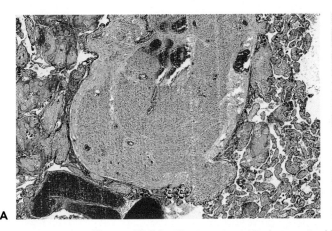

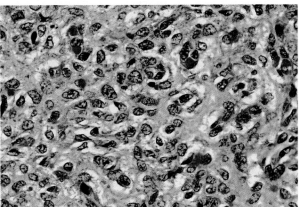

Figure 43.54 Chorioangioma (**A**) characterized by hemangiomatous proliferation (**B**) (HPS stain).

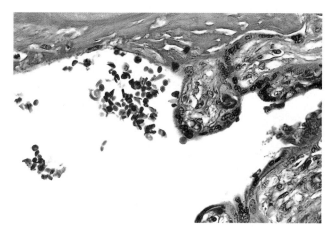

Figure 43.56   Intervillous maternal red cell sickling in patient with sickle cell disease (H&E stain).

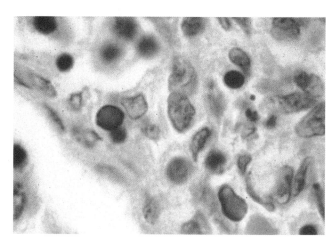

Figure 43.58   Parvovirus B19 infection associated with villous edema and nucleated fetal red cells with characteristic inclusions (H&E).

infiltrates of lymphocytes and plasma cells are found within trophoblastic villi. Special stains may be confirmatory. It is important to distinguish this chronic inflammation from that of the acute inflammatory infiltrate (surrounding villi) associated with acute infarction. An acute inflammatory infiltrate within villi may suggest *Listeria* infection with extensive microabscess formation throughout the placenta. This often can be seen in the gross as innumerable white dots. The odor has been characterized as "sweet" (1). In many instances, inflammatory changes within the villi are limited to an increase in the villous cellularity (increased Hofbauer cells), and no specific infectious disease agent can be identified. Increased numbers of inflammatory cells (without plasma cells) also signify chronic villitis; however, in most instances when this occurs, no infectious disease organism can be identified.

These inflammatory changes within the placenta have been termed "villitis of unknown etiology (VUE)" (64,66) (Figure 43.57A, B). The infiltrate has been identified as maternal in origin (67).

The absence of inflammation does not always coincide with the absence of infection. For example, in parvovirus B19 infection, hydropic villi and the presence of villous vascular nucleated red blood cells (occasionally with "smudged" amphophilic intranuclear inclusion bodies) may herald the presence of severe congenital infection even in the setting of absence of maternal symptoms (1) (Figure 43.58).

Confounding the topic of placental and neonatal infection is the entirely normal placenta, by routine examination. Only special molecular studies will detect antigens and nucleic acids indicating the presence of infectious materials (68) (Figure 43.59A, B).

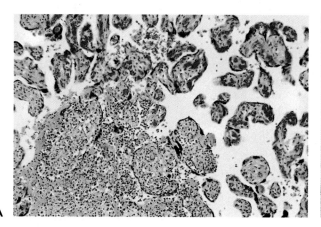

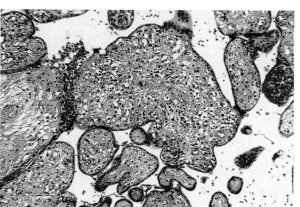

Figure 43.57   Villitis of unknown etiology (VUE) in which a chronic inflammatory infiltrate devoid of plasma cells is present (**A**) and chronic villitis due to known syphilis infection characterized by the presence of a mononuclear infiltrate containing plasma cells (**B**) (HPS stain).

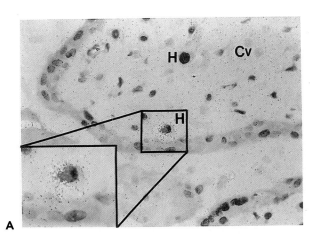
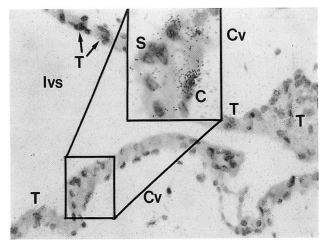

Figure 43.59 In situ hybridization with S^{35} probe detects HIV-1 nucleic acids in Hofbauer (H) cells (**A**) and trophoblast (C,T) of immature villi (Cv) (**B**). Reprinted with permission from: Redline RW, Patterson P. Villitis of unknown etiology is associated with major infiltration of fetal tissue by maternal inflammatory cells. *Am J Pathol* 1993;143:473–479.

DECIDUA

Histology

The hypersecretory glandular epithelium of the endometrium, which is progestationally induced, affords the proper environment for implantation. At times, these hypersecretory glands may exhibit the Arias-Stella reaction in which cytologic atypia is noted (Figure 43.60). In this condition, nuclei are often polyploid. However, nuclear cytoplasmic ratios remain low, distinguishing this normal finding from neoplasia. In this continued progestational influence, endometrial glands become secretorily exhausted. The endometrial stroma has undergone its characteristic "decidualization," and decidual cells of the endometrium are characterized as epithelioid and polygonal. Their small

rounded nuclei are generally situated centrally in abundant pale eosinophilic, often vacuolated, cytoplasm (Figure 43.61). The cytoplasm is rich in glycogen and glycoproteins. In regions of decidual tissue, where trophoblastic derivatives are not present, nuclear content is diploid (69). Ultrastructural examination of the decidua shows that tight junctions separate these cells (70).

In addition to the decidual cells, an admixture of fibroblasts and lymphocytes is also identified. An additional cell type, the "granular cell," has been shown to produce relaxin (71).

The intercellular matrix contains abundant type IV collagen and laminin. Fibronectin and heparin sulfate proteins also have been identified (72). Other collagens are also present throughout the decidual matrix, and these include types I, III, and V.

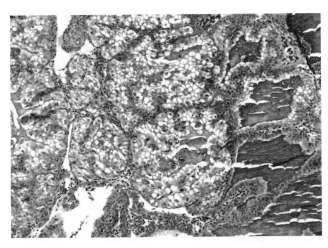

Figure 43.60 Arias-Stella reaction (H&E stain).

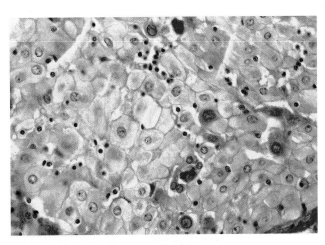

Figure 43.61 Decidua with centrally placed open nuclei and abundant pale cytoplasm with prominent cell borders. Note sparse normal lymphocytic infiltrate and occasional X cell with cytoplasm darker than decidual cytoplasm (HPS stain).

Although prior reports suggested that the secretory activity of the decidua included the production of prolactin and human placental lactogen, it is known that this hormone is produced not by decidual cells but by invading trophoblastic derivatives (principally intermediate trophoblast or X cells) (55). Much of the difficulty in studying decidual tissues and their hormonal production has resulted from the inability of many investigators to distinguish decidual components from invading trophoblastic contaminants (1).

The vascularization of the decidual component of the implantation site is critical to the developing gestation. The major branches of the uterine arteries extend deeply into the myometrial substance, resulting in arcuate arteries that then branch to form radial arteries. These become the spi-

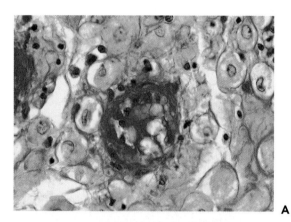

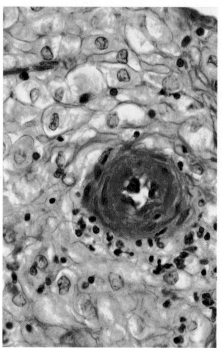

Figure 43.62 Decidual vascular atherosis (**A**) and concentric medial hypertrophy (**B**) from a hypertensive gestation (HPS stain).

ral arterioles, the terminal components of the endometrial vasculature. These spiral vessels have been shown by injection studies to be responsible for the intervillous blood flow within cotyledonary units (73). The precise number of spiral arterioles that serve to perfuse the placenta is a debated topic. Estimates range from 25 to 300 vascular openings (74,75).

That trophoblastic cells invade the underlying decidual vasculate is a well-known phenomenon. This finding has been documented within the decidual bed, as well as in systemic maternal vascular compartments, most notably the lung (76). It is important to distinguish these decidual vascular changes from those abnormalities of the decidual vasculature that indicate pathologic conditions.

Gross inspection of the decidua is generally unrevealing, and important attributes and diagnoses are identified histologically. In through-and-through sections of the placenta disk, which includes the chorionic plate and the villous parenchyma, the underlying decidua is often denuded from the placental implantation site during the delivery process. Therefore, it is not uncommon to find sections of parenchyma devoid of decidual tissue. One region in which decidua is often prominent is on the chorion laeve. Sections of "membrane rolls," which include amnion and chorion, often include sections of adherent decidua, which represent fusion of the decidua capsularis and the decidua vera during development. In some patients in whom decidua abnormalities are suspect, decidual bed biopsies have been performed at the time of delivery. Such biopsies often reveal aberrant vascular relationships of the more proximal vascular tree (radial and basal arteries). The more proximal vessels are characterized by thicker vascular walls, and their arteries often have internal elastic laminae as evidenced by silver stains. The more distal arteries (the spiral arterioles) are thin walled and do not possess any internal elastic lamina.

Histopathology

Principal among decidual pathology is the so-called atherosis of the decidual vascular bed, which is known to accompany preeclampsia and hypertensive conditions of gestation (77). These lesions are characterized by fibrinoid necrosis and hyalinization of the vascular wall along with the deposition of foamy macrophages and should be readily distinguishable from normal trophoblastic vascular invasion. Another abnormality that may characterize hypertensive pregnancies is concentric arteriolar mural hypertrophy (Figure 43.62A, B).

Bleeding (retroplacental) is responsible for premature placental separation or abruptio placenta. This has been related to two maternal conditions: increased maternal blood pressure and decidual vascular necrosis (due to vasculopathies or inflammatory-bacterial decidual infections) (Figure 43.63).

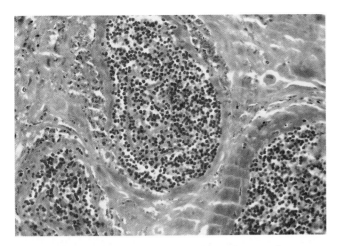

Figure 43.63 Decidual vascular necrosis, in this case due to a severe acute deciduitis. Note vascular wall hyalinization and necrosis, which resulted in adjacent abruptio (H&E stain).

When trophoblastic villi implant directly on myometrial tissue and intervening decidua is absent, the pathologic condition of placenta accreta is present (Figure 43.64). This finding is more common in low implantations of the placenta, especially when prior cesarean sections have been performed. Variations in which trophoblastic villi implanted within the myometrium (placenta increta) and when implantation results in the presence of villous tissue protruding through the uterine serosal surface (placenta percreta) are more severe forms of this condition. Generally, all placental tissue cannot be removed from the uterus at delivery and severe hemorrhage ensues. Heroic measures only rarely save the uterus and may increase morbidity due to persistant hemorrhage (and in latter stages bacterial infection) by delay of definitive therapy, which is hysterectomy. Occasionally, accreta are confirmed by studying the decidua of the chorion laeve. Failure of resolution of villi during capsular expansion may result in myometrial implantation without intervening decidua. Also occasionally, myometrium adherent to frondosum is found without intervening decidua. In both cases the diagnosis of accreta can be made by the pathologist in the absence of the hysterectomy specimen.

Within the decidua attached to the delivered placenta rare leukocytes may be seen. If these cytological constituents are plasma cells, syphilis or CMV infection should be considered.

In the absence of pathologic alterations (placental, maternal or neonatal) these rare leukocytes within the decidua are likely physiologic or nonspecific.

More destinctive inflammatory processes involving the decidua are deciduitis and can be associated with inflammation elsewhere. Acute chorioamnionitis and acute or chronic villitis should be sought in the further examination of the placenta.

GESTATIONAL TROPHOBLASTIC DISEASE

Although the discussion of neoplastic trophoblastic disease is beyond the scope of this chapter, several normal or exaggerated findings of the implantation site or the placenta proper are discussed to distinguish them from more significant pathologic entities.

Degenerative changes of early trophoblastic villi are not uncommon, especially in the presence of incomplete abortus material. Trophoblastic villi from such gestations are often seen in histologic sections to be swollen (hydropic). These findings are distinguished from the gestational trophoblastic neoplasm (complete hydatidiform mole) in several aspects. Principal among these distinguishing characteristics is that no trophoblastic atypia or proliferation is present along the surface of the villi (Figure 43.65A, B). When degenerative changes have taken place and fetal components are blighted, the chorionic vasculature may be absent within the villi. However, if remnants of these vessels persist, the presence of complete hydatidiform mole is essentially not possible. The ease of identifying nucleated hematologic precursors facilitates this observation. Furthermore, should any fetal parts be identified, this too excludes the presence of complete hydatidiform mole. On the other hand, hydropic villi in the presence of fetal parts may herald genotypically abnormal gestations. This form of

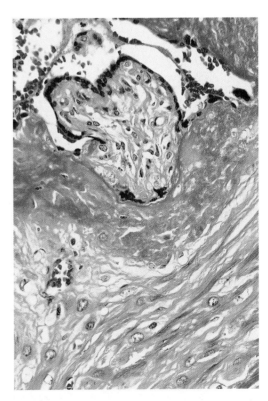

Figure 43.64 Placenta accreta. No decidua is present between the implanting trophoblastic villi and the uterine myometrium. The presence of small amounts of fibrin does not alter the diagnosis.

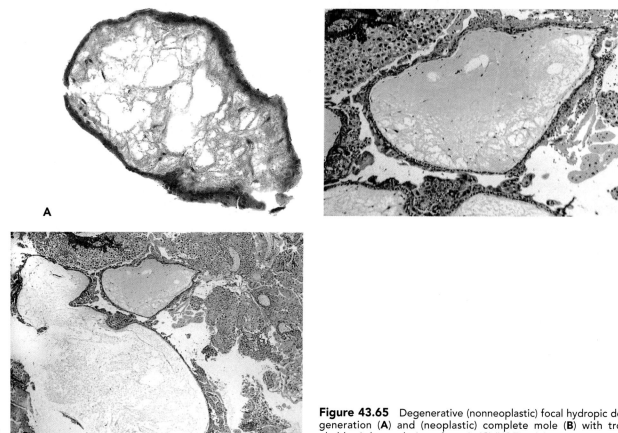

Figure 43.65 Degenerative (nonneoplastic) focal hydropic degeneration (**A**) and (neoplastic) complete mole (**B**) with trophoblastic hyperplasia and atypia (**C**) (H&E stain).

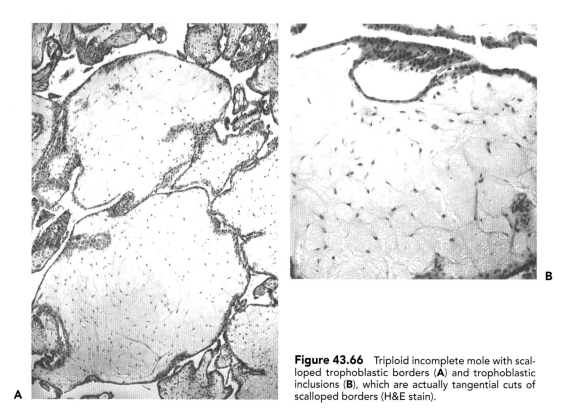

Figure 43.66 Triploid incomplete mole with scalloped trophoblastic borders (**A**) and trophoblastic inclusions (**B**), which are actually tangential cuts of scalloped borders (H&E stain).

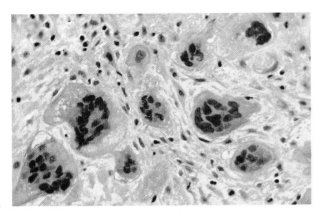
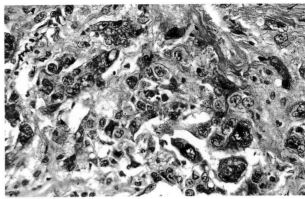

Figure 43.67 Exaggerated implantation site (**A**) and invading choriocarcinoma (**B**) (H&E stain).

incomplete mole, which is rarely neoplastic, is characterized by scalloped trophoblastic borders and occasional trophoblastic island inclusions (representing tangential cuts of scalloped borders within the villous stroma) (Figure 43.66A, B).

Abundant trophoblastic derivates, prominent within the nidus of the implantation site, may from time to time need to be distinguished from choriocarcinoma. The so-called syncytial endometritis—a poor term because it is not an inflammatory or infectious condition—refers to an exaggerated implantation site where syncytiotrophoblastic and other trophoblastic derivative counterparts are prominent (Figure 43.67A, B). In the absence of included trophoblastic villi during examination, the histologic appearance is similar to that of invading choriocarcinoma. The chief distinction is the lack of pronounced cytologic and nuclear atypia that characterizes choriocarcinoma.

Last, an unusual lesion that is neoplastic is the placental site trophoblastic tumor. This neplasm is composed solely of X cells (or, as described by Kurman et al. (55), intermediate trophoblasts) (Figure 43.68).

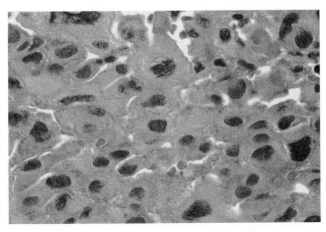

Figure 43.68 Placental site trophoblastic tumor (H&E stain).

REFERENCES

1. Benirschke K, Kaufmann P. *Pathology of the Human Placenta.* 3rd ed. New York: Springer-Verlag; 1995.
2. Lewis SH, ed. *Pathology of the Placenta.* New York: Churchill Livingstone; Elsivier; 1999.
3. Bartholomew RA, Colvin ED, Grimes WH Jr, Fish JS, Lester WM, Galloway WH. Criteria by which toxemia of pregnancy may be diagnosed from unlabeled formalin-fixed placentas. *Am J Obstet Gynecol* 1961;82:277–290.
4. Schremmer BN. Gewichtsveränderungen verschiedener Gewebe nach Formalinfixierung. *Frank Z Pathol* 1967;77:299–305.
5. College of American Pathologists Conference XIX. The examination of the placenta: patient care and risk management. *Arch Pathol Lab Med* 1991;115:660–721.
6. Nuovo G, Richart RM. Buffered formalin is the superior fixative for the detection of HPV DNA by in situ hybridization analysis. *Am J Pathol* 1989;34:837–842.
7. Naeye RL. Umbilical cord length: clinical significance. *J Pediatr* 1985;107:278–281.
8. Lewis SH, Starr C. Cord width. *In Utero* (Unpublished).
9. Grosser O. *Frühentwicklung, Eihautbildung und Placentation des Menschen und der Säugetiere.* Munich: JF Bergman; 1927.
10. Gardiner JP. The umbilical cord: normal length; length in cord complications; etiology and frequency of coiling. *Surg Gynecol Obstet* 1922;34:252–256.
11. Wynn RM, French GL. Comparative ultrastructure of the mammalian amnion. *Obstet Gynecol* 1968;31:759–774.
12. Hoyes AD. Ultrastructure of the epithelium of the human umbilical cord. *J Anat* 1969;105(pt 1):145–162.
13. Moore RD. Mast cells of the human umbilical cord. *Am J Pathol* 1956;32:1179–1183.
14. Nadkarni BB. Innervation of the human umbilical artery: an electron microscope study. *Am J Obstet Gynecol* 1970;107:303–312.
15. Ellison JP. The nerves of the umbilical cord in man and the rat. *Am J Anat* 1971;132:53–60.
16. Lauweryns JM, De Bruyn M, Peuskens J, Bourgeois N. Absence of intrinsic innervation of the human placenta. *Experientia* 1969;25:432.
17. Blanc WA, Allan GW. Intrafunicular ulceration of the persistent omphalomesenteric duct with intra-amniotic hemorrhage and fetal death. *Am J Obstet Gynecol* 1961;82:1392–1396.
18. Priman J. A note on the anastomosis of the umbilical arteries. *Anat Rec* 1959;134:1–5.
19. Arts NF. Investigations on the vascular system of the placenta. I. General introduction and the fetal vascular system. *Am J Obstet Gynecol* 1961;82:147–158.
20. Rana J, Ebert GA, Kappy KA. Adverse perinatal outcome with an abnormal umbilical coiling index. *Obstet Gynecol* 1995;85:573–578.
21. Altshuler G, Hyde S. Meconium-induced vasocontraction: a potential cause of cerebral and other hypoprofusion and of poor pregnancy outcome. *J Child Neurol* 1989;4:137–142.

22. Naeye RL. *Disorders of the Placenta, Fetus and Neonate: Diagnosis and Clinical Significance*. St. Louis: Mosby Year Book; 1992.

23. Vonthobitien N. *Anatomia Suc Undina Human*. 1668.

24. Garza A, Cordero JF, Mulinare J. Epidemiology of the early amnion rupture spectrum of defects. *Am J Dis Child* 1988;142: 541–544.

25. Torpin R. *Fetal Malformations Caused by Amnion Rupture During Gestation*. Springfield, IL: Charles C Thomas; 1968.

26. Danforth D, Hull RW. The microscopic anatomy of the fetal membranes with particular reference to the detailed structure of amnion. *Am J Obstet Gynecol* 1958;75:536–550.

27. Boyd JD, Hamilton WJ. *The Human Placenta*. Cambridge, MA: Heffer & Sons; 1970.

28. Michael H, Ulbright TM, Brodhecker C. Magma reticulare-like differentiation in yolk sac tumor and its pluripotential nature [Abstract]. *Mod Pathol* 1988;1:63.

29. King BF. Developmental changes in the fine structure of rhesus monkey amnion. *Am J Anat* 1980;157:285–307.

30. Mukaida T, Yoshida K, Kikyokawa T, Soma H. Surface structure of the placental membranes. *J Clin Electron Microsc* 1977;10: 447–448.

31. Bourne GL. The microscopic anatomy of the human amnion and chorion. *Am J Obstet Gynecol* 1960;79:1070–1073.

32. Majno G, Joris I. Apoptosis, oncosis, and necrosis. An overview of cell death. *Am J Pathol* 1995;146:3–15.

33. Tsukada T, Eguchi K, Migita K, et al. Transforming growth factor beta 1 induces apoptotic cell death in cultured human umbilical vein endothelial cells with down-regulated expression of bcl-2. *Biochem Biophys Res Commun* 1995;210:1076–1082.

34. Bartels H, Wang T. Intercellular junctions in the human fetal membranes. A freeze-fracture study. *Anat Embryol (Berl)* 1983; 166: 103–120.

35. Robinson HN, Anhalt GJ, Patel HP, Takahashi Y, Labib RS, Diaz LA. Pemphigus and pemphigoid antigens are expressed in human amnion epithelium. *J Invest Dermatol* 1984;83:234–237.

36. Schwarzacher HG, Klinger HP. Die Entstehung mehrkerniger Zellen durch Amitose im Amnionepithel des Menschen und die Aufteilung des chromosomalen Materials auf deren einzelne Zellkerne. *Z Zellforsch* 1963;60:741–754.

37. Schindler PD. Nuclear deoxyribonucleic acid (DNA) content, nuclear size and cell size in the human amnion epithelium. *Acta Anat (Basel)* 1961;44:273–285.

38. Kalousek DK, Fill FJ. Chromosomal mosaicism confined to the placenta in human conceptions. *Science* 1983;221:665–667.

39. Bautzmann H, Hertenstein C. Zur Histogenese und Histologie des menschlichen fetalen und Neugeborenen-Amnions. *Z Zellforsch* 1957;45:589–611.

40. Schmidt W. Struktur und Funktion des Amnionepithels von Mensch und Huhn. *Z Zellforsch* 1963;61:642–660.

41. Schwarzacher HG. Beitrag zur histogenese des menschilichen amnion. *Acta Anat* 1960;43:303–311.

42. Nickell KA, Stocker JT. Placental teratoma: a case report. *Pediatr Pathol* 1987;7:645–650.

43. Salazar H, Kanbour AI. Amnion nodosum: ultrastructure and histopathogenesis. *Arch Pathol* 1974;98:39–46.

44. Bourne GL. *The Human Amnion and Chorion*. London: Lloyd-Luke; 1962.

45. Luckett WP. The origin of extraembryonic mesoderm in the early human and rhesus monkey embryos [abstract]. *Anat Rec* 1971; 169:369–370.

46. Rossant J, Croy BA. Genetic identification of tissue of origin of cellular populations within the mouse placenta. *J Embryol Exp Morphol* 1985;86:177–189.

47. Hoyes AD. Ultrastructure of the mesenchymal layers of the human amnion in early pregnancy. *Am J Obstet Gynecol* 1970;106: 557–566.

48. Hoyes AD. Ultrastructure of the mesenchymal layers of the human chorion laeve. *J Anat* 1971;109(pt 1):17–30.

49. Sala MA, Matheus M. Histochemical study of the fetal membranes in the human term pregnancy. *Gegenbaurs Morphol Jahrb* 1984; 130:699–705.

50. Hessle H, Engvall E. Type VI collagen. Studies on its localization, structure, and biosynthetic form with monoclonal antibodies. *J Biol Chem* 1984;259:3955–3961.

51. Goldstein J, Braverman M, Salafia C, Buckley P. The phenotype of human placental macrophages and its variation with gestational age. *Am J Pathol* 1988;133:648–659.

52. American College of Obstetricians and Gynecologists. ACOG Committee Opinion (Committee on Genetics) no. 160: Chorionic villus sampling; 1995.

53. Pitkin RM, Reynolds WA, Williams GA, Hargis GK. Calcium metabolism in normal pregnancy: a longitudinal study. *Am J Obstet Gynecol* 1979;133:781–790.

54. Tsang RC, Donovan EF, Steichen JJ. Calcium physiology and pathology in the neonate. *Pediatr Clin North Am* 1976;23:611–626.

55. Kurman RJ, Main CS, Chen HC. Intermediate trophoblast: a distinctive form of trophoblast with specific morphological, biochemical and functional features. *Placenta* 1984;5:349–370.

56. Wasmoen TL, Benirschke K, Gleich GJ. Demonstration of immunoreactive eosinophil granule major basic protein in the plasma and placentae of non-human primates. *Placenta* 1987;8:283–292.

57. Wynn RM. Cytotrophoblastic specializations: an ultrastructural study of the human placenta. *Am J Obstet Gynecol* 1972;114: 339–355.

58. Yeh IT, O'Connor DM, Kurman RJ. Vacuolated cytotrophoblast: a subpopulation of trophoblast in the chorion laeve. *Placenta* 1989;10:429–438.

59. O'Connor DM, Kurman RJ. Utilization of intermediate trophoblast in the diagnosis of an *in utero* gestation in endometrial curettings without chorionic villi [Abstract]. *Mod Pathol* 1988;1:68.

60. Redline RW, Patterson P. Pre-eclampsia is associated with an excess of proliferative immature intermediate trophoblast. *Hum Pathol* 1995;26:594–600.

61. Wislocki GB, Dempsey EW. Electron microscopy of the human placenta. *Anat Rec* 1955;123:133–167.

62. Richart R. Studies of placental morphogenesis. I. Radioautographic studies of human placenta utilizing tritiated thymidine. *Proc Soc Exp Biol Med* 1961;106:829–831.

63. Pierce GB Jr, Midgley AR Jr. The origin and function of human syncytiotrophoblastic giant cells. *Am J Pathol* 1963;43:153–173.

64. Altshuler G. Placental infection and inflammation. In: Perrin EVDK, ed. *Pathology of the Placenta*. New York: Churchill Livingstone; 1984.

65. Fujikura T, Froehlich L. Diagnosis of sickling by placental examination. Geographic differences in incidence. *Am J Obstet Gynecol* 1968;100:1122–1124.

66. Knox WF, Fox H. Villitis of unknown aetiology: its incidence and significance in placentae from a British population. *Placenta* 1984;5:395–402.

67. Redline RW, Patterson P. Villitis of unknown etiology is associated with major infiltration of fetal tissue by maternal inflammatory cells. *Am J Pathol* 1993;143:473–479.

68. Lewis SH, Reynolds-Kohler C, Fox HE, Nelson JA. HIV-1 in trophoblastic and villous Hofbauer cells, and hematologic precursors in eight-week fetuses. *Lancet* 1990;355:565–568.

69. Sachs H. Quantitativ histochemische Untersuchung des Endometrium in der Schwangerschaft und der Placenta (Cytophotometrische Messungen). *Arch Gynecol Obstet* 1968; 205: 93–104.

70. Lawn AM, Wilson EW, Finn CA. The ultrastructure of human decidual and predecidual cells. *J Reprod Fertil* 1971;26:85–90.

71. Dallenbach FD, Dallenbach-Hellweg G. Immunohistologische Untersuchungen zur Lokalisation des Relaxins in menschlicher Placenta und Decidua. *Virchows Arch A* 1964;337:301–316.

72. Wewer UM, Faber M, Liotta LA, Albrechtsen R. Immunochemical and ultrastructural assessment of the nature of pericellular basement membrane of human decidual cells. *Lab Invest* 1985; 53: 624–633.

73. Freese UE. The uteroplacental vascular relationship in the human. *Am J Obstet Gynecol* 1968;101:8–16.

74. Borell U, Fernstrom I, Ohlson L, Wiqvist N. The influence of uterine contractions on the uteroplacental blood flow at term. *Am J Obstet Gynecol* 1965;93:44–57.

75. Haller U. Beitrag zur Morphologie der Utero-placentargefaesse. *Arch Gynaekol* 1968;205:185–202.

76. Attwood HD, Park WW. Embolism to the lungs by trophoblast. *J Obstet Gynaecol Br Commonw* 1961;68:611–617.

77. Hertig AT. Vascular pathology in hypertensive albuminuric toxemias of pregnancy. *Clinics* 1945;4:602–614.

ENDOCRINE

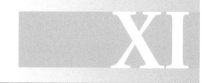

Thyroid

44

Maria Luisa Carcangiu

EMBRYOLOGY

The human thyroid first appears as a median anlage and two lateral anlagen. The median anlage develops in the floor of the primitive pharynx at the foramen cecum (a dimplelike depression at the base of the tongue) from a median ductlike invagination that grows caudally. This formation, known as the thyroglossal duct, contains at its base the developing thyroid gland, which is at first spherical but later, when approaching its final site in front of the trachea at about 7 weeks of gestation, becomes bilobed (1). During this downward migration, the thyroglossal duct undergoes atrophy, leaving as a vestige the pyramidal lobe in about 40% of individuals. Faulty downward migration of the medial anlage or persistence of parts of the thyroglossal duct gives rise to ectopic thyroid tissue, thyroglossal duct cysts, and cervical fistulae.

The initially solid thyroid anlage begins to form cords and plates of follicular cells during the 9th week of gestation. Small follicles appear by the 10th week. Inside these primitive follicles, a finely granular material begins to collect, which by the 20th week acquires the morphologic features of colloid. By week 14 there are well-developed follicles with a central lumen containing colloid. Both the cytoplasm of the follicular cells and the intraluminal colloid are thyroglobulin (TGB)-positive (Figure 44.1A, B). Labeled amino acid studies have shown that TGB synthesis actually begins at a much earlier stage, when the thyroid is still a solid mass at the base of the tongue and long before follicle formation and colloid secretion can be identified morphologically (2,3).

PAX8, a transcription factor expressed in the adult mouse thyroid where it is involved in the maintenance of functional differentiation in follicular cells, has been demonstrated in the human median thyroid anlage, in the tyroglossal duct, and in the ultimobranchial bodies.

Thyroid transcription factor-1 (TTF1), also is expressed in the median thyroid anlage (4,5).

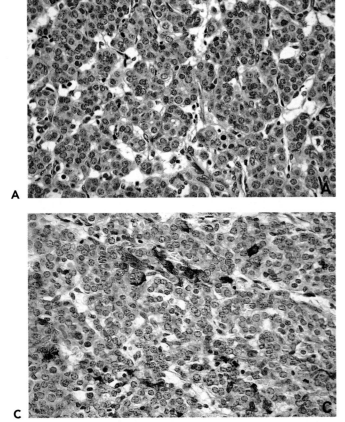

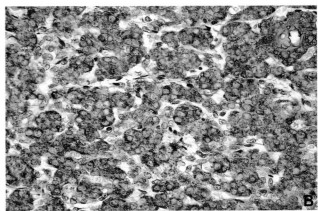

Figure 44.1 Developing thyroid gland in a 14-week fetus. **A.** Rare primitive follicles are seen within a mostly solid proliferation. **B.** The cytoplasm of the follicular cells and the material contained in the lumen of the primitive follicles are immunoreactive for TGB. **C.** C cells, as seen in a CT immunostain preparation, are scattered within follicles.

Immunohistochemically, ghrelin, a growth hormone–releasing hormone, has been shown in the follicular cells of fetal thyroid (from 8 to 38 weeks of gestational age) (6). Fetal thyroid stromal tissue is immunoreactive for galectin 1 but not for galectin 3 (7).

The two lateral anlagen of the thyroid derive from the ultimobranchial bodies (UBBs), which in turn originate from the IVth–Vth branchial pouch complex. UBBs, while still connected to the pharynx, start their migration downward on each side of the neck together with the parathyroid IV anlage. At 7 to 8 weeks they separate from the pharynx and the parathyroid. Their lumens become obliterated by proliferating cells, so that at 8 to 9 weeks they appear as solid masses that fuse with the dorsolateral aspects of the median thyroid anlage and become incorporated into the developing lateral lobes (8).

After its fusion with the medial thyroid (at 9 weeks to term) the UBB enters in the dissolution phase and divides into a central thick-walled stratified epithelial cyst and a peripheral component composed of cell groups dispersed among the follicles: the C cells (9,10) (Figure 44.1C). In postnatal life, the central epithelial cyst largely disappears, its occasional remnants corresponding to the so-called solid cell nests (SCNs).

C cells are thought to derive from the neural crest and to migrate to the UBBs before the incorporation of the latter in the thyroid (11–14). Evidence for a relationship between UBBs and C cells comes from several sources:

1. Patients with Di George syndrome, characterized by complete or partial absence of derivatives of the IIIrd and IVth–Vth pouch complexes, have C cells in their thyroid in only 25% of cases (15,16).
2. C cells are completely absent in thyroglossal duct remnants and cysts, as well as in lingual thyroid (17).
3. In the adult thyroid gland, C cells and follicles carrying such cells in their walls are especially numerous in the vicinity of the UBB remnants (17).

There is some controversy as to whether the role of UBBs in thyroid development is limited to the production of C cells as described above or whether they also contribute to the follicular cell population. Williams et al. (18) described five cases of maldescent of the medial thyroid anlage in which cystic structures were present in the lateral neck in the region of the upper parathyroids. Four of these cystic structures contained intercystic glandular nodules composed of solid areas of irregularly distributed cells that stained positively for calcitonin (CT) and CT gene–related peptide; these cells were intermixed with follicular structures that were immunoreactive for thyroglobin. On the basis of these observations, the investigators concluded that the UBB contributes both C cells and follicular cells to the thyroid gland, and they speculated on the possible role of UBB-derived cells in the genesis of so-called intermediate or mixed medullary and follicular carcinomas. This hypothesis, which was independently postulated by Ljungberg (17), is however contradicted by the observation that in humans with thyroid nondescent (or unilateral aplasia) there are no recognizable thyroid follicles in the usual locations (19).

The fetal thyroid gland develops rapidly until the 4th month of intrauterine growth (crown–rump length 18 mm). After birth the thyroid growth rate parallels that of the body, reaching the normal adult weight at around 15 years of age.

GROSS ANATOMY

The normal adult thyroid has a shape reminiscent of a butterfly, with two bulky lateral lobes connected by a thin isthmus. Each lateral lobe is 2 to 2.5 cm wide, 5 to 6 cm long, and 2 cm deep. Their upper and lower extremities (one having a pointed shape and the other featuring blunt contours) are referred to as upper and lower thyroid poles, respectively. One lobe may be larger than the other, and the isthmus may be exceptionally wide. The pyramidal lobe, a vestige of the thyroglossal duct, is found in about 40% of thyroids; it appears as a narrow projection of thyroid tissue that extends upward from the isthmus to lie on the surface of the thyroid cartilage.

The thyroid gland is located in the midportion of the neck, where it is attached to the anterior trachea by loose connective tissue. The two lateral lobes surround the ventral and lateral aspects of the larynx and trachea, reaching the lower halves of the thyroid cartilage and covering the second, third, and fourth tracheal rings.

The normal weight of the adult thyroid is 15 to 25 g in nongoitrous areas. However, there are significant individual variations, most of them related to gender, age, corporal weight, hormonal status, functional status of the gland, and iodine intake (20). In women, the thyroid volume is known to increase during the secretory phase of the menstrual cycle (21).

A thin fibrous capsule invests the thyroid. Connected to this capsule are numerous fibrous septa that penetrate the thyroid parenchyma and divide it into lobules (so-called thyromeres). The microscopic integrity of the capsule was assessed in a study on 138 thyroid glands from autopsies of adults (age 20–40 years) by Komorowski and Hanson (22). Although grossly all of these capsules seemed complete, microscopically they were focally incomplete in 62% of the cases. Furthermore, thyroid follicles were found within the thyroid capsule in 14% of cases and in the pericapsular connective tissue in 88%. In the latter location, they were mostly seen as nodular aggregates.

The color of the normal thyroid is red–brown. A phenomenon exceptionally seen in normal thyroid glands of elderly individuals is the accumulation in the follicular cells of a melanin-like pigment that imparts to the gland a characteristic coal black stain, easily apparent on gross examination. The terms *melanosis thyroid* and *black thyroid* are used to refer to this phenomenon. These changes are qualitatively identical to those seen in more florid form in thyroids of patients on chronic minocycline therapy (23,24).

Nodularity of thyroid parenchyma is identified grossly in about 10% of the glands of endocrinologically normal individuals (25).

The blood supply of the thyroid gland derives primarily from the inferior thyroid artery (which originates from the thyrocervical trunk of the subclavian artery) and the superior thyroid artery (which arises from the external carotid). A thyroidea ima artery also may be present, which varies widely in size from a small vessel to one the size of the inferior thyroid artery. The superior and medial thyroid veins and the inferior vein drain (via a venous plexus in the thyroid capsule) into the internal jugular and the brachiocephalic vein, respectively (26,27).

An intricate lymphatic network permeates the thyroid gland, encircling the follicles and connecting the two lateral lobes through the isthmus. It empties into subcapsular channels, which in turn give rise to collecting trunks within the thyroid capsule in close proximity to the veins. The lymph vessels draining the superior portion of the thyroid lobes and isthmus collect into the internal jugular lymph nodes, whereas those draining the inferior portion of the gland collect into the pre- and paratracheal and prelaryngeal lymph nodes. The pretracheal lymph node situated close to the isthmus is also known as the *Delphian node* (28). Other lymph node stations are the recurrent laryngeal nerve chain and the retropharyngeal and retroesophageal groups. The anterosuperior mediastinal nodes are secondary to the recurrent laryngeal nerve chain and pretracheal groups; however, injection studies have shown that dye injected into the thyroid isthmus can drain directly into the mediastinal nodes (29).

Some correlations exist between the site of a thyroid tumor within a given lobe and the location of the initial lymph node metastasis. However, the degree of anastomosing between these various nodal groups is such that any of them can be found to be the site of disease regardless of the precise location of the primary tumor.

Vasomotor nonmedullated postganglionic neural fibers originating from the superior and midline cervical sympathetic ganglia influence indirectly the secretory activity of the thyroid gland through their action on the blood vessels. In addition, adrenergic receptors in follicular cells and a network of adrenergic fibers ending near the follicular basement membrane have been demonstrated (30). It has been hypothesized, therefore, that thyroid secretion is regulated

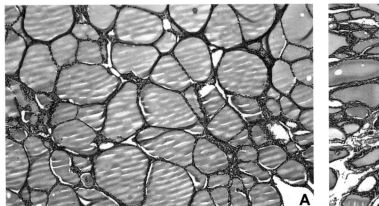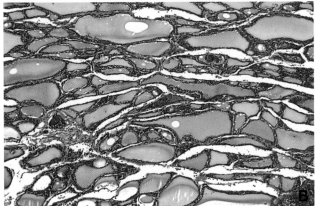

Figure 44.2 **A.** Low-power view of normal adult thyroid gland. The follicles have a round-to-oval shape. **B.** Elongated follicles as a result of compression are seen in the vicinity of an adenoma (not shown in this picture).

both by direct neural signals and by indirect vascular nerve signals (31–33). A role for direct neural influences in the secretion of calcitonin (CT) and other C cell–derived hormones is supported by the demonstration in chickens of a rich cholinergic network encircling the C cells (34).

Small paraganglia are normally present close to the thyroid and are occasionally found beneath the thyroid capsule; their presence explains the rare occurrence of peri- and intrathyroidal paragangliomas.

MICROSCOPIC ANATOMY

The fundamental unit of the thyroid is the follicle, a round to slightly oval structure lined by a single layer of epithelial cells resting on a basement membrane (Figure 44.2A). The lumen of the follicle contains colloid, a viscous material that is mostly composed by proteins secreted by the follicular cells, including TGB. The follicles, which are separated

from each other by a loose fibroconnective tissue, have an average diameter of 200 μm. Their size may vary even within the same gland depending on the functional status of the thyroid and the age of the individual. Variations in the shape of follicles exist, but elongated follicles are a feature of hyperplastic or neoplastic conditions or are the result of compression adjacent to an expansile mass (Figure 44.2B). A characteristic structure present in the normal thyroid but more often seen in hyperplastic conditions, is the Sanderson's polster. (See page 1136.)

The colloid, which is pale eosinophilic in the actively secreting gland, acquires a deeply eosinophilic staining quality in resting follicles. Often, numerous clumps with various shapes appear within the colloid of resting follicles, suggesting an artifactual coagulation-type phenomenon (Figure 44.3). In some follicles the colloid may have an amphophilic or basophilic staining quality, probably the result of an increase in the amount of acidic groups in the TGB molecule (Figure 44.4). In the most advanced expres-

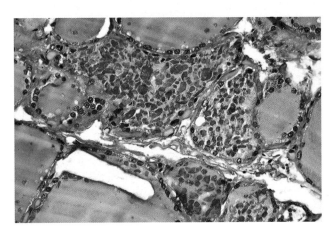

Figure 44.3 Clumps of condensed colloid within follicular lumina.

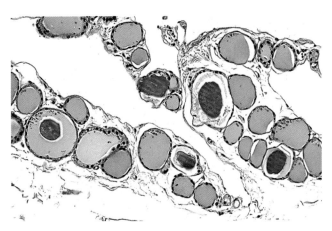

Figure 44.4 The colloid accumulated in these follicles exhibits different densities and tintorial qualities, the latter ranging from acidophilic to basophilic.

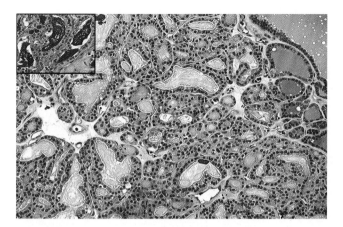

Figure 44.5 The basophilic colloid present in most of these follicles contrasts with the more typical red colloid present in the follicles on the right upper corner. **Inset:** Alcian blue-PAS highlights the mucinous character of the basophilic colloid.

sion of this phenomenon, the intraluminal material acquires a distinct mucinlike appearance (Figure. 44.5).

The glycoproteic material present within the follicles stains for periodic acid-Schiff (PAS) and alcian blue and is immunoreactive for TGB. A row of small vacuoles is seen at the interface between follicular epithelium and the colloid in actively functioning glands; these are referred to as resorption vacuoles. In addition, it is not unusual to find a large round or oval clear space within the colloid; this often appears empty but it may contain birefringent calcium oxalate crystals (See page 1137.)

Another morphologic variation of the colloid is represented by collections of round basophilic corpuscles clustering at one pole of the follicle.

The epithelial glandular cells lining the follicle are known as follicular cells or thyrocytes; among them, there is a second cellular component known as C cells.

FOLLICULAR CELLS

The cells lining the follicles—follicular cells or thyrocytes—show variations in their shape and size according to the functional status of the gland. Three major types, expressions of a morphologic continuum, are described: flattened (endothelioid), cuboidal, and columnar (cylindrical) (Figure 44.6A). Flattened cells are relatively inactive. Cuboidal cells (their height equaling their width) are the most numerous and their major function is to secrete colloid. The rarer columnar cells resorb the TGB-containing colloid, liberate the active hormones, and excrete these hormones into blood vessels; they may feature an apical cuticle, apical lipid droplets, and one or more basilar vacuoles (vacuoles of Bensley).

Functional polarity is apparent at the level of the follicle and the follicular cell. A single follicle may have flattened cells on one side and cuboidal or low columnar cells on the other (Figure 44.6B), the best expression of this phenomenon being the already mentioned Sanderson's polster.

At the cellular level, all follicular cells manifest a definite polarity, resting with their bases on the basement membrane and having the apexes directed toward the lumen of the follicle. Size and position of the nucleus and some components of the cytoplasm may vary considerably. In the resting thyroid, the nucleus is round or oval, is located toward the center of the cell, and usually contains one nucleolus that is eccentrically located. Its chromatin may be finely granular or clumped. In actively secreting cells, the nucleus is enlarged; because of the mostly apical enlargement of the cytoplasm, it acquires a basal position. The cytoplasm is usually weakly eosinophilic; only exceptionally in an otherwise normal thyroid, does it appear granular and intensely eosinophilic; that is, oncocytic (so-called Hurthle cells). In contrast to parathyroid cells, little or no intracytoplasmic glycogen is present. Occasionally, the

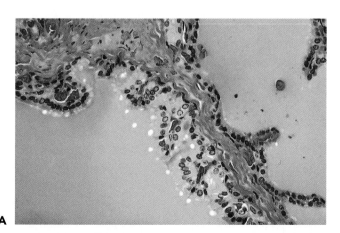
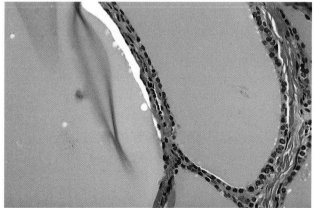

Figure 44.6 **A.** The epithelium of one follicle is low cuboidal and relatively inactive. The adjacent follicle shows a taller epithelium and reabsorption vacuoles. **B.** The epithelium of the same follicle is flattened on one side and cuboidal on the other, as an expression of functional polarization.

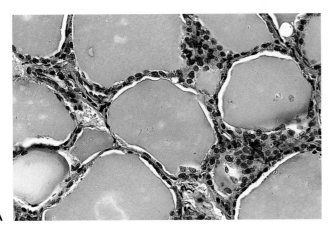
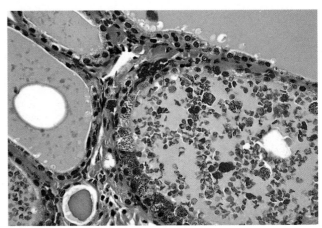

Figure 44.7   A. Lipofuscin in the cytoplasm of the follicular cells. **B.** Granular black pigment in the follicular epithelium and colloid of the thyroid of a 73-year-old patient who was not on minocycline therapy.

follicular cell cytoplasm contains a golden brown pigment of lipofuscin type (Figure 44.7A), which should be distinguished from the melanin-like pigment already mentioned (Figure 44.7B).

Ultrastructurally, the follicular cells are arranged in a single layer around the colloid and rest on a basement membrane, approximately 35 to 40 nm in thickness, that separate them from the interstitial stroma. Microvilli emanate from the surface of the cells, their number being increased and their length greater in actively functioning cells. Cell membranes of adjacent cells interdigitate in a complex fashion and are joined by junctional complexes toward the apex (35,36). The cytoplasm contains variable amounts of endoplasmic reticulum, mitochondria of usually small size, and lysosomes. When the number of mitochondria is highly increased, the cell acquires at the light microscopic level an intensely eosinophilic granular cytoplasmic appearance (corresponding to the above mentioned Hurthle cells).

Immunohistochemistry

A wide variety of markers with various degrees of specificity and diagnostic significance are expressed by the normal adult follicular cells.

Thyroglobulin (TGB)

This is the most specific immunohistochemical marker for normal follicular cells and the tumors composed of them. It can be demostrated with either monoclonal or polyclonal antibodies and the reactivity is both in the cytoplasm and in the colloid (37,38). Oncocytes show a much lesser degree of positivity. Despite its high specificity, TBG can give rise to a common pitfall. Because of its tendency to leak out of the cytoplasm of the follicular cells and to diffuse into the adjacent tissues, where it can then be incorporated into the cytoplasm of other types of cells (e.g., metastatic carcinoma), it can cause a false positivity (39).

Thyroid Transcription Factor-1 (TTF-1)

This is another very useful marker for thyroid follicular cells and tumors composed of them. This nuclear transcription factor, first identified in thyroid follicular cells and later in pneumocytes, is necessary for the development of thyroid and pulmonary tissues. In the normal adult thyroid its distribution is related to that of thyroglobulin and thyroperoxidase (40,41).

Keratins

Normal follicular cells are immunoreactive only for low-molecular-weight keratin, whereas high-molecular-weight types have been found to be expressed in inflammatory and neoplastic conditions (42–44).

Vimentin

Some normal follicular cells occasionally express this intermediate filament in conjunction with keratin, although less commonly than in neoplastic conditions (45).

Epithelial Membrane Antigen (EMA)

Follicular cells are variably positive, with accentuation of the cell membranes.

Triiodothyronine (T3) and Thyroxine (T4)

These hormones can be detected immunohistochemically both in the cytoplasm of the follicular cells and in the intraluminal colloid but their use for diagnostic purposes is negligible.

Estrogen and Progesterone Receptors

Estrogen and progesterone receptors positivity, restricted to the follicular cell nuclei, shows some correlation with the age and sex of the individual (46,47).

S-100 protein

This marker, which is mainly detected in inflammatory/hyperplastic and neoplastic thyroid conditions, is only focally and weakly expressed by normal follicular cells (48,49).

Epidermal Growth Factor Receptor (EGFR)

In normal follicular cells, and because of their functional polarization, the location of this receptor is mainly basal or basolateral (50).

Thyroid Peroxidase

This enzyme is responsible for the oxidation of iodide to iodine. At the immunohistochemical level it shows a pattern of staining correlated with the age of the individual. A cytoplasmic pattern of staining with apical membrane accentuation is seen in children and young adults, and a perinuclear ring distribution is seen in older individuals (51).

Sodium Iodide Symporter

At the immunohistochemical level this molecule, responsible for the active iodide intake into the follicular epithelium, is localized mainly to the lateral basal portion of the cells (52,53).

Physiology

The main function of the thyroid gland is the production of thyroid hormones, the most important being thyroxin (T4) and triiodothyronine (T3). These hormones regulate metabolism, increase protein synthesis in every tissue of the body, and increase O_2 consumption. Thyroid hormones are particularly important for body development and for the normal maturation of the central and peripheral nervous system.

Steps in thyroid hormone biosynthesis include ingestion of iodine ions from water and food, their absorption and transport as iodide into the extracellular fluid and their concentration within the thyroid where their intracellular levels are 30 times higher than in peripheral blood. The active iodide uptake across the basement membrane is mediated by human sodium iodide symporter (hNIS) in a process coupled with the flow of sodium (52). The intrathyroidal iodide is then oxidized to iodine. This last step is dependent on the action of iodide peroxidase, which oxidates the iodine ion to a highly reactive form of iodine, which in turn binds to tyrosine. The results are monoiodotyrosine (MIT) when one iodine molecule is attached, or diiodotyrosine (DIT) when two iodine molecules are attached. The iodotyrosine residues are condensed to form the biologically active thyroid hormones thyroxin (T4) and triiodotyronine (T3). Thyroxin results from the coupling of two molecules of DIT, and triiodotyronine from the coupling of one molecule of MIT with a molecule of DIT (33).

Thyroid hormones are stored in TGB, with numerous iodinated tyrosine residues, including biologically active T4 and T3. TGB, a large protein with a 19 S sedimentation coefficient and a molecular weight of 670,000, is formed by two identical subunits with a 12 S sedimentation coefficient to which many oligosaccharides are linked. Variations in the sugar chains of the thyroglobulin molecule have been evaluated by analysis of reactivity to various lectins and found to differ between the normal gland and various pathologic states, including neoplasms (54).

Thyroglobulin is encoded by a gene spreading over more than 200 kilobases in the bovine genome (55). The molecular mechanisms involved in the tissue-specific and hormone-dependent expression of the thyroglobulin gene have been studied in follicular cells in primary cultures and cell lines (56,57). TGB is collected at the center of the thyroid follicles and is the main constituent of colloid.

Ultrastructural studies have correlated the morphologic changes that accompany thyroid hormone production and secretion. The synthesis of TGB begins in the endoplasmic reticulum and continues in the Golgi apparatus, where the end sugars of the carbohydrate site are incorporated; it is then packaged in small apical microvesicles, the contents of which are discharged into the follicular lumen after fusion of the vesicle membranes with the luminal side of the plasma membrane.

Resorption of TGB takes place through cytoplasmic pseudopodia (streamers) that engulf minute portions of colloid, which are then drawn into the cell in the form of membrane-bound colloid droplets. These subsequently fuse with lysosomes, and their content is digested by the lysosomal enzymes (58–61). The breakdown products, including T3 and T4, diffuse in the blood stream, where they are transported primarily by the specific carrier protein, thyroxin-binding globulin (TBG). TBG normally transports more than 70% of thyroid hormones. Approximately 20% of circulating thyroid hormones is carried by transthyretin (prealbumin) and albumin (62). Only a small portion of circulating thyroid hormones (approximately 0.05% of T3 and 0.015% of T4) is unbound and, therefore, biologically active. Free, circulating, biologically active T3 and T4 are in equilibrium with the hormones bound to the carrier proteins. The amount of circulating T4 is much larger than that of T3; however, T3 is about four times more active biologically; as a result, the final contribution of T3 to the biologic activity of thyroid hormones equals that of T4 (63).

Thyroid hormones stimulate metabolism, increase oxygen consumption, and cause a rise in heat production, cardiac output, and heart rate. They are essential for normal development, growth, and maturation. The acceleration of growth may result from a direct action on the cells to increase their rate of division, by acting permissively for other hormones, or by inducing the synthesis of a variety of growth-promoting hormones (58,62,64–68).

Thyroid biosynthetic and secretory activities are controlled by the blood level of thyroid stimulating hormone (TSH), a glycoprotein synthesized and secreted by the anterior pituitary gland (69). TSH binds to a specific receptor located on the basolateral surface of the follicular cell membrane, and by activating the adenylate-cyclase pathway regulates the complex mechanism responsible for T3 and T4 synthesis (70,71).

Stimulation of the thyroid gland by thyrotropin increases its secretory activity and vascularity and results in both hypertrophy and hyperplasia of follicular cells, accompanied by reduction of colloid storage. At the functional level, this is reflected by an increase in iodide concentration and organic binding, hormone synthesis, and hormone secretion (63,72). TSH release is in turn regulated by a tripeptide secreted by the hypothalamus, thyrotropin releasing hormone (TRH). TSH and TRH release are regulated by the circulating levels of free T3 and T4, via a negative feedback on the pituitary and hypothalamus (low levels of free T3 and T4 stimulate the release of TSH and TRH). In contrast, TSH and TRH releases are inhibited by high levels of circulating free T3 and T4 (69,72,73).

Microscopic Variations

Sanderson's Polster

A characteristic structure, present in the normal thyroid but accentuated in hyperplastic conditions, is the so-called Sanderson's polster. This refers to an aggregate of small follicles lined by flattened epithelium and covered by an undulating layer of columnar epithelium that is seen bulging into the lumina of larger follicles (Figure 44.8). This perfectly benign and to some extent physiologic change, most likely the morphologic expression of the functional polarization of the thyroid follicle, needs to be distinguished from papillary microcarcinoma.

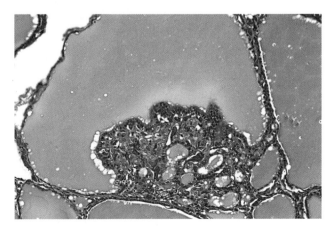

Figure 44.8 Sanderson's polster protruding into the lumen of a follicle.

Granulomas

Granulomas are a relatively common finding in otherwise normal surgically resected thyroids and in autoptic specimens. Both foreign material and colloid may elicit this process. Suture material is the most frequent cause of formation of granulomas in completion thyroidectomy specimens. Larger foreign body granulomas sometimes clinically simulating a thyroid nodule have been reported in thyroids of patients who underwent laryngeal injection of Polytef (polytetrafluoroethylene) (74,75). This material may migrate through the lymphatics into adjacent tissues, where it may start the inflammatory process.

Rarely, interstitial granulomas are seen as a reaction to oxalate crystals that have been released by broken follicles (76).

Granulomatous lesions originated by the rupture of follicles and their invasion by macrophages and leukocytes as a reaction to the extruded colloid are a common incidental finding in surgically resected thyroids. Carney et al. (77) referred to this process as palpation thyroiditis (and also as multifocal granulomatous folliculitis) and attributed it to the minor trauma resulting from physical examination. Support for this interpretation comes from the observation that the number and size of the granulomas is related to the intensity of the palpation and the fact that similar changes have been described in individuals engaged in martial arts (so-called martial-arts thyroiditis) (77,78).

Grossly, a gland affected by palpation thyroiditis appears normal or shows tiny foci of hemorrhage. Histologically, multiple small granulomas centered in a disrupted follicle and composed of histiocytes, lymphocytes, and plasma cells are seen scattered in the thyroid gland (Figure 44.9A). Some of the histiocytes are foamy, while others have the appearance of multinucleated giant cells. The appearance depends on the stage of the process, a common picture being a cluster of foamy macrophages hanging from the follicular epithelium into the lumen (Figure 44.9B). Necrosis, hemosiderin, and iron deposition are seen only rarely. Sometimes up to four or five follicles are involved in a single granuloma.

Immunohistochemically, most of the lymphocytes are T cells; among the plasma cells, K-positive cells predominate (79).

Palpation thyroiditis seems to represent a variation in the theme of colloidophagy, a process described many years ago and characterized by a granulomatous reaction to colloid in follicles allegedly undergoing spontaneous rupture in thyroids affected by goiter or thyroiditis (80).

Palpation thyroiditis needs to be distinguished from interstitial giant cell thyroiditis (in which the granulomas are centered not in the follicles but in the interstitium), necrotizing granulomas following surgical procedures (similar to those more commonly seen in the bladder and the prostate and characterized by a central area of necrosis surrounded by a palisading of epithelioid cells), and aggregates of C cells (which are immunoreactive for CT) (81,82).

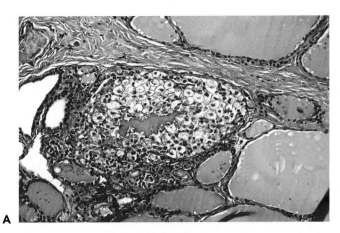

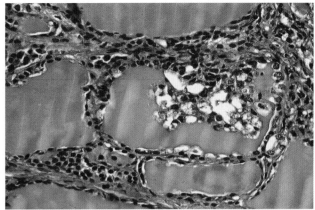

A
B

Figure 44.9 Palpation thyroiditis. **A.** The thyroid follicle in the center is packed with histiocytes and other inflammatory cells, with a clump of residual colloid in the center. The follicular epithelium is barely discernible. **B.** In this case the follicle is only partially involved. Inflammatory cells and desquamated follicular cells protrude into the lumen.

Crystals

Anisotropic crystals of calcium oxalate may be present within the colloid in normal adult thyroid glands. They may be seen in ordinary light, but are more easily identified under polarized light (Figure 44.10). Their shape varies from rhomboid to irregular plaques and their size shows wide variations (83).

In autoptic studies they have been found with a frequency of up to 85% of thyroids examined (84). Their number appears to increase with age; this, together with the observation that the crystals have been found more frequently in colloid with low positivity for TGB, has prompted the suggestion that they result from variations in colloid and calcium concentration in the gland secondary to a low functional state of the thyroid (83–85).

In one study the number of crystals was markedly elevated in glands with subacute thyroiditis, where they were found in the giant cells, in remnants of colloid, and in the thyroid stroma. In the same study crystals were identified only rarely in thyroids with chronic thyroiditis or glandular hyperplasia (86).

Oxalate crystals in the thyroid are also seen in large number in patients undergoing dialysis for renal failure. In this setting, the thyroid is just another site of oxalate deposition, together with the kidney, myocardium, and other sites (87). Rarely, crystals released by follicular breakdown may elicit a granulomatous reaction in the nearby thyroid stroma (76).

At the time of frozen section, their identification within a follicular structure can be useful in distinguishing thyroid from parathyroid gland tissue (88).

Squamous Metaplasia

Benign squamous cells occur as an expression of squamous metaplasia of follicular cells in various benign and malignant thyroid lesions and, under exceptional circumstances, in an otherwise normal thyroid (89–91). They need to be distinguished from transversally cut follicles and from the SCNs of UBB derivation. It also should be mentioned that squamous epithelium is regularly observed as a component of the epithelium of thyroglossal duct cysts.

C CELLS

C cells (parafollicular cells) represent a minor component of the thyroid gland. It has been estimated that they comprise not more that 0.1% of the glandular mass. They have a neuroendocrine function, being responsible for the production of the peptide hormone CT. The term "C cells" was introduced by Pearse (92) to underline their role in secreting and storing this hormone. More recently, other hormones have been found to be produced by C cells, but only in small quantity and not in every cell.

C cells are identified only with difficulty in sections stained with hematoxylin and eosin, where they appear polygonal and with a granular weakly eosinophilic

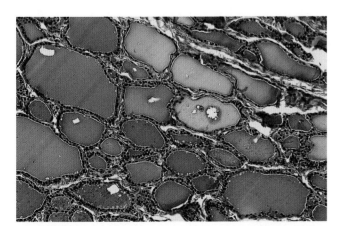

Figure 44.10 Multiple birefringent calcium oxalate crystals are seen in the lumina of normal thyroid follicles (polarized light).

cytoplasm that is larger and paler than that of follicular cells. The nucleus is round to oval, pale, with a centrally located nucleolus.

C cells are located, individually or in small groups, within thyroid follicles. Specifically, most are found at the periphery of the follicular wall (hence the qualifier parafollicular), within its basement membrane and without contact with the follicular lumen. Electron microscopy has shown that C cells occupy an intrafollicular (rather than interfollicular) position, and that they are separated from the thyroid interstitium by the follicular basal lamina. The presence of C cells in the interfollicular stroma has never been convincingly demonstrated ultrastructurally (93).

Occasional C cells have prominent cytoplasmic processes that extend beyond the adjacent follicular cells. In normal adults and neonates, C cells are restricted to the midupper and upper thirds of the lateral lobes of the thyroid, in the area where UBBs (from which they derive) fuse with the thyroid median anlage. The number of C cells varies with the development of the gland, being more numerous in early age. In one study, up to 100 C cells per low-power field were demonstrated in neonates and children; whereas in adults only a maximum of 10 cells per low-power field were counted (94). In another study, no difference in the number of C cells was found between young and middle-aged groups, but in the elderly the number of such cells was variable, with groups of up to 20 or more cells sometimes being observed (95). However, no statistically significant differences among the various age groups in adults were demonstrated. Other studies have since confirmed that normal adult thyroid glands may contain numerous C cells, sometimes in the form of small nodules (22,96) (Figure 44.11). Gibson et al. (96) suggested that such clusters of C cells, in the absence of disturbances in calcium metabolism and of a family history of medullary carcinoma, do not constitute a precursor of medullary carcinoma but may be instead the expression of either a

partial failure of embryonic C-cell migration and dispersion within the gland or of age-related hyperplasia. It needs to be mentioned that C-cell hyperplasia of presumed reactive nature has been observed in the immediate periphery of nonmedullary thyroid neoplasms (97,98), in association with lymphocytic thyroiditis (99–101), and in secondary hyperparathyroidism (102). As already mentioned, C cells tend to aggregate in the vicinity of SCNs.

The main ultrastructural characteristic of C cells is the presence of secretory granules, which range in diameter from 60 to 550 nm (103). Two main types of granules have been identified. Type I granules have an average diameter of 280 nm and a moderately electron-dense, finely granular content which is closely applied to the limiting membranes of the granules. Type II granules are smaller (average diameter of 130 nm) with a more electron-dense content, which are separated from the limiting membranes by a small but distinct electron-lucent space. Most normal C cells are filled with type I secretory granules, with no or few type II granules. Immunocytochemical studies performed at the ultrastructural level have shown that both type I and II secretory granules contain immunoreactive CT (104).

Histochemistry and Immunohistochemistry

Histochemically, normal C cells are characterized by the following:

Argyrophilia
In sections stained with argyrophil techniques such as the Grimelius reaction or analogous stains, the cytoplasm of the C cell is characterized by the deposition of fine silver-positive granules (103).

Lead hematoxylin
The cytoplasm of C cells is selectively stained by this type of hematoxylin (105).

Toluidine blue and coriophosphine 0
These dyes confer marked metachromasia to C cells after acid hydrolysis of tissue sections (105).

Lectin Ulex europaeus agglutinin I
Selective reactivity to this marker has been demonstrated (106).

These methods, widely used in the past for the identification of C cells, have been largely replaced by the use of immunohistochemical techniques.

Immunohistochemically C cells have been found to be reactive to:

Calcitonin (Figure 44.12) (103,104,107,108).
Calcitonin gene–related peptide (CGRP) (109)
Katacalcin (110)
Somatostatin (111–113), *substance P* (114), *helodermin* (115) and ***gastrin-releasing peptide*** (116,117). A small proportion of CT-positive cells are also positive for these neuropeptides.

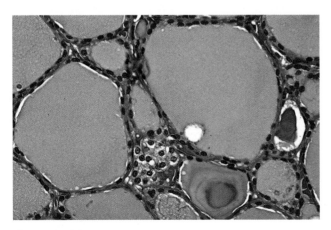

Figure 44.11 Clusters of C cells in the thyroid of an elderly individual with no known clinical or laboratory evidence of calcium disturbance.

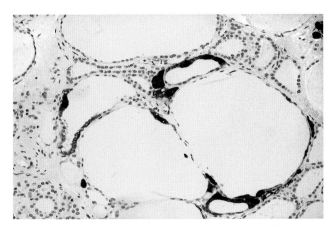

Figure 44.12 Immunoperoxidase stain for CT demonstrates C cells within follicles, arranged either individually or in small groups.

Thyrotropin-releasing hormone. In some species, C cells have been found to contain this hormone as detected immunohistochemically (118).

Serotonin and other biologically active amines (119).

Cytokeratins. C cells are immunoreactive only for low-molecular-weight keratin.

Pan-endocrine markers, such as neuron-specific enolase, chromogranin A, and synaptophysin (120).

Carcinoembryonic antigen (CEA) (103).

It is possible that neuroendocrine cells other than C cells exist in the thyroid and that they represent the cells of origin of the rare thyroid "neuroendocrine carcinomas" having histologic and immunohistochemical features different from those of medullary carcinoma.

Physiology

CT is a 32–amino acid peptide whose main function is the regulation of the level of calcium in the plasma by a feedback mechanism. This is brought about by the inhibition of osteoclastic activity. When calcium plasma levels are increased, CT is released from the thyroid. CT also acts in the kidney to enhance the production of vitamin D.

The major physiological role of CT is most likely the protection of the skeleton during periods of calcium stress such as growth, pregnancy and lactation (121). However, absence of CT is not associated with hypercalcemia, nor does a marked excess of the hormone (as seen in patients with medullary thyroid carcinoma) produce hypocalcemia. In addition to calcium, both gastrin and cholecystokinin induce the secretion of CT, as does the chronic administration of estrogenic hormones.

The CT gene is located on the short arm of chromosome 11 and consists of six axons that encode katacalcin (C-terminal flanking peptide) and CGRP (110,121,122). The primary transcript of the CT gene gives rise to two different mRNAs by tissue-specific alternative splicing events, leading to the production of CT and CGRP mRNAs. The CT-CGRP gene is expressed both in thyroid and nervous tissues, but CT is produced in large quantities only in the thyroid.

In normal male adults, basal CT levels range from 3 to 36 pg/ml (0.9 to 10.5 pmol/L). Plasma levels in females range from 3 to 17 pg/ml (0.9 to 5.0 pmol/L). Normal values after pentagastrin stimulation are less than 106 pg/ml (30.9 pmol/L) for males and less than 29 pg/ml (8.5 pmol/L) for females.

Katacalcin, the C-terminal flanking peptide of CT, is a 21–amino acid peptide that is cosecreted with CT in equimolar amounts (110). Its function, however, is unknown. CGRP is a 37–amino acid peptide that is an extremely potent vasodilator and also serves a neuromodulator or neurotransmitter function (121).

STROMA

Lymphocytes

In thyroids surgically resected because of a mass, it is not uncommon to observe in the interstitium of the normal portion of the gland a few collections of lymphocytes, sometimes admixed with rare plasma cells. Simple chronic thyroiditis and focal lymphocytic thyroiditis are the names given to this process that most likely does not represent a nosologic entity but rather the epiphenomenon of etiologically different conditions. Similar changes may in fact be seen in the proximity of neoplasms, in thyroids of patients taking lithium, or in individuals who have received low-dose external radiotherapy (123).

Fibrous Tissue

The usually thin fibrous septa that separate the thyroid lobules may exhibit microscopic variations. In a study on normal thyroids collected at autopsy from young adults, Komorowski and Hanson (22) found that 8% of the thyroid glands showed extensive fibrosis. According to their description, dense and largely acellular collagen fibers divided the thyroid into small nodules, giving it an appearance akin to micronodular cirrhosis of liver.

Another change that may occur in the interstitium, albeit rarely, is so-called multifocal sclerosing thyroiditis. It is characterized histologically by numerous microscopic foci of stellate-shaped fibrosis composed of cellular fibroblastic tissue frequently entrapping few thyroid follicles in the center. Even if at low power the individual lesions appear similar to those of papillary microcarcinoma, the epithelial component of such lesions lack the cytoarchitectural features of a papillary neoplasm (Figure 44.13A, B). Furthermore, the number of lesions in multifocal sclerosing thyroiditis greatly exceeds that seen in the usual case of papillary microcarcinoma. The etiology and pathogenesis of this process are not known.

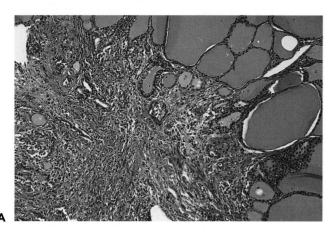
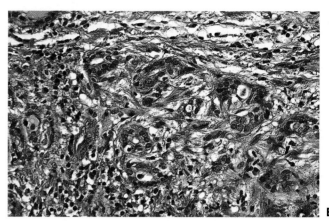

Figure 44.13 **A.** Multifocal sclerosing thyroiditis. On low power, the appearance resembles that of a papillary microcarcinoma. **B.** At higher power, the follicles entrapped in the fibrosis are irregularly shaped but do not show any of the cytologic features of papillary carcinoma.

Adipose Tissue and Skeletal Muscle

Thyroid stroma may undergo adipose metaplasia, resulting in the presence of islands of mature adipose tissue between follicles (Figure 44.14). Mature fat also occasionally may be seen in proximity to the thyroid gland capsule, its presence in this location most likely resulting from the close relationship of fat and thyroid tissue during fetal life (124).

Other tissues that grow in close proximity to the thyroid gland during their development and that can be found within the capsule of adults are cartilage and muscle.

In one study, striated muscle was found within the thyroid parenchyma of 19 glands, usually in the region of the isthmus or in the pyramidal lobe of the gland (22). Conversely, in 10 specimens thyroid follicles were found within fascicles of strap muscle from the same areas (Figure 44.15). Follicles entrapped in perithyroidal skeletal muscle are more easily identifiable when they undergo hyperplastic changes (125).

Calcification

Dystrophic calcifications may be seen in normal thyroid of old age, particularly in relation to vessels. They can easily be distinguished from psammoma bodies because of the lack of laminations and the irregularity of their contours.

Psammoma bodies rarely have been described in benign thyroid lesions but not in normal thyroids (126–128). Finding psammoma bodies in an otherwise normal thyroid or in a cervical lymph node should always prompt a careful search for an occult papillary carcinoma (Figure 44.16).

BRANCHIAL POUCH–DERIVED AND OTHER ECTOPIC TISSUES

Branchial pouch-related structures are found within the thyroid in various forms: solid cell rests (a remnant of the

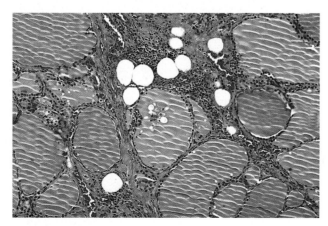

Figure 44.14 Adipose metaplasia of thyroid stroma. Mature adipocytes are seen between follicles.

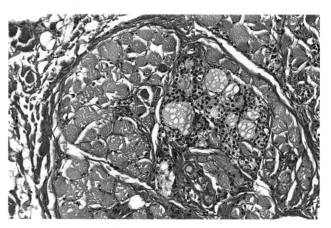

Figure 44.15 Clusters of thyroid tissue intimately admixed with bundles of skeletal muscle adjacent to the thyroid gland.

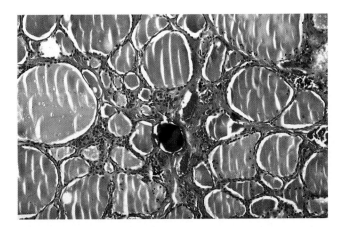

Figure 44.16 Psammoma body in nonneoplastic thyroid tissue adjacent to a papillary carcinoma (not shown in the picture).

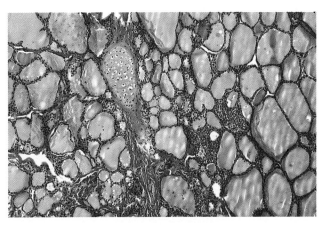

Figure 44.17 Cartilage island is seen in the proximity of SCNs.

ultimobranchial body or branchial pouch complex IV–V), epithelium-lined cysts, parathyroid glands, thymic tissue, salivary gland–type tissue, and heterotopic cartilage.

Solid Ultimobranchial Body Remnants (Solid Cell Nests)

So-called solid cell nests are clusters of epithelial cells interspersed among the follicles. Because they may exhibit squamous differentiation, they have sometimes been misinterpreted in the past as foci of squamous metaplasia in follicles (91). However, a UBB origin, for what in retrospect are clearly the same formations, had already been suggested by Erdheim in 1904 (129) and Getzowa in 1907 (130), following their demonstration of clusters of epithelial cells with solid or rarely cystic appearance in individuals with thyroid aplasia. Additional evidence along these lines was provided by the demonstration of marked similarities of human SCNs with the normal UBB of the rat and the hyperplastic or neoplastic UBB remnants in bulls (131–133).

SCNs are relatively common in normal thyroid, the probability of finding them increasing with the number of sections examined. In one study, SCNs were found in only 3% of routinely examined thyroids but in as many as 61% of specimens when the gland was blocked serially at 2- to 3-mm intervals (134). For unknown reasons SCNs are more common in males than in females. Most SCNs measure an average 0.1 mm in diameter, but occasionally they can reach 2 mm or more. They may be single or multiple. They are usually surrounded by stroma and more or less demarcated by the adjacent thyroid follicles. Adipose tissue and cartilage may be present in their vicinity (Figure 44.17). Most SCNs are found along the central axis of the middle and upper third of the lateral lobes (i.e., in the same area where C cells usually occur); this constitutes additional proof for their origin from the UBB, as it does the fact that the number of C cells is increased in the vicinity of SCNs (135,136).

SCNs are often grouped in clusters featuring a multilobed shape on low-power examination (Figure 44.18A). They have a dual cell population. The main component is made

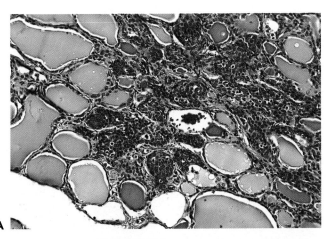
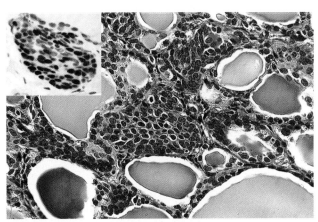

Figure 44.18 **A.** Low-power view shows the multilobed shape often exhibited by groups of SCNs. **B.** SCN in normal thyroid. Note the uniform appearance of the epithelial cells. **Inset:** Strong nuclear immunoreactivity for p63.

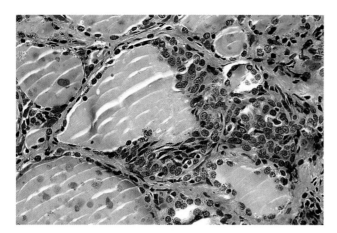

Figure 44.19 So-called mixed follicle. An SCN merges with a follicle lined by a flattened epithelium with colloid in the lumen.

up of cells of polygonal-to-oval shape, elongated nuclei with finely granular chromatin, and acidophilic cytoplasm. Some of these cells show clear-cut squamous differentiation. Immunohistochemically, they are reactive for high- and low-molecular-weight keratins, carcinoembryonic antigen (CEA) and p63 (Figure 44.18B). Ultrastructurally they feature bundles of tonofilaments, desmosomes, and intraluminal cytoplasmic projections (137–139). The positivity for p63 (a p53 homolog that is expressed in basal/stem cells of stratified epithelia), together with the expression of basal cell-type keratins (such as 34betaE12), telomerase and bcl-2, is compatible with a basal/stem cell phenotype for this cellular component (140,141). The second cell population, numerically less conspicuous, is characterized at the light microscopic level by clear cytoplasm and round nuclei, at the ultrastructural level by dense-core secretory granules, and at the immunohistochemical level by immunoreactivity to CT, CGRP, and chromogranin (135,137,138,142). All of these features are indicative of a C-cell nature for this population

and constitute a further link between SCNs and the UBBs. Cystic cavities containing acid mucin are frequently observed in association with SCNs (see next section). A variation in the theme is represented by the admixture of SCNs (pure or admixed with a cystic component) with groups of small follicles lined by low cuboidal TGB-immunoreactive epithelium, forming the so-called mixed follicles (Figure 44.19). The fact that a similar admixture is seen in mixed medullary-follicular carcinomas has led some investigators to suggest that these rare tumors may arise from uncommitted stem cells of the UBBs that have the potential to differentiate into C cells, follicular cells, or both (143).

SCNs need to be distinguished from collections of C cells, follicles with squamous metaplasia, and tangential sections of normal follicles (Figure 44.20).

Cystic Ultimobranchial Body Remnants

UBB remnants also may take the form of cysts. These occur most commonly in the soft tissues of the neck adjacent to the thyroid. Indeed, it is possible that some of the clinically evident branchial pouch cysts located in close proximity to the thyroid gland and sometimes confused clinically with thyroid lesions or lymph nodes are of UBB origin.

Cystic UBB remnants may also develop within the thyroid itself (144). In the latter instance, they may occur by themselves, may be adjacent to SCNs, or may be intimately admixed with them (Figure 44.21). The cysts are lined most frequently by a flattened multilayered epithelium of squamous type, and less commonly by a ciliated columnar epithelium (Figure 44.22) and often contain clumps of eosinophilic material in their lumen. They are especially common in neonates. Cystic UBB remants may have an associated lymphoid component (lymphoepithelial cysts) and are more commonly seen in glands with Hashimoto's thyroiditis (145–148). Pancreatic tissue, a representative of foregut remnants, has been described in the wall of perithyroidal epithelial cysts by Langlois et al. (149).

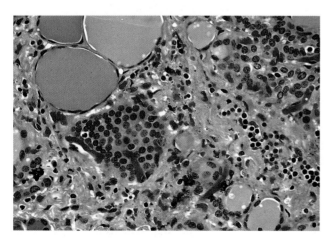

Figure 44.20 Tangential cut of a follicle. This should not be misinterpreted as an SCN.

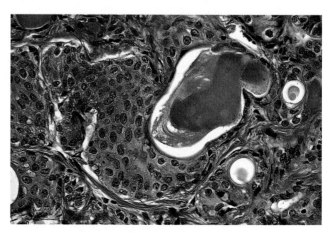

Figure 44.21 SCN with associated cystic formation. A dense eosinophilic material fills the lumen of the cyst.

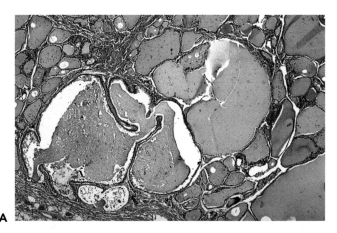

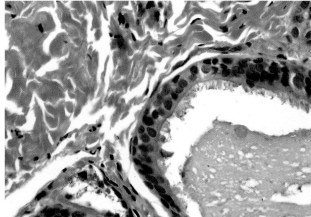

Figure 44.22   A. Intrathyroidal cyst of probable branchial pouch derivation. **B.** Higher-power view showing ciliated epithelium.

Parathyroid Tissue

The development of the parathyroid glands and the thymus from the branchial pouches in close proximity to the thyroid gland explains why these organs occasionally may be found adjacent to the thyroid capsule or even within the thyroid itself (Figure 44.23).

True intrathyroidal parathyroid glands in adults are rare. However, in a study where 58 human fetal thyroid glands obtained at autopsy were systematically studied for the presence of intrathyroidal parathyroid tissue, the latter was found in 13 thyroid lobes from 12 fetuses (22.4%). It was located subcapsularly in nine of 58 cases (15.5%), and it was lying deep in thyroid tissue in four (68%) (150). These intra- and perithyroidal parathyroid structures can be affected by primary or secondary chief cell hyperplasia, adenoma, or carcinoma and represent an often overlooked cause of surgical failure in primary hyperparathyroidism (151).

Thymic Tissue

Most of the thymus derives embryologically from the third branchial pouch, together with the lower pair of parathyroid glands. There is also a small and inconstant portion that derives from the fourth branchial pouch together with the upper pair of parathyroid glands and the UBB, which form the lateral thyroid anlage. It is from the latter source that the islands of thymic tissue occasionally found in or around the thyroid are thought to derive (Figure 44.24) (152). The fact that ectopic thymic tissue is observed more frequently in neonates and infants supports this hypothesis. Harach and Vujanic (153) searched systematically for the presence of intrathymic tissue in 58 thyroid glands obtained at autopsy from fetuses with proven retrosternal thymus. Subcapsular thymic tissue was found in two cases (3.4%) and intrathyroid thymic tissue in one (1.7%). An entire thymic gland within the thyroid of an infant has been described by Neill (154). Mizukami et al. (155) reported thymic tissue in the interlobular septum of the thyroid of a patient with Graves disease. Damiani et al. (156) found thymic rests in 1.4% of 2,575 adult thyroid glands that they examined.

Ectopic thymic tissue may show cystic changes and present clinically as a cystic neck mass. It also may be the source of peri- and intrathyroidal thymomas (157).

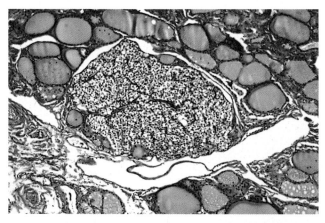

Figure 44.23   Parathyroid gland entirely located within thyroid.

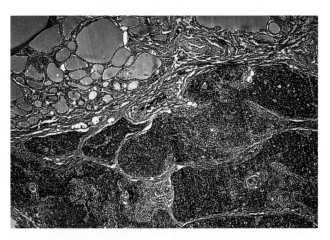

Figure 44.24   Intrathyroidal thymic tissue.

Salivary Gland–Type Tissue

Rarely salivary gland–type tissue has been found within the thyroid. Most of the reported cases have been seen in association with a benign thyroid condition, such as multinodular goiter (158).

Heterotopic Cartilage

Most intrathyroidal islands of mature cartilage probably represent remnants of the branchial pouch apparatus (18,159).

THYROID TISSUE IN ABNORMAL LOCATIONS

The presence of nonneoplastic thyroid tissue outside the normal anatomical confines of the gland may be caused by a variety of mechanisms, ranging from congenital abnormalities to acquired processes. Their main practical interest resides in the fact that lack of knowledge of their occurrence may lead to a mistaken diagnosis of metastatic thyroid carcinoma.

In Midline Structures

Ectopic thyroid is derived from abnormalities in migration patterns of the medial anlage and is therefore more commonly found in the neck in a midline position, at any point in the normal pathway of descent of the thyroglossal duct from the foramen cecum to the lower neck (160–162). In most cases the ectopy is partial, clinically insignificant, and discovered accidentally. The base of the tongue (lingual thyroid) and the hyoid bone and its surroundings (as a component of a thyroglossal cyst) are the most common sites. The opposite phenomenon is represented by exaggerated descent of the median anlage into the mediastinum, which may lead to location of thyroid tissue substernally in the preaortic area, in the pericardial cavity, and in the substance of the heart (163–165). However, the majority of mediastinal goiters represent a dislocation downward of normal glands that have been pulled down by the hyperplastic changes that occurred in them.

Lingual thyroid is a relatively common incidental microscopic finding. The follicles appear normal but because of their intimate relationship with the surrounding skeletal muscle they may raise the differential diagnosis with carcinoma (166). Sauk (167) and Baughman (168) found thyroid tissue in the tongue in 10% of individuals examined at autopsy, with the sex distribution being equal. The tongue is the most common location of ectopic thyroid tissue in the rare cases of total ectopy (169). In this condition ectopic glands are prone to functional insufficiency, frequently followed by compensatory hyperplasia, which may be the cause of dyspnea or dysphagia. Acute hypothyroidism may follow the removal of this ectopic tissue.

The other site where ectopic thyroid tissue is found more commonly is the wall of thyroglossal duct cysts. It appears in the form of small groups of follicles and is present in 25% to 65% of cysts examined histologically, its frequency being related to the number of sections submitted for histologic examination (170). The medial location and the presence of thyroid tissue in the wall distinguish thyroglossal duct cysts from the rarer branchial pouch cysts. Ectopic thyroid derived from abnormalities in migration of the medial anlage typically does not contain C cells. In one study of median anlage anomalies including 23 cases of thyroglossal cysts with adjacent thyroid tissue and one case of lingual thyroid, not a single C cell was found in either the thyroid tissue or the epithelium lining the cysts (17).

In Pericapsular Soft Tissues and Skeletal Muscles

As already discussed, the presence of thyroid tissue in these locations is not a rare event. It most likely results from the intimate relationship of the thyroid gland with the mesodermal structures of the neck during development.

In the Lateral Neck

This phenomenon, frequently referred to as lateral aberrant thyroid, has different pathogeneses. It has been suggested that surgery and trauma may cause implantation of thyroid tissue in the lateral neck. Typically when this is the case, a few nodules of normal-appearing thyroid tissue, always of microscopic size and frequently surrounded by a fibrous capsule, are seen in the lateral neck close to the cervical lymph nodes (171–173). History of previous trauma or surgery on the neck, the presence of suture material (in cases of previous surgery), and the benign appearance of the dislocated thyroid tissue are useful in distinguishing them from metastatic carcinoma. It has to be kept in mind that the latter may appear deceptively benign on microscopic examination. Spontaneous separation of thyroid tissue with subsequent implant in the lateral neck may occur in nodular goiter or Hashimoto's thyroiditis (174,175). In both of these conditions, nodules of thyroid tissue extrude and separate from the surface of the gland and deposit in the extrathyroidal soft tissue, where they may acquire an autonomous blood supply (so-called parasitic nodules). The differential diagnosis with metastatic lymph nodes may be very problematic, especially in the presence of Hashimoto's thyroiditis.

In Cervical Lymph Nodes

Normal-appearing thyroid tissue in medially located cervical lymph nodes is rarely the result of a developmental

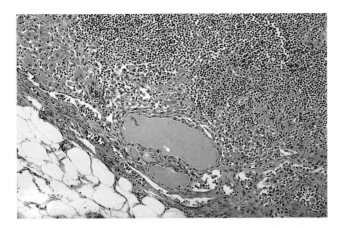

Figure 44.25 A group of benign-appearing thyroid follicles is seen close to the marginal sinus of a cervical lymph node. This patient did not have a carcinoma in the thyroid gland.

anomaly (176). When this is the case, a few microscopic nests of benign-looking follicles are seen in the marginal sinus of the lymph node (Figure 44.25). The follicular cells that compose them should lack all of the cytologic features typical of papillary carcinoma (177). Psammoma bodies and papillae should also be absent. Numerous sections are sometimes needed to rule out a metastasis from a papillary microcarcinoma, which is by far the most frequent cause of thyroid tissue in cervical nodes.

In Other Sites

Rarely, one can find thyroid tissue in locations outside its place of embryonic development and occasionally quite distantly from it. These locations include the sella turcica, larynx, trachea, esophagus, heart, diaphragm, gallbladder, common bile duct, region of the porta hepatis, retroperitoneum, inguinal region, adrenal gland, uterus, vagina, and—last but not least—the ovary. In the latter site, the thyroid tissue represents a component of a teratoma and sometimes is the only evidence for it *(struma ovarii)* (178–185).

REFERENCES

1. Hoyes AD, Kershaw DR. Anatomy and development of the thyroid gland. *Ear Nose Throat J* 1985;64:318–333.
2. Shepard TH. Onset of function in the human fetal thyroid: biochemical and radioautographic studies from organ culture. *J Clin Endocrinol Metab* 1967;27:945–958.
3. Gitlin D, Biasucci A. Ontogenesis of immunoreactive thyroglobulin in the human conceptus. *J Clin Endocrinol Metab* 1969;29: 849–853.
4. Pasca di Magliano M, Di Lauro R, Zannini M. Pax8 has a key role in thyroid cell differentiation. *Proc Natl Acad Sci U S A* 2000;97: 13144–13149.
5. Trueba SS, Auge J, Mattei G, et al. PAX8, TITF1, and FOXE1 gene expression patterns during human development: new insights into human thyroid development and thyroid dysgenesis-associated malformations. *J Clin Endocrinol Metab* 2005;90:455–462.
6. Volante M, Allia E, Fulcheri E, et al. Ghrelin in fetal thyroid and follicular tumors and cell lines: expression and effects on tumor growth. *Am J Pathol* 2003;162:645–654.
7. Savin SB, Cvejic DS, Jankovic MM. Expression of galectin-1 and galectin-3 in human fetal thyroid gland. *J Histochem Cytochem* 2003;51:479–483.
8. Norris EH. The parathyroid glands and the lateral thyroid in man: their morphogenesis, histogenesis, topographic anatomy and prenatal growth. *Contrib Embryol Carnegie Inst* 1937;159: 249–294.
9. Chan AS, Conen PE. Ultrastructural observations on cytodifferentiation of parafollicular cells in the human fetal thyroid. *Lab Invest* 1971;25:249–259.
10. Sugiyama S. The embryology of the human thyroid gland including ultimobranchial body and others related. *Ergeb Anat Entwicklungsgesch* 1971;44:3–111.
11. Le Dourain NM, Teillet MA. The migration of neural crest cells to the wall of the digestive tract in avian embryo. *J Embryol Exp Morphol* 1973;30:31–48.
12. Le Douarin N, Fontaine J, Le Lievre C. New studies on the neural crest origin of the avian ultimobranchial glandular cells— interspecific combinations and cytochemical characterization of C cells based on the uptake of biogenic amine precursors. *Histochemistry* 1974;38:297–305.
13. Nadiz J, Weber E, Hedinger C. C-cell in vestiges of the ultimobranchial body in human thyroid glands. *Virchows Arch B Cell Pathol* 1978;27:189–191.
14. Ito M, Kameda Y, Tagawa T. An ultrastructural study of the cysts in chicken ultimobranchial glands, with special reference to C-cells. *Cell Tissue Res* 1986;246:39–44.
15. Conley ME, Beckwith JB, Tenckhoff L. The spectrum of the DiGeorge syndrome. *J Pediatr* 1979;94:883–890.
16. Burke BA, Johnson D, Gilbert EF, Drut RM, Ludwig J, Wick MR. Thyrocalcitonin-containing cells in the DiGeorge anomaly. *Hum Pathol* 1987;18:355–360.
17. Ljungberg O. *Biopsy Pathology of the Thyroid and Parathyroid.* London: Chapman & Hall; 1992.
18. Williams ED, Toyn CE, Harach HR. The ultimobranchial gland and congenital thyroid abnormalities in man. *J Pathol* 1989;159: 135–141.
19. Harada T, Nishikawa Y, Ito K. Aplasia of one thyroid lobe. *Am J Surg* 1972;124:617–619.
20. Hegedus L, Perrild H, Poulsen LR, et al. The determination of thyroid volume by ultrasound and its relationship to body weight, age, and sex in normal subjects. *J Clin Endocrinol Metab* 1983;56:260–263.
21. Hegedus L, Karstrup S, Rasmussen N. Evidence of cyclic alterations of thyroid size during the menstrual cycle in healthy women. *Am J Obstet Gynecol* 1986;155:142–145.
22. Komorowski RA, Hanson GA. Occult thyroid pathology in the young adult: an autopsy study of 138 patients without clinical thyroid disease. *Hum Pathol* 1988;19:689–696.
23. Bell CD, Kovacs K, Horvath E, Rotondo F. Histologic, immunohistochemical, and ultrastructural findings in a case of minocycline-associated "black thyroid." *Endocr Pathol* 2001;12:443–451.
24. Landas SK, Schelper RL, Tio FO, Turner JW, Moore KC, Bennett-Gray J. Black thyroid syndrome: exaggeration of a normal process? *Am J Clin Pathol* 1986;85:411–418.
25. Brown RA, Al-Moussa M, Beck J. Histometry of normal thyroid in man. *J Clin Pathol* 1986;39:475–482.
26. Imada M, Kurosumi M, Fujita H. Three-dimensional imaging of blood vessels in thyroids from normal and levothyroxine sodium-treated rats. *Arch Histol Jpn* 1986;49:359–367.
27. Imada M, Kurosumi M, Fujita H. Three-dimensional aspects of blood vessels in thyroids from normal, low iodine diet-treated, TSH-treated and PTU-treated rats. *Cell Tissue Res* 1986;245: 291–296.
28. Feind C. The head and neck. In: Haagensen CD, Feind C, Herter FP, Slanetz CA Jr, Weinberg JA, eds. *The Lymphatics in Cancer.* Philadelphia: WB Saunders; 1972:59–222.
29. Crile G Jr. The fallacy of the conventional radical neck dissection for papillary carcinoma of the thyroid. *Ann Surg* 1957;145: 317–320.

30. Uchiyama Y, Murakami G, Ohno Y. The fine structure of nerve endings on rat thyroid follicular cells. *Cell Tissue Res* 1985;242: 457–460.

31. Melander A, Ericson LD, Sundler F, Ingbar SH. Sympathetic innervation of the mouse thyroid and its significance in thyroid hormone secretion. *Endocrinology* 1974;94:959–966.

32. Tice LW, Creveling CR. Electron microscopic identification of adrenergic nerve endings on thyroid epithelial cells. *Endocrinology* 1975;97:1123–1129.

33. Ingbar SH. The thyroid gland. In: Wilson JD, Foster DW, eds. *Williams Textbook of Endocrinology*. 7th ed. Philadelphia: WB Saunders; 1985:682–815.

34. Kameda Y, Okamoto K, Ito M, Tagawa T. Innervation of the C cells of chicken ultimobranchial glands studied by immunohistochemistry, fluorescence microscopy, and electron microscopy. *Am J Anat* 1988;182:353–368.

35. Heimann P. Ultrastructure of human thyroid. A study of normal thyroid, untreated and treated diffuse goiter. *Acta Endocrinol (Copenh)* 1966;53(suppl 110):1–102.

36. Klinck GH, Oertel JE, Winship T. Ultrastructure of normal human thyroid. *Lab Invest* 1970;22:2–22.

37. Kurata A, Ohta K, Mine M, et al. Monoclonal antihuman thyroglobulin antibodies. *J Clin Endocrinol Metab* 1984;59:573–579.

38. Stanta G, Carcangiu ML, Rosai J. The biochemical and immunohistochemical profile of thyroid neoplasia. *Pathol Annu* 1988; 23(pt 1):129–157.

39. Rosai J, Carcangiu ML. Pitfalls in the diagnosis of thyroid neoplasms. *Pathol Res Pract* 1987;182:169–179.

40. Katoh R, Kawaoi A, Miyagi E, et al. Thyroid transcription factor-1 in normal, hyperplastic, and neoplastic follicular thyroid cells examined by immunohistochemistry and nonradioactive in situ hybridization. *Mod Pathol* 2000;13:570–576.

41. Lau SK, Luthringer DJ, Eisen RN. Thyroid transcription factor-1: a review. *Appl Immunohistochem Mol Morphol* 2002;10:97–102.

42. Miettinen M, Franssila K, Lehto VP, Paasivuo R, Virtanen I. Expression of intermediate filament proteins in thyroid gland and thyroid tumors. *Lab Invest* 1984;50:262–270.

43. Miettinen M, Kovatich AJ, Karkkainen P. Keratin subsets in papillary and follicular thyroid lesions. A paraffin section analysis with diagnostic implications. *Virchows Arch* 1997;431:407–413.

44. Fonseca E, Nesland JM, Hoie J, Sobrinho-Simoes M. Pattern of expression of intermediate cytokeratin filaments in the thyroid gland: an immunohistochemical study of simple and stratified epithelial-type cytokeratins. *Virchows Arch* 1997;430:239–245.

45. Viale G, Dell'Orto P, Coggi G, Gambacorta M. Coexpression of cytokeratins and vimentin in normal and diseased thyroid glands. Lack of diagnostic utility of vimentin immunostaining. *Am J Surg Pathol* 1989;13:1034–1040.

46. Bur M, Shiraki W, Masood S. Estrogen and progesterone receptor detection in neoplastic and non-neoplastic thyroid tissues. *Mod Pathol* 1993;6:469–472.

47. Kawabata W, Suzuki T, Moriya T, et al. Estrogen receptors (alpha and beta) and 17beta-hydroxysteroid dehydrogenase type 1 and 2 in thyroid disorders: possible in situ estrogen synthesis and actions. *Mod Pathol* 2003;16:437–444.

48. McLaren KM, Cossar DW. The immunohistochemical localization of S100 in the diagnosis of papillary carcinoma of the thyroid. *Hum Pathol* 1996;27 633–636.

49. Nishimura R, Yokose T, Mukai K. S-100 protein is a differentiation marker in thyroid carcinoma of follicular cell origin: an immunohistochemical study. *Pathol Int* 1997;47:673–679.

50. Westermark K, Lundqvist M, Wallin G. EGF-receptors in human normal and pathological thyroid tissue. *Histopathology* 1996;28: 221–227.

51. Lima MA, Gontijo VA, Schmitt FC. Thyroid peroxidase and thyroglobulin expression in normal human thyroid glands. *Endocr Pathol* 1998;9:333–338.

52. Lin JD, Hsueh C, Chao TC, Weng HF. Expression of sodium iodide symporter in benign and malignant human thyroid tissues. *Endocr Pathol* 2001;12:15–21.

53. Ringel MD, Anderson J, Souza SL, et al. Expression of the sodium iodide symporter and thyroglobulin genes are reduced in papillary thyroid cancer. *Mod Pathol* 2001;14:289–296.

54. Maruyama M, Kato R, Kobayashi S, Kasuga Y. A method to differentiate between thyroglobulin derived from normal thyroid tissue and from thyroid carcinoma based on analysis of reactivity to lectins. *Arch Pathol Lab Med* 1998;122:715–720.

55. de Martynoff G, Pohl V, Mercken L, van Ommen GJ, Vassart G. Structural organization of the bovine thyroglobulin gene and of its 5'-flanking region. *Eur J Biochem* 1987;164:591–599.

56. Christophe D, Gerard C, Juvenal G, et al. Identification of a cAMP-responsive region in thyroglobulin gene promoter. *Mol Cell Endocrinol* 1989;64:5–18.

57. Lee NT, Nayfeh SN, Chae CB. Induction of nuclear protein factors specific for hormone-responsive region during activation of thyroglobulin gene by thyrotropin in rat thyroid FRTL-5 cells. *J Biol Chem* 1989;264:7523–7530.

58. Green WL. Physiology of the thyroid gland and its hormones. In: Green WL, ed. *The Thyroid*. New York: Elsevier; 1987:1–46.

59. Bjorkman U, Ekholm R, Elmqvist LG, Ericson LE, Melander A, Smeds S. Induced unidirectional transport of protein into the thyroid follicular lumen. *Endocrinology* 1974;95:1506–1517.

60. Ericson LE, Engstrom G. Quantitative electron microscopic studies on exocytosis and endocytosis in the thyroid follicle cell. *Endocrinology* 1978;103:883–892.

61. Ide M. Immunoelectron microscopic localization of thyroglobulin in the human thyoid gland. *Acta Pathol Jpn* 1984;34: 575–584.

62. Sterling K. Thyroid hormone action at the cell level (first of two parts). *N Engl J Med* 1979;300:117–123.

63. Liddle GW, Liddle RA. Endocrinology. In: Smith LH, Thier SO, eds. *Pathophysiology: The Biological Prinicples of Disease*. Philadelphia: WB Saunders; 1981.

64. Müller MJ, Seitz HJ. Thyroid hormone action on intermediary metabolism. Part I. Respiration, thermogenesis and carbohydrate metabolism. *Klin Wochenschr* 1984;62:11–18.

65. Müller MJ, Seitz HJ. Thyroid hormone action on intermediary metabolism. II. Lipid metabolism in hyper- and hypothyroidism. *Klin Wochenschr* 1984;62:49–55.

66. Müller MJ, Seitz HJ. Thyroid hormone action on intermediary metabolism. Part III. Protein metabolism in hyper- and hypothyroidism. *Klin Wochenschr* 1984;62:97–102.

67. Oppenheimer JH. Thyroid hormone action at the nuclear level. *Ann Intern Med* 1985;102:374–384.

68. Oppenheimer JH, Samuels HH, eds. *Molecular Basis of Thyroid Hormone Action*. New York: Academic Press; 1983.

69. Larsen PR. Thyroid–pituitary interaction: feedback regulation of thyrotropin secretion by thyroid hormones. *N Engl J Med* 1982;306:23–32.

70. Davies T, Marians R, Latif R. The TSH receptor reveals itself. *J Clin Invest* 2002;110:161–164.

71. Farid NR, Szkudlinski MW. Minireview: structural and functional evolution of the thyrotropin receptor. *Endocrinology* 2004;145: 4048–4057.

72. Pittman JA Jr. Thyrotropin-releasing hormone. *Adv Intern Med* 1974;19:303–325.

73. Wilber JF. Thyrotropin releasing hormone: secretion and actions. *Annu Rev Med* 1973;24:353–364.

74. Walsh FM, Castelli JB. Polytef granuloma clinically simulating carcinoma of the thyroid. *Arch Otolaryngol* 1975;101:262–263.

75. Sanfilippo F, Shelburne J, Ingram P. Analysis of a polytef granuloma mimicking a cold thyroid nodule 17 months after laryngeal injection. *Ultrastruct Pathol* 1980;1:471–475.

76. Chaplin AJ. Histopathological occurrence and characterization of calcium oxalate: a review. *J Clin Pathol* 1977;30:800–811.

77. Carney JA, Moore SB, Northcutt RC, Woolner LB, Stillwell GK. Palpation thyroiditis (multifocal granulomatous folliculitis). *Am J Clin Pathol* 1975;64:639–647.

78. Blum M, Schloss MF. Martial-arts thyroiditis. *N Engl J Med* 1984;311:199–200.

79. Harach R, Jasani B. Thyroid multifocal granulomatous folliculitis (palpation thyroiditis): an immunocytochemical study. *Endocr Pathol* 1993;4:105–109.

80. Hellwig CA. Colloidophagy in the human thyroid gland. *Science* 1951;113:725–726.

81. Manson C, Cross P, De Sousa B. Post-operative necrotizing granulomas of the thyroid. *Histopathology* 1992;21:392–393.

82. Harach HR. Palpation thyroiditis resembling C cell hyperplasia. Usefulness of immunohistochemistry in their differential diagnosis. *Pathol Res Pract* 1993;189:488–490.

83. Richter MN, McCarty KS. Anisotropic crystals in the human thyroid gland. *Am J Pathol* 1954;30:545–553.

84. Katoh R, Suzuki K, Hemmi A, Kawaoi A. Nature and significance of calcium oxalate crystals in normal human thyroid gland. A clinicopathological and immunohistochemical study. *Virchows Arch A Pathol Anat Histopathol* 1993;422:301–306.

85. Reid JD, Choi CH, Oldroyd NO. Calcium oxalate crystals in the thyroid. Their identification, prevalence, origin, and possible significance. *Am J Clin Pathol* 1987;87:443–454.

86. Gross S. Granulomatous thyroiditis with anisotropic crystalline material. *AMA Arch Pathol* 1955;59:412–418.

87. Fayemi AO, Ali M, Braun EV. Oxalosis in hemodialysis patients: a pathologic study of 80 cases. *Arch Pathol Lab Med* 1979;103:58–62.

88. Isotalo PA, Lloyd RV. Presence of birefringent crystals is useful in distinguishing thyroid from parathyroid gland tissues. *Am J Surg Pathol* 2002;26:813–814.

89. Klinck G, Menk K. Squamous cells in the human thyroid. *Mil Surgeon* 1951;109:406–414.

90. Harcourt-Webster JN. Squamous epithelium in the human thyroid gland. *J Clin Pathol* 1966;19:384–388.

91. LiVolsi VA, Merino MJ. Squamous cells in the human thyroid gland. *Am J Surg Pathol* 1978;2:133–140.

92. Pearse AG. The cytochemistry of the thyroid C cells and their relationship to calcitonin. *Proc R Soc Lond B Biol Sci* 1966;164:478–487.

93. Teitlebaum SL, Moore KE, Shieber W. Parafollicular cells in the normal human thyroid. *Nature* 1971;230:334–335.

94. Wolfe HJ, DeLellis RA, Voelkel EF, Tashjian AH Jr. Distribution of calcitonin-containing cells in the normal neonatal human thyroid gland: a correlation of morphology with peptide content. *J Clin Endocrinol Metab* 1975;41:1076–1081.

95. O'Toole K, Fenoglio-Preiser C, Pushparaj N. Endocrine changes associated with the human aging process. III. Effect of age on the number of calcitonin immunoreactive cells in the thyroid gland. *Hum Pathol* 1985;16:991–1000.

96. Gibson WCH, Peng TC, Croker BP. Age-associated C-cell hyperplasia in the human thyroid. *Am J Pathol* 1982;106:388–393.

97. Albores-Saavedra J, Gorraez de la Mora T, de la Torre-Rendon F, Gould E. Mixed medullary-papillary carcinoma of the thyroid: a previously unrecognized variant of thyroid carcinoma. *Hum Pathol* 1990;21:1151–1155.

98. Scopsi L, Di Palma S, Ferrari C, Holst JJ, Rehfeld JF, Rilke F. C-cell hyperplasia accompanying thyroid diseases other than medullary carcinoma: an immunocytochemical study by means of antibodies to calcitonin and somatostatin. *Mod Pathol* 1991;4:297–304.

99. Libbey NP, Nowakowski KJ, Tucci JR. C-cell hyperplasia of the thyroid in a patient with goitrous hypothyroidism and Hashimoto's thyroiditis. *Am J Surg Pathol* 1989;13:71–77.

100. Biddinger PW, Brennan MF, Rosen PP. Symptomatic C-cell hyperplasia associated with chronic lymphocytic thyroiditis. *Am J Surg Pathol* 1991;15:599–604.

101. Guyetant S, Wion-Barbot N, Rousselet MC, Franc B, Bigorgne JC, Saint-Andre JP. C-cell hyperplasia associated with chronic lymphocytic thyroiditis: a retrospective quantitative study of 112 cases. *Hum Pathol* 1994;25:514–521.

102. Tomita T, Millard DM. C-cell hyperplasia in secondary hyperparathyroidism. *Histopathology* 1992;21:469–474.

103. DeLellis RA, Wolfe HJ. The pathobiology of the human calcitonin (C)-cell: a review. *Pathol Annu* 1981;16(pt 2):25–52.

104. DeLellis RA, Nunnemacher G, Wolfe HJ. C-cell hyperplasia. An ultrastructural analysis. *Lab Invest* 1977;36:237–248.

105. Pearse AG. Common cytochemical and ultrastructural characteristics of cells producing polypeptide hormones (the APUD series) and their relevance to thyroid and ultimobranchial C cells and calcitonin. *Proc R Soc Lond B Biol Sci* 1968;170:71–80.

106. Gonzalez-Campora R, Sanchez Gallego F, Martin Lacave I, Mora Marin J, Montero Linares C, Galera-Davidson H. Lectin histochemistry of the thyroid gland. *Cancer* 1988;62:2354–2362.

107. Bussolati G, Pearse AG. Immunofluorescent localization of calcitonin in the 'C' cells of pig and dog thyroid. *J Endocrinol* 1967;37:205–209.

108. McMillan PJ, Hooker WM, Deptos LJ. Distribution of calcitonin-containing cells in the human thyroid. *Am J Anat* 1974;140:73–79.

109. Schmid KW, Kirchmair R, Ladurner D, Fischer-Colbrie R, Bocker W. Immunohistochemical comparison of chromogranins A and B and secretogranin II with calcitonin and calcitonin gene-related peptide expression in normal, hyperplastic and neoplastic C-cells of the human thyroid. *Histopathology* 1992;21:225–232.

110. Ali-Rachedi A, Varndell IM, Facer P, et al. Immunocytochemical localization of katacalcin, a calcium-lowering hormone cleaved from the human calcitonin precursor. *J Clin Endocrinol Metab* 1983;57:680–682.

111. Van Noorden S, Polak JM, Pearse AG. Single cellular origin of somatostatin and calcitonin in the rat thyroid gland. *Histochemistry* 1977;53:243–247.

112. Yamada Y, Ito S, Matsubara Y, Kobayashi S. Immunohistochemical demonstration of somatostatin-containing cells in the human, dog and rat thyroids. *Tohoku J Exp Med* 1977;122:87–92.

113. Kusumoto Y. Calcitonin and somatostatin are localized in different cells in the canine thyroid gland. *Biomed Res* 1980;1:237–241.

114. Kakudo K, Vacca LL. Immunohistochemical study of substance P-like immunoreactivity in human thyroid and medullary carcinoma of the thyroid. *J Submicrosc Cytol* 1983;15:563–568.

115. Sundler F, Christophe J, Robberecht P, et al. Is helodermin produced by medullary thyroid carcinoma cells and normal C-cells? Immunocytochemical evidence. *Regul Pept* 1988;20:83–89.

116. Kameya T, Bessho T, Tsumuraya M, et al. Production of gastrin releasing peptide by medullary carcinoma of the thyroid. An immunohistochemical study. *Virchows Arch A Pathol Anat Histopathol* 1983;401:99–107.

117. Sunday ME, Wolfe HJ, Roos BA, Chin WW, Spindel ER. Gastrin-releasing peptide gene expression in developing hyperplastic, and neoplastic human thyroid C-cells. *Endocrinology* 1988;122:1551–1558.

118. Gkonos PJ, Tavianini MA, Liu CC, Roos BA. Thyrotropin-releasing hormone gene expression in normal thyroid parafollicular cells. *Mol Endocrinol* 1989;3:2101–2109.

119. Nunez EA, Gershon MD. Thyrotropin-induced thyroidal release of 5-hydroxytryptamine and accompanying ultrastructural changes in parafollicular cells. *Endocrinology* 1983;113:309–317.

120. DeLellis RA. Endocrine tumors. In: Colvin RB, Bhan AK, McCluskey RT, eds. *Diagnostic Immunopathology*. New York: Raven Press; 1988.

121. MacIntyre I. Calcitonin: physiology, biosynthesis, secretion, metabolism and mode of action. In: DeGroot LJ, ed. *Endocrinology*. 2nd ed. Vol 2. Philadelphia: WB Saunders; 1989:892–901.

122. Amara SG, Jonas V, Rosenfeld MG, Ong ES, Evans RM. Alternative RNA processing in calcitonin gene expression generates mRNAs encoding different polypeptide products. *Nature* 1982;298:240–244.

123. Kontozoglou T, Mambo N. The histopathologic features of lithium-associated thyroiditis. *Hum Pathol* 1983;14:737–739.

124. Carpenter GR, Emery JL. Inclusions in the human thyroid. *J Anat* 1976;122(pt 1):77–89.

125. Gardiner WR. Unusual relationships between thyroid gland and skeletal muscle in infants; a review of the literature and four case reports. *Cancer* 1956;9:681–691.

126. Klinck GH, Winship T. Psammoma bodies and thyroid cancer. *Cancer* 1959;12:656–662.

127. Batsakis JG, Nishiyama RH, Rich CR. Microlithiasis (calcospherites) and carcinoma of the thyroid gland. *Arch Pathol* 1960;69:493–498.

128. Dugan JM, Atkinson BF, Avitabile A, Schimmel M, LiVolsi VA. Psammoma bodies in fine needle aspirate of the thyroid in lymphocytic thyroiditis. *Acta Cytol* 1987;31:330–334.

129. Erdheim J. I. Uber Schilddrusenaplasie. II. Geschwulste des Ductus Thyreoglossus. III. Uber einige menschliche Kiemenderivate. *Beitr Pathol Anat* 1904;35:366–433.

130. Getzowa S. Zur Kenntnis des postbranchialen Korpers und der branchialen Kanalchen des Menschen. *Virchows Arch* 1907;88: 181–235.

131. Calvert R, Isler H. Fine structure of a third epithelial component of the thyroid gland of the rat. *Anat Rec* 1970;168:23–41.

132. Black HE, Capen CC, Young DM. Ultimobranchial thyroid neoplasms in bulls. A syndrome resembling medullary thyroid carcinoma in man. *Cancer* 1973;32:865–878.

133. Ljungberg O, Nilsson PO. Hyperplastic and neoplastic changes in ultimobranchial remnants and in parafollicular (C) cells in bulls: a histologic and immunohistochemical study. *Vet Pathol* 1985;22:95–103.

134. Harach HR. Solid cell nests of the human thyroid in early stages of postnatal life. Systematic autopsy study. *Acta Anat (Basel)* 1986;127:262–264.

135. Janzer RC, Weber E, Hedinger C. The relation between solid cell nests and C cells of the thyroid gland: an immunohistochemical and morphometric investigation. *Cell Tissue Res* 1979;197: 295–312.

136. Chan JK, Tse CC. Solid cell nest–associated C-cells: another possible explanation for "C-cell hyperplasia" adjacent to follicular cell tumors. *Hum Pathol* 1989;20:498–499.

137. Cameselle-Teijeiro J, Varela-Duran J, Sambade C, Villanueva JP, Varela-Nunez R, Sobrinho-Simoes M. Solid cell nests of the thyroid: light microscopy and immunohistochemical profile. *Hum Pathol* 1994;25:684–693.

138. Mizukami Y, Nonomura A, Michigishi T, et al. Solid cell nests of the thyroid. A histologic and immunohistochemical study. *Am J Clin Pathol* 1994;101:186–191.

139. Yamaoka Y. Solid cell nest (SCN) of the human thyroid gland. *Acta Pathol Jpn* 1973;23:493–506.

140. Reis-Filho JS, Preto A, Soares P, Ricardo S, Cameselle-Teijeiro J, Sobrinho-Simoes M. p63 expression in solid cell nests of the thyroid: further evidence for a stem cell origin. *Mod Pathol* 2003;16:43–48.

141. Preto A, Cameselle-Teijeiro J, Moldes-Boullosa J, et al. Telomerase expression and proliferative activity suggest a stem cell role for thyroid solid cell nests. *Mod Pathol* 2004;17:819–826.

142. Martin V, Martin L, Viennet G, Hergel M, Carbillet JP, Fellmann D. Ultrastructural features of "solid cell nest" of the human thyroid gland: a study of 8 cases. *Ultrastruct Pathol* 2000;24:1–8.

143. Ljungberg O, Nilsson PO. Intermediate thyroid carcinoma in humans and ultimobranchial tumors in bulls: a comparative morphological and immunohistochemical study. *Endocr Pathol* 1991;2:24–39.

144. Beckner ME, Shultz JJ, Richardson T. Solid and cystic ultimobranchial body remnants in the thyroid. *Arch Pathol Lab Med* 1990;114:1049–1052.

145. Louis DN, Vickery AL Jr, Rosai J, Wang CA. Multiple branchial cleft–like cysts in Hashimoto's thyroiditis. *Am J Surg Pathol* 1989;13:45–49.

146. Apel RL, Asa SL, Chalvardjian A, LiVolsi VA. Intrathyroidal lymphoepithelial cysts of probable branchial origin. *Hum Pathol* 1994;25:1238–1242.

147. Streutker CJ, Murray D, Kovacs K, Higgins HP. Epithelial cyst of thyroid. *Endocr Pathol* 1997;8:75–80.

148. Ryska A, Vokurka J, Michal M, Ludvikova M. Intrathyroidal lymphoepithelial cyst. A report of two cases not associated with Hashimoto's thyroiditis. *Pathol Res Pract* 1997;193:777–781.

149. Langlois NE, Krukowski ZH, Miller ID. Pancreatic tissue in a lateral cervical cyst attached to the thyroid gland—a presumed foregut remnant. *Histopathology* 1997;31:378–380.

150. Harach HR, Vujanic GM. Intrathyroidal parathyroid. *Pediatr Pathol* 1993;13:71–74.

151. Spiegel AM, Marx SJ, Doppman JL, et al. Intrathyroidal parathyroid adenoma or hyperplasia. An occasionally overlooked cause of surgical failure in primary hyperparathyroidism. *JAMA* 1975;234:1029–1033.

152. LiVolsi V. Branchial and thymic remnants in the thyroid and cervical region: an explanation for unusual tumors and microscopic curiosities. *Endocr Pathol* 1993;4:115–119.

153. Harach HR, Vujanic GM. Intrathyroidal thymic tissue: an autopsy study in fetuses with some emphasis on pathological implications. *Pediatr Pathol* 1993;13:431–434.

154. Neill J. Intrathyroid thymoma. *Am J Surg Pathol* 1986;10: 660–661.

155. Mizukami Y, Nonomura A, Michigishi T, et al. Ectopic thymic tissue in the thyroid gland. *Endocr Pathol* 1993;4:162–164.

156. Damiani S, Filotico M, Eusebi V. Carcinoma of the thyroid showing thymoma-like features. *Virchows Arch A Pathol Anat Histopathol* 1991;418:463–466.

157. Miyauchi A, Kuma K, Matsuzuka F, et al. Intrathyroidal epithelial thymoma: an entity distinct from squamous cell carcinoma of the thyroid. *World J Surg* 1985;9:128–135.

158. Cameselle-Teijeiro J, Varela-Duran J. Intrathyroid salivary gland-type tissue in multinodular goiter. *Virchows Arch* 1994;425: 331–334.

159. Finkle HI, Goldman RL. Heterotopic cartilage in the thyroid. *Arch Pathol* 1973;95:48–49.

160. Guimaraes SB, Uceda JE, Lynn HB. Thyroglossal duct remnants in infants and children. *Mayo Clin Proc* 1972;47:117–120.

161. Ellis PD, Van Nostrand AW. The applied anatomy of thyroglossal tract remnants. *Laryngoscope* 1977;87(pt 1):765–770.

162. Larochelle D, Arcand P, Belzile M, Gagnon NB. Ectopic thyroid tissue—a review of the literature. *J Otolaryngol* 1979;8: 523–530.

163. De Andrade MA. A review of 128 cases of posterior mediastinal goiter. *World J Surg* 1977;1:789–797.

164. de Souza FM, Smith PE. Retrosternal goiter. *J Otolaryngol* 1983;12:393–396.

165. Kantelip B, Lusson JR, De Riberolles C, Lamaison D, Bailly P. Intracardiac ectopic thyroid. *Hum Pathol* 1986;17:1293–1296.

166. Wapshaw H. Lingual thyroid. A report of a case with unusual histology. *Br J Surg* 1974;30:160–165.

167. Sauk JJ Jr. Ectopic lingual thyroid. *J Pathol* 1970;102:239–243.

168. Baughman RA. Lingual thyroid and lingual thyroglossal tract remnants. A clinical and histopathologic study with review of the literature. *Oral Surg Oral Med Oral Pathol* 1972;34:781–799.

169. Ulrich HF. Lingual thyroid. *Ann Surg* 1932;95:503–507.

170. LiVolsi VA, Perzin KH, Savetsy L. Carcinoma arising in median ectopic thyroid (including thyroglossal duct tissue). *Cancer* 1974;34:1303–1315.

171. Block MA, Wylie JH, Patton RB, Miller JM. Does benign thyroid tissue occur in the lateral part of the neck? *Am J Surg* 1966;112: 476–481.

172. Klopp CT, Kirson SM. Therapeutic problems with ectopic noncancerous follicular thyroid tissue in the neck: 18 case reports according to etiological factors. *Ann Surg* 1966;163:653–664.

173. Moses DC, Thompson NW, Nishiyama RH, Sisson JC. Ectopic thyroid tissue in the neck. Benign or malignant. *Cancer* 1976;38: 361–365.

174. Hathaway BM. Innocuous accessory thyroid nodules. *Arch Surg* 1965;90:222–227.

175. Sisson JC, Schmidt RW, Beierwaltes WH. Sequestered nodular goiter. *N Engl J Med* 1964;270 927–932.

176. Meyer JS, Steinberg LS. Microscopically benign thyroid follicles in cervical lymph nodes. Serial section study of lymph node inclusions and entire thyroid gland in 5 cases. *Cancer* 1969;24: 302–211.

177. Frantz VK, Forsythe R, Hanford JM, Rogers WM. Lateral aberrant thyroids. *Ann Surg* 1942;115:161–183.

178. Donegan JO, Wood MD. Intratracheal thyroid—familial occurrence. *Laryngoscope* 1985;95:6–8.

179. Kaplan M, Kauli R, Lubin E, Grunebaum M, Laron Z. Ectopic thyroid gland. A clinical study of 30 children and review. *J Pediatr* 1978;92:205–209.

180. Kurman RJ, Prabha AC. Thyroid and parathyroid glands in the vaginal wall: report of a case. *Am J Clin Pathol* 1973;59:503–507.

181. Rahn J. Über eine eigenartige. Heterotopie von Schilddrüsengewebe. *Zentralbl Allg Pathol* 1958;99:80–86.

182. Ruchti C, Balli-Antunes H, Gerber HA. Follicular tumor in the sellar region without primary cancer of the thyroid. Heterotopic carcinoma? *Am J Clin Pathol* 1987;87:776–780.

183. Sekine S, Nagata M, Hamada H, Watanabe T. Heterotopic thyroid tissue at the porta hepatis in a fetus with trisomy 18. *Virchows Arch* 2000;436:498–501.

184. Shiraishi T, Imai H, Fukutome K, Watanabe M, Yatani R. Ectopic thyroid in the adrenal gland. *Hum Pathol* 1999;30:105–108.

185. Yilmaz F, Uzunlar AK, Sogutcu N. Ectopic thyroid tissue in the uterus. *Acta Obstet Gynecol Scand* 2005;84:201–202.

Parathyroid

45

Sanford I. Roth   Nicole A. Belsley
Graziella M. Abu-Jawdeh

INTRODUCTION

The surgical pathology of the parathyroid glands largely involves interpretation of their histology in patients with hyperfunction due to neoplastic or primary hyperplastic processes;[1] that is, primary hyperparathyroidism (1–7). Secondary hyperparathyroidism, in contrast, is a consequence of stimulation of parathyroid gland growth (secondary hyperplasia) and hormone secretion by hypocalcemia due to diseases of other organs, such as renal insufficiency, malabsorption (8–10), or genetic defects in the parathyroid or other organs (11). Secondary hyperplasia is histologically indistinguishable, but clinically easily distinguishable from primary hyperplasia. Since other disorders, such as hypoparathyroidism, pseudohypoparathyroidism, and familial hypocalciuric hypercalcemia (12), are not treated surgically and neonatal severe hyperparathyroidism (12) is rare, the parathyroid glands are rarely available for examination in these diseases. In order to adequately interpret the pathology of the parathyroid glands, the surgical patholo-

gist must have a thorough knowledge and understanding of calcium metabolism, the biochemistry of the parathyroid glands, the differential diagnosis and pathobiology of parathyroid disease, and the normal and pathologic anatomy of the glands (13). This chapter presents the normal histology, the embryology and its molecular biology, the alterations of the parathyroid glands that occur with age, and a brief discussion of normal calcium metabolism.

HISTORICAL REVIEW

In 1850 Professor Richard Owen (14), before the Royal College in London, first described the parathyroid glands in the Indian rhinoceros as "a small, compact yellow glandular body . . . attached to the thyroid at the point where the veins emerge." Interestingly this paper (14) was not published for twelve years after its initial presentation. Remak (15) in 1855 and Virchow (16) in 1863 described similar glands in cats and humans, respectively. However, it was not until 1880 that the anatomy and histology of the parathyroid glands of several species, including humans, were clearly established by a medical student, Ivor Sandström (17,18). He demonstrated that the glands, which he named "glandulae parathyroidae," were structures separate from the thyroid. He used this terminology to suggest the physical, as well as the

---

[1] Though hyperplasia is commonly used to describe the pathology of primary hyperplasia involving all four glands, studies of patients with multiple endocrine neoplasia and familial disease (2) demonstrate that these are in fact neoplastic diseases.

possible embryologic, relationship to the thyroid. Kohn (19,20) proposed the term *Epithelköperchen* after he demonstrated by animal experiments that the glands originated independently from the thyroid. However, this terminology has survived only in the German literature.

EMBRYOLOGY

Although an ectodermal origin of the glands has been suggested (21,22), the consensus is that the glands arise from the endodermal region of the branchial pouch (23). Neural crest cells participate in the formation of the mesenchyme of the glands (24). Embryonic parathyroid hormone production has been demonstrated by immunohistochemical studies (Roth, unpublished data). At $8^{3}/_{7}$ weeks gestational age (3.1 cm crown-rump length) a few positive cells are seen in the glands. By 17 to 20 weeks (Figure 45.1) (25-30) abundant parathyroid hormone is present in the glands.

The parathyroid glands arise as diverticula of the endoderm of the third and fourth branchial pouches (31-34). They make their first appearance as bilateral localized proliferations along the anterodorsal surface of pouch III and the lateral portion of the dorsal extremity of pouch IV during the 5th week of gestation (9-mm embryo). The glands are thus referred to as parathyroid III or parathyroid IV, depending on their pouch of origin (the singular is used because of the symmetrical growth). Parathyroid III, along with the thymus, forms as the third pouch separates from the pharynx. At this stage parathyroid III lies cephalad and lateral to parathyroid IV, and the two are separated by the medial thyroid. Differential growth rates of the thymus and the adjacent medial structures determine the final position the glands occupy after birth. The thymus, the most lateral of these structures, attaches to the pericardium and comes to lie largely in the thorax. The attached parathyroid III also develops a more caudad position as the more medial structures grow cepha-

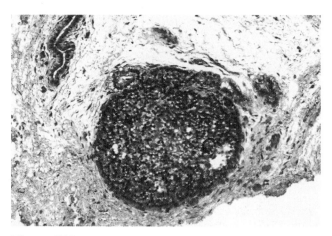

Figure 45.2 An embryonic parathyroid gland still attached to the remnant of the branchial pouch. The chief cells are closely packed and uniform. No stroma is visible.

lad. In the 18 mm embryo, when parathyroid III is at the level of the lower pole of the thyroid, it usually separates from the thymus, forming the lower parathyroid gland. Variations in the level at which this separation takes place are frequent and account for the marked anatomic variations in the final position of the adult glands. Parathyroid IV and the lateral thyroid (the ultimobranchial or postbranchial body) derive from the caudad part of the fourth branchial pouch (Figure 45.2). Together they form a bilobate complex and, as they separate, parathyroid IV acquires its adult position as the upper gland, near the intersection of the recurrent laryngeal nerve and the medial thyroid artery. Due to its medial position, closer association with midline structures, and shorter embryonic migrations, parathyroid IV has a more constant location and is usually cephalad to parathyroid III. During development, small portions of the gland may become separated from the main gland or a gland may separate into two or more parts (see below).

MOLECULAR BIOLOGY

The successful differentiation, development, and migration of the parathyroid glands require multiple genetic events. These events, though not fully understood, are largely known by identification of the genetic defects in various forms of human hypoparathyroidism, particularly DiGeorge Syndrome/velocardiofacial syndrome[2], and by studies on mouse animal models (35–55). Though early studies (53) proposed an origin of the parathyroid glands from neural crest cells migrating into the pharyngeal pouches, it is now recognized that parathyroid epithelial

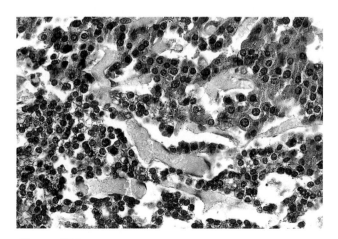

Figure 45.1 Immunohistochemical stain demonstrating PTH in the gland of a 20-week fetus.

---

[2] Result of a hetologous deletion of a portion of the long arm of chromosome 22(del22q11.2), containing *Tbx1*.

cells develop from the third pharyngeal pouch endoderm. Gene products from neural crest cells in the parathyroid mesenchyme are required for modulation of the branchial cleft endoderm into the parathyroid cells (53,54). The development and migration of the parathyroid glands requires a proper balance between epithelial cell death (apoptosis) and proliferation, as well as the appropriate interaction of endoderm with the associated mesenchyme.

Several genes and their products have been identified which are required for normal differentiation, development, and migration of the parathyroid glands (37–52,55), though undoubtedly there are many other not yet identified genes and signaling factors vital to these events. The known factors include genes encoding transcription factors, *Hoxa3*, *Pax9*, *Tbx1*, *GATA3*, *Glial cell missing (Gcm) 2*, and *Eyes absent (Eya)1*, as well as genes encoding secreted signaling molecules, *fibroblast growth factor (Fgf) 8*, *Chordin (Chrd)*, *bone morphogenetic proteins (BMPs)*, *TGFβ(A)* and *Sonic hedgehog (Shh)*. The signaling molecules act by modulating the expression of the respective transcription factors. In homozygous mutant mouse models for many of these genes, amongst multiple pharyngeal and cardiac developmental anomalies, the parathyroids are often aplastic or hypoplastic (37–53).

Hoxa3, a member of the *Hox* family, is a gene that encodes a transcription factor present in the third pharyngeal pouch endoderm as well as the neural crest cells. Mice knockout studies for *Hoxa3* highlight its function in the development of the organs arising from the third and fourth pharyngeal pouches and their dependence on mesenchymal neural crest cells for differentiation (38–40). *Hoxa3* mutants develop multiple anomalies involving the throat, heart, and thyroid and fail to develop the thymus and parathyroids. The failure to develop parathyroids is thought to stem from a defect in the neural crest cells' ability to induce proper differentiation of the pharyngeal pouch endoderm (38,39).

Mammalian *gcm2* (*GCMB* in humans) encodes a transcription factor also found in the third pharyngeal pouch endoderm, but is specifically expressed in a domain restricted to the parathyroid. *Gcm2* deficient mice lack parathyroid glands, demonstrating the crucial role of *gcm2* in the differentiation and function of the parathyroid (41). Interestingly, although *gcm2* expression is restricted to the parathyroid, *gcm2* knockout mice showed parathyroid hormone production originating in the thymus driven by *gcm1*, another homolog of the Drosophila gcm family that functions in placental development. Expression of *gcm* is absent in *Hoxa3* mutant mice, suggesting it acts downstream of *Hoxa3* (41,42).

GATA-3 and *Pax9*, additional transcription factors expressed in the third pharyngeal pouch, also result in hypoparathyroidism when absent. In humans with mutations in *GATA-3*, the resulting disease includes hypoparathyroidism manifest by hypocalcemia and low parathyroid hormone (43). Mice deficient for *Pax-9* show initial formation of the pharyngeal pouches, but have arrested formation of the epithelial buds of the third pharyngeal pouch (44).

Eya1 is expressed in the third pharyngeal endoderm, mesenchyme and ectoderm as well as the organs derived from these structures. In order to investigate the role of *Eya1* in animals, mice knockout experiments were carried out and studied at gestational days 11.5–12.5 (45). In contrast to the wild-type embryos that formed epithelial buds of the thymus and parathyroid primordia at gestational day 12, the *Eya1*$^{-/-}$ mice failed to form these epithelial buds. In addition, *gcm2* expression was down-regulated, suggesting an upstream control by *Eya1*. *HoxA3*, *Pax1* and *Pax9* expression were not affected. Since *HoxA3* and *Pax1* have been shown to regulate *Gcm2* expression (45), the control of *Gcm2* by *Eya1* suggests *Eya1* may lie in a pathway downstream from *HoxA3* and *Pax1* (46).

The close relationships of the endoderm, ectoderm and neural crest cells are demonstrated by the signaling protein FGF8. The protein is expressed in the pharyngeal endoderm and ectoderm; however, the severe developmental anomalies caused by its deficiency are a result of its effect on the neural crest cells (47,48). Decreased FGF8 causes increased apoptosis of the cranial and cardiac neural crest cells, resulting in improper development of the heart and pharynx, mimicking DiGeorge syndrome (48). Studies showed dependence of this secreted molecule on the transcription factor *Tbx-1*, a gene mapped to the microdeletion of chromosome 22 associated with DiGeorge syndrome (49,50).

Antagonistic secreted signaling molecules, *Chrd* and the *BMPs*, regulate the dorsal and ventral developmental organization respectively. *Chrd* is present in the pharyngeal endoderm and acts antagonistically by binding the *BMPs*. Loss of *Chrd* results in an expansion of the allantois (ventral) and reduction in the embryonic mesoderm (dorsal). In addition, the mutant mice show features similar to those found in DiGeorge syndrome, including parathyroid hypoplasia, indicating a role of *Chrd* in not only positioning information but differentiation as well (51). Its role in parathyroid development may be due to decreased expression of *Tbx1* and *Fgf8* caused by loss of *Chrd* (49). An additional gene, *Sonic hedgehog (Shh)*, also contributes to the balance between *Chrd* and *BMPs*. *Shh* encodes a secreted protein expressed in the pharyngeal endoderm that acts as a negative regulator. *Shh*$^{-/-}$ mutant mice showed abnormal third pouch development thought to be due to an overexpression of *Bmp4* (52). The normal repression of *Bmp* by *Shh* in the third pharyngeal pouch is lost in the mutant mice, upsetting the dorsal/ventral balance in favor of ventral expansion of the thymus and absence of the dorsal parathyroid. Although the gland primordium initially formed appropriately, *Gcm* expression was later absent in these mice, correlating with the lack of parathyroid glands (52).

Aside from organogenesis, numerous genes have been implicated in parathyroid disease (55–61). Most neoplastic diseases of the parathyroid, primary chief cell hyperplasia, adenomas and carcinomas, result from alterations in tumor suppressor genes, including *Rb*, *p53*, and *HRPT2*, or cell cycle regulators such as *cyclin D1* (55–59). In addition, genetic mutations involving proteins specific to the parathyroid gland's role in calcium homeostasis have been identified (60), specifically the calcium receptor gene which encodes a gene located in the parathyroid as well as the kidney (61). Although not located in the parathyroid, mutations in vitamin D receptors and PTH receptors indirectly affect the proper functioning of the parathyroid, leading to alterations in calcium homeostasis (62).

CALCIUM AND PARATHYROID METABOLISM

Calcium is one of the most closely controlled ions in mammals (63). Ninety-nine percent (99%) of the calcium is in the hydroxyapatite of the bones and 1% is in the extracellular fluids and soft tissues (64). The serum level of ionized calcium (Ca^{2+}) is maintained within the limits of laboratory error in most individuals. The serum calcium concentration ($[Ca^{2+}]$) is commonly measured as the total calcium, although it is the ionized calcium, approximately 50% of the total serum calcium (64), that is meaningful. In normal humans, calcium ions are bound, primarily to proteins (~40%) such as albumin, but also to chelating agents such as citrate. The serum $[Ca^{2+}]$ is regulated through five organs: the parathyroid glands, the C cells of the thyroid (probably of minimal importance in humans), the bones, the kidneys, and the gastrointestinal tract (65). In humans the two primary hormones responsible for control of $[Ca^{2+}]$ are the parathyroid hormone (PTH) and the metabolites of vitamin D, primarily $1\alpha,25$ ($OH)_2$ vitamin D (66).

Acute control of the serum $[Ca^{2+}]$ is the primary responsibility of PTH (31). PTH operates through a cell surface receptor, primarily found in the proximal convoluted tubule of the kidney and the osteoblasts of the bone. PTH acts to increase the serum calcium. It promotes tubular reabsorption of calcium in the kidney, increases the activity of the 1α vitamin D hydroxylase [thus increasing the synthesis of the active form of vitamin D ($1\alpha,25$ ($OH)_2$ vitamin D) and increasing bone resorption and gastrointestinal calcium transport]. The effect on bone requires the osteoblasts and the osteoclast precursors (see Chapter 4), which have PTH receptors. These cells produce paracrine factors that stimulate osteoclastic bone resorption since the osteoclasts lack PTH receptors. PTH also operates through the osteocytes, resulting is osteocytic osteolysis of the perilacunar bone.

The most active metabolite of vitamin D, $1\alpha,25$ ($OH)_2$ vitamin D, increases calcium resorption from the gastrointestinal tract and acts in synergy with PTH to increase bone resorption (67). $1\alpha,25$ ($OH)_2$ vitamin D also acts as a negative feedback on PTH synthesis and secretion. This action is mediated by inhibiting translation of prepro-PTH messenger through a vitamin D–responsive element related to an upstream promotor of the PTH gene (68).

PTH synthesis and secretion are controlled by the ambient $[Ca^{2+}]$. Increased ambient $[Ca^{2+}]$ decreases PTH synthesis and secretion and intracellular $[Ca^{2+}]$, whereas decreased serum $[Ca^{2+}]$ increases PTH synthesis and secretion. This is in contrast to other organs, where increased intracellular $[Ca^{2+}]$ increases hormone synthesis and secretion, whereas decreased $[Ca^{2+}]$ decreases synthesis and secretion.

A calcium ion–sensing cell surface receptor has been identified (69–71). This receptor is a member of the superfamily of guanine-nucleotide-regulatory G proteins. The gene for this receptor is located on the long arm of chromosome 3 (69–71). The receptor has been identified on the cell membrane of the parathyroid glands and is thought to be responsible for mediating the effect of calcium on the synthesis and secretion of PTH, much as vitamin D acts through its receptor.

Mutations of the calcium receptor gene have been identified in familial hypocalciuric hypercalcemia and severe neonatal hyperparathyroidism (69,72–74). These heterozygous and homozygous mutations result in inactivation of the receptor. The chief cell is thus stimulated to hypersecrete. In some cases of hypoparathyroidism, hyperactivity mutations have been identified in this gene (75), resulting in decreased synthesis and secretion of PTH.

Paracrine control of PTH secretion has been demonstrated in tissue culture, with decreasing cell density resulting in decreasing hormone secretion (76). Chromogranin A, which is cosecreted with PTH and its proteolytic products pancreastatin and parastatin, also inhibit PTH secretion (77–79).

NUMBER AND LOCATION

Ninety percent (90%) to 97% of patients have four parathyroid glands (80–86). However, the number has been reported to vary between two and 12 glands (80,81). The incidence of supernumerary glands in adults varies between 2 and 6.5% (86). Supernumerary glands are most commonly intrathymic and are thought to result from embryonic division of one or more glands (Figure 45.3). Small accumulations of parathyroid tissue as a result of parathyroid cell dispersion during embryonic migration may result in the presence of numerous small nests of cells. Proliferation of these nests, especially in the presence of secondary hyperparathyroidism, [i.e., parathyromatosis (88)], results in multiple accumulations of parathyroid "implants" that

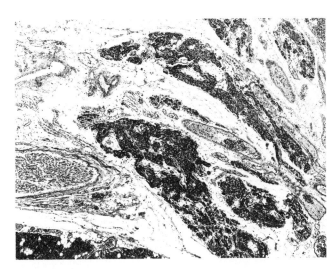

Figure 45.3 Parathyroid gland from a 60-year-old female, divided into several portions by the vascular bundle and recurrent laryngeal nerve.

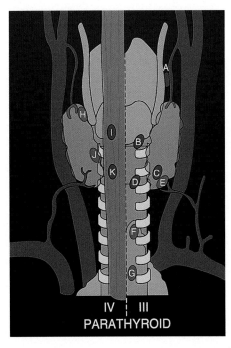

Figure 45.4 Diagram demonstrating the location of the parathyroid glands. (Modified with permission from: Gilmour JR. The gross anatomy of the parathyroid glands. *J Pathol Bacteriol* 1938;46:133–149 and reprinted with permission from: Roth SI. Parathyroid glands. In: Damjanov I, Linder J, eds. *Anderson's Pathology.* 10th ed. St. Louis: Mosby-Year Book; 1966:1980–2007.)

must be distinguished from metastatic implants from a carcinoma. Ectopic glands are one of the factors responsible for persistent hyperparathyroidism after surgical therapy of primary hyperplasia of the parathyroids (86,87) and must be distinguished from other causes of recurrent or persistent hyperparathyroidism such as parathyroid carcinoma and parathyromatosis (88). It is probably rare for there to be less than four glands in the absence of other abnormalities such as thymic aplasia. Because studies of the number of glands are based on autopsy material, we feel that most of the cases with fewer than four glands are due to failure to locate aberrant glands in unusual locations. Despite the known variation in the adult position of the parathyroid glands (20,28–30,69,70), there is a definite pattern in their anatomic distribution, which is related to their embryonic derivation (Figure 45.4). The most common location of the upper or superior (parathyroid IV) glands (77%) is at the cricothyroid junction posteriorly or just above the intersection of the recurrent laryngeal nerve and inferior thyroid artery (70%) (70,82). The second most common location is behind the upper pole of the thyroid (22%) (82), in which case the glands are often within the surgical capsule of the thyroid (Figure 45.5). Other uncommon locations include a more caudad position near the inferior thyroid artery, within the thyroid capsule or parenchyma (Figure 45.5), within or near the pharyngeal wall, a retropharyngeal or retroesophageal position, or within or near the carotid bifurcation. Abnormal upper glands can descend into ectopic locations as low as the posterior mediastinum (70).

The lower or inferior parathyroid glands (parathyroid III) have a more diverse distribution but are most commonly located between the lower pole of the thyroid and the thymus (Figure 45.6). They can occur as high in the neck as the hyoid bone, the pharynx, or the pyriform sinus,

or as low as the pericardium (89,90). In 42 to 61% of the cases they are located on either side of the lower thyroid or in a juxtathyroidal location. Another common location is the "thymic tongue" or "cervical extension of the thymus." Uncommon locations are the mediastinal thymus and the anterior mediastinum (82–86). Ectopic intravagal parathyroid tissue has been reported (91). The gland locations are symmetrical in 80% of patients.

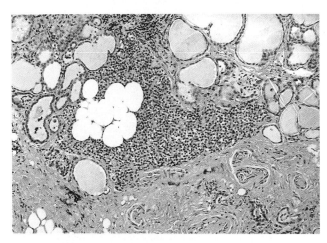

Figure 45.5 A parathyroid gland from a 21-year-old male just below the thyroid gland capsule in the thyroid parenchyma. A large accumulation of adipocytes is present within the parathyroid. Only chief cells are seen within the parathyroid.

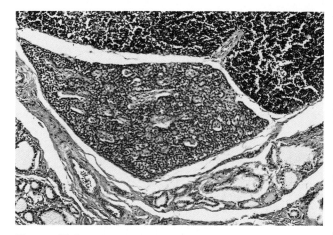

Figure 45.6 A fetal parathyroid (33 weeks' gestation) is seen between the thymus (top) and lower edge of the thyroid (*bottom*). A small amount of stroma surrounds the parathyroid vessels. The gland is composed of pure tightly packed chief cells.

GROSS APPEARANCE, SIZE, AND SHAPE

Each adult gland measures 3 to 6 mm in length, 2 to 4 mm in width, and 0.5 to 2.0 mm in thickness (Figure 45.7). The shape of the gland varies because it is molded by the adjacent structures. The glands are a flattened, ovoid pancake with "sharp" edges. The capsule is grey and almost transparent often with a fine network of small vessels. The underlying parenchyma is yellow to orange–tan, depending on the amount of stromal fat, the number of oxyphil cells, and degree of vascularity (5). The glands are soft and malleable, although they may show a marked increase in firmness, swelling, and a dark red color if surgical manipulation

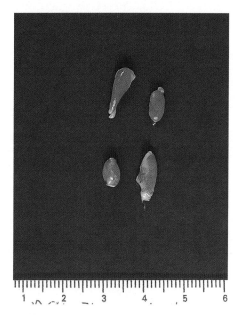

Figure 45.7 Four normal parathyroid glands removed at autopsy from a 53-year-old man.

causes intraglandular hemorrhage. Abnormal glands are usually more bulbous, with rounded edges, and have a firmer consistency and a darker red–tan color (5).

Gland weight and parenchymal cell content are important parameters used in the histopathologic assessment of the parathyroid gland (92–102), and all parathyroid glands or part of glands removed at surgery must be carefully dissected free of capsular fat or thymic tissue, measured and weighed to the nearest milligram. The total parathyroid weight gradually increases throughout embryonic life, reaching a mean total of 5 to 9 mg at the postpartum age of 3 months (97–99). This is followed by a steep linear increase in total parathyroid weight until the third or fourth decade of life, when it levels off at a mean of 120 ± 3.5 mg in men and 142 ± 5.2 mg in women (5). The mean weight per gland is 31.1 mg in men and 29.8 mg in women (100). The lower parathyroid glands are larger then the upper glands (97,101). The parenchymal cell content of the glands is extremely variable and difficult to evaluate. It is reported to average 74% of the weight of the gland in adults (85). It is a somewhat better indicator of gland function than gland weight alone but requires careful morphometric analysis in conjunction with careful evaluation of the total gland weight. The average parenchymal weight per gland is 21.6 mg for men and 18.2 mg for women (100), whereas the mean total parenchymal weight for four glands is 82.0 ± 2.6 mg for men and 88.9 ± 3.9 mg for women (96–98). The total gland weight has been reported to be higher in blacks than in whites (102). In a selected series of patients with primary hyperparathyroidism due to a single adenoma, who had a second gland totally removed because the surgeon felt the gland was enlarged, 15 histologically normal glands weighed over 60 mg (103). The largest gland weighed slightly over 160 mg. The total (10) and parenchymal (101) gland weight are inversely related to serum calcium concentration in patients with secondary hyperparathyroidism. In these patients a direct relationship has been found between the total gland weight and the serum phosphorus and renal function as expressed by serum urea nitrogen (10).

HISTOLOGY

The normal parathyroid gland has a thin fibrous capsule that separates it from the adjacent thyroid thymus or adipose tissue (Figures 45.8 and 45.9), which, except for those glands embedded in the thyroid or its capsule, is adipose tissue or thymus. At the vascular pole, an artery and vein are present surrounded by fibrous tissue. These branch into smaller arteries and veins, which form a complex readily visible in the capsule. The capsular arteries and veins are connected by arterioles, capillaries, and venules located in

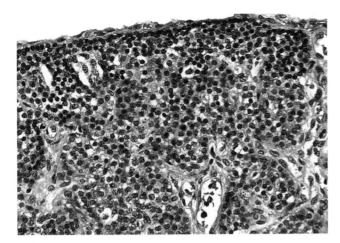

Figure 45.8 A parathyroid gland from a 7.5-month-old girl. The chief cells are the only cell type seen and are arranged in sheets, between the large vascular channels. The capillaries are present between individual chief cells. The chief cells show central regular nuclei and a clear amphophilic cytoplasm. A thin fibrous capsule separates the gland from the stroma.

the fibrous septa between the parenchymal cells (102). This capillary network abuts every chief cell. Due to the rich capillary network, the cut surface bleeds readily, providing an easy way for the surgeon to distinguish the parathyroid from lymph nodes, adipose tissue, thymus, and thyroid, which do not show such prominent bleeding from their cut surfaces. The capillary endothelial lining cells have pores or fenestrations resembling those seen in other endocrine glands (104,105). Dense bodies, Weibel-Palade bodies, pinocytotic vesicles, tight junctions, or zonulae occludens are constituents of the parathyroid capillary endothelium. Two interconnecting plexuses of lymphatic capillaries in the capsule surround the parathyroid glands. From the inner plexus, loops of lymphatics dip into the gland

parenchyma, whereas the efferent lymphatics arise from the outer plexus via special lymphatics or those of the thyroid (106). The interstitial space is limited by the basement membranes of the chief cells and capillaries and contains collagen bundles and elastic fibers (104). Nerve bundles in close proximity to chief cells suggest autonomic innervation (107–110). In the rabbit the nerves have been shown to originate in the medulla oblongata, the dorsal nucleus of the vagus, and the vagus nerve (107,110).

In infants and children the interstitium consists only of the capillary network and the extracellular space. Little or no collagen or stroma is present (Figure 45.8). With age, there is focally increasing collagenization of the perivascular stroma. This forms a delicate fibrous septa in adult glands, imparting to them a somewhat lobulated appearance. Surrounding the capillaries and lymphatics are interstitial cells that consist of fibroblasts, pericytes, mast cells, and a few lymphocytes. Adipocytes are sparse in the stroma of infants and children. Stromal fat cells begin to appear late in the first decade of life and increase throughout life. At puberty, especially in women, there is an increased rate of accumulation of adipocytes. Stromal fat cells increase in number with increasing age, reaching a maximum in the third to fifth decades of life. There is a marked variation in the amount and distribution of stromal fat within a single gland, between glands in the same individual, and among individuals of the same age (Figures 45.8–45.15). Recent studies (96,111,112) confirmed the initial reports of Gilmour (32) that, in adults, adipocytes occupy an average of 50% of the stromal volume rather than of the total parathyroid volume. Women have a higher percentage of stromal fat than do men. The amount of stromal fat is affected by the same factors that affect total body fat; for example, diet, nutrition, chronic illness (such as malignancy), and genetics. These variations make interpretation of the level of parathyroid function difficult to assess on the

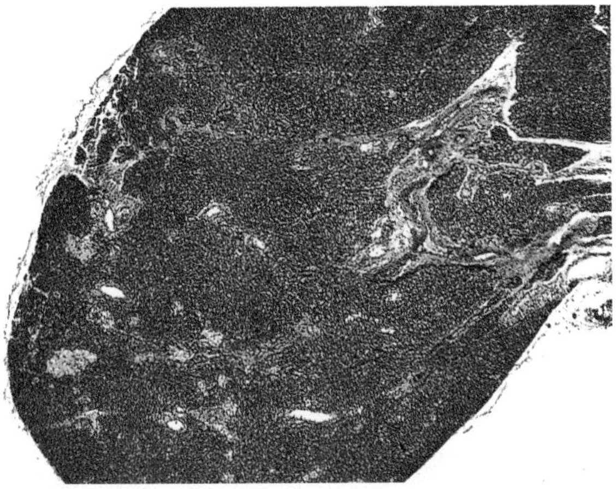

Figure 45.9 A parathyroid from a 27-year-old woman showing only sheets of chief cells and no stromal fat. The vascular pole can be seen at the right margin of the micrograph. A thin fibrous capsule is seen.

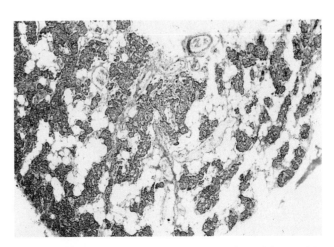

Figure 45.10 Photomicrograph of a parathyroid from a 39-year-old man. There is abundant stromal fat separating the cords of chief cells.

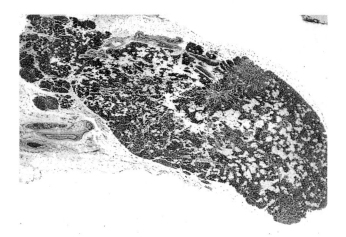

Figure 45.11   A parathyroid from a 69-year-old woman. There is a moderate amount of stromal fat, largely concentrated in the center of the gland. A few small oxyphil nodules can be seen in the parenchyma.

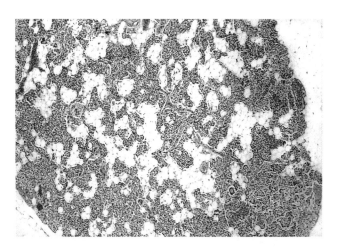

Figure 45.12   A parathyroid from a 76-year-old man. There is a moderate amount of stromal fat, largely in the center of the gland. Small oxyphil nodules are present.

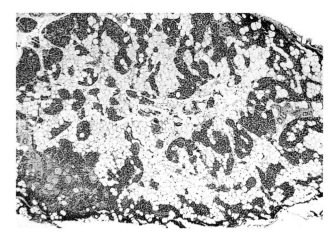

Figure 45.13   A parathyroid from a 77-year-old man with abundant stromal fat. The parenchyma is composed entirely of chief cells.

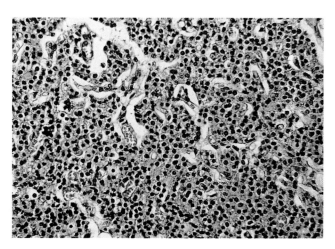

Figure 45.14   A normal parathyroid from a 70-year-old woman showing almost no stromal fat or oxyphil cells.

basis of the stromal fat. In normal glands, the stromal fat appears to "compress" the surrounding parenchyma; whereas, in hyperplastic or adenomatous glands, the fat cells appear scattered among the parenchymal cells. In the fourth decade there is a relative decrease in parenchymal adipocytes.

Each parenchymal cell is separated from the stroma by a prominent basement membrane. The parenchymal cells are arranged in irregular sheets without prominent stroma in infants and prepubertal children. In infants and young children only one type of cell is present, the chief cell. The chief cells of the newborn and infantile parathyroid gland are small and regular, measuring 6 to 8 μm in diameter (Figure 45.16). The chief cell membranes are poorly demarcated, and the cytoplasm is amphophilic, relatively lucent, and occasionally vacuolated. Intracellular fat in the chief cells of children is low compared with the adult gland, with only 30 to 40% of the chief cells of children containing large intracellular fat droplets on fat stains (113). The

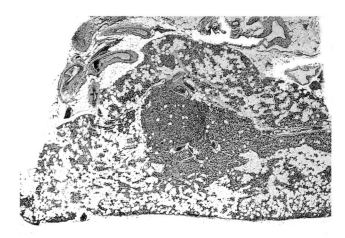

Figure 45.15   A parathyroid gland of a 77-year-old man. The stroma is almost completely replaced by adipocytes. There is a large oxyphil cell nodule in the center of the gland.

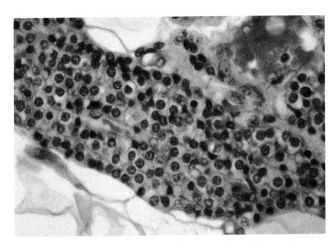

Figure 45.16 Sheets of chief cells in a newborn. The stroma has little collagen and is outside the large sheet. The cell membranes are poorly demarcated. The cytoplasm is eosinophilic.

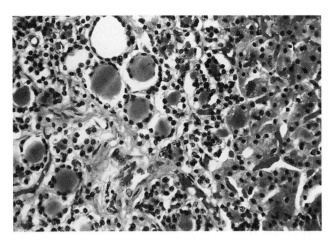

Figure 45.18 Numerous pseudofollicles in a normal parathyroid of a 58-year-old white man. Lining the pseudofollicles are chief cells. At the right of the micrograph is the edge of an oxyphil cell nodule.

nuclei are often molded and they overlap. The nuclei are centrally located, with uniform chromatin and small, inconspicuous nucleoli.

In the adult, the parenchymal cells are arranged in solid nests, rounded or lobulated masses and trabeculae, or a combination of these (Figures 45.8–45.17). A pseudofollicular pattern also has been described in normal glands (Figure 45.18) (114–116). Ultrastructural evidence indicates that follicle formation in the parathyroid is the result of a proliferation of parenchymal cells, with ischemic necrosis and degeneration of those cells separated from their blood supply by other parenchymal cells.

These pseudofollicles are usually filled with cellular debris and a pink eosinophilic homogeneous material resembling the colloid seen in thyroid follicles (Figure 45.18) (114). This material contains glycoproteins, as evidenced by the positive periodic acid-Schiff (PAS) reaction, and PTH

as evidenced by immunostaining. Several investigators have further reported that it stains with Congo red and shows the apple-green birefringence characteristic of amyloid (115). A similar finding has been reported in the follicles of pathologic parathyroid glands (116,117). Cinti et al. (114) were unable to confirm either the presence of amyloid or glycoproteins in the follicles of a series of normal parathyroids removed at the time of thyroidectomy. However, electron microscopy of follicles in a pathologic parathyroid gland did demonstrate fibrils closely resembling those of amyloid in pseudofollicles (113).

There are two types of parenchymal cells recognized by light microscopy in the adult normal parathyroid gland. These are the chief cells (Figures 45.15, 45.18–45.20), in their active and inactive forms, and the oxyphil cell (Figures 45.15, 45.18–45.20) (19,118,119). In adults the chief cells are arranged in sheets, cords, trabeculae, and small

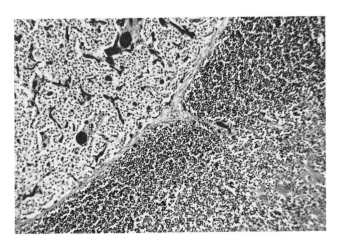

Figure 45.17 Sheets of parathyroid chief cells showing amphophilic clear cytoplasm, adjacent to the thymus. The prominent vascularity of the gland is visible.

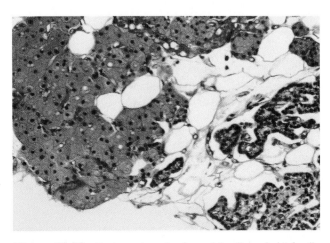

Figure 45.19 Nests and cords of oxyphil cells and chief cells among the adipocytes of the stroma.

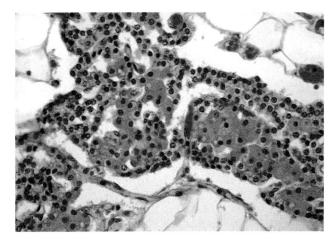

Figure 45.20 Trabecula of parathyroid showing mixture of oxyphil and chief cells.

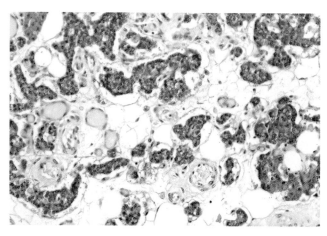

Figure 45.22 Chief cells showing abundant PTH in the parathyroid gland. Note the variation in the amount of hormone in various chief cells. (Immunoperoxidase stain for PTH, hematoxylin counterstain.)

nodules. They are spherical and measure 8 to 12 μm in diameter. The cell borders are poorly defined. The cytoplasm is amphophilic or faintly eosinophilic, with 70 to 80% of the chief cells containing large prominent fat droplets, (Figure 45.21) (5,17), corresponding to the lipid bodies seen in the resting chief cells by electron microscopy (120). It is of interest that these lipid droplets were first recognized in human chief cells by Sandström (17,18), although he did not appreciate their significance. By ordinary light microscopy, the active chief cell may be difficult to identify. The inactive chief cell may be recognized by the vacuolated clear appearance of the cytoplasm that is filled with lipid, glycogen, and lysosomes (120–123). Deposition of silver particles on the secretory granules is responsible for the argyrophil reaction seen in normal parathyroid glands using the Grimelius silver nitrate stain (120,124–126). The granules correspond to the location of PTH (Figure 45.22) (127–131) and chromogranin (Figure 45.23) (128). Differ-

ences in the parathyroid and chromogranin content of the chief cells indicate a variation in the secretory granule content and supports the presence of a secretory cycle in the parathyroid chief cell. The nuclei are round, centrally located, have a sharp nuclear outline, even chromatin, and small rare nucleoli (5,113).

Ultrastructural features of the chief cell correlate with its functional activity (120–122,129–135). The chief cell, considered the basic functional unit of the parathyroid gland, is responsible for the production and secretion of PTH and, in turn, in the maintenance of the homeostasis of ionized calcium (136–139). To achieve this, each individual chief cell undergoes a secretory cycle (120–122,129–133) (Figure 45.24) similar to that of the follicle of the thyroid. Each chief cell is polarized with the Golgi apparatus and granular endoplasmic reticulum farthest from the basement membrane–lined perivascular surface (140).

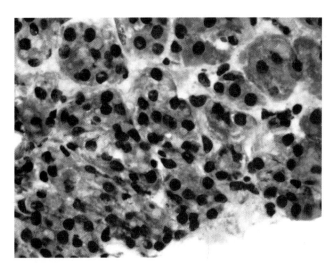

Figure 45.21 Chief cells with intracytoplasmic lipid droplets (Oil-Red-O stain, hematoxylin counterstain).

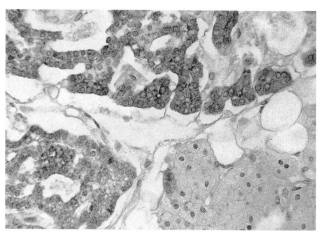

Figure 45.23 Parathyroid gland showing abundant chromogranin in the chief cells. The chief cells have different amounts of chromogranin. The oxyphil cells are free of chromogranin.

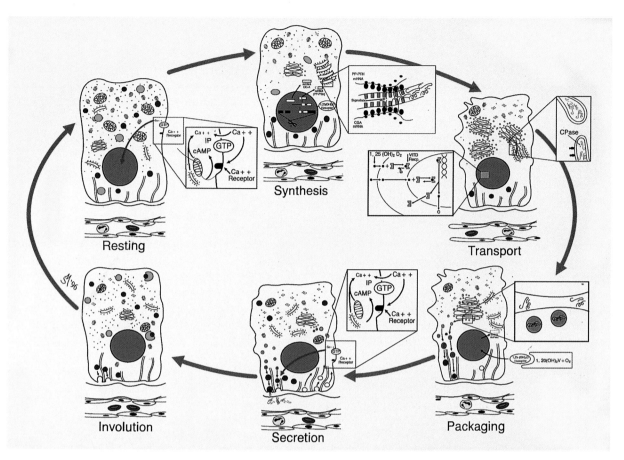

Figure 45.24 Diagram of the secretory cycle of the parathyroid chief cells (derived from electronmicroscopic studies (9). Although these comprise a continuum, typical stages have been recognized ultrastructurally. During the resting phase, the cells are rich in glycogen and lipid bodies with dispersion of the granular endoplasmic reticulum (GER) and free ribosomes. Dense-core secretory granules are relatively uncommon and scattered throughout the cytoplasm. Rare lysosomes are seen. The Golgi apparatus is small and inconspicuous, with few vesicles and vacuoles. The cell membranes are relatively straight with few interdigitations. At the end of the resting phase, presumably due to decreased cytoplasmic [Ca^{2+}] and release of vitamin D, metabolite from the upstream promotor site, the cell begins the process of PTH synthesis. As the synthetic phase begins, transcription of the gene for PTH begins with production of the complimentary RNA for prepro-PTH and presumably accompanied by a similar transcription of chromogranin. The mRNA is produced by removal of the introns and splicing of the exons. The mRNA moves to the granular endoplasmic reticulum, which aggregates [the perinuclear body of Pappenheimer and Wilens (48)]. This is accompanied by aggregation of the free ribosomes to polysomes. The preprohormone crosses into the lumen of the GER, where the preportion of the molecule is removed by a ligase. Other alterations include depletion of the dense-core granules, lysosomes, glycogen, and lipid bodies. The cell membrane increases in tortuosity, probably due to loss of cytoplasmic volume. The synthesis and secretion of hormone is halted, presumably by the action of 1α,25 dihydroxyvitamin D on the upstream promotor region of PTH and the cytosolic [Ca^{2+}]. In the transport phase, the hormone, supposedly accompanied by chromogranin, is transported through the cisternae of the GER to the Golgi apparatus as the pro segment is removed by a "clipase." The hormone is conveyed to the Golgi vesicles. Further depletion of lipid bodies, glycogen, and secretory granules occurs, and the cisternae of the GER disperse. In the packaging phase, the hormone is bundled along with chromogranin into dense-core granules and the Golgi apparatus begins its involution. Secretion occurs as the dense-core granules containing PTH and chromogranin move along the microtubules, fuse with the cell membrane, and release the hormone into the pericapillary extracellular space. Depending on the ambient [Ca^{2+}], the granules are rapidly passed along the microtubules and secreted (low [Ca^{2+}]) or left free in the cytoplasm (high [Ca^{2+}]), to be destroyed by lysosomes or to be secreted at a later time. The Golgi continues to decrease in size and complexity. The free ribosomes disaggregate. The cells begin to involute toward the resting phase with gradual loss of secretory granules and further involution of the Golgi apparatus. The cells begin to accumulate glycogen and lipid bodies and approach the resting phase. Lysosomes containing acid phosphatase accumulate in the cells. These presumably serve to destroy excess hormone and unsecreted secretory granules. (Modified with permission from: Roth SI. Parathyroid glands. In: Damjanov I, Linder J, eds. *Anderson's Patology.* 10th ed. St. Louis: Mosby-Year Book; 1966:1980–2007.)

The resting phase, which corresponds to the inactive chief cell, is characterized by accumulation of glycogen and large lipid bodies that correspond to the lipid seen by light microscopy (see Figure 45.21). The rest of the cell organelles, the Golgi apparatus, the granular endoplasmic reticulum, and secretory granules are small and inconspicuous. This is best seen in the chronically suppressed cell in atrophic parathyroid glands (120–122,129,132,134,135). During this stage, lysosomes (141) as well as variable numbers of small dense-core secretory granules are present, the latter being peripherally located. Sacs of granular endoplasmic reticulum are dispersed throughout the cytoplasm, whereas free ribosomes are only partially aggregated into polysomes. The Golgi apparatus is small and inconspicuous, with few vacuoles and prosecretory granules. The cell membranes are straight with few interdigitations (104).

The synthetic phase is marked by the parallel aggregation of the cisternae of rough granular endoplasmic reticulum and is noted at the light microscopic level by the presence of the body of Pappenheimer and Wilens (120,142). Free ribosomes aggregate into polysomes. It is during this phase that prepro-PTH and chromogranin (120,134) are synthesized within the granular endoplasmic reticulum. During the next phase, the prohormone is split and transferred to the Golgi apparatus which begins to enlarge with increases in smooth membranes, vesicles and vacuoles, and prosecretory granules of different electron densities. As the packaging phase emerges, the granular endoplasmic reticulum disperses throughout the cytoplasm, and larger dense-core secretory granules appear in the Golgi region, gradually moving to the periphery. PTH and chromogranin A are present in the aggregated granular endoplasmic reticulum and dense core granules (128,129). As the secretory granules progress along the microtubules toward the cell surface, there is an involution of the Golgi apparatus; acid phosphatase appears at the secretory face and eventually is transferred into large lysosomes (141). Separation of the secretory granules from the microtubules into the cytoplasm could account for the second compartment of PTH storage postulated by Cohn and MacGregor (136). The cell cytoplasm in the synthetic and secretory phases becomes depleted of glycogen and lipid bodies. During the last phase, there is margination of the lysosomes and secretory granules, fusion of the plasma membrane with that of the secretory granules, and emptying of the products into the extracellular space. The membranes of the secretory granules and lysosomes are probably recycled (143). Shannon and Roth (141) and Hashizume et al. (144) demonstrated that the stored parathyroid secretory granules fuse with lysosomes which provide a mechanism for intracellular degradation of PTH. The chief cell returns to the resting phase with a resultant accumulation of glycogen and complex lipid bodies, which are the best indicators of the resting or functionally suppressed cell. In chronically suppressed nor-

mal glands adjacent to a hyperfunctioning adenoma, 90 to 95% of the chief cells are inactive. In comparison, the normal adult gland has 70 to 80% of the chief cells in the resting phase, and the normal prepubertal gland has 30 to 40% in the resting phase (113,121).

Correlative morphologic studies in normal, adenomatous, and hyperplastic glands have shown that the intracellular content of fat in the chief cells is inversely related to its endocrine activity and is a better indicator of hormonal function than is the stromal fat. An increased cytoplasmic lipid content is a feature of a functionally suppressed chief cell (120,121,145–150), whereas hormonally active cells of adenoma and hyperplasia are largely in the active stages of hormone synthesis and secretion and thus are fat depleted. Based on this fact, evaluation of intracellular fat content by Oil-Red-O stain (Figure 45.21) has been demonstrated to be useful in differentiating between normal and adenomatous or hyperplastic parathyroid glands (141–150). Care must be taken in interpreting these fat stains because some areas of adenomas and hyperplasias may contain intracellular fat (151–154).

Cell culture studies (155,156) using a sequential hemolytic plaque assay confirm the cyclical secretion of both PTH and chromogranin A by individual parathyroid cells. Roth and Raisz (134) demonstrated that the ambient ionized [Ca^{2+}] controls the length of the resting phase of the chief cell cycle. Proliferation of parathyroid chief cells is also controlled by the ambient ionized [Ca^{2+}] (157). Molecular studies (158) have shown that the mechanism of this control may be via depression of cyclins D1 and D2.

The second cell type in the adult gland is the oxyphil cell (see Figures 45.9, 45.12, 45.15, 45.17, 45.19, and 45.25). These are felt to be derived from the chief cells (99,159–162), although the stimulus for the development of oxyphil cells has not yet been identified. Before puberty, only extremely rare oxyphil cells are present in the glands. Beginning at puberty and increasing throughout life, increasing numbers of these cells appear (159). They are distributed among the chief cells as individual cells, sheets, and small or large nodules (5,113), indicating that there is both a continual transformation (see Figures 45.19, 45.20, and 45.24) from the chief cells and clonal proliferation of the oxyphil cells (160). Rarely, these nodules enlarge enough to be visible grossly. When this happens, it is not possible to differentiate these presumably nonfunctioning oxyphil nodules from functioning oxyphil adenomas (5). The normal oxyphil cells contain only minimal PTH or chromogranin (see Figure 45.23).

Oxyphil cells in multiple organs, including abnormal parathyroid glands, have been demonstrated to contain decreased cytochrome oxidase (163). Studies on oncocytic salivary gland tumors (164) manifested decreased concentrations of mitochondrial enzymes when measured against the amount of mitochondrial protein. This is in contrast to histochemical studies showing marked increases in mitochondrial enzymes (165–167). These studies, along with the fact that oxyphil cells increase with age, suggest that there is a mitochondropathy, which may lead to the proliferation of the mitochondria within the cells. PTH-related peptide has been described in oxyphil cells (168), although its function is not clear.

The oxyphil cell measures 12 to 20 μm in diameter and has a clearly demarcated cell membrane, a pyknotic nucleus, and abundant eosinophilic granular cytoplasm (Figure 45.25), rich in mitochondria and resembling the Hürthle cells of the thyroid or the oncocytes of other endocrine organs (159–162). Ultrastructurally, their cytoplasm is completely filled with mitochondria, often with a bizarre shape and size, as well as occasional lysosomes and lipofuscin granules (120). Their function is unknown; however, the oxyphil cells in normal glands do not seem to contain the organelles responsible for PTH synthesis and secretion [i.e., granular endoplasmic reticulum, Golgi apparatuses, and secretory granules (119,120)], as indicated by electron microscopy and the absence of PTH and chromogranin (see Figure 45.23). However, cases of functioning oxyphil cell adenomas (5,6,169) and chief cell hyperplasias (121) have been reported. Protein secretory and synthetic organelles and dense core granules have been demonstrated in these tumor cells.

Transitional oxyphil cells may be recognized by light microscopy by the decreased density of their cytoplasmic eosinophilia. By electron microscopy, these cells have lesser numbers of mitochondria and some of the organelles associated with PTH synthesis and secretion, such as granular endoplasmic reticulum, Golgi apparatuses, and dense-core secretory granules. Both forms of oxyphil cells contain sparse amounts of lipid droplets (150,151).

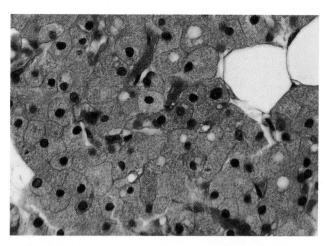

Figure 45.25 Oxyphil cells of the parathyroid in an 80-year-old woman. The centrally located, variably sized, pyknotic nuclei are seen within the granular eosinophilic cytoplasm. The cell membranes and the vascular channels are easily visible.

Cytology of previously localized tumors has been proposed as useful in the preoperative identification of parathyroid neoplasms (170–173). Intraoperative imprints of tumors and normal glands may allow differentiation of adenomas and hyperplasia (174–176). Touch preps or smears from normal glands (Figure 45.26) show small nests or flat sheets of chief cells, with attached stromal fat, as well as naked nuclei in the background. Microfollicles may be present. The nuclei are round to oval and slightly pleomorphic with granular chromatin. The chief cells have pale vacuolated cytoplasm, some with intracytoplasmic lipid droplets (Figure 45.26). Oxyphil cells, with abundant cytoplasm and small, centrally located nuclei, may be

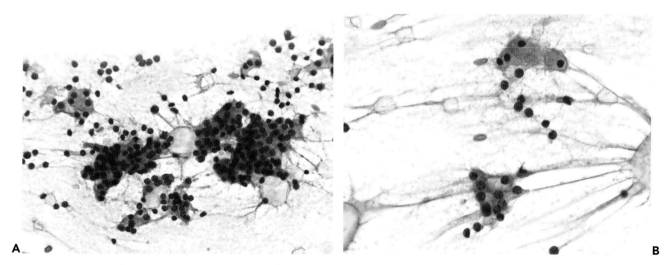

Figure 45.26 **A.** Parathyroid gland smear preparation obtained at autopsy, showing sheets and nests of parenchymal chief cell with attached stromal fat and naked nuclei in the background. **B.** Intracytoplasmic lipid droplets can be seen as well (Hematoxylin and eosin).

identified as well. In contrast, the cytology of parathyroid adenomas shows large dense clusters of crowded cells with increased pleomorphism and decreased intracytoplasmic lipid. (177).

The use of pure histologic criteria in the estimation of the functional or hormonal activity of the gland and in the differentiation between normal, hyperplastic, and adenomatous glands is difficult. The gland size and weight, the shape, and the relative proportion of stromal adipocytes and chief cells are all important criteria in making these distinctions. Account must be taken of the number of oxyphil cells because in normal glands, but not adenomas or primary hyperplastic glands, oxyphil cells are nonfunctional. We have found that the appraisal of these elements, along with the patient's clinical history, and evaluation of cellular cytology and intracellular fat content of the chief cells, all must be carefully considered in arriving at a proper pathologic diagnosis.

REFERENCES

1. Mallette LE. Review. Primary hyperparathyroidism, an update: incidence, etiology, diagnosis, and treatment. *Am J Med Sci* 1987;293:239–249.
2. Cope O, Keynes WM, Roth SI, Castleman B. Primary chief-cell hyperplasia of the parathyroid glands: a new entity in the surgery of hyperparathyroidism. *Ann Surg* 1958;148:375–388.
3. Cope O. Hyperparathyroidism: diagnosis and management. *Am J Surg* 1960;99:394–403.
4. Aurbach GD, Potts JT Jr. The parathyroids. *Adv Metab Dis* 1964;1: 45–93.
5. Castleman B, Roth SI. Tumors of the parathyroid glands. In: *Atlas of Tumor Pathology.* 2nd series, fascicle 2. Washington, DC: Armed Forces Institute of Pathology; 1978:1–94.
6. DeLellis RA. Tumors of the parathyroid gland. In: *Atlas of Tumor Pathology.* 3rd series, fascicle 6. Washington, DC: Armed Forces Institute of Pathology; 1993:1–102.
7. O'Malley BW, Kohler PO. Hypoparathyroidism. *Postgrad Med* 1968;44:71–75, 77–81, 182–186.
8. Hanley DA, Sherwood LM. Secondary hyperparathyroidism in chronic renal failure. Pathophysiology and treatment. *Med Clin North Am* 1978;62:1319–1339.
9. Katz AI, Hampers CL, Merrill JP. Secondary hyperparathyroidism and renal osteodystrophy in chronic renal failure. Analysis of 195 patients, with observations on the effects of chronic dialysis, kidney transplantation and subtotal parathyroidectomy. *Medicine (Baltimore)* 1969;48:333–374.
10. Roth SI, Marshall RB. Pathology and ultrastructure of the human parathyroid glands in chronic renal failure. *Arch Intern Med* 1969;124:397–407.
11. Yagi H, Ozono K, Miyake H, Nagashima K, Kuroume T, Pike JW. A new point mutation in the deoxyribonucleic acid-binding domain of the vitamin D receptor in a kindred with hereditary 1,25-dihydroxyvitamin D-resistant rickets. *J Clin Endocrinol Metab* 1993;76:509–512.
12. Roth SI. Parathyroid glands. In: Damjanov I, Linder J, eds. *Anderson's Pathology.* 10th ed. St. Louis: Mosby-Year Book; 1966: 1980–2007.
13. Roth SI, Wang CA, Potts JT Jr. The team approach to primary hyperparathyroidism. *Hum Pathol* 1975;6:645–648.
14. Owen R. On the anatomy of the Indian rhinoceros (Rh. unicornis, L). *Trans Zool Soc (Lond)* 1862;4:31–58.
15. Remak R. *Untersuchungen über die Entwickelung der Wirbelthiere.* Berlin: G. Reimer; 1855:3–40, 122–124.
16. Virchow R. *Die krankhaften Geschwülste.* Vol 3. Berlin: Hirschwald; 1863:13.
17. Sandström I. Om en ny Körtel hos menniskan och ätskilliga däggdjur. *Upsala Lakaref Forh* 1880;15:441–471.
18. Seipel CM. An English translation of Sandström's "Glandulae Parathyroideae" with biographical notes by Professor J August Hammar. *Bull Inst Hist Med* 1938;6:179–222.
19. Kohn A. Studien über die Schilddrüse. *Arch f Mikr Anat* 1895;44: 366–422.
20. Kohn A. Die Epithelkörperchen. *Ergeb Anat Entwicklungsgeshch* 1899;9:194–252.
21. Pearse AG, Takor TT. Neuroendocrine embryology and the APUD concept. *Clin Endocrinol (Oxf)* 1976;5(suppl):S229–S244.
22. Merida-Velasco JA. Experimental study of the origin of the parathyroid glands. *Acta Anat (Basel)* 1991;141:163–169.
23. Graham A. Development of the pharyngeal arches. *Am J Med Genet A* 2003;119:251–256.
24. Le Lievre CS, Le Douarin NM. Mesenchymal derivatives of the neural crest: analysis of chimaeric quail and chick embryos. *J Embryol Exp Morphol* 1975;34:125–154.
25. Norris EH. Anatomical evidence of prenatal function of the human parathyroid glands. *Anat Rec* 1946;96:129–142.
26. Nakagami K, Yamazaki Y, Tsunoda Y. An electron microscopic study of the human fetal parathyroid gland. *Z Zellforsch Mikrosk Anat* 1968;85:89–95.
27. Ishizaki N, Shoumura S, Emura S, et al. Ultrastructure of the parathyroid gland of the mouse fetus after calcium chloride or ethylenediaminetetraacetic acid administration. *Acta Anat* 1989;135:164–170.
28. Leroyer-Alizon E, David L, Anast CS, Dubois PM. Immunocytological evidence for parathyroid hormone in human fetal parathyroid glands. *J Clin Endocrinol Metab* 1981;52:513–516.
29. Scothorne RJ. Functional capacity of fetal parathyroid glands with reference to their clinical use as homografts. *Ann N Y Acad Sci* 1964;120:669–676.
30. MacIsaac RJ, Heath JA, Rodda CP, et al. Role of the fetal parathyroid glands and parathyroid hormone-related protein in the regulation of placental transport of calcium, magnesium and inorganic phosphate. *Reprod Fertil Dev* 1991;3: 447–457.
31. Welsh DA. Concerning the parathyroid glands: a critical anatomical and experimental study. *J Anat Physiol* 1898;32: 292–307.
32. Gilmour JR. The embryology of the parathyroid glands, the thymus and certain associated rudiments. *J Pathol Bacteriol* 1937;45: 507–522.
33. Weller GL Jr. Development of the thyroid, parathyroid and thymus glands in man. *Contr Embryol Carnegie Inst* 1933;24 (141):95–138.
34. Norris EH. The parathyroid glands and the lateral thyroid in man: their morphogenesis, histogenesis, topographic anatomy and prenatal growth. *Contrib Embryol Carnegie Inst* 1937;26:247–294.
35. Trump D, Dixon PH, Mumm S, et al. Localization of X linked recessive idiopathic hypoparathyroidism to a 1.5 Mb region on Xq26-q27. *J Med Genet* 1998;35:905–909.
36. Kelly T, Blanton S, Saif R, Sanjad S, Sakati N. Confirmation of the assignment of the Sanjad-Sakati (congenital hypoparathyroidism) syndrome (OMIM 241410) locus to chromosome 1q42–43. *J Med Genet* 2000;37:63–64.
37. Wurdak H, Ittner L, Lang K, et al. Inactivation of TGFbeta signaling in neural crest stem cells leads to multiple defects reminiscent of DiGeorge syndrome. *Genes Dev* 2005;19:530–535.
38. Kameda Y, Arai Y, Nishimaki T, Chisaka O. The role of Hoxa3 gene in parathyroid gland organogenesis of the mouse. *J Histochem Cytochem* 2004;52:641–651.
39. Manley N, Capecchi M. Hox group 3 paralogs regulate the development and migration of the thymus, thyroid, and parathyroid glands. *Dev Biol* 1998;195:1–15.
40. Su D, Ellis S, Napier A, Lee K, Manley NR. Hoxa3 and pax1 regulate epithelial cell death and proliferation during thymus and parathyroid organogenesis. *Dev Biol* 2001;236:316–329.
41. Gunther T, Chen Z, Kim J, et al. Genetic ablation of parathyroid glands reveals another source of parathyroid hormone. *Nature* 2000;406:199–203.

42. Hogan B, Hunter M, Oates A, et al. Zebrafish gcm2 is required for gill filament budding from pharyngeal ectoderm. *Dev Biol* 2004;276:508–522.

43. Nesbit M, Bowl M, Harding B, et al. Characterization of GATA3 mutations in the hypoparathyroidism, deafness, and renal dysplasia (HDR) syndrome. *J Biol Chem* 2004;279:22624–22634.

44. Peters H, Neubuser A, Kratochwil K, Balling R. Pax9-deficient mice lack pharyngeal pouch derivatives and teeth and exhibit craniofacial and limb abnormalities. *Genes Dev* 1998;12: 2735–2747.

45. Manley N, Capecchi M. The role of Hoxa-3 in mouse thymus and thyroid development. *Development* 1995;121:1989–2003.

46. Xu P, Zheng W, Laclef C, et al. Eya1 is required for the morphogenesis of mammalian thymus, parathyroid and thyroid. *Development* 2002;129:3033–3044.

47. Frank D, Fotheringham L, Brewer J, et al. An Fgf8 mouse mutant phenocopies human 22q11 deletion syndrome. *Development* 2002;129:4591–4603.

48. Abu-Issa R, Smyth G, Smoak I, Yamamura K, Meyers EN. Fgf8 is required for pharyngeal arch and cardiovascular development in the mouse. *Development* 2002;129:4613–4625.

49. Vitelli F, Taddei I, Morishima M, Meyers EN, Lindsay EA, Baldini A. A genetic link between Tbx1 and fibroblast growth factor signaling. *Development* 2002;129:4605–4611.

50. Packham EA, Brook JD. T-box genes in human disorders. *Hum Mol Genet* 2003;12:R37–R44.

51. Bachiller D, Klingensmith J, Shneyder N, et al. The role of chordin/Bmp signals in mammalian pharyngeal development and DiGeorge syndrome. *Development* 2003;130:3567–3578.

52. Moore-Scott B, Manley N. Differential expression of Sonic hedgehog along the anterior-posterior axis regulates patterning of pharyngeal endoderm and pharyngeal endoderm-derived organs. *Dev Biol* 2005;278:323–335.

53. Le Lievre CS, Le Douarin NM. Mesenchymal derivatives of the neural crest: analysis of chimaeric quail and chick embryos. *J Embryol Exp Morphol* 1975;34:125–154.

54. Le Douarin NM, Dupin E. Multipotentiality of the neural crest. *Curr Opinion Genet Dev* 2003;13:529–536.

55. Nosé V, Khan A. Recent developments in the molecular biology of the parathyroid. In: Lloyd RV, ed. *Endocrine Pathology: Differential Diagnosis and Molecular Advances.* Totowa, NJ: Humana Press; 2004:131–151.

56. Cryns VL, Thor A, Xu HJ, et al. Loss of the retinoblastoma tumor suppressor gene in parathyroid carcinoma. *N Eng J Med* 1994;330:757–761.

57. Cryns VL, Rubio MP, Thor AD, Louis DN, Arnold A. p53 abnormalities in human parathyroid carcinoma. *J Clin Endocrinol Metab* 1994;78:1320–1324.

58. Hsi E, Zuckerberg LR, Yang WI, Arnold A. Cyclin D1/PRAD1 expression in parathyroid adenomas: an immunohistochemical study. *J Clin Endocrinol Metab* 1996;81:1736–1739.

59. Vasef MA, Byrnes R, Sturm M, Bromley C, Robinson RA. Expression of cyclin D1 in parathyroid carcinomas, adenomas, and hyperplasias: a paraffin immunohistochemical study. *Mod Pathol* 1999;12:412–416.

60. Pollack MR, Brown EM, Chou YH, et al. Mutations in the human Ca^{2+}-sensing receptor gene cause familial hypocalciuric hypercalcemia and neonatal severe hyperparathyroidism. *Cell* 1993;75:1297–1303.

61. Janicic N, Soliman E, Pausova Z, et al. Mapping of the calcium-sensing receptor gene (CASR) to human chromosome 3q13.3–21 by fluorescence in situ hybridization, and localization to rat chromosome 11 and mouse chromosome 16. *Mamm Genome* 1995;6:798–801.

62. Thakker RV. The molecular genetics of hypoparathyroidism. In: Bilezikian JP, Marcus R, Levine MA, eds. *The Parathyroids: Basic and Clinical Concepts.* 2nd ed. San Diego: Academic Press; 2001:779–790.

63. Brown EM. Physiology of calcium homeostasis. In: Bilezikian JP, Maarcus R, Levine MA, eds. *The Parathyroids: Basic and Clinical Concepts.* 2nd ed. San Diego: Academic Press; 2001:167–182.

64. Broadus AE. Mineral balance and homeostasis. In: Favus MJ, ed. *Primer on the Metabolic Bone Disease and Disorders of Mineral Metabolism.* 5th ed. Washington, DC: American Society for Bone and Mineral Research Press; 2003:105–11.

65. Brown EM. Homeostatic mechanisms regulating extracellular and intracellular calcium metabolism. In: Bilezikian JP, Levine MA, Marcus R, eds. *The Parathyroids: Basic and Clinical Concepts.* New York: Raven Press; 1994:15–54.

66. Bringhurst RF, Demay MB, Krane SM, Kronenberg HM. Bone and mineral metabolism in health and disease, Part 14, Endocrinology and metabolism, Sect 2, Disorders of bone and mineral metabolism. In: Kasper DL, Braunwald E, Fauci AS, Hauser SL, Longo DL. Jameson L, Isselbacher KJ, eds. *Harrison's Principles of Internal Medicine.* 16th ed. 2005 [cited 1 June 2006]; New York: The McGraw-Hill Companies [117 lines, 2 figures]. Available at: http://www.accessmedicine.com.ezp1.harvard.edu. Also available in paper copy from the publisher.

67. Adams JS, Hollis BW. Vitamin D: Synthesis, metabolism, and clinical measurement. In: Coe FL, Favus MJ, eds. *Disorders of Bone and Mineral Metabolism.* 2nd ed. Philadelphia: Williams & Wilkins; 2002:157–174.

68. Silver J. Naveh-Many T. Parathyroid hormone-synthesis and secretion. In: Coe FL, Favus MJ, eds. *Disorders of Bone and Mineral Metabolism.* 2nd ed. Philadelphia: Williams & Wilkins; 2002: 74–101.

69. Brown EM, Pollack M, Seidman CE, et al. Calcium-ion–sensing cell-surface receptors. *N Engl J Med* 1995;333:234–240.

70. Thompson MW, Gauger PG. Ectopic locations of parathyroid glands. In: Bilezikian JP, Maarcus R, Levine MA, eds. *The Parathyroids: Basic and Clinical Concepts.* 2nd ed. San Diego: Academic Press; 2001:499–514.

71. Brown EM, Pollak M, Chou YH, et al. The cloning of extracellular Ca^{++}-sensing receptors from parathyroid and kidney: molecular mechanisms of extracellular Ca^{++}-sensing. *J Nutr* 1995;125 (suppl 7):1955S–1970S.

72. Pollak MR, Chou YH, Marx SJ, et al. Familial hypocalciuric hypercalcemia and neonatal severe hyperparathyroidism. Effects of mutant gene dosage on phenotype. *J Clin Invest* 1994;93: 1108–1112.

73. Chou YH, Pollak MR, Brandi ML, et al. Mutations in the human Ca^{2+}-sensing-receptor gene that cause familial hypocalciuric hyperpercalcemia. *Am J Hum Genet* 1995;56:1075–1079.

74. Pollak MR, Brown EM, Chou YH, et al. Mutations in the human Ca^{2+}-sensing receptor gene cause familial hypocalciuric hypercalcemia and neonatal severe hyperparathyroidism. *Cell* 1992; 75:1297–1303.

75. Pollak MR, Brown EM, Estep HL, et al. Autosomal dominant hypocalcaemia caused by a Ca^{2+}-sensing receptor gene mutation. *Nat Genet* 1994;8:303–307.

76. Sun F, Maercklein P, Fitzpatrick LA. Paracrine interactions among parathyroid cells: effect of cell density on cell secretion. *J Bone Miner Res* 1994;9:971–976.

77. Cohn DV, Fasciotto BH, Reese BK, Zhang JX. Chromogranin A: a novel regulator of parathyroid gland secretion. *J Nutr* 1995; 125(suppl 7):S2015–S2019.

78. Zhang JX, Fasciotto BH, Darling DS, Cohn DV. Pancreastatin, a chromogranin A-derived peptide, inhibits transcription of the parathyroid hormone and chromogranin A genes and decreases the stability of the respective messenger ribonucleic acids in parathyroid cells in culture. *Endocrinology* 1994;134:1310–1316.

79. Fasciotto BH, Trauss CA, Greeley GH, Cohn DV. Parastatin (porcine chromogranin A347–419), a novel chromogranin A-derived peptide, inhibits parathyroid cell secretion. *Endocrinology* 1994;133:461–466.

80. Gilmour JR. The gross anatomy of the parathyroid glands. *J Pathol Bacteriol* 1938;46:133–149.

81. Vail AD, Coller FC. The number and location of parathyroid glands recovered from 202 routine autopsies. *Mo Med* 1966;63: 347–350.

82. Wang CA. The anatomic basis of parathyroid surgery. *Ann Surg* 1976;183:271–275.

83. Alveryd A. Parathyroid glands in thyroid surgery. I. Anatomy of parathyroid glands. II. Postoperative hypoparathyroidism—identification and autotransplantation of parathyroid glands. *Acta Chir Scand* 1968;389:1–120.

84. Åkerström G, Malmaeus J, Bergström R. Surgical anatomy of human parathyroid glands. *Surgery* 1984;95:14–21.

85. Grimelius L, Åkerström G, Johansson H, Bergström R. Anatomy and histopathology of human parathyroid glands. *Pathol Annu* 1981;16(pt 2):1–24.

86. Hooghe L, Kinnaert P, Van Geertruyden J. Surgical anatomy of hyperparathyroidism. *Acta Chir Belg* 1992;92:1–9.

87. Edis AJ, Purnell DC, van Heerden JA. The undescended "parathymus." An occasional cause of failed neck exploration for hyperparathyroidism. *Ann Surg* 1979;190:64–68.

88. Fitko R, Roth SI, Hines JR, Roxe DM, Cahill E. Parathyromatosis in hyperparathyroidism. *Hum Pathol* 1990;21:234–237.

89. Halstead W, Evans H. The parathyroid glandules. Their blood supply and their preservation in operation upon the thyroid gland. *Ann Surg* 1907;46 489–506.

90. Brewer LA. The occurrence of parathyroid tissue within the thymus: report of four cases. *Endrocrinol* 1934;18:393–408.

91. Lack EE, Delay S, Linnoila RI. Ectopic parathyroid tissue within the vagus nerve. Incidence and possible clinical significance. *Arch Pathol Lab Med* 1988;112:304–306.

92. Åkerström G, Grimelius L, Johansson H, Lundqvist H. Estimation of the parenchymal-cell content of the parathyroid gland, using density-gradient columns. Preliminary report. *Acta Pathol Microbiol Scand A* 1977;85:555–557.

93. Åkerström G, Grimelius L, Johansson H, Pertoft H, Lunqvist H. Estimation of the parathyroid parenchymal cell mass by density gradients. *Am J Pathol* 1980;99:685–694.

94. Åkerström G, Grimelius L, Johansson H, Lunqvist H, Pertoft H, Bergstrom R. The parenchymal cell mass in normal human parathyroid glands. *Acta Pathol Microbiol Scand A* 1981;89:367–375.

95. Grimelius L, Åkerström G, Johansson H, Lundqvist H. Estimation of parenchymal cell content of human parathyroid glands using the image analyzing computer technique. *Am J Pathol* 1978;93:793–800.

96. Dufour DR, Wilkerson SY. The normal parathyroid revisited: percentage of stromal fat. *Hum Pathol* 1982;13:717–721.

97. Gilmour JR, Martin WJ. The weight of the parathyroid glands. *J Pathol Bacteriol* 1937;44:431–462.

98. Parfitt AM. Parathyroid growth: normal and abnormal. In: Bilezikian JP, Maarcus R, Levine MA, eds. *The Parathyroids: Basic and Clinical Concepts*. 2nd ed. San Diego: Academic Press; 2001:293–330.

99. Roth SI. Recent advances in parathyroid gland pathology. *Am J Med* 1971;50:612–622.

100. Dufour DR, Wilkerson SY. Factors related to parathyroid weight in normal persons. *Arch Pathol Lab Med* 1983;107:167–172.

101. Matsushita H, Hara M, Shishiba Y, Nakazawa H. An evaluation of the size of the parathyroid glands. *Endocrinol Jpn* 1984;31:127–131.

102. Ghandur-Mnaymneh L, Cassady J, Hajianpour MA, Paz J, Reiss E. The parathyroid gland in health and disease. *Am J Pathol* 1986;125:292–299.

103. Yao K, Singer FR, Roth SI, Sassoon A, Ye C, Giuliano AE. Weight of normal parathyroid glands in patients with parathyroid adenomas. *J Clin Endocrinol Metab* 2004;89:3208–3213.

104. Thiele J. Human parathyroid gland: a freeze fracture and thin section study. *Curr Top in Pathol* 1977:31–80.

105. Mazzocchi G, Meneghelli V, Frasson F. The human parathyroid glands: an optical and electron microscopic study. *Lo Sperimentale* 1967;117:383–447.

106. Balashev VN, Ignashkina MS. Lymphatic system of parathyroid glands in man. *Fed Proc Transl Suppl* 1965;24:603–604.

107. Altenähr E. Electron microscopical evidence for innervation of chief cells in human parathyroid gland. *Experientia* 1971;27:1077.

108. Yeghiayan E, Rojo-Ortega JM, Genest J. Parathyroid vessel innervation: an ultrastructural study. *J Anat* 1972;112(pt 1):137–142.

109. Isono H, Shoumura S. Effects of vagotomy on the ultrastructure of the parathyroid gland of the rabbit. *Acta Anat (Basel)* 1980;108:273–280.

110. Shoumura S, Iwasaki Y, Ishizaki N, et al. Origin of autonomic nerve fibers innervating the parathyroid gland in the rabbit. *Acta Anat (Basel)* 1983;115:289–295.

111. Saffos RO, Rhatigan RM, Urgulu S. The normal parathyroid and the borderline with early hyperplasia: a light microscopic study. *Histopathology* 1984;8:407–422.

112. Dekker A, Dunsford HA, Geyer SJ. The normal parathyroid gland at autopsy: the significance of stromal fat in adult patients. *J Pathol* 1979;128:127–132.

113. Roth SI. The parathyroid gland. In: Silverberg SG, ed. *Principles and Practice of Surgical Pathology*. 2nd ed. Vol 2. New York: Churchill Livingstone; 1989:1923–1955.

114. Cinti S, Balercia G, Zingaretti MC, Amati S, Osculati F. The normal human parathyroid gland. A histochemical and ultrastructural study with particular reference to follicular structures. *J Submicrosc Cytol* 1983;15:661–679.

115. Anderson TJ, Ewen SWB. Amyloid in normal and pathological parathyroid glands. *J Clin Pathol* 1974;27:656–663.

116. Lieberman A, DeLellis RA. Intrafollicular amyloid in normal parathyroid glands. *Arch Pathol* 1973;95:422–423.

117. Leedham PW, Pollock DJ. Intrafollicular amyloid in primary hyperparathyroidism. *J Clin Pathol* 1970;23:811–817.

118. Gilmour JR. The normal histology of the parathyroid glands. *J Pathol Bacteriol* 1939;48:187–222.

119. Roth SI, Olen E, Hansen L. The eosinophilic cells of the parathyroid (oxyphil cells), salivary (oncocytes), and thyroid (Hürthle cells) glands. *Lab Invest* 1962;11:933–941.

120. Munger BL, Roth SI. The cytology of the normal parathyroid glands of man and Virginia deer: a light and electron microscopic study with morphologic evidence of secretory activity. *J Cell Biol* 1963;16:379–400.

121. Roth SI, Munger BL. The cytology of the adenomatous, atrophic, and hyperplastic parathyroid glands of man. A light- and electron-microscopic study. *Virchows Arch Pathol Anat Physiol Klin Med* 1962;335:389–410.

122. Roth SI, Capen CC. Ultrastructural and functional correlations of the parathyroid gland. *Int Rev of Exp Pathol* 1974;13:161–221.

123. Capen CC, Roth SI. Ultrastructural and functional relationships of normal and pathologic parathyroid cells. *Pathobiol Annul.* 1973;3:129–175.

124. Frigerio B, Capella C, Wilander E, Grimelius L. Argyrophil reaction in parathyroid glands: a light and electron microscopic study. *Acta Pathol Microbiol Immunol Scand A* 1982;90:323–326.

125. Weymouth RJ, Baker BL. The presence of argyrophilic granules in the parenchymal cells of the parathyroid glands. *Anat Rec* 1954;119:519–527.

126. Weymouth RJ. The cytology of the parathyroid glands of the rat after bilateral nephrectomy, administration of parathyroid hormone and hypophysectomy. *Anat Rec* 1957;127:509–525.

127. Futrell JM, Roth SI, Su SP, Habener JF, Segre GV, Potts JT Jr. Immunocytochemical localization of parathyroid hormone in bovine parathyroid glands and human parathyroid adenomas. *Am J Pathol* 1979;94:615–622.

128. Ravazzola M, Orci L, Habener JF, Potts JT Jr. Parathyroid secretory protein: immunocytochemical localization within cells that contain parathyroid hormone. *Lancet* 1978;2:371–372.

129. Stork PJ, Herteaux C, Frazier R, Kronenburg H, Wolfe HJ. Expression and distribution of parathyroid hormone and parathyroid hormone messenger RNA in pathological conditions of the parathyroid [abstract]. *Lab Invest* 1989;60:A92.

130. Personal communication, Komminoth P, Wolfe H (13).

131. Kendall CH, Potter L, Brown R, Jasani B, Pringle JH, Lauder I. In situ correlation of synthesis and storage of parathormone in parathyroid gland disease. *J Pathol* 1993;169:61–66.

132. Thiele J. The human parathyroid chief cell—a model for a polypeptide hormone producing endocrine unit as revealed by various functional and pathological conditions. A thin section and freeze-fracture study. *J Submicrosc Cytol* 1986;18:205–220.

133. Thiele J, Kärner J, Fischer R. Ultrastructural morphometry on human parathyroid tissue. Morphological and functional implications. *J Submicrosc Cytol Pathol* 1988;20:491–500.

134. Roth SI, Raisz LG. The course and reversibility of the calcium effect on the ultrastructure of the rat parathyroid gland in organ culture. *Lab Invest* 1966;15:1187–1211.

135. Altenähr E. Ultrastructural pathology of parathyroid glands. *Curr Top Pathol* 1972;56:2–54.

136. Cohn DV, MacGregor RR. The biosynthesis, intracellular processing, and secretion of parathormone. *Endocr Rev* 1981;2:1–26.

137. Habener JF, Rosenblatt M, Potts JT Jr. Parathyroid hormone: biochemical aspects of biosynthesis, secretion, action, and metabolism. *Physiol Rev* 1984;64:958–1053.

138. MacCallum WG, Voegtlin C. On the relation of tetany to the parathyroid glands and to calcium metabolism. *J Exp Med* 1909;11:118–151.

139. Patt HM, Luckhardt AB. Relationship of low blood calcium to parathyroid secretion. *Endocrinology* 1942;31:384–392.

140. Svensson O, Wernerson A, Reinholt FP. The parathyroid glands in the rat as seen by ultrathin step and serial sectioning. *Bone Miner* 1989;6:237–248.

141. Shannon WA Jr, Roth SI. An ultrastructural study of acid phosphatase activity in normal, adenomatous and hyperplastic (chief cell type) human parathyroid glands. *Am J Pathol* 1974;77: 493–506.

142. Pappenheimer AM, Wilens SL. Enlargement of the parathyroid glands in renal disease. *Am J Pathol* 1935;11:73–91.

143. Wild P, Schraner EM, Eggenberger E. Quantitative aspects of membrane shifts in rat parathyroid cells initiated by decrease in serum calcium. *Biol Cell* 1984;50:263–272.

144. Hashizume Y, Waguri S, Watanabe T, Kominami E, Uchiyama Y. Cysteine proteinases in rat parathyroid cells with special reference to their correlation with parathyroid hormone (PTH) in storage granules. *J Histochem Cytochem* 1993;41:273–282.

145. Roth SI, Gallagher MJ. The rapid identification of "normal" parathyroid glands by the presence of intracellular fat. *Am J Pathol* 1976;84:521–528.

146. Sasano H, Geelhoed GW, Silverberg SG. Intraoperative cytologic evaluation of lipid in the diagnosis of parathyroid adenoma. *Am J Surg Pathol* 1988;12:282–286.

147. Ljungberg O, Tibblin S. Preoperative fat staining of frozen sections in primary hyperparathyroidism. *Am J Pathol* 1979;95: 633–642.

148. King DT, Hirose FM. Chief cell intracytoplasmic fat used to evaluate parathyroid disease by frozen section. *Arch Pathol Lab Med* 1979;103:609–612.

149. Bondeson AG, Bondeson L, Ljungberg O, Tibblin S. Fat staining in parathyroid disease—diagnostic value and impact on surgical strategy: clinicopathologic analysis of 191 cases. *Hum Pathol* 1985;16:1255–1263.

150. Monchik JM, Farrugia R, Teplitz C, Teplitz J, Brown S. Parathyroid surgery: the role of chief cell intracellular fat staining with osmium carmine in the intraoperative management of patients with primary hyperparathyroidism. *Surgery* 1983;94:877–886.

151. Alpern HD, Roth SI, Olson JE. Intracellular lipid droplets in functioning transitional parathyroid oxyphil adenomas. A caveat. *Arch Surg* 1990;125:410–411.

152. Chen KTK. Fat stain in hyperparathyroidism. *Am J Surg Pathol* 1982;6:191–192.

153. Kasdon EJ, Rosen S, Cohen RB, Silen W. Surgical pathology of hyperparathyroidism. Usefulness of fat stain and problems in interpretation. *Am J Surg Pathol* 1981;5:381–384.

154. Dekker A, Watson CG, Barnes EL Jr. The pathologic assessment of primary hyperparathyroidism and its impact on therapy. A prospective evaluation of 50 cases with oil-red-O stain. *Ann Surg* 1979;190:671–675.

155. Ritchie CK, Cohn DV, Maercklein PB, Fitzpatrick LA. Individual parathyroid cells exhibit cyclic secretion of parathyroid hormone and chromogranin-A (as measured by a novel sequential hemolytic plaque assay). *Endocrinology* 1992;131:2638–2642.

156. Fitzpatrick LA. Heterogeneous secretory response of parathyroid cells. *Recent Prog Horm Res* 1993;48:471–475.

157. Lee MJ, Roth SI. Effect of calcium and magnesium on deoxyribonucleic acid synthesis in rat parathyroid glands in vitro. *Lab Invest* 1975;33:72–79.

158. Bianchi S, Fabiani S, Muratori M, et al. Calcium modulates the cyclin D1 expression in a rat parathyroid cell line. *Biochem Biophys Res Commun* 1994;204:691–700.

159. Hamperl H. Über das Vorkommen von Onkocyten in verschiedenen Organen und ihren Geschwülsten (Mundspeicheldrüsen, Bauschpeicheldrüse, Epithelkörperchen, Hypophyse, Schilddrüse, Eileiter). *Virchows Arch f Path Anat* 1936;25:327–375.

160. Hamperl H. Onkocyten and Onkocytome. *Virchows Arch Pathol Anat Physiol Klin Med* 1962;335:452–483.

161. Tremblay G. The oncocytes. *Methods Achiev Exp Pathol* 1969; 4:121–140.

162. Christie AC. The parathyroid oxyphil cells. *J Clin Pathol* 1967;20: 591–602.

163. Müller-Höcker J. Random cytochrome-C-oxidase deficiency of oxyphil cell nodules in the parathyroid gland. A mitochondrial cytopathy related to cell ageing? *Pathol Res Pract* 1992;188: 701–706.

164. Tandler B, Hoppel CL. *Mitochondria*. New York: Academic Press; 1972:1–59.

165. Balogh K Jr, Cohen RB. Oxidative enzymes in the epithelial cells of normal and pathological human parathyroid glands: a histochemical study. *Lab Invest* 1961;10:354–360.

166. Fischer R. Über den histochemischen Nachwies oxidativer Enzyme in Onkozyten verschiedener Organe. *Virchows Arch A* 1961;334:445–452.

167. Tremblay G, Cartier GE. Histochemical study of oxidative enzymes in the human parathyroid. *Endocrinology* 1961;69:658–661.

168. Kitazawa R, Kitazawa S, Fukase M, et al. The expression of parathyroid hormone-related protein (PTHrP) in parathyroid: histochemistry and in situ hybridization. *Histochemistry* 1992;98: 211–215.

169. Wolpert HR, Vickery AL Jr, Wang CA. Functioning oxyphil cell adenomas of the parathyroid gland. A study of 15 cases. *Am J Surg Pathol* 1989;13:500–504.

170. Shapiro MJ, Batang ES. Needle aspiration biopsy of the thyroid and parathyroid. *Otolaryngol Clin North Am.* 1990;23:217–229.

171. Bergenfelz A, Forsberg L, Henderström E, Ahren B. Preoperative localization of enlarged parathyroid glands with ultrasonically guided fine needle aspiration for parathyroid hormone assay. *Acta Radiol* 1991;32:403–405.

172. Halbauer M, Crepinko I, Tomc Brzac H, Simonovic I. Fine needle aspiration cytology in the preoperative diagnosis of ultrasonically enlarged parathyroid glands. *Acta Cytol* 1991;35:728–735.

173. Tikkakoski T, Stenfors LE, Typpo T, Lohela P, Apaja-Sarkkinen M. Parathyroid adenomas: pre-operative localization with ultrasound combined with fine-needle biopsy. *J Laryngol Otol* 1993; 107:543–545.

174. Silverberg SG. Imprints in the intraoperative evaluation of parathyroid disease. *Arch Pathol* 1975;99:375–378.

175. Geelhoed GW, Silverberg SG. Intraoperative imprints for the identification of parathyroid tissue. *Surgery* 1984;96:1124–1131.

176. Roth SI. The parathyroid gland In: Silverberg SG, DeLellis RA, Frable WJ, eds. *Principles and Practice of Surgical Pathology and Cytopathology*. 3rd ed. New York: Churchill Livingstone; 1997: 2709–2750.

177. DeMay RM. Parathyroid. In: *The Art and Science of Cytopathology. Volume II: Aspirate Cytology*. Chicago: ASCP Press; 1996:648–649.

Adrenal

J. Aidan Carney   Ricardo V. Lloyd

INTRODUCTION

The paired adrenal glands are a composite of two endocrine organs—one steroid producing, the other catecholamine producing—that are located in the retroperitoneum, superomedial to the kidneys. The two organs have a different embryonic origin, histology, and function.

ANATOMY

The main portions of the adrenal gland are easily recognized on the fresh or formalin-fixed cut surface (Figure 46.1). Externally, a relatively thick yellow layer is applied to a narrow dark brown band that abuts on a solid, pearly gray interior. The former two zones correspond histologically to the zona fasciculata and zona reticularis of the cortex, and the latter to the medulla of the organ.

The anatomic location of the human adrenal glands, which sandwiches them between several organs, is responsible for their particular shape: pyramidal on the right and crescent shaped on the left. The depression and ridge (crest) on the posterior surfaces (Figure 46.2) result from their close relationship to the kidneys. When a kidney is congenitally absent, the corresponding adrenal is round and the characteristic longitudinal ridge on the posterior surface is missing (1).

EVOLUTION

The anatomic relationship of the adrenal cortex to the medulla that exists in mammals is not found in lower animals. In the shark, for example, the cortex and medulla are topographically completely separate; in amphibians, the two structures are in close contact; in birds, they are

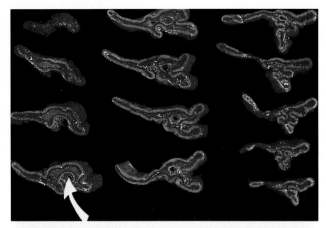

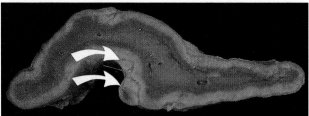

Figure 46.1 Normal adrenal gland. **Top:** Fresh gland sliced from head (*upper left*) through body (*center*) to tail (*lower right*). The yellow cortex and pearly gray medulla are visible in the head (*left*). Yellow zona fasciculata surrounds dark brown zona reticularis in the tail (*right*), where medulla is absent. The gland can be identified as the left adrenal because on this side the adrenal vein runs in a well-developed groove on the surface of the gland at the junction of the head and body (*arrow*). Invaginated cortex surrounds the central vein in the interior of the body. **Bottom:** Slice of formalin-fixed adrenal gland showing, from exterior inward, cortical zona fasciculata (yellow), zona reticularis (brown), and medulla (gray). The cortex is about 1 mm in thickness. Dilated tributaries of the central vein are seen in the medulla. The adrenal vein has been removed from its groove. Nodules of accessory cortex are present (*arrows*).

intermingled. Only in mammals does the intimate proximity seen among the human adrenal cortex and medulla occur. In a prototypic mammal (e.g., the rat), the medulla forms a central core that is uniformly surrounded by the cortex. The distribution of the two zones in the human adrenal is different. In the human adrenal (Figure 46.3), most of the medulla is in the head of the gland (medial), some occurs in the body, and there is usually none in the tail (lateral) (3). Two bands of cortex applied one to the other form the alae of the glands.

DEVELOPMENT

Cortex

The adrenal cortex is of mesodermal origin. Its primordia appear at the 9-mm embryo stage (6th week of gestation) as bilateral cellular aggregations (Figure 46.4) at the mesenteric root, medial to the developing gonad and anterior to the kidney (mesonephros) (4,5). These primordia are composed of two groups of mesenchymal cells: one destined to be the precursor of the transitory provisional or fetal cortex, the other to become the adrenal capsule and its supporting connective tissue framework (5). By the 7th week of gestation, the primordia have become more defined, have separated from the coelomic lining, and include polyhedral cells with eosinophilic, lipid-poor cytoplasm. These cells increase in size and proliferate rapidly, forming a series of parallel columns and cords of cells that ultimately compose the bulk of the provisional cortex. External to this dominant mass, a thin subcapsular

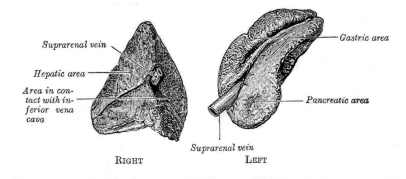

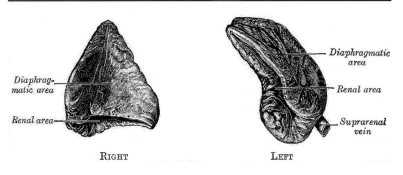

Figure 46.2 External appearance of anterior (*above*) and posterior aspects (*below*) of right and left adrenal glands. The right gland is pyramidal, and the left is crescent shaped. The right adrenal vein is short. The left vein is longer and lies in a groove on the anterior surface of the gland. (Reprinted with permission from: Goss CM, ed. *Gray's Anatomy of the Human Body.* 29th ed. Philadelphia: Lea & Febiger; 1973.)

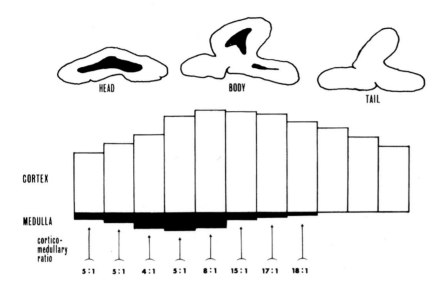

Figure 46.3 Diagrammatic illustration of the distribution of medulla (black) in the head, body, and tail of the adrenal gland (*above*) and corresponding corticomedullary ratios (*below*). (Reprinted with permission from: Symington T. *Functional Pathology of the Human Adrenal Gland.* Baltimore: Williams & Wilkins; 1969.)

rim of smaller cells (the precursor of the permanent or adult cortex) appears (Figure 46.5). These cells are arranged in nests and arches that cap the columns of deeper cells. They have hyperchromatic, closely packed, overlapping nuclei. The nuclei are larger, more vesicular, and less hyperchromatic in the cords. Continuous, spottily distributed degeneration of the cells is found in the cords, and dead cells (apoptosis) are continuously replaced by the proliferation of cells in the narrow subcapsular band. Growth of the developing cortex is therefore centripedal (from outside inward).

At the end of gestation, the provisional cortex accounts for the bulk of the gland (Figure 46.6). Within hours of birth, it becomes acutely congested and starts to degenerate. At the end of 7 to 10 days, the provisional cortex is largely disorganized and necrotic. The narrow peripheral band of cell clusters survives and becomes the source of the permanent cortex.

Medulla

The adrenal medulla is of neuroectodermal origin (5). Precursor cells originate in the neural crest and migrate from primitive spinal ganglia (sixth thoracic to first lumbar) to form the primitive sympathetic nervous system situated dorsal to the aorta. Sympathogonia cells (from the sympathetic anlagen) migrate farther into nerves that sprout from the sympathetic chain, then move alongside large blood vessels that penetrate into the (as yet) unencapsulated fetal adrenal cortex, primarily at its caudal pole (head). [This very likely explains the nonuniform distribution of medulla in the adult adrenal mentioned previously.] The neural cells enter the adrenal primordium as fingerlike processes and pass among the fetal cortical cells. In this manner, sympathogonia and a plexus of nerves are initially scattered among fetal cortical cells (Figure 46.7). Two sets of progeny of the sympathogonia evolve: the majority, small cells with little cytoplasm and

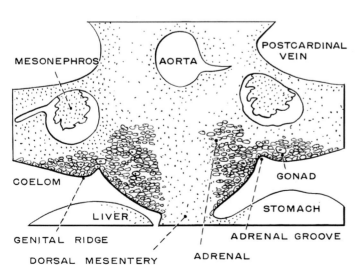

Figure 46.4 Diagrammatic representation of a human embryo at 6 weeks' gestation showing the anatomic relationship of developing adrenal gland to coelomic cavity, gonad, and kidney (mesonephros). (Reprinted with permission from: Dahl EV, Bahn RC. Aberrant adrenal cortical tissue near the testis in human infants. *Am J Pathol* 1962;40:587–598.)

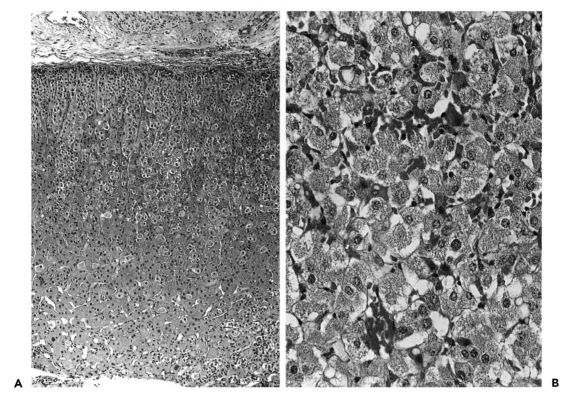

Figure 46.5 Provisional (fetal) cortex (29 weeks' gestation, stillborn infant). **A.** Cortex is dominated by large cells with eosinophilic cytoplasm in vague columns and solid sheet with prominent capillaries. Just beneath the tenuous capsule, there is a rim of smaller cells, the source of the permanent cortex. A sympathetic ganglion and a small nerve are present in the periadrenal connective tissue. **B.** Large, liverlike cells with cytoplasm that is voluminous, eosinophilic, and granular. Nuclei are vesicular with a single small nucleolus. Vascularity is prominent.

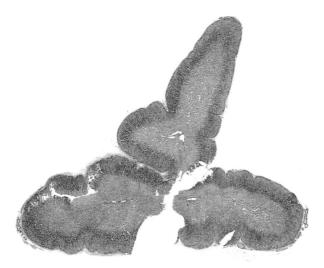

Figure 46.6 Adrenal cortex at birth (35 weeks' gestation; infant died at 2 days). The central, degenerating, eosinophilic provisional cortex is surrounded by the developing, darkly staining outer rim of permanent cortex.

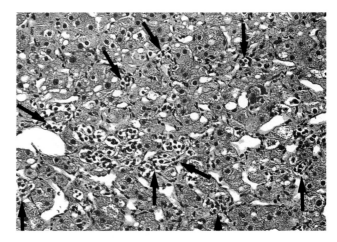

Figure 46.7 Developing adrenal medulla (29 weeks' gestation, stillborn infant). Clusters of small medullary cells with deeply staining nuclei (*arrows*) irregularly distributed in very vascular provisional cortex. When the latter degenerates, the clusters of medullary cells survive and, lacking the support of the cortical cells, aggregate together.

a darkly staining nucleus (neuroblasts); the minority, larger cells with a vesicular nucleus and basophilic cytoplasm (pheochromoblasts). At birth, the medulla comprises a central, very thin core of these cells with offshoots stretching a short distance into the peripheral degenerating provisional cortex. The medullary cells are arranged in irregularly sized clumps containing both cell types, the larger cells now predominating. The postnatal collapse of the provisional cortex and its stroma removes the framework that supported the medullary offshoots and their associated nerve plexus in the cortex (3). With this loss of scaffolding, these structures coalesce around the central veins.

GLAND WEIGHT AND CORTICAL THICKNESS

Although not a structural feature of the adrenal, the weight of the glands is important because assessment of the adrenal normalcy takes this feature into account. Information on truly normal adrenal weight is difficult to obtain because the organ (specifically the cortex) responds rapidly to stress by an increase in mass. Therefore, accurate normal adrenal weight can be determined only from selected autopsy material (e.g., healthy individuals who die suddenly). The combined adrenal weight in these circumstances is about 8–9 g (1). Exceptionally, a gland weighs as little as 2 g or as much as 6 g. Sex differences are not apparent. Formalin fixation has little effect on the gland weight.

Relative to body weight, the adrenals are actually largest at the 4th month of gestation (2). In unselected autopsy cases, the combined average weight of the glands at birth is about 20 g. By the end of the 1st week of life, this mass has decreased (as a result of involution of the provisional cortex) to about 12 g, and a further small decrease occurs during the 2nd week, such that each gland comes to weigh approximately 5 g. Total gland weight then remains constant for 2 years, then gradually rises to the adult postmortem weight of about 13 g between 15 and 20 years of age (3).

The thickness of the normal adult adrenal cortex is approximately 1 mm and ranges from about 0.7 to 1.3 mm. For accuracy, the thickness should be determined microscopically with an ocular micrometer; it is impractical to detect small alterations in the thickness using a metric scale.

ADRENAL GLANDS FOR HISTOLOGIC STUDY

Ideal Material

Ideally, for the reasons already mentioned, adrenal glands used for study of normal histology of the organ should be obtained from healthy patients. Results obtained from the study of glands of patients with primary adrenal disease or disorders that might affect the adrenal histology secondarily should be used with caution. Nevertheless, because the two portions of the adrenal gland, cortex and medulla, are separate functional units that apparently do not affect each other, we think that it is not unreasonable (until shown to be otherwise) to study, for example, the histology of the adrenal medulla (thinking of it as being normal) in a gland surgically removed for a clinically and biochemically nonfunctioning small adrenocortical adenoma. Similar considerations apply to the cortex.

For study of cytologic detail, material should be fresh and not autolysed and therefore obtained at surgery or shortly after death. The zona reticularis of the cortex quickly begins to show the effects of anoxia (degeneration). However, glands that are less than optimally preserved for study of the cell details are satisfactory for determination of general microanatomy of the organ. In practice, fresh (and to a variable extent "normal") adrenal is most often available at the time of radical nephrectomy, in the course of which a gland is removed with the kidney. However, many such glands are torn during the surgical procedure, limiting to some extent their use for study of normal histology. Their usefulness is also limited in that they are representative only of the gland appearance in a particular age range (middle-aged or older patients). In practice, it is difficult to get the complete range of normal adrenal specimens (fetal to aged) that would be ideal for study of normal histology.

Actual Material

The actual tissue used for the histologic description that follows included adrenals from all the foregoing categories. Autopsy material was obtained from individuals (mostly male) who died suddenly (homicide, suicide, or traumatic injury). For some cases there was minimal or no medical history available, and the autopsy protocol and other autopsy slides could not be reviewed. Thus, the state of health of these patients and the condition of other organs could not be determined. A number of normal glands were available from patients undergoing nephrectomy. Also, opportunity was taken to study apparently normal extratumoral medulla and cortex in cases of adrenalectomy for certain primary adrenal neoplasms that were small or relatively small (adrenocortical adenomas producing aldosterone, nonfunctioning adrenocortical adenomas, and pheochromocytoma).

HISTOLOGY

Blood Vessels

The blood supply of the adrenal gland has been studied mostly from the anatomic point of view, often by observing

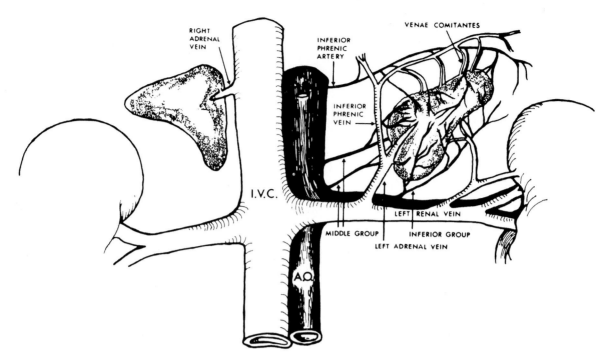

Figure 46.8 Diagrammatic representation of the arterial supply (black) and venous drainage (light and hatched) of the left adrenal gland. (Reprinted with permission from: Symington T. *Functional Pathology of the Human Adrenal Gland.* Baltimore: Williams & Wilkins; 1969.)

the distribution of injected material in the vasculature. The tone of the subcapsular vascular plexus controls circulation through the organ. The histologic appearance of the vessels distal to the plexus suggests that the intravascular pressure in the organ is low.

Arteries

Three separate groups of arteries—superior, middle, and inferior—arising from the inferior phrenic artery, the aorta, and the renal artery, supply each adrenal gland (Figure 46.8). The main vessels divide into 50 to 60 small feeder vessels that penetrate the anterior and posterior surfaces of the glands and form a plexus beneath the capsule of the gland. The former are commonly encountered close to the capsule of the gland; in older patients, they frequently exhibit atherosclerotic changes. The subcapsular plexus, important in regulation of the circulation in the gland, as has just been indicated, is not conspicuous in routine histologic preparations.

Intraglandular Vasculature

Capillary loops from the subcapsular plexus surround the cells of the zona glomerulosa (see "Zona Glomerulosa"), then extend toward the interior of the organ between the columns of cells of the zona fasciculata, and ultimately open into wide interconnecting channels in the zona reticularis to form a second vascular plexus. This ends abruptly

in a vascular dam at the corticomedullary junction that finally drains into the sinusoids of the medulla by relatively fewer channels. The marked vascular congestion commonly seen at the corticomedullary junction of adrenal glands obtained at autopsy may be a reflection of this vascular barrier. Although the medulla receives some arterial blood supply, most of its vascular supply has already nourished the cortex.

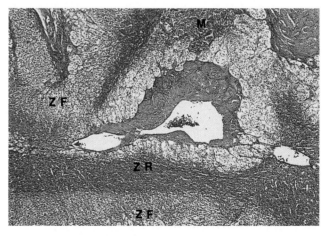

Figure 46.9 Central adrenal vein. Low-power view of the vein surrounded by an invaginated cuff of cortical cells with clear cytoplasm (zona fasciculata type). Distribution of smooth muscle in the vein wall is uneven. The zona fasciculata (ZF) and zona reticularis (ZR) of the cortex are evident, and there is a small amount of basophilic medulla (M).

The venous drainage from the organs occurs via a single vein that emerges from the anterior surface of each gland (Figure 46.2). Inside the organs, the central adrenal vein (which ultimately becomes the adrenal vein as it leaves the organ) and its tributaries have a unique muscle coat, 2 to 6 longitudinally running muscle bundles, varying in size and eccentrically situated around the vein lumen (Figure 46.9). The bundles are heavily laden with elastic fibers that extend into tributaries of the larger central veins and in some instances outline clusters and trabeculae of medullary cells.

The eccentricity of the muscle bundles results in a vein wall that varies greatly in thickness and focally is devoid of muscle. In the zones where the muscle bundles are deficient (and these may be extensive), medullary cells (and sometimes cortical cells) are separated from the bloodstream by intima and a minimal amount of subintimal connective tissue only. This peculiar anatomic structure permits medullary cells or cortical cells to occasionally form polypoid endothelium-covered projections into the lumen of the central vein (Figure 46.10). (This ready access of pheochromocytes to the venous lumen explains the occasional finding of an intravenous tumor plug of pheochromocytoma.) A thick cuff of invaginated cortical cells surrounds the intramedullary central vein and its larger tributaries (Figure 46.10). (Development of a neoplasm in this "displaced" cortex probably explains the occasional

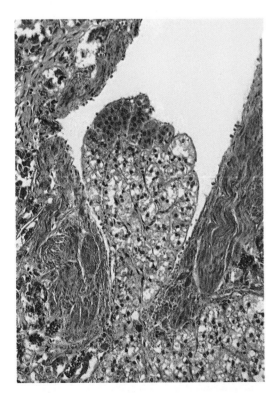

Figure 46.10   Central adrenal vein. Intraluminal protrusion of endothelium-covered adrenocortical cells between the discontinuous muscle bundles of a tributary of the central adrenal vein.

cortical neoplasm that appears to have developed in the medulla of the organ. As explained later, there is another possible source for a cortical neoplasm in this location—from cortical cells that occur among cells of the medulla.)

Veins

The left adrenal vein, 2 to 4 cm in length, initially lies in a groove on the anterior surface of the gland and terminates in the left renal vein (Figures 46.2 and 46.8). The right adrenal vein is short (1–5 mm) and drains into the inferior vena cava (Figures 46.2 and 46.8). Histologically, the extra-adrenal and immediately intra-adrenal portions of the veins have a muscular coat composed of large, similarly sized, evenly disposed smooth muscle bundles, arranged side by side—a structure found in other veins of this size.

Nerves and Ganglia

The innervation of the adrenal gland, specifically of the medulla, emanates from the lower thoracic segments of the spinal cord and passes through the greater splanchnic nerve and the upper lumbar sympathetic ganglia via the celiac plexus. This nerve supply forms a plexus of medullated and nonmedullated nerves on the capsule of the gland, primarily on its posterior aspect. Thus, the largely preganglionic nerve fibers pass into the medulla following either the course of emerging or penetrating vessels or connective tissue trabeculae. Occasionally, a large nerve penetrates directly into the medulla. The number of nerves visible in the medulla varies greatly from case to case; some feature a perineurium, whereas others do not; frequently, they have associated ganglion cells (Figure 46.11). Ganglion cells are also commonly seen singly or in clusters among the pheochromocytes (Figure 46.12). The cells of the cortex do not have a nerve supply.

Lymphatics

Injection studies have demonstrated that there is a rich plexus of lymphatic channels in the capsule of the gland (3). Lymphatics are distributed to the adventitia of the central vein and its main tributaries. There is no lymphatic supply to the cortex. The lymphatics drain into aortic lymph nodes.

Capsule

The capsule of the adrenal gland is composed of hypocellular fibrous tissue in the form of coarse, hyalinized collagen bundles and elastic fibers (Figure 46.13). Usually, the capsule is thin, but it varies considerably in thickness from gland to gland and even within the same gland (Figure 46.14). It is tough and hard to cut but tears easily and does

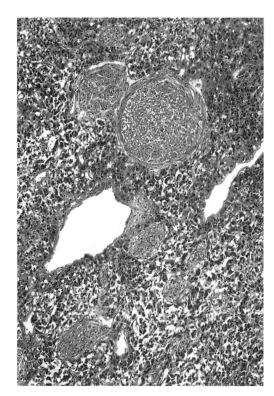

Figure 46.11 Adrenal medulla. Unusual concentration of nerves, some with perineurium and others without.

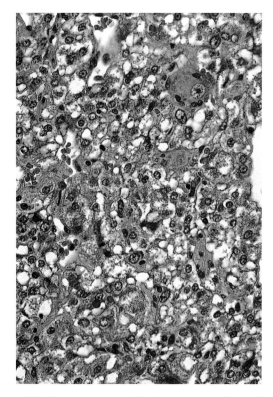

Figure 46.12 Adrenal medulla. Sheet of medullary cells with cytoplasm that is nonhomogeneous, variably basophilic, granular, and vacuolated, resulting in a mottled appearance. A ganglion cell is present among the pheochromocytes.

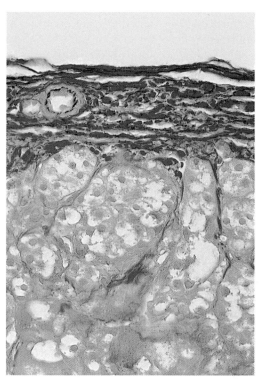

Figure 46.13 Adrenal capsule. Elastic–van Gieson stain shows collagen bundles (red) and intermingled elastic fibers (black). A small artery is present in the capsule.

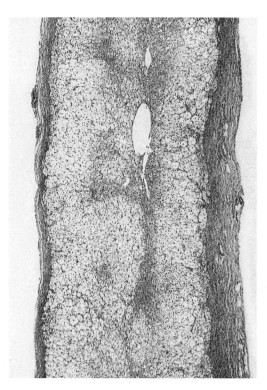

Figure 46.14 Adrenal capsule. Four-fold variation in the thickness of the capsule, which at its maximum thickness measures 0.3 mm.

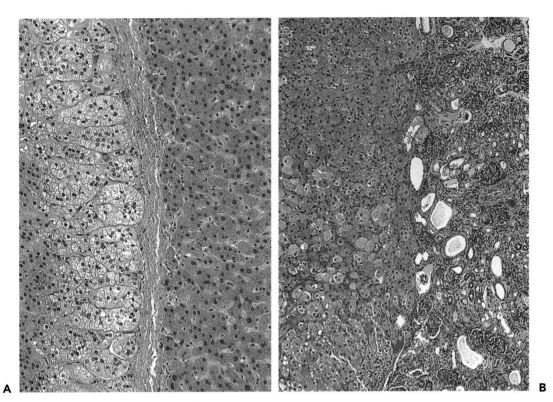

A　　　　　　　　　　　　　　　　　　　　　**B**

Figure 46.15　Adrenal capsule. **A.** Common capsule of adrenal (*left*) and liver (*right*). Note that a zona glomerulosa is not evident in the adrenal cortex. **B.** Absence of an adrenal and kidney capsule results in direct contact of adrenal cortex (provisional) and renal parenchyma.

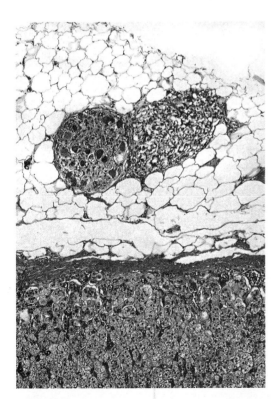

Figure 46.16　Normal adrenal gland. Juxtaposed sympathetic ganglion (*above left*) and paraganglion (*above right*) in periadrenal adipose tissue. The adrenal cortex features cells with clear cytoplasm (zona fasciculata). Zona glomerulosa is not evident.

not support the unfixed gland, which is limp and readily bends. The soft consistency of the fresh glands makes them difficult to section; cooling them for 15 minutes in a refrigerator facilitates this operation.

Because of the propinquity of development of adrenals and kidneys and the liver (on the right side), there is occasional fusion or sharing of a common capsule among the adrenal and kidney and the adrenal and liver (Figure 46.15). The common capsule may be deficient focally, and then parenchymal cells of two organs come into direct contact. The adrenal capsule is surrounded by adult-type fat (brown fat in the fetus and newborn) that features small arteries, veins, nerves, accessory cortex, excrescences of cortex, sympathetic ganglia, and an occasional paraganglion (Figure 46.16).

The capsule is penetrated by blood vessels supplying and draining the gland, the nerves to the medulla, and lymphatic channels. In random sections of the glands, only the site of exit of the adrenal vein is regularly encountered (because of its relatively large size); occasionally, the site of penetration of a large nerve is seen; the entry sites of the small arteries into the glands are also sometimes seen. Commonly found are narrow (occasionally wide) defects in the capsule through which the cortex protrudes into the periadrenal fat to form small nodules of cells that are sometimes delimited by a distended and attenuated adrenal capsule, sometimes not (Figure 46.17).

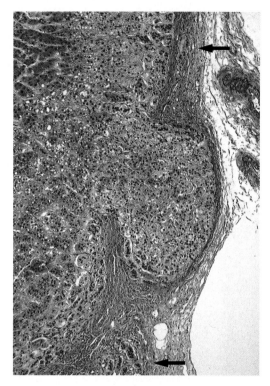

Figure 46.17 Normal adrenal gland. Protrusion of cortical cells surrounded by attenuated capsule through a "wide" defect in the adrenal capsule. A few cortical cells in rows and small aggregates are present in the capsule (*arrows*). A suggestive zona glomerulosa is present deep to the adrenal capsule (*top*).

These excrescences are composed predominantly of epithelial cells with normal zonation patterns among the cells. The protrusions may contain a connective tissue component, and sometimes there is an equal mixture of cords of epithelial cells and fibrous tissue. Single rows and groups of cortical cells, small and oval or large and round, are commonly found here and there in capsular "pockets" (Figure 46.18). Larger oval aggregates cause a slight depression in, and thinning of, the underlying cortex, so that the total width of the two portions of cortex—that in the capsular pocket and that normally situated—is about normal (Figure 46.18).

Sometimes seen attached to the capsule are wedge-shaped foci of small, plump spindle cells with hyperchromatic nuclei. These protrude into the cortex to varying depths and may be present bilaterally (Figure 46.19). The cells are arranged in interlacing bundles and whorls. Largely because of their light microscopic resemblance to ovarian cortical stroma, these aggregates have been termed "ovarian thecal metaplasia"; an alternative interpretation is that they represent areas of adrenocortical blastema that for unknown reasons have failed to mature (6–8). These foci undergo fibrosis, hyalinization, and sometimes calcification. Nests of cortical cells are occasionally found in the spindle cell proliferation, presumably entrapped.

Exceptionally, the proliferations penetrate into the medulla as increasingly narrow tongues of tissue. Ovarian thecal metaplasia is said to occur in postmenopausal women, occasionally in premenopausal women, and exceptionally in old men. We have not seen it in any of the normal adrenal glands we have examined despite a good search. However, we have encountered it fairly commonly in the extratumoral cortex associated with a range of functioning adrenocortical adenomas and in adrenals removed for other pathology, cortical and medullary, always in peri-menopausal or postmenopausal females. The "lesions" are generally incidental microscopic findings that were not recognized grossly.

Cortex

Traditionally, the cortex has been divided into three areas based on light microscopy findings from the capsule inward—the zona glomerulosa, the zona fasciculata, and the zona reticularis—forming the typical zonation pattern of the adrenal cortex (Figure 46.20). The functional significance of this morphologic separation is questionable, but the zona glomerulosa is the site of aldosterone production and is responsive to angiotensin and potassium, and the zona fasciculata and zona reticularis synthesize glucocorticoids and sex hormones. Cells of all zones respond to adrenocorticotropic hormone (ACTH). Recent studies using monoclonal antibodies have shown some differential staining of the normal human cortical parenchyma (9). Division figures are rare in the normal adult cortex; in fact, the zone(s) of normal proliferation for replacement of effete cells is not known, although it is believed to be near the periphery of the cortex. [Under the influence of increased circulating levels of ACTH (Cushing's disease), mitotic figures may be seen in the zona fasciculata and zona reticularis, indicating that cells in the deeper areas of the cortex are also capable of proliferating.]

A number of modern techniques for studying cell proliferation and programmed cell death (apoptosis), specifically, KI-67 immunostaining and 3'-OH nick end-labeling method, respectively, have been applied to study of the human adrenal cortex (10). Cell proliferation as indicated by KI-67 immunoreactivity occurred principally in the zona fasciculata. Cortical cells positive for nick-end labeling (apoptotic) were uniformly present in the zona reticularis and in the zona glomerulosa in one third of cases. The findings suggest that cortical cells may disperse in two directions, centripetally and centrifugally, from the zona fasciculata to the zona reticularis and from the zona fasciculata to the zona glomerulosa, in some cases. Biochemically, apoptosis features chromatin cleavage. Morphologically, there is shrinkage of cytoplasm, condensation, and fragmentation of nuclei and membrane blebbing. Adrenocortical cells undergoing apoptosis are believed to be phagocytosed by histiocytes and cells lining the sinusoids.

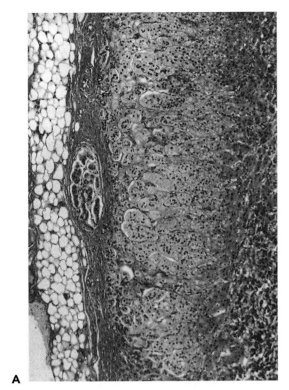

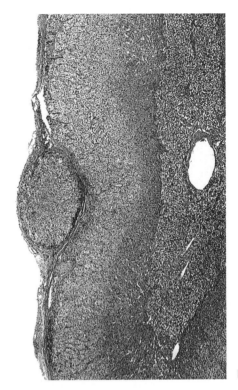

Figure 46.18 Normal adrenal gland. **A.** Aggregate of cells with features of zona glomerulosa type in "pocket" in capsule. **B.** Cortex featuring zona fasciculata (clear cells) and zona reticularis (compact cells) abuts medulla. A larger aggregate of cortical cells with clear (peripheral) and compact cytoplasm (central) is present in a pocket in the capsule. The cortex deep to the pocket is slightly attenuated. A zona glomerulosa is not clearly visible.

Nucleolar organizer regions, loops of ribosomal DNA that appear to be an indicator of cellular and nuclear activity, have been studied to a limited degree in the human adrenal cortex, using a silver technique and formalin-fixed, paraffin-embedded tissue (11).

Zona Glomerulosa

The zona glomerulosa is the narrow, inconstant band of cortex situated immediately beneath the capsule and superficial to the zona fasciculata (Figure 46.21). Sometimes it can be identified throughout a section or over a large portion of one as a distinct rim beneath the capsule; more often it cannot. Where it is deficient, the zona fasciculata extends to the capsule (Figure 46.22). The zone is often easier to identify

Figure 46.19 Ovarian thecal metaplasia (63-year-old woman with a 2-cm aldosterone-producing adrenocortical adenoma). A group of packed spindle cells is attached to the adrenal capsule. Nests of cortical cells are trapped by hyalinized fibrous tissue. A poorly defined zona glomerulosa is present).

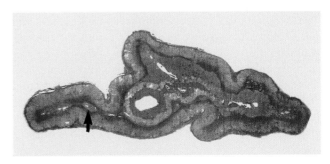

Figure 46.20 Normal adrenal gland. A thick capsule surrounds the adrenal cortex (outer clear zona fasciculata and inner eosinophilic zona reticularis) that encloses the basophilic adrenal medulla. An area of medulla in the ala (*arrow*) is not in continuity with the main mass of medulla. The adrenal vein is surrounded by a cuff of invaginated cortex.

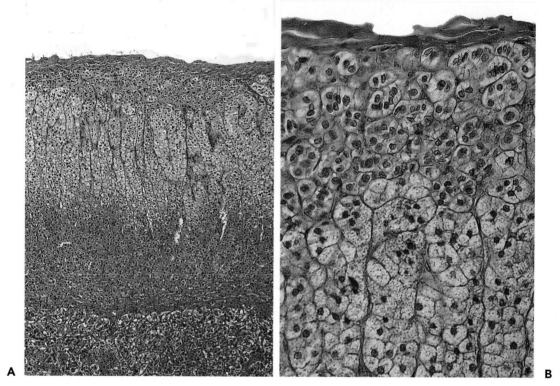

Figure 46.21 Normal adrenal gland. **A.** The normal pattern of zonation of the cortex is seen (clusters of cells with stainable cytoplasm in the zona glomerulosa, columns of cells with clear cytoplasm in the zona fasciculata, and cells with acidophilic cytoplasm in the zona reticularis). There is a sharp interface between the cortex (zona reticularis) and medulla (clusters of cells with basophilic cytoplasm). **B.** Zona glomerulosa composed of packed clusters and short trabeculae of cells beneath the adrenal capsule and superficial to the columns of vacuolated cells of the zona fasciculata. The zona glomerulosa nuclei tend to be oval; those of the zona fasciculata are round.

in autopsy preparations. In routine hematoxylin and eosin preparations, the band may merge with and be separated with difficulty from the outer cells of the zona fasciculata.

The zona glomerulosa cells are well outlined and aggregated into small clusters that are supported by a minimal amount of fibrovascular stroma (Figure 46.21). The clusters occasionally merge into short trabeculae, straight, bent, or hairpin shape. The cells that tend to be columnar also occur in short cords or one-cell rows set parallel to the capsule. The cytoplasm is faintly acidophilic or amphophilic and minimally to distinctly vacuolated. The round nuclei sometimes are indistinguishable from those of the other zones of the cortex, but often they appear slightly smaller and more deeply staining. Commonly, they are ellipsoidal and elongated and display a longitudinal groove, a nuclear configuration not seen in the deeper areas of the cortex (Figure 46.21). The nuclear to cytoplasmic ratio is high.

Zona Fasciculata

The zona fasciculata is a broad band, more than half the thickness of the cortex, that lies between the zona glomerulosa (superficial) and the zona reticularis (deep)

(Figures 46.20, 46.21, and 46.23). The transition between the zones is not sharp. The zona fasciculata cells are large, have distinct cell membranes, are arranged in two-cell wide cords (with the cord axes perpendicular to capsule) and are bounded laterally by parallel-running capillaries. The nuclei are more vesicular and less chromatic than those of the zona glomerulosa, feature a single small nucleolus, and are central in the cells. Especially in the outer two thirds of the zone, the cells are filled with lipid (cholesterol, fatty acids, and neutral fat), much of which is birefringent (Figure 46.24). Because this lipid is dissolved with the usual technical procedures, the fasciculata cells have a spongy, vacuolated, clear appearance and are often referred to as clear cells. When frozen, and sections are stained with a vital dye or stained for fat, the large amount of intracellular lipid can be appreciated (Figure 46.24). The yellow color of the zone seen grossly is due to this high lipid content.

Zona Reticularis

The zona reticularis lies deep to the zona fasciculata, and in the head and body of the gland abuts on the medulla (Figures 46.9, 46.20, 46.21, and 46.23). In the tail of the gland,

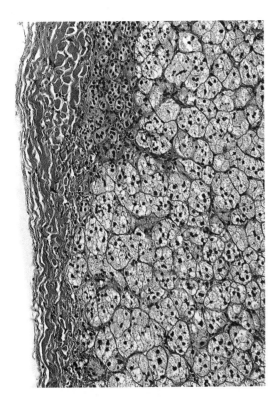

Figure 46.22 Normal adrenal cortex with discontinuity of zona glomerulosa. Zona glomerulosa (*upper half*) composed of clusters of cells with amphophilic cytoplasm forms a distinct band beneath the capsule and is sharply demarcated from the deeper zona fasciculata with its clustered cells having clear cytoplasm. Where the zona glomerulosa is absent (*lower half*), the zona fasciculata extends to the capsule.

where there is no medulla, the zona reticularis is in contact with zona reticularis forming a lateral raphe. It constitutes approximately one quarter of the thickness of the cortex. Zona reticularis cells are arranged in a spongelike mesh-work of gently buckled anastomosing one-cell wide rows of cells that are separated by dilated capillaries. The well-out-lined cells are smaller than those of the zona fasciculata and have cytoplasm that is granular, acidophilic, and rela-tively lipid sparse. The cytoplasm is sometimes referred to as "compact" and the reticularis cells as "compact cells." The deepest cells adjacent to the medulla usually contain yellow lipochrome pigment (lipofuscin), diffusely dis-tributed as coarse granules in the cytoplasm or localized in a single body (Figure 46.25). The yellow pigmentation of the cytoplasm extends outward into the reticularis for a variable distance. The solid granular eosinophilic cyto-plasm and the lipochrome pigment combine to produce the dark brown coloration of the zone seen on cut surface of a fresh or formalin-fixed gland.

Accessory (Heterotopic) Adrenal

The adrenocortical primordium initially is unencapsulated and develops, as has been mentioned, close to the emerging

gonad. Therefore, it is not surprising that (a) some cells of the unencapsulated adrenocortical primordium may become associated with and migrate alongside the gonad (testis or ovary) to be found postnatally distant from the adrenal in the path of gonad descent and (b) cortical cells not sequestered by adrenal capsule formation are subse-quently found in the retroperitoneal fat close to the adrenal glands. In practice, accessory adrenocortical tissue is most often encountered around the adrenal glands themselves (Figure 46.26); it also occurs in the inguinal region and around the ovary, fallopian tube, epididymis, and rete testis. Microscopically, accessory cortex shows normal zonation and responds to ACTH. Rarely, medulla is also present (Figure 46.26).

Adrenocortical Nodules

Adrenocortical nodules, roughly spherical, uncapsulated areas of hypertropic and hyperplastic cortical cells, are not regarded as true neoplasms. They range in size from microscopic to grossly obvious lesions (12). Before the fourth decade of life, they are rare; thereafter, they are encountered with increasing frequency. Although

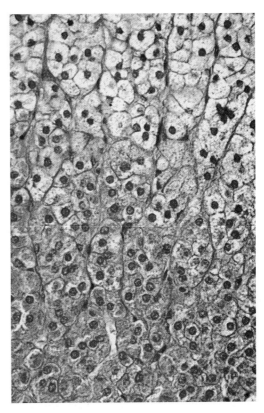

Figure 46.23 Normal adrenal cortex. Zona fasciculata (*upper*) features two-cell wide columns of cells with clear cytoplasm, and zona reticularis (*lower*) consists of cells having acidophilic granular cytoplasm that do not form a distinct pattern. Nuclei are vesicular, and nucleoli are small.

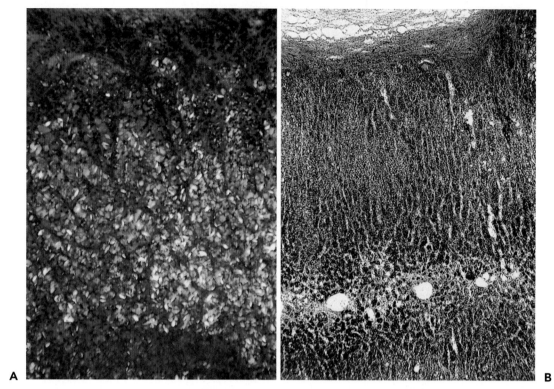

Figure 46.24 Normal adrenal cortex. **A.** Partial polarization shows high lipid content of zona fasciculata and low content of zona glomerulosa (*above*) and zona reticularis (*below*). **B.** Fresh frozen section of adrenal cortex stained with polychrome methylene blue. One complete band of cortex (*above*) and portion of another (*below*) is seen; the junction point between the two is located by the dilated sinusoidal tributaries of the central adrenal vein. Zona fasciculata cells are packed with lipid globules. There are fewer globules in the zona glomerulosa (beneath the adrenal capsule) and in the zona reticularis (on either side of the sinusoidal vessels).

regarded by some as an aging phenomenon, they are not invariably found in older individuals. Usually, multiple nodules commonly consist of large, lipid-laden clear cells; some nodules are composed of clear and compact cells; a minority feature reticularis-type cells only (Figure 46.27). The smallest nodules may be found at any level of the cortex, but usually they occur in the zona fasciculata. Initially, they appear to be the result of hypertrophy of contiguous cells in three or more adjacent cords. The smallest ill-defined nodules thus have the cord structure of the parent tissue. As they enlarge further due to cell proliferation, this organized appearance is lost, and larger nodules are patternless. Large nodules cause compression and distortion of the surrounding cortex.

Medulla

The medulla is situated in the interior of the organ in the head and body of the gland, deep to the zona reticularis (Figures 46.9 and 46.20). Its area and weight are one tenth those of the cortex (1,3). The medulla rarely measures more than 2 mm in thickness. Because of the differ-

ent staining of cells of the two tissues—acidophilia in zona reticularis and basophilia in the medulla—the interface between cortex and medulla is readily visible on low-power microscopic examination. The junction is sharp, with no or minimal intervening connective tissue, leaving cortical and medullary cells in direct contact (Figures 46.20 and 46.25).

The medulla extends to a variable extent into the crest of the gland (the ridge on the posterior surface) and into one or both of the alae (Figure 46.20). Areas of the medulla in the alae are not necessarily in direct continuity with the main mass of the medulla around the central veins. The medulla sometimes extends into the tail of the gland. The finding of medulla in this location therefore does not automatically equate with pathologic abnormality—specifically, medullary hyperplasia. Rarely, a narrow tongue of medulla accompanied by a vessel or nerve or unaccompanied extends through the cortex to contact the capsule of the gland.

The medulla, for practical purposes, is composed of a single cell population, the pheochromocytes (medullary or chromaffin cells) (Figure 46.28). Among the dominant population are scattered small groups of cortical cells and clusters and individual ganglion cells (Figure 46.29). Not

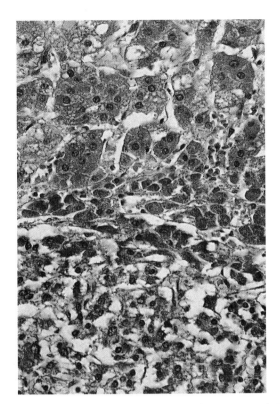

Figure 46.25 Corticomedullary junction. The zona reticularis of the cortex (*upper*) is sharply demarcated from the medulla (*lower*). The deepest cells of the zona reticularis contain granular yellowish pigment (*lipofuscin*).

uncommonly, the ganglion cells feature cytoplasmic, round, lightly acidophilic, hyalin bodies, with concentrically arranged fibrillar appearance, up to 30 μm in diameter (Figure 46.30). Sometimes these bodies appear to be external to the ganglion cells and to indent them; in immunostain preparations (vimentin and S-100) they are separated from the cells by a small amount of intercellular substance. It is unusual to observe these bodies in ganglion cells outside the adrenal medulla. Their nature has not been investigated. The pheochromocytes are arranged in tight clusters and short trabeculae, supported by delicate fibrovascular stroma (Figures 46.28 and 46.31). Sustentacular cells at the periphery of the clusters and trabeculae are not seen in routine histologic preparations (13), but are readily demonstrated by immunostaining for S-100 protein (Figure 46.32).

The pheochromocytes are moderately large cells, polygonal to columnar, and slightly to considerably larger than cortical cells. Poorly outlined, their complete cell borders are visible only occasionally. Although the cytoplasm of most medullary cells is basophilic, finely granular and occasionally vacuolated, sometimes it is amphophilic or slightly acidophilic. Rarely is it partly basophilic and partly acidophilic. The resulting variability and unevenness of medullary cytoplasmic staining and cytoplasmic vacuolization often impart an overall mottled light and dark appearance at intermediate

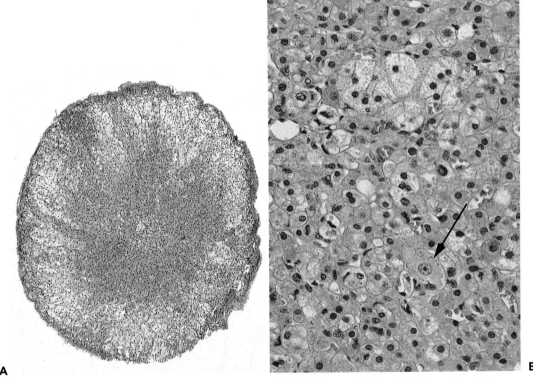

A   B

Figure 46.26 Accessory adrenal cortex in retroperitoneal fat. **A.** Normal zonation is suggested by the narrow rim of cells with clear cytoplasm that surrounds the main mass of cells with light eosinophilic cytoplasm. **B.** Ganglion cell (*arrow*) indicating presence of medulla among cortical "clear" and "compact" cells. The latter contain lipofuscin.

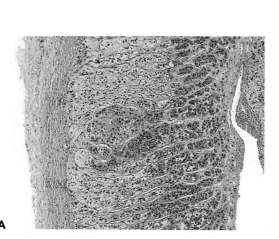

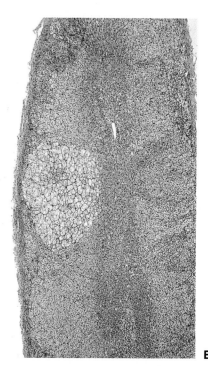

Figure 46.27 Cortical nodules (36-year-old man). **A.** Suggestive nodule in the mid-cortex. **B.** Distinct nodule composed of clear cells in outer cortex.

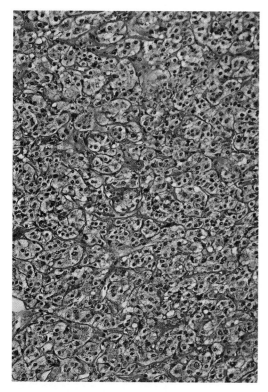

Figure 46.28 Normal adrenal medulla. Clusters of poorly outlined cells with basophilic cytoplasm are separated by a vascularized supporting stroma. There is some variation in nuclear size and shape.

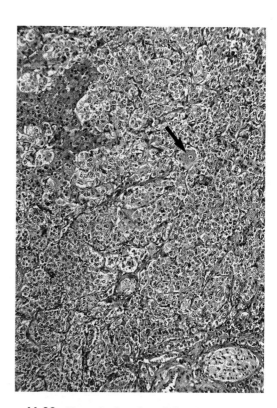

Figure 46.29 Normal adrenal medulla. Pheochromocytes are arranged in poorly delineated clusters. An irregularly shaped group of cortical cells (*upper left*) and an isolated ganglion cell (*arrow*) are present.

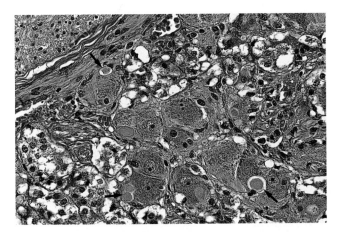

Figure 46.30 Normal adrenal medulla. A group of ganglion cells demarcated by pheochromocytes (*upper right and lower left*) and a nerve (*upper left*). A number of the ganglion cells feature cytoplasmic acidophilic bodies, some outlined by a rim of retracted cytoplasm (*arrows*). There are two such bodies in one cell.

The nuclei of medullary cells characteristically have slight but definite variability of size, shape, and location in the cell. Most pheochromocyte nuclei are slightly larger than those of cortical cells, but nuclei that are larger and smaller than the usual ones are common. The usual nucleus has a finely or coarsely clumped chromatin pattern with a relatively clear nuclear background (Figure 46.31). The chromatin tends to be peripherally disposed and separated into irregular clumps. Larger nuclei often have a prominent eosinophilic nucleolus; smaller nuclei are deeply staining. A rare cell has two or more nuclei.

The nuclei exhibit slight but definite polymorphism. Most are spheroidal, but many are ellipsoidal, and some have other shapes. Large, intensely hyperchromatic and sometimes pleomorphic nuclei are common, usually single and located close to the corticomedullary junction (Figure 46.34). The positions of the nuclei in the cells are not fixed; most are central, but some tend to be eccentric, located away from the vascular pole (Figure 46.35).

The medullary cells have several distinctive histochemical reactions related to their content of secretory granules. The granules contain catecholamines, dihydroxy derivatives of tyrosine, that are converted to colored polymers by oxidizing agents such as potassium dichromate, ferric chloride, ammoniacal silver nitrate, and osmium tetroxide. The oxidized and polymerized derivatives are termed

magnification. A rare normal cell has one or more periodic acid-Schiff positive cytoplasmic colloid droplets (Figure 46.33). The majority of the medullary cells are roughly similar in size, but occasionally standard-sized cells merge with groups of cells that are much smaller or much larger (Figure 46.31).

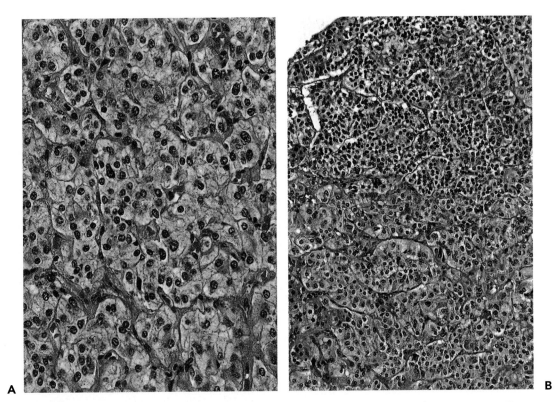

A

B

Figure 46.31 Normal adrenal medulla. **A.** Pheochromocytes arranged in vague clusters. Cell outlines are visible here and there. Nuclear variation in size and shape is typical. The nuclear chromatin is coarsely clumped and often marginated at the nuclear membrane. **B.** Variation in cell size, nuclear size, and cell pattern.

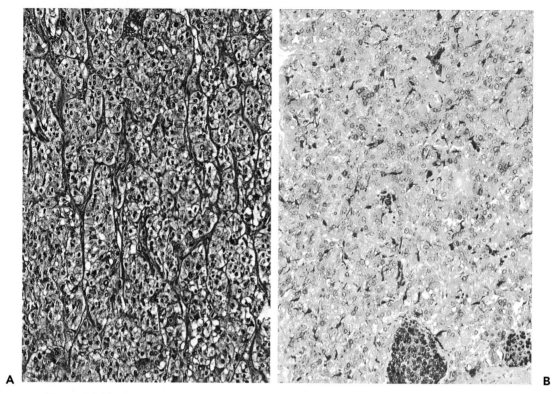

Figure 46.32 Normal adrenal medulla. **A.** Pheochromocytes arranged in trabecular pattern outlined by a delicate vascular supporting stroma. **B.** Sustentacular cells identified by S-100 immunostain that also highlights two nerves.

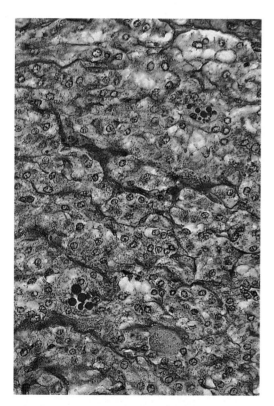

Figure 46.33 Normal adrenal medulla. Cytoplasmic globules, a rare finding in normal pheochromocytes, stained with periodic acid-Schiff. Condensation of the nuclear chromatin at the nuclear membrane is well demonstrated.

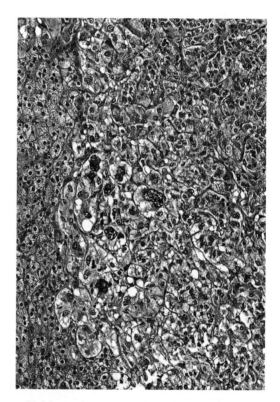

Figure 46.34 Normal adrenal medulla. Pheochromocyte nuclear atypia at the corticomedullary junction. The number of atypical pheochromocyte nuclei crowded together here is unusual; ordinarily, the atypical nuclei are seen one to a medium-power field. The pheochromocytes have basophilic granular cytoplasm. The zona reticularis (*left*) features cells with granular eosinophilic cytoplasm and lipofuscin.

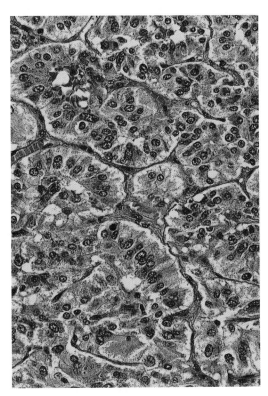

Figure 46.35 Normal adrenal medulla. Uncommon pattern in which pheochromocytes are columnar in shape with nuclei that are located away from the vascular pole. The variations in size and shape of the nuclei are typical. Cytoplasmic staining is uneven and ranges from almost clear to basophilic and granular.

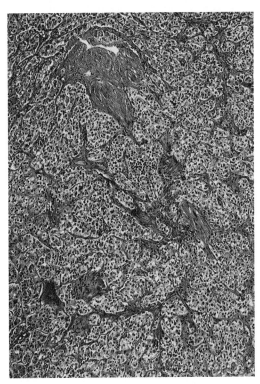

Figure 46.37 Normal adrenal medulla. Bundles and strands of smooth muscle are derived from the smooth muscle of central vein.

adrenochromes. This staining has been called the chromaffin reaction.

Ganglion cells are scattered randomly among the pheochromocytes or in groups, often associated with a nerve (Figure 46.29). Their number varies greatly from medulla to medulla; accordingly, they are found easily or not. Cortical cells also are a regular component of the medulla, found in irregularly shaped groups, sometimes in continuity with the zona reticularis, but more often not (Figure 46.29).

Single or multiple small-to-large accumulations of round cells, plasma cells, and lymphocytes (positive for leukocyte common antigen), often paravascularly located, are common in the normal medulla (Figure 46.36). They have no known significance. The delicate vascular stroma of the medulla is not conspicuous. Sometimes it is augmented focally by prolongations of the musculature of the central veins that separate groups of medullary cells (Figure 46.37).

IMMUNOHISTOCHEMISTRY

Cortex

Cells of the normal adrenal cortex are reported to be immunoreactive against a cytokeratin cocktail and AE1 (14). In our experience, small groups of cells and isolated cells of the three zones have strong reactivity to low- and medium-molecular-weight keratin antibodies (CAM 5.2 and AE1, and MAK 6, respectively). Reactivity is greatest in the zona

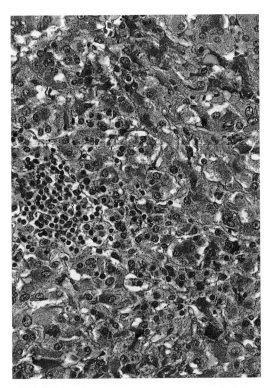

Figure 46.36 Normal adrenal medulla. Aggregates of lymphocytes and plasma cells are often encountered.

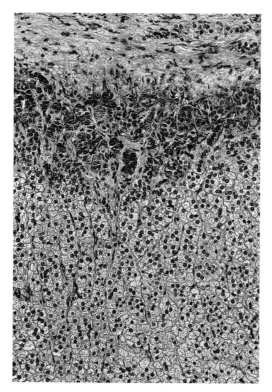

Figure 46.38 Normal adrenal cortex. Zona glomerulosa stains positively for vimentin.

glomerulosa and external zona fasciculata, with some strongly reactive cells in the deep zona reticularis. The character of the staining is variable, membranous, punctate cytoplasmic, diffuse cytoplasmic, and perinuclear, in decreasing order of frequency. There is weak staining to the keratin antibodies, often diffuse, in the zona reticularis. The zona glomerulosa is vimentin positive (Figure 46.38). Cells

of the outer zona fasciculata and the zona reticularis are positive for melan A and inhibin α, respectively (Figure 46.39). Cells of the three zones are variably synaptophysin positive. Cortical cells do not stain with epithelial membrane antigen, chromogranin, or S-100 antibodies.

Medulla

Pheochromocytes stain with antibodies to chromogranin and synaptophysin. The sustentacular cells that mantle the clusters and trabeculae of pheochromocytes are S-100 protein positive (Figure 46.40), as are nerves in the medulla. Some pheochromocytes stain with S-100 antibodies.

ULTRASTRUCTURE

Cortex

There are ultrastructural features shared by the three layers of the cortex relating to their common function—synthesis of steroid hormones. The cells feature voluminous endoplasmic reticulum, stacks of rough endoplasmic reticulum, a well-developed Golgi apparatus, lysosomes, and many mitochondria. The distribution and internal structure of some of the organelles (e.g., the mitochondria) vary from zone to zone. Using the electron microscope, the sometimes distinct transition seen between the zones is not apparent; rather, a gradual alteration from one organelle distribution and type to another being observed. Mitochondria in the zona glomerulosa are round, oval, or elongate, with lamellar infolded cristae, resulting in a ladderlike internal structure, similar to that found in many other

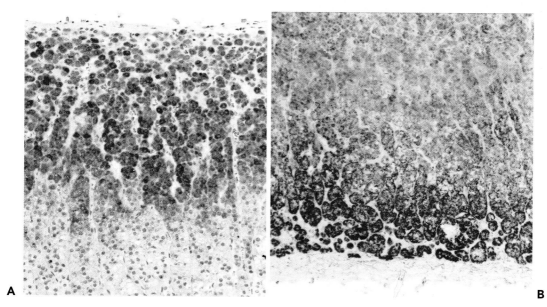

A **B**

Figure 46.39 **A.** Melan A stains the outer zona fasciculata most strongly. **B.** Inhibin α stains the region of the zona reticularis strongly and the remainder of the cortex weakly.

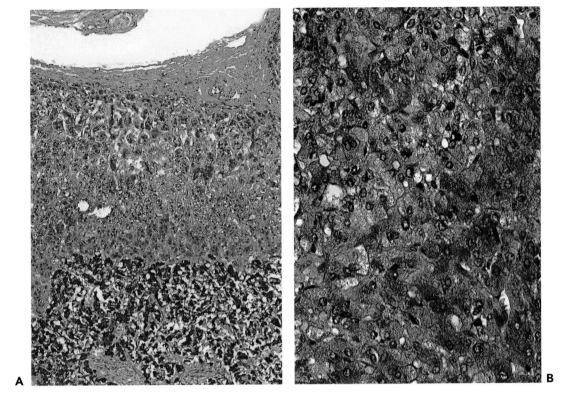

Figure 46.40   Normal adrenal medulla. **A.** Medulla (*below*) stains with chromogranin antibodies; cortex is unstained. **B.** Sustentacular cells and about one half of the pheochromocytes are stained by S-100 protein antiserum.

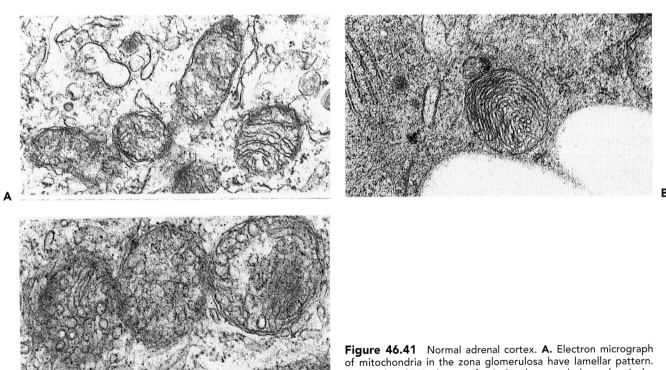

Figure 46.41   Normal adrenal cortex. **A.** Electron micrograph of mitochondria in the zona glomerulosa have lamellar pattern. **B.** Mitochondria in the zona fasciculata have a tubular and vesicular pattern. **C.** Mitochondria in the zona reticularis are elongated and have a vesicular appearance. Bar = 1 μm.

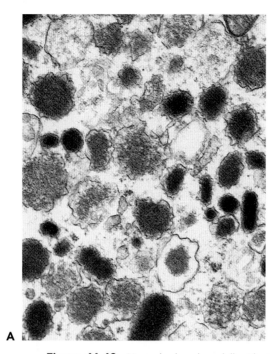
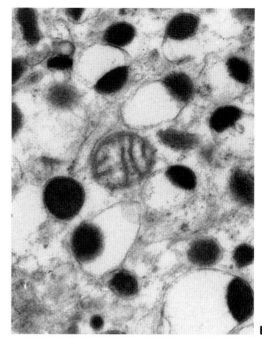

Figure 46.42   Normal adrenal medulla. Electron micrographs of medullary secretory granules. **A.** Epinephrine granules with a variably electron-dense content that fills the majority of the sacs. **B.** Content of norepinephrine granules is electron dense and often eccentrically located. Bar = 1 μm.

tissues (Figure 46.41). In the zona fasciculata, these organelles are large, spherical, and feature tubular cristae (Figure 46.41). Lipid droplets are large and numerous. The mitochondria in the zona reticularis (Figure 46.41) tend to be more elongated and exhibit tubular and vesicular cristae that are a feature of steroid-producing cells. Lipofuscin granules, membrane-bound organelles with a moderately dense matrix that contains dense granules and clear lipid globules are prominent. Glycogen is present.

Medulla

Catecholamine-secreting cells dominate the medulla. Two cell types, epinephrine and norepinephrine, distinguished by granule type are present. In tissue fixed in glutaraldehyde, cells that contain epinephrine feature granules (Figure 46.42) measuring about 190 μm in diameter, with a finely granular texture that is moderately dense but not opaque, and fills the enclosing membrane. Norepinephrine-secreting cells have granules (Figure 46.42) that are electron opaque, often located eccentrically within a dilated sac, and measure about 250 μm in diameter.

REFERENCES

1. Quinan C, Berger AA. Observations on human adrenals with especial reference to the relative weight of the normal medulla. *Ann Intern Med* 1933;6:1180–1192.
2. Ekholm E, Niemineva K. On prenatal changes in the relative weights of the human adrenals, the thymus and the thyroid gland. *Acta Paediatr* 1950;39:67–86.
3. Symington T. *Functional Pathology of the Human Adrenal Gland.* Baltimore: Williams & Wilkins; 1969.
4. Keene MFL, Hewer EE. Observations on the development of the human suprarenal gland. *J Anat* 1927;61:302–324.
5. Crowder RE. The development of the adrenal gland in man, with special reference to origin and ultimate location of cell types and evidence in favour of the "cell migration" theory. *Carnegie Inst Contrib Embryol* 1957;26:193–210.
6. Reed RJ, Patrick JT. Nodular hyperplasia of the adrenal cortical blastema. *Bull Tulane Univ Med Faculty* 1967;26:151–157.
7. Wong TW, Warner NE. Ovarian thecal metaplasia in the adrenal gland. *Arch Pathol* 1971;92:319–328.
8. Fidler WJ. Ovarian thecal metaplasia in adrenal glands. *Am J Clin Pathol* 1977;67:318–323.
9. Backlin C, Juhlin C, Grimelius L, et al. Monoclonal antibodies recognizing normal and neoplastic human adrenal cortex. *Endocr Pathol* 1995;6:21–34.
10. Sasano H, Imatani A, Shizawa S, Suzuki T, Nagura H. Cell proliferation and apoptosis in normal and pathologic human adrenal. *Mod Pathol* 1995;8:11–17.
11. Sasano H, Saito Y, Sato I, Sasano N, Nagura H. Nucleolar organizer regions in human adrenocortical disorders. *Mod Pathol* 1990;3:591–595.
12. Dobbie JW. Adrenocortical nodular hyperplasia: the ageing adrenal. *J Pathol* 1969;99:1–18.
13. Nakajima T, Kameya T, Watanabe S. S-100 protein distribution in normal and neoplastic tissues. In: DeLellis RA, ed. *Advances in Immunohistochemistry* Vol 3. New York: Masson; 1984: 141–158.
14. Gaffey MJ, Traweek ST, Mills SE, et al. Cytokeratin expression in adrenocortical neoplasia: an immunohistochemical and biochemical study with implications for the differential diagnosis of adrenocortical, hepatocellular, and renal cell carcinoma. *Hum Pathol* 1992;23:144–153.

The Neuroendocrine System

47

Ronald A. DeLellis   Yogeshwar Dayal

INTRODUCTION

The results of numerous studies over the past 50 years have established that there are many striking similarities between neurons and neuroendocrine cells. Both cell types have polarized membrane orientations, two separately regulated secretory pathways, neurotransmitter synthesizing enzymes and neural cell adhesion molecules (1). Detailed biochemical and molecular studies have shown a commonality of biosynthetic products that may act as classical hormones, neurotransmitters, and paracrine or autocrine factors. Accordingly, concepts of the endocrine system have been expanded to include not only the traditional endocrine glands but also the peptidergic neurons and the system of neuroendocrine cells that is dispersed throughout many tissues of the body. Although neuroendocrine cells are discussed in the context of other tissues and organs in other chapters of this volume, this chapter will provide a more general overview of this fascinating cell type.

HISTORICAL PERSPECTIVES AND NOMENCLATURE

Current concepts of the neuroendocrine system evolved directly from a series of seminal observations that were initiated more than a century ago. Heidenhain, in 1870, demonstrated a population of chromaffin cells in the gastrointestinal tract and suggested that they might have an endocrine function (2). Pierre Masson (3) later showed that the intestinal chromaffin cells were also argentaffin positive, and subsequent studies by Hamperl (4) using argyrophilic staining techniques led to the identification of a second population of putative endocrine cells within the intestine and a variety of extraintestinal sites. Feyrter, in 1938, suggested that the clear cells (helle Zelle) of the gastrointestinal tract formed a diffuse epithelial endocrine system ("diffuse epitheliale endokrine organe") and that some of these cells might have a paracrine or local hormonal action (5,6). Similar groups of clear cells were illustrated by Frölich within the bronchial tree, and Feyrter also considered them to be a part of the diffuse epithelial endocrine system (7). Ultimately, the argentaffin, argyrophil, and clear cells were recognized as components of a diffusely distributed system of endocrine cells (8).

The modern view of the neuroendocrine cell and neurosecretory neuron stemmed directly from the observations that oxytocin and antidiuretic hormone were synthesized by hypothalamic neurons and were stored within neuronal processes in the posterior pituitary before their release into the circulation (9). Furthermore, the discovery that hormone-releasing and -inhibiting factors were synthesized by hypothalamic neurons, transported via axonal transport to the median eminence, and secreted into the pituitary portal system for interactions with specific adenohypophyseal cell types, established without doubt that neurons could function as endocrine cells (9) (Figure 47.1). These cells essentially could serve as neuroendocrine transducers by converting electrical input directly into chemical or hormonal signals (10).

The discovery that the argyrophil/argentaffin cells and the cells of Feyrter's diffuse epithelial endocrine system did, indeed, have an endocrine function originated from studies conducted in the early to mid-1960s on the source of the hormone calcitonin (11,12). The thyroid glands of many species were known to contain parafollicular cells, which appeared clear in hematoxylin and eosin–stained sections and which showed varying degrees of argyrophilia or argentaffinity (13,14). With immunofluorescence techniques, the parafollicular cells were ultimately shown to be the source of calcitonin, for which they were subsequently renamed C cells (15,16). These studies also led to the discovery that certain endocrine cells shared a series of remarkable functional and morphologic similarities with neurons (15).

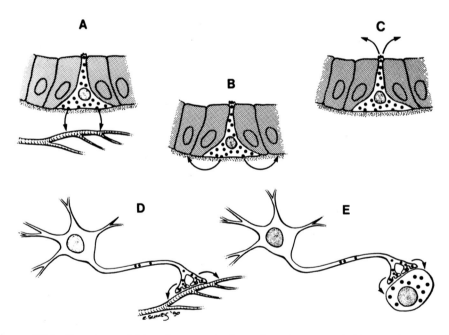

Figure 47.1 Secretory activities of neuroendocrine cells and neurons. **A.** Neuroendocrine cells may secrete their products through the basement membranes into adjacent capillaries for interactions with target tissues at distant sites (endocrine function). **B.** Neuroendocrine cells may secrete their products locally to influence the activities of adjacent epithelial cells (paracrine function). **C.** Neuroendocrine cells may secrete their products within a glandular lumen (luminal secretion). **D.** Neurons may secrete their products into the circulation for interactions with target tissues at distant sites (neuroendocrine function). **E.** Neurons also may secrete products that serve as neurotransmitters or neuromodulators. (Adapted with permission from: Larsson LI, Goltermann N, de Magistris L, Rehfeld JF, Schwartz TW. Somatostatin cell processes as pathways for paracrine secretion. *Science* 1979;205:1393–1395.)

In addition to the presence of calcitonin, C cells had the ability to synthesize and store catecholamines or indolylethylamines after uptake and decarboxylation of precursors of these substances (15). The latter property led to the introduction of the descriptive acronym APUD (amine precursor uptake and decarboxylation) (13). The APUD mechanism was subsequently identified in certain cells of the anterior pituitary and pancreatic islets. Cholinesterase, nonspecific esterases, α-glycerophosphate dehydrogenase, and certain endogenous amines were also noted variably across diverse animal species and among different endocrine cell types (14) (Table 47.1).

In comparing the APUD cells of the thyroid, pancreas, and pituitary to cells of known neural ancestry, Pearse suggested that "the amine storing mechanism and presence of cholinesterase together point towards a common ancestral cell of neural origin, perhaps coming from the neural crest" (15). The list of APUD cells was then expanded to include almost all the peptide- and amine-producing cells throughout the body, including the adrenal medulla, extra-adrenal paraganglia, and parathyroid glands.

As the numbers of candidate APUD cells increased (17), it was recognized that the synthesis of regulatory peptides was a more consistent functional parameter than was synthesis of amines, and amine synthesis was ultimately dropped from the definition of these cells. In view of the many similarities between APUD cells and neurons, the essentially synonymous term, "paraneuron" was introduced by Fujita and Kobayashi (18). Paraneurons, according to Fujita (19), were endocrine and sensory cells that shared structural, functional, and metabolic features with neurons and that produced substances identical with or related to neurohormones and neurotransmitters. The paraneurons also possessed neurosecretory-like granules and synapse-like vesicles, and they recognized stimuli on specific receptors and released their products via the secretory portion of the cell. Many investigators also began to apply the term "neuroendocrine cell" to these cells (17).

EMBRYOLOGY

Embryologic data using the chick–quail chimera system have now refuted the neural crest origin of most neuroendocrine cells (20,21). Currently, the only neuroendocrine cells of proven neural crest origin are those of the adrenal medulla, extra-adrenal paraganglia, cells of the myenteric plexus and sympathetic ganglia, and the thyroid C cells (20,21); however, several studies have questioned the neural crest origin of C cells (22). The peptide- and amine-producing cells of the bronchopulmonary tract and gastroenteropancreatic axis have now been shown to be of endodermal origin.

Studies of normal, chimeric, and transgenic mice have suggested that all gut epithelial cells, including endocrine cells, originate from a single multipotential stem cell present within the base of the intestinal crypts, whereas pancreatic endocrine cells appear to originate from the ductal epithelium. However, those factors responsible for the modulation of ductal epithelium into islets of Langerhans remain largely unknown (23).

Although the neural crest origin of most neuroendocrine cells is no longer tenable, the list of neuroendocrine markers has continued to expand (Table 47.1). In its current context, the term "neuroendocrine" does not imply an embryologic origin from the neuroectoderm but rather implies a shared phenotype characterized by the simultaneous expression of multiple genes encoding a wide variety of neuronal and endocrine traits (24,25).

MOLECULAR ASPECTS OF NEUROENDOCRINE CELL DEVELOPMENT

Although the precise mechanisms for the acquisition of the neuroendocrine phenotype have not been conclusively identified, recent studies suggest an important role for both

---

TABLE 47.1
MARKERS[a] OF NEUROENDOCRINE CELLS

Fluorogenic amine content
Amine precursor (5-hydroxytryptophan and DOPA) uptake
Aromatic amino acid decarboxylase
Nonspecific esterase or cholinesterase
Alpha glycerophosphate dehydrogenase
Cytosolic proteins
    Neuron specific enolase, protein gene product 9.5 (PGP 9.5), histaminase, some enzymes involved in amine synthesis
Secretory Granule/Membrane Proteins
    Chromogranins/secretogranins, prohormone convertases, peptidylglycine alpha amidating monooxygenase and related enzymes, some enzymes involved in amine synthesis, cytochrome b561.
Synaptic vesicle, docking and plasma membrane proteins
    Vesicle membrane protein
    Synaptophysin, synaptic vesicle protein 2, vesicular monoamine transporters, vesicle associated membrane protein (VAMP)/synaptobrevin, Rab3a, synaptotagmin
Plasma membrane
    SNAP-25 (synaptosomal protein of 25kDa), syntaxin
Other markers
    CD56 (NCAM), CD57, transcription factors (TTF-1, CDX2, pit-1, adrenal 4 site/steroidogenic factor), somatostatin receptors (sst2)

[a]The first six markers in this listing were described by Pearse in the original formulation of the APUD concept; however, endogenous amine content and the capacity for amine precursor uptake and decarboxylation are present only in some members of the dispersed neuroendocrine cell system.

positively and negatively acting transcription factors. An important class of regulatory proteins includes those with common DNA binding and dimerization domains, the basic helix-loop-helix (b-HLH) region. The genes encoding these proteins are analogous to the achaete–scute complex, which has been identified during neuronal differentiation in *Drosophila* (26). The homologous mammalial genes have been named mammalian achaete–scute homologs (MASH) while the homologous human genes have been termed HASH. In Drosophila, one group of b-HLH factors encoded by genes such as MASH-1 activates neural differentiation whereas another group of b-HLH factors encoded by Hes1 represses neuronal differentiation. Repressive b-HLH factors such as Hes1 (hairy enhancer of split) appear to be regulated by the Notch pathway (27,28). Known targets of Hes1 mediated silencing include MASH1/HASH1 in the nervous system and lung. Neuroendocrine differentiation in the gastrointestinal tract and pancreas, which are under the control of b-HLH factors, are also inhibited by Hes1.

MASH1 (HASH1 in humans) plays a critical role in the development of the nervous system and neuroendocrine cells of the lung, adrenal medulla, and thyroid (C cells) (29). In the developing mouse lung, MASH1 staining coincides with the appearance of synaptophysin and calcitonin gene related peptide in the neuroendocrine cells. Pulmonary neuroendocrine cells are absent from MASH1 knockout mice while Hes1 knockout mice demonstrate the precocious appearance of neuroendocrine cells, which also are hyperplastic. The results of this study indicate that MASH1 is critical for neuroendocrine differentiation while Hes1 inhibits neuroendocrine differentiation by inactivation of MASH1. Notch receptors, which can activate Hes1, are expressed in nonneuroendocrine cells and are also regulated by Hes1. These observations suggest that Notch receptors can play important roles in differentiation towards nonneuroendocrine cells. In addition to the Notch/Notch ligand pathways, other pathways such as Sonic hedgehog may also play important roles in the differentiation of airway epithelial cells.

LIGHT MICROSCOPY AND HISTOCHEMISTRY

Neuroendocrine cells are difficult to recognize in routinely prepared hematoxylin and eosin–stained sections, where they may appear as oval, pyramidal, or flask-shaped, often with clear cytoplasm (Figures 47.2 and 47.3). In some instances, the cytoplasm may contain fine eosinophilic granules that are often difficult to resolve with usual microscopic preparations. Some neuroendocrine cell types, such as those of the intra- and extra-adrenal paraganglia and gastrointestinal tract, develop a characteristic brown to yellow coloration after primary fixation in potassium dichromate or chromic acid. This pigment results from oxidation of cellular stores of catecholamines (intra- and extra-adrenal paraganglia) or serotonin (gastrointestinal tract and other sites). In the gastrointestinal tract, the chromaffin-positive cells have also been referred to as "enterochromaffin cells" (EC).

Some neuroendocrine cells exhibit a characteristic yellow–green fluorescence after fixation in formaldehyde and other aldehyde fixatives (30) (Figure 47.4). In some instances, the cells may become fluorescent only after administration of L-dihydroxyphenylalanine (DOPA) or 5-hydroxytryptophan. Formaldehyde forms highly fluorescent tetrahydroisoquinoline condensation products with catecholamines and β-carboline derivatives with tryptamines such as serotonin. Occasionally, strong fluorescence may be observed after formalin fixation and paraffin embedding. In other instances, freeze-dried tissues or fresh-frozen sections must be used for the demonstration of cellular stores of amines (30).

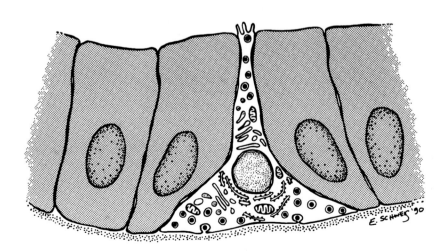

Figure 47.2 Diagram of typical open-type neuroendocrine cell. Secretory granules are concentrated at the basal pole of the cell. Stimulation of such a cell leads to the release of hormonal product by the process of exocytosis. The basal lamina is indicated by the stippled area. Secretory granules are also present in the apical extension of the cell.

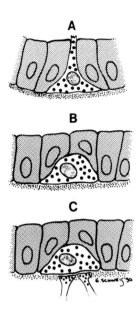

Figure 47.3 Comparison of "open" (**A**) and "closed" (**B** and **C**) neuroendocrine cells. **A**. Open cells may be found within the gastrointestinal tract and other sites. **B**. Closed cells are also widely distributed. The thyroid C cells are typically of the closed type. **C**. The Merkel cells of the skin are innervated closed-type neuroendocrine cells.

Some neuroendocrine cells, including those of the gastrointestinal tract, have the ability to reduce ammoniacal silver to the metallic state (3,4). Such cells are termed "argentaffin cells" (Figure 47.5). In many other neuroendocrine cells, silver positivity is evident only after the addition of an exogenous reducing agent to the staining solution, and such cells are said to be argyrophilic. The chromaffin and argentaffin reactions of neuroendocrine cells in the gastrointestinal tract are due primarily to the

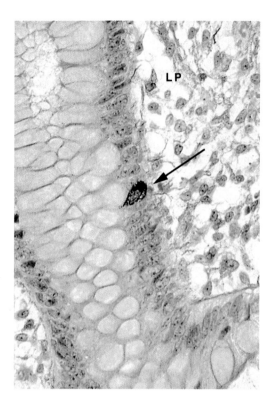

Figure 47.5 Colonic mucosa stained for argentaffin cells with the Masson-Fontana technique and methyl green counterstain. The argentaffin cell (*arrow*) illustrated in this field is characterized by the presence of black cytoplasmic granules. LP, lamina propria.

presence of serotonin. While argentaffin cells are also argyrophilic, only a subset of argyrophil cells is argentaffin positive (31). The chemical basis of the argyrophil reactions (Grimelius, Churukian-Schenk, Sevier-Munger) is unknown, although it is apparent that reduced silver salts have an affinity for a nonamine constituent of neuroendocrine secretory granules (32).

The argyrophil staining techniques have been used extensively for the identification of neuroendocrine cells; however, it should be recognized that these stains are nonspecific. Cellular products such as lipofuscin, glycogen, and certain proteins including α-lactalbumin may be argyrophilic (33). Alternatively, some neuroendocrine cells are argyrophilic only with certain silver staining sequences (Table 47.2).

Most neuroendocrine cells stain metachromatically with toluidine blue and coriophosphine O after acid hydrolysis of tissue sections (34). This property has been referred to as masked metachromasia. Acid hydrolysis not only removes DNA and RNA from the cells but also converts side chain carboxamido groups to carboxyls, which are free to react with the dyes. Both chromogranin proteins and peptide hormones are most likely responsible for the property of masked metachromasia in neuroendocrine cells (34). Lead hematoxylin also has been used for the demonstration of neuroendocrine cells (34).

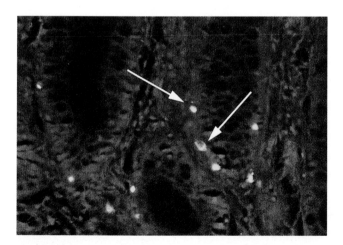

Figure 47.4 Formalin-fixed rectal mucosa photographed in ultraviolet light. The strongly fluorescent cells (*arrows*) correspond to the serotonin-containing enterochromaffin-type cells.

FUNCTIONAL AND MORPHOLOGICAL CHARACTERISTICS OF GUT ENDOCRINE CELLS[a]

Cell Type	Hormone(s)	Granule Size (nm)	Morphology/Histochemistry
G	Gastrin, ACTH	150–400	Round, moderately dense cores; argyrophilic[b]
D	Somatostatin	250–400	Round, moderately dense cores; argyrophilic only by Hellerstrom–Hellerman technique
IG	Gastrin	150–220	Round, dense; argyrophilic
S	Secretin	180–220	Round to slightly irregular; weakly argyrophilic
I	Cholecystokinin	240–300	Round with moderately dense cores; nonargyrophilic
K	GIP	200–250	Round, irregular with dense eccentric cores and less dense matrix which is argyrophilic by Sevier–Munger technique
N	Neurotensin	Up to 300	Round moderately dense; variably argyrophilic
L	Enteroglucagon	250–300	Round, moderately dense; variably argyrophilic
EC$_1$	5-HT, substance P, leu-enkephalin	200–300	Pleomorphic with dense cores and thin halo; argentaffinic
EC$_2$	5-HT, motilin-like, leu-enkephalin	200–400	Pleomorphic, round to irregular, angulated; argentaffinic
EC$_n$	5-HT, unknown	200–300	Elongated or oval, variably electron dense; argentaffinic
ECL	Histamine		Pleomorphic, round to elongated, moderately dense contents; argyrophilic
D$_1$	VIP-like	140–200	Round to pleomorphic granules, moderately to highly electron-dense cores with narrow halo; argyrophilic
P	Bombesin/GRP	90–150	Electron-dense cores; variably argyrophilic
X	Unknown	Up to 250	Round granules, moderately dense cores; argyrophilic

[a]Reprinted with permission from: Dayal Y. Endocrine cells of the gut and their neoplasms. In: Norris HT, ed. *Pathology of the Colon, Small Intestine and Anus.* New York: Churchill Livingstone; 1983:267–300.
[b]Argyrophilia, unless otherwise stated, refers to results with Grimelius technique.

Neuroendocrine cells tend to be dispersed among other cell types as single cells or as aggregates of three to four cells (Figure 47.3). The basal aspects of the cells are closely applied to the subjacent epithelial basement membrane. Processes often extend from the cytoplasm to surround adjacent epithelial cells, and such neuroendocrine cells are referred to as "paracrine cells" (35,36) (Figures 47.6 and 47.7). The products of paracrine cells are thought to be released locally where they influence the activities of adjacent endocrine and nonendocrine cells (35). The apex of the neuroendocrine cell may extend directly to the glandular lumen (open-type cell) or may be covered by the cytoplasm of adjacent epithelial cells (Figures 47.3 and 47.8). The latter cells are referred to as closed neuroendocrine cells (37–39) (Figure 47.3). The products of open endocrine cells may be secreted directly into the lumen of a hollow viscus. In addition, such apical processes may subserve a receptor function. Although the majority of neuroendocrine cells are not directly innervated, some cells, such as those of the skin and bronchial tree, may be innervated (Figure 47.3).

In the gastrointestinal tract, scattered neuroendocrine cells are also found within the lamina propria (40) without attachment to the overlying epithelium. Such endocrine cells are typically surrounded by Schwann cells and unmyelinated nerve fibers to form an enterochromaffin cell (EC)–nerve fiber complex. The EC–nerve complexes are especially prominent in appendices with chronic inflammation and neural hyperplasia (40). Stromal endocrine cells also have been identified in the prostate gland (41).

Phylogenetic and ontogenetic studies have suggested that neurons are the earliest component of the neuroendocrine system because they are present in the most primitive organisms (coelenterates) (42). The next evolutionary step is the appearance of open-type neuroendocrine cells in the gut, which are present in the most highly developed invertebrates. Such cells become extensively diversified in vertebrates. The presence of gastroenteropancreatic neuroendocrine glands of classic solid type (e.g., islets of Langerhans), on the other hand, is a feature that is restricted to true vertebrates (42).

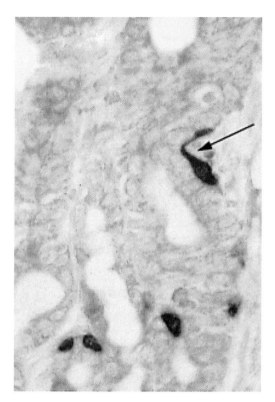

Figure 47.6 Gastric antrum stained for somatostatin using the peroxidase–antiperoxidase technique with diaminobenzidine as the chromogen (no counterstain). A process that extends from the cell body is closely applied to the basal regions of adjacent cells (*arrow*). The somatostatin-positive cells at the lower position of this microscopic field appear to be without processes; however, the processes may be out of the plane of this section.

ULTRASTRUCTURE

The most characteristic ultrastructural feature of neuroendocrine cells is the presence of membrane-bound secretory granules or vesicles, which may vary from 50 to 500 nm in diameter (Figures 47.9 and 47.10). Because of their relatively large size, these structures have also been referred to as large dense core vesicles (LDCV) or large dense core granules (LDCG) (1). Immunoelectron microscopic studies have shown that these granules represent storage sites of peptide and amine hormones. Granules storing different types of hormones are characterized by differences in size, density of contents, and substructure (43) (Table 47.2). Although most neuroendocrine secretory granules are round, others, such as those of the gastrointestinal EC and EC-like cells, are pleomorphic with elongated, reniform, round, oval, or pear-shaped forms. Secretory granules tend to be concentrated at the basal aspects of the cells in relatively close proximity to the basement membrane. Secretory granules are also prominent in cytoplasmic processes and in the apical extensions of the "open" cells. In addition to secretory granules, many neuroendocrine cells also contain small synaptic-type vesicles (SSVs), which have been re-

ferred to as small synaptic vesicle analogs (1). The SSVs are responsible for the release of amino acid neurotransmitters (gamma amino butyric acid, glutamate, glycine) and various biogenic amines in a regulated fashion stimulated by increases in calcium, cAMP and cGMP (1).

APOPTOSIS

Apoptosis plays a critical role in the physiology of many endocrine tissues. For example, deprivation of growth factors, including thyrotropin, epidermal growth factor, and serum from cultures of thyrocytes, leads to DNA fragmentation and morphologic changes of apoptosis (44). Sasano et al. have studied the process of apoptosis in human adrenal cortex using the 3'-OH nick end-labeling or TdT-mediated deoxyuridine triphosphate-biotin nick end-labeling (TUNEL) method (45–48). With this approach, apoptotic cells were present both in the reticularis and glomerulosa, whereas proliferative cells were present primarily in the outer fasciculata. Studies of estrogen-induced prolactin cell hyperplasia in the rat have shown that withdrawal of estrogen results in increased numbers of apoptotic cells (49). This effect is enhanced by the administration of bromocriptine after estrogen withdrawal.

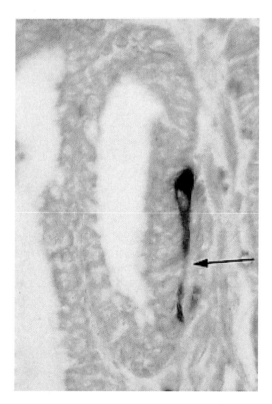

Figure 47.7 Gastric antrum stained for somatostatin using the peroxidase–antiperoxidase technique with diaminobenzidine as the chromogen (no counterstain). The process of this somatostatin-positive cell extends along the basal portion of the gland. A portion of the process is out of the plane of section (*arrow*).

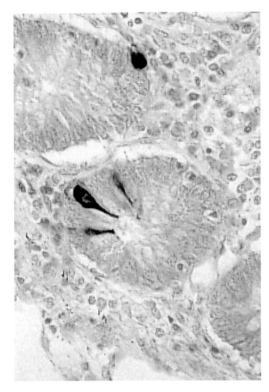

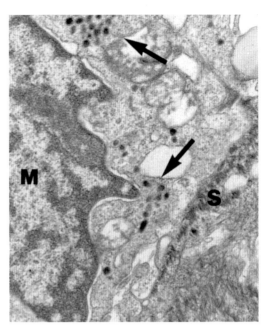

Figure 47.10 Electron micrograph of Merkel cell. Clusters of secretory granules (*arrows*) are present within the Merkel (M) cells. S, squamous cell (original magnification ×27,000).

Figure 47.8 Colonic mucosa stained for serotonin with the peroxidase–antiperoxidase technique with diaminobenzidine as the chromogen and methyl green as the counterstain. A cross section of a gland contains three open-type endocrine cells whose apical processes extend into the lumen.

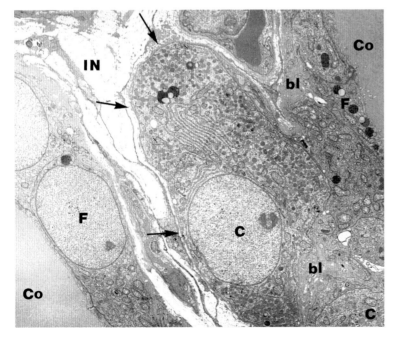

Figure 47.9 Electron micrograph of C cell from a patient with mild C-cell hyperplasia associated with the type II MEN syndrome. The C cell is present at the base of the follicle, where it is in direct contact with the basal cytoplasm of the overlying follicular cell. The basal lamina (bl) is focally thickened at the junction of the C cell and overlying follicular cells. The C cell is separated from the interstitium by the follicular basal lamina (*arrows*). C, C cell; Co, colloid; F, follicular cell; IN, interstitium (original magnification ×14,000).

Although there are few published studies of apoptosis in neuroendocrine cells of the gut and other sites, this process is initiated in neurons when the concentrations of target-derived neurotropic factors are reduced. Garcia and coworkers have demonstrated that overexpression of the bcl-2 protooncogene in cultured sympathetic neurons prevents apoptosis, which is normally induced by deprivation of nerve growth factor (50). It is likely that changes in neuroendocrine cell populations influenced by variations in tropic signals in the gastrointestinal system, pancreas, and other sites may be mediated by apoptosis. However, other mechanisms also may be operative. For example, Kaneto et al. have demonstrated that both exogenous nitrous oxide and nitrous oxide generated endogenously by interleukin (IL)-1 leads to apoptosis of isolated rat pancreatic islet cells. The action of streptozotocin appears to be mediated by a similar mechanism (51). These findings suggest that nitrous oxide–induced internucleosomal DNA cleavage is an important initial step in the destruction and dysfunction of pancreatic β cells induced by inflammatory stimuli or by the action of streptozotocin.

MARKERS OF NEUROENDOCRINE CELLS

Neuroendocrine cells can be classified into those of neural (neurons, paraganglioma cells) and epithelial types. The former contain neurofilaments as their major intermediate filament type while the latter contain cytokeratins with or without neurofilaments. Both cell groups can be identified on the basis of their contents of specific hormones and neurotransmitter substances (52–54), as discussed in other chapters in this volume and by the presence of a variety nonhormonal products. The nonhormonal constituents of neuroendocrine cells include a wide array of cytosolic, secretory granule and vesicle membrane, and plasma membrane constituents. These products can be identified effectively via immunohistochemistry with polyclonal antisera or monoclonal antibodies. This approach is of particular importance when evaluating tissues for the presence of neuroendocrine cells when the specific hormonal product is unknown.

Cytosolic Constituents

A variety of different enzymes can be demonstrated by immunohistochemistry in neuroendocrine cells. Although some of the enzymes are present in most neuroendocrine cells, others have a more restricted distribution. Neuron-specific enolase has been considered as a generic marker both for neurons and neuroendocrine cells (55). The enolases are products of three independent gene loci, which have been designated α, β, and γ (56–58). Nonneuronal enolase (αα) is present in fetal tissues, glial cells, and many nonendocrine tissues. Beta (ββ)-enolase is present in muscle tissue, whereas hybrid enolases (αγ, αβ) have been identified in megakaryocytes and a variety of other cell types. Neuron-specific enolase (γγ) replaces nonneuronal enolase during the migration and differentiation of neurons, and it has been suggested that the appearance of neuron-specific enolase reflects the formation of synapses and the acquisition of electrical excitability. Although the sensitivity of neuron-specific enolase for the detection of neuroendocrine cells is high, its specificity is low.

Seshi et al. have demonstrated a high degree of specificity with monoclonal antibodies to neuron-specific enolase (59). Some of the monoclonal antibodies react predominantly with nerve fibers, whereas others react with the perikaryon exclusively or with the perikaryon and associated nerve fibers. In contrast to the polyclonal antisera that stain a variety of nonneuronal structures, the monoclonal antibodies stain neuronal cells in a more selective fashion. Some monoclonal antibodies also react with normal adrenal medullary cells and with subsets of pancreatic islet cells.

The protein gene product 9.5 (PGP 9.5) is a soluble protein with a molecular weight of 27,000 Daltons (60). PGP 9.5 is a ubiquitin carboxyterminal hydrolase that plays a role in the catalytic degradation of abnormal denatured proteins (61). Immunohistochemical studies have demonstrated that it is present in neurons and nerve fibers at all levels of the central and peripheral nervous system. It is also present in a variety of neuroendocrine cells, except for those in the normal gastrointestinal tract (60). The patterns of staining for PGP 9.5 and neuron specific enolases are generally similar in that positive cells show diffuse cytoplasmic reactivity that is unrelated to the type of hormone produced or to the degree of cellular differentiation. Additional enzymes that have a dominant cytolosolic distribution include histaminase (62) and some of the enzymes involved in catecholamine biosynthesis (54).

Secretory Granule Constituents

The chromogranins/secretogranins (Cg/Sg) represent a widely distributed family of soluble proteins that represent the predominant constituent by weight of neurosecretory granules (Table 47.1 and Figure 47.11) (63–65). Three major chromogranin proteins have been identified and categorized and have been designated chromogranin A, chromogranin B, and secretogranin III. Additional members of the granin family include secretogranins III, IV, and V. The chromogranins are calcium binding proteins that play important roles in the packaging and/or processing of regulatory peptides. These proteins contain multiple dibasic residues that are sites for endogenous proteolytic processing to smaller peptides (66,67). For example, chromogranin A contains 439 amino acids that represent potential cleavage sites by proteases such as the hormone proconvertases.

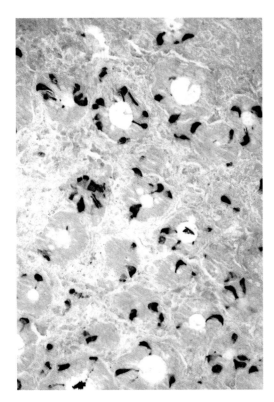

Figure 47.11 Colonic mucosa stained with a monoclonal antibody to chromogranin A (LK2H10) via the avidin-biotin-peroxidase technique using diaminobenzidine as the chromogen and methyl green as the counterstain. This cross section is at the level of the lower third of the mucosa and shows many opened and closed neuroendocrine cells.

Resultant peptides include chromostatin, pancreastatin, parastatin, and vasostatin. Functional roles for these smaller peptides include intracellular binding functions, inhibitory effects on the secretion of other hormones and antibacterial/antifungal effects. Both pancreastatin and chromostatin are present in most neuroendocrine cells, adrenal medulla and anterior pituitary (68,69), while derivatives of chromogranin B (GAWK protein) have been localized to neuroendocrine cells in the pituitary, gastrointestinal tract, pancreas, and adrenal medulla (70).

The Cg/Sg are widely distributed throughout the entire system of neuroendocrine cells and have distinctive patterns of tissue and cellular distribution (71). Although many neuroendocrine cells contain CgA, CgB, and SgII, others contain only one or two of these proteins. For example, thyroid C cells contain CgA and SgII but lack CgB. Parathyroid chief cells, on the other hand, are positive for CgA but lack SgII. The distribution of this family of proteins is reviewed in detail by Huttner et al. (71). The chromogranins are cosecreted with other granule contents, but their replenishment is differentially regulated.

A variety of endopeptidases and carboxypeptidases are required for the formation of biologically active peptides from precursor molecules and are present in the trans-Golgi region and secretory granules of neuroendocrine cells. They include the prohormone convertases, PC1/PC3 and PC2, and carboxypeptidases H & E (72,73). The proconvertases are widely distributed in neuroendocrine cells while other types of endocrine cells (thyroid follicular cells, parathyroid chief cells, adrenal cortical cells, and testis) are negative. Neuroendocrine cells with a neural phenotype (adrenal medullary cells) contain a predominance of PC2 while epithelial neuroendocrine cells contain a predominance of PC1/PC3. With the exception of parathyroid cells, the presence of PC2 and PC3 correlates with the presence of chromogranin and secretogranins. PC2 and PC1/PC3 are present in normal pituitaries and adenomas, with ACTH producing adenomas containing a predominance of PC1/PC3 and other adenomas expressing a predominance of PC2.

Peptidylglycine α-amidating monooxygenase (PAM), peptidyl-glycine α-hydroxylating monooxygenase (PHM), and peptidylamidaglycolate lyase (PAL) are present in neuroendocrine secretory granules (74,75). These enzymes are responsible for the α amidation of the C-terminal regions of peptide hormones, a function which is critical for the biological function of peptides. These enzymes are not restricted in their distribution to neuroendocrine cells. For example, they have also been found in the lung in cells of the airway epithelium and glands, vascular endothelium, some chondrocytes of bronchial cartilage, alveolar macrophages, and smooth muscle cells.

Cytochrome b561 (Chromomembrin B), a neurosecretory granule membrane constituent, is responsible for the transport of electrons into the secretory granule matrix in order to maintain a supply of reduced ascorbic acid, which serves as an electron donor for dopamine β-hydroxylase and for amidases that modify C-terminal portions of certain neuropeptides (76). Antibodies to cytochrome b561 may be useful for the identification of neuroendocrine cells that are engaged in specific functions related to catecholamine synthesis or peptide amidation (77).

Synaptic Vesicle and Docking Constituents

Synaptophysin (molecular weight 38,000) was one of the earliest markers developed to visualize small synaptic vesicle analogs in neurons and neuroendocrine cells (78–80). This protein is widely distributed in nerve terminals in the central and peripheral nervous system and is also present in neuroendocrine cells that are specialized for the regulated secretion of peptide hormones. Synaptophysin is the most abundant integral membrane protein of neuronal vesicles. It is localized in a punctate pattern in synaptic regions of neurons and has a diffuse cytoplasmic distribution in neuroendocrine cells. Ultrastructurally, synaptophysin is present predominantly in smooth-surface synaptic-type vesicles. Although synaptophysin was originally thought to be specific for neuroendocrine cells, it is also expressed in other cell types, including the adrenal cortex (81,82).

Synaptic vesicle protein 2, (SV2), an integral membrane protein, is present in the central and peripheral nervous system and in a wide variety of neuroendocrine cell types (83). This glycoprotein occurs in 3 well-characterized isoforms, which have been designated SV2A, SV2B and SV2C. Immunoreactivity for SV2 is present in neuroendocrine cells in the gastrointestinal tract, pancreas, anterior pituitary, thyroid (C cells), parathyroid, and adrenal medulla. Chief cells of the gastric oxyntic mucosa are also positive for SV2. Interestingly, gastrointestinal stromal tumors have been reported to be positive for SV2 (84). Comparison of SV2, synaptophysin, and chromogranin A immunoreactivities have shown more SV2 and synaptophysin than chromogranin A positive cells in the gastric antrum and pancreas. More SV2 than synaptophysin positive cells were seen in other regions of the gastrointestinal tract and other endocrine organs. Generally, more chromogranin A than SV2 immunoreactive cells were present in the duodenum, colon, and parathyroid.

The vesicular monoamine transporters (VMAT1 and VMAT2) are integral membrane proteins that mediate the transport of amines into vesicles of neurons and neuroendocrine cells (85,86). These two isoforms show broad selectivity for different amines and are distributed differently in various cell types. VMAT1 is expressed in gastrointestinal enterochromaffin (EC) tumors and in the corresponding normal EC cells and the small intensely fluorescent cells of the sympathetic ganglia. VMAT2, on the other hand, is present in histamine producing ECL cells and in central and peripheral neurons. VMAT1 and VMAT2 are both expressed by adrenal medullary cells.

The process of regulated secretion in neurons and neuroendocrine cells is highly complex (1,87,88). According to the SNARE (SNAP-receptor) hypothesis, the selective docking of a transport vesicle with the appropriate target membrane occurs via the formation of a complex between a vesicle membrane protein (v-SNARE) and the corresponding target membrane protein (t-SNARE) (89). The resulting SNARE complex ultimately leads to membrane fusion. Three families of SNARE proteins are currently recognized. They include the VAMP (vesicle associated membrane protein)/ synaptobrevin family of v-SNAREs and two families of t-SNAREs, the syntaxin family and the SNAP-25 family. In the initial phases of exocytosis, N-ethylmaleimide-sensitive factor (NSF) and soluble NSF attachment protein (α-SNAP) act on synaptobrevin, syntaxin, and SNAP-25. This leads to dissociation of the SNARE complexes, activation of the SNARE proteins and removal of the negative regulators of exocytosis. Subsequently, the vesicle protein Rab3 promotes reversible vesicle attachment (tethering) to the presynaptic membrane. Tethering permits the formation of the SNARE complex, which consists of synaptobrevin, syntaxin, and SNAP-25. This series of events brings the vesicle into a docked position, immediately adjacent to the plasma membrane and calcium channels. Docking is an irreversible step in which there is some degree of membrane fusion. At some time during docking, synaptotagmin is recruited to the SNARE complex (89).

Many of the proteins involved in the process of regulated secretion can be visualized in immunohistochemical formats and have been utilized as neuroendocrine cell markers. While some of these proteins are localized within the plasma membranes [SNAP-25 (synaptosomal protein of 25kDa) and syntaxin], others (synaptobrevin, synaptophysin, Rab3a, and synaptotagmin) are present in the synaptic vesicle membranes. The soluble proteins involved in this process include N-ethylmaleimide-sensitive fusion protein (NSF) and soluble NSF attachment proteins (SNAPs).

The vesicle associated membrane proteins (VAMP) play important roles in docking and/or fusion of secretory vesicles with their target membranes. VAMP, which is also known as synaptobrevin, occurs in 3 isoforms, which are designated VAMP-1, VAMP-2, and VAMP-3 (cellubrevin). VAMP-2 and VAMP-3 are expressed in pancreatic islets (90) and are involved in calcium mediated insulin secretion. VAMP-1 is present primarily in pancreatic acinar cells (91).

The synaptotagmins (p65) include a large family of calcium binding proteins that are constituents of the membranes of synaptic vesicles. In the normal pancreatic islets, synaptotagmins are colocalized with insulin in β cells and are involved with calcium induced insulin secretion (92).

Rab proteins are low-molecular-weight GTP binding proteins. The Rab3 isoforms are involved in the exocytosis of synaptic vesicles and secretory granules in the CNS and anterior pituitary. In normal human pituitary, Rab3 isoforms are present primarily within the cytoplasm of growth hormone producing cells with rare expression in other cell types. Among pituitary adenomas, Rab3 is most commonly expressed in growth hormone producing adenomas but also occurs in adenomas of other types (93).

SNAP-25 has been studied most extensively in the pituitary gland. This protein is localized predominantly to the plasma membranes of both normal and neoplastic adenohypophyseal cells (94,95). Similar patterns of localization have been documented in the adrenal and pancreatic islets (96,97).

The presence of certain lymphoreticular antigens in some neuroendocrine cells suggests that these proteins may serve similar functions in endocrine and lymphoid tissues (98–100). These functions potentially include some aspects of cell-to-cell recognition and release of secretory products (e.g., hormones and lymphokines) in response to common microenvironmental signals (98). CD57 (leu 7;HNK-1) recognizes epitopes in natural killer lymphocytes, myelin-associated glycoprotein (MAG), neuronal cell adhesion molecules, and a granule matrix constituent of chromaffin cells (99,100). The largest of the MAGs (MAG-72) is related to the immunoglobulin supergene family proteins as well as neural adhesion molecules. CD57 also reacts with a subset of neuroendocrine cells in the anterior pituitary, pancreatic islets, and gastrointestinal tract (100). In addition, CD57 immunoreactivity has been identified in Schwann cells and other nerve-supporting elements. S-100 protein, which was originally isolated from the brain, is present in cells that serve as a supporting structure in many neuroendocrine tissues, such as the adrenal medulla, paraganglia, and anterior pituitary (101).

The neural cell adhesion molecules (NCAMs) represent a family of glycoproteins that play key roles in cell binding, migration, differentiation, and proliferation (101,102). The NCAM family includes several major peptides that are generated by alternative splicing of RNA from a gene that is a member of the immunoglobulin supergene family. The peptide sequences that are external to the plasma membrane contain five regions that are similar to those present in immunoglobulins. The molecules are modified post-translationally by phosphorylation, sulphation, and glycosylation. The homophilic-binding properties of NCAMs are modulated by differential expression of homopolymers of α2, 8-linked N-acetylneuraminic acid (polysialic acid).

CD57 recognizes a 140kDa isoform of NCAM which is expressed on resting and activated NK cells and a subset of CD3+ cells. Although initial studies had suggested that NCAM was restricted in its distribution to the brain, more recent studies indicate that it is also present in a variety of neuroendocrine cells, including the islets of Langerhans, adenohypophysis, and adrenal medulla, as well as in a variety of nonneuroendocrine cells (103). Komminoth et al. have used a monoclonal antibody reactive with a long chain from of α-2, 8-linked polysialic acid that is present on NCAMs (104). They reported positive staining in cases of familial medullary thyroid carcinoma, both in the neoplastic cells and in hyperplastic C cells adjacent to the tumorous foci. Cases of primary C-cell hyperplasia unassociated with medullary thyroid carcinoma were also positively stained, whereas most normal C cells and C cells in secondary hyperplasia were nonreactive. These findings indicate that determinations of NCAMs may be helpful in distinguishing reactive proliferations of neuroendocrine cells from neoplastic and preneoplastic proliferations of these cells.

Transcription Factors

Transcription factors are proteins that bind to regulatory elements in the promotor and enhancer regions of DNA and regulate gene expression and protein synthesis. They may be cell/tissue specific or may be present in a variety of different tissue types. CDX2 is a transcription factor that has been used extensively as a marker of intestinal adenocarcinoma. In addition to its presence in normal enterocytes, CDX2 is present in all serotonin-producing EC cells,

10% of gastrin-producing G cells, 30% of gastric inhibitory peptide cells, and in a small proportion of motilin-producing cells while other gastrointestinal endocrine cells are negative (105). Thyroid transcription factor-1 (TTF-1) is present both in thyroid (follicular cells and C cells) and in the lung (type II epithelial cells, subsets of respiratory nonciliated bronchiolar epithelial cells and pulmonary neuroendocrine cells) (106). The adrenal 4 site/steroidogenic factor (ad4BP/SF-1) is present in steroid-producing cells and in certain anterior pituitary cell types while the pituitary transcription factor, Pit-1, is present in certain cells of the adenohypophysis and the placenta (107).

Somatostatin Receptors

Somatostatin interacts with specific receptors (sst1–sst5) expressed on target cells (108). These receptors have attracted considerable attention because of novel clinical applications related to their overexpression in certain tumors, including those of the neuroendocrine system. Because of the metabolic instability of natural somatostatin, a number of synthetic analogs (e.g., octreotide) have been developed. Radionuclide conjugates of these analogs have been used successfully for imaging and treatment of tumors. The ability of tumors to express these receptors can be assessed with antibodies to the specific receptors, particularly the sst-2 receptor. Positive staining of normal gastrin-producing cells for sst-2A has been documented in gastric antrum, duodenum, jejunum, and ileum (109). In addition, occasional sst-2A positive cells have been recognized in the basal cell component of bronchi.

FUNCTION OF NEUROENDOCRINE CELLS

The function of neuroendocrine cells has been established by the use of immunohistochemical techniques for the localization of specific hormones and other substances. In many instances, the use of region-specific antisera permits the localization of hormone precursors as well as mature hormones. Proinsulin immunoreactivity in the β cells of normal pancreatic islets is present in a crescent-shaped perinuclear area that corresponds to the Golgi zone (110). Insulin, on the other hand, is present throughout the cytoplasm with a variably stained perinuclear region.

Although initial studies suggested that single neuroendocrine cells were responsible for the production of a unique hormone (one-cell, one-hormone hypothesis), more recent studies indicate that these cells are multimessenger systems (111). The peptide hormones are synthesized within the granular endoplasmic reticulum and are packaged into secretory granules by way of the Golgi region. Multiple different peptide products may be synthesized via this route in single neuroendocrine cells. Other nonpeptide hormone constituents such as catecholamines are synthesized within the cytosol and are then taken up into secretory granules (25). Any individual neuroendocrine cell can, therefore, vary the secretion of its products in response to different signals in normal and pathologic states.

Immunohistochemical and molecular biologic studies have led to many interesting insights into the functional interrelationships of the various components of the neuroendocrine system. For example, peptide hormones first isolated from the gastroenteropancreatic axis have been found subsequently in neurons of the central and peripheral nervous systems, where they may function as neurotransmitters or neuromodulators (10). Other peptides initially isolated from the brain have been localized to the endocrine cells of the gut, pancreas, and lung, where they may have a paracrine function (112). Furthermore, such studies have shown that the microarchitecture of endocrine organs, which may appear homogeneous in hematoxylin and eosin–stained sections, is often organized in a manner that permits paracrine interactions. The somatostatin cells of the pancreatic islets, for example, are located between the insulin and glucagon cells and typically extend short branching processes, which are in apposition to both cell types. Regulation of the secretion of insulin and glucagon may therefore be mediated by the local paracrine effects of somatostatin and by the endocrine effects of somatostatin reaching the islets by the circulation (113,114).

Neuroendocrine cells in different tissues may produce identical peptides. Somatostatin, for example, is present in certain hypothalamic neurons, pancreatic D cells, gastrointestinal D cells, bronchopulmonary endocrine cells, thymic endocrine cells, and a subset of thyroid C cells, where it is colocalized with calcitonin (113–115). Calcitonin is present in thyroid C cells, bronchopulmonary and thymic endocrine cells, and certain urogenital endocrine cells. Gastrin-releasing peptide, a 27–amino acid peptide that is the mammalian homolog of bombesin, is present in thyroid C cells, small intensely fluorescent cells of sympathetic ganglia, neuronal cells of the gastrointestinal myenteric plexus, and bronchopulmonary endocrine cells (116–117).

Neuroendocrine cells may produce multiple distinct peptides from a common precursor molecule. For example, adrenocorticotropin (ACTH) is synthesized from the large precursor molecule pro-opiomelanocortin (POMC) (118). In the adenohypophysis, POMC is processed to yield ACTH, β-lipotropin, and a 16KD N-terminal fragment. In the intermediate lobe, ACTH and β-lipotropin are processed to yield α-MSH and β-endorphin–related peptides, respectively. Hormonal diversity in neuroendocrine cells also may result from alternate splicing pathways that produce different messenger RNAs from a single gene. Both calcitonin and the calcitonin gene–related peptide (CGRP) are produced from a primary RNA transcript that is spliced to produce two different forms of mature messenger RNA

(119). More than one gene may also encode closely related peptides. In anglerfish islets, for example, recombinant DNA techniques have shown two different messages for somatostatin, one of which encodes somatostatin I while the other encodes somatostatin II (120).

DISTRIBUTION OF NEUROENDOCRINE CELLS

The histology of the adenohypophysis, parathyroid glands, intra- and extra-adrenal paraganglia, and pancreatic islets is discussed in separate chapters in this volume. The remaining sections of this chapter review the distribution of neuroendocrine cells in other tissues and organs.

Bronchopulmonary and Upper Respiratory System

The neuroendocrine components of the lung occur singly as solitary neuroendocrine cells and in small aggregates that have been designated neuroepithelial bodies (NEBs) (121) (Figure 47.12). Solitary neuroepithelial cells may be of the opened or closed type. NEBs are composed of

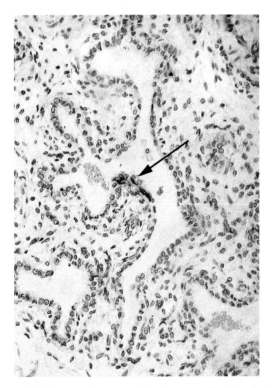

Figure 47.12 Fetal lung stained with a monoclonal antibody to chromogranin A (LK2H10) via the avidin-biotin-peroxidase technique using diaminobenzidine as the chromogen and hematoxylin as the counterstain. A cluster of chromogranin-positive cells (*arrow*) is present just beneath the bronchial epithelium.

clusters of clear to faintly eosinophilic cells that extend from the bronchial basement membrane to the lumen. NEBs are extensively innervated. Although the functions of the two neuroendocrine components are not known with certainty, NEBs most likely act as intrapulmonary chemoreceptors. Solitary neuroendocrine cells most likely subserve a paracrine function.

The secretory granules of neuroendocrine cells in the lung show considerable variation in size and density (122,123). On the basis of granule size, the bronchopulmonary neuroendocrine cells have been divided into three types. The P1 cells have granules that measure 40 to 50 nm in diameter. These cells have been noted in fetal lung. The P2 cells have granules that measure 120 to 130 nm in diameter, whereas the P3 granules measure 180 to 200 nm. The granules of Pa cells, which are found in the adult lung, measure 100 to 120 nm in diameter. Both NEBs and solitary neuroendocrine cells contain serotonin, bombesin/gastrin-releasing peptide (GRP), and calcitonin, whereas the solitary neuroendocrine cells also contain leu-enkephalin (117,121) (Figure 47.13). Severely hyperplastic and dysplastic cells of the NEBs also may produce adrenocorticotropin, vasoactive intestinal peptide, and somatostatin (121). The NEBs are particularly conspicuous in fetal lung tissue but are sparse in the adult (117). The neuroendocrine

components of the lung are also prominent in hypoxic conditions, including high-altitude conditions and chronic pulmonary diseases such as bronchiectasis.

Both in situ hybridization and immunohistochemical studies have shown GRP and its corresponding messenger RNA (mRNA) as early as 8 weeks of gestation in solitary neuroendocrine cells and NEBs, primarily at branch points of bronchioles. The number of cells reach a peak by 16 to 30 weeks of gestation and decline at about 6 months of age. These findings suggest that GRP may be involved in the growth and development of normal lung. Increased numbers of GRP-containing cells have been found in infants with bronchopulmonary dysplasia and in children with cystic fibrosis or prolonged assisted ventilation (117).

Neuroendocrine cells, as defined by their argentaffinity or argyrophilia, are rare in the larynx. Pesce et al. were able to identify scattered argyrophil cells in only two of 43 specimens of larynx within the respiratory epithelium (124). The studies of Torre-Rendon et al. demonstrated occasional argyrophil cells both within the laryngeal squamous and respiratory epithelium (125). Argyrophil cells are also present within adjacent minor salivary glands and the epithelium of the middle ear.

Thyroid and Thymus

In both adult and neonatal thyroid glands, the calcitonin-containing C cells are concentrated in a zone corresponding to the upper to middle thirds of the lobes along a hypothetical central axis (126). The extreme upper and lower poles, as well as the isthmus, are devoid of C cells. The C cells occupy an exclusively intrafollicular position (Figures 47.9, 47.14, and 47.15). In neonates, the C cells are prominent and measure up to 40 μm in diameter. Occasional cells may show branching processes that are closely applied to the follicular basement membrane and the plasma membranes of adjacent follicular cells. Groups of up to six C cells may be present in the thyroids of neonates with up to 100 C cells per single low-power microscopic field. C cells are less numerous in adults than in neonates and appear flattened or spindle shaped. Typically, adult thyroid glands contain fewer than 50 C cells per single low-power field, although occasional normal adult glands may have a higher density of C cells. Rarely, nodules of C cells may be found in normal adult glands, as discussed in the section on aging.

Two types of secretory granule have been observed in normal as well as hyperplastic C cells (127). Type I granules have an average diameter of 280 nm, with moderately dense, finely granular contents that are closely applied to the limiting membranes of the granules. The type II granules, on the other hand, have an average diameter of 130 nm with electron-dense contents that are separated from the limiting membranes of the granules by a small but distinct electron-lucent space. Immunoelectron microscopic

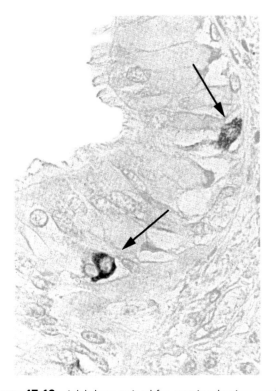

Figure 47.13 Adult lung stained for gastrin-releasing peptide (GRP)/bombesin with an antibody to GRP with the indirect peroxidase-labeled method. Diaminobenzidine was the chromogen with methyl green counterstain. Two GRP-positive cells (*arrows*) are present within the bronchial epithelium. (Courtesy of Dr. Y. Tsutsumi, Tokai University School of Medicine, Japan.)

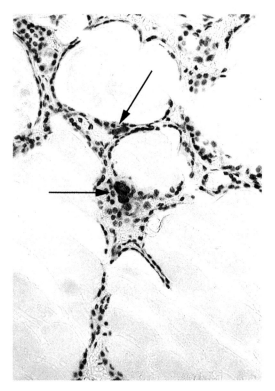

Figure 47.14 Adult thyroid stained with a monoclonal antibody to chromogranin A (LK2H10) via the avidin-biotin-peroxidase technique using diaminobenzidine as the chromogen and hematoxylin as the counterstain. Groups of two to three C cells are present (*arrows*).

studies have shown that both granule types contain immunoreactive calcitonin. Some of the C cells, both in normal adult and in neonatal glands, also contain somatostatin or bombesin/GRP (117,127,128). Approximately 70% of fetal and neonatal C cells contain GRP peptide and mRNA, whereas less than 20% of adult C cells are positive for GRP (46). It has been suggested that GRP may play a role as a thyroid growth factor analogous to its presumed role in the developing lung (117).

Although neuroendocrine cells are found commonly in the thymus glands of many animal species, these cells are sparse in human thymic tissue. In human glands, the neuroendocrine cells may be found within the perivascular connective tissue and in association with Hassall's corpuscles (129).

Skin

The Merkel cells represent the neuroendocrine components of the skin (Figure 47.9). These cells occur singly and in small clusters throughout the epidermis. Merkel cell clusters are particularly prominent in foci of specialized epithelial differentiation, such as the touch domes (130). The cells have elongate processes that surround neighboring keratinocytes. The Merkel cells are characteristically

innervated by long type I myelinated fibers. Secretory granules are abundant and range from 80 to 130 nm in diameter. The granules are particularly prominent in cytoplasmic processes. Aggregates of intermediate filament proteins are predominantly of the cytokeratin type. There is considerable species variation in the content and type of peptide hormone in these cells. The most frequently encountered hormones are met-enkephalin, vasoactive intestinal peptide, and bombesin/GRP (130).

Breast

Although clear cells have been noted in the breast by many observers, the question of whether these cells are neuroendocrine in type has engendered considerable controversy. Bussolati et al. have reported the presence of chromogranin-positive cells in a small number of normal breast samples (131). The cells were present singly or in small clusters in ductules, intralobular ducts of interlobular ducts, and between myoepithelial and epithelial cells. Occasional cell processes extended to the lumen in a manner typical of opened-type neuroendocrine cells. In parallel sections, the chromogranin-positive cells exhibited weak argyrophilia but were negative for a variety of peptide hormones. Chromogranin-positive cells were not identified in cases of fibrocystic disease or in papillomas.

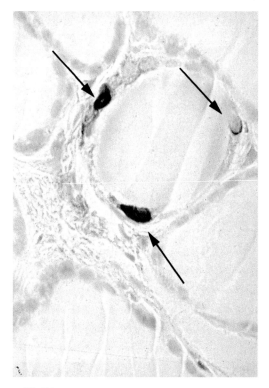

Figure 47.15 Adult thyroid stained for calcitonin via the peroxidase–antiperoxidase technique using diaminobenzidine as the chromogen and hematoxylin as the counterstain. C cells (*arrows*) are present within the follicle as closed-type endocrine cells.

Gastrointestinal System

The gastrointestinal tract, from the esophagus to the anal canal, is extensively populated by a heterogeneous collection of peptide- and amine-producing neurons and neuroendocrine cells (38–40). The gut neuroendocrine cells are responsible for the production of more than 20 different hormones (Figures 47.6–47.8, 47.11, 47.16, and 47.17). Cells of similar morphology and function are also present within the intraextrahepatic bile ducts and the pancreatic ductal system (Figures 47.18 and 47.19). The major products of the gut endocrine cells, together with their morphologic characteristics and distributional patterns, are summarized in Figure 47.16 and in Table 47.2.

In addition to their presence in mucosal and submucosal endocrine cells, peptide hormones also have been identified within submucosal glands. Brunner's glands, for example, contain neuroendocrine cells storing somatostatin, gastrin-cholecystokinin, and peptide YY. Peptidergic nerve structures containing vasoactive intestinal peptide,

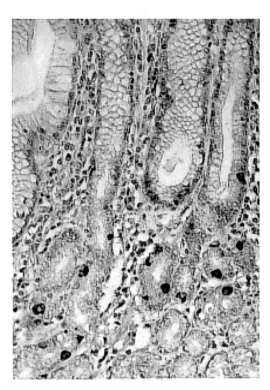

Figure 47.17 Gastric antrum stained for gastrin using the peroxidase–antiperoxidase technique with diaminobenzidine as the chromogen and hematoxylin as the counterstain. The G cells are present primarily within the lower thirds of the gastric glands.

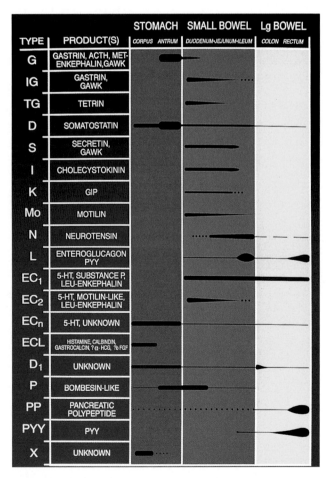

Figure 47.16 Distribution of gastrointestinal endocrine cells. The width of the horizontal bars indicates the number of cells within different portions of the gastrointestinal tract. (Reprinted with permission from: Dayal Y. Endocrine cells of the gut and their neoplasms. In: Norris HT, ed. *Pathology of the Colon, Small Intestine and Anus.* New York: Churchill Livingstone; 1983:267–300.)

peptide histidine methionine, substance P, neuropeptide Y, and gastrin-releasing peptide also have been identified around Brunner's glands. All these peptides, with the exception of gastrin-releasing peptide, have been found in nerve cell bodies of the submucosal ganglia adjacent to the acini of Brunner's glands (40). These findings suggest that multiple peptides may be involved in the control of secretion from these glands.

Urogenital System

Although argyrophil cells are not present in the adult renal parenchyma, rare argyrophilic cells have been reported in the renal pelvis. These cells may be particularly prominent in areas of glandular metaplasia. Neuroendocrine cells, as defined by their argentaffinity or argyrophilia, were first described in the urinary bladder by Feyrter (5,6). Later studies by Fetissof et al. (132) established that the endocrine cells in the urothelium were predominantly of the closed type (Figure 47.20). Immunohistochemical analyses showed that the cells were positive for serotonin but did not contain peptide hormones such as ACTH, gastrin, glucagon, or somatostatin.

The neuroendocrine cells of the prostate include both opened and closed types with a predominance of the latter forms (133–135). As shown in Grimelius-stained preparations, many of these cells have multiple dendritic processes extending between adjacent epithelial cells and occasionally abutting on other neuroendocrine cells. The neuroendocrine cells are more prominent in normal or atrophic prostate than in hyperplastic foci. Most of these cells contain serotonin, and some also contain somatostatin. Both calcitonin and bombesin/GRP also have been observed in the normal prostate, but these hormones are present in considerably less than 5% of the neuroendocrine cells. In contrast to the anorectal canal, which is also derived from the cloaca and contains both pancreatic polypeptide and glucagon immunoreactivities, the prostatic neuroendocrine cells are negative for these peptides.

Ultrastructurally, the cells show considerable pleomorphism in granule morphology (133). The opened cells have basally oriented granules, whereas the closed cells have a more uniform distribution of granules. Prominent lamellar bodies are noted in some cells.

Neuroendocrine cells of both opened and closed types have been demonstrated in the endocervical glandular epithelium and in the exocervical squamous epithelium (136). In both sites, however, the argyrophilic cells are extremely uncommon. However, argyrophil cells have not been identified in the normal ovary, fallopian tube, or endometrium.

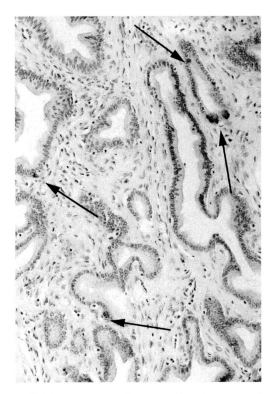

Figure 47.19   Terminal ramifications of bile ducts stained with a monoclonal antibody to chromogranin A (LK2H10) via the avidin-biotin-peroxidase technique using diaminobenzidine as the chromogen and hematoxylin as the counterstain. Both open and closed neuroendocrine cells (*arrows*) are present within the ductal epithelium.

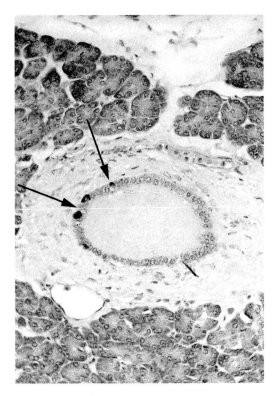

Figure 47.18   Pancreatic duct stained with a monoclonal antibody to chromogranin A (LK2H10) via the avidin-biotin-peroxidase technique using diaminobenzidine as the chromogen and hematoxylin as the counterstain. Occasional closed-type neuroendocrine cells (*arrows*) are present within the ductal epithelium.

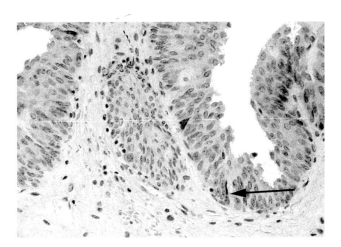

Figure 47.20   Urinary bladder epithelium stained with a monoclonal antibody to chromogranin A (LK2H10) via the avidin-biotin-peroxidase technique using diaminobenzidine as the chromogen and hematoxylin as the counterstain. Neuroendocrine cells are present within the epithelium. A process of another neuroendocrine cell is present at the arrow.

AGING CHANGES

The endocrine system undoubtedly plays an important role in the aging process; however, there have been relatively few systematic studies of the effects of aging in neuroendocrine cell populations in humans. Sun et al. have demonstrated a significant age-related decline in the number and size of growth hormone–producing cells that was most marked in the transition from youth to middle age (137). Pituitary parenchymal cells also decreased in number, but there were no changes in pituitary weight. Prolactin cells, on the other hand, did not show age-related changes. Hypertrophy and relative hyperplasia of thyrotroph cells have been demonstrated in pituitaries from older individuals (138).

O'Toole et al. have studied the effects of the aging process on C-cell populations in the thyroid gland (139). Although C cells appeared to be more numerous in thyroid glands of elderly individuals, as compared with young and middle-aged individuals, the results were not statistically significant because of the large standard deviations. However, C cells more often tended to form clusters or nodules in thyroids from older individuals (140).

Age-related changes in neuroendocrine populations have been characterized in a few other sites, including the prostate. Although the numbers of neuroendocrine cells of the periurethral glands and prostatic ducts remain relatively constant throughout life, those in the peripheral acini are present in highest numbers in the neonatal and post-pubertal periods (41). Cohen et al. have suggested that these variations in prostatic neuroendocrine cells may be mediated in part by the levels of androgenic hormones (41). Bronchopulmonary neuroendocrine cells are considerably more prominent in neonates than in children or adults. In postnatal lungs, there is minimal variation in the numbers of these cells; however, neuroendocrine cells are more likely to be arranged in clusters in younger subjects than in the elderly (141).

SPECIAL PROCEDURES

In addition to the histochemical and immunohistochemical approaches that have been discussed throughout this chapter, molecular methodologies including in situ hybridization provide important approaches for analyzing the distribution and function of neuroendocrine cells (142,143). In contrast to immunohistochemistry, which is dependent on the peptide content of endocrine cells, in situ hybridization techniques permit the identification of cells on the basis of their content's specific mRNAs. For example, endocrine cells that are acutely stimulated or are secreting their products constitutively often produce a negative immunohistochemical signal for the particular peptide. However, studies using nucleic acid probes for the corresponding mRNAs often provide an intensely positive signal in the same cells (142). Extensive posttranslational processing and intracellular degradation of peptide products also may lead to positive hybridization signals with negative immunohistochemical reactions for the corresponding peptides. Additionally, in situ hybridization methods are of particular value for demonstrating hormone receptor mRNAs in target cells and for distinguishing de novo synthesis from uptake of hormonal peptides (142,143,144). The combination of in situ hybridization and immunohistochemistry has the potential for providing the maximal amount of information on the highly dynamic processes of gene transcription and translation (142,144).

The in situ hybridization method also has been combined with polymerase chain reaction (PCR) methods for demonstration of low copy number DNAs and RNAs (145,146). Detection of intracellular PCR products may be achieved indirectly by in situ hybridization using PCR product-specific probes (indirect in situ PCR) or without in situ hybridization through direct incorporation of labeled nucleotides into the PCR amplicants (direct in situ PCR). Although most protocols are designed for the demonstration of DNA, low copy RNA sequences have been demonstrated by the addition of a reverse transcriptase (RT) step to generate cDNA from RNA templates before in situ PCR. This technique, which has been called in situ RT-PCR, may be of particular value when there are fewer than 20 copies of mRNA per cell (118). This technique is of great potential value for the identification of cells with low levels of mRNA-encoding hormones, hormone receptors, cytokines, growth factors, and growth factor receptors. The technical details and potential pitfalls of these methods are discussed in detail in several recent publications (145,147,148).

ARTIFACTS

Because neuroendocrine cells often have a clear appearance, they must be distinguished from a variety of other cell types that also may appear clear in hematoxylin and eosin–stained, formalin-fixed, paraffin-embedded sections. Cytoplasmic clearing may result from intracellular accumulations of lipids or glycogen; alternatively, this change may represent a shrinkage artifact analogous to that seen in the lacunar cells of nodular sclerosing Hodgkin's disease. For example, clear cells in the intestinal epithelium may represent lymphocytes or epithelial cells with retraction of the cytoplasm from the nucleus. In general, this type of artifact is less pronounced in tissues that have been fixed in nonaqueous fixatives. Neuroendocrine cells can be conclusively distinguished from other clear cells by the presence of neuroendocrine markers, including chromogranin proteins or synaptophysin.

Numerous artefacts may be associated with the use of immunohistochemical procedures for the demonstration of peptide hormones and nonhormonal markers. Appropriate positive and negative controls therefore must be used in conjunction with these procedures, as discussed in standard textbooks of immunohistochemistry (149). Nonspecific binding of immunoglobulins to endocrine secretory granules also may result from ionic interactions that may be suppressed to some extent by the use of buffers containing high concentrations of salt (150), as discussed in the chapter on paraganglia. Endogenous biotin-like activity may also contribute to nonspecific staining in neuroendocrine cells and other cell types, particularly following microwave-induced antigen retrieval (151,152). This problem can be circumvented by the use of biotin blocking steps or by the use of biotin free detection systems.

Artifacts also may occur in in situ hybridization procedures. For example, Pagani et al. have demonstrated that oligonucleotides used in in situ hybridization procedures bind to neuroendocrine cells as a result of the presence of endogenous NH_2 groups (153). This type of nonspecific interaction can be blocked effectively by treating the sections with acetic anhydride. Controls for standard in situ hybridization and PCR-based in situ hybridization are discussed in detail in several recent reviews (145,146,148).

DIFFERENTIAL DIAGNOSIS

The differential diagnosis of various neuroendocrine cell populations is discussed in the chapters dealing with the specific organ systems in this volume.

SPECIMEN HANDLING

Most histochemical and immunohistochemical procedures for the demonstration of hormones and nonhormonal constituents of neuroendocrine cells can be performed in formalin-fixed and paraffin-embedded tissues. Other fixatives, including carbodiimide, acrolein, and diethyl pyrocarbonate, also have been used in place of formalin, and these fixatives have been reported to achieve optimal fixation of low concentrations of regulatory peptides such as those occurring in peptidergic nerve fibers (154–157).

The tissue preparative techniques for in situ hybridization studies are discussed in several review articles (142,148). In general, these methods may be performed on frozen samples that are postfixed in paraformaldehyde or in formalin-fixed samples that have been embedded in paraffin.

REFERENCES

1. Wiedenmann B, John M, Ahnert-Hilger G, Riecken EO. Molecular and cell biological aspects of neuroendocrine tumors of the gastroenteropancreatic system. *J Mol Med* 1998;76:637–647.
2. Heidenhain R. Untersuchangen uber den Bau der Labridusen. *Arch Mikrosk Anat Entwicklungsmech* 1870;6:368–406.
3. Masson P. La glande endocrine de l'intestin chez l'homme. *CR Acad Sci (Paris)* 1914;158: 59–61.
4. Hamperl H. Was sind argentaffine Zellen? *Virchows Arch A* 1932;286:811–833.
5. Feyrter F. *Uber Diffuse Endokrine Epithaliale Organe.* Leipzig, Germany: Barth; 1938.
6. Feyrter F. *Uber Die Peripheren Endokrinen (Parakrinen) Drusen Des Menschen.* Vienna: Verlag W. Maudrich; 1953.
7. Frölich F. Die "Helle Zelle" der bronchialschleimhaut und ihre beziehungen zum problem der chemoreceptoren. *Frankfurter Z Pathol* 1949;60:517–559.
8. Polak JM, Bloom SR. Peripheral localization of regulatory peptides as a clue to their function. *J Histochem Cytochem* 1980; 28:918–924.
9. Scharrer B. The neurosecretory neuron in neuroendocrine regulatory mechanisms. *Am Zool* 1967;7:161–169.
10. Snyder SH. Brain peptides as neurotransmitters. *Science* 1980; 209:976–983.
11. Copp DH, Cameron EC, Cheney BA, Davidson AG, Henze KG. Evidence for calcitonin–a new hormone from the parathyroid that lowers blood calcium. *Endocrinology* 1962;70:638–649.
12. Pearse AGE. The cytochemistry of the thyroid C cells and their relationship to calcitonin. *Proc R Soc Lond B Biol Sci* 1966; 164:478–487.
13. Pearse AG. The cytochemistry and ultrastructure of polypeptide hormone-producing cells of the APUD series and the embryologic, physiologic and pathologic implications of the concept. *J Histochem Cytochem* 1969;17:303–313.
14. Pearse AG. 5-hydroxytryptophan uptake by dog thyroid 'C' cells, and its possible significance in polypeptide hormone production. *Nature* 1966;211:598–600.
15. Pearse AG. Common cytochemical properties of cells producing polypeptide hormones, with particular reference to calcitonin and the thyroid C cells. *Vet Rec* 1966;79:587–590.
16. Bussolati G, Pearse AG. Immunofluorescent localization of calcitonin in the 'C' cells of pig and dog thyroid. *J Endocrinol* 1967;37:205–209.
17. Pearse AG. The diffuse neuroendocrine system and the APUD concept: related "endocrine" peptides in brain, intestine, pituitary, placenta, and anuran cutaneous glands. *Med Biol* 1977; 55:115–125.
18. Fujita T, Kobayashi S. Current reviews on the paraneuron concept. *Trends Neurosci* 1979;2:27–30.
19. Fujita T. Present status of paraneuron concept. *Arch Histol Cytol* 1989;52(suppl):1–8.
20. Le Douarin NM, Teillet MA. The migration of neural crest cells to the wall of the digestive tract in avian embryo. *J Embryol Exp Morphol* 1973;30:31–48.
21. Le Douarin NM. *The Neural Crest.* Cambridge, England: Cambridge University Press; 1982.
22. Holm R, Sobrinho-Simoes M, Nesland JM, Sambade C, Johannessen JV. Medullary thyroid carcinoma with thyroglobulin immunoreactivity. A special entity? *Lab Invest* 1987;57:258–268.
23. Vinik AI, Pittenger GL, Pavlic-Renar I. Role of growth factors in pancreatic endocrine cells. Growth and differentiation. *Endocrinol Metab Clin North Am* 1993;22:875–887.
24. DeLellis RA, Dayal Y, Tischler AS, Lee AK, Wolfe HJ. Multiple endocrine neoplasia (MEN) syndromes: cellular origins and interrelationships. *Int Rev Exp Pathol* 1986;28:163–215.
25. Tischler AS. The dispersed neuroendocrine cells: the structure, function, regulation and effects of xenobiotics on this system. *Toxicol Pathol* 1989;17:307–316.
26. Johnson JE, Birren SJ, Anderson DJ. Two rat homologues of Drosophila achaete-scute specifically expressed in neuronal precursors. *Nature* 1990;346:858–861.

27. Ball DW. Achaete-scute homolog-1 and Notch in lung neuroendocrine development and cancer. *Cancer Lett* 2004;204:159–169.

28. Ito T, Udaka N, Yazawa T, et al. Basic helix-loop-helix transcription factors regulate the neuroendocrine differentiation of fetal mouse pulmonary epithelium. *Development* 2000;127:3913–3921.

29. Lanigan TM, DeRaad SK, Russo AF. Requirement of the MASH-1 transcription factor for neuroendocrine differentiation of thyroid C cells. *J Neurobiol* 1998;34:126–134.

30. Falck B, Owman C. A detailed methodological description of the fluorescence method for cellular demonstration of biogenic monoamines. *Acta Univ Lund* 1965;7:5–23.

31. Grimelius L. A silver nitrate stain for A2 cells in human pancreatic islets. *Acta Soc Med Ups* 1968;73:243–270.

32. Grimelius L, Wilander E. Silver stains in the study of endocrine cells of the gut and pancreas. *Invest Cell Pathol* 1980;3:3–12.

33. Aguirre P, Scully RE, Wolfe HJ, DeLellis RA. Endometrial carcinoma with argyrophil cells: a histochemical and immunohistochemical analysis. *Hum Pathol* 1984;15:210–217.

34. Cecilia M, Rost M, Rost FW. An improved method for staining cells of the endocrine polypeptide (APUD) series by masked metachromasia: application of the principle of "fixation by excluded volume". *Histochem J* 1976;8:93–98.

35. Larsson LI, Goltermann N, de Magistris L, Rehfeld JF, Schwartz TW. Somatostatin cell processes as pathways for paracrine secretion. *Science* 1979;205:1393–1395.

36. Dockray GJ. Evolutionary relationships of the gut hormones. *Fed Proc* 1979;38:2295–2301.

37. Fujita T, Kobayashi S. The cells and hormones of the GEP endocrine system. In: Fujita T, ed. *Gastro-entero-pancreatic Endocrine System.* Tokyo: Igaku-Shoin; 1973:1–16.

38. Dayal Y. Endocrine cells of the gut and their neoplasms. In: Norris HT, ed. *Pathology of the Colon, Small Intestine and Anus.* New York: Churchill Livingstone; 1983:267–300.

39. Lechago J. The endocrine cells of the digestive and respiratory systems and their pathology. In: Bloodworth JMB Jr, ed. *Endocrine Pathology: General and Surgical.* 2nd ed. Baltimore: Williams & Wilkins; 1982:513–555.

40. Bosshard A, Chery-Croze S, Cuber JC, Dechelette MA, Berger F, Chayvialle JA. Immunocytochemical study of peptidergic structures in Brunner's glands. *Gastroenterology* 1989;97:1382–1388.

41. Cohen RJ, Glezerson G, Taylor LF, Grundle HA, Naude JH. The neuroendocrine cell population of the human prostate gland. *J Urol* 1993;150(pt 1):365–368.

42. Falkmer S. Phylogeny and ontogeny of the neuroendocrine cells of the gastrointestinal tract. *Endocrinol Metab Clin North Am* 1993;22:731–752.

43. Gould VE, DeLellis RA. The neuroendocrine cell system: its tumors, hyperplasias and dysplasias. In: Silverberg S, ed. *Principles and Practice of Surgical Pathology.* New York: Wiley; 1983:1487–1501.

44. Dremier S, Golstein J, Mosselmans R, Dumont JE, Galand T, Robaye B. Apoptosis in dog thyroid cells. *Biochem Biophys Res Commun* 1994;200:52–58.

45. Sasano H, Imatani A, Shizawa S, Suzuki T, Nagura H. Cell proliferation and apoptosis in normal and pathological human adrenal. *Mod Pathol* 1995;8:11–17.

46. Gavrieli Y, Sherman Y, Ben-Sasson SA. Identification of programmed cell death in situ via specific labeling of nuclear DNA fragmentation. *J Cell Biol* 1992;119:493–501.

47. Hiraishi K, Suzuki K, Hakomori S, Adachi M. Le(y) antigen expression is correlated with apoptosis (programmed cell death). *Glycobiology* 1993;3:381–390.

48. Sasano H. In situ end labeling and its applications to the study of endocrine disease: how can we study programmed cell death in surgical pathology materials? *Endocr Pathol* 1995;2:87–89.

49. Drewett N, Jacobi JM, Willgoss DA, Lloyd HM. Apoptosis in the anterior pituitary gland of the rat: studies with estrogen and bromocriptine. *Neuroendocrinology* 1993;57:89–95.

50. Garcia I, Martinou I, Tsujimoto Y, Martinou JC. Prevention of programmed cell death of sympathetic neurons by the bcl-2 proto-oncogene. *Science* 1992;258:302–304.

51. Kaneto H, Fujii J, Seo HG, et al. Apoptotic cell death triggered by nitric oxide in pancreatic beta-cells. *Diabetes* 1995;44:733–738.

52. Polak JM, Bloom SR. Immunocytochemistry of regulatory peptides. In: Polak JM, Van Noorden S, eds. *Immunocytochemistry: Practical Applications in Pathology and Biology.* Bristol, England: Wright PSG; 1983:184–211.

53. Verhofstad AAJ, Steinbusch HWM, Joosten HWJ, Penke B, Varga J, Goldstein M. Immunocytochemical localization of noradrenaline, adrenaline and serotonin. In: Polak JM, Van Noorden S, eds. *Immunocytochemistry: Practical Applications in Pathology and Biology.* Bristol, England: Wright PSG; 1983:143–168.

54. Lloyd RV. Immunohistochemical localization of catecholamines, catecholamine synthesizing enzymes and chromogranins in neuroendocrine cells and tumors. In: DeLellis RA, ed. *Advances in Immunohistochemistry.* New York: Raven Press; 1988:317–340.

55. Schmechel D, Marangos PJ, Brightman M. Neurone-specific enolase is a molecular marker for peripheral and central neuroendocrine cells. *Nature* 1978;276:834–836.

56. Lloyd RV, Warner TF. Immunohistochemistry of neuron specific enolase. In: DeLellis RA, ed. *Advances in Immunohistochemistry.* New York: Masson; 1984:127–140.

57. Haimoto H, Takahashi Y, Koshikawa T, Nagura H, Kato K. Immunohistochemical localization of gamma-enolase in normal human tissues other than nervous and neuroendocrine tissues. *Lab Invest* 1985;52:257–263.

58. Schmechel D. Gamma-subunit of the glycolytic enzyme enolase: nonspecific or neuron specific? *Lab Invest* 1985;52:239–242.

59. Seshi B, True L, Carter D, Rosai J. Immunohistochemical characterization of a set of monoclonal antibodies to human neuron-specific enolase. *Am J Pathol* 1988;131:258–269.

60. Thompson RJ, Doran JF, Jackson P, Dhillon AP, Rode J. PGP 9.5—a new marker for vertebrate neurons and neuroendocrine cells. *Brain Res* 1983;278:224–228.

61. Li GL, Farooque, M, Holtz A, Olsson Y. Expression of the ubiquitin carboxyl-terminal hydrolase PGP 9.5 in axons following spinal cord compression trauma. An immunohistochemical study in the rat. *APMIS* 1997;105:384–390.

62. Mendelsohn G. Histaminase localization in medullary thyroid carcinoma and small cell lung carcinoma. In: DeLellis RA, ed. *Diagnostic Immunohistochemistry.* New York: Masson; 1981:299–312.

63. Blaschko H, Comline RS, Schneider FH, Silver M, Smith AD. Secretion of a chromaffin granule protein, chromogranin, from the adrenal gland after splanchnic stimulation. *Nature* 1967;215:58–59.

64. Schober M, Fischer-Colbrie R, Schmid KW, Bussolati G, O'Connor DT, Winkler H. Comparison of chromogranins A, B, and secretogranin II in human adrenal medulla and pheochromocytoma. *Lab Invest* 1987;57:385–391.

65. Lloyd RV, Jin L, Kulig E, Fields K. Molecular approaches for the analysis of chromogranins and secretogranins. *Diagn Mol Pathol* 1992;1:2–15.

66. Portela-Gomes GM, Stridsberg M. Selective processing of chromogranin A in the different islet cells in human pancreas. *J Histochem Cytochem* 2001;49:483–490.

67. Portela-Gomes GM, Hacker GW, Weitgasser R. Neuroendocrine cell markers for pancreatic islets and tumors. *Appl Immunohistochem Mol Morphol* 2004;12:183–192.

68. Kimura N, Funakoshi A, Aunis D, Tateishi K, Miura W, Nagura H. Immunohistochemical localization of chromostatin and pancreastatin, chromogranin A-derived bioactive peptides, in normal and neoplastic neuroendocrine tissues. *Endocr Pathol* 1995;6:35–43.

69. Schmidt WE, Siegel EG, Lamberts E, Gallwitz B, Creutzfeldt W. Pancreastatin: molecular and immunocytochemical characterization of a novel peptide in porcine and human tissues. *Endocrinology* 1988;123:1395–1404.

70. Bishop AE, Sekiya K, Salahuddin MJ, et al. The distribution of GAWK-like immunoreactivity in neuroendocrine cells of the human gut, pancreas, adrenal and pituitary glands and its colocalization with chromogranin B. *Histochemistry* 1989;90:475–483.

71. Huttner WB, Gerdes HH, Rosa P. Chromogranins/secretogranins—widespread constituents of the secretory granule matrix in endocrine cells and neurons. In: Gratzl M, Langley K,

eds. *Markers for Neural and Endocrine Cells: Molecular and Cell Biology, Diagnostic Applications.* Weinheim, Germany: VCH; 1991:93–131.

72. Lloyd RV, Jin L, Qian X, Scheithauer BW, Young WF Jr, Davis DH. Analysis of the chromogranin A post-translational cleavage product pancreastatin and the prohormone convertases PC2 and PC3 in normal and neoplastic human pituitaries. *Am J Pathol* 1995;146:1188–1198.

73. Scopsi L, Gullo M, Rilke F, Martin S, Steiner DF. Proprotein convertases (PC1/PC3 and PC2) in normal and neoplastic tissues: their use as markers of neuroendocrine differentiation. *J Clin Endocrinol Metab* 1995;80:294–301.

74. Scopsi L, Lee R, Gullo M, Collini P, Husten EJ, Eipper BA. Peptidylglycine alpha-amidating monooxygenase in neuroendocrine tumors—its identification, characterization, quantification, and relation to the grade of morphological differentiation, amidated peptide content, and granin histochemistry. *Appl Immunohistochem* 1998;6:120–132.

75. Saldise L, Martinez A, Montuenga LM, et al. Distribution of peptidyl-glycine alpha-amidating monooxygenase (PAM) enzymes in normal human lung and in lung epithelial tumors. *J Histochem Cytochem* 1996;44:3–12.

76. Winkler H, Westhead E. The molecular organization of adrenal chromaffin granules. *Neuroscience* 1980;5:1803–1823.

77. Njus D, Knoth J, Cook C, Kelly PM. Electron transfer across the chromaffin granule membrane. *J Cell Biol* 1983;258:27–30.

78. Weidenmann B, Franke WW, Kuhn C, Moll R, Gould VE. Synaptophysin: a marker protein for neuroendocrine cells and neoplasms. *Proc Natl Acad Sci U S A* 1986;83:3500–3504.

79. Gould VE, Lee I, Wiedenmann B, Moll R, Chejfec G, Franke WW. Synaptophysin: a novel marker for neurons, certain neuroendocrine cells, and their neoplasms. *Hum Pathol* 1986;17:979–983.

80. Jahn R, De Camilli P. Membrane proteins of synaptic vesicles: markers for neurons and neuroendocrine cells: tools for the study of neurosecretion. In: Gratzl M, Langley K, eds. *Markers for Neural and Endocrine Cells: Molecular and Cell Biology. Diagnostic Applications.* Weinheim, Germany: VCH; 1991:25–92.

81. DeLellis RA. The neuroendocrine system and its tumors: an overview. *Am J Clin Pathol* 2001;115(suppl):S5–S16.

82. Lloyd RV. Practical markers used in the diagnosis of neuroendocrine tumors. *Endocr Pathol* 2003;14:293–301.

83. Portela-Gomes GM, Lukinius A, Grimelius L. Synaptic vesicle protein 2, a new neuroendocrine cell marker. *Am J Pathol* 2000;157:1299–1309.

84. Nilsson O, Jakobsen AM, Kolby L, Bernhardt P, Forssell-Aronsson E, Ahlman H. Importance of vesicle proteins in the diagnosis and treatment of neuroendocrine tumors. *Ann NY Acad Sci* 2004; 1014:280–283.

85. Jakobsen AM, Andersson P, Saglik G, et al. Differential expression of vesicular monoamine transporter (VMAT) 1 and 2 in gastrointestinal endocrine tumors. *J Pathol* 2001;195:463–472.

86. Rindi G, Paolotti D, Fiocca R, Wiedenmann B, Henry JP, Solcia E. Vesicular monoamine transporter 2 as a marker of gastric enterochromaffin-like cell tumors. *Virchows Arch* 2000;436:217–223.

87. Sollner T, Bennett MK, Whiteheart SW, Scheller RH, Rothman JE. A protein assembly-disassembly pathway in vitro that may correspond to sequential steps of synaptic vesicle docking, activation, and fusion. *Cell* 1993;75:409–418.

88. Elferink LA, Scheller RH. Synaptic vesicle proteins and regulated exocytosis. *J Cell Sci Suppl* 1993;17:75–79.

89. Nicholls JG, Martin AR, Wallace BG, Fuchs PA. *From Neuron to Brain.* 4th ed. Sunderland, MA: Sinauer Associates; 2001:258–265.

90. Regazzi R, Wollheim CB, Lang J, et al. VAMP-2 and cellubrevin are expressed in pancreatic beta-cells and are essential for Ca(2+)-but not for GTP gamma S-induced insulin secretion. *EMBO J* 1995;14:2723–2730.

91. Braun JE, Fritz BA, Wong SM, Lowe AW. Identification of a vesicle-associated membrane protein (VAMP)-like membrane protein in zymogen granules of the rat exocrine pancreas. *J Biol Chem* 1994;269:5328–5335.

92. Brown H, Meister B, Deeney J, et al. Synaptotagmin III isoform is compartmentalized in pancreatic beta-cells and has a functional role in exocytosis. *Diabetes* 2000;49:383–391.

93. Tahara S, Sanno N, Teramoto A, Osamura RY. Expression of Rab3, a Ras-related GTP-binding protein in human nontumorous pituitaries and pituitary adenomas. *Mod Pathol* 1999;12:627–634.

94. Majo G, Ferrer I, Marsal J, Blasi J, Aguado F. Immunocytochemical analysis of the synaptic proteins SNAP-25 and Rab3A in human pituitary adenomas. Overexpression of SNAP-25 in the mammosomatotroph lineages. *J Pathol* 1997;183:440–446.

95. Nishioka H, Haraoka J. Significance of immunohistochemical expression of Rab3B and SNAP-25 in growth hormone-producing pituitary adenomas. *Acta Neuropathol (Berl)* 2005; 109:598–602.

96. Roth D, Burgoyne D. SNAP-25 is present in a SNARE complex in adrenal chromaffin cells. *FEBS Lett* 1994;351:207–210.

97. Sadoul K, Lang J, Montecucco C, et al. SNAP-25 is expressed in islets of Langerhans and is involved in insulin release. *J Cell Biol* 1995;128:1019–1028.

98. Seeger RC, Danon YL, Rayner SA, Hoover F. Definition of Thy-1 determinant on human neuroblastoma, glioma, sarcoma, and teratoma cells with a monoclonal antibody. *J Immunol* 1982;128: 983–989.

99. Lipinski M, Braham K, Caillaud JM, Carlu C, Tursz T. HNK-1 antibody detects an antigen expressed on neuroectodermal cells. *J Exp Med* 1983;158:1775–1780.

100. Tischler AS, Mobtaker H, Mann K, et al. Anti-lymphocyte antibody Leu-7 (HNK-1) recognizes a constituent of neuroendocrine granule matrix. *J Histochem Cytochem* 1986;34:1213–1216.

101. Lloyd RV, Blaivas M, Wilson BS. Distribution of chromogranin and S100 protein in normal and abnormal adrenal medullary tissue. *Arch Pathol Lab Med* 1985;109:633–635.

102. Heitz PU, Roth J, Zuber C, Komminoth P. Markers for neural and endocrine cells in pathology. In: Gratzl M, Langley K, eds. *Markers for Neural and Endocrine Cells: Molecular and Cell Biology. Diagnostic Applications.* Weinheim, Germany: VCH; 1991:203–215.

103. Jin L, Hemperly JJ, Lloyd RV. Expression of neural cell adhesion molecule in normal and neoplastic human neuroendocrine tissues. *Am J Pathol* 1991;138:961–969.

104. Komminoth P, Roth J, Saremaslani P, Matias-Guiu X, Wolfe HJ, Heitz PU. Polysialic acid of the neural cell adhesion molecule in the human thyroid: a marker for medullary thyroid carcinoma and primary C-cell hyperplasia. An immunohistochemical study on 79 thyroid lesions. *Am J Surg Pathol* 1994;18:399–411.

105. LaRosa S, Rigoli E, Uccella S, Chiaravalli AM, Capella C. CDX2 as a marker of intestinal EC-cells and related well-differentiated endocrine tumors. *Virchows Arch* 2004;445:248–254.

106. Hosgor M, Ijzendoorn Y, Mooi WJ, Tibboel D, De Krijger RR. Thyroid transcription factor-1 expression during normal human lung development and in patients with congenital diaphragmatic hernia. *J Pediatr Surg* 2002;37:1258–1262.

107. Lloyd RV, Osamura RY. Transcription factors in normal and neoplastic pituitary tissues. *Microsc Res Tech* 1997;39:168–181.

108. Reubi JC. Somatostatin and other peptide receptors as tools for tumor diagnosis and treatment. *Neuroendocrinology* 2004; 80(suppl 1):51–56.

109. Gugger M, Waser B, Kappeler A, Schonbrunn A, Reubi JC. Immunohistochemical localization of somatostatin receptor sst2A in human gut and lung tissue: possible implications for physiology and carcinogenesis. *Ann N Y Acad Sci* 2004;1014: 132–136.

110. Roth J, Kasper M, Stamm B, et al. Localization of proinsulin and insulin in human insulinoma: preliminary immunohistochemical results. *Virchows Arch B Cell Pathol Incl Mol Pathol* 1989;56:287–292.

111. Hakanson R, Sundler F. The design of the neuroendocrine system: a unifying concept and its consequences. *Trends Pharmacol Sci* 1983;4:41–44.

112. Pearse AG, Polak JM, Bloom SR. The newer gut hormones. Cellular sources, physiology, pathology, and clinical aspects. *Gastroenterology* 1977;72(pt 1):746–761.

113. Reichlin S. Somatostatin. Part 1. *N Engl J Med* 1983;309: 1495–1501.

114. Reichlin S. Somatostatin. Part 2. *N Engl J Med* 1983;309: 1556–1563.

115. Kameda Y, Oyama H, Endoh M, Horino M. Somatostatin immunoreactive C cells in thyroid glands from various mammalian species. *Anat Rec* 1982;204:161–170.

116. Tsutsumi Y, Osamura Y, Watanabe K, Yanihara N. Immunohistochemical studies on gastrin-releasing peptide- and adrenocorticotropic hormone-containing cells in the human lung. *Lab Invest* 1983;48:623–632.

117. Sunday ME, Kaplan LM, Motoyama E, Chin WW, Spindel ER. Gastrin-releasing peptide (mammalian bombesin) gene expression in health and disease. *Lab Invest* 1988;59:5–24.

118. Kruger DT. Pituitary ACTH hyperfunction: pathophysiology and clinical aspects. In: Camanni F, Müller EE, eds. *Pituitary Hyperfunction: Physiopathology and Clinical Aspects.* New York: Raven Press; 1984:221–234.

119. Rosenfeld MG, Mermod JJ, Amara SJ, et al. Production of a novel neuropeptide encoded by the calcitonin gene via tissue-specific RNA processing. *Nature* 1983;304:129–135.

120. Warren TG, Shields D. Cell-free biosynthesis of somatostatin precursors: evidence for multiple forms of preprosomatostatin. *Proc Natl Acad Sci U S A* 1982;79:3729–3733.

121. Gould VE, Linnoila RI, Memoli VA, Warren WH. Neuroendocrine components of the bronchopulmonary tract: hyperplasias, dysplasias, and neoplasms. *Lab Invest* 1983;49:519–537.

122. Bensch KG, Gordon GB, Miller LR. Studies on the bronchial counterpart of the Kultschitzky (argentaffin) cells and innervation of the bronchial glands. *J Ultrastruct Res* 1965;12:668–686.

123. Lauweryns JM, Peuskens JC. Neuro-epithelial bodies (neuroreceptor or secretory organs?) in human infant bronchial and bronchiolar epithelium. *Anat Rec* 1972;172:471–481.

124. Pesce C, Tobia-Gallelli F, Toncini C. APUD cells of the larynx. *Acta Otolaryngol* 1984;98:158–162.

125. Torre-Rendon FE, Cisneros-Bernal E, Ochoa-Salas JA. Carcinoma indiferenciado de células pequeñas de la laringe. *Patologica* 1979;17:47–57.

126. DeLellis RA, Wolfe HJ. The pathobiology of the human calcitonin (C)-cell: a review. *Pathol Annu* 1981;16:25–52.

127. DeLellis RA, Nunnemacher G, Wolfe HJ. C-cell hyperplasia. An ultrastructural analysis. *Lab Invest* 1977;36:237–248.

128. DeLellis RA, May L, Tashjian AH Jr, Wolfe HJ. C-cell granule heterogeneity in man. An ultrastructural immunocytochemical study. *Lab Invest* 1978;38:263–269.

129. Bearman RM, Levine GD, Bensch KG. The ultrastructure of the normal human thymus: a study of 36 cases. *Anat Rec* 1978;190:755–781.

130. Gould VE, Moll R, Moll I, Lee I, Franke WW. Neuroendocrine (Merkel) cells of the skin: hyperplasias, dysplasias, and neoplasms. *Lab Invest* 1985;52:334–353.

131. Bussolati G, Gugliotta P, Sapino A, Eusebi V, Lloyd RV. Chromogranin-reactive endocrine cells in argyrophilic carcinomas ("carcinoids") and normal tissue of the breast. *Am J Pathol* 1985;120:186–192.

132. Fetissof F, Dubois MP, Arbeille-Brassart B, Lanson Y, Boivin F, Jobard P. Endocrine cells in the prostate gland, urothelium and Brenner tumors. Immunohistological and ultrastructural studies. *Virchows Arch B Cell Pathol Incl Mol Pathol* 1983;42:53–64.

133. di Sant'Agnese PA, de Mesy Jensen KL. Endocrine–paracrine cells of the prostate and prostatic urethra: an ultrastructural study. *Hum Pathol* 1984;15:1034–1041.

134. di Sant'Agnese PA, de Mesy Jensen KL. Somatostatin and/or somatostatin-like immunoreactive endocrine–paracrine cells in the human prostate gland. *Arch Pathol Lab Med* 1984;108:693–696.

135. di Sant'Agnese PA. Calcitoninlike immunoreactive and bombesinlike immunoreactive endocrine–paracrine cells of the human prostate. *Arch Pathol Lab Med* 1986;110:412–415.

136. Scully RE, Aguirre P, DeLellis RA. Argyrophilia, serotonin, and peptide hormones in the female genital tract and its tumors. *Int J Gynecol Pathol* 1984;3:51–70.

137. Sun YK, Xi YP, Fenoglio CM, et al. The effect of age on the number of pituitary cells immunoreactive to growth hormone and prolactin. *Hum Pathol* 1984;15:169–180.

138. Zegarelli-Schmidt E, Yu XR, Fenoglio-Preiser CM, et al. Endocrine changes associated with the human aging process. II. Effect of age on the number and size of thyrotropin immunoreactive cells in the human pituitary. *Hum Pathol* 1985;16:277–286.

139. O'Toole K, Fenoglio-Preiser C, Pushparaj N. Endocrine changes associated with the human aging process. III. Effect of age on the number of calcitonin immunoreactive cells in the thyroid gland. *Hum Pathol* 1985;16:991–1000.

140. Gibson WC, Peng TC, Croker BP. C-cell nodules in adult human thyroid. A common autopsy finding. *Am J Clin Pathol* 1981;75:347–350.

141. Gosney JR. Neuroendocrine cell populations in postnatal human lungs: minimal variation from childhood to old age. *Anat Rec* 1993;236:177–180.

142. DeLellis RA, Wolfe HJ. Analysis of gene expression in endocrine cells. In: Fenoglio-Preiser CM, Wilman CL, eds. *Molecular Diagnostics in Pathology.* Baltimore: Williams & Wilkins; 1991:299–322.

143. Lloyd RV. Introduction to molecular endocrine pathology. *Endocr Pathol* 1993;4:64–72.

144. Speel EJ, Ramaekers FC, Hopman AH. Cytochemical detection systems for in situ hybridization, and the combination with immunocytochemistry, "who is still afraid of red, green and blue?" *Histochem J* 1995;27:833–858.

145. Komminoth P, Long AA. In-situ polymerase chain reaction. An overview of methods, applications and limitations of a new molecular technique. *Virchows Arch B Cell Pathol Incl Mol Pathol* 1993;64:67–73.

146. Komminoth P, Long AA. In situ polymerase chain reaction and its applications to the study of endocrine diseases. *Endocr Pathol* 1995;6:167–171.

147. Sällström JF, Alemi M, Spets H, Zehbe I. Nonspecific amplification in in-situ PCR by direct incorporation of reporter molecules. *Cell Vision* 1994;1:243–251.

148. Nuovo GJ. *PCR In Situ Hybridization: Protocols and Applications.* New York: Raven Press; 1992.

149. Taylor CR. Principles of immunomicroscopy. In: Taylor CR and Cote RJ, eds. *Immunomicroscopy: A Diagnostic Tool for the Surgical Pathologist.* 3rd ed. Philadelphia: Saunders Elsevier; 2006:1–45.

150. Grube D. Immunoreactivities of gastric (G-) cells. II. Non-specific binding of immunoglobulins to G-cells by ionic interactions. *Histochemistry* 1980;66:149–167.

151. Bussolati G, Gugliotta P, Volante M, Pace M, Papotti M. Retrieved endogenous biotin: a novel marker and a potential pitfall in diagnostic immunohistochemistry. *Histopathology* 1997;31:400–407.

152. Srivastava A, Tischler AS, DeLellis RA. Endogenous biotin staining as an artifact of antigen retrieval with automated immunostaining. *Endocr Pathol* 2004;15:175–178.

153. Pagani A, Cerrato M, Bussolati G. Nonspecific in situ hybridization reaction in neuroendocrine cells and tumors of the gastrointestinal tract using oligonucleotide probes. *Diagn Mol Pathol* 1993;2:125–130.

154. Kendall PA, Polak JM, Pearse AG. Carbodiimide fixation for immunohistochemistry: observations on the fixation of polypeptide hormones. *Experientia* 1971;27:1104–1106.

155. King JC, Lechan RM, Kugel G, Anthony EL. Acrolein: a fixative for immunocytochemical localization of peptides in the central nervous system. *J Histochem Cytochem* 1983;31:62–68.

156. Pearse AG, Polak JM, Adams C, Kendall PA. Diethylpyrocarbonate, a vapour-phase fixative for immunofluorescence studies on polypeptide hormones. *Histochem J* 1974;6:347–352.

157. Pearse AG, Polak JM. Bifunctional reagents as vapour- and liquid-phase fixatives for immunohistochemistry. *Histochem J* 1975;7:179–186.

Paraganglia

48

Arthur S. Tischler

INTRODUCTION

Paraganglia are anatomically dispersed neuroendocrine organs associated with the autonomic nervous system and characterized by morphologically and cytochemically similar neurosecretory cells derived from the neural crest. For many physiological and pathophysiological purposes, they may be considered to comprise two groups associated with either sympathetic or parasympathetic nerves. Sympathetic paraganglia are distributed along the prevertebral and paravertebral sympathetic chains and along sympathetic nerve branches that innervate the organs of the pelvis and retroperitoneum. The adrenal medulla is the most extensively studied and best understood example of the sympathetic paraganglia. Parasympathetic paraganglia are predominantly distributed along cervical and thoracic branches of the glossopharyngeal and vagus nerves. The prototypical parasympathetic paraganglion is the carotid body.

HISTORY AND NOMENCLATURE

The history of the paraganglia is among the more interesting and controversial in the recent annals of medicine. This material is addressed in detail in several excellent reviews (1–4). The concept of a unitary paraganglionic system was first proposed by Alfred Kohn at the beginning of the 20th century (5). Several earlier investigators had developed histochemical reactions demonstrating that the adrenal medulla contained substances chemically different from those in the adrenal cortex. The reaction that proved most significant from a historical perspective, development of brown coloration in the presence of chromate salts, was apparently first discovered by Bertholdus Werner in 1857 (3). Kohn coined the terms "chromaffin reaction" for the color change and "chromaffin cells" for the reactive cells, which he described in several extra-adrenal locations in the retroperitoneum. He further noted that some cells in the carotid body exhibited a chromaffin reaction, confirming an earlier report by Stilling (3). Kohn believed that the reactive carotid body cells were derived from precursors of sympathetic ganglia and were innervated by sympathetic axons, and he suggested that they were therefore embryologically, histochemically, and functionally comparable to retroperitoneal chromaffin cells. He proposed a new term to encompass all the tissues composed of cells that were analogous to neurons, but not neuronal: "Since the chromaffin tissue complexes form ganglion-like bodies, since their elements are derived from ganglion anlagen, since they are connected to the sympathetic nervous system and still are not genuine ganglia, I have called them paraganglia" (5); translated from German by Dr. Miguel Stadecker).

Obstacles to acceptance of Kohn's concept soon arose from DeCastro's finding that the innervation of the carotid body is primarily derived from the glossopharyngeal nerve (4), and from observations by many investigators that carotid body cells are usually nonchromaffin. Consequently, Watzka (4) divided the paraganglion system into chromaffin and nonchromaffin paraganglia, associated respectively with the sympathetic or parasympathetic nervous systems, and paraganglia of mixed type. Discovery of the chemoreceptor function of the carotid bodies created further difficulties since it implied that the nonchromaffin paraganglia served physiologically in a sensory role, in contrast to the endocrine function of the adrenal medulla. The suggestion was therefore made by Kjaergaard that the parasympathetic paraganglia be referred to by the term "chemodecton" (from the Greek *dechesthai*, to receive). This name was never widely accepted, despite the earlier application by Mulligan of its counterpart, "chemodectoma," to paraganglionic tumors (4).

An additional synonym for the parasympathetic paraganglia is "glomus" (from the Latin *glomus*, ball). This term is a vestige of a 19th-century hypothesis that the carotid body is of vascular origin (4). Although it aptly describes the microscopic *Zellballen* characteristic of paraganglia, it has caused confusion because it is also applied to thermoregulatory structures in the skin and other locations (e.g., glomera cutanea and the glomus coccygeum) and to their corresponding tumors (glomus tumors or glomangiomas). Those structures are modified arteriovenous anastomoses unrelated to paraganglia developmentally or functionally.

It is now possible to return to a unitary concept of paraganglia with a synthesis of new and old data. Paraganglionic neuroendocrine cells are probably all derived from the neural crest (6,7). All produce catecholamines or, in some cases, indolamines (6,8) detectable by more sensitive methods than the chromaffin reaction, and all express multiple additional neuroendocrine markers (9). Recently, chemosensory properties previously considered specific to parasympathetic paraganglia have been documented in cells derived from sympathetic paraganglia as well (10). It is now apparent that the same basic type of neuroendocrine cell may be used differently in different anatomic locations (9,11,12). The term "paraganglion" connotes a constellation of generic characteristics of this type of cell without being dependent on a single histochemical reaction. Since paraganglion was intended by Kohn to imply analogy, rather than merely proximity, to autonomic ganglia, it continues in this context to be both conceptually helpful and literally correct. The chromaffin reaction as a basis for classification of paraganglia is now obsolete. However, reference to the reaction persists for historical reasons. "Chromaffin cell" is the name generally accepted for the neuroendocrine cells of the normal adrenal medulla and sometimes still applied to their extra-adrenal counterparts associated with the sympathetic nervous system. Similarly, "pheochromocytoma" (from the Greek *phaios*, dusky, + *chroma*, color), the name applied by convention to chromaffin cell tumors, refers to the color change imparted by the chromaffin reaction.

SYMPATHETIC VERSUS PARASYMPATHETIC PARAGANGLIA: A CLINICOPATHOLOGIC PERSPECTIVE

Sympathetic and parasympathetic paraganglia differ from a clinicopathologic standpoint despite their similarities at the cellular level. This contrast might result from differences in the type, timing, or intensity of physiological signals to which the two classes of paraganglia are exposed during development or in adult life. The only pathologic changes known to be clinically important in paraganglia are hyperplasia and neoplasia. Several generalizations concerning these proliferative lesions underscore the differences between paraganglia of the sympathetic and parasympathetic classes: when multiple lesions occur within families or individuals, they are usually confined to one or the other class. Although both sympathetic and parasympathetic lesions produce catecholamines, clinical signs of excess catecholamine secretion are usually associated with lesions that are sympathetic, and lesions that produce significant amounts of epinephrine are almost invariably sympathetic. Lesions that occur in patients with prolonged hypoxemia or hypercapnia are almost invariably parasympathetic. In addition, sympathetic paraganglia give rise to tumors of both neuronal lineage (i.e., neuroblastomas, ganglioneuroblastomas, and ganglioneuromas) and neuroendocrine lineage (pheochromocytomas and extra-adrenal paragangliomas), while neoplasms of parasympathetic paraganglia are almost always of neuroendocrine lineage. Neuronal tumors are most common in children, while neuroendocrine tumors usually occur in adults.

Despite the differences in the contexts in which they arise, sympathetic and parasympathetic paragangliomas strongly resemble each other microscopically and are often indistinguishable. They also exhibit a widely overlapping range of secretory products and other neuroendocrine markers, reflecting the similarities of the neuroendocrine cells that are their normal counterparts. A morphologic foundation for the study of paraganglionic pathology therefore requires familiarity with both systemic differences and cellular similarities.

A need for deeper understanding of the differences and similarities between paraganglia in different locations has become apparent as a result of recent advances in characterizing the genetic abnormalities and gene expression profiles of pheochromocytomas and extra-adrenal paragangliomas. Hereditary syndromes now known to be associated with development of pheochromocytomas are Multiple Endocrine Neoplasia (MEN) 2A and 2B, von Hippel-Lindau disease, neurofibromatosis type 1 and familial paraganglioma/pheochromocytoma syndromes, due respectively to mutations of the *RET* protooncogene, *VHL* and *NF1* tumor suppressor genes, and *SDHD*, *SDHB*, and *SDHC* succinate dehydrogenase genes (13,14). Extra-adrenal paragangliomas are rare in MEN2 and neurofibromatosis, and those that occasionally do occur often arise in the vicinity of the adrenal. In contrast, VHL tumors, while predominantly intra-adrenal, are not uncommon in extra-adrenal locations and tumors associated with succinate dehydrogenase mutations are predominantly extra-adrenal (13). The combination of sympathetic and parasympathetic paragangliomas may be particularly suggestive of succinate dehydrogenase mutations (13). Microarray-based gene expression profiling studies complemented by immunohistochemical and/or biochemical analyses have revealed sets of markers that tend to be clustered in tumors with specific genetic backgrounds. For example, genes associated with hypoxia-driven transcription pathways are preferentially expressed in VHL tumors (15). An additional distinctive characteristic of VHL tumors is that they usually produce exclusively norepinephrine, while MEN2 and NF1 tumors produce both epinephrine and norepinephrine (16). Some genotype–phenotype correlations may be accounted for by characteristics of the predominant anatomic sites of tumor origin; for example, the fact that epinephrine production is normally confined to the adrenal medulla. However, the basis for different gene expression clusters in tumors at any given location is for the most part poorly understood. One possibility is that subtle types of cellular heterogeneity within normal paraganglia might allow for different cells of origin predisposed to respond to distinct genetic abnormalities. Alternatively, distinct genetic abnormalities initiating tumors in a single cell type could produce distinct signatures.

DISTRIBUTION OF PARAGANGLIA

Sympathetic paraganglia are found predominantly in the para-axial regions of the trunk along the prevertebral and paravertebral sympathetic chains and in connective tissue in or near the walls of the pelvic organs. In adult humans, they are especially numerous along the fibers of the inferior hypogastric plexuses leading to and entering the urogenital organs, in the wall of the urinary bladder, and among the nerve fibers of the sacral plexus (17–20) (Figure 48.1). They are not generally known by individual names, and their precise locations are variable. Exceptions are the adrenal medulla and the organ of Zuckerkandl, located at the origin of the inferior mesenteric artery (21) (Figures 48.1 and 48.2).

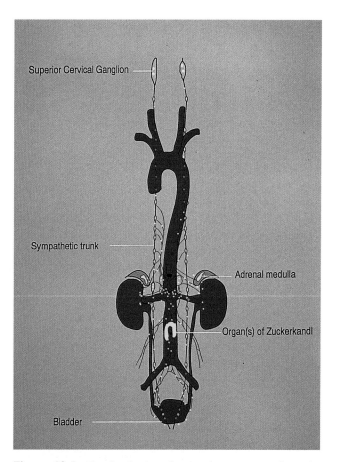

Figure 48.1 The distribution of sympathetic paraganglia in the human fetus. (Adapted with permission from: Coupland RE. *The Natural History of the Chromaffin Cell.* London: Longmans Green; 1965; Glenner GG, Grimley PM. Tumors of the extraadrenal paraganglion system (including chemoreceptors). In: Atlas of Tumor Pathology. 2nd series, fascicle 9. Washington, DC: Armed Forces Institute of Pathology; 1974.)

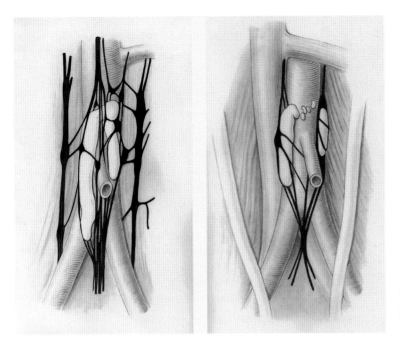

Figure 48.2 Modified renditions of original illustrations by Zuckerkandl (21) representing the anatomic structure that bears his name. The bilobed configuration with a fragmented isthmus (*right*) is the most frequent variation. (Courtesy of Dr. E. E. Lack.)

The distinctive characteristic of the organ of Zuckerkandl is that it is the only extra-adrenal sympathetic paraganglion that is macroscopic. Historically, it is said to have been shown initially to Alfred Kohn as an unusual lymph node by his pupil, Emil Zuckerkandl (4,22). In its most frequent anatomic configuration, it is divided into a set of paired organs (Figure 48.2), and it is therefore often referred to by the plural, "organs of Zuckerkandl" (1). Because its fragmentation and its proximity to numerous smaller paraganglia may make it difficult to identify precisely, some investigators have used the plural to encompass all preaortic paraganglia between the inferior mesenteric artery and the aortic bifurcation (23). However, this chapter maintains the traditional, more specific, macroscopic usage.

Neuroendocrine cells are present both within and adjacent to the ganglia of human sympathetic chains. The former have been referred to in neurobiology literature as small intensely fluorescent (SIF) cells (24), intraganglionic chromaffin cells (25), or small granule-containing (SGC) cells (11,12), depending on the particular technique used to detect them. In pathology literature especially, SIF cells are often regarded as intraganglionic paraganglia (26). In anatomy literature, on the other hand, some investigators reserve the term "paraganglia" for extraganglionic sites (24).

In contrast to sympathetic paraganglia, their parasympathetic counterparts are distributed almost exclusively along the cranial and thoracic branches of the glossopharyngeal and vagus nerves (Figure 48.3). With the exception of the carotid bodies, which are located between the carotid arteries just above the carotid bifurcation (Figure 48.4), parasympathetic paraganglia are highly variable in both number and location (4). Their names refer to general locations, rather than to specific structures. The middle ear, for example, contains 0 to 12 jugular and tympanic paraganglia, with an average of 2.8 (27). The principal paraganglia of the glossopharyngeal nerve are the tympanic paraganglia in the wall of the middle ear and the carotid bodies (4,27). Those of the vagus nerve include the jugular paraganglia in the floor of the middle ear (4,27), the superior and inferior laryngeal paraganglia (4,27,28), and the subclavian and aorticopulmonary or cardioaortic paraganglia near the bases of the great vessels of the heart. They sometimes also may be found in the interatrial septum (4). In addition, "intravagal" paraganglia are located within or adjacent to the vagal trunk in or near the nodose and jugular ganglia (4). These two vagal ganglia are thus the only sensory ganglia known to contain neuroendocrine cells comparable to the SIF cells of sympathetic ganglia. These cells have been described as SIF cells in some publications (29).

Some investigators have classified the parasympathetic paraganglia as "branchiomeric" (26). This nomenclature is based on the suggestion that the branchial arches during embryogenesis are metameric, or serially homologous, structures, each with its own artery, cranial nerve branches, and associated paraganglia. The carotid body would accordingly develop in association with the glossopharyngeal nerve and the third branchial arch artery, which persists as the internal carotid. Subclavian paraganglia would develop with the vagus nerve and the fourth branchial arch artery, and so on. The evolution of this concept is reviewed elsewhere in detail (4). However, the concept does not contribute to the understanding the pathophysiology of paraganglia and may cause confusion by distracting attention from the important differences between parasympathetic

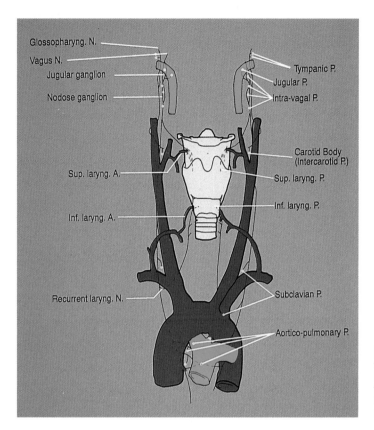

Figure 48.3 The distribution of the principal parasympathetic paraganglia. (Adapted with permission from: Glenner GG, Grimley PM. Tumors of the extraadrenal paraganglion system (including chemoreceptors). In: Atlas of Tumor Pathology. 2nd series, fascicle 9. Washington, DC: Armed Forces Institute of Pathology; 1974.)

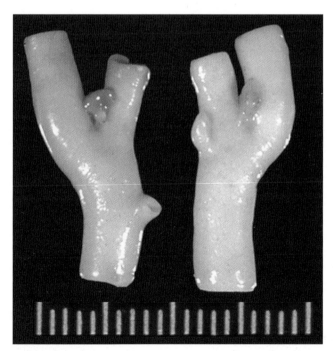

Figure 48.4 Gross specimens from a 5-year-old girl, illustrating normal carotid bodies and their relationship to the carotid arteries. (Courtesy of Dr. E. E. Lack.)

and sympathetic paraganglia, which may occur in close proximity to each other (e.g., the carotid bodies and the SIF cells in cervical sympathetic ganglia). It also is plagued by a number of internal inconsistencies, such as its prediction that the temporal paraganglia should be innervated by the facial nerve (4).

Knowledge of the distribution of normal paraganglionic tissue is important because of its value in predicting the sites of origin of paragangliomas. These tumors have been reported at virtually all locations where normal paraganglia are found during fetal or adult life and tend to be most frequent in areas where paraganglionic tissue is most abundant. For example, in early childhood a high percentage of paraganglionic tissue is extra-adrenal (see "Embryologic Changes" and "Postnatal and Developmental Changes"). Approximately half of all sympathetic paragangliomas in children are also extra-adrenal, most frequently arising in the vicinity of the organ of Zuckerkandl, while only about 10% are extra-adrenal in adults (30). However, it is also important to note that paraganglia may occur in locations outside the well-established sympathetic and parasympathetic distributions, perhaps explaining the existence of paragangliomas in unusual locations. Although intravagal paraganglia in humans have been identified only in the cervical and thoracic portions of the vagus nerve (31), in

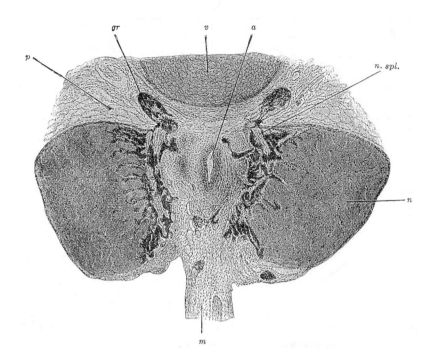

Figure 48.5 Original illustration by Zuckerkandl of a transverse section of a human embryo (17 mm crown–heel length) showing presumed migration of primitive sympathetic cells into the adrenal glands. The darkly stippled masses traversed by nerves are the primitive sympathetic cells. a, aorta; gr, developing sympathetic ganglia; n. spl, splanchnic nerve; v, vertebra; p, peritoneal cushion; m, mesentery; n, adrenals. (Reprinted with permission from: Zuckerkandl E. The development of the chromaffin organs and of the suprarenal glands. In: Keibel F, Mall FP, eds. *Manual of Human Embryology.* Philadelphia: JB Lippincott; 1912.)

rodents they are also present within the abdominal portions (32). It has not been ruled out that some abdominal paraganglia in humans, for example, in the gallbladder (33) (Figure 48.13), may be associated with small abdominal vagus nerve branches. In scattered reports, paraganglia have been described in various sites including the orbit, mandible, and extremities. The validity of some of these reports is questionable (4).

EMBRYOLOGIC CHANGES

During embryogenesis, the paraganglia are first populated by small, primitive cells similar to those in the anlage of the sympathetic ganglia. These cells include precursors of neuroendocrine, neural, and glial cell lineages in adult paraganglia (34,35) (see "Light Microscopy"). They appear to be able to produce some catecholamines at the earliest stages of paraganglionic development (35,36) (see "Function"), and express cytoskeletal or other markers of immature neurons (35), or glia (35) (see "Special Procedures"). They are readily recognized in the paraganglia at about 7 weeks' gestation, although they first arrive somewhat earlier (1), and they are progressively superseded by larger, differentiated, cells. Extra-adrenal sympathetic (1) and parasympathetic (36,37) paraganglia mature cytologically earlier than the adrenal medulla. Primitive cells usually disappear from these locations by week 25 but may persist in small numbers in the adrenal medulla until after birth (1).

Classic, descriptive, embryologic studies (38,39) show primitive sympathetic cells in large numbers around the spinal nerves and branches of the developing sympathetic trunks before the formation of the paraganglia. The cells are also described along the renal and spermatic arteries (39). The adrenal medulla is apparently colonized by invasion of primitive sympathetic cells into the cortex through the medial aspect of the capsule from the contiguous prevertebral and paravertebral sympathetic tissue (Figure 48.5). The invading cells initially form nodular aggregates in the cortex (Figure 48.6) and gradually coalesce around the central vein. They may form rosettes or pseudorosettes early

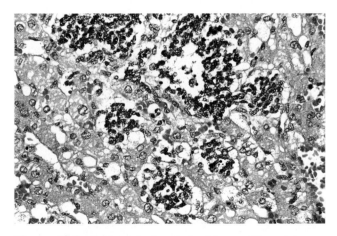

Figure 48.6 Section of adrenal gland from a 16-week human fetus showing typical aggregates of primitive sympathetic cells that are precursors of the medulla. Pyknotic nuclei and nuclei with changes consistent with apoptosis are present within the aggregates. Many of the small cells express immunoreactive tyrosine hydroxylase, the rate-limiting enzyme in catecholamine synthesis, but do not stain for CgA or synaptophysin, which are characteristic of larger, mature, or maturing chromaffin cells (35). Scattered S-100–positive cells consistent with the sustentacular cell lineage are observed at about week 20 (34).

in gestation (1,40). Chromaffin cells are identifiable among these aggregates from about week 8 on (1,40) and gradually increase in number. The centripetal pattern of migration of primitive sympathetic cells into the adrenal may result in subcapsular and intracortical chromaffin cell rests (see Figure 48.25). Although some primitive sympathetic cells appear to penetrate the cortex along sympathetic nerve fibers, some are apparently not associated with nerve fibers (1). Innervation of the presumptive medulla by preganglionic nerve fibers does not appear to be necessary for colonization because experimental studies demonstrate that the medulla can form in adrenal primordia from 4- or 5-day chick embryos explanted to chorioallantoic membranes before the onset of innervation (41).

Nodular aggregates of primitive sympathetic cells, up to 400 μm in greatest dimension, can be demonstrated in the adrenal glands of all human fetuses between the ages of 10 and 30 weeks if the glands are thoroughly sectioned (42). Aggregates with a diameter of over 1 mm may occasionally be observed (40). Nerve fibers may connect intra-adrenal and extra-adrenal aggregates (42). The nodules peak in size and number between the ages of 17 and 20 weeks and then decline. Intranodular cystic degeneration is common from the age of 20 weeks onward (42). Postnatal persistence of the nodules was apparently first described by Wiesel in 1902 (38). These occasional persistent nodules may account for some erroneous diagnoses of "in situ neuroblastoma" (42,43) (see "Differential Diagnosis").

Primitive cells can be observed apparently migrating to developing parasympathetic paraganglia along branches of the glossopharyngeal and vagus nerves as well as from sympathetic nerves (37). The nature, origin, and fate of these cells from different sources and their respective contributions to the mature paraganglia were vigorously debated for more than 70 years (4,37). It is of interest that both the purely morphologic studies of Kohn et al. (38) and later histochemical studies (36) suggest an origin of the neurosecretory cells of the human carotid body, the prototypical parasympathetic paraganglion, from the sympathetic progenitors of the superior cervical ganglion.

POSTNATAL AND DEVELOPMENTAL CHANGES

The amount or distribution of paraganglionic tissue is known to change during development and aging. Sympathetic paraganglionic tissue in fetuses and neonates is primarily extra-adrenal, with the greatest volume in the organ of Zuckerkandl. The organ of Zuckerkandl develops maximally in humans by the age of about 3 years, when its greatest dimension may be more than 20 mm. Thereafter, the organ involutes (1,20), while the adrenal medulla enlarges until maturity. Similarly, SIF cells are present in all human sympathetic ganglia at birth but are rare in adults

(1). Parasympathetic paraganglionic tissue also appears to decrease in some locations and to increase in others. Subclavian and intrapulmonary paraganglia, for example, have been identified in human fetuses but not in adults (4). On the other hand, the number of jugular and tympanic paraganglia apparently increases after birth (27). The carotid bodies, which are the only parasympathetic paraganglia that are macroscopic, increase in size between infancy and adult life, when they are normally about 3 mm in greatest dimension (4) (Figure 48.4).

The mechanisms involved in developmental remodeling of the paraganglionic system may hold a number of clues to the pathobiology of paraganglionic tumors. It is generally accepted that apoptosis plays a critical role in the development of both the central and peripheral nervous systems, where excess neural progenitor cells undergo apoptotic death after failing to establish functional contacts or receive appropriate tropic substances from target tissues (44,45). There have been few studies of apoptosis that are specifically focused on the paraganglia. However, apoptotic bodies can be identified within the aggregates of primitive sympathetic cells in the adrenal medulla (Figures 48.6 and 48.7).

PHENOTYPIC PLASTICITY

Adult human adrenal chromaffin cells are able to "transdifferentiate" into sympathetic neurons when removed from their in vivo environment and exposed to appropriate neurotrophic signals (46) (Figure 48.8). Capacity to undergo this fascinating metamorphosis is retained to varying degrees by developing or adult chromaffin cells from other species (47). The extent to which it is expressed in various extra-adrenal paraganglia has not been fully explored.

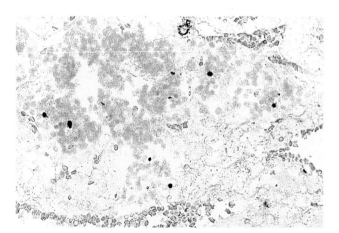

Figure 48.7 Section of the same adrenal as in Figure 48.6 showing terminal deoxynucleotidyl transferase–mediated end-labeling (48) of nuclei within a neuroblastic aggregate (black nuclei). This method, which detects fragmented DNA, can be helpful in locating apoptotic cells. (Courtesy of Dr. Salvador Diaz-Cano.)

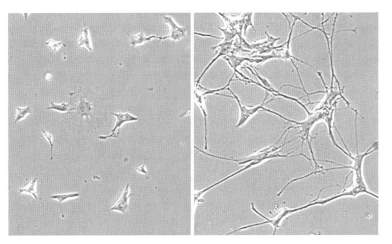

Figure 48.8 Phenotypic plasticity of normal adult human adrenal chromaffin cells demonstrated by acquisition of neuron-like morphology in cell culture. Cells at left were maintained in control medium for 2 weeks and those at right were in medium supplemented with nerve growth factor (46). (Courtesy of Dr. James F. Powers.) Capacity to undergo this "trans-differentiation" is exhibited to varying degrees by chromaffin cells from other species and from other normal or neoplastic paraganglia (47).

GROSS FEATURES AND ORGAN WEIGHTS

The paraganglionic tissue of the grossly identifiable paraganglia is gray or gray–pink. Recognition of this feature is particularly important in the adrenal gland because the medulla is normally confined to the head and body of the gland but extends into the tail and alae in adrenal medullary hyperplasia (49,50). An accurate gross examination requires that the brown tissue of the cortical zona reticularis not be misidentified as medulla.

Because of the anatomic variability of the microscopic paraganglia and the organ Zuckerkandl, meaningful weights can be ascribed only to the adrenal medulla and carotid bodies. Extensive morphometric studies (51) have shown that the neonatal adrenal medulla accounts for approximately 0.4% of the total volume of the gland and weighs approximately 0.012 g. These values increase to 4.2% and 0.08 g at 2 years of age, 7.0% and 0.28 g between the ages of 10 and 13 years, and 9.9% and 0.46 g in adults up to the age of 40 years. After the age of 40 years, there is a small decline in medullary weight and volume. The weight of the carotid bodies appears to correlate more closely with body weight than with age. Lack (52) has proposed an equation to estimate carotid body weight from body weight for any age group: combined weight of carotid bodies (mg) = 0.29 × body weight (kg) + 3.0. Standard deviations for any age group are large (53), but in normal adults the combined weight is usually less than 30 mg. The carotid body increases in size and weight in individuals living at high altitudes (54) and in patients with hypoxemia due to a variety of ailments (55–58).

ANATOMY

All paraganglia are highly vascular, a characteristic that permits them to be localized by leakage of systemically injected dye in animal studies (59). However, the details of their blood supply are highly varied according to their location and function. For example, the adrenal medulla receives arterial blood from three arteries—the inferior phrenic artery, aorta, and renal arteries—and drains via a single adrenal vein that empties into the renal vein on the left and the aorta on the right. The carotid body receives arterial blood from one or occasionally two small arteries arising from the vicinity of the carotid bifurcation and drains via several small veins into the pharyngeal, superior laryngeal, and lingual veins (4).

The innervation of paraganglia is comparably site specific. In general, sympathetic paraganglia receive preganglionic cholinergic sympathetic innervation and variable amounts of noradrenergic and/or peptidergic innervation from intrinsic neurons, nearby sympathetic ganglia, and other sources. Most of the neuroendocrine cells in the adrenal medulla are innervated (60), in contrast to the sparse innervation of extra-adrenal sympathetic paraganglia (1,61), and it has been suggested that the ability of paraganglia to attract or maintain innervation might determine the extent to which they persist or involute at different sites (11). Parasympathetic paraganglia generally receive their innervation from branches of either the vagus or glossopharyngeal nerves but also may receive some sympathetic input. A small percentage of carotid body cells, for example, reportedly synapse with preganglionic sympathetic fibers (62). Some carotid body cells also may lack innervation (63). In addition to innervation that directly involves neuroendocrine cells, paraganglia may receive vasomotor innervation from the nearby superior cervical ganglion and from a small number of intrinsic neurons (62,64). Multiple peptide neurotransmitters have been identified in nerve endings innervating the carotid body, and dynamic alterations of innervation have been reported in response to hypoxic stress (65). Multiple neurotransmitters are also present in adrenal medullary nerve endings and play a variety of roles in regulating both the development and function of adrenal chromaffin cells (66).

The neurovascular relationships of individual parasympathetic paraganglia have been described in great detail by several investigators (4,37). Of particular interest to pathologists are the paraganglia that give rise to glomus jugulare and glomus tympanicum paragangliomas in the floor or the wall of the middle ear. The paraganglia in the human temporal bone are distributed along the auricular branch of the vagus nerve (Arnold's nerve), and the tympanic branch of the glossopharyngeal nerve (Jacobson's nerve) (27). About 70% of paraganglia related to Arnold's nerve occur on the jugular bulb. The remainders follow the nerve through the mastoid canaliculus toward the vertical portion of the facial nerve. Paraganglia along Jacobson's nerve occur anywhere from the origin of the nerve at the petrosal ganglion (10%) to the jugular bulb (28%), tympanic canaliculus (40%), promontory of the middle ear (20%), and beyond (2%). Glomus jugulare tumors may therefore be associated with either Arnold's or Jacobson's nerve, although the former is most likely. Glomus tympanicum tumors are almost always associated with Jacobson's nerve (4).

LIGHT MICROSCOPY

Cell Types

Paraganglia contain two major types of cell: neuroendocrine cells and supporting cells. The former have been referred to in many publications as "granule-containing cells." "chromaffin cells," or "chromaffin-like cells" in sympathetic paraganglia and "glomus cells," "type I cells," or "chief cells" in parasympathetic paraganglia. The latter also have been called "sustentacular cells," "satellite cells," "supporting cells," or "type II cells" (4,26). In addition, there are variable numbers of connective tissue cells, vascular cells, Schwann cells, myelinated or unmyelinated nerve fibers, and intrinsic neurons. An additional commonly encountered cell type is the mast cell, which may be abundant in both ganglia and paraganglia (4,67). In hematoxylin and eosin (H&E) –stained sections, paraganglionic neuroendocrine cells are polygonal cells with amphophilic or basophilic cytoplasm and small, spherical or ovoid, pale-staining nuclei. Immunocytochemical stains for neuroendocrine markers can easily confirm their identity (see "Special Procedures"). Electron microscopy or argyrophil-type silver stains to demonstrate secretory granules or fluorescence methods to demonstrate catecholamines are employed in older publications. The neuroendocrine cells in paraganglia tend to form clusters and cords, described as *Zellballen* and *Zellsträngen* by Alfred Kohn (5), and may be partially or completely surrounded by supporting cells. The latter are usually flattened, with less conspicuous cytoplasm and more deeply basophilic nuclei with coarsely clumped chromatin. They appear to be glial cells, possibly related to non–myelin-forming

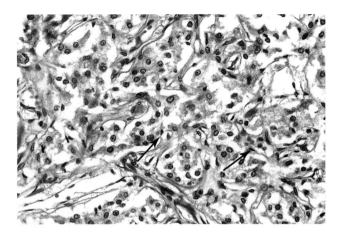

Figure 48.9 Section of organ of Zuckerkandl from a mid-trimester human fetus, demonstrating typical cords and nests of chief cells with rounded or oval nuclei and amphophilic cytoplasm, and occasional interspersed sustentacular cells with flattened nuclei and inconspicuous cytoplasm (*arrows*).

Schwann cells elsewhere in the peripheral nervous system (68), and can be identified by staining for S-100 protein (69) (see "Special Procedures"). Like non–myelin-forming Schwann cells, they have been reported in some instances to also stain for glial fibrillary acidic protein (70). They are present in both parasympathetic (69,70) and sympathetic (71,72) paraganglia but are more numerous in the former, where they cause the *Zellballen* to appear more pronounced (Figures 48.9–48.12).

Lobular Architecture of the Carotid Body

The carotid body is architecturally distinctive in that it consists of lobules separated by connective tissue septa

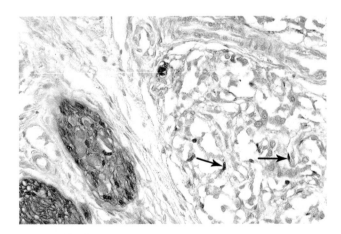

Figure 48.10 Organ of Zuckerkandl and adjacent sympathetic ganglion (same specimen as in Figures 48.20–48.23), stained for S-100 protein. Immunoreactivity for this antigen is typically localized in both nuclei and cytoplasm. Scattered sustentacular cells are stained in the organ of Zuckerkandl (*right, arrows*), where they tend to be located at the periphery of cell nests. Schwann cells are stained in the ganglion (*left*).

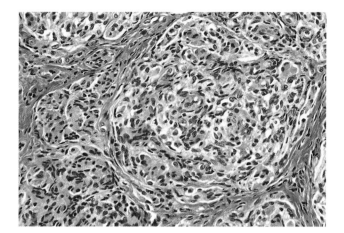

Figure 48.11   Section of carotid body from a 6-day-old infant demonstrating a characteristically more heterogeneous cell population than in Figure 48.9. Small nests of chief cells are highlighted by surrounding sustentacular cells and other cell types.

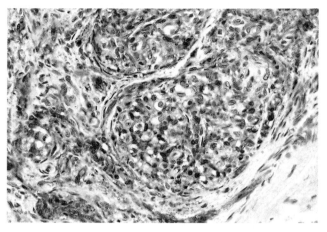

Figure 48.12   Lobule of a carotid body from a 16-day-old infant stained for S-100 protein. In contrast to the relatively sparse S-100–positive cells in the organ of Zuckerkandl (see Figure 48.10), there are numerous stained sustentacular cells within the lobule, accentuating the *Zellballen*, and numerous stained Schwann cells both within and adjacent to the lobule, as diagrammed in Figure 48.17.

(Figure 48.14). Each lobule is individually reminiscent of the microscopic paraganglia that occur in other sites and is composed of nests of chief cells surrounded by other cell types. This lobular arrangement is important to pathologists because carotid body hyperplasia is generally defined as an increase in mean lobule diameter (52–56). The amount of connective tissue between lobules in the carotid body tends to increase with age. Schwann cell proliferation and axonal sprouting also may occur at the periphery of lobules (Figure 48.15). One group of investigators has reported that the latter change is the pathognomonic feature of lobular hyperplasia in elderly patients with emphysema or hypertension (56). Other investigators studying specimens predominantly from patients with congenital heart disease have reported proportional proliferation of sustentacular cells and chief cells (52,53,55), whereas still others have reported chief cell hyperplasia in high-altitude dwellers (54). Lobular architecture similar to that of the carotid body is occasionally observed in other parasympathetic paraganglia, particularly if they are enlarged (53).

ULTRASTRUCTURE

At the ultrastructural level, paraganglionic neuroendocrine cells are characterized by numerous membrane-bound granules or "dense-core vesicles" approximately 60 to 400 nm in greatest dimension. They sometimes also contain small synaptic-like vesicles that may accumulate in clusters near the plasma membrane (73). Neuroendocrine secretory granules may vary in size, shape, and electron density, reflecting differences in the secretory products stored, the functional state of individual cells, and fixation conditions. In the rodent adrenal medulla, where epinephrine and norepinephrine are mostly stored in separate cells, fixation in glutaraldehyde and postfixation in osmium tetroxide cause granules in norepinephrine cells to appear homogeneously electron dense, whereas those in epinephrine cells are lighter and finely particulate. The mechanism for the differentiation involves formation of an insoluble reaction product between glutaraldehyde and norepinephrine, which is subsequently

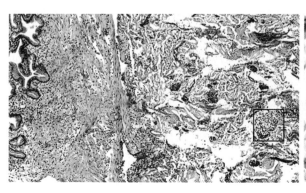
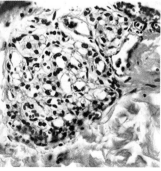

Figure 48.13   A microscopic paraganglion (small, oval, blue structure outlined in box) discovered as an incidental finding in the wall of the gallbladder of a 40-year-old woman. Right panel shows higher magnification of the paraganglion, illustrating prominent capillaries and admixed cell types.

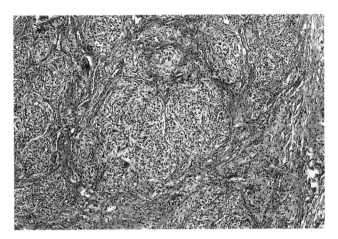

Figure 48.14 Carotid body from a 10-day-old infant, illustrating lobules separated by connective tissue septa.

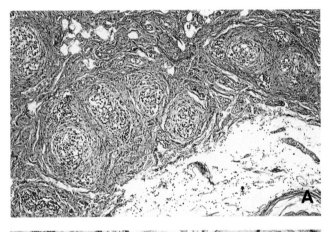

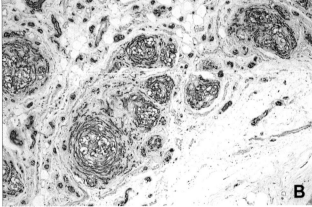

Figure 48.15 **A**. Carotid body from a 55-year-old woman with hypertension and emphysema. Lobules are separated by greater amounts of connective tissue than in Figure 48.14. In addition, there is a circumlobular proliferation of Schwann cells, demonstrable by staining for S-100 protein (**B**). The latter change has been reported by some investigators to be characteristic of lobular hyperplasia in patients with hypertension (56).

darkened by osmium (1,74). Because epinephrine does not similarly react with glutaraldehyde, it diffuses out of the granules, leaving behind other granule constituents that are less osmiophilic. To be successful, this method requires adequate fixation of fresh tissue. Human adrenal medullary cells occasionally exhibit homogeneous populations of epinephrine or norepinephrine-type granules (Figure 48.16), but most cells have mixed granule populations (75) and synthesize both epinephrine and norepinephrine (76). The electron density of most granules in extra-adrenal paraganglia is comparable to that of norepinephrine-type granules in the adrenal.

The ultrastructural organization of paraganglia and the proportions of their constituent cell types vary in different sites, apparently to suit different physiological needs. Both sympathetic and parasympathetic paraganglia contain numerous small capillaries. In the former, portions of the surfaces of neuroendocrine cells closest to these vessels are usually separated from the capillary endothelium only by basal laminae and occasional collagen fibrils, suggesting that sympathetic paraganglia in most instances function as endocrine glands (61). In some locations, their secretory products appear to be provided for local use (9). In contrast, the neuroendocrine cells in parasympathetic paraganglia tend to be separated from the capillary lumina by sustentacular cells, pericytes, or both (Figures 48.17–48.19). It therefore appears that a major role of their

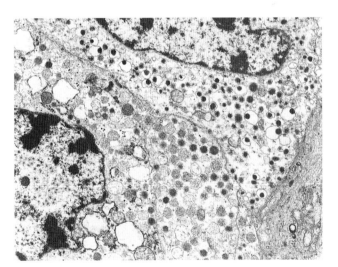

Figure 48.16 Electron micrograph of normal human adrenal medulla fixed in glutaraldehyde and postfixed in osmium tetroxide. Portions of cells at left contain predominantly light, finely particulate epinephrine-type granules, whereas cells at right contain predominantly dark, homogeneously electron-dense norepinephrine-type granules. The eccentric location of the granule cores within their surrounding membranes is a fixation artefact most commonly observed with granules of the latter type (original magnification ×9,677). (Reprinted with permission from: Tischler AS, The adrenal medulla and extra-adrenal paraganglia. In: Kovacs K, Asa SL, eds. *Functional Endocrine Pathology*. Cambridge, MA: Blackwell; 1990.)

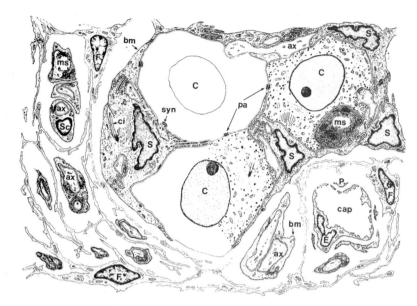

Figure 48.17 Diagram of the architecture of the human carotid body at the periphery of a lobule. Chief cells (C) in a small nest are insulated from the lumen of a nearby capillary (cap) by sustentacular cells (S), fibroblasts (F), and pericytes (P) and form synapses (syn) with parasympathetic axons (ax). They are also joined to each other by simple "puncta adherentia" type junctions (pa). Axons surrounded by Schwann cells (Sc) are present at the periphery of the lobule. Other illustrated structures are basement membrane (bm), endothelial cells (E), cilia (ci), and mitochondrion-rich axonal dilations termed "mitochondrial sacs" (ms). (Reprinted with permission from: Böck P, Stockinger L, Vyslonzil E. The fine structure of the human carotid body [article in German]. *Z Zellforsch Mikrosk Anat* 1970;105:543–568.)

secretory products is to act directly on sensory parasympathetic nerve endings rather than to enter circulating blood (62,73,77,78).

The relationships between individual neuroendocrine cells and nerve endings in paraganglia can be defined as presynaptic, postsynaptic, or reciprocally synaptic, based on the locations of synaptic membrane densities and vesicle accumulations. In the adrenal medulla the chromaffin cells are postsynaptic, consistent with their principal role of secreting hormones in response to neural stimulation. In contrast, numerous reciprocal synapses involving nerve endings and chief cells of the carotid body are consistent with the carotid body's chemosensory functions.

Despite the above generalizations, there is some overlap in the functional organization of sympathetic and parasympathetic paraganglia. This is especially apparent for SIF cells, at least in rodents, where they have been extensively studied. SIF cells are usually related to blood vessels and nerve endings comparably to other sympathetic paraganglionic cells. In some ganglia, however, they are insulated from the capillary lumina (11,12). Generally, they receive preganglionic sympathetic synapses, but in a few locations some may apparently also provide synapses to sympathetic neurons, suggesting a role as interneurons. Some also may be involved in reciprocal synapses with their preganglionic axons, suggesting chemoreceptor functions (79). Different SIF cells within a single small cluster can have different synaptic relationships, and a single process from one SIF cell can both synapse on a neuron and be in direct contact with a capillary basal lamina

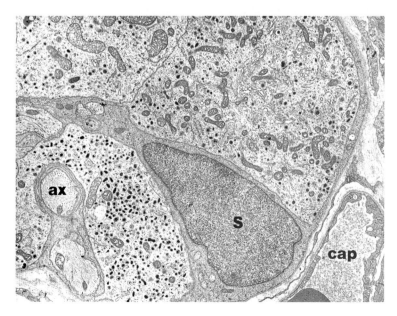

Figure 48.18 Electron micrograph of human carotid body from an area similar to that illustrated in Figure 48.17. S, sustentacular cell; cap, capillary; ax, axon (original magnification ×8,000). (Adapted with permission from: Böck P, Stockinger L, Vyslonzil E. The fine structure of the human carotid body [article in German]. *Z Zellforsch Mikrosk Anat* 1970;105:543–568.)

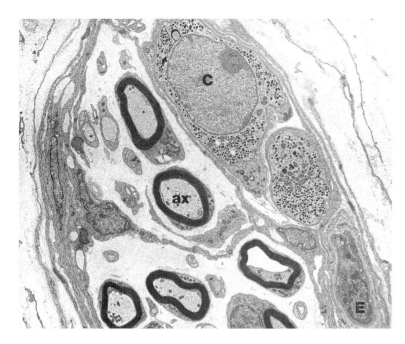

Figure 48.19 Electron micrograph of two chief cells enclosed within the perineurium of a small myelinated nerve in the vicinity of a human carotid body. This configuration has been described for intravagal paraganglia (53). As in the carotid body (see Figures 48.17 and 48.18), the chief cells are separated from the lumen of a nearby capillary (original magnification ×5,400). C, chief cells; E, endothelial cell; ax, axons. (Courtesy of Professor P. Böck.)

(11). It is important to note that two morphologically distinct types of SIF cells have been described in rodents, accounting in part for this functional diversity. "Type I SIF cells," which have ultrastructural features intermediate between neuroendocrine cells and neurons and are possibly interneurons, have not been identified in human ganglia. "Type II SIF cells" which are the only identified human SIF cell, resemble chromaffin cells or chief cells in sympathetic paraganglia (2).

FUNCTION

Physiological Roles

Paraganglia release secretory products in response to neural or chemical stimuli. Those products may be used for endocrine, paracrine, neurotransmitter, or neuromodulatory functions, depending on their anatomic context. Although their secretory products are similar and there is evidence of some functional overlap, sympathetic and parasympathetic paraganglia generally appear to differ in the major types of stimuli to which they respond. Responses to different types of stimuli also may delineate subsets of paraganglia within the sympathetic and parasympathetic groups.

The adult adrenal medulla responds principally to signals derived from neurons via trans-synaptic stimulation. Various physiological stressors reflexly evoke discharges of splanchnic nerve endings that synapse on chromaffin cells, causing release of secretory granules by Ca^{2+}-mediated exocytosis. This secretory response is accompanied by ancillary effects including activation of protooncogenes

(80), activation and induction of enzymes involved in replenishing granule constituents (81), and possibly stimulation of chromaffin cell proliferation (82). Cellular responses to neurally derived signals may be modulated by chemical signals, including corticosteroids and other hormones (81), growth factors (83), and secreted chromogranin fragments (84). Recent studies of the rat adrenal medulla suggest that neurally derived signals may increase the expression of receptors that regulate chromaffin cell function, including the receptor tyrosine kinase RET. The finding that RET expression is not static may help to resolve the conundrum of how that molecule, which is expressed at very low levels in the adult adrenal, contributes to the development of adrenal medullary hyperplasia and pheochromocytoma in MEN2 syndromes (85).

The sparse innervation of the extra-adrenal sympathetic paraganglia (61) suggests that they respond principally to chemical signals, and one possible signal is hypoxemia. It has been suggested that the organ of Zuckerkandl in rabbits and humans secretes catecholamines in response to hypoxemia during development (86,87). In other species, chemoreceptive functions have also been postulated for certain SIF cells (78,87,88), and for the immature adrenal medulla before the establishment of innervation (90).

Chemoreception is best established as a function of parasympathetic paraganglia. It was first shown in the 1930s that the carotid bodies and aortic paraganglia function as portions of reflex loops involving the central nervous system, whereby low pO_2, low pH, and high pCO_2 stimulate breathing (4). However, it was long debated whether the neuroendocrine cells in the carotid body are the primary receptor elements or whether their function is to modulate chemoreceptor properties intrinsic to the sensory nerve endings. Electrophysiological studies of the mechanism of chemoreception have shown that the three major chemosensory stimuli depolarize dissociated carotid body chief cells. This leads to influx of calcium through voltage-gated calcium channels and to calcium-dependent release of secretory products to stimulate sensory nerve endings (10,91). Chemoreceptor reflexes have been postulated for other parasympathetic paraganglia on the basis of their similarities to the carotid body (28,92), but the nature and importance of such reflexes in vivo have not been defined. It may be of interest in this regard that patients who have had their carotid bodies removed exhibit impaired ventilatory reflexes (93), and that carotid body hyperplasia occurs in association with life at high altitude (54), chronic obstructive pulmonary disease, restrictive pulmonary disease, cystic fibrosis, and cyanotic congenital heart disease (52,53,55–58). In contrast, vagal paraganglia only sometimes increase in number or size (55). A tenfold increase in the prevalence of carotid body paragangliomas is reported at high altitudes (94), but this association has not been made for paragangliomas at other sites.

Secretory Products

Although studies using the chromaffin reaction suggested that catecholamines were produced by sympathetic not parasympathetic paraganglia (4), more sensitive methods now available indicate that they are produced by paraganglia of both classes. Those methods include immunocytochemistry to demonstrate both catecholamines themselves and their biosynthetic enzymes (76,95,96), as well as older fluorescence techniques to demonstrate catecholamine stores (97) (see "Special Procedures"). Most of the body's epinephrine production is in the adrenal medulla, where the epinephrine-to-norepinephrine ratio is approximately 4:1 (98). In contrast, over 90% of the catecholamine content of extra-adrenal sympathetic paraganglia is norepinephrine (20). Parasympathetic paraganglia produce almost no epinephrine but may produce significant quantities of dopamine (99). Serotonin has been reported in addition to catecholamines in some human paraganglia (100), but it is not clear in some studies whether the presence of serotonin is due to synthesis or uptake (101).

In addition to producing catecholamines, both sympathetic and parasympathetic paraganglia synthesize regulatory peptides, the most prevalent of which are enkephalins (76,102–105). Regulatory peptides and amines usually coexist in the same cells and in the same secretory granules (105). The granules also contain granin proteins (103,106,107), adenine nucleotides, peptide-cleaving and amidating enzymes, dopamine beta-hydroxylase, and numerous other constituents of both known and unknown function (108). Peptide growth factors that might exert autocrine, paracrine, and neurotropic effects also may be present (108,109). Together these granule constituents comprise a "secretory cocktail," the composition of which can be varied in different physiological and pathological states (81,108).

GENDER DIFFERENCES

Significant gender differences in the histology of paraganglia have not been reported. However, there is some evidence for functional differences. For example, women in general appear to have slightly increased susceptibility to carotid body paragangliomas. This difference is accentuated by life at high altitude, where the tumors have a female-to-male ratio of approximately 8:1 (110).

AGING CHANGES

Aging changes described in human paraganglia are limited to the topographic and involutional changes described in the sections on "Distribution of Paraganglia," "Gross Features and Organ Weights," and "Lobular Architecture of the Carotid Body." Subtle histochemical changes have been described in the composition of adrenal chromaffin granules of rats (111) and also might occur in other paraganglia. Hypertrophy or hyperplasia of extra-adrenal paraganglia also occurs in aging rats (112).

SPECIAL PROCEDURES

Immunohistochemistry

The study of normal and pathologic paraganglia has been greatly facilitated by recent advances in immunohistochemistry. Antibodies that are now commercially available permit identification and functional characterization of specific paraganglionic cell types in sections of formalin-fixed, paraffin-embedded tissue. In addition, the advent of microwave antigen retrieval (113) has both improved the quality of immunohistochemical staining and eliminated some of the variability previously caused by prolonged fixation. Highly sensitive, polymer-based reporter systems have both increased the sensitivity of immunohistochemical staining and eliminated artefact due to endogenous biotin (114). For most purposes, immunohistochemistry can now replace previously useful but more cumbersome or less specific techniques such as electron microscopy, catecholamine fluorescence, or silver stains.

Paraganglia express a plethora of markers shared to varying degrees with other neural and endocrine tissues. A partial categorization includes amines, regulatory peptides, granins and other constituents of the secretory granule matrix, secretory granule membrane and cell membrane components, and cytoskeletal proteins. Proteins known as "SNAP"s and "SNARE"s (SNAP receptors) that are involved in docking of secretory granules at the cell membrane in preparation for exocytosis comprise an important new class of markers. Those proteins include synaptobrevin, synaptotagmin, syntaxin, and SNAP-25 (115).

For pathologists, the major current applications of immunohistochemistry to the paraganglionic system are the diagnosis and functional characterization of paraganglionic tumors. Potential future applications include identification of markers that may be applicable to targeted therapy, such as specific somatostatin receptor subtypes (116), or profiling of tumors for clusters of markers associated with specific tumor syndromes or with malignancy (15) (see "Clinicopathologic Perspective") (76,103,117).

For diagnostic purposes, care must be taken to select from the large number of available markers those that are the most specific. For example, immunoreactivity for synaptophysin, a secretory vesicle membrane protein, is characteristically present in paraganglia but also reported in adrenal cortex (118,119). Similarly, certain SNAP and SNARE proteins are present in normal lymphoid cells (120,121). Reagents that have been particularly valuable in histopathology of paraganglia are antibodies against chromogranin A (CgA), catecholamine biosynthetic enzymes, and S-100 protein.

CgA is an acidic protein that constitutes more than half the weight of many types of neuroendocrine secretory granule. It appears to be present in most or all paraganglionic neuroendocrine cells and is therefore a useful generic marker that can, in most instances, serve to establish the neuroendocrine nature of particular cells or tissues in the paraganglionic system (122,123) (Figures 48.20–48.27). Because it is concentrated mostly in secretory granules, it may fail to stain cells that are degranulated

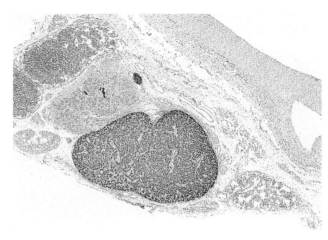

Figure 48.21 Section adjacent to that shown in Figure 48.20, stained for CgA. Staining is intense in the organ of Zuckerkandl and in small nests of neuroendocrine cells within and adjacent to the ganglion, but not in sympathetic neurons.

due to low rates of synthesis, high rates of turnover, or low storage capacity. In sympathetic ganglia, it can be used to conveniently discriminate SIF cells from principal sympathetic neurons, which produce CgA but have few perikaryal secretory granules (124) (Figures 48.21, 48.22, and 48.24). CgA was the first described member of the granin family of proteins, which now includes seven members (CgA and B, secretogranin II and III, 7B2, NESP55, and VGF) (106,107). These proteins are differentially expressed in neuroendocrine tissues of different species. Although most are present in the adrenal medulla, their distributions in other paraganglia are incompletely mapped (107). Their roles include sorting of proteins to the regulated secretory pathway and directing secretory granule biogenesis. In addition, they serve as multifunctional prohormones, giving rise to cleavage fragments that exert a variety of autocrine, paracrine, and systemic effects.

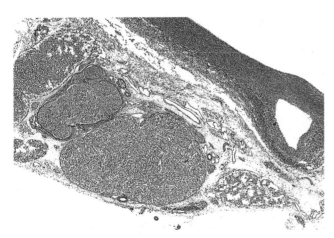

Figure 48.20 Transverse section through the aorta of a mid-trimester human fetus (same fetus as in Figure 48.25) at the level of the inferior mesenteric artery, demonstrating organ of Zuckerkandl and adjacent sympathetic ganglion, related as diagrammed in Figure 48.2.

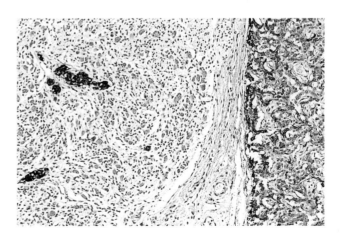

Figure 48.22 Higher magnification of central area of section shown in Figure 48.21. Organ of Zuckerkandl is on right, ganglion on left.

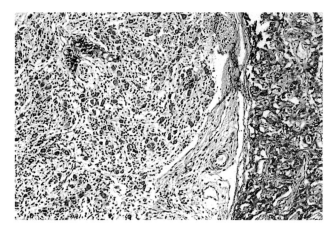

Figure 48.23 Section adjacent to that shown in Figure 48.22, stained for TH. Intense immunoreactivity is present in both sympathetic neurons and paraganglionic neuroendocrine cells.

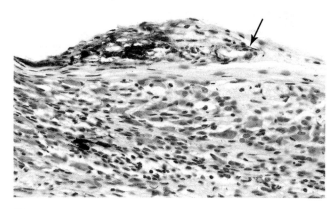

Figure 48.24 Sympathetic ganglion from the paravertebral trunk of a mid-trimester human fetus (same fetus as in Figures 48.20–48.23), stained for CgA. Neuroendocrine cells are identified both within and adjacent to the ganglion. CgA-positive processes, which might be derived from either neurons or neuroendocrine cells, surround a small blood vessel (*arrow*).

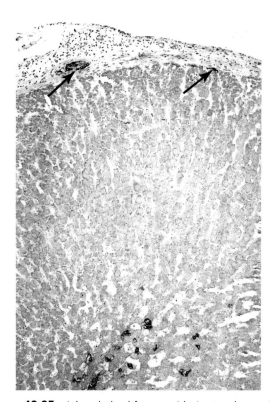

Figure 48.25 Adrenal gland from a mid-trimester human fetus (same fetus as in Figures 48.20–48.23), stained for CgA. The medulla (*bottom*) contains only scattered positive cells, in contrast to the organ of Zuckerkandl (Figure 48.21). Extra-adrenal (*left arrow*) and subcapsular (*right arrow*) paraganglionic cells are also identified by their immunoreactivity.

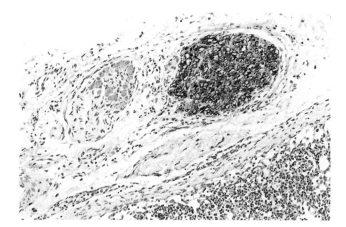

Figure 48.26 A small retroperitoneal paraganglion similar to that in Figure 48.13, incidentally removed along with adjacent ganglion and lymph node from a 5-month-old infant during resection of a Wilms' tumor. Soaking the coverslip off a routine H&E–stained histologic section and restaining for CgA confirmed the identity of the paraganglion. The stability and abundance of this antigen make it particularly suitable for such procedures.

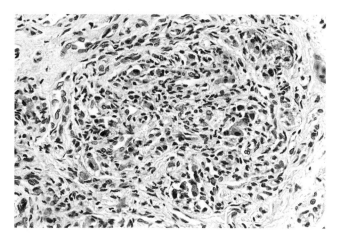

Figure 48.27 Lobule of a carotid body stained for CgA, demonstrating nests of immunoreactive chief cells surrounded by unstained cells of other types.

Perhaps the most important advance in decades from the standpoint of surgical pathology of the paraganglia is the availability of antibodies against the catecholamine-synthesizing enzymes tyrosine hydroxylase (TH), dopamine beta-hydroxylase (DBH), and phenylethanolamine-N-methyltransferase (PNMT). With these reagents, it is now usually possible to infer from a paraffin section not only whether a tumor was catecholamine producing, but also what catecholamines were produced. The need for fluorescence methods that directly detect catecholamine stores but require fresh tissue is therefore, in most instances, eliminated. Tyrosine hydroxylase (TH) is the rate-limiting enzyme in catecholamine synthesis and is therefore found in all catecholamine-producing cells (Figures 48.23 and 48.28), whereas dopamine β-hydroxylase (DBH) is found only in cells that produce norepinephrine, and PNMT is found only in cells that can convert norepinephrine to epinephrine. This immunocytochemical approach provides a cellular correlate to biochemical data by demonstrating that only rarely do extra-adrenal paraganglionic cells stain for PNMT (95), in contrast to the adrenal medulla where the great majority of cells are stained (76) (Figures 48.29 and 48.30). It also has been useful in demonstrating catecholamine-synthesizing ability in pheochromocytomas and extra-adrenal paragangliomas (96,125). Because TH and PNMT are cytosolic enzymes (108), staining is not dependent on storage of secretory granules. Sympathetic neurons, for example, stain strongly for TH (Figure 48.23), in contrast to their weak or absent staining for CgA (Figures 48.21, 48.22, 48.24, and 48.26). In contrast to chromogranins, which are present in many types of neuroendocrine cells, catecholamine biosynthetic enzymes in adult humans are normally present only in paraganglia and neurons (95). In addition to their biosynthetic enzymes, catecholamines themselves may be localized by immunohistochemistry.

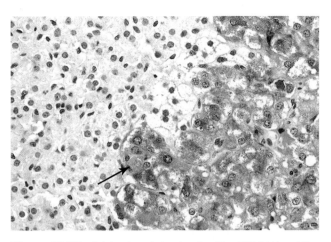

Figure 48.29 Adult adrenal gland stained for PNMT. The ability of almost all neuroendocrine cells in the adrenal medulla to synthesize epinephrine is inferred from their positive staining. Occasional cells are unstained (*arrow*) as previously reported (76) and as suggested by the electron micrograph in Figure 48.16.

However, the presence of catecholamines without biosynthetic enzymes under some circumstances (96) suggests that synthesis cannot be distinguished from uptake by this approach.

S-100 protein was initially described as a calcium-binding dimer consisting of alpha-alpha, alpha-beta, or beta-beta chains and was initially believed to be specific for central and peripheral nervous system glial cells. Subsequent studies showed a wider distribution of immunoreactivity (126). Immunostaining for S-100 nevertheless provides a useful marker in appropriate contexts. Because of their nondescript cytologic characteristics, the sustentacular cells in paraganglia are difficult to identify with certainty in sections stained with hematoxylin and eosin. The intense nuclear

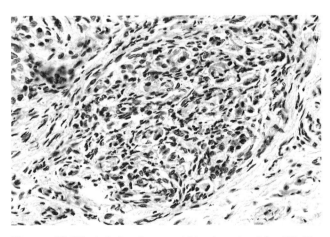

Figure 48.28 Lobule of a carotid body stained for TH. The catecholamine-synthesizing ability of chief cells is inferred by positive staining of chief cell nests, which are surrounded by unstained cells of other types.

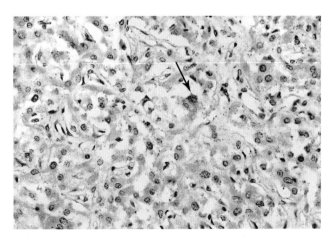

Figure 48.30 Organ of Zuckerkandl (same specimen as in Figures 48.20–48.23) stained for PNMT. Although all the neuroendocrine cells stain for TH and can produce catecholamines (Figure 48.23), only rare cells (*arrow*) contain immunoreactive PNMT. This finding is consistent with the limited ability of extra-adrenal paraganglia to synthesize epinephrine, the final step in the catecholamine biosynthetic pathway.

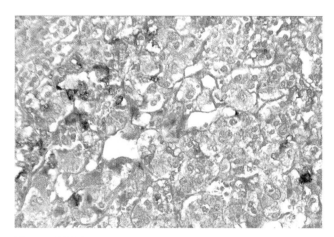

Figure 48.31 Adult adrenal gland stained for somatostatin, illustrating strongly immunoreactive cells scattered among cells with no detectable immunoreactivity. Immunohistochemical staining of paraganglionic neuroendocrine cells for regulatory peptides can suggest functional heterogeneity despite the fact that all of the cells produce catecholamines.

immunoreactivity of these cells for S-100 permits them to be identified in sympathetic and parasympathetic paraganglia (Figures 48.10 and 48.12). Interestingly, they also may be identified in paragangliomas (71,72), a finding that might reflect either ingrowth from nearby normal tissue or bidirectional differentiation. Sustentacular cells must be distinguished from Langerhans cells and interdigitating reticulum cells of the immune system, which also express S-100. Both sustentacular cells and Schwann cells contain predominantly the beta subunit of S-100 (127). The S-100 protein family has now expanded beyond the original alpha and beta subunits to include at least 17 members postulated to play a variety of roles in different cell types (128).

Immunohistochemical studies might help to reveal subtle expressions of functional heterogeneity in normal paraganglia that could contribute to understanding of syndrome-associated phenotypes. Examples might include the absence of epinephrine-synthesizing ability or the expression of particular regulatory peptides in small numbers of human chromaffin cells (76) (Figures 48.29–48.31). Evidence of differential innervation might also provide clues to differential function (103,117).

Immunohistochemical Artifacts

Important artifacts that must be borne in mind in immunohistochemical studies of paraganglia are the nonspecific interactions of some, but not all, antibodies with the secretory granules of mast cells (129,130) and of certain neuroendocrine cells (131). These artifacts may be particularly troublesome because, due to their inconstancy, negative controls consisting of irrelevant antibodies or normal sera are not adequate. The mast cell artifact has undoubtedly resulted in erroneous published reports of neuroendocrine secretory products in nonendocrine tissues, and also could

produce incorrect results in studies of paraganglia because of their sometimes high mast cell content (67). The mechanism of the mast cell artifact is not known (130), but in some cases the staining may be eliminated by dilution in the presence of normal serum proteins (129). Nonspecific binding of immunoglobulins to neuroendocrine secretory granules appears to result from ionic interactions and may be reduced by high concentrations of salt in the buffer (131). A buffer containing 0.5 mol/L NaCl should not interfere with specific high-affinity antigen–antibody interactions and, in many instances, may be used routinely.

Other artifacts that are not specific to neuroendocrine cells may also be encountered in studies of paraganglia. In immunohistochemical protocols that employ a biotin bridge, such as the widely utilized "ABC" technique, artefactual staining may result from the presence of endogenous biotin. This problem may be exacerbated by heat-based antigen retrieval, which can unmask endogenous biotin in addition to specific antigens (132). Commercially available biotin blocking kits offer some remedy, but a preferable solution may be to discontinue the use of biotin-based systems and switch to newer methods that employ secondary antibodies conjugated to polymer-bound reporter enzymes (114). Various types of artifactual staining with less clear mechanisms are also sometimes encountered. In the adrenal gland, for example, some antibodies inexplicably produce spurious staining in the adrenal cortex (114). This particularly tends to occur in the inner portion of the cortex, and might therefore result from nonspecific interactions of some antibodies with lipochrome pigments. Cells that are rich in mitochondria occasionally also show weak nonspecific staining. In addition to spurious staining caused by these and other artifacts, the possibility of actual immunological cross-reactivity of an antibody with different proteins must always be considered.

In general, immunohistochemical studies should be performed with optimally diluted antibodies and verified, when practical, with antibodies from more than one source. Ideally, adsorption controls and immunoblots should also be employed for validation, particularly in research studies or when new markers or antibodies are introduced. Controls consisting solely of primary antibody omission should not be considered adequate even for routine studies. Buffer composition, blocking proteins, and controls are now to some extent becoming standardized in automated staining procedures, but should still be optimized for each new antibody as discussed in many textbooks and reviews (133).

Other Special Procedures

Fluorescence methods for detection of catecholamines or other biogenic amines now have very little use in routine pathology. However, literature searches of PubMed or other databases continue to demonstrate the value of these techniques in occasional research applications.

Catecholamines can be demonstrated in freeze dried or frozen sections or in touch preparations either by formaldehyde vapor– (97,134) or glyoxylic acid–induced (135) fluorescence. The glyoxylic acid method is usually preferable because it produces nondiffusing fluorophores.

Other research applications of histological techniques include the use of in situ hybridization to detect genetic abnormalities in paragangliomas (136–138) or to map the expression of specific mRNAs (139).

DIFFERENTIAL DIAGNOSIS

Paraganglia must be discriminated from normal but similar-appearing nonparaganglionic structures and from a variety of malignant tumors. The ampulloglomerular organ (140), glomus coccygeum, and glomera cutanea are thermoregulatory structures respectively located in the suboccipital and coccygeal regions and in the skin, resembling but unrelated to paraganglia. Lobules of fetal fat may at times appear reminiscent of paraganglia. All of these structures can be readily distinguished from paraganglia by their absence of staining for CgA, TH, or other neuroendocrine markers. Reports of paraganglia in anomalous locations (4) are also now amenable to immunohistochemical verification. Prostatic paraganglia may be misinterpreted as prostatic adenocarcinoma (141), bladder paraganglia may be confused with transitional cell carcinoma (142), and retroperitoneal paraganglia may be confused with metastatic clear cell carcinoma (143). The presence of mitoses, cytologic atypia, glandular or squamous differentiation, or stromal reaction point toward a diagnosis of tumor, and questionable cases can be readily resolved by immunohistochemistry.

More problematic are cases in which paraganglia or paragangliomas must be distinguished from other normal or neoplastic neuroendocrine tissues that express many of the same markers. Knowledge of the distribution and morphology of paraganglia is essential in these cases. In addition, the presence of tyrosine hydroxylase in paragangliomas or of other site-suggestive markers in other types of tumors, for example calcitonin in medullary thyroid carcinoma, may be helpful. Tumors showing glandular or squamous differentiation are almost certainly not paraganglionic.

In the adrenal gland, developmental neuroblastic nests (see "Embryologic Changes") must be distinguished from in situ neuroblastoma (42,43). Cortical invasion, mitoses, and necrosis are all characteristic of normal cells in this instance. Ikeda et al. (40) reported that the nuclei of normal adrenal medullary progenitors are smaller on average than those of neuroblastoma cells, and this might prove to be diagnostically useful. In view of the large potential effect of fixation on nuclear size, however, the problem is more likely to be resolved using molecular techniques (144).

SPECIMEN HANDLING

For most purposes, normal and pathologic paraganglionic tissue may be evaluated histologically and immunohistochemically after routine formalin fixation and paraffin embedding (see "Special Procedures"). In the age of heat-based antigen retrieval, under-fixation may create as many artefacts as the traditional problem of over-fixation. However, some antigens are still irretrievably damaged by excessive fixation. Fixation of thin tissue slices overnight is usually adequate. Electron microscopy, when necessary, is optimally performed after glutaraldehyde fixation and osmium postfixation (see "Ultrastructure"). Catecholamines may be demonstrated in touch preparations or frozen sections using glyoxylic acid–induced fluorescence (see "Special Procedures").

For biochemical analysis, catecholamines may be preserved by freezing small minced tissue fragments or tissue homogenates at $-70\,^\circ$C in 0.4 mol/L perchloric acid in 1 mmol/L ethylene diamine tetra-acetic acid (145). Peptide hormones may be preserved by freezing in 1.0 mol/L acetic acid.

With burgeoning interest in molecular studies of paraganglia, it is increasingly necessary to preserve DNA, RNA, and protein samples. Tissue handling is particularly critical for RNA and protein preservation, and the traditional approach is rapid freezing and storage in liquid nitrogen. However, a number of solutions that are now commercially available provide comparable or superior preservation of both nucleic acids and protein for at least several weeks at room temperature for convenient handling and shipping. This approach may facilitate standardization of noncentralized specimen collection (146,147).

ACKNOWLEDGMENTS

I thank Drs. Peter Böck, Ernest Lack, and James Powers for contributing illustrative material and Dr. Harold Kozakewich for contributing tissue blocks.

REFERENCES

1. Coupland RE. *The Natural History of the Chromaffin Cell.* London: Longmans Green; 1965.
2. Coupland RE. The natural history of the chromaffin cell—twenty-five years on the beginning. *Arch Histol Cytol* 1989; 52(supp l):331–341.
3. Carmichael SW. The history of the adrenal medulla. *Rev Neurosci* 1989;2:83–99.
4. Zak FG, Lawson W. *The Paraganglionic Chemoreceptor System: Physiology, Pathology and Clinical Medicine.* New York: Springer-Verlag; 1982.
5. Kohn A. Die paraganglien. *Arch Mikr Anat* 1903;62:263–365.
6. Pearse AG, Polak JM, Rost FW, Fontaine J, Le Lievre C, Le Douarin N. Demonstration of the neural crest origin of type I (APUD) cells in the avian carotid body, using a cytochemical marker system. *Histochemie* 1973;34:191–203.

7. Le Douarin N. *The Neural Crest.* Cambridge, England: Cambridge University Press; 1982.

8. Hadjiconstantinou M, Potter PE, Neff NH. Trans-synaptic modulation via muscarinic receptors of serotonin-containing small intensely fluorescent cells of superior cervical ganglion. *J Neurosci* 1982;2:1836–1839.

9. Furness JB, Sobels G. The ultrastructure of paraganglia associated with the inferior mesenteric ganglia in the guinea-pig. *Cell Tissue Res* 1976;171:123–139.

10. Spicer Z, Millhorn DE. Oxygen sensing in neuroendocrine cells and other cell types: pheochromocytoma (PC12) cells as an experimental model. *Endocr Pathol* 2003;14:277–291.

11. Matthews MR. Synaptic and other relationships of small granule-containing cells (SIF cells) in sympathetic ganglia. In: Coupland RE, Fujita T, eds. *Chromaffin, Enterochromaffin and Related Cells.* Amsterdam: Elsevier; 1976;131–146.

12. Matthews MR. Ultrastructural studies relevant to the possible functions of small granule-containing cells in the rat superior cervical ganglion. *Adv Biochem Psychopharmacol* 1980;25:77–86.

13. Dannenberg H, Komminoth P, Dinjens WN, Speel EJ, de Krijger RR. Molecular genetic alterations in adrenal and extra-adrenal pheochromocytomas and paragangliomas. *Endocr Pathol* 2003; 14:329–350.

14. Eisenhofer G, Bornstein SR, Brouwers FM, et al. Malignant pheochromocytoma: current status and initiatives for future progress. *Endocr Relat Cancer* 2004;11:423–436.

15. Eisenhofer G, Huynh TT, Pacak K, et al. Distinct gene expression profiles in norepinephrine- and epinephrine-producing hereditary and sporadic pheochromocytomas: activation of hypoxia-driven angiogenic pathways in von Hippel-Lindau syndrome. *Endocr Relat Cancer* 2004;11:897–911.

16. Eisenhofer G, Goldstein DS, Kopin IJ, Crout JR. Pheochromocytoma: rediscovery as a catecholamine-metabolizing tumor. *Endocr Pathol* 2003;14:193–212.

17. Hervonen A, Partanen S, Vaalasti A, Partanen M, Kanerva L, Alho H. The distribution and endocrine nature of the abdominal paraganglia of adult man. *Am J Anat* 1978;153:563–572.

18. Baljet B, Boekelaar AB, Groen GJ. Retroperitoneal paraganglia and the peripheral autonomic nervous system in the human fetus. *Acta Morphol Neerl Scand* 1985;23:137–149.

19. Hervonen A, Vaalasti A, Partanen M, Kanerva L, Hervonen H. Effects of ageing on the histochemically demonstrable catecholamines and acetylcholinesterase of human sympathetic ganglia. *J Neurocytol* 1978;7:11–23.

20. Coupland RE. The development and fate of catecholamine-secreting endocrine cells. In: Parvez H, Parvez S, eds. *Biogenic Amines in Development.* Amsterdam: Elsevier/North-Holland Biomedical Press; 1980;3–28.

21. Zuckerkandl E. Ueber nebenorgane des sympathicus im Retroperitonaealraum des menschen. *Verh Anat Ges* 1901; 15:85–107.

22. Ober WB. Emil Zuckerkandl and his delightful little organ. *Pathol Annu* 1983;18(pt 1):103–119.

23. Lack EE, Cubilla AL, Woodruff JM, Lieberman PH. Extra-adrenal paragangliomas of the retroperitoneum: a clinicopathologic study of 12 tumors. *Am J Surg Pathol* 1980;4:109–120.

24. Helen P, Alho H, Hervonen A. Ultrastructure and histochemistry of human SIF cells and paraganglia. *Adv Biochem Psychopharmacol* 1980;25:149–152.

25. Kohn A. Die chromaffinen Zellen des sympathicus. *Anat Anz* 1898;15:399–400.

26. Glenner GG, Grimley PM. Tumors of the extraadrenal paraganglion system (including chemoreceptors). In: *Atlas of Tumor Pathology.* 2nd series, fascicle 9. Washington, DC: Armed Forces Institute of Pathology; 1974.

27. Guild SR. The glomus jugulare, a nonchromaffin paraganglion, in man. *Ann Otol Rhinol Laryngol* 1953;62:1045–1071; concld.

28. Dahlqvist A, Carlsoo B, Hellstrom S. Paraganglia of the human recurrent laryngeal nerve. *Am J Otolaryngol* 1986;7:366–369.

29. Grillo MA, Jacobs L, Comroe JH Jr. A combined fluorescence histochemical and electron microscopic method for studying special monoamine-containing cells (SIF cells). *J Comp Neurol* 1974;153:1–14.

30. Manger WM, Gifford RW. *Clinical and Experimental Pheochromocytoma.* 2nd ed. Cambridge, MA: Blackwell Science; 1996.

31. Plenat F, Leroux P, Floquet J, Floquet A. Intra and juxtavagal paraganglia: a topographical, histochemical, and ultrastructural study in the human. *Anat Rec* 1988;221:743–753.

32. Goormagtigh N. On the existence of abdominal vagal paraganglia in the adult mouse. *J Anat* 1936;71:77–90.

33. Kuo T, Anderson CB, Rosai J. Normal paraganglia in the human gallbladder. *Arch Pathol* 1974;97:46–47.

34. Cooper MJ, Hutchins GM, Israel MA. Histogenesis of the human adrenal medulla. An evaluation of the ontogeny of chromaffin and nonchromaffin lineages. *Am J Pathol* 1990;137:605–615.

35. Molenaar WM, Lee VM, Trojanowski JQ. Early fetal acquisition of the chromaffin and neuronal immunophenotype by human adrenal medullary cells. An immunohistological study using monoclonal antibodies to chromogranin A, synaptophysin, tyrosine hydroxylase, and neuronal cytoskeletal proteins. *Exp Neurol* 1990;108:1–9.

36. Korkala O, Hervonen A. Origin and development of the catecholamine-storing cells of the human fetal carotid body. *Histochemie* 1973;37:287–297.

37. Kjaergaard J. *Anatomy of the Carotid Glomerus and Carotid Glomus-like Bodies (Non-chromaffin Paraganglia).* Copenhagen: FADL's Forlag; 1973.

38. Zuckerkandl E. The development of the chromaffin organs and of the suprarenal glands. In: Keibel F, Mall FP, eds. *Manual of Human Embryology.* Philadelphia: JB Lippincott; 1912;157–179.

39. Kuntz A. The development of the sympathetic nervous system in man. *J Comp Neurol* 1920;32:173–229.

40. Ikeda Y, Lister J, Bouton JM, Buyukpamukcu M. Congenital neuroblastoma, neuroblastoma in situ, and the normal fetal development of the adrenal. *J Pediatr Surg* 1981;16(suppl 1): 636–644.

41. Willier BH. A study of the origin and differentiation of the suprarenal glandin the chick embryo by chorio-allantoic grafting. *Phys Zool* 1930;3:201–225.

42. Turkel SB, Itabashi HH. The natural history of neuroblastic cells in the fetal adrenal gland. *Am J Pathol* 1974;76:225–244.

43. Beckwith JB, Perrin EV. In situ neuroblastomas: a contribution to the natural history of neural crest tumors. *Am J Pathol* 1963;43: 1089–1104.

44. Garcia I, Martinou I, Tsujimoto Y, Martinou JC. Prevention of programmed cell death of sympathetic neurons by the bcl-2 proto-oncogene. *Science* 1992;258:302–304.

45. Vogel KS. Development of trophic interactions in the vertebrate peripheral nervous system. *Mol Neurobiol* 1993;7:363–382.

46. Tischler AS, DeLellis RA, Biales B, Nunnemacher G, Carabba V, Wolfe HJ. Nerve growth factor-induced neurite outgrowth from normal human chromaffin cells. *Lab Invest* 1980;43: 399–409.

47. Anderson DJ. Cellular 'neoteny': a possible developmental basis for chromaffin cell plasticity. *Trends Genet* 1989;5:174–178.

48. Gold R, Schmied M, Giegerich G, et al. Differentiation between cellular apoptosis and necrosis by the combined use of in situ tailing and nick translation techniques. *Lab Invest* 1994; 71:219–225.

49. DeLellis RA, Wolfe HJ, Gagel RF, et al. Adrenal medullary hyperplasia. A morphometric analysis in patients with familial medullary thyroid carcinoma. *Am J Pathol* 1976;83:177–196.

50. Carney JA, Sizemore GW, Sheps SG. Adrenal medullary disease in multiple endocrine neoplasia, type 2: pheochromocytoma and its precursors. *Am J Clin Pathol* 1976;66:279–290.

51. Kreiner E. Weight and shape of the human adrenal medulla in various age groups. *Virchows Arch A Pathol Anat Histol* 1982;397:7–15.

52. Lack EE. Carotid body hypertrophy in patients with cystic fibrosis and cyanotic congenital heart disease. *Hum Pathol* 1977;8: 39–51.

53. Lack EE. Hyperplasia of vagal and carotid body paraganglia in patients with chronic hypoxemia. *Am J Pathol* 1978;91:497–516.

54. Arias-Stella J, Valcarcel J. Chief cell hyperplasia in the human carotid body at high altitudes; physiologic and pathologic significance. *Hum Pathol* 1976;7:361–373.

55. Lack EE, Perez-Atayde AR, Young JB. Carotid body hyperplasia in cystic fibrosis and cyanotic heart disease. A combined morphometric, ultrastructural, and biochemical study. *Am J Pathol* 1985;119:301–314.

56. Fitch R, Smith P, Heath D. Nerve axons in carotid body hyperplasia. A quantitative study. *Arch Pathol Lab Med* 1985;109:234–237.

57. Smith P, Jago R, Heath D. Anatomical variation and quantitative histology of the normal and enlarged carotid body. *J Pathol* 1982;137:287–304.

58. Heath D, Smith P, Jago R. Hyperplasia of the carotid body. *J Pathol* 1982;138:115–127.

59. McDonald DM, Blewett RW. Location and size of carotid body-like organs (paraganglia) revealed in rats by the permeability of blood vessels to Evans blue dye. *J Neurocytol* 1981;10:607–643.

60. Parker TL, Kesse WK, Mohamed AA, Afework M. The innervation of the mammalian adrenal gland. *J Anat* 1993;183(pt 2):265–276.

61. Hervonen A. Development of catecholamine-storing cells in human fetal paraganglia and adrenal medulla. A histochemical and electron microscopical study. *Acta Physiol Scand Suppl* 1971;368:1–94.

62. McDonald DM, Mitchell RA. The innervation of glomus cells, ganglion cells and blood vessels in the rat carotid body: a quantitative ultrastructural analysis. *J Neurocytol* 1975;4:177–230.

63. Eyzaguirre C, Fidone SJ. Transduction mechanisms in carotid body: glomus cells, putative neurotransmitters, and nerve endings. *Am J Physiol* 1980;239:C135–C152.

64. Kummer W, Habeck JO. Light and electronmicroscopical immunohistochemical investigation of the innervation of the human carotid body. *Adv Exp Med Biol* 1993;337:67–71.

65. Kusakabe T, Hirakawa H, Oikawa S, et al. Morphological changes in the rat carotid body 1, 2, 4, and 8 weeks after the termination of chronically hypocapnic hypoxia. *Histol Histopathol* 2004;19:1133–1140.

66. Holgert H, Dagerlind A, Hokfelt T. Immunohistochemical characterization of the peptidergic innervation of the rat adrenal gland. *Horm Metab Res* 1998;30:315–322.

67. Kraus R, Bezdicek P. The incidence of mastocytes in paraganglia. *Folia Morphol (Praha)* 1988;36:211–213.

68. Mirsky R, Jessen KR. The biology of non-myelin-forming Schwann cells. *Ann N Y Acad Sci* 1986;486:132–146.

69. Kondo H, Iwanaga T, Nakajima T. Immunocytochemical study on the localization of neuron-specific enolase and S-100 protein in the carotid body of rats. *Cell Tissue Res* 1982;227:291–295.

70. Habeck JO, Kummer W. Neuronal and neuroendocrine markers in the human carotid body in health and disease. *Adv Exp Med Biol* 1993;337:31–35.

71. Lauriola L, Maggiano N, Sentinelli S, Michetti F, Cocchia D. Satellite cells in the normal human adrenal gland and in pheochromocytomas. An immunohistochemical study. *Virchows Arch B Cell Pathol Incl Mol Pathol* 1985;49:13–21.

72. Lloyd RV, Blaivas M, Wilson BS. Distribution of chromogranin and S100 protein in normal and abnormal adrenal medullary tissues. *Arch Pathol Lab Med* 1985;109:633–635.

73. Verna A. Ultrastructure of the carotid body in the mammals. *Int Rev Cytol* 1979;60:271–330.

74. Coupland RE, Hopwood D. The mechanism of the differential staining reaction for adrenaline- and noradrenaline-storing granules in tissues fixed in glutaraldehyde. *J Anat* 1966;100(pt 2):227–243.

75. Brown WJ, Barajas L, Latta H. The ultrastructure of the human adrenal medulla: with comparative studies of white rat. *Anat Rec* 1971;169:173–183.

76. Lundberg JM, Hamberger B, Schultzberg M, et al. Enkephalin- and somatostatin-like immunoreactivities in human adrenal medulla and pheochromocytoma. *Proc Natl Acad Sci U S A* 1979;76:4079–4083.

77. Böck P, Stockinger L, Vyslonzil E. The fine structure of the human carotid body [article in German]. *Z Zellforsch Mikrosk Anat* 1970;105:543–568.

78. Hervonen A, Korkala O. Fine structure of the carotid body of the midterm human fetus. *Z Anat Entwicklungsgesch* 1972;138:135–144.

79. Kondo H. Is the SIF cell truly an interneuron in the superior cervical ganglion? *Adv Biochem Psychopharmacol* 1980;25:103–109.

80. Greenberg ME, Ziff EB, Greene LA. Stimulation of neuronal acetylcholine receptors induces rapid gene transcription. *Science* 1986;234:80–83.

81. Sietzen M, Schober M, Fischer-Colbrie R, Scherman D, Sperk G, Winkler H. Rat adrenal medulla: levels of chromogranins, enkephalins, dopamine beta-hydroxylase and of the amine transporter are changed by nervous activity and hypophysectomy. *Neuroscience* 1987;22:131–139.

82. Tischler AS, DeLellis RA, Nunnemacher G, Wolfe HJ. Acute stimulation of chromaffin cell proliferation in the adult rat adrenal medulla. *Lab Invest* 1988;58:733–735.

83. Penberthy WT, Dahmer MK. Insulin-like growth factor-I-enhanced secretion is abolished in protein kinase C-deficient chromaffin cells. *J Neurochem* 1994;62:1707–1715.

84. Mahata SK, Mahapatra NR, Mahata M, et al. Catecholamine secretory vesicle stimulus-transcription coupling in vivo. Demonstration by a novel transgenic promoter/photoprotein reporter and inhibition of secretion and transcription by the chromogranin A fragment catestatin. *J Biol Chem* 2003;278:32058–32067.

85. Powers JF, Brachold JM, Ehsani SA, Tischler AS. Up-regulation of ret by reserpine in the adult rat adrenal medulla. *Neuroscience* 2005;132:605–612.

86. Brundin T. Studies on the preaortal paraganglia of newborn rabbits. *Acta Physiol Scand Suppl* 1966;290:1–54.

87. Hervonen A, Korkala O. The effect of hypoxia on the catecholamine content of human fetal abdominal paraganglia and adrenal medulla. *Acta Obstet Gynecol Scand* 1972;51:17–24.

88. Dinger B, Wang ZZ, Chen J, et al. Immunocytochemical and neurochemical aspects of sympathetic ganglion chemosensitivity. *Adv Exp Med Biol* 1993;337:25–30.

89. Dalmaz Y, Borghini N, Pequignot JM, Peyrin L. Presence of chemosensitive SIF cells in the rat sympathetic ganglia: a biochemical, immunocytochemical and pharmacological study. *Adv Exp Med Biol* 1993;337:393–399.

90. Slotkin TA, Smith PG, Lau C, Bareis DL. Functional aspects of development of catecholamine biosynthesis and release in the sympathetic nervous system. In: Parvez H, Parvez S, eds. *Biogenic Amines in Development.* Amsterdam: Elsevier/North Holland, 1980;29–48.

91. Williams SE, Wootton P, Mason HS, et al. Hemoxygenase-2 is an oxygen sensor for a calcium-sensitive potassium channel. *Science* 2004;306:2093–2097.

92. Howe A, Pack RJ. The response of abdominal vagal fibres in the rat to changes in inspired oxygen concentration [proceedings]. *J Physiol* 1977;270:37P–38P.

93. Honda Y, Myojo S, Hasegawa S, Hasegawa T, Severinghaus JW. Decreased exercise hyperpnea in patients with bilateral carotid chemoreceptor resection. *J Appl Physiol* 1979;46:908–912.

94. Saldana MJ, Salem LE, Travezan R. High altitude hypoxia and chemodectomas. *Hum Pathol* 1973;4:251–263.

95. Hervonen A, Pickel VM, Joh TH, et al. Immunocytochemical demonstration of the catecholamine-synthesizing enzymes and neuropeptides in the catecholamine-storing cells of human fetal sympathetic nervous system. *Adv Biochem Psychopharmacol* 1980;25:373–378.

96. Lloyd RV, Sisson JC, Shapiro B, Verhofstad AA. Immunohistochemical localization of epinephrine, norepinephrine, catecholamine-synthesizing enzymes, and chromogranin in neuroendocrine cells and tumors. *Am J Pathol* 1986;125:45–54.

97. Bjorklund A, Falck B, Lindvall O, Svensson LA. New aspects on reaction mechanisms in the formaldehyde histofluorescence method for monoamines. *J Histochem Cytochem* 1973;21:17–25.

98. Neville AM. The adrenal medulla. In: Symington T, ed. *Functional Pathology of the Adrenal Gland.* Baltimore: Williams and Wilkins; 1969;219–324.

99. Steele RH, Hinterberger H. Catecholamines and 5-hydroxytryptamine in the carotid body in vascular, respiratory, and other diseases. *J Lab Clin Med* 1972;80:63–70.

100. Perrin DG, Chan W, Cutz E, Madapallimattam A, Sole MJ. Serotonin in the human infant carotid body. *Experientia* 1986;42: 562–564.
101. Kent C, Coupland RE. On the uptake and storage of 5-hydroxytryptamine, 5-hydroxytryptophan and catecholamines by adrenal chromaffin cells and nerve endings. *Cell Tissue Res* 1984;236:189–195.
102. Heym C, Kummer W. *Regulatory Peptides in Paraganglia*. New York: Gustav Fisher Verlag; 1988.
103. Heym C, Kummer W. Immunohistochemical distribution and colocalization of regulatory peptides in the carotid body. *J Electron Microsc Tech* 1989;12:331–342.
104. Vaalasti A, Pelto-Huikko M, Tainio H, Hervonene A. Light- and electron-microscopic demonstration of enkephalin-like immunoreactivity in paraganglia of the human urinary bladder. *Cell Tissue Res* 1985;239:683–687.
105. Varndell IM, Tapia FJ, De Mey J, Rush RA, Bloom SR, Polak JM. Electron immunocytochemical localization of enkephalin-like material in catecholamine-containing cells of the carotid body, the adrenal medulla, and in pheochromocytomas of man and other mammals. *J Histochem Cytochem* 1982;30:682–690.
106. Feldman SA, Eiden LE. The chromogranins: their roles in secretion from neuroendocrine cells and as markers for neuroendocrine neoplasia. *Endocr Pathol* 2003;14:3–23.
107. Helle KB. The granin family of uniquely acidic proteins of the diffuse neuroendocrine system: comparative and functional aspects. *Biol Rev Camb Philos Soc* 2004;79:769–794.
108. Winkler H. The adrenal chromaffin granule: a model for large dense core vesicles of endocrine and nervous tissue. *J Anat* 1993;183(pt 2):237–252.
109. Lachmund A, Gehrke D, Krieglstein K, Unsicker K. Trophic factors from chromaffin granules promote survival of peripheral and central nervous system neurons. *Neuroscience* 1994;62: 361–370.
110. Rodriguez-Cuevas S, Lopez-Garza J, Labastida-Almendaro S. Carotid body tumors in inhabitants of altitudes higher than 2000 meters above sea level. *Head Neck* 1998;20:374–378.
111. Santer RM, Hann AC. Quantitative X-ray microanalysis of adrenal medullary cells of young adult and aged rats after glutaraldehyde fixation and potassium dichromate treatment. *Histochemistry* 1993;99:43–48.
112. Yang G, Matocha MF, Rapoport SI. Increased numbers of extraadrenal chromaffin cells in the abdominal paraganglia of senescent F344 rats: a possible role for the glucocorticoid receptor. *Cell Tissue Res* 1990;259:233–238.
113. Shi SR, Cote C, Kalra KL, Taylor CR, Tandon AK. A technique for retrieving antigens in formalin-fixed, routinely acid-decalcified, celloidin-embedded human temporal bone sections for immunohistochemistry. *J Histochem Cytochem* 1992;40:787–792.
114. Powers JF, Brachold JM, Tischler AS. Ret protein expression in adrenal medullary hyperplasia and pheochromocytoma. *Endocr Pathol* 2003;14:351–361.
115. Söllner T, Bennett MK, Whiteheart SW, Scheller RH, Rothman JE. A protein assembly-disassembly pathway in vitro that may correspond to sequential steps of synaptic vesicle docking, activation, and fusion. *Cell* 1993;75:409–418.
116. Mundschenk J, Unger N, Schulz S, et al. Somatostatin receptor subtypes in human pheochromocytoma: subcellular expression pattern and functional relevance for octreotide scintigraphy. *J Clin Endocrinol Metab* 2003;88:5150–5157.
117. Aunis D, Langley K. Physiological aspects of exocytosis in chromaffin cells of the adrenal medulla. *Acta Physiol Scand* 1999; 167:89–97.
118. Komminoth P, Roth J, Schroder S, Saremaslani P, Heitz PU. Overlapping expression of immunohistochemical markers and synaptophysin mRNA in pheochromocytomas and adrenocortical carcinomas. Implications for the differential diagnosis of adrenal gland tumors. *Lab Invest* 1995;72:424–431.
119. Ehrhart-Bornstein M, Hilbers U. Neuroendocrine properties of adrenocortical cells. *Horm Metab Res* 1998;30:436–439.
120. Das V, Nal B, Dujeancourt A, et al. Activation-induced polarized recycling targets T cell antigen receptors to the immunological synapse; involvement of SNARE complexes. *Immunity* 2004;20: 577–588.
121. Prekeris R, Klumperman J, Scheller RH. Syntaxin 11 is an atypical SNARE abundant in the immune system. *Eur J Cell Biol* 2000;79:771–780.
122. O'Connor DT, Burton D, Deftos LJ. Chromogranin A: immunohistology reveals its universal occurrence in normal polypeptide hormone producing endocrine glands. *Life Sci* 1983;33: 1657–1663.
123. Lloyd RV, Wilson BS. Specific endocrine tissue marker defined by a monoclonal antibody. *Science* 1983;222:628–630.
124. Fischer-Colbrie R, Lassmann H, Hagn C, Winkler H. Immunological studies on the distribution of chromogranin A and B in endocrine and nervous tissues. *Neuroscience* 1985;16: 547–555.
125. Takahashi H, Nakashima S, Kumanishi T, Ikuta F. Paragangliomas of the craniocervical region. An immunohistochemical study on tyrosine hydroxylase. *Acta Neuropathol (Berl)* 1987;73: 227–232.
126. Takahashi K, Isobe T, Ohtsuki Y, Sonobe H, Takeda I, Akagi T. Immunohistochemical localization and distribution of S-100 proteins in the human lymphoreticular system. *Am J Pathol* 1984;116:497–503.
127. Iwanaga T, Takahashi Y, Fujita T. Immunohistochemistry of neuron-specific and glia-specific proteins. *Arch Histol Cytol* 1989;52 (suppl):13–24.
128. Schafer BW, Heizmann CW. The S100 family of EF-hand calcium-binding proteins: functions and pathology. *Trends Biochem Sci* 1996;21:134–140.
129. Simson JA, Hintz DS, Munster AM, Spicer SS. Immunocytochemical evidence for antibody binding to mast cell granules. *Exp Mol Pathol* 1977;26:85–91.
130. Spicer SS, Spivey MA, Ito M, Schulte BA. Some ascites monoclonal antibody preparations contain contaminants that bind to selected Golgi zones or mast cells. *J Histochem Cytochem* 1994;42:213–221.
131. Grube D. Immunoreactivities of gastrin (G-) cells. II. Non-specific binding of immunoglobulins to G-cells by ionic interactions. *Histochemistry* 1980;66:149–167.
132. Srivastava A, Tischler AS, DeLellis RA. Endogenous biotin staining as an artifact of antigen retrieval with automated immunostaining. *Endocr Pathol* 2004;15:175–178.
133. van Leeuwen F. Pitfalls in immunocytochemistry with special reference to the specificity problems in the localization of neuropeptides. *Am J Anat* 1986;175:363–377.
134. DeLellis RA. Formaldehyde-induced fluorescence technique for the demonstration of biogenic amines in diagnostic histopathology. *Cancer* 1971;28:1704–1710.
135. de la Torre JC. Standardization of the sucrose-potassium phosphate-glyoxylic acid histofluorescence method for tissue monoamines. *Neurosci Lett* 1980;17:339–340.
136. Decker HJ, Klauck SM, Lawrence JB, et al. Cytogenetic and fluorescence in situ hybridization studies on sporadic and hereditary tumors associated with von Hippel-Lindau syndrome (VHL). *Cancer Genet Cytogenet* 1994;77:1–13.
137. Komminoth P, Kunz E, Hiort O, et al. Detection of RET protooncogene point mutations in paraffin-embedded pheochromocytoma specimens by nonradioactive single-strand conformation polymorphism analysis and direct sequencing. *Am J Pathol* 1994;145:922–929.
138. Hensen EF, Jordanova ES, van Minderhout IJ, et al. Somatic loss of maternal chromosome 11 causes parent-of-origin-dependent inheritance in SDHD-linked paraganglioma and phaeochromocytoma families. *Oncogene* 2004;23:4076–4083.
139. Kimura N, Togo A, Sugimoto T, et al. Deficiency of phenylethanolamine n-methyltransferase in norepinephrine-producing pheochromocytoma. *Endocr Pathol* 1996;7:131–136.
140. Parke WW, Valsamis MP. The ampulloglomerular organ: an unusual neurovascular complex in the suboccipital region. *Anat Rec* 1967;159:193–198.
141. Ostrowski ML, Wheeler TM. Paraganglia of the prostate. Location, frequency, and differentiation from prostatic adenocarcinoma. *Am J Surg Pathol* 1994;18:412–420.
142. Rode J, Bentley A, Parkinson C. Paraganglial cells of urinary bladder and prostate: potential diagnostic problem. *J Clin Pathol* 1990;43:13–16.

143. Makinen J, Nickels J. Paraganglion cells mimicking metastatic clear cell carcinoma. *Histopathology* 1979;3:459–465.

144. Betts DR, Cohen N, Leibundgut KE, et al. Characterization of karyotypic events and evolution in neuroblastoma. *Pediatr Blood Cancer* 2005;44:147–157.

145. Tischler AS, Perlman RL, Costopoulos D, Horwitz J. Vasoactive intestinal peptide increases tyrosine hydroxylase activity in normal and neoplastic rat chromaffin cell cultures. *Neurosci Lett* 1985;61:141–146.

146. Mutter GL, Zahrieh D, Liu C, et al. Comparison of frozen and RNALater solid tissue storage methods for use in RNA expression microarrays. *BMC Genomics* 2004;5:88.

147. Rodrigo MC, Martin DS, Redetzke RA, Eyster KM. A method for the extraction of high-quality RNA and protein from single small samples of arteries and veins preserved in RNALater. *J Pharmacol Toxicol Methods* 2002;47:87–92.

Index

Page numbers followed by an "f" indicate figures; page numbers followed by a "t" indicate tables.